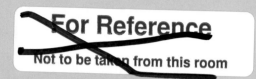
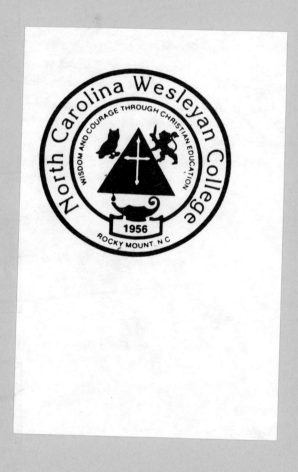

EDUCATIONAL RESEARCH, METHODOLOGY, AND MEASUREMENT: AN INTERNATIONAL HANDBOOK

SECOND EDITION

Resources in Education

This series of Pergamon one-volume Encyclopedias draws upon articles in the acclaimed *International Encyclopedia of Education, Second Edition*, with revisions as well as new articles. Each volume in the series is thematically organized and aims to provide complete and up-to-date coverage on its subject. These Encyclopedias will serve as an invaluable reference source for researchers, faculty members, teacher educators, government officials, educational administrators, and policymakers.

This second edition of *Educational Research, Methodology, and Measurement: An International Handbook* provides an overview of the methods of inquiry that are used in the investigation of problems which arise in the field of education. Since the publication of the first edition of the *Handbook* there have been substantial changes in the conduct of research in education. The issues concerned with the nature of inquiry in the field have been widely debated in terms of the existence of two paradigms and the division between quantitative and qualitative strategies of research.

In addition, on the one hand, research that may be described as participatory or action research, and that leads to the empowerment of individuals and groups has advanced in popularity and acceptance. While, on the other hand, there have been important developments in the techniques of measurement and in the analysis of data which have arisen from the increasing power of and access to desktop computers.

There is now a greatly increased variety in the strategies and tactics employed in research into education problems as well as in the methods, theoretical perspectives, and analytical procedures that are being used to investigate the processes and practices, the context and conditions, and the products and policies which occur in the field of education. However, there is also a growing sense of unity in these scholarly endeavors. It is this emerging unity in the fields that support the use of the term educational research replacing the view that research in education is merely applied research in which knowledge gained in certain disciplines, more especially psychology and sociology, finds application and the advancement of social action.

This *Handbook* presents the view that educational research possesses a unity that extends across different disciplinary perspectives and their methods of inquiry, that rejects the existence of the qualitative and quantitative divide, and that challenges the superficial dichotomies of basic and applied, or conclusion-oriented and decision-oriented, or disciplinary policy research.

This view of the unity of educational research necessarily permeates the methods of investigation employed and the procedures of analysis used that seek confirmation, and test for the coherence. Nevertheless, entries in this *Handbook* are written by a large number of different authors, each of whom has an individual view of the nature of educational research. As a consequence, this *Handbook* seeks to present the different views and perspectives that exist in the field and does not deliberately restrict itself to a single view of research.

Other titles in the series include:

POSTLETHWAITE (ed.)
International Encyclopedia of National Systems of Education, Second Edition

CARNOY (ed.)
International Encyclopedia of Economics of Education, Second Edition

ANDERSON (ed.)
International Encyclopedia of Teaching and Teacher Education, Second Edition

TUIJNMAN (ed.)
International Encyclopedia of Adult Education and Training, Second Edition

PLOMP & ELY (eds)
International Encyclopedia of Educational Technology, Second Edition

DeCORTE & WEINERT (eds)
International Encyclopedia of Developmental and Instructional Psychology

SAHA (ed.)
International Encyclopedia of the Sociology of Education

EDUCATIONAL RESEARCH, METHODOLOGY, AND MEASUREMENT: AN INTERNATIONAL HANDBOOK

SECOND EDITION

Edited by

JOHN P. KEEVES

Flinders University of South Australia, Adelaide, Australia

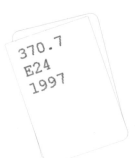
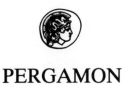

PERGAMON

UK	Elsevier Science Ltd, The Boulevard, Langford Lane, Kidlington, Oxford OX5 1GB, UK
USA	Elsevier Science Inc, 660 White Plains Road, Tarrytown, New York 10591-5153, USA
JAPAN	Elsevier Science Japan, 9-15 Higashi-Azabu 1-chome, Minato-ku, Tokyo 106, Japan

Second edition 1997

Library of Congress Cataloging in Publication Data
Educational research, methodology and measurement : an international handbook / edited by J. P. Keeves. — 2nd ed.
    p.   cm.
   Includes bibliographical references and indexes.
   1. Education—Research—Handbooks, manuals, etc. 2. Educational tests and meaurements—Handbooks, manuals, etc. I. Keeves, John P.
LB1028.E3184 1997
370'.7—dc21   96-52173

British Library Cataloguing in Publication Data
A catalogue record for this book is available from the British Library.

ISBN 0–08–042710–3 (hard : alk. paper)

Printed and bound in Great Britain by Cambridge University Press, Cambridge, UK.

Contents

Contents

Contents

Contents

Contents

Contents

Preface

This second edition of *Educational Research, Methodology and Measurement: An International Handbook* has been prepared to provide an overview of the methods of inquiry that are used in the investigation of problems which arise in the field of education. During the period of ten years since the preparation of the first edition of this *Handbook* there have been substantial changes in the conduct of research in education. The issues concerned with the nature of inquiry in the field have been widely debated in terms of the existence of two paradigms and the division between quantitative and qualitative strategies of research. In addition, on the one hand, research that may be described as participatory or action research, and that leads to the empowerment of individuals and groups has advanced in popularity and acceptance. On the other hand, there have been important developments in the techniques of measurement and in the analysis of data which have arisen from the increasing power of and access to desk-top computers. As a consequence a revised edition of this *Handbook* has become necessary to ensure that graduate students, research workers, teachers at the college and graduate levels, and scholars in allied fields are kept informed of the important changes that are occurring.

There is now a greatly increased variety in the strategies and tactics employed in research into educational problems, as well as in the methods, theoretical perspectives and analytical procedures that are being used to investigate the processes and practices, the context and conditions, and the products and policies which occur in the field of education. However, there is also a growing sense of unity in these scholarly endeavors. It is this emerging unity in the field that supports the use of the term "educational research" replacing the view that research in education is merely applied research in which knowledge gained in certain disciplines, more especially psychology and sociology, finds application and the advancement of social action.

This *Handbook* presents the view that educational research possesses a unity that extends across different disciplinary perspectives and their methods of inquiry, that rejects the existence of the quantitative and qualitative divide, and that challenges the superficial dichotomies of basic and applied, or conclusion-oriented and decision-oriented, or disciplinary and policy research. This unity of the educational research enterprise is presented as having sound epistemological foundations. Positivism is rejected in its various forms, as well as the idea of multiple realities. The purpose of inquiry in educational research is the building of a coherent body of knowledge that has been examined against evidence from the real world, and that is available for transforming the real world through human agency and social action. This view of the unity of educational research necessarily permeates the methods of investigation employed and the procedures of analysis used that seek confirmation, and test for coherence. Nevertheless, entries in this *Handbook* are written by a large number of different authors, each of whom has an individual view of the nature of educational research. As a consequence, this *Handbook* seeks to present the different views and perspectives that exist in the field. It does not deliberately restrict itself to a single view of research, although the editorial role permits presentation with coherence and continuity. The introductions to each of the three major sections of the *Handbook* provide an integration of the entries included in that section and an opportunity for the editor to present his views of the unity in the field of educational research.

The purpose of this Preface is to answer four questions in order to explain the principles that have guided the development of this *International Handbook*. The volume has a strong international perspective. In part, this necessarily arises from the fact that many of the new ideas, methods of measurement and statistical analysis, as well as views of social action have been developed in Europe and Australia and not in North America where it is estimated that approximately 75 percent of the research in education is conducted. This is not to deny the importance of American thought and activity in the field, but rather to emphasize the very powerful contributions that are emerging from Europe, Australia and other parts of the world. As a consequence a strong international coverage is essential if the full range of views and recent developments is to be adequately presented.

1. Why is there a need for a volume concerned with the methods of educational research?

2. What are the relationships between the areas referred to in the title of the volume, namely research, methodology and measurement, and the three sections into which the volume is divided?

3. What are the links between this volume and the second edition of *The International Encyclopedia of Education*, and what principles guided the preparation of this *International Handbook*?

4. How can this volume and the various sources of information incorporated within it be best used?

Prior to any discussion of these four questions it is necessary to acknowledge the marked growth and development that has occurred in the field of educational research from the early 1960s onwards. The injection of financial support for the research enterprise in education initially in North America, and subsequently in Europe and Australasia led scholars from many disciplines to undertake scholarly inquiry into educational problems. They brought with them their theories and their methods of investigation and they greatly enriched the field. These changes occurred at the same time as universities were expanding across the world and teacher training institutions were being incorporated into universities, with an expectation that their staff would engage in research activity. The opening entry in this volume by De Landsheere examines the *History of Educational Research*. During the 1960s and 1970s there was an unprecedented expansion of investigatory activity into educational problems with strong support from both governmental agencies and private foundations.

This expansion of research activity took place not only in the affluent industrialized countries but also in the developing countries that were establishing or rapidly expanding their national educational systems. However, the late 1960s were also marked by the growth of debate in the social and behavioral sciences in reaction to the strident emphasis on a scientific approach that had occurred as a result of access to computers to carry out complex calculations and statistical analyses. In some ways this confrontation damaged systematic research into educational problems and led in some countries to a withdrawal of funding for educational research in the 1980s. Nevertheless, the momentum that was established has been maintained, and the effects of the lack of financial support have been reduced by the increased availability of computers for data storage, data analysis, the transference of information, and the preparation of reports for publication in an attractive form. These developments have benefited research both of a quantitative and non-quantitative kind. The decade from the mid-1980s to the mid-1990s saw very rapid growth in the power of, and access to, desk-top computers that greatly changed the investigatory procedures employed in many educational research studies. As a consequence there is little doubt that research into educational problems proceeds apace, even if financial support for large scale investigations is less readily available.

During the decade since the mid-1980s there has also been a growing realization that a great deal is now known in terms of validated theory about educational processes, and as a result social action can be initiated and maintained in order to change the ways in which education is provided and learning occurs. Furthermore, in addition to the assembling of the substantial body of theoretical knowledge about education that has been presented in the *International Encyclopedia of Education*, initially in the first edition and more recently in a second edition, there is greater recognition and awareness of how education operates to change society. Not only does education work to transmit knowledge to an oncoming generation of students but it also develops in students at all levels the skills involved in the creation and testing of new knowledge. Education differs from the major disciplines in so far as it not only has its own body of knowledge, but it is also concerned with the processes by which it and the disciplines undertake the tasks of transmission of knowledge and the development of the skills of scholarly inquiry. Furthermore, education is concerned with the development of the processes by which the body of knowledge that has been assembled as the fruits of inquiry are employed by human agents through the processes of social action to change society and the real world in which human beings live.

It is these multiple functions of education that have been more clearly recognized during the decade from the mid-1980s to the mid-1990s in the creation, propagation and utilization of knowledge and that have led to the marked expansion of education world-wide, at all levels and in all modes. This expansion has occurred from the years of early childhood, through the primary, secondary and tertiary stages and on to adult recurrent education, as well as in the deliberate employment of the new information technology for educative purposes.

1. The Need for a Single Volume Concerned with the Methods of Educational Research

There are two main perspectives which are employed in the investigation of educational problems. While for some scholars these two perspectives are seen as two distinct paradigms, the entry by Walker and Evers entitled *Research in Education: Epistemological Issues* challenges and rejects the existence of two paradigms. Nevertheless, the existence and operation of two approaches to educational research must be acknowledged. The nature of these two approaches would seem to have been clarified by the distinction made by Dilthey in the 1980s between understanding *(Verstehen)* and explanation *(Erklären)* (see *Research Paradigms in Education*). The humanistic approach places an emphasis on holistic and qualitative information, and the purposes of research are to provide understanding and an interpretative account of educational phenomena. The scientific approach has been developed from the natural sciences and has emphasized the use of empirical and quantifiable observation in order to examine causal explanations of educational phenomena. However, the idea that these two approaches form distinct paradigms must be rejected on the grounds presented by Walker and Evers. Under these circumstances it can be argued that the two approaches enjoy their current strengths as different strategies for the conduct of educational research as a result of the existence of the two cultures that, as C P Snow has pointed out, have been developed in the English-speaking world through specialization at upper secondary school and university levels. These two approaches are not different in purpose in so far as they seek to build a coherent body of knowledge. They supplement each other in the methods employed and the contributions they provide.

There is a third area of research in education that is concerned with the development and analysis of policy, the introduction of change through social action and the evaluation of the outcomes of the changes that have been introduced. It is, however, necessary to recognize that an investigation into educational problems can be undertaken from a perspective that is concerned with either the conservation of an existing situation, and the advancement of knowledge about that problem situation, or alternatively with the promotion of change. In the latter case the purposes of inquiry extend beyond the cumulation of knowledge about educational processes and the explanation or understanding of phenomena. This third area of research which involves an emphasis on change indicates that in addition to research undertaken from either a humanistic or scientific perspective, which can be considered to form a first dimension in the classification of educational inquiry, there is a second dimension present. This further dimension is concerned with the use of educational and social science research in which the advancement or the retardation of change is involved. The emergence of this second dimension and the multiplicity of alternative methods now available for inquiry into educational problems, together with the growing interest in undertaking studies that involve evaluation have since the 1960s led to great diversity in the strategies that are being employed in educational research.

It is argued that the field of inquiry into educational problems and the methods of inquiry now available are a great deal more complex than is considered in many volumes that provide an introduction to educational research from only one of the many perspectives available. The purpose of this volume then is to bring together what is known about the many disparate strategies of research into educational problems into one volume, so that the full diversity of methods is revealed. Nevertheless, it is claimed that there is a unity underlying the different strategies which must be clearly presented to avoid fragmentation and artificial divisions. An emphasis on both the unity and diversity within the field of inquiry into educational problems is seen to meet the urgent need for reconciling the conflicts that currently exist in the field and for the development of a more coherent approach to research. The publication of the many different strategies in a single volume should be seen as a contribution towards this goal.

This *International Handbook* seeks to be a truly international publication, providing coverage of the many different research traditions and strategies of inquiry that are used in different parts of the world, as well as looking forward to the future. It is clear that educational research is a dynamic enterprise. Its methods and procedures are changing, sometimes quite rapidly. This *International Handbook* aims at capturing this changing nature of educational inquiry and in assisting the enterprise to move ahead rapidly and with strength in a way that will contribute both to the creation of knowledge about educational processes as well as to the use of the findings of inquiry in the improvement of both educational policy and practice.

2. *Relationships between areas referred to in the title of the Handbook, namely, research, methodology and measurement and the three sections into which the volume is divided*

The development of the electronic computer has, since the early 1960s, provided a remarkable boost for empirical and quantitative research into educational problems. The sections on measurement and statistical analysis procedures in this *International Handbook* have been assembled after nearly a third of a century of very creative activity in these aspects of the field of educational research. The activity in the area of measurement has resulted in the development of criterion-referenced theory, generalizability theory and more recently item response theory for measurement in the field of education. It is the latter that is now making an important contribution to measurement in psychology and the social sciences. Furthermore, in the area of statistical analysis, techniques of factor analysis, linear structural relations analysis and more recently multilevel analysis have been developed for use in the investigation of educational problems and have found widespread application in other disciplines and fields of inquiry. Of particular significance has been the developmental work in multilevel analysis, which has been recently carried out in the field of education, where students are necessarily investigated in school and classroom groups. There are other fields of inquiry including medicine, sociology, agriculture and forestry where problems of multilevel analysis arise, but have customarily been ignored. In these fields the analytical procedures developed in educational research have started to make very substantial contributions.

Educational problems frequently involve the investigation of learning. The measurement of learning outcomes commonly requires that different instruments must be employed at different points in time, and the measures obtained must be equated for the investigation of change. It is here that item response theory and, in particular, the Rasch measurement model is highly suited for the study of change in outcomes measured over time on a common scale. Multilevel analysis, with the criterion measured over at least three points in time, is a more powerful technique for the analysis of change data than is provided by repeated measures analysis of variance procedures.

It is in the study of learning, which is central to educational research, that these recently developed procedures of educational measurement and statistical analysis combine.

It must be acknowledged that some research workers in education are strongly opposed to the use of procedures of measurement and statistical analysis in the examination of information collected in educational research. Their preferences are sometimes expressed in terms of a rejection of a quantitative approach and an endorsement of a qualitative approach. Such a distinction between quantities and qualities is confounded by the fact, as Kaplan (see *Scientific Methods in Educational Research*) has pointed out, that quantities are of qualities. Moreover, the rejection in the qualitative approach of statistical analysis is contradicted by the powerful procedures of statistical analysis that have been developed in Europe for the examination of qualitative data. However, the critics of the scientific approach would also argue that such an approach is seriously flawed in its orientation, and their views are presented in entries on *Naturalistic and Rationalistic Enquiry* and *Action Research*.

It must also be recognized that over time there have been both tensions and fashions in the adoption of a scientific approach as contrasted with a humanistic approach in educational research. As a consequence of the variations in orientation over time this *International Handbook* seeks to adopt a flexible perspective that takes into account the fluctuations that might be expected to occur in the future in the approaches adopted towards the investigation of educational problems. Since the future cannot be foretold with accuracy, approaches and procedures that have not yet been widely accepted, as well as those that are the subject of some controversy are presented alongside those that are well-established. Thus the traditional approaches and the alternative and the newer approaches, that are being employed by research workers in some parts of the world, are all considered in this volume.

The articles included in this *International Handbook* are assembled into three major sections:

(a) the methods of educational inquiry,

(b) research procedures, and

(c) measurement in educational research.

At the beginning of each major section there is an introduction that not only reviews developments in the area and discusses issues, but also comments on how the entries in the section are clustered together and organized for reference purposes. Thus within each section and subsection the entries are grouped in such a way as to provide a coherent view across the topics presented. In general, a pluralist perspective is adopted with the different approaches being seen as supplementary in nature.

The first section on **The Methods of Educational Inquiry** seeks to provide a broad coverage of topics related to the methods of educational inquiry. The introductory articles are concerned with general research perspectives. They are followed by articles that consider the two major approaches to educational research, namely the humanistic approach and the scientific approach. It is not the purpose of this volume to advocate the use of one approach in preference to the other but rather to present the pluralism of views and perspectives that are employed in educational research. Moreover, this volume, as previously explained, seeks to emphasize the unity and coherence that exists in the field of educational research rather than to emphasize the differences in outlook and the divisions that have arisen.

A fourth part of the first section considers the second dimension of educational research concerned with usage and the orientation towards change. In this section there are entries associated with both the advancement and the containment of change, the examination of the context in which research and change occur, the analysis of policy, and methods of evaluation. The final part of the first section examines several current issues in educational research. Unfortunately space constraints do not permit consideration of those issues related to the creation, diffusion and dissemination of knowledge and the findings of research.

The second section of the *Handbook* includes entries on specific research procedures and techniques with the purpose of advancing the quality of research conducted into educational problems. Consideration is given to both humanistic research procedures and scientific research procedures. The number of entries in the latter part far exceeds the number in the former part. This also reflects the lack of emphasis until relatively recently on the development of specific research procedures within the humanistic approach. Furthermore, there is only one entry associated with the computer analysis of information collected within the humanistic approach in contrast to the many computer based procedures currently employed within the scientific approach.

The third section of this *International Handbook* is concerned with measurement in educational research, and it excludes, because of space requirements, the consideration of issues of measurement that relate specifically to assessment of student performance. The emphasis in this section is primarily on the improvement of measurement which is attainable as a consequence of recent advances in measurement theory. Developments in this field have important applications in the measurement of attitudes as well as achievement, which are the key outcomes of teaching and learning. There are, however, many additional areas where recent developments in both theory and techniques are capable of advancing the quality and the accuracy with which measurements are made in educational research. Some of these areas that are of importance for educational research, such as the use of census data and statistics, environmental measurement, the measurement of social background, classroom observation techniques, and the use of rating scales and questionnaires have also been considered.

The collection of entries assembled in the three sections and their subsections of this *International Handbook* is unique, and the range and depth of treatment of the entries goes well beyond that brought together in other works on educational research, methodology and measurement. Moreover, every effort has been made to include entries which provide information on important new advances in the field.

3. The Preparation of the International Handbook

This *International Handbook* has been developed from the first and second editions of the *International Encyclopedia of Education* which were edited by Torsten Husén and Neville Postlethwaite with the assistance of an editorial board and which were published in 1985 and 1994 respectively. Both editions of the *Encyclopedia* were organized around areas of scholarly specialization related to education. One area was concerned with educational research, methodology and measurement. After the first edition of the *Encyclopedia* was published, it was recognized that there was a need for a series of reference books and text books for university teachers and graduate students, who were reading and studying in different spheres of educational inquiry. Thus it was proposed that a volume should be prepared that was concerned with educational research, methodology and measurement. Between the time of publication of the first edition of the *Encyclopedia* and the first edition of this *International Handbook*, developments in educational research methods proceeded apace and new entries were commissioned and published in the *Handbook*. Likewise in the years between the publication of the first edition of the *Handbook* and the second edition of the *Encyclopedia* developmental work in the field continued and old entries were revised and new entries were written for publication in 1994. Further developments have occurred in the period since the second edition of the *Encyclopedia* was prepared and work was being undertaken for the preparation of the second edition of the *Handbook*. For this volume some new entries have been prepared and many authors have revised their entries before publication. Thus every effort has been made to ensure that the material presented in this volume is as up to date and as relevant as possible.

4. How to Use this International Handbook

Educational research draws on diverse disciplines that have a bearing on problems in the field of education. In addition, over recent decades educational research has built up a body of theoretical knowledge concerned with the processes of education and has developed a battery of methodological strategies, as well as a range of analytical procedures that are particularly suited to the problems encountered in educational research. While it is the editor's contention that there is a unity and coherence running through this volume that is consistent with the unity and coherence that exists in the domain of educational research, this *Handbook* must be seen as a compendium of entries, written by different scholars with different research traditions and drawn from different countries of the world. Thus the volume is intended as a reference or source book for university and college teachers to use in the preparation of lectures; for graduate students to use as a first introduction to a procedure or research technique; and for practising research workers to obtain information on a research strategy or analytical technique that they might employ in their work, or might explore in greater depth in order to tackle their particular research problem. As a consequence of the inclusion of articles on so many topics in a single volume, it is clear that no individual entry can be complete in itself. Thus every entry seeks not only to be relevant and up to date, but also to provide guidance, through a concise set of references and a bibliography to key articles or publications likely to be readily available, from which the scholar, student, teacher or research worker could obtain further information. Furthermore, in order to facilitate the search for information, references are provided within each entry to other entries in the volume where related information has been presented.

In addition, both a detailed Name Index and a Subject Index based on key words or phrases have been compiled to assist the reader in the search for information. As a consequence, the user of this *International Handbook* who wants information on a specific topic could begin by looking up appropriate words in the Subject Index in order either to locate an entry related to the topic or to identify entries where the topic as referenced by the key words is considered. In a similar way, the Name Index can be used to locate references to the writings of a particular author who is known to have made a substantial contribution to a sphere of research related to the topic on which information is sought. In order to facilitate this task, page numbers are given both for the bibliographic reference and for the point at which the reference is cited in the text.

5. Acknowledgments

No work of the size of this *International Handbook* could be published without considerable effort by many people. To several of these people a special debt of gratitude is due. First, I am grateful to Neville Postlethwaite and Torsten Husén who guided the preparation of the first and second editions of the *International Encyclopedia of Education*. Second, I am grateful to the many authors who prepared entries, carefully checked galley proofs, revised their entries and in many cases acted as consultants for other entries in the volume. Third, I am very grateful to Barbara Barrett, Editorial Director of the *Encyclopedia* and to Michele Wheaton who directed the work on the preparation of the second edition of this *Handbook*, as well as to Deborah Wilton and Peter Frank who worked on the many different aspects of the production task. Finally I am grateful to Petra Lietz, Frances Anderson and Susan Malin who have assisted me with the typing of entries in connection with the preparation of this volume. To them all my sincere thanks are offered.

July 1996

JOHN P. KEEVES
The Flinders University of South Australia

The Methods of Educational Inquiry

Introduction: Towards a Unified View of Educational Research

J. P. Keeves

The nature and purpose of educational research is the subject of continuing debate not only in the columns of educational journals but also in seminar rooms and at conferences where the findings of research into educational problems are presented. Furthermore, no systematic review of research in education can fail to grapple with the problem, because of the consequences for funding in comparison with other domains of inquiry. Simple dichotomies of research activity into basic or applied, discipline-oriented or policy-oriented, and conclusion-oriented or decision-oriented do not provide adequately for the complexity of the activities undertaken in educational research. Nevertheless, tensions exist between the proponents of alternative approaches to the investigation of educational problems. These tensions have been known to split schools of education, to lead to marked change in the editorial policy of journals, to prejudice the funding of research in education, and to lead to politicians and senior educational administrators to denigrate the field of educational inquiry. It is an objective of this *Handbook* to present educational research as a unified field that has been remarkably successful over recent decades in the accumulation of a substantial body of knowledge about education. The research enterprise in education draws on many disciplines and employs a wide variety of approaches to investigation, but the research activity has a unity of purpose and a unified epistemological basis that demands the rejection of two or more paradigms of inquiry.

The successes of educational research activity in the past half century since the cessation of the Second World War, and more particularly the three decades since the mid-1960s, are seen in the compilations of knowledge about education that are presented in the first and second editions of the *International Encyclopedia of Education*. This corpus of knowledge is rather more than an accumulated body of wisdom and a related set of practices associated with education. Wisdom no longer refers to 'knowledge of an abstruse kind', but rather to the 'quality of being wise in relation to conduct and the choice of ends and means' in particular situations (*New Shorter Oxford Dictionary*

1994, p. 3700). The knowledge generated by research activity must be debated among scholars and tested against evidence from the real world and stored and structured in a coherent way prior to further review and testing. Failure to view the products of educational research as a coherent body of knowledge would seem to misunderstand the nature of the research enterprise. Educational research, furthermore, has a unique function in this enterprise in so far as it not only involves the construction of a body of knowledge, but it also involves the investigation of the processes by which all knowledge is passed on to successive generations and by which the skills of inquiry are acquired, as well as the processes by which social action is initiated. These ideas about the functions of education and educational inquiry are developed in the pages that follow.

1. Concerning the Nature of Knowledge

Popper and Eccles (1977) have distinguished between three different worlds involved in human inquiry. The entities of the real world which include physical objects, as well as the various structures created by human society and which include schools and universities, form **World 1**. **World 2** is the world of subjective experiences, a world of individual mental states, that comprises the states of conscious thought and psychological dispositions as well as the unconscious states of mind of individuals. Wisdom is an entity in World 2. There is, however in addition, **World 3** which has been created as a new objective world, that is the product of human minds. It should be noted that World 3 not only contains the corporate body of propositional knowledge concerned with causal explanation, but also the works of art, music and literary writings that are all part of the world of shared knowledge. The important point is that World 3 objects have acquired a reality of their own.

The body of propositional knowledge that has been assembled by the natural sciences has been used to transform the real world through technology (Conant

1

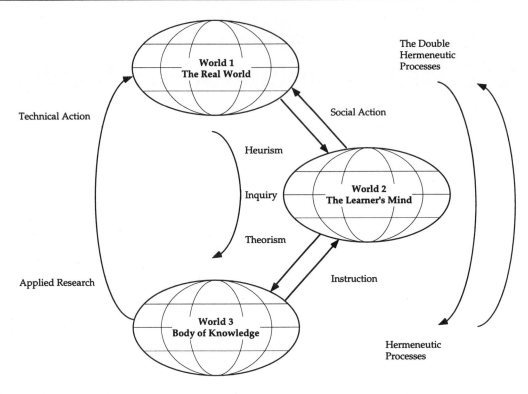

Figure 1
The nature and processes of educational and social inquiry

1947). It has been the marked success of research and development in the physical and biological sciences acting through technology that has advanced the standing of scientific inquiry. Figure 1 presents in diagrammatic form some of the relationships that exist between these three worlds of inquiry and technology.

Research is concerned with the processes of inquiry which involve interactions between World 1—The Real World, World 2—The Learner's Mind, and World 3—The Body of Knowledge. The processes of inquiry involving relationships between World 1 and World 2 in which individuals employ the knowledge they possess to investigate the real world may be referred to as **Heurism**.

Research is also concerned with the processes operating between World 2 and World 3 which may be referred to as **Theorism**. These processes include the formulation of generalizations, the building, testing and revising of models derived from theory and the subsequent advancement or rejection of theory. The skills of theorism are largely taught in universities, while the skills of heurism are taught in schools as well as in higher education. Together heurism and theorism form the processes of inquiry. The manner and the context within which they work, or the manner in which the 'messages of the gods are conveyed to human beings' for the formation of knowledge involve

the **hermeneutic process** as the term hermeneutic implies (see *Hermeneutics*).

The hermeneutic examination of these processes in education and the social sciences has long been established in Continental Europe. It involves the study of meaning and comprises the theory and practice of interpretation and the generation of understanding of the different social contexts in which human beings learn about the world in which they live and work. The hermeneutic method has developed from many different facets of scholarly inquiry in the social sciences, and its goal is that of understanding in the study of human actions within a social context. Moreover, this approach recognizes that in order to obtain meaning with respect to how and why humans act, it is necessary for an investigator to enter into dialogue with the human agents.

Giddens (1984) argues that a double hermeneutic is also involved. There is not only the frame of meaning acquired by individuals in order to view the real world. This involves an interaction between World 2 and World 1 as shown in Fig. 1. There is also a second frame of meaning constructed by the same individuals as they view the world of shared knowledge (World 3) and assimilate the ideas developed by social and behavioral scientists. In Fig. 1 this would require interaction between World 3 and World 2. Thus, it is necessary to consider not only the meanings given by lay persons to the events of the real world (World 1), but also the ideas and relationships that are constructed from the body of knowledge (World 3), which is developed as the result of scholarly inquiry.

The accumulation of wisdom takes place in World 2 and in the minds of those individuals who, as a consequence of experience, develop wisdom which they can apply in particular contexts. Wisdom is fed by knowledge from World 3, but is not necessarily codified and structured as is stored knowledge and is not necessarily subjected to tests of coherence. Wisdom is unique to individuals, is slow to form, and is applied by individuals critically and practically. It is this individual knowledge that constructivist research is investigating.

It should be noted that education plays a highly significant role in these processes. It operates to transmit the essential ideas and relationships held in World 3 to the minds of the individuals who form World 2. However, education is not only involved in transmitting knowledge. Since the body of knowledge contained in World 3 is now so vast, there is the task of selecting or making simple and coherent the extensive and complex ideas and relationships of World 3, for communication in ways that permit the assimilation and structuring of these ideas and relationships in the minds of individuals. Educators are not only the purveyors of knowledge but they are also the gatekeepers of knowledge. Furthermore, they are responsible for training students in the skills of inquiry which include the processes of heurism and theorism.

1.1 The Nature of Social Action

In the first half of the twentieth century research workers in education and the social and behavioral sciences were conducting their inquiries within the perspectives of functionalism, positivism and naturalism. They sought universal generalizations about the social and behavioral world that could be applied to transform society in much the same way that scientific knowledge is applied through technology and technical action to change the physical and biological worlds. The dichotomy widely employed in the classification of research into "pure science" and "applied science" still reflects thinking that is largely inappropriate in education and the social and behavioral sciences. Earlier in this century the dream of many research workers in education and the social and behavioral sciences was that by obtaining knowledge about the processes of human life it would be possible to transform and control the social and behavioral world in much the same way as technology has transformed and controlled the physical world. Furthermore, politicians, administrators and natural scientists continue to accuse educational researchers for their failure to produce results that have direct application, because they view things in this way. This view of educational research is both incomplete and inadequate.

In the mid-1950s and early 1960s it was possible to answer the critics of educational research with proposals for both increased funding and significant expansion of research activity. It was commonly claimed that with increased resources and effort both important generalizations and significant practical applications would emerge. Today, there is widespread realization that such a view was both simplistic and naive. There is no doubt that the increased resources provided for educational research, in particular, transformed this area of inquiry in the period of 20 years from the 1960s to the early 1980s. An immense body of knowledge about educational, social, and psychological processes was assembled, that is only now being assimilated in a coherent and meaningful way. Nevertheless, it is also apparent that few universal generalizations have emerged that can be directly applied to benefit either educational practice or the operation of society.

Giddens (1984) has argued that there has been a failure to understand in an adequate way the nature of social action in the context of changes in social theory. He maintains that the technological view of the application of the findings of educational and social science research is grossly inadequate. Moreover, he contends that there is a sense in which such a view has seriously underestimated the practical impact of research in education and the social sciences on both daily life and on society.

In the quest for universal generalizations in the study of educational processes and in social research there has been a failure to recognize the existence of World 2 and the role of human agents in society. In the study of educational problems and societal processes, human beings as a group do not remain as passive subjects of inquiry. They comprehend the debate which arises during the formulation of ideas, and they not only assimilate these ideas, but they also accommodate to them and are changed. As Fig. 1 shows, World 3, the world of shared knowledge, interacts with World 2, and the world of personal knowledge, to such an extent that the views and perceptions held by human agents of World 1, the world of real things, are also changed.

Since the real world is itself unknowable without these views and perceptions which are held by human beings, the very foundations of human knowledge, are without certainty. Furthermore, a situation arises in which generalizations are advanced, but their existence has been generated from the educational and social theories held by research workers. Thus perceptions of the educational and social world are changed by the theories that have been generated by research, and as a consequence the generalizations that are generated from research are also subject to change and are not universal or permanent laws and principles.

It is clear that Popper and Eccles (1977) are concerned with the same issues, approaching their problems from the perspective of the natural scientist. However, the problems are of greater magnitude in the social and behavioral sciences and in education, because human beings act as social agents. Furthermore, universal schooling and widespread higher and recurrent education have during recent decades facilitated the dissemination of the advances in educational, social and behavioral knowledge through paperback publications, journal articles, and the mass media. As a consequence the rate of change in both educational and social processes has been greatly increased, as has the perceptions and understandings of those processes.

1.2 Using the Findings of Educational Research

There are thus important reasons why it is not possible to point to a substantial number of universal generalizations that have been generated by educational, social and behavioral research. When from a study of human action, new ideas and concepts emerge which explain an educational or social process in a clearer way than members of society were previously able to provide, these ideas are appropriated by those members of society and incorporated back into their thinking and their social lives. These ideas have the effect of changing perceptions of education and social life, as well as the effect of subsequently changing the nature of the ideas and concepts of educational and social theory. Furthermore, the behavior and social actions that follow from these ideas and concepts are also changed, and as a consequence the initial and tentative generalizations that were formed from earlier research no longer hold. Such generalizations may need to be completely reformulated in terms of new ideas and new theory.

In many highly developed countries, including for example, the United States and Australia, the changing concepts of equality of educational opportunity and equity in education, as well as the ideas and theories of the melting pot, cultural mosaic, and multiculturalism, reflect this relative rapid emergence of new ideas of relevance to education. It is not the case that the initial views and generalizations associated with the educational and social processes were necessarily wrong, but rather that the ideas were so powerful that they changed the social processes themselves as well as the perceptions of them. The original ideas were not trivial or of little consequence, but as a result of their formulation, discussion and dissemination by educators, views of society were changed, society itself was changed by consequent social action, and the ideas themselves were subsequently subjected to change.

The impact of new ideas and theories in the social sciences depends upon how human agents assimilate and accommodate to new ideas through education. From these perspectives it would seem likely that educational and social theory may have had a more powerful and more rapid influence on daily life in societies throughout the world than has technological development. Moreover, the task of dissemination and discussion of ideas and developments in educational and social theory falls on education. Thus education

contributes to social change both as a source of ideas, as well as providing the key processes through which such ideas are introduced widely and change is subsequently implemented.

2. The Unity of Educational Research

Since the early 1970s, a conflict has emerged in educational research concerning both the purposes and methods of inquiry. Alternative perspectives have been proposed and accepted by many. The value of alternative approaches is not to be denied, since the scholarly debate that follows and the exploratory use of these alternative approaches adds vitality to the field. The increased resources provided for educational research during the 1960s and 1970s led scholars from many different social science disciplines to study educational problems and to work alongside the historians and philosophers who had over a long period been interested in educational issues. These newcomers brought with them new methods and new perspectives.

Husén (see *Research Paradigms in Education*) argues that these many different perspectives constitute two main paradigms—the scientific and the humanistic which he contends "are not exclusive, but complementary to each other". Nevertheless, a case can be argued that the drawing of a distinction between these two approaches cannot be sustained to the extent that they are to be regarded as two different paradigms. It is necessary to recognize that these perspectives have their origins in long-standing philosophical traditions. Dilthey in the 1890s drew the distinctions, in connection with research conducted in the field of psychology, between interpretation or understanding (*Verstehen*) and explanation in causal terms (*Erklären*). Dilthey suggested that the former was the goal of humanistic research, and the latter the goal of scientific research. Von Wright (1971) subsequently traced the interpretative tradition with its emphasis on understanding back to Aristotle. This approach argued that things happen in the way that they do in terms of intentions, motives and expressed reasons. The alternative tradition of advancing a causal explanation was said by Von Wright to have originated with Galileo.

It must be recognized that these two traditions have been fed during the twentieth century by the specialization that has taken place in upper secondary schools and in universities into two major strands of learning—the humanities and the sciences. Snow (1964) advanced the view that this specialization had led to the formation of 'two cultures', since the burden of developing skills and acquiring foundational knowledge in both areas had become so great that very few students could be expected to develop competence in both areas.

Since these distinctions between the humanistic and the scientific approaches which have emerged in educational research would appear to have had their origins in different philosophical traditions of long standing, it is necessary to ask:

(1) whether it is possible to bring these two traditions together in a unified approach;

(2) whether one approach should be superseded by the other;

(3) whether both must be abandoned, since neither can be meaningfully endorsed; or

(4) whether both should be maintained, because they each have different goals.

The position adopted by De Landsheere (see *History of Educational Research*) and by Husén (see *Research Paradigms in Education*) would seem to be the fourth option in which the two traditions are regarded as complementary. This position permits both lines of research to continue and to contribute. Guba and Lincoln (see *Naturalistic and Rationalistic Enquiry*) would seem to argue for the second position. They draw distinctions between the two paradigmatic approaches in such a way that there is no possibility of reconciliation between their naturalistic paradigm in which there are multiple perceptions of reality and the scientific paradigm, which is translated by them into a positivistic approach.

Walker and Evers (see *Research in Education: Epistemological Issues*) are concerned with the basic question as to whether these two approaches involve 'different ways of knowing or forms of knowledge'. If the two approaches are associated with mutually incompatible ways of investigating World 1, then the educational research worker must of necessity make a choice between the two. In the course of time, it would be expected that one of the two ways of knowing would cease to provide meaningful answers to the problems investigated and the other would survive. In addition, Walker and Evers address the question as to whether or not the two paradigms can both be said to exist. Since each paradigm includes both substantive theories and the methods to be employed for assessing the strength of those theories, there is, unfortunately, no position from which a theory of paradigms could be assessed. The issue could not be resolved by the use of procedures employed by either or both.

If the view is accepted, as has already been done earlier in this entry, that observations of the real world are greatly influenced by the knowledge about that world held by individuals and by groups, then there are no sound epistemological bases for differences between the extreme views of how educational research should be undertaken. If investigators working with both the scientific and humanistic approaches seek to investigate the real world and to build a simple and coherent body of knowledge about education and its processes, then they are engaging in a common

enterprise of inquiry associated with the interactions between World 2 and World 1, and between World 2 and World 3 in order to add to the corpus of knowledge stored in World 3. If they do not seek to add to the knowledge stored in World 3, it might well be argued that they are not engaged in the research enterprise in the field of education.

If, however, they are engaged in adding to the body of knowledge both of the long-standing traditions considered above must be rejected and in addition, the positivist and the naturalistic positions must also be abandoned. Under these circumstances the idea of two or more paradigms can no longer be sustained and the case must be endorsed for unity in educational research. This does not mean a denial of the humanistic and scientific approaches to research. Nor does it imply any rejection of the well established disciplinary methods that are being employed with profit in educational research worldwide. However, it does lead to the adoption of a common approach to educational inquiry in which researchers and practitioners work together to solve educational problems.

Such a perspective, that acknowledges a unified approach, would also permit psychologists to work on educational problems in a laboratory setting and under experimental conditions in the search for a generalization that might be considered to be a universal finding. They would employ procedures similar to those used by the natural scientist. This perspective would also provide for classroom teachers to involve themselves in action research which is directed towards a very practical problem that had arisen in the classroom situation. Furthermore, it would incorporate within the field of educational research the ethnographer who sought an interpretative view of a specific school or classroom situation that would yield a deeper understanding of the school or classroom processes. These educational researchers might not only seek new solutions to practical problems but also new ideas and new knowledge. It is important, moreover, that the ideas developed during such research and the relationships investigated and tested should be incorporated into the body of knowledge relating to education, and should not merely accumulate as the professional wisdom of a few privileged individuals.

3. Coherence—the Test of Knowledge

The issue remaining to be addressed is concerned with the testing, for inclusion in World 3, of the knowledge assembled, in the minds of individual persons in World 2. It is necessary to determine whether the assembled knowledge corresponds with events in the real world—World 1, which is viewed from the perspective of those individuals in World 2 who hold that knowledge. Educational knowledge, like knowledge in other domains, evolves in unsystematic and unplanned ways. In general, knowledge develops with

5

several alternative and competing theories, each with limited usefulness. Sometimes these theories overlap, sometimes they are very different. At different stages in the development of a sphere of knowledge, one theory may be given credence or may hold a dominant position, only to be superseded by an alternative theory as new evidence becomes available. The validation or verification of hypotheses and models derived from theory and subsequently of the theory itself is undertaken to varying degrees with five criteria that have been advanced by Quine and Ullian (1978):

(1) *fruitfulness*, since theory gives rise to explanation and to new ideas;

(2) *testability*, since a theory that cannot be subjected to testing leads nowhere;

(3) *generality*, since a theory must have sufficient generality to address a range of related situations;

(4) *coherence*, since the various parts of a theory must link together to support each other; and

(5) *simplicity*, since a theory must not collapse under its own weight.

It is evident that the purposes of a theory are to unify and systematize knowledge. However, since a theory is never complete, these purposes are never fully achieved. Nevertheless, in the field of education remarkable progress has been made in the 30 years from the mid-1960s.

It is also necessary to ask whether research into educational problems demands an approach to inquiry which is different from that used in other domains of knowledge. Some argue that all knowledge of human activity is essentially subjective, since it involves unique events, the meanings ascribed to those events by individuals, and the responses made by individuals according to the nature of the events and the meanings ascribed. However, educational research is succeeding in building a corpus of theoretical knowledge about educational processes. If this is so, then educational research is now dependent on a quest for evidence that ties the world of theory—World 3 to the real world—World 1, and on the testing of that theory against evidence in order to confirm or reject the theory. The epistemological basis of this process does not differ whether quantitative or qualitative methods of inquiry are employed, whether or not measuring instruments are developed and used, whether or not interaction between the observer and the observed is fostered to increase the richness of the data, and whether an investigation is carefully designed or remains flexible and unconstrained. However, the strength of inquiry may be influenced by these alternative processes.

There is in addition to the humanistic and scientific approaches to educational research a third approach that would seem to be directed towards social action, after taking into account the particular nature of an educational problem. This approach involves what has become known as "critical theory" or critical action research. However, it is primarily engaged in social action and is concerned with the relationships between World 2 and World 1, and the assembling of sufficient supportive opinion in World 2 to effect change in World 1. Ideas may be derived from World 3, but this approach does not always seek to contribute to the body of knowledge in World 3, and sometimes would not seem to acknowledge the body of theory already available in World 3. Lakomski (see *Critical Theory in Education*) challenges very strongly the value of the contribution of critical theory and critical action research to educational inquiry.

4. A Coherent Approach to Educational Research

All research into educational problems lacks secure foundations in the real world, since what is observed is influenced by the theories that direct the observations being made. There is need in educational inquiry to reorient the issues addressed not to the foundations for the observations, but rather to the consequences of the observations. As Kaplan (1964) has pointed out, such an approach is prospective rather than retrospective. If the emphasis in educational research shifts from the foundations to the outcomes of the research, whether in terms of contributing to theory or towards social action or to both, then the choice of problems to be investigated is made in terms of the significance and consequences of the findings rather than the firmness of the foundations. However, in the choice of problems, the part played by values can not be denied. Thus values enter into inquiry not only in the selection of problems, but also in the order in which problems are treated, as well as the resources of time and money spent on their resolution through research (see *Research in Education, Nature, Needs and Priorities*).

In educational research, the conflict between the proponents of the scientific and humanistic approaches to inquiry lacks a sound epistemological basis. Although there are two different traditions involved, each of which is supported by the specialization occurring in schools and universities, a coherentist approach to inquiry rejects any maintenance of these distinctions at the level of two different paradigms. There are, however, a variety of methods that are available for the conduct of research, as well as an emerging synthesis in social theory that could guide research into educational problems. The methods employed in educational inquiry should then be influenced by the nature of the problems being considered. Furthermore, the problems investigated should be those that contribute most both to change in the real world, as well as to the building of a coherent body of knowledge about education and educational processes.

4.1 Concerning the Entries in this Section

The entries in this section are divided into five parts. Collectively, the entries are concerned with the methods of educational inquiry and the issues that emerge from consideration of these methods of research and investigation. In the first part under the heading, **General**, there are five entries. The opening entry considers the *History of Educational Research*, which is followed by the entry on *Research Paradigms in Education*. The third entry provides a response to the question as to whether paradigms may be considered to exist within the field of educational inquiry and is titled, *Research in Education: Epistomological Issues*. The fourth entry is relevant to an *International Handbook* and addresses the problem of *Comparative Methodology in Education*. A final entry involves the construction of theory under the title of *Facet Theory*.

The second part of this section is concerned with **Humanistic Research Methods**. There is an increased number of entries in this area in the second edition compared with the first edition of this *Handbook*. The new entries consider *Anthropological Inquiry; Biographical Research Methods; Educational History in Biographies and Autobiographies; Narrative Inquiry;* and *Semiotics in Educational Research*. Diversification over the period of ten years in the area of humanistic research methods is evident from the new entries.

In the third part of the section are eight entries on **Scientific Research Methods**. The opening entry on *Scientific Methods in Educational Research* is a particularly significant article for those scholars who would wish to equate scientific research methods with positivism. While the entry does not specifically address this issue, it clarifies the nature of the scientific methods that are employed in educational research and leaves no room for a positivistic approach. The inclusion of an entry on *Human Development, Research Methodology* indicates the expanding interest in longitudinal research which follows from the analytical procedures being made available through greater computing power, and appropriate computer programs as well as greater facility for data storage and retrieval. The remaining entries in this section are concerned with well-established procedures within the scientific research tradition, namely: *Cross-sectional Research Methods; Experimental Studies; Longitudinal Research Methods; Simulation as a Research Technique; Survey Research Methods;* and *Twin Studies*. All methods of investigation described in this section have profited greatly in recent decades from the availability of computer programs to undertake the analysis of data in ways that are consistent with the methodology.

The fourth part in the section on research methods involves the uses of educational inquiry with the title: **Critical Theory, Policy Research and Evaluation**. The opening entry on *Critical Theory and Education* provides an examination of the nature of critical theory and questions its epistemological foundations. This entry if followed by several entries that are within the tradition of critical theory, namely *Action Research; Feminist Research Methodology;* and *Participatory Research*, all of which promote change. *Legitimatory Research*, however, is carried out in order for an educational system to contain change. Two entries are concerned with research relating to the making of policy: *Policy Analysis, and Policy-Oriented Research*. However, the entry on *Hermeneutics* involves research of an interpretative nature that examines the context within which research is conducted, how the findings of research are received, as well as how practice is changed as a result of research findings. It is commonly necessary in the wake of change to carry out evaluation studies to examine the consequences of change and entries on *Evaluation Models and Approaches*, and *Evaluation, A Tylerian Perspective* are concerned with these aspects of research.

The final part of this section addresses **Issues in Educational Research**. The opening entry is concerned with important aspects of research planning with the title: *Research in Education, Nature, Needs and Priorities*. Subsequent entries consider *Unintended Effects in Educational Research; Ethics of Educational Research; Politics of Educational Research; Educational Research and Policy Making;* and *Translating Research into Practice*. A final entry in this part involves the issues of *Teachers as Researchers*, implying that research and inquiry in education is not necessarily associated with a program, but is better seen as a way of working and an approach.

Nevertheless, research is a process that is not necessarily concerned with the generation of change, being more concerned with the assembling of a body of knowledge that is examined, tested and integrated in a coherent way with existing knowledge.

References

Conant J B 1947 *On Understanding Science*. Oxford University Press, Oxford [1]

Giddens A 1984 *The Constitution of Society*. Polity Press, Cambridge, and Blackwell, Oxford [2]

Kaplan A 1964 *The Conduct of Inquiry*. Chandler, San Francisco, California [3]

Popper K R, Eccles J C 1977 *The Self and its Brain*. Springer-Verlag, Berlin [4]

Quine M V, Ullian J S 1978 *The Web of Belief*. Random House, London [5]

Snow C P 1964 *The Two Cultures: A Second Look*. Cambridge University Press, Cambridge [6]

Von Wright G H 1971 *Explanation and Understanding*. Routledge and Kegan Paul, London [7]

(a) General

History of Educational Research

G. de Landsheere

Educational research as disciplined inquiry with an empirical basis was first known as "experimental pedagogy." This term was analogous to that of "experimental psychology," an expression coined by Wundt in Leipzig around 1880. Experimental pedagogy was founded around 1900 by Lay and Meumann in Germany; Binet and Simon in France; Rice, Thorndike, and Judd in the United States; and Claparède in Switzerland. Some years earlier, three publications—*Die Seele des Kindes* by Preyer, a German medical doctor, in 1882; *The Study of Children* by Hall in the United States in 1883; and articles by an English psychologist, Sully, in 1884 concerned with children's language and imagination—marked the beginning of the child study movement. Although progress was slow during the 1880s, the foundations were laid through this movement for research into related educational problems. From 1900 onward, in the study of educational problems four movements can be identified: (a) the child study movement, where educational research was associated with applied child psychology; (b) the New Education or progressive movement where philosophy took precedence over science, and life experience over experimentation; (c) the scientific research movement, with initially a positivist approach; and (d) the humanistic research movement which has emerged since the 1960s and draws on the methods of research employed in sociology, anthropology, politics, history, philosophy, and linguistics.

During the first period (1900–30), Cronbach and Suppes (1969) speak of a "heyday of empiricism," empirical educational research focused on rational management of instruction, that challenged the concept of transfer of training, and advanced the development of new curricula, psychological testing, administrative surveys (school attendance, failure rates, etc.), and normative achievement surveys. Descriptive statistics were already well-established, and in the 1920s and 1930s inferential statistics and data analysis developed rapidly.

In the second period (1930 to the late 1950s), however, the strict scientific approach to education lost impetus to make room, practically all over the developed world, for the more philosophically oriented and innovative progressivism. Behind this shift were three factors: (a) the atomistic character of most educational research; (b) a questioning of the scientific approach to the management of education at a time when there was an economic crisis soon to be followed by war; and (c) the charisma of the progressive movement with its combination of empirical research and a social and political philosophy merging free enterprise and liberal spirit with humanistic socialism.

Nevertheless, during this period interest in cognitive development and language studies continued with the work of Piaget in Switzerland, and Vygotsky, who died in 1934, and his associates Luria and Leontief in the Soviet Union. In addition, a new strand of enquiry was opened up in the field of the sociology of education with the publication in 1944 of *Who Shall be Educated?* by Warner et al. (1946) in the United States. These authors brought together a substantial body of research to establish that schooling in the United States favored White children from an urban middle-class background. Studies into adolescence and adolescent development soon followed.

In the third period (1960 and 1970s) a knowledge "explosion" took place and its applications to all fields of research really began. Educational research was soon influenced by this dynamic development. In the United States, challenged by Soviet technological advances (e.g., Sputnik) and being economically affluent, governmental and private agencies supported educational research to an unprecedented extent. A similar development, although not so spectacular, occurred in other highly industrialized countries. During the 1960s the computer added a new dimension to educational research leading to the introduction of sophisticated experimental design and massive national and international surveys, since data processing and data analysis were no longer limited by calculation time as in the precomputer era. From this, new ways of thinking about educational issues developed, which were concerned with assessing probabilities, multivariate analysis of educational outcomes, and the introduction of mathematical and causal modeling to predict and explain educational phenomena (see *Models and Model Buildings*).

The Anglo-Saxon world led the field in educational research while West European countries tended to move more slowly. The profound impact of the Anglo-Saxon research methodology has been felt all over the world since the 1960s. But the 1960s were also marked by the beginning of an epistemological debate in the social sciences, perhaps a reaction to the strident empiricism which had developed. It is now fully realized that the rigid scientific ideal, embodied in the neopositivist approach, cannot take into account the multifaceted aspects of human behavior and all its environment-bound subtle nuances (see *Research Paradigms in Education*).

Confrontation took place. Just as the student movement and revolt can now be considered as part of an emerging, new human culture, the positivistic versus the humanistic or hermeneutic debate can be conceived as the beginning of a new and fourth era in the social sciences. However, the answer to educational researches of the 1990s is not either-or, but both (Husén 1988, Keeves 1988). The scientific approach is seen to be complementary to the anthropological, historical, phenomenological, or humanistic approach.

In tracing the development of educational research this entry examines the successive periods: pre-1900 era, 1900 to 1930s, 1930s to late 1950s, the 1960s and 1970s, and developments in the 1980s and 1990s (see De Landsheere 1982, 1986).

1. Pre-1900

It is not incidental that within a period of about 25 years empirical educational research was born and began to tackle most of the pervasive educational problems which are, in the late twentieth century, still under study throughout the Western world. The foundations for this sudden rise were laid during centuries of educational experience and philosophical thinking, and were inspired by the progress of the natural sciences during the nineteenth century. More specifically, longitudinal observations of individual children were recorded during the nineteenth century and attained a high-quality level with the pioneering study, in 1882, by Preyer, *Die Seele des Kindes* (The Mind of the Child). This was the first textbook on developmental psychology. The idea of experimentation in education is present in the writings of Kant, Herbart, and Pestalozzi, but this idea implied field experience and not experimentation according to an elaborated design.

In the second part of the nineteenth century, several signs show that developments in the natural sciences slowly began to influence psychology and education. In 1859, in *The Emotions and the Will*, Bain considered the construction of aptitude tests. Five years later, Fisher proposed a set of scales for the rating of ability and knowledge in major school subjects including handwriting. Fisher also introduced statistics into educational research by using the arithmetic mean as an index of achievement of a group of students. In 1870, Bartholomäi (1871) administered a questionnaire to 2,000 children entering primary school in order to know the "content of their mind" at that moment. Three years later, the first experimental study of attention was published by Miller in Göttingen. In

1875, James opened the first psychological laboratory in the United States at Harvard in order to carry out systematic observation, but not experimentation. The year 1879 saw the publication of Bain's *Education as a Science*.

The origins of modern educational research and of experimental psychology are not to be found in the emerging social sciences, but in the natural sciences. With his *Origin of the Species* (1859) Darwin linked research on humans with physics, biology, zoology, and geography. Six years later, Bernard published his *Introduction to the Study of Experimental Medicine* —a guide to modern scientific research (see Bernard 1932). In 1869, Galton in *Hereditary Genius*, began his work on the concepts of standardization, correlation, and operational definition by applying statistics to the study of human phenomena. Carroll (1978) sees in Galton's *Inquiry into Human Faculty and its Development* (1883) the invention of the idea of mental testing.

Experimental psychology—soon to be followed by experimental pedagogy—was created in German physics laboratories by scholars with a strong philosophical background. Wundt, a student of one of these scholars, Helmholtz, founded the first laboratory of experimental psychology in Leipzig in 1879. Wundt's laboratory had a considerable impact, and the scientific leadership of the German universities at the end of the 1800s must be recognized in order to understand what happened between 1880 and 1900.

At that time, many students, particularly from the United States, completed their advanced education at the universities of Berlin, Leipzig, Heidelberg, or Jena. This explains the extraordinarily rapid dissemination of Wundt's ideas: Cattell, Stanley Hall, Judd, Rice, and Valentine were among his students. His work was immediately known in France by Ribot and Binet, in Russia by Nestschajeff, in Japan by Matsumoto, and in Santiago, Chile by Mann. Psychological laboratories were soon opened on both sides of the Atlantic.

In the meantime, certain key events were associated with the birth of modern educational research:

1885 Ebbinghaus's study on memory drew the attention of the educational world to the importance of associations in the learning process.

1888 Binet published his *Études de Psychologie Experimentales*; at that time he was already working in schools.

1890 The term "mental test" was coined by Cattell.

1891 Stanley Hall launched the journal *Pedagogical Seminary*.

1894 Rice developed a spelling test to be administered to 16,000 pupils. He published the results of his testing in his *Scientific Management of Education* in 1913.

1895 In the United States, the *National Society for the Scientific Study of Education* was founded (initially called the National Herbart Society for the Scientific Study of Teaching).

1896 In Belgium, Schuyten published a report of his first

educational research study on the influence of temperature on school children's attention. Dewey, a student of Stanley Hall, opened a laboratory school at the University of Chicago.

1897 Thorndike studied under James at Harvard and there discovered the works of Galton and Binet.

Ebbinghaus published his so-called completion test to measure the effect of fatigue on school performance. This can be considered to be the first operational group test.

In the same year Binet began to work on his intelligence scale.

1898 Lay suggested distinguishing experimental education from experimental psychology.

Binet and Henri condemned traditional education in their book *La Fatigue Intellectuelle* and indicated the need for experimental education.

Who is the father of "experimental pedagogy"? The answer to this question differs when the activity covered by the term itself is considered. Empirical research in education definitely existed before 1900. Many American authors regard Rice as the founder because of his research on the effect of spelling drills (1895–97), but other names: Binet, Lay, Mercante, or Schuyten, could also qualify. As for the term itself, it was coined by Meumann (Wundt's former student) in 1900, in the German *Zeitschrift für Pädogogik* where he dealt with the scientific study of schooling. In 1903, Lay published his *Experimentelle Didaktik* where he made his famous statement: " . . . experimental education will become all education." In 1906, Lay and Meumann together published the review *Die Experimentelle Pädagogik*. Subsequently, Meumann's three-volume work *Einführung in die Experimentelle Pädagogik* (1910, 1913, 1914) emphasized both the strict scientific and quantitative side of the laboratory, while Lay continued to emphasize both quantitative and qualitative approaches in classroom research.

When did modern educational research appear in France? There is no doubt that Binet inspired it. In his introduction to *La Fatigue Intellectuelle* (1898) he wrote:

Education must rely on observation and experimentation. By experience, we do not mean vague impressions collected by persons who have seen many things. An experimental study includes all methodically collected documents with enough detail and precise information to enable the reader to replicate the study, to verify it and to draw conclusions that the first author had not identified. (cited by Simon 1924 p. 5)

It is obvious throughout the whole psychological work of Binet that he had a strong interest in all education. In 1905, he founded the School Laboratory in Paris. With him were Vaney, who in 1907 published the first French reading scale, and Simon, the coauthor of the *Intelligence Scale* (1905) and later author of the *Pédagogie Expérimentale*. Binet and Simon's *Intelligence Scale* presented in Rome at the 1905 International Conference of Psychology was the first truly operational mental test covering higher cognitive processes. Like Wundt's ideas, Binet's test became known throughout the world within a few years. Beyond its intrinsic value, this test had a far greater historical significance. It was now acknowledged that a test could be a valid measurement instrument both in psychology and education.

In 1904, Claparède, a medical doctor, founded the Laboratory for Experimental Psychology at the University of Geneva with his uncle Flournoy. In 1892, Claparède had visited Binet in Paris and in the following year was, for a short time, Wundt's student in Leipzig. In 1905, he published the first version of his *Psychologie de l'enfant et pédagogie expérimentale* (1911) that was the only French educational research methods handbook until 1935 when the Belgian Buyse published his *Expérimentation en Pédagogie*. In 1912, Claparède established the J J Rousseau Institute in Geneva which over the next 50 years was to make a marked contribution to child study and education through the work of Piaget. However, Claparède remained mostly psychologically and philosophically oriented. With his theory of functional education, he was the European counterpart of Dewey. Together they were seen as the two main leaders of progressive education.

Among many interesting features in the work of Claparède (following Dilthey's work in 1892 on *Verstehen vs. Erklären*) is his analysis, in 1903, of the explaining (positivist, nomothetic) versus the understanding (hermeneutic) approach. This elicited a debate which still lasts at the end of the twentieth century.

At the end of *Les idées modernes sur les enfants*, Binet (1924 p. 300) mentioned that "it is specially in the United States that the remodeling of education has been undertaken on a new, scientific basis." In fact, at the beginning of the twentieth century, educational research advanced at an extraordinarily quick pace in the United States.

At Columbia University, Cattell, who had obtained his PhD under Wundt and had known Galton in Cambridge, had, in 1890, as mentioned above, coined the term "mental test" in the philosophical journal *Mind*. In 1891, he established his psychological laboratory. Under his supervision Thorndike completed his PhD in 1898 on animal intelligence. Like many psychologists of the time he soon developed a keen interest in education. In this period, so much attention was focused on objective measurement that the experimental education movement was sometimes called "the measurement movement" (Jonçich 1962).

Thorndike can be considered as the most characteristic representative of the scientific orientation in education. During the following decades, he dealt with all aspects of educational research. He was the first person to conceive of teaching methods in terms of an explicitly formulated and experimentally tested learning theory. In so doing, he opened a new teaching era. The influence of Thorndike in the field of educational research can be compared with the influence of Wundt in experimental psychology.

2. The Flourishing of Quantitative Research, from 1900 to 1930

During this period, most educational research was quantitatively oriented and geared to the study of effectiveness. For a while, Taylorism and the study of efficiency became a component of educational thinking. The behavioristic and antimentalist study of human behavior was regarded as the best weapon against the formalism of the past.

The following aspects of research activities are representative illustrations of the era.

2.1 Statistical Theory

It has sometimes been said that there is an inconsistency between the limitations of measurement in the social and behavioral sciences and the rapidly increasing sophistication of the statistical techniques employed. However, it can be argued that many statistical advances were achieved by researchers in education precisely because they were aware of the complexity and the instability of most phenomena they had under study, consequently they had to look for increasingly sophisticated methods of both measurement and statistical analysis to obtain results of sufficient strength or else indicate the limitations of their conclusions.

The applicability of the Gaussian probability curve to biological and social phenomena was suggested at the beginning of the 1800s by Quetelet, who coined the term "statistics." Galton was the first to make extensive use of the normal curve to study psychological problems. Galton also suggested percentile norms. In 1875, he drew the first regression line, and developed the concept of correlation in 1877. In 1896, Pearson, who worked under Galton, published the formula for the product–moment correlation coefficient. In the first decade of the 1900s, the essentials of the correlational method, including the theory of regression, were developed, especially by British statisticians, Pearson and Yule. In the same period, Pearson developed the chi-square technique and the multiple correlation coefficient. Reliability was measured with the Spearman–Brown formula. In 1904, Spearman published his analysis of a correlation matrix to sustain his two-factor theory and factor analysis began to emerge. Researchers were also aware of the statistical significance of differences. In 1908, under the name of Student, Gossett showed how to measure the standard error of the mean and the principle of the t-test was formulated.

Experimental design was also developed. In 1903, Schuyten used experimental and control groups. In 1916, McCall, a student of Thorndike and probably the first comprehensive theorist of experimentation in education, recommended the setting up of random experimental and control groups. In a research study with Thorndike and Chapman (Thorndike et al. 1916), he applied 2×2 and 5×5 Latin square designs.

The contribution of Sir Ronald Fisher was critical. With the publication of his *Statistical Methods for Research Workers* in 1925, small-sample inferential statistics became known, but were not immediately utilized. In the same work, Fisher reinforced Pearson's chi-square by adding the concept of degrees of freedom, demonstrated the t-test, and explained the technique of analysis of variance. In 1935, Fisher published his famous *The Design of Experiments*, originally conceived for agriculture, and not widely applied in educational research before the late 1940s.

A look at some of the statistical texts available in the 1920s is often a surprise for modern students: Thorndike (1913), McCall (1922), Otis (1926), Thurstone (1925) in the United States; Yule (1911), Brown and Thomson (1921) in the United Kingdom; Claparède (1911) in Switzerland; Decroly and Buyse (1929) in Belgium had a surprisingly good command of descriptive parametric statistics and also a keen awareness of the need for testing the significance of differences.

2.2 testing and Assessment

Both mental and achievement tests already existed around 1900. Between 1895 and 1905 tests were administered in schools in the United States, Germany, France, Belgium, and many other countries. Perhaps the critical event was the appearance in 1905 of Binet and Simon's test, the first valid and operational mental measurement instrument. Group testing began in England in Galton's laboratory in 1905, and Burt and Spearman assisted him. In 1911, the United States National Education Association approved the use of tests for school admission and final examinations. A breakthrough occurred with the development and widescale, efficient use of tests by the United States Army, which were quickly constructed in 1917 mostly by drawing upon existing mental tests. Soon after the First World War, these tests were modified for school use (Carroll 1978).

The 1981 *Yearbook* of the National Society for the Study of Education was entirely devoted to the measurement of educational products. In 1928, about 1,300 standardized tests were available in the United States. By the 1930s, normative-test construction techniques were fully developed; item formats, order of items, parallel forms, scoring stencils and machine scoring, norms, reliability, and validity. The psychometric advance of the United States, at that time, was such that standardized tests were often referred to as "American tests."

Mental tests were soon used in all industrialized countries. In particular, Binet's scale was used in Europe, North and South America, and Australia, and was tried out in some African countries. This was far from being the case with achievement tests. Some fairly crude tests were used as research instruments but frequently remained unknown to the classroom teacher. It is, for instance, surprising to observe the lack of sophistication of the achievement tests developed in France after Binet and Simon. This continued until the 1940s, and the situation is particularly well-illustrated in the book by Ferré, *Les tests à l'école*, a fifth edition of which appeared in 1961. It is all the more surprising since in the 1930s traditional examinations (essay and oral tests) were sharply criticized in England and in France where Piéron coined the word *docimologie*, meaning "science of examinations." Lack of validity and reliability, and sociocultural bias were denounced with documented evidence. In Continental Europe, standardized achievement tests were not extensively used in schools.

2.3 Administrative and Normative Surveys

Among educational research endeavors, surveys are the oldest. In 1817, Jullien became the founder of comparative education by designing a 32-page national and international questionnaire covering all aspects of national systems of education. The questions were posed, but unfortunately not answered at that time.

The modern questionnaire technique was developed by Hall at the end of the 1800s to show, among other things, that what is obvious for an adult is not necessarily so for a child.

In 1892, Rice visited 36 towns in the United States and interviewed some 1,200 teachers about curriculum content and teaching methods. Subsequently he carried out a spelling survey (1895–97) on 16,000 pupils and found a low correlation between achievement and time invested in drill. This survey was repeated in 1908 and again in 1911 (Rice 1913). Thorndike's 1906 survey of dropouts was followed by a series of other surveys of school characteristics: differences in curricula, failure rates, teaching staff qualifications, school equipment, and the like. The most comprehensive survey of the period was the Cleveland Schools Survey undertaken in 1915–16 by Ayres and a large team of assistants. The study was reported in 25 volumes each dealing with different aspects of urban life and education.

In Germany, France, Switzerland, and Belgium, similar but smaller surveys were carried out by "pedotechnical" offices such as the one that opened in 1906 in the Decroly School in Brussels.

Several large-scale psychological surveys were undertaken: the Berkeley Growth Study (in 1928), the Fell's Study of Human Development (in 1929), and the Fourth Harvard Study (1929). In 1932, the Scottish Council for Research in Education carried out its first *Mental Survey* on a whole school population which provided a baseline for later surveys and for determining the representativeness of samples of the population of the same age.

A landmark in the history of experimental education was the *Eight-Year Study* (1933–41) conducted

in the United States by the Progressive Education Association. The initial purpose of the study, which was carried out using survey research methodology, was to examine to what extent the college entrance requirements hampered the reform of the high-school curriculum and to demonstrate the relevance and effectiveness of progressive ideas at the high-school level. In this study students from 30 experimental schools were admitted to college irrespective of the subjects they had studied in high school. The by-products of this project were probably more important than the project itself. Tests covering higher cognitive processes and affective outcomes were developed by an evaluation team directed by Tyler. The careful definition of educational objectives was advanced. In 1949, influenced by the *Eight-year Study*, Tyler wrote *Basic Principles of Curriculum and Instruction*, in which he presented his model for the definition of objectives. This was followed by Bloom's first taxonomy in 1956, and this marked the beginning of the contemporary thinking on the definition of objectives and on curriculum development and evaluation.

2.4 Curriculum Development and Evaluation

Curriculum was one focus of attention of empirical educational research from its very beginning. The article, in 1900, in which Meumann used the term *"experimentelle Pädagogik"* for the first time dealt with the scientific study of school subjects. Shortly afterwards, Thorndike introduced a radical change in curriculum development by conceptualizing teaching methods in terms of a "psychology of school branches," and by demonstrating through his work on the transfer of learning the lack of validity of the prevailing theories of formal education, and how it ignored the needs of contemporary society. This methodological approach was perfectly compatible with the new pragmatic philosophy and the attempts to rationalize work and labor. Some years later, Decroly and Buyse hoped to "Taylorize instruction to save time for education." The psychology of school subjects was also dealt with by other leading scholars such as Judd. But, as far as research on curriculum, in the broad sense of the word is concerned, the work of Thorndike on content, teaching methods, and evaluation of material is second to none.

During the same period, the progressive movement, partly inspired by Dewey, remained in close contact with these specific developments, although it soon rejected a strictly quantitative experimental approach to educational phenomena. According to Thorndike's scientific approach, there could be only one standard curriculum at a given time, the best one that scientific research could produce. Most important to the movement was the rejection of formalism for functionality. The main criteria for curriculum content became individual needs in a new society, as conceived by liberal, middle-class educators of the time.

In 1918, Bobbitt published *Curriculum*, soon to be

followed by Charters' *Curriculum Construction* (in 1923). This led to a series of studies with increasingly strong emphasis on a systematic and operational definition of educational objectives. On the European side, the Belgian *Plan d'études* (1936) by Jeunehomme was built on contributions of both strict empirical research and the progressive philosophy.

3. From the 1930s to the late 1950s

The economic crisis of the 1930s made research funds scarce. The Second World War and the years immediately following froze most educational research activities in European countries. Freedom of research was (and still is) not acceptable to dictators. In the former Soviet Union, the utilization of tests (as incompatible with political decisions) and more generally the "pedological movement" were officially banned in 1936 by a decree of the Communist Party, and this situation lasted until Stalin's death. However, other forms of research continued, arising from the publication in 1938 of *Thought and Language* by Vygotsky four years after his death, and the subsequent work of his associates such as Luria and Leontief in the development of Pavlov's ideas. In occupied countries, school reorganization was planned by underground movements which tried to draw conclusions from previous experiments and to design educational systems for peace and democracy. The *Plan Langevin–Wallon*, for the introduction of comprehensive secondary education in France is an example.

Conditions were different in the United States, Australia, and Sweden. Even if no spectacular advances occurred in educational research in those countries, the maturation of ideas went on and prepared the way for the postwar developments. Warfare had again raised problems of recruitment and placement and the role of military psychology and the development of selection tests is exemplified by the work of Guilford (1967) in the United States and Husén and Boalt (1968) in Sweden.

The strong field of interest in the 1940s and 1950s was without doubt in sociological studies. The seminal investigations were those concerned with social status and its impact on educational opportunity. A series of studies in the United States showed the pervasive existence of the school's role in maintaining social distinctions and discriminatory practices. From this research it was argued that schools and teachers were the purveyors of middle-class attitudes and habits. These effects of schooling were particularly evident at the high-school stage, and this trend of research became closely linked to the study of adolescent development. This work spread to the United Kingdom in the mid-1950s and subsequently to other parts of the world and led to challenging the maintenance of selective schools and to establishing comprehensive high schools. This research emphasis on issues associated with educational disadvantage has continued subsequently, with concern for disparities in the educational opportunities provided for different racial and ethnic groups, for inner urban and rural groups and, in particular, for girls.

Educational reforms were launched in several European countries after the Second World War. The structural changes which took place were based on the outcomes, or rather the interpretations of the outcomes, of these research endeavors. In Sweden and the United Kingdom the debate on comprehensive versus selective secondary education was closely connected with several big studies (e.g., Svensson 1962). In Germany, the Max Planck Society decided to establish a research institute for education in Berlin in 1964, an institute which played an important role in the debate on German school reform. Moreover, a Federal Council (*Bildungsrat*) was set up in the 1960s which commissioned a series of studies pertaining to the German school reform.

4. The 1960s and 1970s

During the first part of the 1960s in affluent countries educational research enjoyed for the first time in its history the massive support necessary for it to have a significant impact. This development was particularly marked in the United States. At that time money for research and curriculum development, particularly in mathematics and science, was readily available. In 1954, federal funds were first devoted through the Cooperative Research Act to a program of research and development in education (Holtzmann 1978). The big, private foundations also began to sponsor educational research on a large scale. The civil rights movement, Kennedy's New Frontier, and Johnson's Great Society continued the trend.

In 1965, the Elementary and Secondary Education Act was passed, which authorized funding over a five-year period for constructing and equipping regional research and development (R & D) centers and laboratories. President Johnson implemented developments that had been planned under Kennedy and, in 1968, federal support for educational research reached its peak, with 21 R & D centers, 20 regional laboratories, 100 graduate training programs in educational research, and thousands of demonstration projects, representing a total federal investment of close to 200 million dollars per year. On a much smaller scale, similar developments took place in the United Kingdom and elsewhere.

Expansion also took place in the former Soviet Union. Between 1960 and 1970 the professional staff engaged in educational research increased considerably. The Soviet Academy of Pedagogical Sciences, initially under the name of the Academy of the Russian Republic, was founded in 1943. In 1967, the *Institut Pédagogique National* of France, for the first time, received significant funding for educational research.

By the late 1960s, all highly industrialized countries were in the midst of cultural crises which had a deep impact on scientific epistemology and thus affected the research world. There was also talk about a "world crisis" (Coombs 1968) in education which applied in the first place to the imbalance between demand and supply of education, particularly in Third World countries. Deeply disappointed in their hope for general peace, wealth, and happiness, people realized that neither science and technology nor traditional—mostly middle-class—values had solved their problems. An anti-intellectualist counterculture developed, emphasizing freedom in all respects, rejecting strict rationality, and glorifying community life. The value of "traditional" education was questioned. "Deschooling," nondirectivity, group experience, and participation seemed to many the alpha and omega of all pedagogy. This trend did not leave socialist countries unaffected, and a group of researchers in the former Soviet Union regretted a too rationalistic approach in educational research (Novikov 1977).

At the same time, scholars also began to question science, some with great caution and strong argumentation, others superficially in line with the *Zeitgeist*. Kerlinger (1977) condemned the latter with ferocity: "mostly bizarre nonsense, bandwaggon climbing, and guruism, little related to what research is and should be."

This was not the case in the crucial epistemological debate inspired by scholars like Polanyi, Popper, Kuhn, and Piaget. Fundamentally, the world of learning acknowledged both the contemporary "explosion" of knowledge and the still very superficial comprehensions of natural, human phenomena. Piaget (1972) showed in his *Epistémologie des sciences de l'homme*, that nomothetic and historical (anthropological) approaches are not mutually exclusive but complementary.

In 1974, two of the best-known United States educational researchers, Cronbach (1974) and Campbell (1974), without previous mutual consultation, chose the annual meeting of the American Psychologist Association to react against the traditional positivist emphasis on quantitative methods and stressed the importance of alternative methods of inquiry. Cronbach also emphasized the importance of aptitude-treatment interaction (ATI).

Since the 1960s, the computer has become the daily companion of the researcher. For the first time in the history of humankind, the amount and complexity of calculation are no longer a major problem. Already existing statistical techniques, like multiple regression analysis, factor analysis, multivariate analysis of variance, that previously were too onerous for desk calculation, suddenly became accessible in a few moments. Large-scale research surveys became feasible. Simultaneously, new statistical methods and techniques were developed.

Huge surveys, such as Project Talent in the United States and the mathematics and six subject surveys of the International Association for the Evaluation of Educational Achievement (IEA) would have been unthinkable without powerful data-processing units.

The experience gained in the domain of large-scale achievement evaluation opened the way to systematic monitoring of school systems and to the periodical publication of accountability reports. A pioneer in this kind of evaluation was the United States National Assessment of Educational Progress (NEAP).

Campbell and Stanley's (1963) presentation of experimental and quasi-experimental design for educational research can also be considered to be a landmark. Advances in the field of educational research were not only stimulated by access to funds and to powerful technology, but also by the "explosion" of knowledge in the social sciences, especially in psychology, linguistics, economics, and sociology.

Many scientific achievements in the field of education can be mentioned for the 1960s: the new ideas on educational objectives, the new concepts of criterion-referenced testing (see *Criterion-referenced Measurement*), formative and summative evaluation, teacher–pupil interaction analysis, research on teacher effectiveness, compensatory education for socioculturally handicapped children, the study of cognitive and affective handicaps, research into the importance and methods of early education, social aspects of learning aptitudes, deschooling experiments, adult education, the development of new curricula, empirical methodology of curriculum development and evaluation, and advances in research methodology (Connell 1980, Husén and Kogan 1984).

5. Developments in the 1980s and 1990s

With the advent of the last quarter of the twentieth century, the status of educational research attained a level of quality comparable to that of other disciplines. The epistemological debate of the previous decade classified considerably the relative strengths and weaknesses of the qualitative and the quantitative approaches. It is widely acknowledged in the early 1990s that no one research paradigm can answer all the questions which arise in educational research. Moreover, it is generally recognized that the hardline distinction between quantitative and qualitative methods cannot be sustained since complex statistical procedures have been developed for the analysis of qualitative data (see *Contingency Tables; Correspondence Analysis; Log–Linear Models*). There has also been marked growth of the humanistic research movement which employs the methods of anthropology, sociology, history, and linguistics.

A widely used alternative research strategy is ethnomethodology (Spindler 1988). The way individuals behave in their environment (home, classroom, etc.) is extensively observed (naturalistic observation) and described. Variables are not manipulated. Main research themes are, for instance, the daily life of a class or a school, the observation of classroom processes that may help understanding school failure, and the processes of the latent or hidden curriculum. Ethnography is broadening knowledge of educational processes and phenomena. Unfortunately, this research method takes much time, and since all events are supposed to be observed, accumulated details become hard to interpret.

It is furthermore acknowledged that neither explaining nor understanding paradigms rely on firm empirical foundations. A research method—be it qualitative or quantitative—cannot provide knowledge of the true nature of phenomenon. Contemporary transcendental (or criterial) realism tries to overcome this epistemological difficulty.

A clear impact of this maturity can also be observed in educational practice. Both the scientific quest for the most efficient standard teaching method and the progressive improvisation (for a while replaced by nondirectivity) have been succeeded by subtle classroom management including careful definition and negotiation of objectives, consideration of student and teacher characteristics, of cognitive and affective styles, and of economic and social needs. Thanks to the advancement of developmental and educational psychology it is now understood, for instance, how the Piagetian constructivist theory implies that many crucial educational objectives can only be defined by or with the learner, while interacting with his or her environment. Recent progress in the cognitive sciences, particularly in the study of the functioning of the brain, have opened new research perspectives that are being vigorously pursued.

The frontiers of educational research are constantly changing.

6. Conclusion

Like medicine, education is an art. That is why advances in research do not directly produce a science of education, in the positivist meaning of the term, but yield increasingly powerful foundations for practice and decision-making. In this perspective, it can be said that educational research has gathered a large body of knowledge containing valuable observations and conclusions that have had a very marked impact both on policy-making and practice.

See also: Research Paradigms in Education

References

Ayres L P 1912–16 *Scales for Measuring the Quality of Handwriting. Scales for Measuring the Quality of Spelling.* Russell Sage, New York
Bain A 1859 *The Emotions and the Will.* Parker, London
Bain A 1879 *Education as a Science.* Kegan Paul, London
Bartholomäi F 1871 Psychologische statistik. *Allgemeine Schulzeitung*
Bernard C 1932 *Introduction à l'étude de la médecine expérimentale.* Doin, Paris
Binet A 1924 *Les idées modernes sur les enfants.* Flammarion, Paris
Binet A, Henri V 1898 *La fatigue intellectuelle.* Schleicher, Paris
Binet A, Simon T 1905 Methode nouvelle pour le diagnostic de l'intelligence des anormaux. *L'année psychologique* 11: 191–244
Bobbitt F 1918 *The Curriculum.* Houghton Mifflin, Boston, Massachusetts
Brown W, Thomson G H 1921 *The Essentials of Mental Measurement.* Cambridge University Press, Cambridge
Buyse R 1935 *L'Expérimentation en Pédagogie.* Lamertin, Brussels
Campbell D T 1974 Qualitative knowing in action research. Paper delivered to Annual Meeting of the American Psychological Association, Los Angeles, California
Campbell D T, Stanley J C 1963 Experimental and quasi-experimental designs for research on teaching. In: Gage N L (ed.) 1963 *Handbook of Research on Teaching.* Rand McNally, Chicago, Illinois
Carroll J B 1978 On the theory–practice interface in the measurement of intellectual abilities. In: Suppes P (ed.) 1978 *Impact of Research of Education.* National Academy of Education, Washington, DC
Cattell J M 1890 Mental tests and measurement. *Mind* 15: 373–81
Claparède E 1911 *Psychologie de l'enfant et pédagogie expérimentale. Vol. 2: Les méthodes.* Delachaux and Niestlé, Neuchâtel
Connell W F 1980 *A History of Education in the Twentieth Century World.* Teachers College Press, New York
Coombs P H 1968 *The World Educational Crisis: A Systems Analysis.* Oxford University Press, London
Cronbach L J 1974 Beyond the two disciplines of scientific psychology. Paper delivered to the Annual Meeting of the American Psychological Association, Los Angeles, California
Cronbach L J, Suppes P (eds.) 1969 *Research for Tomorrow's Schools: Disciplined Inquiry for Education: Report.* Macmillan, New York
de Landsheere G 1982 *Empirical Research in Education.* UNESCO, Paris
de Landsheere G 1986 *La recherche en éducation dans le monde.* Presses Universitaires de France, Paris
Decroly O, Buyse R 1929 *Introduction à la pédagogie quantitative: Eléments de statistiques appliqués aux problèmes pédagogiques.* Lamertin, Brussels
Ebbinghaus H 1897 Über eine neue Methode zur Prüfung geistiger Fähigkeiten. *Zeitschrift für angewandte Psychologie*
Ferré A 1961 Les tests à l'école, 5th edn. Bourrelier, Paris
Fisher R A 1925 *Statistical Methods for Research Workers.* Oliver and Boyd, Edinburgh
Fisher R A 1935 *The Design of Experiments.* Oliver and Boyd, Edinburgh
Galton F 1869 *Hereditary Genius: An Enquiry into its Laws and Consequences.* Macmillan, London
Galton F 1883 *Inquiries into Human Faculty and its Development.* Macmillan, London
Guilford J P 1967 *The Nature of Intelligence.* McGraw-Hill, New York

Holtzman W H 1978 Social change and the research and development movement. In: Glaser R (ed.) 1978 *Research and Development and School Change.* Erlbaum, Hillsdale, New Jersey

Husén T 1988 Research paradigms in education. *Interchange* 19(1): 2–13

Husén T, Boalt G 1968 *Educational Research and Educational Change: The Case of Sweden.* Wiley, New York

Husén T, Kogan M (eds.) 1984 *Educational Research and Policy: How Do They Relate?* Pergamon Press, Oxford

Jeunehomme L 1936 *Plan d'études.* Ministère de l'instruction publique, Brussels

Jonçich G 1962 Whither thou, educational scientist? *Teach. Coll. Rec.* 64(1): 1–12

Jullien M-A 1817 *Esquisse d'un ouvrage sur l'éducation comparée,* Colas, Paris

Keeves J 1988 The unity of educational research. *Interchange* 19(1): 14–30

Kerlinger F N 1977 *The Influence of Research on Educational Practice.* University of Amsterdam, Amsterdam

McCall W A 1922 *How to Measure in Education.* Macmillan, New York.

Meumann E 1920 *Abriss der experimentellen Pädagogik,* Nemmick, Leipzig

Novikov L 1977 Probleme der Planung und Organisation der pädagogischen Forschung in der Sowjetunion. In: Mitter W, Novikov L (eds.) 1977 *Pädagogische Forschung und Bildungspolitik in der Sowjetunion: Organisation, Gegenstand, Methoden.* Deutsches Institut für Internationale Pädogogische Forschung, Frankfurt/Main

Otis A S 1926 *Statistical Method in Educational Measurement.* World Books, Yonkers-on-Hudson, New York

Pearson K 1896 Mathematical contribution to the theory of evolution. *Philosophical Transactions* 187: 253–318

Piaget J 1972 *Epistémologie des sciences de l'homme.* Gallimard, Paris

Rice J M 1897 The futility of the spelling grind. *Forum* 23: 163–72

Rice J M 1913 *Scientific Management in Education.* Hinds, Noble and Eldredge, New York

Schuyten M C 1896 Sur les méthodes de mensuration de la fatigue des écoliers. *Archives de psychologie* 2

Simon T 1924 *Pédagogie expérimentale: Ecriture, lecture, orthographe.* Colin, Paris

Spearman C 1904 General intelligence objectively determined and measured. *Am. J. Psychol.* 15: 201–92

Spindler G 1988 *Doing the Ethnography of Schooling: Education and Anthropology in Action.* Waveland Press, Prospect Heights, Illinois

Svensson N-E 1962 *Ability Grouping and Scholastic Achievement; Report on a five-year follow-up study in Stockholm.* Almqvist and Wiksell, Stockholm

Thorndike E L 1906 *The Principles of Teaching Based on Psychology.* Seiler, New York

Thorndike E L 1913 *An Introduction to the Theory of Mental and Social Measurements,* 2nd edn. Teachers College Press, New York

Thorndike E L, McCall W A, Chapman J C 1916 *Ventilation in Relation to Mental Work.* Teachers College Press, New York

Thurstone L L 1925 *The Fundamentals of Statistics.* Macmillan, New York

Tyler R W 1949 *Basic Principles of Curriculum and Instruction.* University Press, Chicago, Illinois

Vygotsky L S 1962 *Thought and Language.* MIT Press, Cambridge, Massachusetts

Yule G U 1911 *An Introduction to the Theory of Statistics.* Griffin, London

Warner W L, Havighurst R J, Loeb M B 1946 *Who Shall be Educated? The Challenge of Unequal Opportunities.* Kegan Paul, London

Further Reading

Boring J 1950 *History of Experimental Psychology.* Appleton-Century-Croft, New York

Galton F 1888 Co-relations and their measurement. *Proceedings of the Royal Society* 45: 35–145

Lay W A 1906 Über Kämpfe und Fortschritte der experimentellen Pädagogik. *Die Experimentelle Pädagogik* 2: 96–117

Vaney V 1909 L'âge de la lecture. *Société libre pour l'étude de la psychologie de l'enfant,* 53

Research Paradigms in Education

T. Husén

Thomas Kuhn, himself a historian of science, contributed to a fruitful development in the philosophy of science with his book *The Structure of Scientific Revolutions* published in 1962. It mapped out how established thinking, research strategies, and methods in a scientific field, in Kuhn's terminology "normal science," were established. It brought into focus two streams of thinking about what could be regarded as "scientific," the Aristotelian tradition with its teleological approach and the Galilean with its causal and mechanistic approach. It introduced the concept of "paradigm" into the philosophical debate.

"Paradigm" derives from the Greek verb for "exhibiting side by side." In lexica it is given with the translations "example" or "table of declensions and conjugations." Although Kuhn himself used paradigm rather ambiguously, the concept has turned out to be useful in inspiring critical thinking about "normal science" and the way shifts in basic scientific thinking occur. A paradigm determines the criteria according to which one selects and defines problems for inquiry and how one approaches them theoretically and methodologically. Young scientists tend to be socialized into the precepts of the prevailing paradigm which to them constitutes "normal science." In that respect a paradigm could be regarded as a cultural artifact, reflecting the dominant notions about scientific behavior in a particular scientific community, be it national or international, and at a particular point in time. Paradigms determine scientific approaches and procedures which stand out as exemplary to the new generation of scientists—as long as they do not oppose them.

A "revolution" in the world of scientific paradigms occurs when one or several researchers at a given time encounter anomalies, for instance, make observations, which in a striking way do not fit the prevailing paradigm. Such anomalies can give rise to a crisis after which the universe under study is perceived in an entirely new light. Previous theories and facts become subject to thorough rethinking and re-evaluation.

In well-defined disciplines which have developed over centuries, such as the natural sciences, it is relatively easy to point out dramatic changes in paradigms, such as in astronomy from Ptolemy through Copernicus to Galileo or in physics from Aristotle via Galileo and Newton to Einstein. When the social sciences emerged in the nineteenth century, people like Comte tended to regard the natural sciences as scientific models, but without awareness that the social scientist is part of a process of social self-understanding. Educational research faces a particular problem, since education, as William James pointed out, is not a well-defined, unitary discipline but a practical art. Research into educational problems is conducted by scholars with many disciplinary affiliations. Most of them have a background in psychology or other behavioral sciences, but quite a few of them have a humanistic background in philosophy and history. Thus there cannot be any prevailing paradigm or "normal science" in the very multifaceted field of educational research. However, when empirical research conducted by behavioral scientists, particularly in the Anglo-Saxon countries, in the 1960s and early 1970s began to be accused of dominating research with a positivist quantitatively oriented paradigm that prevented other paradigms of a humanistic or dialectical nature being employed, the accusations were directed at those with a behavioral science background.

1. The Two Classical Paradigms

The twentieth century has seen the conflict between two main paradigms employed in researching educational problems. The one is modeled on the natural sciences with an emphasis on empirical quantifiable observations which lend themselves to analyses by means of mathematical tools. The task of research is to establish causal relationships, to explain (*Erklären*).

The other paradigm is derived from the humanities with an emphasis on holistic and qualitative information and interpretive approaches (*Verstehen*).

Briefly, the two paradigms in educational research developed historically as follows. By the mid-nineteenth century, when Auguste Comte (1798–1857) developed positivism in sociology and John Stuart Mill (1806–1873) empiricism in psychology, there was a major breakthrough in the natural sciences at the universities with the development of a particular logic and methodology of experiments and hypothesis testing. They therefore came to serve as models and their prevailing paradigm was taken over by social scientists, particularly in the Anglo-Saxon countries (see, e.g., Pearson 1892). However, on the European Continent there was another tradition from German idealism and Hegelianism. The "Galilean," mechanistic conception became the dominant one, particularly with mathematical physics as the methodological ideal. Positivism was characterized by methodological monism. Philosophers at the University of Vienna (such as Neurath), referred to as the "Vienna Circle," developed what is called "neopositivism" or "logical empiricism." Around 1950 they founded a series of publications devoted to the study of what they called "unified science." Positivism saw the main task for the social sciences as being the making of causal explanations and the prediction of future behavior on the basis of the study of present behavior. Neopositivism emanated from the stong influence of analytical philosophy.

There are at least three strands for the other main paradigm in educational research. The Continental idealism of the early nineteenth century has been mentioned. Around the turn of the century it had a dominant influence at German universities with philosophers, such as Wilhelm Dilthey (1833–1911), who in the 1890s published a classical treatise in which he made the distinction between *Verstehen* and *Erklären*. He maintained that the humanities had their own logic of research and pointed out that the difference between natural sciences and humanities was that the former tried to explain, whereas the latter tried to understand. He also maintained that there were two kinds of psychology, the one which by means of experimental methods attempted to generalize and predict, and the one that tried to understand the unique individual in his or her entire, concrete setting. Other philosophers with similar conceptions were Heinrich Rickert and Wilhelm Windelband. A counterpart in France was Henri Bergson (1859–1941) who maintained that the intellect was unable to grasp the living reality which could only be approached by means of intuition. In Sweden, John Landquist advanced an epistemology of humanities.

A second strand was represented by the phenomenological philosophy developed by Edmund Husserl (1859–1938) in Germany. It emphasized the importance of taking a widened perspective and of trying to "get to the roots" of human activity. The phenomenological, and later the hermeneutic, approach is holistic: it tries by means of empathy (*Einfühlung*) to understand the motives behind human reactions. By widening the perspective and trying to understand human beings as individuals in their entirety and in their proper context it also tries to avoid the fragmentation caused by the positivistic and experimental approach that takes out a small slice which it subjects to closer scrutiny.

The third strand in the humanistic paradigm consists of the critical philosophy, not least the one of the Frankfurt school (Adorno, Horckheimer, and Habermas) which developed with a certain amount of neo-Marxism. Marx himself would probably have felt rather ambivalent in an encounter between the two main scientific philosophies. On the one hand, he felt attracted to positivism. On the other hand, Marx belonged to the German philosophical tradition and the neo-Marxists have not had great difficulties in accepting hermeneutics and merging it with a dialectical approach.

The paradigm determines how a problem is formulated and methodologically tackled. According to the traditional positivist conception, problems that relate, for example, to classroom behavior should be investigated primarily in terms of the individual actor, either the pupils, who might be neurotic, or the teacher, who might be ill-prepared for his or her job. The other conception is to formulate the problem in terms of the larger setting, that of the school, or rather that of the society at large. Furthermore, one does not in the first place, by means of such mechanisms as testing, observation, and the like, try to find out why the pupil or the teacher deviates from the "normal." Rather an attempt is made to study the particular individual as a goal-directed human being with particular and unique motives.

The belief that science, particularly social science, would "save us" was expressed as late as in the 1940s by George Lundberg (1947), a sociologist who represented a consistent positivist approach. In the long run, the study of human beings would map out the social reality and provide a knowledge base for vastly improved methods of dealing with human beings, be they pupils in the classroom or workers in the factory. A similar hope still guided the establishment of research and development centers with massive resources at some North American universities in the 1960s. What experience and enlightened empathy could tell was somehow regarded as inferior to the knowledge provided by systematic observations and measurements.

2. A Historical Note

In his *Talks to Teachers on Psychology*, given in the 1890s, James (1899 p. 9) pointed out: "To know psychology . . . is absolutely no guarantee that

we shall be good teachers." An additional ability is required, something that he calls the "happy tact and ingenuity," the "ingenuity in meeting and pursuing the pupil, the tact for the concrete situation." He mentions the demands of making systematic observations that some "enthusiasts for child study" have burdened the teachers with, including "compiling statistics and computing the percent." In order to avoid such endeavors resulting in trivialities they must be related to the "anecdotes and observations" which acquaint the teachers more intimately with the students.

What James refers to is something that in the terminology of the late twentieth century would be seen as a conflict between two main research paradigms. By the end of the nineteenth century, the scientific paradigm emerged that has since then been the prevailing one, at least in the Anglo-Saxon world. It was part of a larger movement toward "scientific management" in industry.

The new scientific approach emerging at the end of the nineteenth century was spelled out by the leading educational psychologist, Edward Lee Thorndike of Columbia University, in the preface to his seminal book *Educational Psychology* in 1903. He set out to apply "the methods of exact science" to educational problems, reject "speculative opinions," and emphasize "accurate quantitative treatment" of information collected (Clifford 1984). He acknowledged the influence on his thinking of people who have advocated the quantitative and experimental approach, like James McKeen Cattell and R S Woodworth in the United States, and Francis Galton and Karl Pearson in England. In a brief concluding chapter he dealt with the problem of education as a science and presented the main characteristics of what he regarded as scientific in education:

> It is the vice or the misfortune of thinkers about education to have chosen the methods of philosophy or of popular thought instead of those of science . . . The chief duty of serious students of the theory of education today is to form the habit of inductive study and learn the logic of statistics. (Thorndike 1903 p. 164)

Part of the new scientific paradigm was to make a clear-cut distinction between the descriptive and the normative. Research conducted according to "logic of science" was supposed to be neutral with regard to values and policy-making.

The prevailing paradigm in North America spelled out by Thorndike was further developed by John Franklin Bobbitt, professor at the University of Chicago, who in 1912 advanced the notion that schools could be operated according to the methods of "scientific management" which had been developed in industry by Frederick Taylor. Bobbitt also played an important role in attempts to determine empirically the content of curriculum by analyzing what people needed as holders of occupations and as citizens in order to arrive at a common denominator of skills and specific pieces of knowledge with which the school had to equip them.

With an eye on the natural sciences, social science has for more than a century made the claim to be an "objective" and "explaining" science. It purported to be able to make a clear-cut distinction between aims and means of achieving these aims. It maintained that in handling social realities it was able to do it without any moral commitments. Its representatives claim like in the natural sciences to reside outside the system they observe. Such a claim has been brought into question. Gunnar Myrdal (1969) did so in a book (first published in Swedish in the 1930s) on science and politics in economics. He showed that the social researcher could not be free from his or her own values and political convictions, but could arrive at more valid conclusions and gain in credibility by making his or her value premises explicit and by making clear what those biases were in describing reality. Thereby the researcher can also give the "consumers" of his or her research an instrument for correction.

Social research, not least that in education, consists of data collection and reflection about societal problems, with their dilemmas and paradoxes, tensions, and so on, as well as alternatives for political action which offer themselves. Not even in the ideal case can a consensus be expected around theoretical paradigms as separated from practical problems. Social science researchers are part of the social process which they set out to investigate. They share social and political values of the surrounding society. In a way, they participate in the process of social self-understanding. This means that there is no such thing as a "social technology" in the same sense as a technology based on natural science. This does not imply, however, that educational research endeavors are of very limited value or entirely futile. The "aloofness" of the researchers in terms of dependence on interest groups and politics with shared social values is a relative matter. The task of the academic of "seeking the truth" can become institutionalized. This is what happens when fundamental, discipline-oriented research is established in institutions where the researchers can pursue their tasks of critical review without jeopardizing their positions.

There were those who, in contrast to William James, thought that it would be possible to make education a science. One of them was Charles H Judd (a student of Wundt), who in *Introduction to the Scientific Study of Education* in 1918, tried to explain how research was related to teacher training and educational practice. In 1909 the Department of Education at the University of Chicago had abandoned course requirements for prospective teachers in the history of education and psychology. These courses had been replaced by one course called "Introduction to Education" and one in "Methods of Teaching." Thereby the teacher candidates could be introduced to the school problems in "a more direct, concrete way."

Each chapter in Judd's book presents practical school problems and gives sources of information for the solution of these problems. Much of this information is very incomplete, but as a whole Judd thinks that it is justified to speak about a "science of education." To use the term "science" he thinks would be justified, even when the information available is very scanty, "for the essence of science is its methods of investigation, not its ability to lay down a body of final rules of action" (Judd 1918 p. 299).

A research paradigm similar to the one advanced by Galton, Pearson, and Thorndike developed in Germany and France under the influence of experimental psychology. Ernst Meumann, a student of Wilhelm Wundt and a leading experimental psychologist, published at the beginning of the twentieth century his monumental three-volume work *Vorlesungen zur Einführung in die experimentelle Pädagogik* (Introduction to Experimental Pedagogy). He meant by "experimental education" largely the application of the systematic, empirical, and statistical methods to educational data. Alfred Binet in France had a similar influence in both child study and intelligence testing.

3. The Two Main Paradigms and Their Compatibility

One can distinguish between two main paradigms in educational research planning with a different epistemological basis (Adams 1988). On the one hand, there is the functional–structural, objective–rational, goal-directed, manipulative, hierarchical, and technocratic approach. On the other hand, there is the interpretivist, humanistic, consensual, subjective, and collegial one.

The first approach is derived from classical positivism. The second one, which in recent years has gained momentum, is partly derived from the critical theory of the Frankfurt school, particularly from Habermas's theory of communicative action. The first approach is "linear" and consists of a straightforward rational action toward preconceived problems. The second approach leaves room for reinterpretation and reshaping of the problem during the process of dialogue prior to action and even during action.

Phillips (1983) has contributed to a valuable conceptual clarification of "positivism." He distinguishes between four varieties of it: (a) the classical Comtean positivism with its belief that the scientific method established in the natural sciences can be applied in the study of human behavior and human affairs in general; (b) logical positivism embodied by the Vienna Circle which had a strong impact among psychologists and sociologists in the middle of the twentieth century with its quest for verification and operational definitions; (c) behaviorism of the Watsonian or Skinnerian type; and (d) positivism as a general label for empiricism, which covers a broad spectrum of epistemological positions.

Phillips (1983) argues that some of the many ardent critics of allegedly positivist researchers are themselves "more positivistic than they recognize," some of them by using an instrumentalistic criterion of truth. They tend to make the mistake of "identifying positivism with particular research methods," such as experimental design or statistical analysis methods. Thus, there is basically not such an unbridgeable gap between the two paradigms as is often purported by representatives of the respective camps.

Keeves (1988) argues that the various research paradigms employed in education, the empirical–positivist, the hermeneutic or phenomenological, and the ethnographic–anthropological are complementary to each other. He talks about the "unity of educational research," makes a distinction between paradigms and approaches, and contends that there is, in the final analysis, only one paradigm but many approaches. The teaching–learning process can be observed and/or video-recorded. The observations can be quantified and the data analyzed by means of advanced statistical methods. Content can be studied in the light of national traditions and the philosophy underlying curriculum constructions. Both the teaching–learning process and its outcomes can be studied in a comparative, cross-national perspective.

Depending upon the *objective* of a particular research project, emphasis is laid more on the one or on the other paradigm. One could quote the following as an example of how quantitative and qualitative paradigms are complementary to each other. It is not possible to arrive at any valid information about a school or national system concerning the level of competence achieved in, for instance, science by visiting a number of classrooms and thereby trying to collect impressions. Even a highly experienced science teacher is not able to gain information that would allow accurate inferences about the quality of outcomes of science teaching in the entire system of education. Sample surveys like the ones conducted by the IEA (International Association for the Evaluation of Education Achievement) would be necessary instruments. But such surveys are too superficial when it comes to accounting for factors behind the differences between school systems. Here qualitative information of different kinds is required.

But the choice or "mix" of paradigm is also determined by what *kind of knowledge* one is searching for. The ultimate purpose of any knowledge arrived at in educational research is to provide a basis for action, be it policy action or methods of teaching in the classroom. The former type of knowledge must by definition be of a more general nature and apply to a lot of local and individual situations, such as reforming the structure of the system or the relationship between home background and school attainments. But the classroom teacher deals with a unique child in a unique teaching–learning situation and is not very much helped by relying on generalized knowledge.

Policymakers, planners, and administrators want generalizations and rules which apply to a wide variety of institutions with children of rather diverse backgrounds. The policymaker and planner is more interested in the collectivity than in the individual child. They operate from the perspective of the whole system. Educational research has made significant contributions to reforms of entire national systems of education. Sweden and Germany are cases in point.

Classroom practioners are not very much helped by generalizations which apply "on the whole" or "by and large" because they are concerned with the timely, the particular child here and now. Research on the teaching–learning process can at best give them a perspective on the particular teaching–learning situation with which they are faced. The pedagogical steps taken have to be guided by the qualitative information that Eisner (1982) refers to as "connoisseurship" which is a body of experiences and critical analysis which may well also be guided by research insights.

4. The Need for Pluralism in Approaches

In the late 1960s and early 1970s critical, dialectical, hermeneutical, and neo-Marxian paradigms were advanced as alternatives or even replacements for the prevailing neopositivist paradigm of quantification, hypothesis testing, and generalizations. The latter had dominated the scene of social science research in the Anglo-Saxon countries for many decades and had taken the lead at many Continental universities as well. The new approaches were espoused by many from these universities to the extent that a group of younger researchers in education even prepared an international handbook of educational research that deliberately challenged the prevailing Anglo-Saxon research paradigms. The behavioral sciences have equipped educational researchers with an arsenal of research tools, such as observational methods and tests, which help them to systematize observations which would otherwise not have been considered in the more holistic and intuitive attempts to make, for instance, informal observations or to conduct personal interviews.

Those who turn to social science research in order to find out about the "best" pedagogy or the most "efficient" methods of teaching are in a way victims of the traditional science which claimed to be able to arrive at generalizations applicable in practically every context. But, not least through critical philosophy, researchers have become increasingly aware that education does not take place in a social vacuum. Educational researchers have also begun to realize that educational practices are not independent of the cultural and social context in which they operate. Nor are they neutral to educational policies. Therefore, dogmatic evangelism for particular philosophies and ideologies espoused as "scientific" and not accessible to criticism is detrimental to the spirit of inquiry. The two main paradigms are not exclusive, but complementary to each other.

See also: Policy-Oriented Research; Hermeneutics; History of Educational Research; Educational Research and Policy-making: Educational History in Biographies and Autoibiographies

References

Adams D 1988 Extending the educational planning discussion: Conceptual and paradigmatic explorations. *Comp. Educ. Rev.* 32: 400–15
Clifford G J 1984 *The Sane Positivist: A Biography of Edward L Thorndike.* Wesleyan University Press, Middletown, Connecticut
Eisner E 1982 *Cognition and Curriculum: A Basis for Deciding What to Teach.* Longman, London
James W 1899 *Talks to Teachers on Psychology: And to Students on Some of the Life's Ideals.* Longmans Green, London
Judd C H 1918 *Introduction to the Scientific Study of Education.* Ginn, Boston, Massachusetts
Keeves J P 1988 The unity of educational research. *Interchange* 19(1): 14–30
Kuhn T S 1962 *The Structure of Scientific Revolutions.* University of Chicago Press, Chicago, Illinois
Lundberg G 1947 *Can Science Save Us?* Longmans Green, London
Meumann E 1911 *Vorlesungen zur Einführung in die experimentelle Pädagogik und ihre psychologischen Grundlagen.* Engelmann, Leipzig
Myrdal G 1969 *Objectivity in Social Research.* Pantheon, New York
Pearson K 1892 *The Grammar of Science.* Adam and Charles Black, London
Phillips D C 1983 After the wake: Postpositivistic educational thought. *Educ. Res.* 12(5): 4–14, 23–24
Thorndike E L 1903 *Educational Psychology.* Scientific Press, New York

Further Reading

Cronbach L J 1975 Beyond the two disciplines of scientific psychology. *Am. Psychol.* (30): 116–27
Eisner E (ed.) 1985a *The Educational Imagination.* Macmillan, New York
Eisner E (ed.) 1985b Learning and teaching the ways of knowing. In: National Society for the Study of Education

1985 *Eighty-fourth Yearbook.* Chicago University Press, Chicago, Illinois
Fritzell C 1981 *Teaching Science and Ideology: A Critical Inquiry into the Sociology of Pedagogy.* Gleerup, Lund
Fromm E (ed.) 1965 *Socialist Humanism: An International Symposium.* Doubleday, Garden City, New York
Gage N L 1989 The paradigm wars and their aftermath: A "historical" sketch of research on teaching since 1989. *Educ. Res.* 18(7): 4–10
Galtung J 1977 *Essays in Methodology, Vol. 1: Methodology and Ideology.* Ejlers, Copenhagen
Guba E 1978 *Toward A Methodology of Naturalistic Inquiry in Educational Evaluation.* University of California, Center for Study in Evaluation, Los Angeles, California
Habermas J 1972 *Knowledge and Human Interests.* Heinemann, London
Heidegger M 1962 *Being and Time.* Harper, New York
Home K R 1988 Against the quantitative–qualitative incompatability thesis or dogmas die hard. *Educ. Res.* 17(8): 10–16
Husén T 1979 General theories in education: A twenty-five year perspective. *Int. Rev. Educ.* 25: 325–45
Husén T 1988 Research paradigms in education. *Interchange* 19(1): 2–13
Husén T 1989 Educational research at the crossroads? An exercise in self-criticism. *Prospects* 19(3): 351–60
Jaeger R M 1988 *Complementary Methods of Research in Education.* American Educational Research Association (AERA), Washington, DC
Landquist J 1920 *Människokunskap.* Bonniers, Stockholm
Lindholm S 1981 *Paradigms, Science and Reality: On Dialectics, Hermeneutics and Positivism in the Social Sciences.* Department of Education, Stockholm University, Stockholm
Landsheere G de 1986 *La recherche en education dans le monde.* Presse Universitaire de France, Paris
Palmer R E 1969 *Hermeneutics: Interpretation Theory in Schleiermacher, Dilthey, Heidegger, and Gadamer.* Northwestern University Press, Evanston, Illinois
Phillips D C 1992 *The Social Scientist's Bestiary.* Pergamon Press, Oxford
Rapoport A 1950 *Science and the Goals of Man: A Study in Semantic Orientation.* Harper, New York
Rizo F M 1991 The controversy about quantification in social research: An extension of Gage's "historical sketch." *Educ. Res.* 20: 9–12
Shulman L S 1986 Those who understand knowledge growth in teaching. *Educ. Res.* 15(2): 4–14
Smith J K, Heshusius L 1986 Closing down the conversation: The end of the quantitative–qualitative debate among educational inquirers. *Educ. Res.* 15(1): 4–12
Soltis J F 1984 On the nature of educational research. *Educ. Res.* 13(10): 5–10
Tuthill D, Ashton P 1983 Improving educational research through the development of educational paradigms. *Educ. Res.* 12(10): 6–14
Wright G H von 1971 *Explanation and Understanding.* Routledge and Kegan Paul, London

Research in Education: Epistemological Issues

J. C. Walker and C. W. Evers

Epistemology is the study of the nature, scope, and applicability of knowledge. Educational research, in being concerned with the conduct of educational inquiry and the development and evaluation of its methods and findings, embodies a commitment to epistemological assumptions—at least it does if its findings are expected to command attention, serve as a sound basis for action, or constitute legitimate knowledge claims. These matters are the subject of epistemological theories which deal more systematically with such general corresponding issues as justification, truth, and the accessibility of reality in the search for knowledge.

In educational research, obviously, there are different methods of inquiry, ranging from controlled laboratory experiments through participant observation to action research, from historical studies to logical analysis. These have been organized in different research traditions, such as "quantitative" and "qualitative," or associated with different theoretical positions, such as behaviorism and critical theory. In practice, the categories of method, tradition, and theoretical position cut across each other to some extent.

The major epistemological question here is whether these distinctions are associated with different ways of knowing or forms of knowledge, which partition educational research so that research traditions, for example, turn out to be radically distinct epistemologically, each having its own theories and rules of justification, meaning, and truth. If so, the next question is whether findings produced by the different traditions can be rationally integrated, rendered coherent, or even compared. For this to be possible, for traditions to be commensurable, there will have to be some shared concepts and standards of justification, meaning, and truth: some epistemological touchstone. If, however, the traditions are so fundamentally disparate that any choice between them in educational research is arbitrary or the result of nonrational commitment—an act of faith—there is no touchstone. The research traditions are incommensurable.

There has long been controversy over these issues, in educational research and the social sciences generally, as advocates of research traditions variously described as "scientific," "humanistic," "quantitative," "qualitative," "positivist," and "interpretative" have tried to sort out the respective epistemological merits of these approaches and the methodological, practical, and even political relations between them.

There are three major views available, which have emerged in educational research in more or less the following historical order. First, it can be asserted that there are epistemologically different paradigms, which are incommensurable in that neither educational research nor any other form of inquiry can provide a rational method for judging between them. Moreover, they are mutually incompatible, competitive ways of researching the same territory. This may be called the "oppositional diversity thesis." Second, it could be decided that there are epistemologically distinct paradigms, but that though incommensurable they are complementary, not competitive: equally appropriate ways of approaching different, overlapping, or perhaps even the same research problems. This may be called the "complementary diversity thesis." The first and second views agree that there is a fundamental epistemological diversity in educational research. The third alternative, the unity thesis, denies this. It disagrees with the view that different research methods can be grouped under incommensurable paradigms, and asserts that the very idea of such paradigms is mistaken, even incoherent. It claims there is touchstone for judging the respective merits of different research traditions and bringing them into a productive relationship with one another. It asserts a fundamental epistemological unity of educational research, derived from the practical problems addressed.

This entry argues for the unity thesis. After a discussion of the term "paradigm," and of the oppositional and complementary diversity theses, it is shown that the theory that there are research paradigms—call it the "P-theory"—is largely responsible for both forms of diversity thesis. Some reasons are offered for believing that P-theory is incoherent, and it is argued that a coherentist epistemology sustains the thesis of the epistemological unity of educational research. A feature of this epistemology is its account of touchstone in educational research.

1. Epistemology and Paradigms

Numerous educational researchers have been drawn to the view that research traditions are best regarded as different paradigms. Indeed, as Shulman (1986 p. 3) observes, in writing about the different research programs of communities of scholars engaged in the study of teaching, "the term most frequently employed to describe such research communities, and the conceptions of problem and method they share is *paradigm*."

As the quantitative/qualitative debate shows, many writers in education distinguish two fundamental paradigms of research: the "scientific" which is often erroneously identified with positivism, and the "interpretative" or "humanistic." Husén associates the distinction with divergent forms of explanation and understanding:

> The twentieth century has seen the conflict between two main paradigms employed in researching educational problems. The one is modeled on the natural sciences with an emphasis on empirical quantifiable observations which lend themselves to analyses by means of mathematical tools. The task of research is to establish causal relationships, to explain (*Erklären*). The other paradigm is derived from the humanities with an emphasis on holistic and qualitative information and to interpretive approaches (*Verstehen*). (1988 p. 17)

In offering a broader, three-way taxonomy of research to account for diversity in inquiry, Popkewitz (1984 p. 35) says: "the concept of paradigm provides a way to consider this divergence in vision, custom and tradition. It enables us to consider science as having different sets of assumptions, commitments, procedures and theories of social affairs." He assumes that "in educational sciences, three paradigms have emerged to give definition and structure to the practice of research." After the fashion of "critical theory" (Habermas 1972), he identifies the paradigms as "empirical-analytic" (roughly equivalent to quantitative science), "symbolic" (qualitative and interpretative or hermeneutical inquiry), and "critical" (where political criteria relating to human betterment are applied in research).

Noting the influence of positivism on the formation of research traditions and the paradigms debate, Lincoln and Guba (1984 p. 15) mention another common three-way distinction, which they apply to "paradigm eras," "periods in which certain sets of basic beliefs have guided inquiry in quite different ways," rather than directly to paradigms as such. They identify these paradigm eras as "prepositivist," "positivist," and "postpositivist." Now the term "positivist" also has a history of varied usage (Phillips 1983) but, because of the practice common among educational researchers of defining their perspectives in relation to one or more of the varieties of positivism, it is important to note some of the issues involved in the transition to postpositivism.

In philosophy of science, views of the nature of science commonly described as positivist have characterized science as value-free, basing its theories and findings on logically simple and epistemically secure observation reports, and using empirical concepts themselves deriving directly from observation (Hooker 1975). Positivism in this sense, as a form of empiricism, involves a foundational epistemology. Knowledge claims are justified when they are shown to be based on secure foundations, which for positivist empiricism are the sense data acquired through empirical observation. Some positivists—the logical positivists—maintained that only the sentences of science thus conceived, and the "conceptual truths" of logic and mathematics, were objectively meaningful, and that therefore here were to be drawn the limits of

genuine knowledge, not simply scientific knowledge. Thus delimited, the domain of knowledge excluded morals, politics, and indeed any field where value judgments were made, which would include much educational research. The movement to postpositivist philosophy of science has occurred because of the undermining of all such doctrines (House 1991).

This use of "positivist" needs to be clearly distinguished from use of the term to describe any view that science (and perhaps conceptual truths of logic and mathematics) is the only way to knowledge, and that the task of philosophy—which is not sharply distinguished from, but continuous with, empirical science —is to find general principles common to all sciences and even to extend the use of such principles to the regulation of human conduct and the organization of society. The move to a postpositivist (in the first sense) philosophy of science is quite compatible with such a view of the nature of science and its role in human affairs.

Unfortunately, this distinction is not always clearly observed in epistemological discussions of educational research. It is one thing to say, with Lincoln and Guba (1984), that since it has been recognized that science is more complex than building on theory-free and value-free observations, qualitative inquiry may be recognized as a legitimate approach; that the latest paradigm era sanctions more than one paradigm. It is another thing to identify science with positivism (in the first sense) and on the basis of this identification to attack all views suggesting an epistemological continuity between the natural and the social sciences including educational research. Ironically, many writers, while they claim to reject positivism (in both senses), retain a positivist (in the first sense) view of natural science (e.g., Habermas 1972). In this entry "positivist" is used in the first sense, to refer to positivistic empiricism, including logical positivism.

In summary, the move from a positivist to a postpositivist philosophy of science has been paralleled by a move from a view of educational research dominated by the quantitative tradition to a more pluralistic view. The advent of the postpositivist era has been characterized by an acceptance of epistemological diversity which, however, insofar as it is formulated in terms of P-theory, leaves educational research epistemologically divided. The question, then, if there are such divisions as have been noted, is whether the diversity must be oppositional, or can it be harmonious?

2. The Oppositional Diversity Thesis

Quantitative researchers have often seen qualitative research as lacking in objectivity, rigor, and scientific controls (Kerlinger 1973 p.401). Lacking the resources of quantification, qualitative research cannot produce the requisite generalizations to build up a set of laws of human behavior, nor can it apply adequate tests for validity and reliability. Moreover, the positivist fact/value distinction is often employed to discredit the claims of qualitative inquiry to produce knowledge, since knowledge is value-free whereas qualitative research is irreducibly value-laden and subjective. In short, qualitative research falls short of the high standards of objectivity and the tight criteria for truth of the quantitative, or "scientific," paradigm. Given the prestige of science, and a positivist view of science, it is easy to see why quantitative researchers have sometimes even seen qualitative research as opposed to sound scientific method.

In reply, many qualitative researchers, invoking the explanation/understanding distinction, claim that the genuinely and distinctively human dimension of education cannot be captured by statistical generalizations and causal laws. Knowledge of human affairs is irreducibly subjective. It must grasp the meanings of actions, the uniqueness of events, and the individuality of persons. From this perspective, it is easy to see the quantitative tradition as an intrusive, even alien and antihuman, approach to the study of education. "Science" may be appropriate to the study of nature, but it distorts the study of human affairs. It is easy to see why, given a perceived *de facto* domination of educational research by the quantitative tradition, qualitative researchers have sometimes seen it in oppositional, even antagonistic, terms.

Thus the debate over whether so-called quantitative research methodology is in conflict with qualitative research methodology does not revolve simply around the use of numbers, of mathematical and statistical procedures. Rather, it concerns the relation of quantification to more basic questions about objectivity, validity, reliability, and criteria for truth. For example, according to Smith and Heshusius (1986 p.9), who have reasserted the oppositional diversity thesis against the increasing popularity of the other two: "For quantitative inquiry, a logic of justification that is epistemologically foundational leads to the position that certain sets of techniques are epistemologically privileged in that their correct application is necessary to achieve validity or to discover how things really are out there." They also state: "From the perspective of qualitative inquiry, this line of reasoning is unacceptable. The assumptions or logic of justification in this case are not foundationalist and, by extension, do not allow that certain sets of procedures are epistemologically privileged." There are two key epistemological distinctions here. First, "logic of justification" (grounds for making claims) is distinguished from research procedures (techniques used to gather, analyze, and interpret data). Second, foundational epistemologies, which provide a logic or justification basing knowledge claims on supposedly secure or certain foundations (such as empirical observations), are distinguished from nonfoundational epistemologies whose logic of justification involves no foundations.

Later in this entry the assumption that quantitative inquiry must be foundationalist is queried.

The key epistemological dilemma posed by Smith and Heshusius is that for the quantitative researcher there exists a mind-independent reality "out there" that is to some extent knowable. Disciplined observation of it provides epistemic foundations. Qualitative researchers, they assert, are committed to denying this. By following certain practices of inquiry that enjoy a cluster of related theoretical advantages—the advantages of internal and external validity, reliability, and objectivity—the quantitative researcher increases the likelihood of discovering something important about that reality. Its properties and the causal structures governing the orderly behavior of its interrelated parts constitute typical goals of quantitative inquiry. What makes these goals possible, and indeed holds together the theoretical features of such inquiry, is a belief that people can know when a correspondence obtains between the sentences of a theory and the world "out there." It is this correspondence that makes knowledge claims true.

It is precisely this belief that is most often questioned by qualitative researchers. Reality, or at least social reality, they frequently maintain, is something constructed with the mind as a product of theorizing. Theorizing shapes reality, rather than the other way around. There is simply no mind-independent or theory-independent reality to match up with or correspond to sentences, to serve as a check on their acceptability. Under this assumption, the theoretical apparatus employed to characterize epistemically virtuous inquiry will apparently have little use for familiar quantitative notions. Instead, distinctly alternative networks of theoretical requirements for qualitative research will need to be devised, tied to procedures for getting at subjective, or intersubjective, symbols, meanings, and understandings.

Critical theorists go one step further in this philosophical opposition to the "intrusion" of the quantitative tradition into the search for knowledge of the "genuinely human." In addition to being unable to capture the necessary relation between the human mind and social reality, critical theorists maintain that the quantitative (or empirical-analytic) tradition cannot capture the essential role of values in that kind of knowledge needed to improve the human condition. Thus Bates (1980) argues that epistemically adequate educational research must be research that makes for "human betterment." The "praxis" tradition in epistemology, well-exemplified in the theoretical writings of Freire (1972), and more particularly in the action research tradition (Carr and Kemmis 1983), provides a rich theoretical context for elaborating further nonquantitative criteria to replace quantitative notions of validity, reliability, and objectivity. In contrast to the usual lines drawn in the quantitative/qualitative debate, the elimination of social injustice, for example, is not merely a matter of constructing alternative realities, or alternative theories. Nor is validity simply a matter of establishing a correspondence between theory and the world, when the goal is social improvement. Rather, what counts as valid inquiry, as epistemically progressive, is limited to what the surrounding epistemology counts as promoting human well-being.

3. The Complementary Diversity Thesis

Within the epistemologically softer climate of the postpositivist era, many educational researchers believe that the various research traditions, even if incommensurable, are equally legitimate and in no necessary conflict. The "scientific" and "humanistic" approaches, "are not exclusive, but complementary to each other" (Husén 1988 p.20). Indeed Shulman (1986 p.4) goes so far as to suggest that "the danger for any field of social science or educational research lies in its potential corruption . . . by a single paradigmatic view." Against what they have regarded as the unwarranted "positivist", quantitative domination of educational research, proponents of the qualitative/interpretative paradigm have succeeded in convincing a number of scholars whose work has been within the quantitative tradition (e.g., Campbell and Overman 1988, Cronbach 1975) that the qualitative approach has its own merits.

Some writers have suggested that complementarity must be recognized in view of various distinct desiderata in educational research, not all of which can be met by any one single paradigm. For example, there are pressing educational and social problems requiring policy and practical responses. The information necessary for policy formulation might not be available for controlled laboratory experiments of limited generalizability (or external validity), but might be provided by "quasi-experiments" (Cook and Campbell 1979) or qualitative research. Moreover, given the rate of social change, or the constant interactive effects of educational treatments and student aptitudes, generalizations yielded by a quantitative approach might become rapidly out of date. The project of developing a stable set of scientific educational laws may not be viable (Cronbach 1975).

For other writers espousing complementary diversity, the multifactorial complexity of educational problems supports epistemological pluralism. Keeves acknowledges that some approaches are more holistic, embracing greater complexity than others:

> The techniques employed in educational research must be capable of examining many variables at the same time, but not necessarily through the use of complex statistical procedures . . . although these have their place. Anthropologists have evolved procedures for analyzing and presenting information from a situation which involves many factors that are very different from those used by psychologists, and different again from those that might be employed by economists and sociologists. (1986 p. 390)

Nevertheless, according to Campbell and Overman (1988), P-theoretical differences are still unavoidable because there remains a need for the kind of research produced by the tools of descriptive science and formal logic, which cannot embrace the value judgments characteristic of much nonquantitative educational inquiry. For other writers, fundamental epistemological differences between explanation and interpretation, of course, remain.

In educational research acceptance of the epistemological integrity of a nonquantitative paradigm has largely been the result of efforts by qualitative researchers to spell out alternative networks of theoretical requirements for qualitative research. These have tended to run parallel to elements in the received epistemological scheme of quantitative research (validity, reliability, etc.). One influential example, elaborated by Lincoln and Guba (1984), employs the notions of credibility, applicability (or transferability), consistency, and neutrality, as analogies respectively for internal validity, external validity, reliability, and objectivity.

The point here, however, is not so much that there is some loose analogical connection between corresponding terms in these sets. Rather, despite détente, the point to note is the persisting apparent epistemological distinctiveness of these theoretically interanimated clusters and their respective embeddings in different epistemologies. Some complementary diversity theorists might think that they can have fundamental epistemological diversity without subscribing to something as strong as the P-theory and its incommensurability doctrine. Here, perhaps, epistemological diversity is being confused with methodological diversity, a diversity of techniques of inquiry. Of course the latter is possible but, in the opinion of the authors, is best underwritten by a "touchstone" account of epistemic justification, not several incommensurable epistemologies. Such an account does not have to be fixed and absolute; it can change. The point is that at any given time it embraces those epistemological commitments that are shared by researchers. This is the unity thesis. If complementary diversity theorists wish to eschew such epistemological touchstone, then they remain committed to P-theory.

It should be noted that many advocates of equal rights for qualitative research have wished to play down the epistemological differences (Lincoln and Guba 1984, Miles and Huberman 1984). It may be that exponents of the complementary diversity thesis who persist with the term "paradigm" do not embrace P-theory's doctrine of incommensurability, although this is rarely made explicit. If they disavow incommensurability, their position would seem to collapse into the unity thesis, with revisionary consequences for the way they draw the distinctions between paradigms. These may be more drastic than at first appears. In the case of the explanation/understanding distinction, for

25

instance, Keeves (1988), in arguing for complementarity, has adopted Giddens's (1984) reworking of this distinction. Not all complementarists have recognized the seriousness of the problem, however. As Smith and Heshusius (1986 p. 7) put it, there has been a tendency to "de-epistemologize" the debate or even ignore paradigmatic differences. Given that paradigms exist, Smith and Heshusius may well be right—but do paradigms exist?

4. Criticisms of the Paradigms Theory

It is apparent that there is some confusion over both the term "paradigm" and the problem of unambiguously identifying paradigms of educational research. Some of the confusion comes from the ambiguity of the term "paradigm" itself. On the one hand, as Husén (1988 p. 17) points out, there would be wide agreement that the most influential use of "paradigm" stems from the work of Kuhn (1970). However, Masterman (1970) identified some 21 different uses of the term in Kuhn's book; Kuhn subsequently published revisions, some substantial, to his original theory (e.g., Kuhn 1974); and finally, not all methodologists embrace Kuhn's ideas uncritically.

Kuhn has also put the principal argument for regarding paradigms as incommensurable, as incapable of being compared or measured against some touchstone standard:

> In learning a paradigm the scientist acquires theory, methods, and standards together, usually in an inextricable mixture. Therefore when paradigms change, there are usually significant shifts in the criteria determining the legitimacy both of problems and of proposed solutions.
>
> That observation . . . provides our first explicit indication of why the choice between competing paradigms regularly raises questions that cannot be resolved by the criteria of normal science . . . will inevitably talk through each other when debating the relative merits of their respective paradigms. In the partially circular arguments that regularly result, each paradigm will be shown to satisfy more or less the criteria that it dictates for itself and to fall short of a few of those dictated by its opponent. (1970 pp. 109–10)

The key claim being made here is that paradigms include both substantive theories and the standards and criteria for evaluating those theories, or paradigm-specific epistemologies. As such, it is also claimed, there is no priviledged epistemic vantage point from which different paradigms can be assessed; there are only the rival epistemic standards built into each paradigm.

Kuhn's early comments on the task of adjudicating the merits of competing paradigms are instructive: "the proponents of competing paradigms practise their trade in different worlds" (Kuhn 1970 p. 150); "the transfer of allegiance from paradigm to paradigm is a conversion experience that cannot be forced" (Kuhn 1970 p. 151); such a transition occurs relatively suddenly, like a gestalt switch "just because it is a transition between incommensurables" (Kuhn 1970 p. 150).

Moreover, the belief that some research traditions are incommensurable can be made to look initially plausible by noting the kind of tradition-specific vocabularies that are used to characterize matters epistemological. As has been seen, methodological reflection on quantitative research commonly trades in such terminology as "scientific," "positivist," "foundational," "correspondence-truth," "objective," "realist," "validity," "reliability," "reductionist," and "empiricist." The qualitative network of such terms includes "nonpositivist," "antifoundational," "interpretation," "understanding," "subjective," "idealist," "relativist," and "antireductionist." The fact that key terms of epistemic conduct in one cluster are formed by negating terms in the other cluster readily suggests no common basis for the conduct and assessment of inquiry, and hence the incommensurability of these traditions.

Clearly, for a defense of the epistemological unity of educational research, the most important obstacle is this P-theoretical analysis of research traditions. So the first point to make in a defense of the unity thesis is that in philosophy, and philosophy of science in particular, P-theory is widely regarded as false. In a major review of the literature following a 1969 symposium on the structure of scientific theories, Suppe (1977 p. 647) remarks: "Since the symposium Kuhn's views have undergone a sharply declining influence on contemporary work in philosophy of science." He goes on to claim that contemporary work in philosophy of science, that is, postpositivist philosophy in science, "increasingly subscribes to the position that it is a central aim of science to come to know how the world *really is*" (Suppe 1977 p. 649). In social and educational research, however, especially among qualitative researchers and critical theorists, antirealist belief in paradigms remains strong. In the authors' opinion, the apparent ubiquity of "paradigms" in educational research occurs because the epistemological assumptions of the P-theory itself, or its P-epistemology, are largely responsible for structuring differences among research traditions into putative paradigms.

Of course epistemologists in general agree that inquiry structures knowledge of the objects of inquiry; this is part of what is involved in maintaining that all experience is theory-laden. Contrary to Smith and Heshusius (1986), it is not a feature peculiar to qualitative inquiry. The interesting question is whether there is any reason to believe that different research traditions partition into paradigms the way P-theory requires. However, it is rarely noted that whether it is even appropriate to give reasons, to marshal evidence, to analyze research practices and inquiry contexts in order to justify such a belief, will depend on whether P-theory is, by its own lights, a paradigm (or part of a paradigm), or not. If it is, then the relevant standards of reasoning, evidence, and analysis will be peculiar to P-theory (or its encompassing paradigm) and so will have rational epistemic purchase on none but the already committed. To the unbeliever, P-theory would literally have nothing to say for itself. For one to believe that educational research comes in paradigms would require an act of faith: to come to believe it after believing the contrary would require a conversion experience.

There are interesting problems with this view. For example, what happens if one is converted to it? Does one then say that it is true that educational research divides into paradigms? Unfortunately the term "true" is P-theoretical and so one needs to determine first whether, for example, the sentences of P-theory correspond to a world of real educational researchers really engaged in incommensurable research practices. If so, then P-theory is not after all a paradigm distinct from those that employ correspondence-truth. If not, then there is a genuine equivocation over the term "true" which will permit the following claims to be made without contradiction: (a) it is correspondence-true that the different research traditions are not epistemologically distinct; and (b) it is P-true that the different research traditions are epistemologically distinct.

In conceding the equal legitimacy of incommensurable rivals (whether oppositional or complementary), however, particularly a correspondence-truth rival, the P-theorist seems to be surrendering the capacity to say anything about actual educational research practices and the historical and theoretical context of current research traditions. Worse still, in eschewing any schema for determining the ontological commitments of P-theory, there seems to be no way of knowing what the P-theorist is talking about. As such, P-theory hardly provides a challenge to a realist view of the unity of educational research.

To avoid the dilemma that threatens when P-theory becomes self-referential, several options are available. Two are considered here. First, a less parsimonious attitude to rival epistemologies can be adopted by maintaining that correspondence-true theories, which caused all the trouble, are false, wrong, or, as hard-hitting relativists are fond of saying, inadequate. Indeed, getting rid of correspondence-truth may be a condition for meaningful P-theoretical claims about theorists' living in different worlds; after all, talk of a real world tends to make other worlds pale into nonexistence. A second, opposite, strategy is to say that P-theory is not a distinct paradigm at all, but rather a set of carefully argued, evidentially supported, correspondence-true claims about the existence of paradigmatic divisions among the major research traditions. It is instructive to note that some methodologists run both these strategies simultaneously (e.g., Lincoln and Guba 1984, Eisner 1979). (For damaging criticism of Eisner's running the two strategies together, see Phillips 1983.)

Arguments for the first option are by now familiar enough. Correspondence-truth is assumed to be located in a network of terms usually associated with the quantitative research tradition. Valid and reliable knowledge about the world is said to be that which is, in some way, derivable from some epistemically secure (or even certain) foundation; in positivistic empiricism usually observations or first person sensory reports. Objectivity consists in intersubjectively agreed matchings between statements and experience. And, of course, these objectively known statements are correspondence-true just in case the required matching occurs (although often the only reality admitted was sense data).

There are many objections to foundational empiricist epistemologies (e.g., Hesse 1974, Churchland 1979), but a version of the earlier argument from self-reference will suffice to illustrate the problems. Although this is not widely recognized in positivistic empiricism, epistemology is a task that requires (as Kant saw) a theory of the powers of the mind. What one can know will depend, to some extent, on what sort of creature one is and, in particular, on what sort of perceptual and cognitive capacities one has. A theory of the mind, however, is something one has to get to know. In the case of empiricist foundationalism, it is necessary to know that one's own sensory experiences will provide one with epistemically secure foundations. Unfortunately for the foundationalist, the theory of mind required to underwrite this claim is not itself an item of sensory experience, nor an observation report. This means that knowledge of how the class of epistemically privileged items is known is not itself epistemically privileged. Indeed, the sophisticated neurophysiological models of brain functioning now typical of accounts of perception and cognition are quite ill-suited to serving the regress pattern of foundational justification. For they so far outrun the purported resources of any proposed foundation that the whole point of foundational justification here collapses. More generally, knowledge of perceptual powers, or possible foundations, like knowledge of everything, is theory-laden. The result is that there is no epistemically privileged, theory-free, way of viewing the world. There is thus no reality that can be seen independent of competing theoretical perspectives. This applies as much to the empirical sciences (and the quantitative tradition in educational research) as to other areas (see Walker and Evers 1982, Walker and Evers 1986).

From the fact that all experience is theory-laden, however, that what one believes exists depends on what theory one adopts, it does not follow that all theories are evidentially equivalent, or equally reasonable. There is more to evidence than observation, or as Churchland (1985 p. 35) argues: "observational excellence or 'empirical adequacy' is only one epistemic virtue among others of equal or comparable importance." The point is that some theories organize their interpretations of experience better than others. A humdrum example employing subjectivist scruples on evidence will illustrate this point. A theory which says that I can leave what I interpret to be my office by walking through what I interpret to be the wall will cohere less well with my interpreted desire to leave my office than a theory which counsels departure via what I take to be the door. It is all interpretative, of course, but some organized sets of interpretations, or theories, are better than others. The theory that enables a person to experience the desired success of departing the perceived enclosure of an office enjoys certain epistemic advantages over one that does not. With all experience interpreted, though, the correct conclusion to draw is not that there is no adequate objective standard of reality, but that objectivity involves more than empirical adequacy. Theoretically motivated success in getting in and out of rooms is about as basic as objectivity ever gets. There are superempirical, theoretical tests which can be couched in a "coherence epistemology." One advocate of coherence epistemology, the postpositivist philosopher Quine, sums up this standard of reality.

> Having noted that man has no evidence for the existence of bodies beyond the fact that their assumption helps him organize experience, we should have done well, instead of disclaiming evidence for the existence of bodies, to conclude: such, then, at bottom, is what evidence is both for ordinary bodies and molecules. (Quine 1960a p. 251)

Quine's point here foreshadows a significant epistemological consequence of this attack on foundationalism. According to Quine, and many coherence theorists, we need to distinguish sharply between the theory of evidence and the theory of truth (Quine 1960a, Quine 1960b, Quine 1969, Quine 1974, Williams 1980). Theory of evidence is concerned with the global excellence of theory, and involves both empirical adequacy, inasmuch as this can be achieved and the superempirical virtues of simplicity, consistency, comprehensiveness, fecundity, familiarity or principle, and explanatory power. Once the best theory according to these coherence criteria has been established, it is the resulting theory itself that is used to state what exists and how the theory's sentences match up with that posited reality. What corresponds to true sentences is therefore something that is determined after the theory of evidence has done its work. It is not something that figures a priori, or in some privileged foundational way in the determination of the best theory.

The evidence suggests that P-theory critiques of foundationalism draw too radical a conclusion. In terms of the quantitative/qualitative debate, for example, the coherence epistemology sanctioned by the most powerful criticisms of empiricist foundationalism cuts across this familiar methodological (putatively paradigmatic) bifurcation. In acknowledging the theory-ladenness of all experience it is nonpositivist and nonfoundational. It agrees that people's window on the world is mind-dependent and subject to the interpretations of theorists. On the other hand, it can be realist, scientific, objective, reductionist, and embrace correspondence-truth. This possibility raises serious doubts about P-theorists' claims concerning the diversity of educational research, whether oppositional or complementary.

A more systematic objection to P-theory can be raised, however, by examining the epistemological warrant for incommensurability. The belief that research methodologies comprising incommensurable networks of theoretical terms are epistemically autonomous is sustained in large measure by a particular theory of meaning, notably that terms gain what meaning they possess in virtue of their role in some network or conceptual scheme. Where conceptual schemes or theories are said to be systematically different, no basis exists for matching the terms of one theory with those of another. So expressions such as "validity" or "truth," which appear as orthographically equivalent across different schemes, are really equivocal, with systematic differences emerging as differences in conceptual role.

Both Kuhn and Feyerabend maintain versions of the conceptual role theory of meaning. The trouble, however, is that they maintain implausibly strong versions of it, for if meaning is determined entirely by conceptual role then incommensurable theories become unlearnable. This all turns on the modest empirical fact that as finite learners people need some point of entry into an elaborate systematically interconnected vocabulary like a theory. In order to learn some small part of the theory, say a handful of expressions, however, P-epistemology requires mastery of the whole theory in order to appreciate the conceptual role played by these expressions. It is at this point that the theory of meaning begins to outrun its own epistemological resources: it posits learned antecedents of learning that cannot themselves be learned. The parts cannot be understood without mastery of the whole, and resources are lacking to master the whole without first scaling the parts. An implicit feature of the epistemology driving P-theory's account of meaning as conceptual role is thus an implausibly strong theory of the powers of the mind. (A P-theoretical attack on correspondence-truth appears to depend on a correspondence-true theory of mind.)

Once again P-theory may be observed getting into difficulty over self-reference. In this case an epistemology should come out knowable on its own account of knowledge. The chief advantage of arguments from self-reference is that they focus directly on the superempirical virtues or weaknesses of a theory.

Inasmuch as one is impressed by such theoretical shortcomings as inconsistency, lack of explanatory power in relation to rivals, use of ad hoc hypotheses, and so on, one is allowing these criteria to function as touchstone in the evaluation of epistemologies and research methodologies. Of course one can ignore these vices in theory-construction: they are not extratheoretical privileged foundations by which all theorizing can be assessed. Methodologists in the main research traditions, however, who expect their inquiries to command attention, serve as a sound basis for action, or constitute a particular or definite set of knowledge claims, have been unwilling to play fast and loose with such virtues as consistency (usually on the formal ground that a contradiction will sanction any conclusion whatever) or simplicity and comprehensiveness (on the ground that ad hoc or arbitrary addition of hypotheses can be used to explain anything whatsoever, and hence nothing at all). Indeed a theory cannot be empirically significant unless it is consistent. With P-theory's theory of meaning exhibiting the superempirical weakness of lack of explanatory power in relation to what it sets itself to explain, and with that weakness being traceable to a theory of mind, it should be observed that whether epistemologies or methodologies are incommensurable turns on such things as empirical theories of mind or brain functioning, or theories of learning and cognition. Epistemology itself is therefore continuous with, and relies upon, empirical science. In Quine's words (1969), epistemology is "naturalized." One consequence is that interpretative theorists, for example, must rely partly on the "scientific" paradigm in order to show the incommensurability of their own paradigm with the "scientific."

5. The Unity Thesis

Although the paradigms perspective is seriously flawed, some account of the kind of unity educational research actually enjoys still needs to be given. In arguing against P-theory, coherence epistemology has already been considered. To conclude this discussion a brief outline will be given of a particular version of coherentism, or epistemological holism, which has achieved considerable prominence in postpositivist philosophy (Quine 1974), has been applied to educational philosophy (Walker and Evers 1982), and systematically to educational administration (Evers and Lakomski 1990) and research methodology (Lakomski 1991).

A more positive epistemological agenda for educational research can be provided by responding to the second strategy a P-theorist can adopt in defending diversity. This strategy involved denying P-theory was a distinct paradigm, conceding correspondence-truth, but arguing that fundamental epistemological diversity still occurred in educational research. In replying to this claim it can be noted that the strategy will need to employ superempirical epistemic virtues to be persuasive. To be effective against a wide range of theoretical perspectives these virtues (consistency, simplicity, fecundity, etc.) will need to be recognized as such by rival epistemologies and hence function as touchstone. As a result the P-theorist's strategy is already compromised. To complete the job, however, a coherence epistemology is needed that yields a touchstone-coherent account of itself and its own epistemic virtues, that is unproblematically self-referential in scope, and that can account for the touchstone-recognized successes of alternative epistemologies and their research extensions.

In the view of the authors, the epistemology that best accounts for knowledge, its growth, and evaluation is a form of holistic scientific naturalism (in Quine's "epistemology naturalized" sense of "naturalism")— a theory that makes ready use of the best or most coherent theories of perception and cognition. According to this view, people are acquiring their knowledge of the world from infancy onward. Indeed, as Quine (1960b) has shown, theory precedes all learning and hence commences with the innate complement of dispositions to respond selectively to the environment. What one can know is dependent on the kind of creature one is and, as human beings, everyone is one kind of creature. Everyone shares genetically derived, though culturally expressed, refined and modified touchstone standards and procedures. Added to these is further culturally produced touchstone that people acquire as social beings sharing material problems in concrete social contexts. Knowledge is made up of theories, whose existence is to be explained causally, as problem-solving devices. There are numerous philosophical accounts (e.g., Laudan 1977) of how theories can be analyzed as problem-solving devices. In the case of epistemological theories, the problems arise from theoretical practice, including empirical (e.g., educational) research. Clearly, there are certain issues concerning whether a theory is addressing the right problems, and a theory is needed of how to distinguish between real problems and pseudoproblems, and between better and worse formulations of problems. Here the epistemology would lean on a theory of evidence and experiment, on the pragmatic relations between "theory" and "practice" (Walker 1985a).

One real problem, shared by all educational researchers, is how best to conduct inquiry into human learning itself. Without this problem there could be no debate about whether educational research is epistemologically diverse. For there to be an issue at all presupposes at least some sharing of language, including general epistemological terminology such as "truth," "meaning," "adequacy," "interpretation," "paradigm," and so on.

Competition remains, of course, but competition between theories, including theories of educational research methodology, not paradigms. Competition arises because, in addition to touchstone, there are unshared (which is not to say incommensurable) concepts, hypotheses, and rules of method. Indeed, this is part and parcel of being able to distinguish one theory from another in a competitive situation. There can be genuine competition between theories, however, only when they have an issue over which to compete, some shared problem(s). Theory A is in competition with theory B when one or more of its sentences is contrary to sentences in theory B. For this situation to obtain, theories A and B must be attempts at solving at least one common problem. To identify a shared problem involves some conceptual common ground and, if only implicitly at first, some shared method; the concepts have to be deployed. Thus one begins to discover and negotiate touchstone theory which, unlike the privileged epistemic units of foundational epistemologies, is merely the shifting historically explicable amount of theory that is shared by rival theories and theorists. Beginning with identification of common problems, one can proceed to identify further touchstone and elaborate the touchstone frameworks within which theories compete.

Having identified common ground between theories, their differences are next rigorously set out and tested against that touchstone by empirical research and theoretical analysis, seeking to identify the strengths and weaknesses of each, and reach a decision on the theory which is strongest under present circumstances (Walker 1985b), taking into account past achievements and likely future problems (Churchland 1979).

Other features of this epistemology include its capacity to survive its own test of self-reference (Quine 1969), its unified account of validity and reliability (Evers 1991), its denial that all science consists of sets of laws, and of any fundamental epistemological distinction between explanation and understanding (Walker 1985c) or between fact and value judgments (Evers and Lakomski 1990).

Finally, although in this entry it has been maintained that such a coherentist naturalistic epistemology is a sound way of underwriting the epistemological unity of educational research, achieved through touchstone analysis, it should be stressed that it is as much a competing theory as any other, and subject to theory testing (Walker 1985a). Granted that it shares touchstone with other epistemologies, arguments can of course be mounted against it; to engage in such arguments, however, all participations would be implicitly conceding the epistemological unity of research.

See also: Research Paradigms in Education; Scientific Methods in Educational Research

References

Bates R J 1980 New developments in the new sociology of education. *Br. J. Sociol. Educ.* 1(1): 67–79

Campbell D T, Overman S E 1988 *Methodology and Epistemology for Social Science: Selected Papers*. Chicago University Press, Chicago, Illinois

Carr W, Kemmis S 1983 *Becoming Critical. Knowing Through Action Research*. Deakin University Press, Geelong

Churchland P M 1979 *Scientific Realism and the Plasticity of Mind*. Cambridge University Press, Cambridge

Churchland P M 1985 The ontological status of observables. In: Churchland P M, Hooker C A (eds.) 1985 *Images of Science: Essays on Realism and Empiricism*. University of Chicago Press, Chicago, Illinois

Cook T H, Campbell D T 1979 *Quasi-Experimentation. Design and Analysis Issues for Field Settings*. Rand McNally, Chicago, Illinois

Cronbach L J 1975 Beyond the two disciplines of scientific psychology. *Am. Psychol.* 30(2): 116–27

Eisner E 1979 *The Educational Imagination*. Macmillan, New York

Evers C W 1991 Towards a coherentist theory of validity. *Int. J. Educ. Res.* 15(6): 521–35

Evers C W, Lakomski G 1990 *Knowing Educational Administration*. Pergamon Press, Oxford

Freire P 1972 *Cultural Action for Freedom*. Penguin, Harmondsworth

Giddens A 1984 *The Constitution of Society: Outline of the Theory of Structuration*. Polity Press, Cambridge

Habermas J 1972 (trans. Shapiro J) *Knowledge and Human Interests*. Heinemann, London

Hesse M 1974 *The Structure of Scientific Inference*. Macmillan, London

Hooker C A 1975 Philosophy and meta-philosophy of science. Empiricism, Popperianism and realism. *Synthèse* 32: 177–231

House E R 1991 Realism in research. *Educ. Researcher* 20(6): 2–9

Husén T 1988 Research paradigms in education. In: Keeves J P (ed.) 1988 *Educational Research, Methodology, and Measurement: An International Handbook*. Pergamon Press, Oxford

Keeves J P 1986 Theory, politics and experiment in educational research methodology. A response. *Int. Rev. Educ.* 32(4): 388–92

Keeves J P 1988 Social theory and educational research. In: Keeves J P (ed.) 1988 *Educational Research, Methodology, and Measurement: An International Handbook*. Pergamon Press, Oxford

Kerlinger F N 1973 *Foundations of Behavioral Research. Educational and Psychological Inquiry*, 2nd edn. Holt, Rinehart and Winston, New York

Kuhn T S 1970 *The Structure of Scientific Revolutions*, 2nd edn. University of Chicago Press, Chicago, Illinois

Kuhn T S 1974 Second thoughts about paradigms. In: Suppe F (ed.) 1977

Lakomski G (ed.) 1991 Beyond paradigms: Coherentism and holism in educational research. *Int. J. Educ. Res.* 15(6): 449–97

Laudan L 1977 *Progress and its Problems. Towards a Theory of Scientific Growth*. Routledge and Kegan Paul, London

Lincoln Y S, Guba E G 1984 *Naturalistic Inquiry*. Sage, Beverly Hills, California

Masterman M 1970 The nature of a paradigm. In: Lakatos I, Musgrave A (eds.) 1970 *Criticism and the Growth of Knowledge*. Cambridge University Press, London

Miles M, Huberman M 1984 Drawing valid meaning from qualitative data. Towards a shared craft. *Educ. Researcher* 13(5): 20–30

Phillips D C 1983 After the wake: Postpositivistic educational thought: The social functions of the intellectual. *Educ. Researcher* 12(5): 4–12

Popkewitz T 1984 *Paradigm and Ideology in Educational Research*. Falmer Press, London

Quine W V 1960a Posits and reality. In: Uyeda S (ed.) 1960 *Bases of Contemporary Philosophy*, Vol. 5. Waseda University Press, Tokyo.

Quine W V 1960b *Word and Object*. MIT Press, Cambridge, Massachusetts

Quine W V 1969 Epistemology naturalized. In: Quine W V 1969 *Ontological Relativity and Other Essays*. Columbia University Press, New York

Quine W V 1974 The nature of natural knowledge. In: Guttenplan S (ed.) 1975 *Mind and Language*. Clarendon Press, Oxford

Shulman L 1986 Paradigms and research programs in the study of teaching. A contemporary perspective. In: Wittrock M C (ed.) 1986 *Handbook of Research on Teaching*, 3rd edn. Macmillan, New York

Smith J K, Heshusius L 1986 Closing down the conversation. The end of the qualitative/quantitative debate among educational inquirers. *Educ. Researcher* 15(1): 4–12

Suppe F (ed.) 1977 *The Structure of Scientific Theories*, 2nd edn. University of Illinois Press, Chicago, Illinois

Walker J C 1985a The philosopher's touchstone. Towards pragmatic unity in educational studies. *J. Philos. Educ.* 19(2): 181–98

Walker J C 1985b Philosophy and the study of education. A critique of the commonsense consensus. *Aust. J. Educ.* 29(2): 101–14

Walker J C 1985c Materialist pragmatism and sociology of education. *Br. J. Sociol. Educ.* 6(1): 55–74

Walker J C, Evers C W 1982 Epistemology and justifying the curriculum of educational studies. *Br. J. Educ. Stud.* 30(2): 213–29

Walker J C, Evers C W 1986 Theory, politics, and experiment in educational research methodology. *Int. Rev. Educ.* 32(4): 373–87

Williams M 1980 Coherence justification and truth. *Rev. Metaphys.* 34(2): 243–72

Further Reading

Chalmers A 1990 *Science and its Fabrication*. Open University Press, Buckingham

Miller S I, Fredericks M 1991 Postpositivistic assumptions and educational research: Another view. *Educ. Researcher* 20(4): 2–8

Phillips D C 1987 *Philosophy, Science and Social Inquiry*. Pergamon Press, Oxford

Salomon G 1991 Transcending the qualitative-quantitative debate: The analytic and systemic approaches to educational research. *Educ. Researcher* 20(6): 10–18

Comparative Methodology in Education

J. P. Keeves and D. Adams

This entry examines the methodologies employed in the making of comparisons in educational research. Scholarly inquiry in the field of education employs two essentially different investigatory strategies. These strategies are referred to as the "holistic" or "systemic" approach and the "comparative" or "analytic" approach. Within the systemic approach the characteristics of the parts are seen to be largely determined by the whole to which they belong. Thus the emphasis in inquiry is on the study of the interrelationships between the elementary parts which are assumed to be interdependent within the whole. Inquiry here involves the study of patterns and processes. The test that is applied is whether the characteristics of an elementary part, a relationship, or a pattern, that is under examination may be considered to exist. Within the comparative approach, characteristics of an elementary part are compared across two or more research situations. Where a difference is observed, a reason for the difference may be sought. Alternatively, where a difference is not observed, the reason for the similarity may be of interest. It is of course possible to apply initially a systemic approach and having established the existence of a pattern or a set of interrelationships between the parts within a whole, to undertake comparisons of the patterns or interrelations observed across two or more research situations. The test that is applied is whether the characteristics of two or more elementary parts, or two or more relationships, or two or more patterns can be said either to differ or to be the same.

Logically, establishing the existence of the characteristics of a part, a relationship, or a pattern, must precede the making of comparisons between two or more such entities. However, one of the tests of existence is whether a difference can be observed in particular research situations. Thus the distinction between the two strategies lies, at least in part, in whether the emphasis is on providing an account of wholes and the need to emphasize holistic qualities, or whether the emphasis is on the decomposition into parts and a comparison and further examination of the characteristics of the parts in two or more situations using analytic procedures.

Comparative studies may be undertaken using either a scientific approach or a humanistic approach. The former commonly involves measurement and statistical analysis, the latter tends to be largely descriptive. Both approaches are considered in this entry.

1. Field of Comparative Education

During the twentieth century travel to other countries has greatly increased, communication with people from other lands has been made much easier, and barriers to cross-national trade have been steadily removed. This has led to increased interest among educators as to how education is provided in different cultures and societies. As a result comparisons have commonly been made between countries with respect to many different aspects of educational provision. A field of scholarly work in education has emerged that is primarily concerned with cross-national comparisons in the provision of education. While initially the work undertaken in this field was solely descriptive and information-seeking, without the explicit making of comparisons between countries, interest in the making of such comparisons increased to such an extent that the field acquired the name of comparative education. The field has identified a founding father in Marc-Antoine Jullien, whose seminal work *L'Esquisse et vue préliminaire d'un ouvrage sur l'éducation comparée* in 1817 emphasized objective observation, the collection of documents, thoroughness, and systematic analysis. The field is also able to trace its roots back into Antiquity (see Brickman 1960, 1966). There are, however, several fallacious ideas concerned with the methods and nature of comparative education that must be dispelled.

1.1 Fallacy of a Single Scientific Method of Comparative Education

In his work *Problems in Education: A Comparative Approach*, Holmes (1965) provided a statement on the scientific method that he advocated for comparative education. He drew on the writings of Dewey (1933) on problem-solving and proposed a sequence of eight major steps in comparative education which for him was both an instrument of reform or planned development in education as well as a method of investigation that led to the production of new knowledge. These steps may be listed as follows: (a) selection of a problem; (b) identification of possible solutions; (c) reflection on the problem, leading to a clearer formulation; (d) analysis of the context of the problem; (e) advancement of hypotheses on policy choices; (f) testing of hypotheses; (g) drawing of conclusions; and (h) reexamination of the processes. The key steps were step (a) which not only involved selection but also analysis; step (b), which involved the formulation of policy proposals; step (d), which involved the identification of relevant factors; and step (f), which involved prediction and the testing of possible solutions against the context analyzed.

In spite of the coherence of Holmes's ideas, educational research workers who are interested in questions that require the investigation of educational provision in one or more countries and who bring to the investigation perspectives drawn from one or more disciplinary areas, such as psychology, sociology, anthropology, geography, economics, history, demography, philosophy, and law, cannot consistently be constrained by a particular sequence of steps in inquiry. Moreover, the conceptual or methodological

problems in comparative research are not unique to a single discipline or investigatory approach. Comparative educators are free to draw on those methods of inquiry that seem most appropriate to them to answer the research questions that have been posed. Frequently, multiple methods are useful in achieving greater understanding. The methods that are chosen may involve perspectives and knowledge drawn from one or more disciplines, as well as the methods of investigation traditionally employed in those disciplines. There is no single scientific method of investigation in comparative education.

1.2 Fallacy of a Choice between Qualities or Quantities

A fallacy widely held among comparative educators is that a choice exists in investigation between, on the one hand, the examination of qualities rather than quantities and, on the other hand, the examination of quantities rather than qualities. Both are misconceived when they are taken to be clear-cut alternatives since quantities are measures of qualities (Kaplan 1964). Moreover, complex procedures of statistical analysis are now available for the rigorous examination of qualitative data, where information is recorded in two or more categories, without any attempt being made to measure, just as there are similar rigorous statistical procedures available for the examination of quantitative data that involve accurate measurement. The issues are simply those concerned with the meaningfulness and consistency of the measurement procedures employed that indicate whether quantitative or qualitative information or both are best used in a particular research situation. Admittedly improving the accuracy of measurement involves refining the abstract concept being measured, and this commonly involves eliminating from consideration certain aspects of the quality under examination. However, increased precision of measurement increases the likelihood of establishing a relationship that may be hypothesized.

1.3 Fallacy of Distinction Between Policy-oriented and Discipline-oriented Studies

While for Holmes (1965) comparative education was an instrument of planned development in education, he also recognized that such inquiry led to a greater understanding of educational systems. The interest shown by politicians and the media in the "horse race" aspects of international studies of educational achievement without concern for developing a coherent explanation of why such differences arise is one consequence of the artificial dichotomy between policy-oriented and discipline-oriented studies or between applied and pure research. Most research workers would wish the results of their research to be useful, but any demand for policy-oriented research at the expense of discipline-oriented research can involve a gross misunderstanding of the nature of social action and the power of ideas. Moreover, it assumes that research in the social and behavioral sciences finds application in the same manner as research in the physical sciences does through technology and applied science. There is, nevertheless, an important role for such institutions as the World Bank, the Centre for Educational Research and Innovation at the Organisation for Economic Co-operation and Development (OECD), and the International Institute of Educational Planning to provide an international platform for discussion, where the results of comparative research studies are translated into terms that policymakers understand. Thus the powerful ideas that emerge from comparative research are made accessible for translation into policy and practice across countries.

1.4 Fallacy Concerning Exclusive Attention to Processes and not Products

In part, in reaction to the interest of policymakers in the outcomes of education and in policy-oriented research, there is a fallacy that comparative research should be concerned with the elaboration and understanding of the processes involved in the provision of educational services. While some naive input–output models of educational provision that are advanced must be cast aside as incomplete and inadequate, so too must the limited study of the processes involved in educational provision. In seeking an indepth understanding of educational provision, it would seem unsatisfactory merely to investigate the processes that operate in a particular educational situation without detailed consideration of the outcomes or products of that system. Thus, in order to achieve greater understanding of education and educational changes, it is necessary to develop and examine models of educational provision and operation that incorporate both the *products* of a system and the *processes* at work as well as the *context* in which the system is set. The methods to be employed in such investigations depend on the nature of the research questions being asked, and on the extent of understanding that has been achieved of the problem situation being investigated.

2. Types of Research in Comparative Education

Research workers in comparative education undertake research studies that involve one or more countries or regions, which can be classified into three types, namely: (a) descriptive studies; (b) developmental studies; (c) analytical, relationship, and process studies. Studies that fall into the second and third categories require theoretical perspectives that are discussed in a later section. In this section the methods employed are considered and examples of such research studies are given.

2.1 Descriptive Studies

An initial and necessary task in the field of comparative education is the development of understanding through studies that provide a descriptive account of the state of education at a specific point in time in generally one, but sometimes more than one country. Examples of these studies are provided by Postlethwaite (1995) for more than 130 countries in the articles on National Systems of Education or in the important series of Studies in Compulsory Education in particular countries which were issued around 1950 as joint publications of the International Bureau of Education (IBE) and UNESCO. A further example involves the examination of the teaching of a school subject, science, in 20 countries, which is provided in a report of the IEA Science Study by Rosier and Keeves (1991) based on case studies conducted in each of the participating countries. Such studies may or may not contain a historical component. Any historical information that might be included is generally more descriptive than explanatory of the provision of education in a particular country. These descriptive studies serve an important purpose since they provide relatively concise accounts of educational policies and practices in a particular country and assist in the building up of an understanding both within that country and outside of the systems of education that operate.

The United Nations Educational, Scientific and Cultural Organization (UNESCO) in Paris, which was established after the Second World War in 1946, and the International Bureau of Education in Geneva, which was established in 1925, have both played an important role over the past half-century in this field. Not only have they published resource material, they have also maintained international surveys on "the condition of education" in each country. In these surveys a questionnaire has been completed by the ministry of education within each country and the responses have been classified and published. Such work is beset with many problems. The major ones are: (a) the absence of a list of the most important educational indicators agreed upon by scholars in the field; (b) the cost and practical difficulties of obtaining data from so many sources; (c) the lack of comparability in the data collected, in spite of efforts made to obtain uniformity; (d) the lack of sufficient analysis of context without which data have limited meaning; and (e) uncertainties about the consistency or meaningfulness of the data returned, because of the tendency for ministry officials to wish to present the conditions of education within their country in the best possible light.

In the later decades of the twentieth century, greatly increased opportunities have become available for travel and study in schools, colleges, and universities outside a person's country of origin, for example, the ERASMUS scheme, which aims to promote student mobility within the European Community and which is also being taken up by countries outside the EC.

There are, however, the very practical problems of: (a) obtaining proficiency in a second language to study effectively; (b) supplying sufficient information on the portability of qualifications; and (c) undertaking meaningful comparisons of the nature and standard of courses. However, problems (b) and (c) listed above are being met by the work of EUROSTAT with benefits both between and within countries. The long-term effects of such student exchange schemes and the increased emphasis on foreign language learning beyond the commercial sphere are difficult to foresee, but are likely to be substantial and highly beneficial. There is, nevertheless, little doubt that descriptive studies in the field of comparative education must play an increasingly important role in the development of a greater understanding of educational provision in other countries. This goes well beyond the aims and purposes of the traditional courses in comparative education that are provided. However, comparative educators led by Kandel (1933), Hans (1949), Bereday (1964), King (1968), and Noah and Eckstein (1969) have all come to recognize that in their field of inquiry both descriptive and historical studies are not enough.

2.2 Developmental Studies

The influence of the social and behavioral sciences on life in different parts of the world is achieved not so much through the implications for policy and practice of a particular research study, but through the power of the ideas and concepts that are generated. In no field of life is this greater than in that of education, where ideas are traded, debated, and successively advanced and promulgated. The remarkable changes in the way of life of both men and women across the world during the past 2,000 years may be ascribed primarily to those ideas that flowed from Greece and Rome, but also from the countries of the Middle East, China, India, and from other centers of learning. In the field of education and through education the changes that have occurred since the mid-nineteenth century have been quite spectacular, particularly in the areas of compulsory education, universal secondary education, the establishment of universities, and more recently in programs of lifelong and recurrent education. The stories of many developments, such as that of the curriculum and methods of science education, remain to be told.

Frequently, accounts of the developments that have occurred in an area of education in a particular country have been merely descriptive and have attributed change to the influence of a certain individual and to the borrowing of particular policies and practices. However, the changes that have taken place have been too rapid and too widespread to be attributed to chance. Kandel (1933) sought to ascribe the developments in education that took place within a particular country to national character. Furthermore, Mallinson (1957) contended that "common identity of interest, that common purpose, leads over the centuries to a

kind of fixed mental constitution" which influenced educational development within a country. While a national mental constitution or culture may be employed to explain certain unique features of German and Japanese education, it cannot be used to explain the widespread commonalities in educational growth that have developed since the mid-nineteenth century.

Hans (1949) moved to a higher level of generality through identifying certain factors that influenced educational development, namely: (a) natural factors (racial, linguistic, geographic, and economic); (b) religious factors (Catholic, Anglican, and puritan); and (c) secular factors (humanism, socialism, nationalism, and democratic ideals). While these factors shift explanation of educational development beyond national boundaries to more widespread regions, they are more concerned with unique factors than with the common or universal factors that would appear to have operated across the world.

Meyer and Hannan (1979) have argued that the thrust for universal primary education, initially in Western Europe from the middle of the nineteenth century onwards, had little to do with national educational policies and must be viewed in a crossnational context. It might be argued that the powerful ideas of this period arose from the Darwinian concept of evolution, the drive to establish a national identity and to strengthen the power of the state, and from the need in an industrialized state for a workforce that could read, write, and count. Likewise, the impact of Marx's ideas influenced educational policies and practices in a substantial region of the world, including the former Soviet Union and China, from early in the twentieth century onward.

More detailed studies into the nature of particular aspects of educational development across countries have also been carried out. For example, the character of an educational system, whether tightly centralized or largely decentralized, Archer (1979) argued, is related to its origins. Those systems with restrictive origins emphasize unification and systematization and those with substitutive origins feature differentiation from other social institutions and a high degree of internal specialization. These characteristics in turn affect the nature and speed of change in an educational system.

Developments that have occurred cross-nationally which particularly warrant examination include: (a) the interaction of educational, social, and economic ideas; (b) the equality of educational opportunity programs built around ideas of social justice; (c) programs for equality between the sexes which have been built from psychological and sociological research into sex and gender differences; and (d) developments in science and mathematics programs that have flowed from a demand for scientific and technological growth to raise standards of living within countries. Studies of the history of education in the twentieth century tend to be encyclopedic and do not seek to reveal how the ideas that have been generated since the mid-nineteenth century have spread across the world to influence the growth and development of education.

2.3 Studies of Relationships and Processes

These studies seek to increase understanding of how variables relate to one another, to explain better the dynamics of learning, teaching, and educational change, and to examine how such relationships and processes vary across systems and countries. The objective frequently is to specify functional or cause-and-effect relationships and outcomes. Such studies often focus on a set of actors (e.g., teachers, students, parents) or roles (e.g., teaching, learning, supporting) to explain the behavior of schools and educational systems. Studies falling within this broad range include input–output studies, production function studies, effective school studies, and process–product studies.

The need and potential for comparative research on educational relationships and processes are reflected in the work of the International Association for the Evaluation of Educational Achievement (IEA). In the late 1950s a group of educational research workers meeting at the UNESCO Institute of Education in Hamburg came to recognize that within a particular country there was commonly insufficient variation in the conditions of education to make it possible to detect by existing methods of statistical analysis the effects of particular factors on learning outcomes. They contended that if research studies could be conducted cross-nationally, then the greater variation that existed across countries could assist in identifying common factors of importance. The feasibility of undertaking research studies across countries into factors influencing educational outcomes was tested through a pilot study (Foshay et al. 1962). The success of this work led to the formal establishment of the IEA. Since that time, the IEA has carried out a series of research studies, primarily survey and cross-sectional investigations, into factors that have an effect on educational achievement, participation rates, and attitudes toward school and school learning. The data collected have been examined across countries, between schools within countries, and between students within countries, and where possible relationships have been sought after controlling for other factors that might affect the educational outcomes under consideration. The specific relationships that have been detected fall into one of several types, namely: (a) relationships between predictor and criterion variables across countries; (b) similar relationships between predictor and criterion variables between students and schools within countries; (c) a relationship between predictor variables and criterion variables and between students and schools within countries that is unique to a particular country or a small group of countries; and (d) the absence of a relationship where current opinion within educational circles believes such a relationship should exist. The extensive body of international research assembled by the IEA has established many generalizations that explain the processes by which education is more or less effective.

The existence of these general relationships involving factors that influence, for instance, science achievement and attitudes, has raised the need to examine in a systematic manner whether similar or different processes operate within schooling in different countries, at different age or grade levels, and across different subject areas. Before the systematic examination of processes can take place, advances must be made along three major fronts. First, it is necessary for theory to be developed and models postulated of specific processes of school learning. One such very influential model in this field has been Carroll's (1963) model of school learning. Second, it is necessary to develop procedures for the collection of data that are sufficiently comparable across countries that the testing of models in a comparative manner is worthwhile. Third, procedures for the testing of models need to be further developed in order to provide better estimates of effects and appropriate estimates of error. Problems arise on all three fronts.

The lack of relevant theory has resulted in the collection of massive amounts of data, in cross-national empirical studies, some of which are never effectively examined, because there is little guidance provided by theory as to what hypotheses or models could be tested or what questions could be asked. However, sometimes models have been advanced long after the data collection and it has been fortuitous that data were available for the testing of a model in secondary analyses. Sometimes, only weak relationships are observed because of bias in samples, or because of marked error of measurement in the data. Such shortcomings generally serve to reduce greatly the possibility of observing an expected relationship within a model, rather than enhancing the possibility of detecting relationships.

Inadequate theory limits all types of studies in the field of comparative education. Naturalistic, ethnographic, and other descriptive techniques have generated rich, detailed analyses of teaching and learning processes and the organizational contexts of education. Yet, generalizations beyond culturally specific meanings are constrained by lack of theory and adequate tests of comparability across countries. However, advances are being made in the requisite conditions for improvements in studies of relationships and processes. Experience in crosscultural ethnographic research and increased sophistication in techniques of interviewing, document analysis, and observation are contributing to more accurate descriptions of schooling and educational activities in their natural or normal setting. Equally significant are the technical advances in analytical methods which have also been made in recent decades, particularly in the areas of multivariate and multilevel analysis. The procedures employed in such statistical analyses are essentially those of making comparisons and testing models when large bodies of data are available.

3. Nature of the Data Collected in Cross-national Statistical Studies

The focus of comparative research in education may be at the individual, institutional (school or classroom) or system level. Yet it is necessary to recognize that the effects of education are experiences in the lives of individual students at a particular point in time. It is, therefore, instructive to consider in greater detail the nature of the data to be collected in crossnational studies, assuming that the basic unit of inquiry is of necessity that of the individual student at a specified time point.

Studies of learning necessarily involve change in student behavior between two or more occasions. Where only one time point is considered, as in a crosssectional study, it must be assumed that the learning being measured has taken place during the life of a student up to that time point rather than change in learning between occasions. (see *Cross-sectional Research Methods*).

It is necessary to recognize that in studies of the effects of schooling, the treatment conditions that operate are provided for some treatments at the level of the school or school district, and for other treatments at the level of the teacher or the classroom. There is thus a series of levels commonly present in the policy-making and practice of education that has to be taken into consideration in both the sampling design and the examination of the effects of treatment conditions. These levels are: (a) within a student between occasions; (b) within a classroom between students; (c) within a school between classrooms; (d) within a school system between schools; (e) within a country between regional or local school systems; and (f) within a sample of countries between countries.

These different levels not only influence the nature of the data to be collected and the drawing of samples of students, but they necessarily also influence how the analyses of data must be carried out to separate the effects associated with differences between occasions, between students, between teachers and classrooms, between schools, between school systems, and between countries. For simplicity a particular level may be ignored; for example, only cross-sectional data may be used and the first level is ignored; or students may be sampled from across classrooms within schools, and the third level is ignored; or the effects of a school system within a country may not be of interest and the fourth and fifth levels are combined.

The statistical significance of the comparisons made between students, or between teachers, or between schools, are only valid and generalizations can only be made to other students, teachers, and schools if random samples have been chosen with a known probability of selection. Where random sampling is not possible (as with occasions, systems, and countries), the nature and magnitude of a relationship can be established as well as its statistical significance but with limited generalization. The other great benefit derived from the use of fully random samples from a defined target population is that the unknown effects of bias arising from the selection procedure employed are reduced (see *Selectional Bias in Educational Research*).

In IEA studies of the 1980s and 1990s (e.g., the Second IEA Science Study— Postlethwaite and Wiley 1992, Keeves 1992), the practice has emerged, largely for administrative convenience in testing in order to avoid the splitting of class groups, of drawing a stratified random sample of schools with a probability proportional to size and with the school as the primary sampling unit. At the second stage of sampling an intact class is drawn from within each school at the specified grade level and all students in that class are tested. Unless at least two classes per school are sampled it is impossible to separate out in statistical analysis the effects of schools in contrast to the effects of classrooms or teachers. A similar difficulty arises if a specified number of students is sampled from across classrooms within the chosen schools, for although some separation of the effects of schools and classrooms is possible, unless large numbers of students are tested the estimates of effect are unlikely to be accurate enough for meaningful findings to be obtained at the classroom level. In part, the limited success of such empirical survey studies, whether cross-sectional or longitudinal in design, to detect strong effects associated with the characteristics of teachers and classrooms, or the characteristics of schools arises from the practical problems of sample design which result in school and classroom effects being confounded with student effects. Moreover, the difficulty of detecting school and teacher effects is due in part to the fact that in most educational systems bad schools and bad teachers are not permitted to operate, and there is limited variation to be explained. However, there are also problems arising in the methods of analysis used with such data (see *Multilevel Analysis*).

The major problem that arises from the existence of the different levels at which data are collected and at which treatment effects operate is that the analysis must be carried out in such a way that the variance is appropriately partitioned between levels. If this is not done then the estimates of effect must be expected to be biased and distorted by the effects of aggregation or disaggregation of data. Furthermore, the significance tests employed must inevitably use incorrect estimates of error unless appropriate partitioning of error into its specific components has been carried out. Consequently care must be taken to partition the effects of error if the significance tests are to be meaningful. Testing for statistical significance is a great deal more complicated than is generally acknowledged and a tendency is emerging merely to consider the magnitude of an effect obtained with a large sample rather than to apply what are considered to be erroneous tests of statistical significance. Such tests are all too commonly based on simple random sampling theory, which clearly does not apply where complex sample designs have been employed and where treatments operate at levels above that of the individual student (see *Sampling Errors in Survey Research*).

An example of the analysis of data collected at the school and student levels on two occasions across eight countries in a three level analysis (see *Hierarchical Linear Modeling* is provided by Lietz's (1996) secondary analysis of the IEA reading achievement data sets assembled in 1970–71 and 1990–91. This study examined models of student, school, and system effects with appropriate tests of statistical significance and with the influence of aggregation bias removed.

4. Quantification of Cross-national Comparisons

In comparative education the typical activity is the drawing of comparisons between national systems. There is, however, the ever-present danger that conclusions are drawn on differences between countries on the basis of observations that are primarily superficial and are largely unrelated to factors that influence learning. For example, age of entry to school differs markedly across countries, largely for historical reasons. However, the effects of age of entry on achievement in reading has proved to be a complex problem to unravel in an appropriate manner unless effective controls are provided for other factors that influence reading achievement (see Thorndike 1973, Elley 1992). As a consequence considerable effort is required in planning the collection and analysis of data to ensure that sound and relevant information is obtained. The second major difficulty encountered in the making of comparisons in cross-national studies of education is that there are many variables involved that interact with each other to influence educational outcomes. The analysis of the data collected must thus proceed through a series of stages to ensure that valid findings are obtained, and this involves multilevel and multivariate analyses.

4.1 Simultaneous Analyses of Data

Powerful statistical techniques have become available that should help to tease out complex relationships between variables at several levels of analysis. One such technique is linear structural relations analysis (Muthén 1991). Linear structural relations analysis now permits the examination of random effects at both micro and macro levels in cases where complex sample designs have been employed, and provides a strategy for the comparison of structural equation models

simultaneously for up to 10 different data sets. These developments (Gustaffson and Stahl 1996) transform the nature of research and analysis into the study of processes across different countries. They provide a strategy by means of which the processes operating within schools and school systems or between sexes can be investigated using structural equation models, and the parameters of the models estimated can be effectively compared across country groups. Reports of crossnational studies have been presented by Yli-Luoma (1990) and Tuijnman and ten Brummelhuis (1993) where up to six countries have been compared in the simultaneous testing of models of educational processes. In these studies the same path model is employed across countries, but with significant differences in the magnitudes of the estimated effects, which would appear to have meaningful explanations in terms of general knowledge and understanding of educational provision within those countries. The methods of analysis employed in these two studies represent a considerable methodological advance in comparative research. Unless it can be shown that similar processes are operating in all countries under survey, it may prove seriously misleading to pool data across countries and merely estimate using least squares procedures the magnitude of national effects using dummy variables. As a consequence, the growing emphasis on the conjoint study of both processes and product, rather than the investigation of product or processes alone is of considerable importance.

5. Theoretical Perspectives

The increased elegance of the quantitative and qualitative methods that can be employed in comparative research studies in education serves to highlight the deficiencies that exist in the theory that might guide cross-national comparative research in the future. Efforts need to be made in the field of new theoretical perspectives if future studies are to achieve their potential. Three areas where developments have occurred recently in this field are provided for purposes of illustration.

5.1 Curriculum Implementation Theory

From the Granna Workshop conducted by IEA in Sweden in 1971, which examined in detail the seminal work *The Handbook of Formative and Summative Evaluation of Student Learning* (Bloom et al. 1971), came the theoretical view of curriculum implementation that has been tested, in part, in reporting the results of the IEA Science Studies and the Second IEA Mathematics Study (Keeves 1974, Rosier and Keeves 1991, Postlethwaite and Wiley 1992, Keeves 1992 Garden and Robitaille 1988).

The curriculum can be considered to exist at three levels: (a) the intended curriculum, (b) the implement-

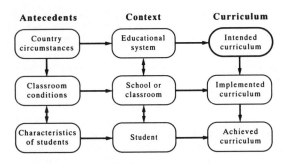

Figure 1
The context and components of the science curriculum

ed curriculum, and (c) the achieved curriculum, which are influenced by the antecedent and the contextual factors operating at the systemic, classroom, and student levels respectively. The *intended curriculum* is usually specified by political bodies and/or authorities in charge of an educational system. However, in some systems the responsibility to specify what is taught resides with the board of an individual school, or with each individual teacher within a school. The *implemented curriculum* is the second level in the curriculum sequence. It is the task of each individual teacher to interpret the intended curriculum by translating it into a set of learning experiences which

are considered appropriate for the particular group of students in a class. The *achieved curriculum* is the third stage. It refers to the extent to which individual students have learnt from the experiences that were planned and organized for them. Figure 1 shows that the intended curriculum is set in the context of the educational system; the implemented curriculum is located in the context of the school or classroom; and the achieved curriculum occurs in the context of the individual student. Moreover, it is clear that the implemented curriculum is dependent on the intended curriculum, and the achieved curriculum upon the curriculum that is implemented in the classroom. A further refinement of this model might include separation of the implemented curriculum into: (a) textbook and materials, and (b) opportunity to learn the items included in a test that is administered. Some work has been done to show the importance of access by students to a textbook (Heyneman and Loxley 1983).

A more detailed discussion of this theory and model is given by Rosier and Keeves (1991). To date the links between the intended and the achieved curricula, and between the implemented and achieved curricula have been examined, but other relationships in the model shown in Fig. 1 remain to be tested.

5.2 A Causal Model of School Learning

The model of school learning advanced by Carroll (1963) has been the source of many theoretical

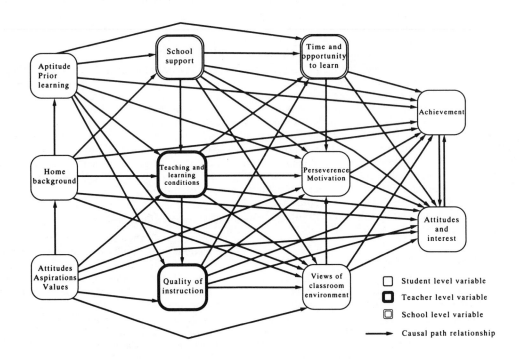

Figure 2
A simplified model of student performance

38

discussions of the factors influencing educational achievement. The IEA studies provide opportunities for such theory and the derived models to be tested empirically (Carroll 1975). In the planning of the Second IEA Science Study a causal model derived from Carroll's model of school learning was advanced in 1981 which was subsequently tested in the analyses of the data collected in that study at the 10-year-old, 14-year-old, and terminal secondary school levels (Keeves 1992). This causal model has also been examined in detail in several doctoral theses.

The model of performance in science is shown in Fig. 2 and its dependence on Carroll's ideas is immediately evident. However, consideration must be given as to the best measurable variables that are manifestations of the latent variables shown in the model. A more detailed discussion of the development of this model is given in Keeves (1992).

5.3 A Cross-national Model of Educational Achievement in a National Economy

In 1967 during the planning phase for the IEA Six-subject Study, a conference was held at Lake Mohonk in the United States which sought to develop "a cross-national model of educational achievement in a national economy." A paper by Dahllöf (1967) developed a scheme for the *educational process* that applied in cross-national settings—see Fig. 3.

Of particular interest for policy-making in education are the frame variables. However, their dependence on: (a) the environment and economy, (b) demand for personnel (c) curriculum content, and (d) objectives cannot be denied.

IEA studies have shown the marked difference in levels of achievement between the developed and the developing countries, with much lesser variation between the countries within each group (Inkeles 1977). Moreover, Lietz (1991) has shown that a causal model that explained well the influence of individual student factors on reading achievement at the 14-year-old level in developed countries was inadequate in two developing countries, India and Iran. Several possible reasons were hypothesized for these results. First, the reading tests employed were possibly inappropriate in the context of developing countries, leading to low scores and reduced variance in the outcome measures. Second, effects of selection probably operated and only students from higher status homes could afford to remain at school to the secondary level. This led to

less variance in explanatory constructs. Selection bias in turn led to less explained variance in the outcome measure. Third, there were the probable effects of limited resources in the homes. The reduced availability of reading resources in the homes of most students in developing countries restricted the explanatory power of this variable. Finally, in many, but not all, developing countries a high proportion of the students were learning and were tested in a language that was substantially different from their mother tongue, and this may also have accounted for the lower average level of performance.

Cross-national studies of educational achievement are, as pointed out above, in need of more highly developed theory and more specific models that can be subjected to testing in order to account for the general uniformity in achievement between developed countries, as well as the marked differences in achievement between developed and developing countries. The Lake Mohonk Conference advanced an input–output–utilization model of education (Super 1967) that included many significant components, namely: (a) inputs (human, financial); (b) production conditions; (c) structure and operations (educational structure, equipment, agents, curriculum, and instructional methods); (d) outputs (knowledge, skills, attitudes, participation, attainment level); and (e) utilization (employment, community involvement, and family activity). While causal influences, student movement, and financial flow were taken into consideration, insufficient thought was given at that stage to the testing of such a complex model. The task still remains for more specific hypotheses and multilevel causal models to be advanced that are amenable to testing, and rejection or refinement.

6. Future Developments

Comparative methodology in educational inquiry reflects both the variety in the disciplinary training of researchers and the limited range of available theories and models that may be examined. Contemporary comparative research in education, following trends in the social sciences, is clearly in a period of methodological diversity. However, a pluralism has emerged emphasizing the complementarity of different research approaches.

In addition to the fundamental need for theoretical developments in the field of comparative education, other advances should be sought. First, there is a need for studies using a multiplicity of methodological approaches. In particular, it should be recognized that the meaning of the context of education and richness of details of educational provision can be provided by painstaking, lengthy, on-site observation and analysis. Second, there is the need for research workers in certain more highly developed countries to adopt more rigorous procedures of sampling, so that

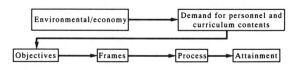

Figure 3
Model of educational process in cross-national settings

genuinely random samples that are representative of a specified target population and that yield unbiased data are studied. Third, there is a need for all countries to recognize the value of complete and high-quality data that are consistent across countries, so that sampling error and systematic bias in data collection are reduced. This requirement also involves a reduction in the amount of erroneously coded data, which can be largely eliminated through the use of appropriate data entry routines. Fourth, there is a need for the employment of computer programs for the analysis of multilevel data that involve latent variables which are fixed or random in nature, and operate at the student, school, and national or sytemic levels. Finally, there is a major need for organizations such as UNESCO and the OECD to continue efforts to develop indicators that can be used in comparative educational studies to assist in the teasing out of cross-national explanatory relationships. The publication of the volume *Education at a Glance: OECD Indicators* (Bottani et al. 1992) is a valuable start in this field. Areas where the information available has been found to be seriously deficient include simple participation rates at the twelfth year of schooling, and in higher education, particularly gender-related participation rates in general and in specific fields. Indexes of the role of women in society and indicators of home learning environments are also needed. Current indicators, while useful for certain planning purposes, fail to provide much insight into the processes of teaching and learning or why educational organizations and systems develop in the way they do. Only when relatively straight-forward but conceptually more meaningful indexes of social and educational change are available will it be possible to examine the effects of change over time both between and within countries.

See also: Research in Education: Epistemological Issues

References

Archer M 1979 *Social Origins of Educational Systems*. Sage, London

Bereday G Z F 1964 *Comparative Method in Education*. Holt, Rinehart, and Winston, New York

Bloom B S, Hastings J T, Madaus G F *Handbook of Formative and Summative Evaluation of Student Learning*. McGraw-Hill, New York

Bottani N, Duchêne C, Tuijnman A 1992 *Education at a Glance: OECD Indicators*. OECD, Paris

Brickman W W 1960 A historical introduction to comparative education. *Comp. Educ. Rev.* 3(3): 6–13

Brickman W W 1966 Prehistory of comparative education to the end of the eighteenth century. *Comp. Educ. Rev.* 10(1): 30–47

Carroll J B 1963 A model of school learning. *Teach. Coll. Rec.* 64(8): 723–33

Carroll J B 1975 *The Teaching of French as a Foreign Language in Eight Countries*. Wiley, New York

Dahllöf U 1967 Relevance and fitness analysis on comparative education. In: Super D E (ed.) 1967

Dewey J 1933 *How We Think*. Heath, New York

Elley W B 1992 *How in the World do Students Read?* IEA, Hamburg

Foshay A W et al. (ed.) 1962 *Educational Achievements of 13-year-olds in Twelve Countries*. UNESCO Institute of Education, Hamburg

Garden R A, Robitaille D F 1989 *The IEA Study of Mathematics 2: Context and Outcomes of School Mathematics*. Pergamon Press, Oxford

Gustaffson J–E, Stahl P A 1996 *STREAMS User's Guide: Structural Equation Modeling Made Simple*. Göteborg University, Göteborg

Hans N 1959 *Comparative Education: A Study of Educational Factors and Traditions*. Routledge and Kegan Paul, London

Heyneman S, Loxley W 1983 The effect of primary-school quality on academic achievement across twenty-nine high and low income countries. *Am. J. Sociology* 88(6): 1162–94

Holmes B 1965 *Problems in Education: A Comparative Approach*. Routledge and Kegan Paul, London

Inkeles T (ed.) 1977 The international evaluation of educational achievement: A review of *International Studies in Education* (9 vols.) by the International Association for the Evaluation of Educational Achievement. *Proceedings of the National Academy of Education* 4: 139–200

Kandel I L 1933 *Comparative Education*. Houghton Mifflin, Boston, Massachusetts

Kaplan A 1964 *The Conduct of Inquiry: Methodology for Behavioral Science*. Chandler, San Francisco, California

Keeves J P 1974 The IEA Science Project: Science achievement in three countries—Australia, the Federal Republic of Germany, and the United States. In: *Implementation of Curricula in Science Education*. German Commission for UNESCO, Cologne

Keeves J P (ed.) 1992 *The IEA Study of Science III: Changes in Science Education and Achievement: 1970 to 1984*. Pergamon Press, Oxford

King E J 1968 *World Perspectives in Education*. Methuen, London

Lietz P 1991 Factors influencing Reading achievement at the 14-year-old level in 15 educational systems (MEd dissertation, The Flinders University of South Australia

Lietz P 1996 *Changes in reading Comprehension Across Cultures and Over Time*. Waxman Publishers, Meunster

Mallinson V 1957 *An Introduction to the Study of Comparative Education*. Heinemann, Melbourne

Meyer J W, Hannan M T 1979 *National Development and the World System: Educational, Economic, and Political Change*. University of Chicago Press, Chicago, Illinois

Muthén B O 1991 Analysis of longitudinal data using latent variable models with varying parameters. In: Collins L M, Horn J L. *Best Methods for the Analysis of Change*. American Psychological Association, Washington, DC

Noah H J, Eckstein M A 1969 *Toward a Science of Comparative Education*. Macmillan, London

Postlethwaite T N (ed.) 1995 *International Encyclopedia of National Systems of Education*, 2nd edn. Pergamon, Oxford

Postlethwaite T N, Wiley D E (eds.) 1992 *The IEA Study*

of Science II: Science Achievement in Twenty-Three Countries. Pergamon Press, Oxford

Rosier M J, Keeves J P 1991 *The IEA Study of Science I: Science Education and Curricula in Twenty-Three Countries*. Pergamon Press, Oxford

Super D E (ed.) 1967 *Toward a Cross-national Model of Educational Achievement in a National Economy*. Teachers College Press, New York

Thorndike R L 1973 *Reading Comprehension Education in Fifteen Countries: An Empirical Study, International Studies in Evaluation 3*. Wiley, New York

Tuijnman A C, ten Brummelhuis A C A 1993 Predicting computer use in six systems: Structural models of implementing indicators. In: Pelgrum W J, Plomp T (eds.) 1993 *Computers in Education: Implementation of an Innovation in 20 Countries*. Pergamon Press, Oxford

Yli-Luoma P V J 1990 *Predictors of Moral Reasoning*. Almqvist and Wiksell, Stockholm

Further Reading

Husén T, Tuijnman A, Halls W D 1992 *Schooling in Modern European Society*. Pergamon Press, Oxford

Purves A C (ed.) 1989 *International Comparisons and Educational Reform*. Association for Supervision and Curriculum Development (ASCD), Alexandra, Virginia

Thomas R M (ed.) 1990 *International Comparative Education: Practices, Issues, and Prospects*. Pergamon Press, Oxford

Øyen E (ed.) 1990 *Comparative Methodology: Theory and Practice in International Social Research*. Sage, London

Facet theory

S. Shye

Facet theory is a general approach—or metatheory—to the design of observations and to the analysis of empirical data for the purpose of formulating and testing theories and conducting measurements. Proposed by Guttman (Guttman 1959, Foa and Turner 1970, Shye 1978a, 1985, Tziner 1987, Shye et al. 1995) as a generalization of Fisher's design of experiments to the design of theories, facet theory has been developed in the context of the behavioral sciences. Facet theory is especially geared to research domains that involve a large number of interdependent variables and hence has been used in studying complex systems and in discovering "structural" theories and laws. Employed in a wide range of behavioral disciplines, its main applications have been in the fields of intelligence research, attitude research, organizational behavior, education evaluation, marketing, and quality of life research.

Facet theory seeks a proper balance between data analysis and conceptual analysis: it is critical of the overdue attention paid to statistical data manipulations, and claims that substantive aspects of behavioral research can and should be formalized. Moreover, it provides the tools and techniques for such formalization, thereby enhancing definitional reliability, scientific communication, and, ultimately, cumulative science. This entry presents briefly the principles of facet theory then illustrates it with some applications.

1. Principles of Facet Theory

1.1 The Role of Questions in Scientific Research

Questions may be thought of as playing two kinds of roles: the role of a "research question" (e.g., "What is the relationship between students' success in English grammar and their success in mathematics?") and the role of an observational question (e.g., "What is Debby's score in her 8th grade English grammar course?"). Often a system of observational questions serves to find the answer to a research question. Indeed, a system of questions of the form:

$$\text{What is the score obtained by 8th grade student}(s_i) \text{ in } \begin{Bmatrix} \text{mathematics} \\ \text{grammar} \end{Bmatrix}?$$

can, under suitable conditions, serve as a basis for assessing the relationship between success in grammar and success in mathematics, provided it is understood that s_i $(i = 1,2, \ldots, N)$ varies over the N students of the investigated class, and that each student is scored with respect to grammar, and with respect to mathematics. In facet theory (s_i) is termed the "focus facet" (or the population facet); and {grammar/mathematics} is termed the "content facet." In the simple design of the present illustration, the system contains, therefore, $N \times 2 = 2N$ observational questions.

Every question, whether it plays the role of a research question or of an observational question, has an intended range of answers which may be implicit or explicit. In facet theory, which generally seeks to increase the level for formalization, that range is made explicit, and is regarded as an inseparable part of the question itself. Thus, a possible range for the above research question concerning the relationship between grammar and mathematics can be {negative, positive} or it may be {very weak, weak, strong, very strong} or {−1.00 . . . 0.00 . . . +1.00} as computed by Pearson correlation coefficient. For the observational questions mentioned above (e.g.,

"What is Debby's score in mathematics?") the intended range of answers could be {0 . . . 100} or {0 . . . 10} or {4, 3, 2, 1, 0} (where $A = 4$, $B = 3$, etc.,); or {1 0} (where Fail = 0, Pass = 1); and so on. An observational question with an explicit range of answers is called a "variable," and a variable which is a part of a system of observational questions is called an "item."

1.2 Common Meaning Range

The range of answers to an observational question may be ordered or unordered ("nominal"), depending not on the set of answers itself but on a substantive (conceptual) specification of the researcher. A seemingly ordered range such as students' height in centimeters may in some research contexts be treated as a nominal characteristic. A person's neighborhood of residence, which *prima facie* is a "nominal" variable, may be regarded in a particular study as an ordered variable—for example, by the neighborhood's proximity to the center of town.

When in a system of variables all variables have answer ranges that are ordered from high to low with respect to a common meaning, it is said that those variables have a "common meaning range" (CMR) or a "common range". To avoid confusion, it is extremely helpful to design the scores, or to recode them, so that a numerically high value would stand for a high measure of the common meaning. For example, if the common meaning by which answer ranges are ordered is "high to low success in school courses," it is useful to assign the numerically high scores to success and the numerically low scores to failure (or the other way around), *uniformally* in all the variables. But, facet design does not require that the ranges be identical and they may have a different number of categories each. For example, look at the answer ranges of (1) below, where it is assumed that students are graded in English grammar by the range {4, 3, 2, 1, 0} and in mathematics by the range {10,9,8, . . . 1,0}. A facet design presentation of the system of observations assigns to each student s_i two scores, one from {4, 3, 2, 1, 0} in grammar, and one from {10, 9, 8, . . . 0}, in mathematics. The system of questions shown above together with the specified ranges of answers (scores), is termed a "Mapping sentence": it "maps" (assigns to) every combination of student (s_i) and school course into a particular value from a pre-specified range of scores. The focus facet and the content facet(s) (of which there may be more than one) define the domain of the mapping and hence are called "domain facets." A mapping sentence is "a verbal statement of the domain and of the range of a mapping including connectives between facets as in ordinary language" (Shye 1978a p. 413).

Focus Facet:	Content Facet:	Range Facets:		
8th Grade Students	School Subjects	Grammar	Mathematics	(1)
The score of (s_i) in	{grammar} {mathematics} (is) $\longrightarrow$	$\begin{Bmatrix} 4 \\ 3 \\ 2 \\ 1 \end{Bmatrix}$	$\begin{Bmatrix} 10 \\ 9 \\ 8 \\ . \end{Bmatrix}$	

Uses of common meaning range include:

(a)   serving as a criterion in selecting or constructing observational items in the study of a trait (such as intelligence, adaptability, etc.), attributable to the investigated population, and in particular, in formulating definitions of investigated concepts;

(b)   serving as a theoretical rationale for hypothesizing positive correlations among observational items and, more generally, as a rationale for "laws of monotonicity";

(c)   serving as a useful criterion in comparing different studies with respect to their design and findings (meta-analysis).

1.3 Mapping Definitions and Laws of Monotonicity

Formal definitions are important for scientific communication. Facet theory offers a technique for defining concepts by specifying the set of all observational items that may serve to assess that concept. This kind of definition, called a "mapping definition," was used to define, for example, the notion of "attitude," thus:

> An item belongs to the universe of attitude items if and only if its domain asks about *behavior toward an object* and its range is ordered from "very positive" to "very negative" toward that object.

The range, of course, need not include the terms "positive" and "negative" verbatim, but rather have the meaning of positive to negative toward the specified object. Unlike other forms of definition, the mapping definition of attitude does not start with "Attitude is . . ." Rather, it characterizes the set of all items of attitude toward a given object in terms of the essential concepts of their domain and the common meaning of their range.

Similarly, a mapping definition of intelligence (based on the observation that intelligence items involve an objectively correct response) would be:

> An item belongs to the universe of intelligence items if and only if its domain asks about *performance relative to an objective rule* and its range is ordered from "very right" to "very wrong" performance, relative to that rule.

In empirical sciences, definitions are evaluated with respect to their contribution to formulating theories or empirical laws. The above two definitions have led Guttman to formulate the law of Attitude Monotonicity and the law of Intelligence Monotonicity. Both laws summarize considerable evidence that has accumulated over many studies. In a simplified form these laws state:

Law of Attitude Monotonicity: If the population observed is not selected artificially, the correlation between any two items of attitude toward an object will be positive or zero.
Law of Intelligence Monotonicity: If the population observed is not selected artificially, the correlation between any two items of intelligence will be positive or zero.

Note that the formulation of these laws is based on the

definitions of attitude items, and of intelligence items, given above.

Laws of monotonicity may be found in other fields of research as well. They are very general and coarse, since they refer to a very general aspect of the data, namely to the correlation sign. Finer laws referring to the relative magnitudes of the intercorrelations among items of a given "content universe" require finer content analysis of the observational items. This is facilitated by the structuring of the domain of the mapping sentence.

1.4 Domain Facets: Population and Contents

One kind of domain facet is the "population facet," or the "focus facet," that defines the objects to be investigated—human subjects, sophomores, classrooms, schools, countries, works of art, and so on. Laws to be inferred may depend, of course, on the specification of the "population." Usually a single population facet is used.

The second kind of domain facet is the "content facet," which makes it possible systematically to extend and deepen the investigated contents. Each content facet constitutes a classification of the observational questions (stimuli) by some content criteria. Facet design of research often strives to formulate content facets whose elements (classes) are exclusive of each other (i.e., facet elements {classes} do not overlap, and are exhaustive, in that all conceivable facet elements {classes} are present). For example, the content facet {grammar/mathematics} in (1) may be used to classify school tests (or test items) into two classes: grammar tests and mathematics tests. "Extension" of a mapping sentence and of the research design is attained by adding facet elements to an existing content facet. Adding "geography" as a third element in the content facet of (1) would extend the mapping sentence, as well as the implied framework for collecting observations. If *all* school subjects taught to the investigated student population were included, that facet would be exhaustive.

The name given to a content facet—"school subject" in the present illustration—is an important feature of the conceptual design because it helps conceptually to clarify what facet elements may or may not be included.

In the present example, is there another, independent way of classifying tests or test items? Cognitive psychologists may be interested in differentiating between test items that require knowledge of facts (definitions, rules), and those that require application of such knowledge to new situations. Such classification into "factual knowledge" and "knowlege application" is independent of the school subject in that it can be relevant, in principle, to every school subject. Hence a second content facet (cognitive task) can be introduced into (1), to form mapping sentence (2), for example:

A. Cognitive Task

The score of (s_i) in $\left\{ \begin{array}{l} a_1 \text{ factual knowledge} \\ a_2 \text{ knowledge application} \end{array} \right\}$ test items in

B. School Subject (2)

$\left\{ \begin{array}{l} b_1 \text{ grammar} \\ b_2 \text{ mathematics} \end{array} \right\} \longrightarrow \left\{ \begin{array}{l} \text{high} \\ \vdots \\ \text{low} \end{array} \right\}$ score

Adding a content facet to an existing mapping sentence is called "intension." It refines and adds a new dimension to the research design. Further intension of the mapping sentence could be effected by further content facets, such as the facet {oral/written}, provided such facets each represent an independent classification of the test items.

Together, the two content facets *A* and *B* of (2) determine four types of test items, each defined by its "content profile." The four content profiles are:

(a) $a_1\ b_1$ factual knowledge in grammar;

(b) $a_1\ b_2$ factual knowledge in mathematics;

(c) $a_2\ b_1$ knowledge application in grammar;

(d) $a_2\ b_2$ knowledge application in mathematics.

Each content profile represents a content sub-universe of the content universe of "success in school studies." Technically, the set of content profiles—here $\{a_1b_1, a_1b_2, a_2b_1, a_2b_2\}$—is a "Cartesian set (product)" of the component sets $A = \{a_1, a_2\}$ and $B = \{b_1, b_2\}$. And, in general, a "profile" (an element of the Cartesian set) is made up by selecting one element from each facet. A facet, then, is simply a set playing the role of a component set of the Cartesian set (Shye 1978b).

1.5 The Use of Facet Theory and Mapping Sentences in Creative Research Design and in the Interpretation of Findings

Facet theory, with its emphasis on Cartesian structure, can enhance creativity in research design and in the interpretation of findings. Some illustrations follow.

1.5.1 Cartesian completion. Suppose that in a study of leisure the following activities are initially considered: reading, TV watching, playing with one's children, discussion groups, hiking, skiing, playing tennis, swimming, folk dancing. These activities may be classified by several independent criteria: by location {indoors, outdoors}; by nature {physical, intellectual}; and by social context {alone, group}. A possible mapping sentence for observations could be:

Facet A: Behavior Modality

The extent to which subject(s) $\left\{ \begin{array}{l} \text{enjoys} \\ \text{actually practices} \\ \text{values} \end{array} \right\}$

B. Location   C. Nature of Activity

an $\left\{ \begin{array}{l} \text{indoor} \\ \text{outdoor} \end{array} \right\}$ $\left\{ \begin{array}{l} \text{physical} \\ \text{intellectual} \end{array} \right\}$ leisure activity which is conducted (3)

D. Social Contex

$$\left.\begin{array}{c} alone \\ in\ a\ group \end{array}\right\} \longrightarrow \left\{\begin{array}{c} high \\ \vdots \\ low \end{array}\right\}$$

After classifying each activity of the initial list by facets *B, C,* and *D* (e.g., TV-watching may be classified as $b_1\ c_2\ d_1$), it may be realized that the combination $b_2\ c_2\ d_1$ (i.e., outdoor intellectual activity conducted alone) is not represented in the initial list. This realization can prompt the researcher to consider what leisure activities belong to this content profile, and include them in the research design (for example, bird watching). Similarly $b_2\ c_2\ d_2$ could be represented, for example, by guided archaeological tours.

In empirical studies, Cartesian completion of this kind not only proves intellectually satisfying but also leads to important insights into the investigated domain.

1.5.2 Cartesian twists, nests, and loops. What may seem "rigid" in the Cartesian design of mapping sentence is so only at a formal level. In fact, this formality allows a surprising flexibility in representing complex structures typical of behavioral reality. Two examples follow.

Example One: Interfacet conceptual dependence. A study of potential work mobility of professionals (e.g., teachers, psychologists) can be based on observations from the following mapping sentence (see Aranya et al. 1976):

The extent to which professional (x) feels certain he or she would change his or her

Facet A: Framework   *Facet B: Incentive*

$$\left\{\begin{array}{l} 1.\ place\ of\ work \\ \\ 2.\ profession \end{array}\right\} \begin{array}{c} if\ were\ offered\ better \end{array} \left\{\begin{array}{l} 1.\ opportunity\ to\ develop\ self \\ 2.\ status \\ 3.\ professional\ freedom \\ 4.\ pay \end{array}\right\}$$

$$\longrightarrow \left\{\begin{array}{l} 1.\ certainly\ would\ change \\ 2.\ probably\ would\ change \\ 3.\ uncertain \\ 4.\ probably\ would\ not\ change \\ 5.\ certainly\ would\ not\ change \end{array}\right\} \qquad (4)$$

Multivariate analysis of the empirical observations by faceted smallest space analysis (see *Smallest Space Analysis*) pointed to an order that exists among the elements of the Incentive Facet, with "pay" being the most extrinsic and "opportunity to develop self" as the most intrinsic incentive. However, the location of the two intermediate elements, "status" and "professional freedom" was not consistent. When "place of work" was specified in the framework in Facet *A,* the order was "pay," "professional freedom," "status," "opportunity to develop"; when "profession" was specified as the framework in Facet *A,* the order was "pay," "status," "professional freedom," "opportunity to develop." Hence the suggestion was made that "status" is more intrinsic than "professional freedom" when change of place of work is considered; whereas "professional freedom" is more intrinsic than "status" when change in the profession is considered. Rewording "place of work" as "organization" and interpreting "status" as "organizational freedom," the following mapping sentence was proposed.

The extent to which professional (*x*) feels certain he or she would change his or her

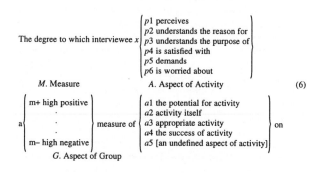

This mapping sentence is for the same observations as the original one. However, in spite of its Cartesian appearance (with its characteristic semantic independence between the content facets), it reflects the conceptual *dependence* between the two content facets—*A*: Framework and *B*: Incentive. This dependence may be thought of as a twist in the original content structure.

Example Two: Recursive mapping sentence. For observing relations among personnel within an organization (e.g., a school) the following mapping sentence was designed (this illustration is taken from Schlesinger 1978):

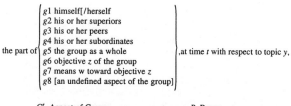

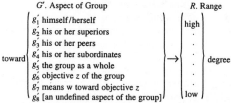

This mapping sentence can be used to analyze innumerable questions in intergroup relations. For example—

Question 1. Are you willing to make efforts on behalf of your friends in the group?

The analysis is (with the style polished a bit): The degree to which interviewee x demands (p_5) a high positive measure ($m+$) of activity (itself: a_2) on the part of himself or herself (g_1) or herself in the future (t), with respect to an undefined topic (y) toward his or her peers (g'_6) $\rightarrow$

And the answer to Question 1 would be selected from the range:

{high degree . . . low degree} of demand.

The topic y has not been specified in Question 1. One advantage of a mapping sentence *after* it has been constructed is that it often requires the reconsideration of the wording of a question: Is it really intended that the topic in the question remain undefined—*Question 2. To what extent is your boss capable of running the firm*? Obviously, this question involves element a_1 ("potential for activity") and g_2 ("superiors"). "The firm" must be analyzed as an element of Facet G', (perhaps as g'_6, or by adding an element). Notice that, in fact, P is the facet to which the range applies. What is the process of interviewee x about which the question is asked? The range pertains to p_1, "perceives": if the interviewee answers "yes" to Question 3, this means that he or she perceives the capabilities of the boss (i.e., they exist, in his or her opinion), and if he or she answers "no," this means he or she does not. Observe that without Facet M the analysis of Question 3 would be indistinguishable from that of the opposite question—*Question 3. To what extent is your boss capable of ruining the firm*? Here, too, it is necessary to ask about the "potential for activity," only this time not, as in Question 2, *on behalf of* the firm. This distinction is incorporated in the positive–negative dimension of Facet M. In other words, Facet M pertains to Facet A (the aspect of the activity of g), whereas the range pertains to Facet P: the degree to which the interviewee perceives, understands, is satisfied with, or worried by an aspect of the activity.

Now consider the following question—*Question 4. Do you think your friends are willing to make efforts on your behalf*? Compare this to Question 1 above. What Question 1 asked about the interviewee is here asked about his or her friends, yet the interviewee must be accounted for. What is needed here is another mapping sentence, containing all the facets of (1) and three additional facets closely parallel to G, P, and M. An abbreviated form of (1) should help to make this clear:

The degree to which x, the interviewee,
p a measure m of a on the part of g at time t,
with respect to y, toward g' $\rightarrow$ r degree of p.

(6a)

For Question 4 the following extended, recursive mapping sentence is needed, which differs from the foregoing only in the addition of the parenthesized expression:

The degree to which x, the interviewee,
p (in regard to g'' *that p'* to degree n)
a measure m of a on the part of g at time t,   (7)
with respect to y, toward g' $\rightarrow$ r degree of p

The new facets G'' and P' include exactly the same elements as G and P, respectively. Facet N contains just the degrees from "high" to "low" (without the positive–negative dimension) of facet M. Question 4 can now be analyzed as follows: The degree to which interviewee x perceives (in regard to his or her peers that they demand to a high degree) a high positive measure of activity on the part of his or her peers in the future, with respect to an undefined topic, toward himself or herself $\rightarrow$

To facilitate comparison with the analysis of Question 1, the elements that have been added or that differ have been italicized here.

Facet N is necessary to distinguish between questions about g'' perceiving, demanding, worrying about, and so on, something (i.e., "to a high degree") and those about g'' *not* perceiving, *not* demanding, or *not* worrying about it (i.e., "to a low degree"). The recursiveness is introduced by the parenthesized expression, which can be repeated an unlimited number of times. For instance, Question 5 will be analyzed as follows—*Question 5. Do you think your superiors expect your friends to be willing to make efforts on your behalf ?* The degree to which interviewee x perceives (*in regard to his or her superiors that they demand to a high degree* {from his or her peers that they demand to a high degree}) that there be a high positive measure of activity on the part of his or her peers in the future, with respect to an undefined topic, toward himself or herself $\rightarrow$

The phrase in which this analysis differs from that of Question 5 is italicized.

In this manner the parenthesized expression can be repeated any number of times. One may want to prove this to oneself by working out examples like the following, which needs a still higher degree of recursiveness—*Question 6. Do you think that your superiors resent your believing that they are unwilling to make efforts on your behalf ?*

Recursiveness is a property of natural languages that facilitates an extension of a mapping sentence. In this instance, then, the English sentence format of mapping sentences, far from obstructing the construction of an adequate conceptual framework, actually leads up to it.

2. The Use of Facet Theory in Formulating Laws and Theories

A "theory" in a substantive domain of research may be defined as "an hypothesis of a correspondence between a definitional system for a universe of observations and an aspect of the empirical structure of those observations, together with a rationale for such an hypothesis (Guttman, in Shye 1978a). A mapping sentence in a particular domain of research does not constitute a theory, but rather provides one of its necessary components, namely the definitional system for the universe of observations. The other component is a "statistic"—a well-defined aspect of reality computed from the collected observations. In principle, that statistic may be of any kind—means, conditional means, (regressions), correlations, features

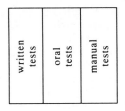
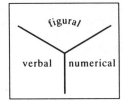
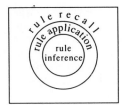

Axial facet:
classification of
tests by mode of
presentation

Angular facet:
classification of
tests by material

Radial facet:
classification of
tests by cognitive
complexity

Figure 1
Pictorial representations of axial, angular, and radial facets

of the correlation matrices, and so on. However, facet theory does prefer a particular kind of statistic, namely the observed pattern of space partition in multidimensional scaling (see *Smallest Space Analysis; Partial Order Scalogram Analysis of Nonmetric Data*). Facet theory anticipates that with respect to *this* multivariate aspect of the empirical observations, behavioral laws are most likely to be discovered.

Facet theory interprets the set of observed variables in a particular content universe (such as achievement motivation, intelligence, etc.) as but a finite sample from the infinite set of variables of that universe. It envisages the concept as a geometric space each of whose points is a possible variable. Observed variables, when processed by smallest space analysis, provide clues as to the structure of the investigated domain (i.e., its dimensionality, its internal components, and the inter-relationships among those components). The conceptual components are represented then by "regions" in the geometric space, while their interrelationships are represented by the spatial orientation of the regions, relative to each other.

A content facet of a mapping sentence is said to be "axial" if the empirical smallest space analysis map can be partitioned by parallel lines into simply ordered striped regions so that variables pertaining to each of the facet elements are all in one region. Thus, a correspondence is established between the facet elements and the ordered regions.

If elements of a content facet are found to correspond to circularly ordered regions (effected by a set of radii emanating from a common center), that facet is said to be "angular." And if elements of a content facet correspond to a set of nested ring-like regions (effected by concentric circles), the facet is said to be "radial" (see Fig. 1).

Two or more facets may correspond to superposed patterns of space partitioning to yield more complex structures—in fact, theories—of the investigated domains (for a systematic review of these patterns see Shye 1978a Chap. 16).

3. Facet Theory in Educational Research

Facet design has been used extensively and profitably in many educational contexts. In particular, in cognitive development (Klauer 1990), intelligence research (Schlesinger and Guttman 1969, Snow et al. 1984, Shye 1988, Guttman and Levy 1991, Klauer and Shye 1991), assessments of school performance (Lewy and Shye 1990), and in content analysis of philosophical approaches to educational evaluation (Lewy and Shye 1978). In the latter work, the operational meaning of "educational evaluation," as advanced by three scholars has been content-analyzed and compared by translating each of the three approaches (Scrivens's, Stakes's, and Stufflebeam's) into a mapping sentence, and then creating a meta-mapping sentence that records the emphases that characterize each approach.

See also: Scaling Methods; Factor Analysis

References

Aranya N, Jacobson D, Shye S 1976 A smallest space analysis of potential work mobility. *Multivariate Behavioral Research* 11(2): 165–73
Foa V G, Turner J L 1970 Psychology in the year 2000: Going structural. *Am. Psychol.* 25(3): 244–47
Guttman L 1959 Introduction to facet design and analysis. In: *Proceedings of the Fifteenth International Congress of Psychology, Brussels, 1957.* North Holland, Amsterdam
Guttman L, Levy S 1991 Two structural laws for intelligence tests. *Intelligence* 15(1): 79–103
Klauer K J 1990 Paradigmatic teaching of inductive thinking. In: Mandl H, De Corte E, Bennett N, Fridrich H F (eds.) 1990 *Learning and Instruction*, Vol. 2.2. Pergamon Press, Oxford
Klauer K J, Shye S 1991 *Formalization of Inductive Reasoning* (technical report). Institute of Applied Social Research, Jerusalem and RWTH, Aachen
Lewy A, Shye S 1978 Three main approaches to evaluating education: Analysis and comparison by facet technique. In: Shye S (ed.) 1978a

Lewy A, Shye S 1990 Dimension of attitude toward higher mental function curricular objectives (HMCO): A partial order scalogram analysis. *Quality and Quantity* 24(3): 231–44

Schlesinger I M 1978 On some properties of mapping sentences. In: Shye S (ed.) 1978a

Schlesinger I M, Guttman L 1969 Smallest space analysis of intelligence and achievement tests. *Psych. Bull.* 71(2): 95–100

Shye S (ed.) 1978a *Theory Construction and Data Analysis in the Behavioral Sciences*. Jossey-Bass, San Francisco, California

Shye S 1978b Achievement motive: A faceted definition and structural analysis. *Multivariate Behavioral Research* 13(3): 327 46

Shye S 1985 *Multiple Scaling: The Theory and Applications of Partial Order Scalogram Analysis*. North- Holland, Amsterdam

Shye S 1988 Inductive and deductive reasoning: A structural reanalysis of ability tests. *J. Appl. Psychol.* 73(2): 308–11

Shye S et al. 1995 *Introduction to Facet Theory*. Sage, Newbury Park, California

Snow R E, Kyllonen P C, Marshalek B 1984 The topography of ability and learning correlation. In: Sternberg S J (ed.) 1984 *Advances in the Psychology of Human Intelligence*, Vol. 2.

Erlbaum, Hillsdale, New Jersey

Tzinner A E 1987 *The Facet Analytic Approach Research and Data Processing*. Peter Lang, New York

Further Reading

Borg I, Shye S in press *Facet Theory: Form and Content*. Sage, Newbury Park, California

Canter D 1985 *Facet Theory: Approaches to Social Research*. Springer-Verlag, New York

Elizur D 1970 *Adapting to Innovation: A Facet Analysis of the Use of the Computer*. Jerusalem Academic Press, Jerusalem

Guttman L 1959 A structural theory for intergroup beliefs and actions. *Am. Sociol. Rev.* 24: 318–28

Guttman L 1965 A faceted definition of intelligence. *Studies in Psychology—Scripta Hierosolymitana* 14: 166–81

Shye S 1980 A structural analysis of achievement orientation derived from a longitudinal study of students in Israeli schools. *Am. Educ. Res. J.* 17(3): 281–90

Shye S 1989 The systemic quality of life model: A basis for urban renewal evaluation. *Social Indicators Research* 21(4): 343–78

(b) Humanistic Research Methods

Anthropological Inquiry

J. U. Ogbu, N. E. Sato, and E.-Y. Kim

Ethnography is a research methodology in anthropology and through this methodology, anthropologists have contributed significantly to the understanding of education and to the development of qualitative research in education. In order to provide rich, descriptive data about the cultures and ways of living of groups of people, long-term residence with and in-depth, contextualized understanding of the participants' views form central features of this research methodology. Different ethnographic approaches have been used by anthropologists to study education and schooling, and a variety of terms have evolved that reveal these differences in topics, theoretical orientations, levels of analysis, and units of study (see Sect. 3).

Because of a sudden rise in interest in employing ethnographic methods in educational research, confusion regarding ethnography has also developed. As an educational research fad, ethnography has been subject to misuse, misinterpretation, and inadequate methodological rigor. Specifically, ethnography has been erroneously equated with "naturalistic inquiry" or "qualitative research" without adequate distinctions drawn between various methodologies. Ethnography evolved within the field of anthropology which distinguishes it from other research traditions that have been labeled "naturalistic," "case study method," and "phenomenological" (see Sect. 2). Ethnography as a methodology must also be distinguished from the specific data-gathering techniques that it employs. Although participant observation and interviews are the main techniques, these are often supplemented by other qualitative and quantitative techniques such as mapping, charting, questionnaires, document and artifact analysis, life histories, narratives, and experiments (Bernard 1988, Berreman 1968, Narroll and Cohen 1970).

Ethnography is a complex subset of qualitative research encompassing a diversity of research traditions, historical roots, philosophical assumptions, and methods. Jacob (1988) presents a discussion of six qualitative research traditions, three of which are ethnographic: holistic ethnography cognitive anthropology, and ethnography of communication. The term "qualitative research" was coined in opposition to the quantitative methods dominating sociology in the early 1900s, and although some proponents eschew any association with quantitative methodologies, others recognize that as an umbrella term, qualitative research encompasses many research traditions and diverse methodologies. Ethnography is one form of qualitative inquiry that has always incorporated diverse data collection strategies because qualitative and quantitative forms of inquiry are seen as interdependent not oppositional. Ethnography is subject to its own rigorous standards of systematic investigation consonant with the nature of the ethnographic research process (see Sect. 4).

Section 1 describes the historical background of ethnography as the fieldwork methodology in anthropology and explores the developments in applying ethnography to the study of schooling and education. Sections 2 and 3 defines ethnography and elaborates upon various ethnographic approaches used by anthropologists in educational studies. Section 4 discusses the strengths and weaknesses of ethnography, and the entry concludes with a brief summary of future trends in educational ethnographic work.

This entry focuses primarily on United States research, which has the most prominent and well-developed educational ethnography research history and tradition. Although other countries have significant and long-standing qualitative research traditions that are not necessarily reported in Western journals and research, they do not have long-standing traditions in educational ethnography. Good examples of educational ethnography are beginning to emanate from these countries (Delamont and Atkinson 1980, *Revue Française de Pedagogie* 1987, Woods 1986), but inhibiting factors are the costly time and labor-intensive nature of ethnographic research.

1. Historical Background

1.1 Development of Fieldwork Traditions in Anthropology in the United States and the United Kingdom

Anthropology was established as a field of study in the United States and Europe in the 1840s. Until the late 1800s, a division of labor existed between those who collected the data and those who analyzed it. Early anthropologists sent questionnaires to those who had regular contact with other cultures (missionaries, travelers, administrators, and explorers), then used their second-hand reports as the basis for their analyses.

The major concerns of early anthropologists were twofold: (a) comparative research whose aim was to create a comprehensive taxonomy of cultures based on an evolutionary scheme of human cultures from "savagery" to "civilization," and (b) salvage work whose aim was to collect data on the "exotic" and "primitive" cultures before they disappeared. These concerns led researchers to focus on collecting as much data on as many societies as possible, without paying proper attention to the methods of data collection.

In the late nineteenth century, increasing concern was expressed about the quality of the data, especially the unsystematic collection and the uncritical and inappropriate use of data. Awareness of the complexity of societies initially considered "simple and primitive" led anthropologists to shift their focus from construction of general evolutionary theory to a more thorough study of particular societies. At the same time, the natural science orientation of scholars influenced data collection procedures. Many scholars, particularly Boas in the United States and Haddon in the United Kingdom, emphasized the need for researchers to collect their own data through direct observation, using systematic terminology and clearly articulating their methodology. Eventually, two major traditions developed in anthropology: historical ethnology in the United States and structural–functionalism in the United Kingdom (Urry 1984).

During the early twentieth century, fieldwork became an essential rite of passage for anthropologists. As a result of his work on Trobriand islanders, Malinowski (1922) enunciated four important principles of ethnographic research, namely, that the ethnographer should (a) learn and work in the native language; (b) live with the people and participate in their activities as much as possible; (c) gather many case examples through actual personal observation; and (d) be prepared to cope with long periods of fieldwork and management of practical problems. These principles still guide ethnographic research in anthropology today. In addition to these principles Malinowski created *a theory of ethnography* in the sense that he was the first anthropologist who clearly articulated the methods of ethnography and how they were related to anthropological theory (Urry 1984). In order to accomplish these principles enunciated by Malinowski, one needed to live with people long enough to contextualize data into a holistic, coherent account and to describe "life as lived."

By the 1930s, anthropologists had shifted their research orientation from salvage work to studying social change, cultural contact, assimilation, and accommodation because they realized that these societies were changing rather than disappearing. At the same time, United States and United Kingdom anthropologists began to study larger, more complex societies and incorporate positivistic techniques, such as statistical procedures, and research instruments from other disciplines, such as psychology, sociology, demography, and economics.

Consequently, various subfields of specialization emerged within anthropology. Studies in culture-and-personality, linguistic analysis, child rearing, and culture transmission grew in popularity. Later in the 1950s and 1960s, variation in ethnographic methods also developed based on different conceptions of culture, such as "old ethnography" and "new ethnography" (see Sect. 3).

1.2 Application of Ethnography to the Study of Education

From the 1930s through the 1950s, the anthropological study of child-rearing practices, enculturation processes, and cultural transmission comprised the earliest forms of studying educational processes of various cultures. For example, Mead (1930) and Williams (1972) focused on life-cycle patterns and culture-and-personality studies, usually studying preliterate, nonindustrialized societies and only indirectly comparing them to the United States during the 1930s. Others studied schools as educational and cultural transmission institutions in those societies (Goetz and LeCompte 1984, Middleton 1970).

Schooling in industrial societies was not studied by anthropologists until the 1950s with research conducted by Henry (1963) from the 1950s to the early 1960s. The interdisciplinary area of educational anthropology was formed by Solon Kimball of Teachers College, Columbia University and George Spindler of Stanford University. As Ogbu notes: "Prior to the 1960s few anthropologists had actually studied formal education, although some had written about it . . . Henry was probably one of the few who had actually studied the schools" (Ogbu 1981 p. 7).

During the 1960s and 1970s, educational ethnography flourished within anthropology. Some continued in the Mead tradition, while others focused on industrialized and industrializing societies, and still others studied subcultural and ethnic enclaves within industrialized societies. Ogbu (1981) cites four factors that influenced what ethnographers have studied about schooling: (a) the traditional anthropological perception of schooling as a social problem; (b) the background of educational ethnographers in culture-and-personality and anthropological linguistic subfields; (c) the birth of educational ethnography in the climate of social and political crisis during the 1960s in the United States; and (d) the patronage of school ethnography by educators resulting in a pressure toward applied research—for example, researchers were usually situated in schools of education as was the research audience, and educators who controlled research funding usually defined the research problems to be studied. Specifically, anthropologists questioned the assumptions of the predominant "cultural deprivation" model for explaining minority and poor students' lack of success in schools and instead developed a cultural difference model (Ogbu 1981, Spradley 1972, Valentine 1968).

A great diversification of educational ethnographies occurred during the 1970s, though the concept of culture remained the unifying construct. Areas of study included language and other formal symbol systems, minority education, desegregation, policy, school and society stratification, social structure, classroom processes, and cultural transmission. Units of analysis varied: for example, career and life histories, small groups within classrooms or schools, single classrooms, classroom scenes or language events, school districts, school–community relations, and conceptually controlled comparisons across numbers of individuals or groups (see Goetz and LeCompte 1984, Green and Wallat 1983, Spindler 1982).

Along with such a diversity of units of analysis, theoretical frameworks, methodologies, topics, and contexts, inevitable problems in the definition of "educational ethnography" developed. Moreover, the intellectual climate, sociopolitical context, research traditions, individual preferences of researchers, ideological and philisophical assumptions, and the nature of the problems studied also affected the kinds of ethnography that evolved.

2. What is Ethnography?

Ethnography is a methodology, a tool for studying and understanding a people's way of life, namely, the "native point of view" (i.e., their ideas, beliefs, values, and assumptions), behavior, and artifacts or things that they make. Ethnographers learn these ways of life through participant observation in a natural setting. Some distinguishing features of this methodology are: (a) long-term residence and interaction with the people (usually at least a year); (b) competence in the native language; (c) empathy to be able to understand life as the people experience it; and (d) a holistic perspective with which to see relationships between different institutions or between observed data and other known facts and ideas, and to discern their relevance and importance.

Good rapport must be established and maintained to ease access to valid and reliable data. Data collection should be as unobtrusive and as naturalistic as possible to minimize the effects of researchers and the research process on the people studied. Manipulation of variables by the researcher is minimized, although researcher effects are never eradicated, and therefore reflexivity is a necessary part of the research process (Hammersley and Atkinson 1983). Since ethnography is "an inquiry process guided by a point of view," rather than "a reporting process guided by a standard technique or set of techniques" (Erickson 1973 p.

10), methodological flexibility and imagination are imperative to be able to construct research instruments or adapt pre-existing ones to unforeseen circumstances in order to increase validity of results. All the above features allow ethnographers access to a much deeper understanding of social phenomena.

The cyclical nature of the ethnographic research process (Spradley 1980) allows for methodological flexibility and distinguishes ethnography from other types of research. In contrast to a positivistic, linear process of research in which the researcher does not alter the original research design during data collection, the cyclical process of ethnographic research assumes that the ethnographer is like an explorer who has an original plan but does not have full knowledge of the field and is therefore prepared to make modifications based on unanticipated discoveries. The ethnographer begins with an original research design, but initial data is collected and analyzed in order to reframe questions, to discover further investigative possibilities, and to revise the original plans if necessary. The ethnographer then returns to the field to collect more data. The process is repeated as often as necessary to create a valid, coherent account. Therefore, during fieldwork there is a continual dialogue between the question and the observed data, and theory may evolve out of this dialogical process.

The role of theory may enter at several points depending on the nature of the study, ranging from exploratory (beginning stages)—defining problems, clarifying concepts, and discovering theories to confirmatory (later stages)—having refined research instruments and clarified concepts to verify hypotheses and theoretical positions. One of the strongest contributions ethnography can make is toward the development of theory.

3. Types of Educational Ethnography

Educational ethnographers use ethnographic research methodology to study the processes of education and schooling (Wilcox 1982). Depending on the criteria for categorizing "ethnographies," various topologies have been generated (see Table 1).

3.1 Explanation of Table 1

The general paradigms of ethnography in anthropology are described by Sanday (1979): holistic includes examination of language, ideas, beliefs, behavior, and artifacts; semiotic focuses on language and ideas; and behaviorist focuses on behavior.

Three orientations in educational ethnography may be discerned based on different levels of analysis and different emphases in their definition of culture: holistic ethnography (also referred to as traditional, "old" ethnography or macroethnography), ethnoscience (also known as "new" ethnography or

Table 1
Types of typologies of educational ethnography[a]

General paradigms of ethnography in anthropology (Sanday 1979)	holistic	semiotic (language)	behaviorist
Orientations in educational ethnography	holistic macroethnography "old" ethnography multi-level (mixed)	ethnoscience cognitive anth. "new" ethnography	ethnog. of communication microethnography
Scope of theory (Hymes 1980)	comprehensive	topic-oriented	hypothesis-oriented
Goals of ethnography	basic research	applied action	basic and comparative
Unit of population or unit of analysis	—culture —community —institution —annual or life cycle	—classroom —neighborhood —family	—individual —selected events, times

a There is no relationship between columns of the different types of typologies, and no significance in ordering of the columns. Different columns just reveal different categories that have been discussed, and the "goals of ethnography" is the only typology with four categories. Units of population could be divided into more categories, but the three columns provide an idea of the range possible and is in no way an exhaustive listing.

cognitive anthropology), and ethnography of communication (microethnography). Holistic ethnographies depict the overall setting or group as a whole, while ethnographies of communication and ethnoscience focus on much smaller units, such as words, individuals, or scenes. Erickson and Mohatt (1982) described this type of ethnography of communication as microethnography, a focused ethnography: that is to say, one that focuses on repeated viewing and detailed analysis of audiovisual records of human interaction in key scenes, accompanied by participant observation of the overall context into which the scenes fit. The multilevel approach proposed by Ogbu (1981) is holistic in nature but includes a mixture of microethnographic techniques along with investigation into the wider societal and institutional context in order to gain greater understanding of complex problems, such as explaining the differential performance of various minority groups. These areas are discussed more fully in Sect. 3.2.

Hymes (1980) classifies ethnography according to scope of theory: comprehensive ethnography (Warren 1967) describes a total way of life of a community; topic-oriented ethnography (e.g., desegregation, cultural transmission, language) focuses on selected topics about target populations; and hypothesis-oriented ethnography (Wilcox 1982) begins with explicitly formulated hypotheses derived from previous research.

Four classifications of ethnography may also be distinguished according to differing goals for ethnographic research: basic research, applied research, action research, and basic and comparative research. Initially, in response to the prevalent cultural deprivation model of the 1960s, ethnography was employed as systematic, basic (descriptive) research into various cultural groups to show that cultural differences and not "deprivation" accounted for less access to learning opportunities for poor and minority children. During the next stage—the early 1970s—case studies thrived in an effort to explain that culture and language discontinuities could be identified as the source of problems in school performance (McDermott 1974, Rist 1970, Rosenfeld 1971). By the early 1970s, two types of research had branched off from the original basic research. One proceeded from basic ethnography toward changing school practices. Ethnography was thus utilized more and more as applied and action research to discover concrete ways to address the cultural discontinuities in practice in order to improve minority student performance (Au and Jordan 1981). In fact, since the 1970s, ethnography has become increasingly popular in applied research, for example, in educational evaluation (Fetterman 1984) and for policy analysis (Goetz and LeCompte 1984). Some researchers (Moll and Dias 1987) prefer action ethnography in which researchers actively engage in school intervention and change as part of the research act.

The second type of research developed in recognition of the variability in school performance among different minority groups. This type is basic research designed to explain the variability by also studying minorities who are relatively successful in spite of culture or language differences. It is comparative research less concerned with direct problem solving or with changing specific school practices. Though the long-range goal may be application to policy and practice, the primary concern is in-depth understanding and explanation of social phenomena. Single classroom research and microethnographies dominated research during this period, which prompted Ogbu's call (1981) for a multilevel approach to relate the microethnographic discoveries to social and institutional structures in the wider societal context.

51

3.2 Examples of Types of Educational Ethnographies

Diverse research traditions exist within each orientation, but major differences between holistic ethnography, ethnoscience, and the ethnography of communication will be clarified through examples in this section. The description of ethnography in Sect. 2 is the more traditional definition and corresponds to the holistic ethnography orientation. It defines culture as consisting of cognition (ideas, beliefs, values, etc.), behavior, and artifacts, and studies all three aspects of culture. Holistic ethnographers aim for understanding the culture of a group or institution from the insiders' points of view and for describing culture as an integrated whole. This approach is useful for understanding a group's way of life in general or a particular aspect of the culture, such as the school system, in relation to the larger society.

Some holistic ethnographers have studied education as one component of their larger studies of a society as a whole. Hostetler and Huntington (1971) focused on the indigenous processes of socialization and formal schooling in Amish culture. They illustrated the cultural context of learning—goals, institutions, practices, and pupil achievement—in relation to the whole of Amish society. Others have focused primarily on schooling. Wolcott (1973) used the holistic approach to study the daily and annual cycles in the life of one elementary school principal and the school in its community setting. Other holistic ethnographers examine the structural relationships between the educational system and other institutions within a given society. Singleton (1967) studied one public (state) school and its relationship both with other organizations and groups operating in the broader framework of a small Japanese community and with the nation as a whole.

The ethnoscience orientation is also called "new" ethnography because it departs from the traditional, holistic ethnography by defining culture primarily as people's cognition. Its basic assumptions are that the content of cultural data consists of rules, codes, and an ideational ordering of society that is organized into different domains of cultural knowledge. Experiences are encoded in lexemes or words; therefore, language is the main source of cultural data, and techniques of language study can be applied to the study of ideational culture or cognition. Consequently, less emphasis is given to participant observation and more emphasis is placed on collection of vocabularies about particular events and on classification schemes. Few educational ethnographies fit into this category compared with the other two paradigms.

Ethnography of communication is an outgrowth of the tendency among anthropologists to "break apart portions of the field of ethnography, to develop new terms, and to apply these to the study of specific aspects of culture" (Heath 1982 p. 42). The emphasis has been on language and language use and to a lesser extent on nonverbal communication. Its methodological and theoretical bases developed from interdisciplinary efforts—anthropology, sociology (particularly ethnomethodology), sociolinguistics, and studies of nonverbal communication—to describe the patterns and processes of face-to-face interaction within and between cultural groups and relate these patterns and processes to larger or "macro" issues of cultural and social processes.

Ethnographers of communication conduct detailed analyses of interpersonal interactions: for example, how students and teachers allocate and negotiate turn-taking (Philips 1972), signal changes in activity (Schultz and Florio 1979), or develop trusting relations (McDermott 1974). Microethnography has enhanced the understanding of mainstream and minority children by examining classroom interactions of specific cultural groups, such as Odawa Indian children, Athabaskan Indians, African Americans, and Mexican Americans. Analysis on the micro level provides an approach and method for understanding differing patterns of social interaction and for analyzing the consequences of these patterns for learning outcomes. For example, Au and Jordan (1981) documented improvements in Hawaiian students' educational performance that resulted from changing classroom social interaction patterns so that they more closely paralleled those the children had learned at home. Heath (1983) showed that questioning patterns in classrooms were more congruent for Whites and less compatible for Blacks, which encouraged Whites to answer more questions. Some researchers study settings other than the classroom, such as educational testing situations (Mehan 1978) and counseling sessions (Erickson and Schultz 1982).

One trend of the 1980s is the development of critical ethnography that integrates theoretical interpretation with practice. Followers of this research area insist that ethnography is not just a methodology but it must be connected to practice and social change. Their work attempts to make a bridge between symbolic interactionist work with its microsociological bias and neo-Marxist work with its macrosociological bias, and thus counterbalance the limitations of each. Since its development is still in its fledgling stage and a variety of examples exist, there is, as yet, no clear definition. However, Gerin-Lajoie (1986) lists three criteria for critical ethnography: that participants' experiences are connected with the larger social structure; that ethnographic accounts help the individuals studied make the connections for themselves; and that critical ethnographers study their own practices.

Regardless of the variety of ways that ethnographic techniques are incorporated into other disciplines and into diverse types of studies in order to serve a variety of purposes, much debate continues regarding the strengths and weaknesses of ethnography.

4. Strengths and Weaknesses

Throughout the debate regarding the utility of ethnography, researchers have raised the issues of reliability (replication of results, i.e., securing the same results with repeated research), internal and external validity (accuracy, credibility), degree of bias (objectivity vs. subjectivity), and individual cases versus generalizability. General questions of methodological rigor are as applicable to ethnography as to any research methodology. They include issues of problem and conceptual definition, research design, operationalization of terms, selecting a representative population, selecting the most appropriate methodology, verification and corroboration of data, and subsequent data analysis, interpretation, and write-up. Simply put, potential methodological problems can be overcome by disciplined inquiry on the part of the ethnographer.

In response to the above criticisms, educational ethnographers have delineated systematic rules of evidence that are necessary to address research design, data reduction, and data analysis issues (Goetz and LeCompte 1984, Spradley 1980). Reliability and validity issues may be addressed in numerous ways and several articles document these methods (Freilich 1970, Goetz and LeCompte 1984, Spindler 1982, Wolcott 1975). Basically, Goetz and LeCompte (1984) advocate using a multimodality approach, that is to say, examining the same issues or problems using multiple modes of information gathering to crosscheck findings. For example, repeated observations of the same phenomenon, repeated interviews of the same informant, interviews with several informants about the same event, and gathering multiple forms of evidence (triangulation) regarding the same phenomenon all help to ensure reliability. In this respect, ethnography has a major advantage over other research methodologies. Living among the people for an extended period, the ethnographer observes the phenomena in its closest state to reality, can detect various unanticipated yet significant features of the setting, and has repeated access to participants under study.

Generalizability is made possible because knowledge is in-depth and contextualized. The comprehensive and detailed ethnographic descriptions allow readers to make reasonable comparisons with other known situations and to make well-informed decisions about generalizability. As Spindler (1982 p. 8) states: " . . . it is better to have in-depth, accurate knowledge of one setting than superficial and possibly skewed or misleading information about isolated relationships in many settings." He believes that research designs which fail to take context and meaning into adequate consideration will produce results that are far less generalizable than those from a good ethnographic study. Finally, ethnography can refine research instruments toward quantitative methods that allow for statistical analysis and generalizability at that level.

The major contributions of ethnography to the study of education have been in revealing misconceptions regarding culture and differing ethnic and minority populations. Previous educational literature (primarily based on quantitative methodologies) often studied isolated variables, and divorced educational processes from their larger social and cultural contexts. Experimental or positivistic research designs may suffer from incomplete explanation, misinterpretation of meaning for those involved, or simply from defining concepts and terms inaccurately and without relevance. Lack of recognition of different goals and different definitions of values, processes, and means for education held by different participants may profoundly affect the definition of the research problem or operationalization of terms and concepts, and prejudice the validity of research results. Educational problems were often considered to be located in the individuals or populations themselves, rather than in the social organization of the school, classroom, or other societal structures. The complexity of interactions, processes, and interrelatedness of discrete variables and parts to wholes was left unappreciated in nonethnographic work.

Strengths of ethnography are diversity, reality, and complexity. Ethnographies provide a voluminous, descriptive data base and a means to comprehend diversity and subtlety in dimensions of meaning for various participants. Vivid descriptions of actual settings enhance reader identification. Its flexibility to entertain new questions, issues, and research design problems during data collection increases validity by verifying contextual influences and by soliciting participant perspectives. As a result, some advantages of ethnography are the rich contextualization of phenomena under study, more complete explanation of concepts and phenomena, and an appreciation of process phenomena and interaction of parts with wholes.

Researchers must continually reflect on the research process and how they are affecting the acquisition of information by being a research instrument themselves. Reflection must include delineating the research process, explicating decision-making junctures, and searching for discrepant cases and data which do not support claims along with the varied data sources that do support claims. Above all, good ethnographies must explain their logic of justification and be faithful to their subject matter (Erickson 1973).

5. Future Trends

As with all research methodologies, continuous assessment of methodological rigor and adherence to standards for quality research, for research design, and for data collection, data reduction, and data analysis will improve ethnographic research. Clarifying various research traditions, historical developments, perspectives, levels of analysis, and theoretical frameworks will also improve the conduct of ethnographic research. As the methodologies and diversity of problems under study evolve and proliferate, the typologies will no doubt change and become more refined. Especially with increased understanding and contributions from scholars beyond the United States and European borders, our conceptions of qualitative research and of educational ethnographies in particular will be broadened and enriched. Hopefully the future will bring an intellectually stimulating dialogue between educational ethnographers from diverse international and cultural backgrounds.

References

Au K H, Jordan C 1981 Teaching reading to Hawaiian children: Finding a culturally appropriate solution. In: Trueba H T, Guthrie G P, Au K H (eds.) 1981 *Culture and the Bilingual Classroom*. Newbury House, Rowley, Massachusetts

Bernard R 1988 *Research Methods in Cultural Anthropology*. Sage, Newbury Park, California

Berreman G D 1968 Ethnography: Method and product. In: Clifton J (ed.) 1988 *Introduction to Cultural Anthropology: Essays in the Scope of the Science of Man*. Houghton Mifflin, New York

Delamont S, Atkinson P 1980 The two traditions in educational ethnography: Sociology and anthropology compared. *British Journal of Sociology of Education* 1(2): 139–52

Erickson F 1973 What makes school ethnography ethnographic? *Anthropology and Education Newsletter* 4(2): 10–19

Erickson F, Mohatt G 1982 Cultural organization of participation structures in two classrooms of Indian students. In: Spindler G D (ed.) 1982 *Doing the Ethnography of Schooling: Educational Anthropology in Action*. Holt, Rinehart and Winston, New York

Erickson F D, Shultz J 1982 *The Counselor as a Gatekeeper: Social Interaction in Interviews*. Academic Press, New York.

Fetterman D M (ed.) 1984 *Ethnography in Educational Evaluation*. Sage, Beverly Hills, California

Freilich M (ed.) 1970 *Marginal Natives: Anthropologists at Work*. Harper and Row, New York

Gerin-Lajoie D 1986 Beyond traditional ethnography. *Rev. Educ.* 13(3–4): 223–26

Goetz J P, LeCompte M D 1984 *Ethnography and Qualitative Design in Educational Research*. Academic Press, Orlando, Florida

Green J, Wallat C 1983 *Ethnography and Language in Educational Settings*. Abtex, Norwood, New Jersey

Hammersley M, Atkinson P 1983 *Ethnography: Principles in Practice*. Tavistock Publications, London

Heath S B 1982 Ethnography in education: Defining the essentials. In: Gilmore P, Glathorn A (eds.) 1982 *Children In and Out of School: Ethnography and Education*. Center for Applied Linguistics, Arlington, Virginia

Heath S B 1983 *Ways With Words: Language, Life and Work in Communities and Classrooms*. Cambridge University Press, Cambridge

Henry J 1963 Attitude organization in elementary school classrooms. In: Spindler G D (ed.) 1963

Hostetler J A, Hungtington G E 1971 *Children in Amish Society: Socialization and Community Education*. Holt, Rinehart and Winston, New York

Hymes D 1980 Ethnographic monitoring. In: Hymes D (ed.) 1980 *Language in Education: Ethnolinguistic Essays*. Center for Applied Linguistics, Washington, DC

Jacob E 1988 Clarifying qualitative research: A focus on traditions. *Educ. Researcher* 17(1): 16–24

Malinowski B 1922 *Argonauts of the Western Pacific*. George Routledge, London

McDermott R P 1974 Achieving school failure: An anthropological approach to illiterary and social stratification. In: Spindler G D (ed.) 1974 *Education and Cultural Process: Toward an Anthropology of Education*. Holt, Rinehart and Winston, New York

Mead M 1930 *Growing up in New Guinea: A Comparative Study of Primitive Education*. Morrow, New York

Mehan H 1978 Structuring school structure. *Harv. Educ. Rev.* 48(1): 32–64

Middleton J (ed.) 1970 *From Child to Adult: Studies in the Anthropology of Education*. The Natural History Press, New York

Moll L, Dias S 1987 Change as the goal of educational research. *Anthropol. Educ. Q.* 18(4): 300–11

Narroll R, Cohen R (eds.) 1970 *A Handbook of Method in Cultural Anthropology*. Natural History Press, New York

Ogbu J 1981 School ethnography: A multilevel approach. *Anthropol. Educ. Q.* 12(1): 1–29 *Revue Française de Pedagogie* 1987 Ethnographic approaches in the sociology of education: Community, school, and classroom. Nos. 78, 80

Philips S U 1972 Participant structures and communicative competence: Warm Springs children in community and classroom. In: Cazden C B, John V P, Hymes D (eds.) 1972 *Functions of Language in the Classroom*. Teachers College Press, New York

Rist R C 1970 Student social class and teacher expectations: The self-fulfilling prophecy in ghetto education. *Harv. Educ. Rev.* 40(3): 411–51

Rosenfeld G 1971 *"Shut Those Thick Lips!": A Study of Slum School Failure*. Holt, Rinehart and Winston, New York

Sanday P R 1979 The ethnographic paradigm(s) In: Van Maanen J (ed.) 1979 *Qualitative Methodology*. Sage, Beverly Hills, California

Singleton J 1967 *Nichu: A Japanese School*. Holt, Rinehart and Winston, New York

Spindler G D 1982 General introduction. In: Spindler G D (ed.) 1982 *Doing the Ethnography of Schooling: Educational Anthropology in Action*. Holt, Rinehart and Winston, New York

Spradley J P 1972 The cultural experience In: Spradley J P, McCurdy D W (eds.) 1972 *The Cultural Experience: Ethnography in Complex Society*. SRA, Chicago, Illinois

Spradley J P 1980 *Participant Observation*. Holt, Rinehart and Winston, New York

Urry J 1984 A history of field methods. In: Ellen R F (ed.) 1984 *Ethnographic Research: A Guide to General Conduct*. Academic Press, London

Valentine C A 1968 *Culture and Poverty: Critique and Counter Proposals*. University of Chicago Press, Chicago, Illinois

Warren R L 1967 *Education in Rebhausen: A German Village*. Holt, Rinehart and Winston, New York

Wilcox K 1982 Ethnography as a methodology and its applications to the study of schooling: A review. In: Spindler G D (ed.) 1982 *Doing the Ethnography of Schooling: Educational Anthropology in Action.* Holt, Rinehart and Winston, New York

Williams T R 1972 *Introduction to Socialization: Human Culture Transmitted.* The C V Mosby Co., St Louis, Missouri

Wolcott H F 1973 *The Man in the Principal's Office: An Ethnography.* Holt, Rinehart and Winston, New York

Wolcott H F 1975 Criteria for an ethnographic approach to research in schools. *Human Organization* 34: 111–27

Woods P 1986 *Inside Schools: Ethnography in Educational Research.* Routledge and Kegan Paul, London

Further Reading

Davis J 1972 Teachers, kids, and conflict: Ethnography of a junior high school. In: Spradley J P, McCurdy D W (eds.) 1972 *The Cultural Experience: Ethnography in Complex Society.* Science Research Associates, Chicago, Illinois

Spindler G D 1963 *Education and Culture: Anthropological Approaches.* Holt, Rinehart and Winston, New York

Wax R H 1971 *Doing Fieldwork: Warnings and Advice.* University of Chicago Press, Chicago, Illinois

Wolcott H F 1971 Handle with care: Necessary precautions in the anthropology of schools. In: Wax M L, Diamond S, Gearing F O (eds.) 1971 *Anthropological Perspectives in Education.* Basic Books, New York

Biographical Research Methods

N. K. Denzin

The biographical method, which is considered in this entry, is defined as the studied use and collection of life documents, or documents of life that describe turning-point moments in individuals' lives. These documents include autobiographies, biographies, diaries, letters, obituaries, life histories, life stories, personal experience stories, oral histories, and personal histories. The subject matter of the biographical method is the life experiences of a person, and biographical methods provide the very foundations for the study of educational processes. When written in the first person it is called "autobiography," life story, or life history. When written by another person it is called a "biography." Sociologist John M Johnson has coined the term "burography" to describe an autobiography that analyzes the intersections of biography, personal experience, and bureaucratic, or organizational structures. An "auto-ethnography" is a partial first-person text, based on the cultural study of the person's own group. There are many biographical methods, or many ways of writing about a life. Each form presents different textual problems and leaves the reader with different messages and understandings. A life or a biography is only ever given in the words that are written about it.

1. Historical Development

The biographical, life history, case study, case history, or ethnographic method has been a part of sociology's history since the 1920s and 1930s when University of Chicago sociologists, under the influence of Robert E Park and others were trained in the qualitative, interpretative, interactionist approach to human group life.

Sociologists in succeeding generations turned away from the method. They gave their attention to problems of measurement, validity, reliability, responses to attitude questionnaires, survey methodologies, laboratory experiments, theory development, and conceptual indicators. Many researchers combined these interests and problems with the use of the life history, biographical method. The result often produced a trivialization, and distortion of the original intents of the method.

In the 1980s and 1990s sociologists and scholars in other disciplines have evidenced a renewed interest in the biographical method, coupled with a resurgence of interest in interpretative approaches to the study of culture, biography, and human group life. In 1978 a "Biography and Society Group" formed within the International Sociological Association (ISA) and met in Uppsala, Sweden. In 1986 that Group became a research committee within the ISA (see *Current Sociology* 1995). The journal *Oral History*, of the Oral History Society, also regularly publishes life history, biographical materials. Within sociology and anthropology *Qualitative Inquiry, Qualitative Sociology*, The *Journal of Contemporary Ethnography*, *Dialectical Anthropology*, and *Current Anthropology* frequently publish biographically related articles, as does *Signs*. The autobiography has become a topic of renewed interest in literary criticism. Feminists and postcolonial theorists (Trinh 1989, 1991) have led the way in this discussion (Personal Narratives Group 1989). Moreover, a number of sociological monographs using the method have appeared. In short, the method has returned to the human disciplines.

Central to the biographical–interpretative view has

been the argument that societies, cultures, and the expressions of human experience can be read as social texts; that is, as structures of representation that require symbolic statement. These texts, whether oral or written, have taken on a problematic status in the interpretative project. Questions concerning how texts are authored, read, and interpreted have emerged. How authors, lives, societies, and cultures get inside interpretative texts are now hotly debated topics.

In 1959 Mills in *The Sociological Imagination* argued that the sociological imagination "enables us to grasp history and biography and the relations between the two within society." He then suggested that "No social study that does not come back to the problems of biography, of history and of their intersections within a society has completed its intellectual journey" (Mills 1959).

A basic question drives the interpretative project in the human disciplines: how do men and women live and give meaning to their lives, and capture these meanings in written, narrative, and oral forms? As Karl Marx observed, men and women "make their own history, but not . . . under conditions they have chosen for themselves; rather on terms immediately existing, given and handed down to them." How are these lives, their histories and their meanings to be studied? Who are these people who make their own history? What does history mean to them? How do sociologists, anthropologists, historians, and literary critics read, write, and make sense of these lives?

2. The Subject and the Biographical Method

From its birth, modern, qualitative, interpretative sociology, which links with Max Weber's mediations on *verstehen* (understanding) and method, has been haunted by a "metaphysics of presence" which asserts that real, concrete subjects live lives with meaning and these meanings have a concrete presence in the lives of these people. This belief in a real subject, who is present in the world, has led sociologists to continue to search for a method that would allow them to uncover how these subjects give subjective meaning to their life experiences. This method would rely upon the subjective, verbal, and written expressions of meaning given by the individuals being studied; these expressions being windows into the inner life of the person. Since Wilhelm Dilthey (1833–1911) this search has led to a perennial focus in the human sciences on the autobiographical approach and its interpretative biographical variants, including hermeneutics (see *Hermeneutics*).

Jacques Derrida has contributed to the understanding that there is no clear window into the inner life of a person, for any window is always filtered through the glaze of language, signs, and the process of signification. Moreover, language, in both its written and spoken forms, is always inherently unstable, in flux, and made up of the traces of other signs and symbolic statements. Hence there can never be a clear, unambiguous statement of anything, including an intention or a meaning. The researcher's task is to reconcile this concern with the metaphysics of presence, and its representations, with a commitment to the position that interpretative sociologists and anthropologists study real people who have real lived experiences in the social world.

3. A Clarification of Terms

A family of terms combine to shape the biographical method. The terms are: method, life, self, experience, epiphany, case, autobiography, ethnography, autoethnography, biography, ethnography, story, discourse, narrative, narrator, fiction, history, personal history, oral history, case history, case study, writing presence, difference, life history, life story, self-story, and personal experience story. Table 1 summarizes these concepts and terms which have historically defined the biographical method.

The above terms require discussion. The word "method" will be understood to refer to a way of knowing about the world. A way of knowing may proceed from subjective or objective grounds. Subjective knowing involves drawing on personal experience, or the personal experiences of others, in an effort to form an understanding and interpretation of a particular phenomenon. Objective knowing assumes that an individual can stand outside an experience and understand it, independent of the persons experiencing the phenomenon in question. Intersubjective knowing rests on shared experiences and the knowledge gained from having participated in a common experience with another person. The biographical method rests on subjective and intersubjectively gained knowledge and understandings of the life experiences of individuals, including a person's own life. Such understandings rest on an interpretative process that leads a person to enter into the emotional life of another. "Interpretation"—the act of interpreting and making sense out of something—creates the conditions for "understanding," which involves being able to grasp the meanings of an interpreted experience for another individual. Understanding is an intersubjective, emotional process. Its goal is to build shareable understandings of the life experiences of another. This is also called creating verisimilitudes or "truth-like" intersubjectively shareable emotional feelings and cognitive understandings.

3.1 Lifes, Persons, Selves, Experiences

All biographical studies presume a life that has been lived, or a life that can be studied, constructed, reconstructed, and written about. In the present context a "life" refers to two phenomena: (a) lived experiences, or conscious existence, and person. A person is a self-conscious being, as well as a named, cultural object or, (b) cultural creation. The consciousness of the person is simultaneously directed to "an inner world of thought and experience and to an outer world of events and experience." These two worlds, the inner and the outer, are termed the "phenomenological stream of consciousness" and the "interactional stream of experience." The phenomenological stream describes the person caught up in thoughts and the flow of inner experience. The outer, interactional stream locates the person in the world of others. These two streams are opposite sides of the same process, or chiasma, for there can be no firm dividing line between inner and

Table 1
Terms/forms and varieties of the biographical method[a]

Term / method	Key features	Forms/variations
1 Method	A way of knowing	subjective/objective
2 Life	Period of existence; lived experiences	Partial/complete/edited public/private
3 Self	Ideas, images and thoughts of self	Self-stories, autobiographies
4 Experience	Confronting and passing through events	Problematic, routine, ritual
5 Epiphany	Moment of revelation in a life	Major, minor, relived, illuminative
6 Autobiography	Personal history of one's life	Complete, edited, topical
7 Ethnography	Written account of a culture, or group	Realist, interpretative, descriptive
8 Autoethnography	Account of one's life as an ethnographer	Complete, edited, partial
9 Biography	History of a life	Autobiography
10 Story	A fiction, narrative	First, third person
11 Fiction	An account, something made up, fashioned	Story (life, self)
12 History	Account of how something happened	Personal, oral, case
13 Discourse	Telling a story, talk about a text a text	First, third person
14 Narrator	Teller of a story	First, third person
15 Narrative	A story, having a plot and existence separate from life of teller	Fiction, epic,
16 Writing	Inscribing, creating a written text	Logocentric, deconstructive
17 *Différance*	Every word carries traces of another word	Writing, speech
18 Personal history	Reconstruction of life based on interviews and conversations	Life history, life story
20 Oral history	Personal recollections of events, their causes, and effects	Work, ethnic, religious personal, musical, etc.
21 Case history	History of an event or social process, not of a person	Single, multiple, medical, legal
22 Life history	Account of a life based on interviews and conversations	Personal, edited, topical, complete
23 Life story	A person's story of his or her life, or a part thereof	Edited, complete, topical, fictional
24 Self-story [mystory]	Story of self in relation to an event	Personal experience, fictional, true
25 Personal experience story	Stories about personal experience	Single, multiple episode, private or communal folklore
26 Case study	Analysis and record of single case	Single, multiple

[a] Adapted from Denzin (1989)

outer experience. The biographical method recognizes this facticity about human existence, for its hallmark is the joining and recording of these two structures of experience in a personal document.

"Epiphanies" are interactional moments and experiences that leave marks on people's lives. In them personal character is manifested. They are often moments of crisis. They alter the fundamental meaning structures in a person's life. Their effects may be positive or negative. They are like the historian Victor Turner's "liminal phase of experience." In the liminal, or threshold moment of experience, the person is in a "non-man's-land betwixt and between . . . the past and the . . . future". These are existential acts. Some are ritualized, as in status passages; others are even routinized, as when a person daily batters and beats his or her spouse. Still others are totally emergent and unstructured, and the person enters them with few—if any—prior understandings of what is going to happen. The meanings of these experiences are always given retrospectively, as they are relived and re-experienced in the stories persons tell about what has happened to them.

There are four forms of the epiphany: (a) the major event which touches every fabric of a person's life; (b) the cumulative or representative event which signifies eruptions or reactions to experiences that have been going on for a long period of time; (c) the minor epiphany which symbolically represents a major, problematic moment in a relationship, or a person's life; and (d) those episodes whose meanings are given in the reliving of the experience. These are called, respectively, the "major epiphany," the "cumulative epiphany," the "illuminative or minor epiphany," and the "relived epiphany."

A "case," as indicated in Table 1, describes an instance of a phenomenon. A case may be even a process or a person. Often a case overlaps with a person; for example, the number of AIDS cases in a local community. "History" is an account of an event and involves determining how a particular event, process, or set of experiences occurred. A "case history" refers to the history of an event or a process; for example, the history of AIDS as an epidemic in the United States. A "case study" is the analysis of a single case, or of multiple instances of the same process, as it is embodied in the life experiences of a community, a group, or a person (see *Case Study Methods*).

An "autobiography," as noted earlier, is a first-person account (which actually takes the third-person form) of a set of life experiences. A "biography" is an account of a life, written by a third party. The poet John Dryden (1631–1700) defined the word biography in 1683 as "the history of particular men's lives." A biographer, then, is a historian of selves and lives. Autobiographies and biographies are structured by a set of literary, sociological, and interpretative conventions. They are formalized expressions of experience. An "autoethnography" is an ethnographic statement which writes the ethnographer into the text in an autobiographical manner. This is an important variant in the traditional ethnographic account, which positions the writer as an objective outsider in the texts that are written about the culture, group, or person in question. A fully grounded biographical study would be autoethnographic, and contain elements of the writer's own biography and personal history. Such an autoethnography would be descriptive and interpretative (see Ellis 1995, 1996).

Several critical points concerning the autobiographical and biographical method may be drawn from these extended excerpts. Autobiographies and biographies are conventionalized, narrative expressions of life experiences. These conventions, which structure how lives are told and written about, involve the following problematic presuppositions, and assumptions that are taken for granted: (a) the existence of others; (b) the influence and importance of gender and class; (c) family beginnings; (d) starting points; (e) known, and knowing authors and observers; (f) objective life markers; (g) real persons with real lives; (h) turning point experiences, and (i) truthful statements distinguished from fictions.

These conventions serve to define the biographical method as a distinct approach to the study of human experience. They are the methods by which the "real" appearances of "real" people are created. They are Western literary conventions and have been present since the invention of the biographical form. Some are more central than others, although they all appear to be universal, while they change and take different form, depending on the writer, the place of writing, and the historical moment. They shape how lives are told. In so doing they create the subject matter of the biographical approach. They were each present in the biographical and autobiographical excerpts just presented. Each is treated in turn below.

Ethnographies, biographies, and autobiographies rest on "stories" which are fictional, narrative accounts of how something happened. Stories are fictions. A "fiction" is something made, or fashioned, out of real and imagined events. History, in this sense, is fiction. A story has a beginning, a middle, and an end. Stories take the form of texts. They can be transcribed, written down, and studied. They are "narratives" with a plot and a story line that exists independently of the life of the storyteller, or "narrator." Every narrative contains a reason, or set of justifications for its telling. Narrators report stories as narratives. A story is told in and through "discourse," or talk, just as there can be discourse about the text of a story. A text can be part of a larger body of discourse

A "life history" or "personal history" is a written account of a person's life based on spoken conversations and interviews. In its expanded form the life history may pertain to the collective life of a group, organization, or community. An "oral history" focuses chiefly on events, processes, causes, and effects, rather than on individuals whose recollections furnish oral history with its raw data. Since oral histories are typically obtained through spoken conversations and interviews, they often furnish the materials for life histories, and case histories. Oral histories should not be confused, however, with personal histories, for the latter attempt to reconstruct lives based on interviews and conversations. Life histories and personal histories may be topical, focusing on only one portion of a life, or complete, attempting to tell the full details of a life as it is recollected (see *Oral History*).

"Life Stories" examine a life, or a segment of a life, as reported by the individual in question. A life story is a person's story of his or her life, or of what he or she thinks is a significant part of that life. It is therefore a personal narrative, a story of personal experience. A life story may be written or published as an autobiography. Its narrative, story-telling form gives it the flavor of fiction, or of fictional accounts of what happened in a person's life.

The life story turns the subject into an author; an author, or authoress being one who brings a story into existence. The subject-as-author is given an authority over the life that is written about. After all it is their life. This means the author has an authority in the text that is given by the very conventions that structure the writing or telling of the story in the first place. But where in the text of the story is the author? Clearly he or she is everywhere and nowhere. For an author is always present in personal name, and signified in the words that he or she uses. But the author is not in those words; they are only signs of the author, the self, and the life in question. They are inscriptions on and of the self or life that is being told about. The author is in the text only through the words and the conventions he or she uses. The languages of biography structure how biographies are written. There is no fixed, ever-present author.

"Self-stories" are told by a person in the context of a specific set of experiences. A self-story positions the self of the teller centrally in the narrative that is given. It is literally a story of and about the self in relation to an experience. The self-story is made up as it is told. It does not exist as a story independent of its telling; although after it has been told, it can take on the status of a story that can be retold. Its narrative form typically follows the linear format; that is, beginning, middle, end. These tellings build on the assumption that each person is a storyteller of self-experiences. These oral histories of self are often mandated by social groups. When a self-story joins with an author's account of popular culture and scholarly discourse on the individual's life experiences it becomes a "mystory"; that is, my story about how my life has been represented by others. ("Mystory" is Gregory Ulmer's term.)

"Personal experience narratives" are stories people tell about their personal experience. They often draw upon the public, oral story-telling tradition of a group. These stories are based on personal experience. They have the narrative structure of a story (i.e., a beginning, middle, and end). They describe a set of events that exist independently of the telling. The experiences that are described draw their meaning from the common understandings that exist in a group, although they do express the "private" folklore, or meanings of the teller. When told, they create an emotional bond between listener and teller. They express a part of the "inner life" of the storyteller.

Personal experience narratives differ from self-stories in several ways. These narratives do not necessarily position the self of the teller in the center of the story, as self-stories do. Their focus is on shareable experience. Personal experience narratives are more likely to be based on anecdotal, everyday, commonplace experiences, while self-stories involve pivotal, often critical life experiences. Self-stories need not be coherent, linear accounts. They need not be entertaining, or recreate cherished values and memories of a group, while personal experience narratives do. Self-stories are often mandated by a group; personal experience narratives are not. Self-stories are often told to groups, while personal experience narratives may only be told to another individual. These two biographical forms are alike, however, in that they both rest on personal experiences.

4. Representing Lives

Lives and their experiences are represented in stories. They are like pictures that have been painted over, and when paint is scraped off an old picture something new becomes visible. What is new is what was previously covered up. A life and the stories about it have the qualities of pentimento: something painted out of a picture which later becomes visible again. Something new is always coming into sight, displacing what was previously certain and seen. There is no truth in the painting of a life, only multiple images and traces of what has been, what could have been, and what now is.

These stories move outward from the selves of the person and inward to the groups that give them meaning and structure. Persons are arbitrators of their own presence in the world, and they should have the last word on this problem. Texts must always return to and reflect the words that persons speak as they attempt to give meaning and shape to the lives they lead. The materials of the biographical method resolve, in the final analysis, into the stories that persons tell one another.

These stories are learned and told in cultural groups. The stories that members of groups pass on to one another are reflective of understandings and practices that are at work in the larger system of cultural understandings that are acted upon by group members. These understandings contain conceptions of persons, lives, meaningful and subjective experience, and notions of how persons and their experiences are to be represented. There are only stories to be told, and listened to. These stories resolve the dilemmas surrounding the metaphysics of presence that haunts the individual as he or she attempts to give shape to this thing called a life and a biography. A person becomes the stories he or she tells. The elusive nature of these stories calls the person back to the understanding that this business of a life story is just that, a story that can never be completed.

Stories then, like the lives they relate, are always open ended, inconclusive, and ambiguous, subject to multiple interpretations. Some are big, others are little. Some take on heroic, folktale proportions in the cultural lives of groups members; others are tragic; and all too few are comic. Some break fast and run to rapid conclusions. Most slowly unwind and twist back on themselves as persons seek to find meaning for themselves in the experiences they call their own. Some are told for the person by others who are called experts, be these journalists, or professional biographers. Some the person keeps to herself or himself and tells to no one else. Many individuals are at a loss as to what story to tell, feeling that they have nothing worthwhile to talk about. Within this group there are persons who have no voice, and no one to whom to tell their story.

This means that biographical work must always be interventionist, seeking to give voice to those who may otherwise not be allowed to tell their story, or who are denied a voice to speak. This is what *écriture feminine* attempts; a radical form of feminist writing which "transgresses structures of . . . domination—a kind of writing which reproduces the struggle for voice of those on the wrong side of the power relationship." This stance disrupts the classic oedipal logic of the life-history method which situates subjectivity and self-development in the patriarchal system of marriage, kinship, and sexuality (Clough 1994). This logic underwrites the scientistic, positivistic use of life histories, and supports institutionalized sociological discourse on human subjects as individuals who can tell true stories about their lives. *Écriture feminine* and certain versions of "Queer theory" (Clough 1994), moving from a deconstructive stance, make no attempt at the production of biographical narratives which fill out the sociologist's version of what a life and its stories should look like. It accepts sociology as fictive writing, and biographical work as the search for partial, not full identities.

Students of the method must begin to assemble a body of work that is grounded in the workings of these various cultural groups. This is the challenge and the promise of this project. In order to speak to the Fourth Epoch, so called by Mills as the "postmodern period," it is necessary to begin to listen to the workings of these groups that make up our time. It is necessary also to learn how to connect biographies and lived experiences, the epiphanies of lives, to the groups and social relationships that surround and shape persons.

5. Personal Writing

As we write about our lives, we bring the world of others into our texts. We create differences, oppositions, and presences which allow us to maintain the illusion that we have captured the "real" experiences of "real" people. In fact, we create the persons we write about, just as they create themselves when they engage in story-telling practices. As students of the biographical method we must become more sensitive to the writing strategies we use when we attempt to accomplish these ends. And, as readers, we can only have trust, or mistrust in the writers that we read, for there is no way to stuff a real-live person between the two covers of a text.

Biographical studies should attempt to articulate how each subject deals with the problems of coherence, illusion, consubstantiality, presence, deep, inner selves, others, gender, class, starting and ending points, epiphanies, fictions, truths, and final causes. These recurring, obdurate, culturally constructed dimensions of Western lives provide framing devices for the stories that are told about the lives that we study. They are, however, no more than artifices; contrivances that writers and tellers are differentially skilled at using. As writers we must not be trapped into thinking that they are any more than cultural practice.

As we learn to do this we must remember that our primary obligation is always to the people we study, not to our project, or to a larger discipline. The lives and stories that we hear and study are given to us under a promise. That promise being that we protect those who have shared with us. In return, this sharing will allow us to write life documents that speak to the human dignity, the suffering, the hopes, the dreams, the lives gained and the lives lost by the people we study. These documents will become testimonies to the ability of the human being to endure, to prevail, and to triumph over the structural forces that threaten, at any moment, to annihilate all of us. If we foster the illusion that we understand when we do not, or that we have found meaningful, coherent lives where none exist, then we engage in a cultural practice that is just as repressive as the most repressive of political regimes.

See also: Hermeneutics; Educational History in Biographies and Autobiographies; Legitimatory Research

References

Clough P T 1994 *Feminist Thought: Desire, Power and Academic Discourse.* Blackwell, Cambridge, Massachusetts
Current Sociology 1995 43(23): Special Issue: Biographical Research
Ellis C 1995 *Final Negotiations.* Temple University Press, Philadelphia, Pennsylvania
Ellis C 1996 Evocative authoethnography: Writing emotionally about our lives. In Lincoln Y S, Tierney W (eds.) 1996 *Representation and the Text: Reframing the Narrative Voice.* SUNY Press, Albany, New York

Mills C W 1959 *The Sociological Imagination.* Oxford University Press, New York

Personnal Narratives Group 1989 *Interpreting Women's Lives: Feminist Theory and Personal Narratives.* Indiana University Press, Bloomington, Indiana

Trinh T 1989 *Women, Native, Other: Writing Postcoloniality and Feminism.* Indiana University Press, Bloomington, Indiana

Trinh T 1991 *When the Moon Waxes Red: Representation, Gender and Cultural Politics.* Routledge, New York

Further Reading

Denzin N K 1987 *Interpretive Biography.* Sage, Newbury Park, California

Denzin N K 1989a *The Research Act:* A Theoretical Introduction to Sociological Methods, 3rd edn. Prentice-Hall, Englewood Cliffs, New Jersey

Denzin N K 1989b *Interpretive Interactionism.* Sage, Newbury Park, California

Feagin J R, Orum A M, Sjoberg G (eds.) 1991 *A Case for the Case Study.* University of North Carolina Press, Chapel Hill, North Carolina

Journal of Applied Behavioral Science 1989 vol. 25 (4) (issue devoted to Autobiography, Social Research, and the Organizational context)

Reinharz S, Davidson L 1992 *Feminist Methods in Social Research.* Oxford University Press, New York

Roman L G 1992 The political significance of other ways of narrating ethnography: A feminist materialist approach. In: LeCompte M D, Millroy W L, Preissle J (eds.) 1992 *Handbook of Qualitative Research in Education.* Academic Press, San Diego

Smith L M 1994 Biographical methods. In: Denzin N K, Lincoln Y S (eds.) 1994 *Handbook of Qualitative Research.* Sage, Newbury Park, California

Case Study Methods

A. Sturman

"Case study" is a generic term for the investigation of an individual, group, or phenomenon. While the techniques used in the investigation may be varied, and may include both qualitative and quantitative approaches, the distinguishing feature of case study is the belief that human systems develop a characteristic wholeness or integrity and are not simply a loose collection of traits. As a consequence of this belief, case study researchers hold that to understand a case, to explain why things happen as they do, and to generalize or predict from a single example requires an in–depth investigation of the interdependencies of parts and of the patterns that emerge.

Kaplan refers to methodology as a "generalization of technics and a concretization of philosophy" (see *Science Methods in Educational Research*). While the techniques relate to the specific strategies that are used in different types of case study, the philosophy is concerned with the place that case study has in educational inquiry, such as the extent to which it can be used to generalize, predict, or explain as opposed to being used to understand or simply to describe.

The following section deals with the philosophical dimension of case study and this is followed by a discussion of the technical dimension.

1. Case Study and the "Concretization of Philosophy"

Diesing (1972) places case study within the holist tradition of scientific inquiry. According to this tradition, the characteristics of a part are seen to be largely determined by the whole to which it belongs. The holist argues that to understand these parts requires an understanding of their interrelationships, and accounts of wholes need to capture and express this holistic quality.

This view is expressed in a different way by Salomon (1991) who has distinguished the analytical and systemic approaches to educational research. The analytic approach mainly assumes that discrete elements of complex educational phenomena can be isolated for study leaving all else unchanged. The systemic approach, on the other hand, mainly assumes that elements are interdependent and inseparable and a change in one element changes everything else. It follows, therefore, that what is required is a study of patterns not single variables.

A holistic or systemic approach quite often entails qualitative techniques in order to tease out the interrelationships of complex variables. Quantitative research also addresses the interrelationships between variables, and statistical modeling procedures enable the testing of complex theories on the way systems operate. While it may be true that much quantitative research has failed to take account of the complexities of human systems and has reduced them to simplistic hypotheses and law-like relations, this is a failure of the research design and not of quantitative research per se. In addition, although holists frequently use qualitative techniques, they are not a distinguishing feature of case study.

While there are those who still argue that qualitative and quantitative approaches are incompatible because of the different philosophical traditions from which they draw their credibility and in particular because of the underlying assumptions that each make about the validity or dependability of findings, in general there is an acceptance that the two traditions can work together. It is accepted that qualitative research is useful both in developing concepts and theories that can be further tested through quantitative approaches —the approach used in the 150 Schools Project, a current Australian study of effective schooling—and also in explaining more fully findings from quantitative research—the approach adopted in the Australian Staffing and Resources Study (see Sturman 1982).

1.1 Case Study and the Development of Theory

Glaser and Strauss (1968) distinguished "grounded theory," that is, theory grounded in the data collected, from theory generated from logical deduction from *a priori* assumptions. They argued that grounded theory is likely to generate more useful hypotheses in that it has been inductively developed from observational research in the real world. Similarly, Wilson (1977) argued that there is room in research for more inductive approaches where the role of preformed hypotheses is reduced to a minimum.

While case study is an ideal methodology for grounding theory, it does not follow that case study researchers approach or should approach settings without guiding theories and hypotheses. In fact, it is unlikely that they would be able to do this even if they wished. Popper (1963) argues that it is impossible to start with pure observation, that is, without anything in the nature of a theory. Selection within observation takes place and this selection is based on conjectures and anticipations and on other theories which act as a frame of reference for investigators.

Glaser and Strauss (1968) also acknowledged that researchers entered settings with a "general sociological perspective." However, what they were warning against was allowing preconceived theories or ideas to dictate relevances in concepts and hypotheses in the conduct of research. Wilson (1977) talked of "suspending" or "bracketing" preconceptions. Researchers should not be expected to be free of conjectures, but these should not preclude other avenues of inquiry.

Where case studies are providing a detailed description and understanding of a case and where researchers are open to new ideas that may challenge existing propositions, they provide not only the means by which existing conjectures and theories can be tested, but also the capacity to develop new theoretical positions. The process involved is what Kemmis (1980) called "iterative retroduction":

> With each cycle of retroduction, new "surprises"[.]are encountered and new hypotheses (interpretations) are

advanced. These, in turn, suggest new implications and avenues for disconfirmation which, when pursued may generate new surprises. (p. 115)

1.2 Case Study and Explanation, Understanding, and Description

Kaplan (1964) has distinguished explanation from understanding: the difference between having an explanation and "seeing" it. He argued that the reason for something is known either when it can be fitted into a known pattern (the pattern model) or when it can be deducted from other known truths (the deductive model). According to the pattern model, something is explained when it is so related to a set of other elements that together they constitute a unified system. In other words, an explanation exists for something when it can be understood.

Case study researchers or holists are more likely to be concerned with pattern explanation than deductive explanation because the pattern model is more appropriate when there are many diverse factors and where the pattern of relations between them is important. To arrive at an explanation, therefore, requires a rich description of the case and an understanding of it, in particular the relationship of its parts.

1.3 Case Study and Prediction and Generalization

Diesing (1972) held the view that because it is not possible to deduce an unknown part of a pattern from a known part, the symmetry of prediction and explanation that occurs in the deductive model, (i.e., in a model where one or more basic factors or laws determine what is to be explained) is not present.

However, this distinction does not always hold. Parsons (1976) commented, for example:

> Interpretation, explanation and understanding in social science contribute to prediction—they are not at odds with it. If one understands, one can attempt prediction and hopefully thereby plan better for the future. Theory organizes description, explanation and prediction in a multi-symbiotic process. (p. 133)

One of the earliest and lingering criticisms of case study methodology relates to the extent that it can be used to generalize to other cases or other settings. In 1975, Campbell referred to this problem in an article entitled *Degrees of Freedom and the Case Study*. The title of his article reflected what was at that time one of the major concerns about case study held by some quantitative researchers. Campbell (1975 p. 175) argued that the difference between qualitative and quantitative research had nothing to do with legitimacy of knowing—he argued that comparative social science engaged in "common-sense knowing" —but was related to confidence in the findings:

> If we achieve a meaningful quantitative 100-nation correlation, it is by dependence on this kind of knowing at every point, not by replacing it with a "scientific" quan-

titative methodology which substitutes for such knowing. The quantitative multination generalization will contradict such anecdotal, single-case, naturalistic observation at some points, but it will do so only by trusting a much larger body of such anecdotal, single-case, naturalistic observations.

The development of multisite case study, where case study methodology is applied to a number of settings or cases, makes such criticism too simplistic but, in any case, the holist argues that even single case study can be used for generalizations.

For example, Diesing (1972) argued that science deals with uniqueness and regularities: if the primary focus is on regularities, the unique shows up, and if it is on particulars, regularities show up. Case study methods include both the particular and the universal instead of segregating the two, and moves from the particular to the universal and back in graded steps.

Stake (1980 p. 69) has also advocated a process of naturalistic generalization arrived at "from the tacit knowledge of how things are, why they are, how people feel about them, and how these things are likely to be, later on or in other places with which this person is familiar." Naturalistic generalization is arrived at, therefore, by recognizing the similarities of the objects and issues in different contexts and "sensing the covariations of happenings." Stake argued that policymakers attain and amend their understandings, for the most part, through personal experience, and knowledge is often transferred through a process of empathetic understanding. Therefore, demands for typicality and representativeness often yield to needs for assurance that the target case is properly described.

For naturalistic generalizations to be possible, it is essential to ensure that the salient features of a case are documented so that a new situation can be illuminated by a very thorough understanding of a known case. This is so whether it is the researcher who is attempting the generalization or practitioners using the description of the known case and applying it to their settings.

2. Case Study and the "Generalization of Technics"

The specific techniques that are employed in case study depend on the type of study that is being conducted. These types can vary considerably, in part because case study embraces both the quantitative and qualitative paradigms.

2.1 Types of Case Study

Leaving aside narrative historical studies, documentary films, and personal case studies such as those used in medical diagnosis and psychology, Stenhouse (1985) has referred to four styles of case study methodology:

(a) Ethnographic case study which involves single in-depth study usually by means of participant observation and interview. An example from the United Kingdom is the study by Hargreaves (1967).

(b) Action research case study where the focus is on bringing about change in the case under study. An example from a developing country is the group of projects initiated under the Collaborative Action Research in Education (CARE) program in Sierra Leone and reported by Wright (1988).

(c) Evaluative case study which involves the evaluation of programs and where quite often condensed fieldwork replaces the more lengthy ethnographic approach. An example from the United States is the study by Stake and Gjerde (1974).

(d) Educational case study which is designed to enhance the understanding of educational action. An example from Australia is the study by Sturman (1989).

While the first and second styles—ethnographic case study and action research case study—are likely, because of the in-depth nature of such research, to be single case study, evaluative and educational case study can involve a single case or can be incorporated into multisite methods. The introduction of multisite methods is particularly noticeable in policy research, which has led Herriott and Firestone (1983) to refer to this as "multisite qualitative policy research."

2.2 Dimensions of Variation in Techniques in Case Study Methods

The degree to which case study research can be structured or unstructured is often ignored in methodological discussions. Louis (1982) has noted:

> In an increasing number of cases, data collected through very unstructured techniques may be transformed through coding into quantitative data bases, which are then analyzed using descriptive or inferential statistical techniques. Conversely, data may be collected through open-ended survey methods and analyzed "holistically" by site. In fact, to understand the variety of methods currently being employed, we must examine the nature of the design and practice at three points in the study: during data collection, during data-base formulation, and during the actual data analysis. (p. 9)

Figure 1, taken from Louis (1982), depicts this. The data collection phase ranges from the unstructured to the structured and can include ethnography, structured or unstructured interviews or surveys, and census data. The data formation stage ranges from the narrative to the numeric and includes the use of field notes; site reports; and nominal, interval, and ratio scales. Similarly, the data analysis phase ranges from

63

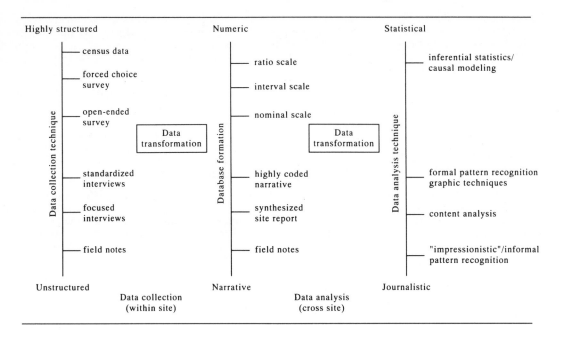

Figure 1
Dimensions of variation in multisite/multimethod studies
Source: Louis K S 1982 Multisite/multimethod studies: An introduction.
American Behavioral Scientist 26(1): 10. © Sage Publications, Inc. (Reprinted by permission of Sage Publication, Inc.)

the journalistic to the statistical and may include impressionistic analysis, content analysis, or inferential statistics and causal modeling.

2.3 Techniques in Multisite Case Studies

Multisite methodology emerged in response to the perceived limitations of much policy and evaluation research for policymakers. Firestone and Herriott (1983 p. 438) have discussed the demands on policy researchers and the implications that these have for case study. They refer to the formalization of qualitative research and they list five major elements of this:

(a) Whereas traditional qualitative research tends to emphasize in-depth description, formalized qualitative research emphasizes explanation.

(b) Whereas traditional qualitative research tends to emphasize the conduct of inquiry by a single individual, formalized qualitative research emphasizes the use of a multiperson team.

(c) Whereas traditional qualitative research tends to emphasize the discovery of relevant questions and variables within the field, formalized qualitative research emphasizes the codification of questions and variables before beginning fieldwork.

(d) Whereas traditional qualitative research tends to emphasize unstructured questioning and observation, formalized qualitative research emphasizes the standardization of data collection procedures through the use of semistructured interview and observation protocols.

(e) Whereas traditional qualitative research tends to emphasize extended presentation of verbal narrative, formalized qualitative research emphasizes the systematic reduction of verbal narrative to codes and categories.

In response to demands of policymakers, one of the major outcomes of such techniques, compared with ethnographic case study, is that researchers engaged in multisite case study usually spend much less time in each site. They trade in-depth inquiry for comparisons across a number of sites.

2.4 Case Study and Credibility

One concern that has been expressed about case study techniques, in particular ethnographic case study, is the credibility of what is seen as subjective research techniques. Although Wilson (1977) has argued that ethnographic case study challenges the traditional stance of the objective outsider, personal judgment forms an essential part of all science and is neither objective or subjective.

An assertion is an act of believing—to this extent it is subjective—but that assertion, whether it emerges from ethnographic research or multivariate statistical modeling, rests on personal judgment which includes an appraisal of evidence within the tenets of acceptable practice as perceived by the research community—to this extent it is objective. To say that science is more than its practitioners and their skills and judgments is a failure to perceive how science and its methods have historically progressed.

At the root of case study research as in all science lays the problem of "justified true belief":

> In every case in which someone would want to claim —however tentatively—to have established a scientific truth, he does so by making one set of assumptions about what counts as justification, along with another set of assumptions about the nature of belief. (Kemmis 1980 p. 102)

The problem of justified true belief is then a double problem which involves reconciling the beliefs (private knowledge) of researchers and readers with the forms of knowledge of public discourse.

Instead of the blanket condemnation of subjectivity or the universal approbation of objectivity, what is needed is an opportunity to appraise those personal judgments being made by scientific colleagues. Case study methodology can achieve its own form of precision. Wilson (1977) has referred to this as "disciplined subjectivity." This requires that evidence must be open to scrutiny, and that the study must be reported in a way capable of "conveying credibility" (Glaser and Strauss 1968) and subjected to standards of "trustworthiness," that is, credibility, transferability, dependability, and confirmability (Guba and Lincoln 1985).

Among the strategies that practitioners have suggested for achieving credibility in case study are the following:

(a) Procedures for data collection should be explained.

(b) Data collected should be displayed and ready for re-analysis.

(c) Negative instances should be reported.

(d) Biases should be acknowledged.

(e) Fieldwork analyses need to be documented.

(f) The relationship between assertion and evidence should be clarified.

(g) Primary evidence should be distinguished from secondary and description from interpretation.

(h) Diaries or logs should track what was actually done during different stages of the study.

(i) Methods should be devised to check the quality of data.

The concept of "triangulation" (Tawney 1975) is central to achieving credibility. Triangulation may involve the use of different data sources, different perspectives or theories, different investigators, or different methods. This process is, according to Diesing (1972), the holist's response to the issue of validity and reliability in survey research. The holist is concerned with contextual validity. This can take two forms: the validity of a piece of evidence which can be assessed by comparing it with other kinds of evidence on the same point, and the validity of the source of the evidence which can be evaluated by collecting other kinds of evidence about that source (see *Triangulation in Educational Research*).

To distinguish contextual validity from the validity important to the survey researcher, Diesing referred to the dependability of a source of evidence.

2.5 Case Study and Data Handling and Retrieval

Where case study involves in-depth observations and interviews, one of the problems faced by the researcher is how to store and retrieve such information.

Examples of how to address these issues come mainly from the fields of information and library science (see, e.g., Levine 1985), although the sourcebook prepared by Miles and Huberman (1984) provides one model for preparing qualitative data for analysis (see *Descriptive Data, Analysis of*).

3. Ethics and the Conduct of Case Study

The problem of ethics is not unique to case study methodology, but where case study involves the portrayal of persons or institutions in forms that may enable recognition, the ethical issues are paramount.

These problems are usually resolved through negotiations between researchers and those researched. This may take the form of an official contract or may be more informal, involving discussions over the content of written reports. While it may not be possible to have one set of rules that governs all situations, there is a responsibility on case study researchers to address in a responsible way ethical issues that emerge in their work.

4. Linking Research Methodologies

While conflicts about different methologies have not disappeared, in recent years there has developed in the research community a suspicion of "scientism," that is, an exaggerated regard for techniques which have succeeded elsewhere in contrast to a scientific temper which is open to whatever techniques hold promise for the inquiry in hand (Kaplan 1964).

There has also developed a recognition of the value of blending different methodologies. In one major study into the characteristics of effective schools in Australia, key concepts and variables were defined through reference both to prior quantitative studies as well as case studies of selected schools. From this a quantitative study of 150 schools is being conducted, but case studies will again complement and help to illuminate the findings from this study. The process is cyclical and case study methodology enters the process at various stages.

See also: Research Paradigms in Education

References

Campbell D 1975 Degrees of freedom and the case study. *Comparative Political Studies* 8(2): 178–93

Diesing P 1972 *Patterns of Discovery in the Social Sciences*. Routledge and Kegan Paul, London

Firestone W A, Herriott R E 1983 The formalization of qualitative research: An adaptation of "soft" science to the policy world. *Eval. Rev.* 7(4): 437–66

Glaser B G, Strauss A L 1968 *The Discovery of Grounded Theory: Strategies for Qualitative Research*. Weidenfeld and Nicolson, London

Guba E G, Lincoln Y S 1985 Naturalistic and rationalistic enquiry. In: Husén T, Postlethwaite T N (eds.) 1985 *International Encyclopedia of Education*, 1st edn. Pergamon Press, Oxford

Hargreaves D H 1967 *Social Relations in a Secondary School*. Routledge and Kegan Paul, London

Herriott R E, Firestone W A 1983 Multisite qualitative policy research: Optimizing descriptions and generalizability. *Educ. Researcher* 12(2): 14–19

Kaplan A 1964 *The Conduct of Inquiry: Methodology for Behavioral Science*. Chandler, San Francisco, California

Kemmis S 1980 The imagination of the case and the invention of the study. In: Simons H (ed.) 1980

Levine H G 1985 Principles of data storage and retrieval for use in qualitative evaluations. *Educ. Eval. Policy Anal.* 7(2):169–86

Louis K S 1982 Multisite/multimethod studies: An introduction. *American Behavioral Scientist* 26(1): 6–22

Miles M B, Huberman A M 1984 *Qualitative Data Analysis: A Sourcebook of New Methods*. Sage, Beverly Hills, California

Parsons C 1976 The new evaluation: A cautionary note. *J. Curric. St.* 8(2): 125–38

Popper K R 1963 *Conjectures and Refutations: The Growth of Scientific Knowledge*. Routledge and Kegan Paul, London

Salomon G 1991 Transcending the qualitative-quantitative debate: The analytic and systemic approaches to educational research. *Educ. Researcher* 20(6): 10–18

Stake R E 1980 The case study in social inquiry. In: Simons H (ed.)1980

Stake R E, Gjerde C 1974 *An Evaluation of T. City*. American Educational Research Association (AERA) Monograph Series in Curriculum Evaluation No. 7. Rand McNally, Chicago, Illinois

Stenhouse L 1985 Case study methods. In: Husén T, Postlethwaite T N (eds.) 1985 *International Encyclopedia of Education*, 1st edn. Pergamon Press, Oxford

Sturman A 1982 *Patterns of School Organization: Resources and Responses in Sixteen Schools*. ACER Research Monograph No.18. ACER, Hawthorn

Sturman A 1989 *Decentralisation and the Curriculum: Effects of the Devolution of Curriculum Decision Making in Australia*. ACER Research Monograph No.35. ACER, Hawthorn

Tawney D A 1975 Evaluation and science curriculum projects in the UK. *Stud. Sci. Educ.* 3: 31–54

Wilson S 1977 The use of ethnographic techniques in educational research. *Rev. of Educ. Res.* 47(2): 245–65

Wright C A H 1988 Collaborative action research in education (CARE)—reflections on an innovative paradigm. *Int. J. Educ. Dev.* 8(4): 279–92

Further Reading

Adelman C, Jenkins D, Kemmis S 1976 Re-thinking case study: Notes from the second Cambridge Conference. *Camb. J. Educ.* 6(3): 139–50

Hamilton D, Jenkins D, King C, MacDonald B, Parlett M (eds.) 1977 *Beyond the Numbers Game: A Reader in Educational Evaluation*. MacMillan Education, Basingstoke

Husén T 1988 Research paradigms in education. *Interchange* 19(1): 2–13

Keeves J 1988 The unity of educational research. *Interchange* 19(1): 14–30

Marshall C 1985 Appropriate criteria of trustworthiness and goodness for qualitative research on education organizations. *Quality and Quantity* 19: 353–73

Simons H (ed.) 1980 *Towards a Science of the Singular: Essays about Case Study in Educational Research and Evaluation*. Occasional Publications No. 10. Centre for Applied Research in Education, University of East Anglia, Norwich

Smith J K, Heshusius L 1986 Closing down the conversation: The end of the quantitative–qualitative debate among educational inquirers. *Educ. Researcher* 15(1): 4–12

Tripp D H 1985 Case study generalisation: An agenda for action. *Br. Educ. Res. J.* 11(1): 33–43

Educational History in Biographies and Autobiographies

T. Husén

In mapping out the intellectual landscape of scholarship in education valuable source material exists in the form of biographies and/or autobiographies of leaders and pioneers in the field. The present entry will refer to some of the more important biographies or autobiographies. Since education as a science to a large extent grew from empirical studies in psychology, several scientists, who are often identified primarily as psychologists, have also been taken into account. The aim of this entry is to show how progress and breakthroughs in educational research have been promoted by certain individuals. It does not pretend to present the emergence or history of educational research.

Systematic and scholarly pursuits in education have a history of about one hundred years which coincides with the emergence of empirical research relevant to educational problems. "Experimental pedagogy" branched off from experimental psychology founded by Gustav Theodor Fechner and Wilhelm Wundt followed by Herman Ebbinghaus and G E Müller toward the end of the nineteenth century. Research with bearings on education in the United States was pioneered by psychologists such as G Stanley Hall and Charles Judd who had their graduate training at German universities, like Leipzig where Wundt had his laboratory. They and their students spearheaded a development that brought the United States to its leadership in the behavioral sciences with scholars like Edward L Thorndike and Ralph Tyler.

In France, experimental psychology was established by Alfred Binet (1857–1911) who came from the fields of physiology and neurology. Binet became the father of intelligence testing and, with Simon, constructed the first standardized individual intelligence test (*échelle métrique*). In the United Kingdom, Francis Galton, anthropologist and biologist advanced the idea of measuring abilities and founded a biometric laboratory in London. His student and successor Karl Pearson was instrumental in developing analytical methods in statistics that were used in dealing with intelligence test data by followers like Charles Spearman, Cyril Burt, and Godfrey Thomson.

Sources for the history of educational research and disciplines relevant to the study of educational problems are to be found in autobiographies and biographies of leading behavioral scientists. This entry will limit itself to those who have either by their own biographies or those of others contributed to the establishment of modern educational research and studies. Such documents can contribute to the casting of light on how new ideas, techniques, and instruments were developed and had a lasting influence on, for instance, school teaching and the conception of how children develop and school teaching should be conducted.

1. Early Educational Psychologists

It is possible to distinguish between three generations of scholars whose influence can be assessed either by their own or by other biographies.

Even though Wilhelm Wundt is rightly known for having, in Fechner's footsteps, established experimental psychology and having taken a negative attitude to practical applications, he came indirectly to play a role through his student Ernst Meumann who wrote a monumental three-volume work on "experimental pedagogy," *Vorlesungen zur Einführung in die Experimentelle Pädagogik* (Introductory Lectures into Experimental Pedagogy), which was published in 1911. Wundt published an autobiography, *Erlebtes und Erkanntes* in 1920, in which he almost entirely deals with the rise of experimental psychology and how it developed from physiology and philosophy.

G Stanley Hall, who studied in Germany, belongs to the same generation and in spite of the fact that he published his main work *Adolescence* in two big volumes in 1904 and founded the journal *The Pedagogical Seminary* in 1893, he can along with William James be seen as the one who established educational psychology in the United States. His autobiography *Life and Confessions of A Psychologist* (1923) is a major source of information both about life in departments of psychology on both sides of the Atlantic and the history of developmental psychology.

Another main source for the history of educational psychology and more importantly, the academic landscape at large in the United States is Geraldine Jonçich Clifford's (1984) biography of Edward Lee Thorndike (1874–1949). In his role as a psychologist at a leading institution, namely, Teachers College at Columbia University, he spearheaded the development of the testing movement, and by his experimental studies of the learning process strongly influenced practical teaching. Clifford's book is without doubt the most exhaustive attempt to describe the early development of educational psychology.

A number of leading contributors to educational psychology during the first few decades of the twentieth century were invited by Carl Murchison to write short autobiographies for his *History of Psychology in Autobiography* which was published in the 1930s in three volumes.

To the same group of scientists whose biographies are relevant belongs Cyril Burt (see Hearshaw 1979).

Hearshaw puts Burt's career and scientific achievements in the context of the Galtonian tradition with its heavy emphasis on heredity and individual differences. Galton's *Memories of My Life* came out in 1908. A more comprehensive and documented biography in four volumes was published by Mark H Haller from 1914 to 1930. All these biographical works give an interesting and illuminating picture of the eugenics movement in the United Kingdom.

David Katz, a German psychologist born in 1884 who had to leave Germany in the early 1930s, became the holder of a combined chair in psychology and education at Stockholm University a few years later. He had been a graduate student and assistant of Georg Elias Müller at Göttingen. Müller in his turn was a former student and assistant of Wundt. At the end of his life Katz was invited to write a contribution to the *History of Psychology in Autobiography*. It appeared in Vol. 4 (see Boring 1952). Katz's assistant during the 1940s, Carl-Ivar Sandström wrote an essay entitled "A Surviving Psychologist: David Katz 1884–1953" which was published in an anthology of psychological essays—*Iakttagelse och upplevelse (Observation and Experience)* (Sandström 1969).

2. Edward L Thorndike—Pioneer in Educational Psychology

Without doubt, the most informative biography ever published about an educational psychologist is the one mentioned earlier by Geraldine Jonçich Clifford, that is *Edward L. Thorndike—The Sane Positivist*. The first edition was published in 1968 followed by a revised edition in 1984. Clifford sets out to report on Thorndike's contributions to the theory and practice of education and psychology. He wanted to be remembered as a scientist with strong regard for the hard sciences. He hoped for the establishment of an experimental science of man which would guide policy-making in all human fields including education. Typically, Woodworth's characterization of Thorndike as a "sane positivist" is taken by Clifford as the subtitle of her biography. Her focus is on Thorndike's time and work more than upon the man himself. In the preface she points out that Ernest Jones in his biography of Sigmund Freud puts the main focus on Freud himself as a person and less upon his work. Thus Clifford's book is a piece of social history where Thorndike is placed within the social and intellectual context of his time. He wanted to be a model of the "educator-as-scientist." The biography therefore is a contribution to the "larger intellectual and social history of the United States" during the first few years of the twentieth century.

The breakthrough of educational psychology occurred during the 1890s with William James lecturing to teachers on psychology, and by the founding of Clark University by G Stanley Hall who, by 1898

(when Thorndike took his PhD at Columbia), had conferred 30 doctoral degrees, more than all other American universities together. In addition to James MacKeen Cattell and William James, both mentors of Thorndike, Charles Judd, trained by Wundt in Leipzig, was the leading scholar in educational psychology, later becoming professor and dean at Chicago and representing a different approach to the study of learning from Thorndike.

Thorndike's approach was the positivist, measuring one. In his *Educational Psychology* of 1903, which became very influential in teacher training, he aphoristically spelled out his firm belief in experimentalism and quantification in research in the exact sciences: "We conquer the facts of nature when we observe and experiment upon them. When we measure them we have made them our servants." In an opening lecture at Columbia University in 1921 which was published in *Teachers College Record* (November 1922) he made another aphoristic statement along the same lines: "Whatever exists, exists in some amount. To measure it is simply to know its varying amounts."

In sweeping over the entire field Clifford is able to show how education as a science, at least as a science of educational psychology, developed with contributions being made by scholars such as Cattell, James, Thorndike, Judd and Hall.

3. Clinical Psychology with Applications in Education

The history of clinical psychology as applied in education in the family and the school can find valuable source material in Sigmund Freud's autobiography *Selbstdarstellung*, first published as a journal article in 1925 and later as a separate monograph by the International Psychoanalytical Publisher in 1936 in Vienna.

Another and by far richer source with bearings on the role of clinical psychology in education is provided by Seymour B Sarason's (1988) autobiography *The Making of An American Psychologist*. In addition to reporting his experiences from clinical work Sarason also has a chapter which deals with "Psychology and American Education." In it he discusses the "low regard in which the field of education (is) held" and the "cyclical bouts of scapegoating" that the American schools are subjected to as well as the "unfortunate example of an educational debate that managed to ignore the obvious" (pp. 333–34).

4. Piaget–Bruner–Skinner

Jean Piaget (1896–1980), along with Bruner, has had a strong influence on how problems of school instruction have been conceived. He started in biology and took his doctorate in zoology at a very young age before embarking upon studies in psychology in Paris. His studies focused on what he called the "genetic", the epistemology of knowledge, and were based on thorough observations of children during various stages of development. He published *Le language et la pensèe chez l'enfant* in 1923 with a Preface by Claparède, the Swiss reform educator who describes Piaget's work as "remarkable." Piaget was also invited to contribute to the series of short autobiographies published by Carl Murchison.

Jerome Bruner started out as a psychologist in the early part of his career, when he dealt with perception and the nature of cognition. When in the late 1950s curricular projects were launched, not least in the United States, there was an approchement between psychology of cognition and classroom didactics. The US National Academy of Sciences in 1959 sponsored a conference at Woods Hole, Massachusetts which was of "seminal" importance and had a historical significance. Bruner wrote a report to the US Office of Education on "The Development of Designs for Curriculum Research" which strongly influenced the agency's policy during the 1960s. In 1960 and 1966 Bruner published his books, *The Process of Education* and *Toward A Theory of Instruction* respectively. Both publications had a strong impact on the thinking about curricular and didactic problems. He and his colleagues thought that they were starting "a new era in education." Psychologists, in particular psychologists of learning, had to tackle the concrete problems of the science of teaching. So far they had tended to be "embarrassed by education."

In his autobiography *In Search of Mind* Bruner (1983) quotes how the Woods Hole Conference was said to "revolutionize" education. The conception of the mind as a method applied to tasks, combined with the Piagetian psychology of the development of abstraction and the emphasis on "generativeness" of knowledge were the basis for *The Process of Education*. The book was also a timely contribution in an era when the knowledge explosion and the new postindustrial technology posed challenges to educators.

Bruner became a member of the President's Science Advisory Committee and thereby gained a strong influence on policymakers in education in Washington, DC.

B F Skinner worked on problems of learning for a long time without making much reference to concrete educational problems. However, like Jerome Bruner he became involved in the debate on the quality and adequacy of American school education that flared up in the 1950s and got quite a lot of fuel from the launching of Sputnik in 1957. By 1954, however, Skinner had participated in a symposium where he demonstrated for the first time a "teaching machine" which could steer the learning process according to the laws and principles that it was subjected to, thus moving

into the realms of educational technology. Already in *Walden Two* (1948) which described a utopian society set up according to the principles of learning that Skinner was espousing he dealt with educational problems not least of upbringing. Later he was critical of Rousseau's educational philosophy of freedom and took up the social philosophy based upon his psychology in *Beyond Freedom and Dignity*, published in 1971. His involvement in the educational debate in the United States is dealt with in the third volume of his autobiography *A Matter of Consequences*, which was published in 1983.

5. Contemporary American Educators

When the Phi Delta Kappan Educational Foundation celebrated its twenty-fifth anniversary it invited 33 distinguished educators to contribute to a *Festschrift* edited by Derek Burleson under the title *Reflections*. The contributors were senior and leading American educators, such as Ernest Boyer, John Brademas, James Coleman, Elliot Eisner, N L Gage, John Goodlad, Harold Howe Jr, and Ralph Tyler. They were asked to bring a historical perspective to their reflections. Generally their essays are more autobiographical than issue oriented. Together, however, they give a good picture of problems that have beset school education in the United States since the Second World War.

6. Contemporary European Educators

European educators who have recently either published autobiographical material or been the subject of shorter or more extensive biographies are Hellmut Becker and Hartmut von Hentig, who have been in the forefront of the educational reform movement in Germany; and Torsten Husén, who entered education from psychology and was closely involved in the research conducted in conjunction with the Swedish school reform. He has dealt with this work in his autobiography *An Incurable Academic* (Husén 1983) and in *Fifty Years as An Educational Researcher* published by the Royal Swedish Academy of Sciences. Recently he has published a series of essays on leading psychologists and educators whom he has met, for instance, James Conant, Benjamin Bloom, Cyril Burt, and Ralph Tyler (Husén 1992).

7. Oral History in Education

Given the new technologies of audiovisual recording, education has started to get its share of oral history. Ralph Tyler, in various capacities as scholar, administrator, and consultant has been perhaps the most influential person in the field of education in the United States in modern time. Since the award of his

PhD at the University of Chicago in 1927, he was at the frontline of educational research and reforms in the United States until his death in 1993. He was extensively interviewed by Malca Chall during three consecutive years from (1985 to 1987). The result goes under the title *Ralph W. Tyler: Education: Curriculum Development and Evaluation* with an Introduction by Carl Tjerandsen. The manuscript covers (apart from family background and university studies) the beginning of curriculum planning and evaluation around 1930; the Eight-Year Study from 1933 to 1941; his time as a professor, university examiner, and dean at the University of Chicago from 1938 to 1953; his directorship at the Center for Advanced Study in the Behavioral Sciences from 1954 to 1967; and subsequently, more than 20 years with special education projects, consultationships in the United States and abroad, and educational commissions. A special chapter is devoted to educational problems in the United States, such as the launching of the National Assessment of Educational Progress (NAEP).

8. Other Sources Providing Biographical Information

Biographical information about many leading educators can be obtained from obituaries published in journals of education and psychology as well as from the proceedings of academies such as the US National Academy of Education.

Some journals have series of "portraits" or "profiles" of educators who have made an impact particularly during the last century. Thus, the UNESCO journal *Prospects*, which is published in several languages, began in the early 1990s to carry one "profile" in each issue. *Revue de psychologie appliqué* published by *Centre de Psychologie Appliqué* in Paris published a series of curriculum vitae plus bibliographies in the early 1960s. Some of these were on educational psychologists. The journal *Biography* 13:1, 1990 had a special issue on leading educators.

See also: Research Paradigms in Education; History of Educational Research

References

Boring E G (ed.) 1952 *History of Psychology in Autobiography*, Vol. 4. Stanford University Press, Stanford, California

Bruner J 1983 *In Search of Mind: Essays in Autobiography.* Harper and Row, New York

Burleson D L (ed.) 1991 *Reflections: Personal Essays by 33 Distinguished Educators*. Phi Delta Kappa Educational Foundation, Bloomington, Indiana

Clifford G J 1984 *A Biography of Edward L. Thorndike: The Sane Positivist*, rev. edn. Weslyan University Press, Middletown, Connecticut

Galton F 1908 *Memories of My Life.* Methuen, London

Hall G S 1923 *Life and Confessions of a Psychologist.* Appleton and Co, New York

Hearshaw L S 1979 *Cyril Burt—Psychologist.* Cornell University Press, New York

Husén T 1983 *An Incurable Academic: Memoirs of a Professor.* Pergamon Press, Oxford

Husén T 1992 *Möten med psykologer, pedagoger och andra* Höganäs, Wiken

Murchison C (ed.) 1930, 1932, 1936 *History of Psychology in Autobiography* Vols. 1–3. Clark University Press, Worcester, Massachusetts

Sandström C I 1969 *Iakttagelse och upplevelse.* Almqvist and Wiksell, Stockholm

Sarason S B 1988 *The Making of an American Psychologist: An Autobiography.* Jossey-Bass, San Francisco, California

Skinner B F 1983 *A Matter of Consequences: Part Three of An Autobiography.* Alfred Knopf, New York

Tyler R W 1987 Ralph W. Tyler: Education: Curriculum development and evaluation. Interviews conducted by Malca Chall in 1985, 1986, and 1987. Manuscript copies. Regional Oral History Office, The Bancroft Library, University of California, Berkeley, California

Wunt W 1920 *Erlebtes und Erkanntes* Kröner, Stuttgart

Further Reading

Allport G W 1942 *The Use of Personal Documents in Psychological Science.* Social Science Research Council, New York

Boring E G, Lindzey G (eds.) 1967 *History of Psychology in Autobiography*, Vol. 5. Appleton, Century, Crofts, New York

Campbell R F 1981 *The Making of A Professor: A Memoir.* Published by author, Salt Lake City, Utah

Lindzey G (ed.) *History of Psychology in Autobiography*, Vol. 6. Appleton, Century, Crofts, Englewood, New Jersey

Lindzey G (ed.) 1989 *History of Psychology in Autobiography*, Vol. 7. Stanford University Press, Stanford, California

van der Meer Q L T, Bergman H (eds.) 1976 *Onderwijskundigen van de twintigste eeuw.* Wolters-Noodrhoff, Groningen

Ethnographic Research Methods

R. Taft

Some educational researchers have advocated the adoption of the ethnographic methods employed by cultural and social anthropologists in their field studies of social groups and communities. These methods are considered to be particularly appropriate for empirical research on the relatively bounded system of a school or classroom but they also have their place in the study of the role of the family, social organizations, or ethnic communities in education. Ethnographic research consists essentially of a description of events that occur within the life of a group with special regard to social structures and the behavior of individuals with respect to their group membership, and an interpretation of the meaning of these for the culture of the group. Ethnography is used both to record primary data and to interpret its meaning. It is naturalistic enquiry as opposed to controlled, and a qualitative as opposed to quantitative, method. In ethnography the researcher participates in some part of the normal life of the group and uses what he or she learns from that participation to produce the research findings. It is consequently often treated as being equivalent to participant observation, in contrast with nonparticipant observation in which the observer as an outsider records the overt behavior of the subjects, but it involves more than that. Participation in a group provides investigators with an understanding of the culture and the interactions between the members that is different from that which can be obtained from merely observing or conducting a questionnaire survey or an analysis of documents. The investigators' involvement in the normal activities of the group may be treated as a case of partial acculturation in which they acquire an insider's knowledge of the group through their direct experience with it. These experiences provide them with tacit knowledge which helps them to understand the significance to the group members of their own behavior and that of others and enables them to integrate their observations about that behavior with information obtained from other sources such as interviews with informants and documentary material.

1. The Development of Ethnographic Methods

Field research was employed by anthropologists and sociologists in the nineteenth and early twentieth centuries, but the first to stress the need for a systematic approach to its conduct was the Polish-British scholar Malinowski, who emphasized the need for ethnographers to employ controls in their assembly of data in a manner that he described as analogous, although by no means similar, to those of the natural scientists.

Malinowski laid down the requirement that observers should tabulate the data on which their conclusions are based, including verbatim statements, and should indicate whether they are derived from direct or indirect sources, a method that he called "concrete statistical documentation" (see the introductory chapter on methodology in Malinowski 1922). He stressed the need for the investigator to establish "trustworthiness" in respect of the study. Malinowski described the goal of ethnographic studies as "to grasp the native's point of view, his relation to life, to realise his view of his world" (p.25). In order to achieve this, the investigator should learn the language of the community being studied, reside for a protracted period in the community—preferably out of contact with "white" people, and use both observation and informed interviews with selected informants from within the community as sources of data.

The field methods laid down by Malinowski have, to a greater or lesser degree, been used in studies of segments of modern, urbanized societies which have provided a model for the application of the methods to educational research. For example, studies were carried out of the unemployed in Austria, industrial organizations (Tavistock Institute), urban areas in the United States (Middletown, Yankee City), hobos, gangs, and dance musicians, to name just a few. These studies each raised their own peculiar problems of research strategy, but what they all have in common is their method of research in which the investigator becomes closely involved over a prolonged period in the everyday life of the members of a designated group or community in order to understand its culture. This contact enables the researchers not only to obtain an intimate and a broad knowledge of the group but also to test and refine hypotheses about the phenomena being studied.

Ethnographic methods of research came to education fairly late. The team of sociologists from the University of Chicago who studied medical students (Becker et al. 1961) were probably the pioneers in the field of education, while Smith and Geoffrey (1968) were the first to base a study of classroom processes on anthropological field studies using a method which they described as microethnography. They stated that their "primary intent was to describe the silent language of a culture, a classroom in a slum school, so that those who have not lived in it will appreciate its subtleties and complexities" (p. 2). Smith observed the classroom every day for one semester and kept copious field notes, which he used as a basis for his daily discussions with the class teacher, Geoffrey, with the purpose of clarifying the intentions and motives behind the teacher's behavior in order to move towards a conceptualization in abstract terms of the teaching process. Both of the investigators were participants in the classroom, although one was more of an observer and the other more of an initiator and an informant.

A word should be added about the terms used in describing ethnographic studies in education. Smith and Geoffrey seem to have simply meant an intensive field study by their term microethnography, while Erickson (1975) confines it more narrowly to studies that use extensive observation and recording to establish the interactional structures in the classroom. For the purposes of this present article, the term ethnography is interpreted liberally to include case studies, the concept preferred by the ethnographers in the United Kingdom. The intensive study of a bounded community is a clear example of a simple case study, even though they are many individuals who make up that community.

2. The Scientific Status of the Ethnographic Method

There is some skepticism about the place of a positivist model or research in the social sciences according to which a detached scholar objectively studies an objective reality. Ethnographers are not detached; they influence their data and they are influenced by it in all stages of observing, interpreting and reporting. Their reports are constructions which are determined by their personal outlook and socio-cultural forces. (The issues are fully discussed in Denzin and Lincoln 1994.) Some scholars argue that the reports of ethnographers should be viewed as "tales" or "narratives" which should be studied for their own sake. In contrast the post-positivist approach adopted here, while it does not ignore the constructionist aspects of ethnographic research, makes the assumption that there is an objective social reality and that ethnography is an appropriate method for studying it.

2.1 The Social Role of the Investigator

The description of the investigator as a participant in the life of the group implies that he or she has some role in it which is recognized by the group. Sometimes this role is simply that of participant observer, a role which does not usually exist in most formal group structures, but one which does have a meaning in many classrooms where outsiders come to observe the class on occasions for one purpose or another. Thus, Louis Smith was introduced to both the children and the teachers as someone from the university who was interested in children's learning, a role which is understood and accepted in modern classrooms. In other cases the investigator fills a normal role in the group other than that of a researcher. For example, the researcher may be a regular classroom teacher

in the school, a situation that represents participant observation in the fullest sense of the word. The role of participant observer has some advantages as a viewing point over that of the participant who plays the additional role of observer. The former is expected by the group to share, probe, ask questions, take notes, and so on because this is consistent with his or her role as an observer whereas the latter has tactical and ethical problems in doing so because of his or her obligations as a participant. On the other hand there is a danger that a participant observer can become so much absorbed into the group after a time that his or her status as an observer may be compromised.

A group member who also acts as a research observer may carry out that latter role overtly or covertly—or as a mixture of both where the member's role as an investigator is known to some but not all members of the group. A participant observer, by definition, plays an obtrusive role in the group process. Where the role of a group member as a researcher is overt, that person's role within the group can be compromised by the other group members' awareness of that fact and the latter are likely to control their behavior in order to enhance or defend their public image. Thus, it can become difficult for the participant observer to carry out either of the roles—participant or observer. For this reason an investigator is tempted to engage in covert observation in which the observer role is not known to the members of the group. This type of research raises serious ethical issues and in many universities and research institutions an application for approval or support for a covert ethnographic study would be subject to rejection on ethical grounds.

2.2 The Inside-Outside View

One of the main advantages of the ethnographic method is that, in the course of becoming involved in the group, the investigator becomes acculturated to it. This means that he or she develops personal knowledge about the rules of the group and begins to perceive the same meanings of events as do the members of the group. The investigator learns what behavior is expected when, where, and in response to what situations. This process of acculturation is sometimes described as transition from the status of a "stranger" to that of "a friend", that is, a person who knows the "silent language" of the group and is in intimate communication with its members. It is, however, significant that a scholar who is studying the subculture of a school in his or her own society is unlikely to be as complete a stranger at the beginning as an anthropologist studying a traditional society.

Nevertheless, being an insider has its drawbacks as a method of studying a group. First, as already indicated, there are constraints imposed by propriety and ethics on an insider revealing to others the secrets of the group. There may, of course, be the same constraints on an outsider but, at least, the group can usually control his or her access to information by barring entry.

Second, the insider may not always have even as much access to information as an outsider. The investigator may have personal knowledge of only a segment of the group's life, sometimes without being aware of the limitation. He or she may even be denied access to the other segments: for example, a teacher may not be permitted to study the classroom of a colleague. In contrast, a stranger who is accepted as an observer may be deliberately informed and invited to observe just because he or she is a stranger. Furthermore, an outsider is more likely to be able to take steps to obtain a respresentative sampling of people, occasions, and settings in the group and thus can help to offset the suspicion of biased observation. A third drawback that may arise as a result of being an insider is that highly salient data may be overlooked just because it is so familiar. Strangers will notice events that stand out as a result of their contrast with the expectations that they have brought with them from their own cultural background and may therefore be better placed to infer their meaning and significance for other events in the group. Some element of surprise aids awareness. A further problem is the one mentioned earlier of the subjects' reactivity to being studied, particularly when the observer is a full participant in the group. Whether or not the observation is obtrusive, it is reactive observation; that is, the observer affects the behavior of the people being studied and consequently will have to take into account his or her own influence when assessing the group. As Everhart puts it "the fieldworker, rather than appearing to be one of many in the audience observing the drama on stage, is himself on stage, interacting with the other actors in 'his' setting and playing a role in the resolution of the production" (1977 p. 14). In order to take into account their own contributions and to assess what the situation would be if it were not for the fact that their presence is influencing the group, investigators need a great deal of self-awareness and a thorough understanding of the group processes. This necessity for playing the dual roles of participant and detached observer can impose a severe strain on the ethnographic investigator and it calls for continual monitoring of the effect the investigator has on others.

2.3 Subjectivity, Reliability, and Validity

The fact that investigators have a role in the group not only requires them to be aware of their own influence but also may give them an emotional stake in a particular research outcome. For example, if the observer is also a teacher, there may be a tendency for observation to be slanted towards a justification of the style of teaching normally used. Since ethnographic researchers use themselves as the instrument through which they observe the group, the method lends itself to extreme subjectivity; that is, the interpretation may be idiosyncratic to the observer with all of the associated limitations, eccentricities, and biases and is not matched by the interpretation of other observers. This raises questions concerning the reliability of the observations and the validity of the conclusions. Observations and interpretations are by their very nature subjective but they still can be made susceptible to reliability checks and it is still possible for the investigation to follow rules that can increase the validity of the conclusions.

Reliability, that is accuracy, of the observations can be enhanced by following the prescription laid down by Malinowski of recording wherever possible the concrete data in the form of a "synoptic chart" on which the inferences are to be based, including verbatim utterances and opinions. Modern methods of recording events so that they can be examined at leisure offer ethnographers unprecedented possibilities of attaining accuracy, but there are still sampling problems in the selection of the data and limitations to accuracy due to bias and lack of opportunity, as well as tactical and ethical considerations in making the recordings.

The reliability of the observations is assisted by the long period of exposure to the data in ethnographic research which provides opportunities for investigators to cross check their observations over time and to reconcile inconsistencies. Cross checks may also be made by triangulation, a procedure in which multiple sources are used to obtain evidence on the same phenomenon. Thus, the observations may be supplemented by interviews, feedback to the members of the group for their comment, and documentary evidence such as school notices, correspondence, minutes, and other archives. An additional source of reliability is to have more than one observer as, for example, in the study by Smith and Geoffrey (1968), a situation which is relatively rare in traditional anthropological studies. In the typical case, the multiple observers may be members of a team who are exposed to the same events and are then able to cross check each other's data.

Validity is a quality of the conclusions and the processes through which these were reached, but its exact meaning is dependent on the particular criterion of truth that is adopted. In ethnographic research the most appropriate criterion is credibility although even that term is subject to fuzziness in meaning. Some authors would add "plausibility" as a further criterion of validity but this is implied by the term "credibility" which is a socially defined concept as far as ethnographic research is concerned. The community of scholars within which an ethnographic researcher operates and to whom the results of the research are communicated has a collective understanding of what makes it acceptable as valid. Credibility is dependent on the apparent accuracy of the data, and all the steps described above that are intended to increase reliability are relevant. Much depends on the way in which the study is communicated to the scientific audience. A report in which the investigator describes the precautions that have been taken to ensure the accuracy of the observations has more credibility than one in which the reader is merely asked top take the data and findings "on faith." The report should contain indications that the investigator is aware of the need to convince the audience of the validity of the study. The interpretations made from the data are more credible when the researcher describes the evidence on which they are based and also any efforts made to test for evidence that would tend to disconfirm any tentative conclusions. One of the procedures that is often followed in ethnographic studies to confirm the validity of interpretations is to feed them back for comment to selected members of the group or to other persons who know the group. If necessary, the interpretations can be "negotiated" with the participants so that the final product is more likely to represent the situation as they see it, but there is always a danger in this procedure that the participants may exercise distortion and cover-up for their own reasons or that the researcher finds it impossible to obtain consensus. Different members of the group may hold different perceptions of the events, for example, teachers and students, or boys and girls. Some researchers have attempted to overcome these problems by setting up small groups of about four participants to engage in discussions towards establishing their shared meanings by acting as "checks, balances, and prompts" for each other, but in practice there are distinct limitations to the possible application of this procedure.

2.4 The Role of Theory, Hypotheses, and Generalization

Malinowski specifically recommends that field workers should commence with "foreshadowed problems" arising from their knowledge of theory, but should not have "preconceived ideas" in which they aim to prove certain hypotheses. The ethnographic method is qualitative and holistic, making use of the investigator's intuition, empathy, and general ability to learn another culture. The investigator is more concerned with discovery than with verification and this requires preparedness to formulate, test, and, if necessary, discard a series of hunches. As investigators develop hypotheses in the course of pursuing a foreshadowed problem they should be alert for data which refute, support, or cast doubts on their hypotheses and should be prepared to alter them in accordance with increased acquaintance with the phenomena. Research workers as they puzzle over the meaning of the behavior of the group, and perhaps seek help from informants, are likely to obtain illumination through a sudden shaft of understanding. Thus there is a continual dialogue between an orientation towards discovery and one towards verification. Gradually a theoretical basis for the understanding of the group processes may emerge through the process often described as grounded theory, that is, grounded in the research process itself. Theory that emerges from exposure to the data is more likely to fit the requirements than theory that is preconceived on an abstract basis. Also the actual data are more likely to produce categories that are appropriate

for describing the particular case. The main problem that arises from grounded theory derived from a case study is that of making generalizations beyond the particular case viewed at a particular time. A straight out description of concrete happenings has some value as an addition to the corpus of information that is available to the investigator and to other interested people—including members of the group itself. However, its value is greatly enhanced when the case can be "located as an instance of a more general class of events" Smith (1978 p. 335). To achieve this, the investigator treats the case in point as either a representative of, or a departure from, a particular type. Sometimes the actual group or groups that are studied have been chosen initially as representatives of a designated type of case and this facilitates generalizations based on it but they should still be treated with reserve.

2.5 Ethnography as a Case Study Method

The problem of the relationship between the One and the Many, a perennial one in philosophy, arises in different guises in the social sciences—idiographic versus nomothetic treatments of data, -emic versus -etic approaches to comparative studies, and the case study versus the sample survey research design. In order to generalize from an individual case study of behavior in one group to behavior in others it is necessary to reach sufficient understanding about the significance of the events in relation to the context in which they occur in order to extend interpretations to other contexts and other groups. In the process of generalizing it is necessary to violate somewhat the full integrity of any one group by describing events in some language that extends beyond the bounds of the culture of that group. Ethnographers are partially acculturated to the group that they are studying, but they are also familiar with other groups with which they compare their experience of the group. To maintain the analogy, an ethnographer is multicultural with respect to the object of study. When an investigator attempts to understand one group, he or she is aided by knowledge of other ones and his or her impressions are partially consolidated with the others. Thus, generalizations are built up through the investigator being able to mediate between one group and others; an ethnographic account of a school, then, derives its value largely from the fact that the investigator—and also the readers—are familiar with other schools, and with schools in general. Diesing refers to this as "pluralism" which he describes as follows: "one might say the method is relativistic in its treatment of individual cases and becomes gradually absolutistic as it moves toward broader generalizations" (1971 pp. 297–98).

In ethnographic studies no generalization can be treated as final, only as a working hypothesis for further studies which may again be ethnographic, or may consist of a survey by means of interviews, questionnaires, or tests. The ethnographic method gains credibility when it combines both subjective and objective methods but it need not be regarded as deriving its value only as a preliminary and exploratory procedure prior to the use of more conventional semiobjective techniques. It can make its own legitimate independent contribution at any stage of a research including the confirmation of hypotheses that have emerged out of other sources provided that the basic principles on which its credibility rests are observed.

References

Becker G S, Beer B, Hughes E, Strauss A 1961 *Boys in White: Student Culture in Medical School.* University of Chicago Press, Chicago, Illinois

Denzin N K, Lincoln Y S (eds.) 1994 *Handbook of Qualitative Research.* Sage, London

Diesing P 1971 *Patterns of Discovery in the Social Sciences.* Aldine-Atherton, Chicago, Illinois

Erickson F 1975 Gatekeeping and the melting Pot: Interaction in counseling encounters. *Harvard Educ. Rev.* 45: 44-70

Everhart R B 1977 Between stranger and friend: Some consequences of "long term" fieldwork in schools. *Am. Educ. Res. J.* 14: 1–15

Malinowski B 1922 *Argonauts of the Western Pacific: An Account of Native Enterprise and Adventure in the Archipelagoes of Melanesian New Guinea.* Routledge, London

Smith L M 1978 An evolving logic of participant observation, educational ethnography, and other case studies. In: Shulman L S (ed.) 1978 *Review of Research in Education,* Vol. 6. Peacock, Ithaca, Illinois, pp. 316–77

Smith L M, Geoffrey W 1968 *The Complexities of an Urban Classroom: An Analysis Toward a General Theory of Teaching.* Holt, Rinehart and Winston, New York

Further Reading

Eisner E W, Peshkin A (eds.) 1990 *Qualitative Inquiry in Education.* Teachers College Press, New York

Wilson S 1977 The use of ethnographic techniques in educational research. *Rev. Educ. Res.* 47: 245–65

Historical Methods in Educational Research

C. F. Kaestle

Historians often observe that their discipline is both a science and an art. When they say that history is a science, they mean that historians adhere to certain procedures of investigation and argument that allow them to agree on some generalizations about the past, even though their personal values and their understanding of human nature may differ. In many cases they can agree simply because the evidence is ample and clear, and because they agree on the ground rules. Factual statements like "Jean-Jacques Rousseau was born in 1712" occasion little debate as long as it is the same Rousseau being spoken about and as long as the surviving records are not contradictory. More complex statements are also capable of verification and may attract wide consensus among historians. Examples are such statements as the following: "The average White fertility rate was declining during the period from 1800 to 1860," or "Most educators in 1840 believed that state-funded schooling would reduce crime."

However, the rules of investigation and analysis help less and less as historians attempt to make broader generalizations about the past, or make judgments about its relation to the present, and this is part of what is meant by saying that history is also an art. Consider such statements as: "Slavery destroyed the American Black family," or "Schooling was a major avenue of

social mobility in France." These claims are not only immensely difficult to study empirically; they also involve problems of definition and problems of implicit value judgments. The process of broad generalization is thus not simply inductive; it remains an act of creative and often normative interpretation, within the limits established by the evidence. To a considerable degree, history remains stubbornly subjective.

The history of education shares the methodological problems of the field of history in general. There is no single, definable method of inquiry, and important historical generalizations are rarely beyond dispute. Rather they are the result of an interaction between fragmentary evidence and the values and experiences of the historian. It is a challenging and creative interaction, part science, part art.

It is important for educators to understand this problematic nature of historical methodology because historical statements about education abound far beyond textbooks or required history courses in schools of education. Beliefs about the historical role of schooling in America are encountered every day as arguments for educational policies. For example, during the debates in America about the decentralization of urban school control in the 1960s, advocates of decentralization argued that centralization was a device by which social elites in the early twentieth century had gained control of urban education, protected the social structure, and tried to impose their particular values on public school children. The decentralizers argued that centralization had been an undemocratic means of social control, and therefore it deserved to be reversed. Opponents of decentralization claimed that it would lead to inefficiency and corruption. Besides, they said, a common, uniform school system has been a successful tool in creating a cohesive, democratic society in America. They too cited history as their authority. Behind these contending positions is a mass of complex evidence and conflicting values. The historian has no magic formula to tell you which analysis is correct.

The uncertain nature of historical generalization has been particularly apparent in the history of education since the early 1960s. During this period the traditional methods and assumptions of educational historians have come increasingly under attack. The controversy has led to fresh insights, new questions and, more than ever, a heightened sense of the precariousness of historical generalizations.

1. The Traditional Framework

Current methodological issues in the history of education are best understood in the light of the assumptions and conclusions of traditional educational historians. Until the 1950s most writers of educational history shared two basic assumptions: first, that the history of education was concerned centrally, indeed, almost exclusively, with the history of school systems; and second, that state-regulated, free, tax-supported, universal schooling was a good thing. These assumptions were largely unquestioned, partly because many educational historians performed a dual role as educational administrators or professors of education, and therefore they had a vested interest in seeing state schooling in a good light. But also there was widespread popular agreement that free, universal schooling was an unquestionably positive institution.

There were several unstated corollaries to these assumptions, and they provided the framework—what some might call the paradigm—for research in educational history. Four elements will be mentioned in this paradigm which helped determine methodology and which occasioned later criticism. The first has to do with the focus on schooling. Because they tended to equate education with schooling, traditional historians rated the educational well-being and enlightenment of earlier societies by assessing how much formal schooling there was, and to what extent it was organized under state control. Because their view of historical development was dominated by their present conception of desirable educational policy, they spent much effort trying to explain the lack of enthusiasm

for state-regulated schooling prior to the 1830s, and they underestimated the importance of the family, the workplace, the churches, and other educational agencies in preindustrial society.

Related to this problem of focus is the problem of intent. Traditional historians of education saw those who favored state-regulated school systems as enlightened leaders working for the common good; they portrayed people who opposed educational reform as ignorant, misled, or selfish. The attribution of human motivation is a very difficult methodological problem in historical writing; it involves careful comparison of public and private statements; and it requires the separation, if possible, of attempts to determine the historical actor's personal motivation from moral judgments on the effects of an event or a policy. Moral judgments may be timeless, but the historical actor's motivation must be understood in the context of the social values and scientific knowledge of the day. The value bias of most traditional educational historians prejudiced them against recognizing self-interest on the part of school reformers or legitimate, principled objection on the part of their opponents. On the other hand, some recent so-called "revisionist" historians have simply reversed the bias, making school reformers the villains and their opponents the heroes. Either value bias tends to collapse the complexity of educational history and to side-step methodological problems in determining intent.

A third corollary of the assumption that state schooling was a good thing is the equation of growth with progress. Methodologically this prompted historians to glory in numerical growth, often without controlling for parallel population growth or monetary inflation, and without taking seriously the differential educational opportunities of different groups. The tendency is seen equally in the traditional history of Roman Catholic schooling, which is largely a chronicle of increasing schools, children, and budgets.

A fourth corollary of the goodness theme is the focus on leadership and organization rather than on the educational behavior and attitudes of ordinary people. The methodological implication of this focus on the governors rather than on the clients of schooling is to give central attention to public records created by elites rather than attempting to tease out of scanty evidence some inkling of the educational lives of the inarticulate, as recent social historians of education have been attempting to do.

The great majority of books and doctoral dissertations written prior to 1950 on the history of education adhered to this paradigm, focusing on the progressive and beneficial evolution of state school systems. There were some notable exceptions, and even within the paradigm, many excellent legal, institutional, and intellectual studies were written. Nonetheless, the traditional framework had long outlived its usefulness by the late 1950s and early 1960s, when it came under attack.

2. Two Strands of Revisionism

The two major thrusts of revision in the history of education resulted from rather distinct critiques of the two major tenets of the traditional paradigm: that is, that the history of education is essentially the history of schooling and second, that state-regulated schooling was benign and desirable. The first critique broadened the focus of educational history to look at various agencies of instruction other than schools in America; it has yielded its finest fruits in the works of Bernard Bailyn and Lawrence Cremin on the colonial period, when schooling was much less important than today in the transmission of knowledge. It remains to be seen whether this broader focus can be applied successfully to the history of education in more recent periods. It will be more difficult to research and construct a coherent account of all the ways children learn in twentieth-century society. Merely broadening the definition to include every aspect of socialization would leave the historian of education hopelessly adrift; each historian must therefore now decide carefully what definition of education lurks in his or her work, and this must depend upon what questions are being asked. If one is asking questions about how children acquire skills and beliefs in a society, then the definition of education must be quite broad indeed. If, on the other hand, one is asking questions about the origins of state policy toward education, it is legitimate to focus on schooling, because past policymakers, like past historians, have equated schooling with education. Society as a whole educates in many ways; but the state educates through schools.

There has been a second, quite different, strand of revision in recent educational history, one which has caused considerable commotion among educators. These revisionists have questioned the assumption that state-regulated schooling has been generated by democratic and humanitarian impulses, and the assumption that it has resulted in democratic opportunity. Their work has emphasized variously the exploitative nature of capitalism and how schools relate to it, the culturally abusive nature of values asserted by the schools, and the negative aspects of increasingly bureaucratic school systems. This reversal of ideological perspective on the development of school systems has not always resulted in methodologically sophisticated work, although as a whole the works labeled "radical revisionism" have raised important questions about the gloomier aspects of educational systems and have made some persuasive statements about the educational failures of state schooling in industrial nations. Since this entry is about methodology, not ideology, it is not the place to argue the merits of the radical view of school history.

3. Quantitative Methods

A newer brand of revisionism has been pursued by historians of various ideological persuasions. Their methods and their subject matter may help answer some of the questions raised by the radicals. These quantitative, social historians have devised the most substantial and problematic methodological innovations. Two aspects of the inadequate traditional framework summarized above were a naive use of numerical data and a focus on the leaders rather than on the clients of educational institutions. Recent social historians of education have taken these problems as their starting-point. They have adopted techniques from sociology and statistics to map out in some detail patterns of literacy, school attendance, years of schooling, school expenditures, voter characteristics on school issues, and other characteristics and have tried to chart changes over time. Much of this work would have been impossible in the early 1960s. It has been made possible by the development of computer programs for social scientists and by the availability of microfilmed sources of information, such as the manuscript United States censuses of the nineteenth century. The inspiration and the models have been provided by historical demographers and by other social historians, who have been charting changing family structures, mobility patterns, wealth distribution, and other phenomena that affect common people. The new emphasis on parents and children in educational history also parallels similar emphases in other fields of educational research: sociologists are studying family background and schooling outcomes, lawyers are studying students' rights, and philosophers are studying the ethics of child–adult relations.

Hopefully, the complex description provided by quantitative historical studies will help develop understanding about educational supply and demand in the past, about the role of schooling in different types of communities, about the different school experiences of different social groups, and about the impact of schooling on later life in different historical periods. The great virtue of quantitative education history is that it places historians in touch with the realities of schooling in the past; it provides a way to start doing history from the bottom up, as it were, and a way to compare popular behavioral patterns with the opinions and policies of educational leaders. However, the quantitative social historian of education also faces problems, problems so numerous and frustrating that they cause some researchers to shun the techniques altogether. Others feel compelled by questions that demand quantitative answers, and they are groping toward a more adequate descriptive social history of education, and to theories that will help explain the patterns they are discovering.

Here is a short list of the problems they encounter. First, statistics and computers are unfamiliar, even alien, to many historians. Even for those who learn the techniques, the work is still very time-consuming and expensive. Experts are constantly devising improved and more arcane statistical techniques. Social historians have trailed along behind sociologists and economists, picking and choosing the techniques that seem most appropriate. Some have moved from simple cross-tabulations and graphs into multiple regression analysis and its various offspring. The social historian who can solve these problems of time, money, and expertise then has to worry about the audience. Most readers of history balk at simple tables; but statistical adequacy demands detailed documentation and detailed presentation of results. This creates problems of style. Methodological sophistication is not worth much if it cannot reach the audience it is aimed at, but it is difficult to serve a technical audience and a general audience in the same work.

As serious as these matters of training and style are, there are more substantive methodological problems in quantitative educational history. First, the data are crude and incomplete. Often the available school and population censuses were ambiguous on crucial matters, or failed to ask the questions that are of most interest now. Most of the data are cross-sectional; they provide only a snapshot of a group at a given moment; but education is a process, and many important questions about educational careers, or the influence of education on people's lives, can be answered only by data that trace individuals over time. Similarly, questions about the role of education in economic development require comparable aggregate data over time. Some historians have taken up this challenge and have developed longitudinal files by linking data from different sources, but that task is prodigious, and the attrition rate in studies of individuals (the cases lost by geographical mobility, death, and the ambiguity of common names) is so great as to render many conclusions dubious. More commonly, historians have tried to infer process from cross-sectional data. For example, they have examined length of schooling among different social groups by calculating the school-entry and school-leaving ages of different individuals in sample years; or, they have made inferences about the impact of industrialization on communities' educational practices by comparing communities at different stages of industrialization in a given year. Although the questions are about process, in neither case do the data trace individual children or communities over time. The logical and methodological problems of inferring process from static information are serious, and they constitute a central problem in quantitative history today.

Even within legitimate cross-sectional analysis—that is, in pursuing questions about a population at a given moment in time—there is a conflict between statistical adequacy and conceptual adequacy. Limits on research resources and on available data often result in small historical samples. In order to attain statistically significant results, it is sometimes necessary to collapse categories that should remain distinct. For example, if an attempt is being made to relate ethnic background and teenage school attendance while controlling for parental occupation, it may

be necessary to combine immigrant groups with quite different cultural and economic features, in order to achieve statistically significant comparisons between children of immigrants and nonimmigrants. The best solution, of course, is to provide the reader with both the significant statistics for the grossly aggregated categories, as well as the descriptively useful information about the smaller subcategories. Here again, though, there are problems of space limits or sheer tedium in presentation.

There are numerous other problems in this new area of research in educational history. For instance, it is difficult to know how conscientiously the data were reported in the first place, or what biases operated; caution on this matter is reinforced when substantial contradictions are found between different sources that claim to measure the same variable in the same population. It is also difficult to create time series on educational variables like attendance, teachers' salaries, educational expenditures, or length of school year, because often the items were defined differently in different periods or omitted altogether.

Despite these many problems, however, some impressive work is beginning to emerge, work which helps to locate the history of education more solidly in the context of social structure and economic development. It is hardly a time for methodological self-congratulation, but neither is it a time for despair. One of the important by-products of this quantitative work in educational history has been to sustain the methodological self-consciousness that began with the critiques of the traditional paradigm in the early 1960s. When the historian does not take methodology for granted, and when his or her methodology is critically scrutinized by other researchers, and when historians are constantly searching for new sources of evidence and techniques of analysis, better work should result.

Not all questions are amenable to quantitative research. It is important to remember that history of education is still vitally concerned with the history of educational ideas. Much good work remains to be done on popular attitudes, on the quality of educational experience in the past, and on the intellectual and institutional history of education. The excitement since the early 1960s has not resulted in a new single methodology, nor in a new, broadly accepted interpretation of educational history. However, the collapse of the old consensus has caused educational historians to explore new questions, discard old assumptions, try new techniques, and attempt to meet more rigorous standards of evidence and argument.

4. Complementary Methods

Many great social theorists, including Karl Marx, Max Weber, Emile Durkheim, Ferdinand Tönnies, and Talcott Parsons, wrote about history. Contemporary theorists from disciplines as diverse as sociology, linguistics, anthropology, philosophy, and statistics also do work that is relevant to historical study. Historians, however, differ in the amount of importance they give to theory, about whether they should attempt to test general theories with historical data, or about whether historians should get involved with theories at all.

There are several reasons why historians should read about theory and think about its relationship to their work. Because historical writing is selective and interpretive, it is necessarily guided by the individual historian's sense of what is important, where to find meaning, and how social change and human motivation work. The answers arise partly from the materials, of course. Although history is not *merely* inductive, it is *partly* inductive. The answers also lie, however, in an individual historian's temperament, convictions, hunches, and theories, whether explicit or implicit. By paying attention to the best theoretical work in related disciplines, historians can better identify their informal, personal theories. More important, they can shape their understanding of human experience by learning from other disciplines. Finally, historical work can reflect back in important ways on social theories, confirming, refuting, or modifying various theoretical statements. A historian need not, therefore, adopt an entire theoretical system in order to profit from theoretical work in other disciplines. Some excellent work has been done from rigorous and systematic theoretical viewpoints, but most historians use theory incidentally and selectively.

Theory has many implications for historical methodology, too numerous to cover in this entry. Theories may influence what sort of evidence we look for, what sort of evidence we will accept, and what sort of arguments we will make from the evidence. For example, if one accepts the Marxist theorem that an individual's relationship to the means of production is crucial to his experience, one will make a concerted effort to determine historical actors' class status and class consciousness, and one will make class a prominent part of the explanation of historical events. If one accepts anthropologist Clifford Geertz's theory that ritualistic or even apparently trivial everyday behavior can symbolize the deeper meaning of a culture, one will devote much attention to developing an interpretation that moves from observed behavior to cultural meaning. Whether a historian accepts a large theoretical system, uses theory incidentally, or resists the mixing of theory and historical writing, each should be conversant with major theoretical positions in related disciplines and self-conscious about their possible relevance for historical methodology.

5. Conclusion: Pervasive Methodological Concerns

There are four key problems to watch for when assessing arguments about the history of education, problems that have been highlighted by recent work in the social history of education, but which are also pertinent to the intellectual history of education, the institutional history of education, and other approaches.

The first problem is the confusion of correlations and causes, a problem particularly salient in quantitative work, but certainly not unique to it. To demonstrate that two phenomena occur together systematically is not, of course, to prove that one causes the other, but historians as well as social scientists are constantly tempted into this kind of argument. For example, Irish families in nineteenth-century urban America sent their children to school less often and for fewer years, on the average, than many other groups. This does not, however, demonstrate that "Irishness" (whatever that is) caused low school attendance. First, it must be asked whether Irish immigrants also tended to be poor, because it might be poverty that caused low attendance. Then it would be necessary to control for family structure, religion, and other factors. If, in the end, after controlling for all other measurable factors, Irish status was independently associated with low school attendance, a causal relationship would still not have been established. It would be necessary to investigate, and speculate on, why and how being Irish affected school-going. Correlations are just concerned with proximate occurrence; causality is about how things work, and correlations do not indicate much about how things work. Because human motivation is often multiple and vague and because society is not very much like a clock, historians must exercise great caution in moving from systematic statistical associations to assertions of causality.

The second problem to which critical readers must give close attention is the problem of defining key terms. The problem of definition can be subdivided into two common pitfalls: vagueness and presentism. As an example of vagueness, the notion that industrialization caused educational reform is commonplace in educational history. However, the statement has almost no analytical value until the meanings of the umbrella terms "industrialization" and "educational reform" are specified. In contrast, consider the statement: "The expansion of wage labor in nineteenth-century communities or regions was followed by an expansion of annual school enrollment." This is much more precise, has important causal implications, and is amenable to empirical research.

By "presentism" is meant the danger of investing key terms from the past with their present connotations, or, conversely, applying to past developments present-day terms that did not exist or meant something else at the time. A classic example in American educational history involves the use of the word "public." In the eighteenth century a "public" educational institution was one in which children learned collectively, in contrast with private tutorial education, and it was one devoted to education for the public good, as opposed to mere selfish gain. Thus the colonial colleges, which were controlled by self-perpetuating trustees and financed mainly by tuition, were thoroughly "public" and were called so at the time, as in England. In today's terminology they would be called "private" in American, but calling them "private" in historical work greatly muddles understanding of eighteenth-century society. Avoiding presentism thus means paying close attention to the etymology of key terms, and it is a methodological imperative in good history.

A third problem that critical consumers of educational history should keep in mind is the distinction between ideas about how people should behave and how ordinary people in fact behaved. Too often evidence of the latter is lacking and evidence of the former is allowed to stand in its place; that is, it is assumed that people did as they were told. The methodological dilemma is posed by the following problem: if the legal and legislative bodies of a society constantly passed rules requiring school attendance, is it evidence that the society valued schooling highly, expressing this value in their legislation, or is it evidence of a society that did not value school-going very much, thus alarming its leaders into coercive efforts? To answer the question, something needs to be known about school attendance patterns by different groups. Here is a more specific example. There was widespread agreement among professional educators and physicians beginning in the late 1830s in the northeastern part of the United States that school attendance by very young children was unwise, even dangerous to their health, as well as being a nuisance to teachers. Parents were constantly urged to keep their children under 5 or 6 at home. This campaign continued throughout the 1840s and 1850s. To infer from this that children normally began school at age 5 or 6 during these decades, however, would be incorrect. Parents resisted the conventional expertise. As is now known from analysis of manuscript censuses and statistical school reports, they persisted in sending 3- and 4-year-old children to school, for reasons that can only be guessed at, until they were coerced to keep them home by local regulations on age of school entry in the 1850s and 1860s. Only then did the aggregate average age of entry rise substantially. Here, then, is an example of the lag between elite opinion and popular behavior, one which warns against equating literary sources with popular behavior. Child-rearing manuals may not cause or even reflect actual child-rearing practices; and exhortations about educational policies often fall on deaf ears.

The fourth and final problem has to do with the distinction between intent and consequences. No matter how wise educational leaders have been, their powers of foresight have rarely equaled the historians' powers of hindsight. It is an inherent advantage in historical analysis—and yet it is a problem too: historians know how things turned out. The problem lies in the danger of assuming that the historical actors could have (and should have) foreseen the full consequences of their ideas and of the institutions they shaped. It is undoubt-edly true that many of the consequences of educational leadership have been precisely as the leaders intended; it does not follow, however, that intent can be inferred from consequences. The fact that large bureaucracies are effective instruments of racial discrimination does not necessarily mean that their creators had a racist intent. The fact that schooling has done an unimpressive job in reducing crime does not mean that school reformers who touted it for that purpose were hypocrites. Intent cannot be inferred from consequences. Direct evidence is needed of intent at the time an act occurred.

No historian can completely transcend or resolve these four problems, but each must recognize the problems and the associated methodological challenges when trying to make meaningful generalizations about the educational past. Historians have always been scavengers. Since history involves all human experience and thought, historians have constantly raided other disciplines for new techniques of analysis and for new insights into society and human nature. This helps explain why there is no single methodology in history, and why historians love their craft so much: because it is so complex and so all-encompassing.

Recent trends in the history of education—the effort to see education as broader than schooling, the effort to see school systems in the context of social and economic development, and the effort to study popular attitudes and behavior as well as the history of elite intentions and actions—have greatly accelerated the borrowing process in this historical subfield. Historians of education have reached out and become involved in the history of the family, of childhood, and of reform institutions, for example, in addition to deepening their traditional commitment to economic and political history as a context for educational development. They have also explored recent sociology, anthropology, psychology, and statistics for new ideas and techniques. Because this period of exploration and revision has resulted in a diverse, eclectic methodology, because no new methodological or ideological consensus has emerged—in short, because there is no successful paradigm in educational history today, it is all the more important that each reader of educational history be critically alert and independent.

See also: History of Educational Research; Oral History; Educational History in Biographies and Autobiographies

Bibliography

Bailyn B 1960 *Education in the Forming of American Society*. University of North Carolina Press, Chapel Hill, North Carolina

Baker D N, Harrigan P J (eds.) 1980 *The Making of Frenchmen: Current Directions in the History of Education in France, 1679–1979*. Wilfred Laurier University Press, Waterloo, Ontario

Butterfield H 1931 *The Whig Interpretation of History*. Bell, London

Carnoy M 1974 *Education as Cultural Imperialism*. McKay, New York

Craig J 1981 The expansion of education. In: Berliner D (ed.) 1981 *Review of Research in Education*. American Educational Research Association, Washington, DC

Cremin L A 1970 *American Education: The Colonial Experience, 1607–1783*. Harper and Row, New York

Cubberley E P 1934 *Public Education in the United States: A Study and Interpretation of American Educational History*. Houghton-Mifflin, Boston, Massachusetts

Dore R F 1967 *Education in Tokugawa, Japan*. Routledge and Kegan Paul, London

Johansson E 1973 *Literacy and Society in a Historical Perspective*. University Press, Umea

Kaestle C F 1992 Theory in comparative educational history: A middle ground. In: Goodenow R, Marsden W (eds.) 1992 *The City and Education in Four Nations*. Cambridge University Press, Cambridge

Kaestle C F 1992 Standards of evidence in educational research: How do we know when we know? *Hist. Educ. Q.* 32: 361–66

Kaestle C F, Vinovskis M A 1980 *Education and Social Change in Nineteenth-century Massachusetts*. Cambridge University Press, New York

Katz M B 1968 *The Irony of Early School Reform: Educational Innovation in Mid-nineteenth Century Massachusetts*. Harvard University Press, Cambridge, Massachusetts

Laqueur T W 1976 *Religion and Respectability: Sunday Schools and Working-class Culture, 1780–1850*. Yale University Press, New Haven, Connecticut

Maynes M J 1979 The virtues of archaism: The political economy of schooling in Europe, 1750–1850. *Comp. Stud. Soc. Hist.* 21: 611–25

Novick P 1988 *That Noble Dream: The "Objectivity Question" and the American Historical Profession*. Cambridge University Press, Cambridge

Rury J 1993 Methods of historical research in education. In: Lancey D *Research in Education*. Longman, New York

Simon B 1960 *Studies in the History of Education, 1780–1870*. Lawrence and Wishart, London

Spaull A 1981 The biographical tradition in the history of Australian education. *Aust. N.Z. Hist. Educ. Soc. J.* 10: 1–10.

Stone L 1969 Literacy and education in England, 1640–1900. *Past and Present* 42: 61–139.

Thaubault R 1971 *Education and Change in a Village Community, Mazières-en-Gâtine, 1848–1914*. Schocken, New York

Tyack D B 1974 *The One Best System: A History of American Urban Education*. Harvard University Press, Cambridge, Massachusetts

Narrative Inquiry

F. M. Connelly and D. J. Clandinin

One of the dilemmas of educational studies is that often the more rigorous and scientific educational research becomes, the less it is connected to human experience. The objectivists sometimes call those who study experience "soft" and "subjective"; conversely experientialists claim that the scientific study of education depersonalizes, dehumanizes, and objectifies people. Narrative and story-telling, two intimately related terms, are increasingly evident in the literature that swirls around these compelling scientific–humanistic modes of inquiry. They are terms representing ideas about the nature of human experience and about how experience may be studied and represented and about which they tread a middle course between the extremes. Narrativists believe that human experience is basically storied experience: that humans live out stories and are story-telling organisms. They further believe that one of the best ways to study human beings is to come to grips with the storied quality of human experience, to record stories of educational experience, and to write still other interpretative stories of educational experience. The complex written stories are called narratives. Properly done these stories are close to experience because they directly represent human experience; and they are close to theory because they give accounts that are educationally meaningful for participants and readers. The creation of these stories in research is based on particular experiential methods and criteria. This entry outlines the theoretical origins of narrative inquiry; gives a brief description of narrative studies in education; describes appropriate methodologies; delineates distinctions between the field, field texts, and research texts; and outlines appropriate research criteria.

1. Theoretical Context for Narrative Inquiry in Education

Narrative has a long history in the study of fictional literature. Perhaps because it focuses on human experience, perhaps because story is a fundamental structure of human experience, and perhaps because it has an holistic quality, narrative is exploding into other disciplines. Narrative is a way of characterizing the phenomena of human experience and its study that is appropriate to many social science fields.

Literary theory is the principal intellectual resource. The fact that a story is inherently temporal means that history and the philosophy of history (Carr 1986), which are essentially the study of time, have a special role to play in shaping narrative studies in the social sciences. Therapeutic fields are also making significant contributions. Psychology has only recently discovered narrative although Polkinghorne (1988a) claimed that closely related inquiries were part of the field at the beginning of the twentieth century but disappeared after the Second World War when they were suffocated by physical science paradigms. Among the most fundamental and educationally suggestive works on the nature of narrative is Johnson's (1989) philosophical study of bodily knowledge and language. Because education is ultimately a moral and spiritual pursuit, MacIntyre's (1984) narrative ethical theory and Crites' (1986) theological writing on narrative are especially useful for educational purposes. (For a review of narrative in and out of education see Connelly and Clandinin (1990), and Clandinin and Connelly (1991).)

2. Related Educational Studies

Berk (1980) stated that autobiography was one of the first methodologies for educational study, though it essentially disappeared until recently (Pinar 1988, Grumet 1988). Autobiography is related to narrative (Connelly and Clandinin 1988a). The focus here is on an individual's psychology considered over a span of time.

Narrative inquiry may also be sociologically concerned with groups and the formation of community (Carr 1986). To date in the 1990's in education, personal rather than social narrative inquiries have been more in evidence. In educational studies a social narrative inquiry emphasis has tended to be on teacher careers and professionalism. It is expected that social narrative will be increasingly emphasized in research.

Some closely related lines of inquiry focus specifically on story: oral history and folklore (Dorson 1976), children's story-telling (Applebee 1978), and the uses of story in preschool and school language experience (Sutton–Smith 1986). Oral history suggests a range of phenomena for narrative inquiry, such as material culture, custom, arts, recollections, and myths. Myths are the storied structures that stand behind folklore and oral history. Van Maanen (1988) provided an introduction to the ethnography of story-telling, both as subject matter and as ethnographers' written form. The best known educational use of oral history in North America is the Foxfire Project (Wigginton 1989). There have been curriculum proposals for organizing subject matter along story lines (Egan 1986). In research on curriculum, teachers' narratives are seen as a metaphor for teaching–learning relationships. In understanding teachers and students educationally, it is necessary to develop an understanding of people with a narrative of life experience. Life's narratives are the context for making meaning of school situations.

Because of its focus on experience and the qualities

of life and education, narrative is situated in a matrix of qualitative research. Eisner's (1988) review of the educational study of experience aligns narrative with qualitatively oriented educational researchers working with experiential philosophy, psychology, critical theory, curriculum studies, and anthropology. Elbaz (1988) focused on teacher thinking studies and showed how feminist studies and studies of the personal are related to narrative. She aligned narrative with many other educational studies which often use participant stories as raw data (e.g., case work research on expert teachers and naturalistic approaches to evaluation).

There is a large literature of teachers' stories and stories of teachers which is narrative in quality but which is not found in standard review documents. This literature refers to accounts of individual teachers, students, classrooms, and schools written by teachers and others.

In this overview of narrative inquiry it is desirable to locate narrative in a historical intellectual context. On the one hand, narrative inquiry may be traced to Aristotle's *Poetics* and St Augustine's *Confessions* (see Ricoeur's [1984] use of these two sources to link time and narrative) and may be seen to have various adaptations and applications in a diversity of disciplines including education. Dewey's (e.g., 1938) work on time, space, experience, and sociality is also central. On the other hand, there is a newness to narrative inquiry as it has developed in the social sciences, including education. The educational importance of this line of work is that it brings theoretical ideas about the nature of human life as lived to bear on educational experience as lived.

3. The Process of Narrative Inquiry

The process of narrative research revolves around three matters: the field, texts on field experience, and research texts which incorporate the first two and which represent those issues of social significance that justify the research. Field, field text, research text, and the relations among them, name primary narrative inquiry decision foci. The relations between researcher and field range from the researcher being a neutral observer to the researcher going native as an active participant. The relations between researcher and field text based on the field experience involve complex questions of the representation of experience, the interpretation and reconstruction of experience, and appropriate text forms. Constructing a research text involves the presence of the autobiographical researcher and the significance of this presence for the research text and for the field it represents. The main point about the transition from field text to research text is that the research text is written for an audience of other researchers and practitioners and must be written in such a way as to go beyond the particulars of experience captured in field texts.

3.1 Working in the Field: Experiencing the Experience

The major issue confronting narrative researchers in the field is their relationship with participants. Traditional methodologies have taught that researchers should be objective and distant from participants, ensuring unbiased results. In narrative research different degrees of closeness with participants are deliberately negotiated with the result that the experience of the researcher becomes intermingled with participants' field experience. The field is no longer being studied in a detached way. It is the field in relation to the researcher that is the object of study. This means that researchers need to pay close attention to their own experience and to the stories of them. They need to understand, document, and think through the consequences of establishing different degrees of closeness with participants.

The second major field concern for a narrative researcher is to look beyond the immediacy of any experience under study. For example, it is not enough to study the opening activities of a school day without understanding that those activities have a history for this teacher, for that class, for this school, and also for the larger history of schooling and culture. Narrative inquiry needs to establish the narrative, cultural history of the events under study for later interpretation in the creation of research texts.

A third major field concern, one which carries through all phases of research including publication, is the negotiation of ethical relationships among researchers and participants (Clandinin and Connelly 1988b). Ethical review protocols for qualitative research are well established in many institutions. Narrative inquiry requires special attention to these matters.

3.2 From Field to Field Texts

What are normally called data (e.g., field notes) are, in narrative research, better thought of as field texts. These are texts created by participants and researchers to represent aspects of field experience. They are called field texts rather than data because texts have a narrative quality. The common notion of data is that they are an objective recording of events. Field texts do not have that quality. They grow out of complex field experience involving relations among researchers and participants and they are selected, interpretative records of that experience. Researchers' relationships to participants' stories shape the field texts and establish their epistemological status. Narrative researchers need continually to monitor and record, the quality of these relationships and their influence on the status of the field texts. In the following section several methods for constructing field texts are outlined.

3.3 Oral History

One method for creating field texts is oral history. There are several strategies for obtaining an oral histo-

ry, ranging from the use of a structured set of questions in which the researchers' intentions are uppermost, to asking a person to tell his or her own story in his or her own way in which the participant's intentions are uppermost. There is a tradition of oral history in the study of culture (e.g., Gluck and Patai 1991). (See *Oral History*.)

3.4 Stories

A closely connected method is the telling or writing of stories. Stories are pervasive in human and social experience. Individuals have stories of their own experience, of school, and of their profession. Furthermore, institutions have a storied quality. For example, teachers, parents, students, and others tell stories about their school. There are also community and cultural stories about schooling generally, and about education and its place in society. Some of these stories take on the quality of myths and sacred stories (Crites 1986).

3.5 Annals and Chronicles

Annals are a simple dated history of significant moments or events for an individual or institution. Annals permit researchers to gain a historical context for the events under study. Chronicles are more thematic representations of the annals. Chronicles represent a thematic aspect of the field of interest (e.g., a chronicle of a school's administration).

3.6 Photographs, Memory Boxes, Other Personal/Institutional Artifacts

Physical artifacts are repositories of experience. The items that a person collects and a school's trophies and mementos can, with discussion with knowledgeable participants, reveal important depths of experience. These items, furthermore, are important triggers for memory.

3.7 Research Interviews

Interviews can be made into field texts by verbatim transcription, note-taking, and the use of interview segments. Interview methodologies range from inquisitional questioning to informal conversation on mutually agreed upon topics to therapeutic methods that shift the focus of inquiry to the participant. Interviews are one of the clearest places for seeing the significant effect that different researcher–participant relationships have on the kind of data collected and field texts written.

3.8 Journals

Journals have been increasingly used for teaching purposes. It is sometimes overlooked that the same qualities that make them an influential teaching tool also make them a valid research tool. Journals provide both a descriptive and reflective record of events, and of personal responses to them. Journals tend to be written in solitude and in a participant's personal time. The energy to write them often flags unless the participant has strong personal reasons for continuing.

3.9 Autobiographical and Biographical Writing

Autobiography and biography are more comprehensive methods than the compilation of journals for interpreting life experience. Narrative researchers commonly think of a life as a story in which a person is the central character and author. Therefore, autobiographical or biographical field texts are interpretative retellings of a story already lived. This interpretative, in contrast to objective, quality applies to other kinds of field texts described in this section. Furthermore, "data" are commonly thought to be true or not. When it can be shown that they "could be otherwise," their validity is undermined. But autobiographical or biographical field texts can always "be otherwise" as they are written for one or other purpose, thereby emphasizing one or other narrative theme. The fact that many autobiographical or biographical field texts may be written for any participant does not undermine the validity of the research provided its purposes are clear and its relationship to the field is established. This point of diversity applies to other field texts though it is most evident in autobiography and biography. (See *Educational History in Biographies and Autobiographies.*)

3.10 Letters

Letters, unlike journals, are written to another person with the expectation of a response. Both letters and journals are used in autobiographical and biographical methods. It is common to write intellectual biographies of key figures in the social and physical sciences (e.g., Charles Darwin), and to base these, in part, on letters. Letters reveal much about the intellectual and social conditions in a person's thought. This applies to the use of letters in narrative research whether or not the research is biographically oriented.

3.11 Conversations

Conversation covers many kinds of activities, including letter writing. Usually conversation refers to nonhierarchical oral exchanges among researchers and participants in collaborative inquiries. Because of the underlying trust in conversation, this methodology may end up probing more deeply than aggressive questioning techniques. Conversations tend to be open-ended and therefore require special attention to methods of recording and interpretation.

3.12 Field Notes and Other Stories from the Field

Field notes are the standard ethnographic method of data collection. Commonly thought to be drafted by researchers, field notes may, in collaborative studies, be written by participants. Field notes may take the form of descriptive records, theoretical memos, points of view, biases, and speculations. Researchers anxious to represent experience truthfully may replace field notes with tape or video recordings. While these time-consuming methods are sometimes warranted, researchers should only use them when verbatim verbal or physical acts are essential.

3.13 Document Analysis

Documents are an easily overlooked source of field texts, particularly in the narrative study of groups and institutions. Documents have a special status because they are public records and often represent an official position. The narrative context in which documents were written and used is crucial to their interpretation and researchers need to collect information on dates, authors, personalities, contextual matters (e.g., board policies as context for a school document), climates of opinion, and so on.

4. From Field Texts to Research Texts

Converting field texts into research texts is a difficult phase of narrative research. Ordinarily the process consists of the construction of a series of increasingly interpretative writings. For instance, a narrative study of the influence of immigration on school opening and closing routines might involve any or all of the above methodologies to construct a second order historical field text. The text might be so compellingly interesting because of its factual and textual liveliness in the form of conversations and personal anecdote that the research might conclude prematurely. This frequently happens with autobiographical and biographical work, where the writing may be so interesting to the researchers that they neglect to consider the social significance of the text or why it might be of interest to others. Field texts tend to be close to experience, descriptive, and shaped around specific events. They have the quality of being a record. Research texts on the other hand tend to be at a distance from the field and from field texts. They are written in response to questions about meaning and significance. It is not enough to write a narrative: the author needs to understand the meaning of the narrative and its significance for others and for social issues. Research texts, therefore, tend to be patterned. Field texts are shaped into research texts by the underlying narrative threads and themes that constitute the driving force of the inquiry.

The intermingling of the researcher's outlooks and points of view which were so central in the field and in the creation of field texts plays an equally important role in the writing of research texts. Relationships established in the field and reflected in field texts are also evident in the thematic reinterpretation of those field texts into research texts. Thus, throughout a narrative inquiry the *researcher's presence* needs to be acknowledged, understood, and written into the final research account. Discovering a researcher's presence in a research text has traditionally been sufficient justification to dismiss the text as inappropriately subjective. But the reverse applies in narrative inquiry: a text written as if the researcher had no autobiographical presence would constitute a deception about the epistemological status of the research. Such a study lacks validity.

Voice and signature are two terms helpful in understanding autobiographical presence. Voice refers to a researcher's sense of having something to say. There is no voice in extreme forms of "objective" research because it is the reliability and validity of the method, and not of the researcher, that is the basis for judgment of the research. But voice creates personal risks for researchers because they must take stands on matters that are only partially supported by field texts. Taken to the extremes, voice is merely an excuse to vent the researcher's biases. Too strong a voice leads to an autocratic subjectivity; too little voice leads to technical objectivity. The dilemma for a researcher is to establish a voice that simultaneously represents participants' field experience while creating a research text that goes beyond the field and its field texts to speak to an audience. There are no formal rules for establishing voice and the matter can only be sorted out judicially study by study.

Signature refers to the writing style that makes it possible to identify a text as an author's work. Developing a signature is difficult, especially for novice narrative researchers. The traditional research signature is impersonal and marked by a well-known structure of problem, literature review, data, etc. But narrative research texts have a personal signature and may be written in seemingly endless literary, poetic, and scientific ways. A word of practical advice for novice narrative researchers is to model their writing on a researcher they admire, just as novice artists become apprenticed to a master painter. The adaptations of a master researcher's work will eventually yield a signature for the apprentice narrative researcher.

Voice and signature come together in the writing of a research text aimed at an audience. The audience redirects a researcher's attention from participant and research self to others and thereby complicates the problem of voice and signature which are more easily established in the field and in the writing of field texts. The researcher now needs to decide on a relationship with the audience. Chatman (1990) described four kinds of research texts which yield four kinds of relationships: descriptive, expositional, argumentative, and narrative. Providing descriptive information differs from explaining (exposition), convincing (argument), or inviting readers into storied meanings with the author (narrative). Each text form can be used in the service of others. For instance, a narrative study

might yield a set of narrative field texts. But the author may wish to influence a policy, school practice, or research direction and decide to write an argumentative "if–then" research text for this purpose. Accordingly, a narrative inquiry may, but need not, be concluded with a narrative research text. Thus, the researcher's intended relationship to an audience complicates the matter of voice and signature since each of these four research text forms has its own qualities independent of the researcher.

5. Notes On Criteria

Because narrative methods in education are so new, and because qualitative methods in general are new and not fully established, in the early 1990s there was much writing on the criteria for judging narrative inquiry. The most important thing to note for this entry is that criteria have been under discussion. In general it may be said that reliability and validity have assumed less importance as matters such as apparentness and verisimilitude have been raised. The mainstay criteria of social science research are overrated and are being supplemented by numerous other considerations (Guba and Lincoln 1989). Narrative researchers are concerned with the representation of experience, causality, temporality, and the difference between the experience of time and the telling of time, narrative form, integrity of the whole in a research document, the invitational quality of a research text, its authenticity, adequacy, and plausibility. Currently, in narrative inquiry, it is important for each researcher to set forth the criteria that govern the study and by which it may be judged. It is also the case that others may quite legitimately adopt other criteria in support of, or in criticism of, the work. The development of narrative inquiry within the social sciences is fascinating to follow as debates rage over narrative inquiry's challenges to traditional research forms.

See also: Biographical Research Methods; Educational History in Biographies and Autobiographies; Oral History.

References

Applebee A N 1978 *The Child's Concept of Story: Ages Two to Seventeen.* University of Chicago Press, Chicago, Illinois

Berk L 1980 Education in lives: Biographic narrative in the study of educational outcomes. *J. Curr. Theor.* 2(2): 88–153

Carr D 1986 *Time, Narrative, and History.* Indiana University Press, Bloomington, Indiana

Chatman S 1990 *Coming to Terms: The Rhetoric of Narrative in Fiction and Film.* Cornell University Press, Ithaca, New York

Clandinin D J, Connelly F M 1991 Narrative and story in practice and research. In: Schön D A (ed.) 1991 *The Reflective Turn: Case Studies in and on Educational Practice.* Teachers College Press, New York

Connelly F M, Clandinin D J 1988a *Teachers as Curriculum Planners: Narratives of Experience.* Teachers College Press, New York

Connelly F M, Clandinin D J 1988b Studying teachers' knowledge of classrooms: Collaborative research, ethics, and the negotiation of narrative. *The Journal of Educational Thought* 22(2A): 269–82

Connelly F M, Cladinin D J 1990 Stories of experience and narrative inquiry. *Educ. Researcher* 19(5): 2–14

Crites S 1986 Storytime: Recollecting the past and projecting the future. In: Sarbin T R (ed.) 1986 *The Stories Nature of Human Conduct.* Praeger, New York

Dewey J 1938 *Experience and Education.* Macmillan, New York

Dorson R M 1976 *Folklore and Fakelore: Essays Toward a Discipline of Folkstudies.* Harvard University Press, Cambridge, Massachusetts

Egan K 1986 *Teaching as Story Telling: An Alternative Approach to Teaching and Curriculum in the Elementary School.* Althouse, London

Eisner E W 1988 The primacy of experience and the politics of method. *Educ. Researcher* 17(5): 15–20

Elbaz F 1988 Knowledge and discourse: The evolution of research on teacher thinking. Paper given at the Conference of the International Study Association on Teacher Thinking, University of Nottingham, September 1988

Gluck S B, Patai D (eds.) 1991 *Women's Words: The Feminist Practice of Oral History.* Routledge, New York

Grumet M R 1988 *Bitter Milk: Women and Teaching.* University of Massachusetts Press, Amherst, Massachusetts

Guba E G, Lincoln Y S 1989 *Fourth Generation Evaluation.* Sage, Newbury Park, California

Johnson M 1989 Special series on personal practical knowledge: Embodied knowledge. *Curric. Inq.* 19(4): 361–77

MacIntyre A 1981 *After Virtue: A Study in Moral Theory,* 2nd edn. University of Notre Dame Press, Notre Dame, Indiana

Pinar W F 1988 "Whole, bright, deep with understanding": Issues in qualitative research and autobiographical method. In: Pinar W F (ed.) 1988 *Contemporary Curriculum Discourses.* Gorsuch Scarisbrick, Scottsdale, Arizona

Polkinghorne D E 1988 *Narrative Knowing and the Human Sciences.* State University of New York Press, New York

Ricoeur P 1984 *Time and Narrative,* Vol. 1. University of Chicago Press, Chicago, Illinois

Sutton-Smith B 1986 Children's fiction making. In: Sarbin T R 1986 *Narrative Psychology: The Storied Nature of Human Conduct.* Praeger, New York

Van Maanen J 1988 *Tales of the Field: On Writing Ethnography.* University of Chicago Press, Chicago, Illinois

Wigginton E 1989 Foxfire grows up. *Harv. Educ. Rev.* 59(1): 24–49

Naturalistic and Rationalistic Enquiry

E. G. Guba and Y. S. Lincoln

Persons concerned with disciplined enquiry have tended to use what is commonly called the scientific paradigm—that is, model or pattern—of enquiry. A second paradigm, also aimed at disciplined enquiry, is currently emerging; this paradigm is commonly known as the naturalistic paradigm, although it is often referred to (mistakenly) as the case study of qualitative paradigm. Its distinguishing features are not, however, its format or methods, or even, as its title might suggest, the fact that it is usually carried out in natural settings. What differentiates the naturalistic from the scientific (or, as it is sometimes referred to, the rationalistic paradigm) approach is, at bottom, the different interpretations placed on certain basic axioms or assumptions. In addition, the two approaches characteristically take different postures on certain issues which, while not as basic as axiomatic propositions, are nevertheless fundamental to an understanding of how the naturalistic enquirer operates.

1. Axiomatic Differences Between the Naturalistic and Rationalistic Paradigms

Axioms may be defined as the set of undemonstrated (and undemonstrable) propositions accepted by convention or established by practice as the basic building blocks of some conceptual or theoretical structure or system. As such they are arbitrary and certainly not "self-evidently true." Different axiom systems have different utilities depending on the phenomenon to which they are applied; so, for example, Euclidean geometry as an axiomatic system has good fit to terrestial phenomena but Lobachevskian geometry (a non-Euclidean form) has better fit to interstellar phenomena. A decision about which of several axiom systems to employ for a given purpose is a matter of the relative "fit" between the axiom sets and the characteristics of the application area. It is the general contention of naturalists that the axioms of naturalistic enquiry provide a better fit to most social/behavioral phenomena than do the rationalistic axioms.

1.1 Axiom 1: The Nature of Reality

Rationalists assume that thee exists a single, tangible reality fragmentable into independent variables and processes, any of which can be studied independently of the others; enquiry can be caused to converge onto this single reality until, finally, it is explained. Naturalists assume that there exist multiple realities which are, in the main, constructions existing in the minds of people; they are therefore intangible and can be studied only in wholistic, and idiosyncratic, fashion. Enquiry into these multiple realities will inevitably diverge (the scope of the enquiry will enlarge) as more and more realities must be considered. Naturalists argue that while the rationalist assumptions undoubtedly have validity in the hard and life sciences, naturalist assumptions are more meaningful in studying human behavior. Naturalists do not deny the reality of the objects, events, or processes with which people interact, but suggest that it is the meanings given to or interpretations made of these objects, events, or processes that constitute the arena of interest to investigators of social/behavioral phenomena. Note that these constructions are not perceptions of the objects, events, or processes but of meaning and interpretation. The situation is very much approximated, the naturalist would say, by the ancient tale of the blind men and the elephant—provided it is conceded that there is no elephant.

1.2 Axiom 2: The Enquirer-Respondent Relationship

The rationalist assumes that the enquirer is able to maintain a discrete and inviolable distance from the "object" of enquiry; but concedes that when the object is a human being, special methodological safeguards, must be taken to prevent reactivity, that is, a reaction of the object to the conditions of the enquiry that will influence the outcome in undesirable ways. The naturalist assumes that the enquirer and the respondent in any human enquiry inevitably interact to influence one another. While safeguards need to be mounted in both directions, the interaction need not be eliminated (it is impossible to do that anyway) but should be exploited for the sake of the inquiry.

Naturalists point out that the proposition of subject-object independence is dubious even to areas like particle physics, as exemplified in the Heisenberg Uncertainty Principle. The effect is certainly more noticeable in dealing with people, they assert. Nor should it be supposed that the interpolation of a layer of apparently objective instrumentation (paper and pencil or brass) solves the problem. Enquirers react to the mental images they have of respondents in developing the instrumentation; respondents answer or act in terms of what they perceive to be expectations held for their behavior as they interpret the meaning of the items or tasks put before them; enquirers deal with responses in terms of their interpretation of response meaning and intent, and so on. Nor, say the naturalists, is interactivity a generally undesirable characteristic; indeed, if interactivity could be eliminated by some methodological tour de force, the trade off would not be worthwhile, because it is precisely the interactivity that makes it possible for the human instrument to achieve maximum responsiveness, adaptability, and insight.

1.3 Axiom 3: The Nature of Truth Statements

Rationalists assert that the aim of inquiry is to develop a nomothetic body of knowledge; this knowledge is best encapsulated in generalizations which are truth statements of enduring value that are context free. The stuff of which generalizations are made is the similarity among units; differences are set aside as intrinsically uninteresting. Naturalists assert that the aim of inquiry is to develop an idiographic body of knowledge; this knowledge is best encapsulated in a series of "working hypotheses" that describe the individual case. Generalizations are not possible since human behavior is never time or context free. Nevertheless, some transferability of working hypotheses from context to context may be possible depending on the similarity of the contexts (an empirical matter). Differences are as inherently important as (and at times more important than) the similarities. Naturalists well-understand the utility of generalizations such as $f = ma$ or $e = mc^2$ in physics, although even in the hard or life sciences, as Cronbach (1975) has pointed out, generalizations are much like radioactive materials, in that they decay and have a halflife. Surely it is unreasonable to suppose that analogous tendencies do not exist in the social and behavioral sciences?

1.4 Axiom 4: Causality

For the rationalist, the determination of cause-effect relationships is of prime importance; for each effect, it is assumed, there is a cause which can, given sufficiently sophisticated enquiry, be detected. The ultimate form for demonstrating cause-effect relationships is the experiment. The naturalist asserts that the determination of cause-effect is often a search for the Holy Grail. Human relationships are caught up in such an interacting web of factors, events, and processes that the hope that "the" cause-effect chain can be sorted out is vain; the best the enquirer can hope to establish are plausible patterns of influence. Naturalists point out that there have been a variety of cause-effect theories proposed since the simplistic "if-then" formulation was critiqued by Hume in the early eighteenth century, including Hume's own constant conjunctions or regularity theory, "law" theories, formulations about "necessary and sufficient" conditions, and more recently, various attributional and semantic theories of causation. All have flaws in the opinion of epistemologists; however, the attributional and semantic formulations provide some insight into the possibility that if the realities with which humans deal are constructed so, most likely, are their ideas of causation. If causality demonstrations are intended by rationalists to be compelling, naturalists feel the best they can do is to be persuasive. Causality can never be demonstrated in the "hard" sense; only patterns of plausible influence can be inferred.

1.5 Axiom 5: Relation to Values

Rationalists assume that enquiry is value free and can be guaranteed to be so by virtue of the "objective" methodology which the rationalist employs. The naturalist asserts that values impinge upon an enquiry in at least five ways, in terms of: the selection made by the investigator from among possible problems, theories, instruments, and data analysis modes; the assumptions underlying the substantive theory that guides the enquiry (for example, a theory of reading or an organizational theory); the assumptions underlying the methodological paradigm (as outlined in the preceding section on axioms); the values that characterize the respondents, the community, and the culture in which the enquiry is carried out (contextual values); and, finally, the possible interactions among any two or more of the preceding, which may be value consonant or value dissonant. Of particular interest is the possibility of resonance or dissonance between the substantive and methodological assumptions which can produce quite misleading results. Naturalists in particular take the position that many of the ambiguities and other irresolutions that tend to characterize social and behavioral research can be traced to such dissonances. So long as methodologies are assumed to be value free, naturalists assert, the problem of dissonance will not be recognized, since by definition it cannot exist. But once the role that values play in shaping enquiry is recognized, the problem becomes very real.

2. Postural Differences Between the Naturalistic and Rationalistic Paradigms

Postures differ from axioms in that they are not logically necessary to the integrity of the paradigm nor are they important to assess in determining fit between a paradigm and the area proposed to be studied. Nevertheless they characterize the "style" of the two positions and are, for a variety of reasons, "congenial" or reinforcing to the practice of each. Some writers who have been anxious to compromise the two paradigms—what might be called an attempt at conceptual ecumenicism—have pointed out that these postures may be seen as complementary, and have urged that both rationalists and naturalists attempt a middle course. But despite good intentions, neither group seems to have been able to respond to this advice, which gives rise to the possibility that, unless one wishes to write off enquirers of both camps as obstinate or intransigent, there must be some more fundamental reason for the failure. That reason is simply that there exists a synergism among the postures as practiced by either camp that virtually precludes compromise. In fact, the arguments that might be made by naturalists, say, in defense of their choices depend in the case of every posture on the choices made among the other postures. And so with rationalists.

Consider first the postures themselves; six are of special importance:

2.1 Preferred Methods

Rationalists tend to prefer quantitative methods probably because of their apparently greater precision and objectivity and because of the enormous advantage of being mathematically manipulable. Naturalists prefer qualitative methods, probably because they appear to promise the most wholistic products and they seem more appropriate to the use of a human as the prime data collection instrument. The distinction between quantitative and qualitative methods is often mistakenly taken to be the chief mark of distinction between the paradigms; in fact, the two dimensions are orthogonal. Either methodology is appropriate to either paradigm, even though in practice there is a high correlation between quantitative and rationalistic, on the one hand, and qualitative and naturalistic on the other.

2.2 Source of Theory

Rationalists insist on a priori formulations of theory; indeed, they are likely to assert that enquiry without a priori theory to guide it is mindless. The naturalist believes that it is not theory but the enquiry problem itself that guides and bounds the enquiry; that a priori theory constrains the enquiry to those elements recognized by the investigator as important, and may introduce biases (believing is seeing). In all events, theory is more powerful when it arises from the data rather than being imposed on them. The naturalist does not, of course, insist on grounding theory afresh in each and every enquiry; what the naturalist does insist on is that the theory to be used shall have been grounded at some time in experience.

2.3 Knowledge Types Used

Rationalists constrain the type of knowledge admissible in an enquiry to propositional knowledge; that is, knowledge that can be stated in language form. In view of their commitment to a priori theory and their interest in shaping enquiry preordinately about particular questions and hypotheses, this is not surprising. The naturalist, often intent on the use of the human-as-instrument, also admits tacit knowledge—insights, intuitions, apprehensions that cannot be stated in language form but which are nevertheless "known" to the enquirer. Of course naturalists seek to recast their tacit knowledge into propositional form as quickly as possible. It is equally clear that rationalists depend upon tacit knowledge at least as much as do their naturalist counterparts; however, the reconstructed logic of rationalism militates against exposing this dependency publicly.

2.4 Instruments

The rationalist prefers nonhuman devices for data collection purposes, perhaps because they appear to be more cost efficient, have a patina of objectivity, and can be systematically aggregated. The naturalist prefers humans as instruments, for reasons such as their greater insightfulness, flexibility, and responsiveness, the fact that they are able to take a wholistic view, are able to utilize their tacit knowledge, and are able simultaneously to acquire and process information. Obviously both sets of advantages are meaningful.

2.5 Design

The rationalist insists on a preordinate design; indeed, it is sometimes asserted that a "good" design makes it possible for the enquirer to specify in dummy form the very tables he or she will produce. The naturalist, entering the field without a priori theory, hypotheses, or questions (mostly), is unable to specify a design (except in the broadest process sense) in advance. Instead, he or she anticipates that the design will emerge (unfold, roll, cascade) as the enquiry proceeds, with each step heavily dependent on all preceding steps. Clearly, the naturalist is well-advised to specify as much in advance as possible, while the rationalist should seek to keep as many options open as possible.

2.6 Setting

The rationalist prefers to conduct studies under laboratory conditions, probably because the laboratory represents the epitome of control. The naturalist prefers natural settings (it is this propensity that has lent its name to the paradigm), arguing that only in nature can it be discovered what does happen rather than what can happen. Moreover, studies in nature can be transferred to other, similar contexts, whereas laboratory studies can be generalized only to other laboratories. Clearly both kinds of studies have utility—it may be just as important to know what can happen as what does happen.

While it might appear that compromise is indeed possible on these six postures, in fact the postures are bound together by a synergism such that each posture requires a counterpart position to be taken on all other postures. Consider rationalists, for example. Begin with a posture, say their preference for a priori theory. Rationalists do not exhibit this preference by accident, however. In part they prefer a priori theory because they deal in propositional language, and theory is the best means for formulating clarifying their propositional statements. The hypotheses or questions are propositional deductions from theory. Because of the precision of these hypotheses or questions it is possible to imagine a design for testing them, and to devise appropriate instruments. Having such instruments makes it unnecessary to interpolate a "subjective" human between data and respondents. Moreover, these instruments can best be used in the highly controlled environment of the laboratory. And precise instruments yield data that can conveniently be expressed in quantitative form, a marked advantage since numbers can be easily manipulated statistically. Hence quantitative methods. And of course numbers can be aggregated and summarized, yielding apparent generalizations, expressions of causality, and so on.

The sum exhibits a synergism such that each posture depends on every other one.

Similar observations can be made about the naturalists' preference. Naturalists are forced into a natural setting because they cannot tell, having no a priori theory or hypotheses, what is important to control, or even to study. They could not set up a contrived experiment because they do not know what to contrive. If theory is to emerge from the data, the data must first be gathered. Since the nature of those data is unknown, an adaptive instrument is needed to locate and make sense of them—the "smart" human. Humans find certain data collection means more congenial than others; hence they tend toward the use of qualitative methods such as observation, interview, reading documents, and the like, which come "naturally" to the human. These methods result in insights and information about the specific instance being studied but make it difficult to produce aggregations, generalizations, or cause-effect statements. Again, the naturalists' behavior demonstrates a kind of synergism among postures which is understandable and defensible only in terms of the totality of positions.

3 The Trustworthiness of Naturalistic Enquiries

Because of its unusual axioms and the apparent "softness" of its postures, naturalistic enquiry is often attacked as untrustworthy, in contrast to rationalistic enquiry which has well-developed standards of trustworthiness.

Recently, serious efforts have been undertaken to develop standards which are parallels of those commonly used by rationalists, that is, counterparts to standards of internal and external validity, reliability, and objectivity. Analogous terms have been proposed, viz., (respectively) credibility, transferability, dependability, and confirmability.

Credibility is seen as a check on the isomorphism between the enquirer's data and interpretations and the multiple realities in the minds of informants. Transferability is the equivalent of generalizability to the extent that there are similarities between sending and receiving contexts. Dependability includes the instability factors typically indicated by the term "unreliability" but makes allowances for emergent designs, developing theory, and the like that also induce changes but which cannot be taken as "error." Confirmability shifts the emphasis from the certifiability of the enquirer to the confirmability of the data.

It is premature to expect that adherents of the naturalistic paradigm would have evolved as sophisticated a methodology for dealing with trustworthiness questions as have the rationalists, who have had centuries of experience to shape their standards. However, some suggestions have emerged for handling trustworthiness questions.

With respect to credibility it is proposed that the

following techniques may be profitably used: (a) prolonged engagement at a site to overcome a variety of possible biases and misperceptions and to provide time to identify salient characteristics; (b) persistent observation, to understand salient characteristics as well as to appreciate atypical but meaningful features; (c) peer debriefing, to test growing insights and receive counsel about the evolving design, discharge personal feelings and anxieties, and leave an audit trail (see below); (d) triangulation, whereby a variety of data sources, different investigators, different perspectives (theories), and different methods are pitted against one another; (e) referential adequacy materials, whereby various documents, films, videotapes, audio recordings, pictures, and other "raw" or "slice-of-life" materials are collected during the study and archived for later use, for example, in member or auditor checks (see below); and (f) members checks, whereby data and interpretations are continuously checked with members of the various groups from which data were solicited, including an overall check at the end of the study.

With respect to transferability, it is proposed to use theoretical or purposive sampling to maximize the range of information which is collected and to provide the most stringent conditions for theory grounding; and thick description, furnishing enough information about a context to provide a vicarious experience of it, and to facilitate judgments about the extent to which working hypotheses from that context might be transferable to a second, similar context.

With respect to dependability, it is proposed to use overlap methods, one kind of triangulation which undergirds claims of dependability to the extent that the methods produce complementary results; stepwise replication, a kind of "split-halves" approach in which enquirers and data sources are divided into halves to pursue the enquiry independently, provided, however, that there is sufficient communication between the two teams to allow for the articulated development of the emergent design, and the dependability audit, a process modelled on the fiscal audit. A fiscal auditor has two responsibilities: first, to ascertain that the accounts were kept in one of the several modes that constitute "good practice," and second, to ascertain that every entry can be supported with appropriate documentation and that the totals are properly determined. The dependability audit serves the first of these functions.

With respect to confirmability it is proposed to use triangulation (as above); to keep a reflexive journal that can be used to expose epistemological assumptions and to show why the study was defined and carried out in particular ways; and the confirmability audit, which carries out the second of the two auditor functions mentioned above.

It is generally understood that the use of even all of these techniques cannot guarantee the trustworthiness of a naturalistic study but can only contribute greatly to persuading a consumer of its meaningfulness.

4. Summary

Naturalistic enquiry is one of two paradigms currently being used by investigators within the framework of disciplined research. While this paradigm has distinguished antecedents in anthropology and ethnography, it is nevertheless relatively emergent and not as much is known about its properties as might be desired.

Naturalistic enquiry differs from rationalistic enquiry in terms of interpretations based on five basic axioms; reality, enquirer-object relationship, generalizability, causality, and value freedom. In addition, a number of salient postures also play important roles; methods, sources of theory, knowledge types used, instruments, design, and setting.

As a relatively new paradigm, naturalism suffers in not having yet devised as solid an approach to trustworthiness as has its rationalistic counterpart. Nevertheless important strides are being made. It seems likely that, given several decades in which to develop, the naturalistic paradigm will prove to be as useful as the rationalistic paradigm has been historically. The major decision to be made between the two paradigms revolve about the assessment of fit to the area under study, rather than to any intrinsic advantages or disadvantages of either.

See also: Ethographic Research Methods; Classroom Observation Techniques; Participant Observation; Hermeneutics

References

Cronbach L J 1975 Beyond the two disciplines of scientific psychology. *Am. Psychol.* 30: 116–27

Further Reading

Cook T D, Campbell D T 1979 *Quasi-experimentation: Design and Analysis Issues for Field Settings.* Rand McNally, Chicago, Illinois

Cook T D, Reichardt C S 1979 *Qualitative and Quantitive Methods in Evaluation Research.* Sage, Beverly Hills, California

Cronbach L J, Suppes P (eds.) 1969 *Research for Tomorrow's Schools: Disciplined Inquiry for Education.* MacMillan, New York

Filstead W J (ed.) 1970 *Qualitative Methodology: Firsthand Involvement with the Social World.* Rand McNally, Chicago, Illinois

Glaser B G, Strauss A L 1967 *The Discovery of Grounded Theory: Strategies for Qualitative Research.* Aldine, Chicago, Illinois

Guba E G 1978 *Toward a Methodology of Naturalistic Inquiry in Educational Evaluation.* Center for the Study of Evaluation, University of California, Los Angeles, California

Guba E G 1981 Criteria for assessing the trustworthiness of naturalistic inquiries. *Educ. Comm. Tech. J.* 29(2): 75–92

Guba E G, Lincoln Y S 1982 *Effective Evaluation.* Jossey-Bass, San Francisco, California

Kaplan A 1964 *The Conduct of Inquiry: Methodology for Behavioral Science*, Chandler, San Francisco, California

Polani M 1966 *The Tacit Dimension*, Doubleday, Garden City, New York

Scriven M 1971 Objectivity and subjectivity in educational research In: Thomas L G (ed.) 1971 *Philosophical Redirection of Educational Research*. University of Chicago Press, Chicago, Illinois

Oral History

B. K. Hyams

Since the early 1960s the oral history approach to general historical enquiry and research has been a burgeoning enterprise. The dramatic growth in this particular facet of scholarship is itself symptomatic of the changing cultural context of the contemporary world. In the first place it is a matter of cultural process. The advent of the postliterate society in this technological age has meant a gradual decline in traditionally important sources of historical evidence—memoirs, diaries, and letters. The eclipse of written communication has added a sense of urgency to the quest to capture the past, and oral history has been the weapon in that quest. In another sense the awakening appreciation of oral history derives from a changing ideology and a changing emphasis. This is encapsulated in the growing interest in the "underclass" in our society—the anonymous, hitherto inarticulate mass, as compared with the concentration on the rulers, the leaders, and the notables. The shift has been characterized as a democratization of emphasis, taking history from the bottom up rather than the top down. Such a focus is of course one which predates the modern use of oral history, for scholars from time to time attended to the mass rather than the elite and based their evidence on various categories of written sources; but the oral history technique has facilitated the popularization of the history of "ordinary" people, and in this new focus mass education looms as an important object of attention. This entry considers oral history, both as a source and as technique of historical evidence, which has assumed greater significance in educational research.

1. Oral History as Technique

The growing maturity of the oral history method has been reflected in two major aspects of development. One is the increased tendency to look beyond what the interviewee merely said, to the way in which questions are answered. All the nuances of testimony and response thus become significant. The nonanswer, the silence, the hesitation, the evasion—all count for interpretation of the evidence being provided. Such reactions and indeed the very tone of voice are features recognized as being relevant to the quality of the evidence. Since these aspects are immediately evident on a tape-recording (but not necessarily in transcript form without special parenthetical provision), oral history sources become more than simply a matter of spoken evidence and more than just the recording of facts.

The other implication of this form of historical evidence is the recognition of its interdisciplinary links. Since memory plays such an important role in oral historical evidence, psychological and sociological theories are applied to structure of memory, based as it is on perception, personal experiences, and on the social environment and the accumulated culture. Recall of the past is, in other words, not simply the regurgitation of facts, either unconnected or occurring in a social vacuum. Similarly pointing to an overlapping of social science genres is the issue of language. Sociolinguistics assumes significant proportions if the interviewer and the interviewee are to collaborate on the basis of a common language understanding, not to be taken for granted even if the two speak the same tongue (Friedlander 1984).

The enlistment of interdisciplinary aid in oral history has been reinforced by this accent on the interviewer–interviewee relationship and by the quest for validity. Refinement of the interview from unstructured monologue to a structured dialogue has brought the oral historian closer to the anthropologist. The oral historian shares with the ethnographer the objective of giving voice to the hitherto voiceless, to the anonymous in the contemporary society as well as that of the immediately past generation. There are also problems in common in dealing with the interviewer's potential ability to influence the informant, a characteristic that is sometimes described as the power relations between the two participants.

In spite of this trend, it appears that the full potential of a fruitful relationship between oral history and anthropology is still far from realized. This is partly due to the fact that the ethnographic technique is the confident instrument of anthropologists, while oral history is still suspect among historians and is as yet a minor methodology of the discipline. This arises from the stronger attraction of historians to quantitative methods (although the balance is shifting) in the borrowings of history from other social sciences. Oral history tends toward intense studies of a limited number of subjects and in any case enjoys far less of the luxury of generalization afforded by quantitative methods. Even when it ventures into the quantitative arena there are often serious difficulties in the matter of sampling. Because oral historians are only interviewing survivors, respondents providing information on some past period may be demographically atypical and the researcher needs to be circumspect in concluding from the evidence (Lumms 1987). Nevertheless, there are ways in which quantitative research and oral history may approach each other more closely. The Q-technique, for example, has been suggested as one means of achieving this. This allows the respondent to make subjective responses to a range of opinions arranged in categories by ranking them; the results may then be quantified. Since this technique focuses on common conversational subjectivity it has potential to share with oral history in the research enterprise (Sharpless 1986).

Subjectivity has, of course, become an important issue in more recent discussions of the oral history technique. It has been argued that oral historians need to turn aside from the emphasis which much of the "new history" gave to demography and quantification, and move more positively toward a concentration on feelings of the individual. This, it is contended, would make the uniqueness of individual testimony an asset in demonstrating the variety of experience stemming from a common culture, instead of appearing as an obstacle to generalization. This emphasis also elevates the subjective in oral evidence: far from detracting from the evidence, emotions, fears and fantasies are thus held to enhance its meaning and its quality (Samuel and Thompson 1990). In this way the mosaic is not totally lost to the macrohistory: the latter will provide the framework, but the dynamics of history must also stem from "the unique subjective meanings humans bring to their lives" (Quantz 1985 p. 441). In this enterprise oral historians may join forces to some extent with psychoanalysts, sociologists, and especially anthropologists. What oral history needs to borrow more extensively from the latter is analysis of behavioral evidence in addition to the narrative. This includes the requirement of careful attention to outcomes of the relationship between the interviewer and the interviewee. What is still to be achieved, probably in general ethnography as well as in oral history, is a thorough discussion in the final text and concluding evaluation in the research work of the ways in which the interview itself affected the narrative (Di Leonardo 1987).

2. Oral History Outside Education

In its early stages of modern application oral history became more than just a method. Although Thompson (1988) has averred that it is a technique, not a compartment of history, it has in addition given rise to new areas of historical inquiry. Even as substance it has several facets. Information gleaned from the oral narrative and interview may be used to supplement and confirm documentary sources, even at times to contradict or correct them. But it may also stand alone as the single source of some historical phenomenon, especially from the hitherto untapped areas which have eluded scholars in the past and would otherwise do so in the future, largely because the subjects involved have not recorded or will not record their narrative and opinions in written form. The singularity of oral history is that it goes beyond collection of data to its deliberate creation through allowing the interviewer to add narrative to the store of factual information and to elicit further information by means of question and cross-examination.

The major periodicals of oral history now offer vivid testimony to the new vistas opened up for the groups whom history formerly disenfranchised. Titles of articles include for example, the world of work, of workers, and the way in which they organized themselves in such studies as that in 1989 of the Lumberjacks of Finnish Lapland, or in an earlier account of union organization in a southern US state. Labor histories based on oral accounts range from expositions of the role of union organizers to that of the rank and file, the latter aspect thus treating the past from the "bottom up." The proliferation of oral history products has proceeded toward those aspects which have always attracted a variety of social scientists, namely the accounts of particular immigrant or ethnic groups in specific locations, ranging from Czech immigrants in Texas to working-class Jews in Amsterdam. Oral history has had an almost explosive effect on the development of general community histories. Beyond that general purpose its advantage is to draw attention to special community groups, for example, those removed by slum clearance in urban renewal projects, where their revealed feelings might not accord with official pronouncements from the authorities (Sharpless 1986). Modern episodes of international conflict have also provided scope for dramatic oral history accounts of crisis situations, such as those of American participants in the Vietnam struggle, memories of the Berlin Wall, or the role of women in the Greek resistance of the Second World War.

The debate which centered on the accumulation of testimonies from the "underclass" is in part due to the lack of clarity of purpose. Tuchman's metaphor of the vacuum cleaner collection of trash finds support if the collections of life stories are deemed to be ends in themselves (Henige 1982). But the charges of trivialization can be met more effectively if the individual accounts are given their due cultural relevance. Although the individual experiences may be unique, they draw on a common culture. This is particularly patent in the oral history interview which has much to do with how the story is told rather than merely what is told. The manner of the narrative or the answers to questioning is important for its silences, evasions, selective and deliberate amnesia, and even lies. It has been suggested that phenomena can often be traced to a dynamic relationship between myth in the personal story and myth in the public tradition (Samuel and Thompson 1990). Passerini has explained this by defining the oral history interview as a record of a cultural form. Hence the individual's accounts, although idiosyncratic, reflect a tradition of story-telling which has been culturally transmitted, manifested in the use of metaphor revealing the accumulation of collective thought processes; and this is done as well even by silences and breaks in the narrative (Smith 1988). The factor of evasion in the interview narrative is one of the features which has made virtually an oral history classic of Passerini's *Facism in Popular Memory*. The analysis of the cultural experience of the Turin working class during that totalitarian regime provides the example of suppression of painful memories. Through emphasis on this and contradictions and other blemishes in the interviews, the study presents cultural concerns and attitudes rather than actions as the historical point of the findings (Smith 1988).

3. Implications for Education Studies

The shifting focus of historical inquiry enhanced by the use of the oral record has direct consequences for research in the history of education, modestly so far in practice but potentially profound. In its earliest modern use in the memoirs of leaders, the oral history thrust had obvious rewards in education in the realm of policy-making which for long had preoccupied historians of education. Hence the traditional interest in biographical studies was boosted by a spate of tape-recorded narratives of educational administrators and other leaders, whose evidence provided accounts of the plans and practices of the recent past. The interviews served to convey motives, attitudes, and reactions of perhaps a university president dealing with a time of student unrest or perhaps of a top bureaucrat at the systems level, handling the implementation of a reform project or responding to changes in the political climate as they impinged on educational policies. The oral interview, as instanced in one Australian study, puts flesh on the bare bones of written documentation in helping to reveal the more subtle aspects of tensions and competing vested interests in the process of public policy development (Hyams 1992). The findings of the oral interview must of course be treated with the same circumspection as the written autobiography, given the propensity of the subject toward apologia. Validation by checking with alternative sources therefore remains an important tool of research.

Institutional history has been another early beneficiary of the oral evidence approach. Recollections of administrators, teachers, and students of individual educational institutions have produced new chapters on the contemporary history of not only nationally prestigious tertiary establishments but also schools or colleges in which the local community has its interest. This type of exercise has special use in elucidating the progress (or decline) both of the typical and also of the unique. The latter category is exemplified in a study entitled, "No Ordinary School, " in which is traced a history of dissent and reform in a radical institution in the United States (Selby 1989).

The value of oral history reaches well beyond the institutional aspect when applied to the broader cultural definitions of education as advanced by Cremin and others in the early 1950s (Butts and Cremin 1953). Informal learning, childhood as a whole, and continuing adult learning are all functions of the cultural context of education to which oral history has direct access. In the process the family emerges as a key object and a readily traceable source of research activity through oral narrative and interview. This medium can assist in revealing the way in which cultural capital is generationally transmitted; it can further probe the nature or interaction between parents, children, and siblings in not only what attitudes and values are developed but in how this proceeds. In general, the value of family studies is to be found in the realm of affective as well as cognitive learning.

4. Grassroots Focus

Public education as an expanding and dominant social institution of the twentieth century is a particularly rich field for examining the underclass, already identified as an object of added prominence through oral history. For the first time scholars can probe into the reactions of the rank and file to the policies and practices of the authorities, and especially the state, in a way hitherto not possible through the written records or even through quantitative, statistical studies, however useful they may be. The family histories will help reveal attitudes of working-class parents to the official conformities of schooling and to the socialization process of formal education. The attitudes of teachers also to the employing authorities and their role expectations in general can be elicited in a much more expansive way than hitherto provided through the limited number of useful autobiographies. The value of teacher studies in this way has been demonstrated in a number of exercises examining industrial action taken by teachers collectively. Hence a description of teacher unionization in Hamilton, Ohio reaches beyond structural causes and examines individual teachers in their construction of cultural concepts (Quantz 1985). Less ambitiously, the use of personal oral reminiscences of teachers also promises to provide a fuller understanding of the implementation of schooling policies. In this way, for example, responses of Hawaiian teachers to official directives in the interwar years add to an otherwise incomplete account of political socialization through schooling (Hyams 1985).

A major aspect of studies of grassroots history of education relates to the notion of resistance. Negative reactions to authority are revealed best by oral history probes into attitudes. Even physical manifestations of reaction are insufficient historical evidence unless assisted by the further dimension of motives and attitudes elucidated by oral interview. A number of important pieces of research of this type indicate clearly the considerable potential of oral history in explicating the unofficial interpretations of noted educational problems or occurrences in modern times. One example of such major exercises was the Humphries study of working-class childhood and youth in the United Kingdom for the 50 years from the end of the nineteenth century. Its relevance to education lay in its focus on the working-class children's resistance to the "content, the structure and the form of the developing state education system" (Humphries 1981 p. 29). The study graphically demonstrated the inadequacy of the written record through testimony of old working-class people which showed that the school log and punishment books failed to record sufficiently the precise nature of misdemeanors committed by students. These gaps were vital since they related to the clash between working-class culture and the contemporary official ideology. Another study of children in revolt was that of the investigation of a 1977 school strike in Southern Italy. The research work not only depicted development of resistance based on a particular grievance with the authorities (about heating the school rooms) but offered insight into the idea of myth as a key to understanding the episodes of the strike and the child interviewees' depictions of it (Basso 1990).

A further development of an education resistance study through oral history is the publication *1968: A Student Generation in Revolt*, in which the respondents include a number of oral historians themselves. The work was greeted as the first large-scale international oral history since the 1948 work of Nevins of Columbia University (Morissey 1988). As a reminder of the salient fact that education is the concern of more than simply the educators and their pupils, political and social controversies arising from formal education issues have been subjected to oral historical inquiry. One of the richest sources of such research is the attempt in the United States at desegregation of schools. A study of that phenomenon in New Orleans which began with an emphasis on archival documentation, progressively resorted to oral interviews as contradictions in the two sets of evidentiary records became more obvious. The result was a fruitful

history of individual and collective experience which also laid bare the underside aspects of community fear and hostility while demonstrating the processes of small group interaction and of politicization as a whole (Rogers 1986).

5. Oral History as a Teaching Device

Although oral history has featured in the work of increasing numbers of scholars and dissertation students, few have attempted to analyze it as an educational method. Nevertheless, findings have suggested that the use of oral history as a classroom exercise has expanded. Part of that expansion could be traced to emulation in the United States and elsewhere following the success of the Foxfire book project which resulted from college students' investigations into their regions' history and folklore. It is also apparent that the popularizing of the approach at university/college level was followed in the 1980s by increasing uses of oral history by high schools. Family, community history, immigration, and ethnic histories have been obvious targets of interest for student exercises. The personalized approach involved is patently an aid to motivation in learning, while topics chosen can well further enhance that motivation through relevance to the student. Pedagogical advantages are also claimed, suggesting that the novice researcher in the classroom will be taken through higher cognitive skill levels of analysis, synthesis, and evaluation (Lanman 1987, 1989). This is not to say that the oral history project has by any means superseded conventional modes of teaching history. Questions of time constraints, cost of equipment or materials, lack of skill and conservative suspicion of educational departures, are impediments to the development of oral history to significant proportions in the school curriculum and the classroom program.

6. Conclusion

Some of these factors may be extended to apply to the enterprise of oral history as a whole. Oral history is still viewed with a degree of suspicion by many historians and is yet to have a major role in the field of historical inquiry. It is, however, indubitably valuable in complementing written records and in opening up otherwise inaccessible sources of information. Just as the rise of technology threatened the literary age of written record, so it has facilitated an alternative through tape-recording of evidence. Researchers have become increasingly aware of the intricacies and subtleties of the interview evidence and are attending much more to the matter of researcher–subject interaction. It may well be that further technological advances such as extended use of audio visual apparatus (i.e., the video recorder) will be harnessed to give further refinement to a relatively new approach to scholarly research in education.

See also: Biographical Research Methods; Historical Methods in Educational Research; Educational History in Biographies and Autobiographies; Narrative Inquiry

References

Basso R 1990 Myths in contemporary oral transmission: A children's strike. In: Samuel R, Thompson P (eds.) 1990

Butts R F, Cremin L A 1953 *A History of Education in American Culture*. Henry Holt, New York

Di Leonardo M 1987 Oral History as Ethnographic Encounter. *Oral History Review* 15: 1–20

Friedlander P 1984 Theory, method, and oral history. In: Dunaway D K, Baum W K (eds.) 1984

Henige D 1982 *Oral Historiography*. Longman, London

Humphries S 1981 *Hooligans or Rebels? An Oral History of Working-class Childhood and Youth 1889–1939*. Blackwell, Oxford

Hyams B K 1985 School teachers as agents of cultural imperialism in territorial Hawaii. *J. Pacific Hist.* 20(4): 202–19

Hyams B K 1992 Towards teacher education autonomy: The interaction of vested interests in Victoria, 1964–1972. *Hist. Educ. Rev.* 21(2): 48–64

Lanman B A 1987 Oral history as an educational tool for teaching immigration and Black history in American high schools: Findings and queries. *Int. J. Oral Hist.* 8(2): 122–35

Lanman B A 1989 The use of oral history in the classroom: A comparative analysis of the 1974 and 1987 Oral History Association surveys. *Oral Hist. Rev.* 17(1): 215–26

Lumms T 1987 *Listening to History: The Authenticity of Oral Evidence*. Century Hutchinson, London

Morissey C T 1988 Oral history as multiple endeavour (editorial). *Int. J. Oral Hist.* 9(3): 195–98

Quantz R A 1985 The complex visions of female teachers and the failure of unionization in the 1930s: An oral history. *Hist. Educ. Q.* 25(4): 439–58

Rogers K L 1986 Decoding a city of words: Fantasy theme analysis and the interpretation of oral interviews. *Int. J. Oral Hist.* 7(1): 43–56

Samuel R, Thompson P (eds.) 1990 *The Myths We Live By*. Routledge, London

Selby J G 1989 Highlander: No ordinary school, Book Review. *Oral Hist. Rev.* 17(1): 195–97

Sharpless R 1986 The numbers game: Oral history compared with quantitative methodology. *Int. J. Oral Hist.* 7(2): 93–108

Smith R C 1988 Popular memory and oral narratives: Luisa Passerini's reading of oral history interviews. *Oral Hist. Rev.* 16(2): 95–107

Thompson P 1988 *The Voice of the Past*. Oxford University Press, Oxford

Further Reading

Cutler W W 1971 Oral history—Its nature and uses for educational history. *Hist. Educ. Q.* 11(2): 184–92

Cutler W W 1983 Asking for answers: Oral history. In: Best J H (ed.) 1983 *Historical Inquiry in Education*. American Educational Research Association, Washington DC

Douglas L, Roberts A, Thompson R 1988 *Oral History: A Handbook*. Allen and Unwin, Sydney

Dunaway D K, Baum W K (eds.) 1984 *Oral History: An Interdisciplinary Anthology*. American Association for State and Local History, Nashville, Tennessee

Ingersoll F, Ingersoll J 1987 Both a Borrower and a Lender be: Ethnography, Oral History and Grounded Theory. *Oral Hist. Rev.* 15: 81–102

Wieder A 1988 Oral history and questions of interaction for educational historians. *Int. J. Oral Hist.* 9(2): 131–38

Phenomenography

F. Marton

"Phenomenography" is the empirical study of the limited number of qualitatively different ways in which various phenomena in, and aspects of, the world around us are experienced, conceptualized, understood, perceived, and apprehended. These differing experiences, understandings, and so forth are characterized in terms of "categories of description," logically related to each other, and forming hierarchies in relation to given criteria. Such an ordered set of categories of description is called the "outcome space" of the phenomenon concept in question.

This entry is concerned with the origins of this approach to research, the nature of experiences, the methods of inquiry employed, and the applications of phenomenography in practice.

1. Origins of Phenomenography

Phenomenography is a research specialization with its roots in a set of studies of learning among university students carried out at the University of Göteborg, Sweden, in the early 1970s. The point of departure for these studies was one of the simplest observations that can be made about learning, namely that some people are better at learning than others. This straightforward observation led to the first question which was to be investigated empirically: (a) What does it *mean* to say that some people are better at learning than others? This in turn led to the second question: (b) *Why* are some people better at learning than others?

The intention from the very start was to take as little for granted as possible. Learning was studied under comparatively natural conditions, and the aim was to describe it through the eyes of the learner. The studies were conducted by holding individual sessions in which a student was asked to read a text which was either taken from a textbook or had a similar character. The students were informed that after reading the text they were going to discuss their understanding of it with the experimenter. Thus, after completing their reading, the students were duly interviewed about what they understood the text to have been about. Sometimes more specific details were also taken up. In addition, they were asked to give as full an account of the text as possible. After that, the interview continued with questions about their experience of the situation and they were specifically asked how they had gone about learning the text.

All the interviews were tape-recorded and subsequently transcribed verbatim. On scrutinizing the transcripts of the students' accounts of how they had understood and remembered the text as a whole, a limited number of distinctively different ways of understanding what the text was about could be identified. Furthermore, these different ways of understanding the text were seen to be in logical relationship to one another, of inclusion or exclusion, for instance. Each of the different understandings was described very carefully, to bring out its special characteristics in relation to the others, thus forming a set of what came to be called "categories of description." By drawing on the logical relationships found between the different ways of understanding the text, a hierarchy was established between categories of description. Such a hierarchically ordered set of categories is called "the outcome space". The outcome space thus depicted the different ways in which the text had been understood; by referring to this outcome space the categories of description could be compared with one another to judge how appropriate, in relation to specified criteria, was the understanding they represented. This line of reasoning applies, of course, not only to the understanding of the text as a whole but also to the various topics dealt with in the text.

The outcome space provided an instrument for characterizing, in qualitative terms, how well learners succeed with their learning task. Thus a way was found of answering the question: What does it mean to say that some people are better at learning than others? (Marton et al. 1984).

The characterization of the qualitative differences in the outcome of learning was based on the students' accounts of their understanding and remembering of the text as a whole, or of certain parts of it. When the transcripts of the students' accounts of how they had experienced the situation and of the way in which they had gone about the learning task were analyzed again, some striking differences were found. For some of the students the text they were reading was transparent, in a manner of speaking, in that they were focusing on what the text referred to; they were trying to understand what it was about. Other students, who recounted experiencing the situation such that they were expected to recall the text after reading it, focused on the text as such, trying to move it into their heads, as it were. The former way of relating to the learning situation was called the *deep approach* and the latter the *surface approach*. It was found that the deep approach was closely associated with "higher" categories of outcome (i.e., better understanding of the text) while the surface approach was associated with "lower" categories of outcome (i.e., more shallow understanding of the text). There was thus a strong relationship between the way in which the students understood the content of learning (the text) on the one hand and the way in which they experienced the learning situation (and their own act of learning), on the other. The two aspects of learning, the content aspect and the act aspect, are, of course, two aspects of the same whole.

Thus the second question posed at the outset of this research enterprise could be answered, at least in part. Some people are better at learning than others because people differ in their approach to learning tasks (Marton et al. 1984). Further research demonstrated that the relationship between approaches to learning on the one hand, and the qualities of the outcomes of learning on the other, is invariant across forms of learning other than learning by reading, even if the specific natures of both the approaches and the outcomes vary both with the type of learning activity —for example, essay writing (Hounsell 1984), listening to lectures (Hodgson 1984), and problem solving (Laurillard 1984)—and with the specific content.

At the focus of this first set of studies was the set of different understandings of some specific content which learners developed in a certain situation; sense was made of these in terms of differences in the approaches the learners adopted to the specific learning task, that is, in terms of differences in their way of experiencing the specific situation. The second step in developing the phenomenographic research orientation was to shift the focus of interest away from that which emerges in a specific situation and toward the learners' preconceived ideas about the phenomena dealt with in the specific situations. The way in which children understand numbers, for instance, is of vital importance to the way in which they deal with arithmetic problems (Neuman 1987, Marton and Neuman 1990). The way in which students understand matter is of vital importance as far as their understanding of chemical reaction is concerned (Renström et al. 1990) and so on. Detailed knowledge of the ways in which learners understand the central phenomena, concepts, and principles within a domain prior to study is believed to be critical for developing their understanding of the central phenomena, concepts, and principles, and hence for their mastery of the domain (Bowden et al. 1992).

That branch of development of phenomenography dealt with the *content* aspect of learning. The *act* aspect of learning was also considered in that, similarly, learners' conceptions of what learning actually is are crucial for the way in which they experience the act of learning, and thus for what approach they adopt in relation to specific learning tasks (Säljö 1982, Marton et al. 1993).

The recurring principle in all the investigations quoted here is that whatever phenomenon or situation people encounter, it is possible to identify a limited number of qualitatively different and logically interrelated ways in which the phenomenon or the situation is experienced or understood. Naturally enough, in subsequent studies this principle was found to be applicable to phenomena and situations well outside the educational context in which the initial studies, described above, had been carried out. Theman (1983) explored conceptions of political power, Wenestam (1984) investigated ideas of death, and Marton et al. (1994) studied the experience of Nobel laureates' views of scientific intuition, for instance.

From some empirical studies of learning in higher education, phenomenography thus evolved as a research specialization aimed at "describing conceptions of the world around us" (Marton 1981). This research specialization is characterized in terms of its object of research on the one hand and in terms of the methods used when studying this research object, on the other.

2. Object of Research

As stated above, phenomenography is the empirical study of the differing ways in which people experience, perceive, apprehend, understand, or conceptualize various phenomena in, and aspects of, the world around them. The words "experience," "perceive," and so on are used interchangeably. The point is not to deny that there are differences in what these terms refer to, but to suggest that the limited number of ways in which a certain phenomenon appears to people can be found, for instance, regardless of whether they are embedded in immediate experience of the phenomenon or in reflected thought about the same phenomenon. The different ways in which a phenomenon can be experienced, perceived, apprehended, understood, or conceptualized according to the way of describing them, are thus independent of the differences between experience, perception, apprehension, understanding or conceptualization.

This point can be illustrated by an example taken from a piece of phenomenographic research. One of the ways in which young children experience numbers is as what Neuman (1987) calls "finger-numbers." According to her, children frequently "lay" the numbers 1 to 10 on their fingers, calling one of the little fingers (usually on the left hand) "1," the ring-finger "2," and so on. Numbers larger than 5 are then understood as 5+ some fingers. In carrying out simple arithmetic tasks children try to keep "the undivided 5" together. Hence when solving problems like 2+7=? they reverse the addends and transform the problem to 7+2=?, where 7 is "undivided 5"+2, and the problem as a whole becomes (5+2)+2=?

What, then, is a conception of something, or a way of experiencing something? (Here, it is noted, the two expressions are being used interchangeably.) It is not a mental representation or a cognitive structure; it is a way of being aware of something. One might be aware of 7 when one perceives it as 5+2 when one looks at one's hands (or as 6+1 or 4+3); it might be an immediate experience of the number 7; it might be the result of reflection; or there are still other possibilities. In all cases, however, 7 is seen as a sum of two parts, 5 and 2 (or 6 and 1, or 4 and 3). Awareness is a relation between subject and object. Furthermore, when something is the object of attention it is always seen, or thought about, or whatever, in some way, by somebody. It is simply not possible to deal with an object without experiencing or conceptualizing it in some way. In this sense, subject and object are not independent, but they form a unity; there is a relation between them which can be called an internal relation. Subject and object are what they are in relation to each other. Following from this, a way of experiencing or understanding a phenomenon says as much about the experienced, understood phenomenon as it says about the experiencing, understanding subject.

Asplund-Carlsson et al. (1992), studying the qualitatively different ways in which secondary school students understood one of Franz Kafka's short stories, argued that their work not only illuminated how young people make sense of literary texts, but was in fact a contribution to research on the interpretation of Kafka's work. In a similar way Lybeck et al. (1988) argued that they had made a contribution to the characterization of the "mole-concept" in chemistry through their study of secondary school students' differing understanding of that concept.

2.1 The Nature of Experience

An experience or a conception of a phenomenon—the internal relation between subject and object—is a way of delimiting an object from its context and relating it to the same or other contexts, and it is a way of delimiting component parts of the phenomenon and relating them to each other and to the whole (Svensson 1984). The delimitation from and relating to a context is the "external horizon" of the phenomenon. The delimitation and relating of parts is the "internal horizon" of the phenomenon. The external and internal horizons together make up the "structural aspect" of the experience. There is a corresponding "referential aspect" in the meaning inherent in the experience. Consider an example taken from Neuman's (1987) work, where the relation between the structural and the referential aspects of two different ways of understanding numbers is illustrated through the description of a change from one to the other. A 7-year-old boy, just started at school, solved the problem "If you have two kronor (crowns) and you get seven more, how much money have you then altogether?" in the following way.

He started off with a counting-on procedure, saying "2 . . . 3, 4 . . ." The idea is, of course, to add 7 units of which "3" is the first, "4" is the second, and so on. As he did not use any procedure for keeping track he could not possibly know when he had uttered exactly seven number words. He simply could not hear "the seven-ness" of seven. Now, what in actual fact happened was that he paused upon saying "7" and then said "8, 9" and declared that the result was 9 (the full sequence reads as follows: "2 . . . 3, 4, 5, 6, 7 . . . 8, 9"). An interpretation—in our view highly reasonable—is that although this little boy was trying to add seven units to two to begin with, when he said "7" he realized all of a sudden that this "7" could be seen as the last unit in the addend "7," if only "7" was placed as the first addend, instead of seeing the same unit as being some way through the second addend.

It is now possible to see how the structure of the sum, as experienced, changes from "1,2 . . . 3,4,5,6,7,8,9" to "1,2,3,4,5,6,7, . . . 8,9." Here it is the internal structure of the sum that changed. (No obvious change in the external horizon can be noticed. The little boy was probably delimiting this problem from the situation at large and related it to other number problems.) Corresponding to the change in the structural aspect of the experience there is a corresponding change in its referential aspect. The meaning of each number changes, the meaning of "1" and "2" changes from being the first and second unit in 2 to being the first and second unit in 7. The meaning of "3," "4" and so on change from being the first, second and later corresponding units in 7 to being the third, fourth and so on units in 7. The meaning of "8" and "9" changes from being the last two units in 7 to being the two units in 2.

The structural changes cannot come about without the changes in meaning. Nor can changes in meaning come about without changes in structure. The structural and the referential aspects thus dialectically constitute each other. Neither is prior to the other.

2.2 Hierarchy of Capabilities

The different ways of experiencing a certain phenomenon, characterized by corresponding categories of description, represent different capabilities for dealing with (or understanding) that phenomenon. As some ways of experiencing the phenomenon are more efficient than others in relation to some given criterion, it is possible to establish a hierarchy of categories of description. It is better to have developed the idea of addition's commutativity and realize that 2+7=7+2, as in the above example, than not to have developed it. To see immediately that 2 and 7 are simply two parts of 9, their order being immaterial, is an even more efficient way of understanding numbers and number relations from the point of view of developing arithmetic skills. In this view, then, it is the way of understanding those phenomena which skills have to handle and which knowledge is about, that is the most critical aspect of skills and knowledge.

2.3 Awareness

A certain way of understanding something is a way of being aware of it. Awareness is seen as a person's total experience of the world at a given point in time. Following Gurwitsch (1964), awareness is not seen in terms of the dichotomy aware/unaware or conscious/subconscious, but as being characterized by an infinitely differentiated figure-ground structure. Certain things or aspects are in the foreground: they are explicit and thematized. Other things are in the background: they are implicit and unthematized. There is, however, no dichotomy between two classes of things or aspects but rather a more or less continuous variation.

When students deal with a mathematical problem, they are presumably aware of the quantities involved, the relations between them and the operations they may need to carry out. More vaguely, they are presumably aware of different parts of mathematics in general; it is through their previous mathematical experience that they make sense of the problem. At the same time they are aware of things which are not immediately relevant to the problem, but surround it in space and time. There is the experience of the situation of the world outside this situation, of what happened before they embarked upon the problem and of what is going to happen afterwards. The external horizon of the situation extends in space and time indefinitely. In this sense they are aware of everything all the time. But they are surely not aware of everything in the same way. Every situation has its own "relevance structure." The world is seen from the point of view of that specific situation. At the same time the situation is seen through all of their experiences of the world. They are aware of everything all the time and they are aware of everything differently all the time. In a phenomenographic study it is possible to explore the different ways in which they can be aware of a certain phenomenon or situation. It is necessary to find out the differences in the structure of awareness and in the corresponding meaning of the phenomenon or situation.

3. Methods of Research

3.1 Collecting Data

As mentioned above in Sect. 1, the dominant method for collecting data has been the individual interview. How something is experienced can of course be expressed in many different ways, not least the ways in which people act expresses how things appear to them. In accordance with this, there are phenomenographic studies where group interviews, observations, drawings, written responses, and historical documents have been used as the main source of information. On the collective level, it is also possible to examine artifacts —historically or comparatively, for example—from the point of view of the different ways of understanding the surrounding world that are embedded in those artifacts (Marton 1984). A piece of equipment for programmed learning from the late 1960s, for instance, might convey a great deal about the view of learning embedded in that equipment.

In spite of the variety of ways of collecting data, the preferred method is the individual interview. The reason for this has to do with what has been said about the object of research above, and especially about the structure of awareness. The more it is possible to make things which are unthematized and implicit into objects of reflection, and hence thematized and explicit, the more fully can awareness be explored. There is an interesting parallel here to the phenomenological method as described by Edmund Husserl.

Phenomenology, too, makes human experience its research object. It is, however, a philosophical method, an enterprise in the first person singular. The philosophers themselves reflect on their way of experiencing the world, or rather specific phenomena in the world. It is not introspection, they are not trying to look into themselves; they are looking at the world, but they are trying to step out of "the natural attitude," in which their way of experiencing the world as individuals is taken for granted. By "bending back" awareness—in a manner of speaking—its focus becomes the way of experiencing something.

It is a similar shift that the phenomenographic interview is trying to bring about in the person who is the subject of the interview. As phenomenography is empirical research, the researcher (interviewer) is not studying his or her own awareness and reflection, but that of the subjects. The interview has to be carried out as a dialogue. It should facilitate the thematization of aspects of the subject's experience not previously thematized. The experiences and understandings are jointly constituted by interviewer and interviewee. These experiences and understandings are neither there prior to the interview, ready to be "read off," nor are they only situational social constructions. They are aspects of the subject's awareness that change from being unreflected to being reflected.

This type of interview should not have too many questions made up in advance, and nor should there be too many details determined in advance. Most questions follow from what the subject says. The point is to establish the phenomenon as experienced and to explore its different aspects jointly and as fully as possible. The starting question may aim directly at the general phenomenon such as, for instance, when asking the subject after some general discussion, "What do you mean by learning, by the way?" Alternatively, it is possible to ask the subject to come up with instances of the general phenomenon, asking for example, "Can you tell me about something you have learned?" Most often, however, a concrete case makes up the point of departure: a text to be read, a well-known situation to be discussed, or a problem to be solved. The experimenter then tries to encourage the subjects to reflect on the text, the situation, or the problem, and often also on their way of dealing with it. The interview thus aims at making that which has been unthematized into the object of focal awareness. This is often an irreversible process. This kind of research interview thus comes very close to a pedagogical situation.

3.2 Analysis

As was pointed out above, in the course of the interviews the participants in the research are invited to reflect on their experience of the phenomena dealt with. They are supposed to adopt an attitude which is similar to that of philosophers who exercise the Husserlian method of phenomenological research. When the interviews have been transcribed verbatim, and the analysis has begun, it is the researcher who is supposed to bracket preconceived ideas. Instead of judging to what extent the responses reflect an understanding of the phenomenon in question which is similar to their own, he or she is supposed to focus on similarities and differences between the ways in which the phenomenon appears to the participants.

As the same participant may express more than one way of understanding the phenomenon, the individual is not the unit of analysis. The borders between the individuals are temporarily abandoned, as it were. The transcripts originating from the different individual interviews together make up undivided—and usually quite extensive—data to be analyzed. The first way of reducing the data is to distinguish between what is immediately relevant, from the point of view of expressing a way of experiencing the phenomenon in question, and that which is not. (Such decisions may, of course, be reconsidered subsequently in the continued course of analysis.) It might sometimes be found that different topics or phenomena have been dealt with in the interviews. In that case the data have to be organized according to topic or phenomenon to begin with, and the analysis has to be carried out for each topic or phenomenon, one at a time. The next step is to identify distinct ways of understanding (or experiencing) the phenomenon. There are two mechanisms through which a certain understanding appears. One is based on similarities: when it is found that two expressions which are different at the word level reflect the same meaning, there is awareness of a certain way of understanding the phenomenon. When two expressions reflect two different meanings, two ways of understanding the phenomenon may become thematized due to the contrast effect. At this point the analysis boils down to identifying and grouping expressed ways of experiencing the phenomenon (literally or metaphorically making excerpts from the interviews and putting them into piles). In order to do this it is necessary to aim at as deep an understanding as possible of what has been said, or rather, what has been meant. The various statements have to be seen in relation to two contexts. One of the contexts is "the pool of meanings" that derives from what all the participants have said about the same thing. The other context is—and here it is necessary to reintroduce the individual boundaries again—what the same person has said about other things. Thus it is necessary to make sense of particular expressions in terms of the collective as well as of the individual context. This is the hermeneutic element of the phenomenographic analysis.

After the relevant quotes have been grouped, the focus of attention is shifted from the relations between the quotes (expressions) to the relations between the groups. It is necessary to establish what the critical attributes of each group are and what features distinguish the groups from one another. In this way the set of "categories of description" is developed, characterized in terms of the variation in which a certain phenomenon is experienced, conceptualized, and understood. There are logical relations to be found between the categories of description and, as they represent different capabilities for seeing the phenomenon in question, in relation to a given criterion a hierarchy can be established. This ordered complex of categories of descriptions has been referred to above as the "outcome space."

The different steps in the phenomenographic analysis have to be taken interactively. As each consecutive step has implications not only for the steps that follow but also for the steps that precede it, the analysis has to go through several runs in which the different steps are considered to some extent simultaneously.

The categories of description and the outcome space are the main results of a phenomenographic study. Once they are found they can be reapplied to the data from which they originate. There will thus be a judgment made in each individual case concerning what category—or categories—of description is (or are) applicable. It is then possible to obtain the distribution of the frequencies of the categories of description.

3.3 Reliability

The question is often raised as to whether another researcher examining the same data would come up with the same results. Such a question implies a view of the analysis as a kind of measurement procedure. And repeated measurements should yield similar results, of course. The analysis is, however, not a measurement but a discovery procedure. Finding out the different ways in which a phenomenon can be experienced is as much a discovery as the finding of some new plants on a distant island. The discovery does not have to be replicable, but once the outcome space of a phenomenon has been revealed, it should be communicated in such a way that other researchers could recognize instances of the different ways of experiencing the phenomenon in question. After having studied the description of the outcome space, another researcher should be able to judge what categories of description apply to each individual case in the material in which the categories of description were found. As far as such a judgment is concerned there should be a reasonable degree of agreement between two independent and competent researchers. The expression "reasonable degree of agreement" is used to refer, somewhat arbitrarily, to cases where the two researchers agree in at least two-thirds of the cases when comparing their judgments and where they reach agreement in two-thirds of the remaining cases after discussion.

4. Applications of Phenomenography

As was pointed out earlier, phenomenography developed from empirical studies of learning in higher education. Although the interrelated nature of the act and the outcome of learning was emphasized in these early studies, in quite a few investigations the experience of the act of learning, problem solving (Laurillard 1984), and so on, and the understanding of the phenomenon of learning, understanding, and so on (Marton et al. 1993, Helmstad and Marton 1992) have been held in focus.

In other studies, the major focus has been on finding critical differences in which central phenomena, concepts, and principles in specific domains are understood (e.g, Linder 1989, Renström et al. 1990). There is an idea that this may be the most powerful way of finding out how the development of knowledge and skills within these domains can be facilitated. Research on learning form a phenomenographic perspective has been brought together by Marton and Booth (in press).

There is a pure phenomenographic "knowledge interest" that transcends the educational context. By describing the different ways in which individuals can experience, or understand, the world around them, they are characterizing the world as it appears to them, which is tantamount to characterizing "the collective mind" encompassing the different ways in which people are capable of making sense of the world (Marton 1981).

References

Asplund-Carlsson M, Marton F, Halász L 1992 Readers' experience and textual meaning. *J. Lit. Semantics*

Bowden J et al. 1992 Phenomenographic studies of understanding in physics: Displacement, velocity and frames of reference. *Am. J. Physics* 60(3): 262–69

Gurwitsch A 1964 *The Field of Consciousness*. Duquesne University Press, Pittsburgh, Pennsylvania

Helmstad G, Marton F 1992 Conceptions of understanding. Paper presented at the Annual Meeting of the American Educational Research Association, San Francisco, California, April 20–24

Hodgson V 1984 Learning from lectures. In: Marton F, Hounsell D, Entwistle N J (eds.) 1984

Hounsell D (1984) Learning and essay-writing. In: Marton F, Hounsell D, Entwistle N J (eds.) 1984

Laurillard D (1984) Learning from problem-solving. In: Marton F, Hounsell D, Entwistle N J (eds.) 1984

Linder C J 1989 A case study of university physics students' conceptualizations of sound. Unpublished doctoral dissertation. University of British Columbia, Canada

Lybeck L, Marton F, Strömdahl H, Tullberg A 1988 The phenomenography of "the mole concept" in chemistry. In: Ramsden P (ed.) 1988 *Improving Learning—New Perspectives*. Kogan Page, London

Marton F 1981 Phenomenography—describing conceptions of the world around us. *Instruc. Sci.* 10(2): 177–200

Marton F 1984 Toward a psychology beyond the individual. In: Lagerspetz K, Niemi P (eds.) 1984 *Psychology in the 1990s*. North-Holland, Amsterdam

Marton F, Booth S in press *Learning and Awareness*. Lawrence Erlbaum Associates, Mahwah, New Jersey

Marton F, Hounsell D, Entwistle N J (eds.) 1984 *The Experience of Learning*. Scottish Academic Press, Edinburgh

Marton F, Neuman D 1990 The perceptibility of numbers and the origin of arithmetic skills. *Report from the Department of Education and Educational Research, University of Göteborg*, No. 5

Marton F, Dall'Alba G, Beaty E 1993 Conceptions of learning. *Int. J. Educ. Res.* 19(3): 277–300

Marton F, Fensham P, Chaiklin S 1994 A Nobel's eye view of scientific intuition: Discussions with the Nobel prize-winners in physics, chemistry, and medicine (1970–1986). *Int. J. Sci. Educ.*

Neuman D 1987 *The Origin of Arithmetic Skills. A Phenomenographic Approach*. Acta Universitatis Gothoburgensis, Gothenburg

Renström L, Andersson B, Marton F 1990 Students' conceptions of matter. *J. Educ. Psychol.* 82(3): 555–69

Säljö R 1982 *Learning and Understanding. A Study of Differences in Constructing Meaning from a Text*. Acta Universitatis Gothoburgensis, Gothenburg

Svensson L 1984 Människobilden i INOM-gruppens forskning: Den lärande människan. *Rapporter från Pedagogiska institutionen, Göteborgs universitet*, No 3

Theman J 1983 *Uppfattningar av politisk makt* Acta Universitatis Gothoburgensis, Gothenburg

Wenestam C-G 1984 Qualitative age-related differences in the meaning of the word "death" to children. *Death Educ.* 8(5–6): 333–47

Self-report in Educational Research

R. Säljö

Since the late 1960s there has been a growth of research into education using so-called qualitative methods in which data are generated through interviews, written protocols, participant observation, and similar approaches. This entry discusses selected aspects of the value and problems of research focusing on self-reports and the role of such findings in furthering the understanding of educational processes.

1. The Collective Nature of Research

To conduct research is to be involved in a collective and institutionalized activity. This means that there are rules and traditions for what counts as valid modes of conducting investigations if these are to qualify as instances of research. The rules that researchers follow, however, are not universally shared amongst all scholars. In fact, there are constant, and sometimes heated, debates about whether a particular result or finding can be considered as scientifically proven or not and whether a particular methodology can be accepted. Self-report data, which are people's accounts of their own behavior and thinking collected through interviews or, sometimes, through written sources, have been the object of much discussion in education and other areas of social inquiry. Questions that have been raised concern the control and objectivity of research procedures when data are generated as well as when they are analyzed. Will two researchers analyzing the same interview protocol come up with the same findings? How does the sex, age, race, social standing of the interviewer and interviewee affect the outcome of interviews? Does it matter whether participants in studies are voluntary or not? Some of these issues have been discussed and analyzed in a very interesting way (see Rosenthal and Rosnow 1969).

In order to be able to judge the potential and the problems of self-report data, and, perhaps more generally, of qualitative data, it is important to have some insight into the historical background of methodological procedures and perspectives in the behavioral sciences.

2. The Issue of Method in Social Science Research: A Historical Sketch

When the social sciences developed during the latter half of the nineteenth century, powerful ideals concerning what were the appropriate rules according to which scientific inquiries should be conducted were already available. Through the impressive accomplishments within the natural sciences, primarily in physics, the distinctive elements of science could be readily identified. The road to future success would undoubtedly lie in the adoption of experimentation, exact measurement of clearly defined variables, and, in general, in incorporating into social science research the notion of objectivity that had proven so successful in the more advanced disciplines. The French sociologist/philosopher Auguste Comte, for instance, initiated the positivist movement which was to have an immense direct and indirect influence on the development of social science research. By focusing on the "positive," that is, the "real" and the "observable," social scientists would be able to objectify and quantify human phenomena in a way analogous to what was being done in the natural sciences. Only those aspects of life that were accessible to objective observations and measurements should be recognized as appropriate targets for research. There should no longer be any room for speculation and subjectivity.

In a similar vein, the foundations for modern empirical research into mental phenomena were laid by the German psychologist Hermann Ebbinghaus at the end of the nineteenth century when he invented the "nonsense" syllable through which memory (and learning) could be studied in an "objective" way. Since everything individuals learned and remembered was fundamentally influenced by what they already knew, it was very difficult to measure and pursue proper experimentation. By using meaningless learning materials in the form of distinctive units of three- or four-letter syllables, exact measurements were possible and retention could be described in exact percentages of what had been acquired. Furthermore, the differences in previous experiences were neutralized, since the previous knowledge of subjects would not interfere with the remembering of meaningless items. Ebbinghaus's ingenious invention and his incorporation of experimental procedures into studies of memory are very clear examples of how methodological ideals—rather than substantive insights—preceded research on cognitive phenomena. Polemi-

cally expressed, it is possible to say that scholars had strong ideas about how to do research but quite often only weak theories about the phenomena they were studying. This contrasts with the situation in the natural sciences where methods and instruments generally have developed in an intimate interplay with theoretical insight.

3. Qualitative Approaches to the Study of Education

The issue of whether atoms and human beings can, and should, be studied with a similar set of methodological approaches continues to be controversial (see, e.g., *Educational Researcher* [1992] which includes a debate where distinguished educational researchers argue for and against the relative merits of "positivist" and "qualitative" approaches to research). If the conflicts are disregarded, and consideration is given to the development of the social sciences since the early 1940s, it is evident that the growth of research traditions that can be loosely termed as "qualitative" has occurred. Thus, within the field of education, studies using participant observation, interviews, and, more recently, discourse analytical approaches for understanding schooling have become frequent. An increasing number of studies of education are inspired by philosophical positions which rely on qualitative data such as ethnomethodology, phenomenology, symbolic interactionism and a range of social constructivist approaches. Similarly, crossfertilization through contacts with other disciplines such as social anthropology and some sociological traditions has resulted in the incorporation of ethnographic approaches into the study of significant educational phenomena.

A key feature of these approaches to the study of social phenomena is that they use language as data and that meaning plays a prominent role. The assumption is that to understand human action and complex phenomena such as schooling, it is necessary to recognize that human beings—unlike inanimate objects studied in other fields—are agents in social situations. They not only respond and react, but they also interpret and create, and they act on the basis of their interpretations. The ability to reflect and to communicate bestowed upon human beings through their use of language makes the study of social and cultural phenomena different from the study of dead objects. To understand complex activities it is necessary to have insight into the modes of construing reality that people rely on and that guide them in their actions in real life settings. Acquiring knowledge in school is infinitely more complex than the phenomena addressed in the laboratory setting in which the learning experiment is conducted. Unless investigators are willing to adopt more "naturalist approaches" (Shulman 1986) to research in which people appear as informants, and not just as research subjects, they run the risk of learning very little about the intricacies of schooling.

An extension of this kind of argument is that teaching and learning in the context of a formal institution such as the school look very different to different actors. Even the very activity of learning is construed differently by people varying in their educational experiences (see Marton et al. 1993 for an interesting case in point). In order to be able to understand educational processes, it is important to scrutinize in detail what people actually do, and not to assume a knowledge of what teaching and learning is all about. In parenthesis, this general idea of not assuming a knowledge of what teaching is, was a key ingredient in one of the earliest studies into classroom life using qualitative (and quantitative) methods (Waller's classic *The Sociology of Teaching*, 1932). Through his in-depth analyses of what life in school was like, it was possible to see the dilemmas and conflicts of teaching and learning that were so significant for the outcomes of schooling, but which would not appear as evidence in research unless the investigators entered the classroom and were willing to postpone definite judgments until they had shared the daily activities of those who were to be studied.

To summarize the arguments so far, verbal data and self-reports in interviews and written documents have become important sources of information about education. Before attempting to continue illustrating the value and potential of findings from research using such methods, it is important to deal with one persistent misunderstanding regarding the status of self-report data.

3.1 Away from Introspectionism

One of the obvious backgrounds for the distrust among scientists of qualitative data is the tendency to consider people's accounts of the world and their reports of their experiences as introspectionism. The rise of modern social science, in particular within psychology, is to a large extent a reaction against the introspectionism that was practiced in the psychological laboratories in Europe in the nineteenth century. In these traditions people were asked to report on their own mental processes and their own psychological reactions. The assumption behind this work was that individuals had access to their own mental processes and that by having subjects report on their perceptions and thoughts, it was possible to find the building blocks of mental life.

Research studies in the early 1990s using qualitative methods and self-report data, in most cases work from the opposite assumption. It is only by seriously attending to people's accounts of their experiences that it is possible to get to know why they act in the way they do. Thus the object of inquiry is no longer the mental processes per se as was the case in introspectionist studies, but rather how the world appears to people with different experiences and different perspectives. For instance, when Jackson (1968) and Hargreaves

(1993) interviewed teachers about their rationales for teaching in the way they did, they asked teachers to provide personal interpretations of professional life and lived experiences, and not to look into the depths of their own minds. Similarly, when representatives of the influential United Kingdom research tradition referred to as the "new sociology of school" investigated student and teacher strategies in school (Woods 1990), or when Willis (1977) talked with British working-class adolescents about their relation to school life, these scholars used interviews (as well as other methods) to gain access to real life events as perceived by those involved, and did not have people report on the mechanisms of their mind. The tendency to misinterpret qualitative data as introspective is still prevalent. A productive discussion of this issue can be found in two influential articles (see Nisbett and DeCamp Wilson 1977, Ericsson and Simon 1980).

4. Research Findings Based on Self-report Data

The use of self-report data has become so commonplace that it is impossible to form a complete overview. To substantiate the claims about the role and value of outcomes from research using such data, some studies that have contributed to an understanding of schooling are briefly summarized.

4.1 Studies of College Life

In 1968, Perry published a highly original study in which self-report data played a prominent role. After working for many years as a student counselor at Harvard University, Perry began to take an interest in how students dealt with academic life and what produced success and failure in the particular context of an institution of higher learning. The kinds of issues that triggered Perry's interest were concerned with how students coped with academic life and how they developed during the course of their university career. In particular, the modes in which students construed their own experiences, and their interpretations of the wealth of impressions they were exposed to inside and outside classes and seminars, were addressed.

In the systematic and longitudinal study which Perry designed on the basis of his observations as a counselor, open-ended interviews were used. The most important question, given at the end of each college year, was simply phrased as "Would you like to say what has stood out for you during the year?". In order to follow up on the general statements given by the students in response to this question, Perry and his colleagues continued: "As you speak of that, do any particular instances come to mind?" (Perry 1968 p. 7). In all their simplicity these two questions illustrate two important features of this kind of qualitative research. Thus, the first question invites the interviewees to comment on what they construe as significant experiences in a particular context using their own language and their own priorities. The second question requires them to describe the actual events and/or situations that triggered these experiences. Accounts are produced according to the priorities and decisions of the interviewee, but attempts are made to ground these descriptions in data regarding the concrete circumstances which triggered the reactions.

Perry's (1968) results are important for several reasons. He shows that cognitive (and ethical) development is not something that is tied to biological processes as, for instance, scholars doing research from a traditional intelligence theory perspective or from a Piagetian framework had more or less taken for granted. On the contrary, cognitive growth is a sociocultural process and a response to the needs of coping with new challenges. Thus, Perry describes how students when they enter the college context have an interpretation of knowledge as essentially equivalent to static "facts" which they are supposed to memorize during their careers. Faced with the relativism of modern scientific thinking and the conflicting views of how to understand and explain significant phenomena in the world, most students develop and become relativists themselves, that is, they learn to live in a world of apparent contradictions and to accept this as a natural state of affairs. They become acculturated into a world view in which knowledge is always from a certain perspective and in which understandings are continuously revised in response to new insights and arguments. In the final stage of their development, students make "commitments" and, while accepting diversity and conflicting world views, they take a personal stand on what is their own point of view.

Perry's (1968) results are also important since they provide a background for understanding students' difficulties that can assist teachers, counselors, and others in the attempts to remedy problems and prevent academic failure. For someone who assumes that knowledge can be conceived as a clear and static entity that is true without qualifications, a context for learning such as a modern university might be quite confusing. In view of these findings, learning problems may not necessarily be construed as resulting from intellectual deficiences. Instead they may be conceived as grounded in unfamiliarity with the particular mode in which this social institution construes knowledge.

A similar study of college life was carried out by the United States sociologists Becker et al. (1968). These authors represent what is known as the Chicago school of sociology, a tradition which has been important in furthering qualitative research on schooling as well as on many other important social issues such as deviance and subcultures. In their book they portray college life as it appears from what they call the "student perspective." Thus, what from the teacher's point of view is done from a certain background and with certain intentions, may, and often is, transformed in the

student perspective to be something else. The authors attempt to demystify the college and regard it not as an environment for learning in any neutral sense of this word. Instead, the student perspective helps students identify the particular definitions of learning that are valid in this specific setting and it thus provides a filter through which they can orientate themselves and decide how to go about their daily lives. A key element is what is called the "GPA-perspective," through which all activities and efforts are evaluated. Grades thus take on a position similar to that of money in other sectors of society; it becomes the yardstick of almost everything. "We were also impressed," the authors argue, "when a common . . . answer to our intentionally vague opening question 'How are you doing?' or 'How are things?' was for the student to give his grade point average for the last or the current semester" (Becker et al. 1968 p. 88). The authors then go on to describe how the institutional form of learning to some extent implies a distortion of genuine learning processes in the sense that students learn to "produce the appearance of satisfactory performance without the substance" (Becker et al. 1968 p. 136).

4.2 Illuminating Pedagogical Practices

Self-report data have also played an important role in illuminating concrete pedagogical practices and students' responses to such practices. In an in-depth study of university students' essay writing, Hounsell (1988) showed how the ability to produce high quality work in an educational setting is not necessarily merely a function of the intellectual capacity of a student (as some of their lecturers seemed to take for granted). By interviewing students and by analyzing the essays they wrote during their studies in different academic fields, Hounsell shows how the difficulties students had in producing satisfactory work could be traced back to their lack of understanding of the nature of traditions for argumentation that were characteristic of different fields. Some of the students, for instance, had no clear conception that arguments had to be grounded in data, or they were unclear about what counted as evidence in a particular discipline. The problems of understanding how disciplines constituted frameworks for discourse must be traced back to the fact that the students had never been introduced to these issues during lectures or in their interactions with the teachers. The criteria remained tacit since the teachers did not assume that there were any difficulties in understanding how students should argue in essays.

4.3 Studies of Mastery of Literacy

In a series of studies on how children learned to read, Francis (1982) employed self-report data from children in order to probe into children's growing mastery of literacy and the difficulties they encountered. On the basis of interviews, as a complement to participant observation of classroom life and analyses of writing activities, Francis showed how some children had difficulties in understanding the correspondence between written and spoken words, and even in realizing why reading was important and what it was used for. Under these circumstances, the teaching of literacy skills to a large extent became incomprehensible for the children.

4.4 Issues of Gender and Schooling

Issues of gender and schooling have been addressed through self-report data. Measor (1984), for instance, began a study of how girls and boys reacted to physical science and domestic science teaching respectively by questioning the gender neutrality of learning processes taken for granted in learning theory. By observing teaching and learning and by interviewing students and teachers, Measor showed how these curricular areas were approached with attitudes and assumptions that were clearly gender related and that had obvious implications for the outcome.

4.5 Research into Learning Strategies

Since the late 1960s there has been a rapid growth of research into the learning strategies used in different subject matter areas. Because researchers have questioned and rejected more and more the assumption of identical learning processes in different areas, considerable attention has been given to trying to understand how students acquire subject matter knowledge. In this research, self-report data often play a prominent role in the attempts to gain access to difficulties in understanding intellectually complex tasks. The point of departure of much of this work is precisely the assumption that insight into students' "alternative frameworks" (Driver and Easley 1978) is a vital component when attempts are to be made to improve education. To gain access to students' perspectives, self-report data on the learning and understanding of significant phenomena in the different subjects are now systematically used (Ramsden 1988).

5. Perspectivity and Research in Education

Self-report data that are rigorously analyzed are important in the understanding of a complex social enterprise such as modern education. It is vital to have access to students' and teachers' perspectives and definitions of what goes on in school if education is to develop and meet present and future challenges. It is also necessary to recognize that different actors in the field of education look at teaching and learning from different perspectives, and their needs for knowledge vary. What the teacher in first grade, the mathematics or history teacher in high school, or the university lecturer wants to know about teaching and learning is different from what the administrator or politician needs to know. To the teachers, knowledge about the daily life in school, pupil strategies when learning to read or when struggling with algebra or grammar, is essential when trying to improve the quality of the educational process, while the administrators and politicians are generally primarily interested in a more global picture of "inputs" and "outputs" of schooling. For those who are involved in schooling, the insights from qualitative research are particularly powerful (Entwistle 1984). Teaching is a communicative enterprise and awareness of students' perspectives and thinking is what makes it possible to take informed decisions on how to instruct, explain, and promote understanding. Self-report data—when properly analyzed—sensitize people to what goes on in schools and provide concepts and frameworks through which a qualified debate about the dilemmas of instruction can be openly pursued. This is an important contribution of research to educational practice.

However, self-report data should not be considered as privileged to other sources of information. When students report on how they try to solve a physics problem or how they understand a certain principle in economics, they provide the researcher with data, but they do not give the whole or the final picture. An individual's interpretation of his or her own activities is not a neutral verdict on what happened that can be accepted at face value. Nevertheless in addressing many significant educational issues, the development of an understanding would be hampered if considerable attention was not given to how schooling was construed by those directly involved.

See also: Phenomenography; Research in Education: Epistemological Issues

References

Becker H, Geer B, Hughes E 1968 *Making the Grade*: *The Academic Side of College Life*. Wiley, New York
Driver R, Easley J Pupils and paradigms: A review of literature related to concept development in adolescent science students. *Stud. Sci. Educ.* 5:61–84
Educational Researcher 1992 A debate on positivist and qualitative approaches to research 21(5)
Entwistle N 1984 Contrasting perspectives on learning. In: Marton F, Hounsell D, Entwistle N (eds.) 1984 *The Experience of Learning*. Scottish Academic Press, Edinburgh
Ericsson K A, Simon H A 1980 Verbal reports as data. *Psychol. Rev.* 87(3): 215–51
Francis H 1982 *Learning to Read*: *Literate Behaviour and Orthographic Knowledge*. Allen and Unwin, London
Hargreaves A 1993 Individualism and individuality: Reinterpreting the teacher culture. *Int. J. Educ. Res.* 19(3): 227–46
Hounsell D 1988 Towards an anatomy of academic discourse: Meaning and context in the undergraduate essay. In: Säljö R (ed.) 1968 *The Written World*. Springer-Verlag, Berlin
Jackson P W 1968 *Life in Classrooms*. Holt, Rinehart and Winston, New York
Marton F, Dall'Alba G, Beaty E 1993 Conceptions of learning. *Int. J. Educ. Res.* 19(3): 277–99
Measor L 1984 Gender and the sciences: Pupils' gender-

based conceptions of school subjects. In: Hammersley M, Woods P (eds.) 1984 *Life in School. The Sociology of Pupil Culture.* Open University Press, Milton Keynes

Nisbett R E, DeCamp Wilson R 1977 Telling more than we can know: Verbal reports on mental processes. *Psychol. Rev.* 84(3): 231–59.

Perry W G 1968 *Forms of Intellectual and Ethical Development in the College Years.* Harvard University, Cambridge, Massachusetts

Ramsden P (ed.) 1988 *Improving Learning: New Perspectives.* Kogan Page, London

Rosenthal R, Rosnow R L (eds.) 1969 *Artifact in Behavioral Research.* Academic Press, New York

Shulman L S 1986 Paradigms and research programs in the study of teaching: A contemporary perspective. In: Wittrock M C (ed.) 1986 *Handbook of Research on Teaching.* MacMillan, New York

Waller W 1932 *The Sociology of Teaching.* Wiley, New York

Willis P 1977 *Learning to Labour. How Working Class Kids get Working Class Jobs.* Saxon House, Farnborough

Woods P 1990 *The Happiest Days? How Pupils Cope with Schools.* Falmer Press, London

Further Reading

Eisner E, Pershkin A (eds.) 1990 *Qualitative Inquiry in Education: The Continuing Debate.* Teachers College Press, New York

Säljö R (ed.) 1993 Learning discourse: Qualitative Research in Education. *Int. J. Educ. Res.* 19(3): 199–325 (special issue)

Semiotics in Educational Research

J. Anward

Semiotics is, in the words of its two founders, the Swiss linguist Ferdinand de Saussure (1857–1913) and the United States philosopher Charles Sanders Peirce (1839–1914), the study of "the life of signs within society" (Saussure 1916 p. 33) and "the essential nature and fundamental varieties of possible semiosis" (Peirce Vol. 5 p. 488), semiosis being the process whereby something comes to stand for something else, and thus acquires the status of sign. Since education, like all social activities, is crucially a sign-mediated activity, semiotics has an obvious bearing on the study of educational phenomena. Educational semiotics can be defined as the study of the use of signs and the fundamental varieties of signs employed within education. This entry is concerned with the use of signs in education, and considers the developments, definitions, and research that has been undertaken in the field of semiotics.

1. Signs

Semiotics does not begin with Peirce and Saussure. A theory of verbal signs, chiefly words, was articulated by the ancient Greeks, most notably by the Stoics, who developed a fully modern theory of verbal signs. According to the Stoics, a spoken or written word which is used on some occasion to stand for a particular object, its referent on that occasion, does not relate directly to its referent. It would be misleading simply to regard the word as a name of that referent. A word unites a form—a signifier—and a concept—a signified—and it is through this connection that a word may stand for a referent or, to be more accurate, an unlimited number of referents. Every phenomenon that falls under the concept linked to a certain word form may be a referent of the word constituted by that word form and that concept. To the Stoics, signifiers and referents are "bodies" and "sensible," while signifieds are only "intelligible." In a contemporary operational definition, signifieds are defined as that which the barbarians cannot grasp when they hear Greek, in contrast to signifiers and referents, which are available to both Greeks and barbarians.

The Stoic theory of verbal signs was taken up and elaborated by Peirce and Saussure, and generalized from a theory of verbal signs to a theory of signs in general, which became the founding moves of semiotics. In Peirce's writings, the Stoic triad of signifier, signified, and referent surfaces as a triad of sign (or representamen), interpretant, and object. "A sign stands *for* something *to* the idea which it produces, or modifies . . . . That for which it stands is called its *object*; . . . and the idea to which it gives rise, its *interpretant*" (Peirce Vol. 1 p. 339). Signs are not a discrete class of phenomena, though. Anything can be a sign, provided that it enters a process of semiosis, where it "determines something else (its *interpretant*) to refer to an object to which itself refers (its *object*) in the same way, the interpretant becoming in turn a sign, and so on *ad infinitum*" (Peirce Vol. 2 p. 300). A remarkable feature of this definition is the notion that the process of semiosis does not stop with the immediate interpretant of a sign. An interpretant is itself a sign, with its own interpretant, which in turn is a sign, and so on. Eco (1976 p. 69) states: "the very definition of sign implies a process of *unlimited semiosis*." In fact, it is this process of unlimited semiosis that is the true object of Peircean semiotics, signs being just more or less stable products of this process.

It is in this perspective that Peirce's famous distinction between index, icon, and symbol should be understood. This distinction is an attempt to generalize and solve the classical semiotic problem posed already by Plato in the dialogue *Cratylus*: How is a word related to the things it stands for? Does the word somehow "reside" in the things it names, being, for example, the characteristic sound of these things, or is it just a conventional label for these things? In the dialogue, Socrates explores the view, held by Cratylus, that words have meaning naturally, using analogies between the way sounds are made and phenomena denoted by words containing such sounds as evidence for natural meaning. For example, the *l* sound is motivated in *leios* (slippery), because there is an analogy between the property that the word denotes and the loose and liquid way in which *l* is produced. However, Socrates also notes cases where *l* is out of place, as in *sklérotes* (hardness), and concludes therefore that both convention and nature must be recognized as sources of meaning for verbal signs.

An index is a signifier which is spatiotemporally connected to its referent, the referent often being the cause of the signifier, as when smoke stands for fire, and tracks for an animal. An icon is a signifier that resembles what it stands for in some respect. Photographs and painted portraits are icons, as are pantomimes and onomatopoetic words, such as "cuckoo." Peirce further subdivides icons into images and diagrams. In an image, each part of the signifier, as well as the way the parts are related, should bear some resemblance to its object, while in a diagram, only the relations among the parts need be iconic. Thus, a portrait of a face is an image, while a histogram comparing, say, the amount of literacy in Sweden with the amount of literacy in the United Kingdom is a diagram. A symbol, finally, is a signifier which is only conventionally related to its object, by rule, as Peirce puts it.

Index, icon, and symbol are normally taken as a classification of signs. But that is misleading, and not in line with Peirce's intentions. What Peirce classifies is rather semioses, ways in which something comes to stand for something else. Semiosis can arise through causation (index), through resemblance (icon), or by rule (symbol), and one and the same sign may combine all these kinds of semioses. Consider, for example, a device which signals that there is too little water in a container. Since the signal is caused by the water sinking below a certain level, the device is an index. If furthermore the signal consists in lighting up an image of an empty container, then the device is also an icon. Finally, if the meaning of the device is "fill the container with water, before you go on," as opposed to, say, "Go on!" then the device is also a symbol. In other words, the semiosis which links the device to the water level in the container, combines semiosis through causation, resemblance, and rule. To Peirce, this kind of composite semiosis is the typical case of semiosis.

A number of developments in semiotic theory have underscored the importance of composite semiosis. Peirce extended indexical semiosis to verbal signs, the most typical symbols there are, to account for what is traditionally called deictic expressions, that is, expressions that refer to some aspect of the speech event, such as "I," "you," "here," "there," "now," and "then." Deictic expressions are "shifters": what is described by "here" at one occasion need not be so describable at another occasion. This makes the spatiotemporal link between such signifiers and their referents a necessary component of their semiosis. At the same time, rules are clearly involved, since the form of deictic expressions is conventional. Garfinkel (1967, see also Heritage 1984 Chap. 6) generalizes this idea, arguing that every act of description has an indexical component to it. In fact, it is precisely this indexical component that allows a signifier to stand for a particular referent, through the mediation of a general signified. What "book" stands for on a particular occasion depends on the spatiotemporal context in which it is used.

Jakobson (1971) argues that verbal signs have a significant iconic component, as well. For example, a plural noun is normally marked by a separate affix, as opposed to a singular noun, which has no number affix. This makes pairs of singular and plural nouns, such as "book—books," into diagrams, where a contrast between a lesser and a larger quantity is expressed by a contrast between a shorter and a longer form. Another example are pairs of expressions with the meaning of "here" and "there." There is an overwhelming tendency in the world's languages to use a front vowel, such as *i*, in the word meaning "here," and a back vowel, such as *o* or *a*, in the word meaning "there" (see, e.g., Tanz 1971). German *hier—da* and French *ici—là* exemplify this tendency. This makes diagrams out of "here—there" pairs, the relative distance of the tongue from the speaker's face at their syllable nuclei mirroring the relative distance from the speaker of the indicated place. A word such as *ici* thus resembles the device for indicating water level described above, in that it combines indexical, iconic, and symbolic semiosis.

In the other direction, Eco (1976) argues that there are no pure icons, that resemblances that constitute icons always require correspondence rules to be recognized. For example, whether

U

is to be interpreted as the letter U or as an empty container depends on which correspondence rules are used.

2. Codes

The distinctive contribution of Saussure to semiotics is his demonstration of the role of codes in semiosis. Saussure takes the Stoic model of the verbal sign, including the terminology of sign, signifier, and signified, as his point of departure, but argues that neither signifier nor signified should be regarded as an object or "body." Just as the signified allows a sign to stand for an unlimited number of referents, the signifier allows an unlimited number of forms to stand for such referents. Each production of a word form is unique, but two such productions can nevertheless be interpreted as instances of the same word. So just as the signified is a concept, and not an object, the signifier is a concept, too, a sound concept. Saussure also follows the Stoics in saying that the relation between the signifier and the signified of a particular sign is arbitrary, not motivated by the nature of the signifier and the signified. Verbal signs are thus Peircean symbols, according to Saussure. However, the Saussurean notions of signifier and signified transcend all previous theories of signs. To Saussure, a verbal sign is not a pairing of independently given concepts. On the contrary, a verbal sign can only exist as part of a larger system of signs, a code. And this is because an arbitrary sign can be motivated only by a code. If a sign is not motivated by an inner relation between signifier and signified, or by being grafted onto an already existing code, then the nature of its signifier and signified can only be determined in relation to other signs, through the ways in which the sign differs from other signs, with which it contrasts and combines. For example, in a small subsystem containing only the words "cow," "horse," "moo," and "neigh," cow is defined through its contrast with horse, and its ability to combine with a following moo, but not with anything else.

However, the position of a sign within a system or subsystem of signs does not determine its full meaning, but only its value. The full meaning derives from that value being applied to some domain of reference. In the terminology of Hjelmslev (1969), a content form (the value of a sign's signified) is applied to a content matter (domain of reference), yielding a content substance, that is, the matter organized by the form. For example, when "cow" and "horse" are applied to the domain of domesticated animals, phenomena in this domain will be organized by two broad and nonoverlapping categories. For orthodox structural linguists, such as Saussure and Hjelmslev, content matter is always organized by language. However, more recent research on, among other things, color terms and terms for shapes suggest strongly that many domains are in fact preorganized by language-independent perception and cognition, which means that verbal signs pertaining to such domains become labels of already existing categories, rather than category-creating devices.

The most important relations organizing a system of verbal signs (Saussure's *langue*) are paradigmatic and syntagmatic relations. Paradigmatic relations hold among contrasting items, that is, items which can substitute for each other in a given position. Syntagmatic relations hold among items that can be combined with each other to form a larger unit. Thus, in the small subsystem presented above, there is a paradigmatic relation between cow and

horse, and between moo and neigh, and a syntagmatic relation between cow and moo, and between horse and neigh. As shown by Jakobson (1971), items organized by paradigmatic relations often exhibit a logic of markedness, whereby one of the items, the unmarked item, contrasts with a set of more informative items, the marked items. For example, in Swedish the paradigm *ko* (cow), *tjur* (bull), and *kalv*, (calf), contains the marked items *tjur* and *kalv*, and the unmarked item *ko*. As Jakobson puts it, *ko*, the unmarked item, can be used either to signal the absence of the properties implied by the marked items, "male" in the case of *tjur* and "child" in the case of *kalv*, or the absence of signaling of these properties, in which case the unmarked item is used as a generic term for the domain covered by the entire paradigm. Jakobson also suggests that markedness is normally diagrammatically iconic, the greater semantic complexity of marked items being matched by greater formal complexity. This can be seen clearly in the Swedish paradigm, but not so clearly in the corresponding English paradigm.

Saussure stays within the Stoic theory in that his notion of sign, unlike Peirce's, does not incorporate a process of unlimited semiosis. In later developments of Saussure's theory, by Hjelmslev (1969) and Barthes (1968), the possibility of further semiosis, beyond the primary signified, is introduced. Hjelmslev proposes a process of connotation, whereby an entire sign is made into a signifier that is associated with a new signified, as when the image of a cross, or the word "cross" comes to signify Christianity. Most of what is called symbolism would thus come out as Hjelmslevian connotation, and Peircean unlimited semiosis can be reconstructed as a series of connotations.

The idea that meaning beyond primary signifieds is coded has come under attack. Sperber and Wilson (1986) argue that such meaning is never coded, but always a product of context-dependent inferencing. Thus, the meaning of Heartfield's famous picture where the branches of a Christmas tree are bent to form a swastika, something like "Nazi oppression extends to every aspect of life," would not be a coded meaning, but the result of a complex inferential process, taking the picture and a variety of contextual assumptions as premises. Sperber and Wilson's argument has considerable force, particularly in view of the context-dependency and open-endedness of connotational meanings. There is, however, a residue of coded connotations, where the meaning is too stable to be derivable in the Sperber–Wilson way. The example of a cross signifying Christianity, contrasting with a half-moon, a lotus flower, a wheel, a sun, and so on is a case in point. Such cases are probably best regarded as conventionalized inferences, which short-circuit the normal inferential process. But this residue does not affect the essential point of Sperber and Wilsons argument, which is a generalization of Saussure's ideas about the code dependency of signs to all kinds of signs. In other words, there can be no semiosis without a code. What appears to be semiosis without code is simply inferencing.

3. *Codes in Educational Activities*

The basic point of Peircean semiotics is that anything can be a sign. The basic point of Saussurean semiotics is that being a sign entails being part of a code. The study of the life of signs and the fundamental varieties of semiosis within a particular social activity is thus a study of the various semiotic codes operating within that activity, their nature, function, and interaction. The semiotic codes operative within education are here discussed primarily in relation to the activity of teaching through classroom interaction.

Teaching is the activity of bringing about learning with respect to something (Hirst 1973). In classroom inter-action, this activity has the following basic components to it, involving one or more teachers (A), one or more students (B), and some kind of subject matter (C):

(a) A brings it about that

(b) B learns something about C, L(C),

(c) by presenting L(C) to A.

(d) B demonstrates that

(e) B has learnt L(C),

(f) by presenting L(C) to A.

Semiotic codes are called on to ensure presentation of the subject matter, to display what is to be learnt or has been learnt about it, and to maintain the frames of the activity itself, differentiating it from other activity types and identifying it as teaching. Semiotic codes provide for these functions by securing the intelligibility of states and events in the activity as signs that stand for some aspect of the subject matter at hand, mark some aspect of the sub-ject matter as involved in learning, and/or indicate some aspect of the encompassing activity. Signs which stand for some aspect of the subject matter at hand elaborate the *topic* of teaching; signs which mark some aspect of the subject matter as something which is to be learnt or has been learnt elaborate the *text* of teaching; finally, signs which indicate some aspect of the activity in which it is embedded elaborate the *activity* itself (Anward 1996).

The simplest elaboration of the activity of teaching is the signification of "this is teaching." This message is indexically signified by the presence of certain persons and objects at a certain place at a certain time, as well as by the spatial organization of these persons and objects at that place at that time. Consider the following quotation from Byers and Byers (1972 p. 19):

> At another time, in the same school, there were two boys who, at the beginning of the year, often behaved wildly and "tore up the classroom." By midyear their relation to the other people in the classroom was proceeding more peacefully. Then, one morning the two boys suddenly swept all the large building blocks off the shelf onto the floor. The teacher recalls asking herself, "Why did they do that? What is different in the room today?" When she looked around the room she saw an adult

who was new and a stranger to the class. So she went up to the boys and said, "Do you want to know who that person is?" They nodded yes. The teacher said, "I think you know the words to ask that question. Now please put the blocks back, come over and sit down, and I'll tell you who she is." The boys put the blocks back and went to the teacher, and she introduced them to the newcomer.

Two things are important in this example. First, the presence of an unintroduced person in the classroom was sufficient to change a signifier of teaching into a signifier of something else, at least for the two boys. Second, this does not mean that the signifier of teaching could not be changed. It was changed, to include the newcomer, but that had to be made in the proper way, by the teacher.

The spatial organization of persons and objects in the classroom is not only a conventional index of the activity of teaching, but also a diagram of the relations of power and distance that hold between teachers and students. Elevation of the teacher's desk, orientation of students toward that desk, significant tools within the reach of the teacher, but not of the students, are among those relations that diagram teacher control over students and tools, and these relations are also typically manipulated in pedagogical experiments of various kinds. The outcome of such experiments is crucially dependent on whether relations of power and distance in the classroom are shaped by the spatial organization of persons and objects in the classroom or have an independent basis, that is, whether the content matter is preorganized or not. If it is preorganized, if power relations depend on other things than spatial organization, then making the signifier of teaching less iconic of such relations will have little effect on teaching itself, although it may have some effect on learning.

Another elaboration of the activity of teaching is provided by signifiers which elaborate the temporal organization of a lesson. Framing markers (Sinclair and Coulthard 1975) index its beginning, its end, and the boundaries between its various phases. The school bell is the most salient framing marker, but a framing marker may also be a shift of position or gaze, a gesture, possibly involving a tool, such as a chalk or a pointer, a word such as "OK," "well," and "now," or some combination of these devices. Another aspect of the temporal organi-zation is turn-taking. There are conventional signifiers to indicate a wish to take a next turn, at speaking or at some other kind of task, such as raising a hand and/or uttering a vocative, and there are conventional signifiers to nominate the one whose turn it is: looking, pointing, uttering "yes," and/or uttering a vocative.

The activity of teaching is also elaborated through rep-resentational means. Both the identity and the temporal organization of teaching can be the topic of classroom talk, as when students are told that they are at school and nowhere else, and entire lessons, as well as phases of lessons, are overtly structured by introductions and summaries. Furthermore, the identity and the temporal organization of teaching are also connoted by classroom talk. An utterance such as "open your books at page 46!"

indexes both a preceding temporal boundary and, by soliciting a teaching-specific action, the very activity of teaching.

Topic is elaborated by a web of signifiers from a wide variety of semiotic codes: gesture, pantomime, nonverbal sound, picture, film, sign language, spoken language, and written language. Consider, for example, a possible lesson on Columbus's voyage to America. Besides a substantial amount of talk on Columbus and related issues, the lesson involves a written text, which is required reading before the lecture, as well as a self-instructing work sheet. The teacher introduces the topic by asking questions about the written text, then moves on to a lecture phase, which is illustrated by pictures in the textbook, and by a short animated sequence shown on video, where Columbus's three ships are seen moving across the Atlantic Ocean. The teacher's talk is accompanied both by gestures, as when a flat horizontal right hand, with the palm down, illustrates a flat earth, and a sphere made by two cupped hands, with palms down, first separating, then moving in downward half-circles, and finally meeting, with palms up, illustrates a round earth, and by a pantomime, including a variety of nonverbal sounds, which illustrates the restlessness of the crew. In the final phase of the lesson, the students work through the self-instructing work sheet, writing answers to print-ed questions, making a few calculations, and drawing Columbus's route on a printed map. For some further relevant examples, see Beckmann (1979) on graphic methods of proof in mathematics, and McNeill (1979) on gestures accompanying talk about mathematical issues.

Assessing the roles of the various codes in the didactic web involves at least two basic issues. The first issue concerns the expressive efficacy of the various codes. This issue is a tangled one (see Goodman 1969, 1978, Benveniste 1981, Baron 1981, Nadin 1984, and Sonesson 1989 for discussion), but some results apparently stand, the most important of which is that verbal codes (sign language, spoken language, and written language), but not nonverbal codes (gesture, pantomime, nonverbal sound, picture, film), have the capacity to establish secondary deictic centers, at which represented events can be located. In other words, only the verbal codes can provide for equivalents of the following opening of a story:

> It *was* a cold night *in Lisbon, Portugal, in 1492. If* the full moon *had not been* shining, *it would have been pitch dark.*

The nonverbal codes generally have no equivalents of the italicized portions of this opening, and it is precisely these portions of the opening that locate the represented event in time (in 1492), physical space (in Lisbon, Portugal), and "logical space" (as the real alternative of an unreal possible world, where the moon was not shining and it was pitch dark). This suggests not only that the verbal codes are indispensible in any kind of topic-elaborating teaching, but also a very specific role for these codes in such teaching, namely the role of anchoring code, that

code which is used to establish the topics which are elaborated by the didactic web.

The role of anchoring code is not the same as the role of interpreting code, introduced by Benveniste (1981). An interpreting code is a code in which all messages of all codes can be interpreted. For Benveniste, the verbal codes are interpreting codes of all semiotic codes, including the verbal codes themselves. Within a particular social activity, such as teaching, an interpreting code is designated as that code in the web of codes of that activity, in which all messages emanating from the entire web can be interpreted. While the verbal codes are cast in the role of anchoring code in teaching, it is not clear that they always constitute the interpreting code. There is pictorial information, involving, for example, design and architecture, that is quite impossible to capture verbally. For relevant discussion, see Nadin (1984).

The second basic issue relating to the composition of the didactic web is the issue of didactic efficacy. What is the optimal composition of the didactic web for various combinations of subject, background, and goal? In the studies reviewed by Beckmann (1979), for example, it was found that graphic methods of proof facilitated learning of mathematics for students with a humanistic background. This may suggest that, for these students, the graphic code took on the roles of anchoring code and interpreting code, with respect to the mathematical code.

The issue of didactic efficacy is intimately connected with the third function of signs in teaching, that of elaborating the text of teaching. In practice, multiple coding of a certain message is often used to mark that message as part of what is to be learnt, as opposed to what is just said or shown during a lesson. A very simple technique is to repeat a spoken message at least once, and then present a record of that message, in the form of a written message or a picture, on the blackboard or on an overhead projector (Anward 1996). Thus, in actual teaching, requirements of multiple coding arising from considerations of didactic efficacy may be superseded by the text-marking function of multiple coding. To complicate things further, explicit text-marking may itself be an essential factor in didactic efficacy.

A series of didactic texts established about a topic organize that topic into a subject part and a non subject part, sustaining a pattern of classification and framing, in the sense of Bernstein (1977). Signs used to establish a certain subject, for example, scientific terms, sentences expressing laws and facts, and graphic representations of various kinds, then come to index that subject, and, since the subject is itself an index of teaching, the very activity of teaching. Thus, a piece of talk or writing containing "species" connotes "this is biology," which in turn connotes "this is teaching." Furthermore, elaboration of a nonsubject topic, or elaboration of a subject topic through nonsubject signs is taken as signifying non teaching.

References

Anward J 1996 Parameters of institutional discourse. In: Gurmarson B-L, Linell P, Nordberg B (eds.) 1996 *The Construction of Professional Discourse*. Addison Wesley Longman, London

Baron N 1981 *Speech, Writing, and Sign: A Functional View of Linguistic Representation*. Indiana University Press, Bloomington, Indiana

Barthes R 1968 *Elements of Semiology*. Hill and Wang, New York

Beckmann P 1979 Iconic elements in mathematics education. *Ars Semeiotica* II(1): 49–78

Benveniste E 1981 The semiology of language. *Semiotica* (special supplement): 5–23

Bernstein B 1977 *Class, Codes and Control. Vol. 3: Towards a Theory of Educational Transmissions*, 2nd edn. Routledge and Kegan Paul, London

Byers P, Byers H 1972 Nonverbal communication and the education of children. In: Cazden C B, John V P, Hymes D (eds.) 1972 *Functions of Language in the Classroom*. Teachers College Press, New York

Eco U 1976 *A Theory of Semiotics*. Indiana University Press, Bloomington, Indiana

Garfinkel H 1967 *Studies in Ethnomethodology*. Prentice-Hall, Englewood Cliffs, New Jersey

Goodman N 1969 *Languages of Art. An Approach to a Theory of Symbols*. Oxford University Press, London

Goodman N 1978 *Ways of Worldmaking*. Harvester Press, Hassocks

Heritage J 1984 *Garfinkel and Ethnomethodology*. Polity Press, Cambridge

Hirst P H 1973 What is teaching? In: Peters R S (ed.) 1973 *The Philosophy of Education*. Oxford University Press, London

Hjelmslev L 1969 *Prolegomena to a Theory of Language*. University of Wisconsin Press, Madison, Wisconsin

Jakobson R 1971 *Selected Writings. Vol. 2: Word and Language*. Mouton, The Hague

McNeill D 1979 Natural processing units of speech In: Aaronson D, Rieber R W (eds.) 1979 *Psycholinguistic Research. Implications and Applications*. Erlbaum, Hillsdale, New Jersey

Nadin M (ed.) 1984 The semiotics of the visual: On defining the field. *Semiotica* 52:(3–4): 165–377 (whole issue)

Peirce C S 1931–1958 *Collected Papers*. Harvard University Press, Cambridge, Massachusetts

Saussure F de 1966 *Course in General Linguistics*. McGraw-Hill, New York

Sinclair J McH, Coulthard R M 1975 *Towards an Analysis of Discourse. The English Used by Teachers and Pupils*. Oxford University Press, London

Sonesson G 1989: *Pictorial Concepts*. Lund University Press, Lund

Sperber D, Wilson D 1986 *Relevance. Communication and Cognition*. Blackwell, Oxford

Tanz C 1971 Sound symbolism in words relating to proximity and distance. *Language and Speech* 14: 266–76

(c) Scientific Research Methods

Scientific Methods in Educational Research

A. Kaplan

Methodology as a discipline lies between two poles. On the one hand is technics, the study of specific techniques of research—interpreting a Rorschach protocol, conducting a public opinion survey, or calculating a correlation coefficient. On the other hand is philosophy of science, the logical analysis of concepts presupposed in the scientific enterprise as a whole —evidence, objectivity, truth, or inductive inference. Technics has an immediate practical bearing, but only on the use of specific techniques. Philosophy of science, though quite general in application, has only remote and indirect practical bearings. Though philosophy is much exercised about the problem of induction, for instance, educational researchers and behavioral scientists would be quite content to arrive at conclusions acceptable with the same confidence as the proposition that the sun will rise tomorrow.

Methodology is a generalization of technics and a concretization of philosophy. It deals with the resources and limitations of general research methods —such as observation, experiment, measurement, and model building—with reference to concrete contexts of inquiry. No sharp lines divide methodology from technics or from philosophy; particular discussions are likely to involve elements of all three.

The concern with methodology has lessened: more and more the researchers do their work rather than working on how they should do it. There has been a corresponding lessening of belief in the myth of methodology, the notion that if only the student of adult education could find "the right way" to go about research, the findings would be undeniably "scientific."

Anxious defensiveness heightened vulnerability to the pressure of scientific fashions. Scientism is an exaggerated regard for techniques which have succeeded elsewhere, in contrast to the scientific temper, which is open to whatever techniques hold promise for the particular inquiry at hand. Computers, mathematical models, and brass instruments are not limited to one subject matter or another; neither is their use necessary for scientific respectability.

Methodology does not dictate that the educational disciplines be hardened or abandoned. Neither does methodology exclude human behavior from scientific treatment. The task is to do as well as is made possible by the nature of the problem and the given state of knowledge and technology.

Fashions in science are not intrinsically objectionable, any more than fashions in dress, nor are they intrinsically praiseworthy. What is fashionable is only one particular way of doing things; that it is in the mode neither guarantees nor precludes effectiveness. Cognitive style is a characteristic way of attaining knowledge; it varies with persons, periods, cultures, schools of thought, and entire disciplines. Many different styles are identifiable in the scientific enterprise; at different times and places some styles are more fashionable than others. Successful scientists include analysts and synthesizers; experimenters and theoreticians; model builders and data collectors; technicians and interpreters. Problems are often formulated to suit a style imposed either by fashion or by personal predilection, and are investigated in predetermined ways. Scientism is marked by the drunkard's search— the drunkard hunts for the dropped house key, not at the door, but under the corner streetlamp, "because it's lighter there." Widespread throughout the sciences is the law of the instrument: give a small child a hammer and it turns out that everything the child sees needs pounding. It is not unreasonable to do what is possible with given instruments; what is unreasonable is to view them as infallible and all-powerful.

1. Scientific Terms

Closely associated with the myth of methodology is the semantic myth—that all would be well in (adult) educational research if only their terms were defined with clarity and precision. The myth does not make clear precisely how this is to be done. Scientists agree that scientific terms must bear some relation to observations. There is no consensus on exactly what relation, nor even on whether a useful scientific purpose would be served by a general formulation of a criterion of cognitive meaning. In particular cases the issue is not whether a term has meaning but just what its meaning might be.

For some decades education was dominated by operationism, which held that terms have meaning only if definite operations can be performed to decide whether the terms apply in any given case, and that the meaning of the terms is determined by these operations. "Intelligence" is what is measured by an intelligence test; "public opinion" is what is disclosed in a survey. Which details are essential to the operation called for and which are irrelevant presupposes some notion of what concept the operations are meant to delimit. The same presupposition underlies attempts to improve adult literacy tests and measures. A more serious objection is that the validation of scientific findings relies heavily on the circumstances that widely different measuring operations yield substantially the same results. It is hard to avoid the conclusion that they are measuring the same magnitude. Most operations relate terms to observations only by way of other terms; once "symbolic operations" are countenanced, the semantic problems which operationism was meant to solve are reinstated.

Ambiguities abound in the behavioral sciences, as in the field of education. The behavioral scientist is involved with the subject matter in distinctive ways, justifiably so. The involvement makes for widespread normative ambiguity, the same term being used both normatively and descriptively—"abnormal" behavior, for example, may be pathological or merely deviant. Also wide spread is functional ambiguity, the same term having both a descriptive sense and an explanatory sense—the Freudian "unconscious" may be topographical or dynamic. Ambiguity is a species of openness of meaning, perhaps the most objectionable. Vagueness is another species. All terms are more or less vague, allowing for borderline cases to which it is uncertain whether the term applies—not because what is known about the case is insufficient, but because the meaning of the term is not sufficiently determinate. All terms have some degree of internal vagueness, uncertainties of application, not at the borderline but squarely within the designation; some instances are better specimens of what the term designates than others (closer to the "ideal type"), and how good a specimen is meant is not wholly determinate. Most terms have also a systemic vagueness: meanings come not singly but in more or less orderly battalions, and the term itself does not identify in what system of meanings (notably, a theory) it is to be interpreted. Significant terms are also likely to exhibit dynamic openness, changing their meanings as contexts of application multiply and knowledge grows.

As dangerous as openness is the premature closure of meanings. The progressive improvement of meanings—the semantic approximation—is interwoven with the growth of knowledge—the epistemic approximation. The advance of science does not consist only of arriving at more warranted judgments but also of arriving at more appropriate concepts. The interdependence of the two constitutes the paradox of conceptualization: formulating sound theories depends on having suitable concepts, but suitable concepts are not to be had without sound theoretical understanding. The circle is not vicious; it is broken by successive approximations, now semantic and now epistemic.

Meanings are made more determinate by a process of specification of meaning. This is sometimes loosely called "definition"; in a strict sense definition is only one way of specifying meanings—providing a combination of terms, whose meaning is presumed to be already known, which in that combination have a meaning equivalent to that of the given term. Definitions are useful for formal disciplines, like mathematics; for empirical disciplines, their usefulness varies inversely with the importance of the term.

In simple cases, meanings can be specified by ostension: making what is meant available to direct experience. Empiricism regards ostensions as the fundamental anchorage for theoretical abstractions. Meanings in the educational and behavioral sciences are often specified by description of the thing meant, especially when this is included in or is close to everyday experience. Most scientific terms have a meaning specified by indication: a set of indexes, concrete or abstract, often the outcomes of specified tests and measures, which constitute, not *the* meaning of the term, but some of the conditions which provide ground for applying the term. Each index carries its own weight; each case exhibits a profile, whose weight is not necessarily the sum of the weights of the constituent indexes. As contexts of application change as well as what knowledge is available, so do the indications and their weight, and thereby also the meaning specified. Premature closure of meaning by definition is likely to provide false precision, groundless or unusable.

Which type of specification is appropriate depends on the scientific purposes the term is meant to serve. Observables, terms denoting what can be experienced more or less directly, invite ostension. Indirect observables lend themselves to description of what would be observed if our senses or other circumstances were different from what they are: such terms are sometimes known as "intervening variables." Constructs have meanings built up from structures of other terms, and so are subject to definition. Theoretical terms have a core of systemic meaning which can be specified only by an open and ever-changing set of indications. Many terms have sufficient functional ambiguity to exhibit characteristics of several or all of these types of terms; they call for various types of specification of meaning. "Lifelong learning" is a good example of such an ambiguous, all-encompassing concept.

2. Classes

Empirical terms determine classes; because of openness of meaning these classes are only approximations to well-defined sets in the sense of mathematical logic, where everything in the universe of discourse definitely belongs to or is excluded from the class. The approximation to a set can be made closer (the term made more precise) by restricting its meaning to what is specifiable by easily observable and measurable indices. The danger is that such classes are only artificial, delimiting a domain which contributes to science little more than knowledge of the characteristics by which it is delimited. Natural classes correspond to an articulation of the subject matter which figures in theories, laws, or at least in empirical generalizations inviting and guiding further research. Artificial and natural classes lie at two poles of a continuum. A classification closer to being artificial is a descriptive taxonomy; one closer to being natural is an explanatory typology. Growth of concepts as science progresses is a movement from taxonomies to typologies—Linnaeus to Darwin, Mendeleef to the modern periodic table, humors to Freudian characterology.

3. Propositions

Knowledge of a subject matter is implicit in how it is conceptualized; knowledge is explicit in propositions. Propositions perform a number of different functions in science.

First are identifications, specifying the field with which a given discipline deals, and identifying the unit elements of the field. In the behavioral sciences "idiographic" disciplines have been distinguished from "nomothetic," the former dealing with individuals, the latter with general relationships among individuals (history and sociology, for instance, or clinical and dynamic psychology). Both equally involve generalizations, because both demand identifications—the same "state" with a new government, or different personalities of the same "person": sameness and difference can be specified only by way of generalizations. Which units are to be selected is the locus problem; political science, for instance, can be pursued as the study of governments, of power, or of political behavior. What is to be the starting point of any given inquiry cannot be prejudged by other disciplines, certainly not by methodology. It is determinable only in the course of the inquiry itself—the principle of the autonomy of the conceptual base.

Other propositions serve as presuppositions of a given inquiry—what is taken for granted about the conceptual and empirical framework of the inquiry. Nothing is intrinsically indubitable but in each context there is always something undoubted. Assumptions are not taken for granted but are taken as starting points of the inquiry or as special conditions in the problem being dealt with. Assumptions are often known to be false, but are made nevertheless because of their heuristic usefulness. Hypotheses are the propositions being investigated.

4. Generalizations

Conclusions of an inquiry, if they are to be applicable to more than the particular context of the inquiry, are stated as generalizations. According to the logical reconstruction prevailing in philosophy of science for some decades (but recently coming under increasing criticism), generalizations have the form: "For all x, if x has the property f, then it has the property g." The content of the generalization can be specified only in terms of its place in a more comprehensive system of propositions.

A simple generalization moves from a set of propositions about a number of individual cases to all cases of that class. An extensional generalization moves from a narrower class to a broader one. Both these types are likely to be only descriptive. An intermediate generalization moves from propositions affirming relations of either of the preceding types to one affirming a relation of both relata to some intermediate term. It begins to be explanatory, invoking the intermediate term to account for the linkage recorded in its premises. A theoretical generalization is fully explanatory, putting the original relata and their intermediates into a meaningful structure. The conclusion of a successful inquiry may produce any of these types of generalization, not only the last.

All empirical findings, whether appearing as premises or as conclusions, are provisional, subject to rejection in the light of later findings. Philosophy of science divides propositions into a priori and a posteriori; for methodology it is more useful to replace the dichotomy by degrees of priority, the weight of evidence required before a finding is likely to be rejected. In increasing order of priority are conjectures, hypotheses, and scientific laws. A law strongly supported by theory as well as by the empirical evidence may have a very high degree of priority, often marked by calling the law a principle. In a logical reconstruction of the discipline in which it appears it may be incorporated in definitions, and so become a priori in the strict sense.

5. Observations and Data

Unless a proposition is a definition or a logical consequence of definition, it must be validated by reference, sooner or later, to observations. Reports of observation—data—must themselves be validated; what was reported might not in fact have been observed. A magician's performance can never be explained from a description of the effect, for the effect is an illusion; a correct description would not call for an explanation.

Errors of observation are virtually inevitable, especially in observations of human behavior; in the fashionable idiom, there is noise in every channel through which nature tells us something. In some contexts, observation can be insulated, to a degree, from error—it might be made, for instance, through a one-way mirror, so that data would not be contaminated by the intrusiveness of the observer. Error can sometimes be cancelled—reports from a large number of observers are likely to cancel out personal bias or idiosyncrasy.

In special cases error can be discounted: its magnitude, or at least its direction, can be taken into account in drawing conclusions from the data—memories are likely to be distorted in predictable ways.

There is a mistaken notion that the validity of data would be guaranteed if interpretations were scrupulously excluded from reports of what is actually seen. This mistake has been called "the dogma of immaculate perception." Observation is inseparable from a grasp of meanings; interpretation is intrinsic to perception, not an afterthought. It has been well said that there is more to observation than meets the eye.

Two levels of interpretation can be discriminated (in the abstract) in behavioral science. First is the interpretation of bodily movements as the performance of certain acts—the grasp of an act meaning. Raised hands may be interpreted as voting behavior rather than as involuntary muscular contractions (such contractions may be act meanings for a physiologist). A second level of interpretation sees observed acts in the light of some theory of their causes or functions—the grasp of an action meaning. Dress and hairstyle may be seen as adolescent rebelliousness.

Both levels of interpretation are hypothetical in the literal sense—they rest on hypotheses as to what is going on. Such hypotheses in turn rest on previous observations. This is the paradox of data: hypotheses are necessary to arrive at meaningful data, but valid hypotheses can be arrived at only on the basis of the data. As with the paradox of conceptualization, the circle is broken by successive approximation.

Because observation is interwoven with interpretation, what is observed depends on the concepts and theories through which the world is being seen. Whatever does not fit into the interpretive frame remains unseen—invisible data, like pre-Freudian male hysteria and infantile sexuality. The data may be noted but be dismissed as meaningless—cryptic data, like dreams and slips of the tongue. Observation also depends on what instruments of observation are available. Techniques like mazes, projective tests, and opinion surveys have had enormous impact on research.

6. Experiments

Creating circumstances especially conducive to observation is an experiment. Not all experiments are probative, meant to establish a given hypothesis or to select between alternative hypotheses (crucial experiment). Some may be methodological, like pilot studies or the secondary experiments performed to determine factors restricting the interpretation of the primary experiment. Heuristic experiments may be fact finding or exploratory. Other experiments are illustrative, used for pedagogy or to generate ideas, a common function of simulations.

The significance of experiments sometimes appears only long after they were performed. Experiments have meaning only in a conceptual frame. Scientific advance may provide a new frame in which the old experiment has a new and more important meaning. The secondary analysis of an experiment already performed may be more valuable than a new experiment.

Experiments in education and the behavioral sciences have often been criticized on the basis of an unfounded distinction between the laboratory and "life." There are important differences between the laboratory and other life situations—for instance, significant differences in scale. Only moderate stresses are produced—subjects may be given, say, only a small amount of money with which to play an experimental game, whose outcome may therefore have only questionable bearings on decisions about marriage, surgery, or war. Secondary experiments may be useful to assess the effect of the differences in scale. All observations, whether in the laboratory or not, are of particular circumstances; applying the findings to other circumstances always needs validation.

Not all experiments are manipulative; in some, the manipulation is only of verbal stimuli—administering a questionnaire can be regarded as an experiment. Events especially conducive to observation even though they were not brought about for that purpose are sometimes called nature's experiments—disaster situations or identical twins separated at birth. The relocation of workers or refugees, school bussing, and changes in the penal code are instances of social experiments. Experimentation and fieldwork shade off into one another.

7. Measurement

The more exact the observations, the greater their possible usefulness (possible, but not necessary). Widespread is a mystique of quality—the notion that quantitative description is inappropriate to the study of human behavior. True, quantitative description "leaves something out"—precision demands a sharp focus. But what *is* being described is more fully described by a quantitative description. Income leaves out of account many important components of a standard of living, but a quantitative description says more about income than "high" or "low."

There is a complementary mystique of quantity—the notion that nothing is known till it has been weighed and measured. Precision may be greater than is usable in the context or even be altogether irrelevant. Because quantitative data are more easily processed, they may be taken more seriously than the actually more important imponderables. The precision may be spurious, accurate in itself but combined with impressionistic data. Fashion in the behavioral sciences may invite the use of quantitative idioms even if no measurements are available to determine the implied quantities.

Measurement is the mapping of numbers to a set of elements in such a way that certain operations on the numbers yield results which consistently correspond to certain relations among the elements. The conditions specifying the mapping define a scale; applications of the scale produce measures which correspond to magnitudes. Just what logical operations on the numbers can be performed to yield empirical correspondence depends on the scale.

Numbers may be used only as names—a nominal scale—in which case nothing can be inferred about the elements save that they are the same or different if their names are such. The numbers may be used so as to take into account relations of greater and less—an ordinal scale—allowing the corresponding elements to be put into a definite order. An interval scale defines a relation of greater and less among differences in the order. Operations may be defined allowing measures to be combined arithmetically, by which magnitudes can be compared quantitatively—a ratio or additive scale. Scales can be freely constructed, but there is no freedom to choose what they logically entail. Equally restrictive are the empirical constraints imposed by the operations coordinating measures and magnitudes.

One measuring operation or instrument is more sensitive than another if it can deal with smaller differences in the magnitudes. One is more reliable than another if repetitions of the measures it yields are closer to one another. Accuracy combines both sensitivity and reliability. An accurate measure is without significance if it does not allow for any inferences about the magnitudes save that they result from just such and such operations. The usefulness of the measure for other inferences, especially those presupposed or hypothesized in the given inquiry, is its validity.

8. Statistics and Probability

No measures are wholly accurate. Observations are multiple, both because data are manifold and because findings, to be scientific, must be capable of replication by other observers. Inevitably, not all the findings are exactly alike. Inferences drawn from any measure are correspondingly inconclusive. Statistics are the set of mathematical techniques developed to cope with these difficulties.

A problematic situation is one inviting inquiry. The situation itself does not predetermine how the problem is to be formulated; the investigator must formulate it. A problem well-formulated is half solved; badly formulated, it may be quite insoluble. The indeterminacy of a situation, from the point of view of statistics, is its uncertainty. When a specific problem has been formulated, the situation is transformed to one of risk. A card game involves risk; playing with strangers, uncertainty. Moving from uncertainty to risk is the structuring problem; it may be more important than computing and coping with risk once that has been defined. How to compute risk is the subject matter of the theory of probability; how to cope with it, the theory of games, and more generally, decision theory.

The calculation of probabilities rests on three different foundations; alternatively, three different conceptions of probability may be invoked. Mathematical probability is expressed as the ratio of "favorable" cases (those being calculated) to the total number of (equally likely) cases. Statistical probability is the (long-run) frequency of favorable cases in the sequence of observations. Personal probability is an expression of judgments of likelihood (or degree of confidence) made in accord with certain rules to guarantee consistency. For different problems different approaches are appropriate. Mendelian genetics or the study of kinship systems makes use of mathematical probability. Studies of traffic accidents or suicides call for statistical probabilities. Prediction of the outcome of a particular war or labor dispute is a matter of personal probability.

Statistics begin where assignment of probabilities leaves off. A multiplicity of data are given. The first task is that of statistical description: how to reduce the multiplicity to a managable unity with minimal distortion. This is usually done by giving some measure of the central tendency of the data, and specifying in one way or another the dispersion of the data around that central measure (like the mean and the standard deviation). Inferences drawn from the data are statable as statistical hypotheses, whose weight is estimated from the relation between the data and the population about which inferences are being made (sampling theory). Depending on the nature of the sample and of its dispersion, statistical tests assign a measure of the likelihood of the hypothesis in question. Explanatory statistics address themselves to the use of statistical descriptions and hypotheses in formulating explanations (for instance, by way of correlations).

9. Theories and Models

Once a problematic situation has been structured and the data measured and counted, a set of hypotheses may be formulated as possible solutions to the problem. Generalized, the hypotheses are said to constitute a theory. Alternatively, it is possible to begin with a set of hypotheses formulated in the abstract, then interpret them as applying to one or another problematic situation. Such a set is called a model.

Often the result of structuring the problematic situation is called a model. Structure is the essential feature of a model. In an interpretation of the model, a correspondence is specified between the elements of the model and those of some situation, and between certain relations holding within each set of elements, so that when two elements of the model are in a certain relation the corresponding elements stand in the corresponding relation, and vice versa. A set of elements related in certain ways is a system; a structure is what is shared by corresponding systems (or it may be identified with the set of all possible systems corresponding to a given one and thus to each other).

A model can be a physical system (like an airplane model in a wind tunnel), in which case it is an analog. An analog computer is a device which allows such systems to be easily constructed—systems consisting, for instance, of electrical networks with certain voltages, resistances, and current flow. Operations on the analog which preserve its structure show what would happen in any other system having the same structure. If the model is a system of symbols it may be called a map. Behavioral science models are maps of human systems.

When the correspondences are only suggested rather than being explicitly defined, the symbolic system is an extended metaphor; intermediate between a metaphor and a model is an analogy, in which correspondences are explicit but inexact. All three have roles in the actual conduct of inquiry; the view that only models have a place in science makes both terms honorific.

In another honorific usage "model" is a synonym for "theory" or even " hypothesis." The term is useful only when the symbolic system it refers to is significant as a structure—a system which allows for exact deductions and explicit correspondences. The value of a model lies in part in its abstractness, so that it can be given many interpretations, which thereby reveal unexpected similarities. The value lies also in the deductive fertility of the model, so that unexpected consequences can be predicted and then tested by observation and experiment. Here digital computers have already shown themselves to be important, and promise to become invaluable.

Two dangers in the use of models are to be noted. One is map reading, attaching significance to features of the model which do not belong to its structure but only to the particular symbolization of the structure (countries are not colored like their maps; psychoanalytic models do not describe hydrodynamic processes of a psychic fluid: "psychic energy" is not equal to mc^2).

The other danger is, not that something is read into the map which does not belong to the structure, but that something is omitted from the map which does. This error is called oversimplification. All models simplify, or they would not have the abstractness which makes them models. The model is oversimplified when it is not known by how much nor even in what direction to correct the outcomes of the model so that they apply to the situation modeled. In an economic model, ignoring differences in the worth of money to the rich and to the poor is likely to be an oversimplification; ignoring what exactly the money is spent on may not be.

Theories need not be models; they may present a significant content even though lacking an exactly specified structure—as was done by the theory of evolution, the germ theory of disease, and the psychoanalytic theory of the neuroses. A theory is a concatenation of hypotheses so bound up with one another that the proof or disproof of any of them affects that of all the others. The terms in which the hypotheses are couched are likely to have systemic meaning, specifiable only by reference to the entire theory. Knowledge may grow by extension—applying a theory to wider domains. It may also grow by intension—deepening the theory, specifying more exactly details previously only sketched in or even glossed over.

Theory is not usefully counterposed to practice; if it is sound, a theory is of practice, though the theoretical problems may be so simplified that the theory provides only an approximate solution to the problems of practice, and then only under certain conditions. A theory, it has been said, is a policy, not a creed. It does not purport to provide a picture of the world but only a map. It guides decisions on how best to deal with the world, including decisions on how to continue fruitful inquiry. It raises as many questions as it answers; the answers themselves are proposed directives for action rather than assertions for belief.

10. Explanation, Interpretation, and Validation

Validation of a theory is a matter, first, of coherence with knowledge already established. A new theory may raise difficulties of its own, but it must at least do justice to the facts the older theory accounted for. Validation means, second, a certain correspondence with the world as revealed in the continually growing body of data—it must successfully map its domain. Validation, finally, lies in the continued usefulness of the theory in practice, especially in the conduct of further inquiry.

A valid theory provides an explanation of the data, not merely a shorthand description of them. The latter, even if comprehensive, is only an empirical generalization; a theory gives grounds for expecting the generalization to be indefinitely extendable to data of the same kind. A dynamic tendency is quite different from a statistical trend. The theory may allow the prediction of data not yet observed, though it may be valid without successful prediction if this is precluded by the intervention of factors outside the theory, or by cumulation of the inexactness to be found in all theories when applied to empirical findings. Conversely, an empirical generalization may suggest successful predictions even though it is unable to say why the predictions should succeed.

Deductive explanation deduces predictions from the premises postulated by the theory (together with the initial conditions of the particular situation). This type of explanation is characteristic of models. Pattern explanation makes the data intelligible by fitting them into a meaningful whole (predictions might then be made of what would fit the gaps). This is characteristic of disciplines concerned with action meanings.

Behavioral interpretation is grasping such meanings, as distinguished from model interpretation, which is setting up correspondences that give content to an abstract structure. In behavioral interpretation actions are understood as purposive, goal directed. Goals need not be conscious, deliberate, intentional—in short, motivational; they may be purely functional, as are the telic mechanisms of cybernetic systems. Interpretation in the behavioral sciences often suffers from mistaking functions for motives, then introducing abstract agents to have the putative motives—neuroses are said to defend themselves, ruling classes to perpetuate a social order, economies to seek to expand.

All explanations, at best, leave something to be desired. They are partial, dealing with only a limited class of situations. They are conditional, depending on special circumstances in those situations. They are approximate—no explanation is wholly precise. They are indeterminate, having only a statistical validity—there are always apparent exceptions. They are inconclusive, never validated beyond any possibility of replacement or correction. They are intermediate, pointing always to something which needs to be explained in turn. They are limited, serving in each instance only some of the purposes for which explanations might be sought—a psychologist's explanation of a death (as, say, a suicide) is very different from a pathologist's explanation (as, say, a poisoning). Both explanations may be equally valid. All this openness of theory corresponds in the epistemic approximation to the openness of meaning in the semantic approximation.

11. Values and Bias

Inquiry itself is purposive behavior and so is subject to behavioral interpretation. The interpretation consists in part in specifying the values implicated in specific processes of conceptualization, observation, measurement, and theory construction. That values play a part in these processes does not in itself make the outcomes of these processes pejoratively subjective, nor otherwise invalidate them. A value which interferes with inquiry is a bias. Not all values are biases; on the contrary, inquiry is impossible without values.

A distinction between facts and values remains; the distinction is functional and contextual, not intrinsic to any given content. Descriptions may be used normatively. They are also shaped by norms which guide not only what is worth describing but also what form the description should take—for instance, the degree of precision which is worthwhile, the size of sample which is worth taking, the confidence level to be demanded, and the like. Values play a part not only in choosing problems but also in choosing patterns of inquiry into them. The behavioral sciences have rightly become concerned with the ethics of the profession, as bearing, for instance, on experimentation with human beings.

A myth of neutralism supposes that scientific status requires rigorous exclusion of values from the scientific enterprise. Even if this exclusion were desirable (a value!), it is impossible. The exclusion of bias, on the other hand, *is* an operative ideal. Bias is only hidden by the pretense of neutrality; it is effectively minimized only by making values explicit and subjecting them in turn to careful inquiry.

The danger that values become biases is especially great when values enter into the assessment of the results of inquiry as distinct from what is being inquired into and how. A truth may be unpleasant, even downright objectionable, yet remain true for all that. Science must be granted autonomy from the dictates of political, religious, and other extra scientific institutions. The content of the pursuit of truth is accountable to nothing and no one not a part of that pursuit.

All inquiries are carried out in specific contexts. Validation of the results of any particular inquiry by reference to the outcomes of other inquiries is important. How important varies with the distance between their respective subject matters, concepts, data, and other components of the process of inquiry. The behavioral sciences have become increasingly willing to affirm their autonomy with respect to the physical and biological sciences. Science suffers not only from the attempts of church, state, and society to control its findings but also from the repressiveness of the scientific establishment itself. In the end, each scientist must walk alone, not in defiance but with the independence demanded by intellectual integrity. That is what it means to have a scientific temper of mind.

See also: Research in Education: Epistemological Issues; Participatory Research; Human Development, Research Methodology

Bibliography

Bailey K D 1978 *Methods of Social Research*. Free Press, New York
Black J A, Champion D J 1976 *Methods and Issues in Social Research*. Wiley, New York
Braithwaite R B 1953 *Scientific Explanation: A Study of the Function of Theory Probability and Law in Science*. Cambridge University Press, Cambridge
Campbell N R 1928 *Measurement and Calculation*. Longman, New York
Durkheim E 1950 *The Rules of Sociological Method*, 8th edn. Free Press, New York
Ellingstad V S, Heimstra N W 1974 *Methods in the*

Study of Human Behavior. Brooks Cole, Monterey, California

Gellner E 1973 *Cause and Meaning in the Social Sciences*. Routledge and Kegan Paul, London

Hanson N R 1972 *Observation and Explanation: A Guide to Philosophy of Science*. Harper and Row, New York

Hempel C G 1965 *Aspects of Scientific Explanation, and Other Essays in the Philosophy of Science*. Free Press, New York

Kaplan A 1964 *The Conduct of Inquiry: Methodology for Behavioral Science*. Chandler, New York

Kuhn T S 1970 *The Structure of Scientific Revolutions*. University of Chicago Press, Chicago, Illinois

Lachenmeyer C W 1973 *Essence of Social Research: A Copernican Revolution*. Free Press, New York

Myrdal G 1969 *Objectivity in Social Research*. Pantheon, Westminster, Maryland

Nachmias D, Nachmias C 1976 *Research Methods in the Social Sciences*. St. Martin's Press, New York

Nagel E 1961 *The Structure of Science: Problems in the Logic of Scientific Explanation*. Harcourt Brace, and World, New York

Neale J M, Liebert R M 1973 *Science and Behavior: An Introduction to Methods of Research*. Prentice-Hall, Englewood Cliffs, New Jersey

Popper K R 1959 *The Logic of Scientific Discovery*. Basic Books, New York

Popper K R, Eccles J C 1983 *The Self and its Brain*. Routledge and Kegan Paul, London

Quine W V, Ullian J S 1978 *The Web of Belief*, 2nd edn. Random House, New York

Runkel P J, McGrath J E 1972 *Research on Human Behavior: A Systematic Guide to Method*. Holt, Rinehart and Winston, New York

Weber M 1949 *Methodology in the Social Sciences*. Free Press, New York

Cross-sectional Research Methods

P. Lietz and J. P. Keeves

There is a strong and growing demand from national authorities, educational administrators, and the wider community for detailed comparative information on the organization and operation of educational systems within their own and kindred countries (Bottani et al. 1992). A cross-sectional study is required to provide such information that is concerned with the existing conditions, processes, and outcomes of an educational system at a particular point in time. However, cross-sectional studies are not limited to nation-level investigations but can range from the collection of information in a classroom, school, or school district through to a state or province, a country, or a group of countries with common characteristics that would make comparisons meaningful. Moreover, cross-sectional studies are not necessarily comparative in nature, although comparisons are commonly informative. Sometimes information on the state of affairs within a single unit is meaningful and of value and such information, in general, is obtained from a cross-sectional investigation.

Inevitably after information has been assembled, which relates to the conditions at one point in time with respect to characteristics of interest, there is concern as to whether such characteristics exhibit stability or change over time. Thus there is a second type of study, which is commonly contrasted with cross-sectional investigations in which stability and change in particular characteristics are examined over time. Such studies are referred to as longitudinal research studies (see *Longitudinal Research Methods*). The distinction between the two types of studies is more a matter of degree than of kind, and warrants further consideration because it involves an examination of the strengths and weaknesses of the two different types of investigations.

This entry considers initially the different types of research studies that can be carried out in educational research, and their relationship to cross-sectional studies, the advantages and disadvantages of cross-sectional studies, the usefulness of cross-sectional studies, the different kinds of research studies that are essentially cross-sectional in nature, as well as the gradations in types of investigation between cross-sectional and longitudinal research studies. In addition, this entry discusses issues concerned with the design of a cross-sectional study, the role of sampling, the methods of data collection, the value of pretest and pilot studies, and the major sources of error in such studies. Further important issues, which are addressed, involve the analysis of data and the problems of explanation associated with the relationships reported from cross-sectional studies in contrast to longitudinal and experimental studies. While studies of change are necessarily longitudinal in nature, and experimental studies remain the ideal types, the difficulties encountered in such studies in the investigation of educational problems are of sufficient magnitude that studies of a cross-sectional type are likely to continue for the foreseeable future as the major source of information to guide both policy and practice and from which to build theory.

1. Strategic Choices in Research Design

Kish (1987) has identified three kinds of strategic choices that must be made in the design of a research study, whether in education or in other fields of inquiry. These choices involve: (a) representation of the target group, (b) realism, and (c) control of treatment conditions. The importance of these strategic choices in the present context is that they permit the drawing of useful distinctions and identify the strengths and weaknesses of different approaches, and are concerned with the quality and nature of inferences that can be drawn from different types of investigations.

1.1 Representation

The first major decision that must be made in the design of an investigation is the nature and extent of the generalizations that are to be drawn from the analysis of the evidence. This decision leads to the identification of the investigation's domain and of the population to which generalization will apply. The ideal is to investigate a complete population or target group, but this is rarely possible although a national census, which is a cross-sectional study, seeks information from a complete population. It is generally necessary to draw a random sample of elements from a defined target population with a known positive probability of selection. There are two main advantages of random selection of elements with known positive probability. They ensure that strong inferences can be drawn at the conclusion of the investigation with respect to the population under investigation. First, because the elements in the sample are chosen at random from the target population, the sample is unbiased and is truly representative of that population. Second, because the sample is a random sample with a known positive probability of selection of each of the elements, estimates of sample statistics for the parameters associated with characteristics of the population can be calculated together with the estimates of the sampling errors linked to these statistics. With knowledge of the sampling error, confidence limits can be specified for the statistics that are estimated, and tests of statistical significance applied. Without the use of random probability sampling there is no guarantee of representativeness or lack of bias, and there is no information about the size of the sampling errors. It is, however, necessary to recognize that the magnitude of sampling error is not related to the probability of selection but to the effective size of the sample. For a simple random sample the effective size is the number of sampling units. For a random sample of complex design, allowance must be made for the *design effect* of the sample in calculating the effective sample size. The need to guarantee representativeness or lack of bias applies with equal strength to experiments as to surveys. However, randomization serves a further purpose in experimentation.

1.2 Realism

The second major decision concerns whether or not the investigation involves subjects in a natural setting and whether a contrived situation is desirable, admissible, or indeed possible. In the investigation of some issues in education it is not acceptable to diverge too far from an existing setting, insofar as it is the lives of individuals that are being changed by the experiment. Thus it is generally necessary to undertake an investigation in a natural setting. This may not only rule out an experimental study, but may also prevent the following of individuals over time, since repeated examination of the same individual may interfere with, or distort the life of, that individual. Under many circumstances, all that is possible is a cross-sectional investigation that studies an individual once and once only in a natural setting, rather than a longitudinal study in which not only is the behavior of the individual likely to be changed but the realism of the investigation is also in jeopardy.

1.3 Treatment Control

The purpose of research is not merely to describe but also to understand and explain. Understanding and explanation are derived from the examination of the effects of treatment factors whether acting in a natural setting, through intervention, or within a designed experiment. In a longitudinal study the effects of treatment factors operating in a natural setting, or of interventions in a quasi-experimental setting are under investigation. However, in such studies the operation of divers other factors may confound the changes observed. Only by the random selection of subjects for study and the random allocation of subjects to treatment and control groups can the effects of these divers other factors be brought under control, so that cause can validly be imputed, and strong generalizations made to a population under investigation. Thus experiments have three major advantages. First, the bias from disturbance factors can be eliminated by the randomization of subjects to treatment and control groups. Second, control can be exercised over the treatment factors, so that their effects can be more strongly inferred. Third, through statistical analysis confidence can be assigned with accuracy to the probability of whether or not the results occurred by chance. Longitudinal studies lack the first advantage. However, in longitudinal studies procedures of statistical analysis seek to employ statistical controls in place of randomization to adjust for the effects of disturbance factors. There is, nevertheless, no guarantee that spurious effects are not present. Cross-sectional studies can also employ statistical controls. Nevertheless, as explained in a later section, the effects of disturbance factors are less readily eliminated in such studies.

In addition to the three strategic choices listed by Kish (1987) there is a fourth choice involving time.

1.4 Time

Time has a central role in the investigation of stability and change. Both experiments and longitudinal studies, in general, require repeated measurement, and the use of repeated measurement extends the duration of an investigation. The exception occurs in situations where the treatment and control groups may be considered to be equal prior to the operation of the treatment condition. In experiments and longitudinal studies time may also become a treatment condition whose effects can be examined. However, in cross-sectional studies the effects of time can at best be only indirectly assessed, because repeated measurements are not made.

The restriction on time and the limitation of a study's duration are generally associated with the availability of personnel over an extended period and the costs of a longitudinal study. No research worker in education can ignore these two questions of personnel and costs. While an experiment or a longitudinal study may be considered desirable in many investigations into specific problem situations, the undertaking of a longitudinal study must frequently be abandoned because of cost and personnel constraints, and a study of a cross-sectional type undertaken.

It is important to recognize that cross-sectional studies do not necessarily involve sample surveys, although such procedures are often employed. It is also possible for a cross-sectional study to be: (a) a local study, in which a representative group is investigated; or (b) a census, in which data are collected for a complete population; or (c) a register study, in which data held on file in a register at a particular time point are examined; or (d) a controlled inquiry where data are collected, with care, although without random selection from a population, and without randomization to treatment and control groups, but at a particular point in time, in order to study a clearly identifiable problem.

2. Four Major Cross-sectional Studies

Cross-sectional studies serve many purposes, although the interest is primarily in providing information on the conditions of education at a particular point in time. Where such studies have been successfully conducted, and have given rise to findings of considerable usefulness, a follow-up or repeat study is sometimes undertaken. Four major cross-sectional studies are considered in the paragraphs that follow, to illustrate the variety of uses to which such studies have been put.

The purpose of a cross-sectional study may be largely descriptive. The purpose, for example, of the first Scottish Mental Survey, carried out in 1932, was initially to ascertain the distribution of intelligence among children aged 11 years in Scottish schools. This study tested a complete population, and reported that the spread in IQ scores was greater than had been expected, and was greater among boys than among girls. In a second survey conducted in 1947, the purpose of the study was to ascertain whether IQ scores were declining and whether the national average of intelligence was falling. Whereas in the first cross-sectional survey in 1932 the difference between boys and girls in IQ was less than one point, in the second survey a difference of four points of IQ in favor of girls was recorded. This difference, while of statistical significance, was not of marked practical significance. However, it helped to account for the small gain in average IQ of the 11-year-old population between the surveys (Scottish Council for Research in Education 1949). In addition, in the second study the opportunity was taken to examine the intercorrelations between IQ scores and a number of sociological variables that were measured.

The crossnational studies conducted by the International Association for the Evaluation of Educational Achievement (IEA) were not designed to provide "league tables" of educational achievement in different school subjects, but to relate these measures of achievement to a wide range of home, student, classroom, school, and system-level variables, describing the conditions of education in the countries involved. These studies, in general, have employed large national probability samples of students at three age levels, namely, near the end of primary schooling, near the end of the period when schooling is mandatory in most countries, and at the preuniversity or terminal stage of secondary schooling.

The IEA surveys are examples of studies that have had goals of both describing and explaining educational outcomes. Sometimes specific hypotheses were tested. In other cases more general models developed from theory were examined. The usefulness of these studies, as evidenced by the publications they produced, the debate that followed the release of the publications, and the changes to policy and practice induced in different parts of the world, cannot be denied. Nevertheless, such studies can be hazardous undertakings and prone to methodological errors in execution and errors in interpretation.

Two other cross-sectional studies have been of great importance for the conduct of educational research. The first study was undertaken in the United States under Section 402 of the 1964 Civil Rights Act, the Equality of Educational Opportunity Survey, which provided the evidence for a report to the President and Congress (Coleman et al. 1966). Not only was this survey of major policy importance, giving rise to widespread debate on the effectiveness of schools and programs for the bussing of students between schools, it also established the feasibility of large-scale surveys in the United States, raised numerous issues about the analysis of data, and indirectly drew attention to the problems of causal inference from cross-sectional studies.

Likewise, the Plowden Report (Central Advisory Council 1967) provided information from a number of surveys carried out in 1964 into the condition of different aspects of education in England and Wales. One study of particular significance was a survey of parents of school children, which established the importance of parental attitudes and addressed major issues of statistical analysis. A follow-up study was carried out four years later (Peaker 1971), and in the report of this study the first use of path analysis was made in the field of education. Other surveys in the Plowden Report were concerned with the standard of reading achievement, child development, and school facilities.

Both sets of studies were conducted by, or on behalf of, governments, in order that statistical accounts of the educational systems in the two countries would be available. However, cross-sectional research studies are not necessarily large-scale surveys. The analysis of data held in the register of a school can sometimes provide valuable information for the administration of that school without need to resort to the use of advanced statistical techniques or elaborate data collection methods.

3. Cross-sectional and Longitudinal Methods

Some of the cross-sectional studies referred to in the previous section involved investigations that were repeated over time, others involved the investigation of two or more age groups at the same time, with inferences being drawn regarding the differences between age levels. There are thus three classes of cross-sectional studies, namely, (a) single cross-sectional studies, (b) simultaneous cross-sectional studies, and (c) trend studies. Classes (b) and (c) may also be considered to be longitudinal studies (see *Longitudinal Research Methods*). Each of the three classes of studies is discussed below.

3.1 Single Cross-sectional Studies

These research studies consider one target population at one point of time only. The limitation to one target population and one time point is primarily determined by considerations of personnel and cost, which require that such studies can be completed relatively quickly at modest cost. While a description of conditions is readily provided by such a study, the nature and quality of the inferences derived from statistical analysis may also be modest.

3.2 Simultaneous Cross-sectional Studies

In a research study of this type, measurements are made at only one point in time and thus personnel and cost considerations are reduced. But two or more related target populations or two or more fields of inquiry are investigated simultaneously with large random samples, so that the samples may be considered both accurate and fully representative of the populations being investigated. In such studies, different age samples may be drawn from the same larger population, but each sample is drawn independently. Likewise, some surveys conducted by the IEA were designed to investigate two or more subject areas in parallel studies in order to examine differences in the conditions under which different school subjects were taught. Since information on similar predictor and criterion variables is also collected, parallel analyses can be carried out to examine differences between age levels or differences between subject fields.

A longitudinal or time dimension in the design of studies of this type is achieved through comparisons of the data for the different age samples. Not only can growth between age levels be estimated, but factors influencing growth can also be examined. The design is simple to execute, and since only one point in time is involved, the confounding effects of environmental influences are reduced. The IEA studies of science (Comber and Keeves 1973, Keeves 1992) have shown clearly the effects of differences in retention rates across countries on growth in science achievement between age levels at different measurement times. Likewise, in a study of French as a Foreign Language, Carroll (1975) showed that the effects of years spent in learning accounted for growth between age levels. The conclusions that can be drawn from this design are only valid if it can be assumed that: (a) the age samples have been drawn from the same common population; and (b) the factors influencing change in the criterion variables and their effects have remained constant across the time span during which the different age samples were exposed to those factors.

3.3 Trend Studies

In this type of study either a single cross-sectional study or a simultaneous cross-sectional study is replicated on a second or further occasion with identically defined target populations. Notable examples of trend studies are those carried out by the Assessment of Performance Unit (APU) in England and Wales (Black et al. 1984), the Australian Studies of School Performance (Bourke et al. 1981) and the National Assessment of Educational Progress. These studies have all been concerned with changes in educational achievement and have not sought to provide explanations of why the changes recorded had occurred. Two sets of problems arise in such studies of educational achievement. First, in circumstances where school curricula change over time with new curricular emphases evolving, it is difficult to design tests that assess achievement validly on two or more occasions. A second problem concerns the strength of the statistical procedures that are employed to scale the achievement test scores on the different occasions to obtain valid and reliable measures that can be compared. The first and second IEA science studies (Keeves 1992) sought to develop item response theory scaling procedures to measure change over time and to account for observed changes in educational achievement in terms of the changes in the conditions for learning science that had occurred between occasions. It should be noted that some research workers in the United States refer to such studies as a "cohort design" (Karweit 1982). Whether studies of this type are cross-sectional or longitudinal in nature is a question for debate, but they avoid the troublesome aspect of maintaining contact over a period of several years with a sample of students and the dangers of heavy attrition that could seriously bias the findings.

4. The Design and Conduct of Cross-sectional Research Studies

In many respects cross-sectional studies are similar in kind to surveys. However, the two types of studies are not necessarily synonymous. Furthermore, both types of studies do not necessarily require the drawing of random or probability samples from specified populations. Not only can a cross-sectional survey study take the form of a census in which a complete population is surveyed, but a cross-sectional study may also involve an investigation of material held in a register, from which a sample of data may be drawn. The decision on which type of cross-sectional study to employ depends on the importance of obtaining highly accurate data. In some cases a census may be preferred to a survey, because of the elimination of sampling error. However, the attempt to conduct a census may result in a high proportion of missing or incomplete data, whereas a well-conducted survey with little missing data may yield data of higher quality, without bias, and with known sampling error. Issues of both time and cost ultimately determine the choice of type of study to be employed. The planning of a cross-sectional study is similar to the planning of a survey (see *Survey Research Methods*).

There is interest in a wide range of measures and indicators concerned with the conditions, causes, and outcomes of education that can be collected from cross-sectional studies. The publication *Education at a Glance* (Bottani et al. 1992), which presents information on indicators of interest to OECD countries in 1988, illustrates this range. Of particular importance, however, since the 1960s, when Coleman et al. (1966) conducted the Equality of Educational Opportunity Survey in the United States and the IEA carried out the first IEA mathematics study in 12 countries (Husén 1967), are measures of educational achievement outcomes. The collection of data in cross-sectional surveys of educational achievement presents particular problems, which are discussed in the two sections that follow.

4.1 Methods of Data Collection in Achievement Surveys

Probably the most common method of data collection in cross-sectional studies of educational achievement is through requiring students to answer tests and respond to self-completion questionnaires and attitude scales. Access to the school system has long been the privilege of the researcher. Teachers in some countries have willingly agreed to supervise students while they respond to tests and questionnaires. Increasingly, however, teachers are seeking some remuneration for this work, or it is necessary to employ testers or to require district educational officers to undertake the testing of students. Interviewing is necessary in some studies where the information is too detailed or complex for students to provide written responses. The interviews may be carried out by teachers, school psychologists, or social workers. However, the use of interviewers trained to work on a particular study can prove especially useful for obtaining data on family background or for probing into the students' thought processes.

Particular problems arise in situations where the target population involves young people of school-going age who no longer attend school regularly. A study of literacy and numeracy among 17-year old youth would require a household survey since many young people who are unable to read and write are likely, by the age of 17 years, to have dropped out from school, even in countries with relatively high retention rates. In such a study it would be necessary for trained interviewers to undertake a household survey and to test the young people sampled in their homes.

In a follow-up study to obtain further information about the activities of students who were tested at school, but who have since left, a postal or telephone survey is likely to prove worthwhile. However, it should be recognized that not all young people are likely to be accessible by telephone, and in order to get people to respond to a telephone or postal survey some rapport must already have been established.

4.2 The Pretest and Pilot Studies

It is important that where achievement tests, attitude scales, and questionnaires have been developed for a study, they should be administered to a trial group as similar as possible to the population under survey in order to check, and if necessary revise, the final form of the instruments. Such a test will also provide estimates of the reliability of the instruments that are independent of the main study. A pretest study provides an opportunity to detect and remove ambiguities, to ascertain the range of possible responses (especially important for open-ended items, from which data may be processed automatically), and to ensure that the questions asked are yielding the information sought.

The pretest of instruments should not be confused with a pilot study. In a pilot study the instruments should be in their final form. The pilot study is used to test all procedures employed in the collection of data, coding, and recording of data and the initial processing of the data. Thus the pilot study also provides an opportunity to learn what the results of the main study are likely to be. Unfortunately, even where a pilot study has been scheduled it is not uncommon for delays to have occurred so that the pilot study is reduced in scope or even eliminated, in order to save time and money. This is generally false economy, since the mounting of a pilot study helps to avoid expensive mistakes in the main study. All cross-sectional investigations should include a pilot study.

5. Sources of Error

Three main types of error can be expected to arise in cross-sectional studies, namely: (a) errors of nonobservation, (b) errors of measurement, and (c) sampling errors. Sampling errors are, however, different in kind from the other two types of error, since they are a necessary consequence of, and obtainable through, the employment of a random probability sample (see *Sampling Errors in Survey Research*).

5.1 Errors of Nonobservation

The extent to which the achieved sample falls short of the designed sample arises from several sources. First, the information on which the sample was designed may have been deficient. Second, some people who were required to respond may have declined or been unable through absence to do so—this applies whether or not a sample is drawn from the population under survey. Third, some respondents may have chosen not to reply to specific questions. Fourth, some respondents may have deliberately or unintentionally provided information that is clearly erroneous. Such errors must be reduced or removed by the wild code checks and the consistency checks that are applied at the stages of data entry or data cleaning (see *Data Management in Survey Research*). Various compensatory procedures are available, such as drawing a replacement sample, using strategies for the estimation of missing data, and compensation through the weighting of the available data. All such procedures require certain assumptions that may or may not be valid. As a consequence, all these procedures introduce some bias into the estimates made, through displacing the mean or changing the variance of the estimates. There is no substitute for a well-planned investigation and a pilot study to reduce the effects of nonobservation. Elaborate procedures for compensation may help, but generally it is not possible to tell whether or not they have been effective (see *Missing Data and Nonresponse*).

5.2 Errors of Measurement

Errors of measurement arise from a variety of sources. They may stem from poorly designed instruments (see *Questionnaires*), from variability in the respondents, or from errors made by the researcher in the collection and recording of data. If items are open-ended then responses have to be coded before data are recorded, and

this may be a source of error. If precoded responses are used the respondent may be careless, or may give a socially desired response, or an acquiescent response as a result of a tendency to avoid conflict. Efforts should be made to increase the reliability of the instruments employed and to obtain sound estimates of reliability with a corresponding sample. Compensation for measurement error can be made by the combination of measures, preferably in ways that will maximize the reliability of the compound measure, such as with principal components analysis and the calculation of principal component scores. Alternatively, measurement error can be modeled in certain procedures of statistical analysis, such as are employed by LISREL programs (Jöreskog and Sörbom 1989) (see *Path Analysis and Linear Structural Relations Analysis*). In addition, estimates can be corrected for attenuation if the reliabilities of the measures are known (see *Reliability*). In general, separate measurement of response variance is not possible, and the response variance has served to inflate the estimated sample variance, with the consequent effects of reducing the magnitude of estimated correlations.

5.3 Sampling Errors

The topic of sampling error is too large to be considered here. Techniques of stratification can be employed to reduce the sampling error of a mean value. This, however, requires that the effects of stratification must be removed by statistical control in estimating the magnitude of relationships through the introduction of the stratification variable into multivariate analyses. The size of sampling errors can also be reduced by efficient design in the case of cluster samples, and by increasing the number of primary sampling units in multistage samples. Where cluster samples have been employed it is necessary to proceed with great caution in all types of statistical analyses, because nearly all computer programs that provide tests of statistical significance assume that the data are associated with a simple random sample. It should be noted that procedures of multilevel analysis are now available that not only permit the estimation of unbiased effects at the different levels of treatment, but also calculate more efficient estimates of sampling error for complex sample designs (see *Multilevel Analysis*).

6. The Analysis of Data

Four problems arise in the analysis of data from cross-sectional studies where the purposes of such statistical analyses are not merely descriptive. These problems exist in addition to the calculation of appropriate sampling errors and the testing of the parameter estimates for statistical significance in comparisons between groups. In such descriptive analyses the estimates of parameters are customarily means and standard deviations. However, most educational researchers are rarely satisfied with analyses that do not present relationships between variables considered to be of interest and importance. Here problems arise because such relationships either tacitly or explicitly involve considerations of causal influence. Two approaches can be taken in the examination of these relationships. These approaches are either exploratory or confirmatory.

6.1 Exploratory Analyses

In the exploratory analysis of data, the researcher rarely postulates a model, and simply lists variables of possible interest, largely on the basis of intuition. He or she employs contingency tables and correlation matrices to screen the data for both practically and statistically significant relationships. Where one or more antecedent factors are known to be of primary importance, it is sometimes considered desirable to examine the relationships between independent and dependent variables after the effects of these antecedent factors have been removed. This is generally achieved by regressing the dependent variable on both the independent variable and the antecedent factors, under the assumption that the antecedent factor may have influenced both the independent and dependent variables. This treatment differs from a covariance adjustment which is generally inappropriate because it assumes an effect only on the dependent variable and not on the independent variable. A further exploratory strategy is to employ stepwise regression in order to select a subset of independent variables that each have a significant unique contribution to accounting for the variance of the dependent variable. In such regression analyses, causal relationships are tacitly assumed and rarely made explicit. However, these stepwise regression analyses serve the valuable purpose of identifying variables that warrant further consideration (see *Exploratory Data Analysis; Multivariate Analysis; Regression Analysis of Quantified Data*).

6.2 Confirmatory Analyses

In confirmatory analyses hypotheses and causal models are advanced—generally ones derived from theoretical considerations—and are tested with recognized procedures of statistical analysis. In general in such analyses there are several independent variables and commonly several dependent variables. Procedures of multivariate analysis must be employed (see *Multivariate Analysis; Path Analysis with Latent Variables; Path Analysis and Linear Structural Relations Analysis*). There is much to be gained from making the multivariate models developed as explicit and as fully specified as possible. Errors of specification, which involve the omission of key factors, are of considerable importance because they lead to the generation of biased estimates of effects.

The danger in nonexperimental research is that the causal models developed may not have allowed for a factor that influences both the independent and dependent variables. The observed relationships are spurious, being confounded by unobserved and unknown factors. In experimental studies the random allocation of subjects to the treatment and control groups serves to annul the effects of such unknown confounding factors. Furthermore, the administration of a specific treatment to the experimental group and not to the control group serves to identify the factor that may cause a detected relationship.

Likewise, in longitudinal studies, through the measurement of change over time in the same subjects it is possible to eliminate the effects of a large number of factors that may have in the past influenced educational outcomes, and to focus attention on those factors that have produced change. Intervention studies in which a treatment is administered to one group and not to another permits testing for the effects of the intervention within a natural setting. However, such studies do not necessarily eliminate confounding effects, since full randomization of subjects to treatments has not occurred. Even in the most elaborate longitudinal studies it is impossible to separate and test fully for the interactions of chronological age, time of measurement, and the time of birth of the cohort that are considered to be primarily and respectively associated with genetic or biological effects, environmental effects that are common to all subjects being studied, and environmental effects that operated prior to the first time point of an investigation (see *Longitudinal Research Methods*).

Furthermore, in longitudinal studies unless the *change* in the criterion or dependent variable is measured with a high degree of reliability there is little chance of detecting the factors that have caused change. This can rarely be achieved through measurement at only two points in time in educational studies, and measurement at four or more time points is to be recommended (see *Change, Measurement of*). Moreover, the analysis of change data is not without its many problems (Collins and Horn 1991). Procedures for the analysis of data at three levels are now available. These permit the investigation of intra-individual growth, of between-individual effects, and of between-class or school group effects (see *Hierarchical Linear Modeling; Multilevel Analysis*). As a consequence more appropriate analyses can now be carried out on longitudinal data sets in educational research studies.

7. Conclusion

There are many limitations associated with cross-sectional studies, particularly in the analysis of data and in the drawing of inferences about causal effects that have not taken into consideration spurious influences. Furthermore, such studies can only investigate factors that influence learning from birth up to the time of data collection, and not the learning that occurs in a particular educational situation, although it may be assumed that current factors are more powerful than those that operated in previous years. In spite of these limitations and the problems of execution of large cross-sectional surveys, it seems likely that cross-sectional research studies will continue to play a major role in educational research.

See also: Sampling in Survey Research; Sampling Errors in Survey Research; Regression Analysis of Quantified Data

References

Black P, Harlen W, Orgee A 1984 Standards of performance-expectation and reality. *J. Curric. St.* 16(1): 94–96
Bottani N, Duchêne C, Tuijnman A 1992 *Education at a Glance: OECD Indicators.* OECD, Paris
Bourke S F, Mills J M, Stanyen J, Holzer F 1981 *Performance in Literacy and Numeracy 1980.* Australian Government Publishing Service for the Australian Education Council, Canberra
Carroll J B 1975 *The Teaching of French as a Foreign Language in Eight Countries.* Wiley, New York
Central Advisory Committee for Education 1967 *Children and their Primary Schools. Vol. 2: Research and Surveys.* HMSO, London
Coleman J S et al. 1966 *Equality of Educational Opportunity.* Ayer and Co., Salem, New Hampshire
Collins L M, Horn J L (eds.) 1991 *Best Methods for the Analysis of Change: Recent Advances, Unanswered Questions, Future Directions.* American Psychological Association, Washington, DC
Comber L C, Keeves J P 1973 *Science Education in Nineteen Countries: An Empirical Study.* Wiley, New York
Husén T (ed.) 1967 *International Study of Achievement in Mathematics: A Comparison of Twelve Countries.* Almqvist and Wiksell, Stockholm
Jöreskog K G, Sörbom D 1989 *LISREL 7: A Guide to the Program and Applications*, 2nd edn. SPSS Publications, Chicago, Illinois
Karweit N L 1982 Survey research methods. In: Mitzel H E (ed.) 1982 *Encyclopedia of Educational Research*, 5th edn. Free Press, New York
Keeves J P 1992 *The IEA Study of Science III. Changes in Science Education and Achievement: 1970 to 1984.* Pergamon Press, Oxford
Kish L D 1987 *Statistical Design for Research.* Wiley, New York
Peaker G F 1971 *The Plowden Children Four Years Later.* NFER, Slough
Scottish Council for Research in Education 1949 *The Trend in Scottish Intelligence: A Comparison of the 1947 and 1932 Surveys of the Intelligence of Eleven-Year-Old Pupils.* University of London Press, London

Experimental Studies

M. J. Lawson

At a very broad level all research activity can be argued to be concerned with the development of knowledge about some part of the world (Chalmers 1990) or, as Strauss (1987 p. 24) put it, with attempts to "uncover the complexity of the reality we study." In any research activity the researcher is engaged in a voyage of discovery to establish something about the nature of some phenomenon. An educational researcher is attempting to uncover the complexity of some aspect of education in order to increase knowledge of the educational world. Experimental studies are one of the major types of research used to develop that knowledge. Through use of the special features of the experiment the researcher attempts to make precise statements about part of that world, or about the nature of relationships between one part and the other.

Experiments have the purposes of elucidating the nature of the phenomenon, and of establishing patterns of relationships or causality. The special features of the experiment reside in the greater extent of control and precision afforded to the researcher. This should not be taken as reason to elevate the experiment to a place of preeminence over other research techniques. It is more appropriate to take the position that it is when the researcher wishes to identify the effect of some intervention, and is able to exercise greater control in a research situation, that the experiment offers advantages of precision over other research methods. It is discussion of issues of control and precision in the design of experimental studies that can be seen as the focus of this article.

1. Preparation for Research

The design of any experiment emerges from consideration of two distinct bodies of knowledge. The first of these, knowledge related to the substantive research issue, provides the conceptual framework used in generation of the research questions and in interpretation of the pattern of results observed. It is this framework that drives the research process, and which is in turn confronted by the findings. The quality of the analysis and interpretation carried out using this conceptual framework is the first major influence on the outcome of the experimental study.

The second influence on the study outcome is the quality of the experimental design, that design being broadly concerned with the manner of arrangement of the procedures used to pursue the research questions established for the study. Decisions made in establishing these procedures are also influenced by a body of knowledge that is the principal concern of discussion here.

2. *Experimental and Quasi-experimental Research*

In 1963 Campbell and Stanley produced a short monograph that has had considerable influence on the design of much experimental research in the behavioral sciences. The monograph is still rewarding reading and its content has been paraphrased in many texts on research design. Four features are important for the discussion here.

First, Campbell and Stanley introduced a distinction between two types of studies in educational research, experimental and quasi-experimental studies. In an experimental study the researcher has control over the assigning of participants to different conditions, or treatments, in order to set up a comparison of the effects of these conditions. This freedom is not available in quasi-experimental research, where the researcher can organize procedures and materials for the research but is unable to decide how subjects will be allocated to conditions.

In a typical quasi-experimental research design the researcher may have access to an appropriate number of participants but is unable to disturb their existing grouping. The researcher may, for instance, be provided with a group of three intact classes for a study of the effects of two different methods of presenting diagrams in science instruction. The restriction on disturbance of these groupings means that the group membership must be considered a possible source of influence on the outcome of the treatments, an influence that is extraneous to the researcher's principal focus on the effect of the different methods. Random assignment of subjects to conditions provides a means of effecting a considerable reduction in the number of such extraneous factors whose influence must be considered by the researcher in discussion of the research outcomes. Randomization increases the likelihood that these factors will not constitute a systematic source of influence on outcome, so that experimental groups are, in a probabilistic sense, comparable prior to the intervention. Differences in outcome should therefore reflect the systematic influence of the experimental treatments. Without freedom to assign subjects to conditions at random the experimenter must consider a range of alternative explanations for any difference in outcome.

However, as Campbell and Stanley (1963) and Cook and Campbell (1979) have shown, it is not the case that sound interpretations are not possible in quasi-experimental designs. In all research the researcher is concerned with consideration of possible explanations for a finding, and must attempt to establish a basis for ruling out competing explanations. In research where it is possible, the random assignment of participants to conditions reduces the range of alternative explanations that needs to be examined. Although, as will be seen later, simple random assignment of subjects to groups may not always be the most appropriate procedure, randomization does constitute one of the key control procedures available to the experimenter.

Campbell and Stanley (1963) also introduced a system of notation that has proved useful in organizing the discussion of experiments. The essence of this is shown in Table 1. The design shown here—one of a number of experimental designs—is useful for discussion because it is frequently used in educational research. The control that can be exercised by the experimenter in allocating subjects according to some form of randomization is represented by R. The observations, or measures, used to gain information about subject characteristics, including their performance on the dependent variables of interest in the experiment, are signaled by the Os. In this design the first occasion of measurement provides information about the pretreatment state of the groups. The subsequent time of measurement provides an indication of the level of posttreatment performance. The differences in the procedures used with the two groups in this design are represented by the X_1 and X_2, and would commonly refer to experimental and control treatments.

The notation makes clear the elements of the experimental study: randomization of participants to conditions, and controlled presentation of measures and forms of treatment. As the notation makes clear, the difference in experience for the two groups of subjects is focused on the difference between the conditions—the Xs. A study set up in this manner is designed to allow the researcher to make statements about the effects of the different conditions, as indexed by the measures. It is the quality of these statements that comes under examination in an experiment, and it is this quality that the researcher tries to maximize

Table 1

The Campbell and Stanley form of notation for research designs

The pretest -posttest control group design

Experimental group	R	O	X_1	O
Control group	R	O	X_2	O

R = random assignment of subjects to groups   O = a time of measurement of subjects in a group X_1 = an experimental treatment or form of intervention X_2 = either no intervention or a standard condition
Source: Campbell and Stanley 1963

in setting up the design of the experiment. Ideally the researcher can attribute differences in outcome to the difference in the Xs. In practice, because of the imprecision inherent in both the researcher's theoretical framework and in the procedures and measurement used in the experiment, and the heterogeneity of the subjects participating in the study, the actual situation is less than ideal. The difference in the Xs therefore constitutes only one of the influences on the outcome, albeit a major one. The aim of experimental design is to maximize the degree of influence of the Xs and to minimize the influence of other, extraneous factors. To achieve this the researcher must attempt to maximize the validity and sensitivity of the design.

3. Validity

A third continuing influence of the discussion of research design issues developed by Campbell and Stanley (1963) is concerned with the qualities they described as the validity of the experimental design. Following Cook and Campbell (1979) it is possible to identify four components of validity, qualities that different experimental designs can be seen as possessing to differing degrees.

3.1 Construct Validity

An experiment's construct validity is affected by the quality of the researcher's theoretical framework, that framework being a specification of the nature and relationships between a set of theoretical constructs. It is the validity of the links between experimental procedures, experimental outcomes, and the study's conceptual framework that is referred to as an experiment's construct validity. The more complete and precise the specification of that framework, and the more precisely the experimental procedures and measures reflect the nature of that framework the greater is the validity of statements about that framework that can be derived from the experimental outcomes. The cost of low precision in this sense is the maintenance of uncertainty about the nature of constructs and the confounding of relationships among constructs. Where confounding of constructs is decreased the greater is the likelihood that the nature of these relationships can be elucidated, and the greater is the construct validity of the experiment.

3.2 Internal Validity

Internal validity is a quality of causal explanation emerging from the design, and is brought into focus by the question: "What confidence can be placed in the argument that the treatment (X) produced the effect that was observed?" The greater the justifiable confidence of the researcher in establishing a relationship between treatment and effect, the greater the internal validity of the design. This component of validity is internal in the sense that what is being examined is the validity of the procedures developed in the experiment to link the treatment and the outcome.

Campbell and Stanley (1963), and later Cook and Campbell (1979), identified a range of factors that constitute potential influences on the outcome that are additional to that of the treatment. These they referred to as "threats" to the internal validity of the design, because they represent extraneous factors that constitute possible sources of influence on the experimental outcome, influences additional to that of the Xs which "threaten" to weaken the chain of inference linking treatment and effect. Space is not available here to consider each of these threats to internal validity, but the sense in which they constitute a potential source of influence on outcome can be gained by considering one, the history of the groups.

In a two-group study, such as that shown in Table 1, the researcher would try to ensure that the experience of the groups during the experiment was identical except for the different experimental treatments (Xs). Any other difference in experience, in the history of the groups during the time of the experiment, could be seen as having the potential to exert an influence on the experimental outcome, and so would threaten the validity of the researcher's claim that the effect was due to the treatment. In designing the experiment the researcher's task is to attempt to rule out this and other threats as alternative sources of influence to the focus of interest, the experimental treatment.

3.3 External Validity

In a similar manner the researcher can ask questions about the degree of external validity, or generalizability, of the outcome, given that there is a strong basis of support for the researcher's statement about the influence of the treatment. Now the concern is with the extent to which this effect is likely to be observed in situations and with subjects not included in the original experiment. Educational researchers have a major interest in whether the same treatments will have the same effect if used by different teachers, or in different areas of a city with different students. External validity is therefore a quality characterizing statements about the applicability of experimental outcomes in situations different to the experimental situation. If an experiment is carried out for the purpose of informing future practice, then its design must be compatible with the set of circumstances obtaining in that target situation or group. It should be clear that the development of sound generalizations from an experimental outcome requires clear specification of the derivation and composition of the sample, the procedures, and the conditions involved in the study. Bracht and Glass (1968) developed the analysis of a range of threats to external validity arising from sampling and context factors (see *Sampling in Survey Research*).

3.4 Statistical Conclusion Validity

The final component of validity identified by Cook and Campbell (1979) concerns the quality of argument based on use of statistical procedures, which they termed "statistical conclusion validity." Statements made about the effect of an intervention on a sample of subjects included in the experimental groups are derived from use of a particular statistical test. The use of this test rests on a set of decisions about such things as the nature of the measures used and the size and composition of the groups. It is the quality of these decisions and the conclusion reached following use of the test that are referred to as statistical conclusion validity. Because it is frequently possible to identify more than one statistical test that can be used for a given set of results, it is important to consider the basis for use of the chosen test. Statistical conclusion validity is considered under the heading of sensitivity later in this entry. The works of Campbell and Stanley (1963), Bracht and Glass (1968), and Cook and Campbell(1979) provide checklists useful in considering threats to validity in each of the four senses identified here (see *Hypothesis Testing*).

3.5 Other Considerations

In a field that has had increasing impact on research in educational psychology, namely that involving strategy training research where it is common to assess the effects of different instructional treatments, Lysynchuk et al. (1989) have established a set of criteria for assessing the adequacy of a range of features of research design and for identifying possible confounding factors that could either threaten the validity of the experimental procedure or compromise the argument developed in discussion of the results. In addition to the concerns raised in sources cited above, these authors make clear the importance of controlling for Hawthorne effects, of equating the nontreatment experience of different groups, of attending to possible confounding of teacher and treatment effects, of checking that instructions were used, that ceiling and floor effects are avoided, and that the appropriate unit is used in analysis of data. These concerns may also arise in other fields of educational research (see *Unintended Effects in Educational Research*).

4. Sensitivity of an Experimental Design

Closely intertwined with a concern for the validity of an experimental design is the sensitivity of that design. Whereas validity is primarily concerned with the soundness of the researcher's theoretical analysis and of the argument concerning the cause of an experimental effect, sensitivity "refers to the likelihood that an effect, if present, will be detected" (Lipsey 1990 p. 12). Consideration of sensitivity is based upon a distinction between the "true," but unknown, state of affairs in a population and the state that is observed by the researcher in the experiment. A design is sensitive to the extent that the researcher's conclusion reflects the "true" state. If any difference between the true and experimental states is considered as error or variability then anything that reduces this error will increase a design's sensitivity. Lipsey (1990) identified a range of factors that may be considered as likely sources of error.

4.1 Subject Heterogeneity

In much educational research, such as investigations of the effects of teaching methods that employ designs like that in Table 1, there is a degree of variability in outcome attributable to the heterogeneity of members of experimental groups. This within-group variability, while desirable when the researcher wishes to investigate effects not limited to very narrowly defined populations, needs to be considered carefully when the major effect of interest is the amount of variability between groups that can be attributed to the experimental arrangements. As will be clear from the design of commonly used statistical tests, the likelihood of detection of an experimental effect is increased as the ratio of between-group to within-group variability increases. The greater the extent of variability due to individual differences of members within the groups, the more difficult it will be to detect the influence of the experimental effect.

One strategy available to the researcher for decreasing subject variability is to restrict the range of subjects included in the study. If the target population for the research is males, then only males need be included in the sample. If the research questions of interest involve the behavior of students with learning difficulties, then students can be screened to ensure that only students with such characteristics are involved.

Simple random assignment may not be the most suitable procedure for dealing with within-group variability, which may reflect the influence of an extraneous factor that the researcher would wish to be able to discount. Simple random assignment can still result in groups whose characteristics differ markedly along a dimension that can contribute to differences in outcome. Where it is possible to identify factors likely to play this role, usually from past research or from observation, a number of procedures are available to the researcher for reducing the variability due to subject heterogeneity. The use of such a factor as a blocking variable in the design is one procedure. In this case a measure that is strongly related to the response measure is obtained and subjects are then grouped on this variable, perhaps into groups high and low on this measure, so that the variability attributable to subjects' membership of a block can be systematically identified in the analysis. In this way, the previously unknown effect of this blocked factor on the extent of response variability can now be identified.

Analysis of covariance (ANCOVA) provides an alternative use of the measure used as a blocking variable. In this case the entire range of variability on the covariate is used in the statistical analysis. The logic of this procedure is that, through regression, the variability of the outcome measure that is predictable from each subjects' standing on the related extraneous variable can be identified and "removed." A third alternative designed to reduce the variability in outcome attributable to subject heterogeneity is, in the two-group situation, formation of pairs of subjects based on standing on a measure argued from previous research to be likely to exert an influence that it would be desirable to control. In a study of vocabulary learning, for instance, it might be argued that subject's existing verbal fluency might exert an influence on the outcome measure. In this case measures of verbal fluency can be obtained for all subjects, and these can be used to produce a set of ranked pairs of subjects. Random assignment of subjects is then carried out within the ordered pairs. Statistical analysis could then be carried out using a correlated, or paired sample, t-test procedure in which the lack of independence between the set of measurements is taken into account. The choice of covariate or blocking variable must be made carefully so that the nature of the relationship between the treatment and outcome is not compromised, as might occur when either measurement of the covariate or the blocking variable itself influences the administration of the treatment. In such circumstances procedures of regression analysis might be employed (see *Regression Analysis of Quantified Data*).

The repeated measures design, in which the repeated measurement of each subject across all treatments of interest, also aims to reduce the influence of subject heterogeneity. This reduction arises from the fact that the involvement of subjects in all treatments removes variability due to subject differences within groups, so that subjects are said to "act as their own controls." This variability due to differences among subjects is identified in the analysis and so does not remain as "unidentified" variability (Brown and Melamed 1990). Lipsey (1990) provided a useful discussion of the specific qualities of each of these different procedures for handling variability due to subject heterogeneity.

4.2 Experimental Variability

One of the advantages of experimental research has been identified as the degree of control that can be exercised by the researcher. Careful control of experimental arrangements and procedures can also reduce the variability in the outcome that should rightly be considered as error. Such variability can arise, for example, from lack of clarity in instructions given to subjects, or from inconsistency in application of these instructions, or from any variation in use of measuring instruments. The first of these can contribute to subtle variations in the subjects' interpretations of the nature of any task or materials. This introduces a degree of variability that can be minimized through piloting the instructions with students comparable in nature to those to be involved in the experiment. The development and use of standard instructions and procedures can minimize the effects of the second and third problems just noted.

Large-scale studies may require the use of several experimenters so that variability in outcome—which must be considered as possible error—might arise from slight differences in emphasis or procedure associated with each experimenter, even when standard sets of instructions have been prepared. In many cases it would be possible to include an experimenter variable in the analysis to assess the extent of this variability. Lysynchuk et al. (1989) argued that, where possible, such variability can be reduced by ensuring that each experimenter is involved to the same extent with each treatment group.

4.3 Measurement Error

Measurement error contributes to the overall variability of the outcome. Like the other sources of error affecting the sensitivity of the design, this is a feature that cannot be removed, though it is possible to reduce its affect by attention to the reliability and appropriateness of measures. Procedures for assessing and modifying the reliability of measuring instruments are discussed elsewhere (see *Reliability*). Consistency of application, discussed above, will assist reliability of measurement, and may require periods of training and piloting prior to initiation of the experimental procedures. In some circumstances, where established measures are not available, or where naturalistic observations are gathered, it may be necessary to use more than one measure or to apply a measure on several occasions.

The appropriateness of measures refers not only to their conceptual status, but also to their suitability for detecting the effects that are of interest in the study. A measure may prove too easy for subjects, or may be too difficult. In both cases such a measure lacks the sensitivity required for detection of the effect of interest. It is also possible that a measure may be too coarse. For example, in a study of mathematical problem-solving a standardized test of mathematical achievement provides a set of scores distributed across a wide range. However, it is possible that this measure does not detect changes in understanding or problem-solving skills at a level of detail that is of interest to the researcher. A more sensitive measure may need to be developed. The coarser measure may not only mask the effect of interest to the researcher but is also likely to increase within-group variability which the researcher wishes to minimize. Consideration of this problem makes clear one important feature of the relationship between validity and sensitivity: the researcher's conceptual analysis needs to be sufficiently complex to allow specification of the nature of measuring instruments required to identify the effects of interest.

4.4 Statistical Power

Statistical power is a central feature of overall experimental sensitivity, and in some discussions power and sensitivity are used as synonyms. There is however a special sense of power associated with the use of statistical tests in experimental research. These investigations typically culminate in the testing of statistical hypotheses concerned, for example, with the identification of an effect of a treatment when compared with a control condition. Statistical power in this situation is the likelihood of detecting a significant treatment effect when the effect is present. A design with greater statistical power is more likely to detect such a difference than one with lower power. Low power can lead to an erroneous conclusion that the treatment did not have an effect. Cohen (1977) identified four components of statistical power that require the attention of the researcher. (See *Hypothesis Testing*.)

4.4.1 The statistical test.
Different statistical tests have different statistical power for detecting effects. Choice of test, therefore, rests not only on consideration of the assumptions of the test and the nature of the data but also on the power of the test to detect a treatment effect. Lipsey (1990) provided a detailed discussion of power differences associated with three alternative tests applied to data derived from a comparison of experimental and control groups. The differences were ones that arose from ways in which the error variance was partitioned in these tests. In this case the statistical power for a one-way ANOVA was 0.2, rising to 0.5 when a blocking variable was used in an ANOVA, and rose further to 0.96 when the same variable was used as a covariate in a one-way ANCOVA.

Power differences arise not only within parametric tests such as the ones just mentioned. In general, these tests have higher power than nonparametric alternatives that are based on use of subject ranks derived from outcome performance rather than use of the subject scores on a given measure. Tests that use more of the information available in the measurements are, in principle, more powerful than those relying on reductions in detail of those measurements. Siegel (1956) provided estimates of the power of different nonparametric tests. Directionality of a test also affects power. Directional or one-tailed tests— that is, those based on the prior specification of the expected direction of the difference between groups —are more powerful than nondirectional, or two-tailed tests, provided that the difference observed is in the predicted direction. For the latter tests the researcher does not specify the expected direction of any difference in level of observed outcome. The different conclusions to be derived from one and two-tailed tests at a given alpha (α) level are apparent from inspection of the size of critical values required for significance in the one- and two-tailed cases for the t-test.

4.4.2 Alpha level (α).
Use of a statistical test requires specification of statistical hypotheses. In seeking evidence of a treatment effect, the researcher can specify and test two hypotheses, a hypothesis of no effect or null hypothesis, and a hypothesis that an effect does exist in the population from which the experimental sample is drawn. A decision about the unknown state of the population on the basis of data derived from a sample involves inference, and this inference has associated risks of error. One error could be a decision to reject the null hypothesis when in fact there is no treatment effect, no difference between groups in the population. The probability of this error, known as Type I error, is set by the researcher. This level of risk is known as the alpha level (α) and is conventionally set at levels such as 10, 5, or 1 percent. Another error possible in decision-making, Type II error, is associated with a decision not to reject the null hypothesis when an effect does exist in the population. The probability of this error is β. The power of a statistical test, the probability of detection of this true effect, is then $1-\beta$. Ideally the researcher would wish to minimize the extent of both types of error, though this is in practice difficult to do since the level of β is not directly under the control of the researcher.

The greater the alpha level the more likely it is that a treatment effect will be identified, and, where that is the true state of affairs in the population, the higher the statistical power of the design. Put another way, the smaller the alpha level the more rigorous is the test of the existence of the effect. From this it can be seen that, if the effect exists in the population, the lower the alpha level the lower the likelihood of detecting that effect—that is the lower is the power of the design and the greater the risk of Type II error (β). With other parameters of power analysis held constant, selection of a low alpha level reduces the risk of Type I error and also reduces power.

Lipsey (1990) argued that in basic research there is a strong case for keeping alpha levels at lower levels because of the requirement to be conservative in situations influencing the development of theory. In more applied situations, especially in treatment effectiveness research, Lipsey argued that the alpha level could be increased to avoid the false rejection of effective methods, especially in cases where the range of such methods may well be limited.

4.4.3 Sample size.
The importance of sample size can be recognized if it is remembered that design sensitivity depends on amount of error or variability. The smaller the sample, the greater the degree of sampling error. As the sample size is increased the extent of sampling error is decreased. In general terms therefore larger samples are to be preferred to smaller ones, though it is not the case that a small sample

is of no use to the researcher. Different research situations impose different limits on the availability of subjects, and in many clinical situations it may be necessary to work with single cases – see Barlow and Hersen (1984) (see *Single Case Research: Measuring Change*). Kraemer and Thiemann (1987) provided an alternative procedure for calculation of sample size to that advanced by Cohen (1977), and showed that in the two-group comparison power is maximized by use of equal size groups. The question of appropriate sample size is intricately tied to the final aspect of power, the effect size.

4.4.4 Effect size. Estimations of the size of an experimental effect, or of a difference between conditions, is a major concern for the researcher. If this question is considered in terms of a real difference existing between conditions in the population, then in the experiment the larger this difference is the more likely that the difference is significant in a statistical test, and the greater the power of the design.

When the effect size is considered in a comparison of a control and an experimental treatment group, then attention is focused on the size of the difference in mean level of performance on one or more measures as an estimate of the effect size. This difference may be thought of as the effect of the experimental intervention. Obviously the magnitude of this difference is affected by the nature of the measure being used, so that its size differs between different experimental situations, even those in the same area of interest. To allow comparison of the size of the effect across different studies a form of standardization is used, and in the situation considered above this standardization is achieved by seeing how large is the difference in means relative to the spread of scores in the groups. A common representation of effect size for the t-test is the ratio of the difference between means to the common standard deviation of the groups (Cohen 1977), so that effects across studies may then be compared in terms of standard deviation units. Cohen's work provides procedures for calculation of power using effect size indices appropriate for a range of statistical tests.

Estimation of effect size is relevant both prior to the finalizing of an experimental design and again when the results of the experiment are being evaluated. To establish the basis for the first of these claims it is necessary to consider statistical power. Statistical power is defined as the likelihood that a true effect is detected, or that a difference between groups is judged significant when there is a difference in the population. A large effect is more likely to be detected than a smaller one, and so the more likely is the attaining of statistical significance for a given test. As was noted previously, the judgment of statistical significance is based upon choice of alpha level and sample size. The critical value of the difference for acceptance or rejection of the statistical hypotheses varies according to these choices. This suggests that it is easier to develop an experimental design that allows detection of a large effect, and more challenging to design one that detects smaller effects. The latter design must be more sensitive. Sensitivity is increased by procedures that reduce the size of unexplained variance, and reduce the degree of error in the experimental design. The greater the reduction in this error, the higher the probability of a smaller effect being detected.

How does the researcher make a judgment about the magnitude of an effect as "large" or "small." Cohen (1977) argued for rule-of-thumb values of 0.20 as small, 0.50 as medium, and 0.80 as large values that conform quite closely to the spread of effect sizes observed in a meta-analysis of treatment effectiveness research (Lipsey 1990). Related research in an area can provide an indication of the range of effects associated with a given treatment; this information can then be used as a basis for the researcher's decision about sample size and power. Cohen (1977) provided a full discussion of these issues for a range of statistical tests and designs.

Cohen (1977) has also provided discussion of procedures for the interrelationship of these four parameters of statistical power, procedures that are of immediate practical significance in, for example, determination of the power of a design, or in determination of the number of subjects needed to attain a certain level of power. Power charts for specific tests are available that allow the researcher to establish a relationship among the four factors involved in power analysis: sample size, alpha level, power, and effect size. Knowledge of three of these parameters allows the researcher to determine the value of the fourth. Lipsey (1990) provided useful guidelines for researchers in considering trade-offs among these factors where, for instance, sample size is limited.

On completion of an experiment the researcher can calculate the size of the effect that could have been detected. For the two-group study discussed above the researcher can identify the difference between group means and relate this to the common standard deviation. The expression of an effect size in this manner is likely to provide an indicator of the practical significance of the treatment, and an indicator of the likely effects when the experimental design is replicated. Replication provides a means of assessing the robustness of the treatment effect, and a sounder basis for decisions about use of an experimental treatment with a larger population.

5. The Analysis of Change

The preceding discussion has been based on the use of a simple two-group design in which control and experimental groups are compared. While this is a frequently used design in experimental research in the behavioral sciences there are good reasons for use of augmented designs for situations that arise commonly in educational research. One of the most common, and most important, educational questions concerns change, or growth, over time. The question of analysis of change is considered at length in another entry (see *Change, Measurement of*) so only the general issues are noted here.

Willett (1988) argued convincingly that, in general, the primary interest of the educational researcher studying change is change across extended time, and that the most suitable strategy for this study is observation of performance in *multiwave* (or multiple occasion) designs rather than observation on just two occasions. Willet (1988) noted that the restriction of observation to two occasions provides a poor estimate of the trajectory of individual growth across time, and that this estimate is improved as the number of points of observation, or waves of data collection, is increased. Willett's 1988 work is also important for its discussion of the status of difference scores and its discussion of multilevel analysis techniques (see *Multilevel Analysis; Hierarchical Linear Modelling*).

6. Classroom Research Designs

Experimental and quasi-experimental research in school classrooms involving the investigation of the effects of different teaching conditions provide some problems for the researcher in arranging research procedures. Here again the researcher finds valuable instruction in the sources discussed in the previous sections where the strengths and weaknesses of a range of research designs are discussed. Some situations require use of independent groups in a project allowing use of a between-subjects analysis. In other situations, for example, where examination of the extent of change or growth is the research objective, it is more appropriate to measure the same group of subjects on several occasions, allowing for use of a repeated-measures or within-subjects design. In still other projects the researcher may wish to look at the interaction of measures in a mixed, between- and within-subjects design.

In some projects it is possible to set up a laboratory situation in part of a school, in a place where individual students or groups can take part in the designated activities. In this case it is possible to execute experimental designs for comparison of effects under different conditions. The same arrangements can be made in observational studies where the choice of the individual or group involved is under the control of the researcher, or in studies where the researcher can establish the sampling design.

Experimental designs may also be implemented within classrooms without the withdrawal of students from those classes. The use of such a design depends on the amenability of the treatment to presentation in forms such as text or computer programs. If the instructions given to groups can be arranged in such a format, the assignment of students to different conditions can be under the control of the researcher.

7. Conclusion

The discussion in this entry has been designed to emphasize the systematic nature of educational research. However, as was indicated in the definitions of research provided in the introduction, it is also important to remember that research is above all a creative activity. In pursuing the voyage of discovery the researcher is developing a new appreciation, a new interpretation that, in Chalmers' (1990) terms, can be pitched against the world. The researcher is required to be creative in all phases of the project, in establishing a conceptual framework, in devising research procedures, in analysis of data, and in developing an interpretation of the results. The procedures discussed in this chapter are intended to provide a sound basis for this creative activity based on the notions of control exercised in order to maximize the validity and sensitivity of the design. As Lipsey (1990) pointed out, it is not helpful to attend only to validity of a design so that extraneous sources of influence can be ruled out, while neglecting the capacity of the procedures to detect the presence of the effect of interest. Experimental design requires juggling of ideals and practicalities, demonstrated in consideration of the relationship between sample size and power. Resources are not always available to recruit sufficient subjects in order to attain a high level of power. A trade-off must be made. Fortunately principles that can inform decisions about trade-offs are now becoming more accessible in sources such as those noted in this article.

References

Barlow D H, Hersen M 1984 *Single Case Experimental Designs*, 2nd edn. Pergamon Press, New York

Bracht G, Glass G 1968 The external validity of experiments. *Am. Educ. Res. J.* 5(4): 437–74

Brown S R, Melamed L 1990 *Experimental Design and Analysis*. Sage, Newbury Park, California

Campbell D T, Stanley J C 1963 Experimental and quasi-experimental designs for research on teaching. In: Gage N (ed.) 1963 *Handbook of Research on Teaching*. Rand McNally, Chicago, Illinois

Chalmers A 1990 *Science and its Fabrication*. Open University Press, Buckingham

Cohen J 1977 *Statistical Power Analysis for the Behavioral Sciences*, 2nd edn. Erlbaum, Hillsdale, New Jersey

Cook T D, Campbell D T 1979 *Quasi-experimentation: Design and Analysis Issues for Field Settings*. Rand McNally, Chicago, Illinois

Kraemer H C, Thiemann S 1987 *How many subjects?: Statistical Power Analysis in Research*. Sage, Newbury Park, California

Lipsey M 1990 *Design Sensitivity: Statistical Power for Experimental Research.* Sage, Newbury Park, California

Lysynchuk L, Pressley M, d'Ally H, Smith M, Cake H 1989 A methodological analysis of experimental studies of comprehension strategy instruction. *Read. Res. Q.* 24(4): 458–70

Siegel S 1956 *Nonparametric Statistics for the Behavioral Sciences.* McGraw-Hill, New York

Strauss A L 1987 *Qualitative Analysis for Social Scientists.* Cambridge University Press, New York

Willett J 1988 Questions and answers in the measurement of change. In: Rothkopf E 1988 *Review of Research in Education.* American Educational Research Association, Washington, DC

Human Development: Research Methodology

A. von Eye and C. Spiel

Developmental research investigates constancy and change in behavior across the human life course. This entry discusses the methods used to arrive at clear-cut statements concerning human development, specifically, methods for data collection, data analysis, and interpretation. Examples are drawn from educational and psychological research.

1. Fundamental Methodological Paradigms

1.1 The Univariate Developmental Paradigm

One of the simplest methodological paradigms in social science research (Baltes et al. 1977) involves the mechanistic or deterministic assumption that observed behavior depends on or can be predicted from causal or independent variables. In brief, this assumption is that $D = f(I)$ where D denotes the dependent variable, for example, performance in school, and I denotes the independent variable, for example, social climate in class.

From a developmental perspective the prediction of constancy and change is important. Dynamic variants of the univariate developmental paradigm predict a variable, observed at later points in time, from the same variable, observed at earlier points in time. For example, a typical question is whether high achievement motivation in the first grade allows one to predict high achievement motivation in later grades. Developmental changes are inferred if prediction equations, for example, regression equations, involve parameters that indicate change, for example, average increases.

Other variants of this paradigm predict changes in behavior from variables other than the dependent ones. For example, changes in behavior in puberty are predicted from changes in hormone levels (Paikoff et al. 1992). To be able to depict changes in behavior within individuals, at least two observations of the dependent variable are required.

1.2 The Multivariate Developmental Paradigm

In a most general sense, multivariate research involves two or more variables on the dependent variable side and two or more variables on the independent variable side (Baltes et al. 1977). In developmental research, one observes two or more variables and predicts constancy or change in these variables from earlier observations of the same variables (dynamic modeling) and/or from other variables.

There has been an intense debate as to what design for data collection is the most suitable. The following sections present the basic research designs, give an overview of this discussion, and summarize conclusions from this discussion.

2. Designs for Human Development Research

There are three basic designs for developmental research: the cross-sectional, the longitudinal, and the time-lag designs. The advantages and drawbacks of each of these will be discussed. The basic assumption that underlies each of these designs is that individuals who participate in investigations are all drawn from the same population.

2.1 The Cross-sectional Research Design

In cross-sectional designs, researchers observe one or more variables at one point in time and in two or more groups of individuals differing in age. The use of cross-sectional designs is by far the most popular research strategy in developmental psychology, for the following reasons: most importantly, only one observation point is necessary, so that studies using cross-sectional observations take little time compared to studies using repeated observations. In addition, financial costs are typically relatively low. There are also benefits on the interpretational side. Because observations are made at only one point in time, sample fluctuations are, by definition, not a problem. Researchers can assume that samples are constant.

However, cross-sectional research also has a number of specific deficiencies, most of which result from using only one observation point. Specifically, for conclusions from cross-sectional research to be valid one has to accept a number of assumptions. Some of these assumptions are strong, that is, they are difficult to satisfy, for example: (a) age samples ("cohorts") are drawn from the same parental population at birth. (If this is not the case there is no way to discriminate between developmental processes and cohort differences); (b) differences in behavior that are related to age, that is, differences between individuals from different age groups, are stable over historical time. (Again, if this is not the case there is no way to discriminate between changes in development that are caused by secular, historical changes, or by cohort differences); (c) differences between individuals from different age cohorts can be interpreted as indicating developmental changes that would occur within individuals as they move from one age group to the other.

If these assumptions do not hold, there is no reasonable way to assign developmental changes to such causes as age or historical time in a clear-cut way. Indeed, there is an abundance of literature showing that cohorts are different from each other (see Baltes et al. 1978). For example, researchers have suggested that the phenomenon of mid-life crisis may be less prevalent in the cohorts born around 1950 than in cohorts born in the time around the Great Depression (see Rybash et al. 1991). Thus, the development of a mid-life crisis may be viewed as a secular phenomenon rather than a ubiquitous developmental phenomenon.

Selection of methods for statistical data analysis depends on the type and distribution of data. Classical statistical methods for analysis of quantitative cross-sectional data include analysis of variance, multivariate analysis of variance, and discriminant function analysis. For qualitative data chi-square decomposition, log-linear analysis, prediction analysis, and configural frequency analysis are often recommended (see von Eye 1990a, 1990b; Rovine and von Eye 1991).

2.2 The Longitudinal Research Design

In longitudinal designs, researchers observe one or more variables at two or more points in time and in one cohort. Variation over time occurs when individuals grow older during the course of the investigation.

Longitudinal studies have a number of advantages over cross-sectional studies, (Baltes et al. 1977, de Ribaupierre 1989, Schaie 1983). One of the most important advantages is that only longitudinal investigations allow one to describe intra-individual development, that is constancy and change within the individual across time. In cross-sectional research intra-individual development must be inferred under strong assumptions. Results from cognitive studies suggest that growth curves derived from cross-sectional data do not necessarily have the same shape as curves derived from longitudinal data (Salthouse 1991).

In addition, interindividual differences in intra-individual development, that is, differences between individuals' developmental patterns, can be depicted only by observing the same individuals more than once. A typical research question is whether students from disadvantaged social backgrounds derive greater benefit from attempts to teach learning strategies than students from other social backgrounds. The description of such differences is important for a researcher interested in homogeneity of development. Homogeneity of development can be investigated at the variable level; for instance, by asking whether certain cognitive abilities decline in adulthood more rapidly than others. Homogeneity can also be investigated at the differential level; for example, by asking whether (and why) individuals display different developmental trajectories.

Another major advantage of longitudinal studies is that the constancy and change in relationships among variables can be investigated. For example, one could ask whether the relationship between school achievement and cognitive capacity changes during puberty. One of the most important preconditions for age, cohort, and time comparisons is what has been termed "dimensional identity" (Schmidt 1977). A set of variables is considered to show dimensional identity if the interrelations among variables remain unchanged over all observation points. When variable interrelations differ in cross-sectional studies, it is impossible to determine whether these differences are due to age or group differences. When variable interrelations change in longitudinal studies they reflect developmental processes. However, in both cases changes in variable interrelations render comparisons of results from different age groups or cohorts difficult.

A last advantage of longitudinally collected data concerns the investigation of causes for constancy and change. A general assumption is that causes occur prior to effects. Thus, causes for development must be observed before developmental changes occur. This observation is obviously possible only in longitudinal research. Causal analysis is of concern in education, prevention, and clinical behavior modification.

The desirable properties of longitudinal research are offset by a number of shortcomings. The first of these is that the wrong choice of the number and spacing of observations may prevent researchers from adequately assessing underlying processes of change. Thus, researchers may miss critical periods or events, may fail to depict validly the dynamics of change, or may even completely misrepresent the shape of a growth curve.

A second shortcoming concerns serial effects of repeated measurements, such as "testing effects." For example, when individuals score higher in a particular test (e.g., an intelligence test) in a second measurement, one cannot be sure that the increase in performance reflects an increase in ability rather than an increase due to remembering test items or familiarization with the test situation.

Similar to cross-sectional designs, sample selection may play a critical role in longitudinal studies. There may be specific selection effects, because longitudinal studies require more effort from participants than cross-sectional studies. In addition, longitudinal studies may suffer from attrition; that is, loss of participants due to moving, loss of interest, illness, or, in particular in studies including older adults, death. Each of these problems can lead to invalid description of developmental processes.

Another important shortcoming of longitudinal research is that the costs are higher than in cross-sectional research. In addition, there are interpretational problems. Most important is that of generalizability over samples. Because of cohort differences, growth curves may not be the same for samples from different cohorts (see Baltes et al. 1977). The same applies if selection effects are taken into account.

Selection of statistical methods for analyzing longitudinal data must consider data quality, distributional characteristics, and sample size. Latent class models and structural equation models that allow the explanation of patterns of relationships among variables in nonexperimental environments are becoming increasingly popular (see Bartholomew 1987, von Eye and Clegg 1994). These methods can also be useful for estimating development and change in continuous or categorical data. (For a more detailed overview of statistical methods for analysis of longitudinal data see von Eye 1990a, 1990b.)

2.3 The Time-lag Design

In time-lag designs, researchers observe one or more variables at two or more points in time and in two or more groups of individuals that belong to different cohorts but are of the same age. Variation over time results from the spacing between observation points. Although time-lag designs are far less popular than cross-sectional and longitudinal designs, they are useful in many respects. For example, the finding that there has been a considerable variation in Standard Achievement Test performance in the United States over the last 50 years could only come from a time-lag investigation.

Time-lag investigations are selected when researchers are interested in comparing cohorts. However, time of measurement and historical time are confounded. Therefore, generalizations to other cohorts, other historical times, or other age groups are problematic. As far as costs are concerned, time-lag designs exhibit the same problems as longitudinal designs. As far as sampling is concerned, there are similarities with cross-sectional studies. As far as interpretability is concerned, there are strong constraints resulting from the focus on only one age group. For these reasons, time-lag designs have been the least popular in developmental research.

2.4 The Age × Time of Measurement × Cohort Design

This is the only developmental research design that varies the three aspects of time: age (A), time of

measurement (T), and year of birth (cohort—C). However, there is no way to vary these three aspects independently, which would be necessary to separate their effects. The reason is that the three time variables are linearly dependent on each other. Each can be expressed as a linear combination of the other two, as is shown in the following formulas. (For the following formulas, T and C are expressed in calendar years, e.g., 1951, A is expressed in years, e.g., 40.)

(a) $A = T - C$

(b) $C = T - A$

(c) $T = C + A$

Therefore, research designs have been developed that vary only two of the three variables, A, C, and T. The following designs result: $A \times C$, $A \times T$, and $C \times T$. (For a more detailed description see Baltes et al. 1977, Schaie 1983.)

With regard to $A \times C$, researchers observe two or more cohorts over three or more observation points. At the beginning of the observation of each cohort, the cohorts are of the same age. Thus observations of the younger cohorts begin when they reach the age the older cohorts were when they were first observed. To carry out a study a minimum of three observation points and two cohorts are necessary. At least two age levels must be covered. Schaie and Baltes (1975) argue that the $A \times C$ arrangement is the most useful for ontogenetic research, because this design allows one to depict constancy and change with age; that is, intra-individual change. In addition, it allows one to depict interindividual differences in intra-individual change. However, the authors also claim that using any of the two-dimensional designs is defensible, depending on the purpose of research.

The main problem with treating A, C, and T as explanations for development is that one has to make strong assumptions when one applies the two-dimensional designs. Specifically, when applying the $A \times C$ design one must assume that the effects of T are negligible; for $A \times T$ one must assume that the effects of C are negligible; and for $C \times T$ one must assume that the effects of A are negligible.

3. Special Methods for Developmental Research

This section covers a selection of special methods, including intervention studies, microdevelopmental studies, single case studies, and training studies.

3.1 Intervention Studies

The designs discussed above are typically applied to observe natural behavior. Intervention does not take place. In contrast, research on specific kinds of intervention and its effects is often done using randomized experiments. For example, experiments examine the effects of systematic variations in teaching behavior on student achievement. For studying intervention effects, researchers observe one or more variables in two or more groups of subjects, who are randomly assigned to treatments, at one or more points in time. Whenever they can be realized, randomized experiments are the preferred designs because causal inferences can be drawn from the results. Methods for statistical analysis of data from randomized experiments most often include analysis of variance.

Examples of designs for intervention studies include reversal designs and multiple baseline designs (see Baltes et al. 1977). In reversal designs researchers first establish the rate of spontaneous behavior; that is, the baseline. Then they introduce some treatment (experimental condition) that constitutes the first reversal, and assess the rate of behavior again. The second reversal occurs at the end of the treatment, and so forth. All later assessments are compared with the first, the baseline.

Reversal designs typically are applied in learning studies. One of the basic assumptions of such studies is that it is, in principle, possible that behavior rates return to the baseline after the treatment. If behavior changes are irreversible, as is often assumed of developmental changes, reversal designs become less useful.

3.2 Single Case Studies

Single case studies, also referred to as "single subject studies," involve the detailed investigation of one individual. The primary goals pursued with single case studies include the detailed description of specific processes (e.g., language development) in individuals, the development of skills in individuals with specific deficits, and treatment of behavior disorders. For analysis of single case studies time series analysis, trend analysis, or spectral analysis are most often applied.

3.3 Training Studies

In training studies researchers often combine reversal with multiple baseline designs. Multiple behaviors are trained, assessments occur before and after training periods, but there is no assumption that training affects only one type of behavior. Goals pursued with training studies include the development of skills (e.g., learning skills), the compensation of losses (e.g., memory in old age), and the reversal of decline (e.g., achievement motivation during puberty). A large number of training studies have been concerned with intellectual development (Willis and Schaie 1986, Baltes et al. 1988). Researchers were able to show that intellectual decline in adulthood can typically be compensated by appropriate training (for a detailed discussion see Salthouse 1991).

Statistical analysis of data from training studies typically involves analysis of variance with repeated observations.

3.4 Microdevelopmental Studies

Typically, longitudinal and sequential studies span several years. For instance, Schaie's Seattle Longitudinal Study observes individuals in a 7-year rhythm. However, development also takes place in shorter time frames. Relatively short-term development is termed "microdevelopment." Studies investigating microdevelopment typically are longitudinal in nature and involve a relatively large number of observation points that are spaced in short intervals so that points in time where changes occur will not be missed (see Siegler and Crowley 1991).

An example of a microdevelopmental study is reported by Fischer and Lamborn (1989) who investigated the development of honesty and kindness in adolescents. They reported a sequence of stages. Development that carries individuals from one stage to the next is termed "macrodevelopment." Progress within stages is termed "microdevelopment." The authors specified transformation rules that describe development at the microdevelopmental level.

Statistical methods for analysis of microdevelopment include trend analysis, time series analysis, and structural equation modeling.

See also: Descriptive Scales; Cross-sectional Research Methods

References

Baltes P B, Cornelius S W, Nesselroade J R 1978 Cohort effects in behavioral development: Theoretical orientation and methodological perspectives. In: Collins W A (ed.) 1978 *Minnesota Symposium on Child Psychology*, Vol. 11. Erlbaum, Hillsdale, New Jersey

Baltes P B, Kliegl R, Dittmann-Kohli F 1988 On the locus of training gains in research on the plasticity of fluid intelligence in old age. *J. Educ. Psychol.* 80: 392–400

Baltes P B, Reese H W, Nesselroade J R 1977 *Life-span Developmental Psychology: Introduction to Research Methods.* Brooks/Cole, Monterey, California

Bartholomew D J 1987 *Latent Variable Models and Factor Analysis.* Oxford University Press, Oxford

de Ribaupierre A 1989 Epilogue: On the use of longitudinal research in developmental psychology. In: de Ribaupierre A (ed.) 1989 *Transition Mechanisms in Child Development: The Longitudinal Perspective.* Cambridge University Press, Cambridge

Fischer K W, Lamborn S D 1989 Mechanisms of variation in developmental levels: Cognitive and emotional transitions during adolescence. In: de Ribaupierre A (ed.) 1989 *Transition Mechanisms in Child Development: The Longitudinal Perspective.* Cambridge University Press, Cambridge

Paikoff R L, Buchanan C M, Brooks-Gunn J 1992 Methodological issues in the study of hormone–behavior links at puberty. In: Lerner R M, Petersen A C, Brooks-Gunn J (eds.) 1992 *Encyclopedia of Adolescence*, Vol 2. Garland, New York

Rovine M J, von Eye A 1991 *Applied Computational Statistics in Longitudinal Research.* Academic Press, Boston, Massachusetts

Rybash J W, Roodin P A, Santrock J W 1991 *Adult Development and Aging*, 2nd edn. Brown and Benchmark, Dubuque, Iowa

Salthouse T A 1991 *Theoretical Perspectives on Cognitive Aging*. Erlbaum, Hillsdale, New Jersey

Schaie K W 1983 What can we learn from the longitudinal study of adult psychological development? In: Schaie K W (ed.) 1983 *Longitudinal Studies of Adult Psychological Development*. Guilford, New York

Schaie K W, Baltes P B 1975 On sequential strategies in developmental research: Description or explanation. *Hum. Dev.* 18(5): 384–90

Schmidt H D 1977 Methodologische Probleme der entwicklungspsychologischen Forschung. *Probleme und Ergebnisse der Psychologie* 62: 5–27

Siegler R, Crowley K 1991 The microgenetic method: A direct means for studying cognitive development. *Am. Psychol.* 46(6): 606–20

von Eye A (ed.) 1990a *Statistical Methods in Longitudinal Research. Vol. 1: Principles and Structuring Change*. Academic Press, Boston, Massachusetts

von Eye A (ed.) 1990b *Statistical Methods in Longitudinal Research, Vol. 2: Time Series and Categorical Longitudinal Data*. Academic Press, Boston, Massachusetts

von Eye A, Clegg C C (eds.) 1994 *Latent Variables Analysis. Applications for Developmental Research*. Sage, Newbury Park, California

Willis S L, Schaie K W 1986 Training the elderly on the ability factors of spatial orientation and inductive reasoning. *Psychology and Aging* 1(3): 239–47

Longitudinal Research Methods

J. P. Keeves

Longitudinal research studies, that is, investigations conducted over time, are of growing importance in the social and the behavioral sciences and, in particular, in the field of education. In the past, investigations conducted over time have been relatively rare, although some important studies have been undertaken. In Sweden, the Malmö study conducted by Husén and his colleagues has been in progress for nearly 60 years. Data were initially collected in 1928 and many reports from this study have been published (Husén 1969, Fägerlind 1975, Tuijnman 1989). In the United Kingdom, two major series of studies have been conducted. The first investigation was started shortly after the Second World War, when all children born in one week in March 1946 formed the sample and detailed medical records as well as information on their educational development were collected (Douglas 1964). The second investigation is the ongoing National Child Development Study which was started 12 years later with a sample of all children born in the United Kingdom during the first week of March 1958 (Davie et al. 1972, Fogelman 1983, Butler and Golding 1986). In the United States, there have been at least eight major longitudinal studies that have investigated well-defined samples of children and that have sought to obtain a large variety of measurements on different characteristics of human development: these particular studies have been reviewed by Bloom (1964).

In all these studies, which have collected data at many points in time, significant problems have inevitably been encountered in maintaining contact or tracing the members of the chosen samples. These investigations are therefore sometimes referred to as tracer studies. This name emphasizes the strategies that are employed for preventing bias which would distort the findings of an investigation as a consequence of substantial losses over time from the sample. In recent years, there has been an increased interest in the problems associated with the design of longitudinal research studies, the selection of a sample, and the strategies used in the analysis of the data collected, as well as with the sources of bias that could invalidate the findings. This work has led to significant advances in the methodology associated with such investigations, particularly in the areas of design and analysis.

Educational research is concerned with the processes of constancy and change, and such a study requires that observations are made for at least two points in time. While it is possible to describe the practice of education by means of a cross-sectional study undertaken at a single point in time, it is necessary to conduct investigations that are longitudinal in nature in order both to describe and explain the influence of educative processes on the constancy and change of related outcomes. Thus the methods of longitudinal research are central to the empirical study of education, whether there is concern for individuals, classrooms, schools, social subgroups, or educational systems. Although there are substantial problems associated with the investigation of change (see *Change, Measurement of*), the importance to education cannot be denied of providing a detailed description of patterns of stability and change and a coherent explanation of how and why change has occurred or failed to occur.

This entry is concerned with the methods employed in longitudinal research and addresses the problems associated with the investigation of both stability and change. It is important to recognize that, while longitudinal methods are frequently contrasted with cross-sectional methods, a detailed comparison between the two methods is largely inappropriate. This is because constancy and change can only be examined through the repeated observations that are the basis of the longitudinal method. Moreover, with increasing interest in multilevel analysis, this entry does not restrict discussion in longitudinal research to the study of individuals, but considers change at all levels, within individuals, between individuals. and between schools and school systems (see Goldstein 1987, Bryk and Raudenbush 1989, Muthén 1991).

1. Explaining Stability and Change in Human Development

Three major systems of influence can be identified in the field of education which affect stability and change in human development (see Baltes and Nesselroade 1979). Using these systems an explanation or causal analysis of human development can be attempted. While educational research is commonly concerned with the investigation of educational processes at the classroom, school, social subgroup, or systemic levels, it is necessary to recognize that the investigation of stability and change in human development must be carried out at the individual level at which the three types of influence operate. The three sets of influences on human development have their origins in: (a) biological factors, (b) environmental factors, and (c) planned learning experiences or interventions. These three sets of influences interact with each other in significant ways. In particular, each individual has the opportunity to choose, at least to some extent, whether or not response will be made to both environmental and intervention influences. However, such choices may in part be biologically determined. Thus the nature and extent of interactions between the three sets of influences are highly complex. As a consequence these three types of influence warrant further consideration.

(a) *Biological influences.* These refer to those determinants that show a strong correlation with chronological age both across historical periods and across a wide range of individuals from different social groups. Development under these influences is ontogenetic and age graded. Normative age-related developments should be seen as largely biological in origin.

(b) *Environmental influences.* These refer to non-biologically based determinants of development that have a pervading effect on those individuals experiencing a particular environment. Bloom (1964) has considered the meaning of the term "environment" and has suggested that it refers to:

> . . . the conditions, forces and external stimuli which impinge on the individual. These may be physical, social, as well as intellectual forces and conditions. We conceive of a range of environments from the most immediate social interactions to the more remote cultural and institutional forces. We regard the environment as providing a network of forces and factors which surround, engulf and play on the individual. (p. 187)

The environment as conceived by Bloom is the total stimulus situation, both latent and actual, that interacts, or is capable of interacting with the individual. Thus, while individuals experience common environments, significant variations also occur as individuals interact with their environments. As a consequence, invariant sequences of development are not observed. Development under environmental influences is largely non-normative, although common patterns occur insofar as a common environment is experienced.

(c) *Intervention influences.* These include those planned learning experiences provided by a wide range of educational institutions that are deliberately designed as part of the educative process. They differ in kind from the pervasive influences of the environment, insofar as they are designed for a particular stage of development and are directed toward highly specific outcomes. The effects of planned learning experiences are assessed in terms of the achievement of particular outcomes rather than in terms of normative and non-normative development. Whereas biological and environmental influences may result in either stability or change in specific characteristics, intervention influences, if successfully administered, may lead to change. Constancy in characteristics involves lack of success in the administration of the intervention.

The interaction between these three types of influence gives rise to analytical problems when attempts are made to identify the effects of particular influences over time. The administration of an intervention under experimental conditions, in which subjects have been randomly assigned to treatment groups and control groups, provides the most appropriate methodology for the investigation of the effects of an intervention, insofar as the cause of change can be identified. However, in many situations within which educational research is conducted, either it is not possible to undertake random allocation to treatment or control groups, or alternatively, randomization and the application of the intervention so affect the educational process that significant distortion from the natural setting occurs. In addition, it must be recognized that even where random assignment to treatment and control groups takes place, prior experiences, as well as genetic and environmental influences, can so interact with the administration of the intervention that the nature of the intervention is changed significantly by these prior and concurrent influences. Some interactions of this type are amenable to analysis where the models being examined can be derived from theoretical considerations (Campbell and Stanley 1963). However, other interactions, particularly those between biological and environmental influences, would not appear to be amenable to rigorous analysis except in the particular circumstances of twin studies (see *Twin Studies*).

A specific problem which arises involves the confounding of biological age-graded effects and environmental non-age-graded effects as a result of a changing environment across the different time periods or age levels at which biological influences are being investigated. Moreover, insofar as some environmental influences may be age related, a similar confounding can arise between different classes of environmental effects. Attempts to unravel such interactions have given rise to specific designs in the conduct of longitudinal investigations. It will be evident from the above comments that, while investigation at different points in time is the key characteristic of longitudinal research, from which it gains its strength, the use of different time points gives rise to certain problems in the conduct of longitudinal studies and the subsequent analysis of the data collected.

2. The Status of Time in Longitudinal Research

Baltes and Nesselroade (1979 p. 2) have stated that "the study of phenomena in their time-related constancy and change is the aim of longitudinal methodology." Furthermore, where repeated observations are made of individuals or groups in order to describe or explain both stability and change, time acts not only as the logical link between the repeated observations, but also as a variable that is a characteristic of the individuals or groups.

Thus the use of time in longitudinal research studies takes place in two distinct ways. First, time is used as a subject characteristic. Second, time is used as a design characteristic. Examples of the first usage occur when chronological age is employed as the basis for the selection of an individual or a group for study, or when the members of an age cohort are studied at successive intervals during their lifespan. In addition, in retrospective studies, events that occurred at particular times in the life of an individual are not only readily identified, but also have special significance. A major limitation on the use of time in this way is that it is not a manipulable variable and subjects cannot be randomly assigned to different time values.

The second use of time is as a design characteristic, which occurs in learning studies, when the extent of learning is measured after successive time periods. Fortunately, in this use of time in a longitudinal study, time is an alterable variable and the effects of time are amenable to analysis. The strength of time in longitudinal studies as a design characteristic arises from the role played by time in the underlying substantive theory. Increasingly, there is recognition that the effects of environmental and biological influences are also time related, insofar as exposure to the environment and biological growth have significant consequences for the magnitudes of measurable outcomes. Nevertheless, length of exposure to an intervention is only one of many factors: for example, the intensity of exposure, or the nature and intensity of opposing forces which can influence educational outcomes. Thus the effects of time are commonly confounded with the effects of these alternative forces.

Time is not only a continuous variable, but equal time intervals are also readily determined. In addition, in many situations a starting point at which time is zero can be identified. Thus it is possible to collect data in the form of a time series, and to examine the constancy or change in particular characteristics with respect to time as recorded on an interval or a ratio scale. Moreover, because time is also a continuous variable, it is commonly possible to investigate time samples of behavior in order to study and compare practices which occur under different conditions. In the investigation of classroom behavior extensive use is made of time samples in order to compare the practices of different teachers, or the effects of different teaching and learning conditions on student behaviors.

Perhaps the most significant characteristic of time lies in its relationship to causal influence, since earlier events influence later events but not vice versa. Thus while it cannot be assumed that measurements made on a variable obtained at an initial point in time can be causally related to an outcome measure obtained at a later time, it is clear that unless the appropriate time sequence exists it is not possible to argue logically for a possible causal relationship. The possibility of investigating causal relationships between variables measured at different points in time is the important contribution that longitudinal research methods have made to the exploration of causal explanations based on theory and the testing of path models and structural equation models. Developments in the methods of analysis used for testing such models has led to an increased emphasis on longitudinal research in education since the 1970s.

3. Types of Longitudinal Research

Inferences concerning the nature and extent of change over time and the factors influencing change are obtained from five design strategies (Kessler and Greenberg 1981): simultaneous cross-sectional studies, trend studies, time series studies, intervention studies, and panel studies.

3.1 Simultaneous Cross-sectional Studies

Within this strategy, two or more related cross-sectional studies are conducted at the same point in time with different age-groups being sampled by each cross-sectional study (see *Cross-sectional Research Methods*). The same predictor and criterion variables are observed for each age sample. Moreover, the age samples are each drawn from the same larger population. However, each sample is drawn independently of the other. Table 1 shows the data matrix for the simultaneous cross-sectional design where there are *m* groups of subjects (i.e., *m* age samples) which are

Table 1
Simultaneous cross-sectional data matrix

Age-group	Sample	Time point	Observed variables
A_1	S_1	T_1	$V_1, V_2, V_3 \ldots \ldots \ldots V_e$
A_2	S_2	T_1	$V_1, V_2, V_3 \ldots \ldots \ldots V_e$
...	...	...	...
...	...	...	...
...	...	...	...
A_m	S_m	T_1	$V_1, V_2, V_3 \ldots \ldots \ldots V_e$

Source: Adapted from Schaie (1965)

observed with respect to e variables. The longitudinal dimension in the design of studies of this type is achieved by consideration of the different chronological ages associated with the independent samples.

This design has been employed in the studies carried out by the International Association for the Evaluation of Educational Achievement (IEA). However, only a few of the many reports issued by IEA have made significant use of the longitudinal element in this design (Comber and Keeves 1973, Carroll 1975, Keeves 1992). In these studies three age-groups were tested: the 10-year old, the 14-year old, and the terminal secondary-school levels; therefore, it was not possible to employ identical tests at each age level. However, overlapping tests were administered and scaling procedures were employed to bring the achievement outcomes to a common scale. In such studies, comparisons across age levels which involved the longitudinal component of the design, employed items that were common to the different age-groups tested. The scaling and measurement issues associated with such comparison are considered in Sect. 5. This design is both simple and economical to execute and, since only one point in time is involved, the confounding effects of environmental influences are reduced and the effects of intervention influences on retention differences across countries (Keeves 1992) and years spent in foreign language learning (Carroll 1975) are more clearly evident. Nevertheless, there are some specific deficiencies in this type of design which arise from the fact that only one time point is employed (see *Cross-sectional Research Methods*). The conclusions which can be derived from this design are only valid under the following assumptions: (a) the age samples have been drawn from the same common population, and (b) the factors influencing change in the criterion variables and their effects have remained constant across the time-span during which the different age samples have been exposed to those factors.

3.2 Trend Studies

Within this strategy, two or more related cross-sectional studies are conducted with identical age-groups at points of time that are sequential. Similar sampling procedures are employed at each time, so that sound comparisons can be drawn over time, and identical or related measures are employed on each occasion. Perhaps the strongest and most widely discussed set of trend data has been associated with the scores on the Verbal and Quantitative Scholastic Aptitude and Achievement Tests in the United States (Donlon 1984). To obtain these sets of data, common test items were employed across occasions, so that the data could be accurately chained from one occasion to the next. Widespread debate has taken place in attempts to explain the highly significant decline in Scholastic Aptitude Test (SAT) scores and the subsequent changes that occurred. However, while many competing explanations have been advanced, none has gained clear support over the others.

In Table 2 the data matrix associated with trend studies is presented. It illustrates that at successive points in time new samples are drawn. In addition, the age-group under survey remains constant and the same variables are observed, so that constancy and change in characteristics of interest in the changing populations can be examined. Further examples of research studies which have investigated trends in educational achievement are those carried out by the National Assessment of Educational Progress (Mullis and Jenkins 1988). Two sets of problems arise in such studies. First, there are the problems of the meaningfulness and validity of achievement test items in circumstances where the curriculum of the schools is changing and new curricular emphases are evolving. These problems can be allowed for in part by the removal of obsolete test items and their replacement with new and more appropriate items. Nevertheless, uncertainties remain as to whether the reduced number of test items, common across occasions, are equally valid for successive samples of students over time. A second set of problems is concerned with the statistical procedures that are employed to scale a constantly changing sample of test items in order to obtain a reliable measure of educational achievement. Item response theory or latent trait scaling techniques have been developed (see Beaton 1987, 1988, Keeves 1992) and have been employed for this purpose. However, the issue remains as to whether, with a changing curriculum, a single latent trait can be considered to exist that covers an area of the school curriculum and that remains unchanged across time.

The major shortcoming of the trend studies referred to above has been that they were not designed initially in such a way as to permit any trends which might have been detected to be explained by biological, environmental, or intervention factors. A study which has been conducted by the International Association for the Evaluation in Educational Achievement in ten countries in the curriculum field of science in 1970 and 1984, provided the opportunity to examine the changes in educational achievement over time which were

Table 2
Trend data matrix

Age-group	Sample	Time point	Observed variables
A_1	S_1	T_1	$V_1, V_2, V_3. . . . . .V_e$
A_1	S_2	T_2	$V_1, V_2, V_3. . . . . .V_e$
. . .	. . .	. . .	. . .
. . .	. . .	. . .	. . .
. . .	. . .	. . .	. . .
A_1	S_e	T_e	$V_1, V_2, V_3. . . . . .V_e$

accounted for by changing educational influences (Keeves 1992).

3.3 Time Series Studies

This type of longitudinal study had its origins in developmental psychology over a hundred years ago. Many such studies have been reported from different parts of the world. These longitudinal studies assume that human development is a continuous process which can be meaningfully examined by a series of "snapshots" recorded at appropriate points in time. They do not necessarily involve equal time intervals between successive observational points. Development can be examined in a valid way through the use of the continuous timescale which has strong metric properties. In Table 3 the research data matrix for such longitudinal studies has been recorded, from which it is seen that the same sample is followed at successive time points with corresponding increases in the age of the group under survey. Information is collected on a range of variables relevant to the aspects of human development being investigated.

There are five advantages which this type of design has over the simultaneous cross-sectional design and the trend design referred to above. First, it is possible to identify intra-individual constancy or change directly, thereby reducing the confounding that arises from

Table 3
Time series data matrix

Age-group	Sample	Time point	Observed variables
A_1	S_1	T_1	$V_1, V_2, V_3. . . . . .V_e$
A_2	S_1	T_2	$V_1, V_2, V_3. . . . . .V_e$
. . .	. . .	. . .	. . .
. . .	. . .	. . .	. . .
. . .	. . .	. . .	. . .
A_m	S_1	T_m	$V_1, V_2, V_3. . . . . .V_e$

changing environmental circumstances, since repeated observations are made of the same subjects. Evidence supporting this advantage has been found repeatedly in the differences in the growth curves obtained from time series longitudinal designs compared with those obtained from simultaneous cross-sectional designs. Second, by observing more than one individual or one group of individuals, differences between individuals or groups in the intra-individual sequences of development become clear. This enables homogeneity or variability in development to be examined between individuals or groups. Third, each group of individuals possesses characteristics that are used to identify individuals as members of the group. As a consequence, the time series design permits the constancy or change in these characteristics of the group to be examined. Moreover, it permits the investigation of relationships associated with such characteristics both within groups as well as between groups.

The two further advantages of the time series design both involve the identification of time-related influences on development. Since this design does not include the examination of the effects of time-specific interventions on development, only those influences that occur naturally over time are involved. The fourth advantage is associated with the study of linkages between such influences and intra-individual or intragroup constancy, or change in particular characteristics. Finally, the fifth advantage is concerned with the investigation of relationships between time-based influences on interindividual and intergroup constancy or change in specific characteristics.

The conduct of time series studies is expensive since it is commonly very costly to maintain contact with a significant number of sample members over an extended period of time, and sample losses can give rise to substantial distortions of observed relationships. A further problem is that a limited sequence of observations might mean that critical information is not available to reveal either a coherent pattern of development or to identify the effects of factors that influence development. Such limitations of a sequence of observations may arise, either through starting with an age-group at some time after birth, or through premature termination of the observation sequence.

The costs associated with the conduct of forward looking or prospective time series studies have led many research workers to employ a retrospective or backward looking time series design. In the latter, a sample is selected and the members of the sample are invited to recall events in their lives at particular times or when they were at specific ages. Retrospective studies suffer from two major shortcomings. First, the sample selected is necessarily biased, because only those who have survived are available for interrogation, and the losses through death, migration, and residential mobility might distort in significant ways the relationships that are derived from the data. Second, the recall by subjects of events that took place at earlier stages in their lives can also be distorted either deliberately or unintentionally. This is because under changing circumstances individuals prefer to present a favorable view of their past lives.

The study of the development of talent in young people reported by Bloom (1985) presents striking findings of how 120 young men and women who reached the highest levels of accomplishment in their chosen fields as Olympic swimmers, world-class tennis players, concert pianists, sculptors, research mathematicians, and research neurologists, were influenced by their homes and educative processes. This study made use of the retrospective time series design, but inevitably was unable to include those who aspired toward such goals, but did not achieve them.

3.4 Intervention Studies

Intervention studies involve a variation of the time series design, but differ with respect to the insertion of a planned learning experience or intervention at a selected time or across a period of time in the lives of individuals. Such intervention designs may involve the selection of probability samples or the random allocation of subjects or groups to treatments. In addition, they commonly involve the administration of experimental and control treatments and the monitoring of treatment conditions. In Table 4 the data matrix for a simple intervention design has been presented. There are of course a large number of variations on the basic design shown in Table 4 that might have been employed and Kratochwill (1978) presents the range of design variations for single-subject and multiple-subject time series investigations.

In the design in Table 4 the samples associated with both the experimental and control groups remain constant throughout the investigation. Initial data on sets of predictor and criterion variables, including pretest performance, are obtained at time T_1 when all subjects are at age A_1. Between times T_1 and T_2 the treatment

conditions are administered to the experimental group and no treatment is given to the control group. At time T_2, when subjects are at age A_2, immediate post-tests are given to both the experimental and the control groups. Again at time T_m delayed post-tests are given to both the experimental and the control groups. Many studies have employed the intervention design in the field of educational research. Important studies to use this design have been: (a) the Ypsilanti Perry Pre-School Project with a long-term follow-up, conducted by the High/Scope Educational Research Foundation and reported by Weikart and his colleagues (Schweinhart and Weikart 1980, Weikart 1984) to evaluate Head Start Programs in the United States; (b) the Sustaining Effects Study concerned with the evaluation of Title I Programs for the educationally disadvantaged in the United States (Carter 1984); and (c) the Mount Druitt Study supported by the Bernard Van Leer Foundation and a study that involved the evaluation of early childhood intervention programs in disadvantaged schools in Sydney, Australia (Braithwaite 1983).

There are many problems associated with the analysis of data from such studies, since few major investigations of this type are able to allocate subjects randomly to experimental and control groups, or to constrain the administration of the intervention or treatment so that characteristics of the experimental group do not influence the nature of the treatment applied. Thus, biological and environmental influences can interact with intervention influences in these studies to such an extent that the assumptions associated with analysis of variance or analysis of covariance procedures are not sustained. As a consequence, such analytical procedures cannot always be safely used in the examination of the data collected through intervention designs. Greater use has been made during recent years of structural equation models to tease out the complex interrelationships which exist within the bodies of data collected in such studies. In spite of these analytical problems, it must be recognized

Table 4
Intervention data matrix

Age	Experimental group	Control group	Sample	Time point	Observed variables
A_1	E_1	C_1	S_1	T_1	$V_1, V_2, V_3. \ldots \ldots V_e$
	Treatment	No Treatment			
A_2	E_1	C_1	S_1	T_2	$V_1, V_2, V_3. \ldots \ldots V_e$
A_m	E_1	C_1	S_1	T_m	$V_1, V_2, V_3. \ldots \ldots V_e$

that through the administration of a treatment to an experimental group and the withholding of a treatment from a control group, it is possible to make stronger inferences about the influence of factors associated with such intervention designs than could be achieved from studies in natural settings.

3.5 Panel Studies

In trend studies, relationships associated with time of measurement are examined while the age of the group under investigation is held constant. In simultaneous cross-sectional studies, the time of measurement is held constant and the age of the group being surveyed is allowed to vary. In the time series design a single cohort is selected and the time of measurement and the age of the cohort are allowed to covary together. All three designs have their shortcomings, insofar as effects associated with time of measurement, age of group being investigated, and the cohort chosen cannot be completely separated from each other. This has led to the development of what are known as "panel studies" in which an attempt is made to unravel the effects of factors associated with age, time of measurement, or cohort.

Schaie (1965) has advanced a general model for the study of longitudinal bodies of data that combines the three aspects of time: cohort (C), time of measurement (T), and age (A). In this model, a measure obtained on variable V is a function of cohort, time of measurements, and age, that is, $V = f(C,T,A)$. This function includes the interactions between the three aspects of time, $C \times T$, $T \times A$, $C \times A$, and $C \times T \times A$. In Fig. 1, the design of a panel study in which the ages of five-year cohorts which are measured at five-year intervals has been presented. The entries recorded in each column correspond to the simultaneous cross-sectional design. The entries in the constant-age diagonals correspond to the trend design, and entries in each row correspond to the time-series design.

In time-sequential analyses, chronological age (A) and time of measurement (T) are combined. In such studies at least three cohorts have to be measured in one investigation (see rectangular boxed data points for years of measurement of 1995 and 2000). In this way complete data are obtained for two time points, 1995 and 2000, and two age levels, 10 years and 15 years, so that an $A \times T$ interaction can be tested. However, the cohort factor (C) is confounded with age and time of measurement.

A similar problem arises in a cohort-sequential analysis in which chronological age and cohort are considered as independent factors. In this case three separate time points are required for the collection of data (see diamond boxed data points for years of measurement 1980, 1985, and 1990). Here the 1980 and 1985 cohorts are being investigated at ages of 0 years and 5 years, and the $A \times C$ interaction can be tested, but it follows that time of measurement is confounded. In a similar way the replicated cross-sectional analysis permits the study of the $C \times T$ interaction, but three age levels have to be investigated (see square box for the 1990 and 1995 cohorts which are surveyed in years 2005 and 2010). Here the age factor is confounded with cohort and time of measurement.

Schaie (1965) considered that age factors were primarily concerned with biological influences associated with ontogenetic development, and that cohort factors involved environmental influences which operated prior to the first time point of an investigation. The time factors were considered to involve environmental effects which were common to all subjects being studied. The interaction effects arose from interactions between the environmental factors and genetic factors. However, if the assumption of a common population was violated, then cohort factors could include genetic differences between cohorts together with the more commonly accepted environmental differences.

Baltes et al. (1979) have proposed a modified version of Schaie's General Developmental Model which is presented in Fig. 2. The figure shows the birth cohorts at five-year intervals from 1980 to 2010 for ages 0 to 30 years and at times of measurement from 1980 to 2040. The simple designs are shown in Fig. 2a, namely: (a) the simultaneous cross-sectional, conducted in year 2010; (b) the trend, for age 30 years; and (c) the time series for the 2010 cohort. A second strategy is presented in Fig. 2b, where simultaneous cross-

Time of birth (C)	Chronological age (A)									
1980	0	5	10	15	20	25				
1985		0	5	10	15	20	25			
1990			0	5	10	15	20	25		
1995				0	5	10	15	20	25	
2000					0	5	10	15	20	25
Time of measurement (T)	1980	1985	1990	1995	2000	2005	2010	2015	2020	2025

Figure 1
Panel design showing ages of five-year cohorts measured at five-year intervals
Source: Adapted from Schaie (1965)

Cohort	\\multicolumn{7}{c}{Age in years}						
	0	5	10	15	20	25	30
							SCª
1980	1980	1985	1990	1995	2000	2005	2010
1985	1985	1990	1995	2000	2005	2010	2015
1990	1990	1995	2000	2005	2010	2015	2020
1995	1995	2000	2005	2010	2015	2020	2025
2000	2000	2005	2010	2015	2020	2025	2030
2005	2005	2010	2015	2020	2025	2030	2035
2010	TS 2010	2015	2020	2025	2030	2035	2040
							TR

Figure 2a

A modified version of Schaie's General Development Model illustrating simultaneous cross-sectional (SC, diagonal band), trend (TR, upright rectangle) and time series (TS, horizontal band) designs

sectional sequences, trend sequences, and time-series sequences are shown. Each involves a replication of a basic design illustrated in Fig. 2a. The simultaneous cross-sectional sequence involves the collection of replicated information on each age-group, while the time series sequences involve the examination of two cohorts.

Whereas the basic designs were considered to be primarily descriptive in nature, the sequence designs were seen by Schaie (1965) also to permit explanation. The distinction between description and explanation is recognized as an important one. Nevertheless, it is clearly not possible to test, in the one analysis, all three factors, cohort, age, and time of measurement. Nor is it possible to examine the three-way interaction, however extensive the data collection might be. The explanatory analysis of data would seem to involve rather more than the investigation of the three factors and their two-way interactions. It would appear to be necessary to construct structural equation models from theory and to test the models using data that permits

Cohort	\\multicolumn{7}{c}{Age in years}						
	0	5	10	15	20	25	30
							SCSª
1980	1980	1985	1990	1995	2000	2005	2010
1985	1985	1990	1995	2000	2005	2010	2015
1990	1990	1995	2000	2005	2010	2015	2020
1995	1995	2000	2005	2010	2015	2020	2025
2000	2000	2005	2010	2015	2020	2025	2030
2005	2005	2010	2015	2020	2025	2030	2035
2010	TSS 2010	2015	2020	2025	2030	2035	2040
							TRS

Figure 2b

Simultaneous cross-sectional sequences (SCS), trend sequences (TRS), and time series sequences (TSS) design strategies.

Source: Based on Baltes et al. 1979 p. 64

(a) Cell entries refer to dates of measurement to be written after both figs 2a, 2b

the examination of cohort-related influences, age-related influences, and time of measurement effects. Where the same cohort is involved in the collection of data at different time points, the different time points can be incorporated into the model. However, the explanation of trends and relationships exhibited across simultaneous cross-sectional studies would appear to demand new analytical strategies. As increasingly large bodies of data become available, for example in the Sustaining Effects Study (Carter 1984), the reduction with age in the magnitude of such influences as those of the effects of school factors on achievement observed in this study, which employed a simultaneous cross-sectional design, clearly warrants more thorough investigation.

In the field of education, relatively few panel studies have been undertaken over time periods that are long enough for age and cohort effects to be distinguished. The Plowden Follow-up Study (Peaker 1971, Marjoribanks 1975) was an important study that involved three grade groups which were investigated on two occasions. Moreover, Peaker (1971) was the first educational research worker to use path analysis as a technique for the examination of longitudinal data using causal models. Subsequently, Marjoribanks (1975) undertook a further examination of the same body of data using more elaborate path models.

4. Validity Issues in Longitudinal Studies

The complex nature of longitudinal studies makes them particularly vulnerable to uncontrolled factors that can threaten their experimental validity. Like other empirical investigations, longitudinal studies can yield meaningful results only insofar as the measurements recorded and the data analyzed are both valid and reliable, and the samples employed are both randomly generated and remain representative of the populations from which they were derived. Without the maintenance of these essential conditions sound generalizations cannot be made beyond the particular groups under investigation. While the pattern of results associated with both the descriptive and explanatory analyses of data from nonrepresentative samples could appear informative, unless these findings were generalizable beyond the situation in which the data were generated, the effort involved in collecting and analyzing the data would be largely wasted.

Kratochwill (1978) has identified two classes of validity—internal and external—and has listed the different types of threat that are likely to occur in longitudinal studies and which arise from these two sources. Internal validity is concerned with the degree of certainty with which measurements associated with the predictor or explanatory variables are capable of accounting for the observed constancy or change in the criterion variables. It will be evident that high levels of consistency and meaningfulness of the predictor variables are necessary preconditions for the interpretation

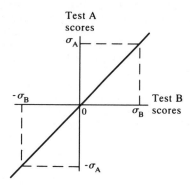

Figure 3a
Line of equivalence for linear scaling

and explanation of time-related observations. External validity refers to the manner and extent to which the findings from the analyses carried out could be generalized to different situations beyond those in which the specific body of data was collected. Kratochwill (1978) notes that the quest for both high internal and external validities can operate against each other. The requirement to obtain a high level of internal validity can demand the exercising of tight experimental controls on the collection of data. However, this might so distort the natural setting in which development occurs that the external validity of the investigation is threatened. The development and testing of causal models derived from theory and the exercising of statistical controls that are consistent with the structure of these models have greatly reduced the demand for rigid experimental designs. As a consequence, the random allocation of subjects to experimental and control groups and the administration of treatment conditions according to rigid specifications are no longer considered to be as important as they were in former decades.

5. Analysis of Longitudinal Research Data

The analysis of the data collected in a longitudinal research study has two primary aims: descriptive analysis, and explanatory analysis. However, before any analysis can be undertaken attention must be given to the problems of measuring attributes on appropriate scales.

5.1 Measurement of Change

The particular problem encountered in educational research studies that employ a longitudinal design is that it is commonly inappropriate to use the identical instrument across different age-groups and at different points in time. The procedures employed for equating the measurements obtained using two different instruments by bringing the scores to a common scale require either that: (a) the two instruments are administered to a common sample; or that (b) the two

instruments contain common components or common items when administered to different samples. Three procedures are employed to bring these scores to a common scale.

(a) *Linear scaling*. In this procedure it is assumed that both the test items and the persons tested represent appropriate samples in the measurement of an underlying trait that is normally distributed with respect to both test items and persons. The scores are standardized, commonly to a mean of zero and a standard deviation of one, and the line of equivalence is used to equate one set of scores with the other. Figure 3a illustrates the use of this procedure (see Thorndike 1971).

(b) *Equipercentile scaling*. In this procedure it is similarly assumed that both the test items and the persons tested represent appropriate samples for the measurement of an underlying trait. In using this procedure cumulative frequency distributions are calculated, scores are obtained at equal percentile points for each test, and a line of equivalence is plotted (see Thorndike 1971). Figure 3b illustrates the use of this procedure which has the advantage over the linear scaling procedure that no assumptions need be made with respect to the shape of the distributions.

(c) *Item response theory (IRT) scaling*. It is also possible to employ models based on the assumption of an unobservable but underlying latent trait which exhibits a relationship with age, for example, as represented by a logistic function. One-parameter (Rasch (1960), two-parameter (Birnbaum 1968) and three-parameter (Lord 1980) models have been developed. The one-parameter model involves item difficulty; the two-parameter model also allows for variability in item discrimination, and the three-parameter model further allows for guessing in multiple-choice items where several alternative responses are provided.

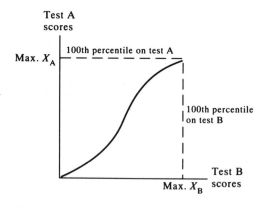

Figure 3b
Line of equivalence for equipercentile scaling

Linear scaling was used by Comber and Keeves (1973) in the development of an international scale for achievement in science across 10-year old, 14-year old, and terminal secondary-school age-groups. A variation of the equipercentile scaling technique was used in the scaling of Scholastic Aptitude Test (SAT) scores over time in the United States (Donlon 1984) and latent trait measurement procedures using a modified three-parameter model have be employed in the scaling of scores in the National Assessment of Educational Progress (NAEP) in the United States (Beaton 1987, 1988). In addition, Keeves (1992) used both the one-parameter model to scale achievement test scores in the study of change in science achievement over time, and linear scaling in the examination of growth across age levels in science achievement.

5.2 Univariate Models of Change

Statistical time series models have been used to describe a great variety of patterns of change in which measurements have been related to age or to another timescale. Goldstein (1979) has listed procedures for the fitting of growth curves to individual records. The most widely used model assumes that relative rate of change in size decreases proportionately to increases in size. Thus where size is very small the relative growth rate is high, but the actual growth rate is low because of small size. However, as size increases the growth rate increases, and when size approaches the final size, the relative and actual growth rates slow down.

The equation for rate of growth is expressed in the following form:

$$\frac{k}{y}\frac{dy}{dt} = b(k - y) \tag{1}$$

where b is a constant, and k is the final size (a constant).

The equation for the growth curve is given by the logistic function:

$$y = c + \frac{k}{1 + \exp(a - bt)} \tag{2}$$

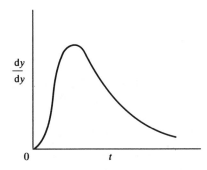

Figure 4a
Curve for rate of growth

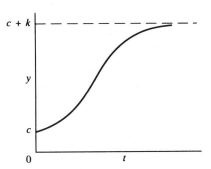

Figure 4b
Curve for growth

where a is a constant, and $y = c$ is the value of the lower asymptote and $y = c + k$ is the value of the upper asymptote.

The curves for rate of growth and growth are shown in Fig. 4a and 4b respectively.

An alternative model for the measurement of growth is provided by the Gompertz curve in which the relative rate of change in size decreases exponentially with time, and thus in equally small intervals of time there are equal proportional decreases in relative growth rate.

The equation for rate of growth is expressed in the following form:

$$\frac{1}{y}\frac{dy}{dt} = \exp(a - bt) \tag{3}$$

where a and b are constants, and the equation for growth is given by:

$$y = k \exp[-\exp(a - bt)] \tag{4}$$

Although research workers in the fields of child and adolescent development have considered the use of other types of curves, the logistic and the Gompertz curves have found most extensive use, including the combining of curves across different age ranges. Burt (1937) found, for example, that the growth in the height of girls from birth to 18 years could be represented by the sum of three logistic curves.

More powerful mathematical models are likely to be used in the analysis of data in educational research as the accuracy of measurement increases and thus the quality of the data included in the analysis increases. Overviews of the mathematical models and statistical procedures which might be used to describe change in longitudinal research studies have been provided by Goldstein (1979), Nesselroade and Baltes (1979), Coleman (1981), Collins and Horn (1991).

5.3 Multivariate Models of Change

In longitudinal research, the costs of carrying out the processes of data collection and maintaining contact with the sample under survey are so great that, in general, there is little to be gained by collecting data on only one criterion measure. As a consequence, data are commonly obtained on a wide range of characteristics rather than on an isolated variable. Under these circumstances multivariate procedures of analysis are widely used in longitudinal research studies. This has also led to the use of techniques to condense the large bodies of data into more simplified data structures and to examine these for change. Techniques that are widely used include factor analysis, multidimensional scaling, cluster analysis, and configural frequency analysis. Variations in the factor patterns or cluster patterns over time are taken to indicate change and development, while stability in factor and cluster patterns over time would seem to imply the measurement of a dimension that is unaffected by environmental or biological influences.

5.4 Explanatory and Causal Analyses

In empirical research in education two strategies are available for the investigation of causal relationships and, in general, both involve the use of longitudinal designs. First, in experimental studies in which subjects are randomly selected from a population and are randomly assigned to experimental and control groups, multivariate analysis of variance techniques are appropriate. Such studies which demand the collection of data at two points in time are common in the investigation of educational processes. Second, in intervention studies where some degree of randomization in the allocation of subjects to treatments has been achieved, it may be possible to use multivariate analysis of covariance techniques in the examination of data. However, it is necessary to establish that antecedent conditions are unrelated both logically and empirically to the application of the intervention before covariance procedures can be safely employed. Moreover, since time and time-related factors cannot be manipulated under experimental conditions and applied as interventions or treatments in studies where more than one time-related variable is being investigated, analysis of variance and covariance techniques cannot be employed because such effects remain confounded.

A variety of techniques is, however, available for the examination of data to provide explanation in terms of causal relationships. These techniques make full use of the time relationships which are present in longitudinal designs. The analytical procedures which are employed require the development of causal models from prior research studies and established theory, and the testing of these models for fit using the available data. Among the procedures now available which are capable of analyzing complex bodies of scaled data are Linear Structural Relations Analysis (LISREL) and Partial Least Squares Path Analysis (PLS). For the examination of bodies of categorized data log–linear modeling and configural frequency analysis techniques are gaining acceptance. In addition, where repeated measures over time on an outcome or criterion variable have been obtained, multilevel analysis

techniques have provided a new approach (Goldstein 1987, Raudenbush and Bryk 1988, Muthén 1991, Gustafsson and Stahl 1996)

6. Conclusion

During the 1980s the advances in techniques of statistical analysis, particularly those concerned with multilevel analysis, have led to renewed interest in the problems associated with the analysis of change. In this entry the emphasis in the discussion has been on the study of groups rather than individuals. The reader is referred to other entries (see *Single Case Research: Measuring Change; Change, Measurement of*) for discussion of the issues concerned with the study of change at the individual level. In addition, recent advances, unanswered questions, and future directions for research in this field are discussed in Collins and Horn (1991), and the methodological issues involved are also considered by Mason and Fienberg (1985).

The use of these new explanatory analytical procedures requires that a longitudinal study should be designed with a clearly stated theoretical formulation from which causal hypotheses and causal models involving structural relationships between variables are developed for testing. These hypotheses and models are either tested and accepted as plausible explanations of the available evidence, or rejected. The incorporation of accepted models into substantive theory that is coherent and useful for further explanation is seen as the outcome of enquiry. Longitudinal research has an important role to play in this regard within the field of educational research.

Educational research is primarily concerned with stability and change in human characteristics, particularly those characteristics that are influenced by learning experiences provided by education in schools and homes. Consequently, the marked advances made in the 1980s and early 1990s suggest that longitudinal research studies will assume growing importance in the last decade of the twentieth century and into the early decades of the twenty-first century.

See also: Cross-sectional Research Methods

References

Baltes P B, Cornelius S M, Nesselroade J R 1979 Cohort effects in developmental psychology. In: Nesselroade J R, Baltes P B (eds.) 1979
Baltes P B, Nesselroade J R 1979 History and rationale of longitudinal research. In: Nesselroade J R, Baltes P B (eds.) 1979
Beaton A E 1987 *Implementing the New Design: The NAEP 1983–84 Technical Report.* National Assessment of Educational Progress/Educational Testing Service, Princeton, New Jersey

Beaton A E 1988 *Expanding the New Design: The NAEP 1985–86 Technical Report*. Educational Testing Service, Princeton, New Jersey

Birnbaum A 1968 Some latent trait models and their use inferring an examinee's ability. In: Lord F M, Novick M (eds.) 1968 *Statistical Theory in Mental Test Scores*. Addison-Wesley, New York

Bloom B S 1964 *Stability and Change in Human Characteristics*. Wiley, New York

Bloom B S (ed.) 1985 *Developing Talent in Young People*. Ballantine, New York

Braithwaite J 1983 *Explorations in Early Childhood Education*. Australian Council for Educational Research, Hawthorn, Victoria

Bryk A S, Raudenbush S W 1989 Towards a more appropriate conception of research on school effects: A three-level hierarchical linear model. In: Bock R D (ed.) 1989 *Multilevel Analysis of Educational Data*. Academic Press, New York

Burt C B 1937 *The Backward Child*. University of London Press, London

Butler N R, Golding J (eds.) 1986 *From Birth to Five: A Study of the Health and Behaviour of Britain's Five Year Olds*. Pergamon Press, Oxford

Campbell D T, Stanley J C 1963 Experimental and quasi experimental designs for research on teaching. In: Gage N (ed.) 1963 *Handbook of Research on Teaching*. Rand McNally, Chicago, Illinois

Carroll J B 1975 *The Teaching of French as a Foreign Language in Eight Countries*. Wiley, New York

Carter L F 1984 The sustaining effects study of compensatory and elementary education. *Educ. Res.* 13(7): 4–13

Coleman J S 1981 *Longitudinal Data Analysis*. Basic Books, New York

Collins L M, Horn J L (eds.) 1991 *Best Methods for the Analysis of Change*. American Psychological Association, Washington, DC

Comber L C, Keeves J P 1973 *Science Education in Nineteen Countries: An Empirical Study*. Wiley, New York

Davie R, Butler N, Goldstein H 1972 *From Birth to Seven: A Report of the National Child Development Study*. Longmans, London

Donlon T F 1984 *The College Board Technical Handbook for the Scholastic Aptitude Test and Achievement Tests*. College Entrance Examination Board, New York

Douglas J W B 1964 *The Home and the School: A Study of Ability and Attainment in the Primary Schools*. MacGibbon and Kee, London

Fägerlind I 1975 *Formal Education and Adult Earnings: A Longitudinal Study on the Economic Benefits of Education*. Almqvist and Wiksell, Stockholm

Fogelman K (ed.) 1983 *Growing up in Great Britain: Collected Papers from the National Child Development Study*. Macmillan, London

Goldstein H 1979 *The Design and Analysis of Longitudinal Studies: Their Role in the Measurement of Change*. Academic Press, London

Goldstein H 1987 *Multilevel Models in Educational and Social Research*. Griffin, London

Gustafsson J-E, Stahl P A 1996 *STREAMS User's Guide: Structural Equation Modeling Made Simple*. Göteborg University, Göteborg

Husén T 1969 *Talent, Opportunity and Career*. Almqvist and Wiksell, Stockholm

Keeves J P (ed.) 1992 *The IEA Study of Science III: Changes in Science Education and Achievement: 1980–1984*. Pergamon Press, Oxford

Kessler R C, Greenberg D F 1981 *Linear Panel Analysis: Models of Quantitative Change*. Academic Press, New York

Kratochwill T R (ed.) 1978 *Single Subject Research: Strategies for Evaluating Change*. Academic Press, New York

Lord F M 1980 *Applications of Item Response Theory to Practical Testing Problems*. Erlbaum, Hillsdale, New Jersey

Marjoribanks K 1975 Cognitive performance: A model for analysis. *Australian Journal of Education* 19(2): 156–66

Mason W M, Fienberg S E 1985 *Cohort Analyses in Social Research*. Springer-Verlag, New York

Muthén B O 1991 Analysis of longitudinal data using latent variable models with varying parameters. In: Collins L M, Horn J L (eds.) 1991

Mullis I V S, Jenkins L B 1988 *The Science Report Card*. ETS, Princeton, New Jersey

Nesselroade J R, Baltes P B 1979 *Longitudinal Research in the Study of Behavior and Development*. Academic Press, New York

Peaker G F 1971 *The Plowden Children Four Years Later*. National Foundation for Educational Research, Slough

Rasch G 1960 *Probabilistic Models for some Intelligence and Attainment Tests*. Danish Institute for Educational Research, Copenhagen

Raudenbush S W, Bryk A S 1988 Methodological advances in analyzing the effects of schools and classrooms in student learning. *Rev. Res. Educ.* 15: 437–75

Schaie K W 1965 A general model for the study of developmental problems. *Psych. Bull.* 64: 92–107

Schweinhart L J, Weikart D P 1980 *Young Children Grow Up: The Effects of the Perry Preschool Program on Youths through Age Fifteen*. High Scope Press, Ypsilanti, Michigan

Thorndike R L (ed.) 1971 *Educational Measurement*, 2nd edn. American Council on Education, Washington, DC

Tuijnman A 1989 *Recurrent Education, Earnings and Well-being*. Almqvist and Wiksell, Stockholm

Weikart D P (ed.) 1984 *Changed Lives: The Effects of the Perry Preschool Program on Youths through Age Nineteen*. High Scope Press, Ypsilanti, Michigan

Simulation as a Research Technique

R. R. Wilcox

Simulation studies are a relatively simple way of getting approximate solutions to many statistical and related problems that are difficult to analyze using conventional techniques. The best way to describe how simulations work is to give some examples of how they are applied.

In research settings, simulations have two major components. The first is a *system* that is of interest to the investigator, and the second is a *model* that represents the system. The system can be almost any set of interrelated elements. For example, it might be the traffic flow in a city, or the operations of a large computer. In education, the system might be an individual learning a skill, or perhaps an examinee responding to an item. The corresponding model can be descriptive, but usually it is mathematical. For instance, in the traffic flow example, the Poisson distribution is frequently used to represent the probability that an automobile will arrive at an intersection during a particular time interval. Learning models are sometimes based on a probability model known as a Markov chain (see *Social Network Analysis*), and several mathematical models have been proposed for describing the probability that an examinee will give a correct response to a test item (see *Classical Test Theory*).

Models have been classified in several ways, but for present purposes the most important distinction is deterministic versus stochastic. "Deterministic models" refer to situations where all mathematical and logical relationships among the elements of a system are fixed. In a "stochastic" model, at least one variable is random. In education, stochastic models are by far the most common, but deterministic models are important in certain situations.

1. Monte Carlo Studies

Simulating a stochastic model is often referred to as a Monte Carlo study. Recently, however, the term "Monte Carlo" has been disappearing from use, and instead they are simply called "simulation studies." The term Monte Carlo was originally a code used for the secret work on the atomic bomb during the Second World War; the goal was to simulate actions related to random neutron diffusion in fissionable materials. Although a Monte Carlo study generally requires a high-speed computer to be of any practical use, the idea is not a modern one. In fact, it can be traced as far back as Babylonian times (Hammersley and Handscomb 1964).

Whether addressing a deterministic or stochastic problem, all Monte Carlo studies require a set of observations generated according to some probability function. The most basic and commonly used probability function is the uniform distribution over the unit interval. This means that a sequence of real numbers between zero and one must be generated such that for any generated number, say x, the probability that x is less than or equal to x_0 is x_0, where x_0 is any constant between zero and one. Symbolically, $Pr(x \leqslant x_0) = x_0$ is required for any x_0, where $0 < x_0 < 1$.

In practice, generating truly random numbers is impossible, and so approximations are used instead. One of the earliest approximations was proposed by von Neumann and his colleagues (von Neumann 1951). Later, however, congruential generators were typically used. These procedures produce a nonrandom sequence of numbers according to some recursive formula. Generally, this formula is given by $x_{i+1} = ax_i + c - mk_i$, where k_i is the largest integer that is less than or equal to $(ax_i + c)/m$, and where the constants a, c and m are chosen so that the sequence has certain optimal properties. For binary computers, $m = 2^{35}$, $a = 2^7$, and $c = 1$ are known to yield good statistical results (Hull and Dobell 1964, MacLaren and Marsagli 1965, Olmstead 1946). Congruential generators are deterministic in the sense that a fixed starting value or seed, and a specific generator will always produce the same sequence of numbers. This is contrary to commonsense notions about randomly generated numbers, but it can be shown that the sequence appears to be uniformly distributed and statistically independent (Knuth 1969). Also, this reproducibility of a sequence facilitates the "debugging" of a computer program designed to simulate a particular model. Currently, there are several pseudorandom number generators to choose from, but none of these dominates all others in terms of the various criteria used to judge their adequacy.

2. Some Illustrations

Monte Carlo procedures have been applied to problems in numerous fields including quantum mechanics, cell population studies, operations research, combinatorics, and traffic flow problems. This section illustrates how Monte Carlo studies can be applied to problems in mental test theory.

Understanding why and how Monte Carlo studies work requires an understanding of the weak law of large numbers. Suppose, for example, a probability model is being investigated where the probability of observing a value x is determined by some unknown parameter, say τ. Further suppose that a statistic $\hat{t}$, which is a function of x, has been proposed for estimating τ. The question arises as to how accurately $\hat{t}$ estimates τ for various values of τ. The law of large numbers says that if observations are randomly generated according to the probability model and a particular value of τ, and if the process is repeated yielding a sequence of $\hat{t}$ values, say $\hat{t}_1, \hat{t}_2, \ldots$, then $\sum_{i=1}^{k} \hat{t}_i/k$ approximates the expected (or average) value of $\hat{t}$. If, for example, $\hat{t}$ is intended to be an unbiased estimate of τ, $\tau - \sum \hat{t}_i/k$ gives a reasonably accurate estimate of the bias, assuming that k is large. By repeating this process with various τ values, an investigator can approximately determine how well $\hat{t}$ estimates τ no matter what τ happens to be. Many related problems can be solved, and some illustrations are given below.

A relatively simple example will help clarify matters. Suppose an examinee reponds to n dichotomously scored test items. Further assume, as is frequently done, that the probability that the examinee gets x items correct is

$$\binom{n}{x} p^x (1-p)^{n-x} \tag{1}$$

where

$$\binom{n}{x} = \frac{n(n-1)\ldots(n-x+1)}{(n-x)(n-x-1)\ldots 2}, \tag{2}$$

and p is the unknown probability of a correct response to a randomly selected item. The most common estimate of p is $\hat{p} = x/n$, which is known to have several optimal properties.

Suppose an investigator is interested in determining how well $\hat{p}$ estimates p. As a measure of accuracy, suppose $E(\hat{p} - p)^2$ is used. In other words, accuracy is measured as the average squared difference between $\hat{p}$ and p, the average being taken over an infinite sequence of independent random samples of n items. It is known that $E(\hat{p} - p)^2 = p(1-p)/n$, but for the sake of illustration, suppose this is not known. For any n and p, the value of $E(\hat{p} - p)^2$ can be approximated as follows:

(a) *Step 1*—Generate a random number between zero and one, that is, a number from the uniform distribution on the unit interval. If this number is less than p, set $y_1 = 1$; otherwise, $y_1 = 0$. Repeat this process n times yielding a sequence of y_i's ($i = 1, \ldots, n$).

(b) *Step 2*—Let $x = \sum_{i=1}^{n} y_i$. It is known that the probability function of x is given by Eqn. (1).

(c) *Step 3*—Compute $\hat{t} = (\hat{p} - p)^2 = (x/n - p)^2$. Since n and p are chosen by the investigator, $\hat{t}$ can be determined.

(d) *Step 4*—Repeat steps 1 through 3 until k values of $\hat{t}$, say $\hat{t}_1, \ldots, \hat{t}_k$ are available. Because the $\hat{t}_i$ values are independent, the weak law of large numbers implies that $k^{-1}\sum \hat{t}_k$ approaches $E(\hat{p} - p)^2$ (in probability) as k gets large. Thus $E(\hat{p} - p)^2$ can be approximated for any n and p that is of interest to the investigator.

There remains the problem of deciding how large k should be. For Monte Carlo studies in general, a conservative choice, one that is frequently recommended, is $k = 10,000$. In practice, however, this can be costly in terms of computer time, particularly when the probability model is complex. To minimize the chances of highly erroneous results, k is usually chosen to be at least 1,000, but there are studies reported in the statistical literature where k is as small as 100.

As another illustration, suppose that a randomly sampled examinee responding to an n-item test gets x items correct with probability

$$\binom{n}{x} = \frac{B(r+x, s+n-x)}{B(r,s)}, \tag{3}$$

where B is the beta function given by

$$B(r\,s) = \int_1^0 t^{r-1}(1-t)^{s-1}\,dt, \tag{4}$$

and where $r, s > 0$ are unknown parameters. This model might appear to be somewhat complex, but it is fairly easy to apply, particularly with the aid of a computer, and it has proven to be very useful in practice.

To apply this model, it is necessary to estimate the parameters r and s. Skelam (1948) proposed an estimate based on the method of moments, and Griffiths (1973) suggests an approximation to the maximum likelihood estimate. The accuracy of both procedures has not been determined analytically, and Griffiths' procedure appears to be particularly intractable when trying to determine its accuracy via standard techniques. This suggests, therefore, that Monte Carlo procedures be used to compare the two estimates for various combinations of r, s and n. This can be done by following the steps in the previous illustration. However, Step 1 requires that observations be generated according to Eqn. (3), and this can be accomplished via the inverse transform method.

3. The Bootstrap Method

Simulations have taken on new importance through a technique called a bootstrap. Ordinarily, simulation studies consist of generating observations from a specified distribution, and determining the characteristics of a particular statistic. The goal is to determine whether a statistic has good properties for a range of distributions that an investigator suspects might occur in applied work. In contrast, the bootstrap procedure provides a tool for analyzing data where simulations are performed on the data at hand. That is, observations are randomly sampled with replacement from the data collected, the statistic that is of interest is computed, and this process is repeated many times in order to gain information about the population of subjects under study. One important feature of the bootstrap is that it can address certain problems for which conventional methods are known to be inadequate. There are many important problems where the bootstrap gives good results, but there are also situations where little or no improvement is obtained over standard techniques.

Two situations are described to provide a better understanding of the bootstrap. The first considers a basic problem in statistics where the standard methods provide an exact solution, but it provides a relatively simple description of how the bootstrap works. The second situation illustrates how the bootstrap can be used to solve a nontrivial problem.

The first situation is unrealistic in the sense that observations are randomly sampled from a known distribution. In particular, suppose $n = 10$ observations are randomly sampled from a normal distribution with mean 0 and variance 16. From standard results, the sample mean, $\bar{X}$, has a normal distribution with mean 0 and variance $\sigma^2/n = 1.6$, and the standard error is 1.6 = 1.265. If this is not known, how else could the standard error of $\bar{X}$ be estimated? One way is to repeatedly sample $n = 10$ observations, and then compute the sample standard deviation of the sample means obtained, and this would estimate $\sigma_{\bar{x}} = \sigma/n$, the standard error of $\bar{X}$. Suppose this is done 15 times. That is, randomly sample $n = 10$ observations, compute the mean, randomly sample another $n = 10$ observations, compute the mean, etc. The 15 sample means obtained might be:

1.4, 0.58, –0.68, –0.66, 0.58, 0.71, 0.40, –0.5,

1.15, –1.7, 0.78, –0.52, –1.47, 1.73.

(These values were generated from a normal distribution using the Minitab command RANDOM.) The sample standard deviation of these 15 values is 1.04, while the actual standard error is 1.265. Thus, the estimated standard error is a bit different from the actual value, but with 100 sample means, rather than 15, the estimate would be fairly close to the correct value.

One difficulty with the illustration that causes problems when dealing with more complicated situations is the assumption of sampling from a normal distribution. In general, the distribution from which observations are sampled is unknown, but it can be estimated with the data available from a particular study. For example, suppose the values obtained are:

9, 9, 10, 12, 10, 1, 9, 11, 8, 10.

Then the estimate of the probability function is $P(X = 1) = 1/10$, $P(X = 8) = 1/10$, $P(X = 9) = 3/10$, $P(X = 10) = 3/10$, $P(X = 11) = 1/10$, and $P(X = 12) = 1/10$. That is, the estimate is based on the observed relative frequencies. Sampling with replacement from this empirical distribution is called generating a bootstrap sample. Generating a large number of bootstrap samples, and computing the sample variances of the resulting sample means, yields an estimate of the squared standard error of $\bar{X}$. It can be shown that this is tantamount to the usual estimate, except that when computing the sample variance, division is made by n rather than $n - 1$. That is, the estimated sample variance is

$$\sum (\bar{X}_i - \bar{X})^2/n, \tag{5}$$

rather than

$$\sum (\bar{X}_i - \bar{X})^2/(n - 1)n. \tag{6}$$

Thus the standard error of more complicated measures of location can be estimated as well, and it is possible to test hypotheses in situations where other procedures are unsatisfactory. Suppose the goal is to compare two methods for teaching reading. If one group of students receives method 1, and the other method 2, the most common approach to comparing the groups is to test

$$H_0 : \mu_1 = \mu_2, \tag{7}$$

the hypothesis that the two groups have identical means. One criticism of this approach is that highly skewed distributions are common in applied work, so the population mean, μ, might be an unsatisfactory measure of location. Another concern, especially with small or moderate sample sizes, is that slight departures from normality, toward a distribution with heavy tails, can spell disaster in terms of power or Type II errors (e.g., Yuen 1974, Wilcox 1994). Moreover, heavy-tailed distributions appear to be quite common in applied work (e.g., Micceri 1989, Wilcox 1990). One way of dealing with this problem is to replace the sample means with a measure of location that has a standard error less affected by heavy-tailed distributions. One such estimate is the Harrell and Davis (1982) estimate of the median given by

$$\hat{\theta} = \sum w_i X_{(i)}, \tag{8}$$

where

$$X_{(1)} \leqslant X_{(2)} \leqslant \ldots \leqslant X_{(n)} \tag{9}$$

are the observations written in ascending order, and

$$w_i = \frac{1}{B(r, s)} \int_{(i-n)/n}^{i/n} y^{(n+1)/2 - 1} (1 - y)^{(n+1)/2} dy \tag{10}$$

An estimate of the squared standard error of $\hat{\theta}$ can be obtained with the bootstrap. Generate a bootstrap sample, compute the estimate of the median, and call the result $\hat{\theta}^*$. Repeat this process N times yielding $\hat{\theta}^*_1, \ldots, \hat{\theta}^*_N$. Usually $N = 100$ will suffice. An estimate of the squared standard error of $\hat{\theta}$ is

$$V = \sum (\hat{\theta}_b - \bar{\theta}^*)^2 / (N - 1). \tag{11}$$

A statistic for testing the hypothesis of equal medians is

$$U = \frac{|\hat{\theta}_1 - \hat{\theta}_2|}{\sqrt{V_1 + V_2}}, \tag{12}$$

where $\hat{\theta}_j$ and V_j are the estimates of the median and squared standard error for the jth group. In order for the test statistic U to have any practical value, an appropriate critical value is required, and again simulations, via the bootstrap procedure, can be used. Compute

$$U_b = \frac{|\hat{\theta}^*_{1b} - \hat{\theta}^*_{2b} - \hat{\theta}_1 + \hat{\theta}_2|}{\sqrt{V_1 + V_2}}, \tag{13}$$

where $\hat{\theta}^*_{jb}$ is the bth bootstrap estimate of the Harrell–Davis estimate of the median for the jth group, $b=1,,,=N$. Now, however, larger values for N are typically required; usually $N = 400$ provides good results. The point is that the U_b values provide an estimate of the null distribution of the test statistic, u, so an estimate of the $1 - \alpha$ critical value is

$$c = U_{((1-\alpha)N)}, \tag{14}$$

where $U_{(1)}, \ldots U_{(N)}$ are the U_b values written in ascending order. There are slight but important refinements of this procedure, but the details are not given here. (For an elemetary description of these refinements, plus an easy-to-use Minitab macro for applying this procedure, see Wilcox 1994). Two points should be stressed. First, the procedure just described provides good control over the probability of a Type I error for $\alpha = 0.05$, but it can be a bit unsatisfactory when $\alpha = 0.01$. Second, the increase in power over the usual t-test can be substantial. For example, with a very slight departure from normality, there are situations where the median procedure has power 0.64, while the t-test has power 0.16! Moreover, reanalysis of data from actual studies has turned up significant results in situations where the t-test is highly nonsignificant.

To elaborate on the increase in power that is possible, suppose a comparison is made between two normal distributions with variance 1 and means 0 and 1. With α 0.05, the power of Welch's test (see Welch 1937) for comparing means is approximately 0.93, which is nearly equal to the power of Student's t-test, while comparing medians with the Harrell–Davis estimator, it is 0.87. Suppose instead that observations come from a contaminated normal distribution given by $H(x) = .9 \, \Phi(x) + .1\Phi(x/10)$, where $\Phi(x)$ is the standard normal distribution. An important point is that the difference between the normal and contaminated normal is very small. In fact, $|H(x) - \Phi(x)| \leqslant$

.04 for any x, and a graph of these two distributions shows that they are nearly indistinguishable. However, the variance of the standard normal distribution is 1, while the variance of the contaminated normal is 10.9! Consequently, the power of both Student's t-test and Welch's method is substantially affected. For example, Welch's procedure has power 0.28, but the method for comparing medians has power 0.78. The reason for the difference in power is that the method for comparing medians is based on a measure of location with a standard error that is relatively unaffected by heavy-tailed distributions. Simulations are important because they provide the only known method for controlling the probability of a Type I error when comparing medians via the Harrell–Davis estimator (see *Significance Testing*).

4. Conclusion

The bootstrap seems to be very useful in situations where the goal is to compare robust measures of location and scale, as well as in robust regression, but when trying to correct problems associated with conventional methods for comparing groups, the bootstrap appears to fail in providing a useful solution. For example, it has been shown that under general circumstances where the sample sizes are unequal, the t-test for two independent groups is not even asymptotically correct. That is, no matter how large the sample sizes might be, the confidence intervals computed cannot be trusted. Attempts at correcting this problem with the bootstrap have failed (Wilcox 1990). Methods for comparing variances are known to be highly nonrobust under nonnormality, and the bootstrap does not improve matters. Inferences about the correlation coefficient are also nonrobust, and again the bootstrap does not provide a practical solution, although early results were very encouraging (Wilcox 1991). Perhaps some improvement of the bootstrap will provide more satisfactory results, but this remains to be seen. However, these negative results should not detract from the important point that for robust measures of location, scale, and association, the bootstrap provides an important and useful tool. Due to the highly nonnormal distributions occuring in practice, robust methods are taking on increasing importance, so the bootstrap promises to be an important tool in the future (see *Sampling Errors in Survey Research*).

See also: Significance Testing; Sampling Errors in Survey Research

References

Griffiths D A 1973 Maximum likelihood estimation for the beta-binomial distribution and an application to the household distribution of the total number of cases of a disease. *Biometrics* 29(4): 637–48

Hammersley J M, Handscombe D C 1964 *Monte Carlo Methods.* Methuen, London

Harrell F E, Davis C E 1982 A new distribution-free quantile estimator. *Biometrika* 69(3): 635–40

Hull T E, Dobell A R 1964 Mixed congruential random number generators for binary machines. *Journal of Association for Computing Machinery* 11(1): 31–40

Knuth D E 1969 *the Art of Computer Programming. Vol. 2: Seminumerical Algorithms.* Addison-Wesley, Reading, Massachusetts

MacLaren M D, Marsagli G 1965 Uniform random number generators. *Journal of Association for Computing Machinery* 12: 83–89

Miccceri T 1989 The unicorn, the normal curve, and other improbable creatures. *Psych. Bull.* 105(1): 156–66

Olmstead P S 1946 Distribution of sample arrangements for runs up and down *Ann. Math. Stat.* 17(1): 24–33

Skellam J G 1948 A probability distribution derived from the binomial distribution by regarding the probability of success as variable between the sets of trials *J. Royal. Stat. Soc.* B10(2): 257–61

Von Neumann J 1951 Various techniques used in connection with random digits. *Applications Maths. Series* 12: 36–38

Welch B L 1937 The significance of the difference between two means when the population variances are unequal. *Biometrika* 29: 350–62

Wilcox R R 1990 Comparing the means of two independent groups. *Biom. J.* 32: 771–80

Wilcox R R 1991 Bootstrap inferences about the correlation and variances of paired data. *Br. J. Math. S.* 44: 379–82

Wilcox R R 1994 *Statistics for the Social Sciences.* Academic Press, New York

Yuen K (1974) The two-sample trimmed t for unequal population variances. *Biometrika* 61(1): 165–70

Further Reading

DiCiccio T J, Romano J P 1988 A review of bootstrap confidence intervals. *J. Royal Stat. Soc.* B50(3): 338–54

Epron B, Tibshirani R J 1993 *An Introduction to the Bootstrap.* Chapman Hall, New York

Noreen E W 1989 *Computer Intensive Methods for Testing Hypotheses: An Introduction.* Wiley, New York

Rubinstein R Y 1981 *Simulation and the Monte Carlo Method.* Wiley, New York

Survey Research Methods

M. J. Rosier

Survey research methods in education describe procedures for the collection of information associated with education. This information is used to extend understanding of educational issues and to assist in the development of educational policy. General works on survey research methods include Fowler (1988), Karweit (1982), and Miller (1991).

Three developments have influenced the methodology of survey research. First, the technology of sampling has reached a high level. Second, many techniques have been developed for collecting valid and reliable information from survey respondents. Third, the availability of computers and survey research software have facilitated the analysis of this information.

This entry is concerned with the purposes of surveys, the distinction between a census and a sample survey (which, while alternatives, are also complementary in nature), and the steps taken in the conduct of survey research. These steps form a cycle of activities, which involve: (a) formulation of the research questions, (b) definition of a conceptual framework, (c) development of survey instruments, (d) collection of data, (e) preparation of the data for analysis, (f) conduct of analyses, and (g) reporting the findings from the survey. In the fourth step attention is given in sample surveys to the problems of sampling and the problems of ensuring the participation and cooperation of the respondents. Subsequently in the analysis stage, the data in a sample should be adjusted to compensate for different response rates and the characteristics of the sample design.

1. Purpose of Surveys

Surveys are conducted to accomplish two main purposes. First, descriptive or enumerative surveys are used to obtain descriptive information. Second, analytic, explanatory or comparative surveys are designed to examine relationships between measures and variables in the survey. The users of surveys for these two purposes are characterized by Groves (1989 p. 3) as "describers" and "modelers."

There are, in general, two types of surveys. First, there is the complete census of all members of the target population. Second, there is a sample survey in which a known proportion of the target population is under survey. The collection of data from a complete population is generally both costly and a burden on the people involved. Thus a sample survey not only reduces costs, but may ensure that the data collected are of high quality. However, the major limitation of a sample survey is the inability to provide detailed information for all members of particular subgroups when needed. A census can achieve better coverage and response rates than sample surveys, although this is not always true. With a well-designed sample, and high-quality procedures of data collection, it may be possible to allocate resources so as to obtain a very high level of response and a greater range of information.

A third source of survey data exists and may be accessed from administrative registers. The "annual census" of the population of most school systems is not so much a census but more a collection and compilation of information that is necessarily held in a standard form in administrative registers. Such information is inexpensive to collect, available when required, and generally accurate and detailed.

Sample surveys and population censuses must be seen to be complementary rather than alternatives, for sometimes within a census it is desirable to include a component that is a sample survey. In this way it is possible to obtain rich and complex data from only a known fraction of a population at the same time as obtaining a complete enumeration of the entire population with respect to a limited amount of information (see Kish 1987).

When a sample is selected for a descriptive survey, the results obtained from the sample must be generalized to the population from which the sample was drawn (the target population). One example is a survey to measure student achievement in literacy and numeracy. Such surveys can be conducted at various levels: school, school district, region, country, or cross-national. Another example is a survey to provide norms for standard tests for students at specified grades or ages, or for specified subgroups of the population defined in terms of sex or locality.

Analytic surveys typically collect information on a range of predictor or explanatory variables that are hypothesized to influence the criterion variables of interest. For example, the main criterion in the Second Science Study of the International Association for the Evaluation of Educational Achievement (IEA) was the science achievement of the students in the participating countries. However, rather than merely reporting the mean levels of science achievement, the data were analyzed to investigate how differences in the science achievement of students were explained by factors such as their home background and their school experiences (Keeves 1992, Postlethwaite and Wiley 1992, Rosier and Banks 1990). Underlying surveys of this type are conceptual models which the researchers wish to examine, in order to improve understanding of the network of factors influencing educational processes. In general, in these survey studies, a sample was drawn, but in some school systems a complete population was tested.

As in the IEA studies, the descriptive and analytic purposes of surveys are not mutually exclusive, since researchers in education commonly wish to fulfill both purposes in a single survey. Although a dual-purpose survey may be less expensive than conducting two separate studies, such a survey may be more complicated, especially in terms of sampling designs and analyses. An efficient sample used to provide descriptive characteristics of a population (population parameters) may not be as efficient for estimating the strength of the relationships in an explanatory model (Kish 1987 p. 46).

Reasons for undertaking surveys vary. Some are undertaken by researchers to investigate a scientific hypothesis, perhaps with funding from individual universities or national research funding agencies. Some are carried out under the auspices of government agencies to evaluate educational and social policy programs. Some, such as the studies carried out by the IEA or the United States National Assessment of Educational Progress (NAEP), aim to monitor levels of achievement, making comparisons across countries or national regions and across time.

The purposes of a survey influence the formulation of the research questions to be examined, the way it is conducted, and the presentation and dissemination of the findings. Many surveys are proposed or sponsored by those responsible for the administration of educational systems. In this case the aims of the study are largely determined by the sponsoring agency, often for the purpose of evaluating some aspect of educational policy. The researchers and the administrators may need to negotiate in order to reach agreement about the aims of the survey so that the intentions of the administrators may be met by the survey.

Most surveys are "cross-sectional," measuring the population at one point in time. However, the major weakness of a cross-sectional survey is that it is not possible with data from such a survey to establish causal relationships. To examine such relationships with data from a cross-sectional survey requires the assumption that variables measured at one point in time may be ordered in a causal sequence. An untestable assumption that a spurious correlation is not present must be made.

This problem of making causal statements from cross-sectional studies may be remedied by taking repeated measures from the same respondents in a "longitudinal" study (Menard 1991). For example, a longitudinal study is required to measure the effectiveness of individual teachers in enhancing the achievement of their students. The students' achievement is measured at several points in a period of time (such as several weeks or months). Any changes in achievement may then be linked directly to the contribution of their teacher over that time period.

A key task of analytic studies is to examine causal paths, where the explanatory factors that influence outcomes are identified. A significant path can provide an empirical justification for interventions to change behavior associated with that variable. For example, if it can be shown that a more structured curriculum leads to higher achievement in elementary school science classrooms, this can provide the basis for policy decisions about the development of science curricula.

A variation on the simple cross-sectional survey involves "replication," where the same basic survey is carried out in several regions or countries, as in the IEA studies. This permits stronger generalizations of relationships to be made across the range of different educational environments represented by the regions or countries. As another form of replication, the study may be repeated at a later stage, to strengthen the generalizability of the results across time. This also enables trends to be monitored.

2. Survey Research Cycle

One helpful way to understand the range of components of a typical survey is in terms of a "survey research cycle." A detailed description of the series of steps involved in surveys is given in Runkel and McGrath (1972). Thinking about survey research in terms of a cycle highlights the need to consider a survey project as an entity which is repeated after an interval of time. Each stage has implications for later stages, and in practice there is feedback from the later stages to modify earlier stages. Both in its planning and execution a survey may be conducted more effectively by reference to the logical demands of the cycle, as is summarized in Fig. 1.

3. Research Questions

The starting point for a survey is a clear statement of the research questions it is designed to answer. The finishing point is a set of results which addresses these research questions. In defining the questions it is customary to identify the relevant demographic, social, and administrative contents. The questions should preferably be stated in "normal" language rather than in "statistical" language. As the study proceeds through its cycle it becomes necessary to adopt the procedures and terminology of statistics, but ultimately the survey

should provide responses to the original research questions in normal language. Especially for sponsored surveys, it is often necessary to convert the general aims of the survey into specific research questions that are amenable to investigation by survey research methods.

4. Conceptual Framework

At the second stage of the cycle, the ideas or components included in the research questions should be specified more precisely in conceptual terms. Where an explanatory survey is being undertaken, the hypothesized relationships between concepts should be expressed in terms of a "conceptual framework," from which models to be examined can be derived. The conceptual framework should be based on a review of previous research studies.

Educational researchers operate in an incremental way in which each survey adds its contribution to what was previously known. Where the basic conceptual framework is complex it may be desirable to proceed by forming a series of reduced frameworks. The incremental approach could operate here as well, by enabling a complex model to be examined in stages corresponding to the simpler frameworks or models.

5. Survey Instruments

The term "instruments" refers to the range of questionnaires, interviews, tests, and attitude scales used for the collection of data in a survey. The instruments should be linked to the concepts included in the conceptual framework. They should be designed for the collection of data that are suitable for conversion into variables for subsequent analysis. The numbers associated with a variable represent a quantification of the underlying concept. The subsequent statistical analyses do not involve the concepts themselves, but the quantified abstractions associated with the concepts.

The researcher has the choice of using existing instruments or of developing new instruments to measure and to collect data (De Vellis 1991). The advantage of using existing instruments is that the work of development and validation has generally been undertaken and published. On the other hand, these instruments may not adequately operationalize the concepts needed for the particular study. Although more work is involved in creating new survey instruments than in using existing instruments, the researcher may have greater confidence in the ability of the new instruments to measure the concepts.

5.1 Types of Survey Instruments

Instruments for use in analytic surveys may be classified into four broad categories, dealing with the meas-

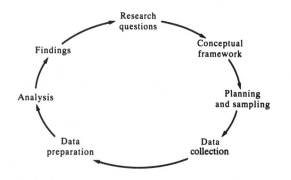

Figure 1
Survey research cycle

urement of (a) background characteristics, (b) subject matter achievement, (c) attitudes, and (d) behavior. The term "background characteristics" refers to the range of personal, social, economic, and demographic measures that are typically used as explanatory variables in research on educational outcomes; for example, the sex of a student, the educational level of a parent, the age of a teacher, the enrollment of a school, or the population of a town.

In educational settings, subject matter achievement is typically measured by tests requiring written answers, although other measures of performance are possible; for example, inquiry skills in science may be measured by means of practical laboratory exercises requiring manipulation of equipment. Attitudes and opinions are often measured by setting out a range of statements on a topic, and asking the respondents to indicate the extent to which they agree or disagree with the statements. Attitudes and knowledge may both manifest themselves in behavior. The measurement of behavior usually requires direct observation, with the respondent's acts being rated according to a defined protocol. In this area, for example, instruments have been developed for measuring the behavior of teachers and students during their lessons as in the IEA Classroom Environment Study (Anderson et al. 1989).

5.2 Development of Survey Instruments

The development of a new survey instrument starts with a statement about the scope and purpose of the instrument in terms of its operationalization of a key concept, such as science achievement or attitude to science. After the initial trial version has been prepared, there will be a cycle of pretesting using respondents similar to those who will be included in the final survey, revising the structure or wording of the instrument, and repeating the pretesting and revision until the instrument is appropriate for its designed purpose, with satisfactory levels of reliability and validity.

Pretesting also provides the opportunity to check that the respondents understand the meaning of the questions or statements (Converse and Presser 1986), to gauge whether test items are at an appropriate level of difficulty, to develop suitable code values for responses, and, generally, to ensure adequate reliability and validity of the instruments. Even where existing instruments are to be used in a survey they should be pretested to ensure that they are suitable. Where possible, the pretesting should be extended as a pilot study to follow the complete cycle, so that procedures for data collection, data preparation, and analysis can be refined prior to the commitment of resources to the main data collection program.

6. Data Collection

The data collection stage of the survey research cycle involves identifying the survey respondents and collecting the desired information from them.

Survey information is collected from people in their natural surroundings; for example, from students in their normal classes. In this way surveys differ from experiments in which the participants are assigned to specified treatment and control groups for the purposes of the research. It is possible to link studies involving other research methods to a survey. For example, information from a survey may be used to identify members of the survey sample for use in a case study requiring detailed qualitative observation.

The data collection stage of a survey is usually the most time-consuming and expensive. If it is not done well the time and resources expended on the survey research study have been largely wasted.

6.1 Populations under Survey

Kish (1987) identified four populations involved in a survey: (a) survey population, (b) frame population, (c) target population, and (d) inferential population. The "inferential population" is that population about which inferences are drawn from the data collected and to which generalizations that are made will apply; for example, all 14-year old students in a country or school system. There may, however, be some students in the inferential population who are inaccessible in a survey, because they are unable to read and write, being in certain special schools, and are unable to respond to an achievement test or questionnaire. Such students must be deliberately excluded from a survey, and the "target population" is formed after their exclusion. The target population may, however, not be fully accessible, because of errors in listings of schools and students. The population which in practice can be investigated, because of being in an incomplete frame and missing units is called the "frame population."

Finally there is the "survey population," which is less than the frame population because of lack of responses and incomplete or missing data. It is the relationship between the survey population and the inferential population and the extent of the discrepancies between them that determines the strength of the inferences that may be drawn from the survey data. The specification of these four distinct populations serves to clarify the sources of error in the drawing of inferences and the steps that must be taken in order to collect sound data.

In the specification of the population to be surveyed, Kish (1987) identified four different characteristics that must be considered. These are: (a) content, for example, student achievement in science; (b) units of investigation, for example, students, teachers, schools; (c) extent of domains in subclasses that are compared, for example, schools, school districts, boys and girls; and (d) period, for example, 10-year old students and 14-year old students, or 1970–71 compared with 1983–84, as in the Second IEA Science Study (Keeves 1992). Only after these characteristics of the populations have been specified is it possible to proceed with the design of a study.

6.2 Sample Surveys

Irrespective of whether a census or a sample survey is carried out, the four populations need to be considered and the four characteristics of the populations to be surveyed need to be specified. The costs, in terms of money, and the labor, in terms of human resources, are typically so high for a census that a sample survey must of necessity be conducted. Sample surveys differ from investigations in so far as probability samples are drawn with a known probability of selection of the units into the sample. Investigations on the other hand are carried out—possibly with care and often with considerable control—so that groups can be meaningfully compared, but without the random allocation that is required by experiments or the random selection with a known probability as required by sample surveys.

The advantages of undertaking a sample survey over an investigation are that the population parameters that are estimated have a known error of sampling and as a consequence inferences can be drawn as to the probability that a parameter is significantly greater than zero, or that the estimates of the parameter for two subgroups are different from each other. It is the known probability of selection of the elements in the sample from the populations under survey, together with the lack of bias, that is the result of discrepancies between the populations, that permits inferences to be made from the sample data to the inferential population. In statistical writing the term "probability sampling" is generally considered to be synonymous with the term "random sampling," although in common usage random sampling tends to be used loosely to imply the taking of *any* part (Kish 1965).

Since the drawing of samples is so widely employed in educational research there are special entries in this *Handbook* that consider both survey sampling and sampling errors (see *Sampling in Survey Research*). As a consequence the material contained in these entries is not replicated here, and the reader is referred to these entries. There are, however, several general principles of importance that need to be emphasized (Skinner et al. 1989).

(a) In educational research it is rarely possible to draw a simple random sample of students, and a two-stage sample (of schools at the first stage of sampling and students within schools at the second stage) is commonly drawn. This cluster design of schools and students within schools must be taken into consideration in the estimation of sampling errors.

(b) In any analysis of data the cluster design of sample data and indeed of census data, which the sample data seek to mirror, must be modeled in the data analysis. Thus multilevel strategies of analyses must be employed (see *Multilevel Analysis; Hierarchical Linear Modeling; *).

(c) More efficient estimates of parameters, such as population mean values, can be achieved by stratification of the sample design, if the stratifying variables are strongly related to the parameter being estimated. However, only a limited number (<10) of stratification categories is effective for each stratifying variable employed in sample surveys.

(d) Where sample survey data are subjected to multivariate analysis, it is necessary to control for the effects of stratification by the inclusion of the stratifying variable in the analysis.

(e) Since there are always administrative and cost constraints on the size of a sample to be drawn in a sample survey study, the design of the sample is necessarily influenced by the need to minimize the errors of sampling within the constraints of cost and sample size on which costs depend. Sample design takes into consideration both the use of cluster sampling and stratification.

(f) Since some losses commonly occur in sample surveys there is a need to compensate for such losses, by either the weighting of data or by replacement of missing data by inferred values (see *Missing Data and Nonresponse*).

6.3 Conduct and Cooperation in a Survey

In addition to the development of the sample design, there are many practical aspects involved in the conduct of the data collection stage of a survey. At an early stage, the appropriate administrative authorities should be approached for their support for the survey, which may also require their permission to collect data. It may also be necessary to approach regional or local administrative units for their support. The authorities should also be asked for relevant census data, since these data are generally necessary for the preparation of the sampling frame, for the choice of a sample design, and for subsequent testing of the adequacy of the achieved sample.

The funding for the study should entail adequate resources for obtaining the cooperation of the authorities who provide the support and of the respondents who provide the data. Both the authorities and the respondents should be persuaded that the survey is relevant and important. Their cooperation is crucial since the value and credibility of surveys depend on high response rates: that is, the percentage of units from whom data are actually obtained. Surveys also depend on the quality of the data, in the sense that the respondents must cooperate in responding to the instruments.

One of the problems with longitudinal survey studies is the need to maintain contact with the members of the original group over the duration of the study. This problem increases as the time gap between data collection stages increases. It is necessary to check that the characteristics of the reduced groups at the later stages are similar to the characteristics of the original group. In planning longitudinal survey studies, it is advisable to collect a variety of contact information from the members of the original group surveyed. For example, it is desirable to collect the names and addresses of the members of the original group to assist in locating them at a later stage.

For surveys where data are collected from students in schools, the data collection procedures should be designed to be interesting for the students and to minimize disruption to the normal school program. Considerable effort and resources should be expended to provide useful feedback to the students and schools about the results of the survey; for example, details about the performance of the students on achievement tests included in the survey.

6.4 Ethical Considerations

An important aspect of the contact with respondents is the assurance that the information provided would be used only for the stated purposes of the survey, with any published reports presenting findings in a manner that would prevent the identification of individual respondents. This is not the same as advocating that all information should be collected anonymously. Where the names of respondents are known, it is much easier to apply follow-up procedures to urge nonrespondents to reply.

Increasingly, countries and institutions are controlling the kinds of research data that may be collected, and the procedures to be followed for maintaining the privacy of the records and for enabling research workers to receive access to the data. In addition, many institutions and funding agencies require that the proposal for a study should be reviewed by an "Ethics Committee" or similar body to ensure that the confidentiality and privacy provisions are adequate. In any case, it is advisable to keep all identifying data, such as the names and addresses of respondents, separate from files containing the other data collected from the respondents.

The students included in a survey, and their parents, should be fully informed about the nature of the study. They should be told who is sponsoring the study, who is conducting it, the amount of time to be taken in participating, and the likely benefits arising from the study. This is often achieved by means of a letter sent to the parents of the students. Many educational systems require that the parents should have the option of withholding permission for the participation of their children. Indeed, especially for studies seeking information of a more sensitive nature, the active written consent of the students and their parents may be required.

6.5 Quality of Data Collection

The final task in the process of collecting data is to assess the adequacy of the procedures employed. In practice there are usually differences between the plans for the survey as originally developed and the actual administration. Reports of a survey should contain a comparison of the designed and achieved numbers of respondents, from which response rates can be calculated. If the response rates differ across strata, the balance may be restored by weighting procedures, although weighting procedures cannot fully compensate for data lost due to different and reduced response rate. Reports of the study should always include details of the different populations, the designed sample, the achieved sample, the response rates, and the weights employed in the analysis of the data.

The adequacy of an achieved sample may also be examined by comparing known characteristics of the population with corresponding characteristics of the sample. Such marker variables may include the percentage of male students, the mean enrollment of schools, or the level of teacher qualifications.

No item of information should be collected in a survey without a clear idea of where it fits into the logic of the research questions or conceptual framework guiding the study. Each item of information collected should have a specified place in the analyses that are linked to the original research questions posed by the survey. It is easy to distort a survey by attempting to collect too much information, which may alienate the respondents and hence reduce the validity and reliability of their responses.

7. Data Preparation and Management

The data preparation stage of the cycle starts with the raw information as collected from the respondents, and concludes with the data carefully organized as computer files ready for analysis. This stage is concerned with checking and coding data, and building the data files. The intended answers of the respondents must be transferred as accurately as possible into a form in which they may be analyzed.

7.1 Coding

Most of the data collected in educational survey research are derived from the respondent's written responses to the survey instruments. Often the items in the questionnaires are precoded, so that the respondent selects one of the options presented, as in multiple-choice items for achievement tests. Otherwise, respondents may write their own responses which are subsequently coded by the researchers. For most survey studies, numerical code values are used so that quantitative analyses can be conducted. A codebook is prepared which specifies the location of each item of the data on the computer file, together with a description of characteristics of each variable: the name of the variable, the valid code values, and the code values for missing data.

In association with the coding of responses, it is necessary to include an editing stage, when anomalies and omissions may be detected. It may be possible to return to the respondents for the resolution of anomalies, or for the completion of omitted items. More commonly, the researcher develops a set of rules to resolve these problems at the coding stage.

7.2 Data Entry

After coding, the responses are normally transferred to a computer file. This is commonly accomplished by typing the coded responses from the survey instrument into a computer file using a program designed for data entry.

Procedures are available to circumvent this labor intensive data entry. For example, the respondent may mark sheets or cards that can be read by optical scanning methods with the coded values being transferred directly to the computer files, although this method will involve some additional human editing where the equipment has not been able to read the marks properly. Alternatively, the respondent's answers may be entered directly into the computer, as in computer-aided telephone interviews.

7.3 Checking and Verification

Once the initial data file has been established, further checking and verification procedures should always be carried out. At one extreme this may involve an independent punching of all responses with a comparison of the two versions in order to resolve any discrepancies. More commonly, a sample of the completed instruments is selected for independent verification. An important check is to ensure that all data have been entered into the correct column locations on the computer file. The actual responses from some of the questionnaires should be compared to the data in the variables on the computer file.

For each variable there will be a range of valid values. An initial stage of checking involves detecting and correcting any values outside the valid range. It is then necessary to return to the original questionnaire completed by the respondent to find the valid value. It is also desirable to include checks of logical consistency; for example, to ensure that educational qualifications are consistent with stated occupations.

Further consideration, in terms of the technology now available, of the tasks of code book preparation, data entry, data clearing, and database design and management are considered in the entry on data management in educational survey research (see *Data Management in Survey Rersearch*). There are relatively few published accounts of the practical aspects of data preparation and management, and notable treatments of this field are provided in Rossi et al. (1983) and Sonquist and Dunkelberg (1977).

8. Analysis

Analysis can commence once the data file has been adequately prepared. In terms of the logic of the survey research cycle, the earlier stages of the cycle should anticipate the analysis stage. The construction of instruments and the coding of responses should anticipate the manipulation of numerical data. The sample design should also ensure that there are sufficient cases or respondents for the planned analyses.

8.1 Variable Construction

An initial stage in analysis is to construct new variables from the basic data. For achievement test data this may involve the development of test scores according to defined rules. For attitude scales this may result in scale scores, often based on factor analysis. For questionnaires, a typical constructed variable would be an index of socioeconomic status of the student's home.

8.2 Univariate Analysis

The plans for a survey will include a description of the analyses to be undertaken. The analyses may be classified in terms of the number of variables involved. "Univariate" analysis deals with the variables individually. "Bivariate" analysis involves pairs of variables. "Multivariate" analysis is concerned with the simultaneous effects of more than two variables.

For all surveys, the initial analyses involve examining the basic univariates for all variables. For data recorded at the categorical level, the univariates would display the frequency of the number of cases for each code value for each variable. For continuous data, such as test scores, the corresponding basic univariates would be the mean, number of cases, standard deviation, skewness, and kurtosis for each variable. The univariates enable the researcher to gain an initial view of the data for each variable. This should be done before submitting data to further analysis. Weaknesses such as highly skewed variables, and variables with large amounts of missing data, may distort the results of more complex analyses.

Where univariates derived from a sample are published, they should incorporate estimates of the sampling errors (standard errors of sampling). Where the data from a sample are used to estimate parameters in a population, the sampling errors indicate the degree of uncertainty associated with the estimates of the corresponding parameters in the population. Data derived from complex samples or stratified sample designs that depart from simple random sampling procedures should be adjusted to compensate for the "design effect" which measures the extent to which the complex sample is less efficient than a simple random sample, with the same number of cases (see *Sampling Errors in Survey Research*).

8.3 Bivariate Analysis

The main bivariate statistics are "cross-tabulations" and "correlation coefficients." With modern computers it is tempting to generate large numbers of cross-tabulations, often involving several nested levels. Classification of data by using cross-tabulations may assist the researcher to gain a good overview of the data, but the method is very inefficient for examining relationships. Most situations in education are complex, involving many interrelated variables.

Matrices of correlation coefficients are useful for summarizing bivariate relationships. In particular they provide an initial opportunity to assess which explanatory variables are strongly associated with each other and with dependent variables. From the correlation matrix it is easy to identify variables that are only weakly linked to a criterion. There is little value in including these variables in explanatory analyses. The correlation matrices may also provide the starting point for multivariate analyses.

8.4 Multivariate Analysis

The multivariate stage of the analysis is designed to unravel the complex interrelationships between the variables. The analysis is guided by the conceptual framework which has identified the likely patterns of relationship.

Many multivariate analysis techniques are available, of which Stevens (1986) provides an overview. One of the most common techniques used in the analysis of survey data is multiple regression analysis, which is used to estimate the relative strengths of several explanatory variables acting simultaneously on a criterion. Underlying the regression analysis should be a statistical model of the relationships between the explanatory variables and the criterion, derived from the conceptual framework on which the study is based.

An extension of multiple regression is the development and estimation of structural equation models (Bollen 1989) in which the explanatory variables may be arranged in a causal sequence. For example, the significant paths associated with achievement indicate where policy changes may most fruitfully be introduced to enhance the levels of achievement.

The use of multistage sampling reflects the hierarchical nature of most educational settings, with students in classes in schools in school districts, and so on. Multilevel analysis is a form of multivariate analysis that takes account of the differences between students within classes and between classes (Raudenbush and Willms 1991). For example, it shows the extent to which differences in achievement depend on the students' membership of a given class or school, and isolates the relative contribution of the individual and the group to the criterion under consideration. This procedure may also be used to estimate the sampling errors and design effects associated with multistage sampling (see *Multilevel Analysis; Hierarchical Linear Modeling*).

In some larger surveys, the researcher may carry out analyses separately for each strata or group of strata, particularly where these strata or groups represent independent administrative units. In effect, each separate analysis is itself a replication. Stronger gener-

alizations may be made where patterns of relationships occur across the replicated analyses.

The ultimate purpose of the analysis stage is to produce sets of statistics that summarize the data: frequencies, proportions, percentages, means, standard deviations, correlation coefficients, regression coefficients, and so on. These should relate to the original conceptual framework or models. The statistics serve to confirm or negate the models and the associated propositions that were to be examined. Reports of the survey should contain sufficient information to enable interested readers to make their independent judgments about the reliability of the data that were collected, the appropriateness of the analysis that was undertaken, and the statistical conclusions that were drawn.

9. Findings

The last stage of the survey research cycle involves the presentation of the findings, which should link to the original questions. This final stage should also include a discussion of the strength of the findings, and of the extent to which they may be generalized. Distinctions should be made between findings that are strong and those that are tentative, and between findings of high generalizability and those that are limited in scope.

The ways in which the findings are disseminated may depend on the sponsorship of the study. Findings couched in statistical language may be appropriate for a scientific audience. For surveys dealing with public policy, every effort should be made to present the findings in language suitable for policymakers who may not have a strong statistical background. It is difficult to present complex findings in a form that can be reported in the print and electronic media without being distorted, but strenuous efforts should be made to do so.

10. Documentation and Secondary Analysis

There is increasing recognition that carefully documented data files, especially from larger surveys, should be lodged in data archive systems. Some funding agencies require the archiving of data as a condition of the grant. National centers for data archives exist in most countries, and there are also international networks for social science data, such as the Inter-University Consortium for Political and Social Research based at the University of Michigan. The lodging of data files with a data archives system facilitates the use of the data by other researchers for secondary analysis. The usefulness of the data for any particular secondary analysis depends on the quality of the associated documentation, so that the secondary analyst can gain a full understanding of the original data collection process, and the relevance of the variables in the survey to the aims of the secondary analysis.

11. Conclusion

The underlying theme of this entry is that the conduct of survey research should follow a logical process, interpreted here as a cycle. The success of a study is not guaranteed by following the cycle, but it may enhance confidence in the management of the survey. No single study can ever identify all the important research questions or find all the answers, so that one cycle may lead to another as findings from one survey lead to new questions for future surveys.

See also: Cross-sectional Research Methods; Data Banks and Data Archives; Longitudinal Research Methods; Secondary Data Analysis; Sampling in Survey Research

References

Anderson L W, Ryan D W, Shapiro B J (eds.) 1989 *The IEA Classroom Environment Study.* Pergamon Press, Oxford
Bollen K A 1989 *Structural Equations with Latent Variables.* Wiley, New York
Converse J M, Presser S 1986 *Survey Questions: Handcrafting the Standardized Questionnaire.* Sage, Beverly Hills, California
De Vellis R F 1991 *Scale Development: Theories and Applications.* Sage, Beverly Hills, California
Fowler F J Jr 1988 *Survey Research Methods*, 2nd edn. Sage, Beverly Hills, California
Groves R M 1989 *Survey Errors and Survey Costs.* Wiley, New York
Karweit N L 1982 Survey research methods. In: Mitzel H E 1982 *Encyclopedia of Educational Research*, 5th edn. Free Press, New York
Keeves J P (ed.) 1992 *The IEA Study of Science III: Changes in Science Education and Achievement: 1970 to 1984.* Pergamon Press, Oxford
Kish L 1965 *Survey Sampling.* Wiley, New York
Kish L 1987 *Statistical Design for Research.* Wiley, New York
Menard 1991 *Longitudinal Research.* Sage, Newbury Park, California
Miller D C 1991 *Handbook of Research Design and Social Measurement.* Sage, Beverly Hills, California
Postlethwaite T N, Wiley D E (eds.) 1992 *The IEA Study of Science II: Science Achievement in Twenty-three Countries.* Pergamon Press, Oxford
Raudenbush S W, Willms J D (eds.) 1991 *Schools, Classrooms, and Pupils: International Studies of Schooling from a Multilevel Perspective.* Academic Press, San Diego, California
Rosier M J, Banks D K 1990 *The Scientific Literacy of Australian Students.* Australian Council for Educational Research, Hawthorn
Rossi P H, Wright J D, Anderson A B 1983 *Handbook of Survey Research.* Academic Press, New York
Runkel P J, McGrath J E 1972 *Research on Human Behavior: A Systematic Guide to Method.* Holt, Rinehart and Winston, New York
Skinner C J, Holt D, Smith T M F (eds.) 1989 *Analysis of Complex Surveys.* Wiley, New York
Sonquist J A, Dunkelberg W C 1977 *Survey and Opinion Research: Procedures for Processing and Analysis.* Prentice Hall, Englewood Cliffs, New Jersey
Stevens J 1986 *Applied Multivariate Statistics for the Social Sciences.* Erlbaum, Hillsdale, New Jersey

Twin Studies

S. Fischbein

It is necessary to differentiate between the study of twins as a subject of interest in itself, and as a research method for investigating heredity and environment interaction and its implications for education. The former type of study is concerned not only with comparisons of twins and singletons in different respects, but also with the specific relationship that a twin pair possesses both before and after birth (Bryan 1983, 1992a, 1992b).

In the second type of study, which will be the main topic of this entry, within-pair differences of monozygotic (MZ) and dizygotic (DZ) pairs are compared for different variables and ages. Reduced to its simplest form, the twin method thereby assumes that any difference within MZ pairs must be due to environmental or at least nongenetic causes, whereas differences within DZ pairs are due to both environmental and genetic factors.

Twin studies are of course not the only method used to investigate genetic and environmental influences on behavior and development. Animal studies as well as the study of human individuals with more or less genetic material in common, for instance, parents and children or nontwin siblings, have been the object of study (Plomin et al. 1990). Of special interest has also been the study of twins reared apart (Bouchard et al. 1990, Pedersen et al. 1991). Biological and adoptive family members have also been compared in different respects (Corley and Fulker 1990, Scarr and Wrinberg 1983, 1994, Weinberg et al. 1992).

1. Fields of Research

Twin studies have been of major interest in different research fields, such as medical science, epidemiological studies, and behavioral sciences, as well as the collaborative field for behavioral scientists and geneticists in behavioral genetics.

1.1 Twin Biology and Multiple Pregnancy

This field of study examines the incidence and factors of twinning, embryology of twinning, and multiple pregnancy. In recent years a general increase in multiple births has been found due to artificial ovulation–induction as well as better life-saving techniques of prematurely born infants (Webster and Elwood 1985, Levene and Wild 1992).

Many studies in this field have also examined the effects of multiple pregnancy on the mother and her offspring. Bryan (1983 p. 32) concludes that "the high prenatal mortality associated with twinning is largely due to complications of pregnancy, such as premature onset of labor, fetal intra-uterine growth retardation and difficulties of delivery." Low birth weight and prematurely born twins have also been shown to be at a disadvantage concerning both physical and mental growth during childhood and adolescence (Alin Åkerman and Fischbein 1991, Alin Åkerman and Thomassen 1992). This type of research might have methodological as well as educational implications when the twins are beginning school(Alin Åkerman 1996).

1.2 Epidemiological and Clinical Studies

In previous studies in this field the twins have often been used as matched pairs. This implies selecting pairs where the twins differ on a recognized experience, exposure or trait.

Epidemiological and clinical studies have been particularly concerned with health risk factors such as smoking, drinking, or substance exposure. Twin studies thereby help clarify the different roles played by genes and the environment in the variation of these habits and the contribution they make to different types of diseases, for instance cancer, coronary heart disease or dementia (Gatz et al. 1992, Lichtenstein et al. in press, Pederson et al. 1995).

1.3 Behavioral Sciences

The study of twins in the behavioral sciences has been specifically used as a method to estimate heritability, "the proportion of phenotypic variance attributable to genotypic variance" (Plomin et al. 1990 p. 252). These studies have encompassed different areas, such as personality, school achievement, and studies of intelligence. The results have mostly shown a higher within-pair similarity for MZ in comparison to DZ twins, suggesting the importance of genetic factors.

The use of heritability estimates as a measure of genetic influences is controversial. Among other things this has to do with the difficulty of generalizing results from one twin population to another, the necessity of taking interactional and correlational as well as additive effects into account and the definition and measurement of environmental concepts in estimating heritability. In the following section, some of these questions will be further elaborated and attempts to tackle these problems will be presented.

2. Methodological Problems

The additive model for interpreting twin data implies that an environmental change will contribute to a comparable change in all genotypes. Interactional effects, on the other hand, will lead to different reactions in genotypes exposed to the same environmental impact. Heredity–environmental correlation "describes the extent to which individuals are exposed to environments as a function of their genetic propensities." In recent years, advances in quantitative genetic analyses have increased possibilities for delineating the importance of such effects (Plomin et al. 1990 p. 251).

Of particular interest to education is the recent debate on the definition and measurement of environmental influences in twin research (Plomin and Daniels 1987, Plomin 1994, Lichtenstein 1994).

2.1 Genotype–Environment Interaction

Genotype–environment interaction can be estimated within quantitative genetic designs, preferably employing adoption data (Plomin et al. 1990). This type of interaction implies, for instance, that individuals high in a trait will react differently from individuals low in a trait. It is thus connected to genotypic level, which presupposes a quantification of genetic contribution. It is interesting to notice that quantitative genetic studies incorporating environmental measures very seldom have found significant genotype–environment interaction effects (Bergeman et al. 1988, Plomin and Hershberger 1991). These results could perhaps be compared to educational research on ability–treatment interactions, which has also found disappointingly few significant interactions (Fischbein and Gustafsson 1979).

There is an obvious difference between the above-mentioned population concept and the organismic type of interaction, which presupposes a reciprocal relationship and focuses upon the psychological environment and the individual as these affect and are affected by each other. Results from adoption/twin studies concerning genetic influences on environmental measures provide evidence for such interactions (Plomin et al. 1990).

2.2 Genotype–Environment Correlation

Genotype–environment correlations, like genotype–environment interactions, can be of different kinds.

Plomin et al. (1990) have defined the following types.

(a) *Passive G × E correlation*. This is present when endowment and environment covary in such a way that, for instance, bright children tend to live in a home conducive to their intellectual development. This type of correlation is called "passive" because it occurs independently of the activities of the individual in question. Analyses of genotype–environment correlation suggest that this type of correlation may be important for intellectual development (Plomin et al. 1988).

(b) *Reactive G × E correlation*. This signifies that people can react differently to persons of different genotypes, thus creating conspicuously dissimilar environmental circumstances. An example of this type of correlation is when certain personality traits are reinforced by particular persons in the environment (Plomin and Daniels 1987).

(c) *Active G × E correlation*. This occurs as a result of the individual's own action. People tend to create for themselves different environments related to their genetic potentials. For instance, in the same home a brighter child may choose to read more books than a less bright child, thereby creating for himself or herself a more stimulating environment (Scarr and McCartney 1983).

There are obvious difficulties in distinguishing between the active type of *G × E* correlation and dynamic *G × E* interaction. This is a matter of definition, and it is probably impossible to maintain a clear-cut distinction between these two concepts. A definition of interaction in the dynamical sense, would be as follows: "Genotypes can be shown to interpret the same environmental treatment in different ways." A definition of the active type of correlation, on the other hand, would be: "Genotypes can be shown to react to the same environmental impact in different ways thereby creating different environments for themselves."

2.3 Shared and Nonshared Environmental Variation

Traditionally, environmental influences studied in twin research have been defined as the portion of variance that cannot be accounted for by heredity. Recently, however, a distinction has been made between shared and nonshared environmental influences (Plomin et al. 1990). The former are those that make members of a family similar to each other. The remainder of the environmental variance, the portion not shared by family members, is called nonshared. Plomin and Daniels (1987) have shown that this type of environmental influences is probably of considerable importance for individual development. Thus,

environmental factors relevant to differences in behavioral development lie, not between but *within* families. If children with different genotypes, such as siblings or DZ twins, create different individual environments for themselves within the same family environment, this could be classified as nonshared environmental variance.

2.4 Genetic Influence on Environmental Measures

Genetic influence can affect measures of environment in two ways. First, genetically influenced characteristics can affect ratings on environmental measures (Plomin 1994, Saudino et al. in press.) Second, individual endowment can affect environmental treatment (Plomin and Bergeman 1991).

Results from twin studies indicate substantial genetic influence on some environmental measures but not on others (Plomin et al. 1988). The most general implication of these results is that labeling a measure environmental does not necessarily make it an environmental measure in origin.

3. Model-fitting Approaches

One of the most recent developments in behavioral genetics has been the application of model-fitting approaches, especially as applied to longitudinal data. This expansion has a promising future due to advances in structural modeling (Jöreskog 1978). With the application of model-fitting procedures to longitudinal twin data it has been possible to test different hypotheses concerning the influence of genetic and environmental covariance components on multiple behavioral measures (Neale and Cardon 1992).

Model fitting basically involves solving a series of simultaneous equations in order to estimate genetic and environmental parameters that best fit observed familial correlations. The main analytic procedure most often used to solve a complex series of equations is called "maximum-likelihood model fitting," which employs computer programs that maximize the fit between the model and the data by finding the set of parameter estimates that yield the smallest possible discrepancies with the data (Plomin et al. 1990). One of the most widely used programs is LISREL, which stands for LInear Structural RELations. Several articles on the application of LISREL to twin analyses have been published (Boomsma et al. 1989).

A rapidly expanding field in twin research is the application of behavioral genetic methods to longitudinal data (Pedersen 1991, Boomsma et al. 1991, Pederson 1993). At each time of measurement the importance of genetic and environmental influences (both shared and nonshared) for interindividual variation in a behavioral measure may be estimated. A number of models are available today which describe the relationship of the parameters at time 1 to those at subsequent time points. It is, however, not within the limits of this short overview to describe them in detail (see *Path Analysis and Linear Structural Relations Analysis*).

4. Lifespan Development in Twins

In recent years there has been an increased interest in twin studies covering not only the childhood and adolescence periods but the whole lifespan development from infancy to aging.

There is one major longitudinal twin study covering the *childhood* period, the Louisville Twin Study (Wilson 1983) in which physical and mental development as well as interindividual temperamental variations have been studied (Wilson and Matheny 1986). The results suggest the presence of synchronized physical and mental growth for MZ twins but not for DZ.

Physical and mental growth in *adolescent* twins has been studied both in the above-mentioned project and in a Swedish longitudinal twin study, the SLU-project. Height and weight measurements as well as intelligence and school achievement test scores were collected at regular time intervals. A more detailed description of this project has been given by Ljung et al. (1977). The intrapair correlations for height growth in MZ and DZ twins show a parallel trend, so that MZ correlations are very high and DZ correlations considerably lower during puberty. For weight, the correlations for MZ tend to be as high as for height. For the DZ pairs, however, there seem to be a divergent trend so that DZ pairs become less similar during this period. This is especially evident for girls (Fischbein 1977). This trend has also been found in a Polish study of physical growth in twins during puberty (Bergman 1988). Sharma (1983) has presented similar data from India, where neither height nor weight correlations show a divergent trend (Fischbein 1991).

In the SLU-project, verbal and inductive reasoning ability was measured at ages 12 and 18 for the boys. For verbal ability there is a divergent trend so that MZ twins become more similar and DZ twins less similar during this period. Possibly, the increasing MZ and decreasing DZ correlations often found for physical and mental growth in twins are due to the interaction and correlation of hereditary and environmental influences.

The examples selected so far have illustrated heredity–environment influences for *different* characteristics. It is also of interest, to study the *same* characteristic in different types of environments. In the SLU-project a standardized achievement test in mathematics has been given to the twins in Grades 3 and 6. The correlations for the total group show a divergent trend, so that the correlation increases for MZ twins and decreases for DZ twins. When socioeconomic background is taken into consideration, however, the divergent trend is much more conspicuous for working-class children than for the other group. This indicates a more "restrictive" environment as regards school achievement for the children coming from higher socioeconomic strata (Fischbein 1979).

Another interesting field in twin research pursued in the SLU-project has been to explore the origin of gender differences. This was done by the inclusion of a substantial sample of opposite-sex twin pairs. An analysis of ability and achievement test results for this group indicates interaction effects for sex and social background so that boys and girls in the same family tend to be more similar, particularly for verbal ability, in higher compared to lower socioeconomic stratas (Fischbein 1990).

A follow-up has been made of the SLU-sample. They are now in their mid-thirties (Lange and Fischbein 1992). Life-situation, health and coping ability have been investigated and related to data collected during adolescence. The results indicate that the disadvantage found for MZ female twins at school age is still present at mid-life. Also, teacher ratings of school behavior are related to coping ability later on in life, particularly for the male twins (Lange and Fischbein in press).

In the middle of the 1980s, a longitudinal study of "aging" Swedish twins (SATSA) was initiated. This project has a very powerful design for separating hereditary and environmental influences since it includes not only MZ and DZ twins being raised together but also a large sample of twins being separated at an early age (Pedersen et al. 1991).

The SATSA study has already contributed very valuable information concerning genetic and environmental influences on variation in cognitive abilities and personality measures, physical and self-rated health, as well as environmental circumstances reported by the respondents. An example of the latter are data on occupational status and educational level (Lichtenstein et al. 1992). The results indicate that, for both education and occupation, environmental effects are more important among women and genetic effects more important among men. Also, genetic influences seem to have a greater impact on education for the younger age-group (<60) compared to the older group (≥60). These results have been compared to the SLU-sample and the hypothesis was that sex differences would be less conspicuous at mid-life. This was corroborated, and a reasonable interpretation is that societal conditions tend to be less restrictive for women at mid-life compared to the older cohort (Fischbein et al. in press).

Only a few of the very interesting and valuable results published from the SATSA project can be commented on here. It is, however, worth mentioning a recently published article concerning genetic effects on individual differences in cognitive abilities later in life (Pedersen et al. 1992). Genetic influences seem to be more pronounced for general cognitive ability in these older twins compared to earlier in life. SATSA has also contributed to a more profound understanding of the psychology of aging from a genetic perspective (Pedersen 1996).

In summary, longitudinal twin research throughout the lifespan has increased impressively. The results are also very interesting and have already demonstrated far-reaching implications for a better understanding of the origins of variations in physical and mental growth as well as health and well-being.

5. Conclusion

It is evident from this entry, that there has been a trend toward more developmental twin studies comprising the entire lifespan. These studies have demonstrated the importance of genetic factors on development. It is also evident that longitudinal studies will be necessary to investigate different types of heredity–environment interaction and correlation.

This field of research has been largely dominated by biologists and behavior geneticists, which has resulted in a certain neglect of environmental factors that have been treated as unspecified sources of variation. Environmental distinctions beyond a separation of shared and nonshared environmental influence are rarely observed in twin studies. What seems to be a fruitful approach by natural and behavioral scientists in this field, however, is to incorporate more refined environmental dimensions into the model building and testing of specific hypotheses.

References

Alin Åkerman B 1996 Eight-year follow-up of cognitive development in 33 twin pairs. *Acta Genet. Med. Gemellol.* 44(3–4): 179–88

Alin Åkerman B, Fischbein S 1991 Twins: Are they at risk? A longitudinal study of twins and nontwins from birth to 18 years of age. *Acta Genet. Med. Gemellol.* 40(1): 29–40

Alin Åkerman B, Thomassen P A 1991 Four-year follow-up of locomotor and language development in 34 twin pairs. *Acta Genet. Med. Gemellol.* 40(1): 21–8

Alin Åkerman B, Thomassen P A 1992 The fate of "small twins": A four-year follow-up study of low birth-weight and prematurely born twins. *Acta Genet. Med. Gemellol.* 41(2–3): 97–104

Bergeman C S, Plomin R, McClearn G E, Pedersen N L, Friberg L T 1988 Genotype-environment interaction in personality development: Identical twins reared apart. *Psychology and Aging* 3: 399–406

Bergeman C S, Plomin R, Pedersen N L, McClearn G E, Nesselroade J R 1990 Genetic and environmental influences on social support: The Swedish Adoption/Twin Study of Aging (SATSA). *Journal of Gerontology: Psychological Sciences* 45: 101–06

Bergman P 1988 The problem of genetic determination of growth in adolescence (in Polish). *Materialy i prace antropologiczne* 108: 165–216.

Boomsma D I, Martin N G, Neale M C 1989 Structural modelling in the analysis of twin data. *Behavior Genetics* 19: 5–8

Boomsma D I, Molenaar P C M, Dolan C V 1991 Individual latent growth curves: Estimation of genetic and environmental profiles in longitudinal twin studies. *Behavior Genetics* 21: 241–53

Bouchard T J Jr, Lykken D T, McGue M, Segal N L, Tellegen A 1990 Sources of human psychological differences: The Minnesota Study of Twins Reared Apart. *Science* 250(4978): 223–28

Bryan E M 1983. *The Nature and Nurture of Twins*. Baillère Tindall, London

Bryan E 1992a *Twins and Higher Multiple Births. A Guide to their Nature and Nurture*. Licensing Agency, London

Bryan E, 1992b *Twins, Triplets and More. Their Nature, Development and Care*. Clays Ltd., London

Corley R P, Fulker D W 1990 What can adoption studies tell us about cognitive development? In: Hahn M E, Hewitt J K, Hendersson N D, Benno R H (eds.) 1990 *Developmental Behavior Genetics: Neural, Biometrical and Evolutionary Approaches*. Oxford University Press, New York

Fischbein S 1977 Intra-pair similarity in physical growth of monozygotic and of dizygotic twins during puberty. *Annals of Human Biology.* 4(5): 417–30

Fischbein S 1979 *Heredity–Environment Influences on Growth and Development During Adolescence: A Longitudinal Study of Twins*. Liber Läromedel, Lund

Fischbein S 1990 Biosocial influences on sex differences for ability and achievement test results as well as marks at school. *Intelligence* 14(1): 127–39

Fischbein S 1991 Heredity–environment influences on growth and maturation during puberty: A cross-cultural comparison. *Anthropologiai Közlemények* 33: 273–81

Fischbein S, Gustafsson J-E 1979 Differences in achievement at school. Results from a twin study (in Swedish). Report No. 14 from the Department of Educational Research. Stockholm Institute of Education, Stockholm

Fischbein S, Lange A-L, Lichtenstein P in press Quantitative genetic analyses of gender differences in educational and occupational careers. *Scandinavian Journal of Educational Research*

Gatz M, Pedersen N L, Plomin R, Nesselroade J R, McClearn G E 1992 The importance of shared genes and shared environments for symptoms of depression in older adults. *J. Abnorm. Psychol.* 101(4): 701–08

Jöreskog K G 1978 Structural analysis of covariance and correlation matrices. *Psychometri.* 43(4): 443–77

Lange A-L, Fischbein S 1992 From Puberty to Mid-Life: A Follow-Up Study of Twins and Controls. *Acta Genet. Med. Gemellol.* 41: 105–12

Lange A-L, Fischbein S in press Life situation, self-reported health and coping ability of 35-year old twins and controls. A follow-up of a longitudinal Swedish twin study at adolescence. Acta Genet. Med. Gemellol.

Levene M, Wild J 1992 Higher multiple births and the modern management of infertility in Britain. *American Journal Obstet. Gynecol.* 99: 607–13

Lichtenstein P, Pedersen N L, McClearn G E 1992 The origins of individual differences in occupational status and educational level: A study of twins reared apart and together. *Acta Sociol.* 35: s13–31

Lichtenstein P, Gatz M, Pedersen N L, Berg S, McClearn G E in press A cotwin-control study of response to widowhood. *Journal of Gerontology: Psychological Sciences*

Ljung B-O, Fischbein S, Lindgren G 1977 A comparison of growth in twins and singleton controls of matched age followed longitudinally from 10 to 18 years. *Annals of Human Biology*. 4: 405–15

Neale M C, Cardon L R 1992 *Methodology for Genetic Studies of Twins and Families*. Kluwer, Dordrecht

Pedersen N L 1991 Behavioral genetic concepts in longitudinal analyses. In: Magnusson D, Bergman L R, Rudinger G, Törestad B (eds.): *Problems and Methods in Longitudinal Research: Stability and Change*. Cambridge University Press, New York

Pedersen N L 1993 Genetic and environmental continuity and change in personality. In: Bouchard T J Jr, Propping P (eds.) 1993 Twins as a tool of behavioral genetics. John Wiley, New York

Pedersen N L 1996 Gerontological behavior genetics. In: Birren J E, Schaie K W (eds.) 1996 *Handbook of the Psychology of Aging*, 4th edn. Academic Press, San Diego, California

Pedersen N L, McClearn G E, Plomin R, Nesselroade J R, Berg S, DeFaire U 1991 The Swedish adoption twin study of aging: An update. *Acta Genet. Med. Gemellol.* 40(1): 7–20

Pedersen N L, Plomin R, Nesselroade J R, McClearn G E 1992 A quantitative genetic analysis of cognitive abilities during the second half of the life span. *Psychol. Sci.* 3(6): 346–53

Pedersen N L, Posner S F, Gatz M 1995 Twin Studies as a tool for bridging the gap between genetics and epidemiology of dementia. In: Finkel S I, Bergener M (eds.) 1995 *Treating Alzheimer's and Other Dementias*. Clinical application of recent research advances. Springer, New York

Plomin R 1994 *Genetics and Experience. The Interplay between Nature and Nurture*. Individual Differences and Development Series. 6. Sage, Thousand Oaks, California

Plomin R, DeFries J C, Loehlin J C 1977 Genotype-environment interaction and correlation in the analysis of human behavior. *Psych. Bull.* 84: 309–22

Plomin R, Daniels D 1987 Why are children in the same family so different from one another? *Behavior and Brain Sciences* 10: 1–16

Plomin R, DeFries J C, Fulker D W 1988 *Nature and Nurture in Infancy and Early Childhood*. Cambridge University Press, New York

Plomin R, McClearn G E, Pedersen N L, Nesselroade J R, Bergeman C S 1988 Genetic influence on childhood family environment perceived retrospectively from the last half of the life span. *Dev. Psychol.* 24: 738–45

Plomin R, DeFries J C, McClearn G E 1990. *Behavioral Genetics: A Primer*, 2nd edn. Freeman, New York

Plomin R, Bergeman C S 1991 The nature of nurture: Genetic influence on "environmental" measures. *Behavior and Brain Sciences* 14(3): 373–427

Plomin R, Hershberger S 1991 Genotype–environment interaction. In: Wachs T O, Plomin R (eds.) 1991 *Conceptualization and Measurement of Organism–Environment Interaction*. American Psychological Association, Washington, DC

Saudino K J, Pedersen N L, Lichtenstein P, McClearn G E, Plomin R in press Can personality explain genetic influences on life events? *J. Pers. Soc. Psychol.*

Scarr S, McCartney K 1983 Now people make their own environments: A theory of genotype → environment effects. *Child Dev.* 54: 260–67

Scarr S, Weinbert R 1983 The Minnesota adoption studies: Genetic differences and malleability. *Child Dev.* 54: 260–67

Scarr S, Weinbert R 1994 Educational and occupational achievements of brothers and sisters in adoptive and biologically related families. *Behavior Genetics* 24: 301–25

Sharma J C 1983. *The Genetic Contribution to Pubertal Growth and Development Studied by Longitudinal Growth Data on Twins*. Department of Anthropology, Punjab University, Chandigarh

Webster F, Elwood J M 1985 A Study of the Influence of Ovulation Stimulants and Oral Contraception on Twin Births in England. *Acta Genet. Med. Gemellol.* 34(1–2): 105–08

Weinberg R, Scarr S, Waldman I D 1992 The Minnesota Transracial Adoption Study: A follow-up of IQ test performance at adolescence. *Intelligence* 16(1): 117–35

Wilson R S 1983 The Louisville Twin Study: Developmental synchronies in behavior. *Child Dev.* 54(2): 298–316

Wilson R S, Matheny A P Jr 1986 Behavior-genetics research in infant temperament: The Louisville Twin Study. In: Plomin R, Dunn J F (eds.) 1986 *The Study of Temperament: Changes, Continuities and Challenges* Erlbaum, Hillsdale, New Jersey

(d) Critical Theory, Policy Research, and Evaluation

Critical Theory and Education

G. Lakomski

Among the various theories competing for acceptance, if not dominance, in the field of education, critical theory is a vigorous and ambitious contender. It is the purpose of this entry to ask just how serious a contender critical theory is by examining its validity as a theory and its usefulness as an approach to educational research.

As a relative newcomer to education theory, the critical theory of society—whether in its original, or later Habermasian, form—has already marshaled significant support and won over a dedicated group of educators. Its arrival in educational research was greeted enthusiastically by writers such as Bredo and Feinberg (1982), for example, who believe that critical theory is able to transcend the distance between the dominant positivist school and its challenger, the interpretivist paradigm. Both schools of educational research have come under attack. Positivist research has been challenged both from within analytic philosophy of science and from interpretivists who criticize its reductionism, while the implicit relativism of the interpretivist approach is said to make it an unsuitable successor to positivism. Critical theory, as seen by its advocates, promises to solve the problems of both schools in a higher order synthesis which allocates the empirical–analytical and the historical–hermeneutic sciences to their own, mutually exclusive, object domains, complete with their respective methodologies.

In addition to relegating the sciences to their respective spheres of influence and thus deflating any claims for the superiority of one or the other methodology, critical theory has a distinctive political orientation. It suggests that the dominance of science and the rise of technology and bureaucracy are developmental tendencies of late capitalism which increasingly encroach on the domain of social life (Habermas 1976b). As a result of such imperialism which is accompanied by the decline and erosion of traditional institutions and legitimations, the legitimatory vacuum thus created is filled by the new belief in science (Habermas 1972c). What is obliterated in this process, according to Habermas, is the possibility of raising questions about social norms and values, and questions about "the good life" in the public domain. Where they are raised, they can only be perceived through the distorting lens of instrumental action, or the technical interest, which makes them appear solvable by the applica-

tion of Weber's means–end scheme. Unmasking the illegitimate intrusion of science into the realm of social norms, Habermas believes, makes critical theory "critical" in the sense Marx understood the term, since science and technology have thus been shown to be ideological. The perspective which makes such insight possible is that of critical reflection which liberates or emancipates actors from false beliefs and subsequently leads to concrete proposals for overcoming oppression.

It is not difficult to see the attraction of critical theory for a number of educators who, critical of positivism, wary of the implicit relativism and conservatism of the interpretive school, and disenchanted with the so-called "economism" of Marxist education theory (e.g., Bowles and Gintis 1976), have been searching for a more appropriate foundation for a socially just educational theory and practice. Critical theory, consequently, has found application in, for example, curriculum theory (Apple 1982, Van Manen 1977), educational administration (Foster 1980, 1986, Bates 1983, Giroux 1983), action research (Carr and Kemmis 1986), teacher education (Baldwin 1987), educational policy analysis (Prunty 1985) and planning (Weiler 1984), educational theory (Young 1989), and adult education (Mezirow 1985). It has also been used to explain the crisis in formal schooling (Shapiro 1984). (For a more comprehensive list see Ewert 1991).

Applying critical theory to curriculum making, Van Manen (1977 p. 209) notes that "Curriculum is approached as a nexus of behavioral modes which must be monitored, objectified, rationalized, and made accountable." Questions about the practical relevancy of, for example, teacher education programs, in Van Manen's view are then directly translatable into demands for increasing teacher competency and curriculum effectiveness.

In educational administration, writers such as Bates, Foster, and Giroux argue that the administration of schools, when carried out from within the scientific theory of administration (which they equate with positivism), merely emphasizes the technical–procedural aspects of their operations which are then taken as the only relevant and legitimate focuses of analysis. They contend that schools ought to be studied in all their interactional complexities. This is to be done by the method of "cultural analysis" with its emphasis on understanding and critical reflection. The rationale for cultural analysis is that, in Giroux's words, "the notion of culture . . . a political force . . . a powerful moment in the process of domination" (Giroux 1983 p. 31).

The advantage of critical theory as seen by those who adopt its central concepts are, as Foster (1980 p. 499) notes, that "it is possible to have a social science which is neither purely empirical nor purely interpretative," on the assumption that critical theory thus escapes the criticisms leveled at positivism and interpretivist theory respectively. The stakes, then, are high, and the goal ambitious, for if critical theory could achieve what is claimed on its behalf, and what it claims for itself, then it would indeed be an outstanding candidate for a new, comprehensive social theory in general, and for education in particular.

The version of critical theory considered here is that presented in the work of Habermas, since it is his version which provides the source material for most educators interested in critical theory, Giroux's emphasis on the older school notwithstanding. The task is then not only to examine critical theory's central claims, but also to explicate briefly what it sets itself to achieve. This is important since critical theory is presented by its advocates as both theoretically superior to positivist social and educational theory and as practically and politically more desirable. While neither claim is considered justified, the first will be examined since the validity of any theory depends on the justification not only of its claims to knowledge, but also on the grounds on which these claims are made. If these are inadequate, then any claims derived from them, be they "practical" or "political," are equally unjustified. If critical theory turns out to be incoherent, so is any educational theory which seeks to derive its justification from it.

This entry examines two central doctrines of the theory: (a) the conception of interests, and (b) the notion of communicative competence which culminates in the "ideal speech situation." The first concept provides the justification of the theory as knowledge, and the second is Habermas's proposed solution to the "theory–practice" problem, that is, the proposal for overcoming domination.

1. Habermasian Interests

Central to understanding Habermas's approach to social theory is what he takes to be the fundamental problem of contemporary social science: the relationship between theory and practice (Habermas 1974). He means by this that the connection between knowledge and social action has become an instrumentalist one, a relation which assumes the neutrality of science. Science is considered to be free of values and cannot, therefore, give people any guidance on how to conduct their lives. This development is the result of the victory of "scientism," or positivism, which, Habermas argues, presents itself as the only valid form of knowledge. As a consequence, it has become impossible, he suggests, to reflect critically on current forms of domination since even they appear as problems which are solvable by technical means. Habermas's aim is to restore to theory the dimension of reflection eclipsed by positivism and present a social theory which, as "ideology–critique," reunites theory with practice.

The quest for a comprehensive theory of social evolution as a theory of rationality leads Habermas to examine recent developments in the social sciences and in the analytic philosophy of science on the one hand (Habermas 1985b), and investigations in the field of philosophy of language and theoretical linguistics on the other (Habermas 1972a, Habermas 1972b, Habermas 1976a, Habermas 1979). In addition, he also re-examines the crisis potential of late capitalism (Habermas 1976b, Habermas 1976c) and the foundations of the older school of critical theory (Habermas 1982). These issues are outside the scope of this entry. For present purposes, the concept of "interests" (*Interessen*) is most important since it is the cornerstone of critical theory, aiming as it does at the re-examination of the connection between knowledge and human interests in general.

Interests, Habermas contends, are not like any other contingent empirical fact about human beings; neither are they rooted in an ahistorical subjectivity. Rather, they are grounded in the fundamental human conditions of work (following Marx) and interaction. What Habermas also calls a "cognitive" interest is consequently:

a peculiar category, which conforms as little to the distinction between empirical and transcendental or factual and symbolic determinations as to that between motivation and cognition. For knowledge is neither a mere instrument of an organism's adaptation to a changing environment nor the act of a pure rational being removed from the context of life in contemplation. (1972a p. 197)

Cognitive, or knowledge-constitutive, interests are hence ascribed a "quasi-transcendental" status, an ascription Habermas acknowledges as being problematic (1974 pp. 8 ff.). Critical theory claims three such interests: the technical, the practical, and the emancipatory. These three are asserted to correspond to the three types of sciences. The natural sciences, in Habermas's view, incorporate a technical interest; the historical–hermeneutic sciences the practical interest; and the critical sciences (such as sociology and Freudian psychoanalysis) the emancipatory. The technical interest guides work, the practical guides interaction, and the emancipatory guides power. Work, or purposive–rational action, is defined as:

either instrumental action or rational choice or their conjunction. Instrumental action is governed by technical rules based on empirical knowledge. In every case they imply conditional predictions about observable events, physical or social. These predictions can prove correct or incorrect. The conduct of rational choice is governed by strategies based on analytic knowledge. They imply deductions from preference rules (value systems) and decision procedures; these propositions are either correctly or incorrectly deduced. Purposive rational action realizes defined goals under given conditions. But while instrumental action organizes means that are appropriate or inappropriate according to criteria of an effective control of reality, strategic action depends only on the correct evaluation of possible alternative choices, which results from calculation supplemented by values and maxims. (Habermas 1972c pp. 91–92)

The second cognitive interest—the practical—enables the grasping of reality through understanding in different historical contexts (Habermas 1972a Chaps. 7, 8). It involves interaction patterns which provide a reliable foundation for communication. What Habermas terms "interaction" or "communicative action" is, like the technical interest, a distinct, nonreducible kind of action which demands specific categories of description, explanation, and understanding. It is this conception which provides the justification for the method of "cultural analysis" employed by some writers in education.

Habermas argues that just as human beings produce and reproduce themselves through work, so they shape and determine themselves through language and communication in the course of their historical development. While he emphasizes with Marx the historically determined forms of interaction, he nevertheless insists that symbolic interaction, together with cultural tradition, forms a "second synthesis" and is the "only basis on which power (*Herrschaft*) and ideology can be comprehended" (1972a p. 42). Marx is accused of not understanding the importance of communicative action since it does not play a separate role in, and is subsumed under, the concept of social labor which Habermas claims fits his own notion of instrumental action. Nevertheless, undistorted communication which, in Habermas's view, is the goal of the practical interest inherent in the hermeneutic sciences, requires the existence of social institutions which are free from domination themselves. On Habermas's own admission, these do not yet exist. By adding the model of symbolic interaction, he wishes to expand epistemologically Marx's conception of labor.

Finally, the notion of the emancipatory cognitive interest leads one to the most fundamental, yet also derivative, interest. It must be understood in the context of the German idealist tradition whose underlying theme, Habermas asserts, is that reason, once properly understood, "means the will to reason. In self-reflection knowledge for the sake of knowledge attains congruence with the interest in autonomy and responsibility. The emancipatory cognitive interest aims at the pursuit of reflection as such" (1972a p. 314). It is this interest which provides the epistemological basis for Habermas's notion of critique which is alleged to be the function of the critical social sciences.

Consequently, this interest is of equal importance for educational theory which aims to be "interested" in just this way.

2. Interests and Their Epistemological Status

Habermas's conception of interests was developed in critical response to positivism. The peculiar status of the interests resulted from his desire to avoid a naturalistic reduction of quasi-transcendental interests to empirical ones. Habermas wants to say, on the one hand, that humans have transformed nature, built social systems, and developed science in the course of their evolution, a process which is analogous to the evolution of claws and teeth in animals (1972a p. 312). On the other hand, he is not content with such naturalism and claims that these achievements of human evolution are not merely accidental or contingent but have developed the way they have because of a priori knowledge–constitutive interests. These cognitive interests are described as being of "metalogical necessity . . . that we can neither prescribe nor represent, but with which we must instead come to terms" (p. 312). They are "innate" and "have emerged in man's natural history" (p. 312) and are located in "deeply rooted (invariant?) structures of action and experience—i.e., in the constituent elements of social systems" (p. 371). From the observation that humans have in fact transformed nature, built social systems, and created science it does not follow that they have done so because of transcendental interests. In other words, there is no equivalence between asserting that the technical, practical, and emancipatory interests have emerged in human natural history, and asserting that they are true and provide the transcendental framework for all human knowledge. How could such a transcendental framework be justified?

Two alternatives are possible. Habermas can resort to another transcendental framework or, alternatively, concede that there is a framework which exists a priori. In the case of the first alternative, Habermas argues that cognitive interests are rooted in the depth structures of the human species. This is merely another transcendental, anthropological concept which is itself in need of justification. This solution leads to an infinite regress of transcendental frameworks since one can press the point of justification with each new framework. This means that in the end, no justification is provided. If this regress is to be avoided one would need to fall back on an a priori framework, a solution Habermas wants to avoid. It would seem that no matter which of these two alternatives is chosen, the status of interests which are neither amenable to empirical demonstration nor to be sought in the transcendental realm (being "*quasi*-transcendental" entities) remains unclear. If the epistemological status of the interests remains in such jeopardy, the consequences for critical theory are serious, since the interests were meant to provide the foundation for the claims made on behalf of the sciences. This means that Habermas's assertion of the existence of two categorically distinct forms of knowledge and inquiry lapses for want of adequate justification.

In the light of various criticisms of the epistemological status of the interests (e.g., McCarthy 1981, Evers and Lakomski 1991, in particular Chap. 7), Habermas felt compelled to note: "My view is today that the attempt to ground critical theory by way of the *theory of knowledge*, while it did not lead astray, was indeed a round-about way" (1982 p. 233). This assessment leads him to ground his theory in the theory of language instead (Habermas 1979, 1985a).

3. Communicative Competence and the Ideal Speech Situation

The concept of communicative competence culminating in the ideal speech situation is the centerpiece of critical theory, since here the various strands of Habermas's investigations are drawn together. Parallel to Marx's critique of political economy, Habermas attempts to elucidate contemporary forms of alienation expressed in distorted communication. He wants to show that the potential for emancipation inheres in ordinary language which both presupposes and anticipates an ideal speech situation in which communication free from domination is possible. The full impact of Habermas's theory of communicative competence cannot be grasped adequately without taking recourse to its three underlying tenets which need further explication: (a) the notion of discourse and its relation to interaction, (b) the consensus theory of truth, and (c) the conception of an ideal speech situation.

Habermas argues that one can proceed from the fact that functioning language games, in which speech acts are exchanged, are based on an underlying consensus which is formed in the reciprocal recognition of at least four claims to validity. These claims comprise the "comprehensibility of an utterance, the truth of its propositional component, the correctness and appropriateness of its performatory component, and the authenticity of the speaking subject" (Habermas 1974 p. 18, 1979 Chap. 1). Habermas contends that in normal communication these claims are accepted uncritically. Only when a background consensus is challenged can all claims be questioned. Their justification is subject to "theoretical discourse" which is an intersubjective enterprise within a community of inquirers. This concept is adapted from Habermas' interpretation of Peirce's model of empirical science (Habermas 1972a Chaps. 5, 6). Although theoretical discourse demands the "virtualization of constraints on action," it still remains implicitly presupposed in interaction because Habermas assumes that the subjects are in fact capable of justifying their beliefs discursively. Such a capability is characteristic of a functioning language game. Yet he is also aware of the fact that there is no complete symmetry of power among the partners of communication.

If one considers a consensus to be rational and discovers after further reflection and argumentation that it is not, how is one to decide what does constitute a rational consensus? Habermas claims that the only recourse one has is to discourse itself. He is aware that this answer might lead into a vicious circle and contends that not every achieved agreement is a consensus, that is, can be considered a criterion for truth. If, for example, an agreement is reached on the basis of what Habermas calls (covert or open) "strategic" action, then that consensus is a "pseudo-consensus" (Habermas 1982 p. 237). Strategic action is that which is undertaken primarily to safeguard an individual's personal success by means of conscious or unconscious deception. In the case of systematically distorted communication (i.e., unconscious deception), Habermas believes that "at least one of the participants is deceiving *himself* or *herself* regarding the fact that he or she is actually behaving strategically, while he or she has only apparently adopted an attitude orientated to reaching understanding" (p. 264). Even in this case, he contends, the actors themselves can know—even though only "vaguely and intuitively"—which of the two attitudes they were adopting. Both kinds are seen as "genuine types of interaction" and may be mixed up with each other in practice. As a result, Habermas asserts: " . . . it is often difficult for an observer to make a correct ascription" (p. 266). If one wants to reach a true (or "founded") consensus, he argues, one must admit as the only permissible compulsion the force of the argument, and consider as the only permissible motive the cooperative search for truth (1972a p. 363).

An argument, then, qualifies as rational when it is cogent and motivates one in one's search for truth. Implicit in this thesis is Habermas's belief that there must be increased freedom for discourse to reach higher levels, that truth claims and claims to correctness of problematic statements and norms must be able to be assessed discursively, and in the course of assessment, also be able to be changed or rejected. The conditions under which such freedom can be attained are, in Habermas's view, given in the "ideal speech situation" because "the design of an ideal speech situation is necessarily implied with the structure of potential speech; for every speech, even that of intentional deception, is oriented towards the idea of truth" (1972b p. 144). The ideal speech situation is attained when the requirements of symmetrical relations obtain which involve all speakers having equal chances of selecting and employing "speech acts" and their being able to assume interchangeable dialogue roles. Since practical discourse is generally distorted, according to Habermas, and since the ideal speech situation can only be anticipated, it is difficult to assess empirically whether or not, or to what extent, the conditions of an ideal speech situation actually obtain. This problem,

Habermas contends, cannot be solved in any a priori way. There is no single decisive criterion by which one can judge whether a consensus reached is "founded," even under ideal conditions; one can only determine in retrospect whether the conditions for an ideal speech situation obtained. This difficulty resides in the fact that:

> the ideal speech situation is neither an empirical phenomenon nor simply a construct, but a reciprocal supposition or imputation (*Unterstellung*) unavoidable in discourse. This supposition can, but need not be, contra-factual; but even when contra-factual it is a fiction which is operatively effective in communication. I would therefore prefer to speak of an anticipation of an ideal speech situation[.]. This anticipation alone is the warrant which permits us to join to an actually attained consensus the claim of a rational consensus. At the same time it is a critical standard against which every actually reached consensus can be called into question and checked. (Habermas in McCarthy 1976 p. 486)

What, exactly, does this notion amount to? Stripped of its abstractions, one is left with a procedural model of negotiation which has the following characteristics in practice: (a) not everyone can participate in a given negotiation because of the existing power differential in society; (b) even when one reaches agreement practically, one is not sure whether it really is a consensus, nor does one have the means to check this (presuming that that is a worthwhile thing to do in the first place); and (c) the language one uses to reach consensus is itself a carrier of ideology. While Habermas emphasizes that his model is only an "anticipation" possessing the status of a "practical hypothesis" which does not refer to any historical society (Habermas 1982 pp. 261–62), one is nevertheless entitled to press the point regarding its potential for realization in the here and now. Recall that the solution to this dilemma is that one can only determine with hindsight whether or not its conditions obtained. Recall further that these are the postulates of symmetrical relations in which all speakers have equal chances of "selecting and employing speech acts." This still does not solve the problem because one has to repeat the question of how one would ever know that these "equal chances" did obtain. Since all one has to go by are self-reports which may be consciously or unconsciously misleading, or even false, even a retrospective assessment would not avoid the skeptical regress.

Habermas calls his model a "constitutive illusion" and an "unavoidable supposition of discourse" which, however, is possibly always counterfactual. From this, McCarthy draws the conclusion that: "Nonetheless this does not itself render the ideal illegitimate, an ideal that can be more or less adequately approximated in reality, that can serve as guide for the institutionalization of discourse and as a critical standard against which every actually achieved consensus can be measured" (1981 p. 309).

While this is not an uncommon defence of the ideal

speech situation, it is nevertheless invalid. This is so because the ideal speech situation is in principle unrealizable. It cannot be "more or less" adequately approximated in reality because the condition of retrospectivity does not get Habermas out of the problem of stopping an infinite skeptical regress, as was argued above. It follows that one cannot even achieve what self-reflection and the emancipatory interest promised: the liberation from dogmatic attitudes which is, in any case, only the formal precondition for practical, political action in Habermas's scheme of things. For his theory to work, one must assume as already given, what, on his own account, does not yet exist but is supposed to come into existence as the result of the theory: namely, a world in which power and control are equalized. On the issue of social change then, this theory, which makes so much of its historical–materialist heritage, is silent. (For further critical comment on this aspect see Evers and Lakomski 1991 Chap. 7).

4. Conclusion

It is perplexing that this model of rationality (i.e., rational persons discussing their differences in an ideal speech situation) has been hailed as at least potentially the solution to the so-called "theory/practice problem" which holds that traditional (positivist) theory is incapable of informing and guiding practice. If the preceding analysis is correct, it seems that critical theory is similarly incapable of doing so. While the reasons outlined above go a considerable way toward explaining the problems of the theory of communicative competence, and hence critical theory, it finally fails because truth-as-consensus is removed from direct confrontation with the "objects of possible experience." In other words, the consensus theory of truth rules out the possibility of making true statements about empirical reality. If one cannot, in principle, know whether or not there is, as Habermas asserts, distorted communication and oppression in contemporary society, then one is left with mere speculation. However intuitively convincing this may be, speculation comes a poor second to knowledge. These fundamental problems need to be resolved if the critical theory of society is to be relevant for this world.

See also: Action Research; Participatory Research; Research Paradigms in Education

References

Apple M W 1982 *Education and Power*. Routledge and Kegan Paul, London

Baldwin E E 1987 Theory vs. ideology in the practice of teacher-education. *J. Teach. Educ.* 38(1): 16–19

Bates R J 1983 *Educational Administration and the Manage-*

ment of Knowledge. Deakin University Press, Geelong

Bowles S, Gintis H 1976 *Schooling in Capitalist America*. Basic Books, New York

Bredo E, Feinberg W (eds.) 1982 *Knowledge and Values in Social and Educational Research*. Temple University Press, Philadelphia, Pennsylvania

Carr W, Kemmis S 1986 *Becoming Critical: Education Knowledge and Action Research*. Falmer Press, London

Evers C W, Lakomski G 1991 *Knowing Educational Administration*. Pergamon Press, Oxford

Ewert G D 1991 Habermas and education: A comprehensive overview of the influence of Habermas in educational literature. *Rev. Educ. Res.* 61(3): 345–78

Foster W P 1980 Administration and the crisis of legitimacy: A review of Habermasian thought. *Harv. Educ. Rev.* 50(4): 496–505

Foster W P 1986 *Paradigms and Promises: New Approaches to Educational Administration*. Prometheus, Buffalo, New York

Giroux H 1983 *Critical Theory and Educational Practice*. Deakin University Press, Geelong

Habermas J 1971 *Toward a Rational Society*. Heinemann, London

Habermas J 1972a *Knowledge and Human Interests*. Heinemann, London

Habermas J 1972b Towards a theory of communicative competence. In: Dreitzel H P (ed.) 1972 *Recent Sociology, No. 2: Patterns of Communicative Behavior*. Macmillan, New York

Habermas J 1972c *Toward a Rational Society*. Heinemann, London

Habermas J 1974 *Theory and Practice*. Heinemann, London

Habermas J 1976a Systematically distorted communication. In: Connerton P (ed.) 1976 *Critical Sociology*. Penguin, Harmondsworth

Habermas J 1976b *Legitimation Crisis*. Heinemann, London

Habermas J 1976c *Zur Rekonstruktion des historischen Materialismus*, 2nd edn. Suhrkamp, Frankfurt

Habermas J 1979 *Communication and the Evolution of Society*. Beacon Press, Boston, Massachusetts

Habermas J 1982 A reply to my critics. In: Thompson J B, Held D (eds.) 1982 *Habermas: Critical Debates*. Macmillan, London

Habermas J 1985a *The Theory of Communicative Action I: Reason and the Rationalization of Society*. Beacon Press, Boston, Massachusetts

Habermas J 1985b *Zur Logik der Sozialwissenschaften*. Suhrkamp, Frankfurt

McCarthy T A 1976 A theory of communicative competence. In: Connerton P (ed.) 1976 *Critical Sociology*. Penguin, Harmondsworth

McCarthy T A 1981 *The Critical Theory of Jürgen Habermas*. MIT Press, Cambridge, Massachusetts

Mezirow J 1985 Concept and action in adult-education. *Adult Educ. Q.* 35(3): 142–51

Prunty J J 1985 Signposts for a critical educational policy analysis. *Aust J. Education.* 29 (2): 133–40

Shapiro S 1984 Crisis of legitimation: Schools, society and declining faith in education. *Interchange* 15(4): 26–39

Van Manen M 1977 Linking ways of knowing with ways of being practical. *Curric. Inq.* 6(3): 205–28

Weiler H N 1984 The political economy of education and development. *Prospects* 14(4): 467–77

Young R E 1989 *A Critical Theory of Education: Habermas and Our Children's Future*. Harvester Wheatsheaf, New York

Further Reading

Carr W 1995 *For Education. Towards Critical Educational Inquiry*. Open University Press, Philadelphia, Pennsylvania

Maddock T 1995 The light of redemption -Adorno and the task of critical reason. *Arena* 219–37

Action Research

S. Kemmis

The lively debates about educational research methodology in the 1970s and 1980s raised fundamental questions about the connections between educational theory and educational practice, between the conduct of research and the improvement of educational practice, and between researchers and teachers and learners. Around the world, a number of theorists of educational research have fostered the development of action research as an approach that provides ways of making these connections. Action research aims to help practitioners investigate the connections between their own theories of education and their own day-to-day educational practices; it aims to integrate the research act into the educational setting so that research can play a direct and immediate role in the improvement of practice; and it aims to overcome the distance between researchers and practitioners by assisting practitioners to become researchers.

This entry outlines a view of action research as a form of participatory and collaborative research aimed at improving educational understandings, practices, and settings, and at involving those affected in the research process. It describes a variety of international perspectives on educational action research, linking it to participatory action research for community development and ideas about critical social and educational science. Some of the contemporary contests about how action research is to be understood are described in terms of a debate between two main schools of thought about action research, one (more collaborative) based on the idea of a critical educational science and the other (more individualistic) based on ideas about practical reasoning and "the reflective practitioner."

1. Definition of Action Research

Kemmis and McTaggart (1988) defined action research as a form of *collective* self-reflective enquiry undertaken by participants in social situations in order to improve the productivity, rationality, and justice of their own social or educational practices, as well as their understanding of these practices and the situations in which the practices are carried out. Groups of participants can be teachers, students, principals, parents and other community members—any group with a shared concern. Kemmis and McTaggart stress that action research is *collaborative*, though it is important to realize that the action research of a group depends upon individual members critically examining their own actions. In education, action research has been employed in school-based curriculum development, professional development, school improvement programs, and systems planning and policy development (e.g., in relation to policy about classroom rules, school policies about noncompetitive assessment, regional project team policies about their consultancy roles, and state policies about the conduct of school improvement programs).

Based on the work of Kurt Lewin, frequently described as "the father of action research," Kemmis and McTaggart (1988) presented an introductory sketch of the process of action research, outlining a spiral of cycles of reconnaissance, planning action, enacting and observing the planned action, reflecting on the implementation of the plan in the light of evidence collected during implementation, then replanning (developing a changed or modified action plan), taking further action and making further observations, reflecting on the evidence from this new cycle, and so on. These steps are (of course) far too mechanical and procedural to be more than a starting point: they are best thought of as tips for beginners.

Kemmis and McTaggart also set out some possible questions to be asked by intending action researchers as they plan and conduct their enquiries, linking each stage of the process (reconnaissance, planning, enacting and observing, reflecting) to three interdependent domains of social and educational life: (a) language and discourse, (b) activities and practices, and (c) social relationships and forms of organization. The first of each of these pairs of terms relates to events and states of affairs in the lifeworld of a setting; the second to its more formal, institutional, systemic aspects (on the distinction and relationships between lifeworld and system, see Habermas 1984, 1987). To address the complexity of the relationships within

and between these pairs of terms requires reflective and critical judgment—a kind of judgment incompatible with a mechanical view of the action research process.

In action research, teachers (and others) are encouraged to treat their own educational ideas and theories, their own work practices, and their own work settings, as objects for analysis and critique. On the basis of careful reflection, it is argued, teachers may uncover theoretical ideas or assumptions that turn out to be unjustified and liable to lead them astray in their teaching (e.g., if they hold too rigid assumptions about the nature of students' innate abilities). Similarly, concerning their practices, teachers may find ways in which practices shaped by habit or tradition have become irrelevant or useless (e.g., finding that practices of classroom discipline, formerly seen as appropriate, may now be unacceptable or even counterproductive). Similarly, concerning the educational settings in which they practice, teachers may discover how the structure of the settings may place obstacles in the way of attaining educational goals (e.g., that the physical structure of the conventional classroom may hinder mixed ability grouping or the use of new technologies, or the management structure of a school may mitigate against new forms of curriculum organization).

The activities in this spiral of cycles aim at the *improvement* of practices, understandings, and situations, and at the *involvement* of as many as possible of those intimately affected by the action in all phases of the research process. Especially when they collaborate with other teachers in action research focused on their ideas, practices, and settings, teachers regularly find new ways of thinking, practicing, and structuring educational settings that will allow them to overcome obstacles and difficulties. In this way, action research contributes directly to the improvement of practice.

The involvement of teachers and others in the action research process—in data-gathering, analysis, and critique—creates an immediate sense of responsibility for the improvement of practice. Participation in action research is thus a form of professional development, linking the improvement of practitioners with the improvement of practices. It enhances the professional role of the teacher, even where beginning teacher–researchers are assisted by outside consultants or facilitators.

Many of the improvements that have flowed from teacher action research, in Australia and elsewhere, have escaped notice in the conventional educational research literature. Teachers have not generally been comfortable in contributing to educational research journals, nor are they frequent readers of such journals. Nevertheless, there is a growing body of action research work authored by teachers. It remains fugitive largely because its justification is the improvement of practitioners' own practices, and writing for others is seen as secondary to this purpose. Moreover, the action research "movement" has contributed to a subtle change in the educational research literature; as a consequence there are many more references to the research work and research problems of teachers in the "official" research literature, and there is a growing number of citations of work on the theory and practice of educational action research. A number of the journals of learned societies for educational research in Australia, Spain, the United Kingdom, and the United States of America, for example, have become more "teacher friendly," making particular efforts to carry reports of teachers' action research projects. Moreover, some specialist action research journals have sprung up (e.g., *Educational Action Research*), and some more conventional research journals have offered special issues on action research (e.g., the *Peabody Journal of Education*, which offered two special issues on action research in 1989). Nowadays, educational researchers outside schools also seem less likely to regard the teacher as "other" or "object" in their reporting of educational research, and are more likely to regard teachers as readers of and contributors to the improvement of education through research. This may be only a subtle effect, but it is an important one in the realignment of the relationship between educational research and educational practice.

2. *Key Points about Action Research*

Kemmis and McTaggart (1988) outlined a number of key features of action research:

(a) Action research is an approach to improving education by changing it and learning from the consequences of changes.

(b) Action research develops through a self-reflective spiral of cycles of planning, acting (implementing plans), observing (systematically), reflecting, and then replanning, further implementation, observing, and reflecting. It is a systematic learning process in which people act deliberately, though remaining open to surprises and responsive to opportunities.

(c) Action research is participatory: it is research through which people work toward the improvement of their own practices.

(d) Action research is collaborative: it involves those responsible for action in improving it, widening the collaborating group from those most directly involved to as many as possible of those affected by the practices concerned. It establishes self-critical communities of people participating and collaborating in all phases of the research process.

(e) Action research involves people in theorizing about their practices—being inquisitive about

circumstances, action, and consequences, and coming to understand the relationships between circumstance, action and consequence in their work and lives.

(f) Action research requires that people put their practices, ideas, and assumptions about institutions to the test by finding out whether there is compelling evidence that could convince them that their previous practices, ideas, and assumptions were false or incoherent (or both).

(g) Action research is open-minded about what counts as evidence (or data), but it always involves keeping records, and collecting and analyzing evidence about the contexts, commitments, conduct and consequences of the actions and interactions being investigated. It involves keeping a personal journal recording progress in, and reflections about, two parallel sets of learnings: learnings about the practices being studied, and learnings about the process of studying them (the action research process itself).

(h) Action research allows participants to build records of their improvements: (a) records of changes in activities and practices; (b) records of changes in the language and discourse in which practices are described, explained, and justified; (c) records of changes in the social relationships and forms of organization which characterize and constrain practices; and (d) records of change and development in the action research process itself. It thus allows participants to provide reasoned justifications of their educational work because it allows them to show how evidence and reflection have provided a basis for a developed, tested, and critically examined rationale for what is being done.

(i) Action research starts small. It normally begins with small changes which even a single person can try, and works toward more extensive changes; with small cycles of planning, acting, observing, and reflecting which can help to define issues, ideas, and assumptions more clearly so that those involved can define more powerful questions for themselves as their work progresses; and it begins with small groups of collaborators at the beginning, but widens the community of participating action researchers so that it gradually includes more and more of those involved in and affected by the practices in question.

(j) Action research involves people in making critical analyses of the situations (classrooms, schools, systems) in which they work—situations that are structured socially, historically, and institutionally. Critical analyses aim to recover how a situation has been socially and historically constructed, as a source of insight into ways in which people might be able to reconstruct it.

(k) Action research is a political process, because it involves making changes in the actions and interactions that constitute and structure social life (social practices); such changes typically have effects on the expectations and interests of others beyond the immediate participants in these actions and interactions.

3. International Perspectives on Action Research

One view of educational action research is associated with the work of a group at Deakin University in Australia. The views of this group derive from the ideas of social psychologist Lewin (1946), the thinking of Stenhouse and his colleagues at the University of East Anglia in the United Kingdom (e.g., Stenhouse 1975, Elliott 1978), and the ideas of the Frankfurt School in critical social science (see Carr and Kemmis 1986). This view of action research emphasizes the importance of collaboration, believing that some action research work of the past has been rather too individualistic, too little aware of the social construction of social reality, and too poorly attuned to the social processes and politics of change. It also understands action research to be a cultural process, in similar terms to Freire's (1970) notion of "cultural action for freedom." On this view, action researchers are understood as groups of people who participate systematically and deliberately in the processes of contestation and institutionalization which are always at work in social and educational life, aiming to help in the improvement of social or educational life by the reflective and self-reflective ways they participate in it.

This Australian view of action research is far from being the only extant view of action research, however. There are many other groups around the world with different views about the development of the theory and practice of action research; indeed, it has become something of a worldwide movement.

A great deal of action research work goes on in the United Kingdom, for example—much of it inspired by Stenhouse's (1975) notion of the teacher as researcher. The Ford Teaching Project of Elliott and Adelman (1973) broke new ground in action research in education in the 1970s, and their work has spawned a great diversity of action research work in schools and colleges around the United Kingdom—some of which can be accessed through publications and conferences of the Classroom Action Research Network based initially at the Cambridge Institute of Education and now at the University of East Anglia. British action research work ranges from the enquiries of individual teachers into their own practice to shared work by groups of teachers (e.g., Hustler et al. 1986, McKernan 1991); from work focused on the analysis of contradictions in practitioners' own theories and practices (Whitehead

1989) to work more critically relating these to wider social, cultural, and political trends (Elliott 1991); and from work informed by practical and interpretative views of social science and its possibilities for professional development (Nixon 1981) to work more closely allied with reflexive sociology and critical theory (Winter 1987, 1989). Despite Stenhouse's (1975) disquiet about "movements" and the possibility of a curriculum development movement based on the notion of teachers as researchers, there can be no doubt that there is an action research movement in the United Kingdom, nor can there be any doubt that it has provided an important source of professional inspiration for teachers and school administrators throughout the country.

There has also been a resurgence of interest in action research in the United States and Canada. Early United States views of action research in education were inspired by the work of Corey (1949); later it was influenced by Schwab's (1969) ideas about practical reasoning, by Schön's (1983) ideas about "the reflective practitioner," by concerns to recognize and develop teachers' craft knowledge, by the desire of university educational researchers to employ field methods that engage teachers in research for their own professional development (Oja and Smulyan 1989), and by teacher educators committed to exploring action research in pre-service and in-service teacher education (Zeichner and Liston 1987). In general, educational action research in the United States has been less responsive to the arguments of critical social and educational theory, but the themes of critical theory have been taken up by a number of American advocates of action research (Noffke and Brennan 1988, Noffke 1991). In addition to this critical work in education, there is a strong tradition of critical action research for community development in the United States, exemplified by the work of Horton, Gavena, and their colleagues at the Highlander Center in Tennessee (Gaventa 1991, Horton and Freire 1990).

In Canada, one strong current of educational action research is based in the phenomenological tradition (Van Manen 1990), and there is also a strong movement in participatory action research in adult education and community development which shares the critical communitarian commitment of the participatory action research of Gaventa in the United States and of Freire and others in Central and South America (see *Participatory Research*).

By the beginning of the 1990s there were many European advocates of educational action research, for example in Germany (Klafki 1988a, 1988b, Finger 1988), Austria (Altrichter and Posch 1990), and Asturias, Spain (Rozada et al. 1989, Cascante 1991). Some of these theorists have been influenced by the ideas of Habermas (1972, 1974) about "sciences of social action" (now known as critical social science), though others have clearly been influenced by the

British action research movement, and others by phenomenological approaches.

In Central and South America there has been a tradition of participatory action research work which has been strongly influenced by Freirean ideas, in Mexico, Colombia, Venezuala, Nicaragua, Brazil, and elsewhere. The social and political commitments of the participatory action research movement in these countries (see Fals Borda 1990, Fals Borda and Rahman 1991, Serra 1988) have extended from community development to popular education and action research in education. The extent to which the forms and content of these community development efforts through action research are realizable in the reconstruction of institutionalized schooling in the developed industrial nations of the West is, of course, a matter for continuing exploration, but the communitarian ethic they embody provides a powerful model of ordinary people reconstructing the circumstances of their own lives.

The Central and South American tradition of participatory action research in community development has spread, through the work of Freire, to other parts of the world; for example, to Africa, India, Nepal, the Philippines, Sri Lanka, and Thailand. There is now a substantial tradition of action research in community development in India (Tandon 1988, Handay and Tandon 1988), and in Southeast Asia (e.g., in Singapore, Malaysia, and Thailand). Some of this work is associated with nongovernment organizations, while other work is associated with official educational projects. In the Southeast Asian context, for example, there has been an exploration of action research for community development through adult education and the Freireian participatory action research movement, on the one hand, and a somewhat separate development of action research in institutional contexts of school improvement and evaluation on the other (a good example of the latter being a project in the initial and postinitial education of nurses; see Chuaprapaisilp 1989). The latter trend seems more closely aligned with the kinds of interests in the educational profession that inspired the British action research movement in its early days.

As this brief review suggests, there is a wide diversity of motivations, forms, and contents of action research around the world. It would be mistaken, therefore, to regard educational action research as expressing a single school of thought or as embodying a coherent and unified point of view on social or educational research.

4. Contest over the Term "Action Research"

Like any significant theoretical term, the idea of "action research" is contested. Its meaning and significance cannot be fixed by any one person or group. It is the subject of continuing argument and debate within and outside the relevant traditions and professions.

There is an internal debate between two main contemporary "schools" of action research internationally, one adopting a critical social science view of action research, while the other draws more on the Schwabian tradition of practical reasoning and, more recently, on Schön's (1983) notion of "the reflective practitioner." The debate between these two schools of thought may have reached the point where they now relate to one another as "external" critics of each other's positions, rather than as "internal" critics who share broad agreements about the nature and conduct of action research, though they also keep these agreements under critical review. When there is uncertainty about whether participants in the field share a common system of beliefs, values, and commitments, it is uncertain whether they are members of and participants in a single tradition. As disagreements about fundamental issues in a field accumulate, it is pushed toward a division into two or more new and opposed traditions. Perhaps it is already true that debates previously regarded as "internal" debates within the field of action research—clarifying and continuously revitalizing a more or less coherent tradition—are now "external" debates between advocates of opposed traditions.

Since the early 1980s, the critical social science view of action research has been subjected to sharp criticism (e.g., Gibson 1985, Elliott 1991). This reaction was partly caused, no doubt, by the drawing of distinctions between "technical," "practical," and "emancipatory" (or critical) action research (Carr and Kemmis 1986), and the insistence of advocates of "emancipatory" view that action research undertaken primarily by individual teacher–researchers was less significant than action research undertaken by collaborating groups in "self-critical communities." Reaction was further fanned by advocacies (like those of McTaggart and Garbutcheon-Singh 1988, Kemmis and Di Chiro 1989) of connections between action research groups and the critical efforts of activists in broader social movements. While at first such advocacies were treated as "utopian" and "idealistic," and as attempting to "capture" action research to a particular view of critical educational science and a particular understanding of the relationship between theory and practice (see, e.g., Gibson 1985, Lewis 1987), they have since been regarded by some as "dangerous" (Elliott 1991). Arguably, some of these criticisms are based on a misunderstanding of critical social science and the possibility of a critical educational science.

A key element of the difference between the two main contemporary schools in educational action research lies in how the aspirations of action research are to be interpreted: whether (on the one hand) they are to be interpreted as a means of improving professional practice primarily at the local, classroom level, within the capacities of individuals and the constraints of educational institutions and organizations, or (on the other) whether they are to be interpreted as an approach to changing education and schooling in a broader sense. Like other choices of principle, this is a choice between different views of human nature and different views of the good for humankind. Like other such debates, it will be resolved not by argument alone, but by the judgment of history.

5. Shortcomings of Some Contemporary Advocacies for Action Research

The critical social science view of action research emphasizes the connections between particular elements of action research in theory and practice, not the separations between them, regarding these elements as dialectically related, not as dichotomies. In particular, the critical view has sought to emphasize the connections between:

(a) the individual and the social (the social construction of social realities and practices) in the practice of action research and in the practice of education (see, e.g., Kemmis and McTaggart 1988);

(b) the cognitive (practitioners' ideas) and the theoretical (formal discourses, whether employed by researchers or by others involved in education; see, e.g., Kemmis 1990);

(c) theory and method in action research practice (the role of action research as a systematic social practice that provides a way of formulating and attacking educational research problems in an educational and social context; see, e.g., McTaggart and Garbutcheon-Singh 1988).

When these terms are regarded as dichotomies, not as dialectically related, advocates and practitioners of action research may be led into fallacies of dualistic, black and white reasoning. Some of these fallacies arise when advocates and practitioners of action research believe, or appear to believe:

(a) that action research can involve the work of individuals without being, simultaneously, intrinsically social (rooted in the fundamental connections between individuals embodied in and shaped by the social media of language, work, and power, though social practices of communication, production, and organization);

(b) that action research can deal with practitioners' ideas without simultaneously recognizing that these ideas are theoretical (or at least pretheoretical or protetheoretical), in the sense that they draw on public discourses which give meaning and significance to their work as educators or as researchers;

(c) that action research is a relatively "neutral"

research technology which can be separated from particular intellectual traditions, involving particular notions and theories about society, education, and social and educational change (especially participatory views about social practices, education, democracy, and change).

When views of action research become structured by dichotomized thinking about these relationships, their advocates may fall into the trap of focusing too much on the individual action researcher and her or his development (e.g., as an individual professional) without also taking a critical view of the social context in which the individual works. They may focus too much on individuals' ideas and thinking without giving sufficient critical attention to the ordinary language and formal discourses that give form and content to individual thinking. Moreover, they may focus too much on action research as a method or procedure without giving critical attention to the social framework in which the procedure operates, and to the way the procedures of action research actively connect with and coordinate processes of change in history —which is to say, politically. Some contemporary action research literature seems to have fallen into these traps.

6. Conclusion

Understanding of action research has been, and will continue to be, reconstructed anew for changing times and circumstances. The idea of action research may be no more perfectible than the idea of the perfectibility of humankind, but over 50 years it has offered and demonstrated possibilities for linking social research and social action, and it has made worthwhile contributions to the improvement of education, science, and society. As Sanford (1970) argued, action research is a social practice that still contains possibilities that may prove useful in addressing the social, cultural, and educational problems of contemporary times.

The notion of action research is just that: it is a notion, not a thing. As a notion, it does no more than give form to a particular kind of democratic aspiration to engage in changing the world as well as interpreting it. It offers an embryonic, local form of connecting research with social, educational, and political action in complex practical circumstances. In this, it is similar to the aspiration sloganized by the environmental movement in the words "think globally, act locally," and, as such, it may be a social form that can help educators address the contradictions, constraints, and limitations of their theories and practices, of their words and our world.

See also: Research in Education: Epistemological Issues; Research Paradigms in Education; Participatory Research; Scientific Methods in Educational Research

References

Altrichter H, Posch P 1990 *Lehrer Erforschen Ihren Unterricht. Eine Einführung in die Methoden der Aktionforschung.* Klinkhardt, Bad Heilbrunn

Carr W, Kemmis S 1986 *Becoming Critical: Education, Knowledge and Action Research.* Falmer, London

Cascante Fernandez C 1991 Los ámbitos de la práctica educativa: Una experiencia de investigación en la acción. *Revista Interuniversitaria de Formación del Profesorado* 10: 265–74

Chuaprapaisilp A 1989 Critical reflection in clinical experience: Action research in nurse education (Doctoral dissertation, University of New South Wales)

Corey S 1949 Action research, fundamental research and educational practices. *Teach. Coll. Rec.* 50: 509–14

Elliott J 1978 What is action-research in schools? *J. Curric. St.* 10(4): 355–57

Elliott J 1991 *Action Research for Educational Change.* Open University Press, Milton Keynes

Elliott J, Adelman C 1973 Reflecting where the action is: The design of the Ford Teaching Project. *Education for Teaching* 92: 8–20

Fals Borda O 1990 Social movements and political power: Evolution in Latin America. *International Sociology* 5(2): 115–28

Fals Borda O, Rahman M A 1991 *Action and Knowledge: Breaking the Monopoly with Participatory Action-Research.* Apex, New York

Finger M 1988 Heinz Moser's concept of action research. In Kemmis S, McTaggart R (eds.) 1988

Freire P 1970 *Cultural Action for Freedom.* Center for the Study of Change, Cambridge, Massachusetts

Gaventa J 1991 Toward a knowledge democracy: Viewpoints on participatory research in North America. In: Fals-Borda O, Rahman M A (eds.) 1991

Gibson R 1985 Critical times for action research. *Camb. J. Educ.* 15(1): 59–64

Habermas J 1972 *Knowledge and Human Interests.* Heinemann, London

Habermas J 1974 *Theory and Practice.* Heinemann, London

Habermas J 1984 *The Theory of Communicative Action. Vol.1: Reason and the Rationalization of Society.* Beacon, Boston, Massachusetts

Habermas J 1987 *The Theory of Communicative Action. Vol.2: Lifeworld and System: A Critique of Functionalist Reason.* Beacon, Boston, Massachusetts

Handay G, Tandon R 1988 *Revolution through Reform with People's Wisdom.* (videotape) Society for Participatory Research in Asia, Khanpur, New Delhi

Horton M, Freire P 1990 *We Make the Road by Walking: Conversations on Education and Social Change.* Temple University Press, Philadelphia, Pennsylvania

Hustler D, Cassidy A, Cuff E (eds.) 1986 *Action Research in Classrooms and Schools.* Allen and Unwin, London

Kemmis S 1990 Some Ambiguities of Stenhouse's Notion of "the Teacher as Researcher": Towards a New Resolution. 1989 Lawrence Stenhouse Memorial Lecture to the British Educational Research Association, School of Education, University of East Anglia, Norwich

Kemmis S, Di Chiro G 1989 Emerging and evolving issues of action research praxis: An Australian perspective. *Peabody Journal of Education* 64 (3): 101–30

Kemmis S, McTaggart R (eds.) 1988 *The Action Research Reader*, 3rd edn. Deakin University Press, Geelong

Klafki W 1988a Decentralised curriculum development in the form of action research. In: Kemmis S, McTaggart R (eds.) 1988

Klafki W 1988b Pedagogy: Theory of a practice. In: Kemmis S, McTaggart R (eds.) 1988

Lewin K 1946 Action research and minority problems. *J. Soc. Issues* 2(4): 34–46

Lewis I 1987 Encouraging reflective teacher research: A review article. *Br. J. Sociol. Educ.* 8(1): 95–105

McKernan J 1991 *Curriculum Action Research: A Handbook of Methods and Resources for the Reflective Practitioner.* Kogan Page, London

McTaggart R, Garbutcheon-Singh M 1988 A fourth generation of action research: Notes on the Deakin seminar. In: Kemmis S, McTaggart R (eds.) 1988

Nixon J (ed.) 1981 *A Teachers' Guide to Action Research.* Grant McIntyre, London

Noffke S E 1991 Hearing the teacher's voice: Now what? *Curriculum Perspectives*

Noffke S E, Brennan M 1988 Action research and reflective student teaching at U W -Madison: Issues and examples. Paper presented at the Annual Meeting of the Association of Teacher Educators, San Diego, California

Oja S N, Smulyan L 1989 *Collaborative Action Research: A Developmental Approach.* Falmer, London

Rozada Martínez J, Cascante Fernández C, Arrieta Gallastegui J 1989 *Desarrollo Curricular y Formación del Profesorado.* Cyan Gestión Editorial, Gijón

Sanford N 1970 Whatever happened to action research? *J. Soc. Issues* 26(4): 3–23

Schön D A 1983 *The Reflective Practitioner: How Professionals Think in Action.* Temple Smith, London

Schwab J J 1969 The practical: A language for curriculum. *Sch. Rev.* 78: 1–24

Serra L 1988 Participatory research and popular education. Paper presented to the North American Adult Education Association Research Conference, University of Calgary

Stenhouse L A 1975 *An Introduction to Curriculum Research and Development.* Heinemann, London

Tandon R 1988 Social transformation and participatory research. *Convergence* 21(2,3): 5–18

Van Manen M 1990 *Researching Lived Experience: Human Science for an Action-Sensitive Pedagogy.* State University of New York Press, Albany, New York

Whitehead J 1989 Creating a living educational theory from questions of the kind, "How do I improve my practice?" *Camb. J. Educ.* 19(1): 41–52

Winter R 1987 *Action-Research and the Nature of Social Inquiry.* Gower, Aldershot

Winter R 1989 *Learning from Experience: Principles and Practice in Action-Research.* Falmer, London

Zeichner K, Liston D P 1987 Teaching student teachers to reflect. *Harv. Educ. Rev.* 57(1): 23–48

Feminist Research Methodology

B. D. Haig

Since the 1960s feminist scholars have made significant contributions to educational and social science research methodology. These contributions are varied in nature and wide-ranging in scope. This entry describes and evaluates some of the central developments in feminist methodology that are relevant to educational research. These include: (a) the feminist critique of standard empiricist research, (b) a consideration of methods used by feminist researchers, (c) the three major feminist epistemologies and their methodological implications, and (d) the relevance of pragmatist thought for the further development of feminist methodology.

1. Is There a Distinctive Feminist Methodology?

A number of feminist researchers have debated the issue of whether there is a distinctive feminist methodology. Interestingly, few feminists have claimed that there is, or could be, though Reinharz (1983) has developed a communal approach to research called "experiential analysis," contending that it is distinctively feminist in character. However, most feminists appear to accept the view that it is a mistake to portray feminist methodology as distinctive. Clegg (1985) contends that there is no unified feminist methodology and that attempts to suggest otherwise run the risk of missing the real value of feminist contributions. Peplau and Conrad (1989) evaluate a number of proposals for distinctively feminist methods and conclude that any method can be misused in sexist ways. Similarly, Harding (1989) argues that attempts to identify a distinctively feminist method are misguided. She contends that feminist researchers use a variety of existing research methods, adapted to their own purposes, and that the arguments against a specifically feminist methodology are largely beside the point.

2. Common Features of Feminist Methodology

Although feminist methodology comprises a diversity of offerings, a number of common themes have been identified in presentations of feminist methodology (e.g., Cook and Fonow 1986, Mies 1983). The following features are often included in these presentations:

2.1 The Rejection of Positivism

Despite their many disagreements, feminist methodologists appear united in their opposition to the many positivist strands of orthodox educational and social science research.

This opposition ranges from efforts to improve on standard empiricism's positivist image by the development of a feminist empiricism, through the endorsement of extant postempiricist methodologies such as the "new" social psychology of Harré and Secord (Wilkinson 1986), to the extreme postpositivism of skeptical postmodernism (Rosenau 1992). The common features of feminist methodology mentioned immediately below are a part of its postpositivist commitments.

2.2 The Pervasive Influence of Gender Relations

Probably the most central feature of feminist methodology is its ubiquitous concern with gender. It is because of differences in the social position and power of women and men that gender relations are held to pervade social life. For this reason feminist researchers are committed to describing, explaining, and otherwise interpreting the female world. From these considerations feminist methodology has urged researchers to acknowledge and portray women's experiences, to identify the patriarchal bias of orthodox research and, relatedly, to assess the ways in which gender relations impact on the conduct of research (Cook and Fonow 1986).

2.3 The Value-ladenness of Science

The persistent positivist myth that science is value-free has never been true to science and has been repeatedly challenged by feminist scholars. From their belief that science is a human social endeavor, feminists maintain that such inquiry takes on the values of the people who do the research as well as the values of the institutions that sustain it. Positivist empiricist research has been undertaken to produce secure factual knowledge bereft of explanatory power, which has served to maintain the status quo in respect of women's oppression. In stressing the value-ladenness of research, feminist methodologists have also been concerned to articulate a feminist ethic (Cook and Fonow 1986) that is concerned with the way gender-biased language subordinates women, the fairness of practices which prevent the publication of feminist research and stifle career opportunities, and problems of researcher intervention into participatory research relationships.

2.4 The Adoption of Liberatory Methodology

The feminist movement characterizes itself as being primarily concerned with the emancipation of women from oppression. In consequence, it is often claimed that research-based knowledge should be employed to help liberate women from their oppression. Mies (1983) forcefully expresses this view by claiming that, in order to change the status quo, feminists must integrate their research with an active participation in the struggle against women's oppression. Consistent with this, Mies claims further that the worth of a theory is to be judged, not through the application of methodological principles, but on its ability to assist the emancipatory process.

Liberatory methodologists are often critical of the use of attitude surveys in gathering knowledge about women on the grounds that they tell us little about women's true consciousness. In formulating a liberatory methodology, feminists have sometimes insisted that the research process must become a process of "conscientization" in Freire's (1972) sense (Mies 1983, Lather 1988). This process involves "learning to perceive social, political, and economic contradictions, and to take action against the oppressive elements of reality" (Freire 1972 p. 15). As a problem-solving methodology, conscientization involves the study of oppressive reality by the subjects of oppression, where the social science researchers give their research resources to the oppressed so that they can formulate and come to understand their own problems. In these ways feminist liberatory methodology is seen to issue in action research.

2.5 The Pursuit of Nonhierarchical Research Relationships

A fifth common feature of feminist methodology is its strong endorsement of a nonhierarchical relationship between the researcher and the researched. This contrasts with positivist empiricism's penchant for assigning the researcher a position of epistemic privilege. In particular, feminist methodology seeks to replace the epistemic privilege of the professional researcher by democratic participatory inquiry where the researcher and researched enter into a social relationship of reciprocity in which there is a complementary recognition of their equal agency. The establishment of a relationship of nonhierarchy also requires the replacement of a spectator view of knowledge with "conscious partiality" (Mies 1983) which the researcher achieves by partially identifying with the researched. Because the identification is not complete, the mutual correction of distortions remains possible.

3. Research Methods

The conclusion that there are no distinctively feminist research methods is borne out by the widespread use of a variety of existing research methods by feminist researchers. However, feminist researchers tend to view these methods critically and deploy them in the light of their particular value commitments.

3.1 Experimentation

Feminists have criticized the use of experimental methods in the social sciences, both for assigning power and privilege to experimenters in their relationships with subjects, and for the artificiality of the laboratory experiment with its simplification of context (e.g., Parlee 1979). For these reasons, feminist methodologists have tended to favor nonexperimental methods in natural settings. However, it should be noted that a plausible case has been advanced by Greenwood (1989) for the constructive use of role-playing experiments in social psychological contexts in a way that can avoid the artificiality of altered social relations in laboratory experiments.

3.2 Meta-analysis

The extended history of research on gender differences has entered its latest phase with the adoption of meta-analytic procedures to summarize the disparate findings of numerous empirical studies in this controversial area. Meta-analysis is a recently developed approach to research integration that involves the statistical analysis of the results of data analyses from many individual studies in a given domain in order to synthesize those findings. Some (e.g., Hyde 1990) see meta-analysis making a significant contribution to feminist research by providing strong quantitative conclusions about the extent and magnitude of gender differences. However, the empiricist basis of its most popular form should temper the widespread view that meta-analysis is a powerful method of research synthesis.

3.3 Ethnography

With the tendency of feminist methodologists to recommend qualitative methods over quantitative alternatives, ethnographic methods have frequently been used by feminist researchers. Such methods are attractive because they acknowledge the importance of the research context, focus on the experiential reports of women, and seek collaborative relationships between the researcher and researched. Glaser and Strauss's grounded theory perspective on ethnography (e.g., Strauss 1987) has been used by a number of feminist social science researchers. Their approach to qualitative research breaks from the prevalent hypothetico-deductive practice of testing existing theories and encourages researchers to generate their own theories inductively to explain patterns in systematically obtained data. However, while acknowledging the methodological advantages that accrue to such ethnographic perspectives on the research process, some feminists worry about the possibilities of serious exploitation, betrayal, and abandonment of the research subject by the researcher in their collaborative relationship (e.g., Stacey 1988).

4. Methodology and Epistemology

In the early 1980s feminism seemed more willing to spell out its methodology than develop its theory of knowledge. However, since then developments in feminist methodology have proceeded more slowly than advances in feminist epistemology. Indeed, much of the content in feminist methodological writings has come to focus on general epistemological issues implicated in the feminist critiques of positivist research and the proposed alternatives. A consideration of feminist methodology, therefore, requires one to attend to the relevant epistemological literature. Harding (1986) distinguished three major alternative feminist epistemologies: feminist empiricism, feminist standpoint epistemology, and feminist postmodernism. A good deal of debate in feminist methodology in the early 1990s involved the ongoing elaboration and evaluation of these positions.

4.1 Feminist Empiricism

Although some feminist scholars have criticized the positivist features of traditional science and sought to replace postpositivist science with a feminist successor, others have looked to reshape traditional science in the belief that it can serve feminist ends. "Feminist empiricism," as the modified account has been called, contends that the sexism and androcentrism evident in much research are social biases that result from doing bad science, but that they can be overcome, or minimized, by following the methodological norms of good orthodox science.

The attainment of these norms has been sought by the construction of guidelines for the conduct of gender-fair research (e.g., Eichler 1988), and by efforts to identify and guard against gender differences in the sex composition of research participants as well as assessment of treatment conditions for gender neutrality.

Feminist research has sanctioned the continued use of many standard experimental, quasiexperimental, and observational methods, as well as a variety of qualitative methods, but with a heightened appreciation of the importance of bias in the deployment of these methods. New methods have also been enthusiastically accepted as improvements on the acknowledged limitations of older methods. For example, meta-analytic review procedures have been employed as a more effective gauge of gender differences than traditional tests of statistical significance (Hyde 1990).

Although research from a feminist empiricist perspective helps to include women in science and can contribute to the improvement of conventional science, it has been criticized for improving the "masculinist conception of objectivity" (Heckman 1990 p. 129) and for ignoring the important connection between science and politics.

4.2 Feminist Standpoint Epistemology

Feminist standpoint epistemologies are seen by their adherents to undergird a successor science that overcomes the inadequacies of both traditional empiricist

science and its feminist improvement. In contrast to feminist empiricism, feminist standpoint theorists contend that the characteristics of researchers are crucial determinants of their understanding of reality. Drawing from Marxist, and/or psychoanalytic theorizing about gender, feminist standpoint epistemologies regard the subjugated social position of women as a privileged vantage point from which to view social reality. One explanation for women's epistemic privilege draws from object relations theory within psychoanalysis and claims that the formation of a distinctively female identity in infancy leads to a distinctive and superior form of knowing than that of men. However, the idea that women have a superior ability to reflect on and comprehend reality has been criticized by feminists and nonfeminists alike. For example, object relations theory has been judged to have weak evidential support, while the general claim of women as better knowers has been criticized as an untenable endorsement of cognitive privilege (Chandler 1990).

4.3 Feminist Postmodernism

Feminist postmodernism rejects the epistemological assumptions of modernist, Enlightenment thought. Thus, it stands opposed to the foundationalist grounding of knowledge, the universalizing claims for the scope of knowledge, and the employment of dualistic categories of thought. By contrast, postmodern feminism is an epistemology that is non-foundationalist, contextualist, and nondualist, or multiplist, in its commitments.

Feminist postmodernists sometimes maintain that language cannot really be used to refer, predicate, identify, and individuate an extralinguistic reality. This view of language underwrites an approach to discourse analysis research which substitutes the study of texts for the broader study of social reality.

Critics of postmodern feminism (e.g., Hawkesworth 1989) argue that this flight to the text is inconsistent with its radical political aspirations. To shift the focus from the study of oppression suffered by women to the interpretation of texts is to abandon the real world for a relativist world of ideas. It is maintained that such a retreat can only serve to reinforce the status quo.

5. A Pragmatist Turn

Harding (1986) believes that because of the unstable nature of the categories they use, feminists should accommodate the tensions between these alternative epistemologies for now. However, Nelson (1990) has combined important insights from Quine's influential philosophy of science with feminist criticisms of science, to formulate an enriched feminist empiricism that she believes has the ability to resolve the differences among these epistemologies. With Quine,

Nelson rejects foundationalist thinking and maintains that science should justify its claims in accordance with a coherence theory of evidence. While foundationalism maintains that theories are justified by being appropriately related to some privileged source, such as observation statements, coherentism maintains that knowledge claims are justified in virtue of their coherence with other accepted beliefs.

Relatedly, Nelson's neo-Quinean perspective regards knowledge as a seamless web with no boundaries between science, metaphysics, methodology, and epistemology. Thus, philosophy does not lie outside science, but is instead contained in, and is interdependent with, other parts of science. From this perspective it can be appreciated that epistemologies and methodologies do not function in isolation, but actually make metaphysical commitments. Traditional empiricist methodology, for example, regards the knower as an abstract and autonomous individual. However, Nelson breaks with Quine at this point and, by joining science and politics, she insists that it is communities rather than individuals who know; that it is the standards of a community that determines what counts as evidence for a knowledge claim.

Feminist scholars have been criticized for seeking distinctively feminist conceptions of science. Lakomski (1989), for example, has criticized Harding for pursuing such a project and suggests that progress in feminist theorizing will come from a consideration of mainstream epistemology and philosophy of science. Indeed, Nelson's radical feminist empiricism may be viewed in part as an advancement of the feminist understanding of science by exploiting Quinean epistemology.

6. Pragmatist Realist Methodology

Seigfried (1991) has lamented the fact that United States feminists have not appropriated their own country's philosophy of pragmatism, a philosophy that has resources suitable for the development of feminist theory. Of importance, however, is the fact that a number of writers in a pragmatist realist tradition have made significant contributions to methodology that are suitable for appropriation by feminist and other postpositivist researchers. This section of the entry outlines some of these developments and briefly links them to feminist concerns about methodology.

6.1 Research Problems

In her forceful plea for overcoming the uncritical employment of method, Daly (1973) suggests that the common practice of having the research problem determined by the method should be reversed so that the method is chosen to fit the problem. However, this reasonable suggestion fails to depict research adequately as a problem-solving enterprise.

Nickles (1981) has developed a constraint inclusion theory of problems which assigns to scientific problems a positive methodological role. On this account a problem is taken to comprise all the constraints on the solution (plus the demand that the solution be found). With this theory the constraints do not lie outside the problem, but are constitutive of the problem itself; they actually serve to characterize the problem and give it structure. This constraint inclusion account of problems stresses the fact that, in good scientific research, problems typically evolve from an ill-structured state and eventually attain a degree of well-formedness, such that their solution becomes possible. Incorporating such an account of problems into research method itself allows the problem to guide inquiry and explain how it is possible.

6.2 Generative Methodology

Most traditional philosophies of science have insisted on drawing a strong distinction between the context of discovery and the context of justification. The context of discovery is concerned with the origin of scientific hypotheses and is thought to be a psychological, but not a methodological, affair. The context of justification is concerned with the validation of hypotheses and is the domain to which methodology properly belongs. Some feminist methodologists such as Harding (1989), for example, have argued that understanding the origin of scientific hypotheses requires one to admit that methodology can rightly operate in the context of discovery. Other advocates of discovery have argued for the same conclusion. This traditional methodological distinction, combined with the dominance of the hypothetico-deductive method, has resulted in a half methodology whereby researchers evaluate knowledge claims solely in terms of their consequences.

However, a methodology adequate to the full range of scientific reasoning must supplement consequentialism with a conception of methodology that is also generative in nature. In contrast to consequentialist thinking, generative methodologies reason to, and accept, the knowledge claims in question from warranted premises (Nickles 1987). The widely used procedure of exploratory factor analysis serves as an example of a method that facilitates generative reasoning by helping to reason forward from correlational data to the plausible factorial theories that they occasion. The endorsement of generative methodologies will be an essential part of feminist methodologists' resolve to acknowledge and scrutinize the entire research process.

6.3 Heuristics

Feminists have frequently criticized positivist empiricism for its rather idealized portrayal of the researcher as a computationally adept being whose behavior is strongly guided by rules. However, this unrealistic picture has been rejected by pragmatist methodologists in favor of a more modest conception of themselves as knowers. A view of the researcher as a "satisficer" has been influential in this regard. The rational behavior of the satisficer is bounded by temporal, computational, and memorial constraints and, as a result, involves the frequent use of heuristic procedures. Heuristic procedures are "rules of thumb" which have the following characteristics (Wimsatt 1981): (a) the correct use of heuristics does not guarantee a correct solution, nor even that a solution will be found; (b) heuristics are cost-effective procedures, making considerably fewer demands on time, effort, and computation than equivalent algorithmic procedures; (c) errors made in using heuristic procedures are systematically biased. Glaser and Strauss's grounded theory perspective on ethnographic methodology, which has been endorsed and used by a number of feminist methodologists, makes considerable use of heuristic procedures.

6.4 Coherence Justification

Feminist scholars have frequently attacked positivist empiricism for justifying its knowledge claims by appealing to a privileged base of observational data. However, foundationalist theories of justification have been widely rejected in contemporary philosophy, and coherentist approaches to justification are being presented as an attractive option. As noted above, Nelson's (1990) neo-Quinean framework for feminist science explicitly adopts a coherence perspective on justification. Also, coherence justification has begun to receive consideration within educational research methodology (Lakomski 1991). And in an important contribution to scientific methodology, Thagard (1989) has developed a new theory of explanatory coherence that is capable of evaluating competing hypotheses in science as well as in everyday affairs. Based on principles that establish the local coherence between a hypothesis and other propositions, Thagard's approach is able to integrate considerations of explanatory breadth, simplicity, and analogy into an overall gauge of explanatory coherence. Thagard's view of theory appraisal as explanatory coherence is a significant postpositivist contribution to a neglected aspect of research methodology that can be implemented widely in areas of research that boast competing explanatory theories.

These are just some of the features of a contemporary pragmatic realist methodology. A comprehensive formulation of such a methodology has been outlined by Nickles (1987) and is exemplified in Wimsatt's (1981) study of reductionism in biology. With its rejection of the methodologies of positivist empiricism, naive realism, and strong versions of social constructivism, pragmatic realism recommends itself as an attractive option. The feminist research enterprise stands to strengthen its hand by taking the pragmatic realist turn in methodology. For its part, pragmatic realism would be enriched by assimilating the gains made by feminist methodology since the late 1970s.

7. Conclusion

Feminist social science research in the 1970s operated largely from the confines of positivist empiricist methodology, but since that time virtually all developments in feminist methodology have been critical of positivism. The feminist methodology of the early 1990s is postpositivist in a number of ways. Although some feminists sought to develop a distinctively feminist approach to methodology, most adapted existing research methods to their own purposes. Feminist methodology broadened to include discussion of the three epistemologies of feminist empiricism, feminist standpoint epistemology, and feminist postmodernism. In the light of criticisms of these theories of knowledge, a pragmatic realist perspective on science recommends itself with a methodology that is appropriate for advancing feminist inquiry and social science research generally.

See also: Research in Education: Epistemological Issues

References

Chandler J 1990 Feminism and epistemology. *Metaphilosophy* 21(4): 367–81

Clegg S 1985 Feminist methodology: Fact or fiction? *Quality and Quantity* 19(1): 83–97

Cook J, Fonow M 1986 Knowledge and women's interests: Issues of epistemology and methodology in feminist sociological research. *Sociological Inquiry* 56(1): 2–29

Daly M 1973 *Beyond God the Father: Toward a Philosophy of Women's Liberation.* Beacon Press, Boston, Massachusetts

Eichler M 1988 *Nonsexist Research Methods.* Allen and Unwin, Boston, Massachusetts

Freire P 1972 *Pedagogy of the Oppressed.* Penguin, Harmondsworth

Greenwood J 1989 *Explanation and Experiment in Social Psychological Science.* Springer-Verlag, New York

Harding S 1986 *The Science Question in Feminism.* Cornell University Press, Ithaca, New York

Harding S 1989 Is there a feminist method? In: Tuana N (ed.) 1989 *Feminism and Science.* Indiana University Press, Bloomington, Indiana

Hawkesworth M 1989 Knowers, knowing, known: Feminist theory and claims of truth. *Signs* 14(3): 533–57

Heckman S 1990 *Gender and Knowledge: Elements of a Postmodern Feminism.* Polity Press, Cambridge

Hyde J E 1990 Meta-analysis and the psychology of gender differences. *Signs* 16(1): 55–73

Lakomski G 1989 Against feminist science: Harding and the science question in feminism. *Educ. Phil. Theor.* 21(2): 1–11

Lakomski G (ed.) 1991 Beyond paradigms: Coherentism and holism in educational research. *Int. J. Educ. Res.* 15(6): 499–597

Lather P 1988 Feminist perspectives on empowering research methodologies. *Women's Studies International Forum* 11(6): 569–81

Mies M 1983 Towards a methodology for feminist research.

In: Bowles G, Klein R D (eds.) 1983 *Theories of Womens Studies*. Routledge and Kegan Paul, London

Nelson L 1990 *Who Knows: From Quine to a Feminist Empiricism*. Temple University Press, Philadelphia, Pennsylvania

Nickles T 1981 What is a problem that we might solve it? *Synthese* 47(1): 85–118

Nickles T 1987 Methodology, heuristics and rationality. In: Pitt J, Pera M (eds.) 1987 *Rational Changes in Science*. Reidel, Dordrecht

Parlee M 1979 Psychology and women. *Signs* 5(1): 121–33

Peplau L, Conrad E 1989 Beyond nonsexist research: The perils of feminist methods in psychology. *Psychol. Women Q.* 13(4): 379–400

Reinharz S 1983 Experiential analysis: A contribution to feminist research. In: Bowles G, Klein R D (eds.) 1983 *Theories of Womens Studies*. Routledge and Kegan Paul, London

Rosenau P 1992 *Postmodernism and the Social Sciences*. Princeton University Press, Princeton, New Jersey

Seigfried C 1991 Where are all the pragmatist feminists? *Hypatia* 6(2): 1–20

Stacey J 1988 Can there be a feminist ethnography? *Women's Studies International Forum* 11(2): 21–27

Strauss A 1987 *Qualitative Analysis for Social Scientists*. Cambridge University Press, Cambridge

Thagard P 1989 Explanatory coherence. *Behavioral and Brain Sciences* 12(3): 435–67

Wilkinson S 1986 Sighting possibilities: Diversity and commonality in feminist research. In: Wilkinson S (ed.) 1986 *Feminist Social Psychology*. Open University Press, Milton Keynes

Wimsatt W 1981 Robustness, reliability, and overdetermination. In: Brewer M, Collins B (eds.) 1981 *Scientific Inquiry and the Social Sciences*. Jossey-Bass, San Francisco, California

Further Reading

Fonow M, Cook J (eds.) 1991 *Beyond Methodology*. Indiana University Press, Bloomington, Indiana

Jayaratne T E 1983 The value of quantitative methodology for feminist research. In: Bowles G, Duelli Kline R (eds.) 1983 *Theories of Women's Studies*. Routledge and Kegan Paul, London

Lather P 1991 *Getting Smart: Feminist Research and Pedagogy with / in the Postmodern*. Routledge, New York

Reinharz S 1992 *Feminist Methods in Social Research*. Oxford University Press, New York

Stanley L, Wise S 1983 *Breaking Out: Feminist Consciousness and Feminist Research*. Routledge and Kegan Paul, London

Tomm W (ed.) 1989 *The Effects of Feminist Approaches on Research Methodologies*. Wilfrid Laurier University Press, Waterloo

Hermeneutics

P-J. Ödman and D. Kerdeman

Until the nineteenth century, "hermeneutics" was commonly defined as "the art (or science) of interpretation (especially of the Bible)." As a consequence of contributions by Schleiermacher, Dilthey, and late existential philosophers such as Heidegger and Gadamer, the meaning of the term has changed. No longer does hermeneutics refer solely to methods of textual exegesis and interpretation. Hermeneutics also describes a philosophical position which regards understanding and interpretation as endemic to and a definitive mark of human existence and social life.

For this entry hermeneutics will be defined as the theory and practice of interpretation and understanding (German, *Verstehen*) in different kinds of human contexts (religious as well as secular, scientific, and quotidian). Several different topics fall under the rubric of this definition. Hermeneutics embraces discussions about: (a) the methodological foundation of the human sciences (German, *Geisteswissenschaften*); (b) the phenomenology of existence and existential understanding; (c) systems of interpretation, used by people to reach the meaning behind myths, symbols, and actions (Palmer 1969). To this list might be added debates concerning: (d) theories of the process of interpretation and the validity of interpretative claims; (e) empirically oriented schools of research that study people in social contexts. It should be noted, however, that many still define hermeneutics as the theory of biblical exegesis, general philological methodology, and the science of linguistic understanding (Palmer 1969).

1. Differences in Relation to Other Traditions of Thought

Hermeneutics is not the only philosophical tradition that regards understanding and interpretation as central to social life. During the twentieth century, a number of other philosophies have come to embrace this position. While they and hermeneutics share many of the same assumptions, it is helpful to sketch some of the differences that make hermeneutics unique.

1.1 Phenomenology

Like hermeneutics, phenomenology is concerned with the structure of understanding. Phenomenology, however, construes understanding primarily in terms of cognitive constructs and functions. For hermeneutics, by contrast, understanding is not only a cognitive function: it also is the ontological condition of human existence. Moreover, while hermeneutics stresses the social nature of meaning, it is not altogether clear whether meaning for phenomenology is primarily subjective or social.

1.2 Wittgenstein's Later Philosophy

Both hermeneutics and the later philosophy of Ludwig Wittgenstein (1889–1951) posit that meaning resides in the conventions and practices of ordinary social life. Meaning, in other words, is not fixed by the rules of an ideal grammar or calculus but instead is negotiated, conditioned, practical, and fluid. Wittgenstein, however, believed that there is no structure common to all "language games" which philosophical analysis could uncover and use to mediate between different life-forms. Hermeneutics, by contrast, holds that mediation between different life-forms is possible. Indeed, articulating the conditions that make mediation or translation possible constitutes a central problem of hermeneutics. Additionally, hermeneutics looks upon language as the mode by which Being is revealed. No such concern for Being characterizes linguistic analysis.

1.3 Critical Theory

Both hermeneutics and critical theory maintain that understanding and meaning are constitutive of social life. Hermeneutics, however, holds that since one's present situation always is involved in any process of understanding, it is impossible to grasp in any final or definitive form all of the meanings embedded in a tradition. Hermeneutics thus eschews the quest to ground understanding in a theoretical framework or method and concentrates instead on interpreting cultures from within given situations and contexts. Critical theory, by contrast, regards understanding as only one interest in the constitution of culture. It aims, therefore, to situate understanding within a broader or more universal explanatory framework, the purpose of which is to make transparent the ways in which ideology informs and conditions not only understanding but all of the interests and relations that constitute social life. (see *Critical Theory and Education*)

1.4 Marxism

Unlike Marxism, the underlying theory of hermeneutics is not primarily materialistic. Moreover, hermeneutics does not focus on the question of historical determinism. Rather, several branches of hermeneutics emphasize freedom in human action.

2. Purpose of Hermeneutics

The purpose of hermeneutics is to increase understanding as regards other cultures, groups, individuals, conditions, and life-styles, present as well as past. The process must be mutual, implying an increase in self-understanding on the part of subject and interpreter alike. Moreover, hermeneutics aims to clarify its own working principles, to "understand understanding." This goal is realized not through the application of method but by bringing into focus the deep assumptions and meanings that inform everyday existence.

Hermeneutics can contribute much to both the practice of education and to educational research. A hermeneutically oriented educator would endeavor, for example, to interpret the meaning that educational practices and conventions hold for those who experience and participate in them. Such an educator might also try to understand various groups of pupils and their life-styles. Additionally, he or she would accentuate the significance of mutual understanding, such as that between teachers and pupils or between pupils of different backgrounds.

Insofar as research is concerned, hermeneutics can deepen the understanding of education by focusing on the meanings that underlie specific educational strategies and practices. A hermeneutic approach to inquiry would explore questions such as the following. How should certain administrative practices be understood? What are their hidden meanings? How might phenomena such as time-scheduling or the separation of learning into different subject-areas be interpreted in a broader cultural and historical context? By means of which educational and teaching strategies is cultural reproduction realized (Bourdieu and Passeron 1970)? Answers to such questions often are given as interpretations through which understanding is promoted.

3. Understanding, Preunderstanding, and Interpretation

The concept of "understanding" can only be defined with the help of analogies and synonyms. The original literal meaning of the term may have been, "to stand close to or under something," or "to place something close to or under oneself." To stand close to something breeds a sense of familiarity. One knows well that to which one is close; one is understanding it. In other words, one is seeing it. The analogy with seeing is appropriate, because it coincides with linguistic practice. In many languages, "to see" connotes "to understand." Often, in fact, the two verbs are used interchangeably.

According to hermeneutics, the idea of familiarity is essential to the interpretative process. Insofar as familiarity obtains, a person to some extent already has understood that which he or she is trying to interpret. This preliminary understanding is known in the hermeneutic tradition as "preunderstanding."

To illustrate the notion of preunderstanding, it is helpful to think about how sense is made of problematic sections in texts. When a difficult passage or word in a narrative is encountered the reader tries to see how that particular part of the text fits within the pattern of the work as whole. Now, the reader may not completely understand the whole text. Indeed, insofar as he or she finds certain passages opaque, understanding is precluded from being complete or absolutely clear. Nonetheless, on some level the reader already does understand the text, albeit in a preliminary way. For without at least a dim sense of familiarity with the work as a whole, there would be no context within which to make sense of or relate individual parts. In this respect, preunderstanding makes reflective understanding possible: it functions as a structure, a whole within the limits of which reflective understanding evolves.

If preunderstanding of an entire text makes it possible to grasp its parts, so the clearer the reader becomes with respect to its parts, and the more clearly the whole narrative will be understood. New dimensions of the text may be noticed. Thus in coming reflectively to understand the parts, the sense of the whole is revitalized.

In short, hermeneutic understanding begins with an inchoate sense of a text in its entirety. At the same time, it is only by probing and analyzing its parts that the whole of a text can be constituted. In this respect, preunderstanding and understanding mutually inform and refine each other. The dialectical relationship of preliminary and reflective understanding is known as the "hermeneutic circle." By means of the hermeneutic circle, texts are clarified or interpreted. According to contemporary hermeneutics, the circular process of preunderstanding, understanding, and interpretation describes more than a method of textual exegesis. Insofar as understanding is central to human existence, the hermeneutic circle captures how ordinary people experience and make sense of life.

4. Historical Background

The word "hermeneutics" derives from Greek antiquity. The Greek verb *hermeneuein* (to interpret) and the noun *hermeneia* (interpretation) are the sources of the modern concept. Additionally, hermeneutics is associated with Hermes, who was both the messenger of and interpreter for the Greek gods. Hermes is also associated with the discovery of language and writing, the most important tools for grasping meaning and conveying it to others (Palmer 1969).

4.1 Hermeneutics as Biblical Exegesis

Biblical exegesis has a very long tradition, dating back to the time of the Hebrew Bible. Indeed, canons for interpreting the Hebrew Bible already had been developed by the first century AD. By the Middle Ages, two main approaches to interpreting both the Hebrew and Christian Bibles had come into use. One approach endeavored to interpret the text literally, spelling out meanings that were already more or less explicit. Over time the literal approach to biblical exegesis became more directed toward reconstructing the historical meaning of biblical texts. The second approach was more concerned with symbolic content. Since the text was regarded as a message from God, it had to be interpreted allegorically. The purpose of allegorical interpretation was to reconstruct or uncover divine meanings not literally apparent.

With the Enlightenment, the scope of hermeneutics broadened. Entering the field of philological research, hermeneutics took a critical first step into the world of modern science. This move had important consequences for biblical exegesis. As an object of philological interpretation, the Bible became simply one among many objects of interpretation; classical and legal texts also were subjected to interpretative philological exegesis. In this respect, literal interpretation constituted an important bridge between interpretation as biblical exegesis and interpretation as a tool for scientific purposes.

4.2 Hermeneutics as "The Art of Understanding"

The German theologian and philosopher Friedrich Schleiermacher (1768–1834) was the first to formulate a new direction for hermeneutics. In Schleiermacher's view, understanding was not automatic: it was an achievement, a coming to grips with meaning which was opaque and problematic. Accordingly, Schleiermacher did not focus on hermeneutics as a body of practical rules: his aim, rather, was to examine the conditions that make understanding possible. How was it, Schleiermacher wondered, that understanding was accomplished? Answering this question, Schleiermacher hoped to establish hermeneutics as the discipline of understanding.

For Schleiermacher, understanding consisted of two elements, one grammatical and one psychological. The relationship between these two elements is dialectical. In grammatical interpretation, the work is interpreted in terms of its linguistic principles, while psychological interpretation aims to interpret a text with regard to the thoughts and feelings of its author. The interpreter does this by identifying with the author's life and situation.

Schleiermacher's conception of understanding was rooted in the principle of the hermeneutic circle. In grammatical interpretation, a work is regarded as a context of meaning. Within this context, specific parts are elucidated, even as the explication of parts makes the entire context intelligible. For its part, psychological interpretation is founded on intuition. In the act of divining an author's intended meaning, the interpreter grasps an inchoate sense of the whole text which he or she will subsequently refine.

4.3 Hermeneutics as the Theoretical Foundation of the Human Sciences

The German philosopher Wilhelm Dilthey

(1833–1911) extended the application of hermeneutics from the interpretation of texts to the whole field of human studies. His line of thought led in ontological as well as methodological directions. Dilthey's thinking can be summarized as an enormous widening of the hermeneutic circle. His central concepts were experience (*Erlebnis*), expression (*Ausdruck*), and understanding (*Verstehen*). Experience for Dilthey had a much broader connotation than it has today: "one may call each encompassing unity of parts of life bound together through a common meaning for the course of life an 'experience'—even when the several parts are separated from each other by interrupting events" (Palmer 1969). Dilthey, in other words, held that people understand discrete life-experiences by assigning them a special place within an experiential whole. At the same time, one singular experience can change the way a person understands himself or herself and his or her life. The very experience of life, in short, is characterized by Dilthey as a continuous interaction between "wholes" and "parts."

The following example illustrates Dilthey's ideas. A teacher wishes to understand why a certain pupil is having difficulty. In order to make sense of the phenomenon, the teacher situates the problem within the context of his or her experience as an instructor. The teacher has previously seen that lack of interest on the part of parents greatly influences a child's progress in school. This understanding prompts the teacher to ask the child how he or she gets along at home; the teacher learns that relations between the child and the parents are very cold. By drawing on his or her experience to clarify the child's situation, the teacher achieves a better understanding of how to help the student. By the same token, understanding the situation of this particular student refines and enriches the teacher's entire instructional experience.

By "expression" Dilthey had in mind all the manifestations or "objectifications" of human experience, even those that are unintentional and nonverbal. Life-expressions, in other words, objectify or make concrete a person's understanding of life. Although expressions of meaning are personal, they are not created in a vacuum, Dilthey says. It is only by drawing on the common stock of meanings embedded in one's culture that an individual is able to express what experience means to him or her.

According to Dilthey, reflective understanding or "interpretation" consists in recovering the intimate connection between experience and expression. In explicating the meaning of a concrete expression, the interpreter brings to light not only the way a particular individual has understood his or her life-experience: because life-expressions are embedded in historical contexts, the interpreter illuminates a cultural milieu as well. As a consequence, an otherwise distant world comes alive in the present. The following example illustrates Dilthey's theory.

A Swedish educational historian seeks to interpret the meaning of some financial accounts which a gymnasium student in the seventeenth century gave to his headmaster. The accounts tell how much money the student collected during one of his wanderings. (Wanderings were common during this period and formed an important source of income for Scandinavian schools.) The interpreter's first task is to clarify the expressions; that is, the meaning of the symbols used in the student's accounts. Second, an attempt should be made to detect the personal experiences that these particular accounts express. Finally, the interpreter must reconstruct the context of forgotten meanings which characterized the practice of wandering and shaped the lives of Scandinavian students during the seventeenth century. In so doing, the interpreter unites the past (the student and his historical context) with the present world of contemporary readers and their preunderstandings.

In extending the hermeneutic circle to the domain of life experience, Dilthey at once both deepened and broadened the concept of "understanding." In particular, Dilthey's vision underscored the situational nature of the interpretative precess. This insight profoundly influenced the development of existential hermeneutics in the twentieth century. No longer was understanding seen as the result of interpretation: with Dilthey, ordinary understanding was transformed into the existential ground from which reflective interpretation derives.

Dilthey hoped to demonstrate how the understanding that occurs in quotidian experience could ground a theory of human science. For Dilthey, however, the scientific study of social life posed an intractable dilemma. Ordinary understanding makes use of part–whole relations conditioned by particular historical contexts. Science, however, demands objectivity, the overcoming of situation. Can an interpretation be at once historically conditioned and also objectively valid? To avoid the threat of relativism, Dilthey felt he had to forgo the condition of historicity. In so doing, he gave up his most profound and influential insight.

5. Hermeneutics as a Phenomenology of Existence

With the German philosophers Martin Heidegger (1889–1976) and Hans-Georg Gadamer (1900–), the existential implications latent in Dilthey's thought became fully developed. According to Heidegger and Gadamer, understanding and interpretation denote how human beings define themselves as beings in the world. In understanding, self and world emerge together: they are fundamentally related.

Understanding is relational in another way as well. Understanding constantly refers to the future. At the same time, it is conditioned by a person's situation: it operates within a totality of already interpreted relations. This relational totality Heidegger called the "world." A teacher entering a classroom can serve as an example. The teacher's understanding of the situation is referenced toward the future: he or she anticipates, for instance, how the pupils will respond to instruction and fears that some of them may cause trouble. Understanding for the teacher also is conditioned by his or her former experience of this class, or by earlier experiences he or she had during the day. In this respect, the teacher's present understanding at once calls up the future and recalls the past.

The linguisticality of understanding is a point stressed by Gadamer (1975). According to Gadamer, language is like a storehouse of assumptions or "prejudices." In this respect, language forms a parameter or "horizon" of possible understandings. This does not mean that language confines individuals to the meanings of particular times and places. Indeed, by means of language, past and present understandings are mediated. Gadamer calls the mediation of past and present a "fusion of horizons."

For Gadamer, a "fusion of horizons" is an interpretative event which demands an attitude of openness on the part of the interpreter. This openness is similar to the kind of attitude with which a person confronts great art. In Gadamer's view, both the encounter with art and the interpretation of historical texts are marked by genuine questioning, founded on a sense of expectancy and a readiness to be changed or transformed by the meaning of a work.

An historian trying to understand a diary written by an elementary school teacher in the nineteenth century illustrates this principle. Based on the way the teacher describes himself in his diary, the historian initially concludes that the teacher was a nice man. As the historian reads further, however, she discovers that in some passages of the the diary, the teacher discusses how he used corporal punishment to discipline his students. When confronted with this information, the historian experiences a clash between her "horizon" of understanding and the world of the teacher. The historian could react by shutting off further efforts to understand. Or, she could ask herself: "How is it possible to make sense of these actions when performed by such a nice person?" In order to reduce her conflict, the historian reads books about the role of corporal punishment in earlier eras of education. Gradually, she comes to see that the teacher in the past was only doing what other teachers and school authorities of his day thought best. The historian also learns that children in the late nineteenth century were not looked upon in the same way as they are in her time. Through a series of questions, then, for which there is a real need to know answers, the historian develops new understanding. In so doing, she extends the limits of her meaning-horizon and lays the groundwork for future understanding.

According to Gadamer, every hermeneutical endeavor proceeds from a stance of openness. In this respect, the interpreter does not "take possession" of the text that he or she interprets. Rather, the interpreter must let the text reveal its world.

6. The Model of the Text

The contribution of the French philosopher Paul Ricoeur to interpretative theory is all-encompassing. It can be described as an effort to synthesize the problems and insights of hermeneutics from Aristotle to the late twentieth century. In one of his definitions, Ricoeur calls hermeneutics "the theory of rules that governs an exegesis, that is to say, an interpretation of a particular text or collection of signs susceptible of being considered as a text" (Palmer 1969 p. 43). For Ricoeur, the literal meaning of a text or system of symbols constitutes a closed world. This view parallels that of structural analysis, which studies language as a closed system of signs. A text also represents an open system, Ricoeur explained, because it refers to a world that exists outside of itself. In this respect, texts-as-discourse are similar to oral discourse, which is characterized by nonverbal signs and cues that direct the attention of the participants to circumstances and facts beyond the immediate discourse situation (Ricoeur 1971). Unlike oral discourse, however, texts are not limited to particular contexts. This is because texts refer not to situations but to worlds.

Texts, therefore, can be regarded in two different ways. First a text can be viewed as representing a closed system of signs. From this perspective, the aim of interpretation is to clarify the meaning inherent in words. Ricoeur calls this the "archaeological" aspect of hermeneutics. Owing to the referential function of words, however, texts also can be viewed as pointing to an existential space. Thus, once the meaning of a text's words has been made evident, the interpreter can focus on the existential world to which the text points. Put differently, once the "what" of the text has been explicated, the "about what" of the text can be sought.

According to Ricoeur, the interpreter in this way moves from what the text says to what it is talking about. This movement, Ricoeur stressed, does not result in an identification with an unknown mentality through acts of empathy (as Schleiermacher thought). On the contrary, the interpreter confronts a world: the world about which the text is talking. Interpretation for Ricoeur is thus not a matter of detecting secrets behind a text. Rather, interpretation is a process of reading the references that constitute a text's existential space. This often entails confronting new perspectives on life through the life-styles of other existential worlds. As a consequence of interpretation and understanding, something heretofore alien becomes part of the interpreter's world, and the interpreter comes to understand himself or herself in a new way. The hermeneutic circle is moving between the interpreter's way of being and the being disclosed by the text.

In Ricoeur's view, all aspects of human communication and activity, including cultural products and

189

artifacts, are analogous to texts. Accordingly, Ricoeur conceived his interpretative schema as pertaining not only to literature but also to the human sciences.

7. Hermeneutic Social Science

Since the late 1960s philosophers and practitioners alike have joined Ricoeur and Gadamer in exploring the implications of hermeneutics for the investigation of social life. A particularly influential contribution was advanced by Taylor (1971). Taylor's conception of human inquiry is anchored by a crucial premise of existential hermeneutics: meaning is not located in the minds of individuals. Rather, meaning consists in matrices of specific intersubjective agreements and understandings which are both constitutive of and expressed in social institutions and practices. Meaning, in short, is not private or subjective in Taylor's model: it is public, relational, and contextual.

This premise, Taylor argues, implies that the logic of hermeneutic inquiry is fundamentally different from the logic of positivistic science which has dominated social research since the nineteenth century. These differences become salient when one compares how hermeneutic and positivistic social science conceive the data of inquiry, the interpretation or explanation of data, and the justification and assessment of interpretative claims.

In the positivist model, physical behavior is distinguished from values, intentions, and goals. The former is observable and "brute identifiable"; the latter are hidden within the psyche, unavailable to sight. Positivist social science, Taylor said, strives to correlate public behaviors with subjective states of mind (Taylor 1971 pp. 18–21). When a significant convergence obtains, events and phenomena are said to be explained.

Such a science is extremely limited, Taylor declares. Because the positivist model regards meaning as hidden and subjective, it vastly underestimates and often just misses the import of social events. Breakdowns in fundamental institutions and practices such as voting, negotiation, and work, for example, represent more than the "public eruption of private pathology." These breakdowns, Taylor says, signal deep crises which represent "a malady of society itself, a malaise which affects its constitutive meanings" (Taylor 1971 p. 41). Like Ricoeur, Taylor argues that changes and crises of meaning per se are not grasped through acts of empathy. Nor can they be explained by subsuming observable sequences of "brute" behavior under general laws. Insofar as the data of social science express "a certain vision of the agent and his relation to others and to society" (Taylor 1971 p. 26), such a science will be unavoidably hermeneutic, less an application of theory and law than a reading of social meaning.

According to the hermeneutic model of inquiry, the only way researchers can justify their interpretations is by pointing to other readings. Man "is a self-interpreting animal," Taylor writes. "He is necessarily so, for there is no such thing as the structure of meanings for him independent of his interpretation of them . . . already to be a living agent is to experience one's situation in terms of certain meanings" (Taylor 1971 p. 16). For Taylor, in short, the justification and acceptance of interpretative claims—no less than their formulation—cannot appeal beyond the hermeneutic circle. Failure to grasp an interpretation is not due to an insufficiency of evidence or an inability to follow the logic of an argument. Inability to see instead derives from a fundamental inadequacy of self-definition which marks out the parameters of possible understanding. It follows, Taylor concludes, that in a hermeneutical science, "a certain measure of insight is indispensable" (Taylor 1971 p. 46). Some interpretations, as a consequence, simply will be "nonarbitrable."

8. Hermeneutics and Validity

The idea that interpretations may resist arbitration is disputed by a number of hermeneuticists. Betti (1967), for example, holds that without theoretical rules of verification, interpretation becomes anarchic. Betti tries to define a method that would allow interpretations to be assessed with "relative objectivity." Since human expressions are objectifications of the human spirit, Betti reasons that it is possible for an interpreter to reconstruct the meaning an author intended. The principle of authorial intention also is propounded by Hirsch (1967). It stands in clear contradiction to the view of Ricoeur, who argues that the author's intention is of secondary interest. This is because texts, when completed, must be regarded as autonomous from their authors.

Whether or not one agrees with Hirsch and Betti, the problem with which they wrestle is crucial. As Heidegger and Gadamer have noted, interpretation is a function of situated engagement: without a context of already interpreted meanings, understanding is impossible. At the same time, emphasis on the situatedness and finitude of interpretative understanding raises the question of whether or not interpretations in principle are decidable (Connolly and Keutner 1988). Is it possible for a hermeneutic philosophy to stay within a historically conditioned circle of understanding and at the same time posit rational principles as conditions for the possible validity or truth of particular claims to understanding (Hoy 1978)? Unless such principles can be articulated, is it clear how competing or conflicting interpretations can be adjudicated, or how the specter of relativism can be avoided?

9. Criteria of Interpretation

One important response to the above questions has

been put forward by Ricoeur. In an essay on the relation between explanation and understanding, Ricoeur argues that the contradiction between the natural and human sciences to a great degree is an artifact (Ricoeur 1986). Texts and other human products can be subjected to explanation in a way similar to that used by the natural sciences. In fact, understanding is impossible without explanation, and, of course, vice versa. Interpretation and understanding are thus promoted by means of logic and argumentation. Moreover, interpretation and understanding often play important roles in the introductory and final stages of scientific research.

The question regarding situatedness and rationality therefore may be wrongly put. Because of its dependence on interpretation and understanding, physical science, no less than hermeneutic philosophy, is always situated within a particular time and place. As Gadamer has stated, there is no position outside our historicity. Humans, therefore, must make themselves aware of their historical situatedness and the preunderstandings that attend this condition (Gadamer 1975). Canons of interpretation, Gadamer maintains, help to achieve this awareness. In Gadamer's view, interpretative processes employ the very rationality and reason that contributed to the birth of the natural sciences.

The main interpretative principle, of course, is that of the hermeneutic circle: the parts of a text and its whole must be checked against each other. By means of the hermeneutic circle, a text can be interpreted mainly in two ways. It can be interpreted literally; or an attempt can be made to reconstruct the world of the text. With respect to literal interpretation, the logic of sentences and actions is often rather strict. It is therefore possible to apply strict logic to check interpretations. One such logical canon holds that an interpretation of phenomena and actions cannot be accepted unless it explains all available relevant information (Trankell 1972). If some important action or meaning in the text as a whole is excluded or only vaguely taken into consideration, the interpretation must be rejected. A second canon holds that an interpretation cannot be fully accepted unless it is the only one that explains the meaning of a research object. In many cases, this second criterion is difficult to satisfy. Even in those successful situations where only one interpretation remains after scrutiny in light of other competing interpretations, there is no guarantee that the interpretation will remain the correct one.

With respect to reconstructing the world to which a text or text-analog refers, the canon of the hermeneutical circle functions as a contextual criterion. According to this principle, every single interpretation must be checked against all available relevant facts, sources, and circumstances in connection with the interpreted object. If knowledge of those facts, sources, and circumstances contradicts the interpretation, it must be rejected or modified. By creating alternative interpretations of the same phenomena, cultural products, actions, or events from the very start, the interpretative process can be systematized. Concomitant with testing his or her main interpretation, then, the interpreter also can judge the validity of alternative interpretations. He or she thereby gradually refines his or her conceptions of the interpreted object.

10. The Position of Hermeneutics

The explosion of existential hermeneutics in the twentieth century has served to challenge a number of dualisms that are deeply rooted in modern epistemology and scientific method. Distinctions between facts and values, explanation and understanding, knowledge and self-knowledge, theory and practice were once regarded as inviolable; now these basic categories are being reconceptualized (Bernstein 1978, Dallmayr and McCarthy 1977). In the process, the relationship between hermeneutics and science with respect to the definition and determination of knowledge has been undergoing change. Some, such as Taylor (1971), have held that the logics driving hermeneutics and science are separate and incompatible. Others, such as Rorty (1979) and Gadamer (1975), have held a very different view. Overturning the old positivist position regarding the universality of science, Rorty and Gadamer have maintained that all knowledge is interpretative. There thus is no essential distinction between science and hermeneutics. Still others, such as Habermas (1973) and Apel (1973), have argued for the integrity of each domain but have posited a dialectical relationship between them.

Within the world of education, hermeneutics has flourished since around 1970, particularly with respect to educational research. The rise of so-called qualitative methods has broadened not only the scope and aim of educational research: it has also prompted investigators to reexamine the principles and aims of social inquiry (see, e.g. Erickson 1986 and the *International Journal of Education Research* 1991.) A surge of interest in interpretative inquiry has prompted a number of important debates with the education community. Issues that have been discussed include the nature of the relationship between interpretative inquiry and more traditionally scientific designs; standards for adjudicating competing or conflicting interpretative claims; and the continued development of interpretative methods.

See also: Research in Education: Epistemological Issues

References

Apel K-O 1973 *Transformation der Philosophie*. Suhrkamp Verlag, Frankfurt
Bernstein R J 1978 *The Restructuring of Social and Political*

Theory. University of Pennsylvania Press, Philadelphia, Pennsylvania

Betti E 1967 *Allgemeine Auslegungslehre als Methodik der Geisteswissenschaften.* Mohr, Tübingen

Bourdieu P, Passeron J-C 1970 *La Reproduction: éléments pour une théorie du système d'enseignement.* Editions de Minuit, Paris

Connolly J M, Keutner T (eds.) 1988 *Hermeneutics versus Science? Three German Views.* University of Notre Dame Press, Notre Dame, Indiana

Dallmayr F R, McCarthy T A (eds.) 1977 *Understanding and Social Inquiry.* University of Notre Dame Press, Notre Dame, Indiana

Erickson F 1986 Qualitative methods in research on teaching. In: Wittrock M C (ed.) 1986 *Handbook of Research on Teaching*, 3rd edn. Macmillan Inc., New York

Gadamer H-G 1975 *Wahrheit und Methode: Grundzüge einer Philosophischen Hermeneutik*, 4th edn. Mohr, Tübingen

Habermas J 1973 *Erkenntnis und Interesse*, 6th edn. Suhrkamp Verlag, Frankfurt

Hirsch E D 1967 *Validity in Intepretation.* Yale University Press, New Haven, Connecticut

Hoy D C 1978 *The Critical Circle: Literature, History, and Philosophical Hermeneutics.* University of California Press, Berkeley, California

International Journal of Educational Research 1991 15(6): (special issue)

Palmer R E 1969 *Hermeneutics: Interpretation Theory in Schleiermacher, Dilthey, Heidegger, and Gadamer.* Northwestern University Press, Evanston, Illinois

Ricoeur P 1971 The model of the text: Meaningful action considered as a text. *Soc. Res.* 38 (3): 529–62

Ricoeur P 1986 Essais d'herméneutique, Vol 2: *Du texte à l'action.* Editions du Seuil, Paris

Rorty R 1979 *Philosophy and the Mirror of Nature.* Princeton University Press, Princeton, New Jersey

Taylor C 1971 Interpretation and the sciences of man. *Rev. Metaphysics* 25 (1): 3–51

Trankell A 1972 *Reliability of Evidence: Methods for Analyzing and Assessing Witness Statements.* Beckman, Stockholm

Further Reading

Bauman Z 1978 *Hermeneutics and Social Science.* Columbia University Press, New York

Bernstein R J 1988 *Beyond Objectivism and Relativism: Science, Hermeneutics, and Praxis.* University of Pennsylvania Press, Philadelphia, Pennsylvania

Bleicher J 1980 *Contemporary Hermeneutics: Hermeneutics as Method, Philosophy and Critique.* Routledge, Chapman and Hall, New York

Bubner R 1981 (trans. Matthews E) *Modern German Philosophy.* Cambridge University Press, Cambridge

Dilthey W 1976 (ed. and trans. Rickman H P) *Selected Writings.* Cambridge University Press, Cambridge

Engdahl H et al. 1977 *Hermeneutik.* Rabén and Sjörgren, Stockholm

Ermarth M 1981 The transformation of hermeneutics: Nineteenth century ancients and twentieth century moderns. *Monist* 64(2): 175–94

Føllesdall D 1979 Hermeneutics and the hypothetico-deductive method. *Dialectica* 33 (3–4): 319–36

Habermas J 1981 *Theorie des Kommunikativen Handelns*, Vol. 1, *Handlungsrationalität und Gesellschaftliche Rationalisierung.* Suhrkamp Verlag, Frankfurt

Habermas J 1981 *Theorie des Kommunikativen Handelns*, Vol. 2, *Zur Kritik der Funktionalistischen Vernunft*, 3rd edn. Surhkamp Verlag, Frankfurt

Heidegger M 1977 *Sein und Zeit.* Klostermann, Frankfurt

Howard R J 1982 *Three Faces of Hermeneutics: An Introduction to Current Theories of Understanding.* University of California Press, Berkeley, California

Gadamer H G 1977 (trans and ed. Linge D E) *Philosophical Hermeneutics: Hans-Georg Gadamer.* University of California Press, Berkeley, California

Mueller-Vollmer K (ed.) 1985 *The Hermeneutics Reader.* Continuum, New York

Ödman P-J 1979 *Tolkning, Förstaåelse, Vetande: Hermeneutik i teori och praktik.* AWE/Gebers, Stockholm

Ödman P-J 1992 Interpreting the Past. *International Journal of Qualitative Studies in Education* 5 (2): 167–84

Ormiston G, Schrift A (eds.) 1990 *The Hermeneutic Tradition: From Ast to Ricoeur.* State University of New York Press, Albany, New York

Rabinow P, Sullivan W (eds.) 1979 *Interpretive Social Science: A Reader.* University of California Press, Berkeley, California

Ricoeur P 1965 *De l'interpretation: essai sur Freud.* Editions du Seuil, Paris

Ricoeur P 1981 (trans. and ed. Thompson J) *Hermeneutics and the Human Sciences.* Cambridge University Press, Cambridge

Ricoeur P 1984–88 (trans. McLaughlin Pellauer D) *Time and Narrative*, 3 Vols. University of Chicago Press, Chicago, Illinois

Taylor C 1985 *Human Agency and Language: Philosophical Papers*, Vol. 1. Cambridge University Press, Cambridge

Taylor C 1985 *Philosophy and the Human Sciences: Philosophical Papers*, Vol. 2. Cambridge University Press, Cambridge

Thompson J B 1981 *Critical Hermeneutics: A Study in the Thought of Paul Ricoeur and Jürgen Habermas.* Cambridge University Press, Cambridge

Wachterhauser B (ed.) 1986 *Hermeneutics and Modern Philosophy.* State University of New York Press, Albany, New York

Legitimatory Research

J. P. Keeves

The rapidly growing interest in policy-oriented research has led to the need to distinguish between those programs of research that are associated with the generation of change, and those research activities that serve to maintain and consolidate existing situations. Educational organizations hold considerable power over the lives of the individuals within them, and it is not surprising that in education there should be a strong reciprocal relationship between power and knowledge. Power on the one hand controls the use and flow of knowledge. On the other hand knowledge is used to support existing arrangements for the exercising of power. Legitimatory research is that type of research which is undertaken to strengthen and maintain existing power structures in educational systems as well as the policies and practices operating within those systems. The term "legitimatory" is used because the research is conducted with the express purpose of legitimating existing arrangements for the exercising of power from the perspectives of the institution supporting the research and controlling the release of the findings.

This entry discusses the characteristics of research carried out within this perspective. It is also concerned with the nature of the legitimatory process, and examines the functions of legitimatory research.

1. Policy-oriented Research

Investigations in the field of education are increasingly being planned with a strong policy orientation. The purpose of such research is to provide information for decision-making with respect to educational policy and practice. Administrators and politicians recognize the usefulness of evidence to which they can add their own value judgments before embarking on a course of action that involves the development and implementation of new policy. When research into an educational problem is designed, conducted, and reported with the specific aim of providing information for the making of policy, or for monitoring the implementation of policy, or for examining the effects of existing policy, then the term "policy-oriented research" is used. Research of this type in the field of education is becoming more common as politicians and administrators seek and achieve greater control over the allocation of the funds available for research and evaluation studies. Consequently it is not surprising that Weiss (1979), in a classification of ways in which social science research might be utilized, has identified a political approach and a tactical approach that are related to the legitimatory research discussed in this entry. Husén

(1984), however, argues that Weiss's seven models may be merged into only two major ones, and that the political and tactical approaches are best combined. It is this combined model that is referred to here as a legitimatory approach to research utilization. In addition, Suchman (1970) has listed the possible misuses of evaluation, which correspond to a legitimatory approach to evaluative research. The growing incidence of such research has led to this more detailed examination of its nature and purpose.

There are types of policy-oriented research in education that have been developed with the particular purpose of introducing change. They combine investigation, educational development, and, in general, the promotion of social change. Two important types of research in this area are known as "action research" and "participatory research." In participatory research, for example, the researcher with specialized knowledge and training commonly joins people in the workplace, and together they undertake an investigation which seeks primarily to improve education and, through education, to improve the lives of those people involved. It is clear that people undertaking this type of policy-oriented research are not neutral in the value judgments which they bring to the conduct of an investigation. Thus, in participatory research in particular, there is a commitment to the processes of change in order to benefit and sometimes emancipate those engaged in the investigation.

It is also possible for research to be carried out with the specific purposes of preventing change, or obtaining evidence to support an existing institution or organization, or to maintain an existing policy. The systematic collection of educational statistics on: (a) the numbers of schools of different kinds; (b) the numbers of enrolled students, teachers and ancillary staff; and (c) the average numbers of students in daily attendance can be seen as simple examples of this type of legitimatory research. Commonly, although such information is collected and tabulated, it is generally published only in part and not in a form that would permit the evidence being used against the educational organization involved. The data are held and employed in situations and in ways that support the organization and do not permit the organization to be challenged.

Giddens (1984) has discussed certain aspects of the dissemination of research findings. He suggests that an investigation can be undertaken from perspectives where

the new knowledge or information is used to sustain existing circumstances. This may, of course, happen even where the theories or findings concerned could, if utilized in certain ways, modify what they describe. The selective appropriation of social science material by the powerful, for example, can turn that material to ends quite other than those that might be served if they were widely disseminated. (p.342)

This type of research that is frequently neither conspicuous nor publicized is commonly undertaken within large educational bureaucracies that have not only the necessary resources to support such research, but also the responsibility to maintain an educational system.

Since, in general, such investigations are carried out to legitimate existing policies and practices, the term "legitimatory research" is appropriate. The findings from research conducted within this perspective are commonly not released as a scholarly publication. They remain as "in house" reports that are summarized in a few pages for administrators and policymakers to read. An example arising from the compilation of educational statistics may contribute to an understanding of how this type of research activity operates. If the information on the average numbers of students by age in daily attendance in some educational systems were examined by critics, they would probably note a very high level of absenteeism at age levels near the end of compulsory schooling. Since it is generally not in the interests of schools and school systems that disruptive students should be present in classrooms, it is considered preferable that this information should not be released, even though it is relevant in a significant way to educational and social problems related to juvenile delinquency. Furthermore, such absenteeism might be perceived to be a consequence of inadequate teaching or of irrelevant curricula.

In some countries, this type of research has very limited visibility, although it is relatively widespread and obtains regular funding at the expense of more impartial and scholarly work. Within most large educational organizations, such as universities, local educational authorities, national and state offices of education and indeed within teacher unions, there are research units that seek to maintain existing policies and support established institutions. The research conducted within these units is largely of a legitimatory nature. A very wide variety of investigatory activity is involved. It may range from the examination of pass rates and studies of prediction of success in universities, to the monitoring of standards of educational achievement in state and national systems, or to studies of teacher stress by teacher unions. The findings from such investigations are only released and widely publicized when it is of value politically to use the information available to support existing policies and practices.

2. Power and Knowledge

Legitimation is a social process. Power and authority are not, in general, assigned or transmitted at a single point in time to an educational organization, or an individual within an organization, but are acquired gradually over time. Power and authority can never be taken for granted. They are constantly being challenged and exposed to competing claims. Consequently, legitimation becomes a continuously operating process. Without legitimation, power and authority are insecure and impermanent.

The concept of legitimation owes much to the writings of Weber, who was concerned with belief in a legitimate order:

Action, especially social action which involves social relationships, may be oriented by the actors to a belief (*Vorstellung*) in the existence of a "legitimate order." The probability that action will actually empirically be so oriented will be called the "validity" (*Geltung*) of the order in question. (Henderson and Parsons 1947 p. 124)

The link between these ideas and the development and use of knowledge was made by Berger and Luckmann (1967 p. 110). They saw legitimation as a "second-order" process that operated on the "first-order" ideas and relationships concerning society and social institutions in such a way as to develop new meanings that would make this knowledge "objectively available and subjectively plausible." In this sense it validates institutionalized knowledge and an institutional order. Thus it is possible to speak not only of the legitimation of a social institution but also of the legitimation of knowledge through the production of new knowledge.

More recently the writings of Habermas (1976) have sounded a warning about the crisis of legitimacy faced by public administration. The argument advanced in *Legitimation Crisis*, is that the increasing intervention of the state in the economy is accompanied by the translation of political issues into technical problems. This leads to greater technical control and the growing dominance of knowledge and information in the service of the state's interests. At the center of this policy of "technocratic consciousness" is what Weber has referred to as "means–ends rationality". As a first step, knowledge is used by the bureaucracy to achieve specific goals. As a second step the criterion of efficiency is employed to choose between competing goals. Subsequently, basic cultural values are evaluated in terms of their efficiency. Finally, the most rational and efficient course of action is identified by recourse to computer analyses. In his writings Habermas postulates four areas of crises: (a) an economic crisis, (b) a rationality crisis, (c) a motivation crisis, and (d) a legitimation crisis. This work has been used to contest established views of institutional governance, particularly in the field of education (see, e.g., Pusey 1979, Hicks 1979, Kemmis et al. 1983).

Research is concerned with organized and systematic activities which are designed to produce knowledge. Consequently legitimatory research involves the compilation of new knowledge that will strengthen a social institution and will validate institutionalized knowledge. In the field of education, research can contribute in a significant way to the legitimation of social institutions and to the support of educational organizations and their policies, programs, and practices. However, educational research is a pursuit that is itself in need of validation, and the support for research provided by educational organizations serves to legitimate research as an activity. Thus educational institutions both validate and are validated by educational research. The dependence of educational research on educational organizations for financial and operational support, together with the contribution that research makes toward maintaining the educational organizations pose certain problems for educational research. Consequently, research that is undertaken at the request of, and with financial support from, an educational organization in order to support the continuance and to maintain the operation of that organization as well as its existing policies and practices, can appropriately be referred to as "legitimatory research."

3. Characteristics of Legitimatory Research

Relatively few studies have been carried out to examine the processes and characteristics of legitimatory research. Although it has had a long-standing presence in many educational organizations, it has only been with the emergence of the field of policy-oriented research that its nature and function have become clear. Some characteristics of legitimatory research and the processes through which such research is conducted are listed below.

(a) The *problem* to be investigated arises from existing policies and practices within an educational organization. This, of course, is not unique to legitimatory research.

(b) The major *aim of the research* is to maintain the existing structure of an educational organization, and the continuance of its existing policies and practices.

(c) Legitimatory research is generally *conducted by people* with competence in research who are employed by the educational organization, so that the organization maintains control over the entire investigation.

(d) In general, *the focus of the research* is on the operation of the organization, on the activities of the people within it, or on the characteristics of those who seek entry into the organization

(e) Central to the operation of legitimatory research is its role in providing information in a concise form for the senior educational administrators in order to *consolidate their position of power* within an organization.

(f) *The release of the findings* of the research is, in general, controlled by a senior administrator to occur at a time to optimize the impact that the findings might have on the legitimation of a particular position, policy, or practice.

(g) It is rare for *the publication* of the findings of legitimatory research to be in a form that would enable both the methods of investigation and the inferences drawn from the research to be examined critically and challenged. The reports are commonly only circulated in summary form on the grounds that the likely readers are interested only in the main conclusions of the investigation, and would not be interested in examining the available evidence in any detail.

(h) Where the investigation is undertaken by research workers who are outside the day-to-day operation of the organization, *a steering committee* is commonly set up to exercise control over the conduct of the investigation.

(i) If the research workers are external to the organization problems may arise over the publication of the reports of a study. Lynn and Jay (1982 pp. 97–99) draw a distinction between the *suppression of a research report* and the making of a decision *not to publish* it. In addition, they list the steps that can be taken to discredit research reports and so prevent their publication.

(j) Frequently, legitimatory research is conducted under the guise of an *evaluation study*, since the need for evaluation is widely acknowledged on the grounds of accountability, yet what is being sought is information to sustain a program or policy in its existing form.

To illustrate these characteristics of legitimatory research an example is provided below.

4. A Study of Staffing and Resources: An Example

In this example, where an independent research organization was commissioned to work with eight educational organizations, some of the problems that can arise in a legitimatory research study were encountered.

The major expenditure in Australian schooling, as in other countries, is on the salaries of teachers, which commonly comprise about 80 percent or more of the total budget allocated to the provision of education in schools. Since education in Australia is a responsibility of the states and not of the commonwealth or federal government, the proportion of the total state budgets allocated to education in schools is high, generally of the order of 25 percent. Overall, approximately 5 percent of gross domestic product (GDP) is spent on education in Australia.

Clearly the total expenditure on the salaries of the teaching service is a matter of considerable economic significance.

Following a long period of militancy by the teacher unions in Australia during the late 1960s and early 1970s directed toward decreasing class sizes, funds were made available for marked reductions in student–teacher ratios and thus class sizes. As could be anticipated, this was accompanied by a very substantial increase in the costs of education that had to be provided at the expense of other activities conducted by the state governments. The ministers of education within New Zealand and each of the Australian state and commonwealth governments, together with their advisers, who are the senior administrators in their educational bureaucracies, meet regularly to develop common policies for the conduct of education in their regions. In the mid-1970s the ministers of education and, to a lesser extent, the directors-general of education recognized that if they were to pursue policies for the broad general growth of their regions as well as for the general development of education, it would be necessary to contain the pressure from the teacher unions for further reductions in class sizes. Thus they were placed in a position of seeking to maintain current policies and practices, and the existing structures of their organizations, without becoming committed to policy changes that would involve a further reduction in student–teacher ratios and class sizes.

As a first step, a review of previous research into class size was commissioned (Lafleur et al. 1974). This review found that little research work had been carried out in Australia, and there were inconclusive findings with regard to the effects of class size on achievement and attitude. However, it should be noted that in Australia the First International Mathematics Study conducted by the International Association for the Evaluation of Educational Achievement (IEA) in 1964, and the First IEA Science Study in 1970 had both found relationships which indicated that, at the 13- and 14-year old levels respectively, the larger the classes the higher the average levels of achievement of the students. These relationships remained significant even after other relevant factors on which data were collected had been taken into account. Although it was difficult to account for these findings, they left much to be explained with regard to the sustained demand for further reductions in class sizes, in terms of effects on achievement outcomes.

In 1978, the results of the meta-analysis by Glass and Smith (1978) into the relationships between class size and achievement were published. The findings from this study received widespread publicity and were hailed with acclaim by the teacher unions. More recently, the criticism of the work of Glass and Smith that have been made by Slavin (1984a, 1984b) have cast serious doubt on the findings of a meaningful relationship between class size and achievement.

However, for a period of several years the work of Glass and Smith was accepted as authoritative throughout Australia and New Zealand.

The Australian Education Council, at its meeting in 1978, expressed interest in the complex questions associated with student–teacher ratios and class sizes and commissioned a study into these problems which would be undertaken in collaboration with the staff of the research branches of the education departments in each of the regions. This study became known as the "Staffing and Resources Study." The initial reports of the work of Glass and Smith had a significant impact on the planning of this study. It was argued by some that further investigations of a nonexperimental kind to examine relationships between class size and achievement were of doubtful value. Nevertheless, it was considered that if a study of teaching behavior could be undertaken which would examine relationships between such behaviors and class size it would be highly relevant. However, it was decided that the main thrust of the study would be to examine general policies and practices at the level of school systems and schools.

The ministers of education sought a study that would examine the costs of education and, in particular, relationships involving the contribution of reductions in class size to the costs and to the benefits, if any, in terms of achievement outcomes and students' and teachers' attitudes. Immediately after work on this study into a highly sensitive area was authorized, pressures were mounted to distort the study and its design so that only peripheral issues would be investigated. Thus the ministers and some of the senior administrators sought a study which would legitimate existing departmental policies. However, the forces for change in Australian education, such as the teacher unions, and some staff at the middle and lower management levels in the bureaucracies sought to modify the plans for the study so that it would generate change. The research workers who were members of an independent educational research organization and who had accepted responsibility for the conduct of the study, were not fully aware at the time the study was commissioned of the tensions that were likely to develop in the study. These tensions were a result of the conflict between the forces of conservatism that sought a legitimatory research study, and innovative educational practitioners who sought to alter the design of the investigation and the conduct of research in ways that focused on the need for change and the directions in which change should proceed.

The legitimatory nature of this study which was carried out at the request of the ministers of education, who were responsible for eight educational systems, led to sustained attacks on the study from both inside and outside these eight systems. While the senior administrators within the eight systems were willing for a detailed examination of policies and practices to be carried out within each system by their own staff, some were unwilling for this information to be made available to the other systems or to external investigators who would be comparing and contrasting the operations of the eight systems. Moreover, in one system a teacher's union prevented the undertaking of a survey of schools in that system.

In due course carefully written reports were prepared and published. The reports covered the following areas: (a) a review of policies in the eight systems (McKenzie and Keeves 1982); (b) a survey of practices in 600 schools (Ainley 1982); (c) a report on critical issues associated with practices in 15 schools that were innovative in their organizational structures (Sturman 1982); (d) a study of relationships between class size, teacher and student behavior, and educational outcomes of achievement and attitudes (Larkin and Keeves 1984); and (e) an executive summary report of the first three volumes listed above (Ainley et al. 1982). In reviewing the study several years after its completion, it was found that many changes flowed from the study. However, the changes introduced were toward an increase in the efficiency of each system rather than educational reform. By and large, the reports of the study were made to serve the purpose of reducing the rate of changes in the eight systems.

Several implications may be drawn from this study for the conduct of legitimatory research in a major policy area.

(a) If the issues being investigated are in conflict with the *policies of the teacher unions*, moves are made by the unions and their members to block the conduct of a study.

(b) If the issues examined by the study challenge aspects of the *operation of the bureaucracies*, then ways are found to distort the conduct of the study.

(c) Legitimatory research is susceptible to interference from administrators and others who wish to *control the investigation.*

(d) The *findings of legitimatory research will* only be used by senior administrators and politicians at times and in ways that will achieve their previously determined purposes.

(e) Major research studies frequently take *several years* to bring to a satisfactory conclusion. During that time both the political and administrative officials who proposed the study may have been replaced and new officials may see issues from very different political perspectives.

(f) Legitimatory research exists because politicians and senior administrators need *evidence to support and legitimate* their policies and the educational organizations in which they work. The

findings from such research are used only if they can be directed toward these ends.

5. Conclusion

It is common for legitimatory research to lead only to a summary report which does not permit an adequate examination of the conduct of the investigation on which the findings are based. As a consequence, although research of a legitimatory nature is relatively widespread within educational bureaucracies, little has been written about this type of research. More detailed analyses of its characteristics and its influence are urgently needed.

See also: Policy-oriented Research; Educational Research and Policy-making

References

Ainley J G 1982 *Six Hundred Schools: A Study of Resources in Australian and New Zealand Government Schools.* ACER, Hawthorn, Victoria

Ainley J G, Keeves J P, McKenzie P A, Sturman A 1982 *Resource Allocation in the Government Schools of Australia and New Zealand.* ACER, Hawthorn, Victoria

Berger P L, Luckmann T 1967 *The Social Construction of Reality: A Treatise in the Sociology of Knowledge.* Penguin, London

Giddens A 1984 *The Constitution of Society: Outline of the Theory of Structuration.* Polity Press, Cambridge UK and Blackwell, Oxford

Glass G V, Smith M L 1978 *Meta-Analysis of Research on the Relationship of Class Size and Achievement.* Far West Laboratory for Educational Research and Development, San Francisco, California

Habermas J 1976 *Legitimation Crisis.* Heinemann Educ., London

Henderson A M, Parsons T 1947 *Max Weber: The Theory of Social and Economic Organization.* Free Press, New York and Oxford University Press, Oxford

Hicks F 1979 Crisis in the Legitimation of Educational Knowledge. In: Pusey M R, Young R L (eds.) *Control and Knowledge.* ANU Press, Canberra

Husén T 1984 Issues and their background. In: Husén T, Kogan M (eds.) 1984 *Educational Research and Policy. How Do They Relate?* Pergamon, Oxford

Kemmis S et al. 1983 *Transition and Reform in the Victorian Transition Education Program.* TAEC, Melbourne

Lafleur C D, Summer R J, Witton E 1974 *Class Size Survey.* Australian Government Publishing Service, Canberra

Larkin A I, Keeves J P 1984 *The Class Size Question: A Study at Different Levels of Analysis.* ACER, Hawthorn, Victoria

Lynn J, Jay A (eds.) 1982 *Yes Minister: The Diaries of a Cabinet Minister by the Rt. Hon. James Hacker M P,* Vol. 2. British Broadcasting Corporation, London

McKenzie P A, Keeves J P 1982 *Eight Education Systems. Resource Allocation Policies in the Government School Systems of Australia and New Zealand.* ACER, Hawthorn, Victoria

Pusey M R 1979 The Legitimation of State Education Systems. In: Pusey M R, Young R E (eds.) *Control and Knowledge.* ANU Press, Canberra

Slavin R E 1984a Meta-analysis in education: How has it been used? *Educ. Res.* AERA 13(8): 6–15

Slavin R E 1984b A rejoinder to Carlberg et al. *Educ. Res.* AERA 13(8): 24–27

Sturman A 1982 *Patterns of School Organization: Resources and Responses in Sixteen Schools.* ACER, Hawthorn, Victoria

Suchman E A 1970 Action for what? A critique of evaluative research. In: O'Toole R (ed.) 1970 *The Organization, Management and Tactics of Social Research.* Schenkman, Cambridge, Massachusetts

Weiss C H 1979 The many meanings of research utilization. *Public Admin. Rev.* 39 426–31

Participatory Research

B. L. Hall

Participatory research has been described most generally as a process that combines three activities: research, education, and action (Hall 1981). Participatory research is a social action process that is biased in favor of dominated, exploited, poor, or otherwise left-out people. It sees no contradiction between goals of collective empowerment and the deepening of social knowledge. The concern with power and democracy and their interactions are central to participatory research. Attention to gender, race, ethnicity, sexual orientation, physical and mental abilities, and other social factors are critical.

With the early support of the International Council for Adult Education, which initiated a global network in participatory research in 1977, and widespread interest over the years, the concept has been elaborated and developed much further. Fals Borda initially referred to a similar process in which he and his colleagues were engaged in Colombia and elsewhere in Latin America in the mid-1970s as "action research" (Fals Borda and Rahman 1991). When Vio Grossi, now of Chile but earlier working in Venezuela, organized a vigorous and dynamic Latin American network under the label "participatory research," Fals Borda joined forces and modified his label to "participatory action research." Both the "participatory action research" of Fals Borda and "participatory research" refer to the same general process. Fals Borda, Rahman of Bangladesh, and scores of other colleagues have been and continue to be central figures in the international participatory research community.

Authors have characterized the nature of participatory research in the following terms:

> Participatory research attempts to present people as researchers themselves in pursuit of answers to the questions of their daily struggle and survival. (Tandon 1988 p. 7)

> Participatory Research is a way for researchers and oppressed people to join in solidarity to take collective action, both short and long term, for radical social change. Locally determined and controlled action is a planned consequence of inquiry. (Maguire 1987 p. 29)

> The final aims of this combination of liberating knowledge and political power within a continuous process of life and work are: (1) to enable the oppressed groups and classes to acquire sufficient creative and transforming leverage as expressed in specific projects, acts and struggles; and (2) to produce and develop socio-political thought processes with which popular bases can identify. (Fals Borda and Rahman 1991 p. 4)

> Participatory research attempts to break down the distinction between the researchers and the researched, the subjects and objects of knowledge production by the participation of the people-for-themselves in the process of gaining and creating knowledge. In the process, research is seen not only as a process of creating knowledge, but simultaneously, as education and development of consciousness, and of mobilization for action. (Gaventa 1988 p. 19)

> Participatory research is collaborative, endogenous, heuristic and experiential. Transculturally, this implies an ability to accept the idea of native science and a sensitivity to the process-oriented, communally-based indigenous methodology. Through joint research projects between equal partners, participatory research can act as a flow-through mechanism for scientific findings from both worlds. (Colorado 1988 p. 63)

> An immediate objective . . . is to return to the people the legitimacy of the knowledge they are capable of producing through their own verification systems, as fully scientific, and the right to use this knowledge, but not be dictated by it—as a guide in their own action. (Fals Borda and Rahman 1991 p. 15).

1. Origins of Participatory Research

It is important to recognize that, while the term "participatory research" may be new, the concerns being expressed have a history and continuity in social science. Many of the ideas that are finding new opportunities for expression can be traced as far back as the early fieldwork of Frederick Engels, who investigated conditions in the early factories of Manchester in the United Kingdom in the mid-nineteenth century. Marx's use of the structured interview—*L'Enquête ouvrière*—with French factory workers is another sometimes forgotten antecedent. In later times aspects of the work of John Dewey, George Herbert Mead, and the Tavistock Institute in London have outlined methods of social investigation that are based on other than a positivistic epistemology.

By the late 1950s and early 1960s, the dominant international research paradigm was a version of the North American and European model based on empiricism and positivism and characterized by an attention to instrument construction and rigor defined by statistical precision and replicability. Through the elaborate mechanisms of colonial and postcolonial relations, international scholarships, cultural exchanges, and training of researchers in Europe and North America, this dominant paradigm was extended to the dependent and poorer nations. Research methods, through an illusion of objectivity and scientific credibility, became one more manifestation of cultural dependency.

The reaction of the Third World—beginning in Latin America—has taken many forms. Dependency theorists, such as Dos Santos, Frank, Amin, and Leys outlined some of the mechanisms of economic and cultural dependency. Hence, in the field of research methods, Third World perspectives have grown in part out of a reaction to approaches developed in North America and Europe; approaches that have not only been created in different cultural settings but which contribute to already existing class distinctions. The Third World's contribution to social science research methods represents an attempt to find ways of uncovering knowledge that can be applied in societies where interpretation of reality must take second place to the changing of that reality.

Practical experience in what was becoming known as participatory research occurred in the work of the Tanzanian Bureau of Research Allocation and Land Use Planning. Here, Marja-Liisa Swantz and teams of students and village workers were involved in the questions of youth and employment in the coast region and later in studies of socioeconomic causes of malnutrition in Central Kilimanjaro. A visit by Paulo Freire to Tanzania in 1971 was a stimulus to many social scientists who might not otherwise have been as impressed by the existing experience of many adult educators or community development workers.

What happened in Tanzania in a small way had already begun in Latin America in the early 1960s. Stimulated in part by the success of the Cuban revolution, Latin American social scientists began exploring more committed forms of research. One of the most useful roles of Paulo Freire has been to bring some of the current ideas of Latin American social scientists to the attention of persons in other parts of the world. His work on thematic investigation, first in Brazil and later in Chile, was an expression of this search. Others, such as Beltran and Gerace Larufa, have

explored alternatives through concepts of horizontal communication (Beltran 1976, Gerace Larufa 1973). Fals Borda (1980) and others in Colombia have been engaged in *investigación y acción* (investigation and action), while the D'arcy de Oliveiras have made people aware of the value of militant observation (D'arcy de Oliveira and D'arcy de Oliveira 1975).

2. Not the Third World Alone

While the specific term "participatory research" developed in the South, consciousness was growing in Europe and North America. Critiques of positivistic research paradigms began to surface in the 1970s. The Frankfurt School was rediscovered through the work of Jürgen Habermas and Theodor Adorno. The International Sociological Association, with encouragement from Peter Park of the United States and Ulf Himmelstrand of Sweden, began to place action-oriented sociology on the agenda of many academic meetings. In Switzerland, researchers in curriculum development adapted methodologies from political research to their needs. In Canada, Stinson developed methods of evaluation along action research lines for community development (Stinson 1979). In the Netherlands, de Vries explored research alternatives as an adult educator. Brown, of the United States, brought participatory research to the world of organizational development (Brown and Kaplan 1981). The National Institute for Adult Education in the United Kingdom pioneered participatory research through its evaluation of the United Kingdom adult literacy campaign (Holmes 1976). In Italy, Paulo Orefice and colleagues at the University of Naples applied the methodology in the context of growing political decentralization (Orefice 1981). In the United States, the Highlander Center in Tennessee has used participatory research for many years to deal with issues of land ownership and use (Horton 1981) and environmental deterioration. In Canada, the Toronto-based Participatory Research Group worked with a wide variety of groups, including First Nations peoples (Jackson 1980, Jackson et al. 1982), adult educators (Cassara 1985), immigrant women (Barndt 1981), and health workers (Hall 1981). The 1991 bibliography on participatory research by the Center for Community Education and Action provides the best perspective on the use and geographic spread of the approach (Center for Community Education and Action 1991). One of the newest books on participatory research reviews the North American experiences during the 1980s (Park et al. 1993).

3. Question of Methods

The literature on participatory research has always been vague on the question of methods. This is so because for participatory research, the most important factors are the origins of the issues, the roles those concerned with the issues play in the process, the emersion of the process in the context of the moment, the potential for mobilizing and for collective learning, the links to action, the understanding of how power relationships work, and the potential for communications with others experiencing similar discrimination, oppression, or violence. In addition, participatory research is based on the epistemological assumption that knowledge is constructed socially and therefore that approaches that allow for social, group, or collective analysis of life experiences of power and knowledge are most appropriate.

This means that for participatory research there are no methodological orthodoxies, no cookbook approaches to follow. The principle is that both issues and ways of working should flow from those involved and their context. In practice a creative and very wide variety of approaches have been used. All approaches have been selected because of their potential for drawing out knowledge and analysis in a social or collective way (Participatory Research Network 1982). They include: community meetings, video documentaries, community drama, camps for the landless in India, use of drawings and murals, photonovels, sharing of oral histories, community surveys, story-telling, shared testimonies, and many more. Even questionnaires have been used at times as a first step in a group-controlled process of reflection. Barndt and the Jesuit Centre for Faith and Social Justice in Canada have developed an approach to social movement research called "Naming the Moment" which offers a method for determining the political space available to them for action (Barndt 1989). Participatory Research in Asia (PRIA) reviewed the methods and results used by 10 different grassroots groups in India (PRIA 1985). The Society for the Promotion of Education and Research (SPEAR) of Belize, Central America, produced a participatory research training guide (SPEAR 1990). Fals Borda, discussed many methodological issues on a videotape produced by the University of Calgary in 1990.

4. Issues and Debates

4.1 The Feminist Advance

Feminist critiques of research have contributed to the understanding and practice of participatory research. Both feminist approaches and participatory research are concerned with knowledge creation in ways that empower those engaged rather than maintaining the status quo. Both feminist research and participatory research seek to shift the center from which knowledge is generated. Spender (1978 pp. 1–2) has described the field of women's studies as follows:

> Its multi-disciplinary nature challenges the arrangements of knowledge into academic disciplines; its methodology breaks down many of the traditional distinctions between

theoretical and empirical and between objective and subjective. It is in the process of redefining knowledge, knowledge gathering and making . . .

In addition, Callaway has demonstrated that women have been largely excluded from producing the dominant forms of knowledge and that the social sciences have been not only a science of male society but also a male science of society (Callaway 1981). Spender urged women "to learn to create our own knowledge." It is crucially important, she states:

> that women begin to create our own means of producing and validating knowledge which is consistent with our own personal experience. We need to formulate our own yardsticks, for we are doomed to deviancy if we persist in measuring ourselves against the male standard. This is our area of learning, with learning used in a widely encompassing, highly charged, political and revolutionary sense. (Spender 1978 pp. 1–2)

Maguire has bridged feminist research approaches and participatory research in her 1987 book which points out what she has called the "Androcentric filter" in participatory research writing (Maguire 1987). Maguire has pointed out the distinct silence around gender and women in the participatory research discourse. She noted that women's ways of seeing were not mentioned until 1981 and that in the general discourse women have been excluded.

Maguire put forward a number of specific guidelines for feminist participatory research:

> (1) the critique is both of positivist and androcentric research paradigms;
> (2) gender needs to be a central piece of the issues agenda;
> (3) integrative feminism which recognizes diversity should be central to theoretical discussions on participatory research;
> (4) the role of gender needs to be taken into account in all phases of participatory research;
> (5) feminist participatory research would give explicit attention to how women and men as groups benefit from a project;
> (6) attention to gender language use is critical;
> (7) gender, culture, race and class all figure in questions about the research team;
> (8) gender should be a factor in considering evaluation;
> (9) patriarchy is a system to be dismantled along with other systems of domination and oppression. (Maguire 1987 pp. 105–08)

Smith has suggested that feminist sociology, like participatory research, must "begin where we are" with real, concrete people with actual lives if it is to do more than reproduce patriarchal patterns of relations (Smith 1979). Oral history as a particular approach to feminist research has been used in participatory research as well (Anderson et al. 1990).

4.2 Question of Voice

Participatory research fundamentally is about who has the right to speak, to analyze, and to act. It is about rural Black women in southern cooperatives in the United States speaking for themselves in obtaining loans for planting. It is about shantytown mothers in Bombay speaking for themselves. It is about citizens of Turkish descent in Germany looking at and articulating their own needs in the face of neo-Nazi revival. It is about women in Thailand's hill country protecting forests. It is about indigenous people of the First Nations of North America researching land rights. It is about people who do not read and write taking control of literacy programs. It is a process that supports the voices from the margins in speaking, analyzing, building alliances, and taking action. As Lourde's (1984) poem "Litany for Survival" says:

> and when we speak we are afraid
> our words will not be heard
> nor welcomed
> but when we are silent
> we are still afraid
> So it is better to speak
> remembering
> we were never meant to survive

According to Hooks, critical theorist and Afro-American woman, "It is our responsibility collectively and individually to distinguish between mere speaking that is about self-aggrandizement, exploitation of the exotic "other", and that coming to voice which is a gesture of resistance, an affirmation of struggle" (Hooks 1988).

Participatory research argues for the articulation of points of view by the dominated or subordinated, whether from gender, race, ethnicity, or other structures of subordination. Participatory research posits that an individual's position in structures of subordination shapes the ability to see the whole. Hooks reflected thus on growing up Black in the United States:

> Living as we did—on the edge—we developed a particular way of seeing reality. We looked both from the outside in and from the inside out. We focused our attention on the center as well as on the margin. We understood both. This mode of seeing reminded us of the existence of a whole universe, a main body made up of both margin and center. Our survival depended on an ongoing private acknowledgment that we were a necessary, vital part of that whole.
> This sense of wholeness, impressed upon our consciousness by the structure of our daily lives, provided us an oppositional world view—a mode of seeing unknown to most of our oppressors, that sustained us, sided us in our struggle to transcend poverty and despair, strengthened our sense of self and our solidarity (Hooks 1984 p. 9)

5. Participatory Research as Counterhegemonic Practice

Disturbed by the fact that dissatisfaction of the working class in Italy produced fascism instead of a socialist transformation as happened in the Soviet Union in 1917, Antonio Gramsci undertook a lengthy study, though this was partly brought about by his imprisonment. The translation of his work into English in the early 1970s allowed greater access to his complex and fascinating ideas (Hoare and Nowell-Smith

1971). Hegemony is one of the major concepts that helps individuals to understand participatory research. According to Gramsci, humans are controlled by both coercion and consent. Laws exist that limit actions that can be taken in redressing structural imbalances, but in fact demand most often "consent" to structures of domination or hegemony. Dominated classes, genders, races, sexual orientations, or different-ability groups internalize the views of what is "acceptable" resistance, "realistic" strategy, their own fault or the natural order of things and thereby participate in the maintenance of hegemony.

But unlike orthodox Marxism, Gramsci saw a more dialectical relationship between consciousness and reality. While not accepting the idealist position that consciousness determines reality, Gramsci allowed that human agency does have a role and that the construction of counterhegemonic patterns was what was needed. In the construction of counterhegemonic ideas there is a role for intellectuals, but new kinds of intellectuals, what he called "organic intellectuals," who are deeply rooted to and part of the class- or other dominated structures from which they come. The knowledge produced in participatory research processes can be seen as part of the counterhegemonic process.

6. Restoration of Ancient Knowledge

The growing awareness globally about environmental and ecological deterioration has reinforced many of the claims and aspirations for participatory research. Shiva of India, for example, has noted that the scientific revolution of Isaac Newton and Francis Bacon was a male, Eurocentric, white science that by its invention immediately created nonscience or ignorance among people or in places that did not share in this particular way of knowing. Western science rendered invisible ancient, feminine, proearth ways of knowing (Shiva 1989).

There is widespread interest in the recovery of ancient ways of knowing that seem more fully integrated into the world and nature as opposed to those ways that view nature as separate and needing to be conquered for human beings to prosper. There is a role for participatory research with people and by people who still have links to ancient knowledge. In this case can participatory research be part of such a recovery or restoration process (Colorado 1988)?

7. Co-optation and the Role of the University

What is the role of the academy in participatory research? What has the academy done with participatory research? What is the status of the knowledge generated in a participatory research process? Participatory research originated as a challenge to positivist research paradigms as carried out largely by university-based researchers. The position has been that the center of knowledge generation needed to be in what dominant society described as the margins: in communities, with women, with people of color, and so forth. Experience has shown that it is very difficult to achieve this kind of process from a university base; hence the need for alternative structures such as community-based networks or centers. But how can this be reconciled with the fact that so many of those who publish are university based?

If the research process is genuinely and organically situated in a community, workplace, or group that is experiencing domination, there is no need to be afraid that the knowledge being generated will be used for purposes that the community or group does not need or wish for. The difficulty arises because there are different uses of knowledge in the academy from those in community or workplace situations. According to the discourse of participatory research, knowledge generated, whether of localized application or larger theoretical value, is linked in some ways with shifts of power or structural changes. But intentions do not always produce desired results, and those who have been working along these lines for a number of years share these assumptions. It is necessary to hope for a fuller understanding of the context and conditions of both work and life.

Knowledge within the academy serves a variety of purposes. It is a commodity by which academics do far more than exchange ideas; it is the very means of exchange for the academic political economy. Tenure, promotion, peer recognition, research grants, and countless smaller codes of privilege are accorded through the adding up of articles, books, papers in "refereed" journals and conferences. Academics in the marketplace of knowledge know that they must identify or become identified with streams of ideas that offer the possibility of publishing and dialogue within appropriate and recognized settings. Collaborative research or at least collaborative publishing is informally discouraged because of the difficulty in attributing authorship. Collaborative research with persons who are not academics by the standards of the academy is uncommon. While academics in fact gain financially through accumulated publications of appropriate knowledge, community collaborators seldom benefit from such collaboration in financial terms. As can be seen, academics are under economic, job survival, or advancement pressures to produce in appropriate ways. It is this structural pressure that plays havoc with academic engagement in the participatory research process. Is it not possible that in spite of personal history, ideological commitment, and deep personal links with social movements or transformative processes that the structural location of the academy as the preferred location for the organizing of knowledge will distort a participatory research process?

Does this mean that there is no role for university-based people to be engaged in participatory research processes? Arguments exist on both sides of this question. Universities or similarly accredited researchers are clearly not *required* to animate a participatory research process. Participatory research is a tool which social movements, activists, trade unionists, women on welfare, the homeless, or any similar groups use as part of a variety of strategies and methods for the conduct of their work. If they wish to invite a university-based group to become involved they need to set up the conditions at the start and maintain control of the process if they wish to benefit as much as possible. Countless groups make use of processes that resemble participatory research without naming it or certainly without asking for outside validation of the knowledge produced.

Participatory research deserves to be taught in universities, and is increasingly being taught. The academic community deserves to discuss and challenge and be challenged by these and other ideas which raise questions of the role of knowledge and power. Adult educators, community workers, social workers, primary healthcare personnel, solidarity cooperators, cooperative movement workers, multicultural workers, teachers, and countless others who begin working after a university education deserve to study, read, and experience the ideas that make up participatory research.

Academics also do not cease to be members of the community by going to work in a university. There are countless community issues, whether related to toxic dumping, homelessness, high drop-out levels in local schools, or unfair taxation policies, that engage us all as citizens. Academics have some skills that can contribute to community action along with the skills of others in the community.

The concern with co-optation is not limited to the academy, but runs through the professional circles of those involved in international development. Rahnema, a former senior Iranian official turned advisor on nongovernmental activities for the United Nations Development Program (UNDP) and visiting university professor, has criticized participatory action research as "The Last Temptation of Saint Development" (Rahnema 1990). He says that in its most generalized form, the call for participation is naı[um]ve and by now accepted by all international agencies. He suggests that participatory research can at best only change external factors affecting people's lives and not touch the deeper conditioning that causes people to do what they do; "It serves no one to make a new fetish out of participation, only because nonparticipatory development has failed in every way" (Rahnema 1990).

8. Historical Materialism, Critical Theory, and Other Philosophical Support

Vio Grossi wrote in 1981 that:

> some . . . understood that participatory research was implicitly rejecting . . . historical materialism. We were accused of integration and reformism. Participatory research

is not, and has never intended to be, a new ideological and scientific holistic system, an alternative to historical materialism. On the contrary, it attempts to start the research from the concrete and specific reality, incorporating the people's viewpoints, in order to contribute to a type of social transformation that eliminates poverty, dependence and exploitation. This assertion requires a further analysis of its components. Historical materialism has been stated as a method for investigating reality with the intent of revealing the main tendencies of changes in order to orient action. (Vio Grossi 1981)

As Gramsci has said:

The starting-point of critical elaboration is the consciousness of what one really is, and in "knowing thyself" as a product of the historical process to date which has deposited in you an infinity of traces, without leaving an inventory. (Hoare and Nowell-Smith 1971 p. 326)

Early efforts to place the evolving practice of participatory research within appropriate or supportive theoretical frameworks focused on debates between pragmatic or historical materialist epistemological frameworks (Kassam and Mustapha 1982). The majority of participatory research writers found themselves agreeing that class, power, ideology, and other social structural elements were critical to understanding change and hence drew upon historical materialist sources. In the mid-1980s, and particularly in North America, contributions linked participatory research to the critical theory streams of Horkheimer, Adorno, and Habermas (Comstock and Fox 1993, Park 1993). Additional linkages were made between the concepts of "critical pedagogy," particularly as both Giroux of the United States and Simon of Canada began to move the focus of their work beyond schooling and into cultural politics and the notions of "border" pedagogies.

It is necessary to stress that the basis for a critical pedagogy cannot be developed merely around the inclusion of particular forms of knowledge that have been suppressed or ignored by the dominant culture, nor can it only center on providing students with more empowering interpretations of the social and material world. Such a pedagogy must be attentive to ways in which students make both affective and semantic investments as part of their attempts to regulate and give meaning to their lives (Giroux and Simon 1992).

9. Local Autonomy and Broader Struggles

Additional debates exist in the field. For example, there is tension between the requirement of local autonomy for a given participatory process and the demand for coordinated social action at the national or regional levels. A national action must be more than an aggregate of local experiences. At certain critical moments, will a local-level participatory research process hinder the progress of broader social

movements by overemphasizing the localized nature of the problem? There is a need to understand the relationships of different kinds of knowledge and information generating from different levels and aspects of society.

10. Question of Power

Emerging from the discussions, debates, and activities of participatory research is the central question of power. Participatory research is intended to contribute to processes of shifting power or democratizing a variety of contexts. Power can be expressed in several ways: A exercises power over B when A affects B in a manner contrary to B's interests; in other words A gets B to do what he or she does not want to do. But A also exercises power by influencing, shaping, or determining B's very wants, by controlling the agenda through a complex interplay of social control (Gaventa 1979).

How, then, can participatory research be useful in shifting power? Practitioners have suggested at least three possibilities.

10.1 Unmasking the Myths

Vio Grossi (1981) has written of participatory research as initiating a process of disindoctrination that allows people to detach themselves from the myths imposed on them by the power structure and which have prevented them from seeing their own oppression or from seeing possibilities for breaking free. Transformative action can be seen as the strategic goal to be reached in the medium or long term. A participatory research process carried out in conjunction with popular groups (and under their control) is designed to facilitate the analysis of stages toward that goal.

10.2 Creation of Popular Knowledge

Fals Borda has contributed to the discussion of popular knowledge in his paper on "Science and the Common People" (Fals Borda 1980). He says the creation of knowledge that comes from the people contributes to the realization of a people's science which serves and is understood by the people, and no longer perpetuates the status quo. The process of this new paradigm involves: (a) returning information to the people in the language and cultural form in which it originated, (b) establishing control of the work by the popular and base movements, (c) popularizing research techniques, (d) integrating the information as the base of the organic intellectual, (e) maintaining a conscious effort in the action/reflection rhythm of work, (f) recognizing science as part of the everyday lives of all people, and (g) learning to listen.

In Gaventa's terms popular knowledge can be seen as a contribution toward limiting the ability of those in power to determine the wants of others, thus in effect transferring power to those groups engaged in the production of popular knowledge (Gaventa 1979).

10.3 Contributing to Organizing

Participatory research is conceived to be an integral process of investigation, education, and action. When the question of power is addressed, it is clearer than ever that the first two aspects are empty without the third. But action must be explained still further. From several years of sharing information and results it has become clear that the most common action and the critical necessity is that of organizing, in its various phases. It has meant building alliances and strengthening links within various progressive sectors.

It would be an error to assume that naive or uncontrolled use of participatory research results in strengthening the power of the powerless at the base of society. Where control over the participatory research process is missing, experience has shown that power can easily accrue to those already in control. There has been ambiguity in some earlier writings on participatory research which has resulted in misunderstanding and manipulation.

References

Anderson K, Armitage S, Jack D, Wittner J 1990 Beginning where we are: Feminist methodology in oral history. In: Nielson J M (ed.) 1990 *Feminist Research Methods.* Westview, Boulder, Colorado

Barndt D 1981 *Just Getting There: Creating Visual Tools for Collective Analysis in Freirean Education Programmes for Migrant Women in Canada.* Par Res Group, Toronto

Barndt D 1989 *Naming the Moment: Political Analysis for Action—A Manual for Community Groups.* Moment Project, Toronto

Beltran L R 1976 Alien premises: Objects and methods in Latin American communication research. *Commun. Res.* 3(2): 107–34

Brown L D, Kaplan R E 1981 Participatory research in a factory. In: Reason P, Rowan J (eds.) 1981 *Human Inquiry: A Sourcebook of New Paradigm Research.* Wiley, London

Callaway H 1981 Women's perspectives: Research as revision. In: Reason P, Rowan J (eds.) 1981 *Human Inquiry: A Sourcebook of New Paradigm Research.* Wiley, London

Cassara B 1985 *Participatory Research: Group Self-directed Learning for Social Transformation.* Adult Education, University of Georgia, Athens, Georgia

Center for Community Education and Action 1991 *Participatory Research: An Annotated Bibliography.* CCEA and Center for International Education, Amherst, Massachusetts

Colorado P 1988 Bridging native and western science. *Convergence* 21(3/4)

Comstock D, Fox R 1993 Citizen's action at North Bonnevile Dam. In: Park P, Brydon-Miller M, Hall B, Jackson T (eds.) 1993

D'arcy de Oliveira R, D'arcy de Oliveira M 1975 *The Militant Observer: A Sociological Alternative.* Institut d'Action Culturelle, Geneva

Fals Borda O 1980 *Science and the Common People.* International Forum on Participatory Research

Fals Borda O, Rahman M A 1991 *Action and Knowledge: Breaking the Monopoly with Participatory Action-Research.* Apex, New York

Gaventa J 1979 *Power and Powerlessness: Quiescence and Rebellion in an Appalachian Valley.* University of Illinois Press, Urbana, Illinois

Gaventa J 1988 Participatory research in North America. *Convergence* 21(2/3): 19–48

Gerace Larufa F 1973 *Comunicación Horizontal.* Librería Studium, Lima

Giroux H, Simon R 1992 Popular culture as a pedagogy of pleasure and meaning: Decolonizing the body. In: Giroux H (ed.) 1992 *Border Crossings: Cultural Workers and the Politics of Education.* Routledge, New York

Hall B 1981 Participatory research, popular knowledge and power. *Convergence* 14(3)

Hoare Q, Nowell-Smith G (eds. and trans.) 1971 *Selections from the Prison Notebooks of Antonio Gramsci.* Lawrence and Wishart, London

Holmes J 1976 Thoughts on research methodology. *Stud. Adult Educ.* 8(2): 149–63

Hooks B 1984 *Feminist Theory: From Margin to Center.* South End, Boston, Massachusetts

Hooks B 1988 *Talking Back: Thinking Feminist Thinking Black.* South End, Boston, Massachusetts

Horton B D 1981 On the potential of participatory research: An evaluation of a regional experiment. Paper prepared for annual meeting of the Society for Study of Social Problems, Toronto, Canada

Jackson T 1980 Environmental assessment in big trout lake, Canada. Paper for International Forum on participatory research

Jackson T, McCaskill D, Hall B 1982 Learning for self-determination: Community-based options for native training and research. *Canadian Journal of Native Studies* 2(1) (special issue)

Kassam Y, Mustapha K 1982 *Participatory Research: An Emerging Alternative Methodology in Social Science Research.* ICAE, Toronto

Lourde A 1984 *Sister Outsider: Essays and Speeches.* Crossing Press, Trumansburg, New York

Maguire P 1987 *Doing Participatory Research: A Feminist Approach.* Center for International Education, University of Massachusetts, Amherst, Massachusetts

Orefice P 1981 Cultural self-awareness of local community: An experience in the south of Italy. *Convergence* 14: 56–64

Park P 1993 What is participatory research? In: Park P, Brydon-Miller M, Hall B, Jackson T (eds.) 1993

Park P, Brydon-Miller M, Hall B, Jackson T (eds.) 1993 *Voices of Change: Participatory Research in the United States and Canada.* Greenwood, Westport, Connecticut

Participatory Research Network 1982 *An Introduction to Participatory Research.* ICAE, New Delhi

PRIA 1985 *Knowledge and Social Change: An Inquiry into Participatory Research in India.* PRIA, New Delhi

Rahnema M 1990 Participatory action research: The "last temptation" of saint development. *Alternatives* 15: 199–226

Shiva V 1989 *Staying Alive: Women, Ecology and Development.* Zed Books, London

Smith D 1979 A sociology for women. In: Sherman J, Bock E (eds) 1979 *The Prism of Sex: Essays in the Sociology of Knowledge.* University of Wisconsin Press, Madison, Wisconsin

SPEAR 1990 *You better Belize It! A Participatory Research Training Guide on a Training Workshop in Belize.* SPEAR and PRG, Toronto

Spender D 1978 Editorial. *Womens Studies International Q.* 1: 1–2

Stinson A (ed.) 1979 *Canadians Participate: Annotated Bibliography of Case Studies*, Centre for Social Welfare Studies, Ottawa

Tandon R 1988 Social transformation and participatory research. *Convergence* 21(2/3): 5–18

Vio Grossi F 1981 The socio-political implications of participatory research. Yugoslavia. *Convergence* 14(3): 34–51

Further Reading

Hall B 1979 Knowledge as a commodity and participatory research. *Prospects* 9(4): 393–408

Hall B, Gillette A, Tandon R 1982 *Creating Knowledge: A Monopoly?* PRIA, New Delhi

Park P, Hall B, Jackson T, and Brydon-Miller M 1993 *Voices for Change: Participatory Research in Canada and the United States.* OISE Press, Toronto

Policy Analysis

M. Trow

Husén (1984) has argued that the relation of research to policy is far more complex, far more indirect than it formerly appeared. Drawing on the informed writings of Weiss (1979) and Kogan et al. (1980) among others, and from rich experience, he dismisses as irrelevant, at least to the field of education, two classical models of the application of research to policy that Weiss lists among seven different models or concepts of research utilization: the "linear" model, which leads neatly from basic knowledge to applied research to development to application, and the "problem-solving" model, in which research is done to fill in certain bodies of knowledge needed to make a decision among policy alternatives. These are dismissed on the grounds that they simply do not even roughly describe what happens in the real world. The remaining models are merged into two. One is an "enlightenment" or "percolation" model, in which research somehow (and just how is of greatest interest) influences policy indirectly, by entering into the consciousness of the actors and shaping the terms of their discussion about policy alternatives. The second, the "political model," refers to the intentional use of research by political decision-makers to strengthen an argument, to justify positions already taken, or to avoid making or having to make unpopular decisions by burying the controversial problem in research.

Of these two models, the first or "percolation" model is the more interesting, since it is the way through which research actually has an influence on policy, rather than merely being used to justify or avoid making decisions. Moreover, the percolation model and its mechanisms and processes are so subtle that they challenge study and reflection.

1. Researchers and Policy Analysts

The decade since the mid-1970s has seen in the United States, and to some extent elsewhere, the emergence of a profession, that of the policy analyst, whose training, habits of mind, and conditions of work are expressly designed to narrow the gap between the researcher and the policymaker and to bring systematic knowledge to bear more directly, more quickly, and more relevantly on the issues of public policy. This entry attempts to compare and contrast the researcher and the policy analyst to see how this breed of staff analyst/researcher, inside as well as outside government, may affect the ways in which research comes to bear on policy. The comparison is not intended to be invidious, that is, there is no implication that the invention of policy analysis has in any way solved the problems of the relation of research to policy that Husén, Weiss, and others have identified. But it may be of interest to see how this emerging profession affects that process, and how it generates new problems —intellectual, political, and moral—as it solves some of the old.

Policy analysis developed as a formal discipline in the mid-1970s through the coming together of a number of strands of work and thought in the social sciences. These included operations research developed during the Second World War on a strongly mathematical basis for improving the efficiency of military operations—the deployment of submarines, bombing raids, and convoy management. Added to this were new forms of microeconomics developed in the 1950s and 1960s; the long-standing tradition of work in public administration; the newer and increasingly strong strain of behaviorism in the political sciences;

organizational theory; certain lines of applied sociology and social psychology; and the emerging interest in the role of law in public policy. Graduate schools of public policy were established in a number of leading American universities around 1970. Some leading universities now have genuine graduate schools of public policy; there are literally hundreds of others which offer programs which include some measure of policy analysis in their schools of management, public administration, or business administration. To the mix of social science and law, some schools have added scientists, engineers, and others interested in public policy problems. These graduate schools for the most part offer a two-year postgraduate professional degree, ordinarily the Master of Public Policy. Their graduates go directly into public service at national, state, or local levels, or get jobs in think-tanks or private agencies concerned with public issues—for example, organizations concerned with the preservation of the environment, with education, overseas trade, and so forth. These latter "private" organizations, however, are directly involved for the most part in public policy —indeed, much of what they do is to try to influence public policy, so the conditions of work for public policy analysts in them resemble those of analysts who enter governmental service itself.

There are several aspects of the training of policy analysts that need to be emphasized. As must already be clear, the training of the policy analyst is intensely interdisciplinary. This is required first because of the diverse nature of its intellectual antecedents; the field itself reflects the coming together of diverse currents in what Lasswell (Lerner and Lasswell 1951) called the "policy sciences." But more important, the training has to be interdisciplinary because that is the way the problems present themselves to decision makers. Real decisions, as we all know, do not respect the boundaries of the academic disciplines: they always have political, economic, and organizational components; they may well also have legal, educational, biological, or other technical implications as well.

Perhaps the most important distinguishing characteristic of policy analysts as contrasted with academic research social scientists is that they are trained, indeed required, to see and to formulate problems from the perspectives not of the academic disciplines, but of the decision makers. In their work, they accept the constraints and values of decision makers—the political pressures on them, the political feasibility of a proposal, its financial costs, the legal context within which it will operate, the difficulties of implementing it, of shaping organizations, and of recruiting, training, and motivating people to work in the service of its purposes. They are, if effectively trained, sensitive to the costs and benefits of programs, to the trade-offs in any decision, and to the alternative advantages of government and the market in achieving social purposes. In a word, they try to see problems from the perspective of the decision maker, but with a set of intellectual, analytical, and research tools that the politician or senior civil servant may not possess. They are, and are trained to be, the researchers in government at the elbow of the decision makers, or if not in government, then serving the "government in opposition" or some think-tank or interest group which hopes to staff the next administration or agency on the next swing of the political pendulum. Of course, not all policy analysts are "researchers," as the university conceives of research. But what they do, bringing ideas and information to bear on social "problems" in a search for "solutions," is the kind of "research" that has the most direct influence on public policy.

By contrast, the faculty members of schools of public policy are not, for the most part, like the students that they train: the former are almost without exception academics with PhDs, trained in and drawn from the social science disciplines, specialists originally who have a particular interest in public policy, and who do research on policy issues, but not on the whole like the research that their students will be doing in their government or quasi-government jobs. The faculty members of these schools are for the most part what Wilson (1981 p. 36) has called "policy intellectuals," while their students are policy analysts—the staff people and bureaucrats serving their policy-oriented clients in and out of governments. The relationship of the policy intellectual in the university to the policy analyst in government bears on the issue of "knowledge creep" and "research percolation" that Husén and Weiss speak of, and to which this entry will return.

Let us look at some of the characteristics of "researchers" as Husén describes them, and at some of the "disjunctions" between research and policy that the nature of the researcher in the university gives rise to. The field of policy analysis and the new profession of policy analyst were, one might say, invented precisely to meet the need of policymakers for analysis and research carried out within the same constraints that the policymaker experiences. Policy analysis thus aims to narrow those "disjunctions" between research and policy of which Husén speaks. He describes three conditions under which researchers work that are different for policy analysts:

(a) Researchers are usually performing their tasks at . . . universities[.]. They tend to conduct their research according to the paradigms to which they have become socialized by their graduate studies. Their achievements are subjected to peer reviews which they regard as more important than assessments made by the customers in a public agency. (Husén 1984 p. 10)

Analysts, by contrast, work for the most part in government or in shadow governmental agencies, or in large private business organizations. The paradigms of research that they acquire in graduate school emphasize the importance of serving the client, of defining or clarifying the nature of the problem, or identifying the policy options available, of evaluating those alternatives in terms of their cost, probable effectiveness, political feasibility, ease of implementation, and the like—the same criteria which the decision maker would use in planning and choosing a course of action. The analyst is trained then to make recommendations among the action alternatives that have been identified, supporting the recommendations made with appropriate arguments and evidence.

Much, perhaps most, of what such analysts do is not published, is not reviewed by peers, and will almost certainly appear, if at all, in greatly modified form, either anonymously or under someone else's name. The analyst's reputation will be made *not* in an academic setting, but in his or her agency, and more importantly among the small but active community of analysts in government agencies, on legislative staffs, in think-tanks, and special interest organizations who know of the analyst's work and its quality. Incidentally, it is in that arena of discussion and assessment—the analyst's analog to the scholar's "invisible college"—that we need to look for the mechanisms of information "drift" and "creep," and for the processes of percolation through which research and evidence come to influence policy.

> (b) Researchers operate at a high level of training and specialization, which means that they tend to isolate a "slice" of a problem area that can be more readily handled than more complicated global problems. (Husén 1984 p. 10)

By contrast, analysts are trained to be as interdisciplinary as possible, to follow the requirements of a problem in their choice of ideas, theories, and research methods, rather than to allow the theories and methods of their discipline select and shape their problems. This is not wholly successful, in part because their teachers in these schools are not themselves equally familiar with the variety of research methods and perspectives across disciplinary lines, and because their students, the fledgling analysts, inevitably come to be more familiar and comfortable with some kinds of analysis rather than others. Nevertheless the requirement that they see problems as the policymakers would were they analysts, requires analysts to transcend the constraints of a single discipline and to tackle problems as wholes rather than by "slices."

> (c) Researchers are much less constrained than policy makers in terms of what problems they can tackle, what kind of critical language they can employ and how much time they have . . . at their disposal to complete a study. (Husén 1984 p. 10)

Analysts, by contrast, ordinarily are assigned their studies, or do them within circumscribed policy areas. That does not wholly preclude their exercise of discretion; and indeed, they may exercise very important amounts of initiative in how they formulate their problems, and in the range of responses to the problems they consider (Meltsner 1976 pp. 81–114). From the researcher's perspective, the captive analyst is merely "a hired gun" doing what he or she is told by political or bureaucratic superiors. But from the perspective of the analyst, discretion, even within the constraints of a given policy problem or area, may be very considerable. How to control air pollution in a given area, for example, allows a variety of regulatory solutions, from setting standards for allowable emissions for different kinds of plants and industries to setting charges on pollutants requiring polluters to pay for each unit of pollutant emitted. The issues are political, technical, economic, legal, and normative—and they are not always decided *a priori* by political or administrative decision-makers.

It is true that analysts are ordinarily held to a closer time frame than are academic researchers; it is not unusual for students to become accustomed to doing analyses of various policy problems, drawing upon the best available data, research, and advice, within 48 or 72 hours, exercises designed to prepare them for the fierce time pressures of legislative hearings or the negotiations that accompany the writing and revision of legislation. Other exercises allow them a week, and a major piece of research equivalent to a master's essay will take up to six months. Time constraints on the job also vary; analysts become skillful in knowing who has been working on a given problem area, and where published or unpublished research or data on the issue can be found. For the analyst, knowledgeable people are a central research resource, and the telephone is part of the student's equipment alongside computers and the library.

But as they develop the skill of rapidly bringing ideas to bear on data, and data on ideas, analysts become heavily dependent upon existing statistics and on research done by others. They are often skillful, and even bold, in drawing analogies between findings in different areas of social life, allowing them thus to use the findings of research in one area for informing decisions in another. These analysts cannot often meet the scholar's standards of depth and thoroughness in their research—for example, in the review of the research literature, or in the critical evaluation of the findings of relevant research. Yet working under time and other pressures in the political milieu, the analysts know that the alternative to what they are doing is not a major university-based research project, but more commonly the impressions, anecdotes, and general wisdom of a staff conference. Their own reports, which include discussions of alternative lines of action based on data regarding their comparative costs and benefits, must, they believe, be better than an unsystematic discussion among friends and advisers.

Policy analysts in government as we have described them have some of the characteristics of researchers, but are more narrowly constrained by their bureaucratic roles. They also have some of the characteristics of Kogan's middle-men, professionals who serve a liaison function (Kogan et al. 1980 pp. 36–38), though they are more active and ready to take research initiatives than the term "middle-man" implies. But they also are not infrequently the decision-makers themselves.

2. *Example from the Field of Education*

One almost always talks about research *influencing* decision makers—and if the researcher is a university social scientist then the decision maker is almost certainly someone a distance away with his or her own concerns, political commitments, interests, and prejudices. But the policy analyst has the advantage of acting within the bureaucracy to make or directly affect a myriad of administrative decisions that rarely get into the newspapers, are not debated by politicians or on floors of legislatures, but nevertheless have very large consequences.

One illustration comes from the University of California, half of whose budget—the half which pays the operating costs of the University, faculty salaries, and the like—comes from the state of California. The preparation of the University's budget and its incorporation into the governor's budget is a complicated procedure. Very substantial parts of the University's budget are governed by formulas, relating, for example, support levels to enrollment levels, that have been negotiated over the years between the budget analysts in the central administration of the University and their counterparts in the State Department of Finance. These formulas, essentially bureaucratic treaties, are mutual understandings which give the university a greater degree of fiscal security and predictability than one would ever guess from reading the newspapers, which almost never report these matters, but only the visible debates in the legislature and speeches by the governor.

The formulas, of course, do not cover all contingencies, especially in an institution as fluid and diverse as the University of California with so many different sources of energy and initiative creating new programs, facilities, and claims on public funds all the time. Claims for resources, old and new, are argued out or negotiated annually between the University analysts and the State Department of Finance analysts; they speak each other's language, and often have been trained in the same graduate schools and departments, not infrequently in Berkeley's School of Public Policy. In these negotiations, "good arguments" by the University are rewarded; that is, requests for additional support funds that are supported by a good bureaucratic argument are often accepted, and new activities are built into the governor's budget. The arguments made for these programs are the arguments of analysts, often based on analogies with existing state-funded activities, and backed by data showing the actual nature of the activity and its costs. For example, the University wants the state to revise the formula allocating funds for the replacement of scientific equipment used in

teaching; it wants more generous provision for teaching assistants; it wants the state to assume the costs of certain athletic facilities; it wants the state to support remedial courses for underprepared students; and so on. In support of these claims the University analysts do research on the actual useful life of laboratory instruments in different scientific departments and on how that record compares with the life of instruments in other universities and in commercial labs; it studies the use and distribution of teaching assistants in the University and how their work contributes to the instructional program; it studies who uses the athletic facilities and for what purposes; and so on. These are not matters of high principle; there exists a broad area of value consensus between the negotiators, but the quality of the research backing those claims is crucial to whether they are accepted, and indeed whether they ought to be accepted. The sums of money that are allocated in these ways are in the aggregate very large. There are many areas of public life in which civil servants exercise wide discretion in decision-making, though they are often wise enough to deny that they are in fact making policy or decisions, but merely "implementing" them. Nevertheless, when we reflect on the influence of research on policy, we should not neglect the realm of bureaucratic and technocratic decision-making in the public sector where researcher and decision maker come together in the person of the policy analyst. University-based researchers need to be reminded that not all research has to percolate down through a complex network of relationships to enter another complex process of "decision accretion"; some research has access to decision-makers quickly and directly, and is done for and by them.

The newly emergent field of policy analysis seems to be thriving in the United States, at least in a modest way, even in the face of budget cuts and hiring freezes in the federal and in many state and local governments. Policy analysts are in demand whether public expenditures are rising or falling; the problems posed to government by budgetary constraints are even more severe than those posed by expansion and the proliferation of public programs and services. And with all the cuts, most governments are not reducing the absolute level of public expenditures on social services, but merely reducing their rates of growth. In any event, public life is becoming increasingly more complex and there is no shortage of work for policy analysts.

3. *Four Problems Facing the Policy Analyst*

It should not be thought that the emergence of policy analysis, and of the infrastructure of graduate schools, journals, professional associations and meetings which give it definition and self-consciousness, solve all the problems of the relation of research to policy. For if policy analysts solve some of those problems, they also create new ones. This section outlines four such problems in the realm of policy analysis as currently practiced, though this does not imply that there are only four. These are all problems which in significant ways affect the quality of the analyst's work and his or her influence on policy and decision-making.

First, and this is a problem that the analyst shares with academic research in education, policy analysis makes relatively little use of ethnographic research methods, the method of direct observation of customary behavior and informal conversation. One consequence of this is that the policy analyst is a captive of existing and usually official statistics; where those statistics are wrong or misleading or inadequate, the analyst's work is flawed, misleading, and inadequate also. By contrast, university researchers are more likely to question the quality of research data, though it is likely that they rarely question the quality of official statistics.

Second, the outcome of public policy analysis, its reports and recommendations, is affected not only by the analyst's own preferences and biases and those of the client, but also by how the analyst bounds the problem, the phenomena and variables that will be taken into account. These boundaries are sharply constrained by the analyst's position within the bureaucratic work setting, more so than for the university-based researcher.

Third, for every policy analyst outside the university there is tension between the needs and requirements of the client, on one hand, and their own professional commitments to intellectual honesty, to the searching out of negative evidence, and to their freedom to speak and publish what is known or has been learnt, on the other. Bureaucratic research settings put severe strains on those scholarly and professional values. Indeed, the moral issue of how policy analysts deal with dual loyalty to their professional identity as analysts and to their political masters and clients is at the heart of policy analysis and not, as moral issues often are, at the margins.

Finally, there is the relation between policy analysts and policy intellectuals which bears on the nature of communication and persuasion in the political arena, and more broadly on the processes of "decision accretion" through enlightenment and the percolation of research findings, ideas, and assumptions in the decision-making process.

4. Policy Intellectuals and Policy Analysts

In his paper identifying several models of connections between research and policy, Husén (1984) is drawn to the enlightenment or "percolation" model. He quotes Weiss to describe research as permeating the policy making process, entering the policy arena not through specific findings or recommendations, but by its "generalizations and orientations percolating through informed publics in coming to shape the way in which people think about social issues" (Weiss 1979).

There is, I think, broad agreement that much of the impact of research on policy (I would not say all) occurs in this subtle, difficult-to-measure way. But is this not at variance with the image of the policy analyst directly at the policy maker's elbow, preparing papers and reports at his or her request, speaking to issues and problems that the policy-maker will be facing even if not yet recognizing their character or the available options? This image of the policy analyst is in fact compatible with the metaphor of the "percolation" of research, and of the notion of research entering into the general debate and discussion about an issue going on among interested publics, an ongoing debate that crystallizes into policy at a moment when a political actor chooses to place it on the agenda for action and not merely discussion. The analyst in government cannot often do basic research or long-range studies; he or she is to a large extent a consumer and adapter of research, part of the attentive audience for research, and among the most active participants in the critical discussion about the issue and the literature that grows up around it. In the United States, analysts who are educated at schools of public policy are especially trained to take part in that discussion because their teachers and their teachers' peers in other policy schools and professional and academic departments do the research and comment on the research of others in such journals as *The Public Interest, Policy Analysts, Public Choice, Policy Studies Journal*, and *The Journal of Policy Analysis and Management*, among others. These university-based writers and researchers, some of whom teach in the schools of public policy, are what Wilson calls "policy intellectuals." And his view of their influence on policy is not far from that of Weiss and Husén's notion of the percolation model. Reviewing the role of policy intellectuals over the past decade, Wilson observes that

> If the influence of intellectuals was not to be found in the details of policy, it was nonetheless real, albeit indirect. Intellectuals provided the conceptual language, the ruling paradigms, the empirical examples . . . that became the accepted assumptions for those in charge of making policy. Intellectuals framed, and to a large degree conducted, the debates about whether this language and these paradigms were correct. The most influential intellectuals were those who managed to link a concept or a theory to the practical needs and ideological dispositions of political activists and governmental officials. (Wilson 1981 p. 36).

Wilson goes further than most of us in downplaying the role of research per se as against the power of the arguments of skillful intellectuals.

> At any given moment in history, an influential idea— and thus an influential intellectual—is one that provides a persuasive simplification of some policy question that is consistent with a particular mix of core values then held by the political elite . . . Clarifying and making persuasive

those ideas is largely a matter of argument and the careful use of analogies; rarely . . . does this process involve matters of proof and evidence of the sort that is, in their scholarly, as opposed to their public lives, supposed to be the particular skill and obligation of the intellectual in the university. (Wilson 1981 p. 36)

The role of the policy intellectual in policy debates, independent of his or her research, is of great importance and deserves to be studied more closely. The influence of such informed discussion and argument will, I think, vary in different policy fields. But of special interest is the combined effect of policy intellectuals based in the universities and the policy analysts whom they have trained, or who were trained to read them, to understand them, and to use their arguments in the preparation of their reports for decision makers in government. These staff papers, reports, and memoranda give the policy intellectuals' ideas and work access, in ways that the intellectuals themselves do not always have, to the committee rooms and governmental conversations where decisions are made.

5. Policy Analysts versus Interest Groups

The structure of government in the United States, both in Washington and in the state capitols, is changing, becoming even more open and responsive than it has been to vocal, well-organized special interest groups, less and less managed by traditional elites. In the field of education, states Murphy,

> State policy systems, no longer the captive of state education establishments, are now far more accessible to interest groups and open to public view. The adoption of a large number of policy reforms reflects a new responsiveness on the part of state government to these groups.
>
> Within government, the most important change is the heavy involvement of legislators and governors in educational matters. Spurred on by worries about money, school quality, and social issues (e.g., integration), general state government has used its new staff and expertise to challenge education professionals and to remove education from its privileged perch "above politics."
>
> There's a different cast of participants outside government as well . . . Some of the new lobbies promote equality, representing such interests as urban areas, the poor, blacks, Hispanics, the disadvantaged, the handicapped, girls. Reform of state school finance laws has been promoted for the past decade by a network of scholars, foundation executives, lawyers, government officials, community organizers, and citizen groups. Other groups work for efficiency and effectiveness, lobbying for comprehensive planning, improved budgeting, accountability laws, standards for graduation, competency tests for students and teachers. More recently, some of these groups have been promoting tax limitation measures and controls on expenditures. Still other lobbies promote "the public interest." (Murphy 1981 p. 128)

All this energy and activity (in part a consequence of mass higher education) generates an extraordinary level of noise, demands, charges and counter-charges, court actions, and so forth. Pressures of every kind are felt by legislators, elected officials, and their staffs. Policy analysts inside government provide some counterweight, some degree of stability, predictability, and rationality through their professional patterns of response to these pressures and demands. This is not to say that the political activists and their pressure groups are not often successful. But how a government agency responds to organized political pressure may well be shaped by the anonymous analysts in the executive and legislative staffs and agencies. And it is through them that a large or at least a different, set of ideas comes into play in these discussions, and these ideas at their best are less narrow and parochial, more likely to be illuminated by historical and comparative perspectives and by the ongoing discussion that policy intellectuals carry on among themselves in the professional journals.

The structure of politics, the character of the policy areas in which discussions and debate about policies are carried on, are quite different in, for example, Sweden than they are in the United States. Careful studies of actual policy formulation and implementation in specific areas must illuminate the patterns of "social interaction" that more often than not are the major determinants of outcomes in the policy arena. In these increasingly complex networks of social interaction, the relations between policy analysts in government and policy intellectuals in the university are of large and growing importance in the United States, with close analogues in Sweden and other western societies.

6. Conclusion: Research and the Rhetoric of Politics

It is natural that members of the research community are concerned that the research they do provides true and illuminating accounts of the institutions and processes that they study. Some researchers are also interested in whether research has any influence on the shaping of policy and the making of decisions, and if it does, how it enters the decision process and affects the outcomes of those decisions.

But it may be useful, and not wholly subversive of the research itself, to reflect that policy research has value independent of its truth or quality or its influence on policy. That is because social research is one of the ways in which political discussions are carried on in democratic societies, a way that is supportive of liberal democratic politics. Political argument is increasingly conducted in the language of research and analysis; concepts like "cost–benefit" and "trade-off" have found their way into the daily language of politicians and bureaucrats. Moreover, social research and democratic politics have some close affinities.

For one thing, like democratic politics, social research is a process not of assertion or demonstration, but of persuasion. Moreover, it is a form of persuasion that appeals to reason and evidence rather than to supernatural authority, or tradition, or the charisma of an individual, or the authority of a legal order. The appeal to research findings is very far from the coercive domination of others by force or threat, and equally far from political manipulations which depend on the exploitation of a differential of knowledge and awareness between manipulator and the manipulated. The appeal to "research findings" is the appeal to the authority of reason, to a rationality that connects means and ends in ways that are consistent with strongly held social values. Max Weber has said that the contribution of sociology to politics is not to affirm ultimate ends, but to help clarify, if possible to "make transparent," the connections between means and ends so that choices can be made in greater awareness of the consistency of the means chosen with the ends intended. Insofar as social science attempts to do that, it becomes part of the persuasive mechanism of politics, rooting politics, at least in part, in persuasion based on an appeal to reason and knowledge. It need not weaken professional concern for the quality and truth of research to suggest that social research makes its largest contribution to liberal society not through its findings, but by its steady affirmation of the relevance of reason and knowledge to the politics of democracy.

See also: Legitimatory Research; Educational Research and Policy-making; Policy-oriented Research; Politics of Educational Research

References

Husén T 1984 Issues and their background. In: Husén T, Kogan M (eds.) 1984 *Educational Research and Policy: How do They Relate?* Pergamon Press, Oxford

Kogan M, Korman N, Henkel M 1980 *Government's Commissioning of Research: A Case Study.* Department of Government, Brunel University, Uxbridge

Lerner D, Lasswell H (eds.) 1951 *The Policy Sciences.* Stanford University Press, Stanford, California

Meltsner A J 1976 *Policy Analysts in the Bureaucracy.* University of California Press, Berkeley, California

Murphy J T 1981 The paradox of state government reform. *Public Interest* 64: 124–39

Weiss C H 1979 The many meanings of research utilization. *Pub. Admin. Review* 39: 426–31

Wilson J Q 1981 Policy intellectuals and 'public policy'. *Public Interest* 64: 31–46

Further Reading

Kallen D B P et al. (eds.) 1983 *Social Science Research and Public Policy Making: A Reappraisal.* NFER–Nelson, Windsor

Policy-oriented Research

J. Nisbet

Policy-oriented research is best defined in terms of its instrumental function rather than by its topics of study. When research in education is designed, managed, and reported with the specific purpose of informing a policy decision, or assisting or monitoring its implementation, or evaluating its effects, the term "policy-oriented" is used to distinguish this approach from "fundamental" research which is designed primarily to extend the frontiers of knowledge. This definition of policy-oriented research may be extended to include research which is closely tied to educational practice as well as policy.

The implicit model is that the function of research is to provide an information base for decision-making, to establish the "facts"; administrators, politicians, or teachers then add the necessary value judgments, supposedly so that policy and practice are firmly based on empirical evidence from experiment and survey. Thus "good" research provides answers to "relevant" problems. In this approach, educational issues which are of current concern are accepted as priority topics for research. This instrumental view of the function of research, however, makes naive and simplistic assumptions about how policy and practice are determined (see *Educational Research and Policy Making*). If adopted uncritically, the emphasis on relevance constrains inquiry within the limits of existing policy and risks a trivialization of research and centralization of control over the choice of topics for inquiry. But with a clearer understanding of the relation of research and policy and with enlightened administration of research funding, the trend toward policy-oriented research could enable research to make a more effective contribution to educational practice.

1. Definitions

The definition of policy-oriented research is usually expressed by contrasting it with fundamental research, on the analogy of pure and applied science. A variety of terms can be used to express the contrast: applied versus basic research, policy-oriented versus curiosity-oriented studies, instrumental versus enlightenment functions, work directed toward decision or action versus work directed toward knowledge or theory. Less charitably, "relevant" research may be contrasted with "academic" research. Cronbach and Suppes (1969) criticized these "popular labels," arguing instead for a distinction in terms of the audience to whom the research is directed. Their concepts of "decision-oriented" and "conclusion-oriented" research have been widely adopted. Decision-oriented research is designed to provide information wanted by a decision-maker; the findings of conclusion-oriented research are of interest primarily to the research community. "The distinction between decision-oriented and conclusion-oriented research lies in the origination of the inquiry and the constraints imposed by its institutional setting, not in topic or technique" (p.23). Thus, Cooley and Bickel (1985) define decision-oriented research as "a form of educational research that is designed to be directly relevant to the current information requirements of those who are shaping educational policy or managing educational systems" (p. xi).

Whichever terms are used, they carry value judgments which can be misleading if they are not made explicit. The distinction between pure and applied research in education is itself misleading, in that theoretical studies provide concepts for the analysis of problems and may even help to identify and define problems. It may be argued that educational research must be set in the context of an educational system: if it is general, it may be better described as psychological or sociological or management research. "From one point of view, *all* educational research is applied research, designed to bring about changes in the way education is carried on, rather than simply to add to our existing stock of knowledge" (Taylor 1973 p. 207). Defined narrowly, policy-oriented research is research which has direct application to current issues in educational policy or practice. A wider definition (and, to anticipate the argument of this analysis, a better one) is that policy-oriented research consists of careful, systematic attempts to understand the educational process and, through understanding, to improve its efficiency.

Listing the procedures involved is one way of defining. Policy-oriented research includes surveys or any comparable data-gathering which enables policymakers or practitioners to base their decisions on evidence rather than on prejudice or guesswork. This includes the search for solutions to pressing educational or social problems, identifying and resolving the problems involved in implementing policy decisions, pilot studies to test new initiatives, monitoring and evaluating initiatives in educational practice, and experimental studies to compare alternative educational methods. It also includes policy studies and retrospective analyses of past policy where the purpose is to help make better policy decisions in the future.

Thus the essential distinction between policy-oriented and other forms of educational research is in terms of purpose, rather than in choice of subject or method. Since the perception of educational issues as being of current concern is subject to volatile popular fashion, an aspect of learning may be regarded as a theoretical issue this year but a topic of policy-oriented research next year. The end products of policy-oriented research are recommendations for decision or action. The products of fundamental research are contributions to knowledge, understanding, or theory. Since decisions and action necessarily imply the adoption of some theory or interpretation, and theory likewise has long-term implications for action, the distinction between the two categories is not as sharp as is sometimes assumed. However, policy-oriented research usually operates within the context of accepted theory: it does not aim to modify theory, though it may do so incidentally. Similarly, fundamental research does not aim to affect practice, but it may do so indirectly. Policy-oriented research is responsive, whereas fundamental research is autonomous.

Autonomous educational research, which does not have to be accountable in the sense of producing useful or usable findings, runs the risk of producing results which are of interest only to other researchers. In its extreme, it is concerned with attacking other people's theories, irrespective of whether the points at issue are of any importance outside the research sphere. Responsive research, designed as a response to a practical need, is no less likely to raise and illuminate fundamental issues, and there is the added bonus that it can be useful at the same time. However, it runs the risk of being left behind by the rapid course of events, since by the time results are available the problem which they were designed to answer is liable to have changed or to be no longer seen as important. The resolution of this dilemma may lie in the concept of "strategic research" (Bondi 1983): "that grey zone of researches that . . . are not immediately of use to the customer, but lay the foundations for being able to answer questions that may be put in the future" (p. 3). Unfortunately, however, the precise nature of strategic research remains uncertain.

Since responsive research operates within the context of existing policy or practice, it is limited in its generalizability, but it is more likely to have an impact on the specific policy or practice for which it is designed. The impact of this kind of research, however, is incremental rather than radical. Policy-oriented research modifies (and hopefully improves) the existing situation, protecting it from running into trouble by identifying or anticipating problems. It may challenge established policy by demonstrating its impracticability, or may develop or explore alternative policies. But it is essentially concerned with movement from a present situation, and therefore it obliges researchers to relate their work to "reality," usually in the form of empirical studies or fieldwork.

2. Trends

Although pressure toward policy-oriented research has increased since the 1970s, many of the early educational research studies had a strong practical orientation. Binet's work, for example, which laid the foundations of psychometry, began with the problem of early identification of slow-learning children. The work of Thorndike and others in the 1920s on the psychology of the elementary school curriculum aimed to influence educational policy and classroom practice. The "scientific movement" in the 1930s envisaged the creation of a science of education based on experimentation, which would be used to improve decision-making at all levels, from day-to-day classroom practice to long-term educational planning. National studies in the 1930s, such as the Eight-year Study to test the feasibility of school accreditation and the international program of research on examinations, were directed to produce practical recommendations for improvement of the system. The distinction between practical and theoretical research was not stressed at this time. The two kinds of research were seen as complementary; and since there was practically no public funding of research, the choice of topic was left to academic researchers in universities and colleges.

The situation changed dramatically in the years after 1950, first with the growth of publicly financed research (1955–65) and a massive expansion of funding in 1965–70, and subsequently with the demand for accountability and a trend toward central control of research. Initially (and relatively slowly) there was acceptance that educational research could make a significant contribution to policy and practice. The social sciences had come of age and their potential value was recognized. (Perhaps it was merely that administrators found themselves at a disadvantage in controversies if they could not produce empirical evidence to support their decisions.) In Sweden, the linking of research to policy began in the 1940s. In the 1960s, in the United States and the United Kingdom (and subsequently in many other countries), formal institutional structures were created for channeling public funds into educational research and development, particularly for curriculum development and intervention programs. As a result, between 1964 and 1969, expenditure on research in education in the United Kingdom multiplied tenfold; and in the United States, expenditure doubled each year from 1964 through 1967. Almost all this funding was for policy-oriented research.

The increase in funding soon led to a demand for accountability, and for a greater say in how the funds were to be spent. Since public funding was for policy-oriented research, policymakers began to demand the right to decide which policy aspects should be researched, and also how the research should be oriented. In 1970 in the United Kingdom,

for example, the Secretary of State for Education and Science demanded that research policy in education "had to move from a basis of patronage—the rather passive support of ideas which were essentially other people's, related to problems which were often of other people's choosing—to a basis of commission . . . the active initiation by the Department on problems of its own choosing, within a procedure and timetable which were relevant to its needs" (DES 1970). This was followed in 1971 by the crude customer–contractor formula of the Rothschild Report (1971): "The customer says what he wants; the contractor (the researcher) does it if he can; and the customer pays" (p. 3). This method of deciding how research should be funded was widely challenged at the time. But the protests could not survive the energy crisis of 1973 and the economic constraints of the years which followed. The need to cut back expenditure made decisions on priorities inevitable, and increasingly these decisions were made by central government. Perhaps too much had been expected, or promised, and disillusionment was allied with suspicion of "academic drift," in which preoccupation with theory was given priority over pressing practical issues. In the 1990s, research which is not linked to policy is at risk of being seen as a dispensable luxury, and major policy issues are seen as the only topics worth studying.

Thus, to quote from a review of developments in eight countries (Nisbet 1981a), "Across the world, educational research is now an integral part of modern administrative procedure. Increased investment in research has led to . . . a concern that the conduct, organisation and funding of research should be directed towards maximising its effect on policy and practice. The major questions to which answers are still sought are, What forms of research should have priority? and, Who is to decide?" (p. 104).

Since then, decisions increasingly have been made centrally by those who control public funds, not only on what should be researched but also on the method and scale (everything short of the results expected), and often with restrictions on the right to publish without official approval. Central decision-making on research priorities runs the risk of restricting the scope of inquiry. The Organisation for Economic Cooperation and Development in a report (OECD 1988 p. 23) expressed its concern at the trend toward a "practical, short-term and commercial orientation" in the national research programs of its member states. However, as Cuban (1992) noted, "the frameworks which educational researchers use . . . often overlook unwittingly the enduring tension-ridden dilemmas that practitioners and policymakers must manage in their organizations" (p. 7). Restrictions on dissemination, though increasingly common in research contracts, run counter to the basic principle of "critical debate," defined in a policy statement of the British Educational Research Association (Bassey 1992) as "opening one's work to the scrutiny of others in order first to search for errors and fallacies, and secondly to seek creative insights into its future development" (p. 8).

If policy-oriented research is to be effective, it needs cooperation between policymakers and researchers; but it also requires a degree of independence. A warning of the danger inherent in central control was given in the United Kingdom in 1982, when a second Rothschild Report (1982) was published on the work of the government-sponsored Social Science Research Council: "The need for independence from government departments is particularly important because so much social science is the stuff of political debate . . . It would be too much to expect Ministers to show enthusiasm for research designed to show that their policies were misconceived. But it seems obvious that in many cases the public interest will be served by such research being undertaken" (p. 12). This raises the issue of how research can best be used in the framing and monitoring of policy.

3. Utilization

How can research best contribute to policy and practice in education? This question is the central theme of the 1985 *World Yearbook of Education* (Nisbet et al. 1985), which reviews contrasting perspectives in 14 countries. People have different expectations of research, and these are often unrealistic. Policymakers and teachers tend to look to research to provide answers to their problems; but research can perform this function only when there is consensus on values, within the framework of accepted policy or in the context of established practice. Researchers are more likely to see the role of research as identifying new problems, or new perspectives on problems—problem-setting rather than problem-solving (Rein and Schon 1977). But implementation will happen only when the findings are seen as relevant to the issues which concern those with the responsibility of action. If it is not to be just an esoteric activity, research in education must have a context. But whose context is it to be?

If research is undertaken in the context of those who are expected to make use of the findings, the likelihood of implementation is much greater. The Australian *Karmel Report* (Karmel 1973) summarized the requirements for impact: "The effectiveness of innovation . . . is dependent on the extent to which the people concerned perceive a problem . . ., are knowledgeable about a range of alternative solutions, and feel themselves to be in a congenial climate" (p. 126). How people perceive a problem is itself influenced by research publications. Thus research shapes people's perceptions, and provides them with concepts to use in thinking about the work they do. In this way, research creates an agenda of concern.

Weiss (1979), reviewing the contribution of social research to public policy, identified seven models of research utilization:

(a) the linear model, which assumes that basic research leads into applied research, followed by development and implementation;

(b) the problem-solving model, in which research identifies the missing knowledge to guide action;

(c) the interactive model, involving researchers and policymakers in constructive cooperative dialogue;

(d) the political model, where research is used to provide justification for an already favored policy;

(e) the tactical model, in which the need for research is used as an excuse to delay decision or action;

(f) the enlightenment model, envisaging research ideas filtering through and shaping how people think;

(g) the intellectual model, by which the activity of research widens horizons and raises the quality of public debate.

The first two models are naive; the third and seventh over-hopeful; the fourth and fifth cynical. In an earlier work, Weiss (1977) argued for the sixth of these models—the enlightenment model—seeing the most important effect of research as indirect and long-term, through "a gradual accumulation of research results" (p. 16), shaping the context within which policy decisions are made. Husén and Kogan (1984) in *Educational Research and Policy: How Do They Relate?*, the most comprehensive review of the issue in the 1980s, accept this "percolation" model, but ask how the percolation of ideas can be engineered. Research can clarify issues, raise awareness, and create space for testing policies before they are put into action; but there is a lack of institutional structures for independent research to have impact on the formulation of policy.

The problem-solving model is implicit in one of the most widely read educational publications of the 1980s, *What Works: Research about Teaching and Learning* (US Department of Education 1986). This 65-page booklet listed 41 research findings about how best to teach and improve learning. Each finding was stated, briefly elaborated, and supported by five references to research literature. In the Preface, the President of the United States commended it as providing practical knowledge based on "some of the best available research for use by the American public." Published in January 1986, 300,000 copies were in circulation within 6 months. Glass (1987) criticized this selection of "useful findings" as "an expression of conservative philosophy" (p. 6), arguing that its popular appeal was due to the possibility of applying the findings within the existing framework of educational assumptions.

Husén and Kogan (1984) identify a major dilemma in the different worlds of policy and research. The two worlds have different and conflicting values, different reference groups and reward systems, and even different languages. Policy decision-making must be firm and authoritative, whereas research is essentially questioning and uncertain.

> A political decision will lead to closure on an issue. Research findings add to, rather than reduce, uncertainty for decision-makers. The interplay between decision-making which must be authoritative and firm and the questioning and uncertainty implicit in the research is an important phenomenon. It leads to a central policy question: can national authorities sponsor the generation of uncertainty? . . . Policy-makers may foreclose on issues too quickly: social science can keep open the space between the dissemination of ideas which might lead to policy changes and their enforcement. (p. 52)

Bell and Raffe (1991) offer a resolution of this dilemma by distinguishing a changing balance between research and policy in three phases of the policy cycle:

(a) recognition of a problem and shaping a policy;

(b) implementing a policy;

(c) evaluating the outcomes and reshaping the policy.

In the first phase, before outlines of a new policy have emerged, "wide-ranging critical research is welcomed, because it will help to win support for change." In the second phase, the government needs to build support for its chosen policy: "research which calls into question the wisdom of the policy or the assumptions on which it is based is not welcome." Here, the policy world is most restrictive and control tightest. In the third phase, "there is a degree of relaxation: the policy is no longer so politically sensitive (it is now the flavour of last month) . . . and critical research findings are less potentially damaging" (p. 141). Bell and Raffe ask why so little policy-related research is commissioned in the first phase of the policy cycle.

The answer lies in who is seen as holding power. The policymakers seek to establish a policy which is acceptable to those with power to influence its implementation. Their concern is not so much a matter of being "right" (for there are different "right" solutions, depending on one's values), but rather of reconciling divergent views in a solution which is seen as "fair" by a maximum number of those affected by it. In this, the aims and values of those with access to power must carry greatest weight.

In the amorphous process of policy-making, there are several functions which research can perform. First, insofar as information conveys power, research strengthens the hand of any group which can produce research findings to support its preferred viewpoint. (Even to describe assertions as "research" strengthens their impact.) Coleman (1984) noted that this strategy "is most often used by those without direct control over policy, who challenge the policies of those in positions of authority" (p. 132); and this may be one reason for policymakers' hostility to research. Administrators commission policy-oriented research to strengthen their hand against the many pressure groups in the policy-making arena. In the view of the administrators, pressure groups are those who seek to further their own policies, whereas administrators see themselves as neutral to the policy they implement. Information thus weakens the power of those who play on ignorance or twist facts to suit their private ends. This, however, assumes that research is value-free, or at least that research makes explicit the values on which it is based.

A second function for research is to ensure that action will achieve what is intended in a policy. For this purpose, research is used to work out the details of how to implement decisions, by identifying obstacles, including the opinions and attitudes of those who might oppose the policy, and by testing out solutions to overcome these obstacles in trials with pilot groups. Using Bell and Raffe's three phases of the policy cycle: in phase 1, surveys gather relevant "facts" as a database for decision; in phase 2, pilot studies establish feasibility and identify likely obstacles; and in phase 3, evaluation provides monitoring and guidance for future decision or modification.

In all three phases, the most valuable research design is one which focuses on analysis of problems, rather than simply seeking to supply answers to questions. There are of course some who still hold the unrealistic expectation that research should provide ready-made incontrovertible solutions. The Secretary of State of the Department of Education and Science for England and Wales, for example, once complained: "It is exceptional to find a piece of research that really hits the nail on the head and tells you pretty clearly what is wrong or what should be done" (Pile 1976 p. 3). Weiss (1977) describes this as the "linear model" of research utilization and criticizes its "instrumental naivety." The sequence implied is: "A problem exists; information or understanding is lacking; research provides the missing knowledge; a solution is reached" (pp. 11–12). There are relatively few situations in which this model is applicable. Halsey's (1972) interpretation is nearer the truth: "Action research is unlikely ever to yield neat and definitive prescriptions from field-tested plans. What it offers is an aid to intelligent decision-making, not a substitute for it. Research brings relevant information rather than uniquely exclusive conditions" (p. 179).

However, the claim that the prime use of research lies in the analysis of problems may be seen only as an academic abdication of responsibility, and may encourage the suspicion that the only ones who derive benefit from investment in research are the researchers themselves. Being isolated from the practical realities of the "real world," as it is termed, they divert public money to academic interests of their own instead of to the problems which require solutions. The solution adopted has been to take the decisions on research priorities out of the hands of the researchers and put them in the hands of the administrators. If research cannot give direction to policy, then the influence should be reserved and policymakers should be given control of research, allowing policy priorities to determine the choice and design of research. If those who are in contact with the "real world" take over the management of research, so the assumption goes, impact will be improved, relevance will be greater, and the risk of wasted money will be avoided.

Consequently, decisions on research priorities are often made by those who are not themselves directly involved in research. This mode of working is familiar to the economist, the engineer, and the agricultural specialist; it is not accepted generally in legal and medical matters. The administrator who controls research funds now expects to be involved in the initial decisions on the topic of inquiry, the design, the time scale, the personnel required, and of course the cost. When a project is funded, there will be continuing interest (or interference, as it may seem to the researcher) in monitoring what is being done through an advisory committee (often designated as a steering committee) and regular reporting on progress. Tighter control may be imposed by "stepped funding," in which funds for each stage are conditional on approval of a report on the previous one. Arrangements for publishing and discussing the findings will be specified in the contract, which may require surrender of copyright and "moral rights" to the sponsor and acceptance of their right of veto should they find the results not to their liking.

It is difficult to stand against these pressures. Not only can sponsors withhold funds: even access to schools is usually made conditional on approval of the research project as a whole and of the research instruments in detail. Thus policy-oriented research can become wholly directed and censored by people who are not themselves researchers and who have a vested interest in the outcomes. Clearly, the dangers here are that criticism of a policy is not likely to be encouraged and that important issues are organized out of debate. Fortunately, many of those responsible for the funding of research are aware of these dangers. In some countries at least, the relationship between researchers and the providers of funds is quite close, both sides understanding the requirements and constraints of the other.

4. Conclusion

Two functions of research in education can be distinguished: one long-term, creating the theoretical context in which day-to-day issues are perceived, writing an agenda of concern; the other more immediate, working out routine problems within the context of the current educational provision and prevailing views. These are the basic and policy-oriented modes of research, but the distinction between them is not as sharp as might appear. The applied sciences have often resulted in significant contributions to theory, and theoretical studies may have profound impact on perceptions of practical needs.

Academic status tends to be accorded to those who make contributions to theory. In the social sciences, their ideas and new concepts are gradually absorbed into popular thought and discussion until they become a new climate of opinion, variously described as a "prevailing view" (Cronbach and Suppes 1969), "a cumulative altering of conceptions of human behavior" (Getzels), "sensitizing" (Taylor 1973), or "ideas in good currency" (Schon). Administrators and politicians respond to the "resonance" of research findings, often to a filtered, out-of-date perception. In the early 1990s, however, research funding is available almost exclusively for policy-oriented studies. Research of this kind can be a powerful instrument of reform, testing out new ideas, modifying them or rejecting them if they are at fault, and if the evidence shows them to be feasible, establishing their credibility all the more widely and quickly. The results are more likely to have impact and thus create in the long term a favorable climate of opinion as to the value of educational research. In a time of financial constraint and accountability, it is difficult to justify the expenditure of public funds on any other kind of research in education.

The danger, however, is that if research is too closely tied to existing educational provision and practice, where the concept of "relevance" implies implementation without radical change, the effects may be only marginal and may even be an obstacle to reform. The restrictions increasingly imposed on researchers in policy-oriented funding are seen by many as running counter to the basic requirement of open, critical study. There is also a danger of accepting a purely technocratic role for research, creating an elite group of researchers in alliance with bureaucrats to manage the system. Though at first sight this may seem an attractive role for the researcher, it is potentially divisive, since it divides the researcher and his or her powerful partner from the teaching profession and the public. An alternative style of research is the "teachers as researchers" movement (see *Teachers as Researchers*) or "action research" (see *Action Research*). In this school-based research, teachers are encouraged to apply the techniques of research to their own work: they define the problems to be researched and they investigate and reflect on their own practice. This style of research also has its risks, of restricting research within the limits of inflexible classroom traditions and narrow professional perspectives. But it could also "be the most fertile soil for educational research to grow in . . . If it can be developed so as to provide teachers (and administrators and parents and all those concerned with education) with the means of improving their own understanding, then its effect will be to put educational studies into a questioning framework" (Broadfoot and Nisbet 1981 p. 121).

216

An interactionist model of this kind for educational research applies also to the relation of research to policy. The association of policy, administration, and research could be developed in such a way that each illuminates the others. Cronbach et al. (1980) argue for an intermediate structure between research and application to promote this interaction, some institutional means of arguing about the policy relevance of ambiguous results in a "context of accommodation" rather than a "context of command" (pp. 83–84). If policy-oriented studies can be developed in this enlightened way, educational research stands to gain from its closer association with both policy and practice. "Two worlds of educational research may be distinguished, the practical and the theoretical, pure and applied; but we are more likely to have a balanced attitude if we have a foot in both worlds" (Nisbet 1981b p. 175). The contributions of research to policy, to practice, and to theory are not easily reconciled; but the research enterprise would suffer if any one of these three is regarded as of lesser importance.

References

Bassey M 1992 Educational research and politics: A viewpoint. *Research Intelligence* 43: 8–9

Bell C, Raffe D 1991 Working together: Research, policy and practice. In: Walford G (ed.) 1991 *Doing Educational Research*. Routledge, London.

Bondi H 1983 Research funding scrutinized. THES August 19: 3

Broadfoot P M, Nisbet J 1981 The impact of research on educational studies. *Br. J. Educ. Stud.* 29(2): 115–22

Coleman J S 1984 Issues in the institutionalisation of social policy. In: Husén T H, Kogan M (eds.) 1984

Cooley W, Bickel W 1985 *Decision-oriented Educational Research*. Kluwer-Nijhoff, Boston, Massachusetts

Cronbach L J, Suppes P (eds.) 1969 *Research for Tomorrow's Schools: Disciplined Inquiry for Education*. Macmillan, New York

Cronbach L J et al. 1980 *Toward Reform of Program Evaluation*. Jossey-Bass, San Francisco, California

Cuban L 1992 Managing dilemmas while building professional communities. *Educ. Researcher* 21(1): 4–11

Department of Education and Science (DES) 1970 Press release December 1, 1970, for speech to National Foundation for Educational Research. In: Taylor W (ed.) 1973 *Research Perspectives in Education*. Routledge and Kegan Paul, London

Glass G V 1987 What works: Politics and research. *Educ. Researcher* 16(3): 5–10

Halsey A H 1972 *Educational Priority*, Vol. 1. HMSO, London

Husén T H, Kogan M (eds.) 1984 *Educational Research and Policy: How Do They Relate?* Pergamon Press, Oxford

Karmel P H (Chair) 1973 *Schools in Australia*. Australian Government Printing Service, Canberra

Nisbet J 1981a The impact of research on policy and practice in education. *Int. Rev. Educ.* 27(2): 101–04

Nisbet J 1981b Educational research and educational practice. In: Simon B, Taylor W (eds.) 1981 *Education in the Eighties: The Central Issues*. Batsford, London

Nisbet J, Megarry J, Nisbet S (eds.) 1985 *World Yearbook of Education 1985: Research, Policy and Practice*. Kogan Page, London

OECD 1988 *Science and Technology Policy Outlook*. OECD, Paris.

Pile W 1976 Some research called "rubbish." THES January 23: 3

Rein M, Schon D A 1977 Problem setting in policy research. In: Weiss C (ed.) 1977

Rothschild Report 1971 *A Framework for Government Research and Development*. HMSO (Cmnd 4814), London

Rothschild Report 1982 *An Enquiry into the Social Science Research Council*. HMSO (Cmnd 8554), London

Taylor W (ed.) 1973 *Research Perspectives in Education*. Routledge and Kegan Paul, London

US Department of Education 1986 *What Works: Research about Teaching and Learning*. Washington, DC

Weiss C (ed.) 1977 *Using Social Research in Public Policy Making*. Heath, Lexington, Massachusetts

Weiss C 1979 The many meanings of research utilization. *Public Administration Review* (Sept/Oct): 426–31

Evaluation Models and Approaches

N. L. Smith

Numerous models and approaches have been developed to define and direct the evaluation of educational programs. The use of these models in evaluation practice has given rise to a variety of theoretical issues and to the development of theories of evaluation. These topics are reviewed in this entry.

1. Early Models and Approaches

The term "model" has been used with wide variability and considerable ambiguity in evaluation practice and literature. Most generally, it refers to particular conceptions, approaches, methods, and even loose theories for thinking about and /or conducting evaluations.

When educational practitioners began conducting widespread, formal evaluations in the mid-1960s, they recognized the need for conceptual overviews to guide the practice of evaluation. The models or conceptual approaches they developed were used to define the nature and purpose of the evaluation they were conducting, to describe the object being evaluated (called the "evaluand"), to structure and guide actual evaluation procedures, and to communicate the nature of their evaluation to clients and audiences.

What started out as simple design heuristics changed, in some cases dramatically, over the next 25 years (see Smith 1992). Alkin (1991) recounts the factors influencing authors to change their conceptions of their own models or approaches: (a) confrontation with others' interpretations of the author's work, (b) confrontation with discrepant positions, (c) incorporation of related work, (d) accumulation of personal research on evaluation practice, (e) increased experience in actually conducting evaluations, (f) personal interactions with colleagues, and (g) public attempts to categorize the attributes of various models. With time, some models became more refined and procedurally specific, while others came to reflect broad philosophical positions. While rapidly evolving from the start, evaluation models have collectively represented the disparate social agendas, philosophical positions, contexts of practice, and methodological predilections of the increasingly diverse participants in the field of evaluation.

The boundaries and components of a particular model are often surprisingly difficult to determine, particularly for evolving approaches to which multiple theorists and practitioners are contributing. Especially in educational evaluation, there is a tendency to equate specific models with particular individuals. For example, both Alkin and Ellet (1990) and Shadish et al. (1991) briefly discuss the problems of delineating which elements belong in a particular model and resolve the difficulty by referring " . . . to 'models' as the largest coherent set of ideas put forward by a particular model builder at a particular time" (Alkin and Ellet 1990 p. 19). Although this is a common way to deal with the problem, it has several limitations, including that it disregards the related work of other theorists, it results in models without highly visible single champions receiving less attention, and it largely ignores the nature of the models as used in practice.

This last point reflects a significant omission since all the so-called evaluation models are prescriptive to the extent that they are based on particular philosophical and methodological positions, provide guiding frameworks for viewing evaluation, and recommend activities or procedures, all directed toward accomplishing a proper evaluation according to that model. Indeed, some writers argue that the so-called models are not actually models at all, but methodological advocacies. "What we have in the evaluation literature are not models but approaches or persuasions . . . evaluation theorists promote their concerns, advocate particular commitments, and emphasize particular purviews. These are persuasions, not prescriptions" (Stake 1991 p. 71; see also House 1980). Worthen and Sanders (1987) concur that the so-called evaluation models are not models in a scientific sense, have little predictive power, and are, as yet, unvalidated

empirically, but they conclude that models have had a significant impact on evaluation practice.

Although evaluators sometimes speak of designing evaluations which follow a particular model, their language generally refers not to instrumental application of procedural specifics, but to the selection of an overall orientation or approach. Because evaluation models are not procedurally prescriptive, are subject to varied interpretations, are mute on many of the details required to implement an evaluation, and must be operationalized within the demands of a specific context of application, many decisions are left to the evaluator's professional judgment in spite of the prior selection of a given model. No one study can thus be argued to be the epitome of a given model, and many quite different studies are arguably appropriate versions of the same model.

Practitioners' use of evaluation models is less a form of instrumental use and more a form of conceptual or enlightenment use. (Shadish et al. 1991 provide a discussion of theories of use within evaluation.) Whether or not evaluators consciously select a particular model in designing a study, their knowledge of alternative approaches helps them frame the study, represent the evaluand, select study procedures, and adopt an appropriate professional role. It is in reconciling the contrasts among competing models, in justifying selections among study alternatives, and in creating designs which are conceptually sound, technically feasible, and situationally useful, that competing models serve to improve professional judgment.

Evaluation models are most appropriately seen, therefore, as general design heuristics which can inform and improve practice, but which are not implementable or testable in discrete, unambiguous ways. These models have been subjected to considerable conceptual analysis and criticism (see Sect. 3), but mature, professional evaluation practice is developed at least as much from practical field experience as from formal training and familiarity with professional literature. If these evaluation models are methodological advocacies, then what is the empirical evidence to support their adoption, even for conceptual use? This is an important issue since the models can be seen as conceptual precursors to empirically validated theories of evaluation practice (see Sect. 4).

2. Selected Models and Approaches

Worthen and Sanders (1987) indicate that between 1967 and 1987 over 50 different evaluation models were developed. Clearly the scope and detail of information available on these alternatives precludes a discussion of each, or more than a brief comment on the ones selected for mention here.

Although usage is inconsistent, the term "model" frequently refers to the work of a single or small number of theorists writing about an orientation which has specific, circumscribed characteristics. "Approach" typically refers to a broader, less focused conceptualization which may include a grouping of several related models. This convention is followed in the inventory of approaches and models presented below. The labeling of a conceptualization as an approach or model is arbitrary and varies with the writer. For example, previous theorists have often mixed both approaches and models within the same classificatory scheme (see Sect. 3.1).

Approaches and models tend to become known by the characteristics which discriminate them most from others. This can underrepresent similarities and highlight specific, oversimplified features, creating model caricatures which make for easy recognition but obscure the real complexity of the model's character. What follows are oversimplifications. Depending on what aspects one wishes to emphasize, different groupings are readily possible. (For more detailed description and discussion of the following models, including references to original sources, see Alkin and Ellett 1990, House 1978, 1980, Scriven 1991, Shadish et al. 1991, Stake 1973, Stufflebeam and Webster 1980, Worthen 1990, and Worthen and Sanders 1987.)

2.1 Testing-Objectives Approaches

The earliest modern approach to evaluating educational programs emphasized the use of educational testing procedures to determine if program objectives were being accomplished. Tyler first formulated this approach in which programmatic objectives were identified, defined in behavioral terms, and student progress on them was then assessed using standardized or locally constructed instruments. This approach and Tyler's writings had considerable impact on initial conceptions of educational evaluation; the Tylerian model is still the most frequently employed approach to evaluation at the local school level.

Subsequent variations on this basic approach were developed by Hammond (EPIC model), who included additional instructional and institutional variables, and Provus (Discrepancy model), who emphasized the comparison of program standards with program performance to provide "discrepancy" information for program improvement. Large-scale testing models of evaluation such as Popham's Instructional Objectives Exchange (IOX), and earlier accountability models of evaluation reflect this basic measurement approach.

2.2 Decision-Management Approaches

Because much evaluation originates to serve decision makers' needs in managing educational programs, models tailored to that specific purpose were soon developed. The earliest such model was Stufflebeam's CIPP model (context, input, process, product) which relied on a modified systems analysis approach to classify the types of decisions managers needed to address and to develop information relevant to each type of decision. Variations included Alkin's CSE model (Center for the Study of Evaluation), which highlighted the distinctions between program implementation and program improvement, and Patton's UFE model (Utilization-Focused Evaluation), which was clearly decision oriented, but more client centered than manager centered. Highly focused on enhancing evaluation utilization, these models remain especially popular among school administrators. For a variety of reasons, the related cost analysis approaches to evaluation (cf. Levin's Cost-Effectiveness model) have not been as widely adopted.

2.3 Research Approaches

Many early specialists conducting educational evaluations approached the task by applying various models of research. For these individuals, evaluation became "evaluative research," a subset of applied social science, employing models of Instructional Research (eg., Cronbach) and Experimental/Quasi-experimental Research (eg., Suchman, Campbell, Cook, Boruch). Although psychologists were initially prominent among this group, other research traditions have been increasingly reflected, for example, Fetterman's Ethnographic Evaluation model. While the testing-objectives and decision-management approaches construe the evaluation enterprise as basically a measurement or decision-making task, the research approaches construe evaluation as a knowledge generation research task.

2.4 Policy Analysis Approaches

Policy analysis approaches are generally employed to deal with national level issues in education. They are used to evaluate policy either directly, or indirectly through the evaluation of programs and projects relevant to specific policy matters. Policy analysis approaches are similar to decision-management approaches in that decision-making is a primary focus, though at the national rather than local level, and are also similar to research approaches in that research methodologies are often advocated.

Over the years, Weiss's analysis has had considerable impact on the theory and practice of this type of evaluation. Shadish et al. (1991) consider Rossi and his Theory-Driven model of evaluation, with its application of social science methods to the evaluation of social policy, to be one of the strongest models of evaluation currently available. Wholey's development of an approach to aid national decision makers has resulted in several unique contributions (eg., Evaluability Assessment, Rapid Feedback Evaluation). Wholey's approach at the national level is reminiscent of Patton's approach at the local level.

2.5 Adversarial Approaches

Adversarial approaches to evaluation are predicated on the assumption that planned, public opposition of alternative positions is an effective means of highlighting the strengths and weaknesses of competing alternatives. When implemented in an open forum, these approaches provide a means for public assessment of relevant positions, counterclaims, and evidence.

Most adversarial approaches used in educational evaluation have been modeled on the legal profession, including the Adversarial models of Levine, and Owens, as well as Wolf's JEM (Judicial Evaluation model). Stenzel developed the Committee Hearings model using congressional committee hearings as a framework. Adversarial approaches are probably the least widely applied of the seven approaches reviewed here.

2.6 Judgment Approaches

The oldest approaches to the evaluation of educational programs have employed the professional judgments of experts. The Accreditation models used by regional and national accrediting bodies have long relied on judgment data provided by site visit panels. At state and national levels, Blue Ribbon Panels have been convened, and Peer Review Panels are frequently used in areas where technical expertise is considered essential in reaching evaluative conclusions.

Stake's early Countenance model emphasized that judgment data were an essential component of any evaluation, and Scriven subsequently pointed out that the source of those judgments is critical (1983). In his Goal-Free model, Scriven argued that evaluative judgments should not be restricted to goals or objectives, but focus directly on program accomplishments and significant side effects.

For Scriven, judgmental conclusions should be consumer oriented, but for Eisner and his Connoisseurial model of evaluation such judgments are expertise oriented. As with Criticism models of evaluation (eg., Kelly, Willis), it is the viewpoint of the expert critic which dominates the evaluation.

2.7 Pluralist-Intuitionist Approaches

A collection of more recently developed approaches to evaluation can be labeled as "pluralist-intuitionist." They share a common commitment to value pluralism, that is, to the identification and preservation of multiple value perspectives. They also rely heavily on a largely intuitive process for collecting and interpreting evaluative information.

Stake's Responsive model of evaluation argues that evaluators should primarily respond to audience concerns and provide information within audience value perspectives. This requires an iterative process with much audience contact. Guba, Lincoln, and others who advocate the Participative model of evaluation go further to argue that evaluation should not be done without "audiences" participating as full partners. Rippey's Transactional model of evaluation focuses on the reactive effects of the evaluation process itself, while MacDonald's Democratic model views evaluation as essentially a political activity. Parlett and Hamilton, in the Illuminative model, argue that evaluation's primary purpose is merely to describe and interpret. All these approaches are highly client centered and share a commitment to subjectivist ethics and epistemology within a liberal ideology (see House 1978).

3. Classifications, Analyses, and Integrations

The varied nature of so many alternative evaluation models and approaches has promoted both a rich methodological diversity and increasing methodological confusion. A number of attempts have been made, therefore, to bring some clarity to what Gephart once called this "multiple model mess." These clarifications have included various classifications of selected models to highlight significant differences of orientation, analyses of underlying principles and ideological or philosophical positions, and preliminary efforts at integrations across models.

3.1 Classifications

Beginning in the early 1970s, theorists have periodically produced classifications of evaluation models and approaches (eg., Stake 1973, Worthen and Sanders 1973, Popham 1975, House 1978, Stufflebeam and Webster 1980, Worthen and Sanders 1987, Worthen 1990). These classifications were designed to clarify distinctions across current approaches, provide a structure for selecting among alternatives, and identify gaps to be filled by new approaches. The intent was not to develop the final, best category scheme, but to record and promote conceptual development in the field. The methods and approaches included in some of the major classifications are listed below in chronological order.

Stake's (1973) classification comprised: Student Gain by Testing, Institutional Self-Study by Staff, Blue-Ribbon Panel, Transaction-Observation, Management Analysis, Instructional Research, Social Policy Analysis, Goal-Free Evaluation, and Adversary Evaluation.

House's (1978) classification comprised: Systems Analysis, Behavioral Objectives, Decision-Making, Goal-Free, Art Criticism, Accreditation, Adversary, and Transaction models and approaches.

Stufflebeam and Webster (1980) used three major categories: (a) political orientation (Politically Controlled Studies, Public Relation-Inspired Studies); (b) questions orientation (Objectives-Based Studies, Accountability Studies, Experimental Research Studies, Testing Programs, Management Information Systems); and (c) values orientation (Accreditation/Certification Studies, Policy Studies, Decision-Oriented

Studies, Consumer-Oriented Studies, Client-Centered Studies, Connoisseur-Based Studies).

Worthen and Sanders (1987) classified the following approaches: Objectives-Oriented, Management-Oriented, Consumer-Oriented, Expertise-Oriented, Adversary-Oriented, Naturalistic and Participant-Oriented.

The models included in these classifications have changed over time, in part to reflect the increasing variety of alternatives. For example, in 1973 Stake categorized the nine approaches listed above, but in 1991 he identified a considerably different list of 11 approaches or persuasions: accountability, case study, decision-oriented, connoisseurship, demographic, ethnographic, experimental, goal-free, illuminative, judicial, and naturalistic. These classifications also evidence a tendency over time to use a slightly smaller number of categories, reflecting both increasing consensus on general groupings and a tendency toward more abstract levels of conceptual analysis.

These classifications have employed different dimensions of contrast. Evaluation models and approaches have been described and classified along such dimensions as: purpose, nature of questions addressed, typical methods, developers and proponents, key elements, major audiences, elements of consensus, case examples, risks, and outcomes. Use of different dimensions has resulted in summaries that are not strictly comparable across classifications.

There are additional difficulties with classification schemes of evaluation models and approaches. For example, the entries do not simply represent alternative evaluation methods, for some entries are identified in terms of purpose (accountability, instructional research, accreditation), some in terms of client (consumer oriented, decision maker oriented), focus (objective focused, transaction focused), or method (goal-free, experimental, case study, adversary). These differences accurately reflect the starting points or primary emphases used in the development of the models and approaches, but make comparative classifications difficult to interpret.

Further, these classifications are both overly simplistic due to the complexity of the models, and overly interpretive due to the inherent ambiguity of many of the models and approaches. Since they are based on textual analysis rather than empirical study (i.e., what proponents say about the models rather than how they are used in practice), it is difficult to determine whether, in a given situation, two models might lead a practitioner to the same design. Such an outcome would suggest that conceptual differences are more apparent than real in practice. These problems have, of course, been long recognized by the theorists who construct such classifications. Stake (1973) states that:

> Of course these descriptive tags are a great oversimplification. The approaches overlap. Different proponents and different users have different styles. Each protagonist recognizes one approach is not ideal for all

purposes. Any one study may include several approaches. The grid is an over-simplification, intended to show some typical, gross differences between contemporary evaluation activities. (p. 305)

These classifications of models and approaches, however, do reflect increasingly sophisticated conceptual and procedural alternatives in evaluation design. They are evidence of movement toward analysis of underlying dimensions and subsequent conceptual integration of evaluation approaches.

3.2 Analyses

The development of models and the construction of classifications have been accompanied by conceptual and empirical analyses of the alternative approaches.

House (1978) analyzed the philosophical assumptions underlying the eight evaluation models listed in his classification with respect to the philosophy of liberalism. He concluded that all the major evaluation models were subjectivist in ethics, although some reflected an objectivist epistemology and others a subjectivist epistemology. He subsequently presented an objectivist ethics approach to evaluation based on justice as fairness (see House 1980). (See Worthen and Sanders 1987 for an updated discussion of this influential analysis.)

Alkin and Ellett (1990 pp. 16, 17) have analyzed the set of principles underlying the dominant evaluation models. They conclude, for example, that the objectives-based approach to evaluation suggests the principle: "The evaluation should judge that a program is good if, and only if, its objectives are achieved." A goal-free evaluation, however, follows the principle: "The evaluation should judge that program X is better than program Y if, all other things being equal, program X's total consequences are on balance better than program Y's total consequences." Similar to House's (1978) analysis, Alkin and Ellett (1990) go beyond surface classification of models to an examination of underlying principles, identification of which could lead to entirely new classes of evaluation approaches. (A different means employed to construct new classes of evaluation approaches was the development of alternative metaphors of evaluation; see Smith 1981b).

Empirical analyses of specific evaluation models have been infrequent, due to the problems discussed above, such as the models' procedural ambiguity. Analyses based on practice have appeared primarily as informal, self-report case studies such as practitioner papers presented at professional meetings. Although there has been formal, systematic study of various aspects of evaluation practice (see Sect. 4.3), studies of specific models have been rare.

Smith (1985) summarized every application of the adversarial/judicial/committee hearings approach to evaluation over a 15-year period and described how the designs differed from formal statements of the model, what problems arose in implementation, and practitioners' conclusions about the feasibility and utility of this approach. Similar "state of the practice" reviews for other models have not been produced, although Shadish and Epstein (1987) and Williams (1989) have done related work.

In a survey of evaluation practitioners, Shadish and Epstein (1987) asked which evaluation literature and theoretical concepts respondents were familiar with and had affected their practice. Some of the literature and concepts were related to evaluation models and were found to relate to aggregated evaluation approaches, but an analysis of specific models was not done. Williams (1989) collected judgments from theorists concerning how similar or dissimilar they perceived their work to be to other theorists'. From these data, she grouped the theorists along four dimensions: (a) qualitative/quantitative, (b) accountability/policy orientation, (c) client participation/nonparticipation, and (d) general utilization/decision-making utilization. Both of these studies collected data on individual theorists rather than on individual models or approaches, a procedure limited by the problems discussed above.

3.3 Integrations

As mentioned above, individual theorists have tended to integrate selected aspects of each others' work into their own over time. For example, more recent statements of Stufflebeam's CIPP model reflect elements of Scriven's and Stake's positions which were not as evident in earlier statements.

In going beyond the analysis of individual models and approaches, both practitioners and theorists have sought rationales for integrating this diversity of evaluation options. The general response has been to advocate the use of multiple alternatives.

The strongest theoretical statement has been Cook's (1985) advocacy of postpositivist critical multiplism:

> The fundamental postulate of multiplism is that when it is not clear which of several options for question generation or method choice is "correct," all of them should be selected so as to "triangulate" on the most useful or the most likely to be true. . . . A similar conceptualization based on multiple verification and the falsification of identified alternative interpretations undergirds all forms of multiplism. . . . Such multiplism can be seen in the advocacy of multiple stakeholder research, multiple competing data analyses and interpretations, multiple definitionalism, multi-method research, multi-task research, multivariate causal modeling, putting multiple plausible hypotheses into competition with each other, and assessing the generality of relationships across multiple populations, settings, and times. (pp. 38, 40, 57–58)

While arguing the epistemological basis for this position, Cook acknowledges that the most difficult problems with the multiplist approach are practical.

Scriven (1983) also supports a multiplist approach, advocating what he calls a "multimodel" in which evaluation is a multifield which is multidisciplinary, multidimensional, multiperspectival, multilevel: " . . . multiple methodologies, multiple functions, multiple impacts, multiple reporting formats—evaluation is a multiplicity of multipliers" (p. 257). Scriven's solution to the practical problems of selecting from so many multiples is the use of his Key Evaluation Checklist (KEC) which focuses the evaluator's attention and assists in the selection of design options.

Practitioners have also increasingly adopted a multiplist position, many advocating the use of multiple methods within a single evaluation. Although there seems to be agreement on the use of multiple techniques (eg., use of a range of types of information, data collection procedures, and analysis procedures), there remains argument about whether the simultaneous use of multiple models in a single study violates the philosophical bases and procedural integrity of the individual models. While theorists have worried about the commensurability of multiple models, practitioners have pushed toward hybrid designs employing whatever methods appear feasible and useful.

Shadish et al. (1991) argue that the most integrated resolution of the problem of selection from multiple evaluation alternatives is evidenced in the work of Rossi and Cronbach, who have developed what Shadish et al. call "contingency theories" of evaluation. These contingency approaches seek to specify the conditions under which different evaluation practices are effective. They assume that each model is effective in dealing with a particular type of evaluation problem, and that the current task is to specify which elements are effective under what conditions.

4. Theories, Metatheories, and Practice

Starting as practical design heuristics, evaluation models proliferated rapidly and could be seen as instantiations of broader, general approaches to evaluation. Concurrent with expanding evaluation practice, efforts were made to classify, analyze, and even integrate the multiplicity of alternatives available to evaluators. This accumulating thought and practice confronts the field with the need for greater clarity about the nature and status of theory in evaluation.

4.1 Theories and Theoretical Issues

The term "theory" is used in evaluation practice and writing as loosely as the term "model," and sometimes synonymously. Three types of theory in evaluation can be identified:

(a) descriptive theory, which describes how a specific type of evaluation is actually conducted; such theory is based on the empirical study of evaluation practice, what is done, why, and with what effect;

(b) prescriptive theory, which specifies how a specific type of evaluation ought to be done; such theory can be based on a definition of social role, an ideological position, or a formal metatheory of evaluation; and

(c) metatheory, which defines the purpose, boundaries, and nature of the evaluation enterprise itself and may thus subsume certain descriptive or prescriptive theories.

Although there have been few well-articulated theories in evaluation in the 1960s, 1970s, and 1980s, there has been extensive writing and discussion of theoretical issues, both foundational and applied. Foundational issues include the following questions:

(a) What is the proper political nature and social role of evaluation?

(b) What is the proper epistemological basis for evaluation (eg., postpositivism vs. phenomenology)?

(c) What is the proper ethical basis for evaluation (eg., subjectivist vs. objectivist ethics)?

(d) What is the proper ontological basis for evaluation (eg., realism vs. relativism)?

(e) What is the proper political basis for evaluation (eg., technocratic, representative democracy vs. pluralistic, participative democracy)?

(f) What is the proper methodological basis for evaluation (eg., causal vs. explanatory vs. descriptive vs. valuational inquiry)?

(g) Are acontextual (i.e., universal) theories of evaluation possible?

(h) Are evaluative conclusions fundamentally a matter of empirical fact, value judgment, or perceptual preference?

(i) Should descriptive or prescriptive value structures form the basis of evaluation judgments?

Applied issues include the following questions:

(a) What is the nature of contextual differences in evaluative practice (eg., federal vs. local, internal vs. external)?

(b) Which is more important, formative or summative evaluation?

(c) Is use of evaluation findings for immediate instrumental use more important than for long-term enlightenment use?

(d) Should evaluators identify and attend to the needs of users, and if so, which users?

(e) Should programs be judged independently, compared to other programs, or compared to absolute standards?

(f) Who should make evaluative judgments: evaluators, decision makers, or stakeholders?

(g) Should evaluations study impact and its causes, or process and its mediating factors? Program outcome or program theory?

(h) Can and should evaluation findings be generalized?

(i) What responsibility does evaluation have for program remediation?

(j) How should an evaluand be analyzed: as a "black box," descriptively, through monitoring, through a process evaluation, with program theory, with substantive theory?

(k) How can cultural differences be appropriately reflected in evaluator selection and study design?

There is extensive literature on many of these issues, which are generally discussed under the topic of evaluation theory. The issues are elements of, and addressable by, well-developed theories of evaluation which only partially exist at present. See Shadish, et al. (1991) for a related, detailed discussion.

4.2 Metatheories

A metatheory of evaluation which specified the purpose, boundaries, and nature of evaluation could resolve a number of the issues identified above. Two of the strongest, most current metatheories of evaluation are summarized below.

Shadish et al. (1991) provide a metatheory of social program evaluation in which they argue that

> "the fundamental purpose of program evaluation theory is to specify *feasible practices that evaluators can use to construct knowledge of the value of social programs that can be used to ameliorate the social problems to which programs are relevant.*" (p. 36)

They specify that an evaluation theory should have a theoretical knowledge base corresponding to each of the following five components of their definition:

(a) social programming: the ways that social programs and policies develop, improve, and change, especially in regard to social problems;

(b) knowledge construction: the ways researchers learn about social action;

(c) valuing: the ways value can be attached to program descriptions;

(d) knowledge use: the ways social science information is used to modify programs and policies;

(e) evaluation practice: the tactics and strategies evaluators follow in their professional work, especially given the constraints they face. (Shadish et al. 1991 p. 32)

This metatheory is restricted by definition to social program evaluation and views evaluation from fundamentally a research perspective. Shadish et al. (1991) employ this metatheory to analyze the accumulated work of seven prominent theorists (Scriven, Campbell, Weiss, Wholely, Stake, Cronbach, and Rossi) to assess the extent to which each has constructed an acceptable theory of evaluation. This metatheory is the most fully developed and applied metatheory currently existent and will undoubtedly receive considerable attention, criticism, and revision.

Scriven (1991) has also proposed a metatheory of evaluation, one profoundly broader and more inclusive than that of Shadish et al. (1991). He argues that evaluation is not merely an area of applied social science, but a:

> key analytical process in all disciplined intellectual and practical endeavors. It is said to be one of the most powerful and versatile of the "transdisciplines"—tool disciplines such as logic, design, and statistics—that apply across broad ranges of the human investigative and creative effort while maintaining the autonomy of a discipline in their own right. (p. 1)

The basis for Scriven's metatheory of evaluation is reflected in two primary claims. The first claim is that there is one and only one discipline of evaluation, a "transdiscipline." It consists of: (a) a wide range of substantial practical applications of evaluation in various fields, some of them long-established primary disciplines, some of them semiautonomous, with a title that includes the term "evaluation"—each of the latter with its own theory and metatheory about a part of evaluation; (b) a nascent core discipline devoted to developing a distinctive and valid logic, general methods for evaluation, and theories about evaluation, its applications and its methods, from various perspectives including ethical, political, psychological, and sociological perspectives; and (c) a metatheory that includes various still more general and less explicit overviews and models or perceptions of evaluation's nature and presuppositions.

The second claim is that:

> the dozen or so fields of evaluation that have achieved some recognition—program, products, policy, and personnel evaluation, for example—and that have developed a healthy repertoire of their own tools can be massively improved by recognizing their connections to the core discipline, to their sibling applications, and to evaluation practices in the primary disciplines. In this direction, it is suggested, lies part of the future of evaluation, the rest lying in improving the work on the core discipline. (Scriven 1991 p. 37)

Thus Scriven's metatheory subsumes the Shadish et al. metatheory. He criticizes past theorists for leaving basic areas of evaluation practice out of their overall consideration of evaluation. For example, discussions of program evaluation rarely treat issues of personnel or product evaluation even though both are essential elements in properly conducted evaluations of programs. It is Scriven's position that there is no fundamental difference in the way one establishes evaluative conclusions, whether evaluating automobiles, student papers, physician performance, or educational programs. A metatheory of evaluation should encompass all these aspects of evaluation.

Scriven's metatheory is broader, but appears to be less thoroughly articulated than that of Shadish et al. (1991), since it is not clear how much of his prior writings on evaluation logic, theory, and procedure he would include under his metatheory. If pursued by contemporary theorists, however, Scriven's metatheory could have a profound impact on the future of evaluation theory and practice.

4.3 Theory and Practice

Evaluation theory and practice have been historically linked in a variety of ways. Initial difficulties in complying with evaluation mandates gave rise to the early evaluation models. Models and approaches continued to be developed as new problems, contexts, and participants influenced the nature of practice. Some theoretical issues arose as a direct result of practical problems. For example, the theoretical and empirical work on factors influencing evaluation utilization (e.g., Alkin, King, Patton) arose from what was happening, or not happening, with evaluation recommendations in the field.

Much of the study of the relationships between evaluation theory and practice has occurred as "metaevaluation," the evaluation of evaluations. Metaevaluations of highly visible, national, educational programs such as Headstart, Follow Through, Push/Excel, and Cities-in-Schools, have highlighted the problems of translating theory into acceptable practice. Most of the writing on metaevaluation has been methodological (eg., Cook and Gruder 1978), with few analytic or comparative studies of actual metaevaluations (cf. Smith 1981a, 1990).

Similarly, the empirical study of other practice-related issues has been sparse, although important, such as investigations of alternative communication strategies (e.g., Brown and Newman), stakeholder participation (e.g., Cousins), and evaluation use in policy formation (e.g., Patton and Weiss).There has been little response to the repeated calls (e.g., Worthen 1990, Scriven 1991) for increased empirical study of evaluation practice to describe the nature of actual practice; to compare the feasibility and effectiveness of alternative methods, models, and theories; to provide a basis for the development of descriptive evaluation theories; and to assess the utility of prescriptive theories. Unfortunately, most justification of evaluation theories is based on self-reported cases of what worked. Shadish et al. (1991) summarize the problem as follows:

To the extent that evaluation theory is still conceptual, a move toward citation of cases to support and illustrate hypotheses is welcomed if for no other reason than to provide these preliminary benefits. In the long run, however, evaluation will be better served by increasing the more systematic empirical content of its theories, by treating evaluation theory like any other scientific theory, subjecting its problems and hypotheses to the same wide scientific scrutiny to which any theory is subjected ... Such efforts have always been relatively rare in evaluation because so little effort is generally put into developing empirically testable hypotheses based in evaluation theory, and because so few evaluators are both interested in the topic and in a position to undertake such studies. (pp. 483, 484)

As important as the conceptual work needed to improve evaluation theory, is the supplementing of evaluators' experiential information with the formal empirical study of their evaluation practice.

References

Alkin M C 1991 Evaluation theory development: II. In: McLaughlin M W, Philips D C (eds.) 1991 *Evaluation and Education: At Quarter Century*. University of Chicago Press, Chicago, Illinois

Alkin M C, Ellett F S Jr. 1990 Development of evaluation models. In: Walberg H J, Haertel G D (eds.) 1990 *The International Encyclopedia of Educational Evaluation*. Pergamon Press, Oxford

Cook T D 1985 Postpositivist critical multiplism. In: Shotland L, Mark M (eds.) 1985 *Social Science and Social Policy*. Sage, Beverly Hills, California

Cook T D, Gruder C L 1978 Metaevaluative research. *Eval. Q.* 2: 5–51

House E R 1978 Assumptions underlying evaluation models. *Ed. Researcher* 7(3): 4–12

House E R 1980 *Evaluating with Validity*. Sage, Beverly Hills, California

Popham W J 1975 *Educational Evaluation*. Prentice Hall, Englewood Cliffs, New Jersey

Scriven M 1983 Evaluation ideologies. In: Madaus G F, Scriven M S, Stufflebeam D L (eds.) 1983 *Evaluation Models*. Kluwer-Nijhoff, Boston, Massachusetts

Scriven M 1991 *Evaluation Thesaurus*, 4th edn. Sage, Newbury Park, California

Shadish W R Jr., Cook T D, Leviton L C 1991 *Foundations of Program Evaluation*. Sage, Newbury Park, California

Shadish W R Jr., Epstein R 1987 Patterns of program evaluation practice among members of the Evaluation Research Society and Evaluation Network. *Eval. Rev.* 11(5): 555–90

Smith N L 1981a Criticism and metaevaluation. In: Smith N L (ed.) 1981 *New Techniques for Evaluation*. Sage, Beverly Hills, California

Smith N L (ed.) 1981b *Metaphors for Evaluation: Sources of New Methods*. Sage, Beverly Hills, California

Smith N L 1985 Adversary and committee hearings as evaluation models. *Eval. Rev.* 9(6): 735–50

Smith N L 1990 Cautions on the use of investigative case studies in metaevaluation. *Eval. Prog. Plan.* 13(4): 373–78

Smith N L 1992 Review of *Evaluation and Education: At Quarter Century. Ed. Eval. Policy Anal.* 14(1): 93–97

Stake R E 1973 Program evaluation, particularly responsive evaluation. In: Madaus G F, Scriven M S, Stufflebeam D L (eds.) 1983 *Evaluation Models*. Kluwer-Nijhoff, Boston, Massuchusetts

Stake R E 1991 Retrospective on "The countenance of educational evaluation." In: McLaughlin M W, Phillips D C (eds.) 1991 *Evaluation and Education: At Quarter Century*. University of Chicago Press, Chicago, Illinois

Stufflebeam D L, Webster W J 1980 An analysis of alternative approaches to evaluation. *Ed. Eval. Policy Anal.* 3(2): 5–19

Williams J E 1989 A numerically developed taxonomy of evaluation theory and practice. *Eval. Rev.* 13(1): 18–31

Worthen B R 1990 Program evaluation. In: Walberg H J, Haertel G D (eds.) 1990 *The International Encyclopedia of Educational Evaluation*. Pergamon Press, Oxford

Worthen B R, Sanders J R 1973 *Educational Evaluation Theory and Practice*. Charles A Jones, Worthington, Ohio

Worthen B R, Sanders J R 1987 *Educational Evaluation: Alternative Approaches and Practical Guidelines*. Longman, New York

Further Reading

Gephart W J 1978 The facets of the evaluation process: A Starter set. Unpublished manuscript. Bloomington, Indiana

Evaluation: A Tylerian Perspective

† R. W. Tyler

The practice of evaluating educational achievement has a very long history, but the systematic study of testing and other forms of educational appraisal is less than 100 years old. Yet in that time profound changes in education have taken place that are greatly influencing the conceptions of educational evaluation. However, the procedures and instruments of evaluation have thus far only partly responded to these changes.

The accepted conceptions of education generally and schooling in particular are changing profoundly, largely in response to the great changes characteristic of modern industrial nations. The increased demand in the economy for educated persons has stimulated an expanded view of universal education. The struggle of the common people for civil rights has fueled their aspirations for education and led schools to focus efforts to educate children from homes where parents have had little or no formal education. The studies that demonstrate that many children previously thought to be uneducable are learning what the schools are teaching has given new meaning to educability and raised serious questions about trying to define the limits of the educational potential of children.

The recognition that modern industrial society is in a state of continuing change has led schools to emphasize new objectives, especially those involving the development of the attitudes, knowledge, and skills required for problem-solving and those central to the development of self-directed learners. At the same time research on learning by cognitive psychologists, and by those concerned with personality development, has helped to construct a model of conscious human learning that furnishes a theoretical basis to guide the development of educational programs to implement the new expectations. Finally, schools, colleges, and educational evaluation practitioners are finding useful tools to assist teachers in the more complex tasks on which many are engaged.

1. Changes in Conceptions of Evaluation

The recent profound changes in the accepted views of education influenced corresponding changes in conceptions of educational evaluation. Standardized testing developed to serve primarily the purpose of sorting students. Sorting for college admission and for other types of selection is still an important function of testing but it is only one of many other purposes for which systematic appraisal could contribute significantly to the improvement of education. The need for comprehensive and dependable appraisals of education programs is widely recognized. Since the late 1950s, massive financial support has been given to projects concerned with the development of new courses in science, mathematics, and foreign languages. Those supporting the construction of the new courses, and teachers and administrators who are considering the use of them in their schools, are contracting for appraisals of these courses in relation to other courses in the same fields. Most tests on the market were not constructerd to furnish relative appraisals of different courses, and they have been found inadequate for the task. Similarly, the evaluation of compensatory educational programs has been handicapped by the lack of instruments and procedures for appraising programmes of this sort.

The recent rapid increase in the number and availability of technological devices in education, such as television, tape recorders, and computers, has brought to attention the need to evaluate the effectiveness of these devices for various kinds of educational tasks. Traditional test theory has not been sufficiently relevant to design evaluative studies of technological devices, nor have the available achievement tests been satisfactory for this purpose.

New knowledge about education is also influencing evaluation. For example, the recent findings of many studies regarding the powerful effects of student's home culture and community environment upon their school learning have revealed the need for assessing these factors in order to guide and improve education. New theories were necessary to rationalize procedures for appraising home and community environment and new instruments had to be developed.

As another illustration, a series of investigations like those of Newcomb (1966) and Coleman (1966) have shown the strong influence of peer-group attitudes, practices, and interests upon the learning of its members. These investigations have also shown the need for evaluating the nature, direction, and amount of peer-group influences in developing effective school programs.

Although from the time that achievement tests were first used, writers have emphasized the need for tests to assist the classroom teacher, few standardized tests have served that purpose. Teachers recognize the need for more dependable appraisals in connection with the planning and conduct of their work. They could use tests or other evaluative procedures for assessing the needs of the students in their classes, for furnishing pretest information for each instructional unit, for unit mastery tests, diagnostic tests, appraisals to be used at the conclusion of several units of instruction, and the like.

Principals and district office personnel are asking for evaluation procedures that enable them to monitor the progress of the students within their area of responsibility in order to identify problems on which assistance and additional resources can be focused. Many parents are asking for information about what their children are learning and what difficulties they are meeting. Many of them ask for evidence that the school is "accountable", a term frequently used in the United States to refer in a general sense to the school's recording and reporting on the educational progress and problems of its students. The general public and particularly those persons who are responsible for educational policies need appropriate and dependable information about educational achievements of students in their area, together with analyses of the data that help them to understand what students are learning and what problems are evident. They need information that serves to identify where, with what kind of students, and under what conditions, the expected achievement levels are not being reached.

One of the most profound changes taking place in educational evaluation is in the increased generalization of meaning attached to this term and others used as synonyms such as educational testing, educational assessment, educational appraisal. It is coming to mean the process of checking the ideas and plans in education with the realities to which these ideas and plans refer. For example, by the end of the third grade, teachers may expect their students to have mastered the mechanics of reading. Tests may be used to find out how many and which children are really able to read simple material. As another example, a new educational program has been developed for the school. It is assumed that the program is being followed in all classes. By using an observation checklist and an interview schedule with teachers, one finds out the extent to which the program is being implemented. As a third example, a remedial reading class is being planned for adolescent students. It is assumed that they will try to read things in which they are interested. An interest inventory or other means for appraising students interests can furnish information about the interests these students really have, and an observation checklist and a self-report schedule can help to find out whether students really do try to read materials that deal with their own interests.

This change to a more generalized meaning has both positive and negative possibilities. On the positive side, it may result in a wider scope for collecting evidence to support or negate ideas that guide us in working in schools and colleges. On the negative side, the terms may be used so vaguely that they are slogans rather than meaningful conceptions of the important process of educational evaluation. Whether the broader scope of meaning will be understood and used thoughtfully will depend on the actions and discussions of evaluation practitioners. Clearly the changing conceptions of education in industrialized societies have influenced many changes in the conceptions of educational evaluation.

2. Paradigm of Early Test Theory

Although group achievement testing is common throughout the western world, and program evaluation is increasing, the evaluation instruments and procedures have changed very little since the 1940s. Among the probable causes for the slow response to the changing conceptions are the continuance of a test theory that is not appropriate to the variety of demands and the continuance of test construction techniques that have not been designed with different particular educational uses in mind. The following examples illustrate these two impediments to the needed changes in practice.

Developing from the original uses of standardized tests for selecting individuals for employment, or for educational or training opportunities, a paradigm that guided the development of testing was formulated. In terms of this paradigm, the function of the testing is to arrange those who take the test along a single continuum from the ones most qualified for the particular selection to those least appropriate. To arrange the

scores on a single continuum it is necessary to summarize an individual's performance on the test exercises in terms of a single score, most frequently the sum of the items correctly answered, although less frequently, weights are used for different items or sections to produce a single score. This score is viewed as a predictor of the individual's success in performance in the job or in the educational or training program. Hence, the validity of the test is estimated by the correlation between the test scores of those taking the test and a criterion which is some obtainable indication of their performance in the job or in the educational or training program. The test can be improved by eliminating items that do not correlate with the criterion and substituting others which, in trials, do correlate positively with the criterion.

There are 18 assumptions that are specified by or associated with the early paradigm guiding test theory but these have been found inadequate to guide the changing roles of educational evaluation. The effort to arrange test takers on a continuum from best performers to the poorest is not required for most of the current uses of achievement tests. Teachers want to know who has learned what has been taught and who had difficulties, and what did they fail to master? Parents want to know what their children have learnd and what they are having difficulties with. The central administrators of the school district want to know in what schools children are making expected progress in learning, in which schools a considerable number of children are failing to reach the goals that have been set, and what kinds of problems these schools are having. The public wants to know what students are expected to learn in the primary grades, the middle grades, and the high school and what proportion of students are learning these things.

None of the answers to these questions require the arrangement of students on a continuum based on the results of a test. In fact, that kind of reporting encourages people to think of schooling as a contest rather than a social institution seeking to help all students learn what is essential or helpful to constructive participation in the society.

The practice of describing a student's test performance by assigning a single score greatly oversimplifies the complexity of the student's behavior and of the learning process. Instead of seeking to aggregate many items of data about the student's test performance, such as the approach he or she used in attacking the problem, the mode of solution, the recall of relevant data, whether or not the answer was checked, and the time required to complete the exercise, a more helpful appraisal provides the teacher with all the relevant information obtained from each student's test performance, and helps him or her to redesign the instructional program to aid the student in learning. Furthermore, a single score does not inform the teacher, the parent, the school administrator, or the public what the students have learned. The score is only an abstract number which is designed to distinguish those who have learned more from those who have learned less but it is not nearly as helpful as a report which informs the user, for example, that this sample exercise represents what 82 percent of the third-grade children were able to do correctly, while this sample exercise represents what only 20 percent of the third-grade children did correctly.

The scoring of a test in terms of numbers of correct answers or some combination of the number of correct and the number of incorrect answers does not provide a defensible basis for assessing most of the kinds of learning that school teaches, and the score sheds little light on the child's pattern of learned behavior. A child's written work can be scored by counting the number of errors he or she has made in the application of the conventions of grammar, spelling, and syntax but, unless each kind of error is reported in relation to the number of opportunities for such an error, very little useful information is provided and such scoring is not appropriate for assessing such things as the comprehensibility, the organization, and the persuasiveness of the writing.

The notion that the validity of a test is shown by the accuracy of its prediction of success in further educational programs or in employment involves two assumptions that are no longer acceptable. One is that the test is designed primarily to serve a static institution (school or employer) and the other is that individuals cannot be expected to change significantly as they encounter environments new to them. In contrast to earlier years, educational institutions are expected to modify their practices so as to reach effectively the wider range of students now seeking admission. The older paradigm assumed a static institution and the test was to identify the students who would get good grades in the static institution. Now the admission tests are expected to identify the range of significant assets that the student has developed and to report these assets to the institution so that the institution can better design its programs to build on their assets. This new view is also spreading through employing institutions. They are increasingly expected to modify their practices so as to capitalize on the assets of new groups of employees and minimize the dependence upon characteristics not possessed in large measure by the new groups.

Evidence obtained from all levels of schooling from preschool to college indicates children and youths can and do change their performance when there are new opportunities for learning which are seen by the learners as challenges. Similar results are being reported in studies of women and minority groups in new employment situations. There is no longer justification to try to validate an aptitude test or an achievement test by correlating its results with success in subsequent educational or employing institutions. A more direct effect to identify the individual's assets and limitations is necessary.

An essential principle in all kinds of testing is that the test be based on a representative and adequate sample of the behavior to be assessed. Representativeness in statistical term means that the sample is either a random sample of the behavior or is a stratified random sample, that is random samples from each stratum of the universe of behavior being assessed. "Adequate" is defined as a large enough representative sample to allow for the estimated variations to be expected among the units of the random sample and still provide a measure that is sufficiently stable to serve the purpose intended. Even when a test is constructed by sampling randomly from the universe of relevant behavior, when it is modified by eliminating items that do not correlate with an external criterion and by adding items that do correlate, then the test items are no longer a representative sample of the test taker's behavior. Hence the results of the modified test no longer provide a reliable description of the individual's behavior.

3. The New Paradigm

The new paradigm of educational evaluation is constructed around the new expectations in education in contemporary society. The old paradigm assumed that educational opportunities had to be rationed because of the limited resources available for schooling. It was also assumed that many children were relatively uneducable and they should be identified early and guided into work at an early age while the more educable should be encouraged to continue their schooling on through high school and college.

The new paradigm assumes that all persons who are not seriously damaged by brain injuries can learn what the schools are responsible for teaching. It recognizes that contemporary society is realizing that its members need increasing amounts of school learning in order that they may become civilized persons, effective citizens, supportive family members, helpful members of their communities, and constructive participants in the economic life of the society.

The old paradigm assumed that the practices of educational institutions were largely static and a role for educational evaluation was to identify persons who would fit into these practices and achieve what the institutions expected of them. The new paradigm assumes that institutional practices can change as the schools and colleges seek to provide real educational opportunities for all of their students. A role of educational evaluation in this connection is to help identify the assets of students on which effective educational programs can be built, and the characteristics which are likely to interfere with the student's learning so that the school or college may help the student overcome these difficulties.

The old paradigm assumed that the task of vocational guidance was to identify the student's present characteristics that most nearly fitted particular job requirements and to advise him or her how to proceed with training which would best prepare the student to fit into this niche. The early slogan was "A round peg should fit into a round hole while a square peg fits into a square hole."

The new paradigm conceives guidance as encouraging and helping students to explore their life options. Every increment of education is viewed as expanding one's life options and increasing one's ability to make wise judgements about the next steps. There are few rigid job characteristics. Most jobs are partly defined by the persons who perform them. Hence, the individual's task in vocational development is continually to learn more about vocations, their missions, their principles, their social conditions, their opportunities for intellectual development and social contributions, and to learn more about himself or herself so as better to estimate performance in these occupational roles. In this connection, educational evaluation seeks to obtain information about significant characteristics of occupations and relevant information about the student.

In brief, this new paradigm conceives the role of educational evaluation to be that of providing information about the realities of the educational arena that can help the institutions to improve the educational opportunities and help individuals gain education of high quality and to become self-directed in continuing their education throughout their life cycle. The phrase, "information about the realities of the educational arena," distinguishes between reality and perceived reality. All human beings appear to have a view of the situations they encounter: they think they usually know what is going on. Some of the notions they have are in harmony with objective reality, but some are not. For instance a teacher thinks he or she has made a clear explanation but a simple questioning of the class may show that few of the students understood it. By the same token a supervisor may think that the curriculum guide is being followed as intended in the classroom but observers may find that the activities in some of the classrooms are quite different from those specified in the guide. Evaluation has become a broader process than simply giving tests or examinations to students. It is now viewed as the process for finding out what is really happening in educational situations to guide plans and actions.

This broader conception means that educational evaluation seeks not only to appraise relevant behavior of the students, their knowledge, skills, attitudes, habits, interests, and appreciations but also to assess the learning activities of the school: What are the learning tasks and their appropriateness both to the learning objectives and to the students present activities? What rewards and feedback does the learner receive as he or she attempts the learning tasks? What are the opportunities for sequential practice? How is transfer assured?

The contemporary view of evaluation also includes assessing the influences on learning outside the classroom. What behavior does the family consider important? How is effective school learning rewarded in the home? What opportunities does the home furnish for transfer of what is learned in school? What opportunities are there in the home for learning some of the behavior which the school emphasizes? This kind of assessment may also be focused on peer-group activities outside the school, and on the other associations and institutions in the community which influence school learning by being supportive or in conflict or by distracting the student's attention from the school learning activities.

Those professionally involved in education are often ignorant of the learning conditions in which students are involved outside the school or the campus so that evaluation, that is, information about relevant realities, can be very helpful in enabling them to build on constructive conditions and seek to change those that interfere with student learning. Sometimes, the research or the experience of other situations can be suggestive about what to evaluate in their own situation to confirm or refute the validity in this situation of the information obtained elsewhere. Thus, in planning an educational program for students from families in which the adults have had very little education, one may learn of a research investigation which reported that most uneducated parents did not value education for their children. This is possible in the educator's own situation but a sample survey found that 85 percent of the parents of the children for which the new program is planned considered education for their children the chief means for the children to survive. They urged their children to work hard and do well in school.

To implement this broader conception of educational evaluation requires a reexamination of purposes, plans, and procedures in order to develop instruments and practices that serve the variety of uses to which evaluation results are to be put. The techniques of instrument construction developed by psychometrists are no longer adequate, because the focus of educational evaluation is now on the individual psyche. The following rationale outlines steps to be taken in developing evaluation instruments that are more nearly adequate to the variety of purposes than the older practices involved in test construction.

4. Rationale for Instrument Construction

This rationale includes the following eight steps:

(a) Identifying the questions to be answered and the relevant information to be obtained from the use of the evaluation procedure and instruments.

(b) Defining the behavior to be appraised in order to obtain the needed information.

(c) Identifying situations in which the persons have opportunity to express the behavior.

(d) Selecting or constructing situations which evoke the behavior.

(e) Deciding on the aspects of the behavior to be described or measured, and the terms or units to be used.

(f) Trying out the proposed procedure and instruments.

(g) Checking on the validity, objectivity, reliability, and practicability of the procedure and instruments.

(h) Revising the procedures and instruments.

The preceding eight steps are suggested as one coherent rationale to guide the development of procedures and instruments for educational evaluation. It is a natural outgrowth from the changing uses of evaluation that are emerging in response to the changes in education that have been evolving with increased rapidity since the end of the Second World War. These educational changes have necessitated changes in the paradigm that has been the intellectual model for test theory.

The systematic study and development of test theory was the work of psychologists who sought to understand the mental activity and processes of individual human beings. Their effort to probe the psyche was guided by the older paradigm which they constructed. It is now becoming increasingly clear that the process of education and the stimulation and guidance of human learning is a practical endeavor. Whatever may be the composition of the psyche, students of all kinds have been learning and becoming educated persons. To guide this practical activity and to understand it more fully is the test of educators. The paradigm to guide them is not the same as the one that is most useful to psychologists.

Correspondingly, the appraisal of student learning and of the aspects of the environment which influence it requires a conception of educational evaluation appropriate to this task. The focus of educational evaluation is not the same as that of psychometrists, and the assumptions that are consistent with educational purposes and programs are different at several major points. If educational evaluation is to serve schools, colleges, and other formal and informal educational institutions, the conceptual paradigm and the rationale guiding the construction of tests and other evaluative devices and procedures must be consistent with the purposes and essential conditions under which education operates. The foregoing discussion is an initial effort to suggest the kind of thinking which needs to become central to developing a sound and useful program of educational evaluation.

Most reports of educational evaluations are not understood by laypeople and are widely misinterpreted. In fact, they are not generally understood by teachers and administrators, and, as a result, the information that could provide a basis for improving the educational program or institution is not communicated. Basic to this failure of communication are several practices devised by psychometrists and adapted without careful consideration by those engaged in educational evaluation.

5. Shortcoming in Reporting Procedures

Psychometrists seeking to measure aspects or factors of the psyche, focus on the appraisal of characteristics of the person rather than on what the person has learned. They hypothesize the existence of abilities, aptitudes, or other factors within the individual, and seek to devise ways of identifying and measuring these characteristics. The teacher is expected to help students of many different backgrounds and with various observable characteristics learn what the schools try to teach, such as to read, write, compute, explain natural phenomena, become interested in intellectual activities and aesthetic objects, perceive things in new perspectives, and so forth. The teacher's task is to help children learn these things as effectively as possible. What the teacher really wants to know from the results of an educational evaluation are the answers to such questions as: What have the students learned? Where are they having difficulty in learning? The teacher is interested in knowing about those hypothetical abilities, aptitudes, and other factors assumed to be within the individual only when they are shown to be causal variables that can be altered by the teacher so as to improve student learning. Otherwise, the report of test results in terms of individual characteristics is not used by the teacher or is misinterpreted as in using aptitude test results to justify the practice of not encouraging students whose scores are low to try to learn.

The focus on individual characteristics leads psychometrists to treat test results as indicators of factors rather than direct evidence of learning. This leads to the prevailing practice of reporting test results in abstract numbers, such as numerical scores, without explaining the concrete referents from which the scores are derived. An even greater source of misinterpretation arises from translating "raw" scores into grade equivalents, or percentiles which have the appearance of clarity, but, in fact, are interpretations of hypothetical referents that are often different from the actual situation.

As an example, the results of standardized tests in the elementary school subjects are usually reported in grade equivalents obtained by translating the raw scores into a scale which is constructed by assuming that the mean of the scores made by students taking the test, who were at the beginning of the first grade, represents the grade equivalent of 1.0. Then, the mean of the scores obtained by students at the beginning of the second grade is called 2.0, and so on, through to the last grade of the elementary school. It is also assumed that the mean scores will progress linearly from grade to grade. For example, it is assumed that the mean scores for students in the middle of the school year will be one half of the difference between the mean scores for the beginning of the next grade and the mean for the beginning of this grade. To illustrate: if the mean score of the students taking a standardized arithmetic test at the beginning of the second grade is 62 and the mean score for students taking the test at the beginning of the third grade is 68, then a score of 65 is assumed to be the mean score that would be attained by students who take the test in the middle of the school year.

Students with the same score often show very different patterns of test performance. They may have answered correctly items that are taught, in later grades, and failed to answer correctly items that are taught in earlier grades. Teachers obtain no information from a grade equivalent score about what the student has learned and with what learning tasks he or she has difficulty. Parents and other laypeople assume that a child whose grade equivalent is 3.2 should, if properly placed, be in the third grade, not realizing the child may already have mastered many of the things taught in Grade 3, while failing to answer correctly items that are taught in other grades.

In high school subjects, the usual practice is to report standardized achievement test results in terms of percentile ranks, based on a hypothetical normal distribution in which all of the scores obtained from the norming administration of the test are placed. A review of typical standardized tests indicates that the items in a test that deals with things taught in any particular school represent only a fraction of what that school is teaching. This is due to the fact that high school courses vary from school to school in the particular content taught. In the construction of a test for national use, the test makers examine textbooks and available curriculum guides to identify topics that are common to many of the books and guides. Test items are then constructed for these common topics. The topics that are not common, however, are more numerous than those for which test items are written. Hence, the report, for example, that the mean of the scores that the student of teacher A obtained on the test was at the 40th percentile of the norming population gives no dependable indication of what these students have learned nor even how well they have learned what they have been taught.

6. Suggested Improvements for Reporting Results of School Learning

It is, of course, necessary to use abstract numbers in studies that seek to identify hypothetical variables that are not directly observable, since their form and extent of functioning must be estimated from observed differences in individual behavior. However, the results of school learning can be much more directly defined, identified, and described in meaningful terms that are relatively concrete.

In reading, for example, learning to comprehend reading material is commonly defined in terms that are easily understood. In the primary grades, comprehension behavior is often defined as reading aloud accurately, or telling in one's own words what the selection says, or doing what the printed directions tell one to do. In the middle grades the definition of "comprehend" takes into account the fact that reading at that level involves getting information from the printed page.

The definition of the reading material which the student is expected to comprehend is also easily understood. In the primary grades the reading material usually includes children's stories, newspaper items, and directions for assembling and using toys and games. If a test in reading for children in the primary grades has been constructed by sampling the kinds of comprehension and the several kinds of reading material, the results can be reported in terms of what the children comprehend: fairy tales, newspaper items, directions for toys and games. If desired, the test could sample several levels of complexity in the reading materials, such as range of vocabulary and complexity of syntax. Then results can be reported in terms of the levels of complexity of the reading materials that each child comprehended. Concrete examples of each level can be included in the report so that the user can make his or her own judgement of what the levels of complexity mean. To take an example in arithmetic, the definition of "computation" with whole numbers is often given as: adding, substracting, multiplying, and dividing with whole numbers; and the content and contexts in which the elementary school child is expected to use computation is often defined as: planning, personal, and group activities in which quantities are estimated, making retail purchases, estimating sales taxes on purchases, and measuring familiar objects and areas.

Levels of complexity in computation behavior are usually defined by increasing numbers of digits in the numbers involved in the computation. Most arithmetic courses do not categorize contents and contexts in terms of difficulty or levels of complexity for children learning to compute. Hence, if a test in arithmetic has been constructed by sampling the kinds of computation and the several contents and contexts in which the students can be expected to use computation with whole numbers, the results can be reported in terms of what kinds of computation they performed accurately —addition, substraction, multiplication, and division —and in which contexts they solved the computational exercises accurately. If desired, the test could sample computation with one-digit numbers, with two-digit numbers, and with numbers of three or more digits. The results could then be reported in these terms representing levels of complexity for children learning to compute.

As an example from another subject and at the high school level, the field of high school biology is typical. One of the major objectives for this subject as presented in curriculum guides is to understand and explain in scientific terms common phenomena of plants and animals. The behavior, understanding and explaining in scientific terms, is often defined as the student's perceiving a biological phenomenon as involving relevant scientific concepts and principles and using them appropriately in his or her explanation. In most biology courses, there are from 20 to 40 concepts used and from 50 to 70 principles presented. The presentations in textbooks and laboratory exercises include several phenomena involving each of the concepts and principles. Students are expected to generalize from these examples and to understand and explain many other biological phenomena encountered in their environment.

An evaluation of student learning in relation to this objective should include test situations in which the student encounters biological phenomena and seeks to explain them in scientific terms. The results of such a test can be reported in terms of the use of each concept and principle if each one has been reliably sampled in the test exercises. More commonly, the concepts and principles will be grouped into classes, each of which is reliably sampled. In that case, the results can be reported in terms of the proportion of the test exercises in each class in which the concepts and principles were appropriately used in the explanations. If desired, the phenomena could be classified into levels of complexity and results reported in terms of the proportion of exercises appropriately explained for each level of complexity.

An evaluation of the products of learning furnishes a somewhat different example of the reporting of results. In evaluating the written work of students, several criteria are usually used, such as clarity, logical organization, and coherence, and each paper is appraised in terms of each criterion. Furthermore, to reduce individual idiosyncrasy in assessment, one or more examples of each level of the criterion are established by a panel of judges and used as a standard to guide all the appraisals. The prevailing practice has been to report the mean levels for each group of students. This furnishes little information of use to teachers, parents, school administrators, and others. A more useful report would present an example of each level for each criterion and state the percentage of the group whose written work was judged to be at that level. To illustrate: in class X, 15 percent of the students' writing was judged to be in the top level in clarity, 60 percent in the middle level in clarity, and 25 percent in the low level in clarity, and so on with the other criteria. By presenting concrete examples of products, parents and other laypeople can understand more clearly what schools are teaching and students are expected to learn than abstract scores can ever provide.

The above examples are by no means exhaustive. They are presented only to illustrate certain major guidelines in reporting the results of an educational evaluation. The first of these is to report results that tell what has been learned and what of the expected learning has not taken place. To report these things there should have been clear definitions of what students are expected to learn. From these definitions, suggestions are obtained about useful terms for reporting the results. Second, since an educational evaluation is focused on what students have learned, one should avoid the use of indicators wherever more direct assessment of the learning can be made, and avoid abstract numbers in reporting wherever what students have learned can be reported more concretely. This reduces the dependence upon untested assumptions in deriving a score. Third, one should present the users of the results with as much information as can be obtained from the evaluation, but in no more detail than they can use. This guideline requires considerable elaboration to suggest its practical employment.

7. Reports for Teachers and Parents

The teacher or parent who works with individual students can use information about each individual whose learning he or she is guiding. Hence, reports of an evaluation for the teacher or parent should not only indicate which children have learned what they have been taught, but also the particular kinds of learned behavior with what content and in what contexts they demonstrated effectiveness, and what difficulties were evidenced.

For a general report to parents, this information needs to be presented clearly but in nontechnical terms. The purpose is two-fold: to give parents information about the particular things the child is expected to learn, and information about what the child is learning and where difficulties are being encountered. Most parents have not understood the test scores that have been reported, and this has led to misinterpretations that have often hampered constructive efforts of the home.

Some test users have reported the results item by item, but this item analysis commonly leads to another misunderstanding. The item analysis reports the number or percentage of test takers who responded to the item is a particular way, usually the percentage who answered the item correctly. However, a single item is rarely, if ever, a representative sample of a defined behavior, or a defined content, or a defined context. Teachers often treat item analyses as though the response to an item indicated probable responses to the kind of behavior that item represents. To draw any dependable inference about a kind of behavior requires information from enough appropriate items to evaluate a representative sample of that behavior. Failing to understand this, some teachers modify their educational efforts to deal with what they thought they could infer from the item analysis.

The reliability of the item analysis is based on estimates of the variability among students responding to the item; it is not an estimate of the variation among items that could be constructed to represent a kind of behavior that can be estimated from actually giving a sample of such exercises to the students.

8. Reports for School Principals

The principal of a school does not usually need to have information about the learning of an individual child. When that is needed on occasion, the teacher can be asked to supply it. The principal needs to know about the progress of learning in each classroom so that assistance can be provided where needed. For example, the principal is usually expected to take the leadership in developing educational goals for each year. These goals should be established after reviewing the educational achievements of the past year; then the school's teaching staff deliberate on goals for the next year which are substantially beyond the achievements of the past year but seem to the teachers to be attainable for the next year. The review of the results of the last educational evaluation will reveal the objectives that were not reached by most students and other indications of problems that need correction and for which the plan for next year represents a substantial improvement over the past year.

For the purposes of setting annual goals, the educational evaluation results can be helpfully expressed in terms of the proportion of the class group who reached or exceeded the goals set for that year. As an example, consider an elementary school enrolling children from homes in which the parents have had little education and where the opportunities to develop and apply what is learned in school are limited. At the end of the third grade, most children from middle-class homes have learned the mechanics of reading; that is, they can get the plain-sense meaning of written material that deals with content and contexts with which they are familiar. However, in the school in the inner city, the educational evaluation showed that only 25 percent of the children at the end of the third grade could read and comprehend this simple material.

After staff discussion and deliberation the goal in reading set for the third grade the following year was for 35 percent of the students to reach this standard. Thus, reporting results—in terms of the percentage of students reaching accepted and defined standards—provided the principal and all the school staff with the information needed to set annual goals and to monitor progress toward them. Reporting the percentage of students exhibiting behaviour that inteferes with school learning can also be useful in goal setting and monitoring. For example, the percentage of students who were absent 5 days, 10 days, 15 days, and 20 days in a term furnishes information helpful in setting goals representing improved attendance.

9. Reports for School Districts

Most local school districts include a number of schools. The district personnel do not need data from an educational evaluation that is as detailed as that needed by the principal of each school. The officers of the district—administrators, coordinators, supervisors, resource persons, and so on—cannot perform the daily functions of teachers, principals, and parents. They must depend on the persons in the local schools to perform these functions. Persons from the district office can stimulate the efforts of the teachers and principals in the schools, they can assist and train local personnel in goal setting, monitoring, and revising goals and plans, they can provide other kinds of assistance, but they cannot take the place of the local school personnel nor depend on their authority to get compliance with their ideas.

To furnish assistance in depth, district personnel need to identify problems serious enough, or opportunities great enough, to justify a considerable commitment of their time. The results of evaluations should indicate what proportion of the students in the local school are attaining the learning objectives and what proportion are having difficulties. The district personnel may ask for breakdowns in these proportions in terms of student demography or sex, or other variables thought to have a causal connection to student achievement. The district personnel also need to know the evidence used by the local school staff in setting the annual goals. However, district personnel do not usually need data on individual students nor even on particular classrooms within the school. The school is the basic unit for monitoring and reporting. Further breakdowns may be needed to guide the appropriate inquiries of the district.

Periodically, the district office needs an appraisal of learning that is independent of the evaluations carried out by personnel in the local school. This is necessary to assure the validity of the data submitted by the school. A few principals may not be able to resist the temptation to doctor results so that their schools will look good. The periodic independent appraisal has the same function in relation to local evaluations that an independent financial audit has to the accounts and accounting activities of an institution. As in the financial audit, only sample checks are made, and if they are not in harmony with the results presented by the local school personnel, a further investigation is undertaken to obtain valid results at the level of detail required.

There are technical problems in conducting an independent appraisal that utilizes a limited amount of students' time, requires modest expenditures, and obtains valid and reliable samples of the various kinds of learning objectives from reliable samples of students from each local school. If only a fraction of the important objectives are sampled, local teachers interpret them as the only ones. So they focus their teaching efforts on these few objectives and neglect the others. If only a fraction of the students are sampled, the reliability of the results may be too low and the reason some students are not tested is not easily explained to the local school staff and parents. An answer to these technical problems is a process often called matrix sampling, as the allocation of test exercises to particular students is often done by making a matrix chart with individual students in the one axis and the test exercises on the other. By the use of matrix sampling, the reliability of the test exercises as representative samples of the learned behavior applied to representative samples of relevant content in representative samples of appropriate context, does not need to be reduced. All of the test exercises constructed for use in making evaluations useful to the local school are presented to the students, but no one student responds to all the exercises. If the completion of all the test exercises would require five hours for one student to do them all, the test can be broken into five subtests each taking an hour of the student's time. One-fifth of the students is given one subtest, another fifth of the students is given a second subtest, and so on. Every student completes test results for the equivalent of one-fifth of all the students in the school.

The results of this independent appraisal can be reported in terms of each kind of educational objective, and the proportion of the students in each school who made expected progress in attaining the objective, and the proportion having difficulty. As with other tests, where representative samples of different levels of behavior are obtained, these can be reported in terms of the percentage of the students reaching or exceeding each level. The report of these results can be compared with the results submitted by each school. Where there are serious discrepancies, inquiries should be undertaken to seek to obtain more dependable data.

10. Reports for State, Regional, and National Agencies

Reports of educational evaluation results that are useful to state agencies, regional organizations, and state and national policymakers need to be even less detailed than those for school district personnel. State, regional, and national groups do not work directly with individual children, and they need no more information about the child's educational progress and problems than the Surgeon General of the United States need to know about the health progress and problems of an individual child. The responsibility for working directly with individual children on their educational progress and problems is that of the teacher and parent.

It is helpful for policy development as well as for state oversight in education to know what children in their area of jurisdiction are learning: what learning is expected of these children at various stages of their development, what progress they are making, and what problems they are encountering. Since the answers to these questions are thought to vary in relation to demographic factors, the questions need to be asked in relation to each major demographic factor. What can the results of evaluation contribute to answering these questions?

In the United States, the constitutional responsibility for public education is left to the government of each state. Most states delegate a great deal of this responsibility to local school districts. Although many of the states have adopted courses of study, none of them defines in clear terms the behavior that students are expected to learn. The courses of study usually specify subjects to be taught, sometimes topics to be covered, but no definition is clearly given as to what students are to learn in these subjects or about these topics. These actual definitions are usually developed by individual teachers, although there is increasing agreement among educators that the teaching staff of a school needs to work as a team to define and agree on the definition of what students are to learn in different subjects and at different levels of their development.

Although in practice, individual teachers or local schools define learning objectives, there is a good deal of agreement among the educated public on the definition of what students should learn in the public elementary and secondary schools. This was documented in the experience of the United States in getting agreement on the learning objectives to be appraised in the National Assessment of Educational Progress (NAEP). In developing an evaluation program to inform policymakers and the public in a state or region, the procedure followed in developing the NAEP is a practicable one. It is also possible to gain a more informed consensus by arranging for discussion groups to discuss at some length the issues of desirable learning goals and to bring together for further discussion and deliberation the reports of the conclusions reached in many smaller discussion groups. One way of doing this is to invite public participants through invitations to many local groups, such as church groups, labor groups. Chambers of Commerce, service clubs, and hobby groups. When the self-selected members come together in a large auditorium, they are presented with an explanation of the project. Then the large group is broken up into discussion groups with about 20 people in each group. Each discussion group is moderated by a person who participated in three brief training sessions. The discussions are directed by a discussion guide who raises the major issues as questions to be discussed and deliberated, and tentative conclusions are reached. The discussion groups usually meet in three or four two-hour sessions. Each discussion group prepares a report of its recommendations which are reproduced for all participants. Then a final meeting is held with the members of all the groups. At this final meeting consensus is sought on the recommendations as they are revised and reformulated to satisfy most participants. This is a time-consuming procedure but it has developed a clearer understanding of what schools are expected to do and thus furnishes a basis for guiding an evaluation and reporting results.

The report of the results of assessments should take into account what the policymakers understand to be the things students are expected to learn. The reports can help further to clarify the meaning of these expectations by presenting an exercise or two that was used to appraise this kind of learning. Where it is appropriate, the report should present examples of different levels of skill, or complexity, or breadth of learning, and for each giving the percent of particular groups who performed at that level or breadth. Where possible, the degree of progress can be reported in terms of the proportion in previous years who performed at that level or breadth. The proportion of students who demonstrated difficulties in performance can be an additional kind of information where this result is obtained from other responses and is not simply the proportion who did not perform at the reported level. Where the learning is thought to be influenced by certain demographic factors, the proportions should be reported for each demographic group for which there was a representative sample taking the test.

11. Conclusion

These examples are not complete; they are presented only as illustrations of efforts to report the results of educational evaluation in terms that are understood by the users as concrete evidence about the learning of clearly defined behavior. From the need for detailed reports by those who work with individual students to the need by policymakers for reports of learning achievements on a large scale, one can select the data and report the results so as to be responsive as far as possible to the kinds of questions different groups are asking.

References

Coleman J S 1966 Peer cultures and education in modern society. In: Newcomb T M, Wilson E K (eds.) 1966 *College Peer Group*. Aldine Publishing, Chicago, Illinois

Newcomb T M 1966 The general nature of peer-group influence. In: Newcomb T M, Wilson E K (eds.) 1966 *College Peer Group*. Aldine Publishing, Chicago, Illinois

Further Reading

Madaus G F, Stufflebeam D L (eds.) 1989 *Classic Works of Ralph W. Tyler*. Kluwer Academic Publishers, Boston, Massachusetts

Tyler R W 1942 General statement on evaluation. *J. Educ. Res.* 35(7): 492–501

Tyler R W 1949 *Basic Principles of Curriculum and Instruction*. University of Chicago Press, Chicago, Illinois

Tyler R W 1951 The functions of measurement in improving instruction. In: Lindquist E F (ed.) 1951 *Educational Measurement*. American Council of Education, Washington, DC

Tyler R W 1983 Educational assessment, standards, and quality: Can we have one without the others? *Educational Measurement: Issues and Practice* 2(2): 14–15, 21–23

Tyler R W 1983 A rationale for program evaluation. In: Madaus G F, Scriven M, Stufflebeam D L (eds.) 1983 *Evaluation Models: Viewpoints on Educational and Human Services Evaluation*. Kluwer-Nijhoff, Boston, Massachusetts

(e) Issues in Educational Research

Research in Education: Nature, Needs, and Priorities

J. P. Keeves and P. A. McKenzie

The major issues for educational research at the end of the twentieth century are those of overcoming the crisis within many countries of the lack of leadership and support for educational research. It is necessary to identify needs and priorities, to publicize the findings of research, to promote and focus debate on the issues confronting policy and practice, and to foster the building of a coherent body of knowledge from current and past research. This entry is concerned with the nature of the research process in education, the utilization of its findings in educational practice and policy-making, and the ways in which the needs and priorities across the whole field of educational research might be identified.

The expansion of teachers' colleges and schools of education in universities that took place in the industrialized countries in the 1950s and 1960s and which was essential to cater for the expanding student population, was followed by marked augmentation of support for educational research. Since then, however, with the decline in school enrollments and financial austerity in most highly developed countries, the expenditure for education had to be reduced, and support for research proved an easy field for a withdrawal of funds. The 1980s saw a crisis situation for educational research in many countries. However, staff and students in universities were often able to devise research activities that did not require heavy sources of funding. These investigators proceeded quietly with their scholarly work within the frameworks of their basic disciplines. Moreover, they often sought to publish the results of their research primarily in journals related to a discipline and not necessarily in ways that would influence educational policy or practice.

In the 1990s most educational research investigations have been conducted within universities by students undertaking studies for higher degrees and by staff who carry out studies to enhance their prospects for advancement, to inform their teaching, and to satisfy both a drive for recognition by their peers and for greater understanding of the field to which they are professionally committed. In addition, staff also supervise their students. Very few universities seek—other than in superficial ways — to publicize the research findings of their own staff and students. Theses and detailed reports of scholarly work commonly remain unpublished and largely inaccessible to all but the most diligent research workers.

The National Academy of Education (1991) report in the United States identified six leading concerns in the organization of educational research that applied in the early 1990s. These concerns are relevant not only to the United States but also to other highly industrialized countries, such as Australia and the United Kingdom.

1 Research on education lacks comprehensive, effective strategies to shape funding . . . . Today a powerful consensus is needed on a strategy of research and development to improve education.
2 Patterns of support for research on education are episodic, buffeted by changing demands, vacillating leadership, unstable commitments and institutional pressures.
3 Studies tend to be small-scale, short term, not interconnected, and rarely longitudinal.
4 Funding is not at a sufficient scale for centers of research to maintain momentum over periods of time long enough to communicate effectively with educational practitioners.
5 Most of the public funding . . . for education research goes into designated studies and research centers regulated more or less overtly by current but rapidly changing political and policy considerations.
6 Too little room is left for coordinating field-initiated ideas, for theory-building and conceptual work to shape new inquiries, and for the cumulative insights of long-term empirical investigations. (National Academy of Education 1991 p. 32)

1. Problems in Educational Research

The problems facing educational research are greater than those of merely identifying a list of priority areas. Educational research as a whole has tended to become highly fragmented and conducted without coherent theory. There is a need to respond to new leads from basic research in allied disciplines, for intensive experimentation, and sustained collaboration with educational practitioners. In addition, there is a need to re-establish active educational research agencies both within large bureaucratic structures and as independent bodies. This demands new and stable sources of funding for educational research, and the identification of fields where the reformed agencies might concentrate their efforts. More research activity is required to support and inform the massive spending that takes place in the field of education than can be provided by the intermittent endeavors of university staff who are also heavily committed to teaching and administration.

2. Dangers of Priority Lists

It is necessary to acknowledge that the establishment of a list of priorities at a national level for the conduct of research in any field carries with it certain dangers. In a review of educational research in Australia in the early 1970s, Radford (1973) argued:

> I do not believe in the laying down of priorities by a central body, and the refusal to support with funds, or staff or interest anything outside that set of priorities. My reason is simple. Such a laying down of priorities to me implies an impossible omniscience, and lays up trouble for itself. But this is not to say that different centres, different units, different institutions, because of their interests, and their perception of priorities should not by their own determination of policy decide to concentrate their efforts rather than disperse them, decide to collaborate with others in an integrated program, and where feelings are strong enough to persuade others to join them. (Radford 1973 p. 120)

The major problem associated with any attempt to establish priorities and to rationalize research effort, whether within a country, an institution, or a small unit comes at the point of making a decision to check the development of one project to the benefit of another, or to transfer support for a research and development enterprise from one institution to another. Snow (1969) has discussed in detail a critical incident that occurred in England in the years immediately prior to and during the Second World War. The incident involved a choice between two research enterprises at a time when resources were very limited: one was concerned with the development of radar, the other with long-range bombing programs. The issues arose from the different views and interpretations of the scientific evidence available, as well as from long-term personal differences between two individuals in key positions. Only by chance was disaster averted, triggered by a sudden and complete change in priorities. The lessons from this incident for the funding and support for research are clear. In an open society, where there are many avenues to be followed to obtain funding for research and many places to be found where the research might be pursued, if one course of action is closed, then it is always possible to turn elsewhere for support. It is apparent that if there is one individual or even one committee with sole power, the situation is potentially dangerous: error of judgment can easily occur. The solution must lie in the provision of alternatives in both sources of funding and in locations where research

might be carried out. Without such alternatives there is no way in which errors of establishing priorities can be exposed. Other problems associated with the setting of priorities are both the possible ossification of research directions, and the risk of being unable to respond quickly to developments that were unknown at the time the priorities were initially set.

These remarks on the rationalization of research effort should not be taken to imply that the setting up of priorities and the need for rationalization from time to time are not important. What is essential is the rejection of a universal listing of priorities and a denial of alternative avenues that might be pursued for the funding and conduct of research. Furthermore, it is important that any groups concerned with the establishment of priorities should be credible bodies, broadly based, and with the authority to implement the results. Moreover, there should be mechanisms for regular reviews of the appropriateness of the priorities that have been laid down.

3. Nature of Educational Research

Superficially it may seem a relatively straightforward task to rationalize research effort in the field of education, to make statements of policy, and to establish a list of priorities. However, the fluctuations in the funding of educational research over the 30-year-period from the mid-1960s to the mid-1990s, and the widespread closure of educational research institutions and research units within bureaucratic organizations clearly indicate the complexity of the tasks involved and the divergent views that have existed. In part, these circumstances have arisen from a failure to reflect on the nature of educational research activity and misunderstanding about how the findings of educational research are applied. As a consequence too much has been expected by politicians and policymakers from educational research too soon after initial studies have been conducted. Moreover, the physical and medical sciences, eager for funds and able to point to the spectacular successes of some of their research efforts, have been all too ready to disparage research in the social and behavioral sciences without consideration of the unique character of such research activity.

3.1 Functions of Research in Education

It is well-established practice in the natural and technological sciences to make distinctions between basic or fundamental scientific research and applied research. Underlying this perspective is the view of a chain of activity starting with basic research, which leads on to applied research, and on again to technological development and the translation of research findings into practice. However, the writings of Conant (1947) and others have gradually influenced understanding of the interrelations between science, technology, and society and while the distinction between basic and applied research may be an administrative convenience in providing support for research in these fields, in practice the strategies and tactics employed in such research are rather more complex than a simple dichotomy would imply.

Coleman (1972) in a discussion of the nature of research in the social sciences distinguished between discipline research and policy research (see *Policy-oriented research*). While there is much to be said in support of Coleman's categorization (see Husén and Kogan 1984), it is important to recognize that educational research cannot be viewed in terms of a single discipline, as an educational science, since educational research frequently draws on many fields from within the social and behavioral sciences as well as from the humanities. Cronbach and Suppes (1969), arguing from the point of view of behavioral scientists, have seen a distinction between conclusion-oriented and decision-oriented educational research as useful. Underlying their perspective is the long-standing view held by psychologists that the field of education is one where the basic findings of psychology may be directly applied. While psychology remains the strongest primary discipline within educational research, it no longer dominates the field to the extent it once did (see, e.g., McGaw et al. 1992). Moreover, the drawing of conclusions in the study of education is enmeshed in a web of belief and the making of decisions is greatly influenced by political expediency. Thus the distinction between basic and applied research is questionable, and other dichotomies that have been proposed must also be challenged.

3.2 Outcomes of Research in Education

It can be argued that educational research and development generate outcomes that fall into three distinct categories. Rich (1977) initially distinguished between the instrumental and conceptual utilization of knowledge in the field of education. Likewise, Fullan (1980) suggested that there are two main ways in which knowledge is used in education. In the first usage, knowledge is applied to a particular problem, and that knowledge may be derived from a particular investigation or from a series of investigations. In the second usage, the knowledge available is cumulative knowledge and action is taken on the basis of cumulative knowledge. There is, however, a third and important form or outcome of educational research and development that involves the preparation of a tangible product for direct use in schools, classrooms, and homes and which incorporates the findings of educational research. In these three types of usage the emphasis is on the outcomes rather than the functions of research. Sometimes in the development of materials, the sequence of basic research, applied research, and materials development might be seen to apply, but this is only one type of usage. The situation is commonly more complex, since when action is taken

implicitly or explicitly on the basis of accumulated knowledge, the applied research stage and the materials development stage are commonly not invoked.

3.3 Nature of Social Action

Giddens (1984) has argued that it is important to recognize that the research and development model that relates to research in the natural sciences has been largely discredited in the social and behavioral sciences. Human beings are agents who are responsible for their own ideas and actions. In the study of educational problems and societal processes, human beings as a group do not remain as passive subjects of inquiry. They understand the debate that occurs during the formulation of ideas in a research study, and they not only assimilate these ideas but they also accommodate to them and are changed. Moreover, the social world is unknowable without using the views and perceptions that are held by human beings. Thus the very foundations of behavioral and social science knowledge lack certainty and the situation arises in which generalizations are advanced from research, but their nature has been influenced by the theories held by the research workers.

Furthermore, universal schooling and widespread higher education have during recent decades greatly facilitated the dissemination of advances in social theory and new educational ideas, through paperback publication, review journal articles, and not the least through the mass media. Consequently, the new ideas arising in the fields of social and educational theory are now quickly fed back into the thinking and actions of human beings and the social and behavioral world is itself changed. As a consequence the social and educational processes that are the subject of investigation are also changed. This does not mean that social or educational inquiry has no utility. Indeed, new ideas and their interrelations, which are the direct products of research, are very powerful initiators of change. Clearly, the nature of social action is very different from the application of scientific knowledge directly through technological development.

3.4 Evaluation and Prospective Inquiry

Educational and social research must not only be concerned with what was, and what is, but also with what might be. Research must help to identify issues and problems before they have emerged. It should also illuminate, employing both theory and pilot programs, the new and alternative pathways that lead toward desired educational and social goals. It has the task of generating new ideas and new ways of doing things from inquiry that is prospective rather than retrospective in orientation. The task for those persons who specify priorities for research is that of identifying those fields where it is possible to generate new ideas and new findings and where it is possible to attain desired goals more satisfactorily than in the past. The danger with a list of priorities identified at a high level by consensus is that problems and issues may be specified at too late a stage, when immediate solutions are required. Time is not available for systematic investigation.

4. Toward a Coherent Body of Knowledge about Education

In educational research a tension exists between responding to the immediate needs of practitioners and the building of a cumulative body of knowledge about educational processes, with recognition that the educational processes themselves are not static and are in a state of change. On the one hand, Tyler (1980) contended that priority should be given to the problems that teachers consider important, and that teachers are, in general, skeptical of problems for research that have been identified by groups outside the schools. On the other hand, Sanders (1981) has argued that educational research has become excessively atheoretical and has not produced an accumulated body of systematic knowledge. There is a danger in viewing these two approaches as alternatives. Unless the attention of research workers in education is focused on problems confronting policymakers and teachers there is the danger that important questions for research will be ignored and that the goodwill of schools and administrators toward research and researchers will disappear. However, unless educational research can add to a cumulative body of knowledge about education, there is the danger that after massive research effort over a long period no progress is made and each new generation of research workers must start afresh.

In the attempts that must be made to build a body of knowledge about the educational process it is important to recognize several key characteristics of research in education.

4.1 Cross-disciplinary Research

The stereotyped view is still held by many that the typical educational research worker has been trained in the discipline of psychology and that he or she prescribes for pedagogical practice the "dos" and "don'ts" that may be derived from the laws and generalizations of psychological theory. The audience for the counsel of the educational research worker and psychologist is seen to be the practicing classroom teacher who seeks to improve the effectiveness and efficiency of his or her daily work (Jackson and Kiesler 1977). It is not surprising that this view should have become established at a time at the beginning of the twentieth century when psychology was developing as a science, and when schools of education were being created. However, a more appropriate perspective is to consider educational research as cross-disciplinary in nature, cutting across and transcending or working at the interfaces between a variety of disciplines in the social and behavioral sciences and the humanities.

It would seem to be unduly restrictive to advance the claim that educational research commands a discipline of its own forming a field of educational or pedagogical science. During the twentieth century most developments in educational research have taken place as a result of thinking about educational problems from the perspectives of the social sciences, the humanities, and the behavioral sciences. Each disciplinary field in these areas can contribute to an examination of educational questions. Furthermore, perhaps the most interesting advances occur at the interfaces between two or more disciplines. Moreover, the educational problems that warrant investigation and for which solutions must be sought are not simply those that occur in the classroom. Education takes place not only in the school, but also within the home and the peer group, and through the mass media, in libraries and museums, at work and at play. The multifaceted nature of education means that there is a very broad variety of groups to whom the findings of educational research are of concern. Those wishing to contribute to educational policy and practice must draw upon the cumulative body of knowledge from many disciplinary areas about many different facets that are relevant to education.

4.2 Variables of the Educational Process

The second key characteristic of educational research is that it must often deal with very complex relationships involving many variables operating simultaneously. It is rare that a high-quality investigation into an educational problem or research situation can be reduced to the examination of a relationship between only two variables. One of the strategies that is commonly employed to investigate the simultaneous action of many variables is to carry out an intensive case study of a situation in which many factors are at work and to report in detail the full complexity and context of the events observed.

A commonly used alternative strategy involves the use of high-speed computers to analyze considerable bodies of qualitative or quantitative data associated with many variables. Because of the capabilities of computers to undertake complex statistical control of specific factors in the analysis of data, it is no longer essential to design an experiment to remove the effects of many variables by random selection procedures. The educational research worker is as a rule not able to design and conduct a controlled experiment to test a specific hypothesis, because it would involve interfering with the lives or schooling of people. The alternative that has emerged is to develop a complex multivariate statistical model, to examine the structure of the model, and then to estimate the parameters of the model through the statistical control of variables rather than through random allocation. Nevertheless, it must be acknowledged that a truly experimental approach, if it were a practicable alternative, would provide more soundly based conclusions than could be obtained from a nonexperimental study in a natural situation.

4.3 Educational Operations on Many Levels

Most educational activity takes place within a social setting where characteristics of the group have influences on the behavior and attitudes of the individual members of the group. For example, student learning and the development of attitudes may be influenced by factors associated with groups, namely: the home, the peer group, the class, the school, and the school system to which the individual student belongs. Moreover, many research problems in the field of education lead to the formulation of hypotheses about the effects of practices and policies implemented at the class, school, district, or national level, since the activities of these organizational units are generally more under the control of educational policymakers than are the practices of families and peer groups. As a consequence data collected in educational research studies associated with some key independent variables are obtained at the group level and others at the student level, while the outcomes of achievement and attitude are necessarily obtained solely at the individual student level. This multilevel nature of educational inquiry must be taken into consideration in the design of a study and the analysis of data. Only comparatively recently has it become possible to undertake the analysis of multilevel data, even where an experimental design is involved. Further developments must also be expected in this field in the future. The potential that now exists for the more effective analysis of multilevel data has important implications for the identification of priorities in educational research (see *Multilevel Analysis; Hierarchical Linear Modeling*).

Failure to recognize the multidisciplinary, multivariate, and multilevel nature of educational problems, in contrast to those research problems commonly encountered in the physical and biological sciences, or those commonly studied in the health and behavioral sciences, can lead funding agencies and committees responsible for the allocation of research grants, especially those comprised of members drawn from noneducational fields, to be uncertain in their identification of priorities for educational research. Even within the field of educational research, an individual steeped in the perspectives of one disciplinary area only, may have restricted views about priorities which result from a failure to understand the nature of educational processes, and the complexity of the issues that must be addressed.

5. Factors Influencing the Directions of Research

Some understanding of the factors that influence developments in educational research has emerged from the studies reported by Suppes (1978). Three factors can be identified, namely: (a) a response to critical issues; (b) the impact of technology and practice; and (c) new ideas and new perspectives that are derived from other disciplinary areas.

5.1 Research in Response to Critical Issues

In the past critical issues have from time to time emerged in education that have changed the direction of educational research while these problems were being investigated. Commonly, public concern for the issues has released funds for such work, but the public debate about the issues has also helped to generate ideas about the nature of the problems involved and to identify aspects that are amenable to research. Persons responsible for the identification of research priorities must attempt to anticipate such problems and to have work at least in progress at the time the issues become critical. As a consequence, in the coordination or rationalization of research in education, there is the danger that priorities are determined solely by what are widely seen to be critical issues at a time when it is too late to conduct systematic research, because immediate solutions are required. Educational research workers ought to become aware of the long-term needs of society, should seek to investigate research issues related to those needs, and should initiate the research activity. There is, however, the danger that some issues that purport to be educational matters are not appropriate or amenable to research in an educational context because the issues are in essence societal problems. If priorities were established solely by a select group who saw educational reform to be the agent of social reform, society would run the risk of being engineered by the select group with evident inherent dangers.

5.2 Impact of Technology on Research and Practice

Since at least the early 1930s, much of the mathematical knowledge necessary for the examination of the interrelations between many predictor variables and many outcome variables has been available. Very little progress was made in developing these ideas for use in the analysis of educational data until the mid-1960s, when advances in technology made widely available increasingly powerful electronic computers. As a consequence of these new procedures for the analysis of large bodies of data, both the types of problems that could be investigated and the ways of thinking about these problems changed. This rapidly led to the development of statistical and mathematical models for the examination of educational questions (see *Models and Model Building*). However, these developments also contributed to a relatively widespread rejection of what was seen to be a positivist approach, and a turning to the use of alternative methods for the investigation of educational problems (see *Action Research; Case Study Methods; Participatory Research*).

Thus advances in technology have had an impact on both how problematic situations in the field of education are conceptualized and on how research is conducted. Moreover, this impact involves not only the use of computers for multivariate analysis, but also a search for other strategies to investigate problems, in which many causal factors may be involved, and which are more exploratory and descriptive and do not demand the use of the computer.

Other advances in educational research may also be traced back to technological development, such as the use of mark-sensed answer sheets which make feasible large-scale cross-national surveys, such as those conducted by the International Association for the Evaluation of Educational Achievement (IEA). A further example is the introduction of the calculator into the classroom which at all levels of schooling makes more time available in the sciences and mathematics for new curricular content and an emphasis on the development of cognitive rather than computational skills, and thus opens up new fields of research, particularly those concerned with the development of cognitive skills and problem-solving.

5.3 Cross-disciplinary Contribution

There is little doubt that new approaches and strategies for educational research will continue to evolve from fertilization across disciplines, as developments in the contributory disciplines are seen to be relevant to educational problems. In identifying priorities for educational research, it is essential that the interdisciplinary nature of research into educational problems should be recognized. There is the danger that certain problems are seen to be not amenable to effective investigation when viewed from the perspective of a single discipline. However, appropriate conceptual theory and methodological approaches can commonly be found if a bridge can be built across several disciplinary areas.

The determination of priorities solely through reference to the magnitude and consequences of the issue involved is unwise. Sometimes it would be of greater benefit to consider the researchability of a problem and whether the development of new technology, or the availability of new methodology or new conceptual frameworks from other disciplines would make the problem more amenable to investigation than it was previously.

6. Determining Priorities for Research

Priorities for research must be identified at many levels. First, there is the individual research worker in a university who must decide what issues should be chosen as worthy of investigation and the devotion of a substantial segment of working time. Second, there is the department or unit in an institution which involves collections of individuals working in collaboration, who must recognize the advantages of

working as a team and focusing the efforts of the group on a particular problem, with different individuals investigating separately or jointly different aspects of the problem. Third, there is the research institution or center which must develop priorities for research and study and submit and argue the case for those priorities to an advisory or governing board. Fourth, there is the foundation that has trust funds to administer, whose priorities for research must be publicly stated as the basis for submissions for funding and support. Finally, there is the research council or board that is provided with substantial sums of public moneys which are to be allocated to research studies either as commissioned investigations, or on the basis of submissions received from research workers seeking support for studies they have chosen to undertake. Since the council must be publicly accountable for the allocation of moneys entrusted to it, there is commonly a need to identify its priorities and make them public both to those seeking funding and to those who provide the moneys.

At each of these levels priorities must be identified. Subsequently, there is the difficult task of making choices between applicants and projects in the light of the quality of the submissions received, the competence of the research workers making the submissions, the assessments of "peers" who have reviewed the research proposals submitted, and the judgments of the panel responsible for advising on the allocation of grants.

6.1 Criteria for Setting Priorities

An Australian Panel for a Strategic Review of Research in Education (McGaw et al. 1992 pp. 72–75) has identified six criteria for setting priorities in a national educational research agenda. However, these six criteria also apply at all levels outlined above.

6.1.1 Social and economic needs. Research into educational problems is conducted within a changing social and economic context and this context must be taken into consideration in identifying problems that warrant investigation. Of particular importance are studies that anticipate changes in the social and economic context. Such research contributes to the capacity of the educational community to think systematically about the effects of change on educational policy and practice.

6.1.2 Equity and social justice. It is important that educational research should contribute to the promotion of social justice and equity in society. The capacity of research to assist in the identification of sources of educational disadvantage, and strategies to overcome barriers to effective participation in society by all social groups are major criteria for advancing priorities for research.

6.1.3 Needs of professional practice. The findings of

educational research must help to meet the needs of professional practice both of those undertaking the research and those who study the findings of research. These contributions may not be immediately obvious, but a long-term influence on human and societal development, including the processes of learning and teaching at all age levels, must be sought.

6.1.4 Existing research strengths. The field of educational activity is so large and so complex that not all areas can be addressed, by an individual, a department, an institution, or even within a country. As a consequence it is desirable to identify existing strengths and to build on such strengths in the hope that significant advances will be made. Research in all fields commonly proceeds by the establishment of a group of scholars and students around an individual or small groups of individuals who have a proven capacity to identify key issues for research, and to deliver useful results from a program of inquiry. However, such centers of excellence are constantly shifting.

6.1.5 Advances in the research field. In the previous section the three main factors seen to influence advances in a field of research were identified and discussed. These three factors either separately or together can be employed to identify priorities.

6.1.6 Important gaps. A major function of identifying priorities is to fill important gaps in existing research programs. By focusing attention on the deficiencies that exist in research programs a more complete view of problem situations is obtained which provides evidence for solving those problems.

7. Statements of Priorities

Statements of priorities for research in education can be made at many levels, including cross-national, national, institutional, and individual research worker levels. In this entry three statements of national research priorities, which were prepared in the early 1990s are briefly presented. These summary statements, however, give some indication of the issues that were seen at that time to be of importance in three different countries in different parts of the world.

The Review Panel for the Strategic Review of Research in Education in Australia in 1992 proposed nine priority areas that it considered should stand for a minimum period of three years before being reviewed (McGaw et al. 1992 pp. 78–81). These may be considered as three groups.

The first group comprises research in areas of continuing importance to education and the improvement of professional practice, in particular: (a) the teaching of thinking skills; (b) learning in the preschool and adult years; and (c) assessment of student learning.

The second group concerns research on the organization and management of educational structures, programs and personnel, and the interrelationship between education and the wider society, in particular: (a) leadership and management in devolved education systems; (b) education, training and work; and (c) teachers' work.

The third group involves research directed towards the revision and improvement of specific areas of the curriculum, in particular: (a) mathematics education; (b) science education; and (c) language and literacy education.

The Institute for Educational Research in The Netherlands in 1991 issued a statement on a research program for the three-year period 1992 to 1995 under the title *Problem-oriented Research: An Agenda for the Future*. It identified seven areas for investigation: (a) vocational qualifications; (b) preparation for participation in society; (c) individual development; (d) the quality of education; (e) evaluation of innovation and developments in education; (f) research as a direct service; and (g) fundamental educational research which included three subprograms: (i) motivation and self-regulation as determinants of achievement; (ii) mother tongue instruction and foreign language learning; and (iii) pupils' school careers. This research program must be viewed in the context of the integration of Europe, where greater mobility is available to those with qualifications and language skills (SVO 1991).

The Report from the National Academy of Education in the United States identified five priority areas in a national research agenda: (a) active learning over the lifespan; (b) assessment; (c) bolstering achievement of historically underserved, "minority" and impoverished groups; (d) school organization; and (e) connection to teachers and teaching. The report argues that the current "research basis is under-funded, limited in focus, and lacks connection to what happens in the classroom" (National Academy of Education 1991).

8. Conclusion

While it is neither possible nor desirable to attempt to develop universal research needs and priorities, there is some commonality between the themes chosen in these three countries from different zones of the developed world. It can be seen that support is advocated for studies that investigate issues that are not only associated with societal problems, but also have a likelihood of contributing successfully to new conceptual knowledge, new policy or practice, or new products for use in educational work. It is, however, important to recognize as Levin (1978) has pointed out after examining certain persistent educational dilemmas, educational research cannot and should not be expected to solve problems that are basically political or social questions.

See also: Politics of Educational Research, Educational Research and Policy Making, Policy Analysis, Policy-oriented Research,

References

Coleman J S 1972 *Policy Research in the Social Sciences.* General Learning Press, Morristown, New Jersey

Conant J B 1947 *On Understanding Science: An Historical Approach.* Yale University Press, New Haven, Connecticut

Cronbach L J, Suppes P C (eds.) 1969 *Research for Tomorrow's Schools: Disciplined Inquiry for Education: Report.* Macmillan Inc., New York

Fullan M 1980 An R & D prospectus for educational reform. In: Mack D P, Ellis W E (eds.) 1980 *Interorganizational Arrangements for Collaborative Efforts: Commissioned Papers.* Northwest Regional Educational Laboratory, Portland, Oregon

Giddens A 1984 *The Constitution of Society: Outline of the Theory of Structuration.* Polity Press, Oxford

Husén T, Kogan M 1984 *Educational Research and Policy: How Do They Relate?* Pergamon Press, Oxford

Jackson P W, Kiesler S B 1977 Fundamental research and education. *Educ. Res.* 6(8): 13–18

Levin H M 1978 Why isn't educational research more useful? *Prospects Q. Rev. Educ.* 8(2): 157–66

McGaw B et al. 1992 *Educational Research in Australia.* National Board of Employment, Education and Training, Canberra

National Academy of Education 1991 *Research and the Renewal of Education: A Report from the National Academy of Education.* National Academy of Education, Stanford, California

Radford W C 1973 *Research into Education in Australia: 1972* Australian Government Publishing Service, Canberra

Rich R F 1977 Use of social science information by federal bureaucrats: Knowledge for action versus knowledge for understanding. In: Weiss C H (ed.) 1977 *Using Social Research in Public Policy Making.* Heath, Lexington, Massachusetts

Sanders D P 1981 Educational inquiry as developmental research. *Educ. Res.* 10(3): 8–13

Snow C P 1969 *Science and Government: With a Postscript.* Oxford University Press, Melbourne

Suppes P C (ed.) 1978 *Impact of Research on Education: Some Case Studies: Summaries.* National Academy of Education, Washington, DC

SVO (Institute for Educational Research in the Netherlands) 1991 *Problem-oriented Research: An Agenda for the Future.* Institute for Educational Research, The Hague (mimeo)

Tyler R W 1980 Integrating research, development, dissemination and practice in science education. Position paper. *Journal Announcement: RIE* July 1991

Unintended Effects in Educational Research

S. Ball

Unintended effects in educational research may stem from influences of the experimental or demonstration situation itself including the measurement procedures. They can also stem from interactions of the researcher with the subjects of the research study.

The size and importance of unintended effects in educational research are, by definition, difficult to estimate. Since they are unintended they are usually unexpected and the researcher therefore has not developed a research design to take them into account. To the extent this occurs, the results of the educational research may lose validity. The best antidote to unintended effects is the careful planning of the research design and of the measurement procedures. This entry considers the main types of unintended effects that occur in educational research studies.

1. Reactive Measurement Effects

Reactive effects in measurement occur when the behavior elicited by the measurement procedures is not characteristic of the behavior that would have occurred in a more typical situation. For example, suppose a researcher wishes to know the impact of a new teaching technique on student behavior, and suppose further that the measurement procedure involves an observer in a classroom using a behavior checklist as the teacher works with the students. The presence of the observer may cause the students to behave differently in comparison to how they would behave with no observer in the classroom. The observer, in this case, has a reactive effect on the evidence obtained.

Distortions due to reactive effects in measurement may be the result of subjects trying to make a good impression on the data gatherer, of personal interactions between interviewer and interviewee (in this case, the sex, race, age, and ethnicity of the interviewer can affect the responses obtained), of response sets (e.g., young children tend to answer "yes" to questions posed by authority figures), of initial questions in a test leading to changes in understanding or to a new appreciation by the test taker of what is considered important and so affecting the way the test taker answers the later questions, and of changes in the environment created by the measurer (e.g., the placing of a videotape machine in a library might affect the way students behave during a library period).

In general, the less obtrusive the measurement procedure, the less reactive it is likely to be. Webb et al. (1966) provide an excellent presentation of unobtrusive measures. An extensive discussion of response sets, reactive effects, and unobtrusive measures is presented by Anderson et al. (1975).

Reactive effects (distortions) due to research evaluation design deficiencies may also lead to erroneous conclusions. Three of the most famous types of reactive design deficiencies that lead to distortions in the conclusions have been labeled the Hawthorne effect, the John Henry effect, and the Pygmalion effect.

2. Hawthorne Effect

The Hawthorne effect refers to the change in behavior that occurs when the subjects in an evaluation or experiment are aware that they are being studied. This awareness is confounded with the independent variable being studied; so any *positive* impact noted in the research can be causally ascribed either to the independent variable or to the awareness of the subjects.

The Hawthorne effect is well-illustrated by the series of experiments (Pennock 1929) which took place at the United States Western Electric Company factory from 1924 to 1927 at Hawthorne, Illinois. The label "Hawthorne effect" was coined by Pennock to describe the unexpected findings noted by him and his colleagues (Snow 1927). Many independent variables were systematically manipulated (e.g., illumination, rest pauses, pay incentives) and the employees were informed of what was happening. The enigma was that productivity tended to increase irrespective of the experimental manipulation. It became clear that the employees' awareness that they were being studied itself had a positive impact on their productivity.

A number of researchers have studied the impact of the Hawthorne effect in educational settings (Cook 1962, 1967), and some have questioned its strength (Bauernfeind and Olson 1973). Nonetheless, there is general agreement among educational researchers that the Hawthorne effect is a potential threat to the validity of educational experiments.

Consider, for example, a situation where a new kind of textbook is being tested in a random sample of classrooms, while another random sample of control classrooms is also being studied for comparison. If the experimenters had no regard for the Hawthorne effect, the experimental classrooms would receive the new kind of textbook, the teachers and students would be allowed to know they were the mediating variables in a textbook experiment, and observers might even

spend time in the experimental, but not the control, classrooms. As a result the teachers and students might work harder; and the positive impact thus seen might then be wrongly ascribed to the new textbook (Trow 1971).

To avoid contamination by the Hawthorne effect, care should be taken with the teachers and students *not* to emphasize the experiment. The control classrooms should be observed as much as the experimental classrooms, and since the experimental classes are receiving new books, the control classes might at least receive new copies of the old text, a "placebo."

The term "placebo" is used mainly in medical research when a chemically inert substance is administered to a sample of subjects in the same manner as a drug or active substance is administered to a different sample of subjects from the same population. This research procedure means that the subjects (and preferably the researchers too) are unaware at the time which subjects receive the experimental treatment and which the placebo. The analogy between this and educational research should be clear (Adair et al. 1989, 1990).

The presence of the Hawthorne effect helps to explain the fads of educational practice. A new idea (e.g., the initial teaching alphabet or i.t.a. approach to reading, or the "open" classroom) is implemented with enthusiasm and with considerable apparent success. Over the following years the fad dies off. It could well be that much of the early success was a manifestation of the Hawthorne effect. As the new treatment becomes routine, the Hawthorne effect and positive impacts accruing therefrom are lost.

The obverse side of the Hawthorne effect is the John Henry effect.

3. John Henry Effect

John Henry effect is an unintended effect in which members of the control group perform better than they typically would perform. The reason why the members of the control group outperform themselves is presumably because they feel competitive about the experimental groups, thereby creating enhanced enthusiasm to do well. This reduces or reverses the effects of a procedure used on an experimental group which may threaten to replace the "control" procedure. The John Henry effect is to the control group as the Hawthorne effect is to the experimental group.

The term "John Henry" is taken from a folk hero of the United States, a black railroad worker who was told that the steam drill would replace human labor in laying railroad tracks. By amazing effort he did better than the machine but the exertion eventually killed him.

The John Henry effect was associated with educational research by Saretsky (1972). He pointed out a peculiar phenomenon with respect to the evaluative research that had taken place on performance contracting. Control groups and experimental groups in school districts had been studied: the control groups had made much greater than anticipated gains though they were presumably receiving no new or different treatment. It seemed, however, that the teachers of the control classes were definitely trying harder than they would normally have worked.

The John Henry effect (improved control group performance), may lead to the wrong conclusion that the experimental treatment, whatever it may be, is ineffective. Frequently the researcher looks at differences between the mean performance of the experimental group and the control group to see if the experimental treatment is effective. The researcher should also ensure there is no unusual change in the untreated control group. Perhaps the most appropriate evaluation (research) design to employ when the John Henry effect is thought likely to occur is a time series design in which measures are taken to provide baseline data before the experiment is introduced. Measurement should also occur after the treatment (experiment) is over. If the John Henry effect has occurred, the control group performance should be enhanced during the course of the experiment and should return to baseline afterward. If the treatment is effective the experimental group, of course, will also show enhanced performance during the experiment. The comparison might then be made with the experimental group's performance and the baseline or projected baseline performance of the control group, thereby discounting the John Henry effect.

Preferably the John Henry effect should not be allowed to occur. Control groups should not be made to feel threatened or in competition with the treatment group just as the experimental group should not be made to feel special and different.

4. Pygmalion Effect

The Pygmalion effect was given emphasis when Rosenthal and Jacobson (1968) published *Pygmalion in the Classroom*. The term "Pygmalion" comes from the Greek myth in which life was infused into an inanimate object by the power of positive thinking. In the Rosenthal studies (Rosenthal and Rubin 1978), expectancies of the experimenter (or teacher) led to improved performance by the subjects (or students). Thus, if a teacher believes a student will do better in the coming year, there is a stronger than chance possibility that this belief will be fulfilled.

The Pygmalion effect, or self-fulfilling prophecy, has been one of the major methodological issues in educational research in the final third of the twentieth century. The original study was heavily criticized (Thorndike 1968), and as well as being the subject of considerable further research, has been generalized to many other areas outside education including business (Eden 1990). A summary of the criticisms is provided by Wineberg (1987) and a response is given by Rosenthal (1987) and by Rist (1987). In general, there

does seem to be a Pygmalion phenomenon (Merton 1987) and its effects *can* be sizable. The generalizable point is that expectations by researcher or participants in a research study can have effects that are unintended by the researcher and thereby cloud the validity of the researchers' conclusions.

Babad et al. (1982) also coined the less used term "Golem effect" after a Jewish myth in which a mechanical creature runs amok and becomes destructive. The Golem effect is a negative expectancy effect (in contrast to the positive expectancy effect called Pygmalion) and is used to explain in part why students about whom teachers have low expectations often perform more poorly than would be likely given their previous school record.

5. Side and After Effects

While reactive measurement and Hawthorne, John Henry, and Pygmalion effects are unintended by the researcher, they are effects which nonetheless are created by the researcher in the process of setting up and executing the research. Other unintended effects may occur through the effects of the treatment. These treatment, side, or after effects can be either positive or negative in impact. In evaluating the treatment they may be crucially important. If the researcher is insensitive to their possibility the research results can be badly contaminated. If the researcher is sensitive to their possibility the research results may become qualified in a number of useful ways.

A side effect is an outcome that is peripherally related to, and *not* the main reason for, the implementation of an experimental program or treatment. Side effects are frequently unintended outcomes; but it is possible that program developers recognize beforehand the possibility of a side effect and plan to have it happen.

An example of an unintended side effect is a foreign-language teaching program that is so heavily structured that the students dislike learning the foreign language. The intended main effect was the learning of the foreign language. The unintended side effect was the development of a distaste for further learning of the language. Certainly the program developers would not want that to happen. Note, then, that in this instance the unintended side effect was negative. It could have been positive. For example, a children's television show might have as an intended main goal that the viewers learn about children in other countries. An unintended positive side effect might be that viewers take out relevant books from the school library and their reading comprehension and vocabulary are thereby improved.

Intended side effects have hoped-for outcomes that usually are outside the domain of the intended main effects. Thus, if the intended main effects are achievement and cognitively oriented, then the intended side effects will usually be attitudinally or affectively oriented. If the major goal is to improve the students' knowledge and skill in mathematics, the intended side effect might be to enhance the students' self-confidence in and liking of mathematics.

Because side effects can be vitally important in evaluating educational programs, Scriven (1972) proposed a goal-free model of program evaluation. He argued that an evaluator who knows the program goals will be too prone to assess only those goal areas, ignoring the unintended side effects. With a goal-free evaluation, however, the evaluator according to Scriven is more likely to assess the full impact of a program whether intended or not.

Evaluators should be aware that sometimes the intended main effects fail to appear, yet positive side effects do occur. For example, innovative educational program A is not superior to traditional program B, but program A does have the positive side effect that students are more motivated to stay on in school. This side effect may itself become the rationale for recommending the substitution of program A for program B.

A difficult question in program evaluation is who decides what side effects to look for. In general, program developers do not want researchers to search for negative side effects. There should be clarity in the contract or the work order specifying the degree of autonomy assigned to the evaluator in making decisions on what side effects to look for given that there could be a multitude of them. Ideally this decision should be arrived at only after full consultation among the program developers, funders, clients, staff, and evaluators.

Another treatment effect that may be unintended has been called "after effect." As the term implies, an after effect is an impact that occurs some time after a treatment has been implemented and assessed. The term "sleeper effect" has also been used instead of after effect. Sometimes an after effect is noted years after the treatment has ended. Most research studies fail to test for the long-delayed after effects because usually the post-test occurs immediately after a treatment is ended. If there is a possibility of an after effect occurring, the research design should include both an immediate post-test (at the end of the treatment) and at least one delayed post-test.

An example of an after effect is provided by Kersh and Wittrock (1962) in their review of research on teaching techniques. They found that "direct" teaching techniques seemed to show a stronger impact than "discovery learning" techniques when the groups were tested immediately after the respective treatment. However, a delayed post-test (some six weeks after the treatment was over) showed the reverse to be true. The discovery learning group had shown little fade out of results and now performed better than the direct teaching group. Presumably an after effect of discovery learning was motivational, causing the students to continue to rehearse and learn to a degree not matched by the direct teaching group.

A controversial but potentially important example of after effect has been noted in the evaluative research on Head Start, a program for disadvantaged preschoolers. In the first decade of Head Start research it was noted that the program had an initial impact on children but that this impact did not seem to be permanent. That is, although the impact was observable when the children started regular school at the age of 5 or 6 years, it seemed to lessen so that there was little or no difference between the erstwhile Head Start participants and their comparable non-Head Start peers by third grade (age 8–9). However, an after effect (sleeper effect) was noted. Children who had been in Head Start seemed to forge ahead of their controls in the middle-school years (Grades 6 and 7).

An after effect should not be confused with a side effect. The side effect happens concurrently with the main, intended effects but the after effect, if it occurs, happens at a time after the main and side effects.

6. Conclusion

Unintended effects in educational research can lead to invalid and therefore misleading results. They may indicate that a given educational treatment is effective when in fact it is simply harnessing in an unintended way, for example, Hawthorne or Pygmalion Effects. It may indicate the treatment is ineffective when in fact the reactivity to the measurement procedures or John Henry Effect worked to mask a true positive impact.

Similarly side effects and after effects can provide additional impact information that a researcher ignores; yet that information may be crucial to the understanding of the treatment's effectiveness.

It is therefore essential that in developing and administering a research design and attendant measurement strategies the researcher should be sensitive to these issues.

See also: Research in Education: Epistemological Issues; Quasi-experimentation

References

Adair J G, Sharpe D, Huynh C-L 1989 Hawthorne control procedures in educational experiments: A reconsideration of their use and effectiveness. *Rev. Educ. Res.* 59(2): 215–28

Adair J G, Sharpe D, Huynh C-L 1990 The Placebo Control Group: An analysis of its effectiveness in educational research. *Experimental Education* 59(1): 67–86

Anderson S B, Ball S, Murphy R T 1975 *Encyclopedia of Educational Evaluation.* Jossey-Bass, San Francisco, California

Babad E Y, Inbar J, Rosenthal R 1982 Pygmalion, Galatea, and the Golem: Investigations of biased and unbiased teachers. *J. Educ. Psychol.* 74(4): 459–74

Bauernfeind R, Olson C 1973 Is the Hawthorne effect in

educational experiments a chimera? *Phi Del. Kap.* 55(4):
271–73

Cook D L 1962 The Hawthorne effect in educational research. *Phi Del. Kap.* 44: 116–22

Cook D L 1967 *The Impact of the Hawthorne Effect in Experimental Designs in Educational Research.* Report 0726. US Office of Education, Washington, DC

Eden D 1990 Pygmalion without interpersonal contrast effects: Whole groups gain from raising manager expectations. *J. Appl. Psychol.* 75(4): 394–98

Kersh B Y, Wittrock M C 1962 Learning by discovery: An interpretation of recent research. *J. Teach. Educ.* 13: 461–68

Merton R K 1987 Three fragments from a sociologist's notebooks: Establishing the phenomenon, specified ignorance, and strategic research materials. *Ann. Rev. Sociol.* 13: 1–28

Pennock G 1929 Industrial research at Hawthorne: An experimental investigation of rest periods, working conditions and other influences. *Personnel Journal* 8: 296–313

Rist R C 1987 Do teachers count in the lives of children? A reply to Wineburg. *Educ. Researcher* 16(9): 41–42

Rosenthal R 1987 Pygmalion effects: Existence, magnitude, and social importance. A reply to Wineburg. *Educ. Researcher* 16(9): 37–41

Rosenthal R, Jacobson L 1968 *Pygmalion in the Classroom: Teacher Expectation and Pupils' Intellectual Development.* Holt, Rinehart and Winston, New York

Rosenthal R, Rubin D B 1978 Interpersonal expectancy effects: The first 345 studies. *Behav. Brain Sci.* 1(3): 377–415

Saretsky G 1972 The OEO PC experiment and the John Henry effect. *Phi Del. Kap.* 53(9): 579–81

Scriven M 1972 Pros and cons about goal-free evaluation. *Eval. Comment* 3(4): 1–4

Snow C E 1927 Research on industrial illumination. *The Tech Engineering News* 8(6): 257–82

Thorndike R L 1968 *Pygmalion in the Classroom* by R Rosenthal and L Jacobson: a Review. *Am. Educ. Res. J.* 5(4): 708–11

Trow M 1971 Methodological problems in the evaluation of innovation. In: Caro F G (ed.) 1971 *Readings in Evaluation Research.* Russell Sage, Rensselaer, New York

Webb E J, Campbell D T, Schwartz R D, Sechrest L 1961 *Unobtrusive Measures: Nonreactive Research in the Social Sciences.* Rand McNally, Chicago, Illinois

Wineburg S S 1987 The self-fulfillment of the self-fulfilling prophecy. *Educ. Researcher* 16(9): 28–37

Further Reading

Adair J G, Sharpe D, Huynh C-L 1989 Placebo, Hawthorne, and Other Artifact Controls: Researchers' Opinions and Practices. *J. Exp. Educ.* 57(4): 342–55

Borg W R, Gall M D 1983 *Educational Research: An Introduction.* Longman, New York

Gay L R 1987 *Educational Research: Competencies for Analysis and Application.* Merrill Publishing Co., Columbus, Ohio

Rosenthal R, Rosnow R L (eds.) 1969 *Artifact in Behavioral Research.* Academic Press, New York

Rosnow R L 1981 *Paradigms in Transition: The Methodology of Social Inquiry.* Oxford University Press, New York

Teachers as Researchers

S. Hollingsworth

The international movement to recognize, prepare, and learn from teachers as researchers has come of age in the years since Elliott's (1985) entry on the topic in *The International Encyclopedia of Education, 1st edn.* This new entry summarizes the breadth, diversity, and significance of the teacher-as-researcher movement across three interrelated areas: curriculum improvement, professional and structural critique, and societal reform. Since teacher researchers are concerned simultaneously with ways to (a) improve their practice, (b) change the situations in which they work, and (c) understand their practices within the larger society, the organization of this entry is not intended to be linear of hiearchical. The discussion, instead, is framed in terms of different organizing focuses.

1. Curriculum Improvement

Curriculum improvement research is a derivative of what was known as "action research" and which led to the conceptualization of teachers as researchers within a process model (Stenhouse 1983). The work in this area produced both immediate curriculum changes on the part of teachers (first-order research), and observations about teacher research from collaborating academics (second-order research).

1.1 Action Research

The use of experimental social science to investigate various programs of social action was popularized in the United States by social psychologist Kurt Lewin (1946). Corey (1953) adapted the concept to improve school practices. He and his faculty colleagues at Teachers College at Columbia University worked cooperatively with public-school personnel on curriculum projects in action. In the post-Sputnik climate of the late 1950s, however, primary funding went to curriculum projects which followed traditional research, development, and dissemination models. Action research, suspect as "unscientific" in such a climate, became "interactive R & D [research and development]," disseminating research results through inservice teacher training. Much of that federally funded work, however, supported regular seminars in which teachers were encouraged to investigate topics related to their practices. It was the curriculum reform movement in the United Kingdom, however, that first popularized teachers as researchers.

1.2 Teachers as Researchers

Stenhouse (1983) is credited with developing the concept of teachers as researchers at the University of East Anglia. As director of the Schools Council's Humanities Project, Stenhouse came to see teachers' authority and autonomy as a basis for curriculum improvement and innovation. Like Corey, Stenhouse used the scientific method of developing and testing curricular hypotheses, but felt that its use to develop replicable results across classrooms was limited. He also questioned the ethical stance of separating the performance from the performer. Stenhouse thus rejected the "objectives model" of curriculum adoption (Tyler 1949) and asked teachers to engage in a "process model" of curriculum innovation where professional and curricular development became part of the same enterprise.

1.3 Developing the Process Model

Three factors made action research in the process model a viable alternative in the late 1970s and 1980s: (a) the difficulties of disseminating quantitative, experimental methodologies to local educational settings; (b) an increasing acceptance of the concept of curriculum as integrated with human deliberation (Schwab 1973); and (c) a professional and political reaction to post-Sputnik accountability as an approach for improving and changing curriculum. Elliott (1991), a colleague of Stenhouse, emphasized the interpretive-hermeneutic nature of inquiry. He saw action research as a pedagogical paradigm—a form of teaching. He argued that educational research should be modeled after action research: "a moral science paradigm to which teacher researchers would be the main contributors, rather than those in academic disciplines" (McKernan 1991, p. 23).

1.4 The Impact of First- and Second-order Research on Curriculum Improvement

First-order research examines changes in the curriculum made by teachers. Examples of such research are included in reports prepared by public-school teachers (Philadelphia Teachers Learning Collaborative 1984), descriptions of university-level teachers' research on their curricular practices (Lampert 1989), and summaries included in texts detailing the action of teacher researchers and academics (Clandinin et al. 1995). Examples of second-order research (that is, discussions about teacher research) can be found in outlines of skills needed by teacher researchers (Hopkins 1985), in discussions of teacher researchers' cognitive

development (Oja and Sumlyan 1989), in descriptions of teacher networks (Smith et al. 1991), and in understandings gained from teacher–university collectives (Carini 1988).

The cumulative effect of this work has changed the manner in which teachers are perceived as professional curriculum developers. It has also influenced collaborative research models and school restructuring plans which emphasize "teacher empowerment." One of the best examples of curriculum-based teacher research, one which improved practice and then led to theoretical, professional, and structural change, is the Bay Area Writing Project (BAWP). Reports from BAWP extensions across the United States range from first-order summaries (Fecho 1992) to second-order analyses of project participants' ideological differences (Schecter 1992).

2. Professional and Structural Critique

Emerging in the 1980s from the success of curriculum improvement research in the United Kingdom and the United States was an attempt to improve social environments and/or conditions of practice through structural and professional critique.

2.1 Structural Critique

Kemmis and his colleagues at Deakin University in Australia and elsewhere have articulated a model of a critical educational science. Their basic premise is that "new ideas are not enough to generate better education. Educational practices and patterns of school and classroom organization must also be changed to secure improvement" (Kemmis and McTaggert 1988, p. 34).

The critical stance of teachers as researchers, focusing on desired and possible changes in the educational structures, has also been noted within the United Kingdom and other countries. Simons (1992), for example, has argued for collaborative partnerships in the teacher research movement, which take into account the practice-oriented views of the curriculum researcher and the structural views of the critical researcher. She points out that reforming schools from the outside cannot work—neither can simple calls for collaboration. Existing structures privilege privacy, hierarchy, and territory within the institution and across collaborative boundaries; thus, structural and professional relationships must change.

2.2 Critiques of Professionalism and Professionalization

Sockett (1989) has drawn educational scholars' attention to the need for professionalism in teaching as well as the professionalization or socialization process by which one becomes a professional. Teacher research is an important part of both processes. Posch (1992) in Austria also speaks of the importance of teacher research for the profession. He argues that teacher professionalism involves teacher research on student professionalism.

Preparing student teachers and experienced teachers to be critical professionals who challenge and change the workplace conditions (including curriculum) is an important part of a professional and structural critique. Feminists involved in teacher education help teachers to develop radical pedagogies or "styles of teaching which help make visible to pupils the structural social inequities which constrain their lives" (Middleton 1992 p. 18).

2.3 Impact on the Workplace and the Profession

Although the preparation of teachers as critical inquirers is not yet widespread, structural and professional changes influenced by this work have been widely noted in new policies for school and professional restructuring. In the United States, a Californian decision to retain and reshape the state-sponsored mentoring project followed teacher research investigations into its possibilities and limitations (see Ashton et al. 1990).

Many of the transformative results from the critical professional and structural stance, however, have been far less public and far more personal. The Boston Women's Teachers' Group (Freedman et al. 1983), for example, met for three years to cope with the isolated struggle of their daily work and to study how their work conditions affected them as teachers. Like other groups who have created similar structures, their professional work was critical rather than curricular. They focused on the creation of conditions under which participants could consider their own interests and develop curriculum innovations.

3. Societal Reform

The focus of teachers as researchers in the societal reform sense is on how schools and teaching are shaped in society and what epistemological views are needed for their transformation. In some countries, the societal focus resulted from an awareness of the increasing gap between the concept of democracy and the reality of domination and oppression. Fueled by the Civil Rights and Women's Movements in the United States, even popular teacher-promoted curricular projects challenging static views of knowledge and societal norms were not free from scrutiny (see, for example, Delpit's (1986) critique of the Bay Area Writing Project). Two broad areas of societal reform are epistemological critique and the problem of gender.

3.1 Epistemological Critique

This view of teachers as researchers developed simultaneously with philosophical critiques of societal positions based on privileged conceptions of knowledge. Bruner (1985), for example, questioned the power ascribed the paradigmatic or "rational" view of knowledge and discussed the power of its antitheses: a narrative view of knowledge. Harding (1991) questioned natural science's position on objectivity as too protective of the power-dominant, White, male society. Belenky et al. (1986) raised questions about alternative ways of knowing which could privilege some women over others. Culturally diverse ways of knowing and representing knowledge, such as those pointed out by Lourde (1984), also critiqued societally accepted knowledge. Finally, many critiques either implicitly or explicitly questioned the separation of hierarchically powered social structures and inquiry methods (Winter 1987).

3.2 The Problem of Gender

Zeichner (1990) challenged the problematic social and epistemological hierarchy by speaking of the importance of teachers as women in the second professional wave of educational reform. Zeichner stressed that "Teaching is not just work; it is gendered work" (p. 366). As he expressed hope for societal reform and emancipation in the press for teacher empowerment, he also offered caution. He pointed out the possibility of curricular reform missions being undermined unless teacher research is incorporated into, instead of added to, teachers' work.

For Hollingsworth (1992), the teacher-as- researcher movement takes on a perspective of feminist praxis. A consciousness of the teacher's personal position within society (i.e., most teachers throughout the world are women), an understanding of research, an appreciation of the teacher's ability to construct and critique knowledge, and the integration of those features in classroom teaching suggests that teaching itself is research. Thus, teachers are the researchers of educational and societal reform—a position Elliott (1991) had endorsed earlier from a curricular stance.

Weiner (1989) contrasts teacher research in the Schools Council Sex Differentiation Project with mainstream professional development or curricular teacher research. Rather than convince teachers of a need to change their practices, gender researchers in the United Kingdom wish to bring about improvements in the social and economic position of women. Similar research is being conducted in the United States (see McIntosh et al. 1992).

3.3 Impact of Societal Reform

Excellent examples of first-order research from the societal reform stance are available (Newman 1990). The publication of such work is indicative of the increasing involvement of teachers in emancipatory work. Further, not only are teacher researchers conducting their own professional meetings, but they are participating at national and international research conferences previously reserved for university researchers. For example, since 1989, the American Educational Research Association has registered a special interest group on teacher research. The National Research Center on Literature Teaching and Learning in the United States sponsored a Teacher Research Institute in 1992. These are but a few examples of how the teacher-as-researcher movement is resulting in societal reform.

The concept of teacher-as-researcher is at the center of international attention to reform in all areas of the educational enterprise: research, teaching, the profession, its moral purpose, and its impact on societies. Some might worry that the political implications of teacher empowerment and societal reform might lead to a new and unknown world with unfamiliar epistemological and social norms. Others might be concerned that the growing popularity of teachers-as-researchers will ensure that it becomes yet another form of power and hierarchy inside schools. If so, the concept may be mandated, measured, and become meaningless to actual improvement of practice. Conversely, it may become a new process for reproducing existing school structures and societal outcomes. The trends found in the literature fail to resolve either of those worries. What is clear is that the movement is part of the larger evolution of society into the postinformation age—and that teachers-as-researchers are no longer marginally involved.

References

Ashton D et al. 1990 *Where Do We Go From Here in the California Mentor Teacher Program?: Recommendations by Seven Mentors*. Stanford/Schools Collaborative, Stanford University, Stanford, California

Belenky M F, Clinchy B M, Goldberger N R, Tarule J M 1986 *Women's Ways of Knowing: The Development of Self, Voice, and Mind*. Basic Books, New York

Bruner J S 1985 Narrative and paradigmatic modes of thought. In: Eisner E (ed.) 1985 *Learning and Teaching the Ways of Knowing, 84th Yearbook of the National Society for the Study of Education*. University of Chicago Press, Chicago, Illinois

Carini P 1988 Prospect's documentary processes. Unpublished manuscript, Bennington, Vermont

Clandinin D J, Davies A, Hogan P, Kennard B (1995) *Learning to Teach: Teaching to Learn Stories of Collaboration in Teacher Education*. Teachers' College Press, New York

Corey S 1953 *Action Research to Improve School Practices*. Teachers College Press, New York

Delpit L 1986 Skills and other dilemmas of a progressive Black educator. *Harv. Educ. Rev.* 56(4): 379–85.

Elliot J 1985 Teachers as researchers. In: Husén T, Postlethwaite T N (eds.) 1985 *The International Encyclopedia of Education, 1st edn*. Pergamon Press, Oxford

Elliott J 1991 *Action Research for Educational Change*. Open University Press, Milton Keynes

Fecho B 1992 The way they talk: An English teacher ponders his role. Paper presented at the Ethnography in Education Research Forum, University of Pennsylvania, Philadelphia

Freedman S, Jackson J, Boles K 1983 Teaching: An imperilled "profession." In: Shulman L S, Sykes G (eds.) 1983 *Handbook of Teaching and Policy*. Longman, New York

Harding S 1991 *Whose Science? Whose Knowledge? Thinking from Women's Lives*. Cornell University Press, Ithaca, New York

Hollingsworth S 1992 Learning to teach literacy through collaborative conversation: A feminist approach. *Am. Educ. Res. J.* 29(2): 373–404.

Hopkins D 1985 *A Teacher's Guide to Classroom Research*. Taylor and Francis, London

Kemmis S, McTaggert R 1988 *The Action Research Planner*, 3rd edn. Deakin University Press, Geelong, Victoria

Lampert M 1989 Research into practice: Arithmetic as problem solving. *Arithmetic Teacher* 36(7): 34–36

Lourde A 1984 *Sister Outsider*. The Crossing Press, Freedom, California

Lewin K 1946 Action research and minority problems *J. Soc. Iss.* 2(4): 24–46.

McIntosh P, Style E, Tsugawa T 1992 *Teacher as Researcher*. National SEED Seeking Educational Equity and Diversity, Wellesley College Center for Research on Women, Wellesley, Massachusetts

McKernan J 1991 *Curriculum Action Research: A Handbook of Methods and Resources for the Reflective Practitioner*. St. Martin's Press, New York

Newman J D (ed.) 1990 *Finding our Own Way: Teachers Exploring their Assumptions*. Heinemann, Portsmouth, New Hampshire

Oja S N, Smulyan L (eds.) 1989 *Collaborative Action Research: A Developmental Process*. Falmer Press, London

Philadelphia Teachers' Learning Cooperative 1984 On becoming teacher experts: Buying time. *Lang. Arts* 61(7): 731–36

Posch P 1992 Teacher research and teacher professionalism. Paper presented at the Int. Conf. Teacher Research, Stanford University, Palo Alto, California

Schecter S R 1992 Ideological divergences in teacher research groups. Paper presented at the Ethnography in Education Research Forum, University of Pennsylvania, Philadelphia

Schwab J 1983 The practical 4: Something for curriculum professors to do. *Curric. Inq.* 13(3): 239–65.

Simons H 1992 Teacher research and teacher professionalism. Paper presented at the Int. Conf. Teacher Research, Stanford University, Palo Alto, California

Smith H, Wigginton E, Hocking K, Jones R E 1991 Foxfire teacher networks. In: Lieberman A, Miller L (eds.) 1991 *Staff Development for Education in the 1990's: New Demands, New Realities, New Perspectives*, 2nd edn. Teachers College Press, New York

Sockett H 1989 Practical professionalism. In: Cass W (ed.) 1989 *Quality in Teaching*. Falmer Press, New York

Stenhouse L 1983 Research as a basis for teaching. In: Stenhouse L (ed.) 1983 *Authority, Education and Emancipation*. Heinemann, Portsmouth, New Hampshire

Tyler R W 1949 *Basic Principles of Curriculum and Instruction*. University of Chicago Press, Chicago, Illinois

Weiner G 1989 Professional self-knowledge versus social justice: A critical analysis of the teacher- researcher movement. *Brit. Educ. Res. J.* 15(1): 41–51

Winter R 1987 *Action-research and the Nature of Social Inquiry: Professional Innovation and Educational Work*. Gower, Brookfield, Vermont

Zeichner K M 1990 Contradictions and tensions in the professionalization of teaching and the democratization of schools. *Teach. Col. Rec.* 92: 363–379

Educational Research and Policy-making

T. Husén

Educational research has two constituencies of practitioners: (a) teachers and school administrators, and (b) policymakers in education. Classroom practitioners expect educational research to help them improve the planning and execution of teaching. At the turn of the century the emerging psychology with its empirical and experimental methods was expected to provide guidelines for educational practice by identifying the facts and laws of learning, and by providing an understanding of individual development and individual differences. In his *Talks to Teachers on Psychology* (1899) William James underlined that education being an art and not a science could not deduce schemes and methods of teaching for direct classroom application out of psychology. "An intermediary inventive mind must make the application by using its originality" (p. 8). In order to bridge the gap between theory and practice, James tried over and over again to make his presentation of psychology less technical. In the preface to his book which appeared several years after the lectures were given for the first time he says: "I have found by experience that what my hearers seem least to relish is analytical technicality, and what they most care for is concrete practical application. So I have gradually weeded out the former, and left the latter reduced: and now that I have at least written out the lectures, they contain a minimum of what is deemed 'scientific' psychology and are practical and popular in the extreme" (p. III).

In general, there is a similar relationship between research and practice in policy-making. For a long time this relationship was, by both partners involved, conceived of in a rather simplistic way. Policymakers wanted research that primarily addressed their pressing problems within the framework of their perceptions of the world of education. They wanted findings that could be more or less directly applied to issues and problems under their consideration. Researches conceived of their role as expert problem solvers who advised policymakers what to do.

The problem of how research in education is related to policy-making was hardly studied before the 1960s. However, after this date, resources given to educational research grew markedly. Governments and private foundations within a period of a decade massively increased the funds for research in education, most of which was conducted by behavioral scientists. Hopes grew correspondingly high about what research might achieve in broadening the knowledge base for educational practice. Research was expected to provide recipes for the successful solution to classroom problems. Policymakers expected educational research to help them in the planning and execution of reforms that would improve the quality of a nation's schools. Typically, the enormous increase of funds for educational research under the provisions of the Elementary and Secondary Education Act passed by the United States Congress in 1965 was part of a big package of legislation on compensatory education being in its turn part of the Great Society program (Husén 1979).

In the 1960s the research and development (R & D) model which had been developed in science and technology was extended to the fields of education and social welfare. The model assumes a linear relationship between fundamental research, applied research, development of a prototype, its mass production, and dissemination in the field. The high hopes easily led to frustrations. Researchers began to be accused of coming up with "findings" which were "useless" to practitioners, be they school teachers or administrators, in schools or governments. There was a growing demand for "relevance."

The simplistic model of "linear" or "direct" application of research does not work in education for two main reasons. In the first place, education is, like other areas in the social realm, imbued with values. Educational research deals with a reality which is perceived differently depending upon ideological convictions and values held by both practitioner and researcher. The way a problem is conceptualized, how it is empirically studied and analyzed, and how the findings from studies are interpreted often depends very much on tacit or overt value assumptions. One typical example is research on bilingual education, the extent to which a minority child in a country with a main language should have an opportunity to be instructed in his or her mother tongue. Second, and often overlooked, are the widely different conditions under which researchers and policymakers operate. Studies of these conditions began in the 1970s.

The value problem in educational research has begun to be analyzed by educational philosophers. It is highlighted by the controversy between logical positivism or neopositivism which has dominated the social science scene since the 1940s and critical philosophies of various brands. The former takes the social reality educational research deals with as a fact and takes for granted that research can advance "objectively" valid statements about that reality. The role of the researcher vis-à-vis the policymaker is that of a technician: he or she provides the instrument or the expertise that policymakers and practitioners "use" in framing and implementing their plans and policies. The latter type of philosophy sees critical studies as a means of changing society and thereby more or less explicitly allows value premises to enter

251

into the research process (see *Research Paradigms in Education*).

In the following discussion, the different conditions under which policymakers and researchers operate will be analyzed and the differences in ethos which guide endeavors in the respective categories will be described. After that, various research utilization models will be dealt with.

1. The Setting for Policy-making

Tensions between researchers and policymakers depend on certain constraints under which policy is shaped and implemented. Some of these have been discussed by Levin (1978) and by Husén and Kogan (1984).

Policymakers are primarily or even exclusively only interested in research that addresses problems which are on their agenda. This means that what researchers conceive as fundamental research which bears no or only a very remote relationship to the issues of the day is of little or no interest, if change in political regime or administration can mean a rearrangement of issues. For instance, the issues of private schools, educational vouchers, and busing took on quite a different importance under the Reagan as opposed to the Carter administration in the United States. In Europe after the Second World War the central issue in many countries was to what extent the structure of the mandatory school should be comprehensive with regard to intake of students and programs. In countries like Sweden, England and Wales, and the former Federal Republic of Germany many studies pertaining to the pedagogical and social aspects of comprehensiveness have been conducted and have been referred to extensively in the policy debate. In England, the 1944 Education Act with its provisions for tripartite, secondary education in grammar, technical, and modern schools, and the selection for grammar school (the so-called "11+ examination") became an issue of the first order and gave rise to a large body of research on methods of selection and their effects. The issue of equality of educational opportunity has been a major one in Europe and the United States since the 1950s and recently in many developing countries as well. It has consequently inspired a large volume of research (Husén 1975).

Politicians have party allegiances which influence not only what they regard as relevant, innocuous, or even dangerous research, but also their willingness to take research findings into account. Research, even if it addresses itself to a major issue on the political agenda, can be discarded or even rejected by one side in a political controversy if it does not support its views. Politicians, in the same way as court advocates, tend to select the evidence which they interpret as supporting their views.

Policymakers have their particular time horizon which in a parliamentary democracy tends to be rather narrow and determined not only by regular general elections, but also by the flow of policy decisions. Research which takes years to complete cannot be considered if the policymaker's timetable requires the outcomes of a research project or program to be available "here and now." Research findings have to be made available in time for the decisions that by necessity have to be taken, irrespective of the nature of the "knowledge base" on which the decision maker stands. He or she needs immediate access to findings. This is a dilemma which planners and policymakers in a government agency continuously have to face. On the one hand, strategic planning with a relatively broad time perspective goes on. On the other hand, operational decision-making is a continuous process which cannot wait for specially commissioned research to produce "relevant facts" of a rather simple, straightforward nature. This had led many administrators involved in policy-making to demand that research should be strictly decision- or policy oriented and address problems "in the field" only.

Policymakers are concerned only with policies in a particular area of their own experience as politicians or administrators. They therefore tend to disregard the connections with other areas. Educational policies have been advanced in order to solve what basically are problems in the larger social context. For example, in the United States in the mid-1960s compensatory education programs with enormous federal funds were made available to local schools. The intention was to "break the poverty cycle" by providing better education and thereby enhancing the employability of the economically disadvantaged (Husén 1979).

Policymakers are in most cases not familiar with educational research or social science research in general. In particular, they are not familiar with the language researchers use in communicating with each other, a language that ideally serves precision in presenting theories and methods, but by laypersons is often perceived as empty jargon. The problem then is to disseminate research findings in such a way that they can be understood by "ordinary people."

2. The Setting for Research

Researchers operate under conditions that in several respects differ from those under which people of practical affairs in politics and administration operate. There are differences of background, social values, and institutional settings.

Researchers in education have traditionally been performing their tasks at teacher-training institutions, most frequently at universities. As a result of growing government involvement, research units have been established by public agencies as instruments of planning and evaluation. Researchers conduct their work according to paradigms to which they have become socialized during their graduate studies (see *Research Paradigms in Education*). They are in the first place anxious to preserve their autonomy as researchers from interferences by politicians or administrators. Second, their allegiance is more to fundamental or conclusion-oriented research than to applied or decision-oriented research. Third, and as a consequence of this orientation, they pay much more attention to how their research is received by their peers in the national or international community of scholars in their field of specialization than by their customers in public agencies. This means, among other things, that once a technical report has been submitted, the researcher tends to lose interest in what happens to his or her findings.

Researchers are much less constrained than policymakers with regard to what problems they can tackle, what kind of critical language they can employ, and, not least, how much time they can use in completing a study. An investigation by the Dutch Foundation for Educational Research (Kallen et al. 1982) found that the great majority of projects financed by the Foundation lagged behind the timetable agreed upon for their completion. In order to conduct an empirical field study properly several years are required. The relevant literature on the "state of the art" has to be reviewed, methods have to be developed, data have to be collected in the field, data have to be processed and analyzed, sufficient time has to be allowed for writing the report, and finally, it takes some time for critical reviews in scholarly journals to appear. This is a process which typically takes about four to six years. Thus, the researcher has a different time horizon to that of the policymaker, both in terms of how much time he or she can allow for a study and in terms of how his or her study fits into the ongoing research in the field. He or she perceives the study as an often humble contribution to an increasingly growing body of knowledge in a particular problem area.

Status in the research system depends upon the reputation that crystallizes from the continuously ongoing review of a researcher's work by colleagues inside or outside his or her own institution. Whereas in an administrative agency status depends on seniority and position in the organizational hierarchy, it is in the long run the quality of a person's research and the recognition of this that determines the reputation in the scholarly community to which the researcher relates himself or herself.

3. Disjunctions between Researchers and Policymakers

The differences in settings and in value orientation between policymakers and educational researchers constitute what could be referred to as different kinds of ethos. It is even possible to speak of "two cultures." The research customers, the politicians, and/or the administrators/planners in a public agency are by necessity pragmatists. They regard research almost entirely as an instrument for achieving a certain policy or for use in planning or implementing certain administrative goals. They want research to be focused on priority areas of current politics.

University-based researchers are brought up in the tradition of "imperial, authoritative, and independent" Research with a capital R. In order to discharge properly what they regard as their task, academics tend to take an independent and critical attitude, not least toward government. They tend to guard anxiously their academic autonomy.

These differences in value orientation and outlook tend to influence the relationship between the policymaker and the researcher all the way from the initiation of a research project to the interpretation of its findings. The "researchworthiness" of a proposed study is assessed differently. The policymaker looks at its relevance for the issues on the agenda, whereas the researcher in the first place tends to assess it on the basis of "research-immanent" criteria, to what extent the proposed research can contribute to fundamental knowledge. The researcher wants to initiate studies without any particular considerations to the applicability of the findings and with the purpose of extending the frontiers of fundamental knowledge.

The fact that education by necessity deals with values anchored in various ideologies easily brings educational research into the turmoil of political controversy. Most regimes and administrations in power tend to perceive social science research with suspicion because of its critical nature. Those who want to preserve the status quo often tend to regard research as subversive radicalism. It is, however, in the nature of research to be in a literal sense "radical," that is to say, to go to the root (Latin *"radix"*).

The close relationship between education and certain political and social philosophies has made it tempting for social scientists to become ideological evangelists. This has had an adverse effect on their credibility. The common denominator of what is understood by "academic ethos" is critical inquiry that does not spare partisan doctrines, not even the ones of the party to which the researcher belongs.

In the 1960s, social science and behavioral research on an unprecedented scale began to be supported by the government in countries such as the United States, Sweden, the United Kingdom, and the former Federal Republic of Germany. Social scientists began to have a strong appeal and provided the arguments liberal politicians needed in favor of programs in education and social welfare. The liberals had a strong confidence in what social science could achieve. This meant that economists, sociologists, and psychologists were commissioned to conduct research that was part of the implementation of various programs in education (Aaron 1978). At the same time, there was a quest for evaluation of these programs and increasingly a component of evaluation was included in planning them.

Soon discrepancies between expectations and actual research performances began to be aired and led to demands for accountability. There have been indications of a decreasing credibility on the part of policymakers vis-à-vis researchers since the early 1970s. Expert testimonies on major policy issues have been seen as inconclusive and inconsistent. Coleman's (1966) survey of equality of educational opportunity was interpreted to support desegregation in the public schools of the United States (Coleman 1966). His subsequent studies of busing were interpreted as providing counterevidence. Policymakers want, as President Truman once expressed it in talking about his economic advisors, "one-handed" advice and are not happy with "on the one hand—on the other hand." Furthermore, the credibility gap has been widened by allegations of ideologically imbued professional advice. In some countries, social scientists working in education have been accused of "Leftist leanings" and subversive intentions. Political preferences among social scientists have even led to the establishment of research institutions with different political orientations, such as Brookings Institution and the American Enterprise Institute in the United States.

There are some inherent difficulties for educational research to prove its usefulness. The committee which at the end of the 1970s evaluated the National Institute of Education pointed out that improvements in the learning and the behavior of students as a result of research endeavors are difficult to demonstrate. The committee gave three main reasons for this: (a) a low level of sophistication in the social sciences in comparison with the physical sciences does not allow "the luxury of predictable results," (b) problems of bringing about and measuring changes in human learning and behavior are "vastly more complex" than those in the field of technological change, and (c) the need for improvement in education is so great that expectations on educational R & D have been set much higher than is possible to achieve.

The crucial problem behind many of the frustrations felt by customers of educational research is that research cannot provide answers to the value questions with which social issues, including those in education, are imbued. This means that research even of the highest quality and "relevance" can only provide partial information that has to be integrated with experience and human judgment. The Australian Minister of Education (Shellard 1979) quoted Glass as saying that there is more knowledge stored in the nervous systems of ten excellent teachers about how to manage classroom learning than what an average teacher could distill from all existing educational research journals.

Implied in what has been said so far are three major reasons for a "disjunction" between policy-making and research.

Research does not "fit" a particular situation. It might not at a given point in time be related to any political issue. Women's equal rights were for a long time a dead issue. But when they became an issue, they rapidly began to spur an enormous amount of research. But research addressing itself to issues on the agenda might come up with evidence that is out of phase with the policy-making process. As pointed out above, policymakers, like advocates, want to use research in order to support or legitimize a "prefabricated position." Often the situation occurs whereby research findings are in contradiction with or at least do not support the policy that a decision-making body or an agency wants to take or has already taken.

Research findings are, from the policymaker's point of view, not particularly conclusive. Furthermore, it is in the nature of the research process that in order to make a public issue "researchable" the overall problem has to be broken down into parts that more readily lend themselves to focused investigations.

A third major reason for the disjunctions between researchers and policymakers is ineffective dissemination. Research findings do not by themselves reach decision-makers and practitioners. Researchers seek recognition in the first place among their peers. They place high premium on reports that can enhance their academic reputation and tend to look with skepticism upon popularization. It has been suggested that this problem can be dealt with by middlepersons who can serve in the role of "research brokers" or policy analysts and can communicate to practitioners what appears to be relevant to them. A particular type of research broker is the one who conducts meta analyses of research, that is to say, reviews critically the existing research in a particular field in order to come up with relatively valid conclusions from the entire body of research (see *Meta-Analysis*).

4. Reviews of the "Utility" of Educational Research

The breakthrough in many countries for educational research with regard to institutionalization and, not least, funding came after the Second World War. Research was expected to serve educational policymakers and practitioners in planning and implementing educational reforms. Countries which provide examples are the United States, the United Kingdom, Sweden, and the former Federal Republic of Germany. However, the expectations bolstered by generous promises often led to disappointments.

Since the late 1970s, achievements of educational research have been reviewed in a spirit of self-criticism and a quest for realism in their promises. It has been pointed out that, until the 1960s, educational research had come up with findings of significance which have had and still have an impact on educational policy and practice. Edward L Thorndike's studies of formal discipline and his establishment of the law of effect made their way into school teaching, as has also Arthur Gate's principle of active learning. The research that Kurt Lewin and his associates made on styles of classroom leadership have had their impact on the training of teachers and administrators. Binet and his successors have strongly influenced the practice in grouping and special education. Recent research which has had an impact is represented by Bloom's on mastery learning, studies of criterion-referenced testing, and the psychology of the reading process.

The National Academy of Education in the United States published in 1991 a report on "Research and the Renewal of Education." It was part of a project on funding priorities for educational research and therefore also reviewed what educational research could achieve. It was underscored that "learning exists outside of schools and that research must embrace education in its broadest contexts—including learning that takes place within families, communities, and in other settings." Research policy should be integrated with the research goals of social, economic, and health services. In proposing a research agenda, the Academy particularly singled out research on active learning over the lifespan, assessment and instructional relevance of testing, historically underserved minority groups, studies of schools as institutions, and the connection between teachers and teaching.

Social science research has been accused of giving divergent and confusing messages, with one researcher refuting the other. Policymakers and practitioners want "one authoritative voice." Coleman (1984) has proposed the setting up of "science courts" as a means of establishing pluralistic policy research. A study could begin by identifying the parties interested in a particular issue, and by describing the vested interests and their legitimacy. The research should be designed so as to address policy-relevant questions and, in doing so, introduce a dialectical element in the research process. The findings could then be subjected to competitive alternative analyses which in their turn could be reviewed by the "science court" which could see to it that the research is presented in an independent report. It should give room for alternative analyses and interpretations.

5. Models of Research Utilization

The way research, in particular social science research, is "utilized" in educational policy-making in general has been studied in the first place by political scientists. Important contributions to the conceptualization have been made by Weiss (1979, 1980), and to the empirical study of the problem by both her and Caplan (1976).

In the first place, Weiss points out that "decisions" on policies or policy actions are not taken in the orderly and rational way that many think, namely that individuals authorized to decide sit down and ponder various options, consider relevant facts, and choose one of the options. Policies are decided upon in a much more diffuse way. What occurs is a complicated dynamic interaction between various interest groups, where, by means of arguments advanced by them, administrative considerations, and, not least, the inertia in the system, guidelines for action begin to emerge. The best way to characterize this process is to talk about "decision accretion."

Not least, researchers have been caught in rational and "knowledge-driven" models of how research findings relate to policy-making. Research findings rather "percolate" through public opinion to policymakers. Instead of the latter taking into consideration particular studies, they tend to be influenced by the total body of research in a particular field. Findings usually do not reach those in positions of influence via scientific and technical reports but to a large extent via the popular press and other mass media. A body of notions that forms a *commune bonum* of "what research has to say" is built up via diverse channels of popularization. Theoretical conceptions and specific findings are "trickling" or "percolating" down and begin to influence enlightened public opinion and, in the last run, public policy.

Weiss (1979) distinguishes between seven different "models" or concepts of research utilization in the social sciences. The first model is the research and development (R & D) model which has dominated the picture of how research in the physical sciences is utilized. It is a "linear" process from basic research via applied research and development to application of new technology. There was a time in the 1960s and early 1970s when the R & D model was expected to apply in education by the development of programmed instruction and material for individualized teaching. Weiss points out that its applicability in the social sciences is heavily limited, since knowledge in this field does not readily lend itself to "conversion into replicable technologies, either material or social" (p. 427).

The second model is the problem-solving one, where results from a particular research project are expected to be used directly in a pending decision-making situation. The process can schematically be described as follows: identification of missing knowledge → acquisition of research information either by conducting a specific study or by reviewing the existing body of research → interpretation of research findings in the context given policy options → decision about policy to pursue.

This is the classical "philosopher-king" conception. Researchers are supposed to provide the knowledge and wisdom from which policymakers can derive guidelines for action. Researchers, not least in Continental Europe, for a long time liked to think of themselves as the ones who communicated to policymakers what "research has to say" about various issues. The problem-solving model often tacitly assumes consensus about goals, but social scientists often do not agree among themselves about the goals of certain actions, nor are they in agreement with the policymakers.

The third model is the interactive model which assumes "a disorderly set of interconnections and back-and-forthness" and an ongoing dialogue between researchers and policymakers.

The fourth model is the political one. Research findings are used as ammunition to defend a standpoint. An issue, after having been debated for quite some time in a controversial climate, leads to entrenched positions that will not be changed by new evidence. A frequent case is that policymakers in power have already made their decision before they commission research that will legitimize the policy for which they have opted.

The fifth model is the tactical one, whereby a controversial problem is "buried" in research as a defense against taking a decision at the present moment.

The sixth model is the "enlightenment" one, which according to Weiss (1979 p. 428) is the one through which "social science research most frequently enters the policy arena." Research tends to influence policy in a much more subtle way than is suggested by the word "utilization," which implies more or less direct use according to the first model. In the enlightenment model, research "permeates" the policy process, not by specific projects but by its "generalizations and orientations percolating through informed publics and coming to shape the way in which people think about social issues." Furthermore, without reference to any specific piece of evidence, research can sensitize policymakers to new issues, help to redefine old ones, and turn "nonproblems into policy problems." Empirical evidence appears to support this model. In a study where she was interviewing 155 policymakers in Washington, DC, Weiss found that 57 percent of them felt that they "used" research but only 7 percent could point to a specific project or study that had had an influence.

The seventh model in Weiss's taxonomy, finally, is referred to as "research-as-part-of-the-intellectual-enterprise-of-society" (research-oriented) model. Social science research together with other intellectual inputs, such as philosophy, history, journalism, and so on, contribute to widening the horizon for the debate on certain issues and to reformulating the problems.

In a presidential address to the American Educational Research Association, Shavelson (1988 pp. 4–5) takes as his point of departure the "uncertainty and the frustrations about the contributions of social science research." He seeks to reframe the issue of "utility" by suggesting "that the contributions lie not so much in immediate and specific applications but rather in constructing, challenging, or changing the way policymakers and practitioners think about problems" (pp. 4–5). He points out that this grows out of a confusion of the two models, science versus social science (see *Research Paradigms in Education*). One

cannot expect education research to lead to practices that make society happy, wise, and well-educated in the same way as the natural sciences lead to a technology that makes society wealthy. Educational research can influence policy and practice by alerting "policymakers and practitioners to problems, increase their commitments to working on a problem area, support a position held, legitimate decisions already made, or be used to persuade others about a position held" (pp. 4–5). The assumption that "educational research should have direct and immediate application to policy or practice rests on many unrealistic conditions" (pp. 4–5). Among these are relevance to a particular issue, provision of clear and unambiguous results, research being known and understood by policymakers, and findings implying other choices than those contemplated by policymakers.

6. Overcoming Disjunctions

The conclusion from analyses and studies of the relationships between research and educational policymaking is that the former has an influence in the long run but not usually in the short term following specific projects at specific points in time. The impact of research is exercised by the total body of information and the conceptualization of issues that research produces. It does not yield "products" in the same way as research in the physical sciences. In spite of misgivings about research as "useless" to practitioners and allegations that it contributes little or nothing to policies and practice, research in the social sciences tends to "creep" into policy deliberations. The "linear" R & D model of research utilization derived from science and technology does not apply in the field of social sciences relevant to educational issues. Nor does the problem-solving model which presupposes either value-free issues or consensus about the values implied.

Research "percolates" into the policy-making process and the notion that research can contribute is integrated into the overall perspective that policymakers apply on a particular issue. Thus the United States Department of Education in 1986 published a brochure under the title *What Works: Research About Teaching and Learning*. Its purpose was to "provide accurate and reliable information about *what works* in the education of our children" (p.V) and it was meant to be useful to all who deal with the education of children, from parents to legislators. It presents, in one or two pages for each problem, "a distillation of a large body of scholarly research" (p.V) by stating findings and spelling out their practical implications. Although most of the research presented relates to classroom practice there is also a considerable body relevant to policy issues. Such research findings contribute to the enlightenment of those who prepare decisions which usually are not "taken" at a given point in time, but are rather accretions (Husén and Kogan 1984).

See also: Politics of Educational Research; Policy-oriented Research; Legitimatory Research; History of Educational Research; Research Paradigms in Education

References

Aaron J H 1978 *Politics and the Professors: The Great Society in Perspective.* Brookings Institution. Washington, DC

Caplan N 1976 Social research and national policy: What gets used by whom, for what purposes, and with what effects? *Int. Soc. Sci. J.* 28: 187–94

Coleman J S 1984 Issues in the Institutionalisation of Social Policy. In: Husén T, Kogan M (eds.) 1984

Coleman J S et al. 1966 *Equality of Educational Opportunity.* United States Department of Health, Education and Welfare, Washington, DC

Husén T 1975 *Social Influences on Educational Attainment: Research Perspectives on Educational Equality.* Organisation for Economic Co-operation and Development (OECD), Paris

Husén T 1979 Evaluating compensatory education. *Proceedings of the National Academy of Education,* Vol. 6. National Academy of Education, Washington, DC

Husén T, Kogan M (eds.) 1984 *Educational Research and Policy: How Do They Relate?* Pergamon Press, Oxford

James W 1899 *Talks to Teachers on Psychology: And to Students on Some of the Life's Ideals.* Longmans Green, London

Kallen D, Kosse G B, Wagenar H C (eds.) 1982 *Social Science Research and Public Policy Making: A Reappraisal.* National Foundation for Educational Research/Nelson, London

Levin H M 1978 Why isn't educational research more useful? *Prospects* 8(2): 157–68

Shavelson R J 1988 Contributions of educational research to policy and practice: Constructing, challenging, changing cognition *Educ. Researcher* 17 (7): 4–11, 22

Shellard J S (ed.) 1979 *Educational Research for Policy Making in Australia.* Australian Council for Educational Research, Hawthorn

United States Department of Education 1986 *What Works: Research About Teaching and Learning.* US Department of Education, Washington, DC

Weiss C H 1979 The many meanings of research utilization. *Public Admin. Rev.* 39: 426–31

Weiss C H 1980 Knowledge creep and decision accretion. *Knowledge: Creation, Diffusion, Utilization* 1: 381–404

Further Reading

Cronbach L J, Suppes P (eds.) 1969 *Research for Tomorrow's Schools: Disciplined Inquiry for Education: Report.* Macmillan, New York

Dutch Foundation for Educational Research 1978 *Programming Educational Research: A Framework for the Programming of Research Within the Context of the Objectives of the Foundation for Educational Research in the Netherlands.* Stichting voor Onderzoek van het Onderwijs (SVO), Dutch Foundation for Educational Research, Staatsuitgeverij, 's-Gravenhage

Her Majesty's Stationery Office (HMSO) 1971 *The Organisation and Management of Government R and D (The Rothschild Report). HMSO, London*

Husén T 1968 Educational research and the state. In: Wall W D, Husén T (eds.) 1968 *Educational Research and Policy-making.* National Foundation for Educational Research, Slough

Husén T, Boalt G 1968 *Educational Research and Educational Change: The Case of Sweden.* Almqvist and Wiksell, Stockholm

Kogan M (ed.) 1974 *The Politics of Education: Edward Boyle and Anthony Crosland in Conversation with Maurice Kogan.* Penguin, Harmondsworth

Kogan M, Korman N, Henkel M 1980 *Government's Commissioning of Research: A Case Study.* Department of Government, Brunel University, Uxbridge

Lindblom C E, Cohen D K 1979 *Usable Knowledge: Social Science and Social Problem Solving.* Yale University Press, New Haven, Connecticut

Rein M 1980 Methodology for the study of the interplay between social science and social policy. *Int. Soc. Sci. J.* 32: 361–68

Rule J B 1978 *Insight and Social Betterment: A Preface to Applied School Science.* Oxford University Press, London

Suppes P (ed.) 1978 *Impact of Research on Education: Some Case Studies: Summaries.* National Academy of Education, Washington, DC

United States Office of Education 1969 *Educational Research and Development in the United States.* United States Government Printing Office, Washington, DC

Ethics of Evaluation Studies

E. R. House

Ethics are the rules or standards of right conduct or practice, especially the standards of a profession. What ethical standards have been proposed for the conduct of educational evaluation? What general principles underlie standards? Are these standards and principles sufficient to ensure an ethical practice? These are the questions this article will address. The extent to which evaluation studies actually meet these ethical standards is not addressed here, except by implication.

The ethics of evaluation studies are a subset of

ethics or morality in general but, of course, ethics applied to much narrower problems than those of general morality. "In the narrow sense, a morality is a system of a particular sort of constraints on conduct—ones whose central task is to protect the interests of persons other than the agent and which present themselves to an agent as checks on his natural inclinations or spontaneous tendencies to act" (Mackie 1977 p. 106).

Thus the task of an ethics of evaluation is to check the "natural inclinations" of evaluators that may injure the interests of another person, a task made all the more formidable by the fact that these inclinations may be unconscious, built into the very techniques and methods employed by the evaluator. Given the relative power of the evaluator over those evaluated, the ethics of evaluation are critical to the establishment of a responsible evaluation practice.

According to Sieber,

If there were a field of applied ethics for program evaluation, that field would study how to choose morally right actions and maximize the value of one's work in program evaluation. It would examine the kinds of dilemmas that arise in program evaluation; it would establish guidelines for anticipating and resolving certain ethical problems and encompass a subarea of scientific methodology for performing evaluation that satisfies both scientific and ethical requirements; and it would consider ways to promote ethical character in program evaluators. (Sieber 1980 p. 52)

There is yet another requirement for an ethics of evaluation: it must be rationally persuasive to evaluators. It seems reasonable to treat evaluators themselves as moral persons. "Thus to respect another as a moral person is to try to understand his aims and interests from his standpoint and try to present him with considerations that enable him to accept the constraints on his conduct" (Rawls 1971 p. 338).

Recently several codes of ethics and standards of practice have been proposed for educational evaluation in particular and for social science research in general. Many of these rules and standards are methodological directives but some are concerned with ethical behavior. For example, in the most elaborate and widely disseminated set of standards, there are four areas of concern—utility, accuracy, feasibility, and propriety. Under propriety the standards are formal obligations, conflict of interest, full and frank disclosure, the public's right to know, rights of human subjects, human interactions, balanced reporting, and fiscal responsibility. These standards relate mostly to privacy, protection of human subjects, and freedom of information. Generally the picture that emerges is that the evaluator should forge a written contract with the sponsor and adhere to that contract. He or she should beware of conflicts of interest in which the evaluator's personal interests are somehow involved. Openness, full disclosure, and release of information are the main ways of dealing with these problems. The limitations on full disclosure are the commonly understood rights of subjects. Ordinarily this means informed consent of the subjects must be obtained. There is also a call for respecting others who are engaged in the evaluation itself, a general admonition to decency.

Anderson and Ball (1978) have compiled a list of ethical responsibilities for the evaluator, as well as a list of ethical obligations for the commissioner of the evaluation. The evaluator is expected to acquaint the sponsor with the evaluator's orientation and values, develop a contract with the sponsor, fulfill the terms of the contract, adhere to privacy and informed consent standards, acquaint the sponsor with unsound program practices, present a balanced report, make the results available to legitimate audiences, allow for other professionals to examine the procedures and data, and publish rejoinders to misinterpretations of the evaluation results. The commissioner of the evaluation has obligations to cooperate in the various tasks of the evaluation. To the degree that they deal with ethics at all, other formal codes of ethics and standards suggest similar ethical principles and sets of problems. Mutual agreement of the evaluator and sponsor is emphasized in most codes.

Ethical issues also emerge from the use of particular techniques in designs, such as the use of control groups. For example, two ethical issues that are of concern in use of control groups are the potential for denying a valuable service to eligible clients who might not be chosen for the beneficial treatment and the equitable allocation of scarce resources to a large group of eligible recipients. acceptance of the clients as equals is one proposed way of dealing with these problems, and multiple treatment groups is another.

A review of the literature suggests four basic ethical problems: (a) withholding the nature of the evaluation research from participants or involving them without their knowledge; (b) exposing participants to acts which would harm them or diminish their self-esteem; (c) invading the privacy of participants; and (d) withholding benefits from participants. These are all intrusions against the individual's person somehow, or infringements against personal rights.

What principles underlie these ethical concerns? The National Commission for the Protection of Human Subjects of Biomedical and Behavioral Research has identified three underlying principles—beneficence, respect, and justice. Beneficence means avoiding unnecessary harm and maximizing good outcomes. In the opinion of the commission this principle is served by the research or evaluation being valid, by evaluators being competent, by the participants being informed, by the results being disseminated, and by the consequences of the evaluation being weighed with others. The evaluation is supposed to be beneficial.

Respect means respecting the autonomy of others by reducing the power differential between the evaluator and participants, having participants volunteer, informing participants, and giving participants a choice in matters that affect them. Justice, in the commission's view, means equitable treatment and representation of sub-groups within society. Justice is operationally defined by equitable design and measurement, and equitable access to data for reanalysis. These three principles constitute the rationale for ethical human research, including evaluation.

For the most part these ethical codes concentrate upon infringements to personal rights. The codes assume that there are inherent individual rights prior to the conduct of the evaluation, that the participants must be accorded these rights, and that the individual must voluntarily agree to participation. Almost all these codes of ethics require that the evaluator enter into a contractual agreement with the sponsor and adhere to the agreement as a matter of ethics. Not adhering to the agreement would be considered unfair. Those who are not a party to the agreement have certain personal rights, such as the rights to be informed about the study and the right to volunteer.

Fairness suggests that people are obligated to uphold their part of an agreement when they have voluntarily accepted the benefits of an arrangement or taken advantage of its opportunities to further their own interests. People are not to benefit from the efforts of others without doing their fair share.

Not just any agreement is considered binding, however. House and Care (1979) have asserted that a binding agreement must meet certain conditions. For example, a party cannot be coerced into signing the agreement. All parties must be rational, equally informed, and have a say in the agreement itself. Only under certain conditions can the agreement be considered an appropriate basis for the evaluation.

The fundamental ethical notion is that of a contractual ethics, the establishment of an implicit or explicit contract as the basis for conduct. This is consistent and, indeed, entailed by viewing society as a collection of individuals. "The essence of liberalism. . .is the vision of society as made up of independent, autonomous units who co-operate only when the terms of cooperation are such as make it further the ends of the parties" (Barry 1973 p. 166). Voluntary consent of the participants is essential to ethical conduct in this framework, and intrusions upon people without their consent is considered unethical and immoral. Individual autonomy is a primary principle within this conceptual framework, and autonomy is reflected in establishment of agreements, informing participants, and requesting consent. The ethics are essentially personal and contractual.

While these principles capture many of the concerns of those who have codified ethical principles for evaluation, other theorists have held that these notions of ethics are too restricted. Ideology plays an important role in how evaluation studies are conducted. In fact Sjoberg contends that evaluation studies usually take for granted the structural constraints of the social system. Evaluations are used for effectiveness, efficiency, and accountability within the dominant bureaucratic hierarchies. The categories used by evaluators are those of the status quo, and the social indicators employed are allied to the political power structure. To the degree to which this is true, the formalized ethics of evaluation are limited to concerns which do not threaten the ideological status quo. Many ethical problems are beyond the recognition of evaluators because they are excluded by the prevailing ideology. People are usually not aware of the limits of this ideological concensus until they step outside it.

For example, MacDonald has carried the principle of autonomy a step beyond the prevailing consensus. He has contended that evaluations usually serve the interests and purposes of bureaucratic sponsors or an academic reference group at the expense of those being evaluated. He has proposed that those being evaluated be shown the information collected from them and be given veto power over what is said about them in the evaluation report. Individual autonomy is carried to the extent that "people own the facts of their lives." This is a right not usually accorded to respondents. Within this framework knowledge of social action is the private property of practitioners, and truth is relative to the different interpretive frameworks by which social agents guide their conduct. This position is too extreme for most evaluators but is based upon an extension of an accepted principle. Another unusual ethical position is that evaluators should make themselves more vulnerable to those evaluated, thus redressing the balance of power between the two parties.

Underlying all these various notions of correct behavior in evaluation are contrasting conceptions of justice. The dominant implicit conception of justice is utilitarian, the idea being to maximize satisfaction in society. Any action which maximizes the total or average satisfaction is the right thing to do. Although such a notion seems remote from the practice of evaluation, indicators such as test scores are often taken as surrogate measures of satisfaction and the right thing to do is determine which educational programs maximize these scores. This thinking ultimately leads to a particular kind of evaluation study and technology, even though evaluators may not be fully cognizant of the underlying philosophical assumptions or ethical implications. For example. Schulze and Kneese have shown that the results of a cost-benefit analysis can vary dramatically depending upon which overall ethical system one adopts. They contrast utilitarian, egalitarian, elitist, and libertarian ethical views. As they note, the philosophical underpinnings of current cost-benefit analyses are utilitarian.

Contrasted to utilitarian justice are pluralist conceptions of justice which presume that there are multiple ultimate principles of justice. Such notions often translate into including the perceptions of various interest groups in the evaluation and distinguishing how different groups are served by the program. Pluralist/intuitionist conceptions of justice hold that there are several principles of justice and no overriding endpoint or measure of the general welfare. In practical terms, evaluations based on pluralist ideas treat interest groups as several in number and as having distinct interests from one another.

From different perspectives some theorists have argued that the interests of the disadvantaged and the lower classes are ordinarily neglected in an evaluation and that such interests should be represented or even given priority as an ethical matter. Such an obligation edges into the political and is quite different from an admonition to respect the rights of individuals. Current formal codes of ethics for evaluators restrict their content to individual rights within a contractual framework.

An expanded view of the ethics of evaluation would be based upon more principles than that of individual autonomy. Autonomy suggests that no-one should impose his or her will upon others by force or coercion or illegitimate means. No-one should be imposed upon against his or her will. Autonomy is intimately tied to the notion of choice and is manifested in the notion of individual rights and the social contract. Presumably a person's autonomy has not been violated if he or she chooses freely what to do.

However, autonomy alone is not sufficient as a moral basis for evaluation. Each person should have an equal right to advance his or her own interests for satisfaction. The fundamental notion of equality is that all persons should be taken as members of the same reference group and consequently should be treated the same. The satisfaction of each person's interests is worthy of equal consideration in the public determinations of wants. Individual rights are a protection against imposition by others but do not guarantee equal consideration. It is here particularly that social-class differences play a most significant but neglected role in evaluation. Often powerless groups are not entitled to consideration or representation of their interests in evaluation. Too often only the interests of the powerful are represented.

Of course, if each individual and group is allowed to advance its own interests, there are inevitable conflicts, and these conflicts must be settled impartially. An evaluation must be impartial, that is, in its procedures it must be fair to all interests. Sometimes impartiality is confused with objectivity, but it is possible to employ an objective procedure which is reproducible but biased against a particular social group. It is possible to have a test which discriminates in a systematic, reproducible but biased fashion against certain social groups. Impartiality is a moral principle that ensures fair consideration.

Impartiality is especially difficult when the evaluator must face a situation in which there are conflicting values. To what degree should the evaluator become involved with the participants? Eraut has suggested two moral principles in such a situation. First, people have a right to know what an evaluation is doing and

why. Second, all those who might be considered as clients have a right to some stake in the evaluation. This position proposes the involvement of participants somewhat beyond the negotiation phase, even to the point of helping with data collection. However, even in such an expanded notion of participant involvement, the evaluator is not expected to side with one group or endorse a particular set of values.

There is one other principle worth considering as a moral basis for evaluation. On the basis of equality, autonomy, and impartiality a person could advance his or her own interests equally, not impose on others, and join others in settling conflicts impartially. Yet what about the losers in such a decision process? The winners have no responsibility for the losers, strictly speaking. Intuitively, a person is disturbed at such a situation. Reciprocity, treating others as you would like to be treated, adds an element of humanity. Reciprocity makes winners at least partially responsible for the losers. Reciprocity is not a primary value of liberalism because it suggests a sense of community which extends beyond the notion of separate individuals who cooperate with each other only to seek their own advantage. One of liberalism's deficiencies is this lack of caring and sense of belonging to a larger community.

Finally, there is the formidable problem of the applications of these principles in the actual conduct of evaluation. Ethical principles are rather abstract notions, and it is not always obvious how such principles should be applied in a given situation. Concrete examples and guidelines are essential if a person is to model his or her behavior on such principles.

Even if a person endorsed all the ethical principles discussed here, their application would not be straight-forward. Some of the most intractable ethical problems result from a conflict among principles, the necessity of trading off one against the other, rather than disagreement with the principles themselves. For example, both liberals and conservatives endorse the principles of autonomy and equality but weigh these principles differently in actual situations. The balancing of such principles against one another in concrete situations is the ultimate act of ethical evaluation.

References

Anderson S B, Ball S 1978 *The Profession and Practice of Program Evaluation.* Jossey-Bass, San Francisco, California

Barry B 1973 *The Liberal Theory of Justice: A Critical Examination of the Principal Doctrines in 'A Theory of Justice' by John Rawls.* Clarendon Press, Oxford

House E R, Care N S 1979 Fair evaluation agreement. *Educ. Theory* 29: 159–69

Mackie J L 1977 *Ethics.* Penguin, London

Rawls J 1971 *A Theory of Justice.* Harvard University Press, Cambridge, Massachusetts

Sieber J E 1980 Being ethical? Professional and personal decisions in program evaluation. *New Directions for Program Evaluation* 7: 51–61

Further Reading

Evaluation Research Society Standards Committee 1982 Evaluation Research Society standards for program evaluation, *New Directions for Program Evaluation* 15: 7–19

House E R 1980 *Evaluating with Validity* Sage, Beverly Hills, California

Joint Committee on Standards for Educational Evaluations 1981 *Standards for Evaluations of Educational Programs, Projects, and Materials.* McGraw-Hill, New York

Politics of Educational Research

P. M. Timpane

A distinct politics of educational research was created worldwide during the 1960s and 1970s, as the support of such inquiry became established government policy in many developed and developing nations (Myers 1981, King 1981). This spread is part—usually a modest part—of the broad development of government support for research in many areas of national significance, ranging from defense and space to physical science, health, agriculture, economics, and other social-policy concerns.

Modern governments support research on education and other social services for a variety of reasons. Policymakers today are more likely to seek and absorb information from research in considering new policies and programs; they understand that information from research can raise important new questions about policies, help improve program performance, and help control program activities; more cynically, they also understand that research results can be used to legitimate policies and vindicate choices—including the choice to delay (Weiler 1983).

At the same time, policymakers have placed only modest confidence in the saving power of educational research. Educational research has been considered a "soft science," unpersuasive either in prospect or product. There were extremely limited numbers of first-rate research scholars or institutions to be enlisted in the enterprise. Equally limited was the political support that educational research enjoyed from the politically more powerful educational associations, such as teachers' unions, associations of administrators, and regional, state, and local educational policymakers (Timpane 1982).

Within this general setting, the politics of educational research operate at three levels: in the establishment of government research institutions and agendas of study, in the selection and conduct of specific research studies, and in the utilization of the results of research. The most visible of these is the first.

1. Establishing Institutions and Agendas

As public institutions and research agendas have emerged in educational research, so has a complicat-ed and fragile politics. A series of related questions are always under political consideration: from what source shall goals and priorities be derived; to whom shall the available resources be allocated; what type of research will best accomplish the agenda? These questions range from the mostly political to the substantially scientific, but politics is absent from none of them.

There is, to start with, no obvious single source from which goals and priorities for educational research may be derived. Goals and priorities may be suggested by government policymakers themselves, but these are multiple in all national political systems. In the United States these include, at least, federal, state, and local officials and officials in the executive, legislative, and judicial branches—and probably more than one agency in each instance. Moreover, the individual researchers and the institutes and universities in which they work have obvious standing to help determine what research is important and possible. So, too, do the field practitioners, such as teachers and local officials, and the concerned publics, for example, parents, taxpayers, and the representatives of special educational interest groups such as the disadvantaged, the handicapped, and the victims of discrimination.

No national government has allocated sufficient resources to carry out any substantial part of the research agenda that these parties of interest might establish in a negotiated political process. Even in the United States with by far the most ambitious educational research program, funding for educational research has never been more than a fraction of that suggested in the initial studies proposing national research agenda. In consequence, the politics of educational research are, at this level, typically a desperate attempt to spread resources too thinly over some representative set of research projects, punctuated by the more or less arbitrary selection of one or two politically and substantively important topics —be they reading or vocational preparation, school finance or organization, bilingual or science education —for concentrated attention and support. The choices made typically disappoint more constituents than they encourage. They also leave government research agencies exposed to continual political attack: for not being "useful to the field" or for "doing bad science"; for being a "tool of the Right" (as Democrats charged during and after the Nixon Administration) or for inveterate "funding of the Left" (as the supporters of President Reagan claimed); for neglecting local realities or for ignoring emerging national problems. The most consistent (and predictable) criticism of the choices that has been made across time and nations is that the research supported is too much applied in character and thereby of too little value with respect to fundamental policy change and to intellectual progress (Nisbet 1982, Kiesler and Turner 1977). Some critics have gone further, to note inherent conflicts between the requirements of politics for timeliness, relevance, and self-protection and the requirements of research for elegance, parsimony, and objectivity, concluding that the research enterprise requires strong protection from the diurnal incursions of public and governmental interest (Coleman 1972, 1978).

2. Selecting and Conducting Studies

The actual conduct of educational research is infested with a similar swarm of political dilemmas. Once governmental research agencies or offices and their priorities are established, there remain a host of questions having no completely "rational" or "scientific" answers. An important set of methodological questions turn out to be political. For the most important areas of educational research, there are no *a priori* grounds for choosing a disciplinary approach; historians, ethnographers, sociologists, and several varieties of psychologists, for example, have important contributions to make in solving education's most vexing riddles. Interdisciplinary and multidisciplinary approaches can bridge some, but only some, of the chasms in perspective among these disciplines. More often, choices must be made among them, and representatives of the disciplines must enter bureaucratic politics to secure consideration of their proposed inquiries. Similarly, proponents of the several functional forms of research must promote their longitudinal and cross-sectional case studies, surveys, experiments, evaluations, ethnomethodologies, data reanalyses, meta-analyses, development activities, or other qualitative and quantitative designs in a context where many arguments are plausible but only a few will be successful. Finally, in many cases, individuals qualified to perform or assist in the research may operate in diverse settings—in colleges and universities, in research institutes, in regional and local agencies, in professional associations, and at the very site of schooling or education. Each institution will provide technical assistance and political support for their candidates seeking to participate in the supported research.

The government research agency has a few strategies available to deal with these political dilemmas; it may adhere to a "free grant" process that distributes resources to traditional places in research, in accordance with the procedures and canons of the disciplines (study groups, peer review, etc.); it may sharply define and manage its research requirements through in-house or contract research; or it may establish a process for negotiation with all or some of the prospective recipients seeking to establish some mix of research activities serving various educational agendas. The selection of any such strategy places the research policymakers and program directors at risk. Each has the goal of sustaining effective research programs, but must do so through the development of successively more imaginative bureaucratic processes involving service to higher political authority, the continual taking of outside advice, the extension of selection and review processes to include all pertinent perspectives, and the creation and administration of justificatory documents—in a context where political support for the entire enterprise is at best unreliable. The result, in the United States at least, has been the segmentation of the research agenda into an array of topically significant programs (reading, teaching bilingual education, desegregation, educational organization, finance, and so forth) within which are nested continuing grant programs for individuals and small groups of investigators and selected directed studies performed mostly by institutions—all undergirded by published research plans and broad field participation in project review and selection. There is important emphasis at every stage on the ultimate significance that the research may have for the national educational enterprise; the basic political objective is to create a balanced portfolio of basic and applied studies of sufficient significance, quality, and utility to satisfy, if not delight, all important constituencies.

3. Utilizing Results

Political perspectives concerning the use of educational research have developed swiftly since the early 1960s. Two developments which precipitated this change were: (a) the collapse of linear models of research, development, testing, demonstration, and evaluation as explanations of the progress of educational research results into program operations (Cronbach and Suppes 1969); and (b) the parallel collapse of systematic planning models as explanations of the progress of educational research results into new educational policy (Cohen and Garet 1975).

Each of these two models has been replaced by a more political view. The delivery of new knowledge to classroom teachers and other educators is now usually understood as part of an extended process of synthesis (where bodies of related research results are gathered and made interpretable) and of introduction into an actual process of classroom or school improvement. The program improvements suggested by the research are considered along with the insights of artful practice and the opinion of respected peers, with the entire process dependent upon consistent administrative encouragement and community support (Mann 1979). The emphasis has shifted from "design" of educational innovation to the "mobilization" of a receptive staff. The process is fundamentally political, and only secondarily technical.

Similarly, new research knowledge enters policy deliberations by the compatible processes of "knowledge creep" and "decision accretion" (Weiss 1980). That is to say, research results from many studies are absorbed irregularly as part, but only part, of the information environment of decision makers, who arrive at their conclusions on given policy issues over an extended period of time, not at one decisive moment. Careful policy analysis may sometimes have a significant impact at an opportune time, but the decision is most often substantially formed by the more gradual process of "accretion" and "creep." In such a view, there is wide play for political forces. The value of research information becomes bound up with the credibility, political influence, and interpretive skill of its bearer.

These new understandings spotlight one of the most important weaknesses in the political system of educational research—the lack of authoritative interpreters who can speak both objectively and practically about both policy and practice from positions grounded in the state of current knowledge (e.g., Wildavsky 1979). These commentators are especially missed because they can simultaneously perform two additional functions essential to the political survival of educational research; to translate many of the significant issues of educational policy and practice into appropriate questions for fundamental and applied research; and to be witness, by their own effectiveness, to the contribution educational research can make to the public interest which supports it.

See also: Educational Research and Policy-making; Policy-oriented Research

References

Cohen D K, Garet M S 1975 Reforming educational policy with applied social research. *Harv. Educ. Rev.* 45(1): 17–43
Coleman J S 1972 *Policy Research in the Social Sciences.* General Learning Press, Morristown, New Jersey
Coleman J S 1978 The use of social science research in the development of public policy. *Urban Review* 10(3): 197–202.
Cronbach L J, Suppes P (eds.) 1969 *Research for Tomorrow's Schools: Disciplined Inquiry for Education: Report.* Macmillan, New York
Kiesler S B, Turner C F (eds.) 1977 *Fundamental Research and the Process of Education.* National Institute of Education, Washington, DC
King K 1981 Dilemmas of research aid to education in developing countries. *Prospects* 11(3): 343–51
Mann D (ed.) 1979 *Making Change Happen?* Teachers College Press, New York
Myers R G 1981 *Connecting Worlds: A Survey of Developments in Educational Research in Latin America.* International Development Research Centre, Ottawa, Ontario
Nisbet J 1982 The impact of research: A crisis of confidence. *Aust. Educ. Res.* 9(1): 3–22
Timpane P M 1982 Federal progress in educational research. *Harv. Educ. Rev.* 52(4): 540–48
Weiler H N 1983 West Germany: Educational policy as compensatory legitimation. In: Thomas R M (ed.) 1983 *Politics and Education: Cases from Eleven Nations.* Pergamon, Oxford, pp. 35–54
Weiss C H 1980 Knowledge creep and decision accretion. *Knowledge: Creation, Diffusion, Utilization* 1(3): 381–404
Wildavsky A B 1979 *Speaking Truth to Power: The Art and Craft of Policy Analysis.* Little, Brown, & Co., Boston, Massachusetts

Translating Research into Practice

F. E. Weinert

After 100 years of systematic research in the fields of education and educational psychology, there is, in the early 1990s, still no agreement about whether, how, or under what conditions research can improve educational practice. Although research and educational practice each have changed substantially since the beginning of the twentieth century, the question of how science can actually contribute to the solution of real educational problems continues to be controversial.

Because there are no general rules or strategies for translating research into practice, the first part of this entry focuses briefly on some of the basic problems concerning the relation between theory and practice in education. Next, six different approaches that attempt in various ways to make research findings relevant to education, particularly in schools, are discussed. These approaches concern: (a) using theoretical knowledge to improve technology for teaching and learning; (b) facilitating teacher expertise as a practical application of research on teaching; (c) using studies on classroom learning to provide the scientific basis for ability grouping, mastery learning, and adaptive teaching; (d) using research on cognitive development and learning as a source of scientific information about how to train student's learning competencies and self-instructional skills; (e) using educational research to design, implement, and evaluate new models of schooling and instruction; and (f) using research findings as a source of background knowledge for practitioners. Suggestions for how research can be made more relevant to educators and for ways in which educational practice can be more research-based are proposed on the basis of these different approaches.

1. The Gap Between Research and Educational Practice

Most research in education and educational psychology is conducted with the explicit or implicit goal of directly or indirectly improving educational practice. As Anderson and Burns (1985) stated, "the primary purpose of classroom research is to help educators to improve the conditions of learning and the quality of learning of increasingly large numbers of students" (p. ix). The kinds of necessary research, the required theoretical insights, and the ways that scientific findings should be translated into practice to attain this goal are issues that have not yet been resolved.

When empirical and experimental research on educational phenomena began, there was a widespread vision, conviction, and expectation that it would generate a scientifically informed basis for educational practice. In 1893, for example, Rein (1893) stated that "there is only one way in teaching that corresponds to nature; to follow carefully the laws of the human mind and to arrange everything according to these laws. The attainment of adequate instructional procedures follows from knowledge of and insight into these laws" (p.107).

When these ambitious hopes did not seem to be realized, there was substantial disappointment among both scientists and practitioners. It was not clear how teachers could use such very general and vague recommendations as those, for example, based on a synopsis of classical learning theories by Thorpe and Schmuller (1954). They concluded that instruction was especially effective when learners were motivated; when task demands matched learners' aptitudes; when learners received sufficient opportunities to relate elements of the learning task to the learning goal; when learners could use external criteria to judge their progress; and when the learning process occurred under conditions that facilitated adaptation to the total situation. Although these conclusions are probably valid, it is not surprising that such nonspecific psychological statements and such obvious educational recommendations

led the educational community to the cynical conclusion that learning theorists were perhaps the only ones who could derive practical uses from learning theory.

Dissatisfaction was not limited to problems in finding practical applications for learning theory. The results from research on teaching also seemed unproductive in providing educators with practical guidance. This can be seen, for example, in Bloom's (1966) summary of the state of research: "large class, small class, TV instruction, audiovisual methods, lecture, discussion, demonstration, team teaching, programmed instruction, authoritarian and nonauthoritarian instructional procedures, etc. all appear to be equally effective methods in helping the student learn more information or simple skills" (p. 217).

The limited applicability of educational science for educational practice has resulted in several metatheoretical debates that have contributed only a little to improving the research situation or to solving practical problems. Some examples of the debated issues are:

(a) Is the gap between scientific and practical work the result of a production deficit in research, a reception deficit in the practitioners, or deficits in translating theoretical knowledge into practical suggestions? This debate has led at least to the insight that scientists and practitioners have different ways of perceiving the world, prefer to define their problems in different ways, and thus speak different "languages."

(b) How relevant is basic, as opposed to applied research, for education? This debate is especially unproductive, both theoretically and practically. On the one hand, it is difficult to differentiate pure or basic research from applied research; on the other hand, it has become clear that findings from both research prototypes have specific advantages and disadvantages with respect to their practical applications.

(c) Is it more appropriate to use quantitative or qualitative methods in educational research? This debate has almost become a religious war for many, even though the theory of science convincingly teaches that both approaches are necessary and complementary components of any system of research.

2. Theory and Research

These metatheoretical debates and the many concrete attempts to derive practical applications from research findings have led to a variety of different proposals for solving the research–practice problem. Two positions are especially characteristic of these proposals: the first is that theory should take precedence; the second is that empirical work should take precedence.

The first characteristic position, that theory should

be preeminent, can be captured by a quotation from Mook (1983), who, in agreement with many other scientists, recalled the truth of the classical adage that nothing is more useful than a good theory.

Ultimately, what makes research findings of interest is that they help us in understanding everyday life. That understanding, however, comes from theory or analysis of the mechanisms; it is not a matter of generalizing the findings themselves. . . . The validity of those generalizations is tested by their success and predictions and has nothing to do with their naturalness, representativeness or even noncreativity of the investigations on which they rest. (p.386)

Examples of the ways in which theoretical models have aided in the solution of practical problems include the use of attribution theory to provide a better understanding of students' intuitive explanations for their success and failure; the use of findings from the expert–novice research paradigm to estimate the relative importance of general abilities and domain specific knowledge in the solution of demanding tasks; and the use of theories of prejudice in the analysis of social conflict.

The second characteristic position, focused on empirical research, is invoked in instances where there are competing theories, where context conditions determine psychological processes, or where descriptive or causal models must be transposed into prescriptive statements. Sequential research strategies are proposed to solve such problems. One example is the description of "six steps on the road from pure learning research to technological research and development in the classroom" suggested by Hilgard (1964): step 1—research on learning with no regard for its educational relevance; step 2—pure research on learning with content that is similar to school subject matter; step 3—research on learning that is relevant to education because the subjects are students, the material learned is school subject matter, and/or the learning conditions are similar to classroom situations; step 4—research on learning and instruction in special laboratory classrooms; step 5—use of experimentally tested learning and teaching strategies in normal classrooms; step 6—developmental work related to advocacy and adoption, for a wider use of the research based educational strategies (p.405–11).

These and similar sequential research strategies are followed in many research and development centers around the world. The differences among the programs are, however, too large to allow conclusions about the success of such a strategy. In principle, the possibilities and limits of this approach also depend on the basic relation between educational research and educational practice. Good educational practice is not simply applied science, nor does it consist in the correct use of findings from applied research. Science can at best only provide an important and useful, but always limited, theoretical basis for the planning, analysis, control, support, reflection, and better understanding of educational practice.

The limits of scientific prediction and explanation of educational outcomes are expressed in the conclusions reached by Haertel et al. (1983) based on a comparison of different psychological models of educational performance. They concluded that:

Classroom learning is the multiplicative, diminishing-returns function of four essential factors—student ability and motivation and quality and quantity of instruction—and possibly four supplementary or supportive factors—the social-psychological environment of the classroom, education-stimulating conditions in the home and peer group, and exposure to mass media. Each of the essential factors appears to be necessary but insufficient by itself for classroom learning; that is all four of these factors appear required at least at minimum levels for classroom learning to take place. It also appears that the essential factors may substitute, compensate, or trade-off for one another in diminishing rates of return. (p.75f)

3. Models for Bridging the Gap between Research and Educational Practice

There is no general rule that specifies correct, expedient, or appropriate ways to use scientific findings to solve the practical problems of education. More importantly, there can in general be no such rule. There are, however, various approaches available that show how research can be used in different ways and the strategies that can be used to translate research into practice.

3.1 From Learning Theories to Teaching Technologies

Educational technology consists of systems of rules, tools, and activities designed to bring students to the point where they can achieve specific learning goals systematically, effectively, and economically. Even more, Glaser and Cooley (1973) perceive technology "as a vehicle for making available to schools what psychologists have learned about learning" (p.855). Such standardized technologies should of course be derived from explicit and tested scientific theory. Although not a necessary component of educational technology, technical devices are frequently used with the purpose of minimizing the negative consequences of fluctuation in attention to errors or mistakes, whether by students or teachers.

The first researcher who, from theoretical grounds, wanted to replace normal instruction in the classroom with almost revolutionary mechanical teaching techniques was Skinner (1954). In the early 1950s Skinner argued that the behaviorist models of learning and conditioning and the psychological laws specifying how to shape behavior through contingent reinforcement of desired reactions were the scientific prerequisites for successful and effective instruction. It was his belief that these principles could not be used in classroom teaching because teachers were not able to present the material to be learned in sufficiently elementary components and were not able to provide the requisite number of reinforcements in the necessary or temporal contiguity to learners' behavior, verbal or nonverbal. Thus, he recommended programmed instruction and the use of teaching machines.

Beyond Skinner's initial attempts, the development of educational technologies made dramatic progress in the 1970s and 1980s. Computer-assisted instruction, integrated learning systems, intelligent tutoring systems, instructional media, and intelligent learning environments are some of the key concepts referring to the development, study, and use of modern technical aids for improving educational practice (for a review see Niemiec and Walberg 1992, Scott et al. 1992)

In particular, modern computer technology offers a variety of possibilities for the technical design of controlled, but flexible, adaptive, and intelligently guided, instructional systems and learning processes. The prerequisites for these systems are general learning theories and domain-specific models of knowledge acquisition that allow the following:

(a) analysis of the learning goal in terms of competent performance (specification of the learning task);

(b) description of the initial state of the learner (specification of individual differences in relevant skills and knowledge);

(c) determination of the methods that effectively lead to knowledge acquisition (specification of instructional methods);

(d) assessment of the effects of these instructional methods (specification and measurement of learning progress).

Although there is no disagreement that educational technologies provide an up-to-date tool for education as well as an excellent opportunity for employing research results in a practical way, the level of these technologies is quite different in developing and developed countries. It is also clear that although such technologies are one way to improve educational practice, they are not the only way.

3.2 Research on Teaching and the Acquisition of Teacher Expertise

A large part of educational research is directed toward investigating educational productivity, teacher effectiveness, and the relation between instructional quality and learning outcomes. Although the empirical findings are very impressive, they are also quite diverse and are not stable across different studies. In a synthesis of the effects of instructional variables on learning, the following rank ordering of noncontent related factors was found (with decreasing effect strength): reinforcement, accelerated learning programs, cues and feedback, cooperation programs, personalized instruction, adaptive instruction, tutoring, and higher order questions (Fraser et al. 1987).

If one considers that the effects of single instructional variables can be masked or mediated by combined, compensatory, and interactive effects from other teaching, student and context variables (Weinert et al. 1989), it becomes apparent that training single teaching skills cannot be a practical implication of these research results.

It seems considerably more effective to provide a combined training program for teachers that uses the results from research on teaching (Tillema and Veenman 1987). The paradigm of the expert teacher provides an interesting theoretical perspective for the practical application of such research findings. Prompted by work in cognitive psychology, this paradigm investigates how experienced and successful teachers differ from inexperienced and/or unsuccessful teachers in their knowledge about education and in their teaching activities (Berliner 1992). The research results from this paradigm have already been applied in the design of teacher training.

This paradigm allows the integration of two research traditions that have been portrayed as alternative approaches (Stolurow 1965): "Model the master teacher or master the teaching model?" (see also Weinert et al. 1992). In the expert teacher paradigm, it is possible to directly and systematically relate research on teaching and learning in the classroom to teacher training. Such training should not be directed toward producing a uniform type of "expert teacher," but should explicitly assume that there are interindividual differences in the teacher competencies to be trained (Anderson and Burns 1985).

3.3 Studies of Classroom Learning

In contrast to the subject pools used in most experimental investigations of learning, the classroom is best described as a group of students with very different learning prerequisites who are to be instructed at the same time in the same place. Massive interindividual differences in cognitive abilities, knowledge, skills, motivation, interests, attitudes, and study habits affect both students' learning behavior and their learning achievements. The relevant research concerning these factors is very extensive. It has led to a large number of psychological theories about how personality states and traits are relevant to learning, and has contributed to the development of measurement models and instruments for diagnosing individual differences in learning prerequisites and learning outcomes.

Carroll (1963) provided an important contribution to the practical application of this psychological research with his "model of school learning." Described simply, Carroll proceeded from the assumption that, given equivalent learning time, students with different aptitudes would diverge in their learning performance: that is, some students would not attain the required performance goal. To avoid this outcome, each learner must be allowed the learning time he or she needs to attain a specific learning goal.

This model has had a strong influence on subsequent research; in many respects it has been further specified, broadened, and extended, and it has also been used for a variety of different practical applications (see Anderson 1984). For example, the following concepts and procedures can be traced to Carroll's original model: time on task (the time during which a student is actually involved in a learning task); the personalized system of instruction; individually prescribed instruction; mastery learning; and, largely independent of Carroll's model of school learning, the aptitude–treatment interaction (ATI) research program (Snow 1989). All these approaches have been concerned with the question of whether and to what extent undesired effects of individual student aptitude differences on learning outcomes can be reduced by variations in instruction.

Research on the dependence of school achievement on aptitude differences and instructional conditions has led to several important practical applications. Three of these are grouping students for learning, mastery learning, and adaptive teaching.

The educational benefits of grouping students for learning are controversial and seem to depend on the effects of a variety of factors. Furthermore, these benefits are both student- and criterion-specific (Slavin 1990). A successful practical application of ATI research has not been made.

Mastery learning is the attempt to ensure that as many students in a class as possible (90–95%) meet a required learning criterion (90–95% correct items in a criterion test). This goal is achieved by a limited increase in learning time (about 20%) and optimal instructional use of the learning time. Although what one can actually expect from mastery learning in normal school instruction is somewhat controversial (Slavin 1987, Kulik et al. 1990), there is no doubt that it is a fruitful model that allows productive research and practical applications.

Adaptive teaching is based on many ideas from Carroll's model of school learning and ATI research. Adaptive teaching

> involves both learner adaptation *to* the environmental conditions presented and teacher adaptation *of* the environmental conditions to the learners' present state, to effect changes in that state. The teacher's goal, in other words, is to make environmental variations 'nurtured' rather than merely 'natural' for each learner of concern. (Corno and Snow 1986 p.607)

"Adaptive teaching" is thus an omnibus term covering a large number of different standardized and informal procedures for adapting teaching in variable, flexible, and dynamic ways to students' individual differences, so that optimal learning conditions can be provided for each student.

3.4 Fostering Students' Learning Competencies and Self-instructional Skills

In the above characterization of adaptive teaching it was noted that the optimization of individual learning requires not only that instruction be compatible with the cognitive and motivational demands of the student, but also that students' learning competencies and learning motivation be explicitly fostered. There is considerable research in cognitive psychology, developmental psychology, and educational psychology that addresses how to promote competencies and motivation. At the forefront are investigations on transfer of training, learning to think, the promotion of metacognitive skills, and the development of self-instructional skills.

Much of the theoretically oriented research also includes suggestions for applying the findings. Relevant support programs have been tried for elementary, secondary, and university students. Although these programs have demonstrated that intellectual skills and thinking performance cannot be arbitrarily trained, they have also convincingly shown that the training of metacognitive competencies and self-instructional skills can result in lasting improvements (Blagg 1991). When such programs have realistic goals, are provided over an extensive time frame, and, if possible, are directed toward the acquisition of domain specific knowledge, all students can profit.

3.5 The Use of Research Findings for New Models of Schooling

Research can be used not only to improve existing educational institutions, school organizations, and instructional conditions, but also to plan new models for schooling. Such an approach to change is needed when it is unclear whether an educational goal can be reached by gradual and piecemeal changes in current activities. Both theoretical discussion and practical experiences are available for using research findings in this way (Salisbury 1993). Such change requires consideration of the factors that must be considered in planning a new educational system, the strategies that should be employed, the problems that must be addressed, and the implementation tasks that must be performed.

3.6 Research as a Source of Background Knowledge for Practitioners

The practical application of research consists of more than the instrumental use of research findings. In addition, science and research have an educational function; that is, they provide individuals with knowledge about themselves and the world, and allow individuals to act rationally.

Because people think, decide, and act primarily on the basis of their available knowledge (whether it is correct or incorrect, complete or incomplete, objective or biased), it is important and necessary for those involved in the educational process (politicians, administrators, principals, teachers, parents, students, and researchers) to be able to change or replace their personal beliefs, intuitive knowledge, prejudices, and suppositions with reliable and valid information. Such a replacement is not only a prerequisite for reflective, responsible, and effective individual action, but also a condition for rational communication and discourse among educational practitioners. Although it is not possible to measure the effectiveness of this function of research, it nonetheless seems plausible and important to translate as many research results as possible into the language of the practitioner.

4. Conclusion

The relation between research and practice is complex and difficult. As a consequence, there is no simple, uniform solution to the problem of translating scientific results into practical suggestions. Nonetheless, some general conclusions can be drawn.

First, many different types of research are applicable to educational practice. The value of a scientific study for educational practice is not in any way directly related to the extent to which it mirrors typical features of an applied educational setting.

Second, research results can be used in educational practice in different ways. Six typical examples have been noted: the development of educational technologies, teacher training, the optimization of instruction, fostering students' learning competencies, the design of new models of schooling, and the use of scientific information as background knowledge for practitioners.

Third, these different strategies for applying research results are not mutually exclusive. Rather, it is desirable to combine several variants to improve the practical situation. Finally, exploring the processes by which theoretical knowledge can be transformed into practical action must itself be an important domain of educational research.

References

Anderson L W (ed.) 1984 *Time and School Learning*. Croom Helm, London
Anderson L W, Burns R B 1985 *Research in Classrooms*. Pergamon Press, Oxford
Berliner D C 1992 The nature of expertise in teaching. In: Oser F K, Dick A, Patry J L (eds.) 1992 *Effective and Responsible Teaching*. Jossey-Bass, San Francisco, California
Blagg N 1991 *Can We Teach Intelligence?* Erlbaum, Hillsdale, New Jersey
Bloom B S 1966 Twenty-five years of educational research. *Am. Educ. Res. J.* 3(3): 211–21
Carroll J B 1963 A model of school learning. *Teach. Coll. Rec.* 64: 723–33
Corno L, Snow R E 1986 Adapting teaching to individual differences among learners. In Wittrock M C (ed.) 1986 *Handbook of Research on Teaching*, 3rd edn. MacMillan Inc., New York
Fraser B J, Walberg H J, Welch W W, Hattie J A 1987 Synthesis of educational productivity research. *Int. J. Educ. Res.* 11: 145–252

Glaser R, Cooley W 1973 Instrumentation for teaching and instructional management. In: Travers R M W (ed.) 1973 *Second Handbook of Research in Teaching*. Rand McNally, Chicago, Illinois
Haertel G D, Walberg H J, Weinstein T 1983 Psychological models of educational performance: A theoretical synthesis of constructs. *Rev. Educ. Res.* 53(1): 75–91
Hilgard E R 1964 A perspective on the relationship between learning theory and educational practice. In: Hilgard E R (ed.) 1964 *Theories of Learning and Instruction*. The National Society for the Study of Education, Chicago, Illinois
Kulik C L C, Kulik J A, Bangert–Drowns R L 1990 Effectiveness of mastery learning programs: A meta-analysis. *Rev. Educ. Res.* 60: 265–99
Mook D A 1983 In defense of external invalidity. *Am. Psychol.* 38(4): 379–87
Niemiec R P, Walberg H J 1992 The effect of computers on learning. *Int. J. Educ. Res.* 17(1): 99–108
Rein W 1893 *Pädagogik im Grundriß*, 2nd edn. Göschen, Stuttgart
Salisbury D F 1993 Designing and implementing new models of schooling. *Int. J. Educ. Res.* 19(2): 99–195
Scott R, Cole M, Engel M 1992 Computers and education: A cultural constructivist perspective. In: Grant G (ed.) 1992 *Rev. Res. Educ.* 18: 191–251
Skinner B F 1954 The science of learning and the art of teaching. *Harv. Educ. Rev.* 24(2): 86–97
Slavin R E 1987 Mastery learning reconsidered. *Rev. Educ. Res.* 57(2): 175–213
Slavin R E 1990 Achievement effects of ability grouping in secondary schools: A best-evidence synthesis. *Rev. Educ. Res.* 60(3): 471–99
Snow R E 1989 Aptitude–treatment interaction as a framework for research on individual differences in learning. In: Ackerman P L, Sternberg R J, Glaser R (eds.) 1989 *Learning and Individual Differences*. Freeman, New York
Stolurow L M 1965 Model the master teacher or master the teaching model? In: Krumbholtz J D (ed.) 1965 *Learning and the Educational Process*. Rand McNally, Chicago, Illinois
Thorpe L P, Schmuller A M 1954 *Contemporary Theories of Learning*. Wiley, New York
Tillema H H, Veenman S A M (eds.) 1987 Development in training methods for teacher education. *Int. J. Educ. Res.* 2(5): 517–600
Weinert F E, Helmke A, Schrader F W 1992 Research on the model teacher and the teaching model. In: Oser F K, Dick A, Patry J L (eds.) 1992 *Effective and Responsible Teaching—The New Synthesis*. Jossey-Bass, San Francisco, California
Weinert F E, Schrader F W, Helmke A 1989 Quality of instruction and achievement outcomes. *Int. J. Educ. Res.* 13(8): 895–914

Further Reading

Bloom B S 1976 *Human Characteristics and School Learning*. McGraw-Hill, New York
Glaser R 1977 *Adaptive Education: Individual Diversity and Learning*. Holt, Rinehart, and Winston, New York
Snow R E, Federico P A, Montague W E (eds.) 1980 *Aptitude, Learning, and Instruction*, Vols. 1, 2. Erlbaum, Hillsdale, New Jersey

Training of Research Workers in Education

K. Härnqvist

Researchers in education are normally trained in graduate schools of education or social science within research universities. Since large-scale educational research puts special demands on that training, several groups and organizations have tried to specify these requirements. This entry presents such attempts and discusses various problems involved in the design and implementation of appropriate training programs.

1. Background

Research training, both generally and in the field of education, has been a minor topic in educational research itself. Most sources of information are of a descriptive or normative kind and little empirical research has explicitly dealt with this advanced level of higher education. This entry focuses on training for educational research workers and places it in the broader context of graduate education in general.

An interest in promoting educational research training developed during the 1960s. It was a consequence of the rapid growth of educational research as an instrument for guiding educational policy and practice. Before that, educational research was an activity of largely academic interest and a by-product of the regular system of degree requirements and academic promotions within universities and schools of education. The need for professional educational research workers grew, arising from the establishment of large funds for contract research, specialized research institutes, and research and development centers for various fields of education. In the United States, for instance, the Office of Education supported research training and the American Educational Research Association (AERA) took on a responsibility for promoting training. In Europe, several national education authorities had similar ambitions and the Council of Europe through its Committee for Educational Research worked out recommendations for research training (Council of Europe 1974). A background paper for that committee (Härnqvist 1973) contains references to the then available documentation.

A renewed search in the Educational Resources Information Center (ERIC) system indicates that the publication of articles and reports on training for educational research was intensive between 1965 and 1974. Sixty references relevant to the topic were found from that period compared with 30 from 1975–84, and only three more through to 1990. Moreover, the emphasis changed from general descriptions of training programs for research and development personnel and their functions in local school systems to studies of more specific aspects such as the involvement of women and minorities in research training.

The major part of this entry deals with research training within the system of advanced academic degrees. In addition, specialized programs for updating or broadening research skills, and for introducing trained researchers from other fields into the field of education, are discussed.

2. Graduate Education: General Considerations

The main instrument for research training in most countries is the program leading up to the award of a PhD, or similar academic degree. This degree usually serves two purposes: the preparation of teachers for higher education and the training of researchers. These two aims may conflict with each other—the former requiring a broad coverage of a discipline, the latter requiring specialization and research expertise. In most fields, however, limitations in teaching facilities and labor market prospects make a combination necessary. Already in 1960, Berelson, in an American setting, discussed this conflict and recommended a specialized training in research and scholarship, providing the skilled specialist with a greater depth of knowledge and understanding.

Another trend observed by Berelson (1960) was the growing professionalization at the doctorate level; that is, using the PhD, program for increasing and specializing competence in professions outside research and teaching. This meant a trend toward skills and technical expertise at the expense of traditional academic values. At the same time the basic disciplines seemed to have strengthened their impact on professional degrees, such as engineering and medicine (see also Halpern 1987).

A third major issue in Berelson's discussion was the place and purpose of the dissertation in the doctoral program. Traditionally the dissertation was supposed to be "an original and significant contribution to knowledge," bearing witness to the student's competence to do independent research. With team research, individual originality had become difficult to evaluate, and the contributions to knowledge had so often been just additions of marginal interest that the fruitfulness of this aim could be questioned. Instead, the dissertation could be seen as a training instrument—a start in research and not, as so often had been the case, both the first and the last contribution to knowledge.

These trends and issues in graduate education appeared first on the North American scene but later spread to other countries as well. One example is found in the Swedish reforms of doctoral programs implemented in the early 1970s, where graduate courses stressing research methods, and increased guidance in the preparation of a dissertation, were recommended.

3. Graduate Education in Education

The target groups for doctoral programs in education and related disciplines are, in principle, the same as those mentioned above: teachers (especially for teacher training), researchers, and professionals in, for instance, educational planning, administration, and evaluation. It is not possible here to give a representative survey of existing programs, but some distinctions of principle can be made.

The focus of educational research is the educational process which is studied in its different stages: from the goals and systems set by society and the input characteristics of the students, through the teaching–learning situation, to the evaluation of outcomes. The different stages are studied at different levels of complexity or aggregation, and from the perspectives of different disciplines. At a macro level, the stress is laid upon education's role in society and upon the structure and functioning of the educational system in relation to the goals set for it and the resources allocated to it. At a micro level, research deals with the development and characteristics of the individual student as well as the basic conditions of learning. At an intermediate level, the teaching situation is emphasized: curriculum, methods of instruction, social interaction in the teaching–learning situation.

Research at these three levels, which roughly correspond to the operations of planning, learning, and teaching, need to be based on theory, concepts, and methods from several disciplines. At the macro level, for instance, economics and sociology as well as history and philosophy have important contributions to make. At the micro level the main scientific support comes from different branches of psychology. At both levels it is important that the contributions of the disciplines be integrated within the context of the study of education. At the intermediate level, educational research is building up its own conceptual and methodological framework within a theory of curriculum and teaching. In a way this is the most characteristic contribution proper of educational research and one through which a better integration between macro and micro levels could be achieved.

The multidisciplinary character of educational research and the need for integration within an educational framework manifest themselves in different organizational structures in different systems of higher education. Such heterogeneity is not unique for educational research but characteristic for the academic profession in general (Clark 1987). In many European countries, education, or pedagogy, is taught as a separate subject at both undergraduate and graduate level, alongside, for instance, psychology and sociology—drawing heavily from these disciplines, from philosophy and history as well, but trying to integrate different kinds of knowledge relevant for education. In United States schools of education the disciplines just mentioned, as well as economics, administration, and curriculum, are taught as educational specialties with their own graduate programs and probably with less stress on integration between disciplines than in the European setting. To some extent this difference is a reflection of differences in resources for graduate education (e.g., a European professor of education is often expected to teach within a broader field than his or her American colleague), but it may also reflect historical and philosophical differences in outlook.

The term "research" can also be given different meanings. A basic line of demarcation exists between different philosophies of science. The dominating tradition, at least in the English-speaking and Scandinavian countries, is an empirical–analytical approach founded on the philosophy of logical empiricism. In fact, it has dominated to such an extent that many researchers only lately have become aware of their affiliation. In countries on the European continent, different approaches to educational research compete (Malmquist and Grundin 1975). Phenomenology, existentialism, hermeneutics, and Marxism are strong alternatives that have a deep influence upon both "knowledge interests" and methodology. These alternative approaches have also seemed to be gaining some ground in the "empiricist" countries.

Even within the empirical–analytical tradition, the term "research" is used with different degrees of strictness—from controlled experimentation and quantitative measurement to naturalistic observations and qualitative analysis of data. This entry largely remains within the empirical–analytical tradition but without any special methodological restrictions as regards "hard" or "soft" procedures. The research ideals adhered to correspond to those of "disciplined inquiry" as defined by Cronbach and Suppes (1969). Such inquiry not only comprises empirical studies within the continuum just indicated but also logical and philosophical analyses and historical studies, provided that they display "the raw materials entering the argument and the logical processes by which they are compressed and rearranged to make the conclusion credible" (p. 15).

Finally, before going into more specific questions, it should be stated that the term research as used here refers to both fundamental and applied research, and to both conclusion- and decision-oriented research (cf. Cronbach and Suppes 1969 pp. 19–27). A research student in education needs preparation for both sides of these continua. Often these distinctions are unclear when it comes to procedures or results even though there is a difference as to where the initiative comes from in a specific study.

4. Two Sets of Recommendations

Writing on behalf of a committee of the United States National Academy of Education, Cronbach and Suppes (1969 pp. 212–13) make the following recommendations for a training program for educational researchers:

(a) full-time study for three consecutive years, preferably at an early age;

(b) training as a part of a student group individually and collectively dedicated to research careers;

(c) participation in research, at a steadily advancing level of responsibility, starting in the first year of graduate school if not earlier;

(d) a thorough grounding in at least one academic discipline, together with solid training in whatever technical skills that discipline employs;

(e) study of the educational process and educational institutions, bringing into a single perspective the social goals of education, the bases on which policy decisions are made, the historical development of the curriculum, the nature of the learners, and other factors.

Another set of recommendations is found in the Council of Europe Committee report (1974 pp. 6–7) where the working party states that the goals of regular research training for education should include:

(a) a thorough knowledge of a discipline, usually one of the social or behavioral sciences;

(b) an integrated understanding of the educational process and of educational institutions, based on historical, philosophical, and comparative considerations;

(c) an understanding of the functions of educational research, acquired against the background of theory and the history of science, and an awareness of alternative methodological processes;

(d) technical research skills of relevance to education and in line with the research style chosen;

(e) direct experience of carrying out and reporting empirical research within a particular area of the educational sciences;

(f) skills in communicating with specialists in other disciplines and with educational practitioners.

Many of these goals can be traced back to the Cronbach-Suppes recommendations but there are some interesting additions too. The most important of these is the explicit reference to alternative methodological approaches and research styles—an emphasis that is probably attributable to the fact that six European countries were represented in the working party.

The two sets of recommendations can be compared with the conclusions from an analysis made by Krathwohl (1965), in which he distinguished between three different orientations among existing empirically oriented training programs:

(a) a professional education orientation with emphasis on curriculum and teaching, and minor importance attached to research methods and own research experience;

(b) a social science orientation with emphasis on a discipline and its research methods as well as on dissertation research;

(c) a methodology orientation with emphasis on design and mathematical statistics, and research experience in addition to the dissertation.

It seems that both sets of recommendations correspond best with the social science orientation. The intermediate location of this orientation lays stress on the skills of communicating with specialists on both sides as well as with other disciplines and educational practice.

5. Recruitment of Students

Candidates for training in educational research are traditionally recruited from two main groups: those who hold a certificate to teach at primary or secondary level, and those who have acquired a first-level university education in the social and behavioral sciences. Some candidates meet both requirements. The proportion coming to research training from each of these groups varies from country to country. In some countries the teacher intake dominates, and may even be the only one permitted; in other countries the intake from the social and behavioral sciences forms the majority.

The type of recruitment has to do with the organizational structure and the location of resources for doctoral programs. Where the graduate programs in education are located in schools of education and similar institutions, a teacher's certificate and a period of teaching practice have often been a formal requirement for entry to the doctoral program. Where education, or pedagogy, is taught as a social science discipline the intake has been more varied—sometimes even with a predominance of those who have a combination of behavioral science courses and no training or experience in teaching.

In empirical studies in the United States (e.g., Buswell et al. 1966, Sieber and Lazarsfeld 1966) it was observed that the research productivity of postdoctoral researchers coming from schools of education was low. In Buswell's study, the average age on completion of the doctoral studies was 39 years. The average age was nearly 10 years less in many science disciplines. Both the low research productivity and the high age were related to the predominance of experienced teachers in the programs—teachers who started their doctoral studies late and completed them in a situation where family and alternative professional aspirations competed for their time and involvement. Sieber and Lazarsfeld eventually recommended that "the requirement of professional experience or of the teaching certificate for admission to doctoral candidacy in education should be eliminated for students who wish to specialize in empirical research." Such a recommendation is also implicit in the list of Cronbach and Suppes (see Sect. 4).

In the late 1960s the low research productivity resulting from existing degree programs in education, and the lack of qualified research personnel in spite of great numbers of people with PhDs, led to the establishment under the United States Office of Education of a support program for graduate research training. Selected graduate institutions received extra funds and the graduate students special stipends. Those recruited during the first years of the program differed strongly from the intake in ordinary doctoral programs in education and were more similar to doctoral students in the sciences.

A development in the opposite direction can be observed in Sweden. During the 1960s, young persons with first degrees in education, psychology, and sociology dominated the intake to graduate programs in education, and many of those now active as professors and researchers in education have this type of background. The introduction of a special degree for professional psychologists in the 1970s, however, led to a decrease in the recruitment from behavioral sciences. At the same time the possibilities increased for teachers to return to universities for further courses in education. The teacher intake to doctoral programs in education then became dominant and the age at entry increased considerably.

These examples have been reported in order to show how sensitive the recruitment situation is not only to formal entry requirements but also to factors over which graduate institutions have little control. Since youth and experience are difficult to combine in one person, it seems that the institutions should strive for a varied intake and adapt their programs individually in order to get most out of the years of research training. Another conclusion is that those funding research must share with the graduate institutions the responsibility for building up the research competence in the field; for instance, through supporting graduate students in their dissertation research and creating positions for postdoctoral research. Otherwise it is impossible for the graduate institutions to compete for competent

students, and for research to compete with alternative professional careers.

Economic incentives, however, are an insufficient means of attracting students to research training. First, for a person not involved in research it is difficult to know what research is like and whether the person's interests and capabilities will meet the demands made by graduate studies and dissertation work. Preferably the prospective research students should already have some experience of research at undergraduate level. This may function both as a recruitment incentive and as an instrument for self-selection. In addition, undergraduate research performances would be one of the best selection instruments for admission to graduate school. It is likely that such early research experience is a more normal part of a first degree in social sciences than in teacher education, and therefore it is desirable to introduce such components in teacher education or arrange an intermediate step of this kind between the teacher certificate and admission to graduate studies. In the 1990s such intermediate courses are being built up in Swedish higher education for professional educators who do not have traditional research experience.

Another aspect of the recruitment problem is to make educational research visible among competing fields of research. These opportunities vary with institutional factors. Where education is studied at undergraduate level only in schools of education and teacher-training colleges, reaching social science students is a difficult task since it will be highly dependent on the interest in educational matters among teachers and researchers in social science disciplines. In this case it seems necessary to establish organized links between education faculties and undergraduate departments in social sciences. The situation may look easier where education is studied as a social science subject, but then it has to compete with other disciplines, and the lack of familiarity among the students with the situation in schools and teaching practice may be a hindrance. Therefore research-oriented departments of education need organized contacts with schools and practical teacher education.

In the late 1970s several affirmative action programs were initiated by universities in the United States in order to recruit more women and minorities into educational research and to support their careers at the postdoctoral stage through fellowships and opportunities for mentor relationships.

6. Degree Programs

The highest university degree in most countries, the doctorate, normally includes research. The programs for this degree vary considerably in length and organization. In many countries there exist intermediate research degrees requiring from one to three years of full-time study after the first university degree.

Examples of such intermediate degrees are masters in English-speaking countries, *"maitrise"* in France, and *"candidate"* in the former Soviet Union. Germany has doctorates at two levels, DrPhil. and *"habilitation."* Where the intermediate degree requires several years of study, course work is often concentrated at this level (in addition to a short thesis), and the only further requirement for the doctorate is research reported in a dissertation.

The Soviet *"candidate"* degree was regarded as the normal research degree and only a small proportion of candidates continued to the doctor's degree. In general, however, the shorter programs are less prestigious and particularly so when the intermediate degree wins a reputation for being used as a "consolation prize" for interrupted doctoral studies. In the American system of graduate education the master's degree exists but seems to have no independent function in a research career. Most researchers take a four-year program for the doctor's degree. On the other hand, in the field of education there exist two doctor's degrees; the doctor of philosophy (PhD) in education or subdisciplines, and the doctor of education (EdD). In general the PhD is more research oriented and the EdD more professionally oriented, but there is great variation between the provisions of graduate schools.

Ideally, research training covers the three to five years that follow the successful completion of a first university degree, but since a great proportion of doctoral candidates do not start directly after their first degree, and often teach or do professional work during their studies, the time lapse between the degrees tends to become at least twice as long as the ideal. Attempts have been made to reduce this interval and to produce postdoctoral researchers at an earlier age. This is important, not least for their future research productivity. Several remedies have been tried: organizing graduate studies in courses, providing more research supervision, reducing the length of dissertations, simplifying publication procedures, and providing economic support in order to recruit more full-time graduate students. In the natural sciences, articles published in refereed journals are often combined to serve as the thesis instead of a dissertation monograph—a procedure that is feasible in fields and countries where an infrastructure of scholarly journals exists.

Criteria for evaluation of a thesis have been formulated by Debeauvais (1986). As a general principle, the dissertation should be a "product of research" and evaluated according to normal academic research criteria. More specifically, these involve a synthetic presentation of theory and previous research on the subject, a contribution of new facts or new interpretations of existing data, a demonstration of appropriate methods for analysis, and originality at least on a modest level.

The regular university programs in education have been criticized not only for producing graduates who are too old and whose productivity in research is low, but also for not having adapted themselves to the needs of large-scale research efforts, particularly of an interdisciplinary character. It has been maintained that admission and degree requirements tend to be too rigid and too influenced by intradisciplinary value systems. Minor research problems with high security are preferred to those that are socially important but involve a high risk. The training takes place in isolation from other disciplines and the field of application.

There is a good deal of truth in this criticism. The stress on regular university programs in this entry, on the other hand, stems from two convictions. One is that educational research is such a difficult and expensive enterprise that it must be based on a thorough grounding in basic disciplines and methodology, which cannot be achieved just through a few research courses or through apprenticeship without the guidance of a basic training program. The other conviction is that universities, in general, are flexible organizations with great potential for adaptation and change in contents and methods, even if their freedom and flexibility now and then seem to be used for rigid decisions. This risk follows from the autonomy they have been granted. According to these convictions, it is better to adjust the regular programs to new needs than to set up basic training programs outside a degree system. The competition for good graduate students calls for such a strategy.

The recommendations quoted in Sect. 4 outlined the main components of a program for research training. More specific requirements have been formulated by an AERA Task Force on Research Training and synthesized by Worthen (1975) in a list of 25 general tasks that researchers and/or evaluators must frequently perform. For most of the tasks, competencies necessary to perform the tasks were also identified. The tasks were listed in a sequence from the search for information on earlier research and formulation of a research problem, through design, instrumentation, and data collection, to analysis, interpretation, and reporting. The competencies involved are important especially for empirical behavioral science research of a quantitative and statistical type, although some of them, especially in the beginning and the end of the sequence, are of a more general nature. The list might be used as a syllabus for an extensive methodology course in the empirical–analytical tradition within a social science-oriented doctoral program. It is, on the other hand, weak on alternative methodological approaches and metascientific background. By definition it does not cover the substantive content of a discipline, nor the broader educational context of the research.

In addition to typical research tasks, the list also comprises tasks that are specific for educational evaluation. This is in line with the fact that evaluation is one of the most important professional specializations for

273

persons with a research training in education. It also fits with the training recommendations in a major book on program evaluation (Cronbach et al. 1980). The authors prefer the doctoral preparation in a social science discipline to specialized programs for evaluation without a disciplinary base.

> Doctoral training in a discipline can be counted on to emphasize competence in research design, data analysis, procedures for collecting data, and tough-minded interpretation. Whatever coloration a particular discipline gives to these topics, thorough training gives a critical perspective that is invaluable in looking at plans and results of evaluations. (Cronbach et al. 1980 p. 344)

The specialization in evaluation then comes through interdisciplinary evaluation seminars, apprenticeship to practicing evaluators, and internship in an agency where policy is formulated.

A specialization that is more difficult to achieve within a social science-oriented program is that of curriculum and teaching methods in nonelementary subject matter areas; for instance, natural sciences and foreign languages. Research with such orientation requires advanced competence in the subject matter in addition to training for empirical educational research. It is unlikely that a social science-oriented postdoctoral researcher will continue with graduate studies in a subject matter area. It may be easier for a subject matter teacher to go in the other direction but this also tends to take too much time to be attractive. In Sweden there is a program that comprises about one year of graduate courses in a subject matter discipline, for example, physics; one year of research methodology and education-oriented courses; and two years of dissertation research.

7. Methods and Institutional Arrangements

The trend in the direction of more organized course work at graduate level should not mean substituting conventional lecturing for the independent study that has predominated. But the expectations put on candidates may become more clearly defined and their studies organized in such a way that they can complete the degree requirements within more reasonable time limits. The methods of instruction, on the other hand, must vary with goals and contents. In some technical parts, lecturing in combination with exercises would be well-adapted to the situation. In others, independent reading followed by seminars or small-group discussions are more appropriate.

The examination procedures, too, should be adjusted to the advanced level of the candidates. Written reports based on the literature can be substituted for conventional examinations. Such reports could also be used as exercises in concise writing, which is a skill that seems to be lacking even among high-level students in many countries. It is then important that the

candidates receive feedback not only on content but also on format and style.

The main instrument for research training is active participation in research in all its phases. Even when regarded as a training instrument, the dissertation should be the central and most exacting requirement for a research degree. The facetious American expression "ABD" ("all but dissertation") indicates what can be a reality for many doctoral candidates. Very often failure begins in the initial phase of the dissertation work when much time and attention ought to be given to the finding and formulation of the research problem.

Research supervision involves a delicate balance between support from the side of the supervisor and freedom on the side of the research candidate. The optimal relation varies from case to case, but in general a nonauthoritarian and nonpatriarchal relationship is preferable where the candidate is treated as a fellow researcher and not as a student. Sometimes emotional support can be as important as intellectual. Under favorable circumstances, the research supervisor may continue to function as a mentor for the new doctoral researcher—become a role model, giving academic advice and assistance in gaining access to the profession (Blackburn et al. 1981). Personal experiences of research supervision and mentorship are reported, for instance, by former students of Lee Cronbach (Snow and Wiley 1990).

One of the most relevant influences in research training is to arrange for candidates to work in a research-oriented setting; that is, in an institution where good research is done and a favorable research climate is created. Learning from models cannot be replaced by methodology courses. An ideal setting would be an apprenticeship in a research group under the guidance of an experienced researcher, working side by side with fellow students. This in turn would be complemented by courses and seminars where methodological and substantive problems can be treated in a more systematic way than with apprenticeship only. The institution within which the research group is located should preferably be big and varied enough to afford communication with groups in other specializations, so that the perspective does not become too narrow (Kaplan 1964 p. 865).

8. Specialized Courses

So far, this entry has focused on the regular degree system. Research training, however, is a continual process; it does not end with a doctorate. Most postdoctoral training is integrated into continued research, but it has to be supplemented with occasional specialized courses.

The AERA Task Force on Research Training identified four objectives for a future inservice training program (Sanders et al. 1970, Dershimer et al. 1973):

(a) upgrade the skills of researchers who are now poorly trained;

(b) maintain the high level of competence of researchers entering the field;

(c) teach new skills made necessary by innovations in educational techniques and products;

(d) broaden the base of personnel engaged in activities calling for the application of educational research skills.

The group also mentioned several "vehicles" for an expanding training program; for instance, courses arranged in connection with the AERA annual conventions; summer institutes, conferences, and workshops; and development of instructional materials.

Professional development and training courses are a regular part of the AERA meetings. In earlier years they emphasized computer applications and methods of quantitative data analysis; for instance, multivariate analysis, structural equation modeling, and item response theory. Later the program became broader, also including ethnographic and other qualitative methods of research, and substantive issues in developing fields of study. Practical skills, such as writing proposals and journal articles, and oral presentations have been regularly represented in the programs.

In Europe several summer Seminars on Learning and the Educational Process (SOLEP), partly staffed with American researchers, were given around 1970, with support from UNESCO and different national foundations. Young researchers from many different countries spent several weeks together discussing research problems and methods. In addition to upgrading research competence, the seminars contributed to the formation of personal contacts among the researchers —the "invisible colleges" that are so important for the infrastructure of a discipline. On the international level also, research projects such as the comparative studies organized by the International Association for the Evaluation of Educational Achievement (IEA) have had important functions in research training and the development of networks among educational researchers.

The Council of Europe Committee on Educational Research has arranged symposia for researchers and practitioners in specialized fields: for instance, preschool education, teacher education, and innovation and change in higher education. Similar activities have been initiated by UNESCO, the Organization for Economic Cooperation and Development (OECD), and other international organizations. Education has also been represented in the postdoctoral program of research courses run in cooperation by the Nordic countries. In general, however, international arrangements decreased during the late 1970s, perhaps as a consequence of a less affluent situation for educational research than a decade earlier.

Another target group for specialized courses have been trained researchers from other fields who enter research in education as partners in interdisciplinary projects or subject matter experts. Some of them may come from the behavioral sciences, having completed doctorates in areas within their own disciplines unrelated to education: for example, psychologists, sociologists, anthropologists, and child psychiatrists. Others have come from linguistics, statistics, economics, political science, philosophy, history, and so on. In all these cases they have brought the methodology of their disciplines with them to be used for educational problems, but they have needed an introduction to the special perspectives of educational study and have been in need of courses in empirical social science methodology. So far such courses have been difficult to find.

See also: History of Educational Research; Politics of Educational Research

References

Berelson B 1960 *Graduate Education in the United States.* McGraw Hill, New York

Blackburn R T, Chapman D W, Cameron S M 1981 Cloning in academe: Mentorship and academic careers. *Res. Higher Educ.* 15(4): 315–27

Buswell G T, McConnell T R, Heiss A M, Knoell D M 1966 *Training for Educational Research.* Center for Research and Development in Higher Education, Berkeley, California

Clark B R (ed.) 1987 *The Academic Profession: National, Disciplinary, and Institutional Settings.* University of California Press, Berkeley, California

Council of Europe 1974 *Report of the Working Party of the Educational Research Committee on the Training and Career Structures of Educational Researchers.* Council of Europe, Strasbourg

Cronbach L J, Suppes P (eds.) 1969 *Research for Tomorrow's Schools: Disciplined Inquiry for Education: Report.* National Academy of Education/Macmillan, London

Cronbach L J et al. 1980 *Toward Reform of Program Evaluation.* Jossey-Bass, San Francisco, California

Debeauvais M 1986 Doctoral theses in France: Can their academic significance be evaluated and compared with those of other countries? In: Postlethwaite T N (ed.) 1986 *International Educational Research: Papers in Honor of Torsten Husén.* Pergamon Press, Oxford

Dershimer R A et al. 1973 *Development of Training Models for Educational Research: A Conceptual Scheme for a Professional Association. Final Report.* AERA, Washington, DC

Halpern S A 1987 Professional schools in the American university. In: Clark B R (ed.) 1987 *The Academic Profession: National, Disciplinary, and Institutional Settings.* University of California Press, Berkeley, California

Härnqvist K 1973 The training and career structures of educational researchers. In: Taylor W (ed.) 1973 *Research Perspectives in Education.* Routledge and Kegan Paul, London

Kaplan N 1964 Sociology of science. In: Faris A E L (ed.)

1964 *Handbook of Modern Sociology*. Rand McNally, Chicago, Illinois

Krathwohl D R 1965 Current formal patterns of educating empirically oriented researchers and methodologists. In: Guba E G, Elam S (eds.) 1965 *The Training and Nurture of Educational Researchers*. 6th Annual Phi Delta Kappa Symposium on Educational Research. Phi Delta Kappa, Bloomington, Indiana

Malmquist E, Grundin H U 1975 *Educational Research in Europe Today and Tomorrow*. Gleerup, Lund

Sanders J R, Byers M L, Hanna G E 1970 A survey of training programs of selected professional organizations. AERA Task Force on Training, Technical Paper No. 11. AERA, Washington, DC

Sieber S D, Lazarsfeld P F 1966. *The Organization of Educational Research in the United States*. Bureau of Applied Research, Columbia University, New York

Snow R E, Wiley D E 1990 *Improving Inquiry in Social Science: A Volume in Honor of Lee J. Cronbach*. Erlbaum, Hillsdale, New Jersey

Worthen B R 1975 Competencies for educational research and evaluation. *Educ. Res.* 4(1): 13–16

SECTION II

Research Methodology

Introduction: Methods and Processes in Educational Research

J.P. Keeves

Research into educational problems had its beginnings a little over 100 years ago, in the mid 1880s, with publications in Germany, the United States, and England that marked the commencement of the child study movement (see *History of Educational Research*). The advent of the electronic computer in the 1960s produced an explosion in empirical research in education, and from this new ways of thinking about educational issues developed. These new ways of thinking were concerned with estimating probabilities and stochastic relationships, the study of the interactions between the many influences on educational outcomes, and the development of mathematical and causal models to explain educational processes. Inevitably, perhaps, tensions developed between those scholars who endorsed and employed these new analytical ways of thinking and those who questioned such analyses and who sought a more holistic approach to inquiry in education. The outcome of these tensions was the proposal for alternative paradigms of inquiry. The debate that has subsequently occurred during the 1980s and 1990s has led to new perspectives that argue cogently for a unified view of educational research.

Many scholars working in the field of education question whether education is a domain with an entity of its own that would permit the term "educational research" to be employed. It is true that many disciplinary areas, such as psychology, linguistics, sociology, demography, history, economics, philosophy, anthropology, and the emerging discipline of cognitive science necessarily contribute to the investigation of educational problems and the building of a body of knowledge about education. However, education holds a unique position among the disciplines, in so far as it not only involves a body of knowledge drawn in part from many disciplines, but it also involves instruction in the processes by which knowledge is acquired, propagated, and used to influence change in the thinking of individual persons as well as change in the structures of society through social action. No other field of inquiry has this dual role, consequently, education is placed in a singular position among the disciplines. Indeed it can also be argued that among

the many great events of the twentieth century, it is the expansion of education worldwide at the primary, secondary, tertiary, and quaternary (adult recurrent education) levels in response to the advancement of knowledge, that is in the long term the most remarkable and most influential of them all. This expansion of education has occurred in recognition of the power of the processes of education and the effects that education has on all aspects of human life.

While a case can be argued for the viewing of research in education as a field of inquiry with an existence both in operation and in the body of knowledge built from investigation and scholarly work that is separate from the other disciplines, it is also necessary to consider whether this field of inquiry involves two or even more than two distinctly different paradigms. It may be argued that the tensions that exist between scholars who are engaged in inquiry into educational problems may be due in substantial part to the education provided at upper-secondary and university levels being split through the two cultures that Snow (1959) identified as operating, particularly in English-speaking countries. As a consequence it can be argued that the distinctions that are commonly drawn between the explanatory or scientific approach and the interpretative or humanistic approach to educational research have arisen from the specialization that occurs in schools and universities after the age of 15 years into the fields of the sciences and the arts. Likewise, the difference between quantitative and qualitative methods and processes of inquiry can be traced to the training received in different disciplines at a university. While it is useful to separate approaches to the conduct of inquiry in education into a scientific tradition and a humanistic tradition, it is important to recognize that such a separation is one of convenience and does not reflect an inherent epistemological difference.

This *Handbook* recognizes the distinction between the scientific approach and the humanistic approach to the conduct of educational research. However, it also seeks to emphasize the supplementary nature of the two approaches and the commonality of purpose in scholarly work in the field of education that is directed towards the building of a coherent body of knowledge. In order to understand the supplementary nature and the commonality of purpose of these two approaches to inquiry in education it is of value to identify what are considered to be the key characteristics of educational research.

1. Key Characteristics of Educational Research

Several key characteristics of educational research must be recognized if the nature of inquiry into educational problems is to be understood. First, the range of problem situations encountered in the field of education can not be viewed in terms of one and only one disciplinary area. Educational research is essentially *multidisciplinary* in nature drawing on many disciplines. There have been times during the twentieth century when psychology can be said to have dominated educational research, many psychological research workers viewing education as the field where generalizations advanced in the discipline of psychology could be applied. However, it is no longer appropriate to view educational research as an area in which the basic knowledge of any one discipline is applied. The current views on the nature of human agency and social action deny such a perspective. Nor is it meaningful to argue that the problems which are to be investigated in the field of educational research should always be tackled from an interdisciplinary perspective, although some inquiries may profit from such an approach. Nevertheless, it is necessary to recognize that research into educational problems are not conducted within a single disciplinary field with the methods of inquiry used within that field.

It is also clear that if many disciplinary approaches can be employed in the investigation of educational problems then many different methods of inquiry are available. Educational research is not only multi-disciplinary but also *multimethod* in the research strategies that are employed. The choice of a method or methods of inquiry to be used in a particular problem situation depends on the nature of the problem, as well as on the skills of the research worker and the disciplinary perspectives from which the problem is viewed. There is clearly no single method of inquiry that should be employed in educational research.

A third key characteristic of most research in education is that it is necessarily *multilevel*. Learning and teaching, in the main, take place in groups. Although it is individuals who learn through the instruction provided, the settings in which the instruction and learning occur are the school, the classroom, the family, the peer group, and the community. As a consequence, any research that involves the effects of teaching, or of the learning that occurs in group settings needs to take into consideration factors operating at the individual and at the group levels. Furthermore, since it is rarely possible in educational research to draw a simple random sample that has any generality across a large population, the samples chosen are, in the main, cluster samples, with schools or classrooms selected at the first stage of sampling and students within schools or classrooms selected at the second stage. In addition, it should be noted that since individuals with like characteristics cluster naturally together in groups, the use of simple random sample estimates of error are commonly grossly inaccurate, to such an extent that the significance tests commonly employed cease to be meaningful. The only resolution to the problem is multilevel analysis.

Failure to design studies and to analyze the information collected in a way that teases out influences at both the individual and group levels has resulted in the past in analyses that have not examined meaningfully the effects operating at either level. In addition, the reported significance of effects in single level analyses must be expected to be in error. One of the consequences of inappropriate design and analysis has been that at the student level, the influences of the classrooms, the teachers, and the schools have been commonly found to be small, compared with the effects of the homes. The answers to these problems of design and analysis lie not only in the collection of information at appropriate levels of inquiry, but also in the systematic analysis of that information at the identified levels in a multilevel analysis, as well as the consideration of cross-level effects.

A fourth characteristic of educational research arises from the complex nature of educational problems. It is rare that a problem in educational research can be reduced in such a way that it can be viewed in terms of only two constructs or variables. Commonly there are many factors operating jointly to influence educational outcomes. Furthermore, it is rare that a large experiment with the power of generalization could be designed in educational research in which, through randomization both to groups as well as the random allocation of groups to treatments, it would be possible to provide effective control over the many factors likely to be involved in learning. Under these circumstances, only by *multivariate* analysis is it possible to exercise statistical control over the factors likely to have influenced the outcomes under investigation.

In general, the analysis of data in educational research must be multivariate in nature, not only to take account of the many predictor variables likely to be operating, but also to take into consideration the many outcomes that need to be examined simultaneously. Some research studies in education seek to remove the problems associated with the many variables involved through a holistic or case study approach, in which the different factors and outcomes are considered together as operating in unison. Within this approach, the whole largely determines the characteristics of the parts which it contains. Consequently it is necessary to provide an account of the whole in order to understand the interrelations between the parts. This approach, in contrast to an analytic approach, is a systemic approach in which the discrete elements that make up the whole are considered to be interdependent and inseparable. Thus this approach involves the study of patterns within the whole and not the study of separate factors or variables.

Fifth, educational research is often concerned with stability and change in human characteristics, since education involves the learning that takes place over time. Any investigation of the factors that influence learning must examine the change that occurs in outcomes over time. While it is of value to measure the outcomes with accuracy and consistency over time, it is the variation in a measure of change that is under examination, and the accuracy and the consistency of the measure of change is not necessarily dependent on the accuracy and consistency of the measures at each time point. Under these circumstances, studies of learning in educational research must employ repeated or *multiple measures*, so that a meaningful and consistent measure of change can be analyzed. Measurement on at least three occasions is required in order to assesss the consistency of a measure of change. Preferably more than three occasions should be employed and sound investigation should involve multiple measures over time.

The sixth and final important characteristic arising from recent developments in educational research involves a change in the type or form of effects investigated in educational research. Prior to the advent of computers the effects of variables that were examined were largely direct and simple. Developments in the analysis of data now permit many different forms of effect to be considered, and educational research has become *multiform*. Not only are direct effects examined, but many other forms of effect can now be tested. Path analysis permits the estimation of indirect or *mediated effects*, with the influence of one variable operating through one or more other variables to influence the outcome. *Reciprocal effects* can also be examined under certain conditions through path analysis, so that the reciprocal relationships between two variables can be estimated. Interaction or *moderator effects* can now be estimated, so that a multiplicative relationship between two variables in their joint influence on an outcome can be readily tested. *Cross-level effects* can also be investigated in multilevel analyses so that the effects of school type, for example, on both the product of individual performance as well as on the processes operating within the groups can be investigated. The influences that can be examined include both *compositional effects* and *contextual effects*. In a compositional effect, characteristics of the group are considered to influence the level of performance of the group as a whole, while in a contextual effect, the characteristics of the group are considered to influence in a differential way the performance of different members of the group. It is evident that no longer is it necessary to limit the analysis of data to effects that are simply linear and additive.

2. Key Characteristics of the Quality of Research in Education

The quality of research undertaken into educational problems is not related to the approach employed, whether scientific or humanistic. Nor is it related to a dependence upon a particular disciplinary field, such as psychology or history. There are, however, several key characteristics of the quality of a research study that influence the weight to be given to the findings in the building up of a body of knowledge about education. These key characteristics may take a different form under different methods and procedures of research. Nevertheless, they are considered to be those aspects of a research study and of its findings on which the quality of the research must be judged.

2.1 Validity

The concept of *validity* is related to the possession of the quality of strength, worth, or value. Kaplan (see *Scientific Methods in Educational Research*), identifies three aspects of validity that are of interest. First, validity involves coherence with knowledge already established. Second, validity indicates a strong correspondence between the result and the real world as represented by some mapping of the domain under investigation. Third, validity is associated with the ongoing usefulness of the findings in practice, as well as in the undertaking of further inquiry. Thus the validity of a theory, a finding, or relationship primarily rests with what can be done with that theory, finding, or relationship, and this depends on the context in which a study is conducted. Furthermore, validity is not necessarily determined by the way the theory, finding, or relationship was obtained, although this may have important implications.

2.1.1 External validity. One of the aspects of validity that is of importance is concerned with the extent to which the findings of a study or the relationships established in an investigation are generalizable beyond the specific set of cases involved, whether they are people, organizations, or events that are under survey. If sampling has occurred from an identified target population, and the sample has been randomly selected, then that sample is representative of the target population and the findings obtained from the sample are generalizable to that population. However, nothing is known about the relevance of the findings to any other target populations. Irrespective of the size of the sample, bias exists to an unknown extent, if there have been losses between the designed sample and the achieved sample. It is generally assumed that the greater the losses the greater the extent of possible bias. However, it is important to note that the magnitude of the error associated with a sample on which observations are made, or through which findings are obtained, is dependent largely on the size of the sample and not to any extent on the sampling fraction employed in the sample design.

In many research and evaluation studies conducted into educational problems the examination of external validity cannot be formal or precise, because the sample must be drawn from a subpopulation of the target group that is accessible to the investigator. Under such circumstances two inferential steps are required in generalization. The first inference is made from the sample to the accessible population, and the second from the accessible population to the target population. The second step does not involve statistical inference that is dependent on sample size. It is, however, dependent on an assessment of the representativeness of the accessible population. A similar problem arises when the researcher seeks to generalize to a different population or subpopulation. In both situations it is necessary for the researcher to provide argument and evidence to support the making of such an inference to a wider population. Here replication in a different setting can be useful.

External validity is also threatened when there is the possibility of an interaction between two or more of: (a) the subjects under investigation; (b) the settings in which a study is conducted; and (c) the times during which the investigation takes place. Thus external validity may be violated if an interaction occurs between the possible effect of a treatment condition across different subjects, settings, or times in the target or accessible population from which the sample is drawn. The problem of such a threat to external validity is overcome if it can be argued from theory that such an interaction can not and does not occur. It is, however, commonly necessary to control for such interactions by representativeness, by randomization, by the administration of the treatment or intervention under controlled conditions, or by the employment of statistical control in data analysis.

2.1.2 Internal validity. Internal validity is concerned with the credibility and authenticity of the findings arising from the manner in which a particular study was conducted. If an intervention or experimental study is undertaken and cases are assigned to experimental or control groups and different groups are assigned to treatment or control conditions then the internal validity of the study is violated unless random assignment has occurred at both the individual case and treatment condition levels. The allocation of cases to the treatment and control groups as well as the assignment of groups to treatment or control conditions are necessary for strong causal inferences to be drawn about the findings of a study. Unless these randomization procedures are employed with sufficiently large groups, there is no guarantee that unknown factors

which are likely to have influenced the outcomes of the experiment or intervention have been brought under control. It is only when unknown factors are controlled by random allocation, that observed effects can be assigned with confidence to the treatment or control condition. Further problems arise in studies of change over time, since in most educational studies the size and completeness of the sample are also difficult to sustain over time with a consequent effect on the internal validity of the findings of the study. Differential attrition between the different groups, as well as atypical behavior between the members of different groups, provide a threat to the internal validity of a study. This occurs because both attrition and atypical behavior may mean that the groups which were initially equivalent are no longer comparable at the end of a study.

Internal validity is also threatened when there is the possibility of interaction between two or more of: (a) the subjects under investigation; (b) the instruments employed in making the observations; (c) the research workers making the observations; and (d) the treatment conditions or the factors influencing the outcomes under consideration. Thus internal validity is violated if an interaction takes place between the possible effect of a treatment condition across different subjects, the operation of the instruments employed, and the makers of the observations with those instruments.

2.1.3 Construct validity. In the planning of a study into an educational problem an initial step commonly involves the consideration of theory and the drawing from theory of a relationship or set of relationships to be examined in the course of inquiry. The relationships generally involve theoretical ideas or constructs that are not directly observable in practice, but which must be operationalized before any observations can be made. For example, many relationships in education involve the construct of social class or of socioeconomic status. Class and status are not directly observable. However, indicators of these constructs that can be examined involve: father's occupation, father's education, mother's occupation, mother's education, ownership of property, and income of family. It is necessary to consider whether such observed variables are meaningful or valid indicators of the constructs of social class and socioeconomic status. Consequently, thought must be given in all cases to the construct validity of the observations and measurements which are made in the course of a study. In some cases a construct might be refined to obtain a more precise definition of the construct for the purposes of measurement of the operationalized variable. In other cases two or more observed variables might be combined to form a latent variable associated with the construct, and in such cases an index of validity can be calculated, which indicates the strength of the relationship between the observed variables and the latent variable or construct.

Threats to construct validity also arise in experimental or intervention studies when the nature of the treatment is inadvertently varied either over subjects, settings, or times. The corruption of a designed treatment condition by different teachers, and for different students over time is a substantial problem in the evaluation of the introduction of any innovative method of teaching or a new curriculum.

The design of a study must be seen, in part, as the work of anticipating different possible threats to the validity of the conclusions to be drawn from a study and taking the necessary steps to eliminate or reduce those threats. Of particular importance at the design stage are threats to the validity of the constructs under investigation through the use of inappropriate or invalid observables, where an observable is defined to be a manifestation of the construct that can be observed. The observable should be defined in such a way that observations can be made with greater precision. However, the refinement of the observable may lead to a gain in precision or fidelity at the expense of a loss in meaningfulness or bandwidth, to employ terms that are now widely used in the recording of sound.

2.1.4 Measurement validity. Much has been written about different aspects of measurement validity in the assessment of educational achievement. The question must be asked whether an instrument measures what it purports to measure and whether the measurements that are obtained are meaningful. Validity of this kind is commonly classified into content, concurrent, and predictive validity and indices that are primarily correlations are widely employed to assess such aspects of measurement validity. Nevertheless, the strength of the measurement ultimately rests on the strength of the relationships that are established and the usefulness of those relationships in prediction and explanation (see *Validity*).

2.2 Triangulation

In holistic or case study research, it is common to employ multisite case studies to establish the generality and validity of the findings. However, the investigation of a single case or a limited number of cases is also of considerable importance. Under the circumstances where a single case is investigated the strength of the findings and relationships advanced lies in consistency with theory as well as in triangulation (see *Triangulation*). In triangulation, confirmation is commonly sought through multiple observations and multiple methods of investigation so that the different perspectives provide support for the findings and observed relationships. In this way triangulation is employed when in a single investigation the researcher combines multiple observers, or multiple methods of inquiry, or multiple sources of information, and the different perspectives obtained provide confirmation and thus strength to the findings and relationships recorded.

2.3 Replication

The quality of research rests in part, but not necessarily under all circumstances, on the replicability of the findings. Repetition is also a procedure that can be employed to improve the quality of observation, but it is the repeatability of the findings under the same or slightly different conditions that provides confirmation of the strength of the research. Nevertheless, sometimes special events can not be repeated and yet they provide important and unique results. However, the search for knowledge is built upon the regularity with which the findings can be replicated.

This commonly leads to the conduct of a series of studies and the subsequent systematic examination of the consistency and coherence of the results. Procedures of analysis (see *Meta-analysis*) have been developed to examine the results obtained from a series of studies in order to consider the regularity of the findings and where possible to remove systematically any bias which exists. In order for a study to be replicated accurately, a high level of documentation must be provided, so that any investigator who seeks to repeat a particular study can do so with accuracy. However, the importance of a repeated study arises from the capacity of replication to convince other investigators that if they were to undertake the same investigation under the same conditions, they too would obtain the same results. The emphasis is on objectivity and the power of persuasion to establish that a general relationship has been found and that a high level of consistency is involved.

2.3.1 Pattern of results. It is not uncommon in the design of an investigation to incorporate replication into the design, so that a variety of conditions are examined. Under these circumstances the pattern of the results obtained is of importance and must itself be subject to examination. The quality of the research rests on the extent to which the research permits the examination of the pattern of the results obtained either in the particular study carried out or in a series of other studies that are directed towards the investigation of the same problem situation. The techniques of meta-analysis enable the pattern of results to be examined in a systematic way.

2.4 Reliability or Internal Consistency of Observations

The quality of research is necessarily dependent on the consistency with which the observations are made. Consistency in turn is dependent on the precision with which an observable is specified. However, an observable can be so refined and the precision of observation increased to such an extent that while consistency is achieved in observation, what is observed has limited meaningfulness or relation to the construct represented by the observable. Estimates of the reliability or consistency of observations are commonly made through the use of a correlation coefficient which is dependent on the variability in the observable under investigation. It is only of value to have a highly reliable measure of an observable with a high degree of internal consistency if and only if it is the variability in a set of observations that is being considered in analysis. The same is true for the set of measures associated with a relationship. Consistency and a high level of reliability exist if the variance associated with the parameter under consideration is large and the error variance is small. However, these are conditions which not only involve the instrument employed, but also the characteristics of the sample on which the observations are made. As a consequence, the reliability of a measuring instrument is not sample free, and situations arise where precision and not variability in parameter estimation is required.

2.5 Dependability or External Consistency of Observations

The idea of the external consistency or dependability of a study involves whether the study was conducted in such a way that the investigation would be consistent over time, across research workers, and across the particular contexts or settings involved. The test is whether a different investigator, observing at a different time, and in a different setting or context would make observations that were consistent with the observations recorded in the particular study under consideration. In order to assess the dependability of observation it is necessary for the investigator to have taken the following steps to achieve external consistency in the observations made and to have recorded the steps taken systematically and with full documentation: (a) the times, settings, and subjects or respondents involved were appropriate and were clearly described; (b) the role and status of the observers were appropriate and were stated explicitly to respondents; (c) where several observers were involved, procedures were adopted and clearly specified that would ensure the obtaining of comparable observations; (d) the making of observations was carried out with appropriate checks taken in both recording and coding; and (e) the observers were required by training and the procedures employed to maintain consistency over time, settings, and respondents.

2.6 Utility

The quality of a study ultimately rests on its utility. However, utility does not necessarily involve direct implications for policy and practice, although these may follow from a study and are increasingly considered to be of importance by funding agencies and administrators. A research study may have clear implications for theory and as such may have a high degree of utility. Alternatively, a study may have important implications for further research and as such may open up a new line of inquiry out of which theoretical advances might be made or changes to policy and practice might follow. Unless a study has implications for theory, further research, or policy and practice it is likely to be ignored and the report of the study relegated to an entry in an information retrieval system. A common index of utility of a report is the number of citations recorded in a citations index, even though such citations are subject to fashion. As a consequence an important study might lie dormant for many years, but in the longer term prove to be very significant. There are two further characteristics of the quality of a research study that relate specifically to investigations in which quantitative estimations of parameters and relationships have been made. These characteristics, consequently, do not apply to research of a more descriptive or qualitative kind. First, there is the statistical significance of a result or relationship. Second, there is the magnitude of an effect or relationship. The former dominates the field of quantitative research. The latter is of growing importance, particularly where the practical implications of the research study for policy and practice are considered.

2.7 Statistical Significance

All measurement has a component of error associated with it. The error may arise from four sources: (a) from the instrument employed; (b) from the object being measured; (c) from the observer making the measurement; and (d) from the fact that commonly it is not possible to make measurements on all existing cases. As a consequence it is sometimes stated that there are two main classes of error namely: measurement error and sampling error. The first three sources listed above relate to measurement error, the fourth source involves sampling error. However, sampling of measurements is sometimes undertaken to allow for variability in the object being measured and for variability that is associated with the observer making the measurements.

Statistics is concerned with errors that occur randomly about a fixed, but commonly unknown value. Bias on the other hand is concerned with systematic error that can sometimes be estimated and removed by an appropriate adjustment. If measurement error can be estimated then it can sometimes be modeled in analysis and its effects allowed for. However, if it cannot be estimated then it must be combined together with sampling error and their effects considered jointly.

In significance testing a researcher advances a model or hypothesis that is examined against observable reality on which a series of measurements has been made. While three alternative approaches involving statistical theory have been advanced to examine whether a hypothesis is consistent with observable reality, a hypothesis can never with certainty be verified because the possibility always exists that data might be observed that contradict the hypothesis (see *Significance Testing*).

If measurement error is of consequence it should be built into the model, and if simple random sampling has not been employed then a multilevel analysis procedure should be used. All three approaches to statistics involve the estimation of the value of a parameter that makes the observed data most probable. Under these circumstances a probability value can be calculated to indicate under the model, the probability with which the data are observed. This level of probability should be reported. However, a low probability associated with a statistically significant finding does not necessarily imply a scientifically important effect, since small and trivial effects can be found to be statistically significant with sufficiently large samples.

2.8 Size of Effect

For 30 years and more, reports of research findings concerned with the difference between two mean values have sometimes recorded the size of an effect in terms of a standardized difference. This standardized difference was subsequently referred to as an *effect size* by Cohen (1969). The effect size is calculated by dividing the difference between the means for two independent groups by the common standard deviation of the two groups, as is employed in the t-test for the difference between the two means. More recently Cohen (1992) has listed effect size indexes for means, correlation coefficients, proportions, contingency tables, one way analysis of variance, and multiple correlations, and has proposed conventions for operational definitions of small, medium, and large effect sizes. The conventions that he proposes contribute in a substantial way to identifying the size of an effect that is worthy of consideration, and that is not dependent on the size of the samples involved.

While there has long been recognition that probabilities employed in statistical significance testing are dependent on sample sizes and that the sample design is largely ignored in commonly available computer programs, there has been a general reluctance in educational research to report and discuss effect sizes and the replicability of results. Recently, however, there has been a shift in emphasis by journal editors towards greater consideration of effect sizes and replicability analysis as well as the testing for statistical significance in the reporting of results of studies in education and psychology.

3. The Supplementary Nature of the Different Approaches

There is growing recognition in educational research that investigation into any particular problem situation which is encountered in research would profit from the examination of the problem through the use of more than one method of inquiry. Different methods of research can build upon each other and can provide

understandings and findings that one method alone could not provide. Furthermore, because different methods are vulnerable to different and commonly unknown biases, only by using different methods would it be possible to undertake triangulation that might confirm or disconfirm the the findings obtained with a particular method.

Miles and Huberman (1984, 1994) have drawn attention to the four ways in which two different research methods can be employed to provide supplementary information. Furthermore, Salomon (1991) has suggested that, in the conduct of research, an analytical approach, in which discrete elements of the problem situation are identified for investigation, may be contrasted with a systemic approach in which it is assumed that the elements are interdependent and inseparable and the problem situation must be viewed in a holistic way. In situations where both approaches could be used it would be possible to employ the two approaches through: (a) an integrated investigation in which both approaches were used simultaneously; (b) the use of a multiwave design in which both methods are employed during each wave of investigation; (c) a sequential design in which systemic methods are employed initially to examine the nature of the problem situation and then analytical methods are used to investigate particular relationships; and (d) a sequential design in which analytic methods of research are first used to establish particular relationships, and subsequently systemic methods of inquiry are employed to elaborate on and provide greater understanding of the relationships observed. The strengths of the first two designs would seem to lie in the triangulation of the findings, and in the second two designs in the better focusing of inquiry on the key issues for investigation.

4. Increasing the Strength of Inference from Evidence

The entries in this section have been grouped under three headings, namely, **Humanistic Analysis Procedures, Scientific Analysis Procedures**, and **Statistical Analysis Procedures**. It should be noted that the entries on procedures of statistical analysis are concerned exclusively with servicing the scientific approach.

4.1 Humanistic Analysis Procedures

A new and important entry in this section is concerned with *Computers and Qualitative Analysis*, in which the techniques are described that have been developed for the examination of data obtained from interviews and case studies and that have been computerized to facilitate both storage and retrieval as well as the crossclassification of such information. The entry on *Interviewing for Clinical Research* presents the procedures that might be used to improve the quality of research that employs intensive interviews to obtain information from individual subjects. The entry on *Descriptive Data, Analysis of* is derived from the work of Miles and Huberman (1984, 1994) and presents the tactics that are employed in humanistic research to derive findings, based on empirical evidence, through the systematic analysis of the available data.

The entry on *Concept Mapping* gives an account of a recently developed procedure that is employed not only in research but also in teaching to investigate the structures employed by students in the storage and retrieval of information. This procedure is believed to have important application in the advancement of the learning of individual students. A similar procedure for the examination of the storage and retrieval of ideas is provided by the *Repertory Grid Technique*.

Three articles are particularly concerned with validity issues. The first is *Participant Observation* where the research worker enters the situation under examination in order to undertake a more valid and more detailed investigation than would be possible from the outside. Under these circumstances the researcher is in a working or participant relationship with those being observed, while evidence is being gathered. In a second article on *Participant Verification* the research worker completes the first phase of an investigation and, having assembled and interpreted the evidence, returns to the situation in which the research is being conducted to confront the participants in that situation with both the evidence on the emerging findings and, where appropriate, the theoretical perspectives that are being derived from the investigation. The aim of the procedure is to validate the evidence, the conclusions drawn, and the theory being developed. A third entry examines the procedures of *Triangulation in Educational Research*, which is the combination and use of several different research methods in the study of the same phenomenon. There are several basic types of triangulation: (a) data triangulation, which involves replication in time and settings but with different subjects; (b) investigator triangulation, which involves the employment of several rather than one observer; and (c) methodological triangulation, which involves the use of two or more different methods of investigation. The aim of the procedure is to validate the evidence, the conclusions drawn and the theory being developed.

4.2 Scientific Analysis Procedures

The entries grouped under this heading are concerned with the general tactics of investigation within the scientific approach rather than the more specific techniques and procedures of statistical analysis. The entries are concerned primarily with the collection of data, whether it is obtained from a census or a survey, from the analysis of text or from observation in a classroom, by interviewing or by questionnaire (see *Census and National Survey Data; Sampling in Survey Research; Content and Text Analysis; Classroom Observation; Interviewing for Survey Research;*

Questionaires). In addition, the issues of the storage and management of data are addressed (see *Data Banks and Data Archives; Data Management in Survey Research*). Furthermore, the issues of secondary data analysis as well as the analysis of the findings from many different studies are also considered (see *Secondary Data Analysis; Meta Analysis*). Important developments have recently occurred in the investigation of change both for individuals and for individuals within groups. These aspects are of considerable relevance to educational research because of the emphasis in education on learning (see *Change, Measurement of; Single Case Research, Measuring Change*). The advances made in the measurement and analysis of change are giving rise to a new wave of studies in educational research concerned with the investigation of learning and growth that leads on to intervention studies and the investigation of school effectiveness (see *Quasi-experimentation; Effective Schools Research*).

4.3 Statistical Analysis Procedures

Data collected in educational research are in three forms. First, there are data in which the characteristic being measured has an underlying continuity and the data recorded are on a scale that has a high degree of precision, so that continuity is assumed in the measurements recorded. Second, while the characteristic being measured has an underlying continuity, the data recorded have been categorized into a limited number of categories. Third, data are collected in many studies that are related to a characteristic or event for which there is no underlying continuity, but categories of response or observation, and the data are categorical or nominal in nature.

With respect to the first type of data, which are continuous, the procedures of maximum likelihood estimation require normality in the distribution of the scores of all variables as well as multivariate normality in the data set. As a consequence there is growing interest in analysis to test for normality and multivariate normality in the data. Where these properties of the data or the underlying variable are not present, generalized least squares procedures are now available for the effective analysis of the data. There is also concern in significant testing for homogeneity of variance and for normality and the absence of outliers in the residuals. Where such problems arise, weighted least squares procedures or robust regression procedures are sometimes employed in the analysis of the data (see *Robust Statistical Procedures*).

With respect to the second type of data which are categorized, the use of procedures that make allowance for the categorization of the data are increasingly being employed (see *Correlational Methods; Path Analysis and Linear Structural Relations Analysis*). Major advances have also been made primarily in Europe in the analysis of categorical data and there is a cluster of analytical techniques that correspond to the procedures employed for the analysis of continuous data, and that are concerned specifically with the analysis of categorical data (see *Configural Frequency Analysis; Contingency Tables; Correspondence Analysis; Event History Analysis; Galois Lattices; Log-linear Models; Logistic Regression; Mobility Tables; Social Network Analysis*). These analytical procedures represent substantial advances in the examination of categorical data.

The second major advance that has occurred in the analysis of data has been in the capacity to model the multilevel structure of the data so that not only unbiased effects at different levels can be estimated, but they can also be examined with appropriate estimates of the error variance which make allowance for the errors operating at the different levels. In addition, cross-level effects, which involve the estimation of interactions between variables at different levels, can now be examined for magnitude and significance (see *Hierarchical Linear Modeling; Multilevel Analysis; Path Analysis and Linear Structural Relations Analyses*).

There are, however, dangers always present with the growing complexity in the statistical techniques that are now readily available on desktop computers, that there is a lack of awareness of the assumptions associated with the use of a particular technique. Consequently a sound understanding of the meaning of the operations employed and the results produced is not always maintained (see *Hypothesis Testing; Significance Testing; Bayesian Statistics*). Of particular importance are the problems of missing data and non-response (see *Missing Data and Non-response*).

These problems, which occur to markedly different degrees in different countries, unless controlled by an adequate level of careful planning, lead to invalidity in the findings of potentially valuable and meaningful studies. Little can be done to rectify a situation where the extent of non-response and the amount of missing data exceed certain critical levels, but strategies are increasingly being employed to make adjustments for missing data and non-response in situations where the problem is not excessive.

The statistical procedures described and discussed in the collection of entries in this section are by no means exhaustive or complete. Indeed, this is a field where new techniques are being developed all the time in order to increase the strength of the inferences which can be drawn from both quantitative and qualitative data.

References

Cohen J 1969 *Statistical Power Analyses for the Behavioral Sciences*. Academic Press, New York

Cohen J 1992 A power primer. *Psych. Bull.* 112(1): 155–59

Miles M B, Huberman A M 1984 *Qualitative Data Analysis*. Sage, London

Miles M B, Huberman A M 1994 *Qualitative Data Analysis*, 2nd edn. Sage, London

Salomon G 1991 Transcending the qualitative-quantitative debate: the analytic and systemic approaches to educational research. *Educ. Researcher* 20(6): 10–18

Snow C P 1959 *The Two Cultures and the Scientific Revolution*. Cambridge University Press, New York.

(a) Humanistic Analysis Procedures

Computers and Qualitative Analysis

L. Richards

Qualitative computing became a recognized field of research and development in the mid-1980's and within a decade was in wide use. Most researchers are aware that a range of programs exists, and increasingly novice researchers assume they should use a computer, although their supervisors have often never done so. To do so no longer seems odd. Just as nobody would think of doing a survey without a statistical package, researchers reach for a qualitative package when faced with unstructured data. For most researchers the question is not why a program but, which program should be used. The first section briefly offers sources of information for those asking that question.

The second section turns to the question not often asked: why compute? Few now ask why should a machine be used in supporting methods traditionally labelled humanistic, holistic, interpretive, idiosyncratic, personal, intuitive. This question should be asked; it is such challenges that drive software development and methodology.

In the third section another question is raised which is rarely asked. What changes does computing bring to methodology? It is a mistake to see qualitative computing as merely facilitating previous techniques. It brings to the qualitative method changes that are both radical and largely ignored.

1. The Challenge of being informed

There is no shortage of sources of information on qualitative computing, but they offer different pictures of a moving target. Most qualitative methods texts have in recent editions added chapters or chapter segments on computers to discussions of techniques for handling data. These vary from serious surveys of available software to addenda to chapters, noting that computers may be used or naming one or a couple of programs, as though the computer merely offers a different container for an unchanging method (Silverman 1993, Coffey and Atkinson 1996).

The now considerable specialist literature on qualitative computing is dominated by collections from conferences (Fielding and Lee 1991, Kelle 1994); surveys of programs (Weitzman and Miles 1995); and stories about using them (Burgess 1995). For the researcher deciding whether to compute, and if so what, these are problematic. Software development has a far more rapid pace than academic publishing, so this literature is inevitably out of date. Objective comparisons are hard to find since researchers see more in the software they use, and/or develop or sell, than in rival packages. Complete coverage is impossible; to do a thorough job of reviewing all examples of all types of qualitative software is a massive task, rapidly growing.

At the time of writing, only one book reviews thoroughly and without partisanship almost all qualitative software available at its time of writing (Weitzman and Miles 1995). There are several recent detailed overviews of the range of programs (Kelle 1995, Richards and Richards 1994). All offer the researcher seeking information the same set of advice: learn about the range currently available for what you want to do and choose on the basis of preferably hands-on trial, taking into account your research method and goals, your computer skills and equipment and your understanding of the range of tools offered by the package. To the researcher wanting to get on with research, this sometimes depressing advice makes the process of choice appear difficult. Qualitative research is a craft, involving working with, feeling through, exploring and building understandings from data. Hence researchers are best able to judge the analysis process when involved with data. The choice is easier if programs are trialed with the researchers own data, to see if the software helps ask the questions to which answers are wanted.

Whilst there is some convergence amongst the software programs that have survived the first generation, each package has different ranges of functions and each has areas of speciality in powerful techniques. For up to date detail about and experience with particular software packages, it is unwise to rely on any printed medium. Information can be obtained from those creating and using the software. Most software is available in demonstration form, from developers or from World Wide Web sites. Internet discussion groups offer a forum for user questions and sharing of experience.

The present author is both user-researcher and part of a software development team (QSR, developers of the NUD.IST software). Hence no claim is made for objectivity in comparing software, and in the scope of this article one could not anyway attempt to review the range or describe in detail what any particular program does. Elsewhere, Richards and Richards (1995) have contributed to a methodological mapping of software architectures and directions. Here, the more generic questions are asked; why compute qualitative work, and what are the results of doing so? The answers to these questions alert the researcher to the main dimensions on which programs differ; particular programs are named only when they typify an approach or have unique capability.

2. *Why compute?*

Nobody asked that question of quantitative research; computers can evidently do more with numbers than the human brain. However, because they are associated with number crunching, rather than with crafting of interpretations, computers seem less obviously attuned to the needs of the qualitative researcher. Qualitative method was assisted by computers in a quite different way from survey research.

The method contains built-in contradictions, and computer software, if directed to this task, can enable their resolution. Researchers working qualitatively are usually handling messy data, usually because their goal is to learn new things, to understand how people see their world, or the complexity of a situation not previously comprehended. So data must be kept messy until it is thoroughly explored. Yet it also has to be managed, to give accurate access to instances, themes, contexts. Manual as well as many computer methods of coding and filing kill richness and complexity.

Most pre-computer (and the "first generation" of post-computer) methods left the researcher on one horn or other of the dilemma: messy rich data or organised storage and accurate access. The goal of sophisticated software is to support efficiency and creativity, to allow accurate access and efficient storage, but also support exploration, discovery and the crafting of theory.

2.1 *Pursuing efficiency*

Computer enhanced efficiency, especially with tasks that are dreary and clerical, has proved a boon to qualitative researchers. However, this side of qualitative computing has tended to dominate the image of computers. Researchers who saw computers as entirely appropriate for quantitative analysis still too often see their relevance to qualitative work only in doing one or more of three survey-like things: coding, storing information, counting. Certainly computers facilitate those tasks, and the earliest programs threw a new emphasis on them. Arguably qualitative researchers have

eschewed such tasks too long. Nevertheless, in supporting such techniques computers also risk distorting the method.

2.1.1 Coding and retrieval. Coding is central to the techniques supported by every qualitative program, just as it has always been central to manual methods. However, there are several meanings of coding in qualitative research. Computers easily support one, the allocating of codes to text so the researcher can retrieve everything coded by one or more codes. This technique, usually referred to as "code-and-retrieve", was pioneered in specialist software with *The Ethnograph*. All qualitative software now will code, in one of several ways, with or without limitations, and permit some sort of retrieval.

These tasks are much easier, quicker and more powerful with computerss. Working with manual filing systems or index cards, reseaerchers had to settle for tight restrictions on extent of information and size and range of categories. Any software softens these restrictions, and researchers requiring removal of limits on number and flexibility of codes will find that some programs support unlimited coding and unlimited code sets, with techniques for managing code sets and storing definitions and ideas about categories. With new emphasis on speed, some programs will automate coding. The swift conduct of coding by computer contrasts dramatically with the old copy/cut/paste/file methods.

Retrieval is the most obvious aspect revolutionised. These tools can permit instantly not only a retrieval of material coded at one category but also explorations of patterns.

2.1.2 Storing information. Some qualitative software can store information about people and sites, and allow this to be used in framing enquiries. Programs differ in the methods used to store information and in the number of item that can be stored and ways they can be used. Some programs allow this information storage to be automated and a few will directly link with statistical programs so that what the program "knows" about a case or a person can be coded to inform the qualitative enquiry.

Used in conjunction with coding of content, this opens up new possibilities for retrieval and inquiry. ("What did the younger women say on this topic? Do those in another age group say different things? Are these attitudes patterned by gender and lifestage?") Some programs will provide a matrix breaking down the segments of text by coding. Several link to statistical packages, either directly or indirectly.

2.1.3 Counting. Counting occurrences, an anathema in much qualitative research, is one of many ways of making sence of complexity, locating and exploring patterns. Almost every qualitative program will count retrievals made by either or both of searches of text and searches of codes and the coding done. Text search programs offer a range of ways of counting occurrences of string of characters and some programs combine this with pattern searching, using wild cards, for alternative words. Researchers whose methods concentrate on these techniques will find a range of increasingly sophisticated and swift text search programs.

2.1.4 Searching text. Text search was not at first included in the functions of qualitative programs; researchers whose manual methods had never been able to use it found it hard to imagine how mechanical searching of text could complement reading and thinking about it. However, there is a wide range of text retrievers available, and most qualitative programs now combine text search with other functions, most commonly coding, and some will code the result of a text search. This ability can be exploited to do "auto-coding" of text, for instance, coding interviews according to the question being asked, or demographic information about the respondent. Moreover, while text search is often not the primary technique of the qualitative researcher, it can also be used as a way of gathering data related to a topic, for further exploration.

2.2 Supporting creativity

In qualitative research an emphasis on efficiency is often inappropriate, and always not enough. This is not merely because it is ideologically unacceptable to see data as "hard", but because the data items are not standardised, so automation of coding, counting and searching tends to address only marginal tasks, not the central goals of theories constructed from data and assessed for their authenticity and credibility (Lincoln and Guba 1985). The future challenges of qualitative computing undoubtedly lie in support for these more elusive goals.

2.2.1 Remaking coding. After the first excitement at being able to code on computer, critics noted a tendency for over-reliance on such mechanical processes (Agar 1991). Overemphasis on coding for retrieval, arguably not a central process for qualitative research, potentially distorts the method if it is regarded as a form of analysis (Richards and Richards 1991, Coffey et al. 1996). Software developments in recent years have emphasized not only the data-disposal techniques of allocating codes to text but also the more creative aspects of the coding process—data exploration and reflection on data, category construction, manipulation, clarification and linking. These are the processes qualitative researchers talk of in sensual terms—feeling through, seeing patterns, hearing noises, in data, processes requiring fluidity, flexibility and multi-task capability.

All qualitative software will allow coding on paper and transferring the coding decisions to the computer.

But coding on-screen has become an expectation in recent years and potentially this remade the task and the results of coding. Ability to do and see several processes simultaneously means coding can become an exploratory process whereby reflections can be stored, categories created, defined and explored, contexts retrieved and comparisons made during the task of deciding the appropriate code for text segments. Recent releases of several packages have emphasized support for recoding, exploration of the results of coding and rethinking of codes, combining them and dimensionalising them. These permit techniques impossible previously; combining and merging coding at diverse categories, testing the patterns resulting, exploring the crosscutting of codes and patterned occurrences in matrices.

2.2.2 Categories and managing them. Software products differ widely in the speed and fluidity of category creation and coding and in ways in which categories can be defined and memos stored about the ideas being developed. This can be a critical issue, as the clerical barrier imposed by coding may block thinking about the data.

Researchers using index cards and filing cabinets had great difficulty in flexibly managing a system of changing categories and discovered subcategories. Computers offer far more storage and far more flexibility, as well as visual display of the growing and changing system of codes. The arrival of graphical user interfaces enhanced this work, as qualitative software permitted researchers to have several windows open on different tasks simultaneously, and to move between them. Packages differ considerably in the handling of categories, the number of categories and richness of coding allowed and modes of managing categories. One, WinMAX, allows numerical loading of coding.

2.2.3 Theory-building: broadening and building on retrievals. Coding always is linked with retrieval. Any qualitative software, or indeed word processor or data base program—unlike card index files, can use retrieval techniques to "get back" the actual text coded. In the near future this will extend to images or sound. Most qualitative programs will do simple retrievals ("get me all the text coded this") or Boolean retrievals ("all the text coded this and that, this or that, this but not that"). Some programs will widen retrievals to show nominated context and some will support returning the researcher to the retrieved extract in its place in the original document.

The most obvious difference between packages that code is what opinions are offered for asking questions about coding in order to support theory-building from coding. In the earliest discussions, this label was applied to any software that could ask questions about coding occuring anywhere in a document. The goals of theory-building are now both more ambitious and more varied, pursuing the central feature of qualitative research that is almost always iterative, rarely a matter of asking one question.

One direction is allowing the researcher to manage codes flexibly, asking questions about context and complex meanings and storing the answers as more coding to build on. The term "system closure" refers to this ability to save the answer as more data, and ask another question (Richards and Richards 1994, Weitzman and Miles 1995) ("Who says this? Those who talked of this and that in the same interview: what did they say on this other topic?"). Researchers constructing an index system in QSR NUD.IST have a toolkit of ways of asking questions of coding and storing the answer as further coding, so another question can be asked.

2.2.4 Linking. Qualitative research is centrally about linking: linking categories to data, and to each other, linking data segments, linking the researcher's ideas to the data and so on. Manual methods normally support only the first sort of links; by coding the data the researcher links category and data segment. Computers are linking machines. "Hyperlinking" of text in one interview with text in another requires the researcher to draw and record mental ribbons; computers can record the researcher's link and return to it at any time. With the arrival of the Hypercard on Macintosh computers, qualitative researchers could purchase tailored software ("Hyper-" names indicate this origin; HyperRESEARCH, Hypersoft, HyperQual) or even create their own. Programs, and researchers, differ on the importance they put on textual or visual links.

2.2.5 Memos and annotations. Computers always supported the researcher's need to record ideas in memos or notes. But recently the memo functions of programs have become more sophisticated. Programs differ on where memos or annotations are stored, the length and variety permitted and whether they can be logged or coded. Some contain their own editors, using these to assist in bringing disparate memos together as understanding of a series of categories or documents develops.

2.3 Diagrams and networks

Qualitative researchers sometimes include the drawing of links and shapes, as a means to the end of understanding and theorising. Programs increasingly support such graphics, in an increasingly wide range of displays. Semantic networks, and the direct manipulation of their parts, were introduced in qualitative computing by ATLASti. Conceptual networks are displayed and explored in a set of programs which include much wider displaying and drawing facilities. Inspiration is one commonly used in conjunction with theory-building programs.

One of the most immediate results of software

shopping expeditions in qualitative analysis is the discovery that most programs assume that the method involves the collection of data records that are or can be typed onto a computer. The techniques of handling these records involve segmenting of text in order to attach a code or codes to the segment.

2.4 Formulating and testing theory

Theory-testing tools address different interpretations of the goals of qualitative research. Hypothesis testing is explicitly supported in quite different ways by AQUAD, which also does cross-case configural analysis, and HyperRESEARCH, which emphasizes replicability of tests. QCA is designed to support the quantified analysis of multi-case studies (Kelle 1995).

3. What did the computer do?

It is seriously misleading to see qualitative computing as merely a new way of doing the same old things with data. The computer changes the method. Much of what computers offer to help with sounds very different from the methods taught a decade ago. However, computing has done more for the method than merely add new techniques.

Methodological changes are not universally welcomed, but are always stimulating. Qualitative computing has been researcher-driven, and accompanied by a growing methodological debate in academic and research circles. Computers have forced clarification of methodological processes, provided entirely new techniques and supported old ones in ways that allow new trajectories of analysis. To take one example, computers have drawn attention to the aesthetics of qualitative research. Interface has emerged as a very significant aspect of methodology. Qualitative researchers think aloud, moving swiftly to follow hunches and record and link growing understandings. Researcher demand has pushed software development towards flexible systems in which interpretations of data are more rapidly reflected on the screen and can be acted on directly. The next generation of software will emphasize user interface.

However undesirable some redirections of method, computing is now inevitable in qualitative research. This raises new issues for research training. Good software seduces the user into doing what it does well. For novice researchers or those unfamiliar with computers they may distract research energy. To take the obvious example, the support computers offer for coding is a particular problem, not because the computer itself demands a distorted method but because insecure researchers unsure what to do fall easily into a mode best described as "if it moves, code it". Then it is a small step to "if it matters I must have a code for it", unless the researcher is equipped with other ways of accessing and exploring data.

All qualitative researchers will be greatly assisted

in some ways by computing: to do qualitative research without a computer now would be rather like doing statistical research with an abacus. But just as statistical packages offered vast possibilities of tests that were meaningless in a particular study, so too qualitative packages must be selectively used. Like innovative cookbooks, software packages should be treated as collections of possibilities, not requirements that you should do everything therein, let alone eat it.

Choice of programs requires a sense of what you want to do. Understanding of the research goals and opportunities offered by computers is essential for sensible desision making. Many of the skills now offered were never used, or even discussed, when manual methods made them unthinkable. Until recently, indeed, it was often hard for novice researchers to find what should be done with the data. The advent of computers has coincided with, and doubtless contributed to, a new trend for methods texts to specify ways of handling data. Pre-computers offered a craft rarely outlined in writing, with an often evangelical literature describing the processes of making data, rather than what should have been done with the data. The best kept secret of qualitative methods pre-computers was the impossibility of managing even small amounts of very rich data without doing damage. Manual methods of handling data offered little support to the skilled researcher in the complex craft of theory construction. Computer software is beginning to support it and theory-crafting has become the target of current software developments.

References

Agar M 1991 The right brain strikes back. In: Fielding N, Lee R (eds.) 1991 *Using Computers in Qualitative Research.* Sage, London

Burgess R (ed.) 1995 *Computing and Qualitative Research: Studies in Qualitative Methodology*, Vol 5. JAI Press, London

Coffey A, Atkinson P 1996 *Making Sense of Qualitative Data: Complimentary Research Strategies.* Sage, Thousand Oaks, California

Coffey A, Holbrook B, Atkinson P 1996 *Qualiative Data Analysis: Technologies and Representations Sociological Research Online* 1:1.

Fielding N, Lee R 1991 *Using Computers in Qualitative Research.* Sage, London

Kelle U (ed.) 1995 *Computer-Aided Qualitative Data Analysis: Theory, Methods and Practice.* Sage, London

Lincoln Y, Guba E G 1985 *Naturalistic Inquiry.* Sage, Beverly Hills, California

Richards L, Richards T 1991 The transformation of qualitative method: computational paradigms and research processes. In: Fielding N, Lee R (eds.) 1991 *Using computers in Qualitative Research.* Sage, London

Richards T, Richards L 1994 Using computers in qualitative analysis. In: Denzin N K, Lincoln Y (eds.) *Handbook of Qualitative Research.* Sage, Newbury Park, California

Richards L, Richards T 1995 From filing cabinet to computer. In: Burgess R, Bryman A (eds.) 1995 *Analysing Qualitative Data.* Routledge, London

Silverman D 1993 *Interpreting Qualitative Data: Methods for Analysing Talk, Text and Interaction.* Sage, London

Weitzman E, Miles M 1995 *Computer Programs for Qualitative Analysis.* Sage, Thousand oaks, California

Concept Mapping

M. J. Lawson

The power of a visual representation of an idea or process is generally accepted in both the wider community and in education. Company logos, maps of subway systems, flow charts, and road signs are seen to be effective forms of representation of ideas of varying complexity in everyday life. Visual representation techniques also constitute one of the major instructional formats available to teachers, ranging from carefully prepared multi-colored diagrams of objects or processes to sketches hastily drawn on paper or even the ground. There is quite strong informal evidence available from both teachers and students that these devices assist learning. Given the long history of use of such devices in teaching it is surprising that there has been relatively little systematic study of their nature and effects. Mayer and Gallini (1990), who have carried out several studies of the effects of illustrations on learning, argue that their potential remains to be fully exploited. In their discussion of different types of illustrations Jones et al. (1988–89) propose that an effective graphical representation allows the development of "a holistic understanding that words alone cannot convey" (p. 21), because the graphical form allows representation of parts and whole in a way that is not available in the sequential structure of text.

An attractive form of visual representation, the "concept map," has emerged in a number of forms in educational research, though the term is most commonly associated with the work of Novak and his colleagues in the science education program at Cornell University (e.g., Novak and Gowin 1984). It is upon this version of concept mapping that this entry will concentrate.

Forms of visual representation have received much

less attention in educational research than have verbal and text-based materials. In part this seems to be related to the lack of availability of a framework for considering ways to structure a complex array of material. While there are well-developed analyses of text structures (e.g., de Beaugrande and Dressler 1981) there is not an analytical scheme of comparable complexity that can be used in description of the structure and components of graphical displays. Kosslyn (1989) has suggested a means for beginning the study of different types of illustrations by setting out a broad framework within which he distinguishes four types of graphic representation of some phenomenon (X)-graphs, maps, charts, and diagrams. In this framework *graphs* are seen as the most constrained form of visual display, involving representation of X in terms of values on at least two axes. The labels and the scales assigned to the axes denote the dimensions of representation of the phenomenon. *Maps* are less constrained in structure than graphs, the central feature of a map in Kosslyn's scheme being its representation of spatial relationships characteristic of X, typically relationships such as size, location, direction and distance. The map need not only be of a static structure such as a city but has also been used as a form of representation for a dynamic system like a brain. The features of charts and diagrams are less firmly established. For Kosslyn the *chart* represents discrete relationships among discrete entities, with relationships such as sequence being typically associated with charts, as in a flow chart. *Diagram* is the least specific of Kosslyn's categories, covering any visual representation not identified in the other categories.

Within Kosslyn's framework the concept map of Novak would not be regarded as a map, for as Thompson (1992) argues it is not a central feature of a concept map that spatial relationships be represented, the more typical focus being the representation of semantic relationships. This entry considers the development and use of the Novak procedure, and some related techniques, for the representation of relationships among ideas in educational research and for ease of reference the term "concept map" will be retained here.

1. The Concept Maps of Novak

Novak's initial interest in the concept map was stimulated by the need to make sense of a large body of data generated through interviews with students in elementary science classes (Novak 1990). The concept map was developed as a means of facilitating analysis of such information by application of a structural device for representing a student's understanding of a complex phenomenon. Novak sought to develop a procedure that would represent that understanding in terms of propositional relationships established among a group of related concepts. Some form of represen-

tation of the structure of student understanding was argued by Novak and Gowin (1984) to be necessary to make progress in identifying areas of difficulty in understanding that might give rise to misconceptions. For Novak a concept map satisfied this need by providing "a schematic device for representing a set of concept meanings embedded in a framework of propositions" (Novak and Gowin 1984 p. 15).

In establishing this representational format Novak drew extensively on the descriptions of learning that had been developed by Ausubel (1968). In Ausubel's theory, the most effective learning, "meaningful learning," involved the establishment of patterns of relationships among concepts with the larger more general patterns coming to *subsume*, or incorporate, the more specific concepts. The establishment of meaningful relationships among concepts was contrasted by Ausubel with "rote" learning in which concepts were not embedded in rich conceptual networks but were left relatively unelaborated and conceptually isolated within the broad conceptual structure. In the Ausubelian view the growth of knowledge in an individual was characterized by the gradual development of more complex and more differentiated structures organized in a hierarchical pattern. The different parts of this structure could be related, or integrated, through the establishment of propositional links. The hierarchical structure of a concept map was seen by Novak as instantiating the process of knowledge growth that Ausubel termed "subsumption." In this process the meaning of a new concept would be assimilated within the sphere of meaning of an existing concept/proposition complex to create a more powerful and coherent structure.

These ideas have been translated directly into the form of a concept map by Novak and his colleagues. In the form developed and used by Novak the concept map is a hierarchical structure, the focal point of which is the superordinate concept, the other concepts of concern being arranged in a manner which indicates their place and semantic relationships within this hierarchy. As noted above the structure is simple with three basic features—a list of concepts, a set of linking relationships among the concepts and, if desired, a set of labels for those relationships. Concepts, or entities, are established in a pattern of relationships. The connection of two concepts in a relationship expresses a proposition. Typically this simple structure is depicted using ellipses to represent concepts and lines to represent the relating links. If required, labels can be assigned to the linking lines in order to express the nature of a proposition.

In its hierarchical form the structure of the Novak concept map bears close similarity to the model of internal semantic network structure developed by memory researchers during the 1960s as a format for representation of long-term memory (e.g., Collins and Quillian 1969). The concept map may be seen as a system for externalizing this internal memory representation. It is not the only technique that has been designed to externalize internal psychological structure. Conceptually it is similar in nature to procedures for structuring conceptualizations that use the multivariate statistical techniques of cluster analysis and multidimensional scaling procedures, some of which are also termed "concept mapping procedures" (see Trochim 1989). The preparation of the typical Novak map does not involve use of these statistical techniques, though such techniques would be quite compatible with the central themes of Novak's work. Repertory grid techniques and semantic differential procedures share essentially the same objective as concept mapping in their concern to produce a representation of the structure of a semantic space. Each of these alternative techniques has been associated with the development of more refined statistical techniques than has Novak's concept mapping. Perhaps because of the close identification of concept mapping with a range of classroom applications its procedures for preparation and scoring have remained less formal than the representational techniques just noted.

The epistemological stance of Novak and other users of the general class of techniques for representation of cognitive structure has been questioned by Phillips (1983). Phillips questions the existence of the relationship between the behavioral representation manifested in the concept map and the internal structural state of the individual. However, as argued by Greeno (1983) in a response to Phillips, it seems that this criticism is overextended by Phillips so that the possibility of the existence of a less than perfect representation of cognitive structure is mistakenly interpreted as lack of such a relationship. Novak (1990) accepts Greeno's view that the outcomes of the use of techniques such as concept mapping do bear a systematic, though perhaps "noisy," relationship to cognitive structure, and so can be used as a basis for derivation of inferences about the state of that structure.

2. Functions of a Concept Map

It is of value to distinguish between the uses of concept maps from teacher and student perspectives.

2.1 Concept Map as Instructional Display

For a teacher the concept map can be used as a means of representing a pattern of relationships in an instructional display, a sort of diagrammatic text. The teacher can propose a structure of relationships in diagrammatic form rather than in verbal, or text, or equation formats. The display is then available for use by the teacher in part or as a whole structure.

For the student the concept map represents a way of introducing structure into the process of knowledge acquisition. This structuring can take two broad forms.

In the first, the instructional display presented by the teacher, or by a text, can be inspected and used by the student to structure the relationships pertinent to the topic under study. The concept map presents a number of propositional relationships for analysis, and would also be expected to influence the form of organization of these propositions in memory. An alternative procedure could require the student to produce the map, from a list of relevant concepts, with one concept being nominated as the focus of the hierarchy. The links established by the students, and the labels assigned to these links, are argued to influence the nature of the understanding of the phenomenon that is developed.

The concept map can also be expected to have the potential to influence events at the time of retrieval of information related to the topic of the hierarchy. The visual character of the map could provide a means of structuring cognitive activity during retrieval, with the concept names and the labels having the potential to act as cues that could guide the search of memory. The use of the map would then be expected to improve the accessing of relevant knowledge because of its potential for influencing both organizational and retrieval events.

A number of researchers have reported positive effects of the use of concept maps as a form of instructional display, the majority of this research involving secondary school science students. In one of the earlier evaluation studies Novak et al. (1983) found that junior high school students who prepared a concept map were able to identify more relevant relationships in reporting on a topic in science than students who were presented with keywords prior to developing their responses. These authors also found that the concept map group solved more problems on a transfer task than did the control group. Okebukola has carried out a number of studies with secondary school science students in which the effectiveness of concept map use during learning for a topic has been evaluated. In a recent study (Okebukola 1990), the effect of adding a concept mapping strategy to discussion and practical sessions in units on genetics and ecology was assessed with students aged 15–22 years. In both units the effect of preparation and the use of concept maps during class sessions was associated with significant improvements in post-test performance. Pankratius (1990) observed a similar pattern of results in a study with high school physics students. The preparation of the maps, and their updating during study, resulted in better performance than did conventional classroom instruction that did not include use of the mapping procedure. Willerman and Mac-Harg (1991) used concept maps as an advance organizer for their eighth-grade science students and found that their mapping group scored significantly higher on a post-test than did the control group that had not used the map organizer.

While these sets of findings indicate that the use of a concept mapping procedure offers an interesting alternative means of instructional presentation to the teacher, it is important to note that not all investigations of the use of concept maps have returned positive results. Lehman et al. (1985) found no differences in achievement in comparisons of mapping and control treatments in biology classes. The results obtained in Prater and Terry's (1988) study of the use of concept maps as an aid to reading comprehension were also equivocal with an advantage for use of concept maps being observed for reading comprehension in only two of the three studies involving fifth-grade students. No advantage for use of the concept mapping approach was obtained on a writing task. Stensvold and Wilson (1990) found that the use of concept maps in chemistry classes resulted in lower scores for high ability students than did the conventional teaching procedure. Heinze-Fry and Novak (1990) noted a similar effect on their higher ability students in initial post-test performance, though this effect was not apparent after a period of five months. In this study no significant effect of concept map use was observed at either immediate or delayed testing.

As is the case for many other instructional techniques the pattern of results for use of concept maps as study devices is mixed. This pattern is not seen here to be sufficient reason to abandon use of concept maps for it is clear that there have as yet been relatively few systematic studies of the use of this form of instructional display. There is such a wide variation in design of concept maps, in manner of presentation of these to students, and in procedures for examining the effects of map use, that it would be premature to argue that a clear picture of concept map use is available. The variation just noted makes clear that it is difficult to assemble very many studies that have involved closely similar conditions, so that precise statements of effects are not available.

2.2 Concept Map as an Evaluation Device

A concept map produced by students is argued by Novak and Gowin (1984) to be as important as an evaluation technique. In very general terms the teacher may identify for a given hierarchy concepts that are incorrectly included in student maps, concepts that are omitted, or valid relationships that are either not justified in the light of current understanding or are missing. Novak and Gowin clearly see this use of the concept map as a valuable alternative to such evaluation devices as objective tests and essays, arguing that in many cases the concept map has greater sensitivity as a measuring device. The strength of this argument rests to a significant extent on the qualities possessed by both the manner of preparation of the map and those of the system used to score the map. At present both these remain issues that require further discussion and investigation before it would be reasonable to claim that the concept map had wide practicability as a formal evaluation device in school or university classrooms. These issues are discussed more fully in a following section.

2.3 Concept Map as Curriculum Organizer

Starr and Krajcik (1990) have used concept maps as a means of developing curriculum plans and sequences, and have found that teachers value the structure which the use of the procedure introduces into planning of lesson sequences. This has involved the structuring of hierarchies based around the major constructs/concepts in a given area and identification of related, subordinate concepts—a process similar to that involved in the use of Gagne's learning hierarchies (Gagne 1968). Both concept maps and learning hierarchies can be used to produce specifications of the content of a teaching/learning sequence, though the learning hierarchies have typically been developed in much greater detail for this purpose than have concept maps. Across a number of sessions Starr and Krajcik (1990) identified the development of a more coherent framework for the presentation of the life science component of the upper elementary curriculum. These authors also saw the process of development of the maps as having the effect of increasing the degree of involvement of these teachers in the curriculum planning process. There is clear scope for the development of more detailed investigation of this use of concept maps.

2.4 Concept Map as Index of Understanding

As indicated earlier the need for a form of representation of student understanding provided the impetus for development of the concept map and this continues to be one of the major uses of the technique (Novak and Musonda 1991; Wallace and Mintzes 1990). Novak and Musonda (1991) used concept maps to document changes in understanding of a wide range of scientific notions in a group of students as they moved from first grade to twelfth grade. In this study the concept maps were developed by the researchers from clinical interviews with students. The procedure used to move from interview to map is not clearly explicated by these authors, though they do claim reasonable validity and reliability for their procedures. Wallace and Mintzes (1990) trained undergraduates to produce concept maps prior to beginning their instructional intervention and then assessed the quality of the student produced maps at preintervention and postintervention times using an "expert-produced" map as a reference point. The training in production of maps followed the procedures set out by Novak and Gowin (1984).

Of these two procedures the latter is more straightforward and appears to be less prone to problems of unreliability. The analysis of interview transcripts requires the interposing of the interpretive framework of the researcher between the consideration of the concept complex and the structuring of the student's map. This places the student at some considerable distance from the process of structuring the map, a disadvantage that is overcome through use of the student-produced maps.

3. Issues

3.1 The Problem of Hierarchical Structure

Novak has maintained hierarchical structure as a central feature of the concept map (Novak 1990), deriving the basis of such a structure from the notion of subsumption as a process of knowledge development and organization. Wandersee (1990) also sees such a structure as being required to represent the "psychological structure" of understanding. It now seems more reasonable to justify the use of a hierarchically structured concept map on practical grounds, rather than arguing for an isomorphism between the structure of the map and psychological structure of meaning. While the early models of semantic memory networks were organized hierarchically (e.g., Collins and Quillian 1969), the psychological evidence for such a pattern of organization is not strong (e.g., Anderson 1990). The recent interest in distributed memory organization moves away from the simple hierarchical pattern of internal representation. Network models, in which the structure of conceptual elements was likened by Anderson (1990) to a massed tangle of marbles with strings attached, are more compatible with current thinking about mental structure. The limited dimensionality of the hierarchy suggests that it is an impoverished representation of memory structure.

Even a limited experience in constructing a concept map within a hierarchical format highlights the problem of variations in degree of generality of a concept that emerge when different features of the concept are highlighted. The analogy drawn by Novak and Gowin between a concept map and a rubber sheet of concepts, part of which (the superordinate concept) is elevated into prominence for purposes of discussion, suggests that they have some appreciation of the limitations of the hierarchical structure. Novak and Musonda (1991 p. 129) acknowledged the difficulty of recognizing hierarchies in a map and scored the maps in their study using level as a broad indicator of hierarchy. The limitations noted here have also been raised in discussions of other hierarchical structures popular in discussions of learning and instruction during the 1970s—Gagne's (1968) learning hierarchies (Merrill and Gibbons 1974). Phillips (1983) has also noted a number of problems that arise in drawing relationships between individual knowledge structures and the structure of a knowledge discipline. A major practical limitation is one concerned with designation of concepts to levels in a hierarchy.

As indicated in Section 2.3, there is value in use of concept maps and like devices for the structuring of a curriculum, or of a lesson. The seeking by a teacher of a clear structure for presentation in an instructional sequence is a necessary activity, and will be of most value when that structure is one that mirrors, at an appropriate level for the particular students, current understanding of the topic. So the seeking of a clear structure is not the problem. The limitation, particu-

larly in a research context, is inherent in a hierarchical representation of knowledge in which complex concepts, or complexes of concepts, are established in a superordinate/subordinate relationship. The concept complexes situated in the subordinate positions are, however, multilevel entities whose constituent parts often relate in a complex manner to the focus concept. As alluded to above, in practice this can mean that the structure being represented in a hierarchy must be accompanied by frequent qualifications that recognize the complexity, the high-level nature, of the entities being placed lower in the hierarchy. Gagne appears to have recognized this limitation in recent discussions of the nature of memory structures such as "schema" (Gagne and Glaser 1987).

Even though the hierarchy may not be a good model of memory organization, and so may be limited as a format for representation of psychological structure, the conventional concept map format, based on establishment of relationships between superordinate and subordinate concepts, may still be useful as a pedagogic device in early stages of use of concept maps. The establishment of a superordinate concept does provide a focus for consideration of relationships of a group of related terms to that focal element which may be easier for students to consider in initial stages of discussion. It seems that this may well be the position adopted by Novak in recent writing (e.g., Novak and Musonda 1991 p. 129). However, once the level of complexity of the representational format increases, the maintenance of a hierarchical format is difficult. It is relevant to note that not all researchers developing concept maps have insisted upon use of the hierarchical structure (Champagne and Klopfer 1981).

3.2 Scoring Concept Maps

One difficulty likely to attend use of concept maps in both classroom evaluation and research is the lack of a common method of scoring of concept maps. The significance of this difficulty can be overstated and it is not suggested that this difficulty is one that should cause teachers or researchers to avoid contact with the concept map. As a measuring instrument the concept map shares with all other instruments the need to provide a set of clear, valid, and consistent procedures that are appropriate for the occasion and which can be understood and applied in the same fashion by other users. The major problems associated with the scoring of concept maps are concerned with the reporting of these procedures in a manner that allows easy application in similar situations.

The basic structure of the concept map suggests a number of these procedures. If the central elements of the concept map are the concept and the relating link then the identification of the presence of concepts and of links suggests a basis for a first-level scoring system. Beyond this the scoring of features of the concept map becomes more complex as judgments are required about such qualities as the suitability of a link or of a label, and the appropriateness of the grouping of a set of concepts. In a research study the development and application of these procedures will require a significant amount of time. In the classroom informal judgments may be made more quickly, though the use of detailed procedures will also be time-consuming.

The scoring of the level structure within the hierarchy is advocated by Novak and Gowin (1984). What is not clear from their scoring procedure is what constitutes a *level*, and it is here that the hierarchy imposes what can be argued to be an artificial restriction on expression of relationships among related conceptual elements. The members of a list of concepts required to be related to a focal concept will not necessarily be intrinsically less general than the focal concept. In establishing these concepts in a network of relationships with the focal concept it seems unnecessary and artificial to insist on a hierarchical form of representation.

Related, but less serious, scoring problems arise in the identification of "segments" of a map, and in the establishment of the soundness of procedures used to justify the scoring of the quality of links within a segment and of those between segments. The problems in this case are regarded as being less serious because they are problems of definition and clarity that attend development of all measuring devices. Stewart (1979) provided an early discussion of the central issues of scoring of concept maps and other representational techniques, while Fisher (1990) has addressed many of these scoring issues in development of the semantic networking computer-based procedure. The scoring of complex relationships remains a challenge for the user of the Novak mapping procedure.

4. Conclusion

The concept map, in both a generic form and in the form developed by Novak, is of contemporary interest in education because the problem of representation tackled by Novak is of central concern to both teachers and researchers. Both groups wish to have access to sensitive indices of the nature of the understandings held by students that is associated with different levels of achievement. The growing body of research on the uses of concept maps by both groups attests to the importance of this need. A review of some of this research suggests that there is good reason to pursue investigation of the design and use of concept maps in order to increase the level of sensivity of the instrument.

References

Anderson J R 1990 *Cognitive Psychology and its Implications*, 3rd edn. W H Freeman, New York

Ausubel D P 1968 *Educational Psychology: A Cognitive View*. Holt, Rinehart and Winston, New York

Champagne A, Klopfer L 1981 *Using the ConSAT: A Memo to Teachers*. Reports to Educators No. R.T.E. 4. Learning Research and Development Center, University of Pittsburgh, Pittsburgh, Pennsylvania

Collins A, Quillian M R 1969 Retrieval from semantic memory. *J. Verbal Learn. Verbal Behav.* 8: 240–57

de Beaugrande R, Dressler W 1981 *Introduction to Text Linguistics*. Longman, New York

Fisher K 1990 Semantic networking: The new kid on the block. *J. Res. Sci. Teach.* 27(10): 1001–18.

Gagne R M 1968 Learning hierarchies. *Educ. Psychol.* 6: 1–9

Gagne R M, Glaser R 1987 Foundations in learning research. In: Gagne R M (ed.) 1987 *Instructional Technology: Foundations*. Erlbaum, Hillsdale, New Jersey

Greeno J 1983 Response to Phillips. *Educ. Psychol.* 18(2): 75–80

Heinze-Fry W, Novak J 1990 Concept mapping brings long-term movement toward meaningful learning. *Sci. Educ.* 74(4): 461–72

Jones B F, Pierce J, Hunter B 1988–89 Teaching students to construct graphic representations. *Educ. Leadership*, 46(4): 20–25

Kosslyn S 1989 Understanding charts and graphs. *Applied Cognitive Psychology* 3(3): 185–225

Lehman J, Carter C, Kahle J 1985 Concept mapping, vee mapping and achievement. *J. Res. Sci. Teach.* 22(7): 663–73

Mayer R, Gallini J 1990 When is an illustration worth ten thousand words. *J. Educ. Psychol.* 82(4): 715–26

Merrill M D, Gibbons A 1974 Heterarchies and their relationship to behavioral hierarchies for sequencing instruction. Paper presented at the Annual Convention of the American Educational Research Association, Chicago, April

Novak J 1990 Concept mapping: A useful device for science education. *J. Res. Sci. Teach.* 27(10): 937–49

Novak J, Gowin D B 1984 *Learning How to Learn*. Cambridge University Press, Cambridge

Novak J, Gowin D B, Johansen G 1983 The use of concept mapping and knowledge vee mapping with junior high school science students. *Sci. Educ.* 67(5): 625–45

Novak J, Musonda D 1991 A twelve-year longitudinal study of science concept learning. *Am. Educ. Res. J.* 28: 117–54

Okebukola P 1990 Attaining meaningful learning of concepts in genetics and ecology: An investigation of the potency of the concept mapping technique. *J. Res. Sci. Teach.* 27(5): 493–504

Pankratius W 1990 Building an organised knowledge base: Concept mapping and achievement in secondary school physics. *J. Res. Sci. Teach.* 27(4): 315–33

Phillips D C 1983 On describing a student's cognitive structure. *Educ. Psychol.* 18(2): 59–74

Prater D, Terry C 1988 Effects of mapping strategies on reading comprehension and writing performance. *Reading Psychology* 9(2): 101–20

Starr M, Krajcik J 1990 Concept maps as a heuristic for science curriculum development: Toward improvement in process and product. *J. Res. Sci. Teach.* 27(10): 987–1000

Stensvold M, Wilson J 1990 The interaction of verbal ability with concept mapping in learning from a chemistry laboratory activity. *Sci. Educ.* 74(4): 473–80

Stewart J 1979 Content and cognitive structure: Critique of assessment and representation techniques used by science education researchers. *Sci. Educ.* 63(3): 395–405

Thompson M 1992 Concept mapping and essay writing in

physics. Unpublished Master of Education thesis, School of Education, Flinders University of South Australia

Trochim W 1989 An introduction to concept mapping for planning and evaluation. *Evaluation and Program Planning* 12(1): 1–16

Wallace J, Mintzes J 1990 The concept map as a research tool: Exploring conceptual change in biology. *J. Res. Sci. Teach.* 27(10): 1033–52

Wandersee J 1990 Concept mapping and the cartography of cognition. *J. Res. Sc. Educ.* 27(10): 923–36

Willerman M, Mac-Harg R 1991 The concept map as an advance organiser. *J. Res. Sci. Teach.* 28(8): 705–12

Descriptive Data, Analysis of

J. P. Keeves and S. Sowden

Much of the evidence collected about educational processes is available in the form of published documents, transcripts of interviews, observations of practice, field notes, tape recordings of oral presentations, and written statements. Such data that are humanistic in nature are of considerable value. They are rich, personal, close to the real world, and contain a depth of meaning that more abstract forms of evidence lack. Nevertheless, substantial difficulties arise in educational research in the collection and examination of data in this form. While bodies of evidence of this kind can provide an understanding of educational phenomena and enable individuals to develop their own personal interpretations of the educational situations in which they work, there are significant problems involved in the assimilation of the evidence into the corpus of knowledge about education and its processes. The collection of such data is labor intensive, lasting sometimes many years. Furthermore, the analysis of the data is time consuming and sometimes very difficult because the evidence has been collected without a recognizable structure. Commonly, sampling has not been employed, and if representative or random sampling were attempted it had been abandoned as rich data became available from other sources. As a consequence the important question of the generalizability of the findings cannot be considered. Furthermore, in general, the procedures by which the evidence has been analyzed have not been reported or discussed.

Miles and Huberman (1984, 1994) have addressed these issues in important publications titled *Qualitative Data Analysis: A Sourcebook of New Methods*. They are specifically concerned with the generalizability of the findings derived from humanistic research and with the replicability of analyses of such data. They have advanced canons for the examination of evidence collected in research investigations that increase the consistency and robustness of the findings. Their proposals cut across the several areas of knowledge that contribute to humanistic research in education, namely the disciplines of sociology, history, law, political science, linguistics, psychology, and anthropology.

Miles and Huberman advance systematic procedures for the drawing of conclusions, testing the conclusions for consistency and coherence, and indeed simplifying the tasks of analyzing large bodies of humanistic data. They argue that in the reporting of research it is essential for the researcher to accept the responsibility of being accountable, and to present clearly a statement on the analytical procedures employed. However, such a strategy demands that there should be agreement about the appropriateness and strength of the particular procedures which have been used. Their practical sourcebook is a highly significant contribution to educational research. This entry draws extensively on their work.

The philosophical and epistemological foundations of Miles and Huberman's work have been subjected to criticism by Donmoyer (1985, 1986), to which Huberman and Miles (1986) have replied. However, in the face of the continuing debate (Gage 1989, Rizo 1991), this entry endorses the view that neither the scientific nor the humanistic research perspectives have a unique advantage and that there is an epistemological unity in educational research (Husén 1988, Keeves 1988). Furthermore, it is recognized that the hardline distinctions that are commonly made between quantitative and qualitative research methods are largely artificial. The difference between quantitative and qualitative data lies in the level of abstraction and the extent of simplification since, as Kaplan (1964 p. 207) has argued, "quantities are of qualities," and the claim that one method is antithetical or alternative to the other is misconceived

In addition, it is necessary to consider the view that all inquiry into educational questions is at least to some extent value-laden. Kaplan (1964) has examined the several ways in which values play a part in inquiry. There are implications for the replicability of the results of inquiry where another investigator with different values conducts a similar inquiry. Kaplan (1964) has also suggested that the only way to avoid subjective relativism in inquiry is to "face the valuations and to introduce them as explicitly stated, specific, and sufficiently concretized value premises." The problem is not whether values are involved in inquiry and whether it is possible to gain access to "reality" independently of values, but "how they are to be empirically grounded." This entry presents procedures

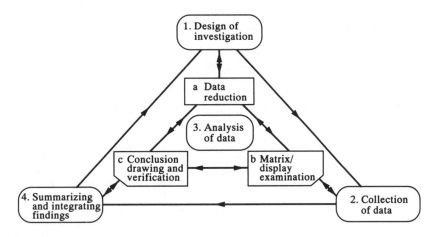

Figure 1
An interactive model of data analysis in humanistic studies

for building the findings of humanistic research studies on empirical evidence through the systematic analysis of the rich and varied data assembled.

1. Strategies of Analysis

The approach to data analysis using these procedures is characterized by strategies that employ both deduction and induction. These procedures are deductive insofar as some orientating constructs—informed by the prior knowledge, the experience, and the values of the investigator—have been put forward and operationalized and matched to a body of field data. This has the advantage of focusing and reducing the data that could be collected. Induction is employed insofar as the gathered data are used to modify and rebuild the original constructs. While deduction and induction are distinct and separate ideas, the difference between the deductive process and the inductive process becomes blurred when it is recognized that the conception of the orientating constructs, which were used in the process of deduction, were themselves a product of induction (Miles and Huberman). The interaction between deductive and inductive processes in the strategy of research where investigation is grounded in empirical evidence and the real world is a key characteristic of the procedures proposed by Miles and Huberman.

There are four major stages in this strategy of research into educational problems, namely: (a) design of investigation, (b) collection of data, (c) analysis of data, and (d) summarizing and integrating the findings. This entry is primarily concerned with the third of these stages: the analysis of data. However, insofar as analysis is dependent on design, collection, and integration, an account must be provided of these three other stages and of their influence and dependence on

the analysis of data. Miles and Huberman have identified three key components of data analysis, namely: (a) data reduction, (b) matrix display and examination, and (c) conclusion drawing and verification. This entry explores in some depth these three components of data analysis. Following Miles and Huberman, an interactive model is presented of the way in which the four stages of a research strategy interact with the three key components of data analysis listed above. In Fig. 1 the four stages and the three key components of data analysis form an interactive and cyclical process. As the research worker progresses through the four stages it is necessary for consideration to be given continuously to the analysis of the data and to the reduction, display, conclusion drawing, and verification components. The whole process is iterative as well as being interactive in a way that only successive iterations permit.

It is important to recognize that this model does not differ greatly from a model that could be constructed to represent the strategy employed in scientific research in education. The major difference is that scientific research commonly starts with a stronger knowledge base, and tends to proceed sequentially in well-defined stages, rather than in the interactive or iterative way that is characteristic of humanistic research, which is more fluid and has a weaker knowledge base. This entry seeks to elucidate the components of the model being advanced for the analysis of humanistic evidence, so that investigations conducted within this context can be more effectively studied.

2. Design of Investigations

The conventional views of both scientific and humanistic investigations in education are that the former involves a highly structured approach while the latter involves a minimal amount of prestructuring and a very loose design. On the one hand, scientific research is seen to involve an identified theoretical perspective, the use of standardized instruments, the testing of prespecified aspects of a conceptual framework, and a high degree of abstraction from the real world. On the other hand, humanistic research is seen to be building theory from observations of the real world, to be loosely structured, and to be very open-ended with respect to the collection of data. It is not surprising that neither description is appropriate. Most scientific research workers in education are more flexible than is suggested above. Likewise most investigators engaged in humanistic research now work somewhere between these two extremes. Humanistic research workers also recognize that a conceptual framework, at least in rudimentary form, is employed to guide an investigation, and that with little effort previous research can generally be found that would account conceptually for the phenomenon under investigation, even if it can not be classed as an established theory. It is this conceptual framework that serves to focus and restrict the collection of data as well as to guide the reduction and analysis of the evidence collected. Thus, those distinctions which are drawn between scientific and humanistic research, and between quantitative and qualitative research cease to be very useful, and much of what follows applies to both approaches.

A conceptual framework serves to describe and explain the major facets of an investigation. It identifies the key factors and the assumed relationships between them. It is not essential that such relationships should be causal. They may simply involve sequences which occur over time, or alternatively there may merely be a pattern in the events or between the factors being observed. If such patterns or time sequences in relationships or causal connections are not assumed to be present, then it is unlikely that the factors being investigated will hold much interest for the research worker. The conceptual framework commonly attempts to state in diagrammatic or narrative form these factors and the relationships between them. Use is made of this conceptual framework in the design of a study. First, it identifies who and what will be examined. Second, it postulates relationships between the persons and the factors being investigated. Such presumed relationships can influence the order in which information is assembled and the type of information collected, as well as the extent of detail obtained.

The conceptual framework also provides a map for the research worker of the field being investigated. Miles and Huberman have made several suggestions with regard to developing a conceptual framework: (a) use a diagrammatical rather than a narrative format; (b) expect to revise the framework successively; (c) encourage each research worker in a team to develop a separate framework, and compare the different versions; (d) avoid a global level of generality that is not specific enough to provide focus and identify bounds, and is not so general that it cannot be proved wrong;

and (e) employ prior theorizing and previous empirical research to test the framework.

Once the framework has been developed it can be used for formulating specific research questions. The process of deduction is commonly involved. Many research workers engaged in humanistic studies reject this step. However, the development of their ideas, while latent and implicit, commonly uses similar processes. Such investigators should be challenged to make as explicit as possible their thought processes. The research questions advanced for a study require successive refinements. Priorities need to be proposed, and the number of questions to which answers are being sought need to be reduced to a manageable size.

Once the research questions have been identified, the collection of evidence must be preceded by identifying cases to be studied. A multi-case design addresses the same research questions in a number of settings using similar data collection and analysis procedures in each setting. It seeks to permit cross-case comparison without sacrificing within-case understanding (Herriott and Firestone 1983). This design rejects the preoccupation with an instance and in contrast concentrates on comparison and generalization across the cases studied (Stenhouse 1983). Some form of sampling is generally involved. One of the great dangers in research is to sample too many cases. The number of cases is limited both by the amount of data that can be processed and by the costs involved. It would seem from experience that 15–20 cases is the maximum amount of evidence that one person can work with for a detailed nonstatistical analysis. Where more cases have been involved in humanistic studies, it is not unusual for much of the available information to be cast aside and only evidence from up to 15–20 cases to be used, at least in the detailed reporting of the study. Alternatively, the research draws on the cases selectively to reduce data complexity or quantify the data from all cases using rigorous coding schemes to allow formal statistical models to be employed in carrying out cross-case analysis. With between 15 and 30 cases statistical methods of analysis can be readily employed, through the use of contingency table analysis and the Fisher Exact Test. Parametric statistical procedures are commonly used where the number of cases is in excess of 30.

Even with up to 15 cases some basis for sampling of cases must be employed, whether the cases are typical, exemplar, random, extreme, innovative, or simply the most accessible. The extent to which the findings can be generalized beyond the single case depends on the basis upon which the cases were selected and the relationship between the selected cases and a wider population. It is important to recognize that sampling can occur of settings, events, and processes as well as of people. In the long term the major constraints on the number of cases to be studied are those of time and cost. Balance must be achieved between the research questions, time, cost, the complexity of the investigation, the number of research workers available to assist, and the number of cases selected.

The extent to which instrumentation is employed likewise depends on the research questions being asked, the number of research workers engaged in the data collection phase, and the level of clarity of the conceptual framework. Arguments can be advanced for both little or no prior instrumentation and for detailed instrumentation. However, failure to develop a conceptual framework, or to identify appropriate research questions, or to construct suitable instruments should not be justified on the grounds of lack of time or lack of effort. Advanced planning usually pays.

3. Data Collection

Miles and Huberman have argued that the preliminary analysis of data should proceed concurrently with the collection of data so that the phase of data collection merges with that of data analysis. There are two important reasons for this. First, there is the very real danger of assembling such a huge amount of evidence that the analysis becomes an overwhelming task. This not only jeopardizes the completion of the work associated with the analysis phase of the investigation, and in some cases has been known to lead to the termination of a study, but more commonly reduces the quality of the work carried out. A second advantage of undertaking the analysis concurrently with the collection of data is both that gaps in the data become apparent, and new hypotheses and relationships emerge before it is too late to collect relevant data. Third, an understanding of the evidence, which commonly takes time to grow, benefits from the longer period available. Sometimes ongoing analysis permits the preparation of an interim report that is reassuring for the client and facilitates the flow of funding for the study.

It is of value to prepare an overall tabular plan for the collection of data to show which items of data are going to be obtained through each particular stage in the inquiry. To some extent such a table serves also as a checklist to ensure that each item of information required for the investigation is collected in the most appropriate way.

It is also important to maintain detailed documented records of the data collected and Miles and Huberman suggest the use of the following forms.

(a)   A contact summary form. This should be used to record the information associated with each contact made in the collection of data, such as an interview with an evaluator or client. In addition, this form would also record memoranda and information of importance to the study which should be noted as they arise.

(b)   A document summary form. This should be employed to maintain a concise record of all documents which are obtained such as newspaper articles, correspondence, agendas and minutes of meetings that provide background information of relevance to the investigation. The documents are often bulky and must be filed separately. However, a file summary, which indicates clearly the relevance of the document to the investigation as well as the location of the document, is of considerable assistance as the volume of such material grows during the course of the study.

(c)   Field notes. These should be compiled daily, if possible, on a standard form and inserted in a looseleaf folder to record information of relevance to the investigation. Such notes are additional to an interview schedule, observation schedule, or tape recording of an interview and serve to record key items of information that are obtained or observed independently of the interview or observation period. Commonly these field notes can contain reflective remarks that arise from watching a situation or talking to people linked to the evaluator or the client. A distinction must be made between the raw field notes, which are rough scribblings and jottings, and the permanent notes that could be read by any reviewer of the work. The permanent notes are more than a sum of the raw notes. They contain reflections and commentary on issues that emerge from a consideration of the raw notes.

(d)   Memos. These are an important additional source of ideas. Field work and coding are absorbing tasks. However, the very intensity of these stages of an investigation frequently gives rise to new and original ideas, which if not recorded in some way as they occur, are lost. The most effective procedure is to have available a standard memorandum form on which these ideas can be recorded as they arise. Probably some sifting of such memoranda is required at a later stage, if a large number are produced. Of particular importance among the memos that are written are ones relating to propositions or relationships to be examined in the course of the investigation.

(e)   Data accounting sheets. These are an essential documentary record of progress on a particular question. If possible the data collected should be related as closely as possible to the major research questions, or if this is not possible, to the areas of the investigation linked to the research questions. On the data accounting sheet a record should be maintained of whether or not a particular source of data relevant to a research question or an area of inquiry has been collected.

4. Analysis of Data

The analysis of the data collected in a study passes through three interrelated stages, namely: data reduction, data display, and conclusion drawing and verification. As already mentioned in an earlier section of this entry these stages are not necessarily sequential, but may form part of an iterative process. Nevertheless, unless the stages are seen as separate there is the danger that they can merge to such an extent that the tasks associated with each are not examined or adequately planned. Each of these three stages is considered in turn.

4.1 Data Reduction

The primary task in data reduction is that of coding the interview record, the observation record, or the document. In order to code evidence obtained by these data collection procedures two approaches are available: the use of key words, or a numerical classification system, which may or may not involve a taxonomy. The development of a taxonomy requires considerable effort in advance of the coding, as well as a detailed understanding of the field. The use of key words has greater flexibility on the surface, but is likely to become complex and confusing unless careful initial planning has occurred. A pilot run through a reduced sample of the evidence, or preferably a pilot study with perhaps three to six cases, should be carried out in order to develop the key words or the taxonomy. The major danger in the development of a numerical coding system or a key word system is that the system will lack the structure necessary to use it systematically in the detailed examination of data. A further relevant aspect is the identification of important quotes that could be used in the reporting of the study. It is common in presenting the findings of an investigation to rely on telling quotes to make an important point and to convince the reader of the report. The process of data reduction should include a starring of codes or key words so that appropriate quotes related to a particular idea or relationship can be readily identified.

One of the most difficult items of evidence to summarize is the taped interview. The use of a tape recording of an interview permits the interviewer to conduct the interview in a relatively relaxed way, without concern that key points are lost. There is, however, always the danger that the interviewee withholds comment because a permanent record is being made. In addition to this, the reduction of the data held on a tape recording poses substantial problems. At one time when taped interview records were less commonly used, it was possible to recommend that each interview record should be typed and hard copy obtained. Today this involves a prohibitive cost for most investigations and procedures have to be employed that minimize cost and yet achieve effective coding of the available evidence.

A suggested set of procedures is described below.

(a) While listening to a tape, a summary of each point made by the interviewee is recorded. These summaries involve paraphrasing responses and are sometimes accompanied by transcriptions of relevant quotations.

(b) A set of key words is developed from the first six interviews that can be used to summarize and reduce further the evidence held. The structure for the key word system is built around the structure of the interview, which is planned in advance.

(c) In order to access the information held both on tape and in the point-to-point summaries, a key word is placed in the left-hand margin of the pages of the summary to provide a reference to the content of each point made in the interview.

(d) In order to access quickly the source material on a tape, the tape counter numbers, giving that section of the tape within which each point is made, are recorded in a second column adjacent to each key word.

(e) Once an interview is coded in the above way, a summary of the themes occurring in the interview is made. The summary is built around the planned structure of the interview.

(f) The interview summaries are examined for inconsistencies, and systematic checks with the tape recording are made to confirm or resolve the inconsistencies.

(g) A summary of the views and perspectives of each interview is prepared and returned to the interviewee with a request to confirm the record that was obtained and where necessary to resolve observed inconsistencies. In this way each interviewee is provided with an opportunity to verify information that is being carried forward to the next stage in the process of analysis.

This sequence of steps, while time-consuming and laborious, ensures that the research worker has assimilated thoroughly the views of each interviewee, and in the processes of condensation and assimilation has not, in an unwarranted way, distorted the evidence provided by the interviewee.

It is important to note that the research worker is not limited to using the information contained in the summary that has been verified by the interviewee. However, the confirmation given by the interviewee, or the correction provided, is evidence that in summarizing the tape recordings significant distortion of the data has not occurred.

In addition, to provide a further check on the reliability of the coding procedures employed, a second person should code a sample of taped interviews using the methods outlined above. The reliability of the coding procedures is estimated using the following formula:

$$\text{Reliability} = \frac{\text{Number of agreements}}{\text{Total number of agreements and disagreements}}$$

A level of intercoder reliability of 80 percent should

be sought. The criteria for agreement are that each of the following three conditions has to be met: (a) the same section of a taped interview is considered to represent a point; (b) for each point summarized the same key word selected from the final listing of key words is used by both coders; and (c) the two summaries of each point have the same meaning.

4.2 Matrix Display and Examination

The use of a matrix display is a valuable procedure for summarizing information so that patterns are evident in a form that can subsequently be used in the presentation of results. Success in the use of a matrix display lies not in whether a "true" or "correct" matrix has been developed, but in whether the use of a matrix display has served the function of providing answers to a research question being asked. Miles and Huberman have listed the key features of a matrix display as well as a set of rules for matrix construction.

The key features of a matrix display are concerned with choices made during the design of a matrix that are associated with ways of partitioning the data.

(a) The first feature relates to whether the matrix has a descriptive or explanatory purpose, and whether an attempt is being made to lay out the data in a manner that might reveal a pattern in the data, or in a way that shows why things happen.

(b) The matrix can be constructed to show relationships within a single case or across cases involved in a study.

(c) The matrix consists of rows and columns and can be constructed in such a way that the categories employed in the rows and columns are ordered or nonordered. Once the development of a matrix has proceeded beyond the initial stages of describing the evidence, it would seem likely that some ordering of categories would be required.

(d) A special case of ordering the information contained in the rows and columns is associated with time ordering. Time sequences are involved in temporal flow, causal chains, or cycles of events.

(e) Sometimes a matrix is constructed with the categories of a particular variable along one axis. Alternatively social units may be placed along an axis where the units commonly used are: students, classrooms, schools, school districts, state systems, and a national system.

(f) The most commonly used matrix is the two-way grid. However, it is sometimes necessary to construct a three-way or four-way matrix, although the latter is hard to use and present. A three-way matrix can be shown diagrammatically by subdividing each column in a parallel fashion, and a four-way matrix can also be shown diagrammatically

by subdividing each row in a similar manner. The pattern involved in the data is usually lost, by using more than a four-way matrix. Greater clarity can be gained by breaking the data down into submatrices.

(g) Furthermore, a choice is available with respect to what is recorded in each cell. Commonly an identifying code is recorded that refers to each case, but sometimes direct quotes or extracts from field notes can be recorded.

(h) Finally, if the set of key words has been carefully developed, or if the taxonomy associated with numerical coding is appropriate, then these coding systems are naturally associated with the categories that are employed in matrix displays.

Miles and Huberman (1984) have advanced nine rules of thumb for the building of matrix displays: (a) keep each display on one large sheet; (b) restrict the number of categories used in each row or column to the range 5 to 15; (c) plan to use a preliminary form of a matrix display and to revise it several times before constructing a final form; (d) encourage members of the research team to develop alternative ways of displaying data in a matrix; (e) transpose rows and columns where appropriate; (f) collapse the categories of a complex matrix, since a reduced form sometimes reveals clearer patterns; (g) be prepared to add new rows and new columns at all times; (h) maintain fine-grained rows and columns so that important differences in the data can be shown; and (i) remember that a particular research question may require a series of matrix displays and be ready to try additional forms.

The development of appropriate matrix displays is an art in research that is acquired with practice and with increased depth of understanding of the issues involved. Miles and Huberman also suggest certain rules of thumb for recording entries in a matrix display so that detail is not lost and yet patterns that exist in the data emerge. In addition, they propose rules for examining a matrix display. It is important to recognize that the tasks of summarizing and of entry of data into a matrix display serve to make the investigator thoroughly familiar with the data, so that some interrelationships between factors operating in the data are held in mind and new relationships emerge. The development of a matrix display thus serves several purposes of familiarization, testing of relationships, providing a basis for speculation on new relationships, and a form of presentation of findings to the reader of a report. Ultimately the purpose of matrix display is the identification of a pattern and the provision of an explanation.

4.3 Conclusion Drawing and Verifying

The crucial stage in the analysis of the data is the drawing of conclusions and the verification of the conclusions. Miles and Huberman have identified 12 tactics for deriving meaning from evidence. The important issue at this stage in the analysis of the data is not one of whether meaning can be found in the evidence available, however chaotic the evidence might seem, but rather whether or not the conclusion is soundly drawn from the evidence available. The checks that can be applied in the drawing of conclusions are whether the results can be presented in a meaningful way to the reader of a research report and whether another person analyzing the same body of evidence would draw the same conclusions. In addition, there is the important question as to whether the research worker is entitled to claim generality for the conclusions beyond the particular body of data that was collected. While the tactics for the deriving of conclusions differ from those of verifying meaning, eliminating possible bias, and confirming the generality of the findings, it is evident that the processes of derivation and verification are interrelated.

4.4 Tactics for Deriving Meaning

(a) Counting. There is a tendency among some research workers to reject counting the number of instances for which a relationship is observed or an event occurs. However, to ignore a count is to overlook the most obvious data. Whether a simple test should be applied to verify that a pattern is unlikely to occur by chance could become more controversial, particularly if little can be said about the nature and quality of the sample.

(b) Noting patterns and themes. Commonly in textural reports or matrix displays recurring patterns of results are quickly seen. A real danger is that of not remaining open to evidence that disconfirms the pattern.

(c) Imputing plausibility. Once a particular result or specific pattern of results has been observed, there is commonly a need on the part of the investigator to consider the plausibility of the result or pattern. The question is asked as to whether the result "makes good sense." There is a very real danger that once a result has been observed, justification will be found, plausibiity is imputed, and the finding is accepted without further checking.

(d) Clustering. Humanistic research lends itself to classifying and clustering events and people into groups. The use of matrix displays greatly facilitates simple clustering. It should be recognized that the outlier or exceptional case can help to provide an understanding of the manner in which a naturally occurring cluster is formed. As a consequence both the outliers and the typical cases should be studied in detail.

(e) Using metaphors. At the analysis stage of an investigation and prior to the reporting of results it can be of considerable value for the researcher to think about the available evidence in terms of metaphors.

The use of analogies and metaphorical thinking not only provides a means for writing a report in an interesting and lively way, but also provides a valuable tactic for seeing through a morass of detail in order to detect new and different perspectives. There is of course the danger for the research worker of developing an analogue ahead of the evidence and failing to test the underlying idea or relationship adequately against the data. Thus "premature closure" of this kind should be avoided. The wisest approach is to seek opportunities to discuss ideas both formally and informally in order to test out such ideas with both colleagues and critics.

(f) Splitting categories. In the planning of the coding and the analysis of the data, categories can be formed that collect a very high proportion of the cases. Classification schemes that fail to discriminate between cases serve little useful purpose. Efforts should be made in such circumstances to use the available evidence, as well as further data that might be obtained to subdivide the category and the associated cases into groups that could add meaning to the analyses and lead to the detection of an important relationship.

(g) Combining categories. The converse to splitting categories is also important. Where there are too few cases in certain categories, these categories serve little purpose in the task of cross-classification. If categories can be combined so that the distribution of cases across categories is more balanced, then it is more likely that meaningful patterns and relationships are observed.

(h) Composition. It is common to include factors in a study that are either conditionally related or have elements in common. There is a danger that the use of too many factors that have fine distinctions between them leads to loss of meaning. The solution is to combine factors and the categories within those factors by procedures of union of sets of elements or intersection of sets of elements in order to form new factors that have greater meaning.

(i) Noting relations. An important step in the analysis of evidence is to examine factors that vary directly (i.e., both increase) or indirectly (i.e., one increases while the other decreases) together. The large amount of evidence which is collected in a humanistic study makes the identification of such relationships extremely difficult. Nevertheless, if the number of likely relationships is restricted on logical grounds then a systematic search is likely to yield valuable results.

(j) Finding mediating factors. It is not uncommon for factors at the beginning and the end of a chain to be found to be related. Such a relationship, while of interest, provides little understanding of the influence of factors that mediate between the two linked concepts. A search for mediating factors might provide the link in a chain of evidence.

(k) Building a logical chain of evidence. The preceding tactic concerned with searching for a factor that is mediated within a logical chain, and this tactic initiates the development of a related chain of factors such that the prior members of the chain are related in a logical way to the subsequent members of the chain.

(l) Constructing a causal chain. A causal chain of factors not only involves a logical sequence as is sought in the preceding two tactics, but also involves a temporal sequence. Since earlier events influence later events and not vice versa the construction of a causal chain must of necessity be governed by a strict time sequence between the operation of the factors in the chain. The evidence might provide tentative support for the existence of mediating factors, logical chains, and causal chains and might indicate whether a link between adjacent factors is present. To proceed beyond a tentative finding requires the employment of related theory, rather than the assembling of further evidence collected from a natural setting and linked in a meaningful way in the concluding stages of an investigation. The approach advanced here is that of induction from the evidence, rather than deduction from theory, although as suggested earlier the processes may not be formally distinguishable in the search for meaning.

5. Confirming Findings

The dangers associated with the pondering over large bodies of evidence are that, while striking relationships may be suggested which are strong in analogy and clearly presented using metaphor, they run the risk of being incomplete, inadequate, and possibly wrong. Another investigator examining the same body of evidence, but without perhaps the same extent of total immersion in the data, may be unable to detect the relationships reported. Alternatively, a research worker investigating the same or similar cases may advance radically different findings. Similar problems arise in studies that employ statistical procedures. However, researchers using nonstatistical methods have, in general, not addressed the question of how to ensure that their findings are replicable and robust, and how to convince other researchers that the tactics they have employed are sound in these respects. Miles and Huberman have identified some of the common sources of error in developing conclusions. These sources of error are listed below.

(a) The holistic fallacy involves ignoring the outlier cases and erratic strands so that events are interpreted as more patterned and with greater congruence than they actually possess.

(b) Elite bias involves giving greater credence to the opinions of high status, articulate respondents than to lower status, less articulate ones.

(c) "Going native" involves accepting the perceptions and explanations of events advanced by the respondents being studied without bringing scholarship and experience in investigation to bear on the work of inquiry.

Miles and Huberman have also advanced 12 tactics that are useful for confirming findings:

(a) Checking the investigation for representativeness. This tactic seeks to avoid the pitfalls of sampling nonrepresentative respondents, observing nonrepresentative events, and drawing inferences from nonrepresentative processes. Nonetheless, it must be recognized that the exceptional case can sometimes reveal more than can be seen from the uniformity of all the representative cases. These dangers are overcome by: (i) searching deliberately for contrasting cases; (ii) sorting the cases into categories in a systematic way; (iii) sampling randomly from within a total universe; and (iv) increasing the number of cases being studied.

(b) Checking for researcher effects. This tactic seeks to diminish in every way possible the influence that the intrusion of an investigator into the situation being studied may have. It is important to recognize that not only may the researcher influence the situation being investigated, but the situation may also have an effect on the perceptions of the researcher in ways that may introduce bias. These problems may be avoided by: (i) spending more time at the site of the investigation; (ii) using unobtrusive observation procedures; (iii) coopting the assistance of an informant to report on the effects of the researcher on the situation being studied; (iv) making sure that misinformation about the investigation does not contaminate the research; (v) undertaking interviews off the site in order to examine the effects the place of interview may have; (vi) reducing emphasis on the role of the investigator; (vii) guarding against identifiable sources of bias (e.g., the holistic fallacy, elite bias, and going native); (viii) avoiding undue concern for individuals by thinking conceptually; (ix) trying to sense if deliberate attempts are being made to mislead; (x) keeping research questions in mind; (xi) discussing field notes with another experienced researcher; and (xii) avoiding the effects on the respondent of knowledge about the issues being investigated.

(c) Triangulation. This involves a range of procedures that the research worker can use to increase the strength of observation. There are four types of triangulation: (i) methodological triangulation which involves the use of more than one method to obtain evidence; (ii) theory triangulation which involves the use of more than one theoretical perspective in the interpretation of phenomena; (iii) investigator triangulation which involves the use of more than one observer; and (iv) data triangulation which involves replication of the investigation in time, in location, or with another sample of persons. The use of more than one method of triangulation is both costly and time-consuming. However, if the issues under investigation are of sufficient importance then the costs of time and money are no doubt worth the increased strength of the findings provided by extensive triangulation (see *Triangulation in Educational Research*).

(d) Weighting the evidence. This is a tactic that can be employed to make allowance for the fact that some data are stronger and other data are more suspect. In order to employ differential weighting of evidence, it is necessary to identify clearly the assessed strength of the data, preferably at the time of collection. This would involve the keeping of a running log on data quality issues and the preparation of a clear summary of information on the relative quality of different items of evidence. There are significant dangers involved in the weighting of data unless it is undertaken on well-argued and rational grounds.

(e) Making contrasts and comparisons. This is a sound tactic for drawing conclusions and presenting results. Contrasts can be made between persons, cases, groups, roles, activities, and sites. However, it is important that the units being compared or contrasted should be identified in some way that is not directly related to the data to be used in the comparisons. Moreover, it is necessary to recognize in advance the extent of a difference that is worthy of consideration.

(f) Examining the outlier case. This is a tactic that can reveal information which would otherwise remain hidden. The temptation is to ignore the outlier and seek uniformity, yet understanding can result from the search for reasons as to why the extreme case has occurred. Outlier cases are not just exceptional people, but can include atypical situations, unique treatments, uncommon events, and unusual sites. Once these exceptional cases have been identified, the characteristics that make them exceptional should be investigated and an explanation as to why the exception has arisen should be sought.

(g) Using the exceptional case to account for regularity. This is the complementary side of identifying, examining, and explaining the outlier. The exceptional case should be seen as not only telling much about itself but also telling something about the group from which it has been drawn.

(h) Searching for a spurious relationship. This tactic is often rewarding. While two factors might be seen to be related in a way that could be interpreted as causal, establishing the existence of a third factor which influences both, commonly leads to a rejection of the causal nature of the observed relationship.

(i) Replicating a finding. Conducting a further separate study or providing an opportunity for an independent investigator to re-examine the available evidence is an important tactic in research, where generality is sought. As indicated above, the exceptional case or the outlier can be of considerable value. However, it is also important to distinguish between those cases where regularities are present and where a nomothetic dimension exists, and those cases which are unique and where and where an idiographic dimension is involved.

(j) Checking out rival explanations. This is an important step in developing a full understanding. While it is important to search for a reasoned explanation of an event or problematic situation, it is also necessary to advance alternative explanations and if possible to resolve between the two or more explanations that have been proposed. Evidence that would help determine which of two alternative explanations is more coherent must be considered to be critical. A greater contribution to understanding is achieved by a resolution between two rival explanations than by merely confirming a well-held explanation or established result. However, confirmation is in itself of consequence.

(k) Looking for negative evidence. This is a useful tactic since it extends the approaches of examining outlier cases, using the exceptional case, and testing out a rival explanation. The search for evidence that could disconfirm an established result can provide opportunities for the development of understanding, whether or not the pursuit of negative evidence is successful. The failure to find negative evidence after a deliberate search does not and cannot establish the "truth" of a result. However, it does increase the probability that the original result is sound.

(l) Getting feedback from respondents. This can provide understanding of both the events being studied and the interpretation or explanation provided for the events. This tactic involves confronting réspondents with emerging theoretical explanations of events and inviting them to report on the validity of the explanations with respect to their knowledge and understanding. The purpose is not one of counting heads to indicate support or rejection of a particular explanation, but rather to obtain additional evidence, to provide new insights, and to learn more about the problematic situation under investigation. Only if the procedures of participant verification are carefully and deliberately planned, with key findings clearly presented together with coherent interpretations of the findings, are the participants able to contribute in a meaningful way.

6. Summarizing and Integrating the Findings

Whereas standard procedures have been developed for the writing of theses, research reports, and journal articles that record the conduct and present the findings of research conducted from a scientific perspective, in the reporting of humanistic research such procedures have not been developed. The dangers are that while an increasing amount of such research is being carried out, either it is not being reported or it is being reported in a way that the research cannot be audited and the conclusions cannot be verified. This gives rise to the anomalous situation that while the evidence is rich and detailed, the very richness and detail of the data collected prevent presentation in a coherent form that would lead to acceptance of the findings as a contribution to scholarly inquiry.

There are few agreed-upon procedures or established conventions for the reporting of humanistic research. As a consequence, the quality of such research cannot be verified because information on the methods employed is lacking. Furthermore, because of the detail in the data, the reports that are prepared are lengthy and time-consuming to read, and as a result the findings from such studies are quickly lost in the growing volume of published research.

There are two important aspects of reporting research. The first involves the presentation of the findings of the research, the second involves reporting on the methods that were employed in the conduct of the research and the analysis of evidence collected. Research in education, irrespective of the nature of the data assembled, is part of the ongoing work of contributing to and building a body of knowledge about educational processes as well as providing guidance for policy-making and practice. Thus any specific piece of research makes contributions, first to theory about educational processes, second to educational practice, and third to the planning of further investigatory activity. It would seem important that, if possible, each of these three aspects should be addressed in the preparation of a report. Nonetheless, the reader of a research report is initially interested in grasping the key findings of the investigation, before examining other aspects relating to theory, practice, and further inquiry.

Two tactics can be suggested to assist in the presentation of the findings of research. After the development of a logical sequence or alternatively a causal chain of factors, it can be of value to present this information in diagrammatic form where a path diagram or schematic model is used to portray the relationships. The path diagram possesses the characteristics of a model in a form that assists comprehension of both the known constructs and their interrelations, and gives rise to the generation of further constructs and relationships that might be examined. Similarly a schematic model is like a map that links the products of analysis and the real world.

A second tactic that is of value in the presentation of results is the formulation of propositions. These propositions can enter into a report in two ways. First, in the opening chapters where a conceptual framework is discussed, propositions can be advanced that can guide the collection and the analysis of data, in a similar way to research questions. Furthermore, in the drawing of conclusions attention can again turn to the propositions stated at the beginning of a study and they can be examined or tested with the evidence available. A second alternative approach involves the developing of a set of propositions using inductive processes and based upon the conclusions that are drawn from the analysis of evidence. In this use the propositions serve to summarize the findings in a form the can be readily comprehended by the reader and tested in subsequent investigations. They provide a clear and concise focus for both the reporter and the reader to use in identifying what a particular investigation has shown.

A further important task involved in the reporting of an investigation that makes use of nonstatistical procedures is the provision of a clear and concise account of how the data were analyzed. Guba and Lincoln (1981) refer to the provision of this type of information as an audit trail. The idea is that another investigator should be able to follow the audit trail step by step in order to verify the procedures employed in the analysis of the data. Miles and Huberman have developed a documentation form for use by research workers to record the procedures used to analyze the data. A separate form is employed for each specific research question. The researcher is required to summarize on the form "what the analysis of the research question was designed to do." The researcher also records on the form the procedural steps taken, the decision rules employed, and the operations of analysis involved in the examination of data with respect to the specific research questions. The form requires at the end a summary of what the analysis found.

The amount of detail included on a form is determined by the nature of the analyses carried out. Miles and Huberman indicate that for the detailed examination of a research question, commonly seven or eight steps are involved and each step or episode requires approximately a page in order to summarize the information. They also suggest that the forms should be completed concurrently with the conduct of the analyses. The use of the form also indicates to the research worker the extent and manner in which the analytical techniques are employed on a specific analytical task. Where too great a reliance is made on a very limited number of analytical techniques the researcher should deliberately seek to increase the range of procedures employed. Miles and Huberman indicate that the completion of the standard form requires something of the order of 20 percent of the time necessary to analyze the data with respect to a particular research question. While these audit procedures are time-consuming to employ, they form part of a deliberate attempt to develop standard procedures for the analysis of data in humanistic research on which consensus might be achieved.

See also: Research in Education: Epistemological Issues; Scientific Methods in Educational Research; Research Paradigms in Education

References

Donmoyer R 1985 The rescue from relativism: Two failed attempts and an alternative strategy. *Educ. Res.* 14(10): 13–20

Donmoyer R 1986 The problem of language in empirical research: A rejoinder to Miles and Huberman. *Educ. Res.* 15(3): 26–27

Gage N L 1989 The paradigm wars and their aftermath: A historical sketch of research on teaching since 1989. *Educ. Researcher* 18(7): 4–10

Guba E G, Lincoln Y S 1981 *Effective Evaluation.* Jossey Bass, San Francisco, California

Herriott R E, Firestone W A 1983 Multi-site qualitative policy research: Optimizing description and generalizability. *Educ. Researcher* 12(2): 14–19

Husén T 1988 Research paradigms in education. *Interchange* 19(1): 2–13

Huberman A M, Miles M B 1986 Concepts and methods in qualitative research: A reply to Donmoyer. *Educ. Res. 15(3)*: 25–26

Kaplan A 1964 *The Conduct of Inquiry.* Chandler, San Francisco, California

Keeves J P 1988 The unity of educational research. *Interchange* 19(1): 14–30

Miles M B, Huberman A M 1984 *Qualitative Data Analysis: A Sourcebook of New Methods.* Sage, Newbury Park, California

Miles M B Huberman A M 1994 *Qualitative Data Analysis: A Sourcebook of New Methods* 2nd edn. Sage, Newbury Park, California

Rizo F M 1991 The controversy about quantification in social research education: An extension of Gage's 'historial' sketch. *Educ. Researcher* 20(9): 9–12

Stenhouse L 1983 School Report: A multi-site case study programme. *Case Study Methods 3*, 2nd edn. Deaking University Press, Geelong Victoria

Further Reading

Denzin N K, Lincoln Y S 1994 *Handbook of Qualitative Research.* Sage, Thousand Oaks, California

Fetterman D M 1989 *Ethnography: Step by Step.* Applied Social Research Methods Series. Vol. 17. Sage, Newbury Park, California

Gladwin C H 1989 *Ethnographic Decision Tree Modeling.* Qualitative Research Methods Series. Vol. 19, Sage Newbury Park, California

Guba E G 1978 *Toward a Methodology of Naturalistic Inquiry in Educational Evaluation.* CSE Monograph Series in Evaluation 8. Center for the Study of Evaluation, UCLA, Los Angeles, California

Quine W V O, Ullian J S 1978 *The Web of Belief*, 2nd edn. Random House, New York

Weitzman E A, Miles M B 1995 *Computer Programs for Qualitative Data Analysis.* Sage, Thousand Oaks, California

Interviewing for Clinical Research

D. M. Keats

Interviewing is used extensively in education for both selection and clinical research. Interviews are frequently employed as the sole means of obtaining information but may also be supplemented by test scores, written reports, and behavioral data.

Selection interviewing is used for selecting staff at all levels; for selecting winners of honors and scholarships; for conducting oral examinations; for determining suitability for entry to various courses, schools, and colleges; for awarding traineeships and apprenticeships; and for assessing would-be immigrants. Selection interviews may be conducted on a one-to-one basis or by an interviewing panel. In some situations the interviewees are assembled in one place to interact with each other while in other cases the interviewee is alone in facing the interviewer or the panel. The dynamics of these situations differ, with consequent effects on potential sources of bias, and on the relationships between interviewer and respondents.

Interviewing in clinical research may be of two types: (a) research interviewing, which uses methods based on individual interviewing with structured interview schedules and probing; (b) research interviewing, based on interviews with clients in counseling or psychotherapy. Interviewing of the first type is frequently found in psychological, educational, anthropological, and sociological research.

Perhaps the most well-known interviewing method is the one that was used by Piaget in which the child's reasoning was explored by intensive questioning. Piaget called this the "clinical method"—this is the sense in which the term is used in this type of research interviewing. Interviewing of the second type is found in research on the efficacy of different methods of counseling and treatment and in diagnostic assessment. Both types are almost exclusively of the one-to-one kind. This entry is concerned with the nature of the interviewing process, how interviews are structured, effective interviewing techniques, the control of bias, the training of interviewers, and the treatment of interview data in research.

1. The Interview: A Complex and Dynamic Process

An interview is a controlled conversation in which the interviewer obtains information from the respondent.

Usually the conversation takes the form of a series of questions asked by the interviewer of the respondent. The mode of interaction is essentially verbal, but nonverbal messages are also present and need to be interpreted along with the verbal elements of the interaction. Complex cognitive, affective, and social processes are involved in the interviewing situation.

Interviews are dynamic situations as both the interviewer and the respondent react to the questions and their answers and to each other. Relationships may change as the interview progresses. The need to maintain consistency in research interviewing means that particular attention must be paid to the control of bias.

In selection interviews the main factors that can produce bias and therefore affect the outcome are the roles of interviewers, the nonverbal factors (including the interviewee's appearance), the influence of verbal fluency over content, the structural properties of the interview, and the use of additional materials supplementary to the interview.

In clinical research, interviewing factors to which special attention must be paid are the relationship between interviewer and respondent; the structure of the interview schedule; the development of skills of listening, probing, and empathy; the control of bias; training of interviewers; and the coding, scoring, and analysis of the responses.

Cognitive skills involved in interviewing are understanding, concept development, reasoning, memory, and interpretation. Verbal skills require attention to pitch, speed of delivery, phrasing, clarity of pronunciation and fluency, and the ability to express ideas in a variety of language styles and with differing levels of abstraction or complexity according to the requirements of the topic and the abilities of the respondent. Listening skills are attentiveness and active construing of the meaning and intention of the respondent, and the ability to refrain from interrupting the flow and to wait until pauses occur. Nonverbal skills are the ability to interpret facial expressions and body positions. Social skills are cultural sensitivity: that is, the ability to interact with respondents who are different from the interviewer and at times displeasing in manners, appearance, and responses. Effective processes encourage the need to be accepted and create favorable rapport between interviewer and respondent.

2. Structure of the Interview

Although it is not always apparent to the interviewer or the respondent, all interviews have a structure of some kind. An effectively structured interview has three main phases. The interview begins with an introductory phase in which the credentials of the interviewer are established and accepted, rapport between interviewer and respondent is developed, and an appropriate language style adopted. This phase is often used to obtain basic nonthreatening background information. In the second phase the main content of the interview is developed. In general, less threatening content will be addressed first, followed by the more detailed exploration of the topic, characterized by probing and elaboration of the interview structure. The third and final phase is the denouement, in which the interviewer concludes the interview and releases the respondent. Courteous thanks for the efforts expended may be sufficient, but in cases where stress and anxiety have been aroused by the interview it is important for the interviewer to make sure that the completion of the interview leaves the respondent in a satisfied state of mind and that high levels of aroused anxiety do not linger.

Within these three main phases the structure of the interview is created by the way in which the interviewer organizes the questions and makes use of the responses obtained. The format of questions may be open or closed: the open question allowing the respondent to create the response; and the closed question asking the respondent to choose from alternatives offered by the interviewer.

In each case the initial response may be followed up by further questioning, termed "probing," which seeks clarification or elaboration. These questions also give feedback because they show that the interviewer has paid attention to the respondent. The probe question may ask for elaboration, as, for example: "Can you tell me more about that?" Clarification may be requested, as in: "Could you explain that to me a little further, I'm not sure that I fully understand?" Probes can also return to a previous question and its response, as in: "You said before that . . . Could you tell me how that connects with what you have just told me?" Nonverbal signs, such as a nod or a pause, can also serve as probes. Probe questions are not independent, but arise from the interview as it proceeds. They can be planned for but only as contingencies. Nevertheless, in research interviewing it is necessary to take the likely contingencies into account when the interview schedule is being prepared.

Groups of questions and their responses produce varying structures. The following are the most frequently found (Keats 1992).

(a) *Independent items: single topic questions.* This structure consists of a series of questions and their responses which appear to have no common thread linking one question to the next. It is more typical of interviews associated with the filling in of forms than with the in-depth exploration of topics. It may sometimes be found in the early fact-finding stage of the first phase of an interview.

(b) *Sequential items: chain structure.* This structure occurs when responses and questions are linked in an associative chain. The response to the first question leads to a second question and the response to that question determines the next question, and so on in a connected chain. The questions are often open-ended. This structure occurs often in probing. It is a structure that is likely to lead the interviewer to stray from the main theme or to concentrate on interpersonal interactions rather than the topic.

(c) *Branching structure with channeling effect.* If the respondent gives more than one response to the question, the chain may begin with only one of these responses, leaving the others neglected. The effect of this is to create a branching structure, but one that will channel the interview in a particular direction.

(d) *Sequential structure with simple feedback loops.* In each of the above structures neither the interviewer nor the respondent returns to a previous question or response. In much skilled interviewing, however, both may refer back to what has been said before, or ignore some aspects of questions and responses deliberately to return to them later. The return is termed "a feedback loop." The simplest form of structure with feedback loops is sequential. In this case a question may lead to a response that has several aspects. The interviewer takes up one aspect after another, probes each response using a chain structure, and returns with a feedback loop referring to the theme of the first response to introduce the sequence of questions on the next aspect. All the feedback loops return to the initial question or response.

(e) *Branching structure with feedback loops.* This is the most complex structure. Both interviewer and respondent move freely from one aspect to another. They may return to questions asked much earlier in the interview, attend to some aspects of the response to probe these, take up the other aspects when each is fully explored, and use each other's questions and responses to pose further questions or qualify earlier responses. There is a dynamic relationship between interviewer and respondent which encourages them both. This structure is the most effective for eliciting the required information, but it places a heavy demand on the cognitive capacity of the interviewer.

(f) *Grouped themes: constellated structure.* Each of the above types of structure may be combined with others to form constellations of questions and responses in which groups of questions on particular themes have their own structures but are linked together under some overriding, more general theme. Thus, for example, a multiple-choice, closed-question format may be combined with a group of open-ended questions with probing, or standardized scales can be combined with individually designed interview schedules.

The interviewer can use the analysis of structure to improve interviewing skills and to assist in the planning of the interview schedule. It can be valuable in finding out where an interview has failed to achieve its objective. For example, a chain structure may reveal a loss of control over the direction of the interview, while channeling after a multiple response without a feedback loop may reveal the presence of bias, memory weakness, poor listening skills, a lack of empathy and/or a failure to recognize the significance of the other aspects of the response.

3. Techniques of Interviewing

Whether for selection or for data-gathering in research, good interviewing requires the development of an integrated repertoire of techniques, which includes speaking skills, listening skills, skills of concept acquisition, and skill in the interpretation of verbal and nonverbal messages. One of the most important attributes of the good interviewer is the ability to show empathy with the respondent. The ability to see a situation from another's point of view is a cognitive ability, but it must be communicated to the respondent to become effective.

As verbal interaction is the principal mode of communication in interviewing, it is necessary for the interviewer to cultivate a mode of speech that is clear, delivered at an appropriate pace, and moderate in pitch and volume. Vocabulary and syntax should be unambiguous and acceptable to the respondent. Within these general requirements it is still possible to develop an interviewing style that builds upon and enhances the interviewer's personal manner and speech characteristics. It is unnecessary and probably impossible to deny one's speech background.

Listening skills are perhaps even more important than speaking skills. Writers on the helping professions (e.g. Carkhuff 1972, Egan 1975, Benjamin 1987) all stress the importance of active as compared to passive listening. Active listening means that the interviewer hears what is said, understands the message, interprets its intent, and demonstrates interest and attentiveness.

Nonverbal behavior can enhance or detract from demonstrating active listening. There are many cultural differences in the nuances of interpreting nonverbal cues. For example, in Western societies a much greater degree of openness is expected than in Asian societies, but there are also differences among Western societies and among Asian societies.

Cultural norms govern the distance between interviewer and respondent that is acceptable. Within the context of the cultural norm, the acceptable distance also varies according to the topic, the genders of interviewer and respondent, the place in which the interview takes place, and the attitudes of the respondent. When the topic is relatively superficial, the distance is increased; when the topic is more involved, the distance is decreased. When the gender of the interviewer differs from that of the respondent, the distance is increased; when it is the same, the distance is decreased. If the interview takes place in a familiar setting in which the respondent is comfortable and in control, such as the respondent's own home, the distance is decreased; when the setting is more comfortable for the interviewer, such as in the interviewer's office, the distance is increased. When attention and participation are fully engaged, the distance decreases; when the attitude of either respondent or interviewer is perceived by the other to be hostile or disapproving, the distance increases. When the placement of furniture makes physical movement impossible for the whole body, the increase in distancing is achieved by such actions as drawing back the head, stiffening the back, and crossing the arms tightly across the chest. The skilled interviewer watches for these nonverbal signs and interprets their intent.

Another important function of nonverbal cues is the expression of feelings. There is cross-cultural evidence of the universality of the meaning of facial expressions of the primary emotions of anger, sorrow, fear, and joy, but cultural differences are found in the more complex emotions and, even more importantly for the interviewing situation, in the degree of openness or inhibition acceptable for their expression. Hostility and anxiety may be revealed nonverbally, especially in cultures that do not encourage the public display of emotion.

4. Bias in Interviewing

A criticism often directed at interviewing as a research tool is that interview data are particularly prone to distortion because of the presence of bias. Bias can be present in the wording of questions and in the manner in which they are expressed. Questions that lead the respondent to be more likely to give one response than another are biased. Such questions may offer alternatives but omit some salient choices, or may subtly suggest that one answer is more acceptable than another.

Bias can be present in the structure of a formal interview schedule but is more likely to occur in the less highly structured interview typified in the chain structure. Biased attitudes can be conveyed by the interviewer's speech style and by the reinforcement given by nonverbal indications of approval for some responses over others. Bias can affect the interpretation of responses and the direction of probing.

When more than one interviewer is used, or when one interviewer must conduct a large number of interviews to meet the sampling requirements of a research study, biases can arise from differences among interviewers and shifts away from the original schedule of questions. Much research has been conducted on the reliability of interviewers in survey research.

In clinical research the interviewer may be working from a theoretical orientation that drives the questioning. Bias occurs if this orientation so limits the scope of questions that it reinforces what the interviewer wants to hear and neglects or misinterprets what does not fit within the expectations of the theory. This type of bias is illustrated in the branching structure with channeling effect.

Bias can be overcome by careful preparation of the interview schedule and the training of interviewers. The clinical researcher needs to be alert for responses that do not fit the preconceptions of theoretical parameters, and for the possible biasing effects of the affective interpersonal relations that develop in the clinical interview. One of the most challenging tasks for the interviewer is to remain unbiased in the presence of biases in the respondents' replies. The known biases of members of selection panels can be utilized to provide a variety of approaches to the selection task. The problem is to avoid biases that prevent applicants from showing their capabilities fully because relevant factors are ignored or treated prejudicially.

5. Treatment of Interview Data in Research

In research interviewing many different statistical treatments are available provided that the responses can be coded satisfactorily into categories that are clearly defined and independent of each other. Theoretically the coding categories should represent the entire range of possible responses. In practice not all possible responses may be obtained, but the coding system should be able to account for all types of response even if a miscellaneous "other" category has to be included. The analysis of such categorized data is considered in other entries (see *Configural Frequency Analysis; Correspondence Analysis; Contingency Tables; Log-Linear Models; Nonparametric and Distribution-free Statistics*).

6. Training of Interviewers

Training is beneficial for all who must use questioning to obtain information from others. For those engaged in selection interviews, training enables prejudicial biases to be controlled and helps to ensure consistency in the treatment of all interviewees. Training is essential for those engaged in research.

Training for selection interviewing is concerned with such questions as: (a) how to manage the time allotted so that the main issues are adequately dealt with; (b) how to put the interviewees at their ease yet encourage them to perform at their best; (c) how to use other supplementary information such as referees' reports; (d) how to detect and counteract bias in questions or responses; (e) what is being conveyed nonverbally; and (f) how to participate in an interview panel.

Training for research interviewing is concerned with developing skills that will produce valid and reliable data in an atmosphere of cooperative effort. Training focuses on: (a) how to establish rapport and maintain motivation; (b) how to listen actively; (c) how to develop speaking skills that ensure clarity and foster understanding; (d) how to avoid bias; (e) how to probe, give feedback, and manage complex question–response structures; (f) how to manage the equipment smoothly and efficiently; and (g) how to conclude the interview, especially if the topic has been a sensitive one. If a team of interviewers is to be employed, or an interviewer has to conduct a number of interviews, training also includes training in consistency. For interviewing across cultures, training should also include attention to relevant aspects of cultural differences; for example, forms of address, response styles, and role relationships.

Effective training tools are video-recording and tape recording of practice interviews. If training is conducted in small groups, the group can provide constructive comment on practice interviews. Video playback is particularly valuable for examining nonverbal behavior and tape recording for concentrating on verbal skills, phrasing of questions to reduce bias, and probing. Analysis of structure reveals biases and failures to follow through with probing. In all cases practice is essential and should not be cut short: it takes time to become a skilled interviewer.

7. Conclusion

Interviews yield data rich in detail and quality in which individual differences are not submerged. They can be used alone or combined with other means of data collection. For example, with young children the use of a doll or puppet play can be very effective. A questionnaire, a video presentation, or a film can be used to focus the questions—a method that ensures consistency in the presentation of stimuli. For many topics of a delicate nature, interviews are the only practical way of obtaining data that are less likely to be distorted by social acquiescence bias and social desirability and hence are likely to be more valid than data from scales and questionnaires. They can take account of cultural differences in response styles and respond flexibly to differences in ability and verbal fluency. If used with skill and care, interviewing can be an extremely powerful research tool.

References

Benjamin A 1987 *The Helping Interview: With Case Illustrations*. Houghton Mifflin, Boston, Massachusetts

Carkhuff R 1972 *The Art of Helping*. Human Resources Development Press, Amherst, Massachusetts

Egan G 1975 *The Skilled Helper: A Systematic Approach to Effective Helping*. Brooks-Cole, Monterey, California

Keats D M 1992 *Skilled Interviewing*, 2nd edn. Australian Council for Educational Research (ACER), Hawthorn, Victoria

Further Reading

Goodale J G 1982 *The Fine Art of Interviewing*. Prentice Hall, Englewood Cliffs, New Jersey

Gorden R L 1969 *Interviewing: Strategy, Techniques and Tactics*. Dorsey Press, Homewood, Illinois

Participant Observation

S. J. Ball

Participant observation is actually a blending of various techniques, a "style or strategy of research, a characteristic type of research which makes use of several methods and techniques organized in a distinctive research design" (McCall and Simmons 1969 p. 341). But the primary tool of participant observation research is the researcher. Face-to-face engagement in the field of study is the simple basis of the participant observation strategy. "Immersion in the setting allows the researcher to hear, see and begin to experience reality as the participants do. Ideally, the researcher spends a considerable amount of time in the setting, learning about daily life" (Marshall and Rossman 1989 p. 79). Entry into the field, the cooperation and trust of respondents, access to events and private arenas, and blending or passing inside the action of the setting all underpin the technicalities of participant observation research and all rely upon a set of interpersonal social relations skills. The participant observer is committed to becoming embedded in the perspectives of those who inhabit the sociocultural world that is to be "captured" and analyzed. The balance between participation and observation, the insider–outsider tension of such research, what Marshall and Rossman call "participantness," varies according to the needs and possibilities of the setting (Gold 1958, Hammersley and Atkinson 1983). Participant observation studies also vary in terms of intensiveness and extensiveness and specificity and diffuseness (Marshall and Rossman 1989). Thus, Wolcott (1988) distinguishes between the active participant, the privileged, and the limited observer. But it is a mistake to see the definition of the research role within the field solely in terms of the preferences of the researcher. Qualitative study of this kind is responsively "designed" to fit or match the vagaries and demands of the setting under study. Instead of emphasizing detailed *a priori* research planning, flexibility is needed to allow the research to "unfold, cascade, roll and emerge" (Lincoln and Guba 1985 p. 210). The conduct of the research must be organized and the researcher role of the fieldworker must be constructed in ways which are acceptable and workable to the actors in the field and the constraints of the setting itself. Thus, the establishment and maintenance of the research self is a deliberate process. It requires careful planning and the researcher will aim for a best compromise between an ideal and practical self-as-researcher. There is no fixed protocol for the conduct of participant observation or the parameters of the research role.

Thus, the key to rigor and the techniques of respondent validation for the participant observer lie not in the application of fixed, abstract procedures but in control over the conduct of the research and the maintenance of a stance of *reflexivity*. "Rather than engaging in futile attempts to eliminate the effects of the researcher, we should set about understanding them" (Hammersley and Atkinson 1983 p. 17). The claims which are made for the adequacy of participant observation data must rest upon a careful monitoring and exposition of the interplay between the social trajectory of the researcher through the field of study, and the social relations developed therein, and the techniques employed to collect, elicit, and analyze data. The researcher must be able both to deconstruct and to control the relationship between fieldwork, data, analysis, and interpretation. The basis for rigor in participant observation is the careful and conscious linking of the social process of engagement in the field with the technical aspects of data collection and *the decisions which that linking involves*. In simple terms the good participant observer is someone who can adapt the research to the constraints of the field of study; understand and demonstrate the effects of those constraints on the adequacy of the data collected; *and* use that understanding, reflexivity, to make informed choices about the process and conduct of the research.

1. The Social Trajectory

Most participant observation research, especially that conducted in formal educational settings, begins with the negotiation of entry into the field. Normally, there are formal channels: the superintendent or principal is approached for permission, which if granted provides entry but perhaps not access. Permission from formal authorities does not always guarantee the cooperation of teachers, students, or others in the setting. Indeed the researcher may actually be "tainted" by the entry process and become indentified with the formal authorities of the institution. This identification may produce reluctance and suspicion on the part of lower participants. Rossman found herself in exactly this situation in a study of school cultures and feared that "continued close association with the power structure might work against her building trust with teachers . . ." (Marshall and Rossman 1989 p. 68). Realistically, in any complex fieldwork setting the researcher is confronted with multiple negotiations of micro-access. Legitimacy frequently has to be won and renewed repeatedly rather than simply being officially granted once and for all time. "Entry negotiation requires time, patience, and sensitivity to the rhythms and norms of a group" (Marshall and Rossman 1989 p. 65). The point is that the means of access may actually constrain the sorts of data and research relationships available to the fieldworker. This is where reflexivity begins. The failure to appreciate how the researcher is perceived and identified by those in the field may inhibit, distort, or channel perception of events. The trust and cooperation of respondents is normally vital to the success of participant observation research. The social relations skills of the researcher will determine the development of "rapport" (an instrumental relationship as far as participant observers are concerned). Researchers "establish rapport to attain ends shaped primarily by their own needs" (Glesne 1989 p. 48). In relation to this, the research must take particular account of the interplay of categorical identities and roles in the research process: that is, for example, age, gender, and ethnic differences between researcher and the researched.

Actors' responses will reflect the researcher's attempt to take or make a research role. Clearly, some educational researchers when faced with this dilemma have sought comfort in taking on a teacher, counselor, or other official role. Other researchers have tried to construct new, idiosyncratic roles that stand outside of available organizational identities (see Peshkin 1984 on being a Jewish researcher in a Christian fundamentalist high school). The role adopted, whatever it is, will influence the kinds of data elicited in the research setting. The taking of a ready-made role may leave the setting relatively undisturbed, and thus much may remain unsaid. The making of a recognizable research role may create disturbance, but in doing so may make the taken for granted more obvious. There are advantages and disadvantages in each case. The key point is that the researcher is aware of the relationships between role and data, and is able to account for these relationships, and that this awareness is used to make tactical decisions about the maintenance of social relations and the organization of data collection within the field. Reflexivity provides for control and for informed decision-making, within the constraints of the field.

The same points can be made about other aspects and phases of the trajectory of fieldwork. The distribution of the researcher's presence (see Sect. 3 below); involvement with social networks; the use of key informants (Ball 1984, Burgess 1985); power, gender, and ethnic relations in the field (Finch 1984, Scott 1984); and even the management of exit from the field all have implications for the possibility and nature of data collected. The researcher should be constantly striving to make sense of the distortions and nuances which these aspects of social relations in the field build into the collection of data, while also seeking to develop fieldwork tactics to counter the effects of these distortions.

2. Triangulation and Types of Data

The participant observer is a research opportunist. Presence in the research setting over a period of time presents opportunities to acquire and use data of all kinds, not just observation data. "Classic participant observation . . . always involves the interweaving of looking and listening . . . of watching and asking— and some of that listening and asking may approach or be identical to intensive interviewing" (Lofland and Lofland 1984 p. 13). In simple terms, four types of data can be identified, some being represented better than others according to different participant observation studies. First, "observation data"—the researcher's own first-hand data—are collected in situ and recorded personally; there are a variety of styles for such data. Second, "respondent data" are usually derived from interviewing or diaries; these data provide respondents' accounts of experiences, events, attitudes, and feelings. Third, "enumeration data" are the counting of events, categories of behavior, types of people, or the use of numerical data already available in the field (see Ball 1981), or the elicitation of questionnaire data. Fourth, "documentary data" are the use of files, records, ephemera, and so on. Access to these different kinds of data provides the researcher with the possibility of triangulation as a way of minimizing the distortions inherent in any one kind of data collection. Triangulation also generates new research questions. In its simplest form, triangulation involves the use of the different forms of data to address one issue, question, or phenomenon in the field. The materials elicited by each technique are compared and offset for differences and inconsistencies. Questions raised or left unanswered by one method and data type may be answered by another. Further, the presence of different kinds of data in relation to key points of analysis will give the reader greater confidence in the researcher's conclusions.

3. Naturalistic Sampling

Participant observation-type research is not normally associated with sampling techniques, and indeed many otherwise well-conducted studies neglect to address sampling issues. However, the significance of sampling in qualitative studies is very different from its use in quantitative ones (see Sect. 4 below). The challenge facing the participant observer, especially when working in complex social institutions, is exhaustive coverage referring primarily to the distribution of people across the field. There are three main dimensions to this "naturalistic sampling" in such settings: time, place, and persons. Basically the claims made by the researcher for the generality of the analysis in relation to particular settings rest upon the adequacy of the database. "Well-developed sampling decisions are crucial for any study's soundness. Making logical judgments and presenting a rationale for these site and sample decisions go far in building the overall case for a proposed study" (Marshall and Rossman 1989 p. 63).

Time is the least well-attended to of these sampling dimensions. This is strange and unfortunate given the temporal complexity of most educational settings and the behavioural variations, related to time, which are often commented upon by practitioners. Most participant observers either fail to use time sampling in the organization of fieldwork or fail to use time as an analytical or descriptive category when presenting data (see Ball et al. 1984). Place is slightly better handled but still remains poorly accounted for in many participant observation studies; action is reported but settings are not. But again the geopolitics of educational institutions are significant and complex. Back-stage and front-stage areas exist for most actors, territorial claims are a fundamental part of the micropolitics of organizations, and social networks often map onto the use of space. Actions also vary across settings. Persons are the final and most obvious focus for sampling decisions made either in terms of their roles or categorical identities or attributes or on the basis of theoretically significant typological properties.

These sampling dimensions provide a spur to the reflexive rigor of the researcher and a simple set of criteria for judgment for the reader of participant observation research.

4. Theoretical Sampling and the Feedback of Data into Analysis

At the heart of the process of participant observation, and fundamental to reflexive practice, is a dynamic, ongoing relationship between data collection and data analysis. That is, the analysis of data alongside the work of data collection allows for the feedback of analytical insights into the organization and conduct of fieldwork. In other words, the analysis of data phase by phase, stage by stage, in relation to fieldwork provides for the making of analytically informed decisions about the collection of new data. This interplay between data collection and data analysis is the basis for the technique of "theoretical sampling" which in turn underpins the development of "grounded theory."

Theoretical sampling occurs when decisions about the selection of new data in the field are based upon conceptual categorizations derived from ongoing analysis. Theoretical sampling also allows for the examination and elaboration of analytical categories and the "testing" of emergent theory (see Strauss and Corbin 1991). The search for, and attempt to incorporate, negative or deviant cases into emerging conceptualizations is a crucial part of this process of constant comparison. As categories are established from the careful coding of data, they are also subjected to interrogation and elaboration from newly collected data. In the course of research, many such tentative categories will be abandoned or significantly amended. Thus, part of the struggle for verification is conducted through the dialectic between interpretation and conceptualization of data. The participant observer is forever distrustful both of the adequacy of data and the sensitivity of theory (see *Triangulation in Educational Research*). As Strauss and Corbin (1991 p. 58) suggest, successful qualitative research rests upon "the attributes of creativity, rigor and persistence, and above all, theoretical sensitivity."

5. Respondent Validation

Respondent validation, respondent verification, or participant verification, is a difficult, and it seems, inevitably limited process of obtaining actors' responses to research materials, what Lincoln and Guba (1985) call "member checking." One form of member checking is simply the feeding back of raw data —observations or interviews—for confirmation. "I shared the transcripts with the relevant interviewees to see if they wanted to add or subtract anything. When they expressed satisfaction that the transcripts were accurate, I began the process of examining my own exaggerated or misplaced fears" (Ely et al. 1991 pp. 116–17). A more demanding exercise is the exposure of the researcher's interpretations to respondents. "Credibility is a trustworthiness criterion that is satisfied when source respondents agree to honor the reconstructions" (Lincoln and Guba 1985 p. 329). There are now several examples of this being done or attempted in participant observation research (Ely et al. 1991 refer to Spitz, Foley, and McGuire, Bloor 1978, and Ball 1984). But it cannot always be assumed that respondents see it in their interests to validate the researcher's account, especially when they feel themselves to be presented as less than perfect.

6. The Research Biography

The reflexive link between the social trajectory of the researcher through the field and the technical procedures of data elicitation and analysis is captured in the writing of a research biography. This informal, experiential account of the research process is increasingly becoming a required component of participant observation theses. It offers the reader a way of understanding the constitutive nature of the fieldwork roles and research self of the participant observer in relation to the data elicited and presented; although in publications the pressures of space frequently mean that this aspect of the research is omitted. Whyte (1955) provides perhaps the definitive version of the research biography in his methodological appendix. Here the crucial role of Whyte's relationships with two key informants and gang rivals is discussed at length, and the nature of the research as a collective endeavor is revealed. But within the process of research, the biography, in the form of a journal, also provides a means of achieving some analytical distance and a reflexive stance. In its final form the research biography provides the grounds for understanding the social production of the research and it offers a link between fieldwork and the interpretative conclusions of the researcher as author.

See also: Research Paradigms in Education

References

Ball S J 1981 *Beachside comprehensive: A Case Study of Secondary Schooling*. Cambridge University Press, Cambridge

Ball S J 1984 Beachside reconsidered: Reflections on a methodological apprenticeship. In: Burgess R (ed.) 1989 *The Research Process in Educational Settings*. Falmer Press, Lewes

Ball S J, Hull R, Skelton M, Tudor R 1984 The tyranny of the "devil's mill": Time and task at school. In: Delamont S (ed.) 1984 *Readings of Interaction in the Classroom*. Methuen, London

Bloor M 1978 On the analysis of observational data: A discussion of the worth and uses of inductive techniques and respondent validation. *Sociology* 12(3): 545–52

Burgess R 1985 In the company of teachers: Key informants and the study of a comprehensive school. In: Burgess R (ed.) 1985 *Strategies of Educational Research: Qualitative Methods*. Falmer Press, Lewes

Ely M et al. 1991 *Doing Qualitative Research: Circles within Circles*. Falmer Press, Lewes

Finch J 1984 It's great to have someone to talk to: The ethics of interviewing women. In: Bell C, Roberts H (eds.) 1984 *Social Researching: Politics, Problems, Practice*. Routledge, London

Glesne C 1989 Rapport and friendship in ethnographic research. *International Journal of Qualitative Studies in Education* 2(1): 45–54

Gold R L 1958 Roles in sociological fieldwork. *Social Forces* 36: 217–23

Hammersley M, Atkinson P 1983 *Ethnography: Principles and Practice*. Tavistock, London

Lincoln Y, Guba E 1985 *Naturalistic Inquiry*. Sage, Beverly Hills, California

Lofland J, Lofland L H 1984 *Analysing Social Settings: A*

Guide to Qualitative Observation and Analysis. Wadsworth, California

Marshall C, Rossman G B 1989 *Designing Qualitative Research*. Sage, Newbury Park, California

McCall G J, Simmons J L (eds.) 1969 *Issues in Participant Observation: A Text and Reader*. Addison-Wesley, Reading, Massachusetts

Peshkin. A 1984 Odd man out: The participant observer in an absolutist setting. *Sociol. Educ.* 57: 254–64

Scott S 1984 The personable and the powerful: Gender and status in sociological research. In: Bell C, Roberts H (eds.) 1984 *Social Researching*. Routledge, London

Strauss A, Corbin J 1991 *Basics of Qualitative Research*. Sage, Newbury Park, California

Whyte W F 1955 *Street Corner Society*: *The Social Structure of an Italian Slum*. University of Chicago Press, Chicago, Illinois

Wolcott H 1988 Ethnographic research in education. In: Jaeger R M (ed.) 1988 *Complementary Methods of Research in Education*. AREA, Washington, DC

Participant Verification

L. Sharpe

The term participant verification refers broadly to the research practice of confronting participants with an emerging theoretical explanation of their actions and inviting them to respond to its status with respect to reality, and then using these responses to refine that explanation. Its purpose as a methodological tool is to explore the links between first order, participants' accounts, and second order, theoretical accounts, as a definite state in the generation of theory (Weber 1949, Schultz 1970).

The investigation in which this method was used was a study of 80 parent couples at a boys' comprehensive school in Greater London (Sharpe 1980). Its intention was to generate a new model of parent-school relations which would remedy weaknesses in existing research, principally by respecting the authenticity of parents' views. To this end a heavy emphasis was placed on interpretive research procedures, especially open-ended interviews, participate observation, and the use of ideal-type constructs. As the research progressed, there was an emerging concern with structural dimensions of parent-school relations and this led to the use of a range of other research techniques and a broadening of the sample to include teachers and pupils. The final model aimed to bring together both action and structural dimensions of parent-school relations to produce an account which though respecting members' definitions went beyond them in certain significant respects.

The first stage in the research involved open-ended interviews with the sample parents in their own homes. These interviews, which were tape-recorded and later transcribed, gave parents an opportunity to talk freely and in an unprompted way about their own understandings of the school and their relationships to it. They produced a wealth of sensitizing data that demonstrated clearly that there were marked differences in the way that parents viewed the school and that these differences in meaning had different consequences for their relationship with the school. Three ideal-type parent figures were constructed to emphasize these differences and to act as heuristic devices for furthering the research. The first was the "agent". This parent figure was constructed so as to hold a view of the school that led to the strategy of lobbying the teachers on behalf of the student, or of engaging in various public relations exercises, at a range of school meetings, all with the intention of marking out the student for special attention by the teachers. The second was the "touchliner" whose view of the school led to the student being encouraged within the home rather than being closely involved with the school. Thirdly, the "absentee" type was constructed whose disillusionment with the school led to the strategy of staying away and encouraging the student to pursue other, nonschool forms of education. These were, in broad outline, the three types constructed to deal with the vast quantity of qualitative material yielded by the interviews. As types, of course, they were not intended as descriptions of particular parents, though the next stage of the research involved using them as classifications.

By the time that the first interviews were completed and the types constructed, the outlines of a new model of parent-school relations were becoming clear. It was apparent that much previous research and policy statements could be grouped together under the heading "hidden-hand" models of parent-school relations: these emphasized that parents' influence on their children's education and schooling occurred in the home and not in the school. Theirs was a hidden-hand at work in the home, providing children with latent culture, such as language skills, encouragement, and the appropriate attitudes—a hidden-hand that had to be grasped in a partnership between teacher and pupils. In contrast, the interviews were suggesting that parents could take a direct hand in school affairs and that the hidden-hand model fitted at best just one type of parent—the touchliner.

The technique of participant verification was used during the next stage of the research which involved subjecting the types to tests of meaning and causal adequacy. Though the tests of meaning adequacy are the major focus here, a brief comment on the tests of causal adequacy is useful. One test involved hypothesizing that parents provisionally classified as agents attended school more regularly than other parents, visits being the lowest common denominator of the agent strategy. Another test sought to establish whether there was any relation between the various strategies and the recognition of parents and students by teachers. These tests generally confirmed the agent and touchliner types, but raised serious doubts about the adequacy of the absentee type, as did the participant verification test. This involved subjecting the parents to a brief description of the emerging model and of the types and inviting them to comment on its validity. For this purpose a second set of interviews was held with a proportion of the original sample, and as before the interviews were tape recorded and later transcribed. The model invited parents to view the school as primarily a differentiating institution, with the process of differentiation giving rise to changes in the official school identities of students as students were moved from band to band in their earlier years at the school before being finally allocated to examination bands. Such changes could give rise to discrepancies between parents' and teachers' definitions of the students' identities, as well as to a concensus of views. The parent-school relations model was essentially a process of negotiation of students' identities occasioned by the process of differentiation, with the types representing distinct ways of dealing with this process.

Participant verification proved to be an important methodological tool in generating theory. Allowing parents an opportunity to verify the emerging theoretical account in terms of their own understandings did much to cast doubt on the adequacy of conventional views of parent-school relations. However, somewhat paradoxically, the process also raised serious doubts about the validity of parents' understandings of parent-school relations. The exercise demonstrated that the social context in which parental strategies are carried out is in many respects beyond the comprehension of the individual parent, whose definition may be a partial one and may even be incorrect in certain respects. So that, although a knowledge of parental meanings and intentions is indispensible, it is necessary to study these as part of a social situation which is defined by others as well, and which has certain nonnegotiable features. Thus, parents' actions can be interpreted by teachers in a way quite unintended by parents. Students can create for their parents a distorted view of the school by selectively delivering information to them. Teachers may only be conscious of a need to encourage, or even contemplate, meetings with parents under certain circumstances, such as when they experience problems with difficult children. Each party may have a vested interest in parent-school relations, and emphasize the aspect which is central to them. Thus there are manifold definitions of parent-school relations, complexly related to each other. The sociological problem for the researcher was to explain how these different definitions were interrelated to form the orderly and unremarkable pattern of parent-school relations found at the school. The final explanation was that the differentiation process at the school was a nonnegotiable fact which gave rise to a common problem for teachers, parents, and students, thus providing a common focus for their interaction. This was the problem of continuity and change in student identities. Whether this explanation is valid is ultimately a matter which rests with sociologists rather than with the parents.

See also: Scietific Methods in Educational Research; Validity; Participant Observation

References

Schultz A 1970 *On Phenomenology and Social Relations: Selected Writings.* Chicago University Press, Chicago, Illinois
Sharpe L 1980 Parent-school relations: A reconceptualization. Unpublished D. Phil Thesis, University of Sussex, Sussex
Weber M 1949 *The Methodology of the Social Sciences.* Free Press, New York

Repertory Grid Technique

R. J. Alban-Metcalf

Repertory grid (repgrid) technique was devised by Kelly (1955) within the context of his "personal construct theory," but has come to be used as a technique in its own right. In essence, it is an approach designed to carry out effectively the everyday process of trying to find out how people view the world from their own perspectives. For this reason, in its simpler forms, repertory grid technique has been compared to a well-structured interview. It can, however, be modified in a wide variety of ways, and can be augmented by sophisticated statistical and other mathematical procedures.

In repertory grid technique, the term "element" is used to denote the persons (including self), things, and events that together constitute an individual's environ-

√ Pole	Me as I am now	Me as I would like to be	Mother	Father	Best friend	Opposite–sex friend	Teacher I like	Teacher I fear	X Pole
Encourages me to work hard	X	√	(√)	(X)	X	X	(√)	√	Doesn't encourage me to work hard
Unfriendly	X	X	(X)	X	X	(√)	X	(√)	Friendly
Can be trusted	(√)	√	√	√	(√)	(X)	√	X	Cannot be trusted
Hardworking		(√)					(√)		Lazy
			◯	◯			◯		

Figure 1

A partially completed repertory grid. Constructs elicited with reference to the triads of elements indicated by the circles

ment. The term "construct" denotes the dimensions or reference axes used by the individual to discriminate between elements. According to Kelly, each person characteristically builds up an internal representation of the world in terms of a finite number of constructs. Constructs are conceived of as being bipolar, for example, "nice to know, versus not nice to know," "interesting, versus boring." Each person's constructs, which are based on the unique way that he or she perceives the world, are themselves unique, though individuals living in the same culture tend to have similar constructs. Unique also is the way that constructs are interrelated to form that person's construct system. Repertory grid technique can be used specifically to determine (a) which constructs an individual uses, (b) how those constructs are used, and (c) the interrelationships between the constructs.

The commonest ways of eliciting constructs are verbal, for example, by an interviewer asking people to indicate what similarities and what differences they see between specified groups of elements, though nonverbal approaches have also been developed. It is important to recognize, however, that a construct is a dimension; it is not a verbal label. Thus, different individuals are likely to have subtly (or in some cases fundamentally) different constructs to which the same verbal label is attached. As an example, the verbal label "funny, versus not funny" may be used to indicate two very different constructs used by a pupil and a teacher. Conversely, though, in the vast majority of instances, people from the same culture use mutually agreed verbal labels to indicate similar constructs. The particular constructs that given individuals use can be determined directly by asking them to verbalize discriminations they make between elements with which they are familiar. How they used these constructs, and the meaning of the constructs, can be inferred by asking the individuals to apply the same constructs to other elements, or exploring the implications of each discrimination. The interrelationships between constructs, and more information about their meaning, can be inferred either by eliciting a series of constructs that the individual sees as being causally related (i.e., laddering), or by recourse to mathematical techniques.

In eliciting constructs from individuals, a number of procedures can be adopted. Of these, the simplest involves presenting the person with combinations of three elements at a time (triads), with the name of each element written on a separate card, and asking for some important way in which two of the elements are similar to each other, and different from the third. The way in which two of the elements are similar is referred as the emergent pole of the construct. The other pole can either be the way in which the third element was different, or be the logical opposite of the emergent pole. As an alternative, the elements can all be presented at the same time, written in a row across the top of a piece of paper marked out into squares, and the constructs elicited by the interviewer directing attention to specified triads (or dyads) (see Fig. 1). After a specified number of constructs has been elicited, and written in columns at each side of the sheet of paper, the person can be asked to construe each of the elements in relation to each of the constructs. Indication of which pole applies to each element can be made either by dichotomous or rated responses, or by rank ordering the elements. A third approach to eliciting constructs is through "free" description, oral or written. "Self-characterization" grids, for example, can be devised by extracting bipolar constructs from individuals' descriptions of themselves. Such descriptions are usually given in the third person, as if they were descriptions of the principal character in a play or film.

Two major developments of the repertory grid have been laddering and pyramid construction. In the first of these, a construct is chosen by the interviewer, and the person asked which pole applies to a given element, say, for example, the element "me as I am now," and why. For example, a teacher might say that the construct pole "like to work in a large school, versus don't like to work in a large school" best describes "me as I am now". In response to a series of "Why?"

questions, the sequence of constructs elicited might be—"like to have lots of other teachers around me" (versus the opposite), "like to have other adults to talk to" (versus the opposite), "like to have my mind stimulated by intelligent conversation" (versus the opposite), and "keeps me sane" (versus the opposite), and "keeps me sane" (versus the opposite). Note (a) that the constructs elicited are related logically to one another (at least from the individual's point of view), and (b) that the sequence of constructs can be thought of as being arranged in an hierarchical manner. Thus, "like to work in a large school" is a relatively subordinate construct, whereas "like to have my mind stimulated by intelligent conversation" is relatively superordinate. Note also, that the teacher could not be expected to give a reasoned answer to the question "Why do you want to remain sane?" "Keeping sane" is a core construct, that is, a construct that is essential to that person's very being as a person.

The elicitation process just described is known as laddering up a construct system. The opposite process of laddering down can be achieved by asking questions of the type, "How do you know that construct pole X applies to element A?", or "What evidence is there that X is true of element A?" In this way, subordinate constructs can be elicited.

In pyramid construction, individuals are asked, first of all, to think of some other element, say, a teacher or a pupil, with whom they feel most relaxed, and to specify an attribute which is characteristic of that element. Second, the request is made to state the kind of element (in this case a person) that would represent the opposite of the selected attribute. Having elicited two poles of a construct, the interviewer inquires what kind of a person the first element is. The third stage involves laddering down each of the opposite poles of the construct, so identifying a "pyramid" of relationships between constructs.

Two principles should govern the choice of elements in the repertory grid technique: (a) the relevance of the elements to the part of the construct system to be investigated, and (b) the representativeness of the chosen elements. Thus, if intimate personal relationships are the focus of interest, then the elements should include persons who correspond to role titles such as, "me as I am now" (and perhaps also "me as I would like to be," "me as my best friend/mother/wife sees me," and so on), members of close family and friends, and "significant" others, such as teachers, and older friends and acquaintances who are loved, admired, or feared. Similarly, if the focus of interest is relationships at school or work, or school subjects, hobbies and interests, careers, or clothes, then representative elements from these areas should be chosen. Relevance of elements selected is important because constructs have only limited ranges of convenience, or appropriateness: thus, the construct "printed, versus not printed" is relevant to construing books and sylla-

bi, and also dresses and skirts, but it cannot be used meaningfully in relation to people, school subjects, or careers. Further, it is likely that a complete range of relevant constructs will be elicited only if the elements constitute a fully representative sample. The number of elements used commonly varies from around 10 to 25. The greater the number of elements, the more likelihood of representativeness being achieved, though in some circumstances, the subject matter may mean that fewer elements are available, or the nature of the sample (e.g., less able pupils) may mean that fewer are desirable.

Just as with elements, the greater the number of relevant constructs that are elicited, the greater their likelihood of being representative. Again, optimal numbers range from around 10 to 25, though most people appear to use fewer than 20 different constructs in relation to people, and some use as few as one or two. Constructs can be classified in a number of ways, such as into physical, for example, "tall" (versus the opposite), situational, for example, "is a pupil from this school?" (versus the opposite), behavioral, for example, "writes quickly" (versus the opposite), and psychological, for example, "is likely to do badly under exam pressure," (versus the opposite); or into vague, for example, "is OK" (versus the opposite), and excessively precise, for example, "is a medical student" (versus the opposite).

Repertory grid data can be analysed in a wide variety of ways, and manipulated using a wide range of procedures. Thus, the interviewer may simply be concerned to note which constructs a given individual uses, and in the case of laddering or pyramid construction, also to infer relationships between constructs. Alternatively, elicited constructs can be used in idiographic or nomothetic instruments, relevant to a particular individual or group of individuals, or to particular elements. In some forms, repertory grid data can be subjected to statistical or other mathematical procedures, or used as the basis for devising interactive computer programs.

Mathematical analyses of repertory grids have been used to calculate a number of "structural" indices concerned with relationships between elements and constructs. Notable among these are cognitive complexity, cognitive differentiation, and articulation, which are measures of tendency to construe elements in multidimensional ways, identification and assimilative projection, which are concerned with perceived similarity between self and others, and constellatoriness and the coefficient of convergence, which measure similarities in the use of constructs. Mathematical techniques commonly applied to repertory grid data include cluster and factor analysis, and on the bases of these, diagrammatic representations of element and construct relationships have been devised. Fansella and Bannister (1977) have written the standard text on the repertory grid technique, and Bannister and Mair (1970) provide a useful treatment of issues of the reliability and validity of repertory grids.

The applications of repertory grid technique fall into two principal groups, "static" and "dynamic." In both groups, repertory grids can either be idiographic, in which case the individual's own constructs (or a mixture of own and provided constructs) are used, or nomothetic, in which case, for purposes of comparison, provided constructs are used commonly (though not exclusively). Examples of the "static" use of repgrid data are determination of a student's (or teacher's) perceptions of, say, self, family, and peers, or perceptions of self in relation to career opportunities in vocational guidance. "Dynamic" use of the repertory grid can involve completion of a comparable grid on two or more occasions, in order to give a measure of the extent to which an individual's construct system changes over time. This can be useful, for example, in studying the development of self-awareness, or friendship development. Alternatively, repertory grid data can form the basis of interactive computer programs, for example, in decision-making exercises.

See also: Questionnaires; Interviewing for Clinical Research

References

Bannister D, Mair J 1970 *The Evaluation of Personal Constructs*. Academic Press, London

Fansella F, Bannister D 1977 *A Manual for Repertory Grid Techniques*. Academic Press, London

Kelly G A 1955 *The Psychology of Personal Constructs*. Norton, New York

Further Reading

Oppenheim A N 1992 *Questionnaire Design, Interviewing and Attitude Measurement*. Pinter, London

Pope M L, Keen T R 1981 *Personal Construct Psychology and Education*. Academic Press, London

Shaw M L G 1981 *Recent Advances in Personal Construct Technology*. Academic Press, London

Triangulation in Educational Research

N. K. Denzin

Triangulation is the application and combination of several research methodologies in the study of the same phenomenon. The diverse methods and measures that are combined should relate in some specified way to the theoretical constructs under examination. The use of multiple methods in an investigation so as to overcome the weaknesses or biases of a single method taken by itself is sometimes called multiple operationalism.

Triangulation can be employed in both quantitative and qualitative studies. Traditionally, in quantitative studies triangulation has been used as a method of validation. That is, the researcher uses multiple methods to validate observations. On the other hand triangulation can be conceptualized as an alternative to validation, and fitted to the particular problems that arise in a purely qualitative inquiry (Stake 1995 pp. 110–11).

The insistence on a multiple operational orientation in the social sciences is commonly associated in the field of psychology with the work of Campbell and his associates (Brewer and Collins 1981). Outgrowths of Campbell's works have included the multitrait-multimethod matrix technique (Campbell and Fiske 1959), (see *Multitrait–Multimethod Analysis*) and the nonreactive, unobtrusive measurement strategies.

The use of multiple measures and methods so as to overcome the inherent weaknesses of single measurement instruments has, however, a long history in the physical and social sciences (Flick 1992, Brewer and Hunter 1989). The commitment to a triangulation strategy also has a long history in feminist social science research (Reinharz and Davidson 1992). The concept of triangulation, as in the action of making a triangle, may be traced to the Greeks and the origins of modern mathematics.

Recently, qualitative researchers have appropriated the concept and fitted it to the problems unique to qualitative research and qualitative approaches to evaluation (Flick 1992, Fielding and Fielding 1986, Guba and Lincoln 1989, Eisner 1991, Pitman and Maxwell 1992).

Interpretative social science scholars who employ the strategy of triangulation are committed to sophisticated rigor, which means that they are committed to making their empirical, interpretative schemes as public as possible. This requires that they detail in a careful fashion the nature of the sampling framework used. It also involves using triangulated, historically situated observations that are interactive, biographical, and, where relevant, gender specific. The phrase "sophisticated rigor" is intended to describe the work of any and all social scientists who employ multiple methods, seek out diverse empirical sources, and attempt to develop interactionally grounded interpretations (Huberman and Miles 1994 p. 438).

1. Need for Triangulation

The social sciences rely, in varying degrees, on the following research methods: social surveys, experiments and quasiexperiments, participant observation, interviewing, case study and life history constructions, and unobtrusive methods (Denzin 1989) (see *Survey Research Methods; Interviewing for Clinical Research; Case Study Methods*). Each of these methods has inherent weaknesses, which range from an inability to enter realistically into the subject's lifeworld in experiments and surveys, to the problems of reflecting change and process in unobtrusive methods, the controlling of rival interpretative factors in participant observation and life histories, or an excessive reliance on paper and pencil techniques in surveys and interviewing.

The realities to which sociological methods are fitted are not fixed. The social world is socially constructed and its meanings, to the observers and those observed, is constantly changing. As a consequence, no single research method will ever capture all of the changing features of the social world under study. Each research method implies a different interpretation of the world and suggests different lines of action that the observer may take toward the research process. The meanings of methods are constantly changing, and each investigator brings different interpretations to bear upon the very research methods that are utilized.

For those reasons, the most fruitful search for sound interpretations of the real world must rely upon triangulation strategies. Interpretations that are built upon triangulation are certain to be stronger than those that rest on the more constricted framework of a single method.

2. Hermeneutics of Interpretation

What is sought in triangulation is an interpretation of the phenomenon at hand that illuminates and reveals the subject matter in a thickly contextualized manner. A triangulated interpretation reflects the phenomenon as a process that is relational and interactive. The interpretation engulfs the subject matter, incorporating all of the understandings the researcher's diverse methods reveal about the phenomenon.

A hermeneutic interpretation does not remove the investigators from the subject matter of study but rather places them directly in the circle of interpretation.

While it is commonplace in the social sciences to place the investigator outside the interpretative process, hence asking the research methods to produce the interpretation that is sought, the hermeneutic interpretation dictates that "what is decisive is not to get out of the circle but to come into it the right way" (Heidegger 1962 p. 195). Triangulation is the appropriate way of entering the circle of interpretation. The researcher is part of the interpretation.

3. Types of Triangulation

While it is commonly assumed that triangulation is the use of multiple methods in the study of the same phenomenon, this is only one form of the strategy. There are five basic types of triangulation: (a) data triangulation, involving time, space, and persons; (b) investigator triangulation, which consists of the use of multiple, rather than single observers; (c) theory triangulation, which consists of using more than one theoretical scheme in the interpretation of the phenomenon; (d) methodological triangulation, which involves using more than one method and may consist of within-method or between-method strategies. There is also multiple triangulation, when the researcher combines in one investigation multiple observers, theoretical perspectives, sources of data, and methodologies (Denzin 1989) and finally; (e) member-check triangulation (Stake 1995 p. 115, Guba and Lincoln 1994 p. 114) where subjects examine and confirm or disconfirm interpretations written about them.

4. Variations on Triangulated Strategies

Flick (1992) and Hammersley and Atkinson (1983) have offered variations on these four main types of triangulation. Hammersley and Atkinson (1983 p. 198) argued that in ethnographic inquiries data source triangulation properly refers to data "deriving from different phases of fieldwork, different points of respondent validation, and accounts of different participants involved in the setting." They introduced the concept of "technique triangulation" to describe data produced by different techniques at different points in the fieldwork process. They stressed that the point of triangulation is not just to combine different types of data, per se; rather, the purpose is to relate different sorts of data in ways that counteract possible threats to validity. They call this strategy "reflexive triangulation" (1983 p. 198).

Fielding and Fielding (1986 p. 34) introduced what may be termed "structural triangulation." This is an approach to data collection that requires one method to explore the structural aspects of a problem and another method to capture the "essential elements of its meaning to those involved."

Flick (1992), arguing for a conception of triangulation explicitly fitted to qualitative studies, introduced the notion of systematic or multipurpose triangulation of micro and macro perspectives. He thus elaborated the Fielding and Fielding position. He illustrated his approach with a study of a counseling center which employed (a) historical documents and subjective theories, at the structural (data) level, (b) interviews and conversation analysis at the micro (method) level, (c) subject-oriented or psychological theories, ethnomethodology and organizational theories at the theory level, and (d) multiple investigators at the investigator level. He termed this "a method-appropriate

319

strategy of founding the credibility of qualitative analyses" (Flick 1992 p. 194.) Conceived in this way, triangulation becomes an alternative to "traditional criteria like reliability and validity" (p. 195).

5. A Case of Multiple Triangulation

The social sciences must move beyond investigations that triangulate only by data source or by research method. Multiple triangulation must become the goal and aim of these disciplines. There are, however, few outstanding illustrations of this commitment. Perhaps Thomas and Znaniecki's publication, *The Polish Peasant in Europe and America* (1918–20) remains the classic in the social sciences.

This five-volume work, which sought to build a social psychology within the nascent field of sociology, utilized personal, historical, religious, and economic documents from and about Polish society, as it was disintegrating and undergoing transition prior to the First World War. The work consists of five documentary volumes which offer a study of the social organization and evolution of the peasant primary groups (family and community) under the influence of industrialization and immigration to America and Germany. Volumes 1 and 2 study the peasant family, the Polish marriage and class system, economic life, religious attitudes, and include correspondence between members of six family groups. Volume 3 is the autobiography of a peasant immigrant. Volume 4 examines the dissolution of primary groups in Poland and Volume 5 is based on studies of the Polish immigrant in America.

Thomas and Znaniecki's investigation used triangulated data, investigators, theories, methods, and member-checks. Life histories, autobiographies, and family letters were at the core of their study yet, in an unparalleled fashion, the research utilized participant observation, interviews, quasicomparative experiments on a grand scale, unobtrusive methods (letters), and surveys. Theoretically, the work wove its way (often implicitly) through the theories of Freud, James, Marx, Spencer, Durkheim, Mauss, Weber, Tonnies, Simmel, Hegel, Mead, Cooley, and Comte.

This study, still a classic and in need of reinterpretation, illustrates the scope and volume that multiple triangulation may assume. Smaller in size, but illustrative and pivotal in importance, stands Geertz's (1972) study on the "Balinese cockfight." This investigation was based on description and interpretation and also triangulated data, investigators, theory, methods.

6. Problems in Designing Multiple-triangulated Investigations

There are at least four basic problems to be confronted in such research. These are: (a) locating a common subject of analysis to which multiple methods, observers, and theories can be applied; (b) reconciling discrepant findings and interpretations; (c) novelty, or the location of a problem that has not been investigated before; and (d) restrictions of time and money.

The location of a common subject of analysis can only be resolved through a clear understanding of the question the investigator wishes to answer. Divergent and discrepant findings are to be expected, for each inspection of the phenomenon is likely to yield different pictures, images, and findings. These differences are not to be ignored, but should be reported so that future investigators can build upon such observations. Novel or new problems are often, upon inspection, not new but merely manifestations of familiar topics previously examined from different perspectives and questions. Restrictions of time and money are the least problematic, for if investigators are thoroughly committed to understanding a problem area they will persist in examining it, even under difficult circumstances.

7. Criticisms of Triangulation

It must be noted that the method of triangulation is not without its critics. Several criticisms have been brought to bear upon the traditional treatments of the triangulation strategy (see Fielding and Fielding 1986, Flick 1992, Lincoln and Guba 1985, Patton 1980, Silverman 1985).

7.1 Data Triangulation

Silverman (1985) has argued that a positivistic bias underlies the triangulation position and that this is most evident in the concept of data triangulation. He argued that a hypothesis-testing orientation is present when authors argue that hypotheses that survive multiple tests contain more validity than those subjected to just one test. He also suggested that to assume that the same empirical unit can be measured more than once is inconsistent with the interactionist view of emergence and novelty in the field situation. If, as Silverman argued, all social action is situated and unique, then the same unit, behavior, or experience can never be observed twice. Each occurrence is unique. Accordingly, data triangulation better refers to seeking multiple sites and levels for the study of the phenomenon in question. It is erroneous to think or imply that the same unit can be measured. At the same time, the concept of hypothesis-testing must be abandoned. The interactionist seeks to build interpretations, not test hypotheses.

Patton (1980 p. 331) has correctly noted that the comparison of multiple data sources will "seldom lead to a single, totally consistent picture. It is best not to expect everything to turn out the same." Patton went on to argue that different types (and levels) of data reveal different aspects of what is being studied. The point is not to ignore these differences, but to attempt to understand and interpret them. Lincoln and Guba (1985 p. 282) extended this point, while stating the general principle that "no single item of information (unless coming from an elite and unimpeachable source) should ever be given serious consideration unless it can be triangulated." This means that the researcher must have multiple occurrences or representations of the processes being studied.

7.2 Investigator Triangulation

No two investigators ever observe the same phenomenon in exactly the same way. Lincoln and Guba (1985 p. 307) suggested that it is a mistake to "expect corroboration of one investigator by another." The argument that greater reliability of observations can be obtained by using more than one observer is thus indefensible. This does not mean, however, that multiple observers or investigators should not be used. When possible, they should be (see Douglas 1976). Their use expands the interpretative base of the research and reveals elements of the phenomenon that would not necessarily be seen by just one researcher. In some cases, a researcher does not have access to a particular site because of gender.

Douglas (1976) has suggested that team research (a similar term for the use of multiple observers) allows an investigator to gain multiple perspectives on a social situation. Members of a research team have a multiplier effect on the research—each adds more than just his or her presence to the knowledge that is gained about the situation being studied. Some team members have special talents that can be drawn upon. They may be good at sociability or at observing people and remembering what they say, or they may be members of the social worlds under investigation (Douglas 1976). These skills can be drawn upon in investigative, team research.

The triangulation of observers may extend, as Patton noted, to triangulating analysts. It is possible to have "two or more persons independently analyze the same qualitative data and then compare their finds" (Patton 1980 pp. 331–32). This approach has been employed in research on alcoholism films (see Denzin 1991). A team of film-viewers have been viewing films together, forming interpretations as they watched the films, checking them out against the film's text, and reformulating them as they watched the films more than once. The intent is not to build a consensual interpretation of the film. Rather, it seeks the multiple meanings that can be located in the viewing experience. In so doing, an adversary-advocacy model of interpretation is adopted (Patton 1980). Each member, working with the same film, marshals evidence to support different, and often opposing, conclusions.

7.3 Theory Triangulation

Lincoln and Guba (1985 p. 307) stated, in regard to theoretical triangulation, that "The use of multiple theories as a triangulation technique seems to us to be both epistemologically unsound and empirically empty." They based this harsh conclusion on a narrow reading of this strategy. As was previously outlined, theoretical triangulation simply asks the researcher to be aware of the multiple ways in which the phenomenon may be interpreted. It does not demand, nor does it ask, that facts be consistent with two or more theories. Such a demand is, of course, absurd.

7.4 Methodological Triangulation

This strategy asks only that researchers use more than one method. It takes the position that single-method studies (that is, only surveys, only experiments, and so on) are no longer defensible in the social sciences. Patton (1980 p. 330) noted that "There is no magic in triangulation." This is true. The researcher using different methods should not expect findings generated by different methods to fall into a coherent picture (Patton 1980, Lincoln and Guba 1985). They will not and cannot, for each method yields a different picture and slice of reality. What is critical is that different pictures be allowed to emerge (Trend 1978). Methodological triangulation allows this to happen.

7.5 Multiple Triangulation

Fielding and Fielding (1986) offered a critical interpretation of this strategy:

> Multiple triangulation, as Denzin expounded it, is the equivalent for research methods of "correlation" in data analysis. They both represent extreme forms of eclecticism. Theoretic triangulation does not . . . reduce bias, nor does methodological triangulation necessarily increase validity . . . In other words, there is a case for triangulation, but not the one Denzin makes. We should combine theories and methods carefully and purposefully with the intention of adding breadth or depth to our analysis, but not for the purpose of pursuing "objective" truth. (p. 33)

The last sentence is accepted. The goal of multiple triangulation is a fully grounded interpretative research approach. Objective reality will never be captured. In-depth understanding, not validity, is sought in any interpretative study. Multiple triangulation should never be eclectic. It cannot, however, be meaningfully compared to correlation analysis in statistical studies.

8. Conclusion

Triangulation is the preferred line of research in the social sciences. By combining multiple observers, theories, methods, and data sources, social scientists can begin to overcome the intrinsic bias that is bound to come from single-method, single-observer, single-theory investigations. There are inherent difficulties in formulating coherent, comprehensive sociological interpretations when only one method is employed. The shifting, conflictual, emergent, constructed nature of the social world, coupled with the unique problems that arise from theories, methods, and observers make the doing of sociology fundamentally difficult.

It is suggested that the resolutions to this difficulty are twofold. First, sociologists must recognize these basic features of the research act. Second, multiple strategies of triangulation must become the preferred line of action when theory-work, research, and interpretation are undertaken. By combining multiple observers, theories, methods, and empirical materials, sociologists can hope to overcome the intrinsic bias and problems that come from single-method, single-observer, single-theory studies.

The triangulated method is not without problems. A number of issues that have been raised about the approach have been discussed above. There is no empirical world independent of observations. No two theories will ever yield completely compatible images of the phenomenon at hand. Every method reveals a different slice of the social world. Every researcher sees different qualities. Triangulation is expensive. Weak designs may result from its implementation. However, its use, when coupled with sophisticated rigor, will broaden, thicken, and deepen the interpretative base of any study.

See also: Research Paradigms in Education; Scientific Methods in Educational Research

References

Brewer J, Hunter A 1989 *Multimethod Research: A Synthesis of Styles*. Sage, Newbury Park, California

Brewer M B, Collins B E (eds.) 1981 *Scientific Inquiry and the Social Sciences: A Volume in Honor of Donald T. Campbell*. Jossey-Bass, San Francisco, California

Campbell D T, Fiske D W 1959 Convergent and discriminant validation by the multitrait-multimethod matrix. *Psych. Bull.* 56: 81–105

Denzin N K 1989 *The Research Act: A Theoretical Introduction to Sociological Methods*, 3rd edn. Prentice-Hall, Englewood Cliffs, New Jersey

Denzin N K 1991 *Hollywood Shot by Shot: Alcoholism in American Cinema*. Aldine de Gruyter, New York

Douglas J D 1976 *Investigative Social Research: Individual and Team Field Research*. Sage, Beverly Hills, California

Eisner E W 1991 *The Enlightened Eye: Qualitative Inquiry and the Enhancement of Educational Practice*. Macmillan, New York

Fielding N G, Fielding J L 1986 *Linking Data*. Sage, Beverly Hills, California

Flick U 1992 Triangulation revisited: Strategy of validation or alternative? *Journal for the Theory of Social Behaviour* 22(2): 175–97

Geertz C 1972 Deep play: Notes on the Balinese cockfight. *Daedalus* 101: 1–37

Guba E G, Lincoln Y S 1989 *Fourth Generation Evaluation*. Sage, Newbury Park, California

Guba E G, Lincoln Y S 1994 Competing Paradigms in Qualitative Research. In: Denzin N K, Lincoln Y S (eds.) 1994 *Handbook of Qualitative Research*. Sage, Thousand Oaks, California

Hammersley M, Atkinson P 1983 *Ethnography: Principles in Practice*. Tavistock, London

Heidegger M 1962 *Being and Time*. Harper, New York

Huberman A M, Miles M B 1994 Data Management and Analysis Methods. In: Denzin N K, Lincoln Y S (eds.) 1994 *Handbook of Qualitative Research*. Sage, Thousand Oaks, California

Lincoln Y S, Guba E G 1985 *Naturalistic Inquiry*. Sage, Beverly Hills, California

Patton M Q 1980 *Qualitative Evaluation Methods*. Sage, Beverly Hills, California

Pitman M A, Maxwell J A 1991 Qualitative approaches to evaluation. In: LeCompte M D, Millroy W L, Preissle J (eds.) 1991 *The Handbook of Qualitative Research in Education*. Academic Press, San Diego, California

Reinharz S, Davidson L 1992 *Feminist Methods in Social Research*. Oxford University Press, New York

Stake R S 1995 *The Art of Case Study Research*. Sage, Thousand Oaks, California

Silverman D 1985 *Qualitative Methodology and Sociology: Describing the Social World*. Gower, Brookfield, Vermont

Thomas W I, Znaniecki F 1918–20 *The Polish Peasant in Europe and America. Monograph of an Immigrant Group*, 5 Vols. University of Chicago Press, Chicago, Illinois

Trend M G 1978 On the reconciliation of qualitative and quantitative analyses: A case study. *Human Organization* 37: 345–54

(b) Scientific Analysis Procedures

Census and National Survey Data

G. Burke

Most national governments conduct a population census every 5 or 10 years. High income countries also carry out sample surveys of the working-age population, on a monthly basis. Annual censuses of particular institutions such as primary and secondary schools and tertiary institutions are also usually conducted. This entry provides an overview of: (a) what is collected; (b) how and when it is published; (c) some of the major uses in research related to planning and policy; and (d) limitations of the data.

The census of a population is an expensive, time-consuming undertaking, carried out by questionnaire delivered to all residences by a national bureau of census and statistics. The aim is to provide basic demographic, social, and economic data for government and private decision-making and research. Between censuses sample surveys are used to obtain up-to-date information and to provide detail on matters not covered in the census. The best known example of the national sample survey is the monthly or current population survey carried out by trained interviewers on a stratified random sample of households: in the United States, 60,000 households; in Canada, 48,000; in Japan, 40,000; and in Australia, 33,000. In a few countries longitudinal studies of a sample population are carried out by national statistical bodies.

Special education collections such as censuses and samples of schools are often handled by a body separate from that concerned with producing social and economic statistics about the national population. For example, in the United States the National Center for Education Statistics was set up to "collect, and analyse and disseminate statistics and other data related to education in the United States and in other nations." In addition, the central administrations of most educational systems assemble a wide range of statistics relating to the supply and demand for schools and teachers, the costs of educational provision, the sizes of classes, the retention, attrition and absentee rates for students and teachers, as well as performance measures of educational outcomes. Such information is commonly made publicly available in annual reports, and is supplied to bodies like the Organization for Economic Co-operation and Development (OECD) and the United Nations Educational Cultural Organization (UNESCO)

The method of undertaking a census or a survey is usually clearly detailed in the publications of the national body that undertakes them. This entry will give only minor attention to these methods and to problems of validity and reliability of the data (see UNESCO 1991; *Quasi-experimentation; Interviewing for Clinical Research*).

1. What is Collected?

Any country's five yearly census will vary over time in size and content. The census collects demographic, economic, and social information by means of a questionnaire from all residents of the country on a particular night. Its range is limited by issues of privacy, the past success in collecting the data and its usefulness, the cost of collection and processing, and the difficulty in obtaining particular information by questionnaire. Examples of problem areas for the census are income and religion and, in some countries, age. The census yields estimates of population by age and sex and region. It usually provides details on employment, educational participation and attainment, main language spoken, ethnicity, housing, mode of transport, and income.

The monthly household population survey is fairly standard in its basic collection of demographic, employment, and unemployment data for persons of working age across the many countries that have adopted most if not all the labor force concepts agreed by the International Labour Organisation (1982), which were based on developmental work carried out in the United States. On an annual or occasional basis, supplementary surveys seek a wide range of information including educational participation and attainment.

National estimates (e.g., of educational participation in postcompulsory education) based on the monthly survey may be provided with an apparently small margin of error. However, the estimates for regions and particular age or social groups are subject to a much larger sampling error. The reliability of estimates may also vary with the way the household questionnaire is administered. If one person answers all questions on behalf of the household there is a tendency on some matters, such as part-time work and part-time study, to underestimate participation compared with the findings of questionnaires administered directly to all members of the household (see, e.g., Freeman and Medoff 1982).

Government censuses of educational institutions always include data on the number and type of institutions, students, and staff. The degree of detail in such collections can vary but student data are usually provided by full-time and part-time status, by age and sex, and by level and type of course. Financial data are sometimes provided in these collections. Comparability across institutions and regions of the data collected in such censuses of educational institutions may be less than desired if (a) common definitions of key concepts such as student, full-time, and teacher are not rigorously defined; and (b) compliance is not assured by institutions surveyed.

Though there may be gaps and deficiencies in the data collected in such censuses of formal educational institutions, they are minor compared with the deficiencies in the data on training in the workplace and on other nonformal types of education. In the 1980s surveys were carried out on modes of training and employee expenditure on training (Australian Bureau of Statistics 1992).

2. Publication of Data

Only part of the data collected by national bodies is published in hard copy. Data from government surveys are increasingly released on CD-ROM and floppy disk as well as on microfiche and tape. The restrictions of confidentiality, and concern about the misuse of estimates for which sampling error may be high, place limits on the data that national statistical bodies are willing to release. Special tables with variables as specified by the user, or unit records, or in the case of the population census the 1 percent sample tapes, may be requested.

These new forms of publication represent a potentially vast increase in access to very detailed information for a wide range of users. This is enhanced by the decline in the costs of computers with their amazingly increased capacity, and improved software. A major concern is the level of charges that governments now make for the data, which may limit access to governments, large companies, and well-funded research institutes. The individual researcher and the interested citizen may find their access limited to the holdings of major libraries.

Sample survey data are often available some months after collection. The release of census data, however, may in some countries be delayed for several years.

3. Major Uses and Limitations

Any government body or private researcher is likely to make use of census and sample survey data from time to time. Use is made of current data and of

time series built up from previous collections, though changes in definitions and in methods of collection may affect comparability over time. The classification of all the uses is an impossible task. As an illustration, attention will be focused on the major use of the national data collections by governments and researchers concerned with policy and planning about education, about education and society, and about education and the economy.

The methods of finance, ownership, and regulation of the education system may be important in determining the type of data that will be needed in policy-making. If education were largely financed and provided in an unregulated private sector then there might seem to be little need for government planning and therefore little need for national and regional data collections. But only the most devout advocates of the free market could believe that a government should accept whatever outcomes the market yields, without concern either for market failure or for social costs and benefits that the market might ignore. The data needs may vary with the type of education system, but the necessity for national monitoring exists even with a market system.

While market elements in the provision of education have expanded since the 1980s, across the world it is still governments that dominate the provision and finance of education. The case is overwhelming that some planning should take place. For example, if schooling is provided free by governments in government schools to all who wish to enroll, then the government needs some means of estimating the numbers wishing to enroll. It needs this information to ensure that schools and teachers are in place when the students seek to enroll.

In order to illustrate the use of national data sets in planning it is necessary to discuss briefly some of the key elements of planning (see *Projections of Educational Statistics*).

3.1 Demography

One of the base elements is demographic analysis. This involves projections of the population and by age and gender and by region based on data collected in the census and supplemented through sample data, migration data, and registrations of births and deaths.

3.2 Demand for Education

A second factor in planning involves the consideration of the demand to participate in any particular sector of education. This is a matter of family income and tastes, of rewards to the particular type of education, and of the costs of that type of education. To some extent these factors are influenced by direct government action on the curriculum and the assessment system; by financial factors such as student financial aid and unemployment benefits; or indirectly by government through the effects of its economic policy on the economy—successful or unsuccessful. The direct action of government, such as provision of financial assistance for students, may stem from concerns for social justice (e.g., reducing youth unemployment) or concern for the needs of industry.

Part, but only part, of the data required for analysis of demand is provided by the national census and sample surveys of the population, and collections from educational institutions. For example, data on trends in enrollments are available from institutions; family income and the recent pattern of earnings by age and qualification level are collected in the national surveys in many countries.

There is often the need to supplement the national collections with administrative data collected within government departments or by sample surveys undertaken by research organizations. This is illustrated by the experience of national or state or provincial committees of inquiry which are regularly established to investigate aspects of education. Almost invariably the nationally compiled census and survey data are inadequate for the particular questions under scrutiny by the inquiry.

Even if the data were apparently adequate, the relationships between the important variables cannot be easily specified. Moreover, relationships estimated on the basis of past data may not hold into the future. A major factor affecting analysis of demand for postcompulsory education in many countries is that enrollments may be determined by the supply of places funded by the government. Current or past enrollments may reflect supply but underestimate demand, leaving the estimation of demand as an extremely difficult exercise.

3.3 Supply of Education by Government

A third factor in planning is the extent to which a government wishes to finance or provide the places to meet demand. Government policy on educational provision is affected by the needs of the economy, its policy on social justice and the environment, and its willingness or capacity to finance the activity. The relevance of national census and survey data to consideration of the needs of the economy and the issue of social justice are briefly considered here.

Governments make judgments on the role of education in meeting the labor force needs of the economy. These judgments are supported through "manpower forecasting," "international comparisons," or through "rate-of-return analysis."

Manpower or labor market forecasting requires detailed data on educational attainment by occupation and by age. Most censuses and some surveys provide data on these. The problem arises from the meaning that attaches to the myriad of qualification levels and the extent to which job skills are represented by educational qualifications. Furthermore, any occupation, even at the finest detail in the census, will nearly always encompass a fairly wide range of qualification levels. Medical practitioners or secondary teachers may be fairly homogeneous groups in many countries and entry to such jobs may be restricted by law to those possessing particular qualifications. However, this is not true of most jobs, and in most jobs there will be persons with little formal education and persons with high levels of qualifications.

Refinement of the data is important. Defining occupations in terms of the type and level of skill they require rather than in historical groupings is important. Similarly, educational qualifications could be defined in terms of sets of competencies in communication, mathematics, and so on. But it must be recognized that the nature of occupations is changing due to technological change and changes in work practices. With almost any form of equipment, alternative forms of job organization may be possible. The mix of persons with high or low qualification levels within an occupation may therefore vary among firms in an industry as well as between industries. An attempt to reach exact correspondence of educational qualifications and occupation may not be desirable either for work or education. So while the inadequacies of data should be diminished, they must always be quite substantial.

Even with good data the task of labor market forecasting is not easy. Changes in key parameters, such as the rate of resignation or retirement from particular occupations, can have drastic implications for the need for new recruits. The effect of apparently small changes is magnified since in most occupations recruits are but a small flow into the large existing stock within the occupation.

International comparisons are frequently used in support of policy changes in education but they remain hazardous. The OECD and UNESCO, the major international organizations with concern for education, are the main compilers of international data (OECD 1990, UNESCO 1991). Where nations differ in demographic structure, level of development, and in structure of the education system comparisons would be difficult to interpret even with similarly defined key concepts such as enrollments, teachers, and expenditure. However, efforts to achieve agreement in definitions and uniformity in data collection are yielding significant results in meeting the need for a set of indicators that will permit effective international comparisons (Bottani et al. 1992, 1993).

Rate-of-return studies and other variants of cost–benefit analysis are advocated as a means of considering the worth of alternative forms of education. The method requires data on education by employment and by earnings as well as cost data. These are rarely collected in the national collections in the detail required for the analysis. In any case there are considerable reservations about the technique (Woodhall 1987).

A government's concern for social justice and related concerns for democracy and for the environment are factors in its willingness to provide or subsidize education. For intervention for these reasons a government needs information on inequalities in education, in work and living standards, and on the connections between them. For example, participation rates by ethnicity and language, region, and socioeconomic background may be obtained from census and in part from survey data. However, these data would need to be supplemented with data from cohorts over time for analysis of the connections between educational inequalities and other inequalities in society and the likely effects of government intervention.

3.4 Resources per Student

Even if a government decides to provide places in schools or postsecondary education for all who wish to attend (at the going structure of fees and student assistance), a fourth step is to determine the level of provision of resources: that is, the rate of staffing of schools, nonstaff resources, and buildings; and the rate of payment to staff relative to the general level of wages in society.

Data relevant to such considerations involve staffing data, some of which will be collected in the census of institutions. Some of the information will be available from other forms of data collection undertaken by national statistical bodies. Data on teachers' salaries relative to other pay rates are usually compiled in national collections on pay rates and form part of the data in cost deflators used in the national accounts on national income and expenditure.

4. Effectiveness Indicators

As a consequence of the marked expansion that has occurred during the latter decades of the twentieth century in the areas of upper secondary, technical and higher education increased concern has developed for the containment of the costs of the provision of education at these levels. There has thus been a growing interest in the identification and use of effectiveness indicators in the economic analysis of educational activities (Windham 1988). The analyses undertaken have distinguished between *input indicators* (teacher qualifications, facilities, equipment, educational materials and the competence of system, district, and school administrators); *process indicators* (student and teacher time allocations, and administrative and supervisory activity); *output indicators* (attainment indicators, achievement measures, equity indices and attitude and behavior indicators) and *outcome indicators* (participation in further education and training rates, unemployment rates, earnings, social mobility indices, the distribution of earnings and incomes, and adult litercy levels). The OECD publication *Education at a Glance* (Bottani et al. 1992,1993) grew from the increased interest in this wide range of effectiveness indicators and has established the value of such information in educational planning. National educational

systems are now collecting data on these indicators with greater care and rigor and are participating in the studies of the International Association for the Evaluation of Educational Achievement (IEA) and the International Association for Educational Assessment (IAEA) in order to obtain information on educational performance that is comparable across countries. The problems encountered in monitoring of the standards of education within and between countries are addressed by Tuijnman and Postlethwaite (1994). Nevertheless, disagreement and disputation have developed between those administrators and politicians who seek to apply economic analyses to educational activities, and those scholars and practitioners who reject what they see to be the gross oversimplification of educational endeavours. Windham (1988) presents the case for the relevance of the range of effectiveness indicators and emphasizes the need for educational policy makers and administrators to be trained to use such information in educational management and decision-making.

5. Conclusion

Data compiled by national statistical bureaus and national educational bodies provide an indispensable input to research for policy and planning in education. However such collections cannot provide all the data required in policy and planning. The national data collections often provide only context data for more basic educational research. Consider, for example, a study on education and ethnicity. Data from the national census and surveys may provide details on the language and ethnicity of persons in the geographical area under consideration, the level of income and unemployment, the type of jobs of the employed, and the particular characteristics of the unemployed compared with the employed. The researcher concerned with the influence of school organization and curriculum or the values and aspirations of young people in various ethnic groups will, however, still have to collect and analyze data relevant to that study. Connections and relationships between the data from national collections and data collected by the researcher still depend on the researcher and the theories by which the research is guided.

See also: Research Paradigms in Education

References

Australian Bureau of Statistics 1992 *Education and Training in Australia.* Australian Bureau of Statistics, Canberra
Bottani N, Duchesne C, Tuijnman A 1992, 1993 *Education at a Glance: OECD Indicators,*1st, and 2nd edns. Organisation for Economic Co-operation and Development (OECD), Paris

Freeman R B, Medoff J L 1982 Why does youth labor force activity differ across surveys? In: Freeman R B, Wise D B (eds.) 1982 *The Youth Labor Market Problem: Its Nature, Causes and Consequences*. University of Chicago Press, Chicago, Illinois

International Labour Organisation 1982 *Statistics of Labor Force, Employment, Unemployment and Underemployment*. Report Prepared for the Thirteenth International Conference of Labor Statisticians. International Labor Office, Geneva

OECD 1990 *Education in OECD Countries 1987–88: A Compendium of Statistical Information*. OECD, Paris

Tuijnman A C, Postlethwaite T N 1994 *Monitoring the Standards of Education*. Pergamon Press, Oxford

UNESCO 1991 *Statistical Yearbook, 1991*. UNESCO, Paris

Windham D 1988 Effectiveness indicators in the economic analyses of educational activities. *Int. J. Educ. Res.* 12(6): 575–665

Woodhall M 1987 Earnings and education. In: Psacharopoulos G (ed.) 1987 *Economics of Education, Research and Studies*. Pergamon Press, Oxford

Further Reading

United Nations 1991 *Demographic Yearbook*. United Nations, New York

United States Department of Education 1991 *Digest of Education Statistics, 1991*. National Center for Education Statistics (NCES), Washington, DC

Change, Measurement of

J. B. Willett

Why is the measurement of change over time so important in educational research? The answer is straightforward. When people acquire new skills, when they learn something new, when they grow intellectually and physically, when their attitudes and interests develop, they are changing in fundamental and interesting ways. By being able to measure change over time, it is possible to map phenomena at the heart of the educational enterprise. Education is intended to foster learning, to bring about changes in attitude, achievement, and values. Only by measuring individual change is it possible to document each person's progress and, consequently, to evaluate the effectiveness of educational systems.

Unfortunately, despite its obvious substantive importance, there has been much controversy over the years about the measurement of change. Influential methodologists concerned about the technical properties of change measurement have argued that it is impossible to measure change well. Empirical researchers were advised to avoid its measurement. Policymakers were told to mistrust research findings based on that measurement.

However, in reality these traditional conclusions and recommendations are incorrect. Change can not only be measured; with a little foresight and planning it can be measured well. Well-publicized false conclusions about the difficulty of change measurement are rooted in a simple misconception: the misconception that individual change should be viewed as an *increment*, as the difference between "before" and "after." Early methodologists and empirical researchers saw each person under study as acquiring a quantum of achievement (or attitude, or value, or whatever) between the "pre" and the "post" measurement. They

thought that investigators should only be concerned with the size of the acquired chunk. This was a mistaken perception. Individual change takes place continuously over time; it is not purely a "before" and "after" phenomenon. The failure to perceive change as a continuous process of development hamstrung the creation of decent statistical methods for its measurement.

However, methodologists have recently modified their position. They have concluded that individual change can be measured well, providing that research moves beyond the limitations of the "before and after," or "two wave," design. They now understand that the continuous process of human development can be easily and efficiently documented if each person is measured repetitively over extended periods of time. In this entry the new "multiwave" perspective is presented, and it is argued that, with a little planning, all questions about change can be answered. Because there has been such controversy, this entry begins by reconsidering traditional methods for the measurement of change.

1. Traditional Methods for Measuring Change

Implicit in any discussion of change are two important kinds of question. The first treats each person as an individual and asks about within-person change. For example, in an evaluation of different reading curricula, it can be asked: Does this person's reading achievement improve over time? Is there rapid improvement, or is improvement more gradual? Does reading achievement grow at a steady rate, or does it level out after one or two years?— and so on for every person in the sample. The second type of question asks about between-person differences in change. Do certain types of people change in different ways? Does the reading achievement of girls change faster than that of boys? Does progress in reading achievement differ by type of first-grade reading program? These are questions about the way in which individual change is related, over people, to background, training, environment, and so forth.

Answering questions about within-person change logically precedes the asking of questions about between-person differences in change. It is necessary to know how each person changes before asking whether the individual changes differ in some systematic way from one person to the next. However, the latter questions about between-person differences in change often have the greatest practical importance in educational research.

Traditionally, in research on change, investigators collected only two waves of data on each person in the sample. They observed each person's "status"—their achievement, attitude, or other attribute, say—at the beginning and the end of the investigation. Then, to answer questions about within-person change, they used the "pre" and "post" data to construct a summary measure of individual change for each person in the study. Subsequently, when questions about between-person differences in change were addressed, the two-wave change summaries were simply regressed on, or correlated with, other variables (the "predictors of change") describing background, training, or treatment.

This seems straightforward, but the apparent simplicity masks serious pitfalls. For one thing, for the strategy to be effective the researcher must be able to use the two waves of data that have been collected to construct a decent measure of change for each person in the sample. Methodologists differ as to how this should be done and psychometric history is littered with strategies proposed for the purpose. Some of these strategies are better than others, but they are all inferior to the multiwave methods introduced in Sect. 2.

The simplest two-wave measure of change is the *observed difference score*, obtained by subtracting the initial measurement from the final one for each person. Originally the difference score was highly favored but then fell into disrepute, being much maligned in the 1960s and 1970s. This led to the birth of a coterie of alternative two-wave measures of change, including *regression-based estimators of true change* and *residual change* scores. Although the use of two-wave change measurement is not advocated in practice, it is desirable to comment briefly below on these measures in order to clarify the continuing controversy.

1.1 Two-wave Measures of Within-person Change

Because of the uncompromising vicissitudes of nature, when a test or rating instrument is administered the obtained measurement combines a measure of the person's true capability and whatever random error happens to accompany measurement. Of course, research interest focuses squarely on *true status*—a commodity that, if *measurement error* is large, may differ considerably from *observed status*. Similarly, when members of a group of people are changing over time on some important attribute, it is not the fallible *observed changes* that are of critical interest but the underlying *true changes*. Measures of observed change simply provide a fallible lens through which the hidden nature of true change may be discerned.

Typically, on the ith occasion of measurement (i.e., at time t_i), methodologists have been content to assume that observed status, Y_{ip}, is simply the sum of true status, η_{ip}, and measurement error, ε_{ip} (the second subscript indicating that the pth person is being referenced). These errors of measurement, ε_{ip}, are usually assumed to be drawn independently from a normal distribution with zero mean and variance σ_{ε}^2. When two waves of data have been collected, observed "pretest" and "post-test" status (measured at times t_1 and t_2) can be represented by their requisite sums: $Y_{1p} = \eta_{1p} + \varepsilon_{1p}$ and $Y_{2p} = \eta_{2p} + \varepsilon_{2p}$. Then, the observed difference score for the pth person, D_p—obtained by subtracting Y_{1p} from Y_{2p}—is the sum of the underlying true change, $\Delta_p = (\eta_{2p} - \eta_{1p})$, and the difference between the two measurement errors, $(\varepsilon_{2p} - \varepsilon_{1p})$.

Statistically speaking, the observed difference score is a reasonable commodity. It is intuitively appealing and easy to compute. It is an unbiased estimator of the underlying true change. Despite these advantages, the difference score has been resoundingly criticized for both its purported unreliability and its correlation with initial status. Although these deficiencies have been shown recently to be largely imaginary, they are discussed here briefly in order to set the record straight.

Some have said that the difference score is always unreliable; others have argued that it cannot be both reliable and valid simultaneously (Bereiter 1963, Linn and Slinde 1977). In general, neither of these claims is correct. They are misconceptions arising from misinterpretation of the concepts of reliability and validity in the context of change over time (Rogosa et al. 1982, Rogosa and Willett 1983, 1985, Willett 1988). Thus, it has been argued that an instrument can only be regarded as measuring the same construct on both occasions of measurement if the correlation of time-1 and time-2 scores is high. This is fallacious. Even when the instrument is perfectly construct-valid, growth may be heterogeneous across people (i.e., different people may be growing at different rates). Then the individual growth trajectories will naturally intersect as time passes, the rank order of people in the group will fluctuate from occasion to occasion, and the between-wave correlation will be less than unity. It is perfectly possible, in the context of highly heterogeneous growth, for the time-1/time-2 correlation to be large and negative even when the instrument is perfectly construct-valid.

As a consequence of misinterpreting the observed pretest–post-test correlation as an index of construct validity in expressions for the reliability of the difference score, authors have misguidedly focused on hypothetical situations in which there is little variation in true change across people. By choosing to examine situations in which the variance of true change is close to zero, they have ensured that the numerator of the expression for the reliability of the difference score (which is defined as the ratio of the variances of true and observed change) is very small and so the reliability is almost zero. In reality, in perfectly ordinary situations, the reliability of the difference score can be quite respectable (Rogosa and Willett 1983). And when variation in true change from one person to the next is large, the reliability of the difference score can even be greater than the reliabilities of the constituent pretest and post-test scores (Willett 1988).

Anyway, even if the difference score were always unreliable, this would not necessarily be a problem for the measurement of within-person change. Low difference-score reliability does not imply unilaterally that within-person change has been measured imprecisely. Low reliability often occurs in practice because most of the people in the sample are changing at about the same rate (especially over the short term). So even though the 20 points (say) that everyone has changed can be measured very precisely, the changes of different people cannot be distinguished from one another and the difference score appears unreliable. This problem of interpretation does not call the difference-score itself into question, since it is possible to know quite precisely that everyone has changed by 20 points. On the contrary, it simply undermines the credibility of reliability as a worthwhile indicator of measurement quality.

The difference score has also been falsely condemned for at least three other reasons, all of which originate in critics' misunderstanding of the association between it and pretest status (Linn and Slinde 1977, Plewis 1985). If there is a positive correlation between change and pretest status, for instance, then people with high initial status will tend to have high gains subsequently. If the correlation is negative, then people with low initial scores will tend to change more rapidly than those with high initial scores. This has led some critics to claim that any measure of change that is not independent of initial status must be unfair because it gives "an advantage to persons with certain values of the pretest scores" (Linn and Slinde 1977 p. 125). But such prejudice is unreasonable: why should change and status be unrelated? The intimate connection between change and status is a consequence of growth history. Current status is a product of prior change; current change determines future status. A correlation between change and status is an almost inevitable fact of life.

Second, numerous investigators have empirically estimated the correlation between change and initial status and have worried because their findings often disagreed. Even when investigating similar populations in similar settings with the same measures, some have found the correlation to be positive, some zero, and some strongly negative. But why should they expect a single value for this correlation? When different people are changing in different ways, individual trajectories are likely to crisscross with time and the correlation between change and initial status can fluctuate markedly as different times are selected as the occasion for "initial" measurement (see Rogosa and Willett 1985). Unless some important occasion can be agreed upon substantively to be *the* initial time, researchers should expect to disagree when they ask: What is the correlation between change and initial status? Because the answer, of course, is, "It depends on the time that you define as 'initial'."

Third, the difference score has been inappropriately criticized because some people have convinced themselves that its correlation with pretest score is always negative. In reality this claim is false (for an example of a positive correlation between the difference score and change see Thorndike 1966). Those who condemn the difference score in this way have usually committed one of two mistakes. Either they have spuriously created the negative correlation themselves by "standardizing" the pretest and post-test scores to the same standard deviation before computing the difference score (an ill-advised process that destroys legitimate growth information). Or they are simply being confused by the vaguenesses of their statistical estimation. In this latter case, they have usually thoughtlessly used the sample correlation of observed initial status and the difference score to estimate the population correlation of true initial status and true change (the real correlation of interest). Unfortunately, because the pretest measurement error appears with a negative sign in the difference score, this estimator is negatively biased. It is often negative even when the underlying true correlation is positive. However, the bias is easily corrected (see Willett 1988) and, anyway, as Rogosa et al. (1982) noted, an unbiased estimate of within-person change—the difference score—should not be rejected because a poorly conceived estimator of the association between true change and true initial status is biased. It is the latter that needs fixing, not the former.

So even though the difference score is not the outcast that many critics have claimed, several modifications of it have been proposed in order to estimate true change, Δ_p, better: for example, Webster and Bereiter's (1963) reliability-weighted measure of change, and Lord's (1956) regression-based estimated true change. These modified estimators improve the measurement of within-person change by trading off unbiasedness for a reduction in mean-squared error. Under very broad assumptions, these modified measures are simply weighted linear combinations of the observed difference score for the particular person and the average observed difference score over the entire group, with weights that depend on the reliability of the difference score. Essentially, the weighting scheme places emphasis on those aspects of the change measurement that are the most "trustworthy" —favoring the difference score when it is reliable but, otherwise, setting each person's change equal to the average change for everyone when there is little real between-person variation in change to be detected. Even though the modified scores are better estimates of true within-person change, they are usually perfectly correlated with the corresponding difference scores and have (almost) identical reliabilities. Therefore, parallel investigations of between-person differences in change using either of these modified scores usually lead to identical conclusions.

The creation of the residual-change score was motivated by an unnecessary desire to create measures of change that were uncorrelated with pretest score. Residual-change scores are obtained by estimating the residuals that would be obtained in the population regression of true final status on true initial status. They are intended to describe the true change that each person would have experienced, if everyone had "started out equal." Various methods have been proposed for their computation (see Rogosa et al. 1982). Much energy has been dissipated in the psychometric literature detailing the properties of the many estimators of residual change and considerable argument has been aroused. When discussing residual-change scores, methodologists disagree as to exactly what is being estimated, how well it is being estimated, and how it can be interpreted. In addition to the many technical and practical problems that arise in the empirical application of residual change scores, there also remain unresolved issues of logic and substance that are too extensive to detail here (but see Rogosa et al. 1982, Rogosa and Willett 1985, Willett 1988). The researcher is strongly advised to avoid these scores as measures of within-person change.

1.2 Detecting Between-person Differences in Change

Once a two-wave measure of change has been computed for each person, the relationship between change and other "background" variables is often investigated by the common methods of correlation and regression analysis. For instance, to find out if changes in achievement are related to gender, the data-analyst might simply correlate pre/post differences in test score with a dummy variable representing gender. Unfortunately, while straightforward, this rudimentary strategy is flawed. As has been seen, the difference score is a *fallible* measure of change that contains both true change and measurement error. This latter random noise attenuates the between-person findings, causing the obtained sample correlations to underestimate the true relationship between change and the covariates. This problem can be avoided by correcting between-person analyses for the fallibility of the difference

score (for methods of correction, see Willett 1988). However, the disattenuation process requires that additional information be available to the data-analyst, usually in the form of an external estimate of the reliability of the difference score. Furthermore, because the disattenuation is sensitive to minor fluctuations in the magnitude of the reliability estimate and because the quality of these estimates themselves is often dubious, there exists the very real possibility of glorious imperfection.

If the difference score is abandoned and an estimate of true change is used instead, information in addition to the pre/post measurement is still required for the estimate of true change to be constructed in the first place. In fact, regardless of the measure of change adopted, acceptable between-person analyses can only be conducted if the researcher possesses information in addition to the pair of pretest and post-test scores. This emphasizes the real and fundamental weakness of the two-wave design: there is insufficient information in two waves of data to measure individual change well. To do a satisfactory job, multiwave data are required.

2. Modern Methods of Change Measurement

Taking a "snapshot" of a person's observed status "before" and "after" is not the best way to reveal the intricacies of their progress. Changes might be occurring smoothly over time with some complex and substantively interesting trajectory. Crude pre/post measurement can never reveal the details of that trajectory. To do a good job of describing individual change over time, a truly longitudinal perspective must be adopted.

2.1 Assembling and Inspecting the Observed Growth Record

People must be followed carefully over time, with multiple "waves" of data collected on their status at sensibly spaced intervals. The investigator must assemble an *observed growth record* for each person in the dataset. If the attribute of interest is changing steadily and smoothly over a long period of time, perhaps three or four widely spaced measurements on each person will be sufficient to capture the shape and direction of the change. But, if the trajectory of individual change is complex, then many more closely spaced measurements may be required (see Willett 1989).

Once collected, preliminary analyses of the observed growth records are aided by plotting an *empirical growth-trajectory* for each person—a graph of observed status displayed against time, perhaps with some type of fitted or sketched trend-line included on the graph to summarize broadly the person's observed growth. Separate inspection of the empiri-

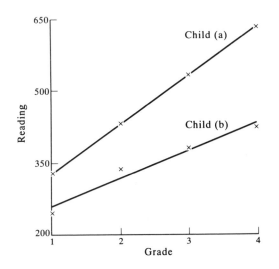

Figure 1
Observed growth records of two children whose reading achievement was measured in Grades 1 through 4. The included trend-lines were fitted by OLS linear regression analysis, conducted separately for each child

cal growth trajectory of each person in the dataset then provides evidence as to whether, and how, each person is changing over time. Fig. 1, for instance, presents the empirical growth trajectories of a pair of children whose reading achievement (scale scores on the Comprehensive Test of Basic Skills) was followed

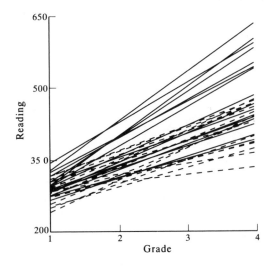

Figure 2
A collection of fitted trajectories summarizing the observed growth in reading achievement between Grades 1 and 4 for 32 children. The fitted trajectories are coded to display reading readiness in kindergarten (solid line for children above the sample median, dashed line for children below the sample median)

yearly from Grade 1 through Grade 4. In both cases, each child's observed growth in reading achievement is summarized by a linear trend-line, fitted by ordinary least-squares regression analysis. Comparing trend-line and data suggests that a straight line is a reasonable summary of the observed growth, although Child (b)'s datapoints are a little more widely scattered around the fitted line than are the datapoints for Child (a). Child (a)'s reading achievement is growing at more than double the rate of Child (b), with the latter child having the additional disadvantage of scoring lower initially.

The empirical growth trajectories of everyone under investigation can also be collected together in a single picture. This provides a simple and straightforward way of exploring questions about between-person differences in change. Eyeball comparisons across people may suggest systematic differences in trajectory—children in a phonics-based reading curriculum may tend to change more rapidly than those using a sight-reading curriculum; girls may be growing faster than boys, and so forth. Fig. 2, for instance, adds the fitted growth trajectories of 30 more children to the two already displayed in Fig. 1. The observed data themselves have been omitted to avoid clutter but the trend-lines have been coded to indicate whether the child was judged "ready for reading" in the kindergarten year (solid line = high reading readiness; dashed line = low reading readiness). Inspection of Fig. 2 suggests that children who were rated highly on reading readiness in kindergarten tended to have both higher reading achievement in Grade 1 and more rapid rates of growth between Grades 1 and 4. Similar plots could be created to display the effects of other interesting predictors.

2.2 Choosing a Statistical Model to Represent Within-person Change

Corresponding to the exploratory inspection of observed growth records and empirical growth-trajectories, a more formal multiwave analysis of change requires that a statistical model be chosen to represent individual change over time. Of course, as has been noted earlier, it is each person's underlying true change that is of critical interest. Consequently, when a statistical model is selected to represent change, it consists of two parts: (a) a "structural" part that represents the dependence of true status on time; (b) a "stochastic" part that represents the random effects of measurement error.

But what does an individual growth model look like? In drawing the empirical growth trajectories in Figs. 1 and 2, a linear or "straight-line" function of time was chosen as a valid representation of individual change in reading achievement between Grades 1 and 4. In this case the observed reading achievement Y_{ip} of child p at time t_i is represented as follows:

$$Y_{ip} = [\pi_{0p} + \pi_{1p}t_i] + \varepsilon_{ip} \tag{1}$$

331

where the structural part of the model, describing the dependence of true reading achievement η_{ip} on time, has been bracketed to separate it from the measurement error ε_{ip}.

The structural part of an individual growth model contains unknown constants called the individual growth parameters. The values of these parameters completely determine the trajectory of true change over time. In Eqn. (1), for instance, there are two individual growth parameters: π_{0p} and π_{1p}. The first parameter, π_{0p}, is the "intercept" of the straight-line growth model, representing person p's true status when t_i is equal to zero (usually defined as the time at which the study began, and therefore π_{0p} represents the true initial status of person p). The second parameter, π_{1p}, is the "slope" of the straight-line growth model, representing the rate at which person p's true status is growing over time. If π_{1p} is positive, then person p's true status is increasing with time; if it is negative then person p's true status is decreasing with time.

Of course, when analyses of multiwave data are conducted, the straight-line model is not the only available representation of individual change. Many different models—perhaps an infinite number—can be hypothesized. Some are simple, like the straight-line model, while others, like the negative-exponential and quadratic curves, are more complex. It is even possible to join several different models together, creating a piecewise individual growth function.

Perhaps the investigator's most important task is to select the individual growth model that will be used. Usually this decision is made via extensive preliminary data-analyses in which the observed growth records are systematically and carefully explored. However, the choice of a particular model for a specific purpose can often be informed by a theory of psychological, social, or educational development. Theory may suggest, for instance, that individual change in a specific domain is constrained to rise to a ceiling. So, by entertaining a growth model that includes an asymptote, the researcher can test this hypothesis and ultimately investigate whether substantively interesting features of the change are associated with differences in people's background, training, and environment. It may be, for instance, that certain background characteristics predict the ultimate limits on growth (the asymptotes), while others predict the rate at which the ceiling is approached. When substantive theory informs model choice, a richer research arena is revealed.

2.3 A Model for Between-person Differences in Change

Once a particular model has been selected to represent true change in a particular domain, everyone in the sample is assumed to have the same generic functional form for their growth. Different people, however, can have different values of the individual growth parameters. For instance, as in the case of

Figs. 1 and 2, when within-person change is linear individuals may differ in intercept and slope. Even more interestingly, the individual growth parameters may differ from person to person in a way that is systematically related to variables describing critical attributes of the people involved (the "predictors of change"). Under the straight-line growth model for reading achievement, for instance, the investigator can ask: Is there a systematic relationship between true rate of change in reading achievement and reading readiness in kindergarten?; between true initial status and reading readiness?; between the individual growth parameters and gender?; home environment?; type of reading program?; and so forth.

Hypothesized relationships between individual growth parameters and predictors of change can be formalized in statistical models for between-person differences in change that are similar to the more familiar regression models (see Rogosa and Willett 1985). Eqn. (2), for instance, presents a pair of between-person models, the true intercepts and true slopes of the straight-line reading achievement growth model in Eqn. (1) as a function of a pair of predictors, FEMALE (0=boy, 1=girl) and READYREAD (teacher rating of reading readiness in kindergarten):

$$\pi_{0p} = \beta_{00} + \beta_{01}\text{FEMALE}_p + \beta_{02}\text{READYREAD}_p + 1\,u_{0p}$$
$$\pi_{1p} = \beta_{10} + \beta_{11}\text{FEMALE}_p + \beta_{12}\text{READYREAD}_p + 1\,u_{1p}$$

$$(2)$$

where u_{0p} and u_{1p} represent residuals (the parts of π_{0p} and π_{1p} that are "unexplained" by FEMALE and READYREAD). In these models, the β coefficients summarize the population relationship between the individual growth parameters and the predictors of change. They can be interpreted in the same way as regular regression coefficients. A nonzero value of β_{01}, β_{02}, β_{11}, or β_{12} indicates that the corresponding covariate is a predictor of true initial status or true rate of change respectively. For instance, if girls tend to grow more rapidly than boys (i.e., if they have larger values of π_{1p}) then β_{11} will be positive. If children who had higher reading readiness scores in kindergarten have higher initial reading achievement in Grade 1, then β_{02} will be positive, and so on. All of the β coefficients in Eqn. (2) are estimated in the between-person phase of a growth study.

One of the main advantages of the longitudinal perspective is that the investigator is not limited to the simple within- and between-person models presented here. Substantively valid curvilinear functions can be used to model within-person growth, and complex between-person models can be used to relate interindividual differences in several growth parameters to many predictors simultaneously. Systematic interindividual variation in the rate parameter of the negative-exponential growth model, or in the acceleration parameter of the quadratic growth model, can be examined. A new universe for measuring change, far from the worlds of the pre/post design, is revealed.

3. Doing the Statistical Analyses

In an investigation of change, within-person and between-person statistical models—like Eqns. (1) and (2)—are fitted to data and their parameters estimated and interpreted. Many methods of model-fitting and parameter estimation are available. Some are very simple and can easily be implemented on the popular commercially available statistical computer packages; others are more sophisticated and require dedicated computer software. In this section, in order of increasing complexity, a taxonomy of such data-analytic strategies is briefly reviewed.

3.1 Estimating the Within-person Growth Parameters by Ordinary Least-squares Regression Analysis

Once a sensible within-person growth model has been adopted, it can be fitted separately to each of the individual observed growth records by ordinary least-squares (OLS) regression analysis (in the same way that the fitted trend-lines were created for Figs. 1 and 2). This person-by-person growth modeling leads to individual estimates of the several growth parameters that can then become the dependent variables in subsequent second-round between- person data analyses. In the case of the straight-line growth model in Eqn. (1), OLS-obtained intercepts and slopes estimate the true initial status and rate of change for each of the people in the sample and can be related directly to background predictors in follow-up correlation or regression analyses corresponding to Eqn. (2). This strategy is straightforward and easy to implement, and the OLS-estimated intercept and growth rates provide more precise measurement of individual change than was possible with the difference score.

3.2 Improving the Between-person Analyses with Weighted Least-squares Regression Analysis

Due to the idiosyncracies of measurement, some people usually have empirical growth records whose entries are smoothly ordered and for whom the growth data fall very close to the underlying true growth trajectory. Other less fortunate people have more erratic growth records and their datapoints are scattered, deviating widely from the underlying growth trajectories. These differences in scatter affect the precision (the standard errors) with which the first-round growth parameter estimation is carried out. People with "smooth and systematic" growth records will have highly precise growth parameter estimates with smaller standard errors; people with "erratic and scattered" observed growth records will have less precise growth parameter estimates with larger standard errors.

Between-person analyses of the relationship between the estimated growth parameters and predictors of change can be improved (made asymptotically efficient) if the precision of the first-round growth parameter estimates is taken into account. To achieve this, weighted least-squares (WLS) regression analysis can be used to fit the between-person models using weights that are inversely related to the square of the standard errors of the first-round parameter estimates. Then, more precisely estimated individual growth parameters (those with the smallest standard errors) will play a more important role in determining the outcomes of the second-phase analyses. Willett (1988) presented an expression for weights that can be used in conjunction with Eqns. (1) and (2).

Any growth analysis will automatically be improved if the first-round estimation of individual growth parameters is more precise. In practice, this is easily achieved by collecting more waves of data on each person in the sample. In the case of straight-line growth, for instance, the standard errors of fitted growth-rates decrease dramatically as extra waves of data are added. It is for this reason alone that multiwave designs provide superior methods for measuring change. Ultimately, researchers can control the quality of their findings; they can simply "add waves" to their design until some desired level of precision is reached (see Willett 1989).

3.3 Estimating the Within-person and Between-person Growth Models Simultaneously Using Dedicated Computer Software

In this entry it has been argued that high-quality measurement of change is possible via the collection of longitudinal data and the fitting of within-person and between-person models such as those in Eqns. (1) and (2). Such models constitute an algebraic "hierarchy" describing the statistical structure of growth data to be analyzed. Methodology for fitting such hierarchical models has advanced rapidly. In the early 1990s there were several dedicated computer programs available for simultaneously estimating all of the parameters of such models, and for providing appropriate standard errors and goodness-of-fit statistics. Kreft et al. (1990) provide a comprehensive description of four of them and compare their workings. They conclude that, in general, "all four programs tend to converge to the same solution" (p. 100). One of them—called "HLM"—has been widely used in the empirical literature and is well-supported (Bryk and Raudenbush 1992). (*See Hierachical Linear Modeling, Multilevel Analysis.*)

3.4 Estimating the Within-person and Between-person Models using Covariance Structure Analysis

There have also been advances in applying the methods of covariance structure analysis to the measurement of change. Covariance structure methods are powerful and general and can be applied easily to many problems in a wide variety of settings. Pioneering work on the application of these methods to the estimation and comparison of mean growth curves was conducted by McArdle and his colleagues (McArdle and Epstein 1987) and other authors have demonstrated how these methods can be used to answer questions about predictors of change (Muthén 1991). Willett and Sayer (1994, 1995) describe how the individual growth modeling framework maps explicitly onto the general covariance structure model and provide detailed examples of how the approach can be applied in practice to a variety of common research questions.

See also: Human Development: Research Methodology

References

Bereiter C 1963 Some persisting dilemmas in the measurement of change. In: Harris C W (ed.) 1963 *Problems in Measuring Change*. University of Wisconsin Press, Madison, Wisconsin

Bryk A S, Raudenbush S W 1992 *Hierarchical Linear Models: Applications and Data-analysis Methods*. Sage, Beverly Hills, California

Kreft I G G, de Leeuw J, Kim K S 1990 Comparing four different statistical packages for hierarchical linear regression: GENMOD, HLM, ML2, and VARCL. Center for the Study of Evaluation, University of California, Los Angeles, California

Linn R L, Slinde J A 1977 The determination of the significance of change between pre-and post-testing periods. *Rev. Educ. Res.* 47(1): 121–150

Lord F M 1956 The measurement of growth. *Educ. Psychol. Meas.* 16: 421–37

McArdle J J, Epstein D 1987 Latent growth curves within developmental structural equation models. *Child Dev.* 58: 110–33

Muthén B O 1991 Analysis of longitudinal data using latent variable models with varying parameters. In: Collins L M, Horn J L (eds.) 1991 *Best Methods for the Analysis of Change: Recent Advances, Unanswered Questions, Future Directions*. American Psychological Association, Washington, DC

Plewis I 1985 *Analyzing Change: Measurement and Explanation using Longitudinal Data*. Wiley, New York

Rogosa D R, Brandt D, Zimowski M 1982 A growth curve approach to the measurement of change. *Psych. Bul.* 93: 726–48

Rogosa D R, Willett J B 1983 Demonstrating the reliability of the difference score in the measurement of change. *J. Educ. Meas.* 20(4): 335–43

Rogosa D R, Willett J B 1985 Understanding correlates of change by modeling individual differences in growth. *Psychometrika* 50(2): 203–28

Thorndike R L 1966 Intellectual status and intellectual growth. *J. Educ. Psychol.* 57(3): 121–27

Webster H, Bereiter C 1963 The reliability of changes measured by mental test scores. In: Harris CW (ed.) 1963 *Problems in Measuring Change*. University of Wisconsin Press, Madison, Wisconsin

Willett J B 1988 Questions and answers in the measurement of change. *Review of Research in Education* 15: 345–422

Willett J B 1989 Some results on reliability for the longitudinal measurement of change: Implications for the design of studies of individual growth. *Educ. Psychol. Meas.* 49: 587–602

Willett J B, Sayer A G 1994 Using covariance structure analysis to detect correlates and predictors of change. *Psych. Bull. 116: 363–381*

Willett J B, Sayer A G 1995 Cross-domain analyses of change over time: Combining growth modeling and covariance structure analysis. In: Marcoulides G A, Schumacker R E (eds.) 1995 *Advanced Structural Equation Modeling: Issues and Techniques*. Lawrence Erlbaum Inc., Hillsdale, New Jersey

Classroom Observation

M. Galton

Structured observation, as used to monitor classroom events, requires an observer to assign such events to previously defined categories. These events may be recorded by mechanical means (e.g., film, audiotape, or videotape) and subsequently coded, or the observer can simultaneously record and code the events while present in the classroom. The three stages of the process therefore involve: (a) the recording of events in a systematic manner as they happen, (b) the coding of these events into prespecified categories, and (c) subsequent analysis of the events to give descriptions of teacher–pupil interaction.

Structured observation is also referred to as systematic observation or more particularly as interaction analysis, although the latter term is more typically applied to observation systems derived from the Flanders Interaction Analysis Category System (FIAC).

According to Flanders (1964), interaction analysis is a "specialised research procedure that provides information about only a few of the many aspects of teaching and which analyses the content-free characteristics of verbal communication" (p. 198). Since, structured observation techniques have also been used to monitor nonverbal behaviors, Flanders's definition of the methodology is now seen to be too restrictive.

1. The Origins of Structured Observation

The origin of these observational techniques arose, in part, from the creation of the Committee of Child Development by the American National Research Council at the beginning of the 1920s. This committee sponsored research into teaching methods in nursery schools and kindergartens. Researchers found it necessary to observe these infants and record their behavior "as it happened." Initially, observers prepared diaries or narrative logs of the activities observed, but the sheer volume of descriptive material collected made the task a very arduous one. Olson (1929) introduced the notion of time sampling, whereby certain categories of behaviors were recorded at specified fixed intervals of time. An essential distinction used to classify behaviors by workers in the child development movement was that between direct teaching, where pupils were told what to do, and indirect teaching, where pupils were consulted and decisions reached by means of discussion and consensus.

By the early 1970s, an anthology of United States observation systems listed 92 instruments (Simon and Boyer 1970), the majority of which were derived from FIAC (Rosenshine and Furst 1973). The Flanders system has been widely criticized, however, for its limited applicability in that it was originally designed for relatively static classrooms where teachers stood in front of pupils who were arranged before them in rows while working on the same subject matter (Hamilton and Delamont 1974). With the increase of "open" or informal approaches to classroom organization, a greater variety of observational methods have been developed. In the 1980s, for example, a review of United Kingdom observation studies (Galton 1979) identified only two systems derived from FIAC. Most of this research had been carried out at the primary stage of schooling where informal approaches are more likely to be found. More recent discussion of the different methodologies can be found in Croll (1986) and Anderson and Burns (1989).

2. Characteristics of Structured Observation

Structured observation involves low-inference measurement (Rosenshine 1970) which requires the development of unambiguous criteria for assigning the various events into categories. Provided that the criteria are sufficiently explicit to be shared by different people, then different observers should arrive at identical descriptions of the same events. Thus an important requirement of a successful systematic observation system is high interobserver agreement.

Although the choice of categories and the definition of the criteria may be highly subjective, reflecting the values of those who construct the system, the technique itself is objective in the sense that the criteria used to describe classroom life are clearly defined. Thus, when the system is used correctly it is unaffected by the personal biases of individual observers. This is in sharp contrast to ethnographic methods where the researcher, although sometimes claiming to take a total view of the classroom before gradually focusing on the more meaningful features (Hamilton and Delamont 1974), in practice can only offer a partial view because

the criteria governing the selection are rarely available for consideration by others.

While Anderson and Burns (1989) contrast a number of approaches based upon different theoretical perspectives, most modern observation schedules are, in practice, combinations of category and sign systems (Croll 1986). The selection of behaviors for use in a sign system is dependent upon those which are thought to be most useful for the particular research purpose. In classroom research, such variables are usually selected because they are thought to be related to learning outcomes or to systematic differences between teachers and their pupils.

3. Data Collection

Galton (1987) lists a number of ways in which a permanent record of classroom events can be obtained, thereby enabling an observer to conduct a subsequent analysis under less pressurized circumstances than those that exist under conditions of live recording. The two most frequently used approaches involve tape and video recorders. There are advantages and disadvantages to such methods.

The availability of relatively cheap hand-held video recorders has increased the popularity of using this method to record classroom events. The method's main advantage is that it supplies permanent visual and sound records which can be played and replayed and then edited. Thus the likelihood of observer agreement during subsequent analysis is increased. Set against this advantage is the highly selective representation of the camera which does not inform the viewer of what is going on in other parts of the classroom. For example, a category such as *target pupil is interested in another pupil's work* would be difficult to code using a video recorder, since the viewer would be uncertain whether the pupil was looking elsewhere in the classroom at what was happening between the teacher and another pupil or whether the pupil was totally distracted.

In an attempt to overcome such difficulties two cameras are sometimes used, one focused on the teacher or pupil and the other using a wide-angle lens to provide a general view of the classroom. Such arrangements, however, can be potential sources of distraction for both pupils and teachers so that what is gained in reliability may be lost in validity.

Another method of producing visual cues is to use stop-frame photography with synchronized sound (Adleman and Walker 1974). The flexibility of such a system has been greatly increased by the use of radio microphones which allow the teacher to move freely around the classroom and reduce the problem of background noise (Bennett 1985). However, the process of transcribing the permanent record from a recording can be very tedious and time-consuming.

It is estimated that to transcribe one hour of audiotape takes nearly a week of an efficient typist's time. Research involving a large number of teachers will, therefore, tend to favor direct observation methods because of the costs of transcribing and processing the data. More importantly, when an observer records events "as they happen," the presence of the observer in the classroom over a period of time has the advantage of enabling him or her to appreciate the shared understanding which exists between pupils and teacher so that certain behaviors can more easily be interpreted. This understanding is particularly important when the investigation concerns aspects of teacher–pupil relationships where private jokes (see Adleman and Walker 1975) are a common feature.

The general view is that it is preferable, at least in the early stages of an investigation, to make use of permanent records only when the focus of interest is in the children's language. Detailed descriptions of the methodology involved in such studies are provided by Edwards and Westgate (1987).

4. Training Observers

According to Flanders (1967), one of the main problems of training observers in the use of systematic observation is "converting men into machines" (p. 158). The usual training technique is to concentrate on a few categories at a time using a teach–test and feedback–reteach cycle. Details of the process are given by Jasman (1980).

Anderson and Burns (1989) provide a number of suggestions for a comprehensive training program. They draw attention, in particular, to the advantage of systematic observation in not requiring highly qualified, experienced observers because the training tends to be more rigorous. The method is, therefore, eminently suitable when employing teachers, who often have greater credibility with colleagues in school.

Usually audiotape and videotape recordings are used to introduce the observer to the problems of classifying particular categories and at the end of a training session another tape can be used to test if the observers can achieve acceptable levels of agreement. It is important to provide simple examples initially, with the guarantee that most observers will obtain total mastery, since observers who fail to identify behaviors correctly during training can often develop hostile reactions to the observation instrument. It is also useful to provide observers with experience of coding under classroom conditions as soon as possible. As stated earlier, it is often difficult to identify the context in which a behavior takes place on videotape which in turn means that the decision about the use of a particular category is not as clear-cut as the trainer might wish.

Once the initial training has been completed, it is important to build into any observation study refresher periods in which the observers go over the categories and check their reliability. These periods protect against what is termed "observer drift," which occurs when observers, who have come to accept criteria which do not conform to their own view of a particular behavior, gradually modify the category definitions over time to fit their own view.

5. Reliability and Validity

Most studies use only observer agreement as a test of reliability. The simplest measure of agreement is the percentage of occasions on which a pair of observers agree. However, this does not allow for the fact that two observers who were coding categories at random would still code the same categories on certain occasions by chance. The Scott (1955) coefficient corrects for this chance effect and is a more rigorous test of reliability. A weakness of this method, however, is that it does not permit study of observer agreement in research using a number of teachers. Medley and Mitzel (1963) offer several designs, based upon analysis of variance, in which each teacher is visited on one occasion by two observers, with the pairing of observers organized so that different observers are paired on each visit. Such a design also allows the teacher stability coefficient to be estimated.

Croll (1986) argues that *absolute agreement*, where the individual coding decisions of the observer are correlated, is preferable to *marginal agreement*, where only the total frequency of each category is compared irrespective of how an observer arrived at this total. Some systems, however, notably those which use broad sampling procedures, prevent any calculation of absolute agreement in the manner recommended by Croll. Croll (1986) also warns against including within a reliability coefficient a number of categories which are described as part of a single variable, but which are not mutually exclusive. If multiple categories can be coded simultaneously, they should be treated as separate variables with separate coefficients (Harrop 1979).

If an observation instrument is to be used by researchers other than those who developed the instrument, then the question of interinvestigator agreement arises, since each group may achieve high levels of observer agreement but interpret the categories differently (Rosenshine and Furst 1973). Anderson and Burns (1989) argue that in certain cases objectivity, expressed as observer agreement, is less important than the question of objectivity viewed as a measure of observer detachment. In some cases differences between observers mask real differences in interpretation and need to be investigated. However, in most cases of structured observation, differences between observers are regarded as error. Some developers of observation systems provide videotape examples already coded so that new users can check their degree of agreement with the developers on a trial tape (Eggleston et al. 1975).

Many researchers concern themselves only with the face validity of the observation instrument, assuming that the definition of the categories is so clear-cut that validity may be assumed providing observer agreement is high. The more complex the observation instrument, however, the less advisable it is to take this face validity for granted. In this case a number of alternative procedures can be employed.

When cluster analysis is used to create a typology of teaching styles or pupil types, observers can be asked to write descriptive accounts (mini case studies) of the teachers and the appropriate pupils. These accounts can then be cross-referenced with the descriptions derived from the clusters. Such descriptions can also be fed back to the observed teachers who can be asked to identify their own particular style or recognize particular types of pupils present in their classrooms.

Where two different observation systems exist having a similar focus, they can be used in the same classroom to compare and contrast results. While this type of cross-validation is recommended by Rosenshine and Furst (1973), only a few studies have attempted this task. In the ORACLE study, however, both the teacher and the pupils were observed using two instruments and the asymmetry of classroom behavior from both the teachers' and pupils' perspective was contrasted (Galton et al. 1980). The same study also made it possible to compare and contrast the "real curriculum" as perceived through both the teachers' and the pupils' activity.

Anderson and Burns (1989) argue that in some contexts, notably the study of different subject matter, it may be more important to investigate the inconsistencies across classrooms rather than seeking to submerge or eliminate these differences. They argue that inconsistencies across occasions are more problematic than inconsistencies across classrooms because of the limited amount of data collected.

Anderson and Burns (1989) conclude that one of the most important tests of validity is the reception of the evidence by teachers. In this regard Anderson and Burns (1984) quote claims that teachers often remarked, after the presentation of the research findings, "You've been in my classrooms." Similar responses have been found in United Kingdom classrooms with respect to reports of research from the ORACLE and PRISMS studies (Galton et al. 1980, Galton and Patrick 1989).

6. Coding and Analysis

In any observation system, discrete analytic units must be used in order to code the behaviors. The simplest division is based on some form of time sampling, where the time unit may vary from three seconds, as used by Flanders, to five minutes as used in Medley and Mitzel's (1958) OSCAR schedule. Every system has its own ground rules which differentiate between the beginning and the end of successive time units and which deal with the problem of behaviors which overlap from one unit to the next. It is important to choose time units so that observed behaviors do not regularly overlap into the next unit since, when this happens, it is found that the degree of agreement between observers decreases rapidly. Observer agreement is also improved when a steady rhythm of recording can be maintained.

Various methods exist for recording behavior and these are discussed in some detail by Croll (1986). These include event sampling (which records a particular event whenever it occurs), instantaneous time sampling (where only events occurring at a particular pretimed interval are recorded), scanning (where the number of individuals within a class who are engaged in a particular activity is recorded at pre-timed intervals), and continuous recording (where an ongoing record is made and the exact time in which a change in activity takes place noted). Finally, there exists a little-used method, one–zero time sampling, where only the first occurrence of a particular event within a given time interval is recorded.

With time sampling methods the extent to which the sample of behavior recorded is representative of the total behavior that occurred during a lesson is clearly dependent on the length of the interval between recordings. If the period is too short, the observers are likely to make mistakes; if the time interval is too long, they may record the behavior accurately but underestimate its overall frequency.

Consequently, when difficult and complex decisions have to be made by the observer, some researchers have preferred to use one–zero time sampling procedure, where the observer records the behavior only once as it occurs within a given time unit. If the time interval is short, then one–zero time sampling approximates to continuous recording of a classroom activity. With longer time intervals—for example, five minute units as used by Eggleston et al. (1975)—only the minimum frequency of occurrence is recorded. Such data, therefore, cannot be used to estimate the overall occurrence of individual categories within the classroom.

Criticisms of one–zero time sampling by Croll (1986) and Dunkerton (1981) are essentially correct in arguing that such systems are unsatisfactory in describing general aspects of classroom behavior. However, in cases where behaviors which discriminate among teachers are very infrequent, as for example in science lessons where it was rare to find teachers encouraging pupils to hypothesize (Eggleston et al. 1975), the method has some advantages in that it discriminates among teachers while, at the same time, allowing the observer sufficient time to recognize and code these infrequent complex interactions.

Critics of this type of coding system have been distracted from its prime purpose because such schedules still retain a number of frequently used categories. The presence of such categories is, however, irrelevant to the purpose for which the schedule is designed. Commonly occurring categories are included primarily to aid reliability, since observers who are not able to code continuously tend to become anxious, with the result that their concentration and reliability decreases. Such systems do, however, have very limited application. They are only preferable in cases where the complexity and variety of behaviors within the observation system require that the observer be given time to reach decisions in more difficult coding areas.

The simplest approaches to analysis operate at a descriptive level and are concerned with an estimation of either the frequency of occurrence of different events or the proportions of time taken up by different activities. The latter analysis is usually the product of time sampling systems.

More sophisticated schedules can be developed which allow the exact moment in time when a particular event occurs to be determined. Time sampling systems, provided the interval is very short, can also be used to determine the sequence of events taking place, since the observer is, in effect, recording a change of category rather than sampling a behavior within a defined period.

Recording a new behavior every time a different category is used employs the use of what are termed "naturalistic units." Here the problem for the researcher is to define a set of rules which will identify the unit of classroom transaction which can be coded under a particular category. Smith and Meux (1962) defined these natural units as "episodes" and "monologues," where an episode involved more than one speaker and a monologue identified a solo performance. The ground rules for identifying the nature of the transaction, however, make it difficult, if not impossible, for an observer to use such a system live in a classroom. For this reason, naturalistic units are most frequently used for the analysis of transcribed recordings. Observers can play and replay recordings until general agreement is obtained on the classification of each transaction.

When naturalistic units are used, the total number of episodes represents the total recorded behavior, since one tally only is made for each episode. In such a case, some record of the sequence of events can be obtained, but the most usual practice is to count the number of recorded tallies for each category and to divide this number by the total number of analytic units observed. With naturalistic units, this ratio closely represents the proportion of the total behavior occurring in a particular category. With longer time units, when a point–time sampling procedure is used, the ratio of the sum of tallies in a particular category compared to the total number of tallies recorded can again be interpreted as a proportion of total behavior.

One–zero time sampling methods in which frequently occurring events may only be coded once during a time unit can give no absolute value for the frequency of the particular behavior. Instead, an estimate of the minimum frequency of occurrence is obtained by dividing the total number of tallies obtained for a category by the total number of observation units.

The simplest analytic approach is that of Flanders (1964). Using a 10×10 matrix, the position of each subsequent event can be coded relative to the preceding interaction. Attempts to extend these procedures beyond the two category model have not been successful. For this reason Croll (1986) suggests the use of developmental profiles.

Anderson and Burns (1989) raise a number of important issues involved in the analysis of quantifiable data such as those obtained from structured observation, specifically the procedures for data aggregation and data reduction and the methods used to establish relationships between different variables. Croll (1986) also discusses a number of multivariate analyses which can be used to interpret observational data, including the use of multiple regression and the analysis of covariance in conducting analysis of the relationships between the observation processes and classroom products such as standardized tests.

With transcribed accounts of lessons, either from videotape or audiotape, greater attention can be paid to the sequential character of exchanges between teacher and pupils. Once suitable units of transcript have been identified, then different patterns in the sequence of these units can be observed. Unfortunately, researchers have tended to use different units for this analysis. The "episode" developed by Smith and Meux (1962) became the "incident" in Nuthall and Lawrence's (1965) study, while others have defined "pedagogical moves" (Bellack et al. 1966). Comparison between different studies is therefore difficult and although it is attractive to believe that effective teaching will eventually be explained in terms of sequential behavior rather than simple frequency units, there has been little progress in this direction since the early 1970s.

7. General Conclusions

In spite of these difficulties, there remains a continued interest in the collection of systematic observational data. Reviews of research on teaching in the United States list a large number of studies which have been carried out since the publication of Rosenshine's review (Rosenshine and Furst 1973). According to Brophy and Good (1986), there is now firm evidence about the most effective teaching strategies for improving pupil performance when measured on standardized tests of reading, language, and mathematical computation. Similar evidence has emerged from studies in the United Kingdom (Galton 1989), although Rosenshine warns that the more complex the intellectual activity the less likely are these direct instructional procedures to be effective. Subsequently (e.g., Galton and Patrick 1990), observational research has concentrated less on teaching behaviors and has instead examined aspects of the curriculum, supporting the view of Anderson and Burns (1989) that the instructional task, particularly the nature of its subject matter, largely determines the frequency and type of teacher–student interaction.

For the future, research is likely to concentrate on two major areas. The first of these concerns itself with models of teacher development. A large amount of research in the 1990s has concentrated on establishing differences between novice and expert teachers (Berliner 1992). However, little information exists about the intervening stages of development. As a consequence, the design and use of structured observation systems which will discriminate between these different stages is likely to assume greater importance. Second, the political attention given to reward systems for teachers based upon related performance criteria means that structured observation systems will increasingly play a part in both systems of appraisal and in school inspection to the neglect of more important issues concerning pupil learning strategies.

References

Adelman C, Walker R 1974 Stop-frame cinematography with synchronized sound: A technique for recording in school classrooms. *Journal of the Society of Motion and Picture and Television Engineering* 83: 189–91

Adelman C, Walker R 1975 *A Guide to Classroom Observation.* Routledge, London

Anderson L, Burns R 1989 *Research in Classrooms.* Pergamon Press, Oxford

Bellack A A, Hyman R T, Smith F L, Kliebard H M 1966 *The Language of the Classroom.* Teachers College Press, Columbia University, New York

Bennett N 1985 Interaction and achievement in classroom groups. In: Bennett N, Deforges C (eds.) 1985 *Recent Advances in Classroom Research* monograph No 2, *British Journal of Educational Psychology.* Scottish Academic Press, Edinburgh

Berliner D 1992 Some characteristics of experts in the pedagogical domain. In: Oser F, Dick A, Patry J (eds.) 1992 *Effective and Responsible Teaching: The New Synthesis.* Jossey-Bass, San Francisco, California

Brophy J, Good T 1986 Teacher behaviour and student achievement. In: Wittrock M (ed.) 1986 *Handbook of Research on Teaching*, 3rd edn. Macmillan, New York

Croll P 1986 *Systematic Classroom Observation.* Falmer Press, London

Dunkerton J 1981 Should classroom observation be quantitative? *Educ. Res.* 23: 144–51

Edwards T, Westgate D 1987 *Investigating Classroom Talk.* Falmer Press, London

Eggleston J F, Galton M J, Jones M E 1975 *A Science Teaching Observation Schedule.* Macmillan, London

Flanders N A 1964 Some relationships among teacher influence, pupil attitudes and achievement. In: Biddle B J, Ellena W J (eds.) 1964 *Contemporary Research on Teacher Effectiveness.* Holt, Rinehart, and Winston, New York

Flanders N A 1967 Problems of observer training and reliability. In: Amidon E J, Hough J E (eds.) 1967 *Interaction Analysis: Theory, Research and Applications.* Addison-Wesley, Reading, Massachusetts

Galton M 1979 Systematic classroom observation: British research *Educ. Res.* 21: 109–15

Galton M 1987 An ORACLE chronicle: A decade of classroom research. *Teaching and Teacher Education* 3(4): 229–312

Galton M 1989 *Teaching in the Primary School.* David Fulton, London

Galton M, Patrick H (eds.) 1990 *Curriculum Provision in the Small Primary School.* Routledge, London

Galton M, Simon B, Croll P 1980 *Inside the Primary Classroom.* Routledge and Kegan Paul, London

Hamilton D, Delamont S 1974 Classroom research: A cautionary tale. *Res. Educ.* 11: 1–15

Harrop L 1990 Unreliability of classroom observation. *Educ. Res.* 21(3): 207–11

Jasman A 1980 Training observers in the use of systematic observation techniques. In: Galton M, Simon B, Croll P 1980

Medley D M, Mitzel H E 1958 A technique for measuring classroom behavior. *J. Educ. Psychol.* 49: 86–93

Medley D M, Mitzel H E 1963 Measuring classroom behavior by systematic observation. In: Gage N L (ed.) 1963 *Handbook of Research on Research on Teaching: A Project of the American Educational Research Association.* Rand McNally, Chicago, Illinois

Nuthall G A, Lawrence P J 1965 *Thinking in the Classroom: The Development of a Method of Analysis.* New Zealand Council for Educational Research, Wellington

Olson W C 1929 *The Measurement of Nervous Habits in Normal Children.* University of Minnesota Press, Minneapolis, Minnesota

Rosenshine B 1970 Evaluation of classroom instruction. *Rev. Educ. Res.* 40: 279–300

Rosenshine B, Furst N 1973 The use of direct observation to study teaching. In: Travers R M W (ed.) 1973 *Second Handbook of Research on Teaching: A Project of the American Educational Research Association.* Rand McNally, Chicago, Illinois

Scott W A 1955 Reliability of content analysis: The case of nominal coding. *Public Opinion Questionnaire* 19: 321–25

Simon A, Boyer E G (eds.) 1974 *Mirrors for Behavior: An Anthology of Classroom Observation Instruments.* Research for Better Schools, Philadelphia, Pennsylvania

Smith B O, Meux M 1962 *A Study of the Logic of Teaching.* Bureau of Educational Research, University of Illinois, Urbana, Illinois

Content and Text Analysis

J. Anderson

Content analysis, sometimes referred to as document analysis, includes the methods and techniques researchers use to examine, analyze and make inferences about human communications. Typically, communications consist of printed or written text but may also comprise photographs, cartoons, illustrations, broadcasts, and verbal interactions. Text analysis, by contrast, has a narrower focus and is restricted to analysis of text features, and usually as these relate to comprehensibility or writing style. The widespread use of computers has seen a resurgence of research studies using methods of content and text analysis.

The techniques of content and text analysis are used by researchers across a range of disciplines: anthropology, psychology, sociology, psychiatry, history, literature, political science, education, linguistics, artificial intelligence. This entry adopts an educational, psycholinguistic perspective and, although there is often overlap, content and text analysis are discussed separately. The focus in this entry is on written communication, on purposes and techniques commonly employed by educational researchers, and on methodological issues.

1. Definitions of Content Analysis

Berelson's chapter in *Handbook of Social Psychology* Vol. 1 (1952) is still regarded as a basic reference for content analysis. (This chapter is a condensed version of Berelson's book *Content Analysis in Communication Research* published two years previously and republished in 1971). Here Berelson defines content analysis as a "a research technique for the objective, systematic, and quantitative description of the manifest content of communication" (p.489). In a further major review of content analysis in the second edition of *The Handbook of Social Psychology*, Holsti (1968) adopts essentially the same definition.

A slightly different interpretation was made by Osgood who defined content analysis as "a procedure whereby one makes inferences about sources and receivers from evidence in the messages they exchange" (Osgood 1959 p. 35). This changed emphasis was taken up by Weber who defined content analysis as "a research methodology that utilizes a set of procedures to make valid inferences from text" (Weber 1985 p. 9). Weber continues: "These inferences are about the sender(s) of message, the message itself, or the audience of the message."

In successive editions of *Foundations of Behavioral Research*, Kerlinger adopts this wider view of content analysis as going beyond description to making inferences about variables. Thus content analysis is defined by Kerlinger (1986 p. 477) as "a method of studying and analyzing communications in a systematic, objective, and quantitative manner to measure variables." While many earlier studies using content analysis focused on descriptions of various communications—for instance, analyzing the content of newspapers, radio and television programs, studies of propaganda, public opinion, bias and prejudice, and studies of literary style, reading difficulty, and error analysis—for Kerlinger, content analysis is also a method of observation and measurement. "Instead of observing people's behavior directly, or asking them to respond to scales, or interviewing them, the investigator takes the communications that people have produced and asks questions of the communications" (p. 477).

2. A Framework for Studies of Content Analysis

A model widely applied to biological, psychological, social, and other systems was that proposed by Shannon and Weaver (1949). Developed to deal with signal transmission, this model incorporates a source, transmitter, channel of communication, noise, receiver, and destination. The model has been adapted to language communication (Anderson 1976), as shown in Fig.1, and provides a framework for studies of content analysis, both in its narrower and wider connotations.

Not only does the language communication model in Fig.1 provide a useful framework for reviewing the field of content analysis, it can also serve as a fruitful source for generating hypotheses. First, studies that focus primarily on the source system typically deal with the psychological states, motivations, or characteristics of encoders and the effects of these upon messages produced. Many of these studies fall into the category of "language style." Second, studies focusing mainly on the receiver system and which investigate attitudes, values, motives, and other psychological characteristics of decoders in relation to messages

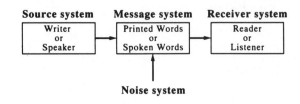

Figure 1
A model for the correspondence of source, message, noise, and receiver systems

received, come into the realm of "audience analysis." Third, other studies where the primary focus is on the *message* itself or on *noise* and the effect of distortion in the message upon receivers belong to the field of content analysis in its narrower sense. Insofar as these three categories of studies involve the message system however, they are all embraced by content analysis in its wider connotation as a method of observation and measurement.

Typical of numerous studies in the first category noted, where the focus of attention is on the message in order to make inferences about encoders of messages, is that of Mahl (1959) who examined the speech of psychotherapy patients in order to assess their anxiety. Exemplifying the second category, where the focus of attention is again on the message but this time to make inferences about decoders, is a study of supporters' and critics' reactions to a television news program aimed at high school students (Wulfemeyer and Mueller 1991). Focusing more directly on the message itself is Anderson and Yip's (1987) study which examined the content of two editions of an Australian reading scheme to see what changes took place in the presentation of sex roles over a decade and a half when the roles of women in western societies changed quite markedly. The numerous investigations into methodological questions relating to "cloze procedure" (a measure of reading comprehension discussed below where subjects attempt to replace deleted parts of text), such as the effect on comprehension of frequency of deletions, type of deletions, and scoring procedures, are illustrative of studies into noise or message distortion.

3. Purposes and Techniques of Content Analysis

The research investigations cited demonstrate the wide range of uses of content analysis. Content analyzed by researchers covers the gamut of human communication: letters, stories, poetry, essays, diaries, obituaries, minutes, biographies, newspapers, radio, television, conversations, cartoons, drawing, photographs, film. As others have remarked, communication content is the *what* in the classic description of communication: *who* says *what* to whom, how, and with *what effect*. The widespread use of computers, together with the increasing ease of inputting text via scanners and text recognition software, are multiplying the number of studies utilizing text analysis.

Although there are several ways to do content analysis, there are, nevertheless, recognized procedures that do not differ markedly from many other procedures in educational research. These procedures are illustrated by reference to specific studies. First and foremost is the need to identify the corpus or universe to be studied. In the investigation cited of sex roles in young children's books (Anderson and Yip 1987), the corpus of reading content for analysis comprised the first nine

books from the *Young Australia Language Scheme* (first published in 1966) and the first nine basic readers from *Young Australia Readers* (published in 1980). These 18 books constituted the content for analysis.

The second essential step is to define the categories into which the universe is to be partitioned. According to Kerlinger (1986), this is the most important part of content analysis because it reflects the purposes of the research and the theory underlying it. Categories must be objectively defined and mutually exclusive. Further, if comparisons are to be made with other studies, generally agreed upon or standard categories need to be adopted. Considerations like these led Stone and his associates to develop *The General Inquirer*, a computerized approach to content analysis (Stone et al. 1966). The bases of this approach are specially developed dictionaries which allow computer tagging of words of text entered into the computer program. The tagged words then serve as indicators of, for example, need-achievement, or discipline, or for whatever the dictionary has been designed.

After defining categories, the next step is to determine units for analysis. In the preceding example, the computer tags words indicating need-achievement. Other units may be themes (often phrases or even sentences), characters, items, or space-and-time measures (like the number of pages in a book or the length of a discussion in minutes). Anderson and Yip (1987) adopted as one form of category the total number of characters (human, animal, fantasy figure, inanimate object) presented in the text and/or accompanying illustrations. Characters were counted for each story in each of the readers, noting the gender of all characters. Where the gender of characters was ambiguous, it was recorded as "other". As another form of category, all activities of male and female characters were categorized under a number of themes established in another study: themes like leadership, triumphing over foe or adversity, rescuing, exploring, showing bravery, showing fear, and so on. The units of analysis determine the level of measurement in statistical analyses.

The techniques of content analysis such as defining categories and determining units for analysis prove useful, too, in a number of investigations where the focus is not primarily on analyzing content. One example is in coding open-ended questionnaire responses. In an evaluation of curriculum materials, for example, rather than ask teachers to tick or otherwise indicate their views by choosing from a series of predetermined responses or multiple-choice questions, Anderson (1981) preferred to ask users to write down their views. The copious detail provided a rich data source, but to capture the depth of detail and allow responses to be analyzed by computer, some data reduction was necessary. Users' comments to individual questionnaire items became the universe. Each universe was examined and a set of categories or a coding scheme developed, as illustrated below in a request for suggestions to produce further language materials.

Code

10–19	Produce materials other than those already available
11	Special materials for "enquiry–approach" projects
12	Materials for infants/younger children
13	Accompanying comprehension exercises or workbooks
14	More evaluation materials
15	Extending the scheme to accommodate advanced students
16	Review workbooks
17	Very basic materials for non-English-speaking children
18	Miscellaneous exercises (e.g., music with sentence drills)

Further codes were for suggestions to expand existing materials (20–29), for suggestions about general presentation (30–39), and for missing data where the question was not answered (99).

Following a decision about units of analysis, a further step is to determine which units may be reliably quantified. In early studies of readability, for instance, researchers looked for factors thought to contribute to reading difficulty, such as sentence complexity, vocabulary load, interest level, and so on. Reliably quantifying the different factors often resulted in a much reduced list. Questions of reliability inevitably raise questions of validity since some argue that there is little use in achieving high reliability if what is left to be measured has little utility or content validity.

Quantification may take the form of a simple "frequency count," as in counting the number of male and female characters per story. Ranking texts in terms of perceived reading difficulty is "ordinal measurement." Space measures like inches of newspaper type, or time measures such as minutes of teacher talk, are "interval measurement."

4. Text Analysis and Comprehensibility

Teachers and librarians have an obvious interest in content analysis since best results in learning are usually achieved by judicious matching of student with appropriate learning materials. This interest has long been manifest, particularly in analyses of characteristics of text as these relate to "comprehensibility." One characteristic of appropriate learning materials in this context is text reading difficulty or "readability." This entry focuses on this aspect, though the interest level of reading materials and students' motivation clearly impact on comprehensibility.

The readability movement was born in the 1920s with the publication of Thorndike's epic work on word frequency, *A Teacher Wordbook of 10,000 Words*. Shortly after this book was published, the first formula for ranking books in relative order of difficulty appeared, a formula based on Thorndike's word list. Since then many readability formulas have been developed for estimating the reading difficulty of texts in English, Japanese, Spanish, French, and other languages. The method used to construct a readability formula essentially comprises four steps, the first two of which are similar to the procedures of content analysis described above. The first is to search for factors thought to contribute to reading difficulty like, for instance, use of affixes, sentence complexity, or unfamiliar vocabulary. This step is what content analysts term "defining the categories." The second step is to determine which of these factors or categories can be reliably quantified. The third, and possibly the most difficult step, is to establish a criterion or exterior measure of reading difficulty against which the quantified factors may be validated. The final step is to incorporate into a regression equation those quantified factors which predict the criterion best. The regression equation becomes the readability formula. Two readability formulas described in Klare (1975) are those by Flesch and Spache:

$$\text{Reading Ease} = 206.835 - 0.846wl - 1.015sl \quad \text{[Flesch]}$$

$$\text{Grade Level} = 0.141 X_1 + 0.086X_2 + 0.839 \quad \text{[Spache]}$$

where wl, sl, X_1, and X_2 are all text factors (different measures of word difficulty and sentence complexity). The widely used Fry readability graph (see Klare 1975) is also a regression equation in graphical form.

The use of computers has had a marked effect on readability measurement, as on measurement generally. Thus, while word length in Flesch's formula (developed in 1948) involved a count of syllables which is relatively easy for human analysts, more recent formulas compute word length by counting characters. Such character counts would rarely have been conceived when analyses were done manually since they were too time-consuming and unreliable. For computers though, character counts are quicker and certainly more accurate than counting syllables.

A research instrument developed at Flinders University for use on microcomputers to analyze text features (Anderson 1992) displays the following text counts when the Text Count icon (the one selected in Fig. 2) is clicked.

Similarly, clicking on the Sentence Profile icon (seen in Fig. 3) displays a sentence profile for a given text.

The same text analysis tool computes an estimate of text reading difficulty, base on the "Rix" index, a measure that traces its origins to an index termed "Lix" which was developed in Sweden by Björnsson (1968). Clicking on the Text Difficulty icon (see Fig. 4) displays information about text difficulty.

Further options compute the reading difficulty of individual sentences and list the number of different words in

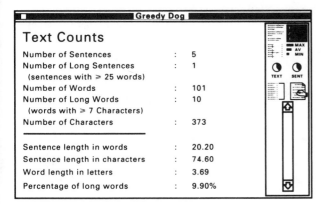

Figure 2
Text counts in Aesop's *The Greedy Dog*

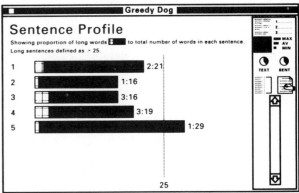

Figure 3
Sentence profile for Aesop's *The Greedy Dog*

a text (ordered alphabetically, by frequency or by word length).

5. Cloze Procedure and Cohesion

Readability measurement as a form of text analysis has obvious advantages and equally obvious shortcomings. Among the advantages are that it is objective and, with computers, quick and easy to apply. Indices such as Flesch, Lix, or Rix provide estimates of readability, that is, predictions of the ease or difficulty that readers are likely to experience in comprehending texts. Herein, however, lies the inherent weakness of such measures because no account is taken of the reader, at least in any direct way.

5.1 Cloze Procedure

Cloze procedure was developed to overcome this precise problem and to involve readers directly. It is basically a straightforward technique, consisting of a set of rules for constructing cloze tests over samples of written (or spoken) materials, administering these tests to subjects and scoring them, and determining from the cloze scores the degree of comprehension of the written (or spoken materials). To construct a cloze test, the words of a passage are systematically deleted in some mechanical way, for example, every seventh word, and replaced by blanks, usually of a standard length (though this condition is not a necessary one). The task for subjects is then to replace the missing words, and their scores, that is, the number of words correctly replaced, is an index of the comprehension of the passage. Thus the technique measures two aspects: the readability or reading difficulty of text and subjects' comprehension of text.

There are many reviews of cloze procedure since it is now included in the repertoire of techniques employed by classroom teachers, as well as being a useful measure in language research. The application of cloze procedure in foreign language testing, and especially with English learned as a foreign language in Southeast Asia as well as with Malay and Mandarin Chinese, is comprehensively reviewed in Anderson (1976).

5.2 Cohesion

"Cohesion" is yet another aspect of text which is receiving increased attention from educational researchers. Cohesion is based on the linguistic concept of cohesive ties, the mechanisms in text that make a text a text, thus differentiating connected discourse from a set of unrelated sentences. The most complete linguistic description of cohesive ties in English is to be found in Halliday and Hasan (1976). Researchers at The Open University in the United Kingdom, in a large-scale longitudinal study and in a series of fine-grained analyses, have tested the educational and psychological validity of cohesion by demonstrating that students' perception of cohesive ties in text is related to other measures of linguistic and verbal ability (see especially Chapman 1983). The *Australian Journal of Reading* (1983) devoted a special issue to the topic of cohesion and the reading teacher.

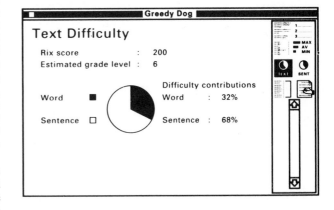

Figure 4
Text difficulty for Aesop's *The Greedy Dog*

6. Content and Text Analysis: Retrospect and Prospect

Content and text analysis deal with essential forms of human interaction, the messages that the human species has developed for communication. As Holsti (1969 p. 1) remarked:

> It therefore follows that the study of the processes and products of communication is basic to the student of history, behavior, thought, art, and institutions. Often the only surviving artifacts that may be used to study human activity are to be found in documents.

Yet, as Berelson (1952 p. 518) even earlier remarked: "Content analysis, as a method, has no magical qualities." The methods of the content or text analyst are open to the same strictures faced by all educational researchers: the need to select the universe of materials for analysis carefully if unwarranted generalizations are not to be made, to select categories that are meaningful, and to pay heed to questions of reliability and validity.

The computer, as a research tool, has had an enormous impact on content and text analysis and this impact is likely to increase even further. Not only does the computer facilitate all statistical analyses, it is a tool that is ideally suited for making routine counts of whatever categories researchers adopt, provided these can be fully defined and therefore quantified. The bottleneck that used to exist when entering text into computers is fast losing force as an obstacle, as scanners linked to computers become more widespread. Improvements in software are making text recognition more rapid and efficient, across a range of languages and alphabets. When voice recognition becomes a reality, the amount of human communication content available for ready analysis will increase even more dramatically.

References

Anderson J 1976 *Psycholinguistic Experiments in Foreign Language Testing.* University of Queensland Press, St Lucia

Anderson J 1981 *A National Survey of User Opinion of Commonwealth-produced Curriculum Materials for Teaching English as a Second Language.* Flinders University, Adelaide

Anderson J 1992 *MacTexan a Tool to Analyze Texts.* Flinders University, Adelaide

Anderson J, Yip L 1987 Are sex roles represented fairly in children's books? A content analysis of old and new readers. *Unicorn* 13(3): 155–61

Australian Journal of Reading 1983 Vol. 6, No. (issue devoted to Cohesian and the Reading Teacher)

Berelson B 1952 Content analysis. In: Lindzey G (ed.) 1952 *Handbook of Social Psychology. Vol. 1; Theory and Method.* Addison-Wesley, Reading, Massachusetts

Björnsson C H 1968 *Läsbarhet.* Bokförlaget Liber, Stockholm

Chapman L J 1983 *Reading Development and Cohesion.* Heinemann, London

Halliday M A K, Hasan R 1976 *Cohesion in English.* Longman, London

Holsti O R 1968 Content analysis. In: Lindzey G, Aronson E (eds.) 1968 *The Handbook of Social Psychology. Vol. 2: Research Methods,* 2nd edn. Addison-Wesley, Reading, Massachusetts

Holsti O R 1969 *Content Analysis for the Social Sciences and Humanities.* Addison-Wesley, Reading, Massachusetts

Kerlinger F R 1986 *Foundations of Behavioral Research,* 3rd edn. Holt, Rinehart, and Winston, New York

Klare G R 1975 Assessing readability. *Read. Res. Q.* 10(1): 62–102

Mahl G F 1959 Exploring emotional states by content analysis. In: Pool I D S (ed.) 1959 *Trends in Content Analysis.* University of Illinois Press, Urbana, Illinois

Osgood C E 1959 The representational model and relevant research methods. In: Pool I D S (ed.) 1959 *Trends in Content Analysis.* University of Illinois Press, Urbana, Illinois

Shannon C E, Weaver W 1949 *The Mathematical Theory of Communication.* University of Illinois Press, Urbana, Illinois

Stone P J, Dunphy D C, Smith M S, Ogilvie D M 1966 *The General Inquirer: A Computer Approach to Content Analysis.* M I T Press, Cambridge, Massachusetts

Weber R P 1985 *Basic Content Analysis.* Sage, Beverly Hills, California

Wulfemeyer K T, Mueller B 1991 Television commercials in the classroom: A content analysis of Channel One ads. *Communication Journalism Education Today* 24(4): 10–13

Data Banks and Data Archives

J. Anderson and M. J. Rosier

Research data are arranged in data sets, defined as organized collections of related data. The term data bank is commonly used to refer to a collection of related data sets, often associated with a single research project or survey. The quantity of data in most data sets or data banks usually necessitates the use of computerized retrieval systems with data stored in machine-readable form. Data archives are places where machine-readable data, such as those contained in data sets, are stored, preserved, and cataloged for access and use by others. Increasingly, educational researchers are making use of data held in data archives to answer questions, for example, about the achievement, attitudes, or attributes of students and schools, or to compare their data with other data collected at a different time or in a different place.

This entry considers the nature of data archives, the necessary documentation for archived data, and problems associated with the organization of data, the coding of data, and the preparation of a codebook. In addition, it identifies the major data archives in the United Kingdom, continental Europe, and the United States and discusses five issues that affect future developments in the field.

1. Data Banks in the Social Sciences

Although the concept of an educational data bank may conjure up visions of vast amounts of information being kept on file about schools, teachers, and students, and thus may be thought of as depersonalizing education, there are reasons that may be advanced for maintaining such data banks.

The collection of research data, particularly from large longitudinal studies or studies conducted nationwide or across countries, is expensive. The possibility that such data may be used by other research workers, for secondary analysis or for providing benchmarks to enable comparisons at some time in the future, helps to justify the expenditure. There is also a certain obligation on the part of researchers to ensure that collections of data, especially if funded by public moneys, are made available as soon as possible to colleagues in the wider research community. This represents an extension of the current practice of the evaluation of the quality of scientific work by means of peer review and thus may lead to better educational research. The analysis of a data set by secondary analysts asking different questions and using a variety of models and statistical techniques should lead to a more robust interpretation of the data, particularly where initial analyses were conducted under severe time constraints imposed by the sponsoring agencies.

The archiving of data and their use by others may also reduce the need to interrupt schools and other educational institutions, which may in turn enhance the response by institutions on occasions when data are collected in the future. This applies particularly to the use of archived data sets for the training of research workers who wish to concentrate their effort on developing a repertoire of statistical techniques rather than on data collection. Part of the justification for establishing the Social Science Research Council (SSRC) Survey Archive in the United Kingdom was that survey data are "a valuable resource in terms of both human effort and cash funds, therefore, to be

protected and utilized so that the gain in knowledge that each individual effort represents is not needlessly dissipated, nor needlessly replicated".

One of the pioneering data banks in education was prepared for the Project TALENT (Tiedemann 1972). Other well-known data banks have been associated with the cross-national studies conducted by the International Association for the Evaluation of Educational Achievement (IEA); for example, the IEA Six-subject Data Bank (Schwille and Marshall 1975, Walker 1976). The IEA Six-subject Data Bank, for instance, holds data collected from approximately 250,000 students, 50,000 teachers, and 10,000 schools in 21 countries as part of six international surveys of achievement in science, reading comprehension, literature, civic education, and French and English as foreign languages. In each of the surveys, student achievement data, as well as information about students' home and socioeconomic backgrounds, attitudes, and interests, together with information from teachers and schools, were gathered by testing students aged 10 years, 14 years, or in the last year or preuniversity year of schooling. The IEA data banks are lodged in data archives at the IEA headquarters in The Hague, The Netherlands, and in the United States (Inter-University Consortium for Political and Social Research, Ann Arbor, Michigan), as well as in other repositories at research centers and universities in Australia, the United Kingdom, Canada, Japan, and New Zealand. The rich IEA data banks have been accessed by research workers from many countries (Degenhart 1990).

The establishment of data banks in the social sciences has been paralleled by the development of refined statistical software packages which facilitate the researcher's task of accessing and analyzing data. Most computer installations have integrated packages of programs for the management and analyses of social science data: for example, the Statistical Package for the Social Sciences, commonly known as SPSS (Norusis 1990) and SAS (SAS Institute 1992). The major packages usually have the facility to access data sets prepared by the use of other packages (see *Secondary Data Analysis*).

2. Data Documentation

Before any use can be made of a particular data set, such as, say, the science survey data set for 10-year-olds in Italy held by the IEA Six-subject Data Bank, it is necessary to have adequate documentation to enable the data to be interpreted.

The documentation requirements are of two kinds. First, there is general documentation providing information about the study for which the data were collected. Second, there is specific documentation describing the format or layout of the machine-readable data. The central requirement is the adequacy of the documentation rather than the particular conventions adopted. The total documentation for any data set would normally contain:

(a) identifying information (e.g., title of study, names of investigator(s), abstract, related publications);

(b) background information (e.g., describing the context within which the study was conducted);

(c) details of design and sampling (of which greater detail may be included in a report cited in the bibliography);

(d) data-gathering information (including test instruments and how these were administered;

(e) information about data organization (e.g., coding of responses and how the response data are stored in the data set).

All or part of this documentation may be located with the data on the computer in machine-readable form. Again, the crucial issue is the availability of this information, rather than how it is stored.

3. Data Organization

In educational research a data set typically comprises measures obtained for a sample of cases. The case, which is the basic unit of analysis, may be some larger unit such as a class of students or a school. Measures might include, for instance, personal characteristics, demographic data, and achievement scores, in which event each case would contain these groups of variables, and the ordering of the variables would be exactly the same for all cases. When all data are being prepared in a form ready for analysis, all variables for each case are organized into a data file. Three steps are involved: coding, entering data, and file building. At the same time a codebook is usually prepared, containing information about the coding scheme adopted for all variables and their location on the data file (see *Data Management in Survey Research*).

3.1 Coding the Data

In entering data into the computer it is usual to code the information collected for each case by assigning symbols to each item on the completed instrument(s). Alphabetic and special characters are generally to be avoided in coding the data, since the computer is able to process numerical data more efficiently. The practice of using multiple codes for a single item, which would involve making several entries in a single column, should also be avoided since many statistical software packages cannot handle this format.

To illustrate the assigning of symbols to items, respondents' names are often coded 001, 002, 003 . . .

while sex might be coded as 1 (male), 2 (female). Coding is thus seen to result in compact storage and, in the case of personal data, helps to preserve confidentiality. Accompanying documentation must clearly indicate the meaning of all assigned codes (though names of respondents or schools are not displayed). This information is commonly included in a codebook.

For open-ended questionnaire items coding must frequently follow the data collection and must take place prior to the entry of data into the computer. There are several good texts (e.g., Johnson 1977) that provide details of coding schemes.

Where possible, the coding of data should preserve the information contained in the original responses, provided that the requirements of anonymity are observed. For example, a variable measuring school size should be coded in terms of the actual enrollments, allowing the investigator or secondary analyst to group the numbers as desired (e.g., less than 600, 601–800, 801–1,000, more than 1,000). Similarly, if the study includes a test, the responses to each test item should be individually coded. Optionally, the data set may contain in addition certain derived scores, such as totals or subscores for groups of items, provided the accompanying documentation details how the derived scores were obtained.

Where respondents fail to answer, or respond "inapplicable" or "don't know," such responses should also be given specific code values. Many of the statistical software packages allow up to three values to be designated as missing: it is thus possible to distinguish between these particular instances of missing data and yet at the same time to process them similarly in any analysis (for example, by excluding all such cases in analyses). If, for instance, two digits have been used to code a given variable then the following codes could be reserved as missing value codes: "97 —inapplicable; 98—don't know; 99—omitted (or not ascertained)." With some analysis packages, problems may occur if missing responses are represented by blanks or spaces on the data file, instead of by alphanumeric symbols. Once the data are coded they may then be entered directly into the computer (see Schleicher 1991).

When the originally coded data on the data file are assembled, and corrected as necessary, a common practice is to create a range of secondary variables from particular original or primary variables. For example, a variable to measure socioeconomic level may be a composite formed from variables measuring occupation, education, and income. The procedures adopted in forming such secondary variables always need to be fully documented.

3.2 Preparing the Codebook

The preparation of a codebook is an essential part of preparing the data file, since the codebook contains details about the characteristics of each variable and its location on the file. The following features are included for each variable in most codebooks.

(a) Variable name: each variable is named or identified by a number or a set of alphanumeric characters. For example, the SPSS system uses a set of alphanumeric characters with a maximum length of eight characters.

(b) Variable label: in general, the variable name is linked to a variable label. Variables to be used in an analysis are usually selected by means of the variable name, while the printout may give both the variable label and the variable name in order to improve readability.

(c) Location: the location of each variable within a given record on a data file must be specified in terms of the numbers of the columns it spans, which is equivalent to giving the number of the first column of the entry for the variable and the width of the entry (the number of columns occupied by the entry).

(d) Format: the format of the variables should be specified in terms of the number of decimal places present or implicit in the data for the variable.

(e) Missing data code(s): where code values have been assigned to missing responses, these should be specified.

(f) Item text: it is also useful to include with each item the actual text of the item used to solicit the data for each variable, even if such information is available in accompanying documentation.

(g) Code values: for each variable with a defined set of code values, the values must be given together with the responses to which they are assigned.

(h) Notes: it is often useful to add notes providing further information about a variable, especially for warnings about problems associated with the data for a given variable.

If the codebook is prepared in machine-readable form, access to data in a data file and statistical analyses of the data are greatly facilitated. Computer software is available for preparing and generating codebooks at most data archives. Because the codebook is accessed directly, accuracy is ensured in locating all variables, variable labels, format specification, missing data values, and value labels.

4. Access to Data Archives

Major data archives have already been established for the social sciences. The archives collect data sets, often reorganizing the data files and documentation before making them available to other users. The archives also provide a range of services to distribute information about the nature and availability of the data sets, and to assist researchers in accessing them. Three major archives are the SSRC (Social Science Research Council) Survey Archive, the Steinmetz Archive, and the Interuniversity Consortium for Political and Social Research (ICPSR).

The first is the national repository of social science data in the United Kingdom. Established in 1967, its brief is "to collect and preserve machine-readable data relating to social and economic affairs from academic, commercial, and government sources and to make that data available for secondary analysis".

The Steinmetz Institute in The Netherlands was established in 1964 and the archives, which are concerned with collecting, documenting, and distributing social science data for secondary analysis, are now part of the Social Science Information and Documentation Center (SWIDOC). The Steinmetz Archive maintains close relationships with other European archives such as Central Archive for Empirical Social Research at the University of Cologne in Germany.

The third archive, the ICPSR, is based at the University of Michigan, and is a major source of archived data sets for universities and other institutions in the United States. The ICPSR also maintains links with universities and national bodies in other countries, such as the SSRC Survey Archive in the United Kingdom, and provides reciprocal borrowing rights.

These archives have produced catalogs describing the data sets that may be borrowed. Researchers normally gain access to the data sets by using the formal channels that have been established between the archives and the institutions participating in the system. Data sets are usually supplied according to the specified technical formats. Documentation in the form of codebooks and test instruments is usually supplied at a nominal cost.

Two international bodies have been established to promote the development and use of data archives. The International Association for Social Science Information Services and Technology (IASSIST) was established in 1976. The International Federation of Data Organizations (IFDO) was started in 1977.

5. Some Issues

Although much progress has been made in establishing good data archives, more work is needed before the level of data archiving can be regarded as satisfactory. Five issues affect future developments.

5.1 Obtaining Data Sets

One of the major problems faced by archives is the difficulty in obtaining data sets. Even where data sets are identified and located, there may be problems in obtaining them for inclusion in the archives. Some researchers are still wary of releasing their data for examination by other persons. Progress in this area will depend largely on a spirit of cooperation between the original researchers and the secondary analysts. One avenue is to encourage the joint authorship by primary and secondary researchers of publications arising from secondary analysis. At the least, the original researchers should be offered the opportunity to make rejoinders in publications that include the results of secondary analysis.

Frequently, there are certain conditions governing access to particular data sets. The SSRC Survey Archive, for instance, has three access categories: (a) unconditional access; (b) access conditional on the depositor being informed of the request; and (c) access conditional on the prior consent of the depositor being obtained. The researcher requesting access to archived data is usually required to sign an undertaking to protect the anonymity of individuals and of institutions supplying the data, to acknowledge indebtedness to the original data collectors and to the archive, and to furnish the archive with any publication resulting from the use of the data.

Some funding agencies are now making it a condition of their grants that any data collected under the grant should be lodged in appropriate data archives. However, the grants should also be large enough so that the researcher has sufficient resources to build good data sets supported by adequate documentation.

5.2 Adequate Documentation

The usefulness of a data set depends largely on the adequacy of the documentation that describes in detail the collection of the data and their characteristics. Good documentation is necessary if for no other reason than that it reduces the costs of secondary analysis by increasing the efficiency with which data can be accessed.

For example, good documentation may include a listing of data for the first few cases on each file. When the secondary analyst first reads an archived file, it is then possible to compare the results from the archived file with the documented listing to ensure that all the data are present, and that the data files correspond to those submitted by the original researcher. In the same way, the codebook entries for each variable should contain a statement about the number of cases (frequency) associated with each value code. The secondary analyst should be able to reproduce these frequencies from the archived data set. As further assistance to the secondary analyst, the set of data-collection instruments could be reproduced with the original responses and the associated coding for one case—say the first case.

5.3 Level of Aggregation of Data

Data are most useful to secondary analysts when they are stored at a minimal level of aggregation (the microlevel). This means that the original responses to questionnaire or test items are retained in a coded form on the data file. The secondary analyst then has the option of changing the level of aggregation; for example, by deriving total test scores from a set of test items, or by deriving a mean school score from the data for students in a given school. If only the aggregated data (total or mean scores) are provided, the option of conducting analyses at the individual level is no longer available. Of course, steps must be taken to ensure that access to microlevel data does not enable the condition of anonymity or confidentiality to be breached.

5.4 Problems of Item Comparability

One of the particularly important uses of data archives is for the study of trends over time, in both national and crossnational studies. There are, however, problems of maintaining item comparability over time in both the wording of questions and the number of response categories employed. Research workers, often on ideological grounds that have uncertain theoretical foundations, change the wording of questions, which are thereby made incomparable with items asked in previous investigations. In other cases, it is contended that a shift has occurred in the distribution of a characteristic—such as the number of books in the home or the number of newspapers read daily in the home—and that the response categories used require alteration. Such changes invalidate comparisons over time, which are clearly of interest. In addition to such obvious removal of comparability, seemingly identical questions can be rendered noncomparable by the use of contingency questions, which precede the specific question for which comparability is sought, or even changing of the context or sequence of survey items which may influence responses. The monitoring and investigation of both stability and change in social science and educational research are now possible through the availability of data banks and data archives. As a consequence consideration needs to be given as to how to optimize the value of such investigations.

5.5 Problems of Sample Comparability over Time

One of the major problems in educational research where the emphasis is on trends and change over time is the gradual change in the structure and composition of the school population. The nature of the school population has been changed considerably by the marked growth in retention rates in all countries throughout the years of secondary schooling, in the second cycle of education, and in some countries by the gradual increase in participation rates at the primary school or first cycle level. Effects also occur as a result of a tendency for students to enter school at an earlier age, or because practices of grade repeating are gradually being eliminated in many school systems. While such changes present problems for simple comparisons of students' achievements and attitudes, or of the conditions of education provided over time, the issues of stability and change in educational provision and outcomes are of sufficient importance to warrant attempts being made to control for changes over time in the composition of the school population both by design and statistical adjustments. More damaging, however, are differences in response rates between occasions, and changes in the definition of the excluded and target populations.

6. Conclusion

Secondary data analysis has recently assumed a key role in educational research. No longer is it possible to encroach on school time or teachers' work within schools through the disrupting effects of small-scale studies. Furthermore, all too often the data collected in large investigations are incompletely analyzed. Moreover, advances in procedures of data analysis are occurring so rapidly that data collected 20 years earlier can now be more effectively analyzed. Theses for graduate degrees at the master's and doctoral levels provide excellent circumstances for careful and systematic secondary analysis, provided the data are held in well-constructed data banks and data archives. Nevertheless, the tasks of developing a data set of high quality that would facilitate secondary data analysis

proves to be both challenging and very demanding (see *Secondary Data Analysis*).

References

Degenhart R E 1990 *Thirty Years of International Research: An Annotated Bibliography of IEA Publications (1960–1990)*. IEA, The Hague
Johnson M C 1977 *A Review of Research Methods in Education*. Rand McNally, Chicago, Illinois
Norusis M J 1990 *SPSS/PC+*. SPSS Inc., Chicago, Illinois
SAS Institute 1992 *SAS User's Guide Version 6 Edition*. SAS Institute Inc., Cary, North Carolina
Schleicher A 1991 *The Data Entry Manager System: A Computer System for Data Entry*. Schleicher Inc., Hamburg
Schwille J, Marshall S 1975 *The IEA Six-subject Data Bank: A General Introduction*. University of Stockholm, Stockholm
Tiedemann D V 1972 *Project TALENT Data Bank: A Handbook*. American Institutes for Research, Project TALENT, Palo Alto, California
Walker D A 1976 *The IEA Six-subject Survey: An Empirical Study of Education in Twenty-one Countries*. Almqvist and Wiksell, Stockholm

Further Reading

Kiecolt K J, Nathan L E 1985 *Secondary Analyses of Survey Data*. Sage, Beverly Hills, California

Data Management in Survey Research

A. Schleicher

Relevant data of good quality are a prerequisite for educational planning, research, and decision-making. Database management systems play an essential role in providing and maintaining accurate and valid educational data.

The purpose of a database management system is to store information relevant to a certain area of activity and to manipulate, analyze, and report that information in order to provide answers to specific questions related to that information. The information can be of any kind that can be recorded within electronic media. It generally involves quantified data which in the educational context often consist of achievement test scores, background questionnaire responses, administrative data, and numerical measurements, but can also include "bibliographic records," citations, abstracts, and graphical data. Database management systems can manage this information in such a way that: (a) the same logical data structure can be used in the context of different applications; (b) the logical data structure

is independent of the physical structure of the database so that the implementation of a database can be modified independently of the logical data structure; (c) data are stored consistently and with a minimum of redundancy; and (d) the information can be retrieved efficiently by a variety of criteria as required by the applications. Applications in the educational context can range from simple datafiles that can, for example, be used to keep track of the enrollment data of students in a school up to complex information management systems which can manage complex structures of textual, graphical, or numerical data, and which permit multiple paths of access to, and a variety of views on the information. Accordingly, database management systems are available on computer systems that range from small micro computers up to large "mainframe" systems.

This entry describes the nature of a database and gives an example of how a database can be used in educational research to provide evidence for policymaking.

1. Main Concepts of a Database Management System

A "database" is a structured aggregation of "data-elements" within a certain area of activity which can be related and linked to other data-elements by a relationship so as to form useful information. These data-elements can then be accessed by the user by specified criteria and the user can exchange information with the database by means of a set of "transaction operations." An example of this is given at the end of this entry. The data-elements in this context involve logical units of information which are assigned a label and which are associated with a set of "data-fields." A data-element can, for example, contain information about a student, a school or any other object of reality. Each of the data-fields describes one attribute of the object, such as the name of a student, his age, or her test score in a mathematics test. For each data-field a data-value is associated with each data-element. One data-field, or a set of data-fields, serves as a classification criterion in the way that each data-element can be distinguished from and located within equally structured data-elements. For example, if the data-elements describe students, then the student's name or matriculation code could serve as their identifier provided it is unique.

The logical unit of a data-element as represented in the conceptual scheme of a database need not necessarily correspond to a physical unit as represented by the internal scheme of a database; on the contrary, it is often advisable to locate the data-elements in different physical units in order to eliminate redundancy.

The bridge between, on the one hand, the data-elements and their conceptual representation in the database and, on the other hand, the views of the users on the database which are represented by the external scheme, is built by a "computer program." The database and this computer program together comprise a "database management system." This program can have either the form of a specific application program or the form of a "query language" as an integral part of the database management system.

Figure 1 presents, in diagrammatic form, the different levels of abstraction of a database ranging from the physical data located in secondary storage and represented by the internal scheme through the levels of logical representation of the data up to the user's view, represented by the external scheme.

A database may be seen from several different viewpoints: (a) from the viewpoint of a functional task as an image of elements of reality; (b) from the viewpoint of the user who is interested in its quality as a system for information retrieval; (c) from the viewpoint of the programmer who is interested in its conceptual design and organization into data-elements; and (d) from the viewpoints of physical and technical conception.

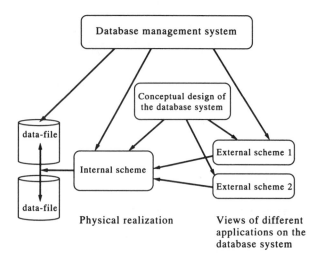

Figure 1
The different levels of abstraction of a database

Databases are often "shared" by multiple users. This means that different users may operate on subsets of the database at the same time. Often a database can be accessed in different ways and the views and purposes with which these users see their subsets of data may be substantially different.

2. Historical Background

"Electronic devices for data storage" became available in the early 1960s. It was at this time that the first database management systems (such as MEDLARS for medical information retrieval or SABRE as an airways reservation system) were developed. The terms "information system" and "database management system," however, were by then used to cover a wide content area and without precise definition.

Examples of early applications could be found: in banking, insurance (Allen 1968), and, related to the educational field, for the management of bibliographic data and text (e.g., the systems SMART [Salton 1968] and LEADER [Hillmann and Kasarda 1969]).

Scientific approaches for analyzing data and data structures were developed in parallel. A major advance in the development of database theory proved to be the introduction of the three levels of abstraction of databases, namely the internal, the conceptual, and the external level. These were first referred to in the Report of the Database Task Group in 1971 (CODASYL 1971). A set-theory approach to the description of data structures (Langefors 1963, Levien 1967) led to the foundation of modern database architecture. In a series of papers published between 1970 and 1975, Codd (1970, 1972, 1975) introduced the "relational algebra" on which the relational data model and data manipulation procedures are based and proved its equivalence to the mathematical tuple relational calculus. These concepts were then generalized to data models such as the hierarchical and the network model (Gallaire and Minker 1978). Since then research has developed in various directions. For example, early attempts were made to use natural language as a query language (Dell'Orco et al. 1977) and to introduce semantic aspects to the relational model (Codd 1979).

The first use of a relational database was the prototype of the "SYSTEM R" which was introduced in 1975 by IBM with the purpose of demonstrating that a relational database management system could satisfy all practical demands on databases (Chamberlin 1981). SYSTEM R was based on the database language SQL which has become the predominant database language since then. The first SQL-based relational database product on the market was ORACLE, introduced in 1980 by Relational Software Inc., followed by SQL/DS introduced by IBM in 1981. In 1990 there were more than 80 SQL-based relational database management systems on the market, the main ones being ORACLE, DB2 (IBM), INFORMIX (Relational Database System), DG/SQL (Data General Corp.), and SYBASE (Sybase Inc.). In the educational field the database management systems dBASE (Ashton Tate Corp.) and ACCESS (Microsoft Corp.) have become widely used systems. When the primary focus of the data management are statistical data analyses, often "statistical packages" are used with integrated database management capabilities such as the SAS Statistical Analysis System (SAS Institute Inc.). These allow the educational researcher to generate and link data structures and to specify data analysis requests, thereby requiring only a minimum of experience in software development and database management.

3. A Database Compared with Traditional Data Archiving

A database has many advantages over traditional paper-based archiving methods. Some of these advantages are given below.

(a) The machine can locate and modify data very quickly in a systematic way (e.g., extract all students from a database who live in a certain district).

(b) While paper-based archives can be ordered, and thus information located, only through a single classification criterion, electronic databases can usually be accessed by a number of classification criteria which themselves can have a complex structure. In this way a query can be answered without a time-consuming manual search.

(c) Since the data-files of a database can be linked

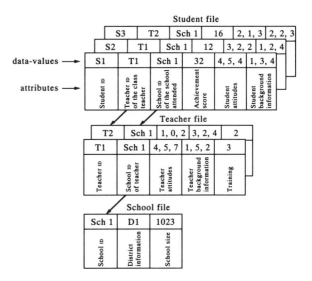

Figure 2
Elimination of redundancy

the information needs to be stored only once. For example, in the data obtained from a large-scale assessment survey which involves achievement data from students and background data from teachers and schools, it would be disadvantageous to store student, teacher, and school information as one unit because many students attend the same school and it would then be necessary to record the same teacher and school information for each student. In order to avoid the redundant storage of teacher and school information the data on students, teachers, and schools could be designed as distinct data-files located in separate physical units. One of the data-fields of the student file could then contain the identification of the school attended so that each student can be associated with the information about that school which is stored separately in the school data-file. Likewise the student may be linked to a teacher, the teacher linked to a school, and the school linked to a school district, and so on. The stepwise elimination of redundancy is called "normalization" and according to the extent or level to which redundancy is avoided the database is said to be in a certain "normalized form." The elimination of redundancy in a database is illustrated in Fig. 2.

(d) Inconsistencies between data-files can occur in traditional non-database filing systems when different data-files with related information are kept for different applications and when changes to the information in one of these data-files are not made correspondingly in the other data-files representing the same information. Such inconsistencies can be consequently avoided in a normalized database. For example, the address of a student might be kept both at the school and at the school district office, but need only be held on one data-file if the school and school district files are linked in a database. When redundancy cannot be avoided, a database management system can still ensure that redundancy does not lead to inconsistency of the data-files by automatically applying a change that is made on one data-value to all other data-values that represent the same information and to all relations that refer to that data-value. In a database management system an update implies all the transactions which are necessary to keep the database consistent.

(e) The data in a database are stored in a way which is basically independent of the application. This implies that the storage is independent of the user's view on the data. Moreover, the database is independent of how the data are physically stored in contrast with a traditional archive in which data storage is organized for a particular task and where the organization of the data and the way in which they can be accessed are inherent in the logic of a particular application. For example, in a paper-based filing system the entries in a student data-file associated with achievement test scores may be sorted by the students' names. For an application in which a student is to be located by his test score (e.g., when the 10 highest achieving students are sought) it would be necessary to re-arrange the whole data-file by sorting the entries according to achievement test scores.

(f) Computerized data which are stored centrally can readily be shared and controlled by a single security system. Problems of both security and confidentiality of information are of growing importance.

4. Basic Types of Database

In some databases the data-elements do not have a unique structure in the sense of a predefined data scheme. For example, they may consist of plain text—as, for instance, in a system for document retrieval in a library—or a graphic image. These data-elements are called "unformatted." The plain text of the unformatted data is usually associated with a structured part for classification purposes (e.g., a subject index, the author's name, etc.). Those words within an unformatted data-element that serve as qualifiers are called "keywords." These keywords may be grouped together in a "thesaurus." The retrieval of information is based on syntactic, or in some cases even on semantic, aspects. The problem of unformatted databases is that they usually contain notable redundancy in the unformatted data-elements.

A database is referred to as "formatted" if the data-elements are associated with a format that is the same for all data elements. Data-elements can, for instance, have a defined length and order in accordance with the syntactic rules of the database management system. The format comprises information on the structure of the data-fields and all information on how the data are modeled together with the transformation rules by which the computer interprets the data-elements.

Different conceptual schemes can be used for the design of a database, dependent on the structure of the information. There are three basic models used to implement the different conceptual schemes which are associated with different functional tasks.

4.1 The Hierarchical Data-model

In hierarchical structured databases the data are organized in the form of a multilevel tree (in which the nodes represent the data-elements and the branches refer to the relations) with fixed relationships between the data-elements. In this way the data-elements are connected through fixed parent–child relationships. The basic operators to access the data in this database structure involve moving up and down in the tree-like hierarchy. This structure requires a close and inflexible relationship between the conceptual scheme and the physical database. Thus, a hierarchical modeled database is closely bound to the application envisaged. Although hierarchical database structures are often not the most efficient way to organize data, many educational databases are based on the hierarchical data model. The data structure is then often used to represent the natural spatial or hierarchical structure of the collected information, such as when students are organized into classes, schools, and districts. A common, but inefficient way to organize hierarchical data in the educational context is to repeat the information for all higher levels in the data-elements at the lower levels, for example, by adding teacher, school, or district information to the data-elements representing the student-level data. A better way is to organize hierarchical data into distinct rectangular data-files which are connected through the identification codes of the corresponding levels of the hierarchy.

4.2 The Network Data-model

This model is related to the hierarchical model, but a data-element can belong to several hierarchies, and thus the database can have several roots.

4.3 The Relational Data-model

This model is based on the set-theory notation of a relation. Its logical data-structure is that of a table with no explicit representation of the relationships between the data-elements and with the data represented as explicit data-values. Each observation can be linked by means of an unique identifier to other data-elements. The basic operators to manipulate data in this data-structure are operators that derive new elements of a table-like structure. This is often a very efficient way for organizing the information, and data of virtually any complexity can be modeled relationally. The relational theory provides methods for the systematic decomposition and normalization of a set of relations, for joining the relations in order to obtain new relations and views of the data, and for defining selections and linkages in order to obtain the required information. The aim of the normalization process is to group the data-elements in such a way that: (a) only one value is assigned to each data-field; (b) each data-field which does not belong to the classification unit is functionally dependent on the classification unit; and (c) each data-field that does not belong to the identification key is transitively dependent on the identification key. In the example considered above, a new data-table might be created when all schools are taken from the district data-file. The schools then represent the rows of the new table and they are combined with the school means of achievement scores derived from the student data-file. The data-tables associated with the relational data-model referred to in the example at the end of this entry are illustrated in Table 1.

An example for a relational data-model

Student file

Student ID	School ID	District ID	Score
S1	SCH1	D1	16
S2	SCH1	D1	12
S3	SCH1	D1	32
S4	SCH2	D2	10
S5	SCH3	D3	34
S6	SCH3	D3	48

District file

District ID	Social Ind.
D1	−3
D2	+6
D3	+2
D4	−5

Students with social indicators

Student ID	School ID	Score	Social Ind.
S1	SCH1	16	−3
S2	SCH1	12	−3
S3	SCH1	32	+6
S4	SCH2	10	+6
S5	SCH3	34	+2
S6	SCH3	48	+2

School mean data

School ID	Mean Social Ind.	Mean Score
SCH1	0	20
SCH2	+6	10
SCH3	+2	41

5. The Structure of a Database

The basic unit of a data-element is the data-field. A data-field has an identifying name and its structure is described by information such as location, format, and data-type. For example a data-field containing achievement scores of students could have the name "SCORE," the data-type integer, and a length of two decimal positions. For each observation within a database a value is assigned to each data-field (e.g., for the first student 16 may be the value for the data-field SCORE). The value together with the information that describes the data-field to which values are assigned constitute a piece of information. The values for a data-field can be taken from a certain set of values for this specific data-field. This set is then called a "domain." For example the data-field "score" may contain a value out of the set {1,2,3, 50} which represents the domain.

A single data-field, however, does not comprise useful information in the sense of an information system. Only when this data-field is linked to other data-fields is a useful piece of information established. For example, only when an achievement score is linked to a student (identified by the field STUDENT ID) is useful information obtained; that is, only when the data-field SCORE is related to the data-field STUDENT ID. Usually several data-fields are combined to form a named unit. If one part of this unit serves as a classification criterion this unit is called a "segment." The classification criterion establishes the identification, characterization, and classification of each observation of a database. For example, the student name may be used as an identification criterion if there are no two students with the same name. The classification criteria determine how data-elements can be linked, ordered, and accessed and thus they form an image of the organizational structure for the task the database is to fulfill.

All data-fields of a database together form a record which represents an observation, such as the data collected for a particular student, teacher, or school. A data-element may be related to other data-elements by a set of single or multiple relationships. Frequently a data-element does not naturally contain an identification data-field. For example, it is possible that two students in a school system have the same name. In this case an "identification key" can often be created from a combination of data-fields. For those data-elements for which no combination of data-fields exists that can be used for a unique identification, an identification key has to be constructed. A variety of "numbering systems" is used for this purpose. Some of these systems are simple sequential numbers which have no data-field that can be used for classification. For example, each student may be associated with a sequential number serving as the student ID which is not associated with any classification scheme. Other numbering systems are hierarchically structured so that parts of the ID at the lower level are derived from the next highest level by increasing the number of confining elements. In this case, each part of the identification key is totally dependent on the preceding part of the ID. Examples are many postal numbering systems, or in the above case, the school ID+student ID+sequential ID, where the sequential ID is a sequential number within those students with the same name within a school. Still other numbering systems have a parallel structure in which each part of the ID has a unique meaning all independent of other parts of the ID and in which operations and transactions can be performed independently. Numbering systems are often combined so as to result in compound numbering systems.

All observations with the same record structure together form a named unit, the database. Again the database must be differentiated from the physical files in which the data may be recorded which may, for example, be coded or crypted or be in a different arrangement than seen by the user or represented by the conceptual scheme.

There are databases in which each data-field can be used for a relationship. There are other systems which have a certain structure permitting only a limited number of predefined data-fields to be used for classification. This, in turn, allows only a limited and predefined number of transactions. In these cases, transactions are usually performed by a specific "transaction code" which in turn calls a corresponding program to execute the transaction.

However, since each data-field can be used as a classification criterion, it is often restrictive to use a predefined set of transactions. A "query language" is therefore often introduced by means of which the user can specify the transactions required. A query asks a particular question about the data in the database (e.g., which students have an achievement score higher than 12). The query is then interpreted by the computer and translated (compiled) into a transaction. In this case the structure of the request becomes apparent

to the computer only at the time of the request. The query's answer consists of all elements that match the query and is called a "dynaset." A query can relate several data-fields and data-elements to each other and analyze the generated construct by a number of functions (e.g., calculate the mean of the achievement test scores for all students that have been taught by certain teachers). A query may thus be very complex.

Simple query languages consist of a number of functions for specific query problems for which the user has to specify parameters. The system will then evaluate and interpret the parameters, possibly ask for further information, and then generate the answer. For example, the function "AVG" may request the specification of a data-field for which to calculate the average, then perform the calculation, and finally return the result.

More complex query languages consist of keywords and a syntax for specification of instructions. Thus, the user can generate a query for a specific query problem which is then translated and executed by the computer. There are many software systems, ranging from formal set-theory based languages to simple structured languages that allow the user to address a request to the database with little attention given to the internal structure of the system. For example a simple request trying to calculate the mean of achievement test scores for all students attending the school with the ID "SCH1" could be stated in the SQL language:

SELECT AVG(score)
    FROM student file
    WHERE school="SCH1"

The system would then return the value 20 if the school mean test score of school "SCH1" is 20.

6. Database Software

The "database software" is the means by which data are assembled and administered. In general, database software consists of the following components.

(a) A first component of the software is used for describing and modifying the format of the data-elements of a database. This component makes the structure of the data known to the computer and thus makes the data manageable for the computer. With the format defined it is possible to create a database from input data or to modify the structure of a database when the format is redefined.

(b) A second component is designed for "maintenance and update" of a database. With this component outdated data-elements can be deleted and new data-elements can be added so that new input data can become part of the operational data of the database. Additionally this component can be used to modify single data-fields within a data-element. Maintenance and update can be performed periodically in an automatic way for all observations (e.g., when a salary is increased for observations which are identified by some formal criterion) or individually (e.g., when the address of an observation is changed).

(c)   The third component is used to derive output data such as messages and reports from the operational data of the database and to analyze these data. This component does not modify the actual data but it produces a report of the data according to the specifications of the query.

7. Application to Education

7.1 Design and Implementation of a Database Management System

The implementation of a verbally formulated task into a computer-manageable database management system is a complex task. It involves the abstraction and structuring of the problem and the implementation of hierarchical and modular concepts to the problem so that the users see a hierarchy of functional entities on which they can operate independently. It involves the principles of localization and standardization since it is desirable that all information relevant to a specific content and all methods required to solve a specific problem are kept at a single location and are presented in a similar way not only in the conceptual design of the database but also in the external scheme. The tasks involved in the design of a database management system are shown diagrammatically in Fig. 3.

Several steps are necessary.

(a)   The task must be defined in a finite and un-equivocal way by stating the purpose and tasks of the system together with the framework within which the database is developed. This should include a detailed analysis of the kind of data which the database management system is meant to handle. The definition should be structured in a way so that the anticipated database operations can be easily decomposed into a number of functional tasks. For example, to design a system that contains student enrolment information we need to decide what information on the students, their classes, and their schools, is required by the different users, how it should be processed; and how it should be accessed, updated and reported.

(b)   The data-elements must be defined, although this may be done in an abstract manner with no regard to the way in which the data will be physically stored. This implies the definition of data-fields, the grouping of similar data-fields to segments, the definition of classification data-fields for each segment, and finally, the aggregation of

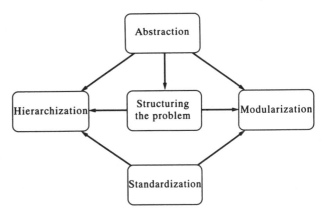

Figure 3
Tasks involved in database design

segments to records. This is usually done by creating a matrix in which each logical data-unit is represented in one row and one column with the elements of the matrix representing the relationships between each pair. Afterwards the matrix is rearranged in such a way that the elements form submatrices which then form the final databases. As indicated above, each data-element must be assigned an identification key which uniquely identifies each observation. The relationships between data-elements should also be defined as data-elements. These relationships may be single (a data-element is related to only one data-element), multiple (a data-element is related to one or more data-elements), or conditional (a data-element can be related to other data-elements according to specified conditions).

(c)   In the normalization of the data-elements the data-fields must be grouped in a way that redundancy is avoided within an aggregation of data-elements. If, for example, data on students and schools are to be managed, then it is useful to store the information on students and schools separately in order to minimize redundancy.

(d)   The design of the transactions is concerned with the ways in which data are accessed and manipulated. In this step the logical relationships for the exchange of information are designed. Great care must be taken in this step since only those operations can be allowed that obey the external and model-inherent conditions of consistency. For example, arbitrary alternation of an identification key is not permitted. The first step in doing this is to analyze quantities and frequencies of handled information and to develop modes of communication.

(e)   The modes of communication differentiate between horizontal and vertical transactions. Horizontal transactions basically involve the shifting and modification of data-elements without changing their structure. Vertical transactions are used to comprise information, to make the characteristics of a large amount of data available to the user and thus provide the basis for decisions. There are several aspects of vertical transactions: (i) information may be filtered, that is only information that is relevant for a certain task is transferred (e.g., it may be necessary to select only certain data-fields for those students of a certain district); (ii) information may be aggregated or summarized to a higher class of information (e.g., it may be necessary to summarize student data to the school or district level); (iii) information may be analyzed and only the results transferred as, for example, by statistical and mathematical operations (e.g., there may be no interest in the data-values but only in their central measure and spread as in the above example with the school mean achievement score).

In the transformation of the conceptual data model into an actual database the definition of the numbering objects and their notation, and the definition and design of the user interfaces by which the user can operate the transactions are required. This includes the design of the database software and the application program or query language.

7.2 An Example

Database techniques are widely applied in the field of educational research, ranging from systems for retrieval of bibliographic information (e.g., ERIC) to the management of large survey data for policy-making.

An example of the latter is a study performed in Australia by Ross (1983) which investigated the use of census descriptions of school neighborhoods in order to develop, validate, and describe the properties of a national indicator of educational disadvantage.

It was considered important that the term "disadvantage" should be associated with schools rather than with individual students, and that the definition was not concerned with the characteristics of the families of the students but rather with the neighborhoods from which the schools obtained their students. This had the following implications for the design of the database.

(a) The schools had to be used as the unit of analysis.

(b) Information describing the neighborhoods from which schools obtained their students was used to describe the schools. For that purpose data from the 1971 Australian national census of population and housing was available so that each student could be associated with the census district data of social indicators.

(c) A criterion measure was required to select appropriate census descriptions of school neighborhoods. The school mean score from a national study conducted in 1975 of educational achievement in Australian schools was taken for that purpose.

This led to the following design of the database. One data-unit contained the student data with one record for each student containing the achievement and background data, an identification of home address, the student ID, and the ID of the school attended. A second data-unit contained the census data with one record for each district and with the social indicators. Both these data-units were designed as separate physical data-units. For the link between the student and census data a relation was established that connected the student's home address to the census district number. Through this connection the census data could be related to the school attended, aggregated over schools, and thus a between school analysis performed.

In conclusion, with computers becoming more extensively used in educational institutions, particularly schools and colleges, it is likely that databases involving storage and management of information across the units of a system will be developed both for the purposes of administration and research.

References

Allen R P 1968 Omnibus, a large data base management system. In: American Federation of Information Processing Societies (AFIPS) 1968 *Proceedings of the 1968 Fall Joint Computer Conference (FJCC)*, Vol. 33. AFIPS, Montvale, New Jersey

Chamberlin D D 1981 A history and evaluation of System R. *Communications for the Association for Computing Machinery (CACM)* 24(10)

Codd E F 1970 A relational model for large shared data banks. CACM 13(6): 377–87

Codd E F 1972 Further normalization of the data base relational model. In: Rustin R (ed.) 1972 *Data Base Systems.* Prentice Hall, Englewood Cliffs, New Jersey

Codd E F 1975 *Recent Investigations in Relational Data Base Systems.* Information Processing, North Holland, Amsterdam

Codd E F 1979 Extending the Database Relational Model to Capture More Meaning. CACM, New York

Conference on Data Systems Languages (CODASYL) 1971 CODASYL Data Base Task Group April 71 Report. CACM, New York

Dell'Orco P, Spadavecchio V N, King M 1977 Using knowledge of a data base world in interpreting natural language queries. In: IFIP 1977 *Proceedings of the 1977 International Federation for Information Processing (IFIP) Congress.* IFIP, Geneva

Gallaire H, Minker J (eds.) 1978 *Logic and Databases.* Plenum Press, New York

Hillman D J, Kasarda A J 1969 The LEADER retrieval system. In: AFIP 1969 *Proceedings of the 1969 Spring Joint*

Computer Conference (SJCC), Vol. 34. AFIP, Montvale, New Jersey

Langefors B 1963 Some approaches to the theory of information systems. *Nordisk Behandlings Informations Tidscrift (BIT)* 3(4)

Levien R E, Maron M E 1967 A computer system for inference execution and data retrieval. CACM 10(11)

Ross K N 1983 *Social Area Indicators of Educational Need.* Australian Council for Educational Research (ACER), Hawthorn, Victoria

Salton G 1968 *Automatic Information Organization and Retrieval.* McGraw Hill, New York

Further Reading

Lochemann P, Schmidt J 1993 *Database Handbook.* Springer-Verlag, New York

Wheeler T 1993 *Open Systems Handbook.* Multiscience Press, New York

Effective Schools Research

J. D. Willms and S. W. Raudenbush

Since the 1960s researchers have been trying to identify the policies and practices that contribute to successful school performance. Research in several countries has shown that schools differ in their outcomes, even after taking account of the characteristics of pupils attending them (Gray 1989, Raudenbush and Willms 1991). But efforts to determine *why* schools differ have been less successful. Some of the early studies in this area suggested that the effects of school resources and organizational factors were weak, and a number of studies produced inconsistent or inconclusive findings (Bridge et al. 1979). Research in this domain entails several complex methodological issues, which probably contributed to the failure to identify the attributes of effective schools. This entry discusses developments in educational measurement, research design, and statistical techniques which have enabled researchers to address these issues.

Research on effective schools has been based on a theory that presumes schooling outcomes are affected by pupils' ability, their family background, and their experiences at school. The goal of the research has been to determine whether schools vary in their outcomes after taking account of ability and background and, if so, whether particular school policies and practices account for these differences. The research has been criticized as being atheoretical because it failed to specify the links between particular school policies and classroom instruction (Barr and Dreeben 1983). Also, the research treated many complex schooling processes as unidimensional concepts, and examined only their direct effects on outcomes. Factors such as "principal leadership" or "teacher morale" are multifaceted and are difficult to define and measure (Anderson 1982, Boyd 1983). Some factors have relatively weak direct effects on schooling outcomes, but are important in that they create a school atmosphere conducive to learning (Rosenholtz 1989). The study of schooling processes requires a multilevel formulation because factors at different levels of the schooling system can affect outcomes, and their effects can interact across levels (Meyer 1980). The identification of schooling outcomes is also problematic. Some educators contend that the emphasis on academic achievement has deterred educators from critically examining the goals of schooling, and how they might best accomplish these goals. Thus, the extent to which research in this domain is productive depends first on the adequacy of theories about how schools work. Valid measurement, strong designs, and powerful statistical techniques require a solid theoretical foundation.

Nearly all studies of school effects have been, in essence, quasi-experiments with pupils receiving different "treatments" in their respective schools. Some of the designs are nested, with sets of schools each applying a certain treatment (e.g., different approaches to school organization, public or private schools). The researcher observes pupil outcomes after treatment, and asks whether differences in outcomes are related to differences in treatment. Such designs are quasi-experimental because pupils are not randomly assigned to schools. Cook and Campbell (1979) described a number of threats to the validity of this and other types of quasi-experiments. The most important threats to the validity of studies of school effectiveness concern the definition and measurement of schooling constructs, the differential selection of pupils into different types of schools, and the nested structure of the schooling system. During the 1980s researchers developed promising techniques for ameliorating these threats. These techniques are discussed below.

1. Definition and Measurement of Schooling Constructs

Many studies of school effectiveness have been based on data collected by school districts or government bodies as part of their general monitoring systems.

These data are often derived from multipurpose surveys designed to serve a number of constituents. Usually these surveys emphasize contextual and setting variables such as school size, pupil–teacher ratio, racial balance, and levels of education of the staff. Generally the information pertaining to school processes has been too "thin" to be useful for explaining why some schools perform better than others. Researchers have recognized the need to collect detailed information on the climate or culture of a school. Recent work has attempted to describe the inner workings of school life: how pupils are organized for instruction, the relationship between curriculum and instructional activities, the formal and informal rules influencing behavior, the interactions between pupils and staff, and the values, expectations, and attitudes they hold. Rather than collecting thin data for a large sample of schools and pupils, some researchers have attempted to obtain detailed information on one or two school processes for a small number of pupils and schools.

Plewis's (1991) study of curriculum coverage in 42 English primary classrooms serves as an example. Results from some national studies had suggested that the match between the intended and enacted curriculum was one of the most important school processes (Lee and Bryk 1989, McKnight et al. 1987). Plewis and his colleagues asked teachers to identify which curricular items in written language and mathematics had been covered by each of the sixth-year (P6) pupils during the year. Plewis's analysis of the pre- and post-test scores in mathematics showed that pupils made more progress when information on their initial achievement was used to group children for instruction, and when the curriculum was closely matched to initial levels of achievement. Because the researchers had collected detailed information on this process, they were able to show that gains in achievement were not simply a function of how much of the curriculum had been covered.

A number of studies have shown the need to control also for the social composition of schools (see Willms 1986 for a review). The aggregate characteristics of a school, such as the average socioeconomic status (SES) of its pupils, have an effect on pupils' outcomes over and above pupils' individual characteristics. This effect, referred to as a "contextual effect," is not fully understood. Researchers are attempting to discern whether there is some critical proportion of high-ability or high-SES pupils necessary for a positive contextual effect, whether the effect is the same for different types of pupils, and whether the effect is confounded by other school factors such as disciplinary climate or teachers' expectations.

Work is also underway to improve the measurement of schooling outcomes. Most previous studies limited their outcome measures to achievement tests of basic skills, often to tests of reading and arithmetic. Few studies employed measures pertaining to the social, personal, and vocational goals of schooling. Many educators have argued that the multiple-choice tests that are commonly used in school effectiveness studies emphasize lower order skills that are isolated from a wider context. These critics have called for more "authentic" forms of assessment based on longer term accomplishments (Wolf et al. 1991). These include, for example, in-depth projects, journals, portfolios, recitals, debates, and oral presentations. The challenge for researchers is to collect data that are more directly related to what is taught and learned in school. These data will inevitably be more expensive to collect, and therefore researchers require designs that are powerful even with small samples of pupils and schools.

2. Promising Approaches to Design

Another major threat to the validity of studies of school effectiveness is selection bias. Selection bias occurs when schools differ in their intakes, such that estimates of the effects of attendance at particular schools are biased by differences in the background and aptitude of the pupils entering the schools. Also, estimates of the effects of particular policies or practices are affected by differences among schools in their intakes (Raudenbush and Willms 1995).

2.1 True Experiments

The best method of controlling for differences among groups is to randomly assign pupils to schools, and schools to treatment conditions. However, "true" experiments of the effects of educational policies and practices are the exception, not the norm. Often political considerations override the desire for valid and reliable assessment. In some settings, though, researchers have been able to conduct true experiments. A notable example in the United States is the Tennessee study of the effects of class size on primary school pupils' achievement, self-concept, and academic motivation (Finn and Achilles 1990). The researchers randomly assigned pupils to one of three types of classes: small (13–17 pupils), regular (22–25 pupils), and regular with a teacher aide. Teachers were also randomly assigned to three class types. Their design ensured that teacher and school effects were not confounded with the effects of class size. Test results at the end of the first grade indicated large and statistically significant effects of class size on achievement. Moreover, the design was powerful enough to detect differences in the class size effect for minority and White pupils.

2.2 Longitudinal Designs with Repeated Measures on Pupils

Without random assignment, researchers can address the problem of selection bias by collecting data on pupils' ability and family background, and making a statistical adjustment for schooling intake. There are several adjustment techniques (Anderson et al. 1980); regression techniques, particularly analysis of covariance, are most common. Researchers have shown that measures of family socioeconomic status (e.g., prestige of parents' occupation, levels of parental education, family income) are by themselves insufficient; measures of pupils' academic achievement or general ability upon entry to school are also necessary. Cross-sectional data tend to yield biased estimates of the effects of schools (Willms 1992). The necessity for longitudinal data that include a premeasure of ability or achievement suggests that most of the earlier studies of school effectiveness produced biased findings. It also implies that many of the comparisons made among schools, districts, or states using cross-sectional data on school performance are misleading and invalid.

In making a statistical adjustment for prior achievement or ability, researchers are attempting to ask whether schools differ in the *rate* at which pupils acquire knowledge and skills, and whether differences among schools are attributable to policy and practice. A more direct way of examining learning rates is to collect data on the same set of pupils on at least three occasions (Bryk and Raudenbush 1987, Willett 1988). With this design, pupils are tested with the same test, or with a parallel form of the test, on each occasion. Alternatively, the researcher can use a set of vertically equated tests which map scores onto a long continuous scale covering several years of schooling.

Designs that provide estimates of individual growth rates have several advantages over cross-sectional or two-time point designs. For example, Bryk and Raudenbush (1988) examined the rate of pupil growth in reading and mathematics from grades one to three for a sample of over 600 pupils in the Sustaining Effects Study. Their research showed that the variation among schools in their pupils' growth rates was considerably larger than in pupils' status at a particular grade level. With a similar design, Willms and Jacobsen (1990) examined pupils' growth in three separate domains of mathematics skills between grades four and seven. The work showed that males and females varied in their patterns of growth in each domain, even though average differences between the sexes were small. Variation in growth rates was related to pupils' age at entry to primary school, their cognitive ability, and the school they attended. Both studies suggested that researchers' attempts to uncover the effects of school policies and practices are more likely to meet with success if they have longitudinal data covering three or four years.

2.3 Longitudinal Designs with Repeated Measures on Schools

Another way of strengthening the quasi-experimental design is to use data describing schooling inputs, processes, and outcomes for successive cohorts of pupils attending the same set of schools. The aim of the design is to determine whether changes in school performance are associated with changes in school policy and practice. The longitudinal design is stronger because each school essentially serves as its own control.

Schools vary in their performance from year to year for a number of reasons. Some of the variation is due to changes in school organization, and to changes in the involvement and effort of school staff. But some of the variation is due to changes in the social and economic conditions of the wider community, or due to measurement error or random fluctuations associated with the interests and abilities of particular cohorts of pupils. In earlier work, the authors set out a design for separating variation due to policy and practice from other sources of variation (Willms and Raudenbush 1989). The design provided estimates of each school's effect on each occasion, and its long-term average effect. It also provided estimates of the effects of policies and practices on changes in school performance. This design was applied to data describing pupils' attainment in one Scottish education authority's secondary schools. The results suggested that the authority's effort to reduce differences among schools in their mean SES resulted in smaller variation among schools in their performance.

3. Multilevel Analysis

The policies and practices that affect schooling outcomes are implemented in organizational settings (e.g., classrooms and schools) which are nested within a hierarchical structure (e.g., school districts or educational authorities). Moreover, the actions of educators and policymakers at one level of the system affect processes at other levels. Researchers have long debated whether the pupil, classroom, or school was the correct unit of analysis for assessing school effects. Most analyses ignored the hierarchical structure of educational data. However, advances in statistics and computing have provided appropriate multilevel statistical methods for analyzing hierarchical data (Aitkin and Longford 1986, Goldstein 1995, Raudenbush and Bryk 1986).

The new statistical and methodological techniques have generated another wave of school effectiveness studies (Raudenbush and Willms 1991). The work has been directed at answering four principal questions, set out by Willms (1992 p. 178): (a) To what extent do schools vary in their outcomes? (b) To what extent do outcomes vary for pupils of differing status? (c) What school policies and practices improve levels of schooling outcomes? (d) What school policies and practices reduce inequalities in outcomes between high- and low-status groups?

The same set of questions can be asked of other organizational units, such as the school district or classroom. The first two questions concern *quality* and *equity.* They require only descriptive techniques; however, they are often extended to ask how much schools vary after adjusting for pupils' family background. The last two questions concern the *causes* of quality and equity.

The underlying logic of multilevel models is that data at one level (e.g., pupils) are fit to a regression model within each of a number of second-level units (e.g., schools). Parameter estimates for the first-level regressions then become dependent variables in second-level regressions fit to data describing the second-level units. The estimation technique combines the regression models for both levels into a single multilevel model, and estimates the parameters simultaneously.

Lockheed and Longford's (1991) study of primary school effectiveness in Thailand provides an example of the basic two-level model. They employed data from the International Association for the Evaluation of Educational Achievement's Second International Math Study, which covered over 4,000 pupils. At the first level they regressed pupils' mathematics scores on a number of pupil-level background variables (mathematics pretest, age, sex, father's occupation, mother's education, and a number of attitudinal variables). The pretest was the most important control variable. Before entering any school-level variables, they addressed the first two questions above. The multilevel model provided estimates of the extent to which background-adjusted school means vary across schools, and the extent to which outcome/pretest regression slopes vary across schools. The background-adjusted means are an indicator of quality: they are the expected score for pupils with average initial achievement and average background. The slopes are an indicator of equity: they show whether schools exaggerate or reduce initial differences in achievement. Lockheed and Longford (1991) found that the schools varied significantly in their background-adjusted means: the highest background-adjusted means were about eight points higher than the lowest adjusted means (standard deviation=2.224) for a test that had a pupil-level standard deviation of about nine points. However, the researchers did not find significant differences among schools in their outcome/pretest slopes.

Variables describing a number of school-level characteristics were then added to the model in an attempt to explain the significant variation among background-adjusted school means. These included a number of variables describing the school setting (e.g., school size, student–teacher ratio, staff qualifications), and process variables describing school organization (e.g., whether the school practiced ability grouping, the time teachers spent on administration) and teacher practices (e.g., time spent on maintaining order, time on seatwork, use of materials). Their model accounted for nearly all of the among-school variation. The most important explanatory variables were the proportion of teachers who were qualified to teach mathematics, whether teachers used an enriched curriculum, and the frequent use of textbooks as opposed to workbooks.

Three-level models can also be constructed to describe effects at three levels, such as pupil-, classroom-, and school-level effects. Moreover, multilevel models can be used to depict pupils' rates of growth, or changes in school performance over time. The combination of longitudinal designs with multilevel techniques could provide a powerful means of overcoming some of the methodological problems associated with the study of schooling.

4. Interpretation

Many of the studies of school effectiveness have found statistically significant effects of certain school factors, but they have not specified the magnitude of the effects. To facilitate interpretation, it is useful to report results both as standardized "effect sizes" (Hedges and Olkin 1985), and in unadjusted units of the outcome variable. The same applies to estimates of the differences among schools or school districts in their outcomes.

5. Conclusions

Most of the research on school effectiveness has been based on quasi-experimental or correlational designs. Therefore, the validity of causal statements about relationships between schooling processes and outcomes has been easily challenged—usually there are a number of rival hypotheses. Measurement problems and selection bias have been endemic. However, the new approaches to examining questions about school effectiveness provide a stronger basis for making causal inferences.

Progress in this area will come first through the development of stronger theories about how processes at each level of the system affect processes and outcomes at other levels. The testing of these theories will require thicker data than have been typically available in large national studies. Recent studies describing school culture and climate have already contributed to our understanding of what constitutes an effective school.

Researchers now have available some powerful methods for the analysis of educational data. These methods enable researchers to study the rate at which pupils acquire skills and knowledge, and to determine the extent to which changes in school performance are related to changes in school policies and practices. The techniques also provide a systematic way to test whether schools differ in their performance, and whether they have differential effects for pupils with differing status.

References

Aitkin M, Longford N 1986 Statistical modelling issues in school effectiveness studies. *Journal of the Royal Statistical Society* A 149(1): 1–26

Anderson C S 1982 The search for school climate: A review of the research. *Rev. Educ. Res.* 52(3): 368–420

Anderson et al. 1980 *Statistical Methods for Comparative Studies: Techniques for Bias Reduction* Wiley, New York

Barr R, Dreeben R 1983 *How Schools Work.* University of Chicago Press, Chicago, Illinois

Boyd W L 1983 What school administrators do and don't do: Implications for effective schools. *The Canadian Administrator* 22(6): 1–4

Bridge R G, Judd C M, Moock P R 1979 *The Determinants of Educational Outcomes: The Impacts of Families, Peers, Teachers, and Schools.* Ballinger, Cambridge, Massachusetts

Bryk A S, Raudenbush S W 1987 Application of hierarchical linear models to assessing change. *Psych. Bull.* 101(1): 147–58

Bryk A S, Raudenbush S W 1988 Toward a more appropriate conceptualization of research on school effects: A three-level linear model. *Am. J. Educ.* 97(1): 65–108

Cook T D, Campbell D T 1979 *Quasi-experimentation: Design and Analysis issues for Field Settings.* Rand McNally, Chicago, Illinois

Finn J D, Achilles C M 1990 Answers and questions about class size: A statewide experiment. *Am. Educ. Res. J.* 27(3): 557–77

Goldstein H 1995 *Multilevel Statistical Models*, 2nd edn. Arnold, London

Gray J 1989 Multilevel models: Issues and problems emerging from their recent application in British studies of school effectiveness. In: Bock D R (ed.) 1989 *Multilevel Analyses of Educational Data.* Academic Press, San Diego, California

Hedges L V, Olkin I 1985 *Statistical Methods for Meta-analysis.* Academic Press, San Diego, California

Lee V E, Bryk A S 1989. A multilevel model of the social distribution of high school achievement. *Sociol. Educ.* 62(3): 172–92

Lockheed M E, Longford N T 1991 School effects on mathematics achievement gain in Thailand. In: Raudenbush S W, Willms J D (eds.) 1991 *Schools, Classrooms, and Pupils: International Studies of Schooling from a Multilevel Perspective.* Academic Press, San Diego, California

McKnight C C et al. 1987 *The Underachieving Curriculum: Assessing U.S. School Mathematics from an International Perspective.* Stipes, Champaign, Illinois

Meyer J W 1980 Levels of the educational system and schooling effects. In: Bidwell C, Windham D (eds.) 1980 *The Analysis of Educational Productivity*, Vol. 2. Ballinger, Cambridge, Massachusetts

Plewis I 1991 Using multilevel models to link educational progress with curriculum coverage. In: Raudenbush S W, Willms J D (eds.) 1991 *Schools, Classrooms, and Pupils: International Studies of Schooling from a Multilevel Perspective.* Academic Press, San Diego, California

Raudenbush S W, Bryk A S 1986 A hierarchical model for studying school effects. *Sociol. Educ.* 59(1): 1–17

Raudenbush S W, Willms J D 1991 The organization of schooling and its methodological implications. In: Raudenbush S W, Willms J D (eds.) 1991 *Schools, Classrooms, and Pupils: International Studies of Schooling from a Multilevel Perspective.* Academic Press, San Diego, California

Raudenbush S W, Willms J D 1995 The estimation of school effects. *J. Educ. and Behavioral Statistics* 20(4): 307–35

Rosenholtz S J 1989 Workplace conditions that affect teacher quality and commitment: Implications for teacher induction programs. *Elem. Sch. J.* 89(4): 421–39

Willett J B 1988 Questions and answers in the measurement of change. In: Rothkopf E Z (ed.) 1988 *Review of Research in Education*, Vol. 15. American Educational Research Association, Washington, DC

Willms J D 1986 Social class segregation and its relationship to pupils' examination results in Scotland. *Am. Sociol. Rev.* 51(2): 224–41

Willms J D 1992 *Monitoring School Performance: A Guide for Educators.* Falmer Press, Lewes

Willms J D, Jacobsen S 1990 Growth in mathematics skills during the intermediate years: Sex differences and school effects. *Int. J. Educ. Res.* 14(2): 157–74

Willms J D, Raudenbush S W 1989 A longitudinal hierarchical linear model for estimating school effects and their stability. *J. Educ. Meas.* 26(3): 209–32

Wolf D, Bixby J, Glenn J III, Gardner H 1991 To use their minds well: Investigating new forms of student assessment. In: Grant G (ed.) 1991 *Review of Research in Education*, Vol. 17. American Educational Research Association, Washington, DC

Interviewing for Survey Research

P. V. Miller and C. F. Cannell

A sample survey is a measurement technique. It consists of a set of interrelated components, each of which is important for the achievement of measurement objectives, and includes conceptualization of the research problem, sample design, questionnaire construction, interviewing, coding, data processing, and analysis. Random and nonrandom errors can intrude on the measurement process at any of these stages. This article focuses on procedures for reducing error in two important survey phases—questionnaire construction and interviewing.

The fact that much is learnt in everyday life by asking people questions leads to the conclusion that framing questions and asking them in surveys are

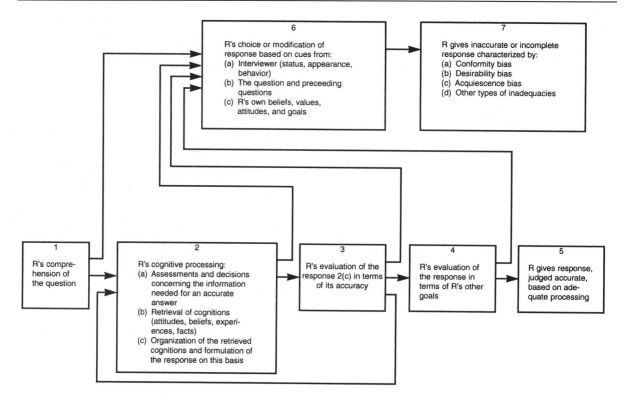

Figure 1
Diagram of the respondent's (R's) question-answering process[a]
a. Source: Cannell et al. 1981 p. 393

simple tasks. Certainly, the gift of language permits information to be gathered from fellow humans by asking questions in surveys, and it is conceivable to believe that their answers reflect the actual conditions of their lives. At the same time, the vagaries of experience and language and the peculiar characteristics of formal interview "conversations" refute the idea of unproblematic data gathering. Writing questions and conducting survey interviews present truly complex problems. The following model of the question-answering process illustrates the issues involved in communication in the interview.

1. Model of the Response Process

The objective of questionnaire construction and interviewing can be seen largely as the creation of "shared meaning" between respondent and interviewer. Simply put, respondents will give accurate information in survey interviews if they are able and willing to do so. Data collection procedures should be designed to increase respondents' ability to meet response objectives and to increase their willingness to expend the necessary effort for response tasks. This can be accomplished by explicit and precise com-

munication of question objectives and of the process which respondents should undertake in formulating their responses.

To exemplify, consider the diagram of the response process in Fig. 1 which begins with comprehending the question (step 1). Comprehension includes issues of vocabulary level, clarity of concept, complexity of sentence structure, and other familiar issues of question wording. In this article, however, the interest lies in broader issues of question interpretation: the respondent's orientation in contemplating a question. When more than one plausible interpretation exists, the respondent needs to consider the various possibilities and must often think up and answer an internal questionnaire to help decide which interpretation to accept. Take, for example, the question: "How many times have you talked to a doctor about your health during the past month?" The respondent may wonder whether to include telephone consultation, whether visits to chiropractors should be included, whether immunizations are part of health, or whether "past month" refers to the past four weeks or to a calendar month. Whether or not the respondent goes through this process explicitly, he or she must proceed on the basis of assumptions concerning the intended meaning of the question.

Step 2 is the stage of information processing that includes the respondent's assessment of what information he or she needs in order to respond accurately and what cues or frames of reference are relevant. Usually this stage involves searching the memory for relevant information and organizing the material to formulate a response.

For step 3 the respondent must evaluate whether the formulated response fulfills the objectives of the question. If the potential response is judged inadequate, the respondent loops back to repeat some or all of the preceding activities (step 2).

At step 4, a second kind of evaluation occurs as the respondent evaluates the psychological meaning of the response in relation to personal goals extraneous to the survey. Some respondents, however well-intentioned, will probably evaluate an intended answer in terms of its potential threat to their personal goals—for instance, self-esteem—in addition to the goal of giving accurate responses. If the potential response is evaluated as non-threatening, the respondent states the response (step 5).

This brief description of the question-answering process, when it is proceeding ideally, illustrates the demands placed on respondents and the potential complexity of responding to questions. Carrying out this process can be difficult, especially when the question requires considerable effort to produce an accurate response as embarrassing or otherwise personally uncomfortable. Undoubtedly, there are respondents who accept this task only provisionally; they will attempt to produce accurate responses as long as this does not require much effort on their part and does not embarrass them.

Figure 1 also suggests ways in which the responding process may go awry. While the ideal respondent follows steps 1 through 4 and eventually produces an adequate response (step 5), at any step he or she may deviate to other response modes (step 6) and produce a response (step 7) that is, to some degree, inadequate.

For the respondent who has not understood the question or is not sufficiently skilled or motivated to go through the retrieval and organizational processes, the extraneous situational cues suggested in step 6 are more likely to be the basis for response selection. Even respondents who proceed adequately through step 3 (that is, who formulate a response they judge to be adequate) will undoubtedly evaluate the response further to determine whether it threatens or is incompatible with some other personal goal (step 4). If a threat emerges at this step, the respondent may deviate (steps 6 and 7) and modify his or her potential response or substitute another.

Once the respondent departs from the appropriate answering process (steps 1 to 5) and relies on other situational cues (steps 6 and 7), the response will exhibit some kind of invalidity (step 7). Researchers have labeled the effects on responses of such situational

cues as social desirability bias, acquiescence bias, and the like. It is sometimes argued that these biases result from the respondent's personality characteristics—such as an "acquiescence trait," a "social desirability trait," or a need for approval—but it must be assumed that the response process is most likely to be shaped by situational cues in the interview itself: from the interviewer, the questionnaire, or the organization for which the research is being conducted. While it may be possible to differentiate people by their willingness to agree to give a socially appropriate response, for the purposes of this article agreeing responses and socially desirable responses are best understood in terms of their perceived appropriateness in the immediate interview situation.

Cognitive and motivational difficulties in answering questions are more common and more serious than is generally realized. Questions are often ambiguous in ways that can have important implications for interpreting research data. Questions may make excessive demands on the cognitive skills of respondents by making unrealistic demands on the respondent's memory or ability to process and integrate retrieved information. Finally, the psychological implication of providing responses that truly reflect the respondent's beliefs or experience may lead to suppressing the information or distorting it into a more acceptable response.

The mechanisms of the responses when adequate processing fails are identified in step 7. Their effect is to distort survey data. That is, the reported information varies from truth in some predictable direction. Perhaps the most common distortion is a failure to report information—that is, making "false negative" reports—because of a failure of retrieval and processing (step 2), which may reflect true memory lapse or carelessness and unwillingness to make the effort necessary to retrieve the information. This form of inadequate response is probably the most frequent in report of past events and behavior.

Another common distortion involves making "false positive" reports—that is, falsely reporting events, behavior, or other information. This distortion may occur frequently when a time reference is specified in the question. For example, in answering a question about events occurring within the past month, the respondent may report things that occurred before that month. Such false reports may reflect faulty recall or may be more purposeful. (The respondent may falsely report information that seems to reflect to his or her credit, for example, or seems to meet some other goal.)

Response problems associated with one or another of these stages have been the focus of a number of methodological studies. For example, consider the problem of the respondent's comprehension of the question (box 1 in Fig. 1). In an investigation of the accuracy with which medical data are reported, the following question was asked: "Last week or the week before, did anyone in the family talk to a doctor or go to a doctor's office or clinic?" The question was intended not only to include routine office visits, but also telephone calls for medical advice and visits for inoculations or other treatments given by a nurse or technician in a doctor's office, and calls and visits by any member of the family whether on his or her behalf or for another. The mother's call to ask the doctor about her child was to be included, whether or not the child was present. From the researcher's viewpoint this single question included all these situations, and an analysis of the words supports the claim in a literal sense. The respondents' frame of reference, however, often produced very different interpretations. Many understood the question to include only personal visits, and then only when the physician was seen. The subsequent inclusion of probe questions asking specifically about these other events resulted in a sizable increase in the number of calls and visits reported (Cannell and Fowler 1965).

Similar problems occur in other content areas, when the researcher fails to take account of the respondent's frame of reference Mauldin and Marks (1950) described efforts to obtain accurate data on education level. For many years the Bureau of the Census interviewers asked the education question in this form: "What is the highest grade of school you have completed?" Interpreted literally, this question should offer no difficulty for the vast majority of people. However, many people heard the phrase "highest grade of school" and immediately thought in terms of the highest grade of the school they "went to." Some people did not even hear the final word in the question, that is, the word "completed." When interviewers obtained answers to the above question and then said, "Did you complete that grade?" a substantial number of respondents answered "No."

In the same study the authors told of asking farmers whether they had any fruit or nut trees or grapevines. Those who answered that they did not were then asked if they had even one or two trees or vines, or whether they had any not now producing fruit. To those probe questions over half the farmers who originally said they had no trees or vines now said that they did. Mauldin and Marks concluded that the farmers took it for granted the census enumerators would not be interested in one or two trees, especially if they were not producing, and were trying to be helpful rather than deceptive.

Bancroft and Welch (1946) showed that respondents answer questions about their labor force status in terms of what they consider to be their major activity, rather than in terms of the actual wording of the question. Even if they were working part time, people who considered themselves primarily students or housewives answered "No" to the question, "Did you do any work last week for pay or profit?" A substantial improvement in the validity of employment estimates was attained by accepting the respondents' frame of reference and building a sequence of questions which first asked for their major activity and then asked students and housewives whether they were also doing any paid work.

These illustrate common comprehension problems for survey respondents. Other investigations demonstrate cognitive processing difficulties in answering survey questions (boxes 2 and 3 in Fig. 1), and offer these generalizations: (a) as the time between the event being investigated and the interview increases, reporting of the event becomes worse; (b) events which are psychologically unimportant to respondents are poorly reported.

The problem caused by time lapse between the event and the interview is exemplified in a study of reported visits to physicians. Failure to report the visit increased over a two-week period from 15 percent in interviews one week after the visit to 30 percent in interviews two weeks after (Cannell and Fowler 1963). Similarly, invalid reporting of hospitalizations increases as the time between the event and the interview increases, from 3 percent for events within 10 weeks of the interview to over 20 percent for episodes which occurred nearly a year prior. Other studies have shown similar findings for reporting of personal finances, household repairs, and household appliance purchases.

The psychological importance (or salience) of the event, as indexed in these studies by the gravity of the illness or the costliness of household goods and repairs, appears to have a marked effect on reporting accuracy, that is, hospitalizations which involved longer stays for respondents were better reported, as were episodes involving surgery (Cannell and Fowler 1963). Major household repairs and purchases were also more apt to be reported than less costly ones.

An adequate job of information retrieval from memory requires effort from the respondent, but many survey tasks ask for greater effort than respondents may be willing to make. Response errors often appear to be the result of the failure of cognitive processing outlined in boxes 2 and 3 of Fig. 1.

Boxes 4 and 5 signal a different reporting problem. Methodologists agree that the respondents' motivation or willingness to report is the most important issue in accuracy of interview data, and that the content of the material sought has a major effect on respondent motivation. The data from methodological research can be interpreted as a postulated need on the respondent's part to maintain self-esteem, to be perceived by the interviewer as a person who does not violate important social norms in thought or act, and to present an image of consistency and worthiness.

Clark and Wallin (1964) describe an example of response bias stemming from a different respondent need. They compared the individual reporting of husbands and wives on the frequency of sexual intercourse and found that the agreement was close for partners who expressed satisfaction with their sexual relations.

Those who expressed dissatisfaction showed a greater discrepancy in report. Those who wanted more frequent sexual contacts tended also to report a lower frequency of marital coitus.

Conversely, voting or being registered to vote was found in several studies to be overreported (Bradburn et al. 1979). Wenar (1963) reported that mothers distort facts of their children's developmental history, and that they do so in ways that make the children appear precocious. Similarly, the reports of mothers regarding their own child-training practices tend to conform more closely to the advice of pediatricians than is justified by data from other sources.

These examples highlight the problem of question threat in survey reporting. As shown in boxes 4 and 5, respondents will often evaluate their answers according to the criterion of whether an answer will make them "look good." Reporting embarrassing events or properties presents considerable difficulty for many respondents, and not being able to report normatively valued characteristics can also cause some psychological discomfort. Therefore, respondents are often apt to censor response intentions which do not meet their preceived standards of social propriety.

2. Some Principles of Question Design and Interviewing

From a model of the question-answering process and data on response errors illustrating how responses can bo awry, the practical implications of these observations from survey practice can now be considered.

2.1 Question Design

The elemental unit of a survey interview is the question. Over the years there has been a good deal of writing on question design, and some general principles have been enunciated (Payne 1951, Kahn and Cannell 1957, Warwick and Lininger 1975). More recently, Schuman and Presser (1981) report experiments on the effects of various question formats. (The various "rules" or folklore of question wording and structure will not be discussed here; they can be found in the sources mentioned above.) The more abstract principles of relating question design to the response process will be discussed.

Survey respondents may be seen as administering an "internal" questionnaire to themselves in order to arrive at a response to a survey question (see Fig. 1). They must decide what sorts of information and experiences are relevant to answering the question and must consider how to organize this material for presentation to the interviewer. They must decide how much effort to put into this process in order to arrive at an adequate answer.

In the ideal case, the survey question should provide the structure needed for the respondent to answer his or her own internal questionnaire. Each question should be specific enough to allow respondents to review thoroughly their own relevant experience and to arrive at an accurate and complete response.

Additionally, the question should communicate some rules about the process of question answering. For example, to find out whether respondents have been the victims of crime in the recent past, it is necessary to ask specifically about the range of incidents which are classified as "crimes" in the survey. If the question were "Have you been a victim of crime in the last six months?" the respondents' "internal questionnaire" would be very complex indeed. They will have to decide what "crime" is, and what it means to be a "victim." Each respondent will use his or her own definition, and what is included in an answer to the question will vary markedly from one respondent to another. Specific cues will help respondents share a common concept and definition. For example, respondents might be asked if they have had things stolen from their mailboxes, whether someone cheated them in a business deal, or whether their automobiles were vandalized. Each specific question, in turn, can be further refined. Respondents could be directed to think about particular kinds of goods which might be stolen or damaged. Specifically, researchers might want crime questions to inform respondents they should mention even incidents which may seem trivial to them. The importance can be stressed of reporting embarrassing or painful events. Each of these cues can help to reduce the complexities of the respondent's "internal questionnaire," and come closer to a shared definition between the interviewer and the respondent.

Questions also can communicate a suggested process for respondents to use in reviewing their experience for relevant material, and for evaluating the adequacy of their intended response. Queries can be prefaced with suggestions that respondents take their time and think carefully before answering or, alternatively, that their first general impressions are all that is required. An exact number can be requested or respondents can be asked to tell in detail about their feelings on a particular issue. These messages about the process of response are intended to answer the questions which people ask themselves when they try to respond to survey items.

In summary, the ideal survey question should clearly communicate a single and common objective for information retrieval. It should also inform respondents on how to produce a response—how much and what kind of effort to invest in answering. Naturally, every questionnaire compromises on the number of questions which can be devoted to a single variable since employing detailed and specific questioning inevitably lengthens the total questionnaire and increases survey cost. The researcher must construct the scope of the survey so that the areas explored can be investigated thoroughly.

3. Interviewing

The process of interviewing—whether face-to-face or over the telephone—involves issues related to question design. Ideally, the information requested in the question would spring from the respondent's psyche directly to the computer input. But since the data collection process has an intervening interviewer, the effects of interpersonal relationship between interviewer and respondent must be a concern. Some rather different models of the interview are described which seek to control "interviewer effects" on responses.

3.1 Rapport

A common belief among survey researchers is that in order to obtain valid information the interviewer must gain the trust (and perhaps affection) of the respondent. Despite much lip-service paid to this concept (termed "rapport"), it is not entirely clear what is meant. However, the manifestations of rapport seeking in interviewer behavior can be identified. Using a clinical approach to interviewing, the survey interviewer seeks to establish rapport and takes a friendly, empathic attitude, he or she is nondirecting—giving the respondent no cues about "correct" answers—and certainly does not express his or her own opinions. A combination of the nondirective approach and a friendly attitude is supposed to decrease response error by relieving the respondent of the pressure to maintain a totally positive self-presentation and by motivating the respondent to reveal him/herself accurately.

The problem is that the neutral or nondirective interviewer style frequently does not sufficiently motivate or inform respondents. A survey interview is a rare experience for most people, and they need guidance to appropriate response behavior. Cues to the respondent for deciding when an adequate response has been rendered are obscure, and they are likely to remain so if the interviewer conforms to the simple rules of being nondirective and friendly. In many studies, respondents may be ignorant of the most simple facts— the purpose of the investigation and the auspices under which the survey is conducted. Following their participation in a National Health Survey interview (Cannell et al. 1968) 45 percent (of 412 respondents) said they did not know what agency was doing the survey or the agency for which it was done; although each respondent had been informed that the survey was being conducted for the United States Public Health Service by the Bureau of the Census: only 11 percent identified the Census Bureau. Other identifications were even more vague—"some government agency," "a state agency." When asked why they thought the information was being collected, more than half said they had no idea. Of those who did report something, most responses were quite general—"for statistical purposes."

The study also examined respondents' perceptions of the interviewers' expectations and goals. Although the questionnaire had been set up to obtain specific and complete reports on specific health conditions (illnesses, days of disability, medication taken, chronic conditions) and health events (physician visits and hospitalizations), only about one-half of the respondents thought the interviewer wanted a detailed report; the rest thought that general ideas were adequate. Three-quarters of the respondents thought the interviewer wanted a report of everything; the rest thought only the important things were to be mentioned. These findings suggest that respondents do not know what is expected of them. They understand neither the general goals of the survey nor what they are supposed to do on a particular question. Apparently "rapport" itself is not sufficient for achieving good interview communication. Moreover, since rapport seeking is an ad hoc procedure, there is considerable variance among interviewers in their approaches to the interview and this introduces error into the data-collection process.

4. Task Orientation and Standardization

A newer model of the interview has been developed which stresses teaching respondents to perform response tasks adequately and motivating them to undertake the effort to answer accurately. More effort also has been spent in attempting to standardize interviewer behavior. While these approaches do not deny the importance of gaining the respondent's cooperation on an affective level, they place considerably more emphasis on "taking care of business" in the interview. They entail a more active role on the part of the study director to specify interviewer behavior. As in question writing, according to this model the investigator must design interview techniques which are scripted in the questionnaire and administered in a standardized manner by all interviewers. As discussed above, such efforts are based on the premise that to achieve accurate measurement, a clear, standard communication environment must be established for the respondent. The specific techniques involved in this approach are elaborated below in discussing commitment, instructions, and feedback.

4.1 Components of Interviewing

The four main components of the interviewer's job are: (a) to introduce the interview to the person and convince him/her to accept it and to apply him/herself diligently to the responding role, (b) to administer the questions using standardized procedures, (c) to follow up those responses which are inadequate—those which fail to fulfill the objectives of the question—using acceptable, nonbiasing techniques, and (d) to record the response accurately and completely. These require the following techniques.

(a) *Introductions.* The purposes of the introduction are to encourage the prospective respondent to agree to be interviewed and to accept the respondent role wholeheartedly. Essentially this means the interview must be perceived as worthwhile, the interviewer as legitimate, and the undertaking as sufficiently valuable to make an effort to respond diligently.

First the interviewer identifies himself or herself, the research agency or university from which he or she comes, and the general topic of the research. He or she explains something of the method by which respondents have been selected and a reference to the amount of time required. How the introduction should be elaborated will depend upon the expressed needs of the respondent or the interviewer's hunches about them, and upon the interviewer's knowledge of the nature and the demands of the interview which is to come. The introduction and any early enlargements on it should make the rest of the interview plausible.

The legitimacy of the research is established by official documents, letters on appropriate stationery, use of the university name, and the like. The interviewer should be able to refer the respondent to a telephone number at which confirming information can be obtained. Sending advance letters or using mass media to announce large-scale data collection is helpful and is increasingly common. The interviewer should be prepared to be explicit as to the uses of the data, the sponsoring agencies, and the kinds of reports to be issued. Reports of similar studies, journal articles, or books can be shown as useful and reassuring evidence of good faith. It is important to disassociate the interview from nonresearch contexts encountered by respondents. Bill collectors and credit investigators ask questions as do welfare officers, police officers, and a whole array of civil servants and private employees, and all are perceived differently by people of different socioeconomic classes. Usually the respondent wants only the assurance that he/she is not being sought for some special and personal reason; a brief description of random and anonymous selection is enough. But, the interviewer should be able to offer an accurate and non-technical account of the sampling process if necessary.

Some studies follow the introduction with a commitment procedure which is often a signed agreement by respondents that they will make an effort to respond carefully and accurately. This shows evidence of improving response quality (Cannell et al. 1981).

(b) *Administering the questionnaire.* Questions often are accompanied by instructions providing cues on the exact kind of information desired and how to be efficient in responding. Including instructions in the questionnaire helps to standardize techniques and is more effective in getting valid reporting than ad hoc instructions or cues devised by the interviewer. Thus, the survey instrument becomes not simply a series of questions but a programmed measurement device including the questions, instructions, and probes. Questions are to be asked exactly as written and, if misunderstood, to be repeated without change. Clarifications or explanations are to be used only when specifically permitted.

(c) *Follow-up of inadequate responses.* If the respondent has performed his or her role properly, the interviewer's task is simply to record the response. At times, however, even after use of probes incorporated into the questionnaire, the response is in some way inadequate. It may be incomplete, irrelevant to the objective, or unintelligible. The interviewer needs techniques which will stimulate further response activity or redirect the communication into relevant channels. Such techniques, designed to accomplish this without influencing the content of the response, are referred to as "nondirective" probes. To request further information they might be: "How do you mean?" "Is there anything else?" "Please tell me more about that." To request specific details, they may include: "Why do you think that is so?" or "When was that?" Training manuals can specify lists of acceptable nondirective probes (Survey Research Center *Interviewer's Manual*, rev. edn. 1976).

Probes (both those incorporated into the question design and those used at the option of the interviewer) are intended to steer the communication and also to motivate respondents to reply adequately. Feedback can both teach respondents what is expected of them and motivate them in task performance. Feedback is used naturally in social communication and serves to inform the other person that the message is being received, attended to, and accepted. Both verbal and nonverbal communication is used in face-to-face interviews; nonverbal is of course absent in telephone interviews. As used in teaching, feedback provides an evaluation to the learner of his/her performance and as reinforcement it rewards good performance and tends to motivate behavior. Feedback may be a simple statement of understanding and interest: "I see, Um-hmm." "I understand." Or it may be more positive in evaluation: "Thanks, that's the kind of information we need." "That will help us in this research." "That's useful." Because of these evaluative and reinforcing properties, feedback can be effective in improving reporting performance. If improperly used, however, respondents will either not learn or will learn the wrong lessons. Consider the following exchange:

Q: How often do you get a dental check-up?
R: Every six months.
Feedback: That's good.

"That's good" is likely to be interpreted as approving of the answer content rather than to give positive support to adequate response behavior. Such misinterpretation by the respondent makes it ineffective in teaching acceptable behavior and may lead to response bias. Therefore, feedback statements must focus on reinforcing hard work by respondents and must avoid expressing approval of the particular response. As survey researchers become more aware of the power and dangers of feedback, they are beginning to include major feedback statements in the questionnaire. They also focus attention on acceptable and unacceptable feedback during interviewer training.

(d) *Recording responses.* Accurate recording of the response is the last component of the interviewing task. For closed questions this usually consists simply of checking the appropriate response category or recording the reply if no box can be checked. The task is more demanding for open questions. This requires recording the respondent's own words and a complete description of the response. Paraphrasing is usually unacceptable since it may miss significant segments—perhaps those of interest to the researcher. Experienced interviewers find that responses can be recorded during the course of the conversation with only minor editing required after the interview. The record should also include any spontaneous probes used by the interviewer, extraneous conversation which occurs during the interview, comments by respondents on questions, and observations about respondents' difficulty in answering questions. All of this information can be coded and used to contextualize the responses to questions in the interview.

4.2 Training and Selection

Research directed at reducing response errors has not been matched with research on procedures to select interviewers or effective techniques for training, supervising, and administering interviews. For example, there are few objective criteria or procedures for selecting competent interviewers. While some selection measures have been tried experimentally, none have demonstrated significant relationships to successful interviewing. Those which are used focus largely on the clerical nature of the interview task. Those studies which have been conducted suggest that interviewing skills can be communicated to a large proportion of the population and that the emphasis needs to be on training rather than on selection of the ideal interviewer types.

This is not to suggest that an interviewer will be equally successful in communicating with all respondents or that all interviewers will attain optimal interviewing skills. Respondent and interviewer differences in age, voice, sex, socioeconomic or cultural background may interfere with accurate reporting when the demographic characteristic is related to the subject of the survey (e.g. when a white interviewer interviews a black respondent about racial attitudes; Schuman and Converse 1971).

The major source of variability in interviewers is, however, probably not in their selection but in variations in techniques from interviewer to interviewer. While there is no training program which is accepted by all survey practitioners, here are some general principles: (a) new interviewers should be provided with the principles of measurement; they should be given

an intellectual grasp of the data-collecting function and a basis for evaluating interviewing behavior; (b) they should be taught the techniques of interviewing; (c) they should be provided with the opportunity for practice and evaluation by actually conducting interviews under controlled conditions; (d) they should be offered careful evaluation of interviews, especially at the beginning of actual data collection. Such evaluation should include review of interview protocols.

Steps (a) and (b) are intended to provide the interviewers with a concept of the goals of interviewing, including the principles of measurement and the exposition of techniques which meet these criteria. Most of the time and attention in training is spent on steps (c) and (d). The assumption underlying technique training is that while it is important to communicate the goals and principles of the research, most of the time needs to be spent in developing the appropriate skills. Simply reading an essay about how to interview will not produce a skilled interviewer. Effective instructional materials must actively involve the trainee in the learning process. The nature of the task dictates the nature of the instruction. Interviewing requires listening, speaking, reading, and writing skills. Therefore, training must incorporate all these modes.

Trainees begin by observing a model of the task they are to learn—they listen to and read along with the tape recording of a skilled interviewer taking an interview. Skills necessary for total task mastery are introduced sequentially throughout a five-day training session. At each skill level, trainees must first recognize appropriate behaviors, then produce them accurately. Providing a model of the desired behavior along with a model of the behavior in which one feature is incorrect highlights the aspect of the behavior to be taught. Standards were gradually built into the head of the learner and self-modification can occur.

Concepts are introduced in self-instructional written materials. Trainees then listen to the tape recording accompanying each section and evaluate the interviewer behaviors which are demonstrated. Role play follows. Lastly, each trainee tape records a sample interview. Then self-evaluation allows the trainee to improve his or her interviewing skills. Practicing those skills in front of the group gives the trainee an opportunity to listen to model behavior, ask questions, and get further feedback on individual performance. Monitoring interviews is an ongoing part of interviewer evaluation.

4.3 Monitoring

Learning and becoming proficient in the skills of interviewing can be enhanced by monitoring of interviewer performance and then using immediate feedback to correct errors. Telephone interviewing from a central location provides opportunity for monitoring and feedback which is more difficult and expensive in field survey. To be most effective, monitoring should consist of the objective coding of interviewer behavior which can identify both good and poor use of techniques based on the principles of interviewing included in the original training. This serves to reinforce training since it can identify the principles which are violated. One system identifies the major categories of interviewer behavior, with the monitor listening to the interview and coding each behavior, identifying it as correct or incorrect. For example, several codes assess the interviewer's delivery of a question: Was it read exactly as written? Read with minor changes without changing the intent of the question? Read with major changes? and so on. Other codes are directed at evaluating the probes used, the feedback, clarifications, the pace with which the interview was conducted, and so on. This results in a sequence of numeric codes for each interviewer behavior for each question. This record is reviewed with the interviewer after the interview to provide immediate feedback and retraining, if needed. Monitoring interviewers in field settings is more cumbersome and expensive. The most efficient procedure has been to make tape recordings of interviews and code behaviors in the office while listening to the tapes. Such monitoring enhances the original training by reinforcing acceptable procedures and correcting poor ones.

5. Issues in Telephone Interviewing

Recent years have seen a growing use of the telephone for survey research. Reduction in survey costs is a primary motivation for the shift from face-to-face contacts to the telephone, and increased household coverage by telephone and techniques for sampling phone numbers through probability methods have made telephone results more comparable to personal interview surveys.

When a survey interviewer makes contact with a respondent by telephone, he or she faces some particular problem of establishing legitimacy and communicating response tasks. Telephone solicitation done under the guise of "doing a survey" hampers the efforts of legitimate survey enterprises to an unknown degree. Survey organizations try to reassure potential respondents by offering toll-free numbers to verify the legitimacy of the contact, and by contacting local police to provide them with information on the survey which can be passed on to inquisitive citizens. "Refusal conversions" are also standard in telephone surveys. An accomplished interviewer calls a respondent who has initially refused to be interviewed and attempts to convince him or her to participate. Such techniques are common in personal interview surveys as well, but they pay off more highly in telephone studies since there are many initial, "soft" refusals in that mode of contact.

5.1 Communication Issues in Telephone Interviews

Some factors which differentiate the style of communication in telephone and face-to-face interviews are obvious. Use of visual cues such as "show cards" is impossible in telephone contacts (unless the materials have been mailed to respondents before the interview and they agree to use them). Therefore, investigators have been concerned about the comprehensibility to respondents of some response tasks when they are presented over the phone. How many scale points can be presented to respondents verbally for their consideration and judgment? Are questions involving a reference period for recall possible to ask effectively without showing the respondent a calendar? The "channel capacity" of the telephone is limited.

Other differences in communication between telephone and face-to-face modes are more subtle, and involve not only perceptual mechanisms but also social custom. Communication by telephone is somewhat less intimate than in-person dialogue. The inability to see conversational partners (facial expressions, gestures, and so forth) may lead to heightened uncertainty about the meaning behind words and about people's ability to understand what is being conveyed. In addition, the pace of dialogue, which is often regulated by nonverbal cues in face-to-face interaction, has to be maintained by verbal or paralinguistic utterances in telephone conversations. Since the household telephone is normally used for speaking with friends and family, and for self-initiated business communication, any call from a stranger is likely to be treated with suspicion. Thus, custom dictates what sorts of telephone contacts are "appropriate," and some people may view any call which does not fall in these categories as an unwarranted intrusion.

In research on mediated communication, investigators have found support for hypotheses that the visual channel is important for conveying affect and evaluation to others (Ekman 1965, Mehrabian 1968) and for regulating conversation flow (Kendon 1967, Duncan 1972). Tasks involving transmission of factual information and cooperative problem solving appear relatively unaffected by whether the participants can see each other or not (Williams 1977). But there is a consistent tendency for subjects to be less confident of their judgments in no-vision conditions, and to express a preference for face-to-face contact (Williams 1977, National Research Council 1979).

The implications of these findings for telephone interviewing are several. In personal interviews, visual communication plus the preinterview acquaintance period allow the interviewer easily and naturally to establish both the legitimacy of the interview and the image of herself/himself as a pleasant, understanding, and safe person with whom to interact. The interviewer's physical presence permits the communication of attention to, interest in, and acceptance of what the respondent has to say, through nonverbal as well as verbal indicators. By contrast, telephone interviews, which may surprise and disturb respondents, lack the sense of legitimacy of the personal contact, and the phone interview may seem somewhat mechanical. The pace of interaction—unregulated by nonverbal cues—may be faster on the telephone, leading to hurried and perhaps less thoughtful responses (Groves and Kahn 1979).

These comparisons imply that the telephone may produce data of lower quality than those collected in person. But it is also possible that the limited channel capacity of the telephone may eliminate distracting or biasing cues from the interviewer, and that phone communication's lack of intimacy may be a boon when the interview questions cover very sensitive matters. Several comparative studies have involved such hypotheses (Colombotos 1969, Hochstim 1967, Bradburn et al. 1979).

In summary, interviewing by telephone has both advantages and disadvantages. In any case, the nature of communication in the interview will be affected by the medium through which it takes place. While research comparing telephone and face-to-face interviews suggests that the differences in data collected via the two modes are generally small (Groves and Kahn 1979), inferences from the research are tentative because most of the studies were not carefully designed to assess the effect of the mode of communication. Interpretation of findings is confounded by the fact that sampling procedures and interviewing styles were not standardized across modes. Miller and Cannell (1982) have reported an experimental study of interviewing procedures for telephone interviews, but more research is needed to develop optimal techniques.

References

Bancroft G Welch E 1946 Recent experience with problems of labor force measurement. *J. Am. Stat. Ass.* 41: 303–12

Bradburn N M et al. 1979 *Improving Interview Method and Questionnaire Design*. Jossey-Bass, San Francisco, California

Cannell C F, Fowler F J 1963 A study of the reporting of visits to doctors in the National Health Survey, Survey Research Center, University of Michigan, Ann Arbor, Michigan

Cannell C F, Fowler F J 1965 *Comparison of Hospitalization Reporting in Three Survey Procedures. Vital and Health Statistics* Series 2, No. 8 Public Health Service, Washington, DC

Cannell C F, Fowler F J, Marquis K H 1968. *The Influence of Interviewer and Respondent Psychological and Behavioral Variables on the Reporting in Household Interviews. Vital and Health Statistics*, Series 2, No. 26. Public Health Service, Washington, DC

Cannell C F, Miller P, Oksenberg L 1981 Research in interviewing techniques. In: Leinhardt S (ed.)pop 1981 *Sociological Methodology 1981*. Jossey-Bass, San Francisco, California

Clark A L, Wallin P 1964 The accuracy of husbands' and wives' reports of the frequency of marital coitus. *Pop. Stud.* 18: 165–73

Colombotos J 1969 Personal versus telephone interviews: Effect on responses. *Public Health Reports* 84: 773–82

Duncan S 1972 Some signals and rules for taking speaking turns in conversations. *J. Pers. Soc. Psychol.* 23: 283–92

Ekman P 1965 Differential communication of affect by head and body cues. *J. Pers. Soc. Psychol* 2: 726–35

Groves R M, Kahn R L 1979 *Surveys by Telephone: A National Comparison with Personal Interviews*. Academic Press, New York

Hochstim J A 1967 A critical comparison of three strategies of collecting data from households. *J. Amer. Stat. Ass.* 62: 976–82

Kahn R. Cannell C F 1957 *The Dynamics of Interviewing*. Wiley, New York

Kendon A 1967 Some functions of gaze-direction, in social interaction. *Acta Psychol.* 26: 22–63

Mauldin W P, Marks E S 1950 Problems of response in enumerative surveys. *Am. Sociol. Rev.* 15: 649–47

Mehrabian A 1968 Inference of attitudes from the posture, orientation, and distance of a communicator. *J. Consult. Clin. Psychol.* 32: 296–308

Miller P, Cannell C F 1982 A study of experimental techniques for telephone interviewing. *Public Opinion Q*. 46: 250–69

National Research Council 1979 *Privacy and Confidentiality as Factors in Survey Response*. National Academy of Sciences, Washington, DC

Payne S 1951 *The Art of Asking Questions*. Princeton University Press, Princeton, New Jersey

Schuman H, Converse J M 1971 The effects of black and white interviewers on black responses in 1968. *Public Opinion Q.* 35: 44–68

Schuman H, Presser S 1981 *Questions and Answers in Attitude Surveys: Experiments on Question Form, Wording, and Context*. Academic Press, New York

Survey Research Center 1976 *Interviewer's Manual*, rev. edn. Survey Research Center, University of Michigan, Ann Arbor, Michigan

Warwick D P, Lininger C 1975 *The Sample Survey: Theory and Practice*. McGraw-Hill, New York

Wenar C 1963 The reliability of developmental histories. Summary and evaluation of evidence. University of Pennsylvania School of Medicine, Philadelphia, Pennsylvania

Williams E 1977 Experimental comparisons of face-to-face and mediated communication: A review. *Psychol. Bull.* 84: 963–76

Meta-analysis

B. McGaw

When any important question has been addressed in a reasonable number of quantitative research studies interpretation involves a synthesis of the findings of the separate studies. The traditional literature review involves careful reading of individual studies and an essentially intuitive integration as patterns in the results are sought. When the number of studies is large, and particularly when the studies vary substantially, the task of narrative synthesis can become overwhelming and will almost inevitably produce a judgment that the findings of the studies do not support any unequivocal conclusions. An important alternative approach is to treat the task of integrating the findings of quantitative research as a quantitative task rather than an intuitive one. Various quantitative procedures were applied over a considerable period before Glass (1976) systematized the approach and applied it first to the large body of studies of the benefits of psychotherapy. He coined the term "meta-analysis" for this approach since it involves an "analysis of analysis," with the findings of separate studies becoming the data for a synthesising meta-analysis. In its earliest applications, the purpose of meta-analysis was primarily to summarise the findings of studies in order to discern any supportable broad generalizations. There has been added, in the late twentieth century the additional, and sometimes alternative, goal of identifying deficiencies in a body of research in order to generate new hypotheses and direct future work.

1. Strategies for Synthesizing Research

One of the most important contributions of meta-analysis is that it has made research synthesis more rigorous and systematic. In the process, it has exposed deficiencies with traditional methods that have not usually been recognized and acknowledged. Cooper and Rosenthal (1980), for example, compared narrative and meta-analytic integrations of the findings of a set of seven studies with a clear overall conclusion and found that narrative reviewers were more likely than meta-analysts to make a Type II error concluding that the results were equivocal and thus missing the clear finding of a significant effect. There are important criticisms of meta-analysis but some that are advanced are not criticisms of its quantitative methods of research synthesis per se but rather of all methods of synthesis.

1.1 Narrative Review

The traditional process of integrating a body of research literature is essentially intuitive and the style of reporting narrative. Because the reviewer's methods are often unspecified, it is usually difficult to discern just how the original research findings have contributed to the integration. Different reviewers can interpret and use the findings of the same research studies quite differently but, because the reviewers' strategies are not explicit, these inconsistencies can be difficult to detect. In extreme cases, careful analysis can reveal that different reviewers actually use the same research reports in support of contrary conclusions (see Miller, cited in Glass et al. 1981 pp. 18–19).

The most serious problem for narrative reviewers to cope with is the volume of relevant research literature that typically needs to be integrated. Most reviewers appear to deal with this problem by choosing only a subset of the studies. Some take the studies they know most intimately. Others take those they value most highly, usually on the basis of methodological quality. Few, however, give any indication of the means by which they selected studies for review (Jackson 1980).

1.2 Early Quantitative Methods

Olkin (1990) and Rosenthal (1991) provide brief summaries of early quantitative methods for synthesising research studies. One approach, dating from the work of Fisher (1932), has been to combine the probabilities associated with reported significance tests. The aggregation produces an estimate of the probability of the observed pattern of individual study results occurring when there is no underlying population effect and so provides a decision rule for acceptance or rejection of the null hypothesis common to the studies. It provides no indication of the magnitude of the effect, nor does it allow any investigation of the relationship between study characteristics and study findings. Rosenthal (1991 pp. 89–99) provides a detailed description of nine different methods for combining probabilities and offers advice about the circumstances in which each is most appropriate.

Another early quantitative approach was to count the relative frequencies with which reported results fall into categories such as statistically significant in one direction, not significant, and significant in the other direction. One serious weakness of this strategy is that the level of significance of a study depends not only on the magnitude of the observed effect but also on the sample size. Trivial findings from large studies will be counted as revealing an effect simply because they achieve statistical significance. More substantial findings from single small studies will be treated as showing no effect simply because they fail to achieve statistical significance.

A further problem with frequency counts arises in setting the decision rule. It is sometimes concluded that there is a significant overall finding if more than one-third of the study findings reveal a significant effect in one direction. Hedges and Olkin (1980) have developed a precise formulation of the probability of significant results occurring in individual studies that shows this simple decision rule to be inappropriate. Where the difference between the population means for the experimental and control conditions is 0.30 of a standard deviation, for example, the probability of means from samples of 20 persons per condition being significantly different at the 0.05 level is only 0.238. The more studies there are to be integrated, the more likely it is that the proportion reporting a significant difference will be close to 0.238 and below the criterion of 0.33. With study sample sizes of 20, the probability of significant results in studies is less than 0.33 for population mean differences as large as 0.50 of a standard deviation. With sample sizes of 50, the probability of significant results is less than 0.33 for population mean differences as large as 0.36. Using the relative frequency of significant findings across studies and a criterion such as 0.33 is, therefore, a misleading way to integrate findings.

1.3 Meta-analysis

An alternative to combined probabilities and frequency counts is aggregation of some index of the size of the effect revealed in each study. For studies making comparisons between experimental and control conditions, Glass (1976) employed as an "effect size" for study i the standardized difference between experimental and control group means

$$d_i = (\bar{Y}_i^E - \bar{Y}_i^C)/s_i \tag{1}$$

where $\bar{Y}_i^E$ and $\bar{Y}_i^C$ are the sample means and s_i the within-group standard deviation. For studies of the relationship between variables, Glass (1976), and Schmidt and Hunter (1977) independently proposed the correlation coefficient as the index for aggregation. In other sets of studies, different common indices, such as proportion of individuals improved due to treatment, may be available.

The term meta-analysis is now generally used to describe any quantitative method for integrating the findings of separate empirical research studies, including those methods developed before the introduction of the term in 1976. Meta-analysis involves quantification of study findings as effect sizes on some common metric, aggregation of effect size estimates across studies, and analysis of relationships between effect sizes and features of the studies. The techniques developed by Glass and his associates are fully described in Glass et al. (1981). Those of Schmidt and Hunter, generalized from their work on correlations to include standardized mean differences, are described in Hunter et al. (1982). Further discussions are pro-

vided in a growing number of publications, including Hedges and Olkin (1985), Cooper (1989), Kulik and Kulik (1989), and Rosenthal (1991).

With the separate study findings quantified and the study characteristics classified, the meta-analyst does not have to hold the complex pattern of study variations in memory for integration as the narrative reviewer does. The pattern is captured and preserved in an explicit fashion, open to both checks and challenges provided that the meta-analytic procedures are well documented. The task of integration is one of data analysis with no necessary limit to the number of studies that might be included.

2. Scope of Literature for Synthesis

2.1 Identification of Studies

For any form of literature review, location of relevant research studies is an important task. Strategies for finding studies are discussed by Glass et al. (1981), and Hunter et al. (1982). Details of the search should be reported to allow others to judge the comprehensiveness of literature included and subsequent reviewers to see most readily where the review might be extended. Jackson's (1980) analysis of 36 published reviews revealed that the reviewers paid little attention to the work of prior reviewers. It may well have been that these prior narrative reviewers gave too little information about their procedures for their experiences to illuminate the path for their successors.

One criticism of meta-analysis is that the capacity it provides to cope with large bodies of literature causes the net to be cast too broadly and encourages the attempted integration of studies which are insufficiently similar. Blind aggregation of studies is certainly not justified in any review but it is appropriate to count "apples" and "oranges" together as long as the concern is with "fruit." In any case, differences among the studies need not be ignored. They can be coded and their relationship with study findings systematically examined in the meta-analysis.

A different consideration is whether the time commitment required for an exhaustive search for relevant literature is justified. An argument in favour can be based on the observation that effect sizes are often larger in the more readily accessible published literature than they are in the more fugitive, unpublished literature and that the general finding will be biased if only the readily accessible literature is used. An argument against is that the task is extremely time consuming and that there are practical limits beyond which time is better spent on duplicate, independent coding of the studies.

2.2 Possibility of Selection of Studies

An important consequence of the meta-analyst's capacity to cope with large volumes of literature is that there is no need for arbitrary exclusion of studies to make the task manageable. There may, however, be grounds for exclusion of some studies from the analysis. Smith and Glass' (1977) early meta-analysis of experimental studies of the efficacy of psychotherapy was criticised because it was based on all available studies and not just the methodologically strongest ones. Smith and Glass had actually first established that methodological quality made no difference to study findings before ignoring it in their aggregation. Several others, using only methodologically sound studies from the total set used by Smith and Glass, subsequently confirmed the correctness of the Smith and Glass estimates of effect size from all the studies. In the body of literature dealing with the effects of class size on learning, the methodological quality of the studies was shown to make a difference to study findings (Glass and Smith 1978, Slavin 1984a, 1984b).

One recommendation, following the early practice of Glass and Smith, has been to treat the influence of methodological quality as something to be examined quantitatively rather than something to be ruled out *a priori*. This at least avoids the potential problem with narrative reviewers who may have a tendency not just to ignore a study judged to be methodologically flawed but to treat it as evidence against the research hypothesis its results apparently support. Hedges (1990 pp. 20–21) reports that, in his experience, studies with poorer designs tend to produce greater variability in results. He does not argue for their automatic exclusion but calls for "*empirical* research that might suggest when research studies are so flawed as to be worthless."

2.3 Sources of Bias in Studies

An important consideration for any reviewer is whether the accessible literature is itself biased. If statistically significant findings are more likely to be published, published studies will be biased against the null hypothesis. The most extreme view is that the published studies are the five percent of studies reflecting Type I errors. Rosenthal and Rubin (1988) provide a method which Rosenthal (1991) illustrates. The strategy is to estimate how many unpublished studies averaging a null result there would need to be to offset a group of published significant ones. For 443 published experiments examining the effects of interpersonal self-fulfilling prophecies and yielding an average effect size of 1.3 standard deviations, Rosenthal shows that there would need to be 122,778 unpublished studies averaging null results if the effects in the published ones were to be due to sampling bias in publication. Rosenthal suggests that, if the number of studies averaging null results required to obliterate the effect size in the number of analysed studies (**K**) exceeds 5**K**+10, then it is reasonable to conclude that such a number of unretrieved studies is unlikely to exist.

Such calculations can dispel much of the doubt about the credibility of published results but cannot dispel all fears of bias in the published literature. Completed meta-analyses have tended to find stronger effects in studies published in journals than in studies reported in theses and dissertations (Glass et al. 1981). It cannot be expected therefore, to summarize adequately what research says on a particular topic by examining only journal articles.

3. Quantification of Study Findings

Once the studies to be dealt with have been identified, the findings of each have to be quantified on a common metric to enable integration of findings across studies and exploration of relationships between the strength of findings and other variables. There is a considerable variety of indices of study findings, or effect sizes, available but the most commonly used have been standardized mean differences and correlations.

3.1 Standardized Mean Differences

The definition of effect size as a standardized mean difference between treatment and control groups, proposed by Glass (1976), is given in Eqn. (1). Glass proposed standardization with the control group standard deviation. Since this standard deviation frequently is not reported, the pooled within-group standard deviation is an alternative. This pooled estimate is actually to be preferred since it has less sampling error and since its use is justified by the assumption of homogeneity of variance required for the original experimental comparison.

The effect size defined by Eqn. (1) is implicitly an estimate of population effect size, defined in terms of population parameters, for study i, as:

$$\delta_i = (\mu_i^E - \mu_i^C)/\sigma_i \tag{2}$$

where μ_i^E and μ_i^C are the population means for the treatment and control conditions and σ_i the common variance within the two populations. Hedges (1981) showed that d_i of Eqn. (1) is a biased estimator of σ_i of Eqn. (2) but that an unbiased estimator d_i^U can be obtained from the approximation:

$$d_i^U \approx d_i\{1 - 3/[4(n_i^E + n_i^C - 2) - 1]\} \tag{3}$$

Since $(n_i^E + n_i^C - 2) > 1$ it can be seen that the unbiased estimate is always smaller than the biased estimate, that is $d_i^U < d_i$ but the correction makes very little difference in practice. If the sample sizes n_i^E and n_i^C are both 20, the unbiased estimate d_i^U will be 0.98 of the biased estimate d_i.

In many research reports the sample means and standard deviations required for direct calculations of d_i are not provided. In some cases, d_i can be obtained directly from reported information such as t or F test values. In others, it can be approximated from information such as proportions of subjects improving under treatment and control conditions. Details of these types of transformations to retrieve effect sizes are given in Glass et al. (1981).

There are some variations among studies, however, which cause the effect size estimates immediately retrievable not to be directly comparable. Some perfectly satisfactory statistical analyses produce arbitrary changes in the metric on which effect sizes are expressed. Covariance adjustments, for example, increase the power of the statistical test but, from the point of view of effect size estimation, arbitrarily decrease the estimate s and thus arbitrarily decrease the estimates d and d^U. The use of change scores, either raw or residual, has the same consequences. Similar lack of comparability occurs with studies which provide, not a simple comparison of experimental and control conditions, but a factorial analysis of variance in which the treatment factor is crossed with other factors. The within-treatments variance is reduced by the removal of main and interaction effects variance attributable to the other factors. As a consequence, the effect size estimate for the experimental treatment is arbitrarily increased. Strategies for adjusting the initial effect size estimates derived from such studies are given by McGaw and Glass (1980) and by Glass et al. (1981).

A further respect in which studies may differ arbitrarily is in the selectivity of the sample investigated. A restriction of range on some selection variable will reduce the variance of criterion scores and lead to an increased estimate of effect size. In the literature on the educational effects of ability grouping, for example, some studies use only gifted children in the homogeneous grouping condition and, from the heterogeneous condition, report data only for the gifted subgroup. If the proportion of the population represented in the sample were the top p, selected on the basis of some variable X, the ratio of the estimated standard deviation on this measure for the full population, s_x, to that for the restricted population, s_x^p, would be

$$u = s_x / s_x^p$$
$$= 1/[1 + \mu_x^p(c^p - \mu_x^p)]^{1/2} \qquad (4)$$

where c^p is the standard score above which the proportion of a normal distribution is p and μ_x^p

is the mean standard score for the segment of the population in the top p, given by

$$\mu_x^p = \varphi(c)p \qquad (5)$$
$$= \{[\exp(-c^2/2]/[(2\pi)^{1/2}]\}/p$$

where $\varphi(c)$ is the ordinate of the unit normal distribution at the point of the cut. The ratio of the estimated standard deviations on the criterion measure Y, for the full and restricted populations, will be

$$s_y / s_y^p = [(u^2 - 1)(r_{xy}^p)^2 + 1]^{1/2} \qquad (6)$$

where r_{xy}^p is the correlation between the selection and criterion variables in the restricted sample. An effect size calculated with s_y^p will be arbitrarily enhanced; s_y should be used as McGaw and Glass (1980) suggest.

The arbitrary differences among studies discussed so far all lead to overestimates of the within-groups standard deviation. Hedges (1981) and Hunter et al. (1982) suggest that the initial effect size estimate, d^U, be corrected for an underestimate due to unreliability of the criterion measure. This unreliability produces an overestimate of the standard deviation. The correction is

$$d^{UR} = d^U / (r_{yy})^{1/2} \qquad (7)$$

where r_{yy} is the criterion reliability. Since $r_{yy} < 1$, then $d^{UR} > d^U$.

The correction in Eqn. (7) expresses the effect size in terms of the estimated standard deviation of true scores instead of that for observed scores. When the observed score values are used, arbitrary differences among studies in the reliabilities of measures cause arbitrary differences in the studies' effect sizes. The sense in which reliability is defined and the way in which it is estimated, however, are crucial to the meaning of corrections of this sort. Information about test reliabilities is needed but similar information is needed for all studies. Different reliability coefficients, such as test–retest and internal consistency, are based on different conceptions of error. Consistent correction of effect size estimates requires a common form of the coefficient.

In an attempt to minimize some of the influence of arbitrary scale variations on effect size estimates, Kraemer and Andrews (1982) proposed a nonparametric effect size estimate. Their procedure requires pretest and posttest scores for individuals in experimental and control conditions or, in some circumstances, for those in the experimental condition alone. They determine the median pretest score for all subjects in a condition, the median posttest score for the subgroup of persons within the range of two distinct scores either side of the pretest median, and then the proportion of all pretest scores $P(D)$ which were exceeded by the subgroup's posttest median. For a study with only an experimental group, the effect size is obtained by re-expressing this proportion as a z-score. This standardizes the difference between the pretest and post–test medians as

$$D_E = \Phi^{-1}[P(D_E] \qquad (8)$$

where Φ is the standard normal cumulative density function. For a study with pretest and posttest scores on both experimental and control groups, separate estimates are derived for both groups and the effect size estimated as

$$D = D_E - D_C \qquad (9)$$

Although the development of a robust nonparametric effect size estimate may prove valuable, the version offered by Kraemer and Andrews is of limited use. In addition to requiring complete individual data for each study, it is likely to give very imprecise estimates of D with extreme proportions $P(D)$. More needs to be known about the standard error of the estimates of D before any serious use of this index can be encouraged. Little further work on nonparametric estimates of effect size seems to have been undertaken.

3.2 Correlations

For some bodies of literature the relationship between a pair of variables is investigated with the correlation coefficient, r, providing an index of effect size. Hunter et al. (1982), who developed their meta-analytic procedures in integrating studies of test validities, suggest that all meta-analyses can be undertaken using correlation coefficients as the index of effect size. Experimental comparisons of treatment and control conditions can be expressed as a point biserial correlation between categorized condition and the criterion measure. For the case with equal experimental and control sample sizes, $n^E = n^C = N/2$,

the relationship between the point biserial correlation coefficient r_{pbis} and the standardized mean difference d, is

$$r_{pbis} = d/[d^2 + 4(N-2)/N] \qquad (10)$$

Procedures for converting from the results of various parametric and nonparametric significance tests to correlation coefficients are summarized by Glass et al. (1981) and Rosenthal (1991). Rosenthal declares, after considerable experience with both forms, a strong preference for the correlation coefficient rather than standardized mean differences. Among his reasons are that there are some studies in which the form of the results will permit only the calculation of r but none for which only d can be determined. Kulik and Kulik (1989), however, point out that Rosenthal's use of correlations computed direct from tests of statistical significance of mean differences takes no account of special features of the statistical test, such as the use of covariance adjustments or factorial analysis of variance designs, that will arbitrarily inflate the effect size estimates.

Schmidt and Hunter (1977) correct the reported correlations for any attenuation due to study artefacts such as unreliability of the variables and restriction in the sample due to selection on one of the variables. Variations in test reliabilities and in the degree of sample selectivity produce arbitrary differences in the reported correlations. Removing these effects is intended to ensure that, however a study is undertaken and reported, its findings will be an estimate of the correlation between true scores on the variables in the whole population.

Where there is a restriction in range, due to the selection of only the top proportion p on the selection variable X, the observed correlation for the restricted sample, r_{xy}^p can be disattenuated by

$$r_{xy} = u r_{xy}^p /[(u^2 - 1)(r_{xy}^p)^2 + 1]^{1/2} \qquad (11)$$

where u is as defined in Eqn. (4).

The correction for unreliability of the variables, using the notions of classical test theory, produces an estimate of the true score correlation, $\rho(T_x, T_y)$, from the observed correlation r_{xy}, as

$$\rho(T_x, T_y) = r_{xy}/(r_{xx}r_{yy})^{1/2} \qquad (12)$$

where r_{xx} and r_{yy} are the reliabilities of the two variables. If the sample is restricted by selection on the basis of observed scores on one of the variables, Hunter et al. (1982) suggest the reliability correction be made only for the other variable. The correction of an observed correlation for unreliability, defined by Eqn. (12), parallels that for correction to a standardized mean difference defined by Eqn. (7). The concern expressed, in connection with that correction, about the need to use comparable definitions of reliability for all studies is also relevant here.

In a study where both corrections are to be applied, the correction for restriction in range, Eqn. (11), is applied before the correction for unreliability, Eqn. (12), unless the reliability estimates are for the restricted subpopulation rather than for the full population.

In practice, many studies do not report data on test reliability or the extent of sample restriction. Adjustments to each finding could be made only if some estimates were used in the absence of information. Hunter et al. (1982) describe an alternative: they use the distributions of reliabilities and range restriction in studies where they are reported to correct estimates of the mean and variance of the correlations obtained from the full set of studies.

For all statistical analyses of effect sizes Rosenthal converts r to z_r using Fisher's transformation

$$z_r = \frac{1}{2} \ln\left[\frac{1+r}{1-r}\right] \qquad (13)$$

This also produces an adjustment for bias in the estimate for cases of high correlation. Hunter et al. (1982) argue, on the other hand, that Fisher's nonlinear transformation gives greater weight to large correlations, appropriately if one is concerned as Fisher was with establishing confidence intervals around individual r's, but inappropriately if one is concerned with estimating the mean of a number of r's (see *Correlational Procedures in Data Analysis*).

3.3 Other Effect Sizes

In some sets of studies other effect size measures than standardized mean differences and correlations can be used. Studies of the treatment of alcoholism, for example, may all express their results as the difference between proportions of individuals in treatment and control conditions reaching some criterion level of improvement. With these studies, this difference could be used as the effect size measure without transformation. In other sets of studies some measure such as IQ may provide a common index for use as an effect size without transformation.

4. Coding Study Characteristics

The ultimate purpose of meta-analysis, in seeking the integration of a body of literature, is both to determine what average effect size is reported in the studies and to establish whether variability in the effect sizes across studies can be accounted for in terms of covariability with characteristics of the studies. The most important study characteristics in terms of refining an understanding of a field are substantive ones but methodological ones also need to be considered to determine whether variations in findings are due to variations in methodology or in methodological quality.

Hunter et al. (1982) suggest that, before any coding of study characteristics is even undertaken, the distribution of effect sizes should be examined to determine whether 75 percent of the observed variance can be accounted for by sampling error and the influences of other artifacts. If it can be, then they claim that the labor of coding can be avoided. Procedures for partitioning variance in study findings into real and artifactual components and the wisdom of such a doctrinaire rejection of further analysis of covariation between study characteristics and findings are discussed in Sect. 5.

Characteristics to be coded should be chosen carefully and clear coding rules should be defined. Coding is time consuming and it is not worth the effort to code trivial study variations though, of course, the value of a characteristic cannot always be anticipated in advance. Another important reason for careful choice of coding categories is that, in the analysis of the covariation between study characteristics and findings, the degrees of freedom are limited. Analyses with many study characteristics run the risk of capitalization on chance variations in the data.

4.1 Substantive Characteristics

Which substantive features of studies are most important to code depends on theoretical considerations. The research literature itself should reveal the characteristics, such as form of treatment, type of population sampled, and type of outcome measured, that are most likely to produce variability in study findings. A helpful initial source of suggestions can be earlier reviews of the same literature. Application of a preliminary version of a coding schedule to key research studies in the field can also facilitate the development of the final version. Some sample coding schemes, developed for a variety of bodies of literature, are given in Glass et al. (1981).

Nonreporting can cause problems for the coding. If variations in a particular characteristic appear to be related to systematic differences in findings, the variations in that characteristic over studies can usefully be coded only if it is reported in a reasonable proportion of the studies. A "not known" category can be used but, if too many studies are coded into it, the characteristic will be doomed to insignificance in the subsequent analysis. Hedges (1990) suggests coding at two levels of specificity with most, if not all, studies being coded at the higher (though vaguer) level to permit analyses in terms of it if too few studies can be coded in the more specific categories. He also suggests the use of other sources such as fuller research reports, program descriptions, and test manuals to provide details not contained in the primary source.

4.2 Methodological Characteristics

For coding of methodological characteristics of studies, previous meta-analyses can be helpful. Characteristics such as type of experimental design, including method of assignment of subjects to treatments, dropout rates of subjects during treatment, and reactivity of the outcome measures, are important for assessing studies in most fields. Samples of coding schemes for such characteristics are included in Glass et al. (1981).

The problem of nonreporting in studies is seldom as great with the methodological as with the substantive characteristics. It is perhaps a sad commentary on the state of the field in such educational and other social research that, in reporting, more attention is given to the methods of research than to the precise conditions of the experiment.

4.3 Reporting Coding Precision

Since much of the explanatory power of a meta-analysis depends on the coding of study characteristics, considerations of validity, and reliability are important. The validity of the codings depends on the definitions of the coding categories and on the objectivity with which they can be used in practice. The definitions can be included in the report of the meta-analysis to allow other reviewers to judge their validity. Even careful definition of the categories, however, cannot avert the precarious inferences about the details of a study which must be made when there is incomplete or imprecise reporting. Decision rules for such inferences can minimize interjudge disagreement but cannot guarantee valid codings.

Lack of agreement among coders and inconsistency of individual coders are the sole sources of unreliability since the objects to be coded are themselves stable. Some index of coder consistency should be reported for any meta-analysis. Even if only one coder is used in a modest review, an index can be obtained from repeated codings of the same studies after a suitable time lapse. Where more than one coder is used, unreliability due to inconsistencies between and within coders can be separately estimated and reported.

5. Combining Study Findings

The primary task of meta-analysis lies in the integration of the findings of separate studies. The purpose may be to seek broad generalizations or to identify inadequacies in the existing research on the basis of which to propose new emphases.

5.1 Averaging Effect Sizes

The first question is whether a nonparametric estimate such as the median or a parametric estimate such as the mean should be used (see *Nonparametric and Distribution-free Statistics*). More powerful statistical analyses can be used in conjunction with parametric estimates, and that is a reason for preferring them, but initial exploratory analyses can give useful information about the distribution of the set of effect sizes and the appropriateness of proceeding with parametric analyses.

A simple mean of the obtained effect sizes takes no account of the variation in precision of the estimates obtained from different studies. A weighted mean of the estimates derived from k studies could be obtained as

$$\bar{d} = \sum_{i=1}^{k} w_i d_i^U / \sum_{i=1}^{k} w_i \qquad (14)$$

Hunter et al. (1982) suggest the use of the sample sizes as the weights, $w_i = N_i$. *Hedges and Olkin (1985) suggest the use of the weights which minimize the variance of $\bar{d}$, that is*

$$w_i = (1/v_i) / \left(\sum_{j=1}^{k} \right) v_j \qquad (15)$$

where v_i is the variance of the estimate d_i^U and can be estimated by

$$v_i = (n_i^E + n_i^C)/(n_i^E n_i^C) + d_i^U/2(n_i^E + n_i^C) \qquad (16)$$

Hedges and Olkin point out that, though the d_i^U are unbiased estimators of δ the weighted mean defined by Eqns. (14) and (15) is not. It provides a consistent but small underestimate but can be improved by a recalculation using weights obtained from Eqn. (16) with the first weighted mean $\bar{d}$ replacing the d_i^U to give a more nearly unbiased estimate $\bar{d}^U$ from Eqn. (14). The adjustment makes little difference. Indeed, use of the N_i as the weights, as Hunter et al. (1982) suggest, is as good in practice as those defined by Eqn. (15).

Where direct effect size estimates are not available for all studies, an overall mean effect size (as a standardized mean difference) can be estimated using only information about the relative frequency of significant findings in the studies (Hedges and Olkin 1980). The method requires the assumption that the sample sizes are the same in all studies and equal for control and experimental conditions. Where they are not the same for all studies, Hedges and Olkin recommend the use of their geometric mean or their square mean root. Although these procedures are not strictly applicable to studies using correlations but reporting only significance levels, because correlation coefficients are not distributed normally, they provide a reasonable approximation. The reporting of significance without the accompanying value of the statistic, however, is less likely with correlation coefficients than standardized mean differences.

5.2 Estimating Variation in Effect Sizes

For an analysis of the variation in effect sizes, the first question is again whether to use parametric or nonparametric procedures. Nonparametric indices such as the interquartile range are less sensitive to skewing of the distribution. Associated exploratory analyses can expose the shape of the distribution and the presence of outliers which might better be excluded as the likely products of error in the original research reports. The more typical procedure in meta-analysis, however, has been to use parametric procedures and to calculate the variance of the effect size estimates and then, in many cases, to establish a confidence interval around their mean.

Where individual studies yield more than one effect size there can be problems because the usual assumptions of statistical independence of data analysis will not be satisfied. The problem also extends across research reports where a common sample yields the data for more than one report. The lack of statistical independence causes no problem with estimation of mean effect sizes but it does with estimation of variance and with significance testing (Rosenthal 1991).

The most conservative approach is to admit only one effect size estimate from each study. Rosenthal (1991) suggests a number of strategies: using a mean or median effect size from each study or, where correlations among the variables are known, creating a composite variable to which the effect size estimate refers. The most liberal approach is to use all effect sizes as though they were independent. Smith and Glass (1977) took the liberal approach in their meta-analysis of the psychotherapy outcome literature but examined the consequences of both methods of analysis in their meta-analysis of the literature examining the effects of class size (Glass and Smith 1978). In this latter case, they found little difference. Subsequent replication of the meta-analysis of the psychotherapy studies showed, for that body of literature also, that essentially the same results were achieved by both methods. Since this early work, however, there is now much more attention being given to the issues of dependency in the total available set of effect sizes for most meta-analyses.

If effect sizes are combined within studies before aggregation, any differences among them in their substantive or methodological characteristics will be lost. If the magnitude of the effect size depends in some way on the type of outcome measure used, that information will be lost in the averaging. The use of more elaborate models of within and between studies variations in effect size will permit better exploration of the meta-analytic data.

From the point of view of variance estimation, the statistical problems of multiple findings from single studies are essentially the same as those of cluster sampling. The standard error of the mean from a cluster sample is larger than that from a simple random sample of the same size. For the case of a meta-analysis, if k studies each yield j effect sizes with a variance of s_d^2, the variance of the mean, treating the effect sizes as simple random sample (SRS), would be estimated as

$$Var(\bar{d}^{SRS}) = s_d^2 / kj \qquad (17)$$

If the effect sizes were treated as a cluster sample (CS), the variance of the mean would be estimated as

$$Var(\bar{d}^{CS}) = Var(\bar{d}^{SRS}) [1 + (j-1)r] \qquad (18)$$

where r is the within-cluster correlation (see *Measures of Variation; Sampling Errors in Survey Research*). Treating the effect sizes as a simple random sample would put too narrow a confidence interval around the mean. Glass et al. (1981) present evidence from six meta-analyses that the average within-cluster correlation of effect sizes was about 0.6. With two effect sizes per study, treating the effect sizes more correctly as a cluster sample would give a standard error estimate 1.26 times that estimated for a simple random sample. With ten effect sizes per study, the cluster sample estimate of standard error would be 2.53 times as large. In a particular meta-analysis, where the number of estimates per study is not constant, Eqn. (18) could be used with j taken as the total number of effect sizes divided by the number of studies. An alternative is to use a jackknife procedure (Glass et al. 1981). Alternatively the methods of multilevel analysis could be employed with empirical Bayes estimation procedures (Raudenbush and Bryk 1985).

Even without common subjects or data, there can be a degree of non-independence among studies conceived under a common influence and using perhaps similar designs and measures. Rosenthal (1991) shows that, at least with one body of literature, the findings of sets of studies completed by different research groups do not differ systematically from each other.

5.3 Analyzing Effect Sizes

Hunter et al. (1982) take the view that, if the effect sizes can be considered a homogeneous sample from a single population, only the estimation of an overall mean effect size is justified. Together with Hedges and Olkin (1985), and Rosenthal (1991), they provide tests of the homogeneity of a sample of effect sizes. These tests are very powerful. With a large body of studies, small variations in study findings will lead to statistical significance and rejection of the null hypothesis of homogeneity.

Hunter et al. (1982) propose an alternative to such significance testing as a way of deciding whether the analysis can stop with the estimate of an overall mean. They estimate the variance in effect sizes which could be due to sampling error, range restriction, and unreliability. Only if it is less than 75 percent of the total do they explore the covariation between effect sizes and study characteristics to account for the remaining variance. This is a hardline position to adopt given the assumptions required for their estimate of sampling error and their adjustments to it for the influence of artifacts. A more flexible position is to allow for the discernment of meaningful covariation even in data where purely statistical considerations such as theirs would provide a counsel of no examination.

Hedges and Olkin (1985) and Hunter et al. (1982) suggest, as a strategy for further analysis, subdivision of the data into subsets on the basis of some characteristic and then testing whether each of the subsets is homogeneous. Hedges and Olkin's (1985) procedure is presented by analogy with analysis of variance and shows how variance components can be obtained for various fixed and random effects using general linear models. They argue that the straightforward use of analysis of variance is inappropriate because the effect size estimates will not have the same distributions within cells of the design and because the analysis provides no assessment of the comparability of effect sizes within cells, or "classes" in their terms. Kulik and Kulik (1989), however, argue for the use of analysis of variance and demonstrate how their approach is equivalent to that proposed by Hedges and Olkin in essential respects.

With this parametric modeling of the effect sizes, several classifications can be used simultaneously to account for variations in effect sizes across studies. If too many classifications are involved there can be problems with empty cells. On the other hand, if factors which have an effective relationship with effect size are excluded, analyses of the remaining factors will be biased if studies in different levels of the excluded factor are unevenly represented.

The use of general linear models opens up the possibilities of all the extensions of that technique developed for the analyses of primary data. In an early example, Miller (cited in Glass et al. 1981, pp. 165–70) estimated main and interaction effects for drug therapy and psychotherapy using the general linear model for a two-way design. The extensions which now need to be made are those that would apply to meta-analysis the hierarchical, or multilevel, models now being used in primary data analysis where data are clustered in different levels (see *Multilevel Analysis; Hierarchical Linear Models*).

The relationship between study characteristics and findings can also be explored by regression procedures (see *Regression Analyses of Quantified Data*). The use of too many study characteristics, however, can result in the traditional problem of capitalization on chance variations in the data (see *Significance Testing*). Where a simple correlation is computed between a study characteristic and effect size, the correlation can be corrected for attenuation due to sampling error in the effect size estimates (Hunter et al. 1982) (see *Reliability in Educational and Psychological Measurement*). The corrected correlation with study feature *f* is given by

$$r_{\tau f} = r_{of} / (s_\tau / s_0) \tag{19}$$

6. Prospects for Meta-analysis

Since its popularization in 1976 with Glass's introduction of the term "meta-analysis" and powerful demonstration of the potential of quantitative synthesis of the findings of separate research studies, meta-analysis has had a considerable impact on the approach to research synthesis in many disciplines. It has brought a rigor to the process and successfully challenged the adequacy of the traditional, narrative review process.

There are important criticisms of meta-analysis though some of them are not unique to it as a strategy. The "file drawer" problem of unpublished and less accessible studies likely to contain less clear-cut findings than published studies is a problem for all reviews. Others, such as the risks of dealing indiscriminately with a large, incoherent body of literature simply because the quantitative strategies facilitate it, are unique to meta-analysis but there is protection in the capacity that the methodology provides to expose the incoherence.

Meta-analysis offers important prospects for educational research. In some substantial bodies of empirical research, it has already exposed consistency of findings where narrative reviewers could discern only enormous variation and, ultimately, equivocation. More was already established by existing research than had been recognized. Meta-analysis may help to re-establish public faith in the efficacy of empirical research in education by making clearer what has already been achieved. It may also expose more clearly the questions for which further research is most needed. The continuing refinement of the methodology of meta-analysis, particularly the recent attention to the final analysis stage with improved methods for dealing with nonindependence of effect sizes, strengthens its claims to be the preferred method of synthesis for quantitative research. The editors of a major review of the methodology of meta-analysis by a specialist group of statisticians conclude that "meta-analysis seems well suited . . . to make a larger and larger contribution to the social and behavioral as well as the medical and natural sciences, and to a broad range of policy-relevant research" (Wachter and Straf 1990 p. 28).

See also: Educational Research and Policy-making; Policy-oriented Research

References

Cooper H M 1989 *The Integrative Research Review: A Social Science Approach*, 2nd edn. Sage, Newbury Park, California

Cooper H M, Rosenthal R 1980 Statistical versus traditional procedures for summarizing research findings. *Psych. Bull.* 87: 442–49

Fisher R A 1932 *Statistical Methods for Research Workers*, 4th edn. Oliver and Boyd, London

Glass G V 1976 Primary, secondary and meta-analysis. *Educ. Researcher.* 5: 3–8

Glass G V, McGaw B, Smith M L 1981 *Meta-analysis in Social Research*. Sage, Beverly Hills, California

Glass G V, Smith M L 1978 *Meta-analysis of Research on the Relationship of Class-size and Achievement*. Far West Laboratory for Educational Research and Development, San Francisco, California

Hedges L V 1981 Distribution theory for Glass' estimator of effect size and related estimators. *J. Educ. Stat.* 6: 107–28

Hedges L V 1990 Directions for future methodology. In: Wachter K W, Straf M L (eds.) 1990 *The Future of Meta-analysis*. Russell Sage Foundation, New York

Hedges L V, Olkin I 1980 Vote-counting methods in research synthesis. *Psych. Bull.* 88: 359–69

Hedges L V, Olkin I 1985 *Statistical Methods for Meta-analysis*. Academic Press, New York

Hunter J E, Schmidt F L, Jackson G B 1982 *Meta-analysis: Cumulating Research Findings Across Studies*. Sage, Beverly Hills, California

Jackson G B 1980 Methods for integrative reviews. *Rev. Educ. Res.* 50: 438–60

Kraemer H C, Andrews G 1982 A nonparametric technique for meta-analysis effect size calculation. *Psych. Bull.* 91: 404–12

Kulik J A, Kulik C C 1989 Meta-analysis in education. *Int. J. Educ. Res.* 13: 221–340

McGaw B, Glass G V 1980 Choice of the metric for effect size in meta-analysis. *Am. Educ. Res. J.* 17: 325–37

Olkin I 1990 History and goals. In: Wachter K W, Straf M L (eds.) 1990 *The Future of Meta-analysis*. Russell Sage Foundation, New York

Raudenbush S W, Bryk A S 1985 Empirical Bayes meta analyses. *J. Ed. Stat.* 10(22): 75–98

Rosenthal R 1991 *Meta-analytic Procedures for Social Research* rev. edn. Sage, Newbury Park, California

Rosenthal R, Rubin D B 1988 Comment: Assumptions and procedures in the file drawer problem. *Stat. Science* 3: 120–25

Schmidt F L, Hunter J E 1977 Development of a general

solution to the problem of validity generalization. *J. Appl. Psychol.* 62: 529–40

Slavin R E 1984a Meta-analysis in education: How has it been used? *Educ. Res.* AERA13(8): 6–15

Slavin R E 1984b A rejoinder to Carlberg et al. *Educ. Res.* AERA13(8): 24–7

Smith M L, Glass G V 1977 Meta-analysis of psychotherapy outcome studies. *Am. Psychol.* 32: 752–60

Wachter K W, Straf M L (eds.) 1990 *The Future of Meta-analysis.* Russell Sage Foundation, New York

Further Reading

Hunter J E, Schmidt F L *Methods of Meta-Analysis, Correcting Error and Bias in Research Findings.* Sage, Newbury Park, California

Microcomputers in Educational Survey Research

A. Schleicher

A microcomputer is an independent computer system with integrated devices for the input and output of data and for data storage, which is based on a microprocessor as the central processing unit. The introduction of microcomputers has brought about enormous changes in the field of educational research, making the possibilities of electronic data processing readily available to educational researchers with different levels of computer knowledge. With microcomputer systems, such persons could obtain as individuals access to the kind of resources that previously were available only to large organizations and manageable only by computer experts.

The applications of microcomputer systems in educational research range from text processing, spreadsheet calculations, graphical design, text analysis, and electronic publishing (usually referred to as "desktop publishing") to data simulation, educational information and expert systems, and the management and statistical analysis of complex data structures from large-scale educational surveys with hundreds of variables and millions of observations. The wide spectrum of potential applications of microcomputer systems is complemented by a variety of degrees of "depths" with which users with different levels of computer knowledge can communicate with a microcomputer. These range from graphical-user interfaces which enable even the inexperienced user to operate the computer without system knowledge, up to programming languages which operate at the system level and require the detailed knowledge of the architecture of the computer.

This entry describes the architecture and the main components of typical microcomputer systems and their major applications in the field of educational research. This includes an overview of: (a) the hardware components of microcomputer systems; (b) basic concepts for microcomputer configurations and computer networks, with a focus on the requirements in large-scale survey research; (c) operating systems and user interfaces; (d) standard software packages and their major applications in educational research for text processing and desktop publishing, spreadsheet calculations, processing of survey data and statistical data analysis, and database management; and (e) the use of programming languages for the creation of tailor-made applications in educational research. This entry takes into account the developments in microcomputer systems up to the beginning of the 1990s. The rapid changes in the technology of microcomputer systems make it difficult to foresee future trends in the field.

1. Historical Background

By building upon the development of the first microprocessors in the early 1970s (such as the models 4004, 8008, and 8080 from Intel Inc.) the history of microcomputers started in 1975 with the Altair-Computer (MITS Inc.). In 1975, the first professional microcomputer system, the model 5100, was introduced by IBM with a system memory of the size of 16 kilobytes ($16 \times 1{,}024$ binary units of information), a tape drive as the external storage device, and an inbuilt interpreter for the programming language BASIC. This model was shortly after succeeded by the models 5110, 5120, and 5150. In 1976, Apple Computer introduced the Apple I, the successor of which, the Apple II, became the first widely used microcomputer system. In 1981, IBM put the IBM personal computer on the market, which, together with its operating system MS-DOS (Microsoft Disk Operating System), has become the most important standard for the microcomputer industry since then. The continuing development of microcomputers has resulted in a large variety of microcomputer systems designed for a wide range of applications and potential users. At the beginning of the 1990s, the most common microcomputer systems in the field of educational research were IBM personal computers and their compatibles and Macintosh computers, both of which were available in a variety of configurations.

2. Microcomputers versus Mainframe and Minicomputer Systems

In the 1960s and 1970s, data processing was mostly undertaken on centralized, large-scale computer systems with which the users interacted through punchcards or through terminals. The level and quality of the services, as well as the costs offered by such systems, were often unsatisfactory. Instead of being in control of the data processing, users were often highly dependent on the type and availability of these mainframe systems; particular problems being: (a) low user-friendliness; (b) an unsatisfactory range of available software; (c) limited availability; and (d) restricted access, both with respect to the amount of computer resources and with respect to the times in which these could be accessed. With the introduction of microcomputers these difficulties could be largely overcome and a broad range of flexible and highly individualized computer resources were made available to computer users without the need for an extensive infrastructure and at comparatively low costs.

The resources offered by microcomputer systems have expanded rapidly to meet the requirements of a growing number of users in the field of educational research. Therefore microcomputers are rapidly replacing mainframe and minicomputer systems in many educational research applications. However, contemporary mainframe systems still considerably exceed the speed of microcomputers. Also the external storage capacities of mainframe systems are usually much greater, and some applications in administrative and survey research require that data are centrally managed and maintained. In the data-processing environments of universities and research organizations, where large quantities of data are collected and analyzed, mainframe systems will therefore not entirely disappear in the near future, but the way in which they are used is changing. An adequate solution to situations where the central management of data is required can be the use of microcomputers as intelligent terminals for mainframe systems which can extract those data from the mainframe system which are relevant to the particular application and then process these locally as required by the user. Another solution lies in networking microcomputers in a distributed processing environment, which can also be linked to mainframe resources, where microcomputer resources are shared by multiple users but each user is still in control of the individual computer resources. The difference to a mainframe system here is that the actual processing is done primarily on the microcomputer with which the user works, whereas in a mainframe system the processing is done centrally for all users.

3. Architecture of Microcomputer Systems

Microcomputers are based on hardware and software components, where the hardware comprises the mechanical and electronic components of a computer, and the software comprises the application programs and the programs that are used to operate the hardware.

3.1 Hardware Components

The hardware environment of a microcomputer is organized into three functional entities which are usually operated and controlled by a single user. The hardware environment of a microcomputer consists of a number of components where each of these is available in a variety of configurations with different capabilities, speed, and power, and which can be employed in a microcomputer system in such a way as to fit both the requirements of the corresponding applications and the demands and abilities of the users.

One component involves the input of data, and typically consists of: (a) a keyboard; (b) a mouse which acts as a pointing device through the translation of two-dimensional movements on, for example, a desk into corresponding movements on the screen; (c) diskette drives and hard disk systems for data input and data storage; (d) a modem through which a microcomputer can be linked to public networks, databases, or other computers; and sometimes (e) a scanner which reads printed text or graphical data and translates these into computer manageable information. Diskette drives, hard disks, and modems serve at the same time as output media.

A second component processes these data according to predefined algorithmic structures, and consists of: (a) the central processing unit (CPU) which forms the core of the computer and which carries out logical and arithmetic instructions, reads and writes to the computer memory, and communicates through input/output ports with external devices; (b) the working memory (random access memory, RAM) which is used by the CPU for reading and writing data and which holds the computer programs and the data; and (c) the permanent system memory (read only memory, ROM) which holds basic instructions related to the system configuration and the hardware environment. The speed and computing power of microcomputer systems is mainly determined by the microprocessor acting as the CPU. The CPU is mainly characterized by: (a) the internal instruction set, (b) the power of the addressbus and the databus (which determine how many distinct storage addresses can be addressed by the CPU and how many binary pieces of information the CPU can transmit in a single operation); and (c) by the speed expressed in terms of how many operations the CPU can perform per time unit. Many CPUs can be supplemented by a coprocessor which can enhance certain arithmetic operations. The size of the working memory that is required in order to operate the computer and to run the application programs depends both on the operating system and the application programs which are used. Microcomputers were, in 1992, usually equipped with a working memory of between 640 kilobytes ($640 \times 1,024$ binary units of information) and 32 megabytes (32,000 kilobytes of information).

A third component generates and provides the output data and typically consists of: (a) a monitor, (b) mass storage devices, and (c) a printer. A variety of graphic standards exists for microcomputers which allow the operation of different monitors ranging from simple TTL-based monochrome monitors up to analog-based high resolution color monitor systems which can handle millions of color shades. Multiscan monitors allow the automatic adaptation of the monitor to the graphic standard provided by the hard- and software. In most microcomputer systems diskette drives and hard disk systems serve as mass storage devices. Diskettes serve as removable media for data storage in the diskette drives and are organized in a number of concentric tracks which in turn are structured into a number of sectors. They are characterized by their physical size (e.g., 5¼" or 3½"), their storage capacity (e.g., 380 kilobytes or 1.44 megabytes), and the number of tracks per side and sectors per track (e.g., 40 tracks and 9 sectors or 80 tracks and 18 sectors). Since diskettes are often used in order to exchange data between computers the user must be aware of the type of diskette used, as well as of the operating system with which the diskettes were initialized by the computer, because only certain types of diskettes and formats are compatible with each other. Hard disks have a much higher storage capacity than diskettes and can usually be accessed faster and more efficiently by the computer than diskettes. Their internal organization is less relevant to the user since the disk is in most cases nonremovable from the drive and less frequently used for the exchange of data, and they are therefore usually only characterized by the storage capacity and the average access time. Further mass storage devices are optical or magneto-optical disks, bernoulli boxes, and, primarily for the purpose of the back-up of data, tape streamers.

Input and output devices are connected to the computer through interfaces. Microcomputers are usually equipped with a standardized parallel and serial interface to which the external devices can be connected. Furthermore, most microcomputers provide a number of expansion slots into which the user can fit expansion cards which can be used in order to expand the capabilities of the computer in various respects as required by the respective application. There are different standards for these expansion slots (such as the Extended Industry Standard Architecture, EISA or the Micro Channel).

Different types of printers are available for different applications. The most common printers for microcomputer systems are dot-matrix printers in which the characters are composed of a matrix of dots which are printed by a set of needles operating through a color ribbon. Matrix printers range from quite simple devices at the lower price range up to high-speed and heavy-duty printers, as they are often required in the field of statistical data analysis and educational research. Operating costs of dot-matrix printers are comparatively low. Ink-jet printers operate in a similar way to dot-matrix printers with a matrix, but instead of using needles and a color ribbon ink is transmitted through a jet on to the paper. The quality of the printout of ink-jet printers is higher compared to dot-matrix printers, but disadvantages are the high operating costs and a comparatively low speed. The highest quality printout can be obtained with a laser printer which operates in a similar way to a photocopier. Laser printers belong to the class of nonimpact printers for which a number of page description standards and page description languages (e.g., POSTSCRIPT and PCL) exist, which provide device independent standards for representing a whole page of a printed document.

3.2 Software Components

The software environment is organized into a hierarchy of four entities, of which the first two are required for the basic operation of the microcomputer and the last two are oriented towards the user and the applications.

At the lowest level of the software environment is the basic input/output system (BIOS) which acts as the interface between the hardware and the software environment, and which is specific for the hardware of the corresponding type of microcomputer.

At the next level is the operating system (OS) which: (a) manages the execution of the application programs; (b) handles the input and output operations between all system components, and between the computer and the application programs; and (c) establishes means for storing, retrieving and documenting data. At the beginning of the 1990s the most common operating systems were: (a) MS-DOS as a single-user and single-task operating system; (b) OS/2 and the Macintosh Operating System as single-user and multitasking operating systems (that is, operating systems in which application programs can be executed in parallel); and (c) UNIX as a multiuser and multitasking operating system (in which additionally multiple users can simultaneous work with the microcomputer). MS-DOS is available on many types of microcomputers with a wide range of capacities, but it is limited to rather small applications, whereas OS/2 and UNIX are most suitable for complex and large scale applications on high-capacity microcomputers. The Macintosh Operating System is specific for Macintosh computers and has been designed mainly to support graphical and text-oriented applications. The computer resources required, the amount of data to be processed, and the application software required all need to be considered when deciding on the use of a particular operating system. This decision is critical since possibilities for information exchange between different operating systems are rather restricted and the investment into a particular operating system and the corresponding applications has therefore often long-term consequences.

Many operating systems interact with the user via a graphical user interface (such as the Macintosh user interface, WINDOWS for MS-DOS, and the PRESENTATION MANAGER for OS/2) in which the different objects, such as applications or the functions of the operating systems, are represented by graphical symbols, or icons, with which the user can interact through dialogue boxes that supply and request information about the particular task the user is performing. Graphical user interfaces represent a more user-friendly approach for interacting with the applications or the operating system because the user does not need to memorize a set of instructions together with a syntax in order to instruct the operating system as is required for the user interfaces of conventional operating systems.

At a third level, the programming languages are used which provide the basis for the writing of both operating systems and application programs.

The highest level is formed by the application programs through which the user performs the tasks for which he or she is using the computer. A great variety of application programs is available and the use of programming languages allows the user to create further applications as required. In modern computer systems the typical user can concentrate on the application level and does not need to be concerned with the technical details of lower levels of the software environment, whereas a programmer usually needs to consider all levels of the software environment.

3.3 Microcomputer Networks

One of the strengths of microcomputer systems is that their resources, such as data files, application programs, peripheral devices, and even computing power can be linked and shared in a microcomputer network without giving up the advantages of configuring each microcomputer with individual hard- and software components as required by the corresponding applications and/or users. Microcomputer networks furthermore allow the different users in a network to communicate in various ways. There are various network topologies for physically linking microcomputers in a network, and various concepts for establishing communication within a network. In some networks one of the microcomputers acts as a dedicated server of resources, whereas in other network systems the microcomputers can mutually share resources. A network administration software is used which manages the resources, and the user sees the resource elements rather as logical entities than as physical elements related to a particular microcomputer in the network. Besides linking microcomputers to other microcomputers of the same or a different type in a local area network, microcomputers can also be linked to: (a) minicomputers or mainframe computers; and (b) through external links to public databases, electronic mailboxes, or other remote services.

Thus in a microcomputer network even large educational research projects become manageable in a microcomputer environment. For example, data from a survey can be acquired and stored centrally on one microcomputer which is configured with large secondary storage devices and can then be accessed, processed, and analyzed in various ways by other microcomputers linked to that network. Similarly, through the linkage of one microcomputer in the network to public databases or mainframe systems, all computers in the network can share such resources. However, network systems often have high demands on the application software. In particular, it is necessary to define which classes of users have access to which kinds of operations and resources, and the application software must ensure that the simultaneous access of multiple users to shared resources does not lead to inconsistencies in the data. For example, if modifications to the data of a student in a database are made by one user, the system must ensure that the data field, record, or datafile which is being modified is not accessible for modifications by other users at the same time.

4. Standard Applications of Microcomputers in Education

4.1 Text Processing

The dominant application of microcomputers in educational research is the electronic processing of written documents which has almost completely replaced the repeated manual cutting and pasting of typewritten documents. Computer programs in this area range from simple text editors (e.g., PERSONAL EDITOR) to sophisticated object-oriented graphical systems for text processing (e.g., MS-WORD or WORDPERFECT FOR WINDOWS). Common characteristic features of text processing systems are: (a) editing commands which allow the user to type, correct, cut, paste, copy, and move textual elements; (b) control commands which allow the assignment of certain attributes to textual elements (e.g., letting them appear bold or underlined); and (c) formatting commands which allow the user to align and structure the textual elements and to design the layout. Many text processing systems also allow the integration of mathematical formulas and graphical elements, and come with features for automatic hyphenation, lexicons and thesauruses for the checking of spelling, facilities for making cross-references and footnotes, commands for creating indexes, tables of authorities, tables of contents, and so on, and macroprogramming facilities which allow the user to preprogram frequently used sequences of commands, and to prepare mail-merge documents. In object-oriented text-processing systems textual elements are defined as distinct objects which are assigned the required textual attributes and which can be individually selected, grouped, modified, and moved.

4.2 Desktop Publishing

An application of growing importance is the integration of textual, tabular, and graphical information in a type-set like fashion using desktop publishing methods. This is of particular importance for the reporting of educational research, because graphical and tabular presentations are extensively used. Desktop publishing systems (such as PAGEMAKER or VENTURA PUBLISHER) support a large variety of design elements and methods, and documents of nearly any kind can be edited and designed with these systems so that the user can see the results of the editing process on the screen in such a way that closely resembles the final printed document. The desktop publishing process thereby comprises the steps of: (a) the creation of the textual and graphical elements which are to be incorporated in the document; (b) the definition of the attributes, position, format, and appearance of these elements in the document; and (c) the integration of the elements and their attributes into the final layout. The use of desktop publishing methods gives the writer of a document the possibility to design the appearance of the document in a creative and interactive way, directly controlling the editing process on the screen which is important for the writing of educational research reports where the adequacy of the design elements can often only be judged by the researcher. It can further help to reduce production times and costs substantially, which is critical because the research results need to be published on time and are often produced only in a limited number of copies which makes type-setting methods costly. Educational journals, curriculum materials, as well as survey research instruments, are examples of documents which are often created with desktop publishing methods.

4.3 Data-oriented Graphics

Frequently micro-computer systems are used for the graphical representation of statistical information in reporting the findings of educational research. Microcomputer software packages (such as HARVARD GRAPHICS or MS-CHART) can commonly represent data in multiple forms, such as: (a) line diagrams, (b) pie-charts, (c) bar-charts or histograms, (d) x-y diagrams, or (e) path diagrams.

4.4 Assistance in Survey Sampling and Survey Fieldwork

Microcomputer system can provide researchers with assistance in the design and execution of efficient probability samples for educational surveys leading the researcher through the steps of: (a) initial planning, (b) constraint recognition, (c) specification of sample selection and estimation techniques, (d) execution of the sample selection, and (e) the calculation of sampling weights. Such systems can be based on interactive knowledge-based software with which the researcher can adequately describe the survey by giving as much and as precise information as possible on the relevant components of the survey and sample design. Computer programs can then develop a sample design by optimizing the balance between the different boundary conditions resulting from the survey

constraints on the basis of prespecified optimization criteria. Selecting the sample from a computerized sampling frame can significantly increase the efficiency of the execution of a survey because the identification of the sample units to be selected, as well as the automatic generation of address labels, personalized cover letters, survey monitoring rosters, and reports can be effected with a single operation. Microcomputers are also of growing importance in conducting the fieldwork. Computerized lists of schools and students can be used for the tracking of respondents and nonrespondents, and to facilitate the later entry and clearing of data.

4.5 Coding of Data, Data Entry, and Data Cleaning

In educational surveys, the coding, entry, and cleaning of the collected information can be greatly facilitated through the use of interactive software systems on microcomputer systems. Microcomputer systems can be used for: (a) data coding, that is, the translation of responses obtained from multiple-choice or open-ended questions into numeric codes on the basis of an electronic dictionary or codebook; (b) the immediate recording of data using optical or magnetic character readers, or optical or magnetic mark readers; and (c) for transcriptive data entry procedures which allow the transcription of the written answers of the respondents either to machine readable form or directly into the computer with a software that provides convenient data entry and editing mechanisms. For some of the systems the data entry procedures are linked to an electronic codebook which contains all information about the variables that make up the datafiles including the validation criteria for the variables. Using such systems, deviations of entered data-values from prespecified validation criteria can be found quickly, and cleaning rules employed efficiently to detect and resolve: (a) inconsistencies in the file structure, (b) duplicate or invalid identification codes, (c) out-of-range values, (d) inconsistencies between the data values of a respondent, (e) inconsistencies between the data of different respondents, and (f) problems in the linkage of related respondents or different levels of data aggregation. Computer programs allow checks that range from simple deterministic univariate checks of data up to complex logical or contingency checks involving multiple variables and conditions. The user can then correct possible errors while the original documents are still at hand. Such systems often also have integrated data and file management capabilities including reporting and quality control procedures and are often conveniently linked to software systems for statistical data analysis.

4.6 Database Management

Microcomputers provide a variety of user-friendly and powerful systems for database management which allow both the newcomer and the professional user easy access to database management methods. The dominant candidates in this field were, in 1992, xBASE related systems (e.g., dBASE or FOXBASE). Such database systems organize the data into a set of related datafiles, each consisting of a number of records which represent the observations, for example, students in a survey or documents in a library. Each record has thereby the same structure and is composed of a set of data fields representing the different pieces of information for each observation that are to be handled by the database system.

Microcomputer-based database systems usually have four components: (a) a component that allows the interactive definition of a database through asking the user questions about the characteristics of the information to be stored, such as the identification, type, and length of the data fields; (b) a component that allows the user to enter, modify, copy, move, and delete individual data fields, sets of data fields, or groups of records; (c) a component that allows the user to relate the different data fields and to search, locate, and retrieve information; and (d) a component for reporting the information in various ways and formats. The applications of database systems on microcomputers can range from a small datafile for storing information on the students in a class up to large and powerful database management systems designed to provide detailed information on whole educational systems involving millions of students and their organization into classes, schools, and other educational structures, or databases that provide access to educational documents and literature references.

4.7 Spreadsheet Programs

For the work on simple statistical problems, or for budget preparation and control, spreadsheet programs (such as MS-EXCEL or LOTUS 1-2-3) are often used, which are based on an electronic "worksheet," the columns and rows of which the user can fill with numbers, text, and formulas, and which then can be manipulated and related in various ways. The columns in this worksheet can, for example, contain the planned expenditures for each month in an educational research project with the rows representing different accounts. Through column-wise operations total and subtotal expenditures can then be calculated for the different months and through row-wise operations total and subtotal expenditures for the accounts can be calculated. Common characteristics of spreadsheet systems are: (a) features for manipulating cells, rows, and columns; (b) features for relating cells, rows, columns, and spreadsheets; (c) features for loading, splitting, joining, and saving spreadsheets; and (d) features for reporting the contents of the spreadsheets in various ways.

4.8 Statistical Data Analyses

One of the key applications of microcomputers in educational research is statistical data analysis. A variety of standard software packages for this purpose exists, ranging from spreadsheet programs with integrated statistical functions up to specialized and complex data analysis systems with which the user communicates through a special command syntax, often assisted through menu systems and contextual help (e.g., SAS or SPSS). Such software systems usually offer a wide range of functions and procedures for: (a) reading and storing data in different formats, (b) data manipulations and transformations of various kinds, (c) statistical analysis, ranging from simple univariate calculations up to the application of complex statistical techniques, and (d) reporting and data representation, ranging from simple tabulations up to enhanced graphical representations of the data. With such software packages an educational researcher can generate, access, analyze, and report data and specify data analysis requests with only a minimum of experience in software development and database management. The computing power and the available storage space of modern microcomputer systems allow the use of advanced statistical procedures with datasets from large educational surveys.

4.9 Programming Languages

Even though a broad range of microcomputer application programs exists that suit the needs of most applications in education, some situations in research and administration demand solutions to problems for which there are no standard software packages. A number of programming languages are available on microcomputers with which specific applications can be created (e.g., ASSEMBLER, BASIC, C, FORTRAN, and PASCAL). These range from languages close to the machine-level, such as ASSEMBLER, up to block-structured high level programming languages such as PASCAL.

5. Conclusion

Microcomputers have made the possibilities of electronic data processing available to a large community of educational researchers, offering a wide range of applications ranging from the preparation of research reports up to the management and analysis of complex survey data. It can be expected that the speed and power of microcomputers will continue to increase dramatically, thus further extending the capabilities and the range of the applications, allowing, for example, educational researchers to perform new and more sophisticated kinds of statistical data analyses on microcomputers which by now are limited to mainframe systems or not manageable at all. At the same time user interfaces will become more user-friendly, supported by a more intuitive graphical representation and new kinds of input/output devices involving spoken language, and so further extend the range of potential users of microcomputers.

Bibliography

Madron T W, Tate C N, Broakshine R G 1985 *Using Micro-computers in Research*. Sage University Paper series on Quantitative Applications in the Social Sciences, 07–052. Sage, Beverly Hills, California

Palmer W J 1983 Micro-computers in survey research. *Interface Age 8* (December): 69–74

Rosenthal L S 1986 *Integrated Software for Microcomputer Systems*. National Bureau of Standards Special Publi-cation 500–135. Institute for Computer Sciences and Technology, Washington, DC

Scholz C 1989 *Einführung in das Personal Computing*. de Gruyter, New York

Schrodt P A 1984 *Micro-Computer Methods for Social Scientists*. University Paper Series, Quantitative Application in the Social Sciences, 07–001. Sage, Beverly Hills, California

Tausworthe R C 1977 *Standardized Development of Computer Software*. Eaglewood Cliffs, New Jersey

Models and Model Building

J. P. Keeves

There is a stage in the conduct of inquiry in any field, after variables have been identified as influencing a particular outcome, or hypotheses have been advanced for explanation in relation to a particular problem, when the interrelations between the elements or the hypotheses which have been formulated need to be combined together into a hypothetical model. The essential characteristic of a model is the proposed structure of the model which is used in the investigation of interrelations between the elements.

Research in education is concerned with the action of many factors, simultaneously or in a causal sequence in a problem situation. Thus it is inevitable that research in the field of education should make use of models in the course of its inquiries to portray the interrelations between the factors involved. This entry is concerned with the types of models that are being employed in educational research and the advantages and the dangers of model building. In addition, the entry gives examples of some powerful models that have been employed in educational research and considers their contribution to the undertaking of inquiry in areas where prediction or explanation is being sought in relation to particular problems.

1. Theories and Models

It is important to recognize that the term "model" is not synonymous with the term "theory." In the investigation of a problem situation a set of hypotheses may be proposed for testing and confirmation or rejection. The hypotheses to be investigated are developed from intuition, from earlier studies, and from theoretical considerations. If they are sustained and can be generalized they will contribute to theory, but until they are confirmed they remain heuristic devices that have been proposed in the course of inquiry. However, as part of an inquiry it may be necessary to consider the hypotheses in abstract and to advance a model that provides a structure for the interrelations which are proposed between the set of hypotheses. The model, like the hypotheses which are contained within it, can be built from accumulated evidence, intuition by analogy, or derived from theory. As Kaplan (1964) has pointed out, a theory may state that the subject matter under investigation should exhibit a certain structure, but the structure is not necessarily part of the theory itself. Kaplan has also stated that the term "model" is useful

only when the symbolic system it refers to is significant as a structure—a system which allows for exact deductions and explicit correspondences. The value of the model lies in part in its abstractness, so that it can be given many interpretations, which thereby reveal unexpected similarities. The value also lies in the deductive fertility of the model, so that unexpected consequences can be predicted and then tested by observation and experiment (see *Scientific Methods in Educational Research*).

To the research worker, model building and the testing of models are merely two of the strategies that can be employed in inquiry. They are not to be confused with either theory or scientific investigation as such.

In order to be useful a model should fulfil the following requirements.

(a) A model should lead to the prediction of consequences that can be verified by observation. This implies that it should be possible to design critical tests of the model using empirical evidence, and if the tests are not sustained, the model should be rejected.

(b) The structure of a model should desirably reveal something of the causal mechanisms which are involved in the subject matter being investigated. Thus the model should contribute not only to prediction, but also to explanation.

(c) Insofar as a model contributes to explanation it should become an aid to the imagination in the formulation of new concepts and new relationships and thus extension of inquiry.

(d) A model should contain structural relationships rather than associative relationships. However, correlational and regression relations which are essentially associative in nature are of value during the early stages of investigation, since they may identify the variables that are important and reveal something about the form of the relationships to be sought. Thus, both correlation and regression can contribute to model building.

It will be clear from the above discussion that a model is explicit and definite. Models can be built, tested, and if necessary rebuilt in the course of inquiry. They relate to theory and may be derived from theory, but they are conceptually different from theory itself.

2. The Shortcomings of Models

Several dangers exist in the use of models. The first danger arises from the fact that the model involves simplification. Without the simplification which is associated with the abstractness of the model, there would be nothing to be gained from building the model. However, one danger that arises lies in oversimplification. Kaplan (1964) in this context refers to the well-known principle of the "drunkard's search," in which the drunkard searches under the street lamp for his house key, when he dropped it some distance away, because "it's lighter here." Thus the danger of oversimplification in the use of a model is not that the model is built incorrectly but, that in the process of abstraction, the model has been built with simplification that has been extended too far.

The second major danger arising from the use of models is that significance might be attached to aspects of the model which do not belong to the structure of the model but to the particular symbols that have been employed in the model. Likewise, there is a danger arising from an overemphasis on the form in which the model is expressed. A forced analogy, an inappropriate metaphor, the unwarranted use of a mathematical formulation, or the inappropriate use of a diagrammatic representation can all, in certain circumstances, serve to conceal rather than reveal the basic structure of the model which holds underlying relationships that could be tested and verified. Nevertheless, the use of a symbolic or diagrammatic form can often serve to make explicit and definite the structure of the model that would otherwise remain hidden in an excess of words.

3. Testing the Model

Perhaps the greater danger that is prevalent in educational research today is that of building or developing a single model, or perhaps alternative models, to serve the purposes of explanation, but without concern for the need for testing the models through the use of empirical evidence. The purpose of building a model, like that of advancing hypotheses, is that the model should be submitted to the test. Consequently, the dangers of model building are not only those of oversimplification or of the inappropriate use of symbols or of form, but rather that the models are not sufficiently specific for their consequences to be worked out with adequate precision and for an appropriate test to be applied. The strength of certain types of models, for example, models expressed in mathematical form, is that they lend themselves more readily to data collection and to testing.

Traditionally, in research in the social and behavioral sciences there has been heavy reliance on the testing of mathematical models by statistical techniques. In the field of educational research the significance test still has an important place (see *Significance Testing*). However, the shortcomings of testing for statistical significance at the expense of recognition of general consistency and pattern in the results obtained is being recognized (Pillemar 1991). Moreover, there is increased interest in assessing the strength of a relationship rather than likelihood of occurrence (Mohr 1990).

In addition, there is another aspect of checking a model against empirical data, namely the estimation of the parameters of the model. From the estimated parameters it becomes possible to make predictions in order to test the generality of the model both from location to location and across time. It is clear that model building, data collection, and the testing of the model must be seen as integrated activities. The structure of the model influences the data to be collected and the data are essential for the verification of the model and the estimation of its parameters. Nevertheless, it should be recognized that the testing of the model may lead to rebuilding or reformulating. The importance, however, of checking a model against empirical evidence must be stressed. Without this step the building of the model has been a pointless exercise. The test against empirical evidence is the only means of establishing the validity of the model, of improving realism, and of making an effective contribution through model building to theoretical knowledge. It is also necessary to recognize that, while the model itself has heuristic value in the development of theory, it is not essential to the establishment of theory in education or any other field of scientific knowledge.

4. Types of Models

Several types of models have been identified by Kaplan (1964) and Tatsuoka (1968), and while the classification that follows draws on both these sources it diverges in certain notable ways from them, in part because of developments that have occurred in education and the social sciences in the years that have intervened since these articles were written.

4.1 Analogue Models

A common and important class comprises those models that are related to a physical system, and it is perhaps not surprising that such models should be widely used in the physical sciences, relatively uncommon in the social and behavioral sciences, and rare in the field of education. Such models are referred to as analogue models. The development of the model of the atom through the successive stages of the "currant bun model" to the "planetary model" to the "wave model" has involved the use of appropriate analogues as were consistent with the evidence available at the time. In advancing such models, correspondences are necessary between the elements of the model and the elements occurring in the problem situation under investigation. Such correspondence which is clear in the use of analogue models, extends to the use of other types of models, although the correspondences may be less explicitly defined. It is important to note the presence of one of the dangers associated with the use of models, namely that there is no guarantee that the correspondences will continue to hold beyond those which have been deliberately introduced by the builder of the model. Clearly such models have limited utility for, while they may furnish the research worker with plausible hypotheses for testing, they generally preclude the making of deductions from the model.

A model of a school population An example of an analogue model used in educational work, which has been taken from the field of demography, is that of a water tank with inlet and outlet pipes to represent the student population of a school system. The inlet pipes correspond to: (a) the intake controlled by the birthrate; (b) the intake as influenced by the rate of immigration, including both external and internal immigration with allowance made for age-specific migration rates; (c) the reception rate into school at ages below the lower age of compulsory schooling; and (d) the return intake to schooling at age levels beyond the upper age of compulsory education, using age-specific return rates. The outlet pipes correspond to: (e) the outflow by emigration, with allowance made for age-specific emigration rates, and (f) the outflow by departure from school using age-specific monthly departure rates. Estimation of the parameters of the model at a particular point in time using data collected over previous years would enable predictions to be made for the size of the school population of the system at a future point in time. The main value of the model that has been developed is for the explanation of changes in the student population and the subsequent predictions that can be made for planning and policy-making. Moreover, the predictions can be used to test

the validity of the model, and the accuracy of the parameters that have been estimated as well as to assess the rates of change in the parameters that are occurring (see *Projections of Educational Statistics*).

4.2 Semantic Models

The essential feature of such models is that they are expressed in verbal form. Frequently such models employ figures of speech or metaphors. Since all language involves the use of metaphors and figures of speech, to a greater or lesser extent, semantic models that are expressed in verbal form can also be referred to as figurative or metaphoric models. However, since the figure of speech is not always explicit, the use of the term "semantic model" would seem preferable for this very common class of model. It should be noted that semantic models provide a conceptual analogue to the subject matter under consideration rather than a physical analogue. A common deficiency of such models is their lack of precision which renders them not readily amenable to testing. However, because they are expressed in verbal form, they provide a valuable explanation of the subject matter that, in general, is readily understood. Semantic models are in common use in the field of educational research. Many are widely disseminated, but few have been subjected to rigorous testing, and hence have failed to serve the heuristic purposes which would justify their construction.

A model of school learning An example of a semantic model that has served an extremely important function since the early 1970s insofar as it has led to extensive and successful attempts to validate relationships within the model is the "model of school learning" proposed by Carroll (1963). The model contains five elements, three of which are associated with the individual student, and two of which arise from external conditions. Carroll initially formulated the model in the following words:

> Factors in the individual are (a) aptitude—the amount of time needed to learn the task under optimal instructional conditions, (b) ability to understand instruction, and (c) perseverance—the amount of time the learner is willing to engage actively in learning. Factors in external conditions are (d) opportunity—time allowed for learning, and (e) the quality of instruction—a measure of the degree to which instruction is presented so that it will not require additional time for mastery beyond that required in view of aptitude. (Carroll 1963 p. 729)

It should be noted that three of the five factors are expressed in terms of time, and it is this property of the factors contained within the model that has made it relatively easy for the constituent relationships of the model to be submitted to verification with empirical data. Carroll, in his presentation of the model, also states that both quality of instruction and ability to understand instruction are quantities that are interrelated to variables that can be measured in terms of time. Consequently they can be submitted to statistical testing. From this model the degree of learning for any individual on a task is tentatively expressed in functional form, as a "ratio of the amount of time the learner actually spends on the learning task to the total amount he needs". Thus:

Degree of learning =
$$f \text{ (time actually spent/time needed)}$$
(Carroll 1963 p. 730).

Initially, this model was not submitted to verification, but in the 1980s a considerable body of research was accumulated to provide support for the general validity of the model (Denham and Lieberman 1980, Anderson 1984). While it is still premature to express the model of school learning in a more precise mathematical form, considerable progress has been made in establishing that the elements of the model are related in the ways that Carroll proposed, thus confirming facets of the structure of the model that Carroll advanced. It is also significant that other research workers in education have used the model as a starting point for the development of theories of school learning. Bloom (1976) has advanced a theory in relation to mastery learning; Cooley and Lohnes (1976) have proposed steps toward a theory in relation to the evaluation of schooling; and Harnischfeger and Wiley (1976) proposed a view of the teaching–learning process in elementary schools based upon the concept of time as part of a more general model of schooling.

It should be noted that both Carroll's model and the Harnischfeger and Wiley perspective identify a set of elements and propose relationships between them. The models do not explain the causal processes which underlie these relationships. Moreover, they do not contribute to the specification of these relationships in precise functional form. Nevertheless, there is the implicit assumption in their presentations of the existence of causal relationships, and the expectation that from further empirical research it will be possible to express the relationships more explicitly in terms of a mathematical model and hence make a significant contribution toward a theory of school learning.

4.3 Schematic Models

A schematic model, as Popper and Eccles (1977) point out, is like a map and generally serves to group and cluster constructs into an ordered relationship. The schematic model serves as a link between theory and the real world. It is like a map that links the world of the products of analysis and investigation with the world of observable objects.

Many psychologists have sought to develop models of intelligence and their investigations have led them to postulate models that can be portrayed in diagrammatic form (Vernon 1950). The most detailed model is that advanced by Guilford (1967) for the "Structure of Intellect." In this schematic model a three dimensional grid has been drawn to show content, products, and operations, and tests have been devised to provide instruments to measure performance in each of the 120 cells of the grid. The quest for a coherent model of intelligence continues (see *Models of Intelligence*).

4.4 Mathematical Models

While mathematical models have been used increasingly since the early 1960s in the behavioral and social sciences, including uses in psychology that have a bearing on educational problems, there have been very few uses of mathematical models directly in the field of educational research. There have, however, been many instances where a measurement model has been used in the field of education, but this involves a generalized model being applied to a measurement problem, rather than the development of a specific mathematical model for use in a particular problem situation. Nevertheless, it is being increasingly recognized in the behavioral and social sciences that mathematical models have an important contribution to make in the advancement of theory, and it would seem likely that there will be greater use made of mathematical models in educational research in the decades ahead.

Tatsuoka (1968) has drawn attention to the fact that before a mathematical model is advanced there must already exist either an informal theory or a semantic model for the problem situation. The building of a mathematical model involves a degree of sophistication and a degree of understanding of the problem that is highly unlikely to arise prior to the establishment of informal theory or the confirmation of a semantic model.

The advantages of a mathematical model are many in addition to elegance and parsimony. The model involves the advancement of basic assumptions and postulates that are made explicit and are thus open to scrutiny and questioning. It permits the derivation of explicit quantitative predictions that can be tested with empirical data, and it lays the foundations for a more formal theory built around the causal relationships that are implicitly or explicitly contained within the model.

The confluence model One application of a mathematical model to an educational problem has been made by Zajonc and his co-workers with respect to the birth order problem. The principle of primogeniture is well-established in most societies, and thus there has been longstanding recognition that the firstborn, especially the firstborn male child, receives preferential treatment. Furthermore, there is worldwide evidence that increasing family size is consistently related to decreasing intellectual performance. Anomalies which have been observed have tended to disappear after controlling for socioeconomic status. However, much of the evidence that has been collected during the twentieth century from educational and psychological research has shown inconsistent findings for birth order and such characteristics as intellectual development. Belmont and Marolla (1973) reported findings from a very large sample of no fewer than 380,000 cases for male youths aged 19 years which showed strong and consistent relationships between birth order and intellectual performance on the Raven Progressive Matrices test for successive family sizes. The magnitude of the effects reported is shown by the fact that the highest of the observed values for the firstborn of a family of two exceeded the lastborn of a family of six by approximately two-thirds of a standard deviation. These data on family size and birth order exhibited five important relationships: (a) intelligence scores decreased with increasing family size; (b) within family size, intelligence scores declined with increasing birth order; (c) with the exception of the lastborn child, there appeared to be a reduction in the rate of decline with higher birth orders; (d) the deceleration in the trend with birth order was not observed for the lastborn who exhibited a discontinuous drop in intellectual performance; and (e) the only child also showed a discontinuity, scoring at a level approximately the same as that of the firstborn of a family of four.

In explaining the effects of family size on intellectual development, the influence of the educational environment of the home on the individual has been commonly used. It has been generally acknowledged that the educational level of the parents and the reading resources of the home contribute to the intellectual home background of the child. Thus, it was within this historical context, based on informal theory concerning the educational environment of the home, that Zajonc and Markus (1975) set out to develop a mathematical model which would account for the strong evidence presented by Belmont and Marolla (1973).

The "confluence model" that Zajonc and Markus (1975) advanced was built around the concept of mutual intellectual influences among family members as children develop within the family environment. The primary emphasis was on the intellectual environment of the child and in particular on the intellectual level of the individual's siblings and parents during the course of development. A reparameterized version of this model was presented by Zajonc et al. (1979) to account for the conflicting results reported in the birth order literature. In the first paper (Zajonc and Markus 1975), it was assumed that the effects of family configuration could be represented by a sigmoid function of age:

$$M_t = 1 - \exp[-k^2 t^2] \tag{1}$$

where t is age in years and k is an arbitrary constant associated with the type of intellectual ability involved. In the reparameterized version (Zajonc et al. 1979), rate of intellectual growth was hypothesized to be a function of intellectual development within the family, α, and a factor λ which was associated with the special circumstances of the last children. Thus the level of mental maturity $[M_{ij(t)}]$ achieved at age t by the *ith* child in a family of j children in a household of n persons was expressed by the equation,

$$M_{ij(t)} = M_{ij(t-1)} + \alpha_i + \lambda_i \tag{2}$$

The two parameters α_i *and* λ_i are expressed as weighted yearly increments of the sigmoid function M_t where

$$\Delta f(t) = (1 - \exp[-k^2 t^2]) - (1 - \exp[-k^2 \{t-1\}^2])$$
$$= \exp[-k^2\{t-1\}^2] - \exp[-k^2 t^2]$$

Then

$$\alpha_i = \omega_1 \Delta f(t) \left[\frac{\sum\limits_{i=1}^{n} M_{in\ (t-1)}^2}{n_{(t-1)} + 1} \right]^{1/2} \tag{3}$$

and

$$\lambda_t = \frac{\omega_2 L_t \Delta(f)\Delta(\tau)}{(n-1)^2} \tag{4}$$

The terms ω_1 and ω_2 are weights associated with the two components; τ is the age of the adjacent younger sibling; and L_t is the last child index.

Using simulation procedures, the confluence model predicted accurately the data recorded in six large national surveys of intellectual performance in relation to family configuration factors when all three parameters k_1, ω_1 and ω_2 were used. When the third parameter ω_2 was held constant, little accuracy was lost. The variations in the estimated values of the parameters that reflected the variations in the patterns of effects could be interpreted in a meaningful way in terms of the psychological theory. Thus the confluence model was found to account for the data available on birth order and intellectual performance. The values of the growth constant k were highest for the American data, were very similar for the Dutch, French, and Scottish data, and were nearly twice the size for the Western Israeli sample as for the Oriental Israeli sample. It should be noted that the three Western European samples were cross-sectional samples from the total national population, while the American and the two Israeli samples were selective and not representative of their respective national populations. The values of best fit for the parameter ω_1 associated with the intellectual environment within the family showed a perfect inverse relationship with the ages at testing of the six samples and were consistent with the assumption that the impact of the family intellectual environment decreased as the age of the child increased and with changes in family structure. The values obtained for the parameter ω_2 associated with the handicap for the last born child, indicated how much elder siblings gained from serving as a resource for the intellectual development of the lastborn. For fuller details of the findings and the interpretation of the results of this study which employed simulation procedures to estimate the parameters of the model, Zajonc and Bargh (1980a) should be consulted. In summary, the findings indicated that when an additional child joined the family, two significant changes could be assumed to take place in the intellectual development of the older child. First, the educative environment of the family was diminished as a consequence of the addition of the new child, and second, the older child acquired a teaching role within the family which had positive consequences for the intellectual development of the older child. It is interesting to note that the decline in the quality of the educational environment as a consequence of the addition of a child to the family initially exceeded the benefits that arose from the teaching role. However, the rate of decline was such that the benefits could surpass the losses and a reversal in intellectual performance could arise. Such reversals were shown to occur before the age of 14 years.

The confluence model advanced by Zajonc and his colleagues has also been used to predict changes in achievement test scores over time. Associated with changes in birthrate there will be changes in average order of birth. An increase in birthrate will be accompanied by larger families and a correspondingly lower average birth order. Since the confluence model predicts a decline in intellectual performance with an increase in birth order, there should be changes in average achievement test scores corresponding to changes in the birthrate and the associated variables, family size, and average birth order. Data from elementary-school populations for the states of Iowa and New York in the United States, confirmed the predicted relationships.

Further confirmation of the confluence model came from the performance of a large sample (nearly 800,000) of high school students on the National Merit Scholarship Qualification Test in the United States. However, an examination of student performance on the Scholastic Aptitude Test, a test employed for admission to college-level studies in the United States with respect to family configuration, has shown that only a negligible proportion of the decline in the Scholastic Aptitude Test scores between 1965 and 1977 could be attributed to birth order and family size. However, it was considered possible that the samples used to test the predictions in Scholastic Aptitude Test scores were both too small and not representative enough of the population to show the trends that were predicted (Zajonc and Bargh 1980b).

The confluence model provides an excellent example of a mathematical model that has been developed in the field of educational research from informal theory and from prior research findings and tested with large bodies of data. The use of computer-based simulation procedures to estimate the parameters of the model and to validate the model is of particular interest. Furthermore, the application of this model to predict trends and to explain fluctuations in achievement test data over time illustrates well the manner in which models can be used. It should be noted that the confluence model is not a theory, but its confirmation does provide strong support for theories of the educational environment of the home.

Nevertheless, the confluence model has been strongly criticized. Galbraith (1982) has drawn attention to mathematical inconsistencies in the model. In addition, Scott-Jones has reviewed reports of studies where the evidence fails to support the model and has contended that "efforts need to be directed toward the study of the specific mechanisms within the child's environment through which family configuration might affect cognitive development" (Scott-Jones 1984 p. 270).

4.5 Causal Models

Since the early 1970s there has been increasing use of causal models in the field of educational research. The employment of causal models derives from work in the field of genetics associated with the analytical technique of path analysis. Rudimentary use was made of path analysis in the field of education by Burks (1928) but the procedure lay dormant for over 40 years in education until used by Peaker (1971) in England. This revival of interest in path analysis was built on the seminal work of Blalock (1961) concerned with the making of causal inferences in nonexperimental research. Subsequent work in sociology drew on earlier developments in the fields of genetics and econometrics and a new approach to models and model building became available for use in educational research.

The procedures employed for the development of causal models enable the investigator to move from a verbal statement or a semantic model of a complex set of interrelationships between variables to a more precise one in which the principles of path analysis and a set of structural equations are employed. The use of diagrams to portray the interrelations are of assistance, but are not essential to the procedures by which the set of linear equations is constructed to specify the relationships between the variables in the causal model. It is the use of the set of structural equations that has led to the introduction of a further name for the procedures, that is "structural equation models."

The essential idea of a causal model involves the building of a simplified structural equation model of the causal process operating between the variables under consideration. The model is constructed using knowledge gained from substantive theory, and from previous research, and the model is written as a set of linear equations each representing a causal relationship hypothesized to act between the variables. From these structural equations the parameters of the model may be estimated and the model and its component parts evaluated. As an outcome the model is either confirmed or rejected for reformulation to provide an alternative that could also be tested with the available data.

For a large class of causal models, such as those

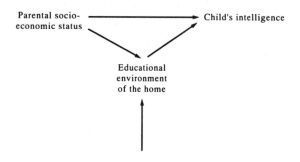

Figure 1
The standard deprivation model

advanced in educational research, in which the model is recursive, the procedures of ordinary least squares regression analysis can be used to obtain solutions to the set of linear equations of a causal model. There are, however, other analytic procedures that can be used to obtain solutions to more complex models.

Models of the home environment. Williams (1976) has made a significant contribution to the understanding of the manner in which the home environment might operate to influence the development of intellectual ability of a child through the construction and estimation of causal models to describe the situation.

The first model shown in Fig. 1 (from Eckland 1971) is the standard deprivation model which is commonly employed to account for relationships between parental socioeconomic status, the educational environment of the home, and the child's intelligence. This model denies the possibility that the child could inherit from its parents genetic material that might influence the growth of the child's intelligence. Thus while this model is widely used in educational research, although rarely in an explicit form, it can be argued to be deficient.

A second causal model is shown in Fig. 2 in which provision is made for the possibility that the child has inherited from its parents genetic material that will affect in part the intellectual ability of the child.

This second model denies the possibility that the

child might influence the type of educational environment provided by the parents as a consequence of the child's level of intellectual ability. A third causal model is shown in Fig. 3 in which provision is made for the reciprocal influence between the educational environment of the home and the child's intelligence. However, in order to solve the linear equations of a causal model in which a reciprocal effect is included it is necessary to introduce into the model an instrumental variable which influences one of the reciprocating variables but not the other. It is not always possible to identify an appropriate instrumental variable. However, in this situation the research on the confluence model considered above would appear to indicate that family size is likely to influence the growth of the child's intelligence only indirectly through the educational environment of the home rather than exert a direct influence on the child's genetic composition. Thus family size can be included in the model as an instrumental variable as shown in Fig. 3.

The models shown in Figs. 1 and 2 are both recursive models and can be readily estimated by ordinary least squares regression analysis. The model shown in Fig. 3, is a nonrecursive model because of the reciprocating effect but the linear equations of this model can be solved by indirect regression analysis or by two-stage least squares regression analysis procedures. Further, with the inclusion of family size as a variable in the model it is questionable whether parental socioeconomic status exerts a direct causal effect on the child's intelligence, or acts only indirectly through family size and the educational environment of the home. However, this issue is perhaps best left to be determined by the magnitudes of the path coefficients which are estimated for the model from empirical data.

Williams (1976) measured the dimensions of the environment of the home of a sample of Canadian children and with data on the other components estimated the parameters of models similar to the ones shown above. He has shown that the environment of the home has a significant influence on the child's intelligence, but more importantly he has shown that

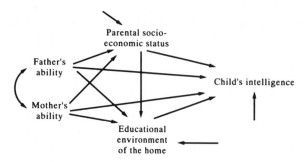

Figure 2
Inheritance of ability model

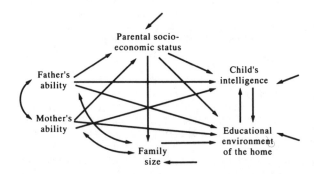

Figure 3
Mutual influence of environment and intelligence model

392

the influence of the child's intelligence back on the environment of the home is too large to be ignored. Thus in Williams's model, which is sustained by the data available, not only is a child advantaged or disadvantaged by the socioeconomic status of the parents as is commonly acknowledged, but the child is further advantaged or disadvantaged by inheritance from the parents. In addition, the child from a high-status home, with parents of high ability, is likely to be further advantaged by the influence that a high-ability child can exert over the level of the educational environment of the home to benefit his or her further intellectual development.

The causal models analyzed by Williams may suffer from oversimplification of an extremely complex problematic situation. Nevertheless, they do provide an enhanced understanding of the factors that contribute to influencing the development of a child's intelligence and they provide the means by which attempts can be made to estimate the effects of the major factors that would seem to contribute to the intellectual ability of a child.

It is important to note that a distinction should be made between causal models that are deterministic in nature and those that are probabilistic or stochastic in nature. In the former case it is assumed that since A causes B, then the manipulation of A leads to the complete prediction of B, from a knowledge of the specified model, provided all other causes of B in the model are held constant. Such models would appear to arise in the physical sciences in some situations but not in others. In education and the social sciences the causal models developed are probabilistic or stochastic in nature, insofar as B cannot be predicted entirely from A, and an error or disturbance term must be introduced into the model. Even if the model were well specified with all appropriate predictors included, the model would remain probabilistic in nature. However, parameters indicating the strength of a relationship can be estimated. The effects of erratic or random disturbances remain and are also estimated.

5. Conclusion

Since the early 1960s there has been an increased use of models and model building in educational research, especially through the use of causal models. These developments have occurred partly as a result of the availability of computers to undertake the extensive calculation necessary to test quantitative relationships in mathematical and causal models, and, in addition, to obtain estimates of the parameters of such models. In part, too, these developments have taken place as the result of work done in other fields, in particular, the social and behavioral sciences. Nevertheless, the use of semantic models still dominates the field of educational research. As a consequence, the use of causal models is still not common and the use

of mathematical models in educational research is extremely rare.

In this entry, models have been referred to that are being investigated in relation to the educational environment of the home, intelligence, and school learning. These are three areas that are central to the process of education, and this work indicates that advances are continuing to be made in the development of theory in these important areas through the use of models and model building. It would seem probable that if further progress is to be made in the development of theory in other areas of the field of education, increased use should be made of mathematical and causal models, and the scientific research methods associated with the use of modeling procedures.

References

Anderson L W (ed.) 1984 *Time and School Learning: Theory, Research and Practice*. Croom Helm, London
Belmont L, Marolla F A 1973 Birth order, family size, and intelligence. *Science* 182: 1096–101
Blalock H M Jr 1961 *Causal Inferences in Nonexperimental Research*. Norton, New York
Bloom B S 1976 *Human Characteristics and School Learning*. McGraw-Hill, New York
Burks B S 1928 The relative influence of nature and nurture upon mental development: A comparative study of foster parent–foster child resemblance and true parent–true child resemblance. *National Society for the Study of Education Yearbook* 17: 219–316
Carroll J B 1963 A model of school learning. *Teach. Coll. Rec.* 64: 723–33
Cooley W W, Lohnes P R 1976 *Evaluation Research in Education*. Irvington, New York
Denham C, Lieberman A (eds.) 1980 *Time to Learn*. National Institute of Education, Washington, DC
Eckland B K 1971 Social class structure and the genetic basis of intelligence. In: Cancro R (ed.) 1971 *Intelligence, Genetic and Environmental Influences*. Grune and Stratton, New York
Galbraith R C 1982 Sibling spacing and intellectual development: A closer look at the confluence models. *Dev. Psychol.* 18(2): 151–73
Guilford J P 1967 *The Nature of Human Intelligence*. McGraw-Hill, New York
Harnischfeger A, Wiley D E 1976 The Teaching–learning process in elementary schools: A synoptic view. *Curric. Inq.* 6(1): 5–43
Kaplan A 1964 *The Conduct of Inquiry: Methodology for Behavioral Science*. Chandler, San Francisco, California
Mohr L B 1990 *Understanding Significance Testing*. Sage, Newbury Park, California
Peaker G F 1971 *The Plowden Children Four Years Later*. National Foundation for Educational Research (NFER), Slough
Pillemer D B 1991 One- versus two-tailed hypothesis tests in contemporary educational research. *Educ. Researcher* 20(9): 13–17
Popper K R and Eccles J C 1977 *The Self and Its Brain*. Routledge and Kegan Paul, London

Scott-Jones D 1984 Family influences on cognitive development and school achievement. *Rev. Res. Educ.* 11: 268–71

Tatsuoka M M 1968 Mathematical models in the behavioral and social sciences. In: Whitla D K (ed.) 1968 *Handbook of Measurement and Assessment in Behavioral Sciences*. Addison-Wesley, Reading, Massachusetts

Vernon P E 1950 *The Structure of Human Abilities*. Methuen, London

Williams T H 1976 Abilities and environments. In: Sewell W H, Hauser R M, Featherman D L (eds.) 1976 *Schooling and Achievement in American Society*. Academic Press, New York

Zajonc R B, Bargh J 1980a The confluence model: Parameter and estimation for six divergent data sets on family factors and intelligence. *Intelligence* 4(4): 349–62

Zajonc R B, Bargh J 1980b Birth order, family size and decline of SAT scores. *Am. Psychol.* 35(7): 662–68

Zajonc R B, Markus G B 1975 Birth order and intellectual development. *Psychol. Rev.* 82(1): 74–88

Zajonc R B, Markus H, Markus G B 1979 The birth order puzzle. *J. Pers. Soc. Psychol.* 37(8): 1325–41

Multilevel Analysis

J. P. Keeves and N. Sellin

Many investigations into educational problems are concerned with two basic types of variables: (a) measures of the properties of individual students; (b) measures of the properties of groups of students. This occurs because students are customarily brought together into classes for the purposes of instruction by teachers; classes are grouped together in schools; and schools are linked together into larger units, such as school districts, for administrative purposes. Problems arise in educational research in the analysis of data collected at two or more levels as a consequence of the fact that it is rarely possible to assign students randomly to treatment or control groups in an experimental study, or to allocate the groups by random selection to receive the treatment or stand as the control. In addition, naturally occurring groups of students are found, in general, to contain members who are more like each other than they are like the members of other groups. The clustering of students into groups with similar characteristics means that, unless it can be shown that the groups do not differ significantly from each other, it is generally inappropriate to pool students from different groups into a combined group for the purposes of analysis. The problems that occur in the analysis of the data do not arise only because it has been necessary to sample first schools or classrooms and then to sample students within schools or classrooms, but also because the characteristics of the students commonly influence the treatments they receive in the groups.

In truly experimental studies, where random allocation of students to treatment and control groups has taken place, analysis of variance and covariance procedures can be employed. However, since random assignment can rarely be fully carried out, in both quasi-experimental studies and those in which data are collected from natural situations, statistical control must be exercised in the analysis of data through regression and related procedures in order to examine the effects of both individual and group level variables.

Formerly the issue associated with the appropriate level of analysis was considered to be influenced largely by the nature of the research questions to which answers were sought (e.g., whether the problem was concerned with individual students or with classroom groups) as well as by the level at which sampling had taken place and at which generalization to other situations was sought. More recently it has become apparent that a multilevel analysis strategy is required if appropriate answers are to be obtained. These issues were raised by Cronbach et al. (1976) and many aspects of this problem have been addressed by Burstein (1980). In addition they were admirably treated by Finn (1974) in the analysis of data from rigorous experimental studies, where unequal numbers of students were clustered in treatment and control groups. However, it is becoming increasingly apparent that strategies of multilevel analysis are required for the effective examination of data collected in schools and classrooms in quasi-experimental studies. This entry seeks to expose the nature of these analytical problems and to develop a multilevel approach to analysis for the examination of such data, where regression and related statistical procedures are involved.

1. Levels of Analysis

Since the publication of the article by Robinson (1950) on the problems associated with ecological correlations and the making of inferences about the behavior of individuals from data analyzed at the group level, there has been a general awareness that consideration had to be given to the appropriate level of analysis to be employed in handling data in which correlation and regression coefficients were reported. Three different levels of analysis have been available, and the question has been which of these three levels should be employed.

1.1 Between Students Over All Groups

At this level of analysis the data from different groups are pooled and a single analysis is carried out between all students in the total sample. In symbols a regression analysis of this type with two predictor variables can be stated as follows:

$$Y_{ij} = b_0 + b_1 X_{ij} + b_2 G_{ij} + \varepsilon_{ij} \qquad (1)$$

where Y_{ij} is the criterion variable, X_{ij} is a student predictor variable, G_{ij} is a group predictor variable (G_j), $j = 1, \ldots, J$ for groups, $i = 1, \ldots, n_j$ for students within groups, $N = \sum_{j=1}^{j} n_j$ for the total number of students, and ε_{ij} is the random error.

It should be noted that the group variable G_j has been disaggregated to the student level. This type of analysis was used exclusively in the First International Mathematics Study (Husén 1967), and was widely used in many investigations during the following two decades.

1.2 Between Groups

In this type of analysis data are aggregated by group, and the mean value for each group forms the criterion variable. Likewise, the student data for each predictor variable are aggregated by group, and group data for a group-level predictor variable need not be disaggregated. In symbols a regression analysis of this type with two predictor variables can be stated as follows:

$$Y_{\cdot j} = c_0 + c_1 X_{\cdot j} + c_2 G_j + \alpha_j \qquad (2)$$

where $Y_{\cdot j}$ is the mean value of the criterion variable (Y_{ij}) for group j, $X_{\cdot j}$ is the mean value for the predictor variable (X_{ij}) for group j, G_j is a group predictor variable, and α_j is the random error.

This level of analysis was used together with the between-students overall analysis in the examination of the data collected in the International Association for the Evaluation of Educational Achievement (IEA) Six Subject Study (Peaker 1975), and has been relatively widely used in other investigations.

1.3 Between Students Within Groups

In this type of analysis the measures for each student are subtracted from the group mean and thus the deviation values from the group mean are employed. Moreover, the data for all groups are pooled for a combined analysis. It is clearly not possible to include group level variables in such analyses. In symbols a regression analysis of this type with two predictor variables can be stated as follows:

$$(Y_{ij} - Y_{\cdot j}) = w_1(X_{1ij} - X_{1 \cdot j}) + w_2 (X_{2ij} - X_{2\cdot j}) + \delta_{ij} \qquad (3)$$

where X_{1ij} and X_{2ij} are two student predictor variables

and δ_{ij} is random error and the remaining symbols are defined above. This type of analysis together with the between groups type of analysis were used in the examination of the data collected in the Plowden National Survey in England (Peaker 1967).

1.4 Grouping Analysis

A fourth mode of analysis is sometimes employed that examines the grouping effect (sometimes erroneously referred to as a contextual effect) of a student-level variable. In this mode of analysis the criterion variable at the student level is regressed on both a student level predictor variable and a variable that involves the mean values of that student predictor variable, that has been aggregated by groups and then disaggregated for analysis to the student level. In symbols a regression analysis of this type can be stated as follows:

$$Y_{ij} = b_0 + b_1 X_{ij} + b_2 X_{\cdot j} + \varepsilon_{ij} \qquad (4)$$

where the symbols employed are as previously defined with $X_{\cdot j}$ being the group-level variable.

Analyses using all four models have been undertaken. Differences were recorded in the magnitudes of the regression coefficients obtained for the same measures analyzed at the different levels of analysis. There is no doubt that errors in the specification of the models used at different levels give rise to biased results (Cooley et al. 1981). Nevertheless, it is also possible that differences in model specification may be appropriate at different levels, according to the differences in the research questions being examined, and may give rise to different estimates of effect for the same variable at different levels. This does not necessarily involve specification error. As Cooley et al. (1981) pointed out, the differences are a consequence of grouping effects, when factors influencing group membership are related to one of the variables involved in the analysis.

Aitkin and Longford (1986) have also examined in some detail the results of analyses employing all four models outlined above. They dismiss the fourth mode of analysis because there is no reliable interpretation of a grouping effect "since it can be arbitrarily large or small." Moreover they state, "It will be found quite generally that the standard errors of individual level variables aggregated to the school level are very large, when the individual level variables are also included" (Aitkin and Longford 1986 p. 12).

2. Grouping Effects

The divergent and sometimes contradictory results that arise in regression and correlation analyses conducted at different levels stem from the effects of grouping. Cheung et al. (1990) have shown that the crosslevel differences between the regression coefficients obtained in analyses at the different levels are, in part, due to the differences between individual level and aggregate level predictors, since the group level variances are necessarily smaller than their individual level counterparts.

It is of interest to examine the relationship associated with the difference between an aggregated group level regression coefficient and the corresponding student level regression coefficient namely (c_1-b_1) when expressed in the symbols of Eqns. (1, 2), and the between-group variance expressed as a fraction of the total variance. The grouping effect is sometimes referred to as "aggregation bias" and the use of this term is probably not inappropriate. In Fig. 1 this relationship is illustrated in a sketched diagram, which shows how aggregation bias will generally tend to change as the proportion of between-group variance to total variance changes.

It will be seen that when the between-group variance is small compared with the total between-student variance then the aggregation bias is small. This corresponds to random grouping. However, the aggregation bias increases as the proportion of variance associated with between-group variance increases to reach a maximum value but falls again to zero as the proportion approaches 1.0. Peaker (1975) has shown, using data from the IEA Six Subject Study (conducted in 13 countries) in three subject areas and at three grade levels that this proportion is commonly of the order of 20 percent. Consequently in most studies undertaken in different parts of the world the existence of such bias must be expected.

For those 12 countries that tested in science at the 14-year old level in 1970, the average aggregation bias for the standardized partial regression coefficients when science achievement was regressed on an index of socioeconomic status at the between-school and student levels of analysis was 0.28. The average proportion of the school variance to the total student variance for science achievement test scores for those 12 countries was 0.21. Generally speaking, the regres-

sion coefficients doubled in size from student to school level of analysis. The average size of the clusters was 24 students per school, and the average values of the design effects were for correlation coefficients—2.6 and for regression coefficients—1.7. This would imply intraclass correlation coefficients for the correlations of 0.07, and for the regression coefficients of 0.03. While these measures of clustering are not large they can be associated with quite substantial proportions of between-school variance to total between-student variance and substantial aggregation bias. Since clustering has such important consequences for the estimates of regression coefficients when aggregated data are used, it would seem essential that work should always be done to assess the extent of clustering associated with particular predictor and criterion variables in the analysis of multilevel data. In addition, it is necessary to caution that the disaggregation of a variable from the group level to the individual student level also gives rise to biased estimates in the analysis of multilevel data.

3. Framework of Multilevel Analysis

The discussion in the previous section leads to the conclusion that for data collected at more than one level, for example, the student and school levels, an analyst must consider the need to examine the data using multilevel analysis. In this treatment of multilevel analysis the formulation advanced by Mason et al. (1983) has been followed. The data are collected at two levels: the student or micro level and the group or macro level.

The micro level equation may be stated:

$$Y_{ij} = b_{0j} + b_{1j}X_{1ij} + b_{2j}X_{2ij} + \varepsilon_{ij} \qquad (5)$$

where Y_{ij} is the criterion variable, X_{1ij} and X_{2ij} are two student predictor variables, and ε_{ij} is random error at the micro level for student i in group j.

At the macro level the equations may be stated:

$$b_{0j} = c_{00} + c_{01} G_{1j} + \alpha_{0j} \qquad (6)$$

$$b_{1j} = c_{10} + c_{11} G_{1j} + \alpha_{1j} \qquad (7)$$

$$b_{2j} = c_{20} + c_{21} G_{1j} + \alpha_{2j} \qquad (8)$$

where G_{1j} is the macro level or group predictor variable and α_{kj} is random error at the macro level for $k = 0, 1, 2$.

These equations are written with the usual assumptions associated with the rank condition, and with the error terms at the micro level independent of the errors at the macro level. Equations (6) to (8) represent the effects of the macro level predictor variable (G_1) on the three parameters of the micro level model and it is assumed that once the systematic component associated with this variable has been removed from b_0, b_1 and

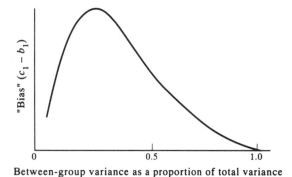

Figure 1
Relationship between aggregation bias and proportion of group variance to total variance

b_2 the resulting variability is strictly random.

A single equation can be stated for the multilevel model by substituting Eqns. (6) to (8) in Eqn. (5).

$$Y_{ij} = c_{00} + c_{01}G_{1j} + c_{10}X_{1ij} + c_{11}X_{1ij}G_{1j} + c_{20}X_{2ij}$$

$$+ c_{21}X_{2ij}G_{1j} + [\alpha_{1j}X_{1ij} + \alpha_{2j}X_{2ij} + \alpha_{0j} + \varepsilon_{ij}] \quad (9)$$

The term in brackets represents a combination of random effects of the micro level variables, namely $\alpha_{1j}X_{1ij}$ and $\alpha_{2j}X_{2ij}$ and random error components, namely α_{0j} and ε_{ij}. The random coefficients associated with X_{1ij} and X_{2ij} require special statistical treatment that will be discussed below in connection with the hierarchical linear model (HLM). If, however, $\alpha_{1j} = \alpha_{2j} = 0$ is assumed, Eqn. (9) reduces to a regression model that has no unusual estimation or computational problems.

4. Conditions for Pooling Data

In research situations where groups form the primary sampling unit and students within groups are studied with or without sampling at a second stage, consideration must be given as to whether it is appropriate to pool data across groups. If, however, sampling has occurred at the individual student level the problems associated with the pooling of data are clearly less acute, since some of the effects of grouping have been reduced by random sampling procedures.

Pedhazur (1982) has argued that the critical issues to consider in the pooling of data for analysis at the level of comparing students across groups or the between-students within-groups level as stated in Eqns. (1) and (3) above are that:

> such an analysis is valid only after it has been established: (1) the *b*'s are not significantly different from each other (the *b*'s are homogeneous); and (2) there are no significant differences among the intercepts of the separate groups. In short, when r_t or b_t is calculated it is assumed that a single regression equation fits the data of all groups. (Pedhazur 1982 p. 537)

Four possible situations arise which influence the analyses. It should be noted that the b_{0j} and b_{1j} coefficients in Eqn. (5) are considered to be random variables whose variability can be examined and tested using the error variance associated with the micro level measures. These situations are as follows:

Case 1: Both the b_{0j} and b_{1j} coefficients are not significantly different from each other.

Case 2: The b_{0j} coefficients are significantly different, but the b_{1j} coefficients are not.

Case 3: The b_{0j} coefficients are not significantly different, but the b_{1j} coefficients are.

Case 4: Both the b_{0j} and b_{1j} coefficients are significantly different from each other.

These four situations can be shown in a 2×2 contingency table (see Table 1).

Table 1
Contingency table for coefficients b_{0j} and b_{1j}

b_{1j}	b_{0j}	Not significantly different	Significantly different
Not significantly different		Case 1	Case 2
Significantly different		Case 3	Case 4

(a)   In Case 1 there are no significant differences between the b_{0j} and b_{1j} coefficients. Since there are no significant differences between groups, and since the b_{0j} coefficients do not differ, analyses at the between-group level are inappropriate. Moreover, the analyses can be carried out by pooling the student data and using the between-students overall groups model since the b_{1j} coefficients are also equal.

(b)   In Case 2 there are significant differences between b_{0j} coefficients and hence between groups. However, there are no significant differences between the b_{1j} coefficients and under these circumstances it is appropriate to pool the data in a between students within groups analysis and obtain an estimate of the b_1 coefficient. Thus a pooled between students within groups analysis can be conducted as suggested by Cronbach and Webb (1975).

(c)   In Case 3 there are no significant differences between the b_{0j} coefficients and under these circumstances a between-groups analysis is inappropriate. However, since there are significant differences between the b_{1j} coefficients it is inappropriate to pool the data at the micro or between-student level and separate analyses for each group should be carried out. Macro level analyses of the b_{1j} coefficients could also be undertaken.

(d)   In Case 4 there are significant differences between the b_{0j} coefficients and the b_{1j} coefficients and under these circumstances a full multilevel analysis should be carried out.

In educational research, where the investigation of differences between schools and classrooms is of primary interest, it would seem that Case 4 would be the situation occurring most frequently in practice. It is, however, unsafe to test simply for statistical significance. Specht and Warren (1976) have warned against unwarranted recognition of differences that are small and which, although statistically significant, are substantively slight. This advice should be heeded if trivial analyses are to be avoided when very large samples are employed.

For simplicity, and without loss of generality, the data for variables at the individual level are commonly subtracted from the corresponding group mean values. Thus deviation scores are employed in the analysis and the micro level equation may be stated:

$$(Y_{ij} - Y_j) = b_{1j}(X_{1ij} - X_{1 \cdot j}) + b_{2j}(X_{2ij} - X_{2 \cdot j}) + \varepsilon_{ij}$$

$$(10)$$

It should be noted that the intercept term b_{0j} is no longer included in the equation. However, this does not prevent a multilevel analysis being carried out. It should also be recognized that while deviation scores have been calculated, the scores have not been standardized, so that metric or unstandardized coefficients are employed which can be compared across groups in the analyses (Keeves and Larkin 1986).

5. *Hierarchical Linear Models* (HLM)

A task facing educational research workers, which is of vital importance in the study of classrooms, schools, and school districts, as well as in crossnational studies of educational achievement, is the development of appropriate procedures for the analysis of multilevel data. The general framework for such procedures is that of multiple regression, with the outcome variables regressed on variables that measure student as well as teacher, classroom, and school characteristics. The procedures must take into consideration the nesting of students within classrooms, and possibly class-rooms within schools, and make full provision for the clustering or grouping effects of the micro units within the macro units. In order to ensure generality of findings it is customary for random sampling of both the macro units and the micro units to take place. Thus where such sampling has occurred the effects at both micro and macro levels should be regarded as "random" rather than "fixed" effects. The general class of models developed for the analysis of multilevel data has become known as "hierarchical linear models" (HLM), although such terms as "variance components analysis models" and "multilevel models" have been used.

A major problem, as can readily be envisaged, is not only that of formulating the analyses to be carried out but also the inversion of large and complex matrices. As a consequence three different algorithms have been developed with different computing routines and with different analytical strategies. These strategies are: (a) a general EM algorithm (Mason et al. 1983); (b) a Fisher scoring algorithm (Aitkin and Longford 1986); and (c) a generalized least squares algorithm (Goldstein 1987). Each approach is discussed below.

5.1 *The General EM Algorithm*

This approach involves a two-stage process. In the first stage a criterion variable at the micro level is regressed on micro level predictor variables. At the second stage the regression coefficients from the micro stage, including the intercept terms, where meaningful, are regressed on the macro level predictor variables. The major difficulty in this strategy is that the estimation of the regression slopes is associated with considerable error. The issue in the macro level analysis is that of separating the variability in the regression coefficients into their "real" and "random error" components. Mason et al. (1983) employed a restricted maximum likelihood empirical Bayes estimation procedure, and Raudenbush and Bryk (1986) have extended and applied this procedure to the reanalysis of the data from the 1982 follow-up of the *High School and Beyond* study. The major problem that Raudenbush and Bryk consider is the error variance in the estimation of the regression coefficients. Since the sampling precision of these regression coefficients varies across units of different sizes and with different extent of variation in the micro level predictor variables, the basic assumptions of ordinary least squares regression analysis would have been violated. Raudenbush and Bryk proposed that the variability in these regression coefficients should be divided into two components, namely, variance due to error and the variance of the parameter itself. Following the partitioning of the variance of these regression coefficients into the error and parameter components, the parameter variance is estimated as accurately as possible. This permits the macro level effects to be more accurately estimated from an analysis using the parameter component of the variance.

An empirical Bayes estimation procedure is employed to obtain values of the micro level regression coefficients with reduced error variance. These weights are obtained by an iterative process in which the initial estimate of each micro level regression coefficient is compared with the mean value of these coefficients. Outlier values that are unreliable are successively weighted down and the group coefficient is weighted down more until convergence is obtained. The procedure "shrinks" these micro level regression coefficients and reduces the variance of the estimates prior to the macro level analysis. Since the micro level regression coefficients have been estimated more accurately, the estimates of the effects of the group level variables on these coefficients might be expected to be stronger. While this procedure is computationally complex, it is relatively straightforward conceptually and can be applied where specific models for micro level and macro level effects are being examined.

This approach to hierarchical linear modeling involves two major assumptions, namely: (a) the criterion variable at the micro level is normally distributed; and (b) the regression coefficients obtained from the analysis at the micro level are normally distributed. The first assumption is generally satisfied when achievement tests are used as criterion measures. However, the second assumption could be more problematic, since little experience has been gained from the examination of the distributions of such coefficients. The other assumptions that are necessary do not differ from those required for ordinary least squares (OLS) regression analyses, which have been found to be generally robust. Indeed it might be asked whether OLS regression analysis could be employed. If the condition of homogeneity of the variances of the micro level regression coefficients is satisfied then it might be expected that the use of OLS regression analyses would yield similar results. One problem encountered in the analysis of the micro level regression coefficients is that the intercept terms (b_{0j}), which are obtained when scaled predictor variables are used (e.g., a pretest score of achievement), have no clear meaning since the position of the axis to obtain the intercept is arbitrary. The situation is simplified if, as Raudenbush and Bryk (1986) proposed, the within-group data for the micro level analyses are centered around either the grand mean or the group mean values of the micro level variables.

5.2 *The Fisher Scoring Algorithm*

Aitkin and Longford (1986) have reported on the use of the Fisher scoring algorithm in the context of statistical modeling problems connected with British school effectiveness studies. The Fisher scoring algorithm provides maximum likelihood estimates and standard errors for the regression coefficients and group parameter effects of the model:

$$Y_{ij} = b_0 + b_1 X_{ij} + d_j + \varepsilon_{ij} \tag{11}$$

where the symbols are defined as in Eqn. (1) except that d_j are the school or group effects assumed to be a random sample from distribution $N(0, \sigma_1^2)$, and σ_1^2 is the group parameter variance.

It should be noted that this model is in many ways equivalent to the inclusion of a dummy variable for each group and the fitting of a single intercept and regression coefficient for the total set of data. Group level predictor variables that explain the variation in the estimates of d_j can subsequently be sought. However, the micro level regression coefficients are assumed not to vary, and this strategy would appear to be a variation of Case 2 rather than a true HLM analysis required by Case 4.

In fitting the model, weights are employed that are estimated from the variance component estimates. As with the previous procedure which used the general EM algorithm, because the within-group observations

are correlated, a coefficient for the ratio of the parameter variance to the sum of the parameter variance and the error variance is obtained from the estimates of the parameter variance and the error variance. The weights are a maximum when the estimates of the parameter variance are zero, and reduce to zero when the parameter variance is large compared to the sampling variance. This model can be extended to include additional "fixed effect" micro level predictor variables.

Aitkin and Longford (1986 p. 16) noted that:

> school level variables cannot reduce the pupil level component since these variables are constant within school. The failure to distinguish between pupil and school variance components has led in the past to attempts to "increase R^2" by including school level variables in individual level regressions. When the school variance component is zero or very small such attempts are bound to be fruitless, when it is appreciable, a serious overstatement of significance of such variables is almost inevitable, because the standard errors of the parameter estimates for such variables are seriously understated by individual level regressions.

While certain points are well made, it has long been recognized that simple random sample estimates of error are inappropriate for the testing of such estimates of not only regression coefficients but also mean values, correlation coefficients, and multiple R's. More appropriate procedures are widely used (see *Sampling Errors in Survey Research*). The variability in the micro level regression slopes across groups would seem to be an issue of greater consequence.

Consequently, Aitkin and Longford (1986 p. 19) extended their model to include a term in the equation to account for variation in the regression slopes:

$$Y_{ij} = b_0 + b_1 X_{ij} + d_j + f_j X_{ij} + \varepsilon_{ij} \tag{12}$$

where b_0 and b_1 are the mean intercept and regression slope and d_j and f_j are the random intercept and slope for group j, and where d_j and f_j are not assumed to be independent of each other.

The data they examined provided an example where one school had a markedly different slope to the others after appropriate adjustments had been made as a result of this analysis. This was a finding of considerable interest.

The general strategies of analysis that they advanced have been employed in the reanalysis of the data obtained in the study of *Teaching Style and Pupil Progress* (Aitkin, Anderson and Hinde 1981, Aitkin, Bennett and Hesketh 1981). The existence of substantial intraclass correlations for the mean score estimates of clustering effects ranging from 0.17 in English to 0.35 in reading indicated the need to undertake a multilevel analytical approach.

Aitkin and Longford (1986) also made the valuable point that the clustering effects are not simply a consequence of the sampling design but result from the inherent nature of the grouping of students with similar characteristics within schools.

5.3 Generalized Least Squares Algorithm

Goldstein (1987) employed the statistical model presented in Eqn. (9) which included an interaction term associated with a micro level predictor variable and a macro level predictor, in order to analyze multilevel data. Moreover, he recognized that if such an approach were adopted, then the number of levels involved in an analysis was not necessarily limited to two. In this way the groupings of students within classrooms, classrooms within schools, and schools within districts could all be taken into account in a single analysis. The overall variance of the criterion variable was partitioned into components for each level in the ensuing analysis; hence the term "variance components model" was used.

Goldstein proposed that iterative generalized least squares procedures should be employed to obtain estimates of the parameters of the model associated with both "fixed" and "random" coefficients. Like the two other procedures described above, generalized least squares weighted the data according to the accuracy of the estimates at the group level. Goldstein argued that this analytic strategy could also be applied to models for time-related data, with a set of measurements for each individual on a particular variable at different ages or time points. Moreover, there is no requirement that the measurements at each time point should involve the same variable. This approach would appear to be a very powerful and highly flexible one for the efficient analysis of data gathered in educational research. In addition, the use of generalized least squares, while yielding estimates equivalent to maximum likelihood estimates in cases with normal errors, also provides efficient estimates for other distributions.

6. Some Analytical Issues

De Leeuw and Kreft (1986) have considered many of the developments discussed in this entry and have raised several analytical issues. In addition they have undertaken the analysis of the same data set using four different approaches: (a) ordinary least squares regression analysis using the two stage estimation procedure represented by Eqns. (5) and (6) to (8); (b) ordinary least squares regression analysis using a one stage estimation procedure represented by Eqn. (9); (c) weighted least squares with Swamy weights; and (d) weighted least squares with maximum likelihood weights.

6.1 Random or Fixed Variables

Many studies have been undertaken that have paid insufficient attention to whether or not the regression coefficients from the micro level analysis should be regarded as random variables or as fixed coefficients. Not only should the nature of the sampling process be taken into consideration, but as Tate and Wongbundhit (1983) have argued: (a) the micro level regression coefficients can reflect particular policies and strategies associated with the groups; (b) they are also influenced by unspecified factors associated with the groups; (c) these disturbance factors are commonly considered as giving rise to random variability; and (d) failure to specify these coefficients as random variables annuls attempts that might be made to adjust for such error. It should be noted that ordinary least squares regression analysis treats these regression coefficients as fixed, when there is clearly a very strong case to consider such measures as random variables.

A further question is concerned with whether or not the micro level and macro level predictor variables should be considered as random regressors or fixed regressors. De Leeuw and Kreft (1986) acknowledged that the models they have employed regard the predictor variables as fixed regressors, when random variables are probably involved. They argue for the development of procedures that deal with both mixed regressor models and fully random regressor models.

6.2 Estimation Procedures

The two important aspects of any consideration of estimation procedures are whether the estimates of the parameters are unbiased and whether the estimates of error are efficient. There are, however, further questions as to whether the sampling distributions of the estimates of error are known so that significance tests can be applied.

6.2.1 Least squares estimation. Ordinary least squares regression procedures are widely used in educational research and have been employed in multilevel analysis. For example, Larkin and Keeves (1984) have used least squares regression analysis without weighting, arguing that the appropriate weights that might have been used would be given by the numbers of cases in each group involved in the analysis at the micro level. Consequently, the use of weighted least squares regression analysis (Chatterjee and Price 1977), would have contaminated the analysis with respect to the variable of interest, namely class size. Under these circumstances it was considered inappropriate to weight the data. While the estimation of parameters by ordinary least squares produces unbiased estimates, the estimation of errors of these estimates is inefficient. Clearly in analysis the most efficient estimation procedures available should be employed. However, De Leeuw and Kreft (1986 p. 72) contended that "the weighted estimate will generally improve on the unweighted estimates, although this is by no means certain."

6.2.2 Weighted least squares.

De Leeuw and Kreft (1986) argued that the weighted least squares estimate has the same asymptotic distribution as the un-weighted separate equation estimate. However, since the weighted estimates are generally more efficient and thus improve on the unweighted estimates, at least with relatively small numbers of groups and group sizes, the use of weighted estimates is to be preferred.

6.2.3 Separate or single equation estimation.

There is little doubt that separate equation analyses are easier to interpret and to understand and are less likely to be contaminated by problems of multicollinearity than are single equation analyses. However, both approaches lead to unbiased estimates.

6.2.4 Maximum likelihood or weighted least squares estimation.

In general, maximum likelihood estimation procedures lead to smaller estimates of error and are thus more efficient, although in the example presented by De Leeuw and Kreft (1986) the gains were slight. It must be recognized, however, that the use of maximum likelihood procedures in general requires that the variables included in the analysis are normally distributed.

6.2.5 Generalized least squares.

Although generalized least squares is an analytic strategy that was advanced more than 50 years ago, and has been treated by Johnston (1972), it would appear that the variance estimates obtained are not distributed as a chi-square distribution and no proper methods are available to provide confidence limits about the values predicted by regression analysis.

6.3 Compositional and Contextual Effects

In order to clarify issues associated with the use of aggregated data it is desirable to distinguish between "compositional" and "contextual" effects (Bryk and Raudenbush 1988). It is, however, necessary to note that the latter term has been used by educational research workers with a variety of meanings.

A compositional effect involves the influence that the average background of the students in a group has on student performance that is distinct from the effect of the background of each individual student on student performance. Thus the compositional effect is associated with the use of an aggregated micro level variable, which varies between the macro level units to account for the intercept term in Eqn. (5).

A contextual effect involves the influence that an aggregated micro level variable has on the slope of the group regression lines which vary about the mean group regression slope. Thus the performance of an individual student is influenced by both that student's relative standing within the classroom group and by the average standing of the students in the group.

In order to show the difference between these two

effects, Bryk and Raudenbush (1988) rewrote Eqn. 5 as centered around the group mean value

$$Y_{ij} = b_{0j} + b_{1j} (X_{1ij} - X_{1\cdot j}) + \varepsilon_{ij} \qquad (13)$$

where $X_{1\cdot j}$ is the mean for variable X_1 in group j. In addition variable $X_{1\cdot j}$ can be centered around the grand mean $(X_{1\cdot\cdot})$ and Eqns. (6) and (7) rewritten where G_{1j} is replaced by the aggregated student level variable $X_{1\cdot j}$

$$b_{0j} = c_{00} + c_{01} (X_{1\cdot j} - X_{1\cdot\cdot}) + \alpha_{0j} \qquad (14)$$

and

$$b_{1j} = c_{10} + c_{11}(X_{1\cdot j} - X_{1\cdot\cdot}) + \alpha_{1j} \qquad (15)$$

By substituting Eqns. (14) and (15) in Eqn. (13)

$$Y_{ij} = c_{00} + c_{01} (X_{1\cdot j} - X_{1\cdot\cdot}) + \qquad (16)$$
$$(c_{10} + c_{11}(X_{1\cdot j} - X_{1\cdot\cdot})) (X_{1ij} - X_{1\cdot j}) + \mu_{ij}$$

By adding and subtracting $c_{10}X_{1\cdot\cdot}$ from Eqn. (16)

$$
\begin{aligned}
Y_{ij} = c_{00} & \\
+ (c_{01} - c_{10})(X_{1\cdot j} - X_{1\cdot\cdot}) & \quad \text{compositional effect} \\
+ c_{11}(X_{1ij} - X_{1\cdot j})(X_{1\cdot j} - X_{1\cdot\cdot}) & \quad \text{contextual effect} \\
+ c_{10} (X_{1ij} - X_{1\cdot\cdot}) & \quad \text{individual effect} \\
+ \mu_{ij} &
\end{aligned}
$$

where the residual term $\mu_{ij} = \alpha_{0j} + \alpha_{ij} (X_{1ij} - X_{1\cdot j}) + \varepsilon_{ij}$

The term $(c_{01} - c_{10}) (X_{1\cdot j} - X_{1\cdot\cdot})$ is the compositional effect since it involves the contribution to variability of the individual score on the criterion measure that comes from the difference between the mean of the predictor variable for the group to which the individual belongs and the grand mean for the predictor under consideration. The compositional effect is given by the between group regression coefficient minus the within group regression coefficient for the predictor variable.

The term $c_{11}(X_{1ij} - X_{1\cdot j}) (X_{1\cdot j} - X_{1\cdot\cdot})$ is the contextual effect. It involves an interaction term associated with the variability of the individual with respect to the group mean, and the variability of the group mean with respect to the grand mean of the predictor variables. It arises from the explanation of the variation of the regression slopes when the criterion measure is regressed on the predictor for each group.

The term $c_{10}(X_{1ij} - X_{1\cdot\cdot})$ is the individual effect where the difference between the individual's standing on the predictor variable with respect to the grand mean is taken into consideration.

6.4 Exploring Different Procedures

Many different analytical procedures have been proposed for the solution of the problems associated with the analysis of multilevel data. Cheung et al. (1990) have systematically explored the different solutions that have been proposed and have compared the results obtained from the HLM procedure with that obtained from the use of iterative generalized least squares (ITGLS). In general, HLM is found to provide a more readily interpreted solution than ITGLS does and the version of the computer programs available was easier to operate. In addition, by using successive HLM analyses it was possible to construct a recursive path model showing micro, macro, and inter-active effects. Nevertheless, the search for appropriate procedures to be used in the analysis of data collected in large-scale surveys of educational achievement must continue if the effects of schools and classrooms on student performance are to be appropriately estimated.

One of the most powerful techniques developed for the analysis of causal path models is linear structural relations analysis. Work by Muthén (1989, 1991) has provided an approach that has been incorporated into the STREAMS computer program (Gustafsson and Stahl 1996).

7. Conclusion

Multilevel analysis is a field in which a number of highly significant papers were published in the 1980s and 1990s. Much has been accomplished toward the solution of a critical problem in the analysis of educational research data in the short period of time since Mason et al. (1983) suggested to research workers in the social sciences that the problem might be addressed using multilevel analysis procedures. Wong and Mason (1985) have also developed a hierarchical logistic regression model for multilevel analysis where a categorial criterion variable is employed. These procedures have now been included in a computer package for hierarchical linear and nonlinear modeling (Bryke et al. 1996). It is necessary to await the applications of these principles and procedures in the detailed analysis of the extensive bodies of data in educational research that are multilevel in nature and which are concerned with real problems that are of importance for educational practice and policy-making. However, attention needs to be given to the effects of model misspecification on HLM estimates at the different levels of analysis.

See also: Models and Model Building; Sampling in Survey Research

References

Aitkin M, Anderson D, Hinde J 1981 Statistical modelling of data on teaching styles. *J. Royal Stat. Soc. A.* 144(4): 419–61
Aitkin M, Bennett N, Hesketh J 1981 Teaching styles and pupil progress: A re-analysis. *Br. J. Educ. Psychol.* 51(2): 170–86
Aitkin M, Longford N 1986 Statistical modelling issues in school effectiveness studies. *J. Royal Stat. Soc. A.* 149(1): 1–2
Bryk A S, Raudenbush S W 1988 Methodology for cross-level organizational research. In: Straw B (ed.) 1988 *Research in Organisational Behavior*, Vol. 10. JAI, Greenwich, Connecticut

Bryk A S, Raudenbush S W, Congdon R T 1996 *HLM Hierarchical Linear and Nonlinear Modeling with the HLM/2L and HLM/3L Programs.* Scientific Software Internatrional, Chicago, Illinois
Burstein L 1980 Issues in the aggregation of data. *Review of Research in Education* 8: 258–63
Chatterjee S, Price B 1977 *Regression Analysis By Example.* Wiley, New York
Cheung K C, Keeves J P, Sellin N, Tsoi S C 1990 The analysis of multilevel data in educational research: Studies of problems and their solutions. *Int. J. Educ. Res.* 14(3): 217–319
Cooley W W, Bond L, Mao B J 1981 Analyzing multilevel data. In: Berk R (ed.) 1981 *Educational Evaluation Methodology: The State of the Art.* Johns Hopkins University Press, Baltimore, Maryland
Cronbach L J et al. 1976 *Research on Classrooms and Schools: Formulation of Questions, Design and Analysis.* Stanford Evaluation Consortium, Stanford University, Stanford, California
Cronbach L J, Webb N 1975 Between-class and within-class effects in a reported aptitude x treatment interaction: Re-analysis of a study by G L Anderson. *J. Educ. Psychol.* 67(6): 717–24
De Leeuw J, Kreft I 1986 Random coefficient models for multilevel analysis. *J. Ed. Stat.* 11(1): 57–85
Finn J D 1974 *A General Model for Multivariate Analysis.* Holt, Rinehart and Winston, New York
Goldstein H 1987 *Multilevel Models on Educational and Social Research.* Oxford University Press, New York
Gustafsson J–E, Stahl P A 1996 *STREAMS User's Guide: Structural Equation Modeling Made Simple.* Göteborg University, Göteborg
Husén T (ed.) 1967 *International Study of Achievement in Mathematics: A Comparison of 12 Countries.* Almqvist and Wiksell, Stockholm
Johnston J 1972 *Econometric Methods*, 2nd edn. McGraw-Hill, New York
Keeves J P, Larkin A I 1986 The context of academic motivation. *Int. J. Educ. Res.* 10(2): 205–14
Larkin A I, Keeves J P 1984 *The Class Size Question: A Study at Different Levels of Analysis.* Australian Council for Educational Research, Hawthorn, Victoria
Mason W M, Wong G Y, Entwisle B 1983 Contextual analysis through the multilevel linear model. In: Leinhardt S (ed.) 1983 *Sociological Methodology 1983–84.* Jossey-Bass, San Francisco, California
Muthén B O 1989 Latent variable modeling in heterogeneous populations. *Psychometri.* 54(4): 557–85
Muthén B O 1991 Analyses of longitudinal data using latent variable models with varying parameters. In: Collins L M, Horn J L (eds.) 1991 *Best Methods for the Analysis of Change.* American Psychological Association, Washington, DC
Peaker G F 1967 The regression analyses of the national survey. In: Central Advisory Council for Education 1967 *Children and Their Primary Schools: A Report of the Central Advisory Council for Education. Vol. 2: Research and Theories.* HMSO, London
Peaker G F 1975 *An Empirical Study of Education in Twenty-One Countries.* Almqvist and Wiksell, Stockholm
Pedhazur E J 1982 *Multiple Regression in Behavioral Research*, 2nd edn. Holt, Rinehart and Winston, New York
Raudenbush S, Bryk A S 1986 A hierarchical model for studying school effects. *Sociol. Educ.* 59(1): 1–17

Robinson W S 1950 Ecological correlations and the behavior of individuals. *Am. Sociol. Rev.* 15: 351–57

Specht D A, Warren R D 1976 Comparing causal models. In: Heise D R (ed.) 1976 *Sociological Methodology 1976.* Jossey-Bass, San Francisco, California

Tate R L, Wongbundhit Y 1983 Random versus nonrandom coefficients models for multivariate analysis. *J. Ed. Stat.* 8(2): 103–20

Wong G Y, Mason W M 1985 The hierarchical logistic regression model for multivariate analysis. *J. Am. Stat. Assoc.* 80(391): 513–24

Further Reading

Bock R D (ed.) 1989 *Multilevel Analysis of Educational Data.* Academic Press, San Diego, California

Bryk A S, Raudenbush S W 1992 *Hierarchical Linear Models: Applications and Data Analysis Methods.* Sage, Newbury Park, California

Raudenbush S W, Willms J D (eds.) 1991 *Schools, Classrooms and Pupils: International Studies of Schooling from a Multilevel Perspective.* Academic Press, San Diego, California

Multivariate Analysis

J. P. Keeves

Educational research is necessarily concerned with many variables in its attempts to predict and explain educational processes. It is rare that attempts are made to explain and predict educational outcomes using only a single variable, and it is rare that there is concern for only one outcome. Likewise in descriptive studies, where attempts are made to describe a body of data in a parsimonious manner, research workers seldom employ only a single variable. The many-faceted nature of educational processes demands that measurements should be made on many variables, and that the analytical procedures employed should be capable of the simultaneous examination and analysis of the many variables on which data have been collected. Until the mid-1960s, educational research workers were largely denied the opportunity to analyze in full the rich bodies of data that they were able to collect. However, with the availability of the high-speed computer, the tedious and repetitive tasks associated with data analysis were largely eliminated and it was possible to undertake the analysis of data that involved a large number of cases and many variables. The mathematical and statistical procedures associated with such analyses had, in general, been available for many years and simply awaited the arrival of the computer to facilitate calculation. However, the widespread use of these procedures has inevitably led to advances in the field of multivariate analysis. Moreover, the availability of powerful desktop computers has supported the further development of multivariate analytical techniques. As a consequence the field of multivariate analysis is clearly one in which marked advances are likely to continue to take place.

Some research workers have, nevertheless, been reluctant to make use of these techniques of multivariate analysis and have continued to employ simpler and frequently inappropriate procedures involving univariate analysis only. Other research workers have rejected the research strategy associated with accurate measurement and the analysis of quantitative data and have endorsed the exclusive use of ethnographic and interpretative approaches. Whilst the use of such approaches in the initial and exploratory examination of a problem is not inappropriate, in general, greater exactness in the making of observations increases their potential usefulness (see *Scientific Methods in Educational Research*).

Multivariate analysis is primarily concerned with the study of relationships between and within one, two, or more sets of variables that are sequentially ordered with respect to time, logic, or theory. The first measured set of variables forms the predictor set; the second measured set forms the criterion set. Where a third set of variables forms the criterion set, the second set, being located with respect to time of measurement between the predictor and the criterion sets, forms a mediating or moderating set. Sometimes a strict time sequence in the measurement of sets of variables cannot be adhered to with two or more variables measured at the same point in time, and a logical sequence, customarily associated with an underlying temporal relationship, is employed to order the sets of variables.

Darlington et al. (1973) have pointed out that certain general types of questions may be asked about sets of variables ordered in this way:

(a) questions about the similarity between variables within one set, which are referred to as the "internal analysis" of a set of variables;

(b) questions about the number and nature of mutually independent relationships between two sets of variables, which are referred to as the "external analysis" of sets of variables; related to these questions are further questions about the degree of overlap or redundancy between the two sets of variables; and

(c) questions about the interrelations between more than two sets of variables, which are referred to as the "structural analysis" of the relationships between the sets of variables.

The different procedures for multivariate analysis are considered in this entry under these three headings, internal analysis, external analysis, and structural analysis.

1. Variates and Variate Values

It has become increasingly necessary to employ, in certain circumstances, a distinction between measures and their values which are observed and recorded and the underlying constructs that are under investigation. This distinction is of particular importance where the observed or manifest measures are combined in analysis to form latent constructs which have greater explanatory power. In the British tradition there is a distinction advanced by Bartlett between using the term "variates" for the observed measures, and the term "variables" for the underlying factors and latent constructs (Bartlett 1947, Ferguson 1989).

In the consideration of variates and variate values, it has also proved useful (see Tatsuoka 1982) to distinguish between *quantified* and *categorized* data and measures. While some oversimplification is necessarily involved in making this distinction, it is important in obtaining data to recognize that sometimes accurate measurement is possible, in other situations whole numbers are assigned where there is an underlying normal or other distribution, and in other situations again the data are simply counts in specified categories.

With the availability of computer programs that calculate very rapidly polychoric and polyserial correlations, consideration can now be given to whether the categorized variate values are associated with an underlying normally distributed variable so that the calculation of a polychoric or polyserial correlation is appropriate. In cases where one variate is quantified and continuous and the other is categorized and is associated with an underlying normally distributed variable, then a polyserial correlation may be appropriately calculated. A computer program for the calculation of polychoric and polyserial correlations (PRELIS) (Jöreskog and Sorbom 1993) is available.

During the 1970s and 1980s two separate sets of analytical procedures were developed which correspond to the distinction between quantified and categorized data, although there are many procedures which have been designed for the analysis of data where one set of variates involves quantified data and another set involves categorized data. In this entry analytical procedures are separated into these two groups, but the distinction between variates and variables is only made where it is necessary to avoid confusion.

2. The Multivariate Analysis of Quantified Data

There are several important issues to be considered in the multivariate analysis of quantified data.

2.1 The Multivariate Normal Distribution

The general theory for the multivariate analysis of quantified data is based upon the multivariate normal distribution. The use of this distribution as the mathematical model for multivariate analysis, together with use of the large sample theory of probability and the multivariate central limit theorem, enable the testing of the significance of relationships between variables obtained from multivariate analyses. While there is much remaining to be learned about the sensitivity of the multivariate model to departures from the assumptions of the multivariate normal distribution, in general, the model would appear to be relatively robust.

As a partial test of multivariate normality it is desirable to examine each variable at a time by constructing normal probability plots or possibly histograms (Norusis 1990). However, positive results do not guarantee that the data are multivariate normally distributed, nor do they guarantee the absence of outliers. More rigorous procedures exist, which involve the calculation of Mahalanobis distances (Jöreskog and Sorbom 1993).

2.2 Major Assumptions in the Use of the Multivariate Normal Model

The major assumptions associated with the use of the model are first, that observations on a predictor set of variates must be independent of one another, with respondents being both independently sampled and providing information without reference to one another. Second, the variance–covariance matrix among the criterion set of variates must exhibit homogeneity regardless of sampling from the population or of the values of the predictor set of variates. While the former assumption cannot wisely be ignored, testing for a violation of the latter assumption is often neglected, It would seem desirable that, in analyzing data, tests should be applied for the homogeneity of the variance–covariance matrix and a warning recorded if departure from homogeneity is large. Commonly, an examination of residuals will provide information on marked departures from homogeneity in the variance–covariance matrix. Standard tests employed in statistical packages include the Bartlett Box–F test, Cochran's C test, and Box–M test (see Norusis 1990).

2.3 Variate Values in Multivariate Analysis

The variates to be examined in the multivariate analysis of quantified data may involve nominal data with two categories (dichotomous data), or with more than two categories (polychotomous data), or the variables may involve ordinal, interval, or ratio-scaled data. Where the variables involve nominal data, they may be submitted to quantification or scaling to permit their examination and analysis. Where the variates involve ordinal data, in addition to the possibility of using a polyserial or polychoric correlation procedure, it is possible to scale the data using rank-scaled scores, through which an appropriate integer score value is assigned to each category. Alternatively, criterion scaling procedures may be used. Commonly in criterion scaling, regression weights are assigned to categories which have been obtained from regression analysis using an appropriate criterion measure (Peaker 1975). It may also be commonly necessary to transform variate values that are members of the criterion set to ensure that they are normally distributed and that the use of the multivariate normal distribution model is appropriate. Where the measures are dichotomous in nature the logit transformation is used (Snedecor and Cochran 1967). In addition, where variates show a high degree of skewness, the variate values are normalized, as the procedure is commonly referred to, or more accurately, transformed using the probit transformation (Fisher and Yates 1963).

A further assumption required for the multivariate analysis of quantified data is that of the homogeneity of the variances (or homoscedasticity) in two or more subpopulations from which the samples were drawn. If a marked degree of heteroscedasticity is observed in the variance–covariance matrix from standard tests or from an examination of residuals, then a weighted least squares (Chatterjee and Price 1977) or generalized least squares (Goldstein 1987) procedure may be employed.

2.4 Tests of Significance

The fundamental question in testing for significance is concerned with calculating the probability that some sample statistic is representative of a particular population parameter. The techniques employed assume both multivariate normality of distribution and homogeneity of the variance–covariance matrix. Several different approaches have been advanced with regard to testing for significance in multivariate analysis. However, the principles of testing employed in multivariate analysis are parallel to those used in univariate analysis (see *Significance Testing*). Nevertheless, there is considerable difference of opinion between statisticians with regard to which multivariate test statistic is the most appropriate one to use in a particular situation. Thus, while there is agreement that Bock's generalized FG statistic and Roy's largest root criterion are of value in the detection of group mean differences along a single dimension, the most commonly used tests for the significance of effects on all criterion measures simultaneously are Wilk's likelihood ratio criterion, Hotelling's trace criterion, and the step-down test (Bock and Haggard 1968).

However, such procedures of significance testing

commonly assume that the sample drawn from the defined population is a simple random sample. This is the exception rather than the rule in educational research, where, in general, schools are first sampled, then classrooms are sampled from within schools and all students in the classroom groups are tested, or students are sampled from within schools across classroom groups for testing. The appropriate modeling of such cluster sample designs poses major problems in multivariate analyses, and only in the late 1980s and early 1990s was the problem sufficiently recognized for work to commence on the development of more rigorous procedures. This topic is considered in Sect. 5 of this entry.

3. Estimation in Multivariate Analysis

Two general approaches to estimation in multivariate analysis have been developed. The one most commonly employed involves the reduction of the ordered collections of numbers in the matrices associated with sets of variates in accordance with certain specified rules, typically with respect to minimizing errors of prediction or description. In this approach, the principle of least squares is used to determine regression weights in multiple regression analysis and canonical correlation analysis, and the initial position of factors in some types of factor analysis. A second approach has been to obtain maximum likelihood estimates. The task is to find a factor matrix in the sample data most like that which exists in the population. Lawley (1940) was the first to derive the necessary equations, but unfortunately the equations could not be solved by direct computation. Subsequently Lawley (1943) proposed an iterative solution to these likelihood equations. The best solution available in the mid 1990s has been developed by Jöreskog (1967). This procedure involves the obtaining of an iterative solution to the complex set of equations based on the assumption that there is a particular number of factors. At the end of the analytic procedure a test is applied to determine whether the solution involving this number of factors is adequate to describe the sample data.

3.1 Internal Analysis Techniques

These techniques seek interrelations between the variables within a single set:

Cluster analysis is a general term for those analytical techniques which seek to develop classifications of variables within a set. The cluster analysis of a set of variables commences with the correlations between the variables, obtained by summing across persons. It is, however, possible to obtain correlations or indices of similarity between persons, summing across variables, and this is the basis for a commonly used form of cluster analysis (see *Cluster Analysis*).

Smallest space analysis is a technique of data analysis for representing geometrically the pairwise similarities between variables in a set as indicated by the correlations or other measures of distance between the variables of the set. However, smallest space analysis is also used to describe the similarities which exist between persons with respect to the measured variables (see *Smallest Space Analysis*).

In principal components analysis, the problem is that of the reduction of the number of measures used to describe a set of persons, by the derivation of a smaller set of significant variables or components that are statistically unrelated (orthogonal) to each other. The extraction of principal components is the first step in one commonly employed form of factor analysis (see *Factor Analysis*).

There are many forms of factor analysis, each employing a different analytical procedure. In one procedure it is possible, following the extraction of the principal components from the data on a set of variates, to rotate the principal axes while keeping them orthogonal, in order to maximize the distribution of variance across the factors (varimax rotation). Rotation of the axes under other conditions is also possible. Through the use of such procedures, sometimes carried out under apparently arbitrary conditions, it is possible to obtain what would seem to be a more meaningful reduction of the original set of measures (see *Factor Analysis*).

3.2 External Analysis Techniques

In general, these techniques seek not only interrelations between the variables within two sets but also the interrelations between the two sets of variables.

Perhaps the most widely used of the multivariate procedures of analysis is multiple regression analysis. Although multivariate regression may be considered to involve more than one variable in the criterion set, the analytical procedures employed when there is only one criterion variable and when there are more are essentially the same. In regression analysis linear combinations of both the variables in the predictor set and the criterion set are sought in order to minimize the residual variance. It is common that there are more variables in the predictor set than are necessary for a parsimonious solution to the problem, and stepwise selection procedures are frequently employed before the inclusion of a variable from the predictor set in the regression equation. Where the predictor variables are polychotomous, dummy variable regression procedures are commonly employed, so that each category is considered as a separate variable in the analysis (see *Regression Analysis of Quantified Data*).

In canonical correlation analysis the nature and number of relationships between two sets of variates are examined. The analysis is carried out in such a way that linear and orthogonal combinations of variates from the set of predictor variates are related to linear and orthogonal combinations of variates from the criterion set. In addition, the analysis provides information on the degree of overlap in variance or redundancy between the variables so formed in the predictor set and the variables in the criterion set. Since the method of analysis maintains full reciprocity between the two sets of variables, in a manner that does not occur in multivariate regression analysis, it is not necessary to identify one set of variables as the predictor set and the other as the criterion set, although it is frequently meaningful to do so (see *Canonical Analysis*).

Multivariate analysis of variance and covariance are analytical techniques that can only be properly applied where subjects have been assigned at random to treatments which form the predictor set of variables. The variables in the predictor set are thus categorized and not quantified variables. Analysis of covariance differs from analysis of variance insofar as the former is associated with the regression of the criterion variable on one or more variables in the predictor set. Thus the variables in the criterion set are adjusted for the effects of the predictor variables which are considered to be covariates. However, it is important to note that such adjustment is inappropriate if the covariates influence systematically the nature of the treatment received by the subjects. Although analysis of covariance is widely used in research in education and the behavioral sciences, its use is sometimes inappropriate, since subjects have not been randomly assigned to treatments and the subject's standing on the covariate may have influenced the treatment given (see *Variance and Covariance, Analysis of*).

In discriminant analysis identification of membership of particular groups is considered to be associated with one set of variates, and measures of the characteristics of the groups provide information on the other set of variates. The analysis seeks to obtain one or more composites of the quantified variates such that the composites show maximum differences between group means with respect to these composite scores and minimum overlap in the distributions of these scores. This technique can also be viewed in such a way that membership of the groups forms the criterion set, and the quantified variates form the predictor set. From this perspective, the analysis seeks to maximize prediction of membership of the criterion groups using information on the quantified variates in the predictor set (see *Discriminant Analysis*).

In factorial modeling the analyst is required to name latent variables or factors and to specify each by means of an exclusive subset of predictor variates. The variance associated with the variates in the criterion set is then partitioned among the latent variables or factors which have been identified. The strength of the technique is in its capacity to partition the criterion variance into independent contributions from uncorrelated factors or latent variables (see *Factorial Modeling*).

As a consequence of the search for interaction effects among predictor variables, the technique known as automatic interaction detection (AID) subdivides persons into groups and subgroups, by successively splitting the total sample so that there is maximum variation between groups and minimum variation within groups with respect to a criterion variable. The criterion variable must be either an interval-scaled quantified variable or a dichotomous categorized variable. The identification of groups of persons who are either high or low on the criterion is frequently of very considerable value (Sonquist et al. 1971).

The technique employed in THAID is similar to that used in automatic interaction detection (AID), except the criterion variable is associated with membership of one of a number of mutually exclusive groups. Again the sample is split into subgroups so that the number of correct predictions of membership of each group is maximized with respect to the proportion of persons in each group category (Morgan and Messenger 1973).

Multiple classification analysis (MCA) uses an iterative procedure to obtain estimates of the effects of several predictor variables, in nominal or ordinal form, on a criterion variable in dichotomous or interval form, so that each of the predictor categories has been adjusted for its correlations with the other predictor categories. The technique does not make provision for the obtaining of information on interaction effects. However, the interaction problem can be handled in appropriate ways, if knowledge of the existence of an interaction effect is available from the use of automatic interaction detection, and the correct crossclassification terms are introduced into the analysis. While this technique is equivalent to the use of dummy variable multiple regression, the procedure would appear to be less vulnerable to multicollinearity problems as well as providing information that is more directly interpretable (Sonquist 1970).

3.3 Structural Analysis Techniques

Path analysis is a technique that in its simplest form employs multiple regression analysis in order to estimate the causal links between a series of predictor and mediating variables and a criterion variable. In the analysis of more complex models which are nonrecursive in nature, the techniques of indirect regression and two-stage least squares regression analysis may be used (see *Path Analysis and Linear Structural Relations Analysis*).

Linear structural relations analysis (LISREL) may be used for the analysis of causal models with multiple indicators of latent variables, measurement errors, correlated errors, correlated residuals, and reciprocal causation. LISREL is based on maximum likelihood statistical theory, and is associated with the analysis of the variance–covariance matrix by maximum likelihood procedures (Jöreskog and Sorbom 1993). If a sound fit of the model to the data is obtained then a highly meaningful interpretation is produced. However, many difficulties are commonly encountered in the use of the procedure and in obtaining a significant solution. In addition, the multivariate normal distribution or some other known distributions must be assumed for the variates included in an analysis (see *Path Analysis and Linear Structural Relations Analysis*).

Partial least squares path analysis (PLS), like LISREL, may be used for the analysis of causal models with multiple indicators of latent variables. However, it does not require such rigid specification of the error terms, and from its use estimates of parameters for a complex model are readily obtained. Since it is a least squares method of analysis, it does not demand the rigid distributional and independence assumptions necessary in maximum likelihood methods. As a consequence the same level of statistical inference cannot be attained with partial least squares path analysis as with linear structural relations analysis (see *Path Analysis with Latent Variables*).

4. Multivariate Analysis of Categorized Data

This is a rapidly developing field of analysis, in which many of the advances made during the 1980s occurred in continental Europe.

4.1 Internal Analysis Techniques

In contingency table analysis, information is obtained on a set of variables within discrete categories with respect to a number of persons or events. Initially the analysis carries out tests for the independence of the categorized variables by means of a chi-square test. Where statistical significance is observed it is then necessary to undertake a more detailed investigation of the reasons for the significant association between the variables (see *Contingency Tables*).

The analytical technique of correspondence analysis seeks to present the relationships between the variables forming the contingency table in a graphical form. It operates by obtaining a set of coordinate values to represent the row and column categories of the contingency table. These coordinates are similar to those obtained from the principal components analysis of quantified data, except that they are derived by partitioning the chi-square statistic for the table instead of the variance (see *Correspondence Analysis*).

In latent class analysis the categorized variates are assumed to involve a number of clusters or latent classes. Within these latent classes the observed categorized variates are independent. The observed associations between the variates are generated by the existence of the latent classes. Conceptually this type of analysis is similar to that of factor analysis with quantified variates.

The purpose of configural frequency analysis is to identify overfrequented or underfrequented cells in multidimensional contingency tables. The overfrequented cells are denoted as "types" and the underfrequented cells are denoted as "antitypes." A cell is overfrequented if the number of cases observed in this cell is significantly greater than is assumed under the null hypothesis of independence. Likewise an underfrequented cell has the number of cases significantly less than would be expected under the null hypothesis. In this way the variables that contribute to the rejection of the null hypothesis are identified (see *Configural Frequency Analysis*).

4.2 External Analysis Techniques

Log–linear models are used in the analysis of contingency tables through the fitting of multiplicative models to sets of data and estimating the parameters of the models. Subsequently, the main effects and interaction effects are tested for significance. These procedures may be extended to use in the analysis of causal models with categorical data, by analyzing change over time, for examining panel data, and for the investigation of Markov chain models. Such uses of log–linear models in essence involve structural analysis techniques (see *Log-Linear Models*).

5. Multilevel Analysis

One of the major problems encountered in educational research, where schools and classrooms are sampled randomly as the primary sampling unit and then students are drawn at random from within these schools and classrooms, is that of the level of analysis. Failure to employ procedures of multilevel analysis in situations where data have been collected at more than one level has two major shortcomings. First, the effects of variables at both the group and at the individual levels are not partitioned, resulting in serious bias in the estimates. Second, the error terms employed in testing estimates of effect for significance are generally inappropriate (see *Multilevel Analysis*). Three solutions to this problem were developed during the 1980s, namely: (a) The Fisher Scoring Algorithm (Aitkin and Longford 1986); (b) Iterative Generalized Least Squares Method (Goldstein 1987); and (c) Hierarchical Linear Modeling which employs empirical Bayes procedures and the EM Algorithm (see *Hierarchical Linear Modeling*). In the early 1990s the uses of these procedures were still being developed, insofar as they could be extended to more than two levels of analysis and could be employed in the analysis of growth, particularly in studies of learning (Bock 1989).

An important development has been made by Muthén, who has built upon earlier work (Muthén 1989, 1991) and combined the two analytical traditions of random effects modeling and structural equation modeling using LISCOMP. However, this approach does not permit the analysis of structural models with randomly varying slopes, although it does permit the analysis of random structural regression intercepts. Furthermore, the variables need not be normally distributed. Muthén's work has been extended

for use with LISREL and multilevel modeling of linear structural relations in the STREAMS computer program (Gustafsson and Stahl 1996) (see *Multilevel Analysis; Path Analysis and Linear Structural Relations Analysis*).

6. Some Problems of Analysis

There are five problems in educational research associated with the analysis of data by multivariate analytic procedures which are both persistent and widespread. It is common in a very high proportion of investigations in educational research to sample first by schools or classrooms and then by teachers or students within schools or classrooms. Furthermore, in quasi-experimental studies the school or classroom becomes the unit of treatment although data are collected from individual students. Unfortunately, students are commonly viewed as the unit of analysis. In this approach to investigation lie the origins of some of the problems (Keeves and Lewis 1983).

6.1 Units of Analysis

The data collected can be analyzed at one of several levels: between schools, between classrooms, between classrooms within schools, between students within classrooms, between students within schools, and between students. Commonly, analyses are carried out at the between-student level only, and biased estimates obtained and inferences drawn that are inappropriate to the school as a whole or to the classroom as a unit. Where analyses are undertaken at the between-school or between-classroom level, it is generally recognized as inappropriate to make inferences that apply to students, but not generally acknowledged that the estimates made are seriously biased. Consequently, it is necessary that greater care should be taken in stating the propositions to be examined and the hypotheses to be tested so that the appropriate multilevel analysis procedures can be employed.

6.2 Effective Number of Units

Even where it is appropriate to undertake analyses at the between-student level, it is important to recognize that, in investigations in natural settings, the student was not the primary unit of sampling and, where the school or the classroom was the primary unit of sampling, effects of sampling may be expected to be substantially greater than if the student was the primary sampling unit. As a consequence of the clustering of students within classrooms and schools, it is inappropriate to use simple random sample formulas for the calculation of errors, and it is necessary to use a correction factor to allow for the design effect of the sampling procedures employed. Fortunately, some procedures are now available for calculating the sampling errors of statistics estimated from complex samples (Ross 1976, Wilson 1983). Moreover, it is now possible to undertake the analysis of data at more than one level of analysis using multilevel analysis models or hierarchical linear models, and the use of such procedures generally produces appropriate estimates of sampling errors (see *Sampling Errors in Survey Research; Multilevel Analysis*).

6.3 The Effect of Prior Performance on Treatment

In investigations in a natural setting, it is frequently inevitable that the prior characteristics of the students should influence the treatment provided by the teacher and by the school. As a consequence, the measures obtained on school and classroom variables can be influenced significantly by such characteristics of the student as prior achievement. Only when there has been fully random assignment of students to class-rooms and to treatments in an experimental study is it likely that the prior achievement of the student will have been adequately controlled. Thus, only when the design of the study makes the necessary provision for random allocation are the procedures of analysis of variance and covariance appropriate. Moreover, it is clear that, where treatment is influenced by prior performance, analysis of covariance provides an unsatisfactory statistical control. Under such circumstances regression analysis should be used.

6.4 Overfitting of Data

The use of a large number of students at the between-student level of analysis frequently conceals the fact that there are insufficient numbers of classrooms and schools from which data have been collected. Thus, in multivariate analysis where data derived from relatively few classrooms and schools are being included in the analysis, the introduction of many classroom or school variables to the analysis is likely to lead to problems in the multicollinearity of the data that are not immediately evident because of the substantial number of students involved.

6.5 Suppressor Variables

One of the signs associated with problems which arise in regression analysis from the overfitting of data or from serious measurement error in the measurement of one or more predictor variables can be observed when an estimate of a partial regression coefficient changes in sign or changes markedly in magnitude as the number of predictor variables in the analysis is measured. The occurrence of such suppressor effects must be viewed with great caution, although sometimes such a change in sign is meaningful (Tzelgov and Herick 1991) (see *Suppressor Variables*).

7. Pictorial Representation

Multivariate analysis procedures are not a collection of unrelated statistical techniques, but rather a family of closely related models. This can be seen not only in terms of the matrix notation employed but also through

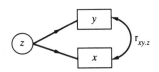

Figure 1
Partial correlation

pictorial representation. It is common for latent variables to be shown by circles and indicated by letters of the Greek alphabet, while observed variates are commonly shown by boxes and labelled with letters of the Roman alphabet. A path of influence is shown by a line with an arrow from the determining variable to the variable which is determined, while an association is shown by a curved line with arrowheads pointing towards the two variables which are related. Mutual determination or a reciprocal relationship is shown by two parallel lines in opposite directions, and a model in which a reciprocal relationship exists is referred to as a "nonrecursive" model (the negative expression is confusing). A model in which there is a consistent unidirectional path of influence or causal structure is referred to as a "recursive" model.

The use of a pictorial representation frequently aids the explanation of relationships in multivariate analysis and is to be encouraged where space is available. The following examples may be of interest (Van de Geer 1971).

(a) *Partial correlation.* In partial correlation analysis, two variables are assumed to be determined by a third variable and their intercorrelation is adjusted to allow for the effects of the third variable (Fig. 1).

(b) *Partial regression, or multiple regression analysis.* In partial regression analysis, two variables are assumed to determine a third variable, and their paths of influence are adjusted to allow for their intercorrelation. A residual or error term is also shown in the model to indicate the existence of error or disturbance terms on the third variable (Fig. 2).

(c) *Path analysis.* Path analysis is best viewed as a series of partial regression analyses. The order of

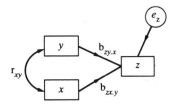

Figure 2
Partial regression

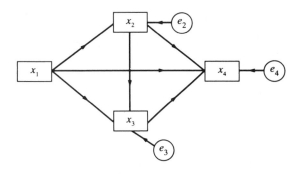

Figure 3
Path analysis[a]
a x_2, x_3, x_4 are endogenous variables

variables in the model is determined as a temporal or logical sequence (Fig. 3).

(d) *Factor analysis.* In factor analysis two latent variables replace or summarize the information contained in three or more observed variates (Fig. 4).

(e) *A nonrecursive path model.* In a nonrecursive path model two variables may be reciprocally related to each other and each determined by other variables in the model. (see Fig. 5). Nonrecursive models, when appropriately specified, can be analyzed by indirect regression, two-stage least squares regression analysis, LISREL, or partial least squares path analysis.

(f) *Canonical variate analysis.* In the analysis of quantified data canonical variate analysis may be considered to be the most general analytical procedure. Other procedures may be viewed as special cases of canonical analysis. In Fig. 6 the x-variates are specified as the predictor set and the y-variates as the criterion set.

The latent variables are indicated by χ_1 and χ_2. It should be noted that the statistical analysis does not

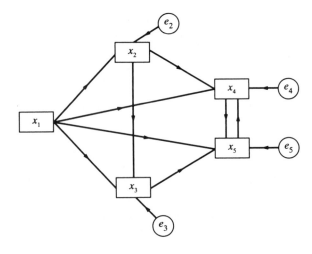

Figure 5
Nonrecursive path analysis

distinguish between the predictor and the criterion sets of variates.

8. Computer Programs

In educational research it is rare to have data sets that can readily be analyzed by hand or by a simple calculator. This has led to reliance on a range of statistical packages. Each of the large commercial packages has advantages and disadvantages for the analysis of multivariate data sets. Comment is provided briefly on the packages that are widely used.

(a) Statistical Programs for the Social Sciences (SPSS) provides a set of interrelated programs that have considerable flexibility of data management, editing, and analysis. The programs are particularly easy to use, and very clear manuals are provided (Nie et al. 1975, Norusis 1990).

(b) The BMDP package provides a set of programs for a wide range of analytical techniques, but the procedures for data management and editing

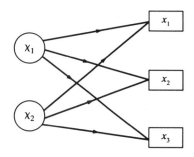

Figure 4
Factor analysis

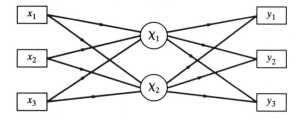

Figure 6
Canonical variate analysis

are not as straightforward as in other packages (Dixon and Brown 1979).

(c) The OSIRIS package was well-designed for use with very large data sets, and is particularly appropriate for the merging of files, and for building files to be used at different levels of analysis. While there is a wide range of multivariate procedures available, and while these programs make economical use of the computer, the individual programs have some deficiencies and are sometimes not particularly easy to use. However, routines are available for the calculation of appropriate sampling errors for some multivariate analyses (University of Michigan 1976).

(d) The SAS package has a variety of programs as well as procedures for matrix manipulation. Although the package requires a greater degree of sophistication in computing from the user than do the three packages mentioned above, the flexibility thus gained is considerable (Helwig and Council 1979).

(e) Generalized Linear Interactive Modeling (GLIM) is particularly useful for the interactive testing of a wide variety of linear and log–linear models. However, considerable mathematical and statistical sophistication is needed in order to utilize its advantages fully (Baker and Nelder 1978).

(f) The MULTIVARIANCE package is particularly suited to the analysis of nested designs by analysis of variance and covariance procedures. The multivariate analysis programs provided are very sophisticated and require considerable statistical skill to use (Finn 1974).

(g) Structural equation modeling can now be undertaken at two levels using the LISREL (Jöreskog and Sorbom 1993), and the STREAMS (Gustafsson and Stahl 1996) computer programs.

In order to analyze large bodies of data it is no longer necessary for the educational research worker to spend long hours on tedious calculations, nor is it necessary to become a master of computer programming. However, it is important to have a firm understanding of statistical principles and to maintain a preparedness to consult an experienced statistician concerning the analyses to be undertaken.

9. Comparisons of Methods of Analysis

The *International Journal of Education Research* in 1986 published a series of articles comparing different methods of analysis, including path analysis, canonical analysis, LISREL, factorial modeling, partial least squares analysis, and multilevel analysis. The differences in the results obtained were very informative (Keeves 1986). In addition, Cheung et al. (1990) have compared the results obtained from the use of the different procedures which have been suggested for multilevel analysis in a later issue of the *International Journal of Educational Research*.

References

Aitkin M, Longford N 1986 Statistical modelling issues in school effectiveness studies. *Journal of the Royal Statistical Society, Series A.* 149 (Part 1):1–26

Baker R J, Nelder J A 1978 *The GLIM System Release 3: Generalized Linear Interactive Modelling*. Numerical Algorithms Group, Oxford

Bartlett M S 1947 Multivariate analysis. *Journal of the Royal Statistical Society, Series B.* 9:176–97

Bock R D 1989 *Multilevel Analysis of Educational Data*. Academic Press, London

Bock R D, Haggard E A 1968 The use of multivariate analysis of variance in behavioral research. In: Whitla D K (ed.) 1968 *Handbook of Measurement and Assessment in Behavioral Sciences*. Addison-Wesley, Reading, Massachusetts

Chatterjee S, Price B 1977 *Regression Analysis by Example*. Wiley, New York

Cheung K C, Keeves J P, Sellin N, Tsoi S C 1990 The analysis of multilevel data in educational research: Studies of problems and their solutions. *Int. J. Educ. Res.* 14(3): 215–319

Darlington R B, Weinberg S L, Walberg H J 1973 Canonical variable analysis and related techniques. *Rev. Educ. Res.* 43(4): 433–54

Dixon W J, Brown M B (eds.) 1979 BMDP-79: *Biomedical Computer Programs*. University of California Press, Berkeley, California

Ferguson G A 1989 *Statistical Analysis in Psychology and Education*, 6th edn. McGraw-Hill, New York

Finn J D 1974 *A General Model for Multivariate Analysis*. Holt, Rinehart and Winston, New York

Fisher R A, Yates F 1963 *Statistical Tables for Biological, Agricultural, and Medical Research*, 6th edn. Oliver and Boyd, Edinburgh

Goldstein H 1987 *Multilevel Models in Educational and Social Research*. Oxford University Press, New York

Gustafsson J-E, Stahl P A 1996 STREAMS *User's Guide: Structural Equation Modeling Made Simple*. Göteborg University, Göteborg

Helwig J T, Council K A (eds.) 1979 SAS *User's Guide*, 1979 edn. SAS Institute, Raleigh, North Carolina

Jöreskog K G 1967 Some contributions to maximum likelihood factor analysis. *Psychometri.* 32: 443–82

Jöreskog K G, Sorbom D 1993 LISREL 8, PRELIS 2 *User's Reference Guide*. Scientific Software International, Chicago, Illinois

Keeves J P 1986 Aspiration, motivation and achievement. Different methods of analysis and different results. *Int. J. Educ. Res.* 10(2): 117–243

Keeves J P, Lewis R 1983 Issues in the analysis of data in natural classroom settings. *Australian Journal of Education* 27(3): 274–87

Lawley D N 1940 The estimation of factor loadings by the method of maximum likelihood. *Proceedings of the Royal Society of Edinburgh* 60: 64–82

Lawley D N 1943 The application of the maximum likelihood method to factor analysis. *Br. J. Psychol.* 33: 172–75

Morgan J N, Messenger R C 1973 THAID: *A Sequential Analysis Program for the Analysis of Nominal Scale Dependent Variables*. Survey Research Center, Institute for Social Research, Ann Arbor, Michigan

Muthén B O 1989 Latent variable modeling in heterogeneous populations. *Psychometri* 54(4): 557–85

Muthén B O 1991 Analysis of longitudinal data using latent variable models with varying parameters. In: Collins L M, Horn J L (eds.) 1991 *Best Methods for the Analysis of Change*. American Psychological Association, Washington, DC

Nie N H, Hull C H, Jenkins J G, Steinbrenner K, Bent D H 1975 *Statistical Package for the Social Sciences*, 2nd edn. McGraw-Hill, New York

Norusis M J 1990 SPSS *Base System. User's Guide*. SPSS, Chicago, Illinois

Peaker G F 1975 *An Empirical Study of Education in Twenty-one Countries*. Almqvist and Wiksell, Stockholm

Ross K N 1976 *Searching for Uncertainty: An Empirical Investigation of Sampling Errors in Educational Survey Research*. Australian Council for Educational Research, Hawthorn

Snedecor G W, Cochran W G 1967 *Statistical Methods*, 6th edn. Iowa State University, Ames, Iowa

Sonquist J A 1970 *Multivariate Model Building*. Institute for Social Research, The University of Michigan, Ann Arbor, Michigan

Sonquist J A, Baker E L, Morgan J N 1971 *Searching for Structure*. Institute for Social Research, The University of Michigan, Ann Arbor, Michigan

Tatsuoka M M 1982 Statistical analysis. In: Mitzel H E (ed.) 1982 *Encyclopedia of Educational Research*, 5th edn. The Free Press, New York

Tzelgov J, Herick A 1991 Suppression situations in psychological research: Definitions, implications, and applications *Psych. Bull.* 109(3): 524–36

University of Michigan Institute for Social Research 1976 *OSIRIS IV Manual*. University of Michigan, Ann Arbor, Michigan

Van de Geer J P 1971 *Introduction to Multivariate Analysis for the Social Sciences*. Freeman, San Francisco, California

Wilson M 1983 *Adventures in Uncertainty*. Australian Council for Educational Research, Hawthorn

Prediction in Educational Research

R. M. Wolf and W. B. Michael

Prediction represents an effort to describe what will be found concerning an event or outcome not yet observed on the basis of information considered to be relevant to the event. Typically, there is a temporal dimension to prediction when, say, ability test scores are used to forecast future achievement in a course of study.

1. Predictor and Criterion Variables

The information that is used to make a prediction is typically referred to as a predictor. In any prediction study there is at least one predictor variable. Predictor variables can be either quantitative—for example, scores on a test—or qualitative—for example, type of course in which enrolled. It is possible to combine qualitative and quantitative variables in a prediction study. The event or outcome to be predicted is typically referred to as a criterion. There are several types of criterion variables. One of the most common is performance on some quantitative continuous variable such as an achievement test or a grade point average. Other criterion variables could be qualitative in nature. When a counselor helps a student make a choice of career or course of study, the counselor is at least implicitly making a prediction about a qualitative variable, career choice, or course of study, in which the student is likely to succeed and from

which he or she can derive satisfaction. The criterion in this case can be regarded as membership in a particular group. In more complex cases, a criterion may be multidimensional in character, as when one is interested in predicting an individual's profile on a number of variables such as a battery of achievement measures. While possible, simultaneous prediction on a number of criterion variables is quite rare.

Prediction studies can be highly varied depending on the nature of the population under study and the number and types of predictor and criterion variables used. However, there are a number of common elements in prediction studies. The first element involves identifying the outcome or event to be predicted. Education, social, or business necessity is usually the basis for such a choice. The second element is to develop or select a measure that will serve as a criterion variable. This crucial step of the process generally receives far less attention than it should. If one decides to use "success in college" as a criterion in a prediction study, then how is success to be defined and measured? Obviously, there are many ways to do this task. Unfortunately, there is no clearly correct way to define and measure success. Any definition of success will have its limitations, and any measure based on a particular dimension will be somewhat deficient. The use of an earned grade point average in college as a measure of success, for example, will only reflect the standards used by a particular group of instructors in a set of courses and will ignore performance in noninstructional aspects of college life. Furthermore, the standards used by a particular set of instructors may not reflect the standards of the institution as a whole. In fact, it is possible that there may be no uniform agreement on a set of standards that will serve to define success across all the instructional areas of the institution. Thus, even a widely used criterion variable such as the grade point average suffers from a number of weaknesses.

The definition and measurement of criterion variables is a formidable challenge. The desired qualities in a criterion variable, whether it is quantitative or qualitative are: (a) *relevancy*: standing on the criterion is determined by the same factors as those that make for success in the situation; (b) *freedom from bias*: the measure of the criterion variable is free from external factors that provide each individual with the same opportunity to achieve a good score on the criterion; (c) *reliability*: the measurement of the criterion variable must be stable or reproducible if it is to be predicted; (d) *availability*: a measure of the criterion should be readily available. Although a number of empirical procedures such as task or job analysis, work-sample tests, and factor analysis can be useful in helping to develop measures of criterion variables, the basic ingredient in the definition of criterion variables is judgment. Considerable background and expertise are required to define and develop adequate measures of criterion variables.

A third element in all prediction studies is the identification and measurement of the variable or variables that will serve as predictors. Again, considerable background and expertise are needed. The fourth element in a prediction study is to collect information on both the predictor variable or variables and the criterion for a sample of individuals, and to subject these data to analysis. The typical kind of analysis involves some form of least squares procedures. The results will provide an estimate of the extent to which the criterion variable or variables can be predicted from the predictor variable or variables. The results, however, will only apply to the sample that was studied. Consequently, it will be necessary to see whether the results obtained with one sample apply to a different sample. This procedure is called cross-validation (Mosier 1951). If it can be shown that the results obtained with one sample apply to a new sample, one can use the results with some confidence. It is necessary, however, to check periodically to see whether the results are holding up. That is, are the level and accuracy of prediction the same for subsequent groups as they are for the initial sample?

Prediction always involves uncertainty. A prediction study is undertaken with a particular sample of individuals, for example, when ability test scores are used to predict subsequent achievement in a learning situation. Once a prediction study has been completed, that is, a group of individuals has been followed and their subsequent performance has been assessed, the real purpose of the study is to be able to use the results with a subsequent group of learners. It is in this sense that prediction contains uncertainty as the intent is to use information derived from the study of one group in a prospective way with another group.

2. Simple Linear Regression or Prediction

The simplest type of prediction study involves the use of a single predictor variable measured on a continuous scale to predict a single criterion variable also measured on a continuous scale. An example of such a study would be the use of an ability test score to predict performance on an achievement test after a period of instruction. To conduct a prediction study involving these two variables would require the administration of the ability test to a group of students prior to the onset of instruction, locking away the results, and the administering of a test of achievement after instruction. Withholding the results of the predictor test until the criterion variable has been obtained is necessary to avoid possible contamination of the criterion either consciously or unconsciously by those people who provide instruction and develop, administer, and grade the achievement test. Once data have been collected, they need to be analyzed. In the elementary example to be described, the usual procedure would be a simple regression analysis of the criterion score on the predictor scores.

3. Regression Equation

The analysis would yield a number of items of information. The first item would be a regression equation of the form:

$$\hat{Y} = a + bX \tag{1}$$

where $\hat{Y}$ is the predicted score on the criterion variable; a is a constant that would represent the expected score on the criterion variable if the value of X, the score on the predictor variable, were zero; b is the regression coefficient that denotes the number of units of increase in Y, the criterion variable, that is associated with one unit of change on the X variable; and X is an individual's score on the predictor variable. In calculating the regression equation, one employs the procedure of least squares. In least squares, the residuals, the sum of squares of the difference between each individual's actual Y score and the score obtained from the regression equation ($Y - \hat{Y}$, an error in prediction) is a minimum. That is, the sum of squares is less than the residuals of errors obtained from any other values of a and b. In most regression analyses, the least squares procedure that is used is ordinary least squares (OLS). Sometimes, however, a weighted least squares (WLS) procedure is employed. This might be used when the error variance is not homogeneous but varies from case to case. In using WLS, one applies to each case a weight proportional to the inverse of the variable (Draper and Smith 1981 pp. 77–81, Judd and McClelland 1989 pp. 19–20).

The regression equation can be used to predict each individual's score on the criterion variable. The chances are that the regression equation will predict few, if any, individuals' criterion scores with perfect accuracy. Thus, it is necessary to have additional items of information to evaluate the goodness or accuracy of prediction.

3.1 The Correlation Coefficient in Simple Regression Analysis

A second item of information that would normally be obtained from a simple regression analysis undertaken in a prediction study would be the correlation coefficient (r) between the two sets of scores. The correlation coefficient is an index number that can take values from −1.0 to +1.0. The magnitude of the correlation coefficient describes the strength of the relationship between the variables while the sign of the correlation describes the direction of the relationship. Correlation coefficients of +1.0 and −1.0 describe a perfect relationship, whereas a correlation coefficient of zero denotes no relationship at all between the variables. The square of the correlation coefficient describes the percentage of the variance in the criterion variable that is accounted for by the variation in the predictor variable. In a prediction study, the higher the value of r and r^2 the better or more accurate the prediction.

It is not easy to say how high the correlation coefficient should be in order to be considered satisfactory for predictive purposes. There are several bases on which the issue can be approached. First, does the use of a particular predictor variable improve prediction over chance levels? If so, there could be a basis for using the particular predictor variable under study. Second, is the use of a particular predictor variable better than that of other currently available predictors? If the answer is affirmative then there is a basis for using the particular predictor variable. Third, does the use of a predictor variable improve prediction over other currently available predictor variables? This last consideration involves the use of multiple predictors. It requires having information about the population of applicants who will be admitted to a training or employment situation (the selection ratio) and the gain in prediction that is achieved by using the predictor variable under study, the incremental validity of the predictor variable (Anastasi 1988).

3.2 Standard Error of Estimate

The third item of information that would result from a simple regression analysis is the standard error of estimate ($S_{y \cdot x}$). The standard error of estimate is defined as follows:

$$S_{y \cdot x} = S_y (1 - r^2)^{1/2} \tag{2}$$

where S_y is the standard deviation of the criterion variable and r is the correlation coefficient between the predictor and criterion variable.

The smaller the value of the standard error of estimate, the more accurate the prediction. It is clear that if the correlation between the predictor and the criterion variable is +1.0, then the standard error of estimate would be zero. If the correlation coefficient was zero, however, the standard error of estimate would be equal to the standard deviation of the scores on the criterion variable. The standard error of estimate is often used in connection with the predicted criterion score ($\hat{Y}$) to establish limits within which an individual's predicted criterion score can be expected to lie with a particular level of confidence. The establishment of such confidence limits is based upon the theory of the normal curve. In much practical prediction work, two standard errors of estimate ($2S_{y \cdot x}$) are added and subtracted from $\hat{Y}$ to establish an interval within which one can be 95 percent confident that an individual's predicted score on the criterion will lie.

3.3 Expectancy Table

The regression equation is one way of using information from a simple prediction study. Another means of using information from a simple prediction study is an expectancy table. An expectancy table is essentially a form of scatter diagram that displays the relationship between the predictor and criterion variables in percentage terms so that it is possible to estimate the chances of obtaining a particular level of performance on the criterion variable given a particular level of performance on the predictor. An example of an expectancy table is shown in Table 1. Thus, if a student scored in the second quarter on the predictor variable, there are 14 chances in 100 that he or she would score in the lowest quarter on the criterion, 26 chances in 100 of being in the third quarter on the criterion, 32 chances in 100 of scoring in the second quarter on the criterion, 28 chances in

Table 1
Expectancy table for predictor and criterion variables ($r = 0.60$)

Quarter on predictor	Quarter on criterion			
	Lowest	3rd	2nd	Top
Top	4	14	28	54
2nd	14	26	32	28
3rd	28	32	26	14
Lowest	54	28	14	4

100 of scoring in the top quarter on the criterion, and 28 + 32, or 60 chances in 100 of a placing in the top half of the criterion scores. An individual as well as a research worker can use an expectancy table to estimate the chances of achieving particular levels of performance on the criterion given a particular level of performance on the predictor variable. The values in the cells of an expectancy table will change with changes in the magnitude of the correlation between the predictor and criterion variable. The example in Table 1 is based on a correlation of 0.60 (validity coefficient) between the predictor and criterion variables (see *Expectancy Tables in Educational Predictions*).

3.4 Additional Considerations

The regression equation and the correlation coefficient in a simple prediction study (one predictor and one criterion variable) are usually estimated by simple linear regression analysis. This statistical procedure assumes that there is a straight line relationship between the two variables. This circumstance has been found to be satisfactory for many purposes. However, there is no requirement that the relationship between the variables should be linear. There are many nonlinear ways of handling the data from even a simple prediction study (Pedhazur 1982). It is usually recommended that an investigator study the shape of the scatter diagram for the predictor and criterion variables and select a statistical model that will best reflect the nature of the relationship between the variables. The introduction of a number of graphical programs on both large computers and microcomputers has made this task quite easy.

4. Multiple Linear Regression Analysis

The example previously described in some detail—a single predictor variable and a single criterion variable—is the simplest of all prediction models. Yet, as can be seen, it can be rather complex. As one moves toward more complex prediction studies, the situation becomes increasingly complicated. In the next level of prediction study, there are several continuous quantitative predictor variables and a single continuous quantitative criterion variable. The basic procedures for conducting such a study are similar to those for a simple prediction study. The two major differences are: (a) information about several predictor variables is gathered, and (b) multiple rather than simple regression analysis procedures is used.

Multiple regression analysis is similar to simple regression analysis except that a weighted composite of the predictor variables is sought that will correlate maximally with the criterion variable. One of the chief tasks in multiple regression analysis is to determine the set of weights which, when applied to the predictor variables, will maximize the correlation between the composite of the predictor variables and the criterion. The analytic procedures for achieving this goal are presented elsewhere (Pedhazur 1982, Thorndike 1949, 1982). Multiple regression analysis is a general-data analytic procedure that can be applied not only to continuous quantitative variables such as test scores but also to quantitative discrete predictor variables such as type of course enrolled in and categories of parent's occupation. The special technique that permits handling of such variables is called dummy variable coding (Pedhazur 1982). Multiple regression analysis makes it possible to estimate the contribution that each predictor variable makes to the estimation of the criterion variable and also allows the development of a prediction equation that will best estimate the criterion variable with the smallest number of predictor variables. The general form of a multiple regression equation is:

$$\hat{Y} = a + b_1X_1 + b_2X_2 + \ldots + b_kX_k \qquad (3)$$

where $\hat{Y}$ and a were defined previously; b_1, b_2, ..., b_k are the regression weights for the various predictor variables; and X_1, X_2, ..., X_k are values of the predictor variables for an individual.

Generally, multiple regression analysis is used to develop a linear prediction of a criterion variable from a set of predictor variables. However, regression analysis procedures can be used when the relationships between variables are nonlinear. Various transformations can be readily applied to handle nonlinear variables (Pedhazur 1982). In addition to the regression equation described earlier, multiple regression analysis will also yield a coefficient of multiple correlation (R) that describes the relationship between the set of predictor variables and the criterion variable, and a standard error of estimate that permits the setting up of confidence limits for the prediction of individual criterion variable scores.

Both simple and multiple regression analysis have as their goal the prediction of an individual's status on a single continuous quantitative criterion variable. The difference between the two procedures hinges on whether there is one or more than one predictor variable (see *Regression Analysis of Quantified Data*).

5. Multiple Discriminant Analysis

In contrast, there are prediction situations in which the criterion variable is categorical in nature. A situation may be considered in which a counselor is advising a student about a career choice. The counselor would have information about the student such as achievement in various courses, some indicator of ability, and

415

perhaps interest test scores. These indicators would serve as predictor variables. The criterion variable—career choice—consists of a set of categories that do not constitute a continuum. Such categories might be medicine, engineering, commerce, architecture, law, and so on. The goal of prediction is to help the student to select a career choice in which he or she is likely to succeed and to achieve satisfaction. Regression analysis procedures would be useless in such a situation because of the categorical nature of the criterion variable. The appropriate statistical procedure for analyzing data from a prediction study in order to estimate an individual's membership in a group is multiple discriminant analysis. This technique uses a set of predictor variables that can be quantitative or categorical to predict the group to which an individual is most likely to belong. These results can then be compared to the group of which the individual has elected to become a member in much the same way that predicted and actual criterion variable scores on continuous quantitative variables can be compared. Although the complexity of the computation of multiple discriminant analysis requires the use of computers, there are standard programs available for such analyses (SPSS 1988).

In general, there is considerably more work in predicting group membership than in predicting status on a continuous quantitative variable. The usual reason given for this differential is that the greater complexity of the computations in the analysis had to await the development of high-speed electronic computers and statistical programs to perform the necessary calculations. The need to make such predictions, however, has long been recognized. Whether there will be more applied work in the area in the future remains to be seen.

One common element in the prediction situations that have been detailed is the existence of a single criterion variable to be predicted. Even in the case of predicting an individual's group membership, there is the single criterion variable, that is, group membership. The specific categories of group membership are somewhat analogous to the different score levels of a continuous quantitative criterion variable (see *Discriminant Analysis*).

6. Canonical Correlation Analysis

In the last situation to be described, there is more than one criterion variable to be predicted. This situation involves the prediction of the profile of an individual on a set of criterion variables on the basis of his or her performance on a set of predictor variables. Such prediction is possible using a statistical procedure called canonical correlation analysis (Cooley and Lohnes 1971). Canonical correlation seeks, by appropriate weighting of both the predictor and criterion variables, to maximize the correlation between the linear composites based on the two sets of variables. The highly complex computations involved in carrying out a canonical correlation analysis require the use of a computer, although a few heroic studies have been done by hand (Thorndike 1949).

In canonical correlation there is concern for predicting an individual's performance on a set of criterion variables. There has generally been little use of canonical correlation in prediction work. Besides the arduous computational burden involved, there appear to be few situations in which it has been considered necessary or desirable to predict performance on a number of criterion variables simultaneously. Rather, the tendency has been to express performance on a single composite criterion and to use this criterion in a multiple regression analysis. This practice is perhaps unfortunate, as the reduction of criterion performance to a single variable undoubtedly results in a loss of information. This loss is especially true when different aspects of a criterion performance are not highly related to one another. On the other hand, inclusion of a number of criterion variables in a prediction situation can lead to rather strange results sometimes, as the weights that are obtained for both the predictor and criterion variables are mathematically derived. If the weights, especially the ones for the criterion variables, do not accord with the weights that would judgmentally be given these variables, then the weights given to the predictor variables can be rather misleading and, in some cases, meaningless. For example, there might be interest in predicting a number of aspects of a student's performance in a mathematics course. As predictor variables these could be measures of various abilities. The criterion variables may be scores on tests of mathematical concepts, mathematical computation, and problem solving. A canonical correlation analysis might result in a high correlation between the two sets of variables but this outcome might be due to a high weight being given to the mathematical computation test score and low weights to the other criterion variables. Thus, there are dangers in the blind use of canonical correlation in prediction research (see *Canonical Annalysis*).

7. Conclusion

Prediction has been a major goal of research in education. Institutions all over the world routinely conduct prediction studies and use the results for selection, placement, and classification. Such work can be expected to continue and expand. The goal of all prediction research is to enable educators to make the soundest possible decisions on the basis of evidence.

See also: Multivariate Analysis; Regression Analysis of Quantified Data

References

Anastasi A 1988 *Psychological Testing*, 6th edn. Macmillan, New York

Cooley W W, Lohnes P R 1971 *Multivariate Data Analysis*. Wiley, New York

Draper N R, Smith H 1981 *Applied Regression Analysis*, 2nd edn. Wiley, New York

Judd C M, McClelland G H 1989 *Data Analysis: A Model-Comparison Approach*. Harcourt Brace Jovanovich, San Diego, California

Mosier C I 1951 Problems and designs of cross-validation. *Educ. Psychol. Meas.* 11(1): 5–11

Pedhazur E J 1982 *Multiple Regression in Behavioral Research: Explanation and Prediction*, 2nd edn. Holt, Rinehart and Winston, New York

SPSS 1988 SPSS-X: Users Guide, 3rd edn. SPSS, Chicago, Illinois

Thorndike R L 1949 *Personnel Selection: Test and Measurement Techniques*. Wiley, New York

Thorndike R L 1982 *Applied Psychometrics*. Houghton-Mifflin, Boston, Massachusetts

Q-Methodology

R. M. Wolf

Q-methodology has its origins in factor-analytic work of the 1930s but did not emerge as a fully developed approach to the study of individuals until the early 1950s when Stephenson published *The Study of Behavior*. This seminal work systematized a considerable body of both conceptual and empirical work and claimed that Q-methodology was " . . . a comprehensive approach to the study of behavior where man is at issue as a total thinking and behaving being" (Stephenson 1953 p. 7).

1. Q-Sorts

While Q-methodology is regarded as a general approach to the study of individuals and consists of a variety of techniques, Q-sorts lie at the heart of the method. A Q-sort consists of a number of stimuli which an individual is called on to sort into piles along some dimension. The stimuli can be verbal statements, single words, pictorial material, or figures. The task for the subject is to sort the stimuli along a particular dimension such as "prefer most" to "prefer least," "most like me" to "least like me," and so forth. Usually, a Q-sort will involve about 40–120 stimulus items and about 7–12 categories into which the stimuli are to be sorted. Often, the instructions to an individual require that a specified number of objects be sorted

into each category. Such prespecified distributions are often quasi-normal distributions. Figure 1 sets forth one possible prespecified distribution for a Q-sort.

The result of a Q-sort is a rank-ordered set of stimuli along a particular dimension. What is done with these statements depends, of course, on the purposes of a particular investigation. The earliest Q-sorts were used to obtain correlations among participants. If several individuals perform a Q-sort, it is possible, using the scale values of the categories, to obtain correlation between individuals' responses to the stimulus items. This is in direct contrast to typical correlations between variables over individuals. The latter correlations, summarized in a matrix are referred to as "R" while the former, to signify the difference, are labeled "Q".

Correlations between individuals can be inspected to identify whether there appear to be clusters of individuals that serve to define particular "types." Correlation matrices have also been subjected to factor analysis for the purpose of analytically identifying clusters or type of people, and such correlation approaches have tended to dominate Q-studies (Wittenborn 1961).

It is also possible to compare a single individual's Q-sort under varying instructions. For example, before beginning therapy, clients might be instructed to rank order a set of statements along the dimension of "most

Categories	Most prefer										Least prefer
	11	10	9	8	7	6	5	4	3	2	1
No. of stimuli	3	4	7	10	13	16	13	10	7	4	3 = 90

Figure 1
Possible prespecified distribution for a Q-sort

like me" in order to describe their perception of themselves. They could then be instructed to sort the same set of statements along the dimension of "what I want to be like" to "what I don't want to be like" in order to describe an ideal self. Finally, the same individuals could be instructed to re-sort the statements along the dimension "how others see me" to "how others don't see me" so as to describe how they perceive themselves to be seen by others. The three sortings can be correlated and represented in a 3×3 correlation matrix for a single individual. Repetition of the procedure over the course of therapy could be used to trace how the relationships between real self, ideal self, and perceived self change over time. As long as the set of stimulus variables are reasonably homogeneous, that is, they measure one broad variable such as "self," they are serviceable in such work.

A distinction is made between unstructured and structured Q-sorts. The Q-sort that was described above is an unstructured one. The stimulus items are selected because they measure a single broad variable. The single variable might be the self, paintings, or adjectives describing an object. In selecting a set of stimuli, the presumption is that the stimuli are representative of the domain of interest.

In a structured Q-sort, the items to be sorted are carefully selected to represent different categories of a particular domain. For example, Stephenson (1953 pp. 69–79) illustrates how a set of 10–15 statements for each of Jung's (1993) four major personality types could be generated and used in a Q-sort. Similarly, Kerlinger (1986 pp. 512–14) shows how a Q-sort could be developed for Spranger's six types of men. In each case, the category values into which statements were classified could be used to produce a mean for each type. The standard deviation for each type can also be computed. Inspection of the means can reveal the individual's relative standing on each type. In addition, Stephenson recommends that analysis of variance be used to test for the significance of difference between types in order to characterize an individual properly.

The above description illustrates what is called a structured one-way Q-sort. Stephenson extended structured Q-sorts into two-, three-, and four-way sorts. Consider the design shown in Fig. 2, in which two traits are represented: dominant–submissive and introvert–extrovert. Stephenson would seek to develop or select an equal number of statements (15–20) with which dominant introverts might describe themselves, and so on, for each cell of the design. More than two levels on a dimension and more than two dimensions may be used. The statements are then assembled into a deck for sorting into a predetermined quasi-normal distribution and administered to a subject. The resulting information can then be analyzed, using a two-way analysis of variance, to test for the main effects of dominance/submission and introversion/extroversion and the interaction between the two according to Stephenson.

Figure 2
Structured two-way Q-sort

Q-methodology relies heavily on comparative judgments and ranking. An individual who is presented with a Q-sort is required to order a set of stimuli along a particular dimension. If a prespecified distribution is used, such as a quasi-normal distribution, the result is a rank-ordered set of statements. Two individuals ranking the same set of statements could obtain the same mean and standard deviation on all dimensions being measured by a Q-sort and yet be markedly different with regard to their actual standing on each dimension. This is due to the comparative nature of the sorting process and the use of a prespecified distribution. For these reasons, some writers have questioned the use of forced distributions, while others have advocated the abandonment of ranking procedures and the use of normative measurements by which an individual is asked to rate stimuli according to particular value labels.

2. Evaluation of Q-Methodology

It is not easy to evaluate the arguments that have swirled around Q-methodology. The reason for this is that Q refers to a loosely related bundle of techniques and not to a single procedure. Thus, if one were to try to evaluate the criticism about the relative nature of rankings in Q and the use of forced distributions, one's position would largely depend on what aspect of Q is being considered and what one will be doing with the resulting data.

For example, if the object of a particular investigation is to compare an individual's ranking of a set of self-descriptive statements with what he or she would like to be (ideal self) then the exact distribution form has little effect on the kinds of analyses which are performed on the data. Correlation coefficients and the factors obtained from them are largely insensitive to changes in distribution shapes.

On the other hand, if one wanted to estimate an individual's actual level of, say, self-esteem, the Q-methodology would be inappropriate. This is not a criticism of Q-methodology. It is simply a recognition of the fact that different procedures are used for different purposes.

Nonetheless, it is possible to make some evaluative comments about Q-methodology. The general approach has been part of the research scene since the 1930s, and a systematic treatment (Stephenson 1953) has been available since the 1950s.

One of the most notable features of Q-methodology is the prominent role given to theory. Any investigator who undertakes to use Q is forced, from the outset, to consider how a theory or aspects of a theory can be expressed in categories or levels, and if stimulus items can be selected or devised to express those categories or levels. In such use, Q can be a powerful way to test theories. Even the most severe critics of Q (Cronbach and Gleser 1954) acknowledge the importance of these newer ways in which questionnaire items can be used. Q simultaneously allows for flexible use of questionnaire items and for the standardization of descriptions of complex phenomena in a theoretically relevant way. Proponents of Q suggest that the attention to theory and the importance of content sampling may be among its most important contributions (Nunnaly 1970). A second major feature of Q is its suitability for the study of the individual. The same individual can be studied under different conditions of instructions (real self, ideal self, etc.), as well as over time, in order to assess the impact of therapy or other program interventions. The approach is not free of pitfalls, however. Although rank ordering is used in connection with forced distribution, the effects of response sets are not totally eliminated.

A third claim regarding Q-methodology regards its use in testing the effects of independent variables on complex dependent variables. The use of structured Q-sorts offers the possibility of sensitively assessing the effects of variables through the use of analysis of variance procedures on an individual-by-individual basis. Although this has been done rather infrequently, the promise remains.

Finally, Q offers considerable promise for exploratory studies as well as for its heuristic value. Intensive study of a single case or a few individuals can help in generating new ideas, formulating hypotheses, and examining relationships. Stephenson's own work (1953) perhaps illustrates this quality better than any treatise can. One gets the impression of a lively mind at work while engaged in working with Q.

3. Criticisms of Q-Methodology

Q-methodology has also drawn strong criticism. One suspects that some of the criticism stems from the way in which Stephenson presented Q. Strong claims were made for Q, yet there was also a general neglect of a number of issues that make Q somewhat methodologically dubious.

One major criticism of Q has been statistical in nature. Since Q-sorts are ipsative in nature and most statistical tests assume independence, there is an inherent conflict between Q-procedures and most forms of data analysis that are used to analyze the data resulting from Q-sorts. Technically, the statisticians are on firmer ground than the proponents of Q. However, the important question is whether the violation of statistical assumptions is serious enough to invalidate the use of factor analysis of variance. Proponents of Q (Kerlinger 1986, Nunnally 1970) say they are not, while critics (Cronbach and Gleser 1954, Sundland 1962) say they are. Given the unresolved nature of the issue, it would seem that caution should be exercised in the use of Q.

A more basic criticism centers on the issue of external validity or generalizability. Studies using Q are invariably based on very small samples, from 1 to 20 individuals. What populations can be generalized from results obtained from such small samples? The small sample sizes simply do not provide the basis for generalizations. Since this is the case, what uses can be made of Q? A partial answer is that Q can be used in exploratory studies. Q can also be used in clinical work in the study of individual cases. Beyond that, normative studies using much larger (and representative) samples are needed to test theoretical propositions adequately.

Other technical issues surrounding the use of Q involve the use of forced versus unforced distributions, and the loss of information through the lack of elevation and scatter because of the ipsative nature of Q-procedures. These issues have received considerable attention in the literature but have not been fully resolved. It is doubtful if they ever will. The issue of lack of elevation and scatter because of the ipsative nature of Q is not an issue that can be resolved. If elevation and scatter are important considerations, Q cannot be used. If they are not, Q can be used.

4. Conclusion

Q-methodology, as a systematic approach to the study of human behavior, has been available in a systematized form since the 1950s. It has taken time for Stephenson's ideas to gain acceptance and they have done so primarily outside psychology. In the 1990s, researchers in political science appear to be making the greatest use of Q-methodology, and there is some evidence that it is being rediscovered in psychology. A recent primer on Q (McKeon and Thomas 1988) may stir additional interest. Also, a journal—*Operant Subjectivity*, devoted almost exclusively to articles about Q and studies that employed Q-techniques—began publication in 1977. Whether this journal will spark new interest in Q remains to be seen.

See also: Factor Analysis

References

Cronbach L J, Gleser G 1954 Book review of William Stephenson's "The study of behavior: Q-technique and its methodology." *Psychometrika* 19: 327–30.

Jung C G 1993 *Psychological Types.* Harcourt, New York

Kerlinger F N 1986 *Foundations of Behavioral Research: Educational and Psychological Inquiry*, 3rd edn. Holt, Rinehart and Winston, New York
McKeon B, Thomas D 1988 *Q Methodology*. Sage, Newbury Park, California
Nunnally J C 1970 *Introduction to Psychological Measurement*. McGraw-Hill, New York
Stephenson W 1953 *The Study of Behavior: Q-technique and its Methodology*. University of Chicago Press, Chicago, Illinois
Sundland D 1962 The construction of Q sorts: A criticism. *Psychol. Rev.* 69: 62–64
Wittenborn J R 1961 Contributions and current status of Q methodology. *Psychol. Rev.* 58: 132–42

Quasi-experimentation

R. M. Wolf

In the mid-nineteenth century, psychology broke off from philosophy and moved from the armchair into the laboratory. In the twentieth century, research in psychology and education moved from the laboratory to field settings. Classical experimental designs of the type developed by R A Fisher were found to be rather limited in dealing with the problems encountered in conducting educational research in field settings. Specifically, it was found that investigators frequently did not have the power to assign subjects at random to different treatment conditions. Quasi-experimentation, which is examined in this entry, was developed as a general approach to conducting research in field settings where the power to randomize was either seriously curtailed or altogether absent. In addition, several specific research designs were developed under the general heading of quasi-experimentation in order to conduct research in field settings where the investigator was not in full control of the situation.

1. Threats to Internal Validity

Classical experimental design depended heavily on sampling theory. If a randomization procedure is correctly implemented, the expected pretreatment difference between experimental and comparison groups is fully known and is zero. When the assumptions of sampling theory are met, random assignment distributes all known and unknown causes of the dependent variable equally over all treatment conditions, thereby eliminating any confounding of the treatment contrast and all theoretically irrelevant causal forces. Campbell (1957) began a career-long quest to develop methods for cause-probing research with long-lasting treatments in open system contexts. He sought to identify the particular alternative causes that random assignment rules out. He used his and others' experience to generate a list of these causes, focusing on those factors that repeatedly produced problems in making causal inferences in the past: he called them "threats to internal validity." The list was begun in 1957 and expanded in Campbell and Stanley (1967) and Cook and Campbell (1979). The list is still being added to (Borg

and Gall 1989 pp. 644–49). The purpose of the list is to enable investigators to examine alternative explanations for results when randomization is not possible. For Campbell, the key to confident causal inferences was the ability to construct a persuasive case that every plausible and identified threat to internal validity had been ruled out in a particular study. This requires assuming that the list of threats to internal validity is comprehensive and that the structural design features, such as the use of a pretest and comparison groups, can support the burden of "falsification" (Karl Popper's use of the term) placed on them.

In this respect, quasi-experimentation is an approach to the conduct of research and the interpretation of results. It represents Campbell's attempt to provide a theoretical justification for the conduct of studies in field settings where the absence of randomization does not necessarily invalidate results.

2. The Interrupted Time Series Design

The other aspect of quasi-experimentation is the development of specialized designs for research. Quantitatively specific causal expectations are promoted in two ways. The first is the "interrupted time series design." A time series is involved when multiple observations are made over time. The observations can be on the same units, as when particular individuals are repeatedly observed; or they can be on different but similar units, as when annual achievement test scores for a particular grade are displayed for a school over a number of years. In the latter case, different students will be in the grade each year. Interrupted time series analysis entails knowing the specific point in the series when a treatment occurred. The inferential key here is that with swift-acting cause–effect links (or when a causal delay period is independently known), a clear expectancy exists about the exact time when a change should occur in the level, slope, or variance of a time series. Thus, the research question is: Do the obtained data match the point-specific time pattern predicted? The statistical analysis of data from a time-series design can be complex and depends heavily on having a sizable number of data points (McCain and McCleary 1979) (see *Change, Measurement of*).

3. Regression–Discontinuity Design

The second design is the "regression–discontinuity design." In this design, the prediction is that a discontinuity should occur at the exact cut-off point that defines treatment exposure, such as eligibility for a remedial program or the grade point criterion for going onto a dean's list. In a regression discontinuity design, all individuals who are eligible for a particular treatment are given it.

Consider the situation when a school decides to institute a remedial program for students who have been found to have deficiencies in reading skills at a particular grade level. A reading test is administered to all students in the school at the grade level in question. A certain score on the test is used as a cut-off, so that all students scoring at or below the cut-off score are placed in the remedial program while students who score above the cut-off score are placed in regular classes of instruction. Strict adherence to the cut-off score is required in a regression discontinuity design.

After the establishment of the groups, remedial and regular, appropriate instruction is dispensed to each group. At the conclusion of the treatment, all students in both regular and remedial groups are again administered a reading test.

The analysis of the data proceeds as follows. First, a regression analysis of post-test scores on pretest scores is carried out and a best-fitting regression line is obtained for the group receiving the experimental treatment. In this case, it is the group of students in the remedial program. Second, a separate regression analysis of post-test scores is carried out and a best-fitting regression line is obtained for the group receiving regular instruction. The term "best-fitting" refers to a regression line that minimizes the sums of squares of deviations of the points from the regression line. Standard least squares regression analysis procedures are used to obtain such lines. While usual practice is to obtain straight lines, there is no reason why this has to be. Curved regression lines may fit the data better than straight lines. The third step in the analysis of data from a regression discontinuity design involves a comparison of the lines at the cut-off point. To accomplish this, the prediction equation produced by each of the regression analyses is used to compute the estimated post-test score for a pretest score at the cut-off point. Since there are two regression equations, there will be two estimated post-test scores, one for each group. In Fig. 1 the results of the discontinuity analyses are shown. The regression line for the students in the regular program is a curved one. The research question here is: Does an inflection in the response variable occur at the cut-off point? In each case, a point-specific hypothesis is under test; matching the data to this

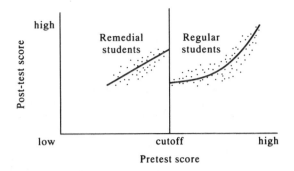

Figure 1
Graph to show results of remedial reading program following regression discontinuity analysis

expectation provides much of the basis for a causal inference.

In this example presented above, the estimated post-test score for the remedial group is higher than the estimated post-test score for the regular group at the cut-off score. The difference on discontinuity at the cut-off point suggests a positive augmenting effect for the remedial program.

4. Conclusion

Quasi-experimentation has come to mean both a general orientation to the conduct of research in field settings and specific designs for the conduct of studies. This entry has attempted to address both aspects of quasi-experimentation, noting the particular features of each aspect.

See also: Experimental Studies; Scientific Methods in Educational Research

References

Borg W R, Gall M D 1989 *Educational Research: An Introduction* Longman, New York
Campbell D T 1957 Factors relevant to the validity of experiments in social settings. *Psych. Bull.* 54: 297–312
Campbell D T, Stanley J C 1967 *Experimental and Quasi-experimental Design for Research.* Houghton Mifflin, Boston, Massachusetts
Cook T D, Campbell D T 1979 *Quasi-experimentation: Design and Analysis Issues for Field Settings.* Rand-McNally, Chicago, Illinois
McCain L J, McCleary 1979 The statistical analysis of the simple interrupted time-series quasi-experiment. In: Cook T D, Campbell D T (eds.) 1979

Further Reading

Cook T D 1991 Qualifying the warrant for generalized causal inferences in quasi-experimentation. In: McLaughlin M, Phillips D C (eds.) 1991 *Evaluation and Education: At Quarter Century* National Society for the Study of Education, Chicago, Illinois,

Questionnaires

R. M. Wolf

A questionnaire is a self-report instrument used for gathering information about variables of interest to an investigator. It consists of a number of questions or items on paper that a respondent reads and answers. The questions or items can be structured or unstructured. That is, the categories of response may be specified or left unspecified. A structured item such as sex would have the two categories, "male" and "female," and the respondent is asked to check the one that describes him or her. An unstructured item, on the other hand, may ask the respondent to describe how he or she spent his or her last vacation.

1. Assumptions in Use of Questionnaires

A questionnaire, as a self-report instrument, is based on three assumptions. These are:

(a) the respondent can read and understand the questions or items;

(b) the respondent possesses the information to answer the questions or items;

(c) the respondent is willing to answer the questions or items honestly.

These assumptions may or may not be warranted for a particular questionnaire in a particular study. Accordingly, the assumptions often have to be tested through adequate developmental work before a questionnaire can be used with confidence. Such developmental work often includes interviewing, piloting, and pretesting.

The variables of interest for which information is sought in a questionnaire can be quite varied. They can include factual questions about the respondent, such as age, sex, and occupation; attitudes, opinions, interests, beliefs, aspirations, and expectations; past, present, and planned activities in particular areas; memberships in various groups; and perceptions of various things. The list of what can be included in a questionnaire is almost without limit. What is included in a questionnaire will obviously be limited by the purposes of a study, what can reasonably be asked in a questionnaire, and time constraints.

An investigator should limit the questions or items in a questionnaire to variables of primary interest. Each question or item should be explicitly or implicitly related to a particular research question or hypothesis. Even when investigators so restrict themselves, they often find it difficult to investigate fully all variables

of interest without making the questionnaire so long as to substantially reduce the likelihood that respondents will answer it. Consequently, even when investigators restrict themselves to variables of interest, decisions still need to be made about what can and should be included in a particular questionnaire.

The second constraint on what will be included in a questionnaire involves the sensitivity or delicacy of the content of particular questions or items. Matters of a personal nature such as sexual behavior and attitudes are a case in point. Many individuals do not wish to reveal their attitudes and behavior in an area that they consider to be a matter of privacy. Respondents may simply refuse to answer such questions, give what they believe to be socially desirable responses or, perhaps even worse, consign the questionnaire to the nearest wastebasket.

It is clear that asking highly personal questions can produce problems in a questionnaire. It is less obvious that apparently straightforward and objective questions can also create problems for the respondent. For example, a question regarding the amount of schooling may pose a problem for a respondent. If the residents of a community have, by and large, earned a university degree, an individual with only a high school diploma may feel threatened by a question regarding the amount of schooling. Similarly, divorced people may feel reluctant to report their true marital status if they view divorce as containing some social stigma. Sensitivity on the part of the individual developing a questionnaire is needed along with considerable developmental work if such problems are to be fully identified and provisions made to deal with them.

The third constraint as to what will be included in a questionnaire is time. Respondents cannot be expected to spend a great deal of time answering a questionnaire. Experience with adults suggests that 30 minutes is about the upper limit that can be expected in the way of answering time when questionnaires are administered in a group setting. When questionnaires are mailed to respondents, about 15 minutes appears to be the limit of respondent time. Questionnaires that are administered to students may need to be shorter and require less time. There are two issues involved here. The first is respondent fatigue. Simply stated, answering questionnaire items requires effort. After a while, respondents will tire and this can lead to careless or inaccurate responses. How much questionnaire material can be presented to a respondent is an issue to be addressed in development work. The second issue is more serious. It is the issue of respondent cooperation. A lengthy, time-consuming questionnaire may cause a respondent to cease to cooperate after a period of answering questions. At best, one will receive an incomplete questionnaire and, at worst, the questionnaire will not be returned. Again, careful developmental work is needed to establish how much questionnaire material can be presented to a particular target group.

2. Developing a Questionnaire

A well-made questionnaire is highly deceptive. It appears to be well-organized, the questions are clear, response options are well-drawn and exhaustive, and there is a natural ordering or flow to the questions that keeps the respondent moving toward completion of the questionnaire. These desirable attributes and the deceptive simplicity of a well-made questionnaire do not spring naturally out of the process of questionnaire construction but are the result of a great deal of painstaking developmental work. The remainder of this entry will describe the steps that are needed to achieve such a result along with some attention to the problems that arise and decisions that are required at each step.

2.1 The Identification of Variables

The first step in developing a questionnaire is the identification of variables to be studied. Such identification will depend on the nature of the research problem to be studied and the specific hypotheses and questions to be investigated. Theory and previous research will be a major guide in this area as well as conversations with knowledgeable individuals. It is also at this initial stage that the population of interest that will be studied needs to be identified.

Once the list of relevant variables has been identified, it is necessary to decide how data will be collected. A questionnaire is only one means of data gathering. Interviews, tests, and observational procedures are some of the other ways in which information can be gathered. A decision about an appropriate method of data collection will depend on: (a) the nature of the variables to be studied, (b) the nature of the target population that is to be studied, and (c) the amount of resources available for the investigation. Kinsey, for example, decided that the nature of the variables he wished to study, that is, sexual behaviors, were of such a delicate nature that only a carefully structured and sensitively conducted interview could elicit the information he needed (Kinsey et al. 1948). Other examples can be cited. The point is that the use of questionnaires as a method of data gathering is neither automatic nor obvious.

2.2 Translation of Variables into Questions

Assuming that a decision has been made to use a questionnaire to gather data as a result of a conscious, deliberate process, it is then necessary to translate the variables into questions that can elicit the desired information. At this early stage it is generally recommended that the questions or items be left relatively unstructured—that is, no attempt be made to provide a set of response categories for the items. The items should then be organized into an order that appears reasonable to the investigator for tryout in an interview format. The investigator and one or two co-workers would then try out the questions in an interview with a few (for example, four or five) respondents from the population that will be studied. The aim of such an exercise is to obtain some information on the comprehensibility of the questions and whether they appear to elicit the desired information. Such an exercise is important in helping to provide a reality base for further development work and to furnish some feedback on how the questions and items are being received and interpreted as well as some idea as to the range of responses.

On the basis of such small tryout work it should be possible to revise the initial set of questions so that both their clarity and the likelihood of eliciting the desired information are increased. While it is expected that the wording of the initial questions will be modified and that additional questions may have to be added, it is possible that other questions will be eliminated. In the case of the tryout of several alternative ways of asking a particular question, it should be possible to decide which of the alternatives is most suitable. Also, it may be found that particular questions fail to elicit the information that is needed with regard to a variable of interest and, consequently, may need to be eliminated.

2.3 The Pilot Stage

While considerable revision can and will take place on the basis of an initial tryout in an interview format, it is premature to structure the items by providing a set of response categories for each item. The information to structure items at this point in the developmental work is too limited. What is recommended rather is that the items and questions be organized into a pilot questionnaire that is reproduced for administration to a group of respondents from the target population. Such a pilot questionnaire would require some introductory statement informing the respondent of the nature of the study being undertaken, why the requested information will be important, a request for cooperation, and a pledge of anonymity and confidentiality in the treatment and use of information supplied by the respondent. This last requirement is the easiest to honor since the information supplied by the respondent will be used solely for further developmental work. Not having the respondent supply his or her name at this stage will usually enhance cooperation. Whether respondents do or do not supply their names in the main collection of data is an ethical issue.

At the pilot stage there are still likely to be many

more questions than will be included in a final questionnaire. This is to be expected since many decisions about the selection of a final set of questions or items will require additional information. Since the tryout questionnaire is apt to contain considerably more questions than a final questionnaire and since questions will be asked in an unstructured or open-ended form, the amount of time that would be required to complete the questionnaire might be considerable. If this is so, the questionnaire could be fractionated into two, three, or even more parts for the tryout. This would reduce the amount of time required for answering since the respondent would be answering only a fraction of the questions. Since the object of the tryout is to find out how individual terms or, at most, groups of items are being answered, such fractionation is not only permissible but probably even desirable. Generally, when fractionating a questionnaire, it is necessary to develop several forms of about equal length or, more important, of equal answering time. In administering the tryout questionnaire(s), it is also necessary to have roughly equivalent groups take one each of several forms. The desired number of respondents for each form should be at least 30 with a goal of about 50 people who are fully representative of the target population.

2.4 Refining the Questionnaire

The results of the tryout will yield a wealth of information. Since this is the first set of results of the questions and items administered in written form, it will be interesting to determine whether the questions provide the desired type of response data or whether further work on the wording of questions is needed. Examination of the response data will also provide a basis for structuring many of the questions or items. For example, if one question asks respondents to indicate the number of books in their home, it will be possible to produce a frequency distribution of books in the home, and, on the basis of that frequency distribution, produce a set of categories that will encompass the distribution and have sufficient variability for later analysis. Other variables that yield quantitative responses can be handled similarly. For qualitative variables, the data should permit the identification of a number of response categories and a frequency count for each category. In this way, it should be possible to structure or "close" many of the items. This will considerably facilitate later coding and analysis in the main study.

It may not be possible to structure all the items in a questionnaire although this remains a goal. For example, items about occupation, either the respondent's or his or her father's and mother's, may require unstructured items in order to obtain sufficient descriptive material to permit classification into an occupational categorization scheme. In such a case, a closed-ended item will not suffice. In addition, unstructured questionnaire items can be a source

of rich and spontaneous response material that can enhance the interpretation of results. On the other hand, unstructured items place an additional burden on the respondent that can result in a reduction of the level of cooperation. Consequently, an investigator needs to achieve a delicate balance between the number of structured versus unstructured items. Information from the next phase of developmental work, pretesting, should furnish some guidance on the appropriate balance between the two types of items.

The results of the questionnaire in tryout form should enable an investigator to produce a penultimate version of the questionnaire. This version should consist largely of items in a structured form. However, since one cannot be sure that the response categories for all structured items are exhaustive, it is common practice to provide an extra category labeled "Other (please specify)" for many items and to allow ample space for the respondent to supply the needed information.

There are a number of other considerations that are necessary at this stage of the developmental work. A short statement of the purpose of the questionnaire needs to be placed at the beginning of the questionnaire along with the specific directions for answering. The material from the tryout version, with appropriate modification, should be used. It is also customary to begin the body of the questionnaire with an item asking the respondent to note the time he or she started to answer the questionnaire, requesting that the questionnaire be answered in a single sitting, and, at the end of the questionnaire, requesting that the ending time be noted. In this way, it is possible to estimate the time required to complete the questionnaire. This is important for two reasons. First, it will enable an investigator to decide whether to further shorten the questionnaire or not. Second, it will furnish a basis for scheduling the administration of the final questionnaire. The last task in the assembly of the questionnaire for pretesting is to affix a short statement at the end of the questionnaire instructing the respondent how to return the questionnaire to the investigator and to thank the respondent for his or her cooperation. Instructions regarding the return of the questionnaire are critical if the questionnaire is to be mailed.

One variable that is critical at this stage of development is the layout of the questionnaire. A good deal of work is required to produce a draft of the questionnaire in which the items are presented in a format that is attractive and will assist the respondent to complete the instrument. Consideration needs to be given to the size of type, sequencing of items, provision of adequate space to answer unstructured items, and other details of presentation. Unfortunately, there are few detailed guides for such work. Experimentation with different layouts and review by a few people from the population on whom the questionnaire will eventually be used are often undertaken for guidance on such matters. It is not necessary that the questionnaire actually be administered at this time, merely that it be reviewed on the basis of layout.

One area in which there has been research and where there is a fair degree of agreement is with regard to classificatory items such as sex, age, race, and the like. It is generally recommended that such items be placed at the end of a questionnaire and be preceded by a short introductory statement that such items are supplementary and will be used for classificatory purposes. The reason for this recommendation is that if the questionnaire began with such items and the stated purpose of the questionnaire was to survey, say, television viewing, a respondent might be put off by the apparent irrelevance of such items and, consequently, not answer the questionnaire. It is better to begin with items that are clearly related to the stated purpose of the questionnaire.

2.5 Field Testing the Questionnaire

The draft questionnaire, reproduced in bulk, should be administered to a sample of individuals from the target population. A sample size of 50 to 100 respondents should be sufficient. Post-administration analysis should focus on producing frequency distributions of responses for each variable. Additional "closing-up" of items should take place, if warranted. The investigator will also need to pay attention to items in which the rate of nonresponse, or of "don't know" responses, exceeds 5 percent of the respondent sample. Such high rates are usually indicative of ambiguities that are still inherent in items or inadequacies in the response categories. Such problems will need to be dealt with in one way or another. If the variable that the item is measuring is central to the study, further developmental work might be needed. Finally, an analysis of the data on time to complete the questionnaire will have to be made to determine whether the questionnaire will have to be shortened or not. Even if the time data indicate that the time needed to answer the questionnaire is reasonable, a suggested time limit needs to be established for purposes of administration. It is generally recommended that a time limit be set at the time corresponding to the 90th percentile in the distribution of time data. This will ensure that virtually everyone will answer the questionnaire.

At this point, a final questionnaire should be ready for use in a study. It should be attractive and present no problems for a respondent. If so, it is the fruit of a long and often painstaking process of development. The questionnaire should consist largely of structured items in which the respondent can easily find and check an appropriate response category. The number of items in which the respondent has to supply an answer in his or her own words should be small. The full questionnaire should require certainly less than 30 minutes to complete and, preferably, less than 15 or 20. It should also be possible to develop a codebook for easy post-administration coding and analysis.

3. Points Requiring Attention

The above presentation is intended to describe the process of questionnaire development. It is by no means exhaustive. Further information about each step can be found in the References and Further Reading sections. Particular attention will also need to be given to question wording so that subtle or not so subtle cues, that suggest responding in a particular way are not supplied. For example, consider the following questions:

(a) Do you approve of school prayer?

(b) You *do* approve of school prayer, don't you?

(c) Don't you disapprove of school prayer?

(d) You don't approve of school prayer, do you?

While the above four questions appear to be asking the same question, they are not. Questions (c) and (d) are highly suggestive and question (b) is rather suggestive. It should not be surprising that if each question was given to an independent random sample from the same population, results would differ. The point is that sensitivity and care are required in question wording if unbiased results are to be obtained. Further information on the specifics of question wording can be found in an excellent monograph by Converse and Presser (1986).

3.1 Validity and Reliability

Two considerations that are considered important in judging the adequacy of measuring instruments are validity and reliability. These are typically applied in the review of tests and scales. Unfortunately, they are not often applied to questionnaires. Too often, investigators assume that respondents possess the information to answer questionnaire items, can read and understand the items, and are answering honestly. Research suggests that these assumptions may not be true and that the validity and reliability of questionnaires need to be established. Wolf (1993) reported a study designed to test the validity of questionnaire items for use with 10-year olds in various countries. A questionnaire was developed and administered to judgment samples of roughly equal numbers of boys and girls from upper, middle, and lower socioeconomic levels in four countries (Australia, Finland, Iran, and Sweden). Subsequently, an interview was conducted with the mother of each student who was tested or a questionnaire was sent to the home to be completed by the mother. In either case, the same questions that were put to the student were put to his or her mother.

The data were then coded and transmitted to a central processing site.

The results of the study were fairly clear-cut. There was a very high degree of agreement between the student and his or her mother to items that asked for a description of present status or home conditions. For example, both student and mother agreed as to the father's occupation, student age, and where the student studied at home. There was considerable disagreement, however, on items that were prospective or retrospective in nature. For example, the median correlation between mother and student on the amount of additional schooling desired was 0.35, while the correlation for length of attendance in a nursery school was 0.44 for those that had attended.

The fact that mother and child agreed in their responses to certain questionnaire items about the home situation is not conclusive evidence of validity. It is, however, a reassuring indicator. On the basis of the results of that study, it was decided that it was indeed feasible to ask 10-year olds to complete questionnaires that asked them to furnish information about their present life situation. However, the number of items that asked the student to furnish information about the past or the future were kept to a minimum.

Reliability of questionnaire information can also be investigated. There are two general approaches to the determination of the reliability and, hence, measurement error present in questionnaires. One approach is to ask the same question that was presented early in the questionnaire in the same or slightly altered form later in the questionnaire. This provides a modest consistency check but does not take into account variations in time of day or day-to-day variations. The second and superior approach is to readminister a questionnaire to the same group of individuals several days later and compare the results that were obtained. This latter approach was used by Munck (1991) in a small study of 9-year olds in Sweden. Munck's results present a striking example of the amount of unreliability inherent in questionnaires. Three items from her questionnaire are presented below along with the "kappa coefficient," the statistic describing the extent of relationship between the responses at the two times.

Item	Kappa
Are you a boy or a girl?	0.98
Do you speak Swedish at home?	0.77
How often do you read for somebody at home?	0.41

The results are quite informative. While a kappa of 0.98 for sex seems high, one wonders why, for such a basic item, it is not 1.00. The results for the other two items are rather disappointing. The kappa for reading to someone else at home is so low that its value in any analysis is highly questionable.

In a similar vein, Witte (1990), in a secondary analysis of data from a major study in the United States, "High School and Beyond" (Coleman and Hoffer 1987), found that the level of mother's and father's occupation reported by the same students at grades 10 and 12 correlated 0.54. While the United States is noted as a country with a relatively high degree of social mobility, it is unlikely that there is that much instability in father's and mother's occupational levels over a two-year period. Correlations of other socioeconomic variables were equally low, suggesting that there is a considerable amount of error in response to questionnaire items. It is important that research workers who develop or plan to use questionnaires investigate for measurement error so that the results obtained from questionnaires can be used with confidence or correction for unreliability made in analysis.

4. Coding Schemes

The use of questionnaires in a study will produce a great deal of information that will need to be analyzed. This is usually done on computers. Investigators will therefore have to develop procedures for coding questionnaire information for entry into a computer. Such a procedure is called a "coding scheme." For many variables of interest, responses to structured questionnaire items can be assigned numerical variables. For example, the sex of the respondent could be coded "1" for female and "2" for male. Missing information can be coded using some other digit. For unstructured items, it is usually necessary to examine data obtained from the tryout stage and develop a set of categories into which responses can be classified and a numerical value assigned to each category. The codes developed for structured and unstructured items in a questionnaire are called a "codebook." This serves as the specifications for translating the responses from a questionnaire into a form that can be readily analyzed by computers. It is strongly recommended that a codebook be prepared before a questionnaire is administered so that any problems in coding can be anticipated and dealt with before the questionnaire is administered to a large group.

5. Conclusion

This entry has attempted to describe what questionnaires are and how they are developed. Well-made questionnaires are somewhat deceptive. They appear to be clear and logical. This appearance, however, is invariably the result of a long and often complicated process of development and tryout. Well-made questionnaires cannot be developed in a short time. They typically require hard and sustained effort over a long period of time.

See also: Self-report in Educational Research

References

Coleman J S, Hoffer T 1987 *Public and Private High Schools: The Impact of Communities.* Basic Books, New York

Converse J M, Presser S 1986 *Survey Questions: Handcrafting the Standardized Questionnaire.* Sage, Beverly Hills, California

Kinsey A C, Pomeroy W B, Martin C E 1948 *Sexual Behaviour in the Human Male.* Saunders, Wayne, New Jersey

Munck I 1991 *Plan for a Measurement Study Within the Swedish IEA Reading Literacy Survey and Some Results for Population A.* Institute of International Education, University of Stockholm, Stockholm

Witte J 1990 Understanding high school achievement: After a decade of research, do we have any confident policy recommendations? Paper presented at the annual meeting of the American Political Science Association, San Francisco, California

Wolf R M 1993 Data quality and norms in international studies. *Meas. Eval. Couns. Dev.* 26: 35–40

Further Reading

Berdie D R, Anderson J F 1974 *Questionnaires: Design and Use.* Scarecrow, Metuchen, New Jersey

Jacobs T O 1974 *Developing Questionnaire Items: How to Do It Well.* Human Resources Research Organization, Alexandria, Virginia

Labaw P J 1980 *Advanced Questionnaire Design.* Abt, Cambridge, Massachusetts

Oppenheim A N 1992 *Questionnaire Design, Interviewing, and Attitude Measurement.* Pinter, London

Payne S L 1951 *The Art of Asking Questions.* Princeton University Press, Princeton, New Jersey

Sudman S, Bradburn N 1982 *Asking Questions: A Practical Guide to Questionnaire Design.* Jossey-Bass, San Francisco, California

Sampling in Survey Research

K. N. Ross and K. Rust

Educational research is aimed at developing useful generalizations about educational environments and the ways in which individuals behave in such environments. However, due to practical constraints on research resources, the educational researcher is usually limited to the study of a sample rather than a complete coverage of the population for which these generalizations are appropriate. Provided that scientific sampling procedures are employed in association with appropriate methods of data analysis, the use of a sample often provides many advantages compared with a complete coverage. These advantages include reduced costs associated with obtaining and analyzing the data, reduced requirements for specialized personnel to conduct the fieldwork, greater speed in most aspects of data manipulation and summarization, and greater accuracy due to the possibility of closer supervision of fieldwork and data preparation.

Kish (1965, 1987) has divided the research situations that arise in the social sciences in which samples are used in three broad categories: (a) *experiments* —in which the treatment variables are deliberately introduced and all extraneous variables are either controlled or randomized; (b) *surveys*—in which all members of a defined population have a known nonzero probability of selection into the sample; and (c) *investigations*—in which data are collected without either the randomization of experiments or the probability sampling of surveys. Experiments are strong with respect to "internal validity" because they are concerned with the question of whether a true measure of the effect of a treatment variable has been obtained

for the subjects in the experiment. In contrast, surveys are strong with respect to "external validity" because they are concerned with the question of whether findings obtained for subjects in the survey may be generalized to a wider population. Investigations are weak on both types of validity and their use is due frequently to convenience or low cost.

1. Populations

The populations which are of interest to educational researchers are generally finite populations that may be defined jointly with the elements that they contain. A population in educational research is therefore, usually, the aggregate of a finite number of elements, and these elements are the basic units that comprise and define the population.

Kish (1965, Chap. 1) states that a population should be described in terms of (a) content, (b) units, (c) extent, and (d) time. For example, in a study of the characteristics of Australian secondary school students, it may be desirable to specify the populations as: (a) all 14-year old students, (b) in secondary schools, (c) in Australia, and (d) in 1992.

In order to prepare a description of a population to be considered in an educational research study, it is important to distinguish between the population for which the results are desired, the "desired target population," and the population actually covered, the "survey population." In an ideal situation, these two populations would be the same. However, differences may arise due to noncoverage; for example, for the population described above, a list may be compiled of schools during early 1992 which accidentally omits some new schools which begin operating later in the year. Alternatively, differences may occur because of nonresponse at the data collection stage. For example, a number of schools having large concentrations of educationally retarded students might be unwilling to participate in the study.

Strictly speaking, only the survey population is represented by the sample, but this population may be difficult to describe exactly, and therefore it is often easier to write about the defined target population (Kish 1965 Chap. 1). The defined target population description provides an operational definition which is used to guide the construction of a list of population elements, or sampling frame, from which the sample may be drawn. The elements that are excluded from the desired target population in order to form the defined target population are referred to as the "excluded population."

For example, during a 1991 UNESCO survey of the reading performance of Grade 6 students in Zimbabwe (Ross and Postlethwaite 1991), the desired target population was centered around a grade description, as distinct from an age description, of students attending schools. After extensive consultations with the Zimbabwe Ministry of Education and Culture concerning the key purposes of the study, it was agreed that the desired target population should be as follows:

> All students at the Grade 6 level in 1991 who are attending registered government or nongovernment schools in the nine educational administration regions of Zimbabwe.

It was also decided that the study should be directed toward primary schooling within the mainstream national education system. Therefore, the term "students" in the description of the defined target population was restricted in its meaning so as to exclude students attending special schools for handicapped students. These students were few in number when compared to the total population of Grade 6 students. The numbers of students and schools associated with the desired, defined, and excluded populations have been presented in Table 1.

2. Sampling Frames

Before selecting the sample, the elements of the defined target population must be assembled into a sampling frame. The sampling frame usually takes the form of a physical list of the elements, and is the means by which the researcher is able to "take hold" of the defined target population. The entries in the sampling frame may refer to the individual elements (e.g., students) or groups of these elements (e.g., schools).

In practice, the sampling frame is more than just a list because the entries are normally arranged in an order which corresponds to their membership of certain strata. For example, in the 1991 International Assessment of Educational Progress in mathematics and science, sampling frames for each of the participating countries were constructed that listed schools according to their enrollment size, school type (e.g., government or nongovernment, comprehensive or selective) and region (urban or rural, geographic region of the country) (Chu et al. 1992).

The use of strata during the preparation of a sampling frame is often undertaken in order to ensure that data are obtained which will permit the researcher to study, and assess more accurately, the characteristics of both individual and combined strata.

Table 1
Zimbabwe Grade 6 pupils: Tabular descriptions of the desired, defined, and excluded populations for the UNESCO Grade 6 survey conducted in 1991

Education region	Desired		Defined		Excluded	
	Schools	Pupils	Schools	Pupils	Schools	Pupils
Harare	222	28,421	214	28,360	8	61
Manicaland	755	46,130	753	46,124	2	6
Mashonaland Central	319	20,780	319	20,780	0	0
Mashonaland East	442	27,776	440	27,774	2	2
Mashonaland West	415	27,752	414	27,708	1	44
Masvingo	665	41,664	662	41,628	3	36
Matabeleland North	530	29,411	525	29,311	5	100
Matabeleland South	421	17,533	421	17,533	0	0
Midlands	718	44,314	716	44,288	2	26
Zimbabwe	4,487	283,781	4,464	283,506	23	275

3. Probability Samples and Nonprobability Samples

There are usually two main aims involved in the conduct of sample surveys in educational research: (a) the estimation of the values of population attributes ("parameters") from the values of sample attributes ("statistics"), and (b) the testing of statistical hypotheses about population characteristics. These two aims require that the researcher has some knowledge of the accuracy of the values of the sample statistics as estimates of the population parameters. Knowledge of the accuracy of these estimates may generally be derived from statistical theory provided that probability sampling has been employed. Probability sampling requires that each member of the defined target population has a known, and nonzero, chance of being selected into the sample. The accuracy of samples selected without using probability sampling methods cannot be discovered from the internal evidence of a single sample.

Nonprobability sampling in educational research has mostly taken the form of judgment sampling in which expert choice is used to guide the selection of typical or representative samples. These samples may be better than probability samples, or they may not. Their quality cannot be determined without knowledge of the relevant population parameters, and if these parameters were known then there would be no need to select a sample.

The use of judgment samples in educational research is sometimes carried out with the (usually implied) justification that the sample represents a hypothetical universe rather than a "real" population. This justification may lead to research results which are not meaningful if the gap between this hypothetical universe and the related real population is too large. Since nonprobability samples are not appropriate for dealing objectively with the aims of estimation and hypothesis testing, they will not be examined in the following discussion.

4. Probability Sampling Methods

There are a number of methods that can be employed to draw probability samples. These methods are often used in combination for a given application. The aims of these methods are to give samples that provide reliable estimates for the population in a manner which is both practical to implement and cost effective. The more widespread techniques are outlined below, followed by a discussion of techniques for comparing alternative sample designs.

4.1 Multistage Sampling

A population of elements can usually be described in terms of a hierarchy of sampling units of different sizes and types. For example, a population of school students may be seen as being composed of a number of classes each of which is composed of a number of students. Further, the classes may be grouped into a number of schools.

The hypothetical population of school students in Fig. 1. shows 18 students distributed among 6 classrooms (with 3 students per class) and 3 schools (with 2 classes per school).

From this population a multistage sample could be drawn by randomly selecting two schools at the first stage, followed by randomly selecting one classroom from each of the selected schools at the second stage, and then randomly selecting two students from each selected classroom at the third stage. This three-stage sample design would provide a sample of four students. It would also provide a sample which is an "epsem sample" (equal probability of selection method) (Kish 1965 Chap. 1). That is, the probability of selecting any student in the population would be the same for all students ($2/3 \times 1/2 \times 2/3 = 4/18$). Similarly, a simple random sample of 4 students from the population of 18 students would also provide an epsem sample in which the probability of selection would be the same for all students (4/18). A simple random sample is one for which each possible sample of four distinct students from the population of 18 students is equally likely to be selected. Epsem sampling is widely used in survey research because it usually results in self-weighting samples. In these samples an unbiased estimate of the population mean may be obtained by taking the simple average of the sample cases.

It is important to remember that the use of probability sampling does not automatically lead to an epsem sample. Probability sampling requires that each element in the population has a known and nonzero chance of selection—which may or may not be equal for all elements. There are many examples in the literature which demonstrate that educational researchers often overlook this point. For example, one popular sample design in educational research has been to select a simple random sample of say, a schools from a list of A schools, and then select a simple random sample of b students from each selected school. The probability of selecting a student by using this design is ab/AB_i, where B_i is the size of the ith school in the population. Consequently, students from large schools

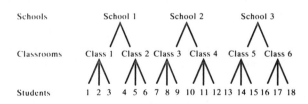

Figure 1

Hypothetical population of 18 students grouped into 6 classrooms and 3 schools have less chance of selection and the simple average of sample cases may result in biased estimates of the population mean—especially if the magnitudes of the B_i values vary a great deal and the survey variable is correlated with school size. Further discussion of issues of analysis of non-epsem samples appears in Sect. 5.

4.2 Stratification

The technique of stratification is often employed in the preparation of sample designs for educational survey research because it generally provides increased precision in sample estimates without leading to substantial increases in costs. Stratification does not imply any departure from probability sampling—it simply requires that the population be divided into subpopulations called "strata" and that the random sampling be conducted independently within each of these strata. The sample estimates of population parameters are then obtained by combining the information from each stratum. It is, however, important to note that gains in sampling precision are only obtained if the stratifying variable is strongly correlated with the population parameters being estimated.

Stratification may be used in survey research for reasons other than obtaining gains in sampling precision. Strata may be formed in order to employ different sample designs within strata, or because the subpopulations defined by the strata are designated as separate domains of study. Some typical variables used to stratify populations in educational research are: school location (metropolitan/rural), type of school (government/nongovernment), school size (large/medium/small), and sex of pupils in school (males only/females only/coeducational).

Stratification does not necessarily require that the same sampling fraction be used within each stratum. If a uniform sampling fraction is used, then the sample design is known as a proportionate stratified sample because the sample size from any stratum is proportional to the population size of the stratum. Such a sample design is epsem. In a stratified sample design of elements, different sampling fractions may be employed in the defined strata of population. If the sampling fractions vary between strata, then the obtained sample is a disproportionate stratified sample. The chance that a given element appears in the sample is specified by the sampling fraction associated with the stratum in which that element is located.

In theory, the precision of sample estimates will increase with increasing numbers of strata. In practice, as the number of strata increases, the additional gains rapidly become minimal, especially if the additional strata are obtained through increasingly finer subdivisions of a single stratification variable. Generally, it is good practice to use several variables for stratification, with only a few categories (say up to five) for each.

4.3 Systematic Selection

A popular, simple, and effective technique to draw the sample of units for a given stage of sampling within a given stratum is that of systematic selection. The method is implemented by first establishing the desired rate of sampling for the stratum f. The population units are ordered, and every F th unit is selected, where F is the reciprocal of f. The initial unit selection is made with equal probability from among the first F units listed. If the units are first ordered randomly, systematic selection provides a convenient means of drawing a simple random sample. More often, and of more use generally, the list is sorted using characteristics of the units that are likely to be related to the survey subject. This procedure will generally increase the reliability of the sample estimates. The variables used for such sorting are often those such as enrollment size or graduation rates that can provide a continuum of different school types within explicit strata. Systematic sampling, as described here, produces epsem samples, although it can be adapted to draw samples with probability proportional to size—this technique will be discussed in the next section.

4.4 Probability Proportional to Size Two-stage Sample Designs

In educational research the most commonly used primary sampling units, schools and classes, are rarely equal in size. If the sizes of the primary sampling units vary a great deal then problems often arise in controlling the total sample size when the researcher aims to select a two-stage epsem sample.

For example, consider a two-stage sample design in which a schools are selected from a list of A schools, and then a fixed fraction of students, say $1/k$, is selected from each of the a schools. This design would provide an epsem sample of students because the probability of selecting a student is $a/(Ak)$ which is constant for all students in the population. However, the actual size of the sample would depend directly upon the size of the schools which happened to be selected into the sample.

One method of obtaining greater control over the sample size would be to stratify the schools according to size, and then select samples of schools within each stratum. A more widely applied alternative is to employ "probability proportional to size" (PPS) sampling of the primary sampling units followed by simple random or systematic sampling of a fixed number of elements within these units. An exact execution of the PPS method provides complete control over the sample size and yet ensures epsem sampling of elements.

For example, consider a sample of m schools selected with PPS from a population of M schools followed by the selection of a simple random sample of $\bar{n}$ students from each of the m schools. Consider student i who attends school j which has n_j members from the total of N students in the defined target population.

The probability of selecting student i, p_{ij}, into this sample may be expressed as:

$$p_{ij} = m \times \frac{\bar{n}_i}{N} \times \frac{n}{nj} = \frac{m\bar{n}}{N} \qquad (1)$$

Since m, $\bar{n}$, and N are constants then all students in the defined target population have the same chance of selection. That is, the PPS sample design would lead to epsem sampling, and, at the same time, fix the total sample size as $m\bar{n}$ students.

When accurate information concerning the size of each primary sampling unit is not available, then PPS sampling is often conducted by using "measures of size" rather than true sizes. That is, at the first stage of sampling, the clusters are selected with probability proportional to their measure of size. The difference between the actual size of a cluster and its measure of size can be compensated for at the second stage of sampling in order to achieve an epsem sample design. Kish (1965 pp. 222–23) has presented formulae which demonstrate how to calculate the appropriate second-stage sampling fractions for these situations.

An often-used technique for selecting a PPS sample of, say, schools from a sampling frame is to employ a lottery method of sampling. Each school is allocated a number of tickets which is equal to the number of students in the defined target population within the school. For example, consider the hypothetical population described in Table 2. Only the first 7 and final 3 schools have been listed. However, the total numbers of schools and students are assumed to be 26 and 4,000 respectively. Each school is allocated a number of tickets equal to the number of students in the defined target population within the school.

If 5 schools are to be selected, then 5 winning

Table 2
Hypothetical population of schools and students

School	Number of students in target population	Cumulative tally of students	Ticket numbers
A	50	50	1-50
B	200	250	51-250
C	50	300	251-300
D[a]	300	600	301-600
E	150	750	601-750
F	450	1,200	751-1,200
G[a]	250	1,450	1,201-1,450
—	—	—	—
—	—	—	—
—	—	—	—
X[a]	100	3,750	3,651-3,750
Y	50	3,800	3,751-3,800
Z	200	4,000	3,801-4,000

a Schools selected into final sample

tickets are required. The ratio of number of tickets to the number of winning tickets is $4,000/5 = 800$. That is, each ticket should have a 1 in 800 chance of being drawn as a winning ticket. The winning tickets are selected by using a systematic sampling procedure. A random number in the interval 1 to 800 is selected from a table of random numbers and a list of 5 winning ticket numbers is created by adding increments of 800. For example, with a random start of 520, the winning ticket numbers would be 520, 1320, 2120, 2920, and 3720. The schools which are selected into the sample have been marked in Table 2. School D corresponds to winning ticket number 520, and so on to school X which corresponds to winning ticket number 3,720. The chance of selecting a particular school is proportional to the number of tickets associated with that school. Consequently each of the five schools is selected with probability proportional to the number of students in the defined target population.

5. Population Inference from Sample Survey Data

5.1 Estimation and Weighting

Once sample data have been collected, an analysis of the data to derive estimates of population parameters must account for the probabilities of selection of the units included in the sample. The reciprocals of the sampling probabilities, which are sometimes called the "raising factors," describe how many elements in the population are represented by an element in the sample. At the data analysis stage either the raising factors, or any set of numbers proportional to them, may be used to assign weights to the elements. The constant of proportionality makes no difference to the sample estimates. However, in order to avoid confusion for the readers of survey research reports, the constant is sometimes selected so that the sum of the weights is equal to the sample size.

For example, consider a stratified sample design of n elements which is applied to a population of N elements by selecting a simple random sample of n_h elements from the hth stratum containing N_h elements. In the hth stratum, the probability of selecting an element is n_h/N_h, and therefore the raising factor for this stratum is N_h/n_h. That is, each selected element represents N_h/n_h elements in the population.

The sum of the raising factors over all n sample elements is equal to the population size. If there are two strata for the sample design then:

$$\left(\frac{N_1}{n_1} + \frac{N_1}{n_1} + \ldots \text{ for } n_1 \text{ elements}\right) + \left(\frac{N_2}{n_2} + \frac{N_2}{n_2}\right.$$

$$\left. + \ldots \text{ for } n_2 \text{ elements}\right) = N \qquad (2)$$

In order to make the sum of the weights equal to

the sample size, n, both sides of the above equation will have to be multiplied by a constant factor of n/N. That is:

$$\left(\frac{N_1}{n_1} \times \frac{n}{N} + \ldots \text{ for } n_1 \text{ elements}\right) \times \left(\frac{N_2}{n_1} + \frac{n}{N}\right)$$

$$+ \ldots \text{ for } n_2 \text{ elements}\right) = n \qquad (3)$$

Therefore the weight for element i in the hth stratum

is $W_{hi} = \frac{N_h}{n_h} \times \frac{n}{N}$

In analyzing survey data stored on computer files, the standard practice is to store the weight associated with each unit as one variable on the data file. Estimates of population parameters are then obtained from the survey data by first multiplying each variable in the analysis by the weight, w, and then deriving the statistic in the same manner as would usually be applied to unweighted data. Thus for example, a sample estimate ($\bar{x}$) of the population mean is given by the following formula, regardless of the methods of probability sampling adopted:

$$\bar{x} = \left(\sum_i w_i x_i\right) / \left(\sum w_i\right). \qquad (4)$$

5.2 Accuracy, Bias, and Precision

The sample estimate derived from any one sample is inaccurate to the extent that it differs from the population parameter. Generally, the value of the population parameter is not known and therefore the actual accuracy of an individual sample estimate cannot be assessed. Instead, through a knowledge of the behavior of estimates derived from all possible samples which can be drawn for the population by using the same sample design, it is possible to assess the probable accuracy of the obtained sample estimate.

For example, consider a random epsem sample of n elements which is used to calculate the sample mean, $\hat{x}$, as an estimate of the population parameter, $\bar{X}$. If an infinite set of independent samples of size n were drawn successively from this population and the sample mean calculated for each such sample, then the average of the sampling distribution of sample means, the expected value, can be denoted by $E(\hat{x})$.

The accuracy of the sample statistic, $\hat{x}$ as an estimator of the population parameter, $\bar{X}$, may be summarized in terms of the mean square error (MSE). The MSE is defined as the average of the squares of the deviations of all possible sample estimates from the value being estimated (Hansen et al. 1953):

$$\text{MSE}[\hat{x}] = E\,[\hat{x} - \bar{X}]^2$$

$$= E[\hat{x} - E(\hat{x})]^2 + [E(\hat{x}) - \bar{X}]^2 \qquad (5)$$

$$= \text{Variance of } \hat{x} + [\text{Bias of } \hat{x}]^2$$

A sample design is unbiased if $E(\hat{x}) = \bar{X}$. It is important to remember that "bias" is not a property of a single sample, but of the entire sampling distribution, and that it belongs neither to the selection procedure nor the estimation procedure alone, but to both jointly.

The reciprocal of the variance of a sample estimate is commonly referred to as the "precision," whereas the reciprocal of the mean square error is referred to as the "accuracy."

For most well-designed samples in educational survey research, the sampling bias is either zero or small. The accuracy of sample estimates is, therefore, in most cases primarily a function of the precision of the estimator ($\hat{x}$) which generally speaking increases with increasing sample size. That is, the sampling variance generally (but not always) decreases with increasing sample size.

As an example, the variance of the sample mean, $\hat{x}_{pps}$ obtained from the PPS sample design described in Section 4.4 may be obtained from the following formula (Cochran 1977):

$$\text{Var}\,(\hat{x}_{pps}) = \frac{S_1^2}{m} + \frac{S_2^2}{m\bar{n}} \qquad (6)$$

where S_1^2 denotes the population variance between the means of the primary sampling units and S_2^2 denotes the population variance within primary sampling units, m denotes the number of primary sampling units selected, and $\bar{n}$ denotes the (common) number of elements selected from within each selected primary sampling unit.

This formula emphasizes two important points. First, the variance of the sample mean may be reduced (for a given population of primary sampling units) by increasing the number of primary selections. Second, the variance of the sample mean may be reduced (for a given number of primary selections) by forming the primary sampling units in a fashion which reduces the variation among the means of the primary sampling units in the population, for example, through the use of schools as the primary sampling unit rather than classrooms. Stratification of the primary sampling units also provides a method of reducing S_1^2, and thus increasing the precision of the sample estimator, $\hat{x}_{pps}$.

5.3 Sample Estimates of Precision

For the probability sample designs used in practice as discussed above, it is generally possible, although not always straightforward, to obtain an expression for the true sampling variance, $\text{Var}\,(\hat{x})$, of an estimator $\hat{x}$ (say) as a function of various parameters in the population. As outlined later, sampling statisticians use these formulae to help in determining the most appropriate design to use in a given application, and to establish sample size requirements. These expressions for the true level of sampling variance are of little use to the analyst of the completed survey since they involve unknown population quantities.

A feature of a well-designed probability sample, however, is that it not only permits accurate estimates to be made of the population parameter of interest, $\bar{X}$ (say), using the estimator, $\hat{\bar{x}}$, but also gives accurate estimates of the quantity Var $(\hat{\bar{x}})$. This is achieved either through the use of an explicit formula for var $(\hat{\bar{x}})$, the sample estimate of Var $(\hat{\bar{x}})$, or through one of the number of replication techniques.

For a simple random sample of n elements drawn without replacement from a population of N elements, the variance of the sample mean may be estimated from a single sample of data by using the following formula (Kish 1965 p. 41):

$$\text{var}(\hat{\bar{x}}) = \frac{(N-n)}{N} \frac{s^2}{n} \tag{7}$$

where $s^2 = \Sigma(x_i - \hat{\bar{x}})^2 / (n-1)$ is an unbiased estimate of the variance of the element values x_i, in the population. Note that for sufficiently large values of N, the variance of the sample mean may be estimated by s^2/n because the finite population correction, $(N-n)/N$, tends to unity.

Explicit formulae for many types of sample design are given in Cochran (1977), and are generally based on an approximation obtained through Taylor series linearization. A general approach is described by Binder (1983). The two most widely used replicated variance estimation techniques are the jackknife technique and balanced repeated replication (BRR). For a full discussion of replication techniques, see Wolter (1985), Kish and Frankel (1974) and Rust (1985). In brief, replicated methods are generally much more computationally intensive than direct estimation via an explicit formula. The advantage that they offer is that a single approach is appropriate for all parameter estimators for a given survey, whereas the alternative is to derive an explicit variance estimator for each parameter type of interest.

Whatever the method of choice for obtaining estimates of the sampling variance, it is important that a method be used that is appropriate for both the form of the estimator and the features of the sample design. In particular, it is not appropriate to use a variance estimator designed for use with simple random samples when in fact a more complex design has been employed. In most applications in educational research this approach will lead to serious underestimation of the level of sampling variance.

In many practical survey research situations, the sampling distribution of the estimated mean is approximately normally distributed. The approximation improves with increasing sample size even though the distribution of elements in the parent population may be far from normal. This characteristic of the sampling distribution of the sample mean is associated with the "central limit theorem" and it occurs not only for the mean but for most estimators commonly used to describe survey research results (Kish 1965 Chaps. 1, 14).

From a knowledge of properties of the normal distribution, it is possible to be "68 percent confident" that the range $\hat{\bar{x}} \pm \sqrt{[\text{var}(\hat{\bar{x}})]}$ includes the population mean, where $\hat{\bar{x}}$ is the sample mean obtained from one sample from the population and var$(\hat{\bar{x}})$ is the estimate of sampling variance. The quantity $\sqrt{[\text{var}(\hat{\bar{x}})]}$ is called the "estimated standard error," se$(\hat{\bar{x}})$, of the sample mean, $\hat{\bar{x}}$. Similarly, it is known that the range $\hat{\bar{x}} \pm 1.96 \ \text{se}(\hat{\bar{x}})$ will include the population mean with 95 percent confidence. The calculation of confidence limits for estimates allows researchers to satisfy the estimation aim of survey research. Also, through the construction of difference scores $\hat{d} = \hat{\bar{x}}_1 - \hat{\bar{x}}_2$, and using a knowledge of the standard errors se$(\hat{\bar{x}}_1)$, and se$(\hat{\bar{x}}_2)$, (and in some cases the covariance of $\hat{\bar{x}}_1$ and $\hat{\bar{x}}_2$ the goal of testing statistical hypotheses may be satisfied.

It should be remembered that, although this discussion has focused on sample means, confidence limits can also be obtained for many other population values. For example, for a parameter θ, estimated from the sample by $\hat{\theta}$ a confidence interval is constructed of the form $\hat{\theta} \pm t \sqrt{\text{var}(\hat{\theta})}$. The quantity t represents an appropriate constant which is usually obtained from the normal distribution or under certain conditions from the t distribution. For most sample estimates encountered in practical survey research, reliance on the assumption of normality leads to errors that are small compared with other sources of inaccuracy. For further discussion of the topic of confidence interval estimation for survey samples, see Skinner et al. (1989 Chap. 2).

5.4 Multivariate Analysis of Complex Survey Data

As well as making estimates of population parameters, analysts of educational survey data often wish to construct models and conduct tests of multivariate hypotheses using survey data. Just as for the more simple case of estimating population parameters, the analyst must consider the impact on the analysis of the use of differential sampling probabilities for the units of the sample, and the use of a complex sample design (i.e., a design other than simple random sample). Consideration should be given not only to the effects of complex sample design on the estimates of standard errors of the mean, but also to whether there is a need to use multilevel analysis procedures and to estimate variance components. These issues have been the subject of much recent debate and are discussed in detail in Skinner et al. (1989) and Lee et al. (1989). These texts also discuss the currently available computer software for use in analyzing complex survey data. Multilevel analysis in educational studies is discussed in, for example, Goldstein (1987), Bock (1989), and Bryk and Raudenbush (1992).

6. Issues in the Design of Survey Samples

6.1 The Comparison of Sample Designs

In a previous section, it was shown that, for the hypothetical population in Fig. 1, either a three-stage sample design or a simple random sample design could be used to select epsem samples of the same size. However, equality of selection probabilities in the two designs provides no guarantee that the variances of sample estimates obtained from each design will be the same.

Fisher (1922) suggested that sample designs could be described and compared in terms of their *efficiency*. For example, one sample design, denoted i, may be compared to another sample design, denoted j, by considering the inverse of the variance of sample estimates for the same sample size. Using *Eff* to represent the efficiency of a sample design for the sample, and n_i to represent the sample size of sample i, the efficiency of these two sample designs can be compared by constructing the following ratio:

$$\frac{Eff_i}{Eff_j} = \frac{\hat{Var}(x_j)}{\hat{Var}(x_i)} \tag{8}$$

More recently, Kish (1965 Sect. 5.4) recommended that the simple random sample design should be used as a standard for quantifying the efficiency of other types of more complex sample designs. Kish introduced the term "Deff" (design effect) to describe the ratio of the variance of the sample mean for a complex sample design, denoted c, to the variance of a simple random sample, denoted srs, of the same sample size ($n_c = n_{srs}$).

$$Deff_c = \frac{Var(\hat{x}_c)}{Var(\hat{x}_{srs})} \tag{9}$$

The values of $Deff_c$ for sample means and multivariate statistics, such as correlation coefficients and regression coefficients, have been found to be substantially greater than unity for many sample designs which are commonly used in educational survey research (Peaker 1975, Ross 1978).

6.2 The Effective Sample Size

Complex sample designs may also be compared to simple random sample designs by calculating the value of the "effective sample size" (Kish 1965 p. 259) or the size of the "simple equivalent sample" (Peaker 1967 p. 149). For a given complex sample, the effective sample size is, for the variable under consideration, the size of the simple random sample which would have the same variance as the complex sample. For example, consider a population of N students. If the complex sample design is used to select an epsem sample of n_c students, then the variance of the sample mean, Var $(\hat{x}_c)$ may be written as:

$$Var(\hat{x}_c) = Deff_c \times Var(\hat{x}_{srs}) \tag{10}$$

Or, alternatively, since $n_c = n_{srs}$, this expression may be written in the form presented by Kish (1965, p. 258):

$$Var(\hat{x}_c) = Deff_c \times \frac{(N - n_c)}{N} \times \frac{S^2}{n_c} \tag{11}$$

where S^2 is the population variance.

Now consider a simple random sample design which is used to select a sample of n^* elements from the same population of students. Let the variance of the sample mean for this sample, Var*$(\hat{x}_{srs})$, be equal to the variance of the sample mean for the complex sample design, Var$(\hat{x}_c)$. That is, Var$(\hat{x}_c) = $ Var*$(\hat{x}_{srs})$.

Substituting on both sides gives the following:

$$Deff_c \times \frac{(N - n_c)}{N} \times \frac{S^2}{n_c} = \frac{(N - n^*)}{N} \times \frac{S^2}{n^*} \tag{12}$$

If N is large compared to n_c and n^*, then $n^* \simeq n_c / Deff_c$ is the effective sample size for the complex sample design.

It is important to recognize that in complex sample designs the sampling precision is a function of the whole sample design and not just the total sample size. In order to make meaningful comparisons of the sampling precision of complex sample designs, the design effects must be compared in association with the total sizes of complex samples. Moreover, it is important to recognize that different design effects arise in practice both for different parameters and the different estimators that are used to estimate such parameters.

6.3 Simple Two-stage Sampling

In educational research, a complex sample design is often employed rather than a simple random sample design because of cost constraints. For example, a two-stage sample consisting of the selection of 10 schools followed by the selection of 20 students within each of these schools would generally lead to smaller data collection costs compared with a simple random sample of 200 students. The reduced costs occur because the simple random sample may require the researcher to collect data from as many as 200 schools. However, the reduction in costs associated with the complex sample design must be balanced against the potential for an increase in the variance of sample estimates.

The variance of the sample mean for the simple two-stage sample design depends, for a given number of selected primary units and a given sample size within each primary unit, on the value of the "intraclass correlation coefficient," rho. This coefficient is a measure of the degree of homogeneity within primary units. In educational research, student characteristics are generally more homogeneous within schools than would be the case if students were grouped at random. The homogeneity of individuals within primary sampling units may be due to common selective factors, or joint exposure to the same influence, or mutual interaction, or some combination of these. It is important to note that the coefficient of intraclass correlation may take different values for different populations, different methods of defining primary sampling units, different parameters, and different estimators.

Consider a population of elements divided into equal-sized primary units. One method of drawing a sample of *n* elements is to draw a simple random sample from the population. A second approach is to use a two-stage sample of the same size, drawn from the population by using simple random sampling to select m primary units, and then for each of the selected primary unit using simple random sampling to select $\bar{n}$ elements, so that the total sample size is given by: $n = m \times \bar{n}$. The relationship between the variances of the sampling distributions of sample means for these two designs is (Kish 1965 p. 162):

$$\text{Var}(\hat{\bar{x}}_c) = \text{Var}(\hat{\bar{x}}_{srs})\,[1 + (\bar{n} - 1) \times \text{rho}] \tag{13}$$

where $\text{Var}(\hat{\bar{x}}_c)$ is the variance of sampling distribution of sample means for the simple two-stage design; $\text{Var}(\hat{\bar{x}}_{srs})$ is the variance of the sampling distribution of sample means for the simple random sample design; $\bar{n}$ is the sample size within each primary sampling unit, and rho is the coefficient of "intraclass correlation."

By transposing the above equation, the value of the design effect from the simple two-stage sample design may be written as a function of the sample size within each primary unit ($\bar{n}$) and the coefficient of intraclass correlation:

$$\text{Deff}_c = \frac{\text{Var}(\hat{\bar{x}}_c)}{\text{Var}(\hat{\bar{x}}_{srs})} = 1 + (\bar{n} - 1)\,\text{rho} \tag{14}$$

Since rho is generally positive (for students within schools and students within classrooms) the precision of the simple two-stage sample design (which uses either schools or classrooms as primary sampling units) will generally result in sample means that have larger variance than a simple random sample design of the same size. The losses in sampling precision associated with the two-stage design must therefore be weighed against the "gains" associated with reduced costs due to the selection and measurement of a smaller number of primary sampling units.

Experience gained from large-scale evaluation studies carried out in many countries (Peaker 1967, 1975) has shown that rho values of around 0.2 provide reasonably accurate estimates of student homogeneity for achievement variables within schools. Higher values of rho for achievement variables have been noted in Australia when considering student homogeneity within classrooms (Ross 1978). These higher values for students within classrooms are sometimes due to administrative arrangements in school systems. For example, students may be allocated to classrooms by using ability streaming within schools, or there may be substantial differences between classroom learning environments within schools.

6.4 Estimation of the Coefficient of Intraclass Correlation

The coefficient of intraclass correlation (rho) was developed in connection with studies carried out to estimate degrees of fraternal resemblance, as in the calculation of the correlation between the heights of brothers. To establish this correlation there is generally no reason for ordering pairs of measurements obtained from any two brothers. The initial approach to this problem was the calculation of a product–moment correlation coefficient from a symmetrical table of measures consisting of two interchanged entries for each pair of measures. This method is suitable for small numbers of entries—however, the number of entries in the table rises rapidly as the number of pairs increases.

Some computationally simpler methods for calculating estimates of this coefficient have been described by Haggard (1958). The most commonly used method is based on using one-way analysis of variance where the clusters which define the first-stage sampling units, for example, schools or classrooms, are regarded as the "treatments." The between clusters mean square, BCMS, and the within clusters mean square, WCMS, are then combined with the number of elements per cluster, $\bar{n}$, to obtain the estimate of rho:

$$\text{estimated rho} = \frac{\text{BCMS} - \text{WCMS}}{\text{BCMS} + (\bar{n} - 1)\text{WCMS}} \tag{15}$$

The application of an alternative formula based upon variance estimates for elements and primary unit means has been discussed by Ross (1983):

$$\text{estimated rho} = \frac{\bar{n}s_c^2 - s^2}{(\bar{n} - 1)s^2} \tag{16}$$

where s_c^2 is the variance of the primary unit means; s^2 is the variance of the elements and $\bar{n}$ is the sample size within each primary unit. This formula assumes that the data have been collected by using simple two-stage sampling, and also that both the number of elements and the number of clusters (primary sampling units) in the population are large.

6.5 Sample Design Tables for Simple Two-stage Sample Designs

The two-stage sample design is frequently used in educational research. Generally this design is employed by selecting either schools or classes at the first stage of sampling, followed by the selection of either students within schools or students within classes at the second stage. In many research situations these sample designs will be less expensive than simple random sample designs of the same size. Also, they offer an opportunity for the researcher to conduct analyses at higher levels of data aggregation. For example, the selection of a sample of students from a first-stage sample of classes would allow the researcher, provided there were sufficient numbers of classes and sufficient numbers of students per class in the sample, to create a data file based on class mean scores and then to conduct analyses at the "between-class" level (see *Multilevel Analysis*).

The previous discussion showed that the precision of the simple two-stage design relative to a simple random sample design of the same size was a function of $\bar{n}$, the second-stage sample size within each primary selection, and rho, the coefficient of intraclass correlation. With knowledge of both of these statistics, in combination with the required level of sampling precision, it is possible to establish a "planning equation" which may be used to guide decisions concerning the appropriate number of first- and second-stage sampling units.

For example, consider an educational research study in which test items are administered to a sample of students with the aim of estimating the item difficulty values and mean test scores for the population. If a simple random sample of n^* students is selected from the population in order to obtain an estimate $\hat{p}$ of the proportion P who have obtained the correct answer on an item, the variance of $\hat{p}$ as an estimate of the population difficulty value may be estimated from the following formula (Kish 1965 p. 46):

$$\text{Var}\ (\hat{p}) = \frac{P(1 - P)}{n^*} \tag{17}$$

This formula ignores the finite population correction factor because it is assumed that the population is large compared to the sample size.

Suppose that it is specified that the standard error of $\hat{p}$ should not exceed 0.025, so that, with 95 percent confidence, $\hat{p}$ will be within approximately 0.05 of P, the true proportion.

The maximum value of P(1–P) occurs for P = 0.5. Therefore, in order to ensure that these error requirements can be satisfied for all items, it is necessary to require that

$$(0.025)^2 \geqslant \frac{0.5\ (1 - 0.5)}{n^*} \tag{18}$$

That is, n^* would have to be greater than or (approximately) equal to 400 in order to obtain 95 percent confidence that $\hat{p}$ will be within 0.05 of P.

Now consider the size of the simple two-stage sample design that would provide equivalent sampling accuracy to a simple random sample of 400 students. That is, it is necessary to discover the numbers of primary sampling units (for example, schools or classes) and the numbers of secondary sampling units (students) that would be required in order to obtain 95 percent confidence that the estimate $\hat{p}$ is within 0.05 of the true proportion P.

From previous discussion, the relationship between the size of a complex sample, n_c, which has the same accuracy as a simple random sample of size $n^* = 400$ may be written as:

$$n^* = \frac{n_c}{\text{Deff}_c} = 400 \tag{19}$$

Since the complex sample is a simple two-stage

sample design, the value of Deff_c may be replaced by $1 + (\bar{n} - 1)\text{rho}$ in the above expression to obtain the "planning equation":

$$n_c = 400\ [1 + (\bar{n} - 1)\text{rho}] = m\bar{n} \tag{20}$$

where rho is the "coefficient of intraclass correlation" for the student measure which is being considered; m is the number of primary selections and $\bar{n}$ is the number of secondary selections within each primary selection.

As an example, consider rho = 0.2 and $\bar{n}$ = 10. Then,

$$m = \frac{400}{\bar{n}}\ [1 + (\bar{n} - 1)\text{rho}]$$

$$= \frac{400}{10}[1 + (10 - 1)0.2]$$

$$= 112$$

That is, for rho = 0.2, a simple two-stage design of 1,120 students consisting of 112 primary selections followed by the selection of 10 students per primary selection would be required to obtain accuracy which is equivalent to a simple random sample of 400 students.

In Table 3, the planning equation has been employed to list sets of values for $\bar{n}$, m, and n_c which describe a group of simple two-stage sample designs that have equivalent sampling accuracy to a simple random sample of 400 students. Two sets of sample designs have been listed in the table corresponding to rho values of 0.2 and 0.4.

The most striking feature of Table 3 is the rapidly diminishing effect that increasing $\bar{n}$, the second stage sample size, has on m, the number of clusters that must be selected. This is particularly noticeable for both values of rho when the second stage sample size reaches 10 to 15 students. For example, when rho = 0.4, the selection of 15 students per primary selection from 176 primary selections would have equivalent sampling accuracy to a design in which 50 students per primary selection were

Table 3
Sample design table for simple two-stage cluster samples having an effective sample size of 400[a]

Students per cluster $\bar{n}$	rho = 0.2			rho = 0.4		
	Deff_c	n_c	m	Deff_c	n_c	m
1	1.0	400	400	1.0	400	400
2	1.2	480	240	1.4	560	280
5	1.8	720	144	2.6	1,040	208
10	2.8	1,120	112	4.6	1,840	184
15	3.8	1,520	102	6.6	2,640	176
20	4.8	1,920	96	8.6	3,440	172
30	6.8	2,720	91	12.6	5,040	168
40	8.8	3,520	88	16.6	6,640	166
50	10.8	4,320	87	20.6	8,240	165

a The values of m, the number of primary sampling units selected, have been rounded upward to the nearest integer value selected from 165 primary selections. The total sample size in these two cases differs by a factor of over three—from 2,640 to 8,240.

It is important to remember that the planning equation is derived with the assumption that the actual sample design fits the model of a simple two-stage sample design. In practical educational research studies sample designs may depart from this model by incorporating such complexities as the use of stratification prior to sample selection, and/or the use of varying probabilities of selection at each of the two stages of sampling. Consequently the planning equation must be seen as a tool which assists with the development of a sample design, rather than a precise technique for predicting sampling errors. The actual sampling accuracy of a sample design must be determined after the sample data become available for analysis.

The selection of an appropriate cluster size for an educational research study usually requires the researcher to reconcile the demands of a set of often competing requirements. A number of authors (e.g., Hansen et al. 1953, Kish 1965, Sudman 1976) have presented descriptions of the use of cost functions to calculate the optimal or most economical cluster size for certain fixed costs associated with various aspects of sampling and data collection. These approaches provide useful guidelines but they must be considered in combination with the need for high validity in the collection of data. For example, achievement tests which are to be administered in schools should preferably be given at one point of time in order to prevent the possibility of those students who have completed the test being able to discuss the answers with students who will be given the test at some later time. Educational researchers generally cope with this problem by limiting the within-school sample size to the number of students who can be tested under standardized conditions in one test administration. In most education systems, this would represent around 20 to 30 students per school when tests can be given by group administration. Much smaller sample sizes may be necessary for tests which require individualized administration unless a large number of test administrators can be assigned at the same time to a particular school.

A further constraint on the choice of the second-stage sample size may occur when analyses are planned for the between-student level of analysis and also at some higher level of data aggregation—for example, at the between-school level of analysis. In order to conduct analyses at the between-school level, data from students are sometimes aggregated to obtain data files consisting of school records based on student means scores. If the number of students selected per school is too small, then estimates of school characteristics may be subject to large within-school sampling errors. The gains to be made in accuracy and precision decrease rapidly for second-stage sample sizes greater than $\bar{n} = 25$ (being related to $1/\sqrt{n}$). Sample sizes of around 20 to 30 students are generally employed at the second stage of sampling not only for administrative convenience and to control cost, but also because they provide adequate estimates at the group level of means, correlations, variances, and covariances.

7. The Problem of Nonresponse

In most educational research studies, there is usually some loss of data due, for example, to the nonparticipation of schools, or the nonresponse of sample members within selected schools. The resulting missing data give rise to differences between the designed sample and the achieved sample.

One of the most frequently asked questions in educational research is: "How much missing data can be accepted before there is a danger of bias in the sample estimates?" The only realistic answer is that there is no general rule which defines a safe limit for nonresponse. The nonresponse bias may be large even if there are small amounts of missing data, and vice versa.

There are two broad categories of nonresponse: total nonresponse and item nonresponse. Total nonresponse refers to a complete loss of data for particular sample members, and is often dealt with by employing weights in order to adjust for differential loss of data among certain important subgroups of the sample. Item nonresponse refers to the loss of a few items of information for particular sample members, and is usually dealt with by the assignment of values which replace the missing data, known as imputation. For a description of the various imputation techniques available, see Kalton (1983).

It is important to remember that the level of bias in sample estimates which may occur through nonresponse generally cannot be overcome by increasing the sample size. The common approach of using random replacement of nonresponders usually provides additional sample members who resemble responders rather than nonresponders. The level of bias which actually occurs in these situations depends upon the variables which are being examined and their relationships with the nature of the nonresponding subgroup of the defined target population.

The problem of nonresponse in educational research appears to have received limited research attention. This is unfortunate because even doing nothing about nonresponse is an implicit adjustment scheme in itself which is based upon the assumption that loss of data is equivalent to random loss of data (*see Missing Data and Nonresponse*).

8. Conclusion

This discussion of sample design for educational research has focused on some aspects of the survey approach and its application to large-scale educational studies. However, the issues that have been raised have direct bearing on the conduct of experimental studies because the distributions of relationships between charateristics in causal systems, like the distributions of these characteristics taken alone, exist only with reference to particular populations. The discussion is also relevant to investigations, as often accuracy and validity can be enhanced by applying sampling methods to a portion of the data collection, even though the study is not a full survey of a population. For example, a researcher may wish to investigate relationships among variables for a convenient group of schools that are not sampled from a population of schools. The study might well be enhanced, however, if sampling methods are used to obtain samples of classrooms, teachers, and students from within those schools.

The techniques of sampling are relatively few, and simple to comprehend. Because in practice these methods must be combined with methods of estimation, analysis, and inference, it is generally not advisable to proceed with conducting a sampling survey without consulting a sampling statistician. At the same time it is important for researchers, analysts as well as those designing surveys, to understand the principles of sample design and thus the impact that decisions about the design will have on the quality of the results obtained from analysis.

See also: Sampling Errors in Survey Research; Survey Research Methods; Multivariate Analysis

References

Binder D A 1983 On the variances of asymptotically normal estimators for complex surveys. *Int. Stat. Rev.* 51: 279–92

Bock R D (ed.) 1989 *Multilevel Analysis of Educational Data.* Academic Press, Orlando, Florida

Bryk A S, Raudenbush S W 1992 *Hierarchical Linear Models: Applications and Data Analysis Methods.* Sage, Newbury Park, California

Chu A, Morganstein D, Wallace L 1992 *IAEP Technical Report. Part 1: Sampling.* Educational Testing Service, Princeton, New Jersey

Cochran W G 1977 *Sampling Techniques,* 3rd edn. Wiley, New York

Fisher R A 1922 On the mathematical foundations of theoretical statistics. *Philosophical Transactions of the Royal Society Series A* 222: 309–68

Goldstein H 1987 *Multilevel Models in Educational and Social Research.* Griffin, London

Haggard E A 1958 *Intraclass Correlation and the Analysis of Variance.* Dryden, New York

Hansen M H, Hurwitz W N, Madow W G 1953 *Sample Survey Methods and Theory,* Vols. 1 and 2. Wiley, New York

Kalton G 1983 *Compensating for Missing Survey Data.* Institute for Social Research, Ann Arbor, Michigan

Kish L 1965 *Survey Sampling.* Wiley, New York

Kish L 1987 *Statistical Design for Research.* Wiley, New York

Kish L, Frankel M R 1974 Inference from complex samples. *Journal of the Royal Statistical Society* B36: 1–37

Lee E S, Forthofer R N, Lorimer R J 1989 *Analyzing Complex Survey Data.* Sage, Newbury Park, California

Peaker G F 1967 Sampling. In: Husén T (ed.) 1967 *International Study of Achievement in Mathematics: A Comparison of Twelve Countries,* Vol. 1. Wiley, New York

Peaker G F 1975 *An Empirical Study of Education in Twenty-One Countries: A Technical Report.* Almqvist and Wiksell, Stockholm

Ross K N 1978 Sample design for educational survey research. *Eval. Educ.* 2(2): 105–95

Ross K N 1983 *Social Area Indicators of Educational Need.* ACER, Hawthorn

Ross K N, Postlethwaite T N 1991 *Indicators of the Quality of Education: A National Study of Primary Schools in Zimbabwe.* International Institute for Educational Planning. UNESCO, Paris

Rust K 1985 Variance estimation from complex estimators in sample surveys. *Journal of Official Statistics* (4): 381–97

Skinner C J, Holt D, Smith T M F (eds.) 1989 *Analysis of Complex Surveys.* Wiley, Chichester

Sudman S 1976 *Applied Sampling.* Academic Press, New York

Wolter K M 1985 *Introduction to Variance Estimation.* Springer-Verlag, New York

Further Reading

Deming W E 1950 *Some Theory of Sampling.* Dover, New York

Foreman E K 1991 *Survey Sampling Principles.* Marcell Dekker, New York

Jaeger R M 1984 *Sampling in Education and the Social Sciences.* Longman, New York

Kalton G 1983 *Introduction to Survey Sampling.* Sage, Beverly Hills, California

Levy P S, Lemeshow S 1991 *Sampling of Populations: Methods and Applications,* 2nd edn. Wiley, New York

Moser C A, Kalton G 1971 *Survey Methods in Social Investigation,* 2nd edn. Heinemann, London

Raj D 1972 *The Design of Sample Surveys.* McGraw-Hill, New York

Scheaffer R L, Mendenhall W, Ott L 1990 *Elementary Survey Sampling,* 4th edn. PWS–Kent, Boston, Massachusetts

Stuart A 1984 *The Ideas of Sampling,* 2nd edn. Griffin, London

Sukhatme P V, Sukhatme B V, Sukhatme S, Asok C 1984 *Sampling Theory of Surveys with Applications,* 3rd edn. Iowa State University Press, Ames, Iowa

Williams W H 1978 *A Sampler on Sampling.* Wiley, New York

Yates F 1981 *Sampling Methods for Censuses and Surveys,* 4th edn. Griffin, London

Secondary Data Analysis

R. A. Reeve and H. J. Walberg

The typical educational researcher collects his or her own data; but potential for conducting original research using precollected data is immense, and has been unexploited by the educational research community. Nevertheless, interest is growing in the reanalysis or secondary analysis of previously collected and analyzed data. The growing availability of large national and international archived data sets of educationally relevant information; the increasing sophistication of bureaucrats and their requests for empirical evidence upon which to base educational policy; the converging interests of sociologists, psychologists, and educational researchers on macro level factors affecting learning and schooling outcomes; the growing familiarity with statistical packages on powerful mainframe computers; and the economic costs of collecting large data sets coupled with the general decline in insufficient financial support for social science research have all contributed to the growing interest in secondary analysis.

The purposes of this entry are to introduce and illustrate the goals, methods, and implications of secondary analysis; to summarize substantive findings; to evaluate present and potential contributions; and to identify some possible limitations of the approach. The theme is that, although secondary analysis is hardly a panacea, funding agencies and research workers have underinvested their money and effort in secondary analysis. Data that may have cost hundreds of millions of dollars lie dormant, waiting to tell their story. In this entry six issues are considered: (a) the relation between secondary and other forms of analysis, (b) common uses of secondary analysis, (c) reasons underlying educators' previous reluctance but growing willingness to use the method, (d) methodological and interpretive issues, (e) applications of the research synthesis methodology, and (f) conclusions and future research directions.

1. Types of Educational Research

Secondary analysis fits into a framework or typology of different forms of educational research (Walberg 1986). The definitions below show how secondary analysis and another related form of analysis, that is, research synthesis, compare to and contrast with traditional primary research and narrative reviews.

Primary research, for the purpose of this entry, involves analyses of original raw qualitative or quantitative data. It may include, or be motivated by, a literature review, a theoretical framework, and explicit hypotheses. Secondary analysis, in contrast, is

the reanalysis of data by the original or, more often, other investigators for similar or different purposes for which the data were collected.

Reviews are narrative commentaries about primary and secondary research findings. They usually summarize and evaluate studies one by one, but rarely quantitatively analyze them. Reviews often contain theoretical insights and practical recommendations, but rarely assess rival theories by the parsimonious accounting of statistical regularities of data in primary studies.

Research synthesis explicitly applies statistical techniques and scientific standards to the evaluation and summary of research; it not only quantitatively summarizes effects across studies, but also provides detailed descriptions of replicable searches of literature, selection of studies, metrics of study effects, statistical procedures, and both overall and exceptional results with respect to experimental conditions, context, or subjects (Wallberg and Haertel 1980, Glass et al. 1981). Qualitative insights may be usefully combined with quantitative synthesis, and results from multiple reviews and synthesis of the same or different topics may be compiled and compared to estimate their relative magnitudes and consistencies (Walberg 1982).

It is also possible to carry out secondary analyses of data using research synthesis procedures. Since the data gathered from original reports may be used to calculate effect sizes, vote counts, or other indices of interest, these data, in turn, may also be reanalyzed by using alternative procedures. Hedges and Stock (1983) pioneered this idea in carrying out what might be called secondary synthesis of class size effects on learning from data originally collected by others; they used alternative mathematical estimators of the effects for better precision.

2. Common Uses of Secondary Analysis

The rationale for using secondary analysis procedures in education has been clarified due to the need to evaluate programs (see evaluations of Sesame Street by Cook et al. 1975, and of Head Start by Magidson 1977 and Barnow and Cain 1977). The exemplary case of secondary analysis, however, is the large-scale multiple-question sociological survey reanalyzed for other than the original purposes or by other than the original investigators. Before secondary analysis of such surveys, academic sociologists could hardly compete with private survey firms who had the organization and resources to conduct political surveys and commercial market research (Hyman 1972). Foundations and government agencies sometimes funded surveys, but were generally interested in quick results and answers to specific questions that were not necessarily of fundamental and enduring importance. In the absence of large-scale survey data, sociologists were restricted to using obviously unrepresentative survey samples of a 100 or so students taking an elementary university course.

One of the earliest and best United States examples of surveys designed to allow secondary analysis of the national adult population is the General Social Survey (GSS) begun in 1972 by the National Opinion Research Center at the University of Chicago. Conducted annually, the GSS includes many of the same questions year after year, or in longer periodic cycles, so that temporal trends in adult opinion can be assessed systematically. In fact, the GSS includes some items on capital punishment that originated in private polls taken as early as 1937.

At an annual cost of roughly $750,000 in 1988, the GSS obtains 90 minutes of face-to-face interview time from about 1,500 survey respondents in a carefully drawn random sample. Earlier in its history the GSS allowed piggy backing, or added extra items, because of their relevance to contemporary topical issues or to the interests of external investigators or organizations. The added cost of special items is small since the cost of administration, sampling, and interviewing is large and fixed. The main constraint on items is the 90 minutes of interview time; and proposed one-time or cycled questions must be approved by a committee responsible for weighing their utility and importance.

The resulting public opinion data (and scores on a short vocabulary test) can be analyzed for time trends, region, and individual characteristics such as age and sex. The answers may be analyzed as discrete responses or composited in various ways using techniques such as Guttman scaling and factor analysis. Responses to multiple questions may also be analyzed to determine, for example, how many women over 40 years of age who favor arms control are against preschools, and how this group has changed its opinion since the questions were first asked.

There are, of course, seemingly infinite combinations of trends, topics, and respondent characteristics that may be analyzed by different procedures. The data have served as a gold mine for academic researchers, mostly sociologists, but also political scientists and a few specialists in communication, education, and law. Approximately 1,000 authors have written about 1,800 publications from secondary analyses of GSS data (GSS News 1987).

It could indeed be said that all GSS analyses are now secondary. As soon as the data are verified they are immediately archived at the University of Michigan's Inter-University Consortium for Social and Political Research in the form of sample and procedural description, codebooks, and computer tapes. They may

be purchased at low cost and are kept at duplicate archives at member universities.

The benefits of this approach are several. The sampling and interviewing for the survey are first rate and the items are repeated year after year to allow comparisons across time of important changes in public opinion; yet the survey can afford to add in some questions of urgent contemporary interest. The annual cost in 1988 of about US$750,000 is worth much more than 10 US$75,000 studies that would be inferior in sample size, geographical coverage, and possibly, methodological rigor. Small surveys, by their nature tend to lack comparability with one another and with past surveys.

The value of secondary analysis is often dependent on the broad national representativeness of information and on the number and variety of comparisons the source data allow. International comparisons are obviously of great interest, and the premier archive for secondary analysis of achievement including students of several ages in many countries at several time points since the mid-1960s is the International Association for the Evaluation of Educational Achievement (IEA). Among the most ambitious of the IEA studies have been those in the areas of mathematics and science (Husén 1967, Comber and Keeves 1973, IEA 1988, Postlethwaite and Wiley 1992, Keeves 1992).

The data for the first IEA study in mathematics was conducted in 1964 using 8th- and 12th-grade students from 12 different countries and assessed several different kinds of mathematical abilities (arithmetic, algebra, geometry, etc.) (Husén 1967). The second IEA mathematics study examined the performance of students from 17 different countries (McKnight et al. 1987). The results of the IEA studies have been particularly distressing for educators in the United States because United States students performed at or below the median level in each of the topic areas evaluated.

The IEA mathematics and science studies have sought to identify influential and uninfluential factors that could help explain cross-national differences in performance. Interestingly, neither class size nor years of teacher training explained differences in performances. On the other hand, the status granted to teachers and the nature of the curriculum disappear to contribute to students' performance. Not surprisingly, the course a student takes affects performance. The IEA data sets are, of course, limited in that they only address a small subset of issues, with cross-cultural performance differences raising more questions than are answered. There are many other aspects of mathematics and science achievement that need to be explored cross-nationally such as teachers', students', and parents' beliefs about mathematics and science learning in particular. Nevertheless, the IEA studies continue to yield insights into the nature of cross-cultural differences in achievement as secondary analysts probe the data.

Another survey that offers rich opportunities for

secondary analysis of international comparisons, not of learning but of public opinion, is the International Social Survey Program (ISSP). Begun several years ago, the ISSP is an annual program of cross-national collaboration of pre-existing social surveys that brings international perspective to national studies. Started by the *Zentrum fuer Umfragen Methoden, und Analysen of Mannheim*, and Chicago's National Opinion Research Center, the ISSP includes other European countries that collaborate in building a longitudinal cross-national data base with special topics covered on an occasional basis.

3. Secondary Analysis and Educational Research

The preference for certain kinds of research techniques have historically limited the use of secondary analysis in educational research. Of the academic disciplines, educational research has traditionally been influenced most heavily by psychology. Psychologists have typically preferred direct observations of small local samples, and have tended to study the more observable and proximal causes of learning. There are, of course, exceptions to this view. Developmental psychologists have long used deliberately gathered longitudinal data sets to answer research questions about growth and development; also, psychologists with interests in individual differences in abilities or in measuring attitudes have often used in their research either questionnaires or precollected data. Economists, sociologists, political scientists, and others, in contrast to the typical psychologist, have more often relied on self-reports and data from organizational records and archives, often collected cross-sectionally at a single point in time, to answer research questions.

Since the focus of much psychological research is on narrow issues where an attempt is made to control experimentally extraneous factors, there is less room for debate about either the choice of appropriate statistical analysis or the kind of conclusions that can be drawn. Immediate measures of learning, for example, are often assessed using analysis of variance techniques, simple planned contrasts or post hoc *t*-tests, comparing the performance of control and experimental groups. Sociologists, on the other hand, have traditionally attempted to control extraneous causes by explicitly measuring them. In particular, hypothetical models of the structural relations among major factors are posited and evaluated using a variety of multivariate statistical techniques (LISREL, loglinear analysis, partial least squares analysis, path analysis, and so on) (see *Multivariate Analysis*). The value of such approaches is that they provide means of assessing some of the multiple macrolevel factors (e.g., income, socio-economic variables) thought to affect learning and other schooling outcomes. A strength of much sociological research, moreover, lies in the generalizability of results from samples

to populations. Random or stratified random samples, which are normally very expensive, permit scientific generalization, even though the measures and causal relations may be more questionable than those used in traditional psychological research.

A further reason for educators' earlier reluctance to engage in secondary analysis may stem from the lack of skill and experience needed to conduct such analyses and from a failure on the part of many universities to endorse such research as an appropriate basis for the preparation of a doctoral dissertation. The accepted apprenticeship model for the educational researcher has traditionally been based on the humanities convention of a solitary investigator carrying out all research tasks alone. Large-scale educational surveys, however, require, in addition to substantive mastery of social science methods and expertise in the subject matter of the survey, skills in research administration, finance and accounting, human relations, politics, sampling, psychometrics, language translation, causal modeling, data analysis, interpretation, and writing. Research training in education has tended to emphasize only a subset of these skills. As marketplace demands for secondary analysis in education increase, it is likely that research training will increasingly accommodate these needs.

4. Methodological and Interpretive Issues

The secondary analysis of existing data involves problems common to all forms of research and problems specific to the particular form of analysis itself. Among other issues, these range from the difficulty of reading computer information, to problems of deriving conceptually meaningful measures from measures that may have been designed to address a completely different issue, to deciding on the use of appropriate statistical procedures.

Archived data sets are typically distributed using magnetic computer tapes. In principle, the data tapes are self-explanatory and even self-reading in that they include files of format information, variable names, and explanations in computer languages such as the Statistical Package for the Social Sciences (SPSS) and the Statistical Analysis System (SAS). The data, their encoding, and explanation, however, may be recorded in various protocols and tape densities that often make it difficult for the secondary analyst to decipher in practice (see *Data Management in Survey Research*).

Even when the data can be read into a computer, secondary analysts must often seek out those who can resolve various discrepancies in source documents before and after encoding the data on tapes. These original encoders may not be found in some cases or they may have forgotten how they constructed the files on tape.

According to a codebook, for example, "sex of respondent" may have been coded "1" for females, "2" for males, and "9" for those who failed to answer the question. However, secondary analysts may find that 5 percent of the data are coded "3" and "4", which, although omitted from the codebook, meant respondents for girls and boys at single-sex schools. It may be that the principal investigator has forgotten this obscure point, and the research assistant who might remember has turned to long-distance sailing. Secondary analysts who wish to take sex differences into account may have to persevere or use other data. Even though the data may be thoroughly described in codebooks and sampling manuals, aspiring secondary analysts have encountered grave difficulties in reading the data into computers and understanding their meaning.

One of the main problems faced by secondary analysts is that the problem or issue they are interested in examining may be poorly represented or even absent from the data archive. Questionnaire data is typically collected to answer specific questions and researchers, who work with the data later, often have to argue that a particular set of responses represents the construct they are interested in examining. There are many issues to be resolved concerning the integrity of the data and the meaning of data. The secondary analysis must provide a comprehensive rationale that a question or set of questions drawn from a secondary source can reasonably be used as a proxy for the particular theoretical construct under examination (e.g., socioeconomic level, educational interest). The lack of sensitivity to this issue has led to the rejection of statistically sound secondary analysis by sophisticated policymakers (Boruch and Pearson 1985). Indeed, as Boruch and Pearson (1985) noted, nearly all questionnaire data is an imperfect representation of reality. However, far too little attention is paid to theoretical questions concerning both the measurement properties and the psychometric validity issues surrounding the secondary analysis of data (Bailar and Lanphier 1978). Needless to say, these issues are often exacerbated by poor questionnaire design and inadequate data-gathering techniques. Boruch and Pearson (1985) have suggested that if there is doubt about the value of particular constructs, small field experiments should be conducted to provide converging evidence of claims.

It is widely recognized that methodological assumptions influence the statistical procedures used by researchers and these, in turn, affect the resulting interpretations, and possible claims that can be made about the research. Since the results of secondary analysis may be used to argue for policy, great care is needed in selecting statistical methods and interpreting the outcomes appropriately. Indeed, statistical jargon itself needs to be correctly understood or explained. The term "independent variable," for example, implies a causal relation that is difficult to demonstrate or disconfirm using correlational data, especially data collected from a single sample at a single point in time. Nevertheless, a causal relation is implicit in claims of educational relevance since the explicit goal is often

to understand the link between efficient means and desirable ends. In practice, of course, most decisions by policymakers and practitioners are based on only partial knowledge of conditions and causes.

To determine policy and practice, it is often worthwhile subjecting data, especially state, national, and international data, to multiple analyses to test the robustness and generalizability of findings rather than accepting the results of a single analysis. As noted earlier, however, inferences about data are constrained by the form of analysis used (Bowering 1984, Keeves 1986b). Indeed, on questions of policy secondary analysis procedures are often disputed by experts representing different political or policy persuasions (Boruch et al. 1981). Campbell and Erlebacher (1970) pointed out that it is possible to make education program interventions look harmful by using commonly used but inappropriate statistical procedures. In short, great care is needed in selecting statistical procedures. An excellent example of the inferences possible from different forms of multivariate analysis techniques is provided by Keeves (1986b).

Keeves (1986b) asked a number of researchers who had statistical expertise in different multivariate techniques to use them in analyzing a specified problem that was based on a precollected data set. Keeves selected the techniques because they are used with frequency in different areas of the social sciences concerned with educational issues (economics, sociology, psychology, and education). The techniques used were regression analysis (Keeves 1986b), canonical correlation analysis (Keeves 1986b), analysis of linear structural relations (McGaw et al. 1986) factorial modeling (Lohnes 1986), and partial least squares analysis (Sellin 1986). A discussion of the technical details of the analyses, and of the interpretive limitations imposed by the assumption underlying the different analytic procedures, is beyond the scope of this entry and is less important than the general issues raised by Keeves (1986a, 1986b).

The data for the analyses were based on a random sample of 1,933 students, who completed their last year of elementary school in the Australia Capital Territory in 1968 and who attended secondary school for the first time in 1969 (see Keeves 1972 for details). Data were obtained from the students in 1968 on general ability and achievement in mathematics and science, on attitudes of self-regard, liking of school, and school learning. Early in 1969 data were gathered on students' attentiveness in science and mathematics classrooms; and late in 1969, data were collected on students' achievement in mathematics and science, and their attitudes of liking mathematics and science. The problem Keeves set for the experts was to use their techniques in interpreting a specific causal path model linking motivation and achievement over the two-year performance cycle (see Keeves 1986a, for details of the model).

Keeves pointed out that each of the techniques

had interpretive strengths and weaknesses, contingent upon the problem being examined, and that a situation could be found where each technique was the most appropriate one to use. In other words, different kinds of effects were noted when using different analysis procedures. The use of regression procedures, for example, allowed a separate analysis of the mathematics and science performance cycles, but the presence of a suppressor effect limited the conclusion that could be drawn. Further, only through using the factor modeling procedure was it possible to identify a relationship between students' self-concept and achievement outcomes. Keeves also pointed out that if the data for the problem were altered slightly, the differential value of the five different statistical techniques would also vary. As Keeves himself noted:

> It is clear that each procedure might be considered to provide identifiable gains at the expense of certain losses. Perhaps a potential user of one or more of the techniques should have regard to the meaning extracted by the alternative techniques, rather than for the ease with which the technique might be employed (Keeves 1986b p. 201).

This is a salutary comment and underscores the importance of applying statistical procedures flexibly to meet the demands of the problem.

A further study of the appropriate use of different statistical procedures is provided by the secondary analysis of data collected in the Second IEA Mathematics Study which explores the use of linear structural relations analysis (LISREL), partial least squares analysis, iterative generalized least squares analysis, and hierarchical linear modeling (HLM) to examine issues associated with the analysis of multilevel data in educational research (Cheung et al. 1990).

5. Research Synthesis

A group at the University of Illinois at Chicago has attempted to build a psychological theory of educational productivity and test it with both experimental and nonexperimental evidence (Walberg 1986). By 1988, they had summarized about 8,000 small-scale experimental studies and also carried out many secondary analyses of large-scale United States national surveys of achievement. Prior psychological theory had suggested that academic achievement is a function of five proximal factors: student age, ability, motivation, the amount and quality of instruction; and four supportive or substitutive factors: the environments of the classroom, home, peer-group outside the school, and mass media, particularly television, to which students are exposed. More than 100 syntheses of small-scale studies of these factors show their consistent association with learning outcomes. Few prior intensive experiments and quasi-experiments, however, are national in scope, and most analyze only one or two of the factors and sample limited populations within a school

or community. They are often strong on observational technique, measurement, verification, and random assignment to treatments—in short, internal validity—but they are often weak in generalizability or external validity, since they do not rigorously sample from large, well-defined populations.

The complementarity of intensive and extensive studies, however, is important. In principle, consistent, powerful effects should consistently emerge from either form of research as well as from case studies. Robust findings give a strong basis for educational policy and practice.

With respect to the productivity theory, indeed, nine regression studies of extensive survey data on 15,802 13- and 17-year old students tested in mathematics, science, social studies, and reading by the National Assessment of Educational Achievement supports the implications of these findings (Walberg 1986). Although the correlations of the factors with achievement and subject-matter interest as learning outcomes varied from -0.45 to $+0.68$, 83 (or 91) percent of the 91 correlations were in the expected direction. Moreover, when the factors were controlled for one another in multiple regressions, 58 (or 91) percent of the 64 coefficients were as expected. The Chicago group extended this work to the original mathematics survey of the International Association for the Evaluation of Educational Achievement with similar results.

6. Summary and Goals for the Future

In summary, secondary analysis has complementary strengths and weaknesses: it often draws on large, stratified, random samples of national and international populations, and measures more factors but sacrifices internal validity since the factors are usually measures cross-sectionally and perhaps superficially with only a few items. Survey research can statistically control to some extent for multiple causes and may be more causally convincing than quasi-experiments controlled only for one or two covariates.

Because large surveys tend to take longer than expected, and because their initial phases are dominated by test and questionnaire constructors and sampling experts, analysis and writing are often given short shrift. The initial report of a national study may come out three or four years after the initial idea of commissioning the study. By this time, policy and interest may have shifted to other matters. The report may gain little attention, and the data may never be thoroughly analyzed. Still, the data may be capable of far better answers to the original question than those yielded by the initial analysis; and they may be able to shed light on other questions of more fundamental or contemporary policy interest.

Although there is a growing awareness of the value of archived data, conducting secondary analysis can be a frustrating experience. More forward planning is needed to ensure the usefulness and easy access to data. There is also a subsequent need to provide full documentation of the planning and conduct of the study so that the work of secondary analysis can be facilitated. Since governments and foundations are increasingly tending to focus on large-scale data sets to answer policy questions, future grantees and contractors will likely be required to archive the data more systematically than in the past, and make it available to secondary analysts by providing codebooks that explain how the data are recorded on computer tapes. Now that large-scale secondary analyses have been made of educational data sets such as the National Assessment of Educational Progress in the United States, and data sets of the International Association for the Evaluation of Educational Achievement from several dozen countries, it is apparent that the previous reluctance to reanalyze data is disappearing.

See also: Meta-Analysis; Data Banks and Data Archives; Survey Research Methods

References

Bailar B A, Lanphier C M 1978 *Development of Survey Methods to Assist Survey Practices.* American Statistical Association, Washington, DC

Barnow B S, Cain G G 1977 A reanalysis of the effects of Head Start on cognitive development: Methodological and empirical findings. *J. Hum. Resources* 12: 177–97

Boruch R F, Pearson R W 1985 *The Comparative Evaluation of Longitudinal Surveys.* Social Science Research Council, New York

Boruch R F, Wortman P M, Cordray D S (eds.) 1981 *Reanalyzing Program Evaluations.* Jossey-Bass, San Francisco, California

Bowering D J (ed.) 1984 *Secondary Analysis of Available Data Bases.* Jossey-Bass, San Francisco, California

Campbell T D, Erlebacher A 1970 How regression artifacts in quasi-experimental evaluations can mistakenly make compensatory education look harmful. In: Hellmuth J (ed.) 1970 *Compensatory Education: A Nationale Debate.* Brunner/Mazel, New York

Cheung K C, Keeves J P, Sellin N, Tsoi S C 1990 The analysis of multilevel data. *Int. J. Educ. Res.* 14(3)

Comber L C, Keeves J P 1973 *Science Education in Nineteen Countries.* Almqvist and Wiksall, Stockholm

Cook T D et al. 1975 *Sesame Street Revisited.* Sage Foundation, New York

Glass G V, McGaw B, Smith M L 1981 *Meta-analysis in Social Research.* Sage, Beverly Hills, California

GSS News 1987 November, No. 1. *General Social Survey.* National Opinion Research Center, The University of Chicago, Chicago, Illinois

Hedges L V, Stock W 1983 The effects of class size: An examination of rival hypotheses. *Am. Educ. Res. J.* 20: 63–85

Husén T (ed.) 1967 *International Study of Achievement in Mathematics.* Wiley, New York

Hyman H H 1972 *Secondary Analysis of Sample Surveys: Principles, Procedures, and Potentialities.* Wiley, New York

International Association for the Evaluation of Educational Achievement (IEA) 1988 *Science Achievement in Seventeen Countries: A Preliminary Report.* Pergamon, Oxford

Keeves J P 1972 *Educational Environment and Student Achievement.* Australian Council For Educational Research, Hawthorn, Victoria

Keeves J P 1986a The performance cycle. *Int. J. Educ. Res.* 10: 143–58

Keeves J P 1986b Testing the model by multivariate analysis. *Int. J. Educ. Res.* 10: 159–73, 200–04

Keeves J P (ed.) 1992. *The IEA Study of Science III: Changes in Science Education and Achievement: 1970 to 1984.* Pergamon Press, Oxford

Lohnes P R 1986 Factor modeling. *Int. J. Educ. Res.* 10: 181–89

Magidson J 1977 Toward a causal model approach to adjusting for preexisting differences in the nonequivalent control group situation. *Evaluation Quarterly.* 1: 399–420

McGaw B, Sorbom D, Cummings J 1986 Analysis of linear structural relations. *Int. J. Educ. Res.* 10: 173–81

McKnight C C et al. 1987 *The Under-achieving Curriculum: Assessing U.S. School Mathematics from an International Perspective.* Stipes Champaign, Illinois

Postlethwaite T N, Wiley D E 1992 *The IEA Study of Science II: Science Achievement in Twenty-Three Countries.* Pergamon Press, Oxford

Sellin N 1986 Partial least squares analysis. *Int. J. Educ. Res.* 10: 189–200

Walberg H J (eds.) 1982 *Improving Educational Performance and Standards: The Research and Evaluation Basis of Policy.* McCutchan, Berkeley, California

Walberg H J 1986 Synthesis of research on teaching. In: Wittrock M C (ed.) 1986 *Handbook of Research on Teaching*, 3rd edn. Macmillan, New York

Walberg H J, Haertel E H (eds.) 1980 Research integration: The state of the art. *Eval. Educ.* 4(1): 1–142

Further Reading

Cook T D, Campbell D T 1979 *Quasi-experimentation.* Houghton Mifflin, Boston, Massachusetts

Hakim C 1982 *Secondary Analysis in Social Research: A Guide to Data Sources and Methods with Examples.* George Allen and Unwin, London

Kiecolt K J, Nathan L E 1985 *Secondary Analysis of Survey Data.* Sage, Beverly Hills, California

Stewart D W 1984 *Secondary Research: Information Sources and Methods.* Sage, Beverly Hills, California

Travers K J, Crosswhite F J, Dossey J A, Swafford J O, McKnight C C, Cooney T J 1985 *Second International Mathematics Study Summary Report for the United States.* Stipes, Champaign, Illinois

Selection Bias in Educational Research

A. C. Tuijnman

In this entry the conceptual and methodological problems arising from the use in educational research of samples drawn from selected or self-selected populations are discussed. The existence of selection bias greatly limits the validity of generalizations that can be drawn from the analysis of data associated with samples where selection has taken place. Moreover, it commonly distorts the findings of educational research, where no allowance has been made for its effects.

This entry provides examples of research studies in which the presence of selection bias can harm the accuracy of the parameter estimates and impair the validity of statistical inference. Methods for detecting and reducing selection bias are also reviewed.

1. Definitions

Wei and Cowan (1988 p. 332) define selection bias as "the bias that occurs in a clinical trial, experiment or sample survey because of the effects of the mechanism used to select individuals or units for inclusion in the experiment or survey." In sample surveys selection bias can influence the estimates of certain parameters because the selection probabilities for inclusion in a survey can be related to the variables being studied. This may be the case if there are unobserved determinants of the probability of inclusion that correlate significantly with unobserved determinants of the criterion variables.

At the core of selection bias is a restriction of range. As a result of the way they were chosen for inclusion in the program, the children enrolled in the Headstart Program, for example, were likely to have restricted ranges on home background measures, scholastic achievement, and many other variables. Much of the research on selection bias has originated from work in the area of social and educational program evaluation. The evaluation of Headstart and public training programs for the unemployed are two examples. The harmful effects of selection bias on the accuracy of mean scores and regression estimates are now widely recognized and documented.

In the case of regression analysis, for example, it is normally assumed that there is no range restriction on the dependent variables. Selection bias in the regressors distorts regression estimates and other statistics only in certain specifiable ways. According to Darlington (1990 p. 198) statistics such as the regression slope b_j, the intercept a, the predicted variance of the dependent variable $\hat{Y}_i$, the residual variance e_i, and the mean square error, MSE, are *not* distorted by a restriction of range. However, statistics such as the multiple correlation R^2, the variance of the dependent variable Y, all values of the correlation r_{yj}, and the values of the partial correlation pr_j for the restricted variables are affected. In general, however, the statistics undistorted by range restriction are those used in causal analysis, whereas the distorted statistics are used in prediction. Therefore, prediction studies are seriously distorted by range restriction more often than regression studies involving causal analysis.

Different concepts exist for describing the phenomenon highlighted above. Statisticians would appear to be neutral; they tend to use the practical term "selection bias." For partly theoretical reasons, the designation "*self*-selection bias" has much currency in the economics of education. By contrast, educational sociologists tend in certain situations to use concepts such as "retentivity" and "selectivity." These are thought to encapsulate the idea that individuals often have no control over the selection mechanism, which may be random or nonrandom. The prefix "self" can be taken as suggesting that participation in an educational program is based on rational choice, and that the people who are *not* selected for enrollment in a program carry responsibility for themselves. Since many people seem to have no such choice, the term "self-selection bias" might well be considered misleading.

2. Selection Bias in Sample Surveys

In survey research methodology, a distinction is often made between the desired target population and the defined target population, from which a sample can be drawn. Differences normally occur between the ideal and the achievable, for example, because it may not be possible to obtain observations for all of the desired units. The accuracy of a sample statistic, $\bar{x}$, based on a probability sample is generally assessed in terms of the variance of $\bar{x}$, denoted $\text{Var}(\bar{x})$, which quantifies the sampling stability of the values of $\bar{x}$ around the expected value $E(\bar{x})$ (Ross 1987). Sampling error, which is a property of the entire sampling distribution, belongs to both the selection and estimation procedures that are employed in obtaining sampled data. Selection bias is therefore a very special case of sampling bias.

The information obtained from a sample is normally used to advance useful generalizations about the defined population. The usefulness of statistical inference depends, among other factors, on how closely the achieved sample reproduces the characteristics of the defined population. Because the exact population parameters are unknown, the influence of sampling error is usually assessed on the basis of the internal evidence of a single sample of data. However, sampling error, conventionally defined, does not necessarily take account of the possible differences between the desired target and the defined target population. The ideal is a population free of any selection mechanism that is related to the variables being studied and that influences the selection probabilities for inclusion in a sample. As the examples given below suggest, this ideal is often unattainable. Hence systematic differences can arise between the desired and defined target populations. Such differences may introduce selection bias in sample surveys. Even if the sampling errors are very small, which is usually the case in well-designed studies, then the presence of selection bias in the data can seriously harm the accuracy of the parameter estimates and impair the validity of statistical inference (see *Sampling in Survey Research; Survey Research Methods*).

3. Examples of Selection Bias and Adjustment Methods

Selection bias is usually not a problem in educational research as long as the defined target population from which a sample is drawn comprises all students in an age group attending compulsory school. Of course, the noncoverage and nonresponse of certain categories of school-age children may introduce threats to accuracy and validity that are, at least conceptually, very similar to problems associated with selection bias. Yet serious selection bias can occur if the enrollment status of students in postcompulsory programs is used as a criterion for sampling, since the mechanisms that impinge on individual choice and the decision to enroll

in a program of postcompulsory education may well determine the characteristics of the target population from which a sample can be drawn. Because the participants in such programs may differ markedly and systematically from those who are not enrolled, studies involving samples drawn from heterogeneous target populations associated with certain postcompulsory school programs can be highly vulnerable to selection bias and other sampling effects. The following examples provide illustration of this.

3.1 IEA *Study of Science Achievement*

In a study of science education in 23 countries conducted in 1983–84 by the International Association for the Evaluation of Educational Achievement (IEA), three target populations were selected in each school system (Postlethwaite and Wiley 1991, Keeves 1992): (a) Population 1—all students aged from 10 years to 10 years 11 months on the specified date of testing, or all students in the grade where most 10-year olds were to be found; (b) Population 2—all students aged from 14 years to 14 years 11 months on the specified date of testing, or all students in the grade where most 14-year olds were to be found; (c) Population 3—all students in the final grade of full-time secondary education in programs leading to entry into higher education.

With the exception of two developing countries, close to 100 percent of an age group was in school at the Population 1 level. In addition, at the Population 2 level nearly 100 percent was in school in the systems of the industrialized countries participating in the survey. However, as can be seen from Table 1, the percentage of an age group attending full-time education at the Population 3 level varied substantially across systems. This table also shows that the mean scores on comparable tests of student

Table 1
Percentage of an age group in school, mean ages (Population 3), grade level, means and standard deviations in chemistry (25 items) and physics (26 items)

Educational system[a]	grade level tested	% in school[b]	mean age[c]	% in school[d]	Chemistry X̄ test score	s.d. test score	% in school	Physics X̄ test score	s.d. test score
Australia	12	39	17.3	12	49.1	19.5	11	48.7	15.2
England and Wales	13	20	18.0	5	69.3	17.9	6	58.4	15.1
Finland	12	41	18.6	16	35.9	15.3	14	37.9	14.1
Hong Kong (Form 6)	12	27	18.3	20	68.2	17.7	20	61.2	14.5
Hungary	12	18	18.0	1	50.2	19.7	4	58.7	17.6
Japan	12	63	18.2	16	55.5	22.9	11	58.5	17.8
South Korea	12	38	17.9	37	30.9	14.8	14	39.8	16.9
Norway	12	40	18.9	6	44.3	18.4	10	54.1	15.9
United States (1986)	12	83	17.7	2	37.7	18.2	1	45.3	15.9

Source: Postlethwaite and Wiley 1991
a Data collected in 1983 and 1984   b Excluding students in vocational education   c Age given in years and months   d Percent of an age group

achievement in chemistry and physics differed across systems.

Inferences based on IEA data, such as that included in Table 1, often involve the making of comparisons across educational systems at the same time. For example, in 1983–84 the physics yield of Japanese schools at the Population 3 level was substantially higher than that of comparable Australian schools. This particular example may either be true, since in both systems 11 percent of an age group take physics, or it may not, since the standard deviations are different. Which inferences can safely be drawn from the data presented in this table remains an open question, but one aspect stands out clearly: there is unwanted variation in variables such as age and percent of an age group in school which can influence the dependent variable being measured, namely, the system mean score on the IEA physics and chemistry tests.

The problem of accounting for undesired but natural variation in age and school enrollment in selective educational systems was clearly recognized at the time the first IEA Mathematics project was carried out in the early 1960s. Walker (1967) developed a mathematical model to represent the effects of selection, which at that time was known as retentivity bias. The basic idea underlying the model is that "each country has the same distribution of mathematical ability in the complete age group and that the differences in means and variances found at the preuniversity mathematics stage are a result of selection procedures" (p. 135). The validity of this assumption can, of course, be questioned but it serves well in demonstrating how the adjustment model works when it uses, as in this case, the formula derived for the truncated normal distribution:

$$E(\bar{x}) = y/q; \text{Var} = 1 - (y/q)\{(y/q) - k\} \quad (1)$$

where $E(\bar{x})$ = expected or adjusted mean score; q = percentage of students selected; y = ordinate of normal curve at point of cut-off; and k = point of cut-off.

Walker used the formula in equation (1) to calculate the expected mean scores for data of the type shown in Table 1. The adjusted mean scores are said to be *unbiased* estimators of some population parameter. After comparing the expected with the observed scores, (Walker 1967, p. 136) concludes: "for such sweeping assumptions as have been made, the agreement between theory and results is moderately good." If Walker's basic assumption concerning the equal and normal distribution of mathematical ability across countries is accepted, then the formula in Eqn. (1) could be used to calculate expected mean scores for the chemistry and physics test results shown in Table 1. Walker also shows (p. 136) how the model (see Eqn. 2) can be adapted to take account of other assumptions or observations, for example, a correlation r between the variable (or possibly variables) representing the selection mechanism and the outcome (see *Models and Model Building*):

$$E(\bar{x}) = r(y/q); \text{Var} = r^2(y/q)\{(y/q-k)\} \quad (2)$$

3.2 Scholastic Aptitude Testing

The selection problems besetting IEA studies that involve sampled data from students in postcompulsory grades of the educational system of course apply equally well to other studies in which the mean scores of selected samples of students are compared across countries and regions. Several examples are known from the United States. A much publicized case concerns the ranking of states by the mean scores obtained by students taking the College Board's Scholastic Aptitude Test (SAT) or the American College Testing program (ACT). Since the proportion of students taking such tests differs from state to state, and also because certain variables such as college requirements and state funding policies influence the selection probabilities for inclusion in a SAT sample, meaningful statistical inferences cannot be made simply on the basis of unadjusted SAT mean scores. The question that has occupied many statisticians for decades is how such an adjustment can be made.

The simplest approach is to adjust for the selection ratio, by covarying out the participation rate. Powell and Steelman (1984 p. 400) conclude on the basis of an analysis that sought to adjust for the selection ratio that "about 82 percent of the variation in states' performance can be attributed to this variable" and that "at best, only 18 percent can be considered 'real' variation." This approach to adjustment is questioned on the grounds that "percentage taking the SAT" can be considered as a posttreatment concomitant variable that itself is influenced by the selection process, the properties of which are unknown (see Wainer 1986 pp. 11–13). Other approaches have been proposed, namely regression adjustment for relevant background variables, and enlarging the SAT pool by means of imputation and other methods. These approaches and methods are discussed in Section 4 below.

3.3 Training Programs for the Unemployed

A third group of researchers developed an interest in the phenomenon of selection bias in connection with the evaluation of public employment training programs. Many governments assigned high priority to the reduction of unemployment, especially in the latter half of the 1970s, the early 1980s, and the mid-1990s. Skills training was considered important, and publicly supported training programs were either set up or, in countries where they already existed, extended.

Especially in Sweden, the United States, and the United Kingdom much effort was devoted to evaluating the effectiveness of public training programs in terms of the postprogram employment status and earnings of the trainees (for an overview, see Barnow 1987). However, the findings of this expanding body of research were inconclusive, in that the expected benefits could often not be demonstrated. The absence of the expected outcomes led some econometricians to suggest that program effectiveness could not be determined because the participants enrolled in employment training programs were negatively self-selected with respect to the important predictors of program success; hence the doubtful or even negative relationships between program treatments and outcomes. This example has become a classic case in the writings on self-selection bias, not so much because a definite methodological breakthrough was reached but rather as a consequence of the energy which economists devoted to the problem.

3.4 Higher and Continuing Education

Even with the recent expansion of intake, enrollment in higher and continuing education remains selective on a number of accounts. Compared with all eligible students, university entrants are likely to be more homogeneous with respect to variables such as cognitive ability, achievement motivation and potential, and expected life career. Both groups are also likely to be more homogeneous than the general population. Selection bias may thus be present in studies in higher education that make use of samples in which students are selected for inclusion on the basis of their enrollment status (see *Validity*).

During the 1980s the research on the effects of education was increasingly focused on the postinitial sector. Because of the magnitude of the social and economic stakes involved, funds for conducting large-scale evaluation studies of continuing education, and especially job training, became accessible in many countries, and relevant data sets were assembled as a result.

Two conclusions soon emerged from this line of work. First, the designs for research have to be developed so that one can distinguish between effects due to initial education and those due to continuing education. The failure to account for previous experience of learning will otherwise result in an upward bias in the parameter estimated for the effect of continuing education. Second, any group of women and men who take part in programs of adult education, public employment training, and human resource development in firms is atypical in some sense. Because of the variety of postinitial educational programs and the heterogeneity of their clientele, the results obtained in evaluation studies of continuing education are seldom comparable and generalizable. Since selection bias obviously operates, doubt is cast on the validity of any statistical inference made.

Tuijnman and Fägerlind (1989) report a longitudinal study of differences between participants and nonparticipants in continuing education at various stages in the lifespan (see *Longitudinal Research Methods*). Table 2 shows that there are marked differences between the two groups on a number of indicators and at different ages. The sheer size of the differences makes it clear that evaluation studies involving data sampled only from program participants are likely to suffer from a very large selection bias. The conclusion seems clear: because participants in postinitial education and training programs tend to differ systematically from nonparticipants in a number of respects, major problems arise in estimating the effectiveness of such programs. The consequences of selection bias can no longer be ignored. Priority may therefore have to be given to the definition of control groups and to the improvement of techniques

Table 2

Differences between participants and nonparticipants in continuing education at different ages with respect to selection-relevant characteristics (*Malmö Study* data [a]; effect size indices [b])

Variable/characteristic	Participation age 30-35	Participation age 36-42	Participation age 43-56
Father's occupation	0.41	0.44	0.38
Cognitive ability measured at age 10	0.44	0.54	0.54
Perception of parental support for schooling	0.50	0.61	0.43
Formal educational attainment	0.63	0.70	0.58
Cognitive ability measured at age 20	0.54	0.54	0.65
Interest in continuing education [c]	0.98	0.83	0.61
Occupational level [c]	0.63	0.82	0.91
Earnings (logarithm)[c]	0.32	0.54	0.68
Job satisfaction[c]	0.04	0.23	0.37
N cases	716	703	671

Source: Tuijnman and Fägerlind 1989, p. 59

a The *Malmö Study* is a longitudinal study of a group of 1,432 Swedish men and women that was begun in 1938. The most recent data collection took place in the early 1990s   b Effect size is the difference between two group means expressed in standard deviation units   c Measured, respectively, at age 35, 42, and 56 years for the sampling of populations representative of the nonparticipant groups in education.

4. Additional Methods

Because of the work carried out by statisticians, economists, and researchers in education, each in his own field, understanding of selection bias has developed rapidly since the mid-1970s. Methods for detecting—and possibly reducing—selection bias have also been developed. The basic approaches were outlined above. Regression adjustment and imputation methods are discussed below.

4.1 Simple Allocation Designs

Allocation methods usually involve the making of assumptions about participation and adjusting for selection by "partialling out" the nonparticipation effect from the data. The simplest approach has been mentioned above, namely to adjust for unequal selection by covarying out participation rates. Many variations on this theme can be found in the research literature.

4.2 Selection Bias as a Specification Error

Another approach is to employ at least one regressor variable measuring an important aspect of program exclusion restrictions or the decision to participate. If such information is available and specified in the equation determining enrollment, then selection bias can be reduced. Regression adjustment methods thus consider selectivity as a specification error (Heckman 1979). The key to this approach is to obtain measures on some or all of the characteristics that make comparisons unfair. By including these measures in the regression equation it is hoped that the biasing effects of selection can be removed from the variables of interest.

This approach is conceptually analogous to the method of handling unwanted design effects in stratified probability samples by carrying the stratification variables through all stages of the data analysis. The application of regression adjustment is straightforward in the case of controlling for design effects, because the stratification variables are known and data on them usually collected. The difficulty of using the method in order to adjust for selection effects is precisely that the variables associated with these effects are mostly unknown and data on them often not available. The method thus stands or falls with the quality of previously validated knowledge and data.

4.3 Selection Modeling

Selection modeling is a methodology proposed by Heckman and Robb (1986) to overcome some of the problems of treating selection bias as a specification error. It can be used to generate artificially the missing scores on the outcome variables for the (nonobserved) nonparticipants by means of a regression imputation technique. The methodology consists of three basic steps (Wainer 1986 p. 3): (a) *observe* the distribution of the outcome variables of interest; (b) *hypothesize* the functional relationship between the likelihood of participation and the variables observed; and (c) *calculate* the distribution of the outcome variables for both those who are observed and those who are not.

Not surprisingly, this method has met with strong criticism. The difficulty is of the same kind as that associated with the approach taken by Walker in the adjustment for selection effects in IEA data: the validity of the minimal identifying assumptions that guide the adjustment usually cannot be fully tested with data. Despite this criticism the method is not completely without merit, as Heckman and Robb (1986) demonstrate on the basis of experiments and simulations.

4.4 Imputation Adjustment

As in the example above, imputation adjustment also involves the making of assumptions about nonobservation. Imputation methods can be used to compensate for the effects of range restriction in ways analogous to the treatment of attrition and selective noncoverage and nonresponse in survey samples (see *Missing Data and Nonresponse*).

4.5 Mixture Modeling

Mixture modeling also considers selection bias as a problem of missing data, that is, nonresponse or nonobservation dependent on the outcome variable. The approach, as its name suggests, uses a combination of methods to predict the scores that are missing in range-restricted, dependent variables. The key assumption in mixture modeling is that the respondents and the nonrespondents form different populations, that a procedure can be designed for the multiple imputation of data values for nonrespondents, and that parameters for nonrespondents can be estimated using assumptions about the relationship between respondents and nonrespondents. In practice this means that the same person is simultaneously observed as a member of the program participant group and the excluded group. If both states can be observed then the selection effect can be identified from the treatment effect and, provided that the data are appropriately weighted, unbiased estimates of program impact may be obtained. Propensity score methodology (Rosenbaum and Rubin 1985) is a related approach.

5. Experimental and Quasi-experimental Designs

It can be inferred from the diversity of available methods to adjust for selection bias that the search for alternatives to rigorous experimental controls in program evaluation has been a long one. Many statisticians and others contend that this effort has not yielded a method that can appropriately be used for inference from nonexperimental data derived from self-selected samples. In the absence of such valid methods, a strong case is made for program evaluation by experimental design. Experimental procedures commonly involve the use of multiple groups that, even though randomized, differ substantially with respect to their background characteristics and the level of program treatment. These groups are then compared in terms of preprogram and postprogram characteristics. However, problems also beset this approach: for example, it may not be possible to employ strict controls in social settings.

An alternative for controlled experimentation is the quasi-experimental or comparison group design. Quasi-experimental methods are often used in program evaluation. In its basic form it requires a preprogram measure, a postprogram measure that can reflect the effect of the program being studied, and a measure describing the status of the persons in the sample, usually whether they took part (treatment group) or did not (comparison group). In educational research the comparison group usually comprises nonparticipants who are assumed or shown to have many characteristics in common with the program treatment group. Bryant (1978) provides an example of how unbiased estimates of program effects might be obtained from a sample of participants and a comparison group drawn from a large household survey. Difficult problems concern both the definition and use of a comparison group, and whether characteristics of the groups influence treatment conditions. Range restriction may also beset quasi-experimental studies employing multiple samples. It may also be impractical or even impossible to identify an appropriate comparison group and collect data on the group members. Estimates of program impact are therefore likely to remain biased, unless an appropriate control group can be identified and sampled, and assuming characteristics of the groups have not influenced treatment conditions.

Unlike the conditions that are specific to an experimental design, the accuracy of parameter estimates in nonexperimental evaluations of program effectiveness depend on the way the program input, treatment, and program outcome equations are specified. Some nonexperimental evaluations of postinitial education have made use of two-wave models or even multiple time–series designs. Although it is acknowledged that these and other adjustment methods are imperfect, nonexperimental evaluation cannot be ruled out, because many complex programs exist where one or more of the following conditions apply: (a) selection mechanisms or voluntary self-selection are a condition for inclusion; (b) it cannot be established with certainty whether and in what respects participants differ from nonparticipants; (c) the program treatments cannot be directly measured; and (d) an adequate comparison group cannot be defined, and characteristics of the groups influence treatment conditions (see *Experimental Studies; Quasi experimentation*).

6. Conclusion

The only way to solve the selection bias problem is to draw a sample in such a way that the enrollment status of program participants becomes irrelevant as a criterion for sampling. An attractive means of overcoming selection and simultaneity problems is presented by longitudinal studies in which an age group is sampled before it leaves compulsory school. Longitudinal data cannot be regarded as a panacea, however. Serious problems of data analysis remain even in cases where some of the data are collected before the treatment and the sample is taken from a population comprising both participants and nonparticipants. If unobserved variables and their errors correlate with the outcome variable, which is often the case, then specification errors may be present and unbiased estimators cannot be obtained. Hence, since their use may yield inconsistent estimates of program effects even in cases where selection bias has been ruled out, regression methods may have limited applicability in program evaluation research (see *Longitudinal Research Methods*).

See also: Regression Analysis of Quantified Data; Sampling Errors in Survey Research; Validity; Sampling in Survey Research

References

Barnow B S 1987 The impact of CETA programs on earnings: A review of the literature. *J. Hum. Resources* 18: 157–93

Bryant E C 1978 Survey statistics in social program evaluation. In: David H A (ed.) 1978 *Contributions to Survey Sampling and Applied Statistics*. Academic Press, London

Darlington R B 1990 *Regression and Linear Models*. McGraw-Hill, London

Heckman J J 1979 Sample selection bias as a specification error. *Econometrica* 46: 931–59

Heckman J J, Robb R 1986 Alternative methods for solving the problem of selection bias in evaluating the impact of treatments on outcomes. In: Weiner H (ed.) 1986

Keeves J P (ed.) 1992 *Changes in Science Education and Achievement: 1970 to 1984*. Pergamon Press, Oxford

Postlethwaite T N, Wiley D E 1991 *The IEA Study of Science II: Science Achievement in Twenty-three Countries*. Pergamon Press, Oxford

Powell B, Steelman L C 1984 Variations in state SAT performance: Meaningful or misleading? *Harv. Educ. Rev.* 54: 389–412

Rosenbaum P, Rubin D B 1985 Constructing a control group using multivariate sampling methods that incorporate the propensity score. *American Statistician* 39: 33–38

Ross K N 1987 Sample design. *Int. J. Educ. Res.* 11(1): 57–75

Tuijnman A C, Fägerlind I 1989 Measuring and predicting participation in lifelong education using longitudinal data. *Scandinavian J. Educ. Res.* 33: 47–66

Wainer H 1986 The SAT as a social indicator: A pretty bad idea. In: Weiner H (ed.) 1986
Walker D A 1967 An attempt to construct a model of the effects of selection. In: Husén T (ed.) 1967
Wei L J, Cowan C D 1988 Selection bias. *Encyclopedia of Statistical Sciences* 8: 332–34

Further Reading

Ashenfelter O 1987 The case for evaluating training programs with randomized trials. *Econ. Educ. Rev.* 6(4): 333–38
Behrman J R 1987 Schooling and other human capital investments: Can the effects be identified? *Econ. Educ. Rev.* 6(3): 301–05
Fraker T, Maynard R 1987 The adequacy of comparison group designs for evaluations of employment-related programs. *J. Hum. Res.* 22(2): 194–227
Glynn R J, Laird N M, Rubin D B 1986 Selection modeling versus mixture modeling with nonignorable nonresponse. In: Weiner H (ed.) 1986
Husén T (ed.) 1967 *International Study of Achievement in Mathematics: A Comparison of Twelve Countries*, Vol.2. Almqvist and Wiksell, Stockholm
Kiefer N 1979 Population heterogeneity and inference from panel data on the effects of vocational training. *J. Polit. Econ.* 87: S213–26
Rubin D B 1987 *Multiple Imputation for Nonresponse in Surveys.* Wiley, New York
Weiner H (ed.) 1986 *Drawing Inferences from Self-selected Samples.* Springer-Verlag, Berlin
Willis R J, Sherwin R 1979 Education and self-selection. *J. Polit. Econ.* 87(5, Pt.2): S7–36

Single Case Research: Measuring Change

C. F. Sharpley

When teachers or researchers begin a new program of instruction, they often want to know how it affects each student in the class or group receiving it. Single-subject experimentation, or single case research, is a field of measurement which focuses upon this issue, and which has developed a nomenclature and data analysis procedures of its own. The problems which arise from this use of only one subject as the unit of analysis are concerned with the gathering of sufficient data to enable reliable conclusions to be drawn regarding the effects of the intervention. Although earlier research used graphed representations of the data gathered from single subjects, since the 1980s there has been a preference for statistical procedures unique to this field.

1. Evaluation Effects: Groups or Individuals?

Research into the outcomes of a particular intervention upon the behavior of a set of subjects may be treated as either a "group-oriented" task or a "single-subject" task. For each of these types of measurement task, there are different perspectives, giving rise to different statistical developments and problems. Group designs will not be dealt with here: they are the focus of a great deal of other work, and information on them may be easily gleaned from a variety of sources. By contrast, there is far less in the educational measurement literature concerning single-subject research, although a few excellent texts are in existence and are listed in the Further Reading section of this entry.

This entry includes the following: an overview of the development of a rationale for examining single-subject data, the history of what has become a major disagreement in this (esoteric) field, some arguments why single-subject data should be examined via statistical procedures (where possible and sensible), and a reference to some of the later developments in the statistical analysis of these data.

2. Why Examine Single Subjects?

When researchers average results from a group of subjects they (perhaps unintentionally) omit a great deal of richness in the data. Group means do tell the overall story, but they do not indicate, for example, how a certain subject reacted to the new teaching strategy just introduced. While the majority of classroom members might react in one direction, there may also be some students who respond differently, or even in an opposite direction to the mean of the group. These students deserve attention just as much as the majority, and educators need to take into consideration these "unusual" responses when evaluating teaching interventions. Thus individual or single-subject research designs have evolved.

Another way in which the focus is turned toward individual subject data is by only using one or two subjects in the research being conducted. In other words when there are a few students in a classroom who do not appear to respond to the general teaching style offered, then some extra or different intervention needs to be developed—and assessed for its effect. Therefore, there is a need to apply the rigors of

451

experimental research design to the individual subject. In their seminal work on this topic, Barlow and Hersen (1984) pointed out some of the limitations of group-designed research and suggested that such research can confuse and even prevent the discovery of causal links between environmental influences (such as teachers) and an individual's behavior.

3. Some of the Nomenclature of Single-subject Design

Single-subject research designs almost completely rely upon what are termed "interrupted time-series" models for their parenthood. Interrupted time-series designs utilize the collection of data over time, with at least one change of environmental conditions during the time period sampled. For example, in trying to reduce the frequency of nocturnal enuresis in an intellectually disabled young female adult, Mohr and Sharpley (1988) collected data on the frequency of night-time wetting over a period when there was no change in the subject's environment. Then, when these "baseline" data had been collected, several different interventions were applied to test for effects of a range of variables upon the behavior which was targeted for change (in this case, reduction or elimination of enuresis). Data from the baseline or nonintervention period are referred to by use of the letter "A". Actual interventions (such as reducing the level of caffeine intake—a procedure which acted to eliminate nocturnal enuresis in the above example) are referred to as "B". Returns to baseline (used to test for the effects of removal of the intervention) are also known as A, but with the use of a number to indicate which in a series of baselines is referred to: hence the designations A1, A2, and so on. The practice is the same with additional and different interventions: B1, B2, and so on. Thus, a typical design might be ABA1B1. Examples of these designs abound in the literature.

Several caveats exist for the reliable application of ABAB type designs (which will henceforth be referred to as "interrupted time-series" designs, or ITS: this latter term is widely used in the literature and familiarity with it will thus be of benefit for future investigation of this topic). First, data must be collected on baseline A *before* there is any suggestion of intervention. In other words, it is unwise to try to recall what the subject was doing before intervention after that intervention has (perhaps unintentionally) begun. Data should be collected by persons who are not aware of the planned intervention if they are also involved in the daily activities of the subject. Conversely, there is also a need to keep any plans for intervention secret from those persons who may come into contact with the subject. For example, telling a teacher that a certain intervention will be commenced in two weeks will almost ensure a change in the subject's behavior *during* baseline, and therefore invalidate any testing

for effects by comparing data from intervention to that from baseline. This may be illustrated by the hypothetical example of a particular student presenting a behavior problem for a teacher, where intervention of the type not uncommon in schools was planned for implementation after two weeks' baseline data had been collected. If the teacher was aware that the student was going to receive points for appropriate behavior during intervention, then there is some likelihood that the teacher would (quite unwittingly, but nevertheless effectively crushing the experimental validity of the research) alter his or her behavior toward the student. This might be in so small a way as to avoid responding to the student's misbehavior because (in the teacher's mind) the "problem" was planned to be "fixed" in two weeks. Such nonattention to misbehavior is actually an intervention which has received a great deal of use and support. The intervention would thus have begun immediately, rather than after two weeks of baseline. Comparison between baseline and intervention would be ineffective in determining the usefulness of the intervention, and thus the research project itself.

A further point to be aware of when applying ITS designs is the need to collect data over a sufficiently long period of time so that a representative sample of the behavior in question is obtained. For readers more familiar with group designs, this is the issue of power, and the issue of number of observations collected is similar to the issue of number of subjects in a group design. Some suggestions as to the minimum number of observations necessary are made in the discussion below.

4. Detecting Change in ITS

The analysis of data from interrupted time-series research has been marked by an ongoing and continuing disagreement between the *visual* analysts and those who maintained that a statistic was necessary to perform reliable assessment of changes (i.e., the *statistical* analysts). Based upon B F Skinner's initial work with animals, where data were very clear and almost an "all or nothing" effect was common, visual analysis was predominant in the laboratory and in classroom research of the period 1940–60. However, after some time, increasing sophistication in behavioral psychology and in the research questions being asked resulted in less obvious effects. In some cases, the "human" factor appeared, leading to variations in data which made interpretation difficult. With this instability in data came the need to decide whether such data were not amenable to clear visual analysis and therefore should be ignored (a perspective taken by visual analysts) or, at best, analyzed by complex visual analysis procedures which ultimately depended upon quite subjective decisions. Conversely, the other side in this debate (the statisticians) considered that these data represented the frontier of investigation simply because they were not so clear-cut. The latter position led to the development of statistical procedures, some of which will be described below.

4.1 Some Problems with Visual Analysis

As suggested above, simple visual analysis (via graphic representation) of ITS data is open to subjectivity and misinterpretation. Much has been written on this issue (e.g., Gottman 1981, Gottman and Glass 1978, Sharpley 1981), and the findings may be summarized as follows.

Graphs themselves can "lie". Campbell (1974) has illustrated how the same data can be graphed in different styles and according to different scales so as to show large effects or virtually no change at all. Thus, both Type 1 errors (assuming that an effect is present when it is not) and Type 2 errors (missing an effect present) are easily made when graphic presentation is used to detect change in behavior. There are some quite compelling data on this issue.

First, White (1972) showed that some visual analysts saw an increase in data when others saw a decrease in the same data. Second, Jones et al. (1978) asked a panel of 11 judges who were familiar with data from ITS research to examine data sets from the *Journal of Applied Behavior Analysis* (a major source of graphed data). This panel comprised " . . . fulltime researchers, university professors, and graduate students with 3 to 17 years of research experience in psychology, including applied behavior analysis" (Jones et al. 1978 p. 278). These experienced researchers agreed only 39 percent of the time, suggesting that even familiar and relatively "expert" visual analysts were unable to determine if typical data represented increases or decreases in behavior. A further study of this type was reported by De Prospero and Cohen (1979), who used 114 reviewers and editors of the *Journal of Applied Behavior Analysis* and the *Journal of the Experimental Analysis of Behavior* to evaluate graphs for change. Agreement in this case was greater (61%), but hardly so high as to inspire confidence in the use of these techniques by the relatively inexpert. De Prospero and Cohen identified a need for a "yardstick" for assessing data from ITS research, one which could be equally applied by the uninitiated as well as the expert. That yardstick was statistical analysis.

5. Statistical Analysis of ITS Data

Traditional statistical procedures are not always applicable to ITS data because of the distorting effects of "autocorrelation." This term refers to the fact that repeated observations taken relatively closely together in time are correlated with each other. The extent of this correlation can be assessed, and is presented as a correlation coefficient (e.g., $r = 0.6$). Sharpley and Alavosius (1988) presented a table of the degree

to which such autocorrelation in ITS data distort the outcome of traditional t-tests or ANOVAS. For example, data which have an autocorrelation of 0.6 will inflate a t or F value by 200 percent, thus arguing strongly against the use of these procedures with ITS data. Recent interchanges on this issue of the presence and effects of autocorrelation upon analysis of ITS data may be found in Busk and Marascuilo (1988), Huitema (1985, 1988), Sharpley and Alavosius (1988), Suen (1987, 1988), Suen and Ary (1987), and Suen et al. (1990). This area is not free from dispute, and the interested reader is advised to gain at least some familiarity with this literature in order to understand the underlying arguments for whichever side of the debate is chosen.

A second major issue in the statistical analysis of ITS data is that concerning the number of observations required for reliable estimation of effects. The principal problem has been assumed to be that of identification of the underlying model of the data. Several such models are possible, for example, the "Autoregressive", the "Moving Averages", the mixed "Autoregressive–Moving Averages", and the "White Noise" models (see Glass et al. 1975 for a clear explanation of these). It is sufficient to note here that it has traditionally been assumed that correct model identification requires between 50 and 100 observations in each phase, a figure well beyond the logistics of most classroom research. However, there is an alternative to this problem.

Working on the assumption that accurate identification of the model is possible, Velicer and Harrop (1983) asked 12 graduate students to identify 32 series of ITS data. These students had had intensive training in model-identification as recommended by Glass et al. (1975). Of 384 models identified (12 students for 32 series of data each), surprisingly only 109 (28%) were correct. Hacker (1986) replicated these results, suggesting that the (necessary) model-identification process may not be possible in many cases.

However, Harrop and Velicer (1985) proceeded to determine if such inaccuracy in model-identification really made any difference to the outcomes from tests of intervention. After an exhaustive treatment of the data, they concluded that "the model identification process might be eliminated altogether" (p. 42) simply by adopting one model and assuming that it was sufficient. This conclusion agrees with Gottman's (1981) finding that, for the two models which were considered to be most different (the Autoregressive and the Moving Averages models), each was able to be modeled in terms of the other.

A third issue which has impeded the ready implementation of statistical procedures with ITS data has been that concerned with the number of observations necessary for reliable use of statistical procedures. Returning to the 50 to 100 observations figure mentioned above (and in most of the early literature), Gottman (1982) performed a Monte Carlo study by generating 5,000 ITS series and then testing for Type 1 error rates (i.e., concluding a significant effect when there was none). Gottman used series of 60 baseline and 60 intervention observations to 5 baseline and 5 intervention observations, with levels of autocorrelation from −0.9 to +0.9. The outcome of this simulation study was that the incidence of Type 1 error was less than 5 percent in most cases (i.e., within the traditional limits), particularly with short series of 5 baseline and 5 intervention observations. Gottman concluded that "sample size makes relatively little difference" (p. 355), and that interrupted time-series "analysis with autoregressive models can be used with confidence even in small samples" (p. 359). Gottman used only Autoregressive models because he had determined that Moving Averages models could be remodeled as Autoregressive models (see above). He cautioned that Type 2 errors (missing a significant effect) usually required more observations, but that the process of testing the null hypothesis was, in itself, quite unattractive simply because of the need to gather a great deal of data to justify accepting such a hypothesis. Thus, long series are only necessary when power is a major consideration. If the effects from a short series are significant, confirming an *a priori* hypothesis, then power is not a problem.

5.1 Attempts at Reliable Statistical Analysis of ITS Data

There is a history of development of statistical yardsticks for use with ITS data. Probably the first widespread computer program for ITS was that developed by Glass and his colleagues (see Glass et al. 1975, for a detailed description). There were some problems with the use of this program (termed "TMS" one of which is that its valid use depends upon the removal of "slope" in the data prior to testing for change due to intervention. Such slope is a gradual increase or decrease in the data over time. The other important parameter for ITS (and TMS addressed this) was the "level" of the data (i.e., the overall score or numerical level which the data possess). Perhaps the most impeding aspect to TMS was the laborious, time-consuming, and inefficient process which the program went through to estimate the degree of autocorrelation in the data before estimating the effects of intervention.

A later development is the program ITSE, developed by Gottman and others (see Gottman 1982 for a comprehensive account of this procedure). It represents a major step in statistical analysis of ITS data because it can be employed legitimately with data which has a slope and because ITSE models the data on the assumption that there is slope. Matrix algebra is then employed to produce a line of best fit for each phase (i.e., baseline, intervention) after the influence of autocorrelation has been removed. The program determines three things: (a) whether the phase 2 (i.e., intervention) line of best fit differs significantly from the extension of the phase 1 (i.e., baseline) line of best fit; (b) whether these lines of best fit have signi-

ficantly different intercepts on the vertical axis; and (c) whether these lines of best fit have significantly different slopes.

Two of the most recent developments in this area are DMITSA2 (see Crosbie and Sharpley 1989 for a detailed description) and ITSACORR (Crosbie 1993), the latter is especially valuable when analyzing very short series of data observations. Both of these programs are easy to use and run on personal computers.

6. Conclusion

The field of analysis of data collected on single subjects moved a long way during the 1980s. In particular, the development of simplified and user-friendly software since then has brought what were quite daunting statistical procedures within the reach of even the most statistically naive researcher. Thus, there is little pragmatic reason for not performing statistical analysis of these data. Another aspect of the increasing use of these techniques is the "flow-on" of rigor in experimental design which usually accompanies the use of statistical procedures. These two developments can only tighten the validity and reliability of single-subject research and render it an even more exciting and evolving field.

See also: Experimental Studies

References

Barlow D H, Hersen M 1984 *Single Case Experimental Designs*, 2nd edn. Pergamon Press, New York
Busk P L, Marascuilo L A 1988 Autocorrelation in single-subject research: A counterargument to the myth of no autocorrelation. *Behav. Assessment* 10(3): 229–42
Campbell S K 1974 *Flaws and Fallacies in Statistical Thinking*. Prentice-Hall, Englewood Cliffs, New Jersey
Crosbie J, Sharpley C F 1989 DMITSA: A simplified interrupted time-series analysis program. *Behav. Res. Meth. Instr. and Comput.* 21(6): 639–42
Crosbie J 1993 Interrupted time-series analysis with brief single-subject data. *J. Consult. Clin. Psychol.* 61(6): 966–74
De Prospero A, Cohen S 1979 Inconsistent visual analysis of intrasubject data. *J. Appl. Behav. Anal.* 12(4): 573–79
Glass G V, Willson V L, Gottman J M 1975 *Design and Analysis of Time-series Experiments*. Colorado Associated University Press, Boulder, Colorado
Gottman J M 1981 *Time-series Analysis: A Comprehensive Introduction for Social Scientists*. Cambridge University Press, Cambridge
Gottman J M, Glass G V 1978 Analysis of interrupted time-series experiments. In: Kratochwill T R (ed.) 1978
Hacker W J 1986 An evaluation of both statistical and visual methods for making inferences of time series data. Unpublished master's dissertation, University of New England, Armidale
Harrop J W, Velicer W F 1985 A comparison of alternative approaches to the analysis of interrupted time-series.

Mult. Behav. Research 20(1): 27–44

Huitema B E 1985 Autocorrelation in applied behavior modification data: A myth. *Behav. Assessment* 7(2): 107–18

Huitema B E 1988 Autocorrelation: 10 years of confusion. *Behav. Assessment* 10(3): 253–94

Jones R R, Weinrott M, Vaught R S 1978 Effects of serial dependency on the agreement between visual and statistical inference. *J. Appl. Behav. Anal.* 11(2): 277–83

Mohr C, Sharpley C F 1988 Multi-modal treatment of nocturnal enuresis. *Educ. and Train. in Mental Retardation* 23(1): 70–75

Sharpley C F 1981 Time-series analysis of counseling research. *Meas. Eval. Guid.* 14: 144–57

Sharpley C F, Alavosius M P 1988 Autocorrelation in behavioral data: An alternative perspective. *Behav. Assessment* 10(3): 243–52

Suen H K 1987 On the epistemology of autocorrelation in applied behavior analysis. *Behav. Assessment* 9(2): 113–24

Suen H K 1988 Agreement, reliability, accuracy, and validity: Toward a clarification. *Behav. Assessment* 10(4): 343–66

Suen H K, Ary D 1987 Autocorrelation in applied behavior analysis: Myth or reality? *Behav. Assessment* 9(2): 125–30

Suen H K, Lee P S C, Owen S V 1990 Effects of autocorrelation on single-subject single-facet crossed-design generalizability assessment. *Behav. Assessment* 12(3): 305–16

Velicer W F, Harrop J W 1983 The reliability and accuracy of the time-series model identification. *Eval. Rev.* 7: 551–60

White O R 1972 Pragmatic approach to the description of progress in the single case. Doctoral dissertation, University of Oregon. *Dissertation Abstracts International* 32/OU-Ap5078

Further Reading

Cook T D, Campbell D T 1979 *Quasi-Experimentation: Design and Analysis Issues for Field Settings*. Rand McNally College Publications, New York

Jones R R, Vaught R S, Weinrott M M 1977 Time-series analysis in operant research. *J. Appl. Behav. Anal.* 10(1): 151–66

Kratochwill T R (ed.) 1978 *Single-subject Research*. Academic Press, New York

McDowall D, McCleary R, Meidinger E E, Hay R A 1980 *Interrupted Time-series Analysis*. Sage, Beverly Hills, California

Williams E A, Gottman J M 1982 *A User's Guide to the Gottman-Williams Time-series Analysis Computer Programs for Social Scientists*. Cambridge University Press, Cambridge

(c) Statistical Procedures

Bayesian Statistics

H. R. Lindman

Bayesian statistics involve both a philosophy and a set of statistical methods. Their main advantages over traditional statistics are that they encourage thinking about the data in new ways, that they bring prior information and informed opinions explicitly into the data analysis, and that they provide a more realistic philosophical position from which to evaluate the results of statistical procedures.

The principal disadvantages of Bayesian statistics are that the mathematical calculations are sometimes more complicated, prior information and opinions are sometimes difficult to assess in a manner appropriate for Bayesian statistics, and the allowance for prior information and opinions can lead to abuses. For these reasons the methods themselves are probably most valuable when two criteria are met. The first criterion is that relatively simple statistical procedures such as t-tests or binomial tests are being used; the second is that decisions have practical consequences that will ultimately affect the person making them (so that there are strong motives to separate true opinions from desires). However, a person may be philosophically a Bayesian even when using traditional statistical techniques as a second-best alternative. The Bayesian philosophy can affect the way the findings are interpreted. In this entry, these issues are discussed more fully after the basic ideas of Bayesian statistics have been presented.

1. Bayes's Theorem

The term "Bayesian statistics" is derived from a theorem first proved by the Revd Thomas Bayes and published posthumously in 1763. Then the theorem was novel; in the early 1990s, it can be easily proved in any beginner's statistics or probability theory class. Let $P(B|A)$ represent the probability of event A, given that event B has occurred, and let B' represent the complement (nonoccurrence) of B. Then Bayes's theorem can be written in any of several forms:

$$P(B \mid A) = \frac{P(A \mid B)P(B)}{P(A)} \tag{1}$$

$$P(B \mid A) = \frac{P(A \mid B)P(B)}{P(A \mid B)P(B) + P(A \mid B')P(B')} \tag{2}$$

$$P(B \mid A) / P(B' \mid A) \tag{3}$$
$$= [P(A \mid B) / P(A \mid B')][P(B) / P(B')]$$

The third equation is called the odds form of Bayes's theorem because it relates the odds of B and B', conditional on A, to the data and the unconditional odds. The first term in brackets on the right side of the third equation is commonly called the "likelihood ratio."

The mathematical correctness of Bayes's theorem is unquestioned. The application of Bayes's theorem distinguishes Bayesian from traditional statistics. In traditional statistics it is an interesting but seldom-used formula. In Bayesian statistics it is central.

To see why, consider an ordinary test of a null hypothesis, using, say, the normal distribution. Let the null hypothesis be H_0: $\mu = 50$, and let the sample mean be 46. Suppose that on the basis of these data the null hypothesis can be rejected at, say, the 0.05 level, one-tailed. What exactly is meant by that? Specifically, it means that if the null hypothesis were true, then the probability of obtaining a sample mean as small as, or smaller than, 46, would be less than 0.05.

This is a complicated concept, as any student of elementary statistics can testify. It also contains some serious weaknesses. First it considers the probability of obtaining data that were not actually obtained (i.e., it considers the probability of obtaining sample means smaller than 46 as well as equal to 46), and that therefore should presumably be irrelevant. Second, it considers only the consequences of rejecting the null hypothesis; it ignores the possibility of incorrectly accepting it. (Lip service is given to beta levels in statistics classes, but in practice they are almost universally ignored because there is no simple, direct way to deal with them.) Third, it purports to test a null hypothesis in which little faith is held to begin with. There is usually confidence that the parameter is not *precisely* equal (e.g., to more than, say, 20 decimals) to the hypothesized value. In most cases a null hypothesis test is actually an artificial way of deciding whether the parameter is really larger or smaller, rather than precisely equal to, the hypothesized value. Fourth, it does not give the likelihood directly that the null hypothesis is true; it tells only how likely the obtained results would be *if* the null hypothesis were true.

The last weakness is especially important. There are times when the data may be unlikely, given a particular hypothesis, but a reasonable decision would be to accept the hypothesis in spite of the data. Suppose, for example, that 50 is the mean score on a standardized achievement test for children of age 12, and that 46 was the mean score of a sample of students in a local, well-respected college or university. In such a case, the researcher's inclination would be to admit that the data are unlikely under H_0: $\mu = 50$, but to conclude nevertheless that the unlikely has occurred. Of course, one way to deal with this problem is to choose a very small significance level for rejection. However, within traditional statistics there is little guidance in choosing a specific significance level. That is why the 0.05 level, a purely conventional value, is so commonly used.

The same problem arises with confidence intervals. A 95 percent confidence interval is constructed in such a way that it will cover the true population mean in 95 percent of the cases for which it is constructed. However, previous information, unrelated to the experimental data, may indicate that the present experiment is one of the unlucky 5 percent (suppose a 95% confidence interval of 100 to 105 were obtained for the mean IQ of Oxford University students). The paradoxical situation then exists of having constructed a confidence interval in which no confidence is held.

Now consider the alternative using Bayes's theorem. Suppose, in the above equations, that B represents any (not necessarily the null) hypothesis, and A represents the obtained sample data. Then the formula indicates that the probability of the hypothesis, conditional on the sample data, should depend in a specific way on the unconditional probability (i.e., the probability before the data were collected). The plausibility (i.e., probability) of the hypothesis can thus be calculated directly, avoiding the roundabout methods of traditional statistics. This will be illustrated later with a specific example, but first the principal objection usually given to this approach must be dealt with.

2. Probability Theory

Although Bayes's theorem is accepted by all statisticians, its application to the above example is not. In traditional statistics, probabilities are assigned to data, but it is not considered legitimate to assign probabilities to hypotheses. The reason lies in the history of probability theory.

Probability theory was first applied to gambling. As in many areas of mathematics, the procedures were used before the philosophy had been worked out. This caused few problems in gambling situations, in which the appropriate probabilities were usually obvious. However, in scientific applications it led to many abuses, perhaps the most famous being due to Laplace. Applying Bayes's theorem (along with some assumptions that were widely accepted in his day) to the known fact that the sun had risen every day for

more than 5,000 years, Laplace stated that the odds in favor of the sun rising tomorrow were higher than 1,826,213 to 1.

The reaction against these abuses came in the form of a theory that assigned probabilities only to the outcomes of rather broadly defined "experiments." An experiment was defined generally as an act or process that led to a single well-defined outcome. Thus the administration of an achievement test to a sample of 12-year olds is an experiment, as is the toss of an ordinary coin.

However, before probabilities can be assigned to these outcomes, the experiment must have a special property; the experiment must be repeatable, at least in principle, an infinite number of times under identical conditions. In practice this is generally interpreted to mean that the outcomes must be generated by some random process whose outcomes and probabilities do not change upon repetitions of the experiment. The 12-year olds must be a random sample from some well-defined population of 12-year olds; the coin must be randomly tossed, and so on.

This new theory of probability corrected the old abuses. It was adopted by Neyman and Pearson, who developed the foundations of the statistical theory and tests commonly used today. However, it has serious weaknesses: it is extremely limiting; it precludes the assignment of numerical values in the most natural way (i.e., by assigning probabilities) to beliefs about hypotheses, because hypotheses are either true or false (i.e., they cannot be "repeated under identical conditions"); and it prevents simple pursuits such as giving odds on horse-races. (Try to imagine a horse-race being repeated an infinite number of times under identical conditions.)

Moreover, the philosophical foundations of this view are shaky. No experiment can really be repeated even a finite number of times under exactly identical conditions, and if it could, it would always lead to the same results. If a coin is tossed in precisely the same way every time, then it could be expected that it would land precisely the same way every time. Probabilities exist to the extent that conditions are nonidentical. However, under nonidentical conditions there is no objective way to determine whether the probabilities have remained constant from trial to trial. In fact the very question may be meaningless.

Alternative approaches to probability were proposed in the first half of the twentieth century. Most important were the personalist and necessarist interpretations of probability. According to both, probabilities are assigned not to events but to propositions—statements of fact. A probability represents a "degree of belief" that the statement is true. The personalist and necessarist views differ in that the personalist believes such probabilities are entirely personal—a given person may have any degree of belief whatsoever in a given proposition—while the necessarist believes that there is a "right" probability (usually unknown and unknowable) that one should have for the proposition. Most applied Bayesian statisticians hold the personalist view because the necessarist view gives little practical guidance in searching for the "right" probability.

The personalist view would seem to lead to chaos, letting anyone assign any probability to any proposition. However, this is not the case, at least for reasonable people. The early personalists—Ramsey (1931), de Finetti (1937), Savage (1954), and others—showed that, to be useful, personal probabilities had to have certain properties.

First, the probabilities had to be realistic in that they had to be tied to possible concrete actions by the individual. (Otherwise the probabilities would be meaningless.) To oversimplify the problem, if there is a probability of 3:4 for a given proposition, then it must be reasonable to give 3:1 odds in a bet that the proposition is true. Second, these theorists showed that probabilities, to be consistent, must satisfy the mathematical laws of probability theory. Violation of the laws could lead to the acceptance of sets of gambles which would necessarily result in loss of money (de Finetti 1937).

Requirements such as these are more restrictive than is supposed. For example, it has been shown that if two reasonable people are exposed to a large amount of unambiguously interpretable data bearing on a certain proposition, then those two people should subsequently finish with approximately the same probability for the proposition, even though they began with very different probabilities (Edwards et al. 1963). These approaches to probability are more sound philosophically than the relative frequency approach, and they have the advantage of allowing the assignment of probabilities to hypotheses as well as to outcomes of experiments.

Note, however, that the word "should" is used in the previous paragraph. The theory of personal probabilities is a normative, not a descriptive, theory. It specifies how rational people should behave, not how they naturally do behave. The purpose of Bayesian statistics, like all statistics, is to approach more closely the rational ideal.

3. Examples

These ideas can now be applied to a relatively simple concrete problem. Consider an abilities test whose scores are known to be normally distributed with a standard deviation of 10, then compare the two hypotheses, H_0: $\mu = 50$ and H_1: $\mu = 55$. Perhaps the typical score for all children at age 12 on this test is 50, while the typical score for children at age 14 is 55.

The sample consists of children of age 12, but the second hypothesis states that their ability level is actually typical of age 14. Suppose that, for whatever reasons, it is believed that they are twice as likely to

have a mean level of age 14 as of age 12. Then a probability of 1:3 should be assigned to hypothesis H_0 and 2:3 to hypothesis H_1.

Twenty-five students are sampled, and the sample mean is 53. The standard error of the mean is then 2, and both hypotheses can be rejected at the 0.05 level. However, if these are the only two plausible hypotheses, it is not possible to reject both.

In this case, with continuous normally distributed data, Bayes's theorem can be modified to read:

$$P(B \mid \bar{X}) = kf(\bar{X} \mid B)P(B)$$

where $\bar{X}$ is the sample mean, $f(\bar{X}|B)$ is the density function of $\bar{X}$, and k is a constant to be determined later. In the above example, $\bar{X}$ has a normal distribution with a standard deviation of 2, and, given that H_0 is true, a mean of 50. Thus the regular formula for the normal distribution is:

$$f(\bar{X} \mid H_0) = \frac{1}{2\sqrt{2\pi}} \exp\left[-\frac{1}{2}\left(\frac{\bar{X} - 50}{2}\right)^2\right] \quad (4)$$

Similarly, $f(\bar{X}|H_1)$ is the same, with 55 substituted for 50 in the exponent. These numbers can be calculated, and the following values are obtained:

$$P(H_0 \mid \bar{X}) = k(0.0648)(1/3) = k(0.0216) \quad (5)$$

$$P(H_1 \mid \bar{X}) = k(0.1210)(2/3) = k(0.0807) \quad (6)$$

In each equation, the first number in parentheses is $f(\bar{X}|H_i)$, and the second is the prior probability for the hypothesis. k can easily be found by noting that the two probabilities must sum to one, giving

$$k = 1/(0.0216 + 1\ 0.0807) = 9.775 \quad (7)$$

$$P(H_0 \mid \bar{X}) = 0.21 \quad (8)$$

$$P(H_1 \mid \bar{X}) = 0.79 \quad (9)$$

After the data have been analyzed, the probability for H_1 has increased from 2:3 to about 4:5; it is thus possible to say that the prior probability (before the experiment) was 2:3 and the posterior probability (after the experiment) is about 4:5.

With a much larger sample, the sample mean would be expected to be very close to either 50 or 55, depending on which hypothesis was actually correct, and the posterior probability for that hypothesis would be very nearly one; then the evidence would be overwhelmingly in favor of the correct hypothesis, and uncertainty would be replaced by near certainty. This is a special case of the earlier assertion that large amounts of unambiguous data should lead to near agreement among reasonable people.

Of course in the above simplified example the possibility that some other hypothesis, such as 52.5, might be correct, is ignored. In practice, any number of hypotheses can be considered at once, with only obvious minor modifications of the procedure just outlined.

Bayesian statistics are most interesting and most useful when all possible hypotheses are considered. In the above example, all points on the real line can be considered as possible values for the population mean. As usual in such a case, the probability that the mean is exactly equal to a particular value can no longer be considered (that probability is always zero), but the probability that the mean is between any two values can be considered. The probabilities can then be described by a density distribution—a curve such that the area under the curve between any two values represents the probability that the mean is between those two values.

To reconsider the previous example, since it is to be expected that the children perform like 14-year olds, suppose it is believed (before gathering the data) that the most likely value for the mean is 55. Suppose, further, that a probability of about 0.34 is assigned to the proposition that the mean is between 50 and 55, and that the same probability is assigned to the proposition that it is between 55 and 60. Moreover, a belief of about 95 percent certainty is held that the mean is between 45 and 65. The probabilities, before the experiment, can then be rather well-represented by a normal distribution having a mean of 55 and a standard deviation of 5.

For this case, Bayes's theorem can be rewritten:

$$f(\mu \mid \bar{X}) = kf(\bar{X} \mid \mu)f(\mu) \tag{10}$$

replacing the probabilities with density distributions. Here $f(\mu)$ is the density distribution representing the probabilities after gathering the data, and k is chosen so that the area under the curve given by $f(\mu|\bar{X})$ is one.

Now the calculations appear even more difficult; two exponential functions are involved and the multiplication must be done symbolically. However, the actual calculations are very simple. If, before the experiment is conducted, opinions about μ can be represented by a normal distribution having a mean of m and a standard deviation of σ, and if the sampling distribution of $\bar{X}$ is normal with a mean of μ and a standard deviation of $s / \sqrt{N}$, then, after the experiment has been conducted, opinions about μ are represented by a normal distribution whose mean m^*, and standard deviation, σ^*, are

$$m^* = \frac{(s^2/N)m + \sigma^2\bar{X}}{(s^2/N) + \sigma^2} \tag{11}$$

$$\sigma^* = \sqrt{\frac{(s^2/N)\sigma^2}{(s^2/N) + \sigma^2}} \tag{12}$$

In the example, the posterior probabilities, after analyzing the data, have a normal distribution with mean $m^* = 53.3$ and standard deviation $\sigma^* = 1.9$. The distribution is now much narrower (i.e., has a much smaller standard deviation), indicating that it is possible to be more sure about the true mean for the students. For example, the probability that μ is between 50 and 55 has increased from 0.34 before gathering the data, to 0.85 after gathering the data.

A curious and important fact is that the posterior distribution would have been approximately normal with a mean close to 53 and a standard deviation close to 2, even if the prior probabilities had not been well-represented by a normal distribution, or if the mean of the prior distribution had been somewhat different from 55. Thus the prior probabilities played a relatively small role, while the data played a large role, in determining the posterior probabilities. This is always the case when strong data are combined with comparatively vague prior opinions. If the sample had been much larger the posterior mean would have been almost exactly equal to the sample mean, and the posterior standard deviation would have been almost exactly equal to the standard error of the sample mean, as can be seen from the above equations. Thus, once again, with strong data the subjectivity of the probabilities in effect disappears, and reasonable researchers will reach near agreement.

Now that the posterior distribution has been calculated, it can be used for a variety of purposes. It is possible to calculate point estimates and confidence intervals, and test hypotheses about μ. The best point estimate, for general purposes, is the mean of the posterior distribution, 53.3. For a 95 percent confidence interval it is possible to cut off the upper and lower 2.5 percent of the posterior distribution (i.e., at $z = \pm 1.96$) in this example, and a 95 percent level of confidence is held that μ is between 49.6 and 56.9.

When hypotheses are tested, Bayesian statistics give a choice. Usually when a null hypothesis is tested, interest does not really lie in the null hypothesis itself. For example, if $H_0: \mu = 50$ is tested, the interest is really in whether μ is larger than or smaller than 50; the sample mean indicates whether it is larger or smaller, and the significance level indicates the degree of confidence that can be had in that conclusion. In Bayesian statistics it is possible to assign a probability directly to the hypothesis that $\mu < 50$;
it is simply the probability that a normally distributed random variable, with a mean of 53.3 and a standard deviation of 1.9, will be less than 50. For the above example, the probability is about 0.04. Note that it is almost, but not quite, possible to reject $H_0: \mu = 50$ by a traditional significance test, at the 0.05 level, one-tailed. With a much larger sample the posterior probability that μ was less than 50 would have been almost exactly equal to the traditional one-tailed p-value. Many Bayesians have argued that the practical value of traditional statistics lies in this fortunate coincidence between traditional and Bayesian results.

Occasionally the interest actually lies in the null hypothesis itself. Perhaps the 12-year olds really are like typical 12-year olds (i.e., have a mean of 50). In that case the odds form of Bayes's theorem is most convenient. However, it is necessary to know the probability of the data given that the null hypothesis is false as well as given that it is true. Here traditional statistics fail because, in essence, the beta level must be known, and that is usually unknown and unknowable.

The Bayesian approach is described in detail in Edwards et al. (1963). For the above example, the likelihood ratio is about 1.14 against the null hypothesis, meaning that the posterior odds against the null hypothesis are equal to the prior odds multiplied by 1.14. If it was previously considered that the odds against the null hypothesis were about 2:1, then the posterior odds are about 2.28:1. Notice that a traditional test would almost reject the null hypothesis at the 0.05 level (one-tailed), yet the data only slightly favor the alternative. The reason is simple. Although these data are not very probable under the null hypothesis, they are not very probable under the alternative either. Therefore they do not give strong evidence for either hypothesis.

The above are just two simple examples of Bayesian procedures. They can be extended to other distributions, such as the binomial and Poisson, with almost equally simple results. They can also be extended to the normal distribution where both the mean and variance are unknown, and to more complicated problems such as analyses of variance and covariance, multiple regression, and so on.

4. Problems

At first the philosophy behind Bayesian statistics met with great resistance from statisticians. Today that resistance is disappearing. However, there are four major difficulties preventing the widespread use of Bayesian statistics today.

The first difficulty is computational—the calculations are more complicated in Bayesian than in traditional statistics. An obvious solution is to develop computer programs. However, none of the commonly used general statistics packages, such as SAS or SPSS, incorporate Bayesian procedures. Perhaps there is a "vicious circle" here. The procedures are not in common use so they are not incorporated into commercial programs. However, if they are not available in commercial programs they are not likely to be in common use.

The second difficulty involves the problem of ascertaining prior opinions in probabilistic terms. With strong data this problem may not exist—the data may overpower any reasonable estimate of the user's prior probabilities. However, for such data traditional statistical methods usually give adequate results.

For more complicated problems, such as analyses of variance, the problem is more difficult. Prior probabilities for several parameters that are interrelated must then be assessed. Suppose, to take a simple example, the scores of 10-, 12-, and 14-year old children are be-

ing assessed on an abilities test. It may not be possible to have a very clear notion of whether the 14-year olds have a high or low mean score, yet it may be possible to be quite sure that the 14-year olds will score higher than the 12-year olds. In such a case it is not sufficient to evaluate prior opinions for each group separately; a joint distribution must be obtained for the means of all three groups. If the standard deviations are also known it complicates the problem still further.

Two solutions have been proposed for this problem. The first is an attempt to remove the subjectivity while retaining the Bayesian mathematics. A set of plausible priors for the parameters is proposed for universal use, relieving the individual researcher of the difficulties of assessing his or her own priors. Sometimes, plausible priors can be generated from previously occurring data; the resulting procedures are called "empirical Bayes procedures." However, some feel that such procedures violate the spirit, at least, of the Bayesian approach, and take away many of its advantages (see *Hierarchical Linear Models*).

The second reduces the more complicated problem to a series of simpler problems. Instead of doing an overall analysis of variance, a number of orthogonal contrasts might be tested, choosing contrasts so that an individual's opinion of the value of each contrast is approximately independent of the individual's opinions of the values of other contrasts. This works well in theory, but the practical problems of choosing contrasts can be difficult.

The third and fourth roadblocks preventing the use of Bayesian statistics are more psychological. The third is that users are reluctant to give up the comfort they receive from having the statistical analyses determine their opinions for them. If the data show without ambiguity whether to accept or reject a null hypothesis, the investigator is relieved of the responsibility of making that difficult decision. The comfort is, of course, illusory—responsibility is accepted when a significance level is chosen. However, many users are unwilling to give up the illusion. It is perhaps significant that Bayesian statistics have been used most widely in business applications, where such illusions cost money.

The fourth is simple inertia. Traditional statistical methods are commonly used. Therefore they must be taught so students can understand the existing literature. People then use the statistics that they have been taught, perpetuating the old traditions.

5. Other Applications

Two other applications of Bayesian ideas should be discussed. The first involves empirical Bayes solutions. This is a somewhat technical application of Bayesian principles to problems of inference. Sometimes, especially when testing mathematical models, the parameters are not simple to estimate. Then ad hoc methods may have to be devised. However, it may be hard to tell whether these methods give even reasonable estimates. If it can be shown that the estimates would have arisen using a Bayesian procedure with a reasonable prior, then the estimates themselves must be reasonable.

The second is a kind of "philosophical Bayesianism." It was seen above that with large amounts of data, the results of certain Bayesian tests are nearly the same as those of traditional tests. The traditional tests can therefore be done and interpreted in a Bayesian manner, that is, in terms of posterior probabilities. With smaller amounts of data, results can still be interpreted in the light of Bayesian concepts. For example, even moderately strong data can be discounted if it supports an implausible hypothesis. However, without explicit Bayesian methods, the interpretations are not always clear, and without explicit Bayesian calculations there is no certainty that they are appropriate.

See also: Significance Testing; Hypothesis Testing

References

de Finetti B 1937 La Prévision: Ses lois logiques, ses sources subjectives. *Annales de l'Institut Henri Poincaré* 7:1–68
1964 Foresight: Its logical laws, its subjective sources. In: Kyburg H E, Smokler H E (eds.) 1964
Edwards W, Lindman H, Savage L J 1963 Bayesian statis-
tical inference for psychological research. *Psychol. Rev.* 70(3): 193–242
Ramsey F P 1931 *The Foundations of Mathematics and Other Logical Essays*. Kegan Paul, London
Savage L J 1954 *The Foundations of Statistics*. Wiley, New York

Further Reading

Kyburg H E, Smokler H E (eds.) 1964 *Studies in Subjective Probability*. Wiley, New York
Lindley D V 1965a *Introduction to Probability and Statistics from a Bayesian Viewpoint. Part 1: Probability*. Cambridge University Press, Cambridge
Lindley D V 1965b *Introduction to Probability and Statistics from a Bayesian Viewpoint. Part 2: Inference*. Cambridge University Press, Cambridge
Novick M R, Jackson P H 1974 *Statistical Methods for Educational and Psychological Research*. McGraw-Hill, New York
Phillips L D 1974 *Bayesian Statistics for Social Scientists*. Crowell, New York
Savage L J 1981 *The Writings of Leonard Jimmie Savage: A Memorial Selection*. American Statistical Association/Institute of Mathematical Statistics, Washington, DC
Schmitt S A 1969 *Measuring Uncertainty: An Elementary Introduction to Bayesian Statistics*. Addison-Wesley, Reading, Massachusetts
Winkler R L 1972 *An Introduction to Bayesian Inference and Decision*. Holt, Rinehart and Winston, New York

Canonical Analysis

J. P. Keeves and J. D. Thomson

During the 1970s and 1980s there was increasing acceptance and use of multivariate analytic procedures that examined the interrelations between the latent variables formed from defined sets of observed variates. Canonical variate analysis was first developed as early as 1935 by Hotelling (1935) and was largely unused because of the complexity of the computations that had to be carried out by hand. With the introduction of the electronic computer, programs which permit its use have become more readily available. However, the power of this analytical procedure is not generally acknowledged. Canonical variate analysis is in fact the general analytic method of which most other parametric statistical procedures, varying from t-tests and analysis of variance through to principal components analysis, factor analysis, and regression analysis and discriminant analysis are but special cases. Both historically and conceptually the basic analytical procedure employed in multivariate analysis is that of ca-

nonical variate analysis. Thus a sound understanding of the ideas and principles involved in canonical variate analysis provides an excellent foundation for the development of an understanding of other analytical procedures, such as partial least squares path analysis (PLS), linear structural relations (LISREL) analysis, and multivariate analysis of covariance (MANCOVA). This entry is concerned with the analytical procedure of canonical variate analysis. In this treatment, following Bartlett (1941), the term "variate" is used to refer to those observed measures that are introduced into the analysis, while the term "variable" is reserved for the latent constructs that are formed as a combination of the observed measures or variates.

1. Introduction

Canonical analysis or canonical variate analysis (CVA) is one of the statistical methods used for studying relations between two sets (X and Y) of variates. Each set may contain one or more than one variate. In this situation, Darlington et al. (1973) envisage three different types of questions that can be asked concerning the correlation matrix of the $(n_x + n_y)$ variates.

(a) Questions about the number and nature of mutually independent relations between the two sets of variates.

(b) Questions about the degree of overlap or redundancy between the two sets. This implies questions about the extent to which one set may be predicted from the other, and vice versa.

(c) Questions about the similarity between the two within-set correlation or covariance matrices.

The use of CVA is often appropriate in answering questions of type (a), sometimes appropriate for those of type (b), and never appropriate for those of type (c).

In order for the purpose of CVA to be more clearly understood, Darlington et al. (1973 p. 439) set out in a table the relationship of CVA to the techniques of analysis of variance, multiple regression analysis, and multivariate analysis of variance. They also point out that by the appropriate use of dummy variables, CVA can perform multiple discriminant analyses and simple contingency table analyses. Canonical variate analysis is thus a technique to be used when either set X or set Y contains one or more variates, and the variates in either set may be continuous, categorical, or mixed.

In canonical variate analysis, the first canonical correlation is the highest correlation that can be found between a weighted composite of the X variates and a weighted composite of the Y variates (the composites being the first pair of canonical variables). The second canonical correlation is the highest correlation that can be found between the X and Y weighted composites which are uncorrelated (orthogonal) with the first pair of canonical variables. The significance of the first, the second, and each subsequent canonical correlation (there being in all n_{min} correlations where n_{min} *is the minimum of* n_x *and* n_y) is tested by Bartlett's chi-square approximation to the distribution of Wilks's lambda or by an F-ratio.

The canonical correlation coefficient (Rc_i) between each pair of variables describes the strength of the relationship between the two variables. The square of this relationship Rc_i^2 describes the proportion of the variance of one variable predictable from the other variable both within the same pair of canonical variables.

2. Relationship of CVA with Regression Analysis and Principal Components Analysis

The description of the first and subsequent canonical

correlations given above can be compared with two other types of analysis.

First, multiple regression analysis where the Y set contains only one variate and a weighted composite of X variates is obtained to maximize the correlation (R_y) between the Y variable (often called the criterion) and the X composite (called the predictor variable). In this situation R_y^2 can be thought of as the proportion of the variance of the criterion that can be "predicted" (or "accounted for," or "explained") from a knowledge of the set of X variates, in particular, the predictor variable.

Second, within each set, the formation of the first, second, and subsequent variables has a univariate analogue in factor analysis, where each factor is a weighted composite of, say, the X variates. In principal components analysis the first composite is formed to maximize the variance extracted. The effect of this first factor is then removed from the original correlation matrix and a second composite formed which is orthogonal to the first composite. The factor loadings of each composite (or variable, or factor), when squared and summed enable the proportion of variance extracted by the factor to be determined. The relationships between regression analysis and CVA, and between factor analysis and CVA, are discussed by Van de Geer who gives two overviews of multivariate models. The first, a pictorial overview, and the second, an overview in terms of operations of matrices, emphasize "that multivariate techniques do not fall into separate categories as special techniques for special situation, but instead form a close family" (Van de Geer 1971 p. 91).

3. A Pictorial Representation of Canonical Variate Analysis

In examining and presenting the results of canonical variate analysis (see Van de Geer 1971) it is generally appropriate to provide a pictorial representation of the results. It is common to indicate observed variates by boxes and latent variables by circles, and to identify

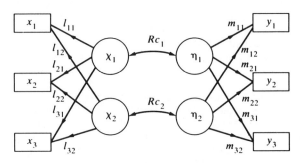

Figure 1
Canonical variate analysis seen as double factor analysis with two orthogonal latent variables.

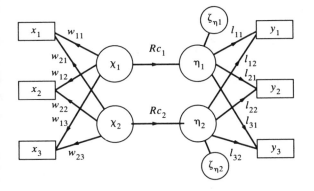

Figure 2
Canonical variate analysis seen as a regression model with two pairs of orthogonal latent variables

the former by normal alphabetical symbols and the latter by Greek alphabetical symbols. If a variable χ is merely considered to be correlated with variable η, the bidirectional nature of the association is indicated by a curved line with arrow heads at both ends. The analytical procedure of canonical variate analysis does not itself distinguish between the different conceptualizations that may be applied to interpret the results of the analysis. These conceptualizations are models derived from theory that have been postulated. The nature of a model is predicated upon theory. If no causal relationship is assumed between the X and Y sets of variates then canonical correlation may be viewed as a double factor analysis. This model is shown pictorially in Fig. 1.

If, however, the variates in set X are viewed as determining the variates in set Y the model is conceptually different and the relationships between the variates and the variables are shown in a different way. This model is shown pictorially in Fig. 2.

For simplicity in pictorial representation the latent

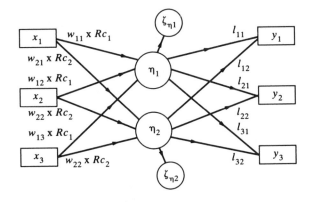

Figure 3
Canonical variable analysis seen as a reduced regression model with two orthogonal latent variables

variables χ and η in Fig. 2 corresponding to the X set of variates and the Y set of variates respectively, can be combined and the model reduces to the simplified or equivalent form shown in Fig. 3.

4. Structure Coefficients and Transformation Weights

Two types of coefficients are available to assist in the interpretation of canonical variate analysis, namely "transformation weights" and "structure coefficients." Sometimes the terms "function coefficient" or "canonical weights" are used instead of "transformation weights," and sometimes the term "standardized canonical loadings" is used instead of "structure coefficients." The interpretation of the factors formed in a canonical variate analysis has traditionally been based on the standardized transformation weights which are analogous to the beta weights in multiple regression analysis and which are assigned to the original variates in forming each latent variable as a linear combination of the variates. Alternatively, the structure coefficients which are the correlations between each of the derived canonical variables and the original variates may be used. From the view of multiple factor analysis these structure coefficients or loadings enable the pairs of canonical variables to be identified and related to the relevant variates in their respective batteries. Moreover, the sum of the squared structure coefficients enables the proportion of variance (V_i) of each set that is extracted by each factor to be determined.

Tatsuoka has commented on the use of structure coefficients:

> That this is a more reasonable approach in attempting to *interpret* the canonical factors (as against assessing the relative contribution of each original variable to the factors) becomes obvious when we recall that the standardized weights (canonical or discriminant) are partial coefficients with the effects of other variables removed or controlled. This is fine when the purpose is to gauge the contribution of each variable in the company of others, but is inappropriate when we wish to give substantive interpretations. (Tatsuoka 1973 p. 280)

Nevertheless, different meanings can be extracted from each set of coefficients with respect to the nature of the model in terms of which the canonical variate analysis is interpreted.

In the path model shown in Fig. 2 it is assumed that the X variates completely determine the latent variables χ_1 and χ_2 and that these latent variables determine, in part, the latent variables η_1 and η_2 with residual error term $\xi_{\eta 1}$ and $\xi_{\eta 2}$. The paths from the X variates to the χ variables are given by the transformation weights (w), while the paths from the η variables to the Y variates are given by the structure coefficients l. The influences of the χ latent variables on the η latent variables are given by the canonical correlations Rc_1 and Rc_2 as shown in Fig. 2.

In Fig. 3 where the χ latent variables are omitted, arrows are drawn directly from the X variates to the two η, latent variables, and the values of the path coefficients are given by the products of the corresponding transformation weights and canonical correlations. The residual error terms also act on the η latent variables as shown in Fig. 3.

In Fig. 1 where the model employed uses canonical variate analysis to examine two sets of variables as a double factor analysis, then the paths from the latent variables to the observed variates are given by the appropriate structure coefficients (l). Thus both the structure coefficients and the transformation weights have different uses in the interpretation of the data depending upon the nature of the model that is postulated from theory.

It should be noted that not all readily available computer programs provide both the structure coefficients and the transformation weights and since the models employed may require for full understanding both sets of coefficients, care must be taken in selecting which computer program is employed for the canonical variate analysis with a particular set of data to test a specific model derived from a relevant theoretical perspective.

5. Variance Considerations

Some computer programs commonly used for canonical analysis, for example, (Cooley and Lohnes 1971) also include in their printout, measures of redundancy. These measures combine the proportion of variance of one canonical variable predictable from the other canonical variable Rc_i^2 and the proportion of variance (V_i) of each test battery is predictable from a knowledge of scores on the variates in the other battery. This is determined for each canonical variable and is called the factor redundancy: $Rc_i^2 \times V_i$. The factor redundancies are totaled to give the total factor redundancy for each battery given the other battery. Thus it is the redundancy (and not Rc_i^2) that describes how much variance is predictable from one battery to another, whereas for the univariable criterion model of regression analysis, the value of R_y^2 describes this proportion of predictable variance. These measures of redundancy tell much more than do the canonical correlation coefficients about the outcome of the canonical analysis. However, Pugh and Hu (1991) endorse avoiding the interpretation of redundancy coefficients because of their lack of multivariate properties.

6. Partitioning of Redundancy

Mayeske et al. (1969) in their re-examination of the data available from the Equality of Educational Opportunity Survey in A *Study of Our Nation's Schools* partitioned the estimates of variance accounted for into unique and joint effects following a procedure

which has been discussed more fully by Wisler (1969) and Mood (1971). This technique had been advanced earlier by Newton and Spurrell (1967) and was employed by Peaker (1971) in the report of the Plowden Follow-up Study. Mood (1971) noted a shortcoming of the measure—under certain circumstances the joint contributions to variance explained could be negative. These effects are similar in kind to suppressor relationships. In spite of this shortcoming in the interpretation of the results of partitioning variance, the technique is a useful one for drawing attention to the confounding that occurs between both individual predictor variates and between domains of predictor variates which account for the variation in the criterion variates.

Subsequently, Cooley and Lohnes (1976) developed procedures for the partitioning of variance in canonical analysis. The unique contribution of a domain of predictors to the multivariate prediction of a set of criterion measures is that part of the variance of the criteria explained by the full model which cannot be obtained without using the particular domain of predictor variables. It is that part of the total redundancy which the particular domain of predictors will account for when these predictors are added to the other predictors included in the canonical analysis. The joint contribution for each predictor domain is the redundancy explained by the full model less the sum of the unique contributions. Thus the total redundancy is partitioned into unique and joint contributions, and the commonality or confounded contribution is separated from the contributions which are not so confounded.

The procedures for partitioning variance and redundancy are simply those of separating quantities associated with overlapping sets. Where there are more than two domains of predictors the possibility exists of partitioning the redundancy into pieces associated with various subsets of the predictors, but where more than four domains exist, the number of possible partitions becomes large and not very meaningful.

Cooley and Lohnes (1976) have propounded the rules for the partitioning of redundancy where $V(j, k, l)$ is the redundancy for a canonical regression model with the predictor sets of J, K, and L. These rules are derived with the use of the Venn diagram shown in Fig. 4.

Two Predictor Sets

Uniqueness for Set 1	$=U(1)$	$=-V(2) + V(1,2)$
Uniqueness for Set 2	$=U(2)$	$=-V(1) + V(1,2)$
Commonality for Set 1 and Set 2	$=C(1,2)$	$=V(1) + V(2) - V(1,2)$

Three Predictor Sets

Uniqueness for Set 1	$=U(1)$	$=-V(2,3) + V(1,2,3)$
Uniqueness for Set 2	$=U(2)$	$=-V(1,3) + V(1,2,3)$
Uniqueness for Set 3	$=U(3)$	$=-V(1,2) + V(1,2,3)$
Commonality C(1,2)	$=-V(3) + V(1,3) + V(2,3) - V(1,2,3)$	
Commonality C(1,3)	$=-V(2) + V(1,2) + V(2,3) - V(1,2,3)$	
Commonality C(2,3)	$=-V(1) + V(1,2) + V(1,3) - V(1,2,3)$	
Commonality C(1,2,3)	$=V(1) + V(2) + V(3) - V(1,2) - V(1,3) - V(2,3) + V(1,2,3)$	

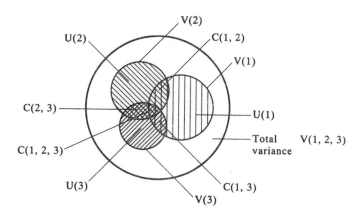

Figure 4
Venn Diagram for three predictor sets

Examples of canonical analysis showing both pictorial representation and the partitioning of redundancy are given by Keeves (1975, 1986). In the latter case the results of the analysis of data using this analytical procedure may be compared with those obtained through the use of alternative procedures.

7. Significance Testing

While significance tests are available for the extraction of latent roots from the complete body of data in canonical variate analysis, which also provide a test for the level of significance of the canonical correlations obtained, such tests assume a simple random sample of cases. However, simple random samples are the exception rather than the rule in the examination of educational data sets. As a consequence the significance tests employed are totally inappropriate. Furthermore, there are no commonly used procedures for testing the significance of transformation weights and structure coefficients or redundancy coefficients. The investigator is thus left to examine critically the magnitudes of these different coefficients and to make a decision regarding which coefficients it is appropriate to include in the interpretation of the data.

8. Some Developments

Pugh and Hu (1991) have reviewed the use and interpretation of canonical analysis. Of particular interest is their discussion of the number of subjects needed in relation to the number of variates included in an analysis. No simple rules seem adequate, and the use of the largest possible sample size to be recommended with a ratio of at least 20:1, for subjects to variates, is necessary for accurate interpretation. Furthermore, they strongly endorse the use of cross-validation to examine the invariance of the analysis.

In both the predictive and descriptive uses of canonical analysis, it is possible to employ stepwise procedures for the inclusion of variables in the analysis. However, where such procedures are used some form of cross-validation is desirable if not essential. In addition, by calculating the appropriate matrices of residual correlations it is possible to undertake a part (or partial) canonical analysis, but such procedures have not been widely used in substantive studies (Thorndike 1978).

In addition, Van de Geer (1971 pp. 169–70) considers the application of canonical analysis procedures in situations when the first and second pairs of canonical variables are considered correlated and not orthogonal. Furthermore, Horst (1965) and Van de Geer (1968) provide treatments of problem situations where there are three or more data matrices which are simultaneously matched by canonical variate analysis. However, the development of LISREL has tended to supplant the use of canonical variate analysis in the testing of these and more complex models.

See also: Regression Analyses of Quantified Data; Factorial Modeling

References

Bartlett M S 1941 The significance of canonical correlations. *Biometrika* 32: 29–38
Cooley W W, Lohnes P R 1971 *Multivariate Data Analysis*. Wiley, New York
Cooley W W, Lohnes P R 1976 *Evaluation Research in Education*. Irvington, New York
Darlington R B, Weinberg S L, Walberg H J 1973 Canonical variate analysis and related techniques. *Rev. Educ. Res.* 43: 433–54
Horst P 1965 *Factorial Analysis of Data Matrices*. Holt, Rinehart and Winston, New York
Hotelling H 1935 The most predictable criterion. *J. Exp. Psychol.* 26: 139–42

Keeves J P 1975 The home, the school and achievement in mathematics and science. *Sci. Educ.* 59(4): 207–18

Keeves J P 1986 Canonical variate analysis. *Int. J. Educ. Res.* 10(2): 164–73

Mayeske G W et al. 1969 *A Study of Our Nation's Schools.* United States Government Printing Office, Washington, DC

Mood A M 1971 Partitioning variance in multiple regression analyses as a tool for developing learning models. *Am. Educ. Res. J.* 8: 191–202

Newton R G, Spurrell D J 1967 A development of multiple regression for the analysis of routine data. *Appl. Stat.* 16: 51–64

Peaker G F 1971 *The Plowden Children Four Years Later.* National Foundation for Educational Research, Slough

Pugh R C and Hu Y 1991 Use and interpretation of canonical correlation analysis. *J. Educ. Res.* Articles: 1978–1989; *J. Educ. Res.* 84(3): 147–52

Tatsuoka M M 1973 Multivariate analysis in educational research. In: Kerlinger F N (ed.) 1973 *Review of Research in Education 1.* Peacock, Itasca, Illinois

Thorndike R M 1978 *Correlation Procedures for Research.* Gardner, New York

Van de Geer J P 1968 *Matching k Sets of Configurations.* University of London, Department of Data Theory, London (Report RN-005-68)

Van de Geer J P 1971 *Introduction to Multivariate Analysis for the Social Sciences.* Freeman, San Francisco, California

Wisler C F 1969 Partitioning the explained variation in a regression analysis. In: Mayeske G W et al. 1969

Further Reading

Pedhazur E J 1982 *Multiple Regression in Behavioral Research.* Holt, Rinehart and Winston, New York

Thompson B 1984 *Canonical Correlation Analysis: Uses and Interpretation.* Sage University Paper Series on Quantitative Applications in the Social Sciences, 07-001. Sage, Beverly Hills, California

Cluster Analysis

B. S. Everitt

One of the most basic abilities of living creatures involves the grouping of similar objects, individuals, and so on, to produce a classification. Prehistoric people, for example, must have been able to recognize that many individual objects shared certain properties such as being edible, or poisonous, or ferocious, and so on. The idea of sorting similar things into categories is clearly a primitive one since classification, in the widest sense, is necessary for the development of language, which consists of words which help in the recognition and discussion of the different types of events, objects, and people encountered. Each noun in a language, for example, is a label used to describe a class of things which have striking features in common. So animals are named as cats, dogs, horses, and so on, and such a name collects individuals into groups. Naming is classifying.

As well as being a basic human conceptual activity, classification is also fundamental in most branches of science, since it involves two basic scientific functions: (a) the description of objects of interest or those under investigation, and (b) the establishment of general laws or theories by means of which particular events may be explained or predicted. Some areas where classification has played an important role are biology, where attempts at the classification of living organisms date from the time of Aristotle, and were a necessary prerequisite to the development of the evolutionary theories of Darwin; chemistry, where the classification of the elements in Mendeleyev's periodic table had a profound influence on uncovering the structure of the atom; and medicine, where a satisfactory classification of diseases is needed prior to investigating etiology and developing treatments. In education, researchers are often interested in producing classifications of both teachers and pupils.

1. Numerical Classification Techniques

Numerical methods for classification have been developed largely since the 1960s, this development clearly paralleling that of the electronic computer, a machine necessary to undertake the prodigious amounts of arithmetic generally associated with such techniques. Most of these methods operate either directly on a matrix of scores on a number of variables for each of the objects or individuals to be classified, or on a matrix of distance or similarities usually derived from the raw data matrix.

Many clustering methods are now available and can be used routinely via their implementation in standard software packages such as BMDP, SAS, or SPSS, or in other more specialized packages such as CLUSTAN, GENSTAT, and S-PLUS. The most commonly used methods can be grouped broadly into three classes, "agglomerative hierarchical," "K-means iterative reallocation," and "mixtures." It is important to remember however, that in some situations, simple graphical approaches may often be sufficient to identify groups or clusters. Suppose, for example, a number of individuals have had their height and weight record-

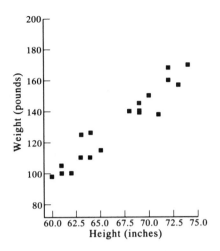

Figure 1
Scattergram of height versus weight

ed. A scattergram of such a data set is shown in Fig. 1. Two distinct "clusters" of points are clearly visible. In one sense the aim of most clustering techniques is to imitate and automate the process that the human observer does so well when the data involve only two variables, and extend it to the more common situation where more than two variable values are recorded on each of the objects or individuals under investigation. A description of several other graphical methods which might be helpful in a clustering context is given in Everitt (1993).

A point which should be noted before proceeding is that clustering is concerned with classifying

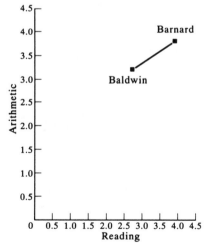

Euclidean distance = $[(2.7 - 3.9)^2 + (3.2 - 3.8)^2]^{0.5} = 1.33$

Figure 2
Euclidean distance in two dimensions

Table 1
Achievement test scores for twenty-five schools[a]

SCHOOL	Fourth Grade Reading	Fourth Grade Arithmetic	Sixth Grade Reading	Sixth Grade Arithmetic
Baldwin	2.7	3.2	4.5	4.8
Barnard	3.9	3.8	5.9	6.2
Beecher	4.8	4.1	6.8	5.5
Brennan	3.1	3.5	4.3	4.6
Clinton	3.4	3.7	5.1	5.6
Conte	3.1	3.4	4.1	4.7
Davis	4.6	4.4	6.6	6.1
Day	3.1	3.3	4.0	4.9
Dwight	3.8	3.7	4.7	4.9
Edgewood	5.2	4.9	8.2	6.9
Edwards	3.9	3.8	5.2	5.4
Hale	4.1	4.0	5.6	5.6
Hooker	5.7	5.1	7.0	6.3
Ivy	3.0	3.2	4.5	5.0
Kimberley	2.9	3.3	4.5	5.1
Lincoln	3.4	3.3	4.4	5.0
Lovell	4.0	4.2	5.2	5.4
Prince	3.0	3.0	4.6	5.0
Ross	4.0	4.1	5.9	5.8
Scranton	3.0	3.2	4.4	5.1
Sherman	3.6	3.6	5.3	5.4
Truman	3.1	3.2	4.6	5.0
West Hills	3.2	3.3	5.4	5.3
Winchester	3.0	3.4	4.2	4.7
Woodward	3.8	4.0	6.9	6.7

a Data used with permission from Hartigan (1975)

previously unclassified material. At the start of the investigation, the number and composition of the classes is unknown. It is this that differentiates the techniques of cluster analysis from those of discrimination where groups are known *a priori*. Such methods are described in Everitt and Dunn (1992).

2. Distance and Similarity Measures

The raw data for clustering is usually a set of scores for a number of individuals or objects. An example is given in Table 1. These data consist of achievement test scores on reading and arithmetic for children in the fourth and sixth grades of 25 schools. Here the interest in clustering the schools might be to identify different levels of performance, and to assess similarities and differences in the patterns of change from fourth to sixth grade.

Many, though not all, methods of cluster analysis operate not directly on the profile of variable values of each object or individual, but on a matrix of interindividual distance or similarity values derived from these. The most commonly used distance measure, for example, is Euclidean. This measure is illustrated in Fig. 2 for the fourth grade scores of the

Table 2
Euclidean distances for first five schools in Table 1[a]

	1	2	3	4	5
1	0.00				
2	2.39	0.00			
D = 3	3.32	1.48	0.00		
4	0.57	2.42	3.21	0.00	
5	1.32	1.12	2.24	1.33	0.00

a Only the lower triangular part of this matrix is given since it is 'symmetric'

first two schools in Table 1.

When more than two variable values are involved the Euclidean distance between two individuals, *i* and *j* is given by

$$d_{ij} = \sqrt{\sum_{k=1}^{p} (x_{ik} - x_{jk})^2} \qquad (1)$$

where p is the number of variables and x_{ik} and x_{ij}, $k = 1, 2 \ldots, p$ are the variable values for the two individuals concerned.

The Euclidean distance matrix for the first five schools in Table 1 is shown in Table 2. Problems with use of the Euclidean distance measure, particularly the scaling of the variables, are discussed in Everitt (1993).

Also familiar in a clustering context are measures of similarity, particularly those for dichotomous, binary variables. To illustrate, consider Table 3 which shows four such variables recorded for five 15-year olds who had been subjected to sexual abuse as young children. Interest in clustering such data might center on determining groups of abused children with different outcome patterns.

An intuitively sensible index of the similarity between two children would be the number of variables on which they were given the same score. In general, however, similarities are scaled to be between zero

Table 3
Binary variables observed on abused children

Child	Variable			
	1	2	3	4
1	0	1	0	1
2	0	1	1	1
3	1	0	1	1
4	0	0	0	0
5	1	1	1	0

Variable 1: Academic performance: below average (0), above average (1)
Variable 2: Child still living with perpetrator: no (0), yes (1)
Variable 3: Age at time of abuse: ≤ 4(0), > 4(1)
Variable 4: Social class: I or II (0), III or IV (1)

and one, so an appropriate index would be simply number of matches divided by number of variables. This index will take the value zero for two children who do not match on a single variable and one for two children who have an identical set of scores. For the data in Table 3, this matching coefficient for each pair of children is shown in Table 4. Many other such coefficients are discussed in Everitt (1993).

3. Agglomerative Hierarchical Clustering Methods

Members of this class of clustering technique are perhaps the most widely used in practice. All operate in essentially the same way, building up clusters by combining one or more individuals at a time, beginning at the stage of separate individuals and ending at the stage where all individuals are combined into a single group. The whole series of steps is conveniently described by means of a diagram known as a "dendrogram," examples of which are given below. Each intermediate stage in the procedure corresponds to a partition of the individuals into a particular number of groups or clusters; choosing the most appropriate or "best" number of groups for a set of data is usually a difficult problem (see Everitt 1979).

A variety of agglomerative hierarchical techniques exist because of the different ways of defining distance (or similarity) between a single individual and a group, or between two groups. This intergroup distance could, for example, be taken as the distance between the closest pair of individuals, one from each group (see Fig. 3) leading to "single linkage" clustering. An alternative is to use the opposite of this, that is, to take the intergroup distance as that between the most remote pair of individuals (see Fig. 4), giving "complete linkage" clustering. Each of these uses only a single interindividual distance measure to define the intergroup measure. A method using all the distances between members of the two groups is "group average," illustrated in Fig. 5.

To describe the operation of an agglomerative hierarchical clustering method, single linkage will be applied to the first five schools in Table 1 using the Euclidean distance matrix shown in Table 2. Initially there are five clusters each containing a single school.

Table 4
Matching coefficient for data in Table 3

	1	2	3	4	5
1	1.00				
2	0.75	1.00			
S = 3	0.25	0.50	1.00		
4	0.50	0.25	0.25	1.00	
5	0.25	0.50	0.50	0.25	1.00

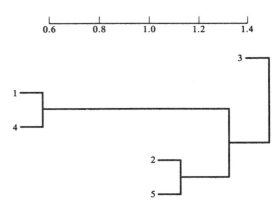

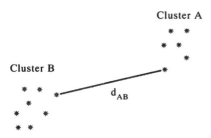

Figure 3
Single linkage distance

The first step is to combine the closest pair of schools. From Table 2 this is seen to be schools 1 and 4. The distance between each of schools 2, 3, and 5 and the two school cluster [1, 4] must now be calculated. The single linkage distance between school 2 and the pair [1, 4] is found as follows:

$$d_{2,[4]} = \min [d_{1,2}, d_{2,4}] = d_{12} = 2.39 \qquad (2)$$

After these new distances are calculated, the smallest value is again used to decide which fusion should take place. Here this involves schools 2 and 5. At this stage there are three clusters, containing schools [1, 4], [3], [2, 5]. The next stage involves the combination of individual 3 with the [2, 5] cluster and the final stage the fusion of clusters [1, 4] and [2, 3,

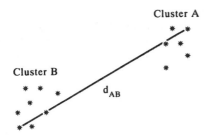

Figure 4
Complete linkage distance

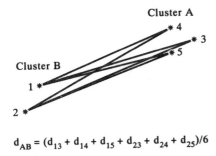

$$d_{AB} = (d_{13} + d_{14} + d_{15} + d_{23} + d_{24} + d_{25})/6$$

Figure 5
Group average distance

Figure 6
Single linkage dendogram for distances in Table 2

5]. The corresponding dendrogram is shown in Fig. 6. Figs: 7 and 8 show the corresponding dendrograms for complete linkage and group average clustering.

The dendrogram from applying complete linkage to all 25 schools is shown in Fig. 9. Details of the three-group solution given by this method are shown in Table 5.

4. K-means Iterative Reallocation Methods

Methods in this class operate by attempting to produce a partition of the individuals or objects into a given number of clusters so as to optimize some index measuring the internal homogeneity of the clusters. One such index, for example, might be the average within cluster distance between individuals. Given the number of groups it appears to be a relatively straightforward task to identify the partition which minimizes this index: simply consider every partition into the requisite number of groups, calculate the index for each, and select the appropriate one. Unfortunately the number of partitions is very large; with 19 individuals and 8 groups, for example, there are 1,709,751, 003,480 distinct partitions. Complete enumeration is

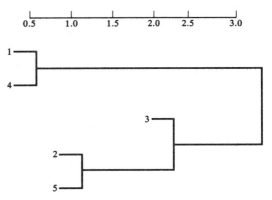

Figure 7
Complete linkage dendrogram for distances in Table 2

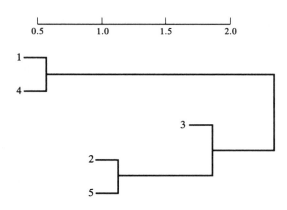

Figure 8
Group average dendogram for distances in Table 2.

clearly out of the question even with the very fastest computers now available. Some restriction is obviously required to reduce drastically the possible partitions that need to be considered. The strategy generally adopted is to begin with some initial, relatively arbitrary partition into the required number of groups, and then consider individuals for re-allocation from their own to some other group, such re-allocation being made if it improves the particular criterion value being used. The process continues until no re-allocation causes further improvement. Such "hill-climbing" algorithms are described in more detail in Everitt (1993).

As with hierarchical techniques, a difficult problem is that of deciding on the number of groups appropriate for the data. Some ad hoc procedures are described in Dubes and Jain (1979), and a detailed investigation of the number of groups problem is undertaken by Milligan and Cooper (1985).

Table 5
Three-group solution given by complete linkage clustering on data in Table 1

Group	Means			
	G4A	G4R	G6A	G6R
1	3.25	3.43	4.65	5.05
2	4.20	4.07	6.28	5.98
3	5.45	5.00	7.60	6.60

Schools in each group:
Group 1: 1, 4, 5, 6, 8, 9, 11, 14, 15, 16, 17, 18, 20, 21, 22, 23, 24
Group 2: 2, 3, 7, 12, 19, 25
Group 3: 10, 13

Iterative relocation methods were used by Bennett (1976) and Galton et al. (1980) to delineate both teacher and pupil types.

5. Mixture Method

Most cluster analysis methods are essentially nonstatistical in the sense that they have no associated distribution theory or significance tests; consequently it is often difficult to know how much confidence to place in any clusters found, and generally impossible to relate from sample to population. For many investigators involved in an initial exploration of their data, this may present no real difficulties. Attempts have been made, however, to develop a more acceptable statistical approach to the clustering problem, using what are generally known as *finite mixture distributions* (see Everitt and Hand 1981). Consider, for example, a set of data consisting of the heights of a number of school children of a particular age. The frequency distribution

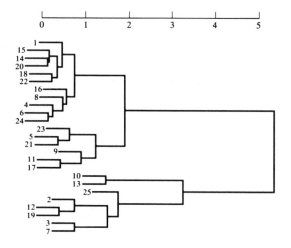

Figure 9
Complete linkage dendogram for Euclidean distances between all schools in Table 1

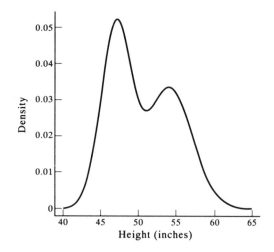

Figure 10
Density function for the heights of school children

of such a data set might look like Fig. 10, and might be described by the sum of two normal distributions with different means and possibly different variances. Here the component distributions are likely to correspond to those well-known clusters "boys" and "girls." The idea can be extended to more than a single variable using "multivariate normal distributions" and to more than simply the two-cluster situation.

An analogous mixture model for categorical (usually) binary variables is the basis of a technique generally known as "latent class analysis." Here a number of clusters or latent classes are assumed present in the data, within which the observed categorical variables are independent. The observed associations between the variables are generated by the presence of the classes. (Compare the factor analysis model for continuous data.) Details of the model are given in Everitt and Dunn (1992). The method has found wide use in education and a number of interesting applications are to be found in the papers by Macready and Dayton (1977, 1980) and Dayton and Macready (1980). A particularly important and influential study was that of Aitkin et al. (1981) into teaching styles and pupil progress using data originally collected and analyzed by Bennett (1976). One part of the investigation involved applying latent class analysis to 468 teachers each described in terms of 38 binary items relating to teaching style. Two and three class models

Table 6
Two-Class parameter estimates for teacher data[a]

	Class 1	Class 2
1. Students have choice in where to sit	22	43
2. Students sit in groups of three or more	60	87
3. Students allocated to seating by ability	35	23
4. Students stay in same seats for most of day	91	63
5. Students not allowed freedom of movement in classroom	97	54
6. Students not allowed to talk freely	89	48
7. Students expected to ask permission to leave room	97	76
8. Students expected to be quiet	82	42
9. Monitors appointed for special jobs	85	67
10. Students taken out of school regularly	32	60
11. Timetable used for organizing work	90	66
12. Use own materials rather than textbooks	19	49
13. Students expected to know tables by heart	92	76
14. Students asked to find own reference material	29	37
15. Students given homework regularly	35	22
16. Teacher talks to whole class	71	44
17. Students work in groups on teacher tasks	29	42
18. Students work in groups on work of their own choice	14	46
19. Students work individually on teacher tasks	55	37
20. Students work individually on work of their own choice	28	50
21. Explore concepts in number work	18	55
22. Encourage fluency in written English even if inaccurate	87	94
23. Students work marked or graded	43	14
24. Spelling and grammatical errors corrected	84	68
25. Stars given to students who produce best work	57	29
26. Arithmetic test given at least once a week	59	38
27. Spelling test given at least once a week	73	51
28. End of term tests given	66	44
29. Many students who create discipline problems	09	09
30. Verbal reproof sufficient	97	95
31. Discipline: extra work given	70	53
32. Smack	65	42
33. Withdrawal of privileges	86	77
34. Send to head teacher	24	17
35. Send out of room	19	15
36. Emphasis on separate subject teaching	85	50
37. Emphasis on aesthetic subject teaching	55	63
38. Emphasis on integrated subject teaching	22	65
Estimated proportion of teachers in each class	0.538	0.462

a Decimal point omitted from class probabilities

were considered. The results for two classes are shown in Table 6, each class being characterized by a set of 38 estimated response probabilities, that is, the probabilities of responding "yes" to each of the 38 binary items. An obvious interpretation of the two classes is that they represent essentially "formal" and "informal" teaching styles.

6. Evaluating and Interpreting Results

There are many problems associated with using clustering techniques in practice. Some have already been mentioned: choosing the number of clusters, the lack of any inferential framework, and the lack of a satisfactory definition of exactly what constitutes a cluster. Others concern the appropriate scaling of variables and how to use both quantitative and qualitative variables in the same analysis. Perhaps of overriding importance is the question of how to evaluate the results of clustering in terms of the stability, validity, and in particular, the usefulness of the clusters found. The latter issue is clearly demonstrated in the following quotation from Needham (1965) discussing the classification of human beings into men and women.

> The usefulness of this classification does not begin and end with all that can, in one sense be strictly inferred from it—namely a statement about sexual organs. It is a very useful classification because classing a person as man or woman conveys a great deal more information about probable relative size, strength, certain types of dexterity and so on. When a statement is made that persons in class *man* are more suited than persons in class *woman* for certain tasks and conversely, then only incidentally is it a remark about sex, the primary concern being with strength, endurance etc. The point is that it has been possible to use a classification of persons which conveys information on many properties. On the contrary a classification of persons into those with hair on their forearms between 3/16 inch and 1/4 inch long and those without, though it may have some particular use, is certainly of no general use, for imputing membership in the former class to a person conveys information on this property alone. Put another way there are no known properties which divide a set of people in a similar manner. (Needham 1965 p. 347)

Clearly a number of questions need to be asked and satisfactorily answered before any given solution can be offered as a reasonable and useful system of classification. Do the members of different groups differ substantially on variables other than those used in deriving them? Do essentially the same groups emerge when a new sample of similar individual is clustered? Are the clusters predictive of outcome, or reaction to treatment? Consideration of such questions may help to curb overenthusiastic researchers making inappropriate claims for the clusters they find.

In summary, the methods of cluster analysis are potentially very useful, but they require care in their application if misleading solutions are to be avoided. Researchers should remember the essential "exploratory" nature of the techniques.

See also: Multivariate Analysis; Scaling Methods

References

Aitkin M, Bennett S N, Hesketh J 1981 Teaching styles and pupil progress: A re-analysis. *Brit. J. Educ. Psychol.* 51(2): 170–86

Bennett N 1976 *Teaching Styles and Pupil Progress.* Open Books, London

Dayton C M, Macready G B 1980 A scaling model with response errors and intrinsically unscalable respondents. *Psychometri.* 45(3): 343–56

Dubes R, Jain A K 1979 Validity studies in clustering methodologies. *Pattern Recognition* 11(4): 235–54

Everitt B S 1979 Unresolved problems in cluster analysis. *Biometrics* 35(1): 169–81

Everitt B S 1992 Examining multivariate data graphically. *Journal of the Royal Statistical Society*, Series A

Everitt B S 1993 *Cluster Analysis*, 3rd edn. Edward Arnold, Sevenoaks

Everitt B S, Hand D J 1981 *Finite Mixture Distributions.* Chapman and Hall, London

Everitt B S, Dunn G 1992 *Applied Multivariate Data Analysis.* Edward Arnold, Sevenoaks

Galton M, Simon B, Croll P 1980 *Inside the Primary Classroom.* Routledge, London

Hartigan J A 1975 *Clustering Algorithms.* Wiley, New York

Macready G B, Dayton C M 1977 The use of probabilistic models in the assessment of mastery. *J. Educ. Stat.* 2(2): 99–120

Macready G B, Dayton C M 1980 The nature and use of state mastery models. *App. Psychol. Meas.* 4(4): 493–516

Milligan G, Cooper M 1985 An examination of procedures for determining the number of clusters in a data set. *Psychometri.* 50: 159–79

Needham R M 1965 Computer methods for classification and grouping. In: Hymes D (ed.) 1965 *The Use of Computers in Anthropology.* Mouton, The Hague

Configural Frequency Analysis

W. Kristof

This entry is intended to introduce the main principles of "classical" configural frequency analysis (CFA) as initially proposed by Lienert (1969) and subsequently presented by Krauth and Lienert (1973). Since then there have been many publications both on theoretical issues and applications. A more recent overview is contained in Lienert (1988).

The general objective of CFA is the analysis of multivariate frequency data typically summarized in the form of multidimensional contingency tables. The key idea is the search for *types* in such a body of data, possibly supplemented by an analysis of the *interaction structure*.

The typical situation is as follows. From some population a sample of n units has been drawn, the units being persons in most instances. There are a number of observable attributes, $A_1, \ldots, A_t$, say, and each attribute A_i is made up of r_i mutually exclusive and exhaustive categories, $C_{i1}, \ldots, C_{ir_i}$. Hence the attributes are assumed discrete. If $r_i = 2$ then A_i is a dichotomy. Any observed unit can be classified according to the categories to which it belongs. An ordered set of such categories is called a "configuration." Obviously, the total of possible configurations is the product $r = r_1 r_2 \ldots r_t$. The above notation will be adhered to throughout. For instance, let A_1 indicate "gender" with categories C_{11} = "male," C_{12} = "female." Similarly, A_2 may denote "age groups" with categories C_{21} = "under 30 years of age," C_{22} = "between 30 and 60," and C_{23} = "over 60." Finally, A_3 may designate "employment" with C_{31} = "self-employed," and C_{32} = "not self-employed." Then the configuration (C_{11}, C_{21}, C_{32}) refers to a male under 30 years of age who is not self-employed.

The frequencies with which each configuration occurs in a sample of observed units are obtained by counting. Configural frequency analysis now purports to identify such configurations that are realized more often than should be expected by chance alone. Such a configuration is called a "type." On the other hand, one may speak of an antitype if a particular configuration occurs with too low a frequency. In most cases, however, interest focuses only on types.

It is necessary to specify exactly the *base model* according to which chance is supposed to operate. The underlying assumption is total independence among all attributes. A different base model of intuitive appeal has been proposed by Victor (1989). This remark may suffice for present purposes. In each event, CFA is a residual analysis after the base model has been taken into account.

1. Statistical Definition of Types

According to the previously introduced notation C_{ij_i} with $i = 1, \ldots, t$ and $j_i = 1, \ldots, r_i$ designates the j-th category of attribute A_i. Let the corresponding marginal probability of observing C_{ij_i} in some population be π_{ij_i}, that is, the probability of C_{ij_i} occurring regardless of the categories of the other attributes to which a unit belongs. On the other hand, let the probability of observing the configuration ($C_{1j_1}, \ldots, C_{tj_t}$) be given by $\pi_{j_1 \ldots j_t}$. For ease of notation the first subscripts $1, \ldots, t$ have been suppressed as the sequence of the second subscripts serves to identify the configuration in question. It follows from the base model of total independence that

$$\pi_{j_1 \ldots j_t} = \pi_{1j_1} \times \ldots \times \pi_{tj_t} \tag{1}$$

If, however, the inequality

$$\pi_{j_1 \ldots j_t} > \pi_{1j_1} \times \ldots \times \pi_{tj_t} \tag{2}$$

holds then ($C_{1j_1}, \ldots, C_{tj_t}$) constitutes a type. It is an antitype if the reverse inequality holds.

The existence of at least one type implies the existence of at least one antitype. For, if a configuration is found that appears more often than chance alone would allow then there must be another configuration with too small a frequency and vice versa.

2. Search for Types

After collection of a body of data as previously described, the researcher will wish to search for such configurations that presumably constitute types. This can be achieved by several methods. It is necessary, however, to distinguish two stages of any such search. During the *exploratory stage* hypotheses about specific configurations being types should be generated. This may be done by inspection of the data. In each event, such hypotheses must be considered preliminary and, strictly speaking, should not be subjected to statistical tests on the basis of the same data that served to suggest them. It appears that this point is often neglected in practice. Statistical tools concerning hypotheses about types make up the *confirmatory stage* of the search process. To this end new data should be employed. They should be independent of the ones already used. Randomly splitting the initial total sample suggests itself. If hypotheses regarding types have been set up independently of the data then the researcher can immediately enter into the second stage. At any rate, when hypothesis testing is intended the following quantities apart from sample size n, that is, the number of observed units, are required.

(a) For each configuration $(C_{1j_1}, \ldots, C_{tj_t})$ the number of units exhibiting this pattern is determined. Let this frequency be $f_{j1} \ldots j_t$. The order of the subscripts is essential, of course. These frequencies may be regarded as the entries of a t-dimensional contingency table, the number of cells being the product $r = r_1 \times \ldots \times r_t$.

(b) For each category C_{ij_i} $i = 1, \ldots, t$, the number of units falling into this category is determined. Let this marginal frequency be $f \ldots j_i \ldots$ in the familiar dot notation.

(c) Under the assumption of fixed marginals and total independence of the attributes the probabilities of observing configurations $(C_{1j_i}, \ldots, C_{tj_t})$ are calculated from the data. From the multiplication theorem of probabilities the result

$$\pi_{1j_1} \ldots \pi_{tj_t} = f_{j1} \ldots \times f_{.j2} .. \times \ldots \times f \ldots j_t / n^t \quad (3)$$

is obtained.

(d) The expected frequency associated with configuration $(C_{1j_1}, \ldots, C_{tj_t})$ under the above assumptions becomes

$$e_{j1} \ldots j_t = n\pi_{1j_1} \ldots \pi_{tj_t} = f_{j1} \ldots \times f_{.j2.} \times \ldots \times f \ldots j_t / n^{t-1} \quad (4)$$

These are the quantities basic to all further calculations. The actual search for types can be performed by a number of methods applicable at both the exploratory and the confirmatory stages of an empirical study involving CFA.

2.1 Lienert's Original Test

According to Lienert's (1969) original proposal the following statistical criterion for a configuration $(C_{1j_1}, \ldots, C_{tj_t})$ to be a type needs to be satisfied apart from $f_{j1} \ldots j_t > e_{j1} \ldots e_{jt}$:

$$L^2 = (f_{j1} \ldots j_t - e_{j1} \ldots j_t)^2 / e_{j1} \ldots e_{jt} \quad (5)$$

when regarded as a chi-square value with $df = 1$ has an upper tail probability less than some prescribed significance level α. It is a prerequisite, however, that for the expected frequency $e_{j1} \ldots j_t \geqslant 5$ should hold. This is a conservative procedure of only heuristic value.

2.2 Kristof's Test

An immediate improvement over L^2 is obtained when in addition to a particular configuration $(C_{1j_1}, \ldots, C_{tj_t})$ the remaining configurations and the associated frequencies are considered. The total of the units can be divided into two classes according to whether a unit exhibits the configuration in question or not. The corresponding frequencies are $f_{j1} \ldots j_t$ and $n - f_{j1} \ldots j_t$, respectively. The expected frequencies under the same assumptions as before are $e_{j1} \ldots j_t$ and $n - e_{j1} \ldots j_t$. It

follows that

$$K^2 = (f_{j1} \ldots j_t - e_{j1} \ldots j_t)^2 \left(\frac{1}{e_{j1 \ jt}} + \frac{1}{n - e_{j1 \ jt}} \right) \quad (6)$$

is approximately chi-square distributed with $df = 1$. Evidently, $K^2 > L^2$. Hence (6) provides a test less conservative than (5). Through personal communication by the author test statistic (6) first appeared in Rittich (1988). With the abbreviations $f = f_{j1} \ldots j_t$ and $\pi = \pi_{1j_1} \ldots \pi_{tj_t}$ this relationship is equivalent to:

$$Z = (f - n\pi) / \sqrt{n\pi(1 - \pi)}, \quad (7)$$

Z being a standard normal. This formula supplemented by the familiar continuity correction was given by Krauth (Krauth and Lienert 1973 p. 44, Krauth 1985a, and elsewhere). As to be expected, $Z^2 = K^2$. Obviously, Z is to be used as a one-sided test statistic.

2.3 Krauth's Test

Test statistic (7) is an asymptotic result for n large. If this condition does not hold so that the approximation by a standard normal is doubtful then Krauth's binomial test is preferable, for example, see Krauth and Lienert (1973) and Krauth (1985a). For a configuration $(C_{1j_1}, \ldots, C_{tj_t})$ with theoretical probability $\pi = \pi_{1j_1} \ldots \pi_{tj_t}$ and observed frequency $f = f_{j1} \ldots j_t$ the value

$$b = \sum_{i=f}^{n} \binom{n}{i} \pi^i (1 - \pi)^{n-i} \quad (8)$$

is calculated. It gives the probability of observing f or an even larger frequency and may be compared with a preassigned significance level α according to a one-sided test.

2.4 Other Approaches

All of the foregoing tests are conservative. This is most pronounced with method (5) and probably least with (8). In each event, the performance of these techniques is generally known. The same cannot be said of Lehmacher's (1981) method. In this case the test statistic resembles (7) but the denominator is calculated in a different way. According to Krauth (1985a) and others it remains unknown whether the performance of Lehmacher's test is conservative or liberal in particular cases. Evidence for liberal performance has been gathered by Lindner (1984), Küchenhoff (1986), and Wüpper (1988).

Lindner's (1984) test is based on a generalization of the exact Fisher–Yates test for fourfold tables such that more than two attributes are admitted. In general the required calculations are too cumbersome to commend themselves despite the exactness of the test.

Wüpper (1988) modified Lehmacher's (1981) approach by the introduction of various continuity corrections, using Lindner's (1984) exact test as a criterion. However, Wüpper has not demonstrated generalizability of his recommendation as regards sample size or number of attributes and categories.

2.5 Alpha Adjustment

The various previously introduced statistical tests may also be employed during the confirmatory stage of the search for types. If just a *single* configuration is of interest then no problem regarding the significance level exists. For any chosen level α the corresponding critical value of chi-square with $df = 1$ or of the standard normal can be read off at once. This does not hold, however, when two or more such tests are to be carried out simultaneously. One must distinguish between a prescribed overall level α and the corresponding nominal level α^* to be used with the single tests so that the given α value for the total test may result.

Suppose it is hypothesized that k explicitly selected configurations qualify as types, and suppose this composite null hypothesis H_0 is tested at the overall level α. Let the required level used with each single test be α^*. Acceptance of H_0 is equivalent to accepting each of the partial null hypotheses. If all the single tests are independent, then by the multiplication theorem for probabilities $1 - \alpha = (1 - \alpha^*)^k$. Since α^* is typically small, $(1 - \alpha^*)^k$ may be replaced by $1 - k\alpha^*$. Hence $\alpha^* = \alpha/k$ results. On the other hand, suppose that the single tests are totally dependent, that is, the same. Then, of course, $\alpha^* = \alpha$. Most cases, however, will assume an intermediate position somewhere between total independence and total dependence so that $\alpha/k \leqslant \alpha^* \leqslant \alpha$. Thus it is on the safe side if

$$\alpha^* = \alpha/k \qquad (9)$$

is always chosen. This is the so-called Bonferroni adjustment of α. It is recommended for general use in the present context. For completeness Holm's (1979) somewhat more complicated method of adjusting α should be mentioned. Details may be found in Krauth (1985a).

There is still another variety of alpha adjustment. As has been said before, (7) is to be used as a one-sided test since only positive values of Z are in favor of $f > n\pi$. In other words, the significance level α is an upper tail probability of the standard normal. For instance, the minimal significant Z at the level $\alpha = 0.05$ is about 1.65 and not 1.96. So, when test (6) is employed, the corresponding minimal significant chi-square is not to be read off for $\alpha = 0.05$ but for $\alpha' = 2\alpha = 0.10$. It is not $3.84 \approx 1.96^2$ but $2.71 \approx 1.65^2$. The same applies when (5) is used. As a consequence, when simultaneous chi-square tests as provided by (5) and (6) are intended then the Bonferroni adjustment (9) should be modified. The previous α^* should be replaced by

$$\alpha' = 2\alpha/k \qquad (10)$$

to be used with each single test so that the chosen overall α may result as a maximum. Employing the previous α^* rather than α' is unnecessarily conservative.

3. Derived Contingency Tables

So far general techniques have been described relevant to the search for types when a multidimensional contingency table is given. The case may arise, however, that new tables derived from the original one appear more adequate for further analysis. Such tables will be called "derived." The general techniques of analysis will remain appropriate nevertheless. In introducing derived tables it is convenient to follow Krauth's (1985a) enumeration of instances and also to adopt his example.

Four ways of obtaining a derived contingency table are presented. By way of illustration, an example with $t = 4$ attributes A, B, C and D, each with two categories, is employed. This yields $r = 2^4 = 16$ different configurations. The initial table is signified by $A \cdot B \cdot C \cdot D$, the dots separating the attributes. Combinations of attributes are indicated by AB, ABC, and so on, the categories by A_1, A_2, B_1, B_2, and so on. It is possible to apply consecutively different ways of getting a derived table.

3.1 Reduction of Dimension

A derived table with fewer dimensions results when the categories are combined across two or more attributes. By this process the total number of cells and the frequencies remain unchanged. In the extreme, all 16 configurations are strung out along one single dimension. For example, attributes A and B may be combined to form a new attribute AB with categories (A_1B_1), (A_1B_2), (A_2B_1) and (A_2B_2). This new table has only three attributes or dimensions but again $4 \cdot 2 \cdot 2 = 16$ cells. It may be signified by $AB \cdot C \cdot D$. Other derived tables of reduced dimensionality may be obtained in the same vein.

3.2 Marginal Tables

Such derived tables result if one or more attributes are deleted. This yields a lower dimensionality and a smaller number of cells. The new configurations are strings of fewer categories. Frequencies of old configurations which differ only with respect to deleted attributes are added and yield the frequencies of the new configurations. The sum of all frequencies remains unaltered. For example, if attribute D is deleted the three-dimensional table $A \cdot B \cdot C$ with $r = 2^3 = 8$ cells obtains.

3.3 Partial Tables

Fixing a category for one or more attributes leads to partial tables. In general, this will lower sample size n because only units that belong to the fixed categories are considered. The dimensionality is reduced as well. For example, if category A_1 of attribute A is fixed then the three-dimensional table $B \cdot C \cdot D \mid A_1$ is generated. It has $r = 2^3 = 8$ cells.

3.4 Anchoring to a Single Configuration

The term "anchor" is introduced here to denote a particular configuration or cell. This configuration consists of a certain sequence of categories pertaining to the attributes. Suppose that the categories not making up the selected configuration are combined attribute-wise so that each attribute is reduced to two categories. This procedure leads to another derived table. It is not applicable to the initial example $A \cdot B \cdot C \cdot D$ because there were only two categories per attribute anyway.

3.5 Interaction Analysis

Krauth and Lienert (1974) proposed procedures for investigating interactions of the attributes in a multidimensional contingency table. It may be interesting, for instance, to determine whether one or more of the initial attributes are immaterial for the existence of types. Let A be the attribute in question and form by reduction of dimension the two-dimensional table $A \cdot BCD$ with $2 \cdot 8 = 16$ cells. Calculate the associated chi-square value with $df = 15$ under the independence hypothesis. A will be retained only if no significant result emerges. Tables $B \cdot ACD$, $C \cdot ABD$, and $D \cdot ABC$ may be treated in the same vein. Suppose that A proves superfluous. Then, in a next step, the marginal table $B \cdot CD$ and so on may be analyzed until all irrelevant attributes have been eliminated.

The interpretability of an initially determined type becomes doubtful if the attributes can be partitioned into seemingly independent subsets of more than one attribute each. For example, the two-dimensional table $AB \cdot CD$ obtained by reduction of dimension with $4^2 = 16$ cells may be considered. There are no clear-cut rules on how to handle the matter, but a caveat is certainly in order.

Certain types may exist in one subpopulation but not in another. For instance, the partial table $B \cdot C \cdot D \mid A_1$ may yield a particular type consisting of categories of attributes B, C, D but the partial table $B \cdot C \cdot D \mid A_2$ may not.

Various procedures utilizing reduction of dimension and marginal and partial tables may be subsumed under the common heading "interaction analysis." The previously presented methods of searching for types remain basic. Interaction analysis is a means toward a better understanding of types although it is not a univocal and easily handled concept.

4. Numerical Example

By way of illustration, real data reported by Rittich (1988) will be used in an exploratory CFA. The area under investigation is complexity of writing styles in essays, the units being samples of such writing. Six dichotomous attributes capturing various aspects of

Table 1
CFA of attributes A_1, A_2, A_3

Configuration	Observed frequency	Expected frequency	Chi-square according to (6)
000	70	39.29	29.9
001	17	30.25	6.8
010	25	29.64	0.9
011	10	22.82	8.1
100	8	25.12	13.3
101	19	19.34	0.0
110	10	18.95	4.7
111	41	14.59	51.6

complexity were originally defined. Three of them will be subjected to a CFA. These are A_1 = simple clause usage with categories 0 = simple clauses preferred, 1 = clauses at higher levels preferred; A_2 = complex sentence usage with categories 0 = no interrelated clauses or more complex sentences used, 1 = one or more such clauses or sentences used; A_3 = end of sentences with categories 0 = simple clauses preferred, 1 = higher levels preferred. There were $n = 200$ units. The CFA is summarized in Table 1. Under the hypothesis of independence of the attributes the total chi-square becomes 101.4 with $df = 2^3 - 3 - 1 = 4$. This is significant at a level α much lower than 0.001. Hence the existence of types (and antitypes) may be anticipated.

This being an exploratory study it is hypothesized that all configurations are either types or antitypes. To ascertain an overall significance level $\alpha = 0.05$, adjustment (9) is in order. This is so because types and antitypes are not specified so that two-sided testing with $\alpha^* = 0.05/8 = 0.00625$ is indicated. The critical chi-square value with $df = 1$ becomes 7.46. It follows from Table 1 that configurations 000 and 111 may be hypothesized to be types whereas 011 and 100 may well be antitypes.

Suppose now that the null hypothesis of independence of the three attributes had been confronted with the above alternative in a confirmatory study using the same data. Then $k = 4$. For overall significance a minimal chi-square of 8.1 is now prescribed. This corresponds to $\alpha' = 0.005$. According to (10), the null hypothesis would be rejected at an overall level $\alpha = 0.01$ in favor of the alternative. Considering the substantive content of the attributes, these results appear perfectly satisfactory.

5. Special Applications of CFA

It appears that most special applications of the general methods are analyses of tables derived from the original table by reduction of dimension, forming marginal or partial tables, anchoring to a single configuration and combinations of these operations. Hence a variety of derived tables are utilized. The methods of ascertaining types previously introduced remain basic.

One example is *prediction* CFA. Here the aim is to predict a certain combination of categories of a set 1 of attributes by means of another combination of categories of a set 2 of other attributes. References to details may be found in Krauth (1985a), for instance.

Another example is *multisample* CFA. One wishes to find *discrimination types* that distinguish between different populations of units. For instance, consider the four-dimensional table $A \cdot B \cdot C \cdot D$, each attribute being a dichotomy. Let D designate gender with categories D_1 = male and D_2 = female. By reduction of dimension the two-dimensional table $ABC \cdot D$ with $8 \cdot 2 = 16$ cells is derived. Suppose it is necessary to know if configuration $(A_1B_2C_1)$ is a discrimination type by which males and females tend to differ. As a first step the table is now anchored to the configuration or cell $([A_1B_2C_1] D_1)$. This yields a fourfold table with categories $A_1B_2C_1$, not $A_1B_2C_1$ and D_1, D_2. Configuration $(A_1B_2C_1)$ will be recognized as a discrimination type as regards gender if the independence hypothesis for the attributes of said fourfold table can be refuted. The appropriate procedure in this case is the familiar chi-square test based symmetrically on all four cells, possibly with a continuity correction. The observed frequency of configuration $([A_1B_2C_1]D_1)$ must exceed its expected frequency and the test should be one-sided. This implies that the critical chi-square value for $df = 1$ and level α' should be read off for $\alpha' = 2\alpha$. As an alternative, the exact Fisher–Yates test is applicable.

A further special application is *longitudinal* CFA as proposed by Krauth and Lienert (1980). Suppose there are a number of initial attributes. All combinations of categories across these attributes are formed and regarded as the categories of a new attribute. The effective attributes in a subsequent CFA are this new attribute observed on a number of units at various points in time. The dimensionality of the resulting table equals the number of time points. The search for *longitudinal types* is effected after anchoring the table to such hypothesized types. For further hints consult Krauth (1985a).

The above enumeration of special applications of the principles of CFA is by no means exhaustive. Rich materials are contained in Lienert (1988).

There are certain peculiarities worth noting as regards a fourfold table. This case has already been encountered in connection with multisample CFA. Consider Table 2. The notation is standard. The cells contain observed frequencies. Let e_{ij} be a typical expected frequency under the hypothesis of independence of the two attributes and fixed marginals. Determining the e_{ij}'s is standard. For configuration $(1,1)$ to be a type it is necessary that $n_{11} > e_{11}$. Easy calculations show that the following equivalences hold:

$$n_{11} > e_{11} \Leftrightarrow n_{22} > e_{22} \Leftrightarrow n_{12} < e_{12} \Leftrightarrow n_{21}$$
$$< e_{21} \Leftrightarrow n_{11}n_{22} > n_{12}\,n_{21} \tag{11}$$

An analogous chain of equivalences results on reversing the directions of the signs. This means that both $(1,1)$ and $(0,0)$ are types and both $(1,0)$ and $(0,1)$ are antitypes or both $(1,0)$ and $(0,1)$ are types and both $(1,1)$ and $(0,0)$ are antitypes if types occur at all. In the first case coefficient phi associated with the fourfold table is positive and in the second case it is negative. Hence both types and antitypes exist only in pairs diagonally arranged that make up the whole fourfold table.

For the search for types in the present situation the exact Fisher–Yates test may be utilized. Alternatively, the difference $(n_{11}/n_{.1}) - (n_{12}/n_{.2})$ may be tested for significance in the familiar way, that is, a one-sided test based on the standard normal results. Or else, the usual chi-square test for independence of the dichotomous attributes may be carried out equivalently. It is necessary, however, to replace α by 2α in order to ensure the required one-sidedness at level α.

6. Relation to Other Methods

There has been an attempt by Blasius and Lautsch (1990) to utilize CFA and correspondence analysis (CA) in a complementary way on the same data set. Correspondence analysis is an exploratory technique for the analysis of mainly two-dimensional contingency tables and has become quite popular. By combining initial attributes any contingency table can be transformed to the required format. Hypotheses may be generated by CA and then CFA may be used to test them. At present, however, any pronouncement as to the fruitfulness of such endeavors would be premature.

The relation of CFA to the analysis of multidimensional tables by log-linear modeling is quite close. The simple CFA model may be viewed as a log-linear model allowing only for main effects but no interaction effects. Configural frequency analysis is a sort of residual analysis that purports to find outliers that contradict the simple model. On the other hand, log-linear modeling is meant to describe the interac-

Table 2
Observed frequencies in a fourfold table

| | | Categories of Attribute 2 | | |
		1	0	
Categories of	1	n_{11}	n_{12}	$n_{1.}$
Attribute 1	0	n_{21}	n_{22}	$n_{2.}$
		$n_{.1}$	$n_{.2}$	n

tion structure as a whole. It is this particular structure which gives rise to types in the sense of CFA.

In an example analyzed by Lienert and Lehmacher (1982) three dichotomous attributes were used and all of the eight possible configurations proved to be types or antitypes. At the same time a log-linear analysis revealed only negligible correlations between any two attributes but a substantial trivariate interaction. This alone gave rise to the types and antitypes found. In a sense, CFA and log-linear modeling are two sides of a coin.

See also: Contingency Tables; Correspondence Analysis of Qualitative Data; Log-Linear Models

References

Blasius J, Lautsch E 1990 Die komplementäre Anwendung zweier Verfahren: Korespondenzanalyse und Konfigurationsfrequenzanalyse. *ZA-Inform* 27: 110–33
Holm S 1979 A simple sequentially rejective multiple test procedure. *Scand. J. Statist.* 6: 65–70
Krauth J 1985a Principles of configural frequency analysis. *Z. Psychol.* 193(4): 363–75
Krauth J 1985b Typological personality research by configural frequency analysis. *Pers. Individ. Diff.* 6(2): 161–68
Krauth J, Lienert G A 1973 *Die Konfigurationsfrequenzanalyse (KFA) und ihre Anwendungen in Psychologie und Medizin.* Alber, Freiburg
Krauth J, Lienert G A 1974 Zum Nachweis syndromgenerierender Symptominteraktionen in mehrdimensionalen Kontingenztafeln (Interaktionsstrukturanalyse). *Biom.* 16(3): 203–11
Krauth J, Lienert G A 1980 Die Konfigurationsfrequenzanalyse. XII. Symptommusterfolgen (Durchgangssyndrome). *Z. Klinische Psychol. Psychother.* 28(4): 302–15
Küchenhoff H 1986 A note on a continuity correction for testing in three-dimensional configural analysis. *Biom. J.* 28: 465–68
Lehmacher W 1981 A more powerful simultaneous test procedure in configural frequency analysis. *Biom. J.* 23: 429–36
Lienert G A 1969 Die Konfigurationsfrequenzanalyse als Klassifikationsmittel in der klinischen Psychologie. In: Irle M (ed.) 1969 *Bericht über den 26. Kongress der Deutschen Gesellschaft für Psychologie in Tübingen, 1968.* Hogrefe, Göttingen
Lienert G A (ed.) 1988 *Angewandte Konfigurationsfrequenzanalyse.* Athenäum, Frankfurt
Lienert G A, Lehmacher W 1982 Die Konfigurationsfrequenzanalyse als Komplement des loglinearen Modells. In: Lienert G A (ed.) 1988
Lindner K 1984 Eine exakte Auswertungsmethode zur Konfigurationsfrequenzanalyse. *Psychol. Beitr.* 26(3): 393–415
Rittich R 1988 Configural Frequency Analysis. In: Keeves J P (ed.) 1988 *Educational Research, Methodology, and Measurement: An International Handbook* Pergamon Press, Oxford
Victor N 1989 An alternative approach to configural frequency analysis. *Methodika* 3: 61–73
Wüpper N 1988 Auffindung und Identifikation konfiguraler Typen in sozialwissenschaftlichen Daten. (Doctoral dissertation, University of Hamburg)

Further Reading

Greenacre M J 1993 *Correspondence Analysis in Practice.* Academic Press, London
Krauth J 1993 *Einführung in die Konfigurartions - frequenzanalyse (KFA).* Beltz, Weinheim
Lautsch E, von Weber S 1990 *Die Konfigurationsfrequenzanalyse (KFA) Methoden und Anwendungen.* Volk und Wissen, Berlin
von Eye A 1990 *Introduction to Configural Frequency Analysis.* Cambridge University Press, Cambridge

Contingency Tables

B. S. Everitt

In an investigation of solvent abuse and examination attainments, Chadwick et al. (1990) considered the influence of a number of background domestic factors. The results for two of these, living with both natural parents and employment status of main breadwinner, are shown in Table 1. Such an arrangement of data, where a number of individuals have been classified with respect to two qualitative variables, is known as a *"contingency table"* and such tables rise very frequently in the social sciences, generally as a result of surveys of one type or another. The entries in the cells of Table are counts or frequencies. These may be transformed into proportions or percentages, but it is important to note that in whatever form they are finally presented the data were originally frequencies or counts rather than continuous measurements.

Table 1 is a 2×2 contingency table since the variables involved each have two categories. Table 2 shows a 3×2 table, also from the solvent abuse study of Chadwick et al., and Table 3 a 4×4 table resulting from the cross classification of 4,353 individuals with respect to occupational group and educational level. Tables 1 to 3 are specifically two dimensional; they involve the classification of the individuals with

Table 1
Living with both natural parents and employment status of main breadwinner

	Controls	Solvent abusers	Total
Living with both natural parents			
No	35	41	76
Yes	68	60	128
Total	103	101	204
Employment status of main breadwinner			
Unemployed	3 (7.77)	12 (7.22)	15
Employed	96 (91.22)	80 (84.77)	176
Total	99	92	191

Table 2
Relationships with teachers

	Controls	Abusers
Gets on with most teachers	92(77.18)	60(74.82)
Some problems with most teachers	4(14.72)	25(14.28)
Marked antipathy toward most teachers	2(6.09)	10(5.91)

respect to two variables. Higher dimensional tables arise when a sample of individuals is cross-classified with respect to more than two variables. Table 4, for example, shows a three-dimensional contingency table displaying data concerned with the examination results of children. The first variable is the verbal reasoning band that the child occupied at age 10 years,

Table 3
Occupational group versus educational level

	Educational level				
	E1(low)	E2	E3	E4(high)	Total
Self-Employed business	239	309	233	53	834
Self-employed professional	6	11	70	199	286
Teacher	1	7	12	215	235
Salaried	794	781	922	501	2998
Total	1040	1108	1237	968	4353

the second is the occupation of the parent when the child was 14 years of age and the third relates to examination results based on O-level passes. The table gives the number of children falling in each of the 18 categories defined by the combination of these three variables.

This entry considers the ways in which contingency tables can be analyzed in educational research studies.

1. Independent Classifications: Association

The question of most interest about contingency table data is usually whether the qualitative variables forming the table are independent or not. To address this question it is clearly necessary to examine just what independence between the classifying variables would imply. In the case of a 2×2 table this is readily seen. Take for example, Table 1. In this table it is clear that if employment status of the main breadwinner is independent of group, then the proportion of controls with unemployed main breadwinners will be the same as the corresponding proportion for solvent abusers. If these proportions differ, unemployment of the main breadwinner tends to be *associated* more with one

Table 4
Examination results

Band	1			2			3		
Occupation of parent	1	2	3	1	2	3	1	2	3
Exam result									
No O-level passes	6	5	2	17	29	35	4	16	21
At least 1 O-level pass	5	6	3	21	22	10	2	2	2

of the groups than with the other. Of course, the two proportions might be expected to differ in some measure due solely to chance factors of sampling and for other reasons which might be attributed to random causes. What needs to be ascertained is whether or not the difference between the observed proportions is too large to be attributed to such causes, and for this purpose the statistical significance test outlined in the next section is used.

2. Chi-Square Test of Independence

To test for an association in a contingency table, the observed cell frequencies must be compared with those frequencies to be expected when the variables forming the table are assumed to be independent. The comparison involves the well-known "*chi-square statistic*". For example, in Table 1, if unemployment status is independent of group then the best estimate of the probability of the main breadwinner being unemployed is obtained from the relevant marginal total as 15/191. So the number of control children with an unemployed main breadwinner would be estimated to be $99 \times 15/191 = 7.77$. Similarly for solvent abusers the corresponding figure w
ould be 7.22. All four estimated expected values are shown in brackets in Table 1. The chi-square statistic is calculated from summing the (observed frequency − expected frequency)^2/expected frequency, for each cell. For Table 1 this gives:

$$X^2 = \frac{(3 - 7.77)^2}{7.77} + \frac{(12 - 7.22)^2}{7.22} + \frac{(96 - 91.22)^2}{91.22}$$
$$+ \frac{(80 - 84.77)^2}{84.77} = 6.61$$

Since, given the marginal totals, only one of the cells of a 2×2 contingency table is not fixed, this statistic is known as a "chi-square with a single degree of freedom." From the appropriate chi-square distribution it is possible to determine that the probability of observing a value as large or larger than 6.61 assuming that the variables forming the table are independent is 0.013. Consequently, there is some evidence that unemployment status and group are not independent. It appears that the proportion of solvent abusing children whose main breadwinner is unemployed is higher than the corresponding proportion for the control children.

The extension of the chi-square test of independence to contingency tables with more than two row and/or column categories is straightforward. Expected values under independence are calculated as row total × column total/total number of individuals, and the chi-square statistic is again calculated as described previously. For a table with r rows and c columns the statistic has $(r - 1)(c - 1)$ degrees of freedom. For example, the expected values for Table 2 are shown

in brackets next to the observed values and the chi-square statistic takes the value 27.2 with 2 degrees of freedom. The associated p value is less than 0.001. It appears that solvent abusing children have more difficult relationships with their teachers.

Similar calculations for Table 3 give a chi-square value of 1,254.1, which with 9 degrees of freedom is highly significant. Clearly occupation and educational level are related.

3. Small Expected Frequencies

The derivation of the chi-square distribution as an approximation for the distribution of the statistic X^2 is made under the rather vague assumption that the expected values are not "too small." This has, for many years, been interpreted by most users of the chi-square test as meaning that all expected values in the table should be greater than 5 for the chi-square test to be valid. But as long ago as 1954, Cochran pointed out that such a "rule" is too stringent and suggested that if relatively few expectations are less than 5 (say 1 cell out of 5), a minimum expectation of unity is allowable. Even this suggestion may be too restrictive since work by Lewontin and Felsenstein (1965) and Larntz (1978) shows that many of the expected values may be as small as 1 without affecting the test greatly.

Nevertheless for small, sparse, or skewed data the asymptotic theory may not be valid, although it is often difficult to predict *a priori* whether a given data set may cause problems. In the case of 2×2 tables, approaches which have been used for many years to overcome this problem have been "Fisher's exact test," and "Yates's correction", both of which are described in Everitt (1992). More recently Mehta and Patel (1983, 1986a, 1986b) have derived methods which allow exact significance levels to be computed for the general $r \times c$ table. To illustrate the differences that can occur between the exact approach and the usual procedure involving the chi-square distribution consider the following 3×9 contingency table:

0	7	0	0	0	0	0	1	1
1	1	1	1	1	1	1	0	0
0	8	0	0	0	0	0	0	0

For this table $X^2 = 22.9$. The corresponding p value from the chi-square distribution is 0.1342. The true p value is, however, 0.0013. The exact analysis indicates that the row and column classifications are not independent. The asymptotic analysis fails to show this relationship. (For interest, the exact p value for Table 1 is 0.014, very similar in this case to the approximate value given earlier.)

A procedure which has been used almost routinely for many years to overcome the problem of small expected frequencies is the pooling of categories. Such a procedure may be criticized on several grounds. First, a considerable amount of information may be lost by the combination of categories and this may detract greatly from the interest and usefulness of the study. Second, the randomness of the sample may be affected. The whole rationale of the chi-square test rests on the randomness of the sample and on the categories into which the observations may fall being chosen in advance. Pooling categories after the data are seen may affect the random nature of the sample with unknown consequences. Lastly, the manner in which the categories are pooled can have an important effect on the inferences drawn. As an example consider the following data set given by Baglivo et al. (1988):

	Column				
	1	2	3	4	5
Row 1	2	3	4	8	9
Row 2	0	0	11	10	11

When this table is tested for independence using the usual approximate methods, the calculated significance level is 0.086 which agrees with the exact probability to two significant figures although a standard statistical package will issue a warning like "some of the expected values are less than 2, the test may not be appropriate." If the first two columns are ignored, however, the p value becomes 0.48; and if the first two columns are collapsed into the third, it becomes 1.00.

The practice of combining classification categories should be avoided and is no longer needed because of the availability of the exact tests referred to previously.

4. Matched Samples

One-to-one matching is frequently used by research workers to increase the precision of a comparison. The matching is usually done on variables such as age, sex, weight, and so forth, and other such variables which might possibly affect the response variable. Two samples matched in this way must be thought of as correlated rather than independent, so the usual chi-square test is no longer strictly applicable.

The appropriate test for comparing frequencies in matched samples is one due to McNemar (1955). The test statistic is given by:

$$X^2 = \frac{(b-c)^2}{b+c}$$

where b is the number of matched pairs where members of sample I have the attribute of interest, and those of sample II do not; and c is the number of pairs where members of sample I do *not* have the attribute while those of sample II do. Under the hypothesis of no difference between the matched samples with respect to the attribute, X^2 has a chi-square distribution with a single degree of freedom.

As an example, consider an investigation of schoolchildren who admit to being smokers. A total of 50

Table 5
Truancy in matched samples of smoking and nonsmoking schoolchildren

		Smokers		
		No	Yes	Total
Nonsmokers	No	30	10	40
	Yes	3	7	10
Total		33	17	50

such children were matched one-to-one on sex, school year, and school with children who claimed to be non-smokers. The children were then asked about various behavioral and emotional problems such as sleeping difficulties, headaches, truancy, and loneliness. The results for truancy, for example, are given in Table 5. The result of McNemar's test is

$$X^2 = \frac{(10-3)^2}{13} = 3.77.$$ The associated p value is 0.052. The data give some fairly weak evidence perhaps that smokers and nonsmokers differ with respect to truancy.

5. Displaying Contingency Tables Graphically —Corespondence Analysis

Recent years have seen a growing interest in a technique which attempts to display the relationship between the variables forming a contingency table graphically. The method, "correspondence analysis," has in fact been known for a long time but its use until recently was, for some reason, largely confined to French data analysts.

Correspondence analysis works by finding a set of coordinate values to represent the row and column categories of the table. These coordinates are analogous to those derived from a principal component's analysis of multivariate, continuous data (see Everitt and Dunn 1992), except that they are derived by partitioning the chi-square statistic for the table rather than variance. A full account of correspondence analysis is given in Greenacre (1984)—here the method will be illustrated by its application to Table 3. The two-dimensional correspondence diagram is shown in Fig. 1. This diagram can be interpreted by noting the positions of the points representing the row and column categories relative to each other *and* relative to the origin. Row and column category points close to each other and relatively far from the origin imply that the frequency in the correspondence cell of the table is larger than would be expected if the two variables were independent. Row and column points distant from one another and from the origin suggest a negative association so that the corresponding cell in the table will have a smaller frequency than expected

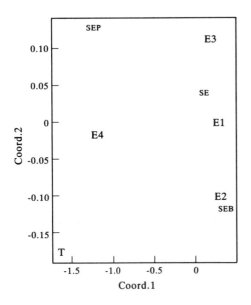

Figure 1
Correspondence analysis of occupation and educational level data:
Two-dimensional solution

under independence. Here the diagram indicates that the individuals in the self-employed business category (SEB) tend to have educational level E2 more than would be expected if occupation and educational level were independent. Similarly teaching (T) and self-employed professional (SEP) are positively associated with educational level E4.

6. Higher Dimensional Contingency Tables

Three and higher dimensional contingency tables arise when a sample of individuals is cross-classified with respect to three (or more) qualitative variables. An example has already been given (see Table 4). The analysis of such tables presents problems not encountered with two-dimensional tables, where a single question is of interest, namely, that of the independence or otherwise of the two variables involved. In the case of higher dimensional tables, the investigator may wish to test that some variables are independent of some others, that a particular variable is independent of the remainder, or some more complex hypothesis. Again the chi-squared statistic is used to compare observed frequencies with those to be expected under a particular hypothesis.

The simplest question of interest in a three-dimensional table is that of the mutual independence of the three variables; this is directly analogous to the hypothesis of independence in a two-way table and is tested in an essentially equivalent fashion. Other hypotheses which might be of interest are those of the partial independence of a pair of variables, and the

conditional independence of two variables for a given level of the third.

A more involved hypothesis concerns whether an association between two of the variables differs in degree or in direction in different categories of the third. All such hypotheses are assessed by comparing the frequencies to be expected under the model with the corresponding observed frequencies by means of chi-square statistic. For some hypotheses, expected values cannot be obtained simply from particular marginal totals but must be calculated interatively (for details, see Everitt 1992 Chap. 5). Such hypotheses are best assessed by the use of the models which are described briefly in the next section.

7. Log–Linear Models for Contingency Tables

A major development in the analysis of contingency tables occurred in the 1960s with the introduction by Birch (1963) of the "log–linear model." Such models propose some conceptual framework for the observations, and the parameters of the model represent the effects that particular variables or combinations of variables have in determining the observed frequencies. Such an approach is commonly used in other branches of statistics, for example, regression analysis and analysis of variance.

To introduce the log–linear model consider a two-dimensional table which, in the population, has frequencies m_{ij} in the ij-th cell. (The expected values met previously may be thought of as estimates of the m_{ij}.) If the two variables forming the table are independent then it is relatively simple to demonstrate that m_{ij} may be expressed in the form

$$\ln m_{ij} = u + u_{1(i)} + u_{2(j)} \tag{1}$$

where u, $u_{1(i)}$, and $u_{2(j)}$ are parameters of the model representing respectively a "grand mean" effect, and "row" and "column" effects (for details, see Everitt 1992 Chap. 5).

If this model fails to provide an adequate fit to the data, an "interaction" term can be added giving

$$\ln m_{ij} = u + u_{1(i)} + u_{2(j)} + u_{12(ij)} \tag{2}$$

The extra term represents discrepancies between the actual cell frequencies and those to be expected under independence. Such a model would provide a perfect fit since the number of parameters is the same as the number of cells in the table. For this reason it is known as the "saturated" model for a two-dimensional table.

For a three-dimensional table the corresponding saturated model is

$$\ln m_{ijk} = u + u_{1(i)} + u_{2(j)} + u_{3(k)} + u_{12(ij)} \tag{3}$$
$$+ u_{13(ik)} + u_{23(jk)} + u_{123(ijk)}$$

In this model the parameters $u_{123(ijk)}$ represent the possibility that associations between a pair of variables

Table 6
Log-linear models for Table 4

Model (terms omitted from saturated model)	G^2	df	Change in G^2 from model 1	df
1. u_{123}	3.84	4	—	—
2. u_{12}, u_{23}, u_{13}, u_{123}	40.14	12	36.30	8
3. u_{12}, u_{123}	12.66	6	8.82	2
4. u_{13}, u_{123}	15.73	6	11.89	2
5. u_{23}, u_{123}	10.37	8	6.53	4

may differ in degree or direction in each category of the third variable. By dropping parameters from Eqn.(3), models corresponding to the mutual, partial, or conditional independence of the variables may be obtained. For example, the model corresponding to the mutual independence of the three variables has the form

$$\ln m_{ijk} = u + u_{1(i)} + u_{2(j)} + u_{3(k)} \qquad (4)$$

When assessing the fit of particular log–linear models, expected and observed frequencies are again compared by the usual chi-square statistic or, more commonly, by a "likelihood ratio" statistic, G^2 given by

$$G^2 = 2 \sum \text{observed} \ln \frac{\text{observed}}{\text{expected}} \qquad (5)$$

where summation is over all cells of the table.

The degrees of freedom of G^2 are the degrees of freedom for the model—that is, the number of independent parameters subtracted from the number of cells in the table. For large sample sizes G^2, like X^2, is distributed as a chi-square variate.

To illustrate the application of log–linear models, several will be applied to the data in Table 4. The results are summarized in Table 6. Clearly a number of models provide an adequate fit and a question that might be asked is how does one choose between models? Differences in fit can be measured by differences in the G^2 statistic. The aim is for the model with the least number of parameters which provides an adequate fit. For example, moving from Model 1—no second order relationship between the three variables, to Model 2—mutual independence of the

three variables, leads to an increase in G^2 of 36.30 and an increase in degrees of freedom of 8. This indicates a significant *decrease* in the ability of the model to account for the data and so Model 2 would not be retained. Judgments between the other models considered in Table 6 can be made in a similar fashion. Model 5 appears to hold most promise—this model implies that, given the verbal reasoning band, parental occupation and examination result are independent.

Log–linear models allow a systematic approach to be taken to discover the relationships that may be present in complex multidimensional tables and provide a powerful addition to methods available for the analysis of contingency table data.

See also: Correspondence Analysis; Log-Linear Models

References

Baglivo J, Oliver D, Pagano M 1988 Methods for the analysis of contingency tables with large and small cell counts. *J. Amer. Statist. Assoc.* 83: 1006–13
Birch M W 1963 Maximum likelihood in three-way contingency tables. *J. Roy. Statist. Soc. B.* 25: 220–33
Chadwick O, Yule W, Anderson R 1990 The examination attainments of secondary school pupils who abuse solvents. *Brit. J. Educ. Psychol.* 60: 180–91
Cochran W G 1954 Some methods for strengthening the common X^2 tests. *Biometrics* 10: 417–77
Everitt B S 1992 *The Analysis of Contingency Tables*, 2nd edn. Chapman and Hall, London
Everitt B S, Dunn G 1992 *Applied Multivariate Data Analysis*. Edward Arnold, London
Greenacre M J 1984 *Theory and Applications of Correspondence Analysis*. Academic Press, London
Larntz K 1978 Small-sample comparison of exact levels for chisquared goodness-of-fit statistics. *J. Amer. Statist. Assoc.* 73: 253–63
Lewontin R C, Felsenstein J 1965 The robustness of homogeneity tests in $2 \times N$ tables. *Biometrics* 21: 88–117
McNemar Q 1955 *Psychological Statistics*. 2nd edn. Wiley, New York
Mehta G R, Patel N R 1983 A network algorithm for performing Fisher's exact test in $r \times c$ contingency tables. *J. Amer. Statist. Assoc.* 78: 427–34
Mehta G R, Patel N R 1986a A hybrid algorithm for performing Fisher's exact test in unordered $r \times c$ contingency tables. *Commun. in Statist.* 15: 387–403
Mehta G R, Patel N R 1986b FEXACT: A Fortran subroutine for Fisher's exact test on unordered $r \times c$ contingency tables. *ACM Trans. Mathemat. Software* 12: 154–61

Correlational Methods

R. M. Thorndike

In its most general sense, the term "correlation" refers to a measure of the degree of association between two variables. Two variables are said to be correlated when certain values of one variable tend to co-occur with particular values of the other. This tendency can range from nonexistent (all values of variable 2(Y) are equally likely to occur with each value of variable 1(X)), to absolute, (only a single value of Y occurs for a given value of X). A correlation coefficient is a numerical index of the strength of this tendency. This entry is concerned with the properties and uses of correlation coefficients.

There are many special types of correlation coefficients. All share the characteristic of being measures of association between two variables. The difference lies in how the variables are defined. What is commonly called the "correlation coefficient" (or, more properly, the "Pearson product–moment correlation coefficient" or PMC) is an index of association between two variables where both variables are considered as single observed variables. The association between scores on a reading readiness test and a later measure of reading achievement is an example of such a correlation. Although each measure is the sum of scores on several items or subtests and represents a complex human characteristic, it is treated as a single undifferentiable variable for the purposes of analysis.

At the other end of the spectrum is a procedure called set correlation (Cohen 1982). Like the ordinary PMC, it is a measure of the association between two variables; however, in this case the association is between two unobservable variables that are weighted additive combinations of multiple measured variables. The unobserved variables are often called latent variables or composite variables. If, for example, the reading readiness and achievement measures each yielded several subscales, the correlation between a weighted combination of one set of subscales and a weighted combination of the other would be a canonical correlation. Set correlation is a generalization of canonical correlation in which additional sets of variables can be statistically removed from one or both of the sets being correlated (see partial correlation below).

1. Mathematical Definition of Correlation

The mathematical definition of an index of correlation is quite straightforward in most cases, although its actual computation may be very involved and time consuming. Adopting the notation conventions that

X_i is the score of individual i on variable X

Y_i is the score of individual i on variable Y

$\bar{X}$ is the mean of X scores = $\Sigma X/N$

$\bar{Y}$ is the mean of Y scores

where X and Y may be measured variables or composites, the variances of X and Y are both of the general form

$$S_X^2 = \sum_{i=i}^{N} (X_i - \bar{X})^2/N \tag{1}$$

For any given set of measurements, the mean of the set is a least-squares description of the entire set. That is,

$$1/N \sum_{i=1}^{N} (Y_i - \bar{Y})^2 = \text{minimum} \tag{2}$$

For a single variable, this is clearly S_Y^2. However, if a second variable (X) is available it may be possible to use that second variable to form subgroups such that some value other than $\bar{Y}$ is a least-squares description within each subgroup. Since for any group or subgroup its mean on the variable in question is the least-squares descriptor, the subgroups must have different mean values if group information is to improve on the overall mean. Letting $\bar{Y}_j$ stand for the mean of group j, an individual's deviation from the overall mean $\bar{Y}$, can be seen as composed of two parts:

$$(Y_{ij} - \bar{Y}) = (\bar{Y}_j - \bar{Y}) + (Y_{ij} - \bar{Y}_j) \tag{3}$$

The deviation of the ith individual in group j from the overall mean is the sum of the deviations of the group's mean from the overall mean and the individual's score from the group mean.

By going through the process of computing a variance, that is, squaring, summing over N cases, and dividing by N, the above equation becomes:

$$\left[\sum \sum (Y_{ij} - \bar{Y})^2\right]/N = \left[\sum \sum (\bar{Y}_j - \bar{Y})^2\right]/N$$
$$+ \left[\sum \sum (Y_{ij} - \bar{Y}_j)^2\right]/N \tag{4}$$

The term on the left is clearly an ordinary variance of the form found in Eqn. (1). The terms on the right are also variances, but the first is the variance of group means around the overall mean and the second is the pooled variance within groups. The numerators of these two terms are the sums of squares between and within groups from the analysis of variance.

Recall that groups were formed on the basis of the other variable, X. The differences among the subgroup means are due to the X variable in the sense that it was the X variable that led to the identification of groups. Therefore, the second term in Eqn. (4) is the variance in Y that is due to X or is related to X. The third term, then, is the variance in Y that is unrelated to X or independent of X. This is sometimes called the "residual variance."

Equation (4) may be rewritten in terms of variances as:

$$S_Y^2 = S_{\hat{Y}}^2 + S_{Y \cdot X}^2 \tag{5}$$

where $S_{\hat{Y}}^2$ is the Y variance due to X. $S_{Y \cdot X}$ is the residual variance and is the quantity to be minimized in Eqn. (2). With these variance terms defined, the general form for an index of correlation is

$$\text{corr} = (S_{\hat{Y}}^2 / S_Y^2)^{1/2} = [1 - (S_{Y \cdot X} / S_Y^2]^{1/2} \tag{6}$$

That is, an index of correlation is the square root of the proportion of Y variance that is related to X. This mathematical definition of correlation is based on the assumption that Y is measured on an interval scale and has a normal distribution, but X can be a nominal variable. The basic definition in Eqn. (6) is called the correlation ratio and is usually given the symbol η (eta).

2. Product–Moment Correlation

The definition given above is a general definition of correlation in which no assumptions are made about the nature of the X variable (Y is assumed to have a normal distribution). It is frequently the case in educational research that both X and Y variables can be assumed to be measured on interval scales with normal or approximately normal distributions. When both variables are continuous, measured on an interval scale, and normally distributed their joint frequency distribution is bivariate normal.

When X is a discrete or group-membership variable, it is clear that the Y scores of people at any given value of X form a frequency distribution and the mean, $\bar{Y}_j$, is the least-squares description for the group. Likewise, when X is continuous there is a distribution of Y scores for people with a particular X score (X_i), and the mean of these Ys (call it $\hat{Y}_i$), is a least-squares description for these individuals taken as a group. The assumption that X and Y have a bivariate normal distribution means that there is a consistent relationship between changes in X and changes in $\hat{Y}$. The graph of X and $\hat{Y}$ is a straight line of the form

$$\hat{Y}_i = B_{Y \cdot X} X_i + A_{Y \cdot X} \tag{7}$$

At any particular value X_i, the variance in Y scores around $\bar{Y}_i$ is the unexplained variance, $S_{Y \cdot X}^2 = \Sigma(Y_i - \bar{Y}_i)^2 / N$. The values of $B_{Y \cdot X}$ and $A_{Y \cdot X}$ are determined such that, across the entire set of data, $S_{Y \cdot X}^2$ is minimum. By the logic used in developing Eqns. (4) and (5), the total variance of Y may be expressed as

$$S_Y^2 = S_{\hat{Y}}^2 + S_{Y \cdot X}^2 \tag{8}$$

It can be shown that the value of $B_{Y \cdot X}$ is given by

$$B_{Y \cdot X} = \Sigma \, x_i y_i \, / \, \Sigma \, x_i^2 = \Sigma \, x_i y_i \, / \, N S_X^2$$

$$A_{Y \cdot X} = \bar{Y} - B_{Y \cdot X} \bar{X} \tag{9}$$

where $x_i = X_i - \bar{X}$ and $y_i = Y_i - \bar{Y}$. When X and Y are expressed in the standard score form

$$B_{Y \cdot X} = \Sigma \, Z_{Y_i} Z_{X_i} \, / N \tag{10}$$

The symbol $r_{y \cdot x}$ is used to represent the slope coefficient in Eqn. (7) when X and Y are expressed in standard scores.

$$r_{Y \cdot X} = \Sigma \, Z_Y Z_X \, / N. \tag{11}$$

This is one of several definitional formulas for the product–moment correlation. Since the intercept (A) must be zero ($\bar{Z}_Y = \bar{Z}_X = 0$), Eqn. (7) may be written as

$$\hat{Z}_{Y_i} = r_{YX} Z_{X_i} \tag{12}$$

Rewriting the least-squares function in Eqn. (2) for Z scores produces

$$1/N \, \Sigma \, (Z_{Y_i} - \hat{Z}_{Y_i})^2$$

$$= 1/N \, \Sigma \, (Z_{Y_i} - r_{YX} Z_{X_i})^2 = \text{minimum} \tag{13}$$

By squaring, summing, dividing by N, simplifying the result, and recalling from Eqn. (3) the expression for the residual variance, the following is obtained:

$$S_{Z_Y \cdot Z_X}^2 = 1 - r_{YX}^2. \tag{14}$$

In terms of the original raw scores, this equation becomes

$$S_{Y \cdot X}^2 = S_Y^2 \, (1 - r_{YX}^2). \tag{15}$$

Solving for r_{YX}^2 yields

$$r_{YX}^2 = [1 - (S_{Y \cdot X}^2 / S_Y^2)] = S_{\hat{Y}}^2 / S_Y^2 \tag{16}$$

which is identical to Eqn. (6). A useful computing formula for r is

$$r = \Sigma \, y_i x_i / N S_X S_Y \tag{17}$$

or its raw-score equivalent

$$r = \frac{N \, \Sigma \, Y_i X_i - \Sigma \, Y_i \, \Sigma \, X_i}{\left[N \Sigma \, Y_i^2 - \left(\Sigma \, Y_i \right)^2 \right]^{1/2} \left[N \Sigma \, X_i^2 - \left(\Sigma \, X_i \right)^2 \right]^{1/2}} \tag{18}$$

To this point, three meanings of the product–moment correlation coefficient have been developed. They are

(a) The slope of the least-squares regression line for standard score variables is r (Eqn. [11]).

(b) The strength of association between two variables $S_{\hat{Y}}^2 / S_Y^2$ is r^2 (Eqn. [16]).

(c) The residual variance in Y, which may be viewed as the inaccuracy of prediction, is $S_Y^2 (1 - r_{YX}^2)$

(Eqn. [15]).

There are several additional interpretations of the PMC that are discussed by Harman (1976), McNemar (1969), or Thorndike (1978). Interested readers should consult these sources for a complete presentation.

3. Other Bivariate Correlations

The product–moment correlation is the most widely used and understood correlational index. It has several advantages, such as its numerous interpretations, that accrue when the conditions for its use are met. However, there are numerous research situations in which not all variables are continuous, represent an interval scale, and have normal distributions. A number of alternative correlation coefficients are available for situations that do not meet all the assumptions of the product–moment correlation.

Perhaps the most common case occurs when one or both of the variables is represented in the data as a set of categories. The correct procedure then depends on the basis for the categorization and the number of categories. If the variable is truly categorical and dichotomous, no special treatment is required. If the measured variable represents a categorization of a variable that could in theory be measured on a continuum, special procedures are needed to estimate what the correlation would be for a continuous variable. Truly categorical polychotomous variables can be analyzed in some situations, but because they seldom possess ordinal properties, measures of association that involve such variables are few and interpretations are severely restricted.

3.1 Special Product–Moment Coefficients

Truly dichotomous variables have two values (male or female) while polychotomous variables have several categories (geographic region). When one or both of the variables in a correlation is truly dichotomous, the analysis results in a special PMC with restricted interpretation and perhaps restricted range. If one variable is polychotomous, eta may be used. Chi-square is the statistic of association for two polychotomous variables. As measures of association, eta and chi-square cannot be used in further analyses.

A correlation between one dichotomous variable and one continuous variable is called a point-biserial correlation (r_{pb}). The correlation between two dichotomous variables is called the "fourfold point correlation" or "phi" (ϕ). Both of these coefficients are PMCs and may be computed by the usual formulas

as well as by special formulas given in some statistics books. They require no special attention on the part of the investigator in that dichotomous variables included in a computer run for correlation analysis will be properly processed by the usual equations and the results will be either r_{pbs} or ϕs. However, the investigator should be aware that neither of these coefficients should be used in Eqns. (11) or (14). They may be interpreted as indicating strength of association and they are the appropriate coefficients to use when truly dichotomous variables such as gender occur in a multivariate analysis. Because they are dichotomous, their variances will be smaller than is the case for continuous variables, and the resulting correlations will also tend to be smaller.

A second situation that is encountered occasionally in educational research is that the data occur as rankings or other ordinal forms of measurement. While several methods exist for analyzing ordinal data, one popular bivariate procedure is the Spearman rank-order correlation (*rho*). This index is a PMC that may be computed from two sets of ranks by the usual formulas for r (Eqns. [17] or [18]) or by the classic formula developed by Spearman and given in most statistics texts. *Rho* is properly interpreted as an index of degree of association only, but it is the appropriate index to use (with caution) when rank variables are included with interval variables in multivariate analyses. When more than one observation occupies the same rank, special procedures are required.

3.2 Estimates of Product–Moment Correlations for Ordered Categories

It is often the case that a categorical variable represents an attribute that may reasonably be considered continuous and normally distributed. A classic example is the multiple-choice test item which dichotomizes the ability continuum into passes and fails. For bivariate situations where it is reasonable to assume an underlying normal distribution in one dichotomous variable and with the other variable measured as a continuum (e.g., 0/1 item scores and total test scores) the appropriate index is the biserial correlation (r_b). This coefficient is an estimate of what the PMC would have been, had the dichotomous variable been measured as a continuous variable. The biserial correlation, using the subscripts 1 and 2 to indicate the higher and lower portions of the dichotomy, is as follows:

$$r_b = (\bar{Y}_1 - \bar{Y}_2)(pq)/hS_Y \qquad (19)$$

where p is the proportion in the upper group, q is the proportion in the lower group, $\bar{Y}_1$ is the mean of the continuous variable in the upper group, $\bar{Y}_2$ is the mean in the lower group, S_Y is the standard deviation of Y, and h is the height of the normal curve at p.

The biserial correlation is an appropriate statistic for certain bivariate applications, but it is not a product–moment correlation. It can, on occasion, exceed unity and is not a directly computable function of the scores themselves. Experience has shown that inclusion of biserial correlations multivariate analysis can result in singular correlation matrices. r_b should be used with caution in multivariate analyses.

A situation that arises with some frequency in educational research is the case of one truly dichotomous variable and one artificial dichotomy: for example, inclusion in a treatment program (1) or not (0) (a true dichotomy) and passing (1) or failing (0) a test (continuous underlying trait). Under these conditions the appropriate index is the biserial-phi coefficient (Becker and Thorndike 1988, Thorndike 1949). For the four-fold table where $a = (1,0)$, $b = (1,1)$, $c = (0,0)$, and $d = (0,1)$ the biserial-phi is given by

$$\phi_{bis} = (bc - ad)/h(pq)^{1/2} \qquad (20)$$

where a, b, c, and d are the frequencies in the four cells; p and q are the proportions of cases in each category of the truly dichotomous variable; and h is the ordinate of the normal curve at p.

Another coefficient, the tetrachoric correlation (r_{tet}), is analogous to ϕ, in that it is based on the assumption that each of two dichotomous variables represents an underlying normally distributed continuous variable. The coefficient estimates what the relationship between two continuous variables would be in order to produce the four-fold pattern found in the data. In some multivariate analyses where tetrachoric correlations have been used they have caused singularity, so they must be used with caution.

Olsson has presented generalizations of the biserial and tetrachoric correlations that are appropriate for the case where one or both variables represent a series of three or more ordered categories (Olsson 1979, Olsson et al. 1982). These coefficients have been called "polyserial" and "polychoric correlations" respectively. Their computation is impractical without a computer, but maximum likelihood estimates of both coefficients are available through the LISREL program (Jöreskog and Sörbom 1989). Experience indicates that when the necessary assumptions are met and the coefficients have been estimated by the algorithm in LISREL the results can be used with confidence in further analyses. However, they may cause singularity of the correlation matrix, which will result in problems with some multivariate analyses.

The primary reason for using polyserial or polychoric correlations (or their special cases, the biserial and tetrachoric) rather than ϕ or r_{pb} (or their multicategory generalizations) is that categorization of a variable reduces its variance. This has the effect of restricting the range of PMCs that involve categorical variables so they underestimate the actual degree of association between the variables when the assumptions necessary for the polyserial and polychoric coefficients are met. Such underestimates can affect the results of factor analyses and other multivariate procedures.

4. Significance Tests

The topic of statistical significance is most fruitfully viewed from the perspective of sampling distributions. Assume that there is a population that reasonably approximates infinite size and that every member of this population has or could have a value on every variable of interest. If random samples are drawn from this population, measured on the variables of interest, and summary statistics computed, it is possible to make frequency distributions of these summary statistics. Such frequency distributions are called "sampling distributions," and they exist for all descriptive statistics.

Of course, the population is never really completely available, and it is unusual to draw more than one sample, but mathematical statisticians have derived theoretical sampling distributions for many statistics. These theoretical distributions form the basis for statistical inference and significance testing.

Tests of statistical significance are usually applied to means, but they may be used with any statistic, such as a correlation coefficient. Suppose, for example, that an investigator wishes to test the hypothesis that the correlation between two variables such as number of books in the home and reading ability at age 10 is greater than zero. This implies a one-tailed null hypothesis of the standard form that ρ (rho, the correlation in the population) is zero or negative ($\rho \leqslant 0$), and this hypothesis creates a hypothetical sampling distribution of the correlation coefficient, r for samples of size N. The investigator obtains a sample, computes r and the appropriate test statistic (described below), determines the probability of obtaining this large a value of the test statistic, and reaches a conclusion. If the value of the test statistics is unlikely, given the hypothesized sampling distribution, the investigator concludes that $\rho > 0$ in the population from which the sample was drawn.

4.1 Tests for a single r

Tests of statistical significance are more complicated for correlation coefficients than for means. With sufficient sample size the sampling distribution of the mean is symmetric around the population parameter regardless of the value of that parameter. For the correlation coefficient the shape of the sampling distribution depends on both ρ and N. When ρ is zero or close to zero, the sampling distribution is symmetric; however, when ρ exceeds about ± 0.25 the sampling distribution becomes skewed with the direction of skew toward zero. The degree of skewness increases as ρ increases.

Asymmetry of the sampling distribution is not a problem for most simple tests of hypotheses because for most cases the null hypothesis is $\rho = 0$. However, for nontypical nulls, such as $\rho = 0.60$, and for confidence intervals on larger correlations, the problem is more serious.

When testing the hypothesis that $\rho = 0$, the appropriate statistic depends upon N. For $N > 50$, the standard error of r is $\sigma_r = 1/(N^{1/2})$ and the statistic $z = r/\sigma_r$ is normally distributed. Smaller samples require that $t = r/[(1 - r^2)/(N-2)]^{1/2}$ with $df = N-2$ be used instead.

The solution to the asymmetry problem for the PMC was derived by R A Fisher. The transformation

$$z_F = ln(1 + r) - ln(1 - r) \tag{21}$$

which is known as Fisher's z, results in a statistic that has a sampling distribution that is very nearly normal in shape for any value of ρ. The standard error of z_F is $1/(N - 3)^{1/2}$, and the statistic $z = (z_F - K)/\sigma_{z_F}$ is a normal deviate. In this case K is the z_F transformed value of ρ specified in the null hypothesis. Tables for transforming r to z_F and back are provided in some statistics texts, such as McNemar (1969), Thorndike (1982), and Hays (1988).

4.2 Significance of r_{pb}, ϕ, r_b, and rho

For small samples ($N < 100$) the best way to test the hypothesis ($\rho = 0$) for r_b and r_{pb} is to test the significance of the difference between group means. If the value of t exceeds the critical value with $N - 2$ degrees of freedom, the correlation is statistically significant. When $N > 100$, r_{pb} may be treated as any other PMC, while the standard error of r_b is approximated by $\{[(pq)^{1/2}/h] - r_b^2\}/N^{1/2}$.

The ϕ coefficient may be tested for significance by the relationship $\chi^2 = N\phi$, where χ^2 has $df = 1$. If the value of χ^2 exceeds the critical value, it is appropriate to conclude that $\phi > 0$. When the sample size is fairly large, the approximate standard error of ϕ is $1/N^{1/2}$.

A word of caution is necessary with regard to tests of significance for these coefficients. If the frequencies in the two categories of a dichotomous variable are very unequal, tests of significance may be inappropriate. McNemar (1969) suggests that when the proportion of cases in either category of a dichotomous variable exceeds 0.90 the significance tests should be viewed with caution. Tests of significance have not been developed for the biserial-phi, polyserial, and polychoric correlation coefficients.

Rank order coefficients such as *rho* are seldom used with large samples because of the difficulty of obtaining a clear ranking of large numbers of observations. Therefore, the statistic for testing significance will usually be a t test of the form $t = \rho/[(1 - \rho^2)/(N - 2)]^{1/2}$, which is identical to the small sample test for r. Tables of critical values for as few as five pairs of ranks are included in several introductory statistics books.

4.3 Testing Differences between r's

The situation occasionally arises when it is desirable to test a hypothesis about the equality of two correlation coefficients. Such tests may take either of two forms. The correlations being tested may be correlations between same variables in different samples, or they may be correlations between one variable and two different variables in the same sample. In the first case, both

rs are transformed to z_{FS}. The standard error of the difference between two z_{FS} is $\sigma(z_{F1} - z_{F2}) = [1/(N_1 - 3) + 1/(N_2 - 3)]^{1/2}$ and the test statistic $z = (z_{F1} - z_{F2})/\sigma (z_{F1} - z_{F2})$ is a normal deviate.

The second situation is a little more complicated. Three variables have been measured on a sample of N individuals, so there are three correlations, r_{12}, r_{13}, and r_{23}. If an investigator wishes to test the null hypothesis that $\rho_{12} = \rho_{13}$, the necessary test is

$$t = \frac{(r_{12} - r_{13})[(N - 3)(1 + r_{23})]^{1/2}}{[2(1 - r_{12}^2 - r_{13}^2 - r_{23}^2 + 2r_{12}r_{13}r_{23})]^{1/2}} \tag{22}$$

with $df = N - 3$.

4.4 Other Uses of z_F

There are two other useful applications of Fisher's z transformation in correlational research. The first of these is averaging correlations. Since the correlation coefficient itself does not represent an interval scale, it is not proper to average correlations directly. However, z_F is an interval scale measure of association, so it is appropriate to compute an average z_F weighted by N. After converting each r to z_F, a mean z_F is found:

$$\bar{z}_F = \frac{(N_1 - 3)z_{F1} + (N_2 - 3)z_{F2} + \ldots + (N_j - 3)z_j}{(N_1 - 3) + (N_2 - 3) + \ldots + (N_j - 3)} \tag{23}$$

The standard error of $\bar{z}_F$, $1/[(N_1 - 3)(N_2 - 3) + \ldots + (N_j - 3)]^{1/2}$, may be used to test hypotheses about $\bar{z}_F$. Once $\bar{z}_F$ has been calculated, the mean correlation, $\bar{r}$, may be found by reversing the original transformation. Finding $\bar{z}_F$ to be statistically significant is equivalent to finding r significant.

An alternative approach that is common in the literature is to use the unweighted median of a set of correlations to represent the central tendency of the set. This procedure is acceptable, but it does not use all the information in the original data. Correlations based on larger samples should ordinarily have greater influence on the average. Also, there is no standard error to use for hypothesis tests.

The second application for z_F is the determination of a confidence interval for ρ. Since the sampling distribution of r is not symmetric except when ρ is zero, the confidence interval for any nonzero ρ cannot be symmetric. However, the sampling distribution of z_F is symmetric. A proper confidence interval for any ρ can be obtained by transforming r to z_F, finding the standard error of z_F, multiplying σ_{z_F} by the appropriate critical values from the normal distribution, adding these products to z_F and finally transforming the resulting limits for z_F back into correlations. For example, if $r = 0.65$ and $N = 19$, then $z_F = 0.775$ and $\sigma_{z_F} = 0.25$. To find the 95 percent confidence interval the critical values are $+1.96$ and -1.96. Multiplying these by 0.25 yields $+0.49$ and -0.49, and adding these values to z_F gives 1.265 and 0.285 as the upper and lower limits for z_F. These are transformed back to correlations, yielding 0.85 and 0.28 as the limits of the 95 percent confidence interval for ρ. Note that this confidence interval is symmetric around r in terms of probability, but not in the scale of r. The procedure for confidence intervals can also be applied to mean correlations.

5. Partial and Semipartial Correlation

There are many occasions in educational research where it is desirable to control or remove statistically the effect of one or more variables. One way by which this can be accomplished is through sampling. A characteristic that is constant for all subjects in a study cannot be a source of variance in the results. The effect of gender can be removed by using only male or only female subjects. Likewise, maturational factors can be controlled, at least in part, by studying children who are all the same age.

However, control at the sampling stage of a study has some definite drawbacks, the most important of which is that the generalizability of the finding may be severely restricted. Also, there are many research situations in which it is impossible to control variables by selection or it may be undesirable to do so because one or more of the questions of interest in the study involves the control variables as independent or dependent variables in the study. For example, in a study of the relationship between pupil attitudes and achievement the investigator might wish to remove or hold constant the effect of differences in age and measured intelligence. Selecting pupils of only a particular age and intelligence level would be wasteful of subjects and might distort the sample on other relevant variables such as socioeconomic status. In addition, the investigator might wish to include one or both of the control variables in a later phase of the analysis.

The solution to this problem is to collect data on an unrestricted sample, a sample that is representative of the population to which generalizations are to be extended, and then remove the control variables statistically. Note that the term "control variable" is being used in a restricted way in this discussion. Some potential variables such as conditions under which measurements are obtained should be held as constant as circumstances allow. It is to other variables, particularly status characteristics of the subjects, such as age, intelligence, and gender, that this discussion is directed. These variables may be measured during the data collection phase, and their effects removed during analysis. It is therefore important to include measures of all relevant variables in the design and data collection stages of a study.

If X is a student motivation variable, Y is a performance measure, Z is ability, and S is sex, then it might be of interest to examine the relationship between motivation and performance both with and without controlling for ability and gender. The effect of one variable on another may be removed by analyzing the residual variance. For example, the residual variance in Y after controlling S is the variance in Y within levels of S, pooled across levels of S. The Y variance is found for males and for females independently, and the weighted average of these two variances is the variance in Y that is independent of S.

The analysis of residual variance is equivalent to using deviation scores of the form $y_{ij} = Y_{ij} - \bar{Y}_j$, or, for continuous variables, $y_i = Y_i - \hat{Y}_i$. Each individual's residual score is his or her deviation from the least-squares prediction made from the variables being removed or controlled. The residual scores are then analyzed like scores on any other variables. For example, the correlation between motivation and performance with the effect of sex differences removed from the motivation variable would involve correlating residual scores on motivation ($x_{ij} = X_{ij} - \bar{X}_j$) with raw scores on performance. It is given the symbol $r_{Y(X \cdot S)}$, where the subscript indicates that S is controlled in X but not in Y. The subscript $YX \cdot S$ would indicate that S is controlled in both Y and X.

Correlations that involve residual variances are called "partial correlations." When residual scores appear on both sides of the equation the term partial correlation is used if the same variable is controlled in both X and Y. Bipartial correlation is used when one variable is controlled in X and a different variable is controlled in Y. Semipartial or part correlations are those that involve residual scores on only one side of the relationship.

While the logic of partial correlations involves residual scores, the computations can generally be performed with the ordinary bivariate correlations themselves. Starting with the definitions of the residual scores as deviations from least-squares predictions, the partial correlation of X and Y with Z removed is

$$r_{XY \cdot Z} = (r_{XY} - r_{XZ}r_{YZ})/[(1 - r_{XZ}^2)^{1/2}(1 - r_{YZ}^2)^{1/2}] \tag{24}$$

There is only one partial correlation between X and Y controlling Z, but there are two possible semipartial correlations, one where Z is controlled in X and one where it is controlled in Y. The formulas for these correlations differ from Eqn. (24) only in the denominator:

$$r_{Y(X \cdot Z)} = (r_{XY} - r_{XZ}r_{YZ})/(1 - r_{XZ}^2)^{1/2} \tag{25}$$

$$r_{X(Y \cdot Z)} = (r_{XY} - r_{XZ}r_{YZ})/(1 - r_{YZ}^2)^{1/2} \tag{26}$$

5.1 Higher Order Partial Correlations

There may be occasions when it is desirable to control more than one variable statistically. The logic is a direct generalization of the case of a single variable. That is, the analysis involves residual scores in one or both of the variables being correlated. The difference is that now the residuals are more complex. For example, the partial correlation between motivation and performance with sex and ability controlled (a second-order partial correlation) would first involve the residual scores on X, Y, and Z from sex. The X and Y residuals would then be entered into analyses with the Z residuals and the residuals of the residuals obtained. Finally, the correlation between second-order X and Y residuals yields the desired second-order partial correlation. Higher order semipartial correlations can be conceptualized in the same way; however, they are very closely related to the standardized regression weights of multiple regression analysis and are usually obtained in that way (see *Regression Analysis of Quantified Data*).

Partial correlations of any order are correlations between residual scores of that order. As was the case with the first-order partial, the analysis may be performed starting with ordinary bivariate correlations. The procedure is a sequential one involving repeated use of Eqn. (24). First, all first-order partials removing one variable (say Z) are computed. Then Eqn. (24) is repeated for a second control variable, but with each term replaced by the appropriate first-order partial.

For problems involving more than two control variables the procedure described is quite cumbersome. Although it would be conceptually and computationally sound to continue in such a sequential fashion, the analysis would almost certainly be performed by one of the computer programs that uses a matrix algebra solution.

5.2 Test of Significance

The statistical significance of a partial correlation may be tested by procedures analogous to those used for simple rs. The z_F transformation is appropriate and with large N the standard error of z_F is $1/(N - p - 3)$ where p is the number of variables being partialled out of the relationship. z_F may be used either to test a hypothesis about the partial correlation or to set up a confidence interval for ρ.

An alternative way to test the hypothesis that $\rho = 0$ for small N is available. The statistic $t = r_p/[(1 - r_p^2)/(N - p - 2)]^{1/2}$, in which r_p is the partial correlation and p is as above, is distributed as t with $df = (N - p - 2)$.

Tests of significance for semipartial correlations are closely related to multiple correlation. In general, the significance of a semipartial correlation is tested by exploring the significance of the difference between the multiple correlation with the relevant variable both included and excluded. If the difference between multiple correlations is statistically significant, the semipartial correlation of the excluded variable with the dependent variable of the multiple correlation analysis is significant.

6. Multiple Correlation

Correlation was defined as an index of the degree of association between two variables. Common bivariate correlations describe the relationship between a pair of observed variables. Partial correlations are PMCs between sets of residual scores after the effect of one or more variables has been removed. In all of these cases the correlation coefficient is an index of maximum relationship in terms of a least-squares criterion.

Multiple correlation extends the concept of least-squares association to the relationship of one dependent or outcome variable with more than one independent or predictor variable. The multiple correlation coefficient is the bivariate product–moment correlation between the outcome variable (Y) and some combination of the set of predictor variables (X_1, X_2, . . . X_p). The combination of X variables (call it P) is determined in such a way that the correlation r_{YP} is the largest possible correlation that could be obtained from the given set of data.

The majority of work with multiple correlation in education and the behavioral sciences defines P as a weighted linear combination of the Xs. That is, if the array (B_1, B_2, . . . B_p) is a set of weights to be applied to the Xs, then P is of the general form

$$P = B_1X_1 + B_2X_2 + \ldots + B_pX_p + A \qquad (27)$$

To say that P is a weighted linear combination of the Xs means that no term in Eqn. (27) involves a product of X terms or any X term other than the first power. The restriction of linearity is not a necessary one, and there are some situations where a particular theory may postulate nonlinear relationships, but for most applications the linear model is best for two reasons: its simplicity and its generalizability.

The definition of the best- or least-squares composite of the set X is relatively simple, but is most easily accomplished if all variables are expressed as standard scores. In standard score form Eqn. (27) becomes

$$z_P = \beta_1 z_{X_1} + \beta_2 z_{X_2} + \ldots + \beta_p z_{X_p} \qquad (28)$$

It can be shown that for the special case of $p = 2$ the values of β_1 and β_2 are given by

$$\beta_1 = (r_{1Y} - r_{2Y}r_{12})/(1 - r_{12}^2) \qquad (29)$$

$$\beta_2 = (r_{2Y} - r_{1Y}r_{12})/(1 - r_{12}^2) \qquad (30)$$

These equations are very similar to semipartial correlations; β_1 represents the contribution of X_1 to P that is independent of X_2, and β_2 is the independent contribution of X_2 to P. They differ from semipartial correlations only by the scaling factor $(1 - r_{12})^{1/2}$ in the denominator. The squared multiple correlation, r_{YP}^2, can be shown to be equal to the sum of products of the βs and the bivariate predictor–criterion correlations, $r_{YP}^2 = (\beta_1 r_{YX_1} + \beta_2 r_{YX_2})$, and the multiple correlation itself is the positive square root of r_{YP}^2.

Generalization to the multivariable case is most easily handled by using matrix algebra. The solution, which is simply a substitute for solving p linear equations in p unknowns, is given by $\boldsymbol{\beta}_p = \boldsymbol{R}_{PP}^{-1} r_{PY}$, where $\boldsymbol{\beta}_p$ is a $p \times 1$ vector of β-weights for use in Eqn. (28),

R_{PP}^{-1} is the inverse of the $p \times p$ matrix of correlations among the p predictors, and r_{PY} is the $p \times 1$ vector of correlations between the predictor variables and Y. The squared multiple correlation is then given by $r_{YP}^2 = \boldsymbol{\beta}_{YP}\boldsymbol{r}_{PY}$.

The β-weights may be expressed in the metric of the original variables appropriate for use with Eqn. (27) by the transformation $B_{X_j} = \beta_{X_j}(S_Y/S_{X_j})$.

The value of the intercept, A, is given by

$$A = \bar{Y} - \sum_{j=1}^{P} B_j\bar{X}_j \tag{31}$$

Of course, the correlation between Y and P is unchanged by this transformation.

6.1 Asymmetry of Multiple Correlation

There is an important restriction on the interpretation of r_{YP}^2. Whereas r_{XY}^2 was a symmetric index of the degree of association between two variables, r_{YP}^2 is not. The simple squared bivariate correlation reflects the proportion of variance in Y that is related to X and the proportion of variance in X that is related to Y. It is bidirectional. The multiple correlation is unidirectional in the sense that r_{YP}^2 is the proportion of variance in Y that is related to the set of X variables but not the proportion of variance in the set of X that is related to Y. The relationship is symmetric in the observed variable Y and the latent variable P.

The reason for this asymmetry is the fact that P does not contain all of the variance of the set X. The correlation of each variable X_j with P is given by $r_{PX_j} = r_{YX_j}(1/r_{YP})$. These correlations of observed variables with a latent variable are factor loadings. The mean of squared loadings

$$\bar{r}_{PX}^2 = \sum r_{PX_j}^2/p$$

is the proportion of X set variance that is related to P, and the product $(\bar{r}_{PX}^2) \cdot (r_{YP}^2)$ is the proportion of variance in the set X that is related to Y.

6.2 Tests of Significance

There are several types of hypotheses that can be tested in a multiple correlation analysis. The most obvious is $\rho_{YP} = 0$. The appropriate test of this hypothesis is an F test of the ratio of the mean square due to the multiple regression equation (MS_P) to the mean square residual (MS_R). Note that the total sum of squares of Y is

$$SS_Y = \sum (Y_i - \bar{Y})^2 \tag{32}$$

and that this is a combination of SS due to regression (SS_P) and residual (SS_R). That is, $SS_Y = SS_P + SS_R$.

It can be shown that these SS terms are given by $SS_P = r_{YP}^2 SS_Y$ and $SS_R = (1 - r_{YP}^2)SS_Y$. Each, divided by its degrees of freedom, is a mean square [$MS_P = SS_P/p$; $MS_R = SS_R/(N - p - 1)$]. The ratio of these MS s canceling where possible, is an F with $df_1 = p$ and $df_2 = N - p - 1$:

$$F = (r_{YP}^2/p)/[(1 - r_{YP}^2)/(N - p - 1)] \tag{33}$$

A second hypothesis of interest relates to the contribution of some subset of the set X. The significance of the contribution of a subset of variables may be determined by the equation

$$F = \frac{[(r_{YP_1}^2 - r_{YP_2}^2)/(p_1 - p_2)]}{[(1 - r_{YP_1}^2)/(N - p_1 - 1)]} \tag{34}$$

where $r_{YP_1}^2$ is the squared correlation between Y and a set of p_1 X variables and $r_{YP_2}^2$ is for some subset of the variables in the first correlation. If F with $df_1 = p_1 - p_2$ and $df_2 = N - p_1 - 1$ is statistically significant, the contribution of the variables that were omitted from p_1 in p_2 is statistically significant. By applying Eqn. (34) repeatedly with each single variable omitted in turn, the significance of each β-weight in Eqn. (28) can be determined. Eqn. (34) is also used with the general linear model to perform tests on hypotheses related to the analysis of variance.

6.3 Stepwise Analysis

When many predictor variables are available, a small subset of these variables will usually account for most of the predictable variance in the outcome variable. It is generally desirable to determine the smallest set of predictors that will do a satisfactory job of prediction for reasons of economy and simplicity. The method by which such a minimum subset is identified is stepwise analysis.

A stepwise analysis may be either a step-up or a step-down procedure. In the former, the analysis starts with the best single predictor and variables are added in order of the magnitude of their contribution. A step-down analysis begins with the complete set of predictors and deletes those variables that make the smallest contribution at each stage. The decision about which variables to add or delete is usually made by selecting the variable that results in the largest (step-up) or smallest (step-down) F as computed by Eqn. (34) (see *Regression Analysis of Quantified Data*).

7. Canonical Correlation

A canonical correlation is the bivariate correlation between two latent variables or composites where each composite has been determined in such a way as to maximize its relationship to the composite of the other set. Given a set of X variables (measures of student achievement, for example) and a set of Y variables (interest or motivation measures) a canonical analysis finds a weighted linear combination, P, of the X set and a weighted linear combination, Q, of the Y set such that the correlation between them, r_{PQ}, is maximized. This is similar to the multiple correlation problem except that it involves the simultaneous solution for two sets of regression weights.

There is an additional complication in canonical analysis. Where there was only one multiple correlation coefficient, there are as many canonical correlations as there are variables in the smaller set. The first canonical correlation (R_{c1}) is the highest possible correlation between composites of the two sets of original variables. The second correlation, (R_{c2}), is the highest possible correlation between composites of the two sets of residual variables with the first pair of composites partialled out. In general, R_{ci} is the correlation between composites of residual variables with all preceding composites partialled out. Thus, each succeeding pair of composites is statistically independent of all other pairs and each R_c describes an independent dimension of association between the sets.

A canonical analysis begins with three correlation matrices: $\boldsymbol{R}_{PP}$, the within set matrix of correlations among the X variables, $\boldsymbol{R}_{QQ}$, *the within set matrix for the Y* variables, and $\boldsymbol{R}_{PQ}$, the between set correlations of the X variables with the Y variables. The solution of a series of complex matrix equations (Tabachnick and Fidell 1989, Thorndike 1978) results in two matrices of standardized regression weights (βs) that define the latent variables for the X and Y sets and the R_cs between the pairs of composites.

However, interpretation of a canonical analysis is complex and requires additional information. While the regression weights indicate the relative contributions of the variables to the composites of their own set, the correlations between the observed variables and the composites, which are akin to factor loadings, may be of greater interest. There are four matrices of such loadings, two matrices of intraset canonical loadings of the X variables on the P composites and the Y variables on the Q composites, and two matrices of interset canonical loadings of the X variables on the Q composites and the Y variables on the P composites. These loadings, both intra- and inter-set, enable the investigator to treat the composites as factors and interpret them in a similar fashion (see *Factor Analysis, Canonical Analysis*).

7.1 Tests of Significance

The statistical significance of canonical correlations is tested sequentially. If there are J canonical correlations (the number of variables in the smaller set), then the first hypothesis tested is that all of them are zero. A significant value of the test statistic (χ^2) implies that at least R_{c1} is nonzero. R_{c1} is removed and the hypothesis that the remaining R_{ci} are zero is tested. The sequence is repeated, removing the largest remaining correlation, until the hypothesis cannot be rejected. The pairs of composites associated with statistically significant correlations may then be interpreted. The test of statistical significance is an aid to the investigator in determining the dimensionality of the space in which the relationships among the variables will be interpreted. Rotation of the composites is sometimes used to aid interpretation.

7.2 Redundancy

The problem of asymmetry in interpreting the relationship described by a canonical correlation is more acute than for multiple correlations because R_c is an index of association between two latent variables, not the observed variables or the sets of variables. Proper interpretation of a canonical analysis requires computation of an index which was given the unfortunate name "redundancy" (see Thorndike 1978).

Although there are alternate ways to conceptualize the redundancy index, perhaps the simplest is in terms of the interset canonical loadings. An interset loading is the correlation between an observed variable of one set and a composite of the other. The square of this loading is the proportion of variance of the observed variable that is related to the composite. The mean of squared loadings across observed variables in the set is the proportion of variance of that set that is accounted for by the composite of the other set. There are therefore two sets of redundancies: those of the X set of variables with the Q composites and those of the Y set of variables with the P composites. The sum of the redundancies for a set is the total redundancy of that set with the other set. In general the redundancy of set X with set Y will not equal the redundancy of Y with X (see *Canonical Analysis*).

8. Set Correlation

Canonical analysis is a general and flexible data-analytic model that has only briefly been described here. It has been shown (Knapp 1978) that most commonly used hypothesis-testing procedures such as analysis of variance are special cases of the canonical model (see *Variance and Covariance, Analysis of*).

Cohen (1982) has provided a more complete generalization of correlational procedures, and therefore a very general model of data analysis which he has called "set correlation." This approach views the covariance matrices of sets of variables in a manner similar to individual variables. It is possible to partial one covariance matrix out of another one, producing a residual covariance matrix which contains partial covariances. For example, given a set of aptitude measures, W, a set of demographic characteristics, X, a set of motivational variables, Y, and a set of achievement measures, Z, one might ask what is the relationship between aptitude and achievement with demographic characteristics partialled out of the aptitude variables and motivational variables partialled out of the achievement measures? The set correlation $r_{(W\,X)(Z\,Y)}$ would be the (bipartial) canonical correlation between the residual part of the aptitude set (demographics controlled) and the residual part of the achievement set (motivation controlled). Semipartial and partial variations are also possible. As Cohen has pointed out, multivariate analysis of covariance is a special case of semipartial set correlation, just as

ANOVA is a special case of multiple correlation analysis and MANOVA and discriminant function analysis are special cases of canonical correlation analysis.

However, proper interpretation of analyses such as these is complex and requires a deeper grasp of their technical aspects than can be developed here. Potential users of canonical analysis should consult a source such as Harris (1985), Tabachnick and Fidell (1989), or Thorndike (1978) for a more detailed explanation and examples. Cohen's (1982) paper is the best source for set correlation.

9. Cross-validation

Whenever an index of relationship is developed on a sample using the least-squares criterion, the result is optimum for that sample. However, a least-squares equation in one sample will not be a least-squares solution for another sample from the same population. In the bivariate case the degree of correlation and the equation of the regression line will fluctuate from sample to sample. In multiple correlation the problem is compounded because the least-squares equation depends not only on the correlations of the predictors with the criterion but also on the correlations among the predictors. To the extent that the pattern of correlations in a sample deviates from the pattern in the population or in other samples—a condition called sample-specific covariation—the equation developed in that sample will give poorer results with new sets of data. Of course, the problem is worse with canonical analysis because two sets of regression weights are being fitted simultaneously.

The tendency of multiple and canonical correlation analyses to capitalize on sample-specific covariation raises two related issues: (a) the degree to which the description (magnitude and pattern) of relationships generalizes to future samples, and (b) the accuracy of predictions made from the regression equation itself. A useful response to both of these issues is the procedure called "cross-validation."

Cross-validation involves applying the least-squares regression equation from one set of data to a new set of data. The correlations between predicted and observed scores provide a good indication of how well "real" predictions would work if the criterion measures were yet to be obtained. Since the regression equation is not a least-squares equation in the new sample, it will be unaffected by sample-specific covariation in the data.

Likewise, the degree and pattern of relationships in the new set of data as described by the multiple or canonical loadings indicates the generalizability of the original equations as a model for new samples. The multiple or canonical correlations in cross-validation provide an index of the degree of fit of the model. A more complete discussion of issues relating to cross-validation may be found in Thorndike (1978).

See also: Multivariarte Analysis; Factor Analysis

References

Becker G, Thorndike R L 1988 The biserial-phi correlation coefficient. *J. Psycholo.* 122(5): 523–26
Cohen J 1982 Set correlation as a general multivariate data-analytic method. *Multivariate Behav. Res.* 17(3): 301–41
Harman H H 1976 *Modern Factor Analysis*, 3rd edn. University of Chicago Press, Chicago, Illinois
Harris R J 1985 *A Primer of Multivariate Statistics*, 2nd edn. Harcourt Brace Jovanovich, San Diego, California
Hays W L 1988 *Statistics*, 4th edn. Harcourt Brace Jovanovich, San Diego, California
Jöreskog K G, Sörbom D 1989 *LISREL VII User's Reference Guide*. SPSS, Chicago, Illinois
Knapp T R 1978 Canonical correlation analysis: A general parametric significance-testing system. *Psych. Bull.* 85(2): 410–16
McNemar Q 1969 *Psychological Statistics*, 4th edn. Wiley, New York
Olsson U 1979 Maximum likelihood estimation of the polychoric correlation coefficient. *Psychometrika* 44(4): 443–60
Olsson U, Drasgow F, Dorans N J 1982 The polyserial correlation coefficient. *Psychometri.* 47(3): 337–47
Tabachnick B G, Fidell L S 1989 *Using Multivariate Statistics*, 2nd edn. Harper Collins, New York
Thorndike R L 1949 *Personnel Selection*. Wiley, New York
Thorndike R M 1978 *Correlation Procedures for Research*. Gardner, New York
Thorndike R M 1982 *Data Collection and Analysis: Basic Principles*. Gardner, New York

Correspondence Analysis

G. Henry

The factorial analysis of correspondence is one of the procedures developed for the analysis of information in the form of contingency tables, where nominal data are presented for examination. This procedure is one of the most efficient for describing and establishing relationships in qualitative data and was initially proposed by Benzecri (1963). It stands alongside contingency table analysis, configural frequency analysis, Galois Lattices, log–linear models and the scaling of nominal data, as one of a battery of new techniques that can be employed for the investigation of qualitative data. This procedure has as its principal

Table 1
Contingency table of numbers of records and buyers

| Type of Music | Buyers | | | | Total |
	Young people	Female adults	Male adults	Old people	
Songs	69	172	133	27	401
Jazz	41	84	118	11	254
Classical music	18	127	157	43	345
Total	128	383	408	81	1,000

Table 3
Contingency table of relative cell proportions (by columns) of records and buyers

| Type of music | Buyers | | | |
	Young people	Female adults	Male adults	Old people
Songs	0.539	0.449	0.326	0.333
Jazz	0.320	0.219	0.289	0.136
Classical music	0.141	0.332	0.385	0.531
Total (N = 1,000)	1.000	1.000	1.000	1.000

characteristic an exchange of the roles of variables and observations and seeks to represent them in the same space. This type of representation was initially suggested by Kendall, but for a long time remained unused.

1. An Illustrative Example

The following hypothetical example was employed by De Lagarde (1983) to illustrate the procedure.

Let us suppose that a store has sold 1,000 records and has filed information on the characteristics of the records (jazz, songs, or classical music) and on the characteristics of the buyers (young people, male or female adults, and old people). It is then possible to construct a contingency table (see Table 1) in order to analyze relationships between age, sex, and type of music.

Let the proportional frequencies of the cells in the contingency table be denoted by f_{ij} for cell (i,j) where $i = 1, \ldots, i, j = 1, \ldots, j$. The marginal frequencies are denoted by

Table 2
Contingency table of cell proportions of records and buyers

| Type of music (i) | Buyers (j) | | | | Total |
	Young people	Female adults	Male adults	Old people	
Songs	0.069 (f_{11})	0.172 (f_{12})	0.133 (f_{13})	0.027 (f_{14})	0.401 (r_1)
Jazz	0.041 (f_{21})	0.084 (f_{22})	0.118 (f_{23})	0.011 (f_{24})	0.254 (r_2)
Classical music	0.018 (f_{31})	0.127 (f_{32})	0.157 (f_{33})	0.043 (f_{34})	0.345 (r_3)
Total (N = 1,000)	0.128 (c_1)	0.383 (c_2)	0.408 (c_3)	0.081 (c_4)	1

$$R_i = \sum_j f_{ij} = r_i \quad \text{for rows, and}$$

$$C_j = \sum_i f_{ij} = c_j \quad \text{for columns.}$$

The values of the proportional frequencies are recorded in Table 2. The variable "type of music" is obviously recorded on a nominal scale. Likewise the variable "buyers" is also on a nominal scale. The aim of correspondence analysis is to represent graphically the data contained in this two-dimensional contingency table.

In this example, it would clearly be possible to use three rectangular axes (songs, jazz, and classical music) to represent the four categories of buyers in this three-dimensional space. However, such a direct representation is limited to small contingency tables and is not very useful. Correspondence analysis permits more complex bodies of data to be represented in simplified form.

Correspondence analysis is based not on the proportional frequencies recorded in Table 2, but on the relative proportions which are obtained by dividing f_{ij} by c_j for columns or f_{ij} by r_i for rows.

The relative frequencies for columns are presented in Table 3.

If we denote f_{ij} divided by c_j as x_i, then $\Sigma x_i, = 1$ for each value of j. Thus it is possible to state this as the equation of a plane

$$x_1 + x_2 + x_3 = 1$$

If we have l dimensions with $(l > 3)$ the equation of the corresponding hyperplane will be

$$x_1 + x_2 + x_3, \ldots, x_l = 1.$$

In this example the four points representing young people, female adults, male adults and old people belong to a plane since their three coordinates will satisfy the first equation. Moreover, this plane will intersect the three axes at points A, B, and C which are

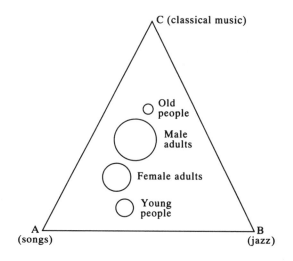

Figure 1
Type-of-music plane with buyer groups shown

at a distance of one unit from the origin of the three-dimensional space. These three points will therefore form an equilateral triangle. As shown in Fig. 1, it is possible to represent the data for each group of buyers by a circle of area proportional to the value of c_j.

The reciprocal analysis is also possible in which the three points (songs, jazz, and classical music) are located on a hyperplane in four-dimensional space. In the reciprocal analysis, Benzecri (1973) weights the values of x_i by (r_i) for the first analysis, and the values of x_j by (c_j) for the reciprocal analysis.
In the first analysis:

$$x_i = \frac{f_{ij}}{r_i(c_j)^{1/2}}$$

and in the reciprocal analysis:

$$x_j = \frac{f_{ij}}{c_j(r_i)^{1/2}}$$

By proceeding in this way, the three poles of the triangle in the first analysis are no longer equidistant from the origin. The perpendicular line from the origin to the four dimensional hyperplane intersects the plane at a point G. Thus, OG becomes the initial axis of the four-dimensional scatter plot. By considering the reciprocal analysis, it is a simple task to identify the second axis. Mathematical procedures have been developed for computing these different axes. In the example concerned with buyers and type of music there are only two axes and the total proportion of variance extracted by these two factors is 100 percent. The four types of buyers and the three types of records can consequently be accurately represented in two-dimensional space as in Fig. 2. It should be noted that G is the centroid at which the proportions would be the same for each buyer or type of music category. When a point is far from G it contributes significantly

to the location of the axes. Distances between points are also meaningful. For instance, in the example, note the relative proximity of the positions of female adults and songs, and between old people and classical music. In addition, it is clearly possible to identify the meaning of the two axes. The horizontal axis (axis 1) in Fig. 2 represents the relationship between young people and old people, while the vertical axis (axis 2) distinguishes between jazz and non-jazz music.

One advantage of this procedure is that more complex mathematical operations can be carried out, but they will not be developed in this entry. For example, it is possible to calculate the relative contribution of each dimension to each of the factorial axes in order to identify more clearly the nature of the axes. It is also of value to calculate the expression.

$$R = \sum_{ij} \left(\frac{f_{ij}^2}{r_i c_j} \right)$$

Since R is distributed with a chi-squared distribution, it is possible to proceed beyond a description of the sample and to employ inferential statistics.

Moreover, it is possible to generalize correspondence analysis to a *m* by *n* table. If *j* is the lowest dimension of the table then *j*–1 axes of reference can be identified, and as with traditional factor analysis, the first two or three axes generally account for a high proportion of the total variance. These features of the procedure will be illustrated in the following example drawn from educational research.

2. A Study of Teaching Behavior

In a study reported by Crahay (1987) of teaching behavior, 21 lessons were observed of one teacher teaching the same sixth grade class. The verbal interactions between the teacher and the students were recorded on audiotape. The tape recordings of the first 20 minutes of each lesson were transcribed for more detailed analysis. Since the extracts of each of the

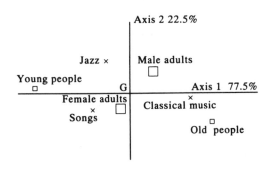

Figure 2
Positions of types of music and buyers represented in two-dimensional space.

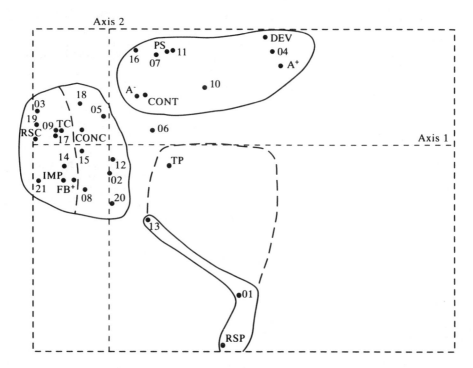

Figure 3
Spatial representation of categories and lessons

lessons sampled and examined are of the same duration, the absolute frequencies of teaching behavior are comparable between lessons.

From an examination of the transcripts, the verbal behavior of the teacher was coded using a nine-category system developed by De Landsheere (De Landsheere and Bayer 1969, De Landsheere et al. 1973). The directions of the teacher–student interactions were also coded, namely, whether the teacher spoke to the whole class or to a specific student. In addition, the verbal participation of the students was coded into one of three categories. In this system of classification of teacher behavior there was thus a total of 14 categories of teacher or student behavior.

Five axes were identified as significant by correspondence analysis. The proportion of the data accounted for by each of the five axes has been recorded in Table 4.

The first two axes account for 63.48 percent of the data, which is sufficient to restrict further analysis to consideration of these two axes only. Distances in this two-dimensional space and the relative contributions of each variable can be calculated, but limitations of space prevent such information being presented here. However, a diagrammatic presentation of the lessons and teaching behavior variables in the two-dimensional space has been recorded in Fig. 3.

In Fig. 3, each of the 21 lessons is indicated by

a number and each of the teaching behaviors by a combination of letters. In the following discussion only those teaching behaviors and lessons which have a relative contribution equal to or greater than 0.20 are considered. Two groups of lessons can be identified and contrasted on the horizontal axis (axis 1). The first group are shown clustered on the left hand side of Fig. 3, namely lessons: 19, 3, 21, 17, 9, 14, and 15. The second group of lessons lie on the right hand side of Fig. 3, namely lessons: 4, 10, 1, 6, 7, and 11. The first group of lessons is associated with five teaching behavior variables: TC (teacher speaks to the whole class); RSC (a student responds to a request that the teacher has addressed to the whole class, without specifying

Table 4
Proportion of data accounted for by each axis

Axis	Proportion of data explained
1	33.07
2	30.41
3	8.05
4	7.47
5	7.01
Total	86.01

who has to respond); IMP (imposed instruction); FB + (positive feedback) and CONC (concretization by the teacher).

The second group of lessons may be characterized by five teaching behaviors: TP (teacher speaks to a specific student); RSP (a student responds to a request that the teacher has addressed specifically to the student); PS (a student spontaneously asks a question or reacts to the teacher's comment without specifically being asked); DEV (content development in the lesson); and A + (positive affectivity).

The first group of lessons reflect a traditional teaching style. During these lessons, the verbal behavior of the teacher is mostly directed toward the whole class (TC). The teacher lectures and frequently asks questions of the whole group without specifying who has to respond. We may assume that those students who participate verbally are those who know the correct answer. This would account for the high level of positive feedback (FB +).

The second group of lessons reflects another pattern of interaction: (a) where a specific student questions the teacher (PS); (b) the student responds (RSP); (c) the teacher's verbal behavior is oriented toward a particular student (TP); (d) the teacher develops (i.e., accepts, classifies, and amplifies what the student says) (DEV); and (e) the teacher gives more positive affect than usual (A +). In the first group of lessons verbal participation by the students is quite different in comparison to the second group of lessons where the students participate spontaneously or respond to questions directed to them personally.

Before discussing the second group of lessons in greater detail, it is necessary to examine the vertical axis in Fig. 3 (axis 2). Few teaching behavior variables show high relative contributions. The axis is clearly polarized on two forms of verbal participation by the students. On the one hand there is a student responding to a request that the teacher has specifically addressed to the student (RSP). On the other hand there is a student spontaneously asking a question or reacting to the teacher's comment without being specifically asked (PS). Four other teaching behavior variables were found to have substantial loadings along this second axis: imposed instruction (IMP) and positive feedback (FB+) on the negative side; and content development (DEV) and controlling function (CONT) on the positive side. However, the roles that these four teaching behavior variables play in the definition of the second axis is slight, since their relative contributions do not exceed 0.28.

Five lessons are located on the negative side of this second axis (namely, 1, 8, 13, 20, 21). On the positive side, four lessons (namely, 4, 7, 11, 16) show a high relative contribution on this axis (greater than 0.44) and three others (namely, 3, 10, 18) show a lower positive loading on this axis (between 0.22 and 0.25). The six lessons which belong to the positive side of the first axis are split into three groups by the second axis. Four lessons (4,7,10,11) are characterized by a high frequency of spontaneous participation by the students, and by a low frequency of personally solicited participation, whereas lesson 1 is characterized by a low frequency of student spontaneous participation, and by a high frequency of personally solicited participation.

3. Conclusion

Correspondence analysis has therefore allowed the construction of a typology of lessons and their characterization according to two main dimensions. These two main dimensions take into account the different types of variables which have been observed. In one sense this technique of correspondence analysis may be compared with factor analysis and the scores assigned along the two axes to the calculation of factor scores, but the mathematical model is very different, and the technique is suitable for use with nominal data, whereas factor analysis is suitable for use with scores associated with an underlying normal distribution. Correspondence analysis seeks to account for the distribution of data in the specified categories, and factor analysis seeks to account for the variance in the scores obtained with respect to specified variables.

See also: Log Linear Models; Galois Lattices; Factor Analysis

References

Benzecri J P 1963 *Cours de linguistique mathématique.* University of Rennes, Rennes
Benzecri J P 1973 *L'analyse des données. Vol. 2: L'analyse des correspondances.* Dunod, Paris
Crahay M 1987 Stability and variability of teachers' behaviors: A case study. *Teaching and Teach. Educ.* 4(4)
De Lagarde J 1983 *Initiation a l'analyse des données.* Bordas and Dunod, Paris
De Landsheere G, Bayer E 1969 *Comment les maîtres enseignent.* Ministère de l'Education Nationale, Brussels
De Landsheere G, Nuthall G, Cameron M, Wragg E, Trowbridge N 1973 *Towards a Science of Teaching.* National Foundation for Educational Research (NFER), London

Further Reading

BMDP Statistical Software Manual 1990. Vol. 2: Procedure CA Parts 1 and 2. University of California Press, Los Angeles, California
Lefebvre J 1976 *Introduction aux statistiques multidimensionelles.* Masson, Paris
SAS/STAT User's Guide 1990. Vol. 1: Anova-freq, Version 6, 4th edn. SAS Institute Inc., Cary, North Carolina
SPSS/PC+ Procedure ANACOR. SPSS, Chicago, Illinois

Data Envelopment Analysis

L. Anderson and H. J. Walberg

1. Introduction and Scope

The chief purpose of schooling is learning; and much quantitative analysis in education is devoted to examining the relation of means and goals. "Means" may be thought of as the actions taken or resources employed to attain educational objectives. Once they are identified, educators can specify the organization, materials, procedures, programs, and other means to bring them about within the context, tradition, and constraints of the setting. To do this, they face two problems—knowing the causal relations between means and ends, and employing limited means or allocating scarce resources to achieve attainment of these objectives. A major purpose of education evaluation therefore is concerned with the degree to which means are combined to achieve educationally relevant ends. In this entry, data envelopment analysis, a relatively new approach to frontier or best-level estimation in public sector evaluation is introduced. Contrasts are made between this new approach and other more conventional ways of carrying out evaluation of educational organizations.

2. Causal Analysis

Most decision situations are characterized by multiple goals and multiple means. One of the largest challenges to analysts is the need to establish the causal relations between these means and goals. In education, considerable progress has been made in this regard: for example, nine psychological factors—student ability, age, and motivation, the quantity and quality of instruction, and the social environments of the home, classroom, peer group, and mass media—have shown powerful and consistent influences on learning (Walberg 1986). Examples of the analytic methods employed to establish the consistency and size of these effects or influences are t-tests, F-tests, and regression weights.

Causality, however, can hardly be taken for granted. Psychologists, for example, have conducted thousands of experiments in which students, classes, or schools are assigned randomly to control groups and to new instructional methods or other educational arrangements to determine which are the most effective. Experiments are hardly foolproof since they may not reproduce natural conditions, nor be generalizable beyond the limited sites in which they are usually conducted. Educational practitioners, moreover, find it difficult to carry out experiments since they require unfamiliar technical procedures and administrative re-arrangements.

Economists, sociologists, and others have employed regression, structural modeling, and other statistical procedures to sort out causal influences from non-experimental observations and other data. Since such data is available on random samples of large universes, sometimes from entire nations, the results are readily generalizable. Still, the traditional means of analyzing such data may not be capable of dealing satisfactorily with measurement error and other data problems that may vitiate causal inferences.

Though no method is foolproof, structural modeling offers some advantages over previous analytic methods. It offers a systematic approach for probing causal theories. When combined with the results of case studies, experiments, and traditional regression analyses of survey data, it helps policymakers and practicing educators better understand educational processes.

3. Prescriptive Analysis

Causal understanding, however, is only part of the analytic solution. In applied fields such as agriculture, education, engineering, and medicine, practitioners must choose what to do. They may seek the most effective treatment—a heroic medical treatment, for example, most likely to save a patient's life without regard to pain or financial costs. Or they may try to choose an efficient combination of means that maximizes values of outcomes subject to costs or resource availability. Decision-making in these contexts can be defined as identifying an efficient allocation of scarce resources such as time and money in order to secure valuable objectives.

Both causality and efficient resource allocation are important in the planning and conduct of education, yet rarely do educational analysts and practitioners comprehensively, rationally, and objectively confront the decision-making problem. Rather they may form impressions of efficiency or follow popular trends, and shift from one program or method to another without explicit analysis.

An elaborate set of methodologies has been available and employed in the military, business, and industry since about 1945 under the name of "operations research." For example, given the availability of inputs and the value attaching to objectives, it is possible to identify the most efficient combination of inputs to achieve stated objectives. Such analyses, which have been extensively used at the macro (international and national) levels of educational planning and finance, have seldom been employed at the micro (state, local, and school) levels of education decision-making because educators are often unclear about their objectives, know neither the costs nor benefits of current programs and methods, and are unsure about the best technology of learning under the varying circumstances.

4. Evaluations in the Public Sector

Public sector provisioning departs from that in the private sector in at least one decisive way: the absence of prices of outcomes with which to carry out evaluation of the decision-making unit such as a local educational authority or school. Without explicit values of outcomes it is impossible to use anything resembling the market mechanism as a model for identifying system or unit performance. The absence of an evaluation mechanism in the form of profits or rate of return leaves public sector organizations without a means for carrying out formative or summative evaluation, since only unsystematic and subjective feedback is possible.

In their extensive review of analytic approaches in the analysis of public sector performance, Johnson and Lewin (1984) identify four broad groups of models which have been used to derive assessment measures. The first, or "goal model," places emphasis on the process of specification of goals. The implication is that in the absence of carefully specified objectives, the organization cannot hope to be efficient in the use of organizational resources. A second model, termed the "system model," places emphasis on design features of the organization. Much work, in both the private and public sectors, has drawn important insights from these two models. A third model, the "decision systems" model is related to the goal model, but places major emphasis on effective decision-making in organizations. The fourth model is subsumed under operations research, derived from a management-science tradition, and is usually geared to the routinized solution of fairly standard problems in the public and private sectors. None of these models solves all the problems associated with operations in the public sector which usually involve multiple and incommensurable outputs and multiple inputs, goal specification problems of proper weighting of public choices, and questionable theories of alternative technologies.

Data envelopment analysis appears to meet the above shortcomings in that it is firmly based theoretically in microeconomics, and it avoids the problems associated with arbitrarily weighting aggregate outputs and inputs. Additionally, it allows for the choice of any common set of objectives recognized by a comparable set of decision-making units, using a common set of inputs as explained below.

5. Educational Productivity

Most economic assessments of educational performance have employed production functions which assume educational output as a function of resources which contribute linearly and additively to the output. An extensive body of research associated with the formulation of an estimation of the educational production function can be identified. A book-length treatment is found in Bridge et al. (1979) (see also Lau 1979, Hanushek 1986). The usual regression analysis or general linear model is the statistical expression of the view of schooling production, and regression coefficients express the sensitivity of outcomes to inputs. Although such a model remains a useful approach to the study of some types of education production problems, such resource-based models limit the range of possibilities for studying education production processes (Miller 1985). In particular, resource-based models, by their logic, identify average performance and relate particular school outcomes to these average performance measures. They do not identify best performance, and measures of best performance are what is needed.

The production function in economics, moreover, relates inputs and outputs in a technological relationship derived from prior optimization efforts. The production functions are therefore supposed to allow for the identification of changes in outputs due to unit changes in independent or input factors. However, such possibilities exist only for efficient education producers and are misleading when applied to efficient as well as inefficient ones. Since the vast majority of education production function studies employ linear regression, the estimated equation is really only an average relationship between inputs and outputs.

Within the regression tradition and still consistent with economic theory, new methods of best performance production functions appear to resolve the several previous limitations by estimating a boundary to the set of data points, such that distance from the estimated boundary becomes a measure of inefficiency defined in terms of cost differentials (Wagstaff 1989). Few reported studies have, however, used this methodology for the analysis of efficiency in education production.

The single-equation regression model is deficient on another count as well. Schooling produces multiple outcomes rather than a single outcome. Regression methods are basically inappropriate for the study of the production of multiple outcomes (Hanushek 1979, Brown and Sacks 1980). A single outcome measure may be derived from prior weighting of separate outcome measures, but such weighting may be arbitrary. This difficulty has been addressed in work in the single-equation tradition through the use of canonical regression methods (Gyimah-Brempong and Gyampong 1991) and appears to be promising.

In a manner typical of organizations in the public sector, schools and other educational units produce multiple outputs using a range of inputs. Carrying out an assessment of the performance of such entities requires a measurement of the efficiency with which these entities use their resources in producing outputs. Schools utilize material resources such as books and equipment, in conjunction with nonmaterial resources, such as teaching and administration, to generate schooling outputs. Efficiency evaluation normally requires an estimate of the best output levels to be compared with actual performance levels. In the case of organizations in the public sector, such evaluations have been difficult. Outputs are often not measurable in ways which would allow for aggregation to a single measure, and production processes are usually not known in the same way that engineering descriptions of production processes in private sector industrial establishments are known and manipulable.

Another limitation in efficiency assessment of public sector organizations resides in the largely nonprice domain in which they operate, making evaluations of social usefulness of specific outputs difficult to achieve. In the case of schools, social usefulness can often be inferred from broad national and local policies, but it is still difficult to weigh each school's outputs in accordance with higher level objectives identified with such policies. This difficulty is therefore inherent in the way such production units are related to higher-order governmental units. Schools could use national and local norms to guide their operations, and much discussion has centered on this mechanism for improving schooling performance. Nonetheless, apart from knowing that in fact they do or do not meet such norms, typical analyses do not provide much guidance as to the reasons for either attainment or nonattainment of such objectives.

One particular problem with such limitations is that production processes are either fixed and nonmanipulable, or are totally unknown. Schooling shows both of these difficulties. For example, some important parts of the production process are fixed either by custom or by some general understanding of what would be minimally necessary. Class size is an obvious case. These issues are important, because such resources are not easily changeable in the short term, and therefore should be combined in the most efficient manner to produce desirable outputs.

Under the above conditions, it would be desirable to discover both efficient production methods and decision-making units. Methodologies to assist in meaningful assessment should allow decision-making units to compare themselves with others that are required to produce similar outputs.

An alternative way of looking at education production processes is to focus on the structure of production rather than simply on the numerical value of resources used in production. In this way, it is possible to identify efficient and inefficient school production technologies, defined in terms of how well resources are combined by individual schools in the production of schooling outputs. Such technologies are discoverable, and identification of efficient technologies should perform a useful service for education managers responsible for producing desirable outcomes as efficiently as possible.

The broad strand of work suggested here concerns the discovery of frontier performance, characterized by a search for efficient schools and other educational decision-making units. It ranks schools ordinally by their level of efficiency by identifying efficient versus inefficient use of resources. More significantly, by its emphasis on how resources are combined in production, such work can lead to the discovery of alternative structural arrangements that result in enhanced output performance even in the absence of increases in school resources.

A robust methodology has been applied to the problem of public sector evaluation, and even in comparing productive efficiency between public and private organizations. The technologies have also been used to evaluate productive efficiency in public education (Bessent et al. 1982, Bessent et al. 1983, Barrow 1991, Jesson et al. 1987).

6. Data Envelopment Analysis

Data envelopment analysis (DEA) is described in earlier work by Charnes et al. (1978), Banker et al. (1984) and by Bessent et al. (1988). A bibliography lists several hundred theoretical and applied works (Seiford 1989). Exhaustive reporting on the DEA model is therefore well beyond the limits of this entry. What is intended here is an explanation of DEA's potential in the analysis of school performance. Graphic illustrations of the analytic method may promote understanding of the analytic techniques. Algebraic formulations and applications are also available in the literature cited that illustrate the potential of the technique for analysis and diagnosis.

At any one time, individual school units are not likely to be operating with the same technology, namely the same ratios of inputs per unit of output. This condition may not so much reflect a disregard by managers for discovering optimal input/output relationships, as point up the fact that in nonprice domains, such as those in which public schools operate, these optimal ratios are not discoverable by ordinary means. Thus production functions and, therefore, efficiency levels are likely to vary from one school to another, with nothing preventing those variances from being fairly wide. In other words, resources are not necessarily utilized efficiently in combination with each other in each individual school.

Economists define "efficient production" in terms of the conditions of Pareto optimality which state that efficiency in production has not been reached if it is possible to increase output(s) without increasing any single input or subset of inputs. On the input side, a decision-making unit is not operating efficiently if it is possible to maintain outputs while decreasing any

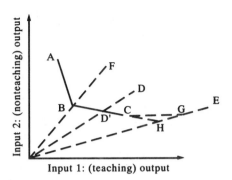

Figure 1
Geometric representation of DEA

single input and not increasing any other input. When considering operations on inputs and outputs, efficiency is attained if and only if both of these conditions do not obtain (Charnes et al. 1981).

Inefficient use of resources means that changes in input levels will not necessarily raise output levels commensurately. In principle, however, DEA points the way to improve efficiency by identifying efficient units and technologies.

7. The DEA Model

The geometric formulation in Fig. 1 of the DEA model shows its properties and utility in the case of a single output and two inputs. The algebraic statement of the

$$\text{Max: } h_k = \frac{\sum_{r=1}^{s} (u_{rk} y_{rk})}{\sum_{i=1}^{m} (v_{ik} x_{ik})} \qquad \begin{array}{l} r = 1, \ldots, s \text{ (outputs)} \\ \\ i = 1, \ldots, m \text{ (inputs)} \end{array}$$

$$\text{S. T. } \frac{\sum u_{rk} y_{rj}}{\sum v_{ik} x_{ij}} \leq 1, j = 1, \ldots n \text{ (dmu's)}$$

$$u_{rk} \geq \epsilon > 0, r = 1, \ldots, s$$

$$v_{ik} \geq \epsilon > 0, i = 1, \ldots, m$$

Figure 2
Algebraic representation of the DEA problem[a]

a Several formulations of the basic DEA model exist in the literature. The equation in Figure 2 is the most transparent form. It seeks the maximization of the ratio of weighted outputs to weighted inputs for each decision-making unit (here a school), subject to the condition that when the derived weights are used for all decision-making units, the ratio of weighted outputs to weighted inputs cannot be greater than unity. The geometric representation given in Fig. 1 is really the dual, in mathematical programming language, of an algebraically transformed Fig. 2 equation.

DEA problem (Fig. 2), generalizes to any number inputs and outputs (see Charnes et al. 1981).

Figure 1 is the geometric representation of a simple DEA problem, one with six schools, each one producing a single output with two inputs, teaching and administrative resources. The axes define input/output space in normalized inputs (per unit of output). The managers of each school are presumed to be attempting to use resources as efficiently as possible, but may not know how other schools use scarce resources. On the basis of actual output levels and known resource availabilities, each school can be located in input/output space for the two inputs.

Figure 1 presents the mathematical programming problem of minimizing input per unit of output. Maximizing output per unit of input is an equivalent way of stating the same decision objective by exploiting the duality relationships of mathematical programming.

Since each school tries to use its resources economically, those schools that in fact have the lowest ratios of inputs to output are by definition the most efficient ones. In Fig. 1, schools A, B, and C can be seen to be efficient. To illustrate, lines are drawn to join school A to school B and school B to school C. The line ABC represents the efficient set of schools and their efficient technologies for producing the single output. Schools F, D, and E all achieve their respective output levels with greater amounts of resource use than is the case with schools A, B, and C. In DEA terminology, schools A, B, and C are efficient, and schools D, E, and F are less than fully efficient. An important benefit of the DEA approach can now be demonstrated since it is possible to calculate precisely the degree of inefficiency of schools F, D, and E.

For example, D's efficiency (or lack of it) can be measured by taking the ratio of OD' to OD. Clearly this ratio is less than unity, which it would be if D were in fact efficient. Since all units on the line ABC are efficient, they form the reference units for the evaluation of inefficient or enveloped schools like D, which in this case is related to its reference school D'.

With respect to school D, it is instructive to note the relationship of the line BC to its evaluation regarding efficiency. Clearly D uses the same ratio of normalized inputs to outputs as reference unit D' which is on the line BC. Since all points on BC can be expressed as linear combinations of the coordinates of the points B and C, D's efficiency can be evaluated using those coordinate values in conjunction with values to be derived from the solution of the implied mathematical programming problem for that unit D. A straightforward statement of the problem in algebraic terms is presented below.

The line from the origin to school F does not cut a line segment but can be related naturally to both of the efficient line segments AB and BC. School E is clearly inefficient and its level of inefficiency must be calculated by other means since line OE does not cut any part of ABC. Schools F and D are enveloped by schools *A*, *B*, and *C* while school *E* is not naturally enveloped by any of the efficient schools.

The fact that unit *E* is not naturally enveloped suggests the need to construct facets with which it could be evaluated for efficiency purposes. Charnes et al. (1978) suggest the construction of a fictitious school *G* which differs from a rightward (horizontal) extension of *C* by an arbitrarily small amount, while Bessent et al. (1988) construct their fictitious school from the extension of the facet *BC* to *OE*. The unit *G* is used by Bessent et al. (1988) to identify upper bounds for *E*, while unit *H* is used to identify the greatest lower bound for such an evaluation. For units that are not naturally enveloped then, upper and lower bounds are computed and become part of the output from the efficiency analysis. The case of the not-naturally enveloped schools turns out to be empirically more the rule than the exception, making this extension of the original DEA model an important one (Bessent et al. 1988).

It should be pointed out that the efficiency concept utilized here is that of technical efficiency. Schools that are evaluated using this methodology are evaluated only on the degree to which they achieve desirable weighted inputs-to-weighted-outputs in natural terms, not in value terms.

Returning to the example, each of the schools *A*, *B*, *C*, *D*, *E*, *F* can be associated with a measure of technical efficiency depending on whether it is on the efficient frontier *ABC* or not. Efficiency levels are constrained to lie within the range from zero to unity with schools on the frontier having levels of efficiency of unity, with those not on the frontier having efficiency levels of less than unity.

It is important to note that the derived indexes of efficiency are measured relative to the reference set. Therefore, a change in the reference set is likely to result in a change in the derived set of efficiency measures. In other words, the efficiency measures derived are interpretable only in the context of the reference set used to derive them. Accordingly, the derived measures of efficiency have greatest evaluative significance in analyzing comparable units.

8. Education Policy Options

Data envelopment analysis has proven to be extremely useful in the assessment of comparable public sector organizations. It has also been found to be a superior assessment tool in situations where the relevant organizational units produce a range of outputs using several resources. As a model for studying school accountability, it has substantial appeal since it now becomes possible simultaneously to include in the usual resource sets facing schools—teacher, administration, and other nonteaching resources—the effects of socioeconomic conditions which are known to have decisive impact on school performance.

The usefulness of DEA in studying changes over time occurring among a set of comparable institutions should also be noted. Over time, the efficient frontier of a set of comparable organizations is likely to change. It should be of some interest to see how the frontier changes by observing which schools, for example, remain efficient from year to year, and which do not. This particular use of DEA highlights the additional potential for combining quantitative assessment with qualitative ones since it is likely that deep understanding of changes over time will require bringing together qualitative and quantitative insights.

The literature cited contains examples of the above applications of data envelopment analysis to public school performance. At the time of writing this entry, the authors are studying Chicago public school performance using the technique in conjunction with qualitative assessments.

9. Conclusion

Throughout the world, citizens, politicians, and policymakers expect more from schools. Data envelopment analysis can show how their expectations might be more fully realized. Making educational goals clear and measurable, setting priorities for their attainment, studying what optimized them effectively and efficiently, implementing systemic solutions, and carefully evaluating progress—these are the major activities that can contribute to effectiveness and efficiency under the DEA framework. They might play a large role in improving educational productivity.

References

Banker R D, Charnes A, Cooper W W 1984 Some models for estimating technical and scale inefficiencies in data envelopment analysis. *Management Science* 30 (7): 1078–92

Barrow M 1991 Measuring local educational authority performance: A frontier approach. *Econ. Educ. Rev.* 10(1): 19–27

Bessent A, Bessent E W, Kennington T, Reagan B 1982 An application of mathematical programming to assess managerial efficiency in the Houston independent school district. *Management Science* 28(12): 1355–67

Bessent A, Bessent W, Charnes A, Cooper W W, Thorgood N. 1983 Evaluation of educational program proposals by means of data envelopment analysis. *Educ. Admin. Q.* 19(2): 82–107

Bessent A, Bessent W, Elam J, Clark T 1988 Efficiency frontier determination by constrained facet analysis. *Operations Research* 36(5): 785–86

Bridge R, Judd C, Moock P 1979 *The Determinants of Educational Outcomes. The Impact of Families, Peers, Teachers, and Schools.* Ballinger, Cambridge, Massachusetts

Brown B W, Saks D H 1980 Production technologies and resource allocation within classrooms and schools. Theory and measurement. In: Dreeben R, Thomas J A (eds.)

1980 *The Analysis of Educational Productivity*, vol 1. Ballinger, Cambridge, Massachusetts

Charnes A, Cooper W W, Rhodes E 1978 Measuring the efficiency of decision making units. *European Journal of Operational Research* 2(6): 429–44

Charnes A, Cooper W W, Rhodes E 1981 Evaluating program and managerial efficiency. *Management Science*, 27(6): 668–97

Gyimah-Brempong K, Gyampong A O 1991 Characteristics of education production functions: An application of canonical regression analysis. *Econ. Educ. Rev.*, 10(1): 7–17

Hanushek E A 1979 Conceptual and empirical issues in the estimation of educational production functions. *Journal of Human Resources* 14(3): 351–88

Hanushek E 1986 The economics of schooling: Production and efficiency in public schools. *J. Econ. Lit*, 24(3): 1141–77

Jesson D, Mayston D, Smith P 1987 Performance assessment in the education sector: Educational and economic perspectives. *Oxford Rev. Educ.* 13(3): 249–66

Johnson R, Lewin A Y 1984 Management and accountability models of public sector performance. In: Miller T (ed.) 1984 *Public Sector Performance: A Conceptual Turning Point*. Johns Hopkins University Press, Baltimore, Maryland

Lau L 1979 Educational production functions. In: Windham D (ed.) 1979 *Economic Dimensions of Education*. Report of a Committee of the National Committee of the National Academy of Education, Washington, DC

Miller T 1985 Structure based changes in performance: The proper focus for social science. Paper presented at the Association for Public Policy and Management Conference

Seiford L M 1989 *A Bibliography of Data Envelopment Analysis (1978–1989) Version 4*. Department of Industrial Engineering and Operations Research, the University of Massachusetts, Amherst, Massachusetts

Wagstaff A 1989 Estimating efficiency in the hospital sector: A comparison of three statistical cost frontier models. *Appl. Econ.* 21(5): 659–72

Walberg H J 1986 Syntheses of research on teaching. In: Wittrock M C (reflx) 1986 *Handbook of Research on Teaching*, 3rd edn. Macmillan, New York

Discriminant Analysis

P. R. Lohnes

Discriminant analysis is the special case of regression analysis which is encountered when the dependent variable is nominal (i.e., a classification variable, sometimes called a taxonomic variable). In this case, either a single linear function of a set of measurements which best separates two groups is desired, or two or more linear functions which best separate three or more groups are desired. In the two-group application, the discriminant analysis is a special case of multiple regression, and in those applications where the criterion variable identifies memberships in three or more groups, the multiple discriminant analysis is a special case of canonical regression. However, because of its focus upon the parsimonious description of differences among groups in a measurement space, it is useful to develop the algebra of discriminant analysis separately from that of regression, and to have computer programs for discriminant analysis which are rather different in their printouts from general regression programs.

1. Aspects and History

Discriminant analysis has had its earliest and most widespread educational research applications in the areas of vocational and career development. Because education prepares people for a variety of positions in the occupational structures prevalent in their societies, an important class of educational research studies is concerned with the testing of theories about the causes of occupational placements and/or the estimation of prediction equations for allocating positions or anticipating such allocations. This research is characterized by criteria which are taxonomies of occupations or other placements, and predictors which are traits of the individuals who have been sampled from the cells of the taxonomy. Thus there are many independent variables which can be taken as approximately multivariate normal in distribution, and a dependent variable which is a nominal identifier of the cells of a taxonomy (or the populations in a universe). The resulting discriminant analysis design may be thought of as a reverse of the simple one-way "MANOVA" (multivariate analysis of variance) design.

Where MANOVA assumes a nominal independent variable and a multivariate normal dependent vector variable, discriminant analysis assumes a multivariate normal independent vector variable and a nominal dependent variable. Both methods share the assumption of equal measurement dispersions (variance–covariance structures) for the populations under study, so that much of the statistical inference theory of MANOVA is applicable to the discriminant design, especially the significance tests provided by Wilks' Λ, Pillai's V, Roy's θ, and the Lawley–Hotelling U statistics (Tatsuoka 1971 pp. 164–68, Timm 1975 pp. 369–82). There is also a formal equivalence of discriminant analysis to the canonical correlation design with dummy variates representing group memberships (Tatsuoka 1971 pp. 177–83). Discriminant analysis is also closely related to the statistical literature on the classification problem, since a discriminant space may be optimal for classification decisions in some situations (Rulon et al. 1967 pp. 299–319, 339–41). However, a good discriminant program will report interpretive results which will not be obtained from a canonical correlation program, and modern computers so easily compute classifications in original measurement spaces of very large dimensionality that the reduction in dimensionality provided by a discriminant space no longer has great utility when the emphasis is on classification.

Discriminant analysis serves primarily to provide insight into how groups differ in an elaborate measurement space. It is most useful when the number of measurement variates is so large that it is difficult for the human mind to comprehend the differentiation of the groups described by a table of means. Usually it will be found that the major differences can be captured by projecting the group means onto a small number of best discriminant functions, so that an economical model of group differences is constructed as an aid to understanding. Often the discriminant functions will be theoretically interpretable as latent dimensions of the manifest variates. It is even possible to make a rotation of the discriminant dimensions to more interpretable locations, once the best discriminant hyperplane has been located. Thus the goals and procedures are not unlike those of factor analysis.

Barnard (1935) seems to have been the first to describe the discrimininant problem clearly. She wanted to classify Egyptian skulls into four dynasties on the basis of four measurements, which was so definitely a discriminant problem that Rao (1952) and Williams (1959) presented her results in their texts. Barnard had the problem but not the optimal solution, as she regressed a single time-line comparison of the skulls on the four measurements, thus making a standard multiple regression. Rao commented:

> Barnard maximized the ratio of the square of unweighted regression of the compound with time. It is doubtful whether such a linear compound can be used to specify an individual skull most effectively with respect to progressive changes, since linear regression with times do not adequately explain all the differences in the four series. (Rao 1952 p. 271)

Fisher (1937) provided the appropriate criterion to be maximized by a discriminant function, as equal to the ratio of the between-groups sum of squares to the pooled within-groups sum of squares on the function. He treated only the two-group case, for which weights which maximize λ depend only on the inverse of the pooled within-group dispersion and can be found by regression. His example used four measurements on 50 flowers from each of two species of iris, and is reproduced in the text by Kendall (1957). Tatsuoka

(1971 pp. 170–77) gives an outstanding treatment of the special two-groups case.

Bartlett (1938) was the first to develop the multiple groups generalization of discriminant analysis. "If the 'most predictable criterion' were to be used as a discriminant function," said Bartlett (1938 p. 36), it would be possible to maximize λ more than once when there were three or more criterion groups, using dummy-coded variates to represent the group membership information. He stated with great clarity and elegance the application of Hotelling's 1935 invention of the canonical correlation method to the multiple discriminant problem. He showed that if there are g groups and p measurements the number of nonzero λs must be the lesser of $g-1$ and p, and for each nonzero λ the corresponding canonical variable of the measurements is a discriminant function. He had no doubt that the desired discriminant functions should be uncorrelated and should span a hyperplane of minimum dimensionality to get the job done. In this time when there is so much hard sell for modeling methods that encourage the use of correlated latent variables, it may be well to consider the motives of the great pioneers, including Pearson, Fisher, Hotelling, and Bartlett, who assumed that well-constructed variables should be uncorrelated among themselves. Bartlett's (1938) paper deserves to be reprinted and read widely as a classic argument for parsimonious and mathematically disciplined modeling methods.

Hotelling's and Bartlett's inventions were destined to lie fallow for two decades for lack of computing machinery capable of evaluating the eigenstructures requiring numerical analysis in most practical applications of canonical and discriminant methods. In the interim there was one more major theoretical invention. Rao and Slater (1949) developed the algebra to generalize Fisher's criterion directly from the customary MANOVA accumulations matrices, rather than by using dummy variates in canonical regression. Since the Rao and Slater algebra is now accepted standard algebra for presenting the mathematics of discriminant analysis, it is reviewed in the next section of this entry. Rao and Slater also originated the mapping of the group centroids in the best discriminant plane which has become the standard display of the model for the data, and is illustrated in the example provided later in this entry, as Fig. 1. Strangely, Rao (1952) did not choose to incorporate these developments in his great pioneering textbook, but instead concentrated on the alternative device of using one classification discriminant function for each group, based only on the inverse of the pooled within-groups dispersion. He did reproduce the Rao and Slater (1949) demonstration of this approach (Rao 1952 pp. 307–29). Anderson (1958) also confined his treatment to classification discriminant functions, while Williams (1959) presented only the Barnard-type generalization to an arranged linear placement of the several groups which is then regressed upon the measurements. Rao's classification discriminant functions are mutually intercorrelated, and while they provide an efficient classification rule they do not provide an elegant and parsimonious descriptive model for the differences among the groups. Kendall seems to have provided the first textbook treatment of Rao and Slater's generalization of Fisher's λ to the multiple discriminants method. Kendall said vividly, "If (the means) are collinear, one discriminator is sufficient; if they are coplanar two are required; and so on" (1957 p. 169).

Perhaps Rao and Anderson ignored the multiple discriminants method in their texts because it is not essentially a statistical method. The interesting statistical issues are subsumed under MANOVA and classification. Discriminant analysis is essentially mathematical and geometric modeling of data on group differences. The model provided is a spatial one. The researcher's decisions about the rank of the model (i.e., the number of discriminant dimensions) and the naming and interpretation of the dimensions, which are so critical to the meanings produced, are based more on theoretical or practical considerations than statistical ones. The special value of the discriminant analysis is heuristic, and as Kendall perceived, in this it "links up with component and canonical correlation analysis and our various topics are to be seen as different aspects of the same fundamental structure" (1957 p. 169). The difference is that discriminant and canonical analyses involve regression structures which are not viewed by principal components.

2. Mathematics

Let

$$\bar{x}_j = \bar{X}_j - \bar{X} \quad (j = 1, 2, \ldots, g) \tag{1}$$

where g is the number of populations sampled (i.e., the number of groups), so that x_j is the vector of deviations of the jth sample means from the grand means

$$y_j = V' \bar{x}_j \tag{2}$$

is the desired discriminant model for the centroids, transforming the centroids into discriminant space. The necessary rank of y is the lesser of p (the number of variates in the measurement vector X) and $g - 1$, but often n (the rank of y) will be even smaller by choice of the analyst. Thus the desired transformation matrix V is a $p \times n$ matrix, each column of which contains the discriminant function weights for one of the functions v_r ($r = 1, 2, \ldots n$). Fisher's (1937) criterion for v_r is

$$\lambda_r = (v_r' \, B \, v_r)/(v_r' \, W \, v_r)|\text{max} \tag{3}$$

where

$$B = \sum_{j=1}^{g} N_j \, \bar{x}_j \, \bar{x}_j' \tag{4}$$

and

$$W = \sum_{j=1}^{g} \sum_{i=1}^{N_j} (X_{ji} - \bar{X}_j)(X_{ji} - \bar{X}_j)' \tag{5}$$

making B the between-groups matrix and W the within-groups matrix. Underlying assumptions are that the populations are multivariate normal with a common dispersion Δ estimated by

$$D_w = W/(N - g) \tag{6}$$

where

$$N = \sum_{j=1}^{g} N_k \tag{7}$$

making N the total sample size. Thus by assumption information about population differences is concentrated in the centroids.

The required maxima are provided by the eigenvalues and eigenvectors of

$$(W^{-1} \, B - \lambda I)v = 0 \tag{8}$$

The resulting discriminant functions are uncorrelated among themselves, but when the column eigenvectors associated with the nonzero eigenvalues are placed in V, V is not column-orthogonal. Tatsuoka (1971 p. 169) shows the angle between two discriminant dimensions has cosine equal to $v_r v_r / v_s$, and he remarks that the discriminants are an oblique rotation of the principal components of X (p. 163).

Since $W^{-1}B$ is nonsymmetric, the numerical analysis of its eigenstructure is complicated. In 1962 Cooley and Lohnes published a practical discriminant analysis program supported by a subroutine called DIRNM (*di*agonalize a *r*eal *n*onsymmetric *m*atrix) which facilitated computation of the eigenstructure of $W^{-1}A$. The DIRNM subroutine lies at the heart of the improved programs for discriminant and canonical analyses that they published later (Cooley and Lohnes 1971 pp. 192–98, 258–60).

The discriminant functions can be scaled to unit standard deviation for the total sample by creating the matrix $T = B + W$ and the matrix $D = T/(N-1)$, then defining the discriminant factors as

$$f_{ji} = (V'DV)^{-\frac{1}{2}}V'X_{ji} \tag{9}$$

$$= C' \, X_{ji} \tag{10}$$

Then

$$S = DC \tag{11}$$

is the very useful matrix of factor structure coefficients (i.e., correlations of the original variates with the discriminant functions). Users wishing to scale the functions to unit variance within groups may substitute D_w in Eqn. (9) and Eqn. (11).

Choice of scale for a discriminant function is arbitrary, since the weights are determined only with regard to their proportionality to each other. Williams (1959 p. 177) suggested that it would be useful to set the variance for the total sample to unity, in order that the pooled-within-groups variance on the discriminant function would decrease as further efficient predictors were added to the measurement vector. The complement of this pooled-within-groups variance provides a useful index of the discriminating power of the function which is both the correlation ratio for the function and the squared canonical correlation coefficient between the discriminant function and the implicit canonical function of the group-identifying dummy variates. This excellent statistic is calculable as

$$R_r^2 = \lambda_r / (1 + \lambda_r) \tag{12}$$

Cooley and Lohnes liked this argument and scaled the discriminant functions produced by their program this way, so that this convention is represented by the example of the next section, and by Fig. 1. Others have argued that the appropriate scaling would set the pooled-within-groups variance to unity, so that the plot of the group centroids in a discriminant plane would display the distances among groups in units of within-groups standard deviation. Isofrequency contours could then be drawn around centroids as circles. Since the model is on the means and is a spatial model, the argument for facilitating the interpretation of distances among centroids is a good one. Bock (1975 p. 405) provides a strong statement of the case for scaling so that the within-groups variance is unity.

Bock (1975) text is especially strong on interpretation of discriminant functions. It asserts that discriminants are most useful when the many measurements available are low in reliabilities and factorially complex in validities. "Working with linear combinations of these variables tends to reduce variation due to measurement error and to enhance the effect of latent sources of variation common to two or more variables" (p. 416). Bock distinguishes between the case where a new measurement increases the reliability of a discriminant function and the case where it sponsors an additional dimension of discrimination. His examples illustrate collinearity of centroids, bipolarity of functions, and suppressor variables. Bock asserts that discriminant functions may be difficult to interpret "until

the results of a number of independent studies utilizing the same set of variables become available" (p. 416). This is so, but it would also be helpful if authors of reviews of research would be alert for the appearance of substantially the same discriminant functions in studies using different mixes of measurements. More research studies should be undertaken in which previously discovered discriminant functions are moved intact to new samples. Many years ago Bartlett remarked about discriminants fitted by Hotelling's method to one sample, that "if a function suitable for discriminating species or groups were so devised, any subsequent use *on further data* would simply conform to orthodox analysis-of-variance lines" (1938 pp. 37–8).

3. Example

Cooley and Lohnes remark that the best discriminant plane is very often an adequate model for the data (1971 p. 244). The resulting reduction in rank, or simplification of the measurement basis, is perhaps the most attractive aspect of discriminant research strategy. In their Project TALENT research study, they found that approximately the same discriminant plane was discovered in a series of 14 analyses using different samples and different taxonomic criteria but a common measurement basis (Cooley and Lohnes 1968 pp. 5–8). One of their analyses can provide an example for this entry.

The current career plans of 9,322 young men were collected by questionnaire 5 years after they left high school. These plans were classified into 12 categories of a careers taxonomy. Table 1 lists the 12 categories, with an acronym for each, and the subsample count. Six years earlier, when they were high school seniors, these men had taken a battery of 60 ability tests and 38 typical performance scales. Lohnes (1966) created a factor analytic solution for these two batteries, and the measurement basis for the discriminant analysis was

Table 1
Career plan groups

Acronym	Group name	Sample size
MED	Medicine and PhD Biology	279
BIO	Medicine and Biology below MD and PhD	438
RES	Physical Science and Mathematics PhD	221
ENG	Physical Science and Engineering MS and BS	939
TEC	Technical worker	1,297
LBR	Laborer with no post-high school training	706
CLK	Office worker with no post-high school training	530
ACT	Accountants and other trained nontechnical	1,430
BUS	Business BA and BS	1,214
MGT	Management post-baccalaureate training	270
WEL	Sociocultural MA and BA	1,183
PRF	Sociocultural research degree	815

Table 2
Discriminant functions

MAP Measurement basics	Discriminant	
	Science-oriented scholasticism	Technical vs. sociocultural
Abilities	$R_c = 0.69$	$R_c = 0.37$
Verbal knowledge	0.62	0.20
Perceptual speed and accuracy	0.02	0.10
Mathematics	0.73	−0.49
Hunting-fishing	−0.10	−0.26
English	0.28	0.23
Visual reasoning	−0.01	−0.43
Color and foods	0.08	0.10
Etiquette	0.05	0.07
Memory	0.00	0.01
Screening	−0.33	−0.25
Games	0.10	−0.05
Motives		
Business interests	−0.04	0.31
Conformity needs	0.21	0.12
Scholasticism	0.78	−0.19
Outdoors and shop interests	−0.41	−0.42
Cultural interests	0.25	0.47
Activity level	−0.22	−0.10
Impulsion	−0.01	0.08
Science interests	0.54	−0.36
Sociability	−0.19	0.47
Leadership	0.28	0.22
Introspection	−0.06	−0.03

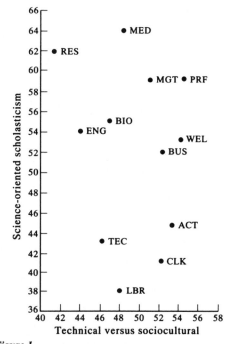

Figure 1
Group centroids in discriminant space

his 22 MAP factors. Table 2 lists these 22 factors and locates the two best discriminant functions by their correlations with the 22 scales of the measurement basis. The major discriminant function, called "science-oriented scholasticism," is oriented toward mathematics and verbal abilities, and scholastic and science interests. The minor discriminant factor is bipolar, contrasting technical abilities and interests with sociocultural abilities. Figure 1 maps the 12 group centroids on this plane. Note how it separates the laborer and office workers from the medical and research doctorates.

See also: Canonical Analysis; Regression Analysis of Quantified Data

References

Anderson T W 1958 *An Introduction to Multivariate Statistical Analysis.* Wiley, New York

Barnard M M 1935 The secular variations of skull characters in four series of Egyptian skulls. *Ann. Eugenics* 6: 352–71

Bartlett M S 1938 Further aspects of the theory of multiple regression. *Proc. Cambridge Philos. Soc.* 34(1): 33–40

Bock R D 1975 *Multivariate Statistical Methods in Behavioral Research.* McGraw-Hill, New York

Cooley W W, Lohnes P R 1968 *Predicting Development of Young Adults: Project TALENT Five-year Follow-up Studies.*

Interim Report 5. American Institutes for Research, Palo Alto, California

Cooley W W, Lohnes P R 1971 *Multivariate Data Analysis*. Wiley, New York

Fisher R A 1937 The use of multiple measurements in taxonomic problems. *Ann. Eugenics* 7: 179–88

Kendall M G 1957 *A Course in Multivariate Analysis*. Griffin, London

Lohnes P R 1966 *Measuring Adolescent Personality: Project TALENT Five-year Follow-up Studies. Interim Report 1*. American Institute for Research, University of Pittsburgh, Pittsburgh, Pennsylvania

Rao C R 1952 *Advanced Statistical Methods in Biometric Research*. Wiley, New York

Rao C R, Slater P 1949 Multivariate analysis applied to differences between neurotic groups. *Br. J. Psychol.* Statistical Section 2(1): 17–29

Rulon P J, Tiedeman D V, Tatsuoka M M, Langmuir C R 1967 *Multivariate Statistics for Personnel Classification*. Wiley, New York

Tatsuoka M M 1971 *Multivariate Analysis: Techniques for Educational and Psychological Research*. Wiley, New York

Timm N H 1975 *Multivariate Analysis with Application in Education and Psychology*. Brooks/Cole, Montery, California

Williams E J 1959 *Regression Analysis*. Wiley, New York

Further Reading

Mueller R O, Cozad J B 1988 Standardized discriminant coefficients: Which variance estimate is appropriate? *J. Educ. Stat.* 13(4): 313–18

Nordlund D J, Nagel R N 1991 Standardized discriminant coefficients revisited. *J. Educ. Stat.* 16(2): 101–08

Effects: Moderating, Mediating, and Reciprocal

A. Russell

This entry discusses two fundamental aspects of educational and psychological research, namely prediction and explanation. It does so through an examination of moderating and mediating effects. The aim is to clarify and illustrate the moderator–mediator distinction and show its importance for psychological and educational research. In addition, it considers some theoretical and data analysis issues associated with attempts to examine such effects. Special attention is given to issues associated with the use of path analysis as the procedure for examining mediating effects. It is shown that while it is comparatively straightforward to demonstrate moderator effects, mediator effects are more complex, if the aim is to discover actual causal mechanisms.

Prediction and explanation "have acquired a variety of meanings and usages, resulting in ambiguities and controversies" (Pedhazur 1982 p. 135). To an extent, the distinction between explanation and prediction is a matter of degree rather than kind as explanation generally enables prediction, and prediction—for instance, in noting that one event (event A) is commonly followed by another event (event B)—might be said to provide an explanation in the sense that event A could be argued as a cause of event B (Nowak 1976). In general, however, it has become customary to argue that prediction involves knowing no more than that two, or more, variables are related, so that given the value or level of one variable (the predictor) it is possible to predict the value or level of another variable (the criterion). For example, learning performance (the criterion) might be related to the size of the class. From this, researchers or educational practitioners could predict what learning outcomes might be expected given knowledge of class size. In a similar exercise, parents might be able to predict what outcomes would occur if they used a given childrearing practice, such as authoritative parenting, from knowledge of the association between childrearing styles and child outcomes. In another example, clinicians may be interested in knowing that nonsynchrony in parent–child interactions predicts conduct disorders in children.

Predictions can be made more specific through the identification of moderating effects. For example, if it is found that the effect of class size differs according to the teaching method used, then the teaching method moderates (changes) the relationships between class size and student learning. Or, the link between nonsynchrony and child conduct disorders may be stronger for children with difficult temperaments. The more moderator effects that can be identified, the more precise the prediction. In each of these cases of prediction, it can be seen that the reasons for the effects occurring does not matter. It does not necessarily matter, for example, what occurs within classes of various sizes that leads to different outcomes. For prediction, it is necessary to know only something about the strength of association between variables, not about how or why the variables are linked. Moderating effects are critical to prediction because they make such predictions more specific and hence accurate. While moderating effects imply differences in causes or processes operating, they do not identify these processes. This is where mediating effects become relevant.

Enhanced prediction does not necessarily yield explanations for the outcome if explanation is seen as requiring information on the causal mechanisms involved in producing the effects. Knowing, for instance, that authoritative parenting produces one set of outcomes for boys and a different set of outcomes for girls does not provide information as to the causal mechanisms or processes that lead to the separate outcomes in boys and girls. Here, what is needed is information on the causal processes occurring within *each sex*. Mediating effects are addressed to this kind of problem, that is, what factors mediate between the input (authoritative parenting) and the outcome for the child. Such mediating effects are important for the explanation of phenomena in education and psychology.

In general, then, mediating effects are aimed more at the identification of actual causal factors leading to the outcome. For example, if some schools are more effective than others, mediating effects attempt to determine what processes occur in different schools that are responsible for the differences in outcomes from schools. If parent–child nonsynchrony predicts conduct disorders in children, it is necessary to know who creates this condition, the parent or the child, and the processes that lead to the establishment of conduct disorders. Overall, then, moderating effects relate more to the enhancement of prediction, and mediating effects more to the task of explanation and the identification of causal processes.

Terminology of one variable "having an influence on," or "affecting" another variable is often used by researchers. Usually, the use of "influence" or "affect" in this way incorporates both moderating and mediating effects, and hence is less precise. For example, a child's attitudes to education, his or her IQ and his or her father's education and occupation may all "influence" the child's educational performance at school. But the notion of influence or affect here is being used loosely, with some of the variables possibly operating more as moderators in the sense of improving prediction, while others may be potential mediators in the sense of being part of causal mechanisms (e.g., the child's attitude to education, which determines how much effort is devoted to study, thereby providing the mediating link between home environment and school performance). The moderator–mediator distinction assists in making clear what kinds of variables are being dealt with. This helps direct not only data analysis strategies, but also an understanding of research findings and hence possibly the world the data are describing.

1. Moderating Effects

A moderating effect occurs when a variable "affects the direction and/or strength of the relation between an independent or predictor variable and a dependent or criterion variable" (Baron and Kenny 1986 p. 1174). Examples of moderating effects were given above. The variable having the moderating effect can be either discrete (such as child sex or family social class) or continuous (such as child IQ or number of years of teaching experience). Moderating effects are shown in correlational studies by differences in zero-order correlations (either in the strength or the direction of the correlation) as a function of the third variable. For example, if the correlation between degree of classroom structure and learning is positive for girls but negative for boys, then child sex moderates the relationship between structure and learning. Alternatively, in a regression analysis, a moderator effect would be shown by a significant difference in the regression coefficients between classroom structure and learning for boys versus girls.

In these examples child sex is selected as the moderator by the researcher, not by the statistical analysis. Which is the primary variable and which the moderator is determined by the focus of the research. If, for instance, the main interest in the research is on the effects of classroom structure, then it is proper to see child sex as the moderator. Equally, however, a researcher may be mainly interested in the effects of child sex on learning in subjects such as reading, mathematics, or science. Here child sex would be seen as the primary variable and classroom structure might moderate the relationship between child sex and learning.

In the case of analysis of variance designs, the moderating effects on an outcome such as student learning is revealed by an interaction between the independent variable (e.g., teaching style) and a moderator such as student anxiety level. Thus, teaching style may affect student learning differently, depending on anxiety level. Again, it needs to be recognized that if the main interest is in the effects of anxiety level, a researcher could show that anxiety level may affect student learning differently, depending on teaching style.

Some properties of a moderating effect are shown in Fig. 1, where there is a predictor (e.g., class size) and a moderator variable (e.g., teaching style). There may be a significant effect of one or both of class size and teaching style on student learning, but a moderating effect occurs when the interaction between class size and

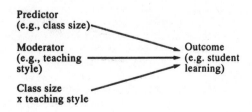

Figure 1
Moderating effects

teaching style is significant (see *Interaction, Detection and its Effects*).

2. Mediating Effects

The nature of mediating effects is given in the following statements: "Whereas moderator variables specify when certain effects will hold, mediators speak to how or why such effects occur" (Baron and Kenny 1986 p. 1176); and " . . . a mediating variable is tested using a path-analytic model" (Quittner et al. 1990 p. 1267). Such path models are usually assumed to depict a causal chain. For instance, in Fig. 2 the independent variable is teaching style and the criterion is student learning. A possible mediator in this situation is time on task. The path model enables a test to be made of whether the principal effects of teaching style on student learning are due to effects of teaching style on time on task, which in turn causes learning. If the effects of teaching style are not mediated by time on task, then in the path model the direct path from teaching to learning would be significant, and the indirect path through time on task would be smaller than the direct path. Alternatively, a comparison of a model with only the direct path with a model containing the mediated path may show that the direct path model provides a better fit for the data. The search for mediators would then need to turn to other possibilities. It can be seen that in the case of the mediating variable here, it is both an effect (of teaching style) and a cause (of learning outcome).

While the path model outlined in Fig. 2 is a good example of testing for mediator variables, it is not the only strategy. For instance, if child sex moderates the relationship between classroom structure and learning outcomes, the issues with a dichotomous moderator such as this would be to determine what mediates between classroom structure and learning outcomes for each sex. This might be done in one of two ways. First, using a correlational design, the researcher could include a range of additional measures such as how boys and girls behave under different conditions of classroom structure, their attitudes to different teaching methods, the behavior of teachers to boys and girls under different levels of classroom structure, and so on. The researcher could then develop different path models for boys and girls in which possible mediating mechanisms were examined in each case.

A second strategy would be to conduct experimental studies testing for the mediating effects of different variables. For example, a researcher might deliberately manipulate the behavior of teachers to boys and girls under different conditions of classroom structure to determine whether changes to teacher behavior were associated with the effects. If, for example, under high structure teachers increased their demands on boys to conform to the tasks set in the curriculum and boys did so conform, and this was associated with better outcomes for boys, then this would indicate that a possible

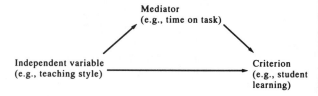

Figure 2
Mediating effects
Note: The path from the independent variable to the criterion estimates the direct effect and the path via the mediator estimates the indirect effect.

causal factor in boys' lower performance under high structure was that they were less inclined to follow instructions and undertake the designated curriculum tasks. Equally, for theoretical reasons the researcher might predict that conformity to the teacher's demands by both boys and girls under high versus low levels of classroom structure is the critical causal mechanism. If observations of boys and girls under different conditions of structure confirmed this, then conformity could be proposed as a mediating variable.

Experimental studies require careful control of the relevant treatment variables and random allocation of subjects to treatments, so that the researcher is sure that any effects that occur are due to the experimental treatment. Because of the demands of such experimental studies, much research in education and psychology is necessarily correlational, based on the measurement of existing or natural conditions. For this reason, the appropriate strategy for the examination of mediating effects is through path analysis. Consequently, it is important to consider the potential and limitations of path analysis as a means of identifying mediating effects, especially because of a tendency to argue that such mediating effects can be taken as revealing causal mechanisms.

3. Path Analysis: Mediating Effects and Causal Processes

There are two main issues associated with the use of path analysis (i.e., LISREL and PLSPATH) in the examination of mediating effects and hence possible causal mechanisms. They are related, and concern whether the path analysis has indeed revealed the mediating effects, and whether these effects can be assumed to constitute causal mechanisms or processes. Together, these issues deal with questions of measurement, data analysis, and theory (see *Path Analysis and Linear Structural Relations Analysis; Path Analysis with Latent Variables*).

While it may be possible to develop a path model that shows statistically that one variable mediates between two other variables, some have claimed that this should be treated in the first instance as no more than a statistical summary of the data. The mediator so identified may not necessarily be assumed as constituting the causal process. For example, a path model may show that time on task mediates between teaching style and student learning, so that it appears that the reason given teaching styles affect learning is because teaching style affects student time on task. With such a causal theory, then increasing time on task should increase learning, because the path model suggests that time on task is the causal process associated with learning.

However, the model in many ways could be said to have provided only a statistical summary of how the variables included in the model are related, without having necessarily established the causal mechanisms. Estimating the magnitude of the indirect effect of teaching style on student learning via time on task (i.e., the role of time on task as a mediating variable) is helpful. It advances understanding of the data and of possible mechanisms involved in the effects of teaching style. The caution needed involves placing too much weight on the finding of a mediating variable as having identified the causal process.

For example, it might be that time on task per se is not the critical causal factor. Rather, the kind of tasks selected by teachers under different teaching styles and the consequent nature of students' engagement with the tasks might be the critical processes. Thus, with certain teaching styles students may spend more time, but more importantly they may see the tasks as more significant, treat the teacher as more knowledgeable, have more positive attitudes to the subject matter, and hence may concentrate more intensely on the academic tasks chosen by the teacher. Thus, while the statistical model suggests that time on task is the causal mediator, it is actually the kind of tasks and the level of student engagement with and concentration on the tasks, not just the amount of time spent on them, that more appropriately could be said to constitute the causal mechanism. Possibilities such as these could, of course, be modeled and tested in subsequent analyses.

There has been some discussion in the literature of the assumption that in revealing mediating effects path analysis is identifying causal processes. Path analysis has often been described as "causal modeling," with an acceptance that path models reveal the "causal processes assumed to operate among the variables under consideration" (Rogosa 1979 p. 266). Steyer (1985), among others (e.g., Freedman 1987, Rogosa 1987), however, points out that path analysis tests only the statistical fit of the model to the data. The analyses "do not test the hypothesis that the model describes the causal mechanisms that generate the data" (Steyer 1985 p. 96). Making a similar point, Freedman (1987 p. 112) said: "A theory of causality is assumed in the path diagram . . . The path analysis does not derive the causal theory from the data, or test any major part of it against the data. Assuming the wrong causal theory

vitiates the statistical calculations." Later he claims that he does "not think there is any reliable methodology in place for identifying the crucial variables in social systems or discovering the functional form of their relationships. In such circumstances, fitting path models is a peculiar research activity: The computer can pass some planes through the data, but cannot bind the arithmetic to the world outside" (p. 120). Rogosa (1987) argues that path models are statistical models and " . . . statistical models may have little substantive meaning or interpretability even when their technical assumptions are satisfied by the data" (p. 186).

This leads to questions about the meaning of "cause" and what is being achieved in path analyses. Many seem to use the "cause" in causal modeling in quite a strong sense, arguing that regression equations or path analyses somehow take us beyond the bidirectional correlation coefficient to indicate causal processes. For example, Cohen and Cohen (1983 p. 353) remark " . . . the simplest regression equation, $Y = BX + A$, is a prototypical causal model with X the causal variable and B the size of its effect. Regression invites causal thinking because, unlike correlation, it is asymmetrical, just as are a cause and its effect" (see *Regression Analysis of Quantified Data*).

Others treat the term "causal" as rather incidental, suggesting that terms such as "process" or "system" modeling might equally well be used (Bentler 1980). Hope (1987) seems to take this kind of view, suggesting that if the path model assists prediction and provides order to complex data it is beneficial, and that there should not be undue concern with so-called "actual causal mechanisms." However, for many researchers, the desire to understand and explain is a more important goal than prediction.

A third alternative is to be critical of any use of "causal" in connection with regression equations or path models (e.g., Freedman 1987, Rogosa 1987). De Leeuw (1985) says: "It is not at all clear if and in how far linear structural models have anything to do with causality" (p. 371). He adds: "I think that the use of causal terminology in connection with linear structural models of the LISREL type means indulging in a modern, but nevertheless clearly recognizable, version of the *post hoc ergo propter hoc* fallacy" (p. 372). This fallacy relates to arguing from mere temporal sequence (one thing occurs in time after another) to cause and effect relationships.

Rogosa sees path model construction as providing parsimonious ways of *describing* correlations in terms of a restrictive model. He and others place most emphasis on the theory or model construction process, and see not enough effort going into model building, conceptual analysis, and understanding. "In most social science situations the true problem is model selection (not necessarily from the LISREL class), and conventional statistical theory has preciously little to say about that problem" (de Leeuw 1985 p. 374).

Hence, from the viewpoint of using path analysis to examine mediational processes, it is true that these models can provide a statistical summary of the relationships among the variables, but much effort has to go into model building and variable selection for one's research if the activity is to be taken as examining causal mechanisms. Even then, if the data are correlational (rather than experimental), Rogosa (1987 p. 193) argues that attempts to answer causal or explanatory questions are "fundamentally askew."

Nevertheless, even the critics see some role for path analysis in the identification of mediating variables and causal processes. For instance, Rogosa (1987) says " . . . path analysis (causal) models may be useful until a field acquires some insights into what's going on and then moves to appropriate models and methods" (p. 186). This suggests a role for path analysis in the testing of hypotheses and in the generation of theory about mediating or causal processes.

4. Bidirectional or Reciprocal Effects

Another difficulty with assuming that by identifying mediating effects in path models causal processes have also been identified is that the path models are generally unidirectional or recursive. Actual causal processes are in many cases unlikely to be only unidirectional. For example, learning performance may affect time on task as well as time on task affecting learning, so that as students master the material they become more involved and more confident with the subject matter, and as a consequence spend more time on task. In the case of Olweus (1980), it was found that mothers' permissiveness of aggressive behavior apparently mediated the effects of boys' temperament on boys' aggression. Presumably, mothers of sons who were more temperamentally difficult were more permissive of aggression. However, it was also likely that reciprocal influence processes existed, so that if boys were more aggressive, mothers were more permissive of aggression. When considered in this light, the relatively simple causal model of the effects of temperament on aggression being mediated by mothers' permissiveness must seriously be questioned. However, such nonrecursive models, whether with simultaneous or longitudinal data, can be tested.

For example, reciprocal (or nonrecursive) effects can be included in path models, with the statistical process requiring estimations of paths in opposite directions (e.g., examining the influence of boys' aggression on mothers' permissiveness of aggression as well as the influence of mothers' permissiveness on boys' aggression). Such reciprocal influences can be estimated in LISREL and in PLS using two stage

least squares. Estimating bidirectional effects is clearly a helpful advance in attempts to identify causal processes. The critics, however, focus again on the limitations of path analysis of the kind already outlined. Noting, for example, that while a path analysis might reveal reciprocal effects among the variables, inferences about the reciprocal effects depend for their validity on the validity of the model on which the analysis was based. This is a somewhat circular dispute, as the validity of the model is also partly assessed through the size and direction of the reciprocal effects shown in the analysis (see *Path Analysis with Latent Variables*).

5. Conclusion

Olweus (1980) provides a useful summary of much of the above argument in claiming "causal relations can never be definitely proven but only inferred, with greater or lesser certainty, on the basis of theoretical considerations and analysis of conditions surrounding the assumed causal connections" (p. 654). This emphasizes the close relationship between theory and data analysis. Bentler (1980) makes a similar point in noting that the application of path analysis would be improved if there were better databases and better substantive theories. The implication is that in most cases where path analyses show mediating variables there is need for caution and the results should be assessed critically in the light of the data used and existing theory. On the other hand, in terms of the potential contribution to the development of such theory, there can be no doubts about the benefits of path analysis. These analytical techniques provoke researchers to make hypotheses about potential causal processes, enable them to assess the strength of the hypotheses, and estimate the magnitude of the postulated effects.

References

Baron R M, Kenny D A 1986 The moderator–mediator variable distinction in social psychological research: Conceptual, strategic, and statistical considerations. *J. Pers. Soc. Psychol.* 51: 1173–82

Bentler P M 1980 Multivariate analysis with latent variables: Causal modeling. *Annu. Rev. Psychol.* 31: 419–56

Cohen J, Cohen P 1983 *Applied Multiple Regression/Correlation Analysis for the Behavioral Sciences*, 2nd edn. Erlbaum, Hillsdale, New Jersey

Freedman D A 1987 As others see us: A case study in path analysis. *J. Ed. Stat.* 12: 101–28

Hope K 1987 Barren theory or petty craft? A response to Professor Freedman. *J. Ed. Stat.* 12(2): 129–47

de Leeuw J 1985 Reviews. *Psychometrika* 50(3): 371–75

Nowak S 1976 *Understanding and Prediction: Essays in the Methodology of Social and Behavioral Theories*. Reidel, Dordrecht

Olweus D 1980 Familial and temperamental determinants of aggressive behavior in adolescent boys: A causal analysis. *Dev. Psychol.* 16: 644–60

Pedhazur E J 1982 *Multiple Regression in Behavioral Research: Explanation and Prediction*, 2nd edn. Holt, Rinehart and Winston, New York

Quittner A L, Glueckauf R L, Jackson D N 1990 Chronic parenting stress: Moderating versus mediating effects of social support. *J. Pers. Soc. Psychol.* 59(6): 1266–78

Rogosa D 1979 Causal models in longitudinal research: Ra-

tionale, formulation, and interpretation. In: Nesselroade J R, Baltes P B (eds.) 1979 *Longitudinal Research in the Study of Behavior and Development*. Academic Press, New York

Rogosa D 1987 Causal models do not support scientific conclusions: A comment in support of Freedman. *J. Ed. Stat.* 12: 185–95

Steyer R 1985 Causal regressive dependencies: An introduction. In: Nesselroade J R, Von Eye A (eds.) 1985 *Individual Development and Social Change: Explanatory Analysis*. Academic Press, Orlando, Florida

Event History Analysis

J. B. Willett and J. D. Singer

An important class of educational research questions contains the words "Whether?" and "When?" Researchers investigating the student career ask, for instance, *whether* a student has mastered an important skill and, if so, *when* that mastery occurred. Alternatively, questions are asked about whether, and when, students are identified as remedial or whether, and when, students drop out of school, begin to smoke, go to college, get pregnant, graduate with a diploma, obtain employment, and so forth. The potential topics are seemingly boundless. Indeed, many similar questions arise when the careers of teachers and administrators are also investigated.

Questions that ask "Whether?" and "When?" are enquiring about the timing and occurrence of critical events in a person's life or career. Unfortunately, such questions can be difficult to answer using familiar statistical techniques because the value of the conceptual outcome—time—may not be known for everyone under study. No matter how long data collection continues, some participants will never experience the target event while the researcher watches: some students will not drop out; some children will not reach the stage of formal operations and some teachers will not quit. These people have "censored" event times.

Censoring creates a dilemma for the analysis of event occurrence: What should be done with the censored cases? Although the researcher knows something about them—if they ever experience the event, they do so after data collection ends—this knowledge is imprecise. However, these cases cannot be ignored because they are usually the "longest-lived" people in the study.

Sound investigation of the occurrence and timing of educational events requires analytic methods that deal evenhandedly with censoring. Biostatisticians have developed such techniques in the service of modeling human lifetimes (Cox 1972). These methods —known variously as "survival analysis," "event his-

tory analysis," or "hazard modeling"—prove valuable in educational research too because they provide a sound mathematical basis for exploring whether, and when, events occur—even in the face of censoring (Singer and Willett 1991, Willett and Singer 1991).

This entry provides a conceptual introduction to survival analysis. First, discrete-time and continuous-time survival analysis are distinguished from one another—a distinction critical for understanding the concepts underpinning the methodology. Second, the hazard and survivor functions—two important quantities that summarize the pattern of event occurrence over time—are defined. Third, statistical models linking the pattern of temporal risk to predictors are introduced. Throughout, comment is made on the practicalities of data analysis and interpretation.

1. Distinguishing Discrete-time and Continuous-time Survival Analysis

When event occurrence is investigated, times-to-event must be measured for everyone in the sample. As the label implies, continuous-time survival analysis requires that these measurements be recorded as continuous data. Discrete-time survival analysis, on the other hand, requires only that the investigator know in which of several discrete time-periods the event of interest occurred. Typically, these intervals may each represent a day, a week, a month, or whatever time-period is prudent for the process under investigation.

This entry begins by describing discrete-time survival analysis because this particular methodology has advantages for educational research. First, discrete-time methods are more appropriate for much event history data collected in educational research because, for logistical and financial reasons, observations are often made in discrete time. Second, discrete-time survival analysis is intuitively more comprehensible than its

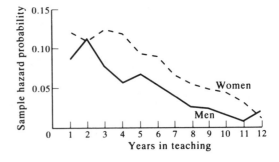

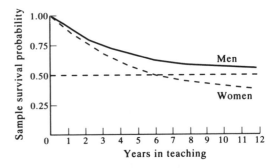

Figure 1
Sample hazard and survival probability plotted against years of teaching completed for 3,941 special educators hired in Michigan, by sex

continuous-time cousin and mastery of its methods facilitates the transition to continuous-time (if required). Third, both "time-invariant" and "time-varying" predictors can easily be included in discrete-time survival analyses, whereas the inclusion of the latter can be more intractable under the continuous-time approach. Fourth, discrete-time survival analysis fosters inspection of how the pattern of risk shapes up over time. The most popular continuous-time survival analysis strategy ("Cox regression"; Cox 1972) ignores the shape of the temporal risk profile entirely in favor of estimating the influence of predictors on risk, under a restrictive assumption of "proportionality." Fifth, under the discrete-time approach, the proportionality assumption is easily checked—and "nonproportional" models fitted. Finally, in discrete-time survival analysis, all statistical analyses can be conducted using standard logistic regression analysis. This avoids reliance on the dedicated computer software that is usually required for continuous-time survival analyses.

2. Introducing the Hazard and Survivor Functions

The "hazard function" and the "survivor function" are two important quantities that summarize and describe the occurrence and timing of critical events. Broadly speaking, estimates of these functions answer the related descriptive questions: When is the event of interest likely to occur? How much time must pass before people are likely to experience the event?

2.1 The Hazard Function

When the occurrence of a specific educational event —such as "leaving teaching"—is examined for a particular group of people—such as "high school science teachers"—then it becomes interesting to examine the pattern of event occurrence over time. It might be asked, for instance, if high school science teachers are more likely to quit teaching in their first year of service than in their second year, or in their third year, and so forth. When such questions are asked the "risks" of event occurrence across time periods are being compared. Knowing how the risk of leaving teaching fluctuates over the years of a high school science teacher's career, for instance, allows research questions about the "Whether?" and "When?" of quitting high school science teaching to be answered.

But what statistic should be computed to summarize these "risks" in the sample, especially in the face of censoring? In discrete-time survival analysis, the fundamental quantity that represents the risk of event occurrence in each time period is the "hazard probability." Its computation in the sample is straightforward: in each time period, identify the pool of people still at "risk" of experiencing the event (the "risk set") and compute the proportion of this group that leaves during the time period. Notice that this definition is inherently "conditional"; once someone has experienced

the event (or been censored) in one time period, he or she no longer qualifies as a member of the risk set on which some future hazard probability is computed (Kalbfleisch and Prentice 1980).

Not only is the hazard probability a substantively meaningful quantity, but the "conditionality" of its definition is critical. It ensures that everyone remains in the risk set until the last time period for which they were available (at which point they are either censored or experience the event of interest). Therefore, by definition, sample hazard probability is a statistic that "deals evenhandedly" with censoring. Consequently, data analyses based on the hazard probability make use of all the information available in the sample event histories. This is why hazard forms the conceptual cornerstone of survival analysis.

Plotting the hazard probabilities against time provides the "hazard function," a chronological summary of the risk of event occurrence. By inspecting the sample hazard function, it is possible to pinpoint when events are most likely to occur. In the top panel of Fig. 1, data describing the careers of 3,941 special educators hired in Michigan in the early 1970s are used to illustrate this (see Singer 1992). The panel presents sample hazard functions, computed separately for men and women, describing the risk of leaving teaching in the first year of teaching, the second year, and so on, up to the twelfth year. Notice that both men and women are most likely to quit teaching during their first few years on the job but, except for the second and twelfth years, women appear to be at greater risk of quitting than men.

2.2 The Survivor Function

In addition to using the hazard function to explore the risks of event occurrence in any given time period, it is useful to cumulate these period-by-period risks into an overall display of the proportion of the original group that "survive" through each time period. The term "survival probability" refers to this proportion, and the term "survivor function" refers to plots arraying the survival probabilities against time. Sample survivor functions provide summaries of the career in aggregate. They are easily computed by cumulating the entries in the sample hazard function over time periods (Willett and Singer 1993).

In the bottom panel of Fig. 1, the survivor function is illustrated. The panel presents sample survivor functions indicating the proportion of the entering cohorts of women and men who "survived" through their first year of teaching, their second year, and so on. The curves slope steeply downward in the beginning and then level off as time passes. When the teachers are newly hired, they are all surviving by definition and the survival probabilities are 1.00. As the career progresses, teachers leave their jobs, and the survivor functions drop. Because not everyone leaves before data collection is over, the curves do not reach zero.

All sample survivor functions have a similar shape —a monotonically nonincreasing function of time. The rate of decline, however, can differ across groups and even small differences in shape can yield large differences in aggregate career duration. For example, although the two sample survivor functions in Fig. 1 have similar shapes, the sharper decline among women suggests that, on average, they leave teaching more readily and consequently have shorter careers.

It is possible to summarize how long the "average" person "survives" before the event of interest occurs by using the sample survivor function to estimate a "median lifetime"—the amount of time that passes until half the sample has experienced the event of interest. In the bottom panel of Fig. 1, for instance, a horizontal dashed line is constructed where the survival probability equals 0.5 and the median lifetimes of men and women special educators are imputed by projection onto the horizontal "Years in Teaching" axis. Notice that the answer is about 6 years for women and over 12 years for men. Because of the censoring— more than half the men are still teaching after 12 years —it is not possible to estimate their median lifetime precisely; but it exceeds 12 years.

3. Detecting Predictors of Event Occurrence and Event Timing

Estimated hazard functions, survivor functions, and median lifetimes describe when (and whether) a group of people is likely to experience a critical event. These descriptive statistics can also be used to answer questions about differences between groups. Do girls become formal operators before boys? Do science teachers tend to quit teaching before teachers of other subject specialties? Are students who were raised in poverty, or by a single parent, more likely to drop out of school?

Each of these examples implicitly uses other characteristics—child gender, teacher subject specialty, poverty, and family status—to predict variation in the risk of event occurrence. When the pair of sample hazard and survivor functions displayed in Fig. 1 are examined, teacher sex is implicitly being treated as a predictor of the career profile. But such descriptive comparisons are limited. How can the effects of continuous predictors using such plots be examined? Is it possible to examine the effects of several predictors simultaneously, or explore statistical interactions among predictors? Can inferences be made about the population from which the sample was drawn? With survival analysis, these queries are answered by fitting and testing statistical models of the hazard function.

3.1 Specifying a Statistical Model for the Hazard Profile

Statistical models of discrete-time hazard express hypothesized population relationships between entire hazard profiles and predictors. To motivate that representation of these models, examine the two sample hazard functions in the top panel of Fig. 1 and imagine teacher gender as the dummy variable, FEMALE, which can take on two values (0 for men, 1 for women). In this case, the entire hazard function is the conceptual "outcome" and FEMALE is a potential "predictor."

How does the predictor affect the outcome? When FEMALE=1, the sample hazard function is "higher" than when FEMALE=0. So conceptually, the predictor FEMALE "shifts" one sample hazard profile vertically relative to the other. A population hazard model formalizes this conceptualization by ascribing the vertical displacement to predictors in much the same way as an ordinary linear regression model ascribes differences in mean levels of any continuous noncensored outcome to predictors.

The difference between a hazard model and a linear regression model is that the entire hazard profile is no ordinary continuous outcome. The discrete-time hazard profile is a set of conditional probabilities, each bounded by 0 and 1. Statisticians modeling a bounded outcome as a linear function of predictors generally transform the outcome so that it is unbounded. This prevents derivation of fitted values that fall outside the range of permissible values—in this case, between 0 and 1. When the outcome is a probability, the "logit" transformation is normally used. If p represents a probability, then *logit (p)* is the natural logarithm of $p/(1-p)$

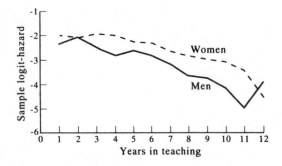

Figure 2
Sample logit-hazard versus years of teaching completed for the special educators in Fig. 1

and, in the case of the teaching career for instance, can be interpreted as the log-odds of leaving teaching (Hanushek and Jackson 1977).

The effect of the logit transformation on a hazard profile is illustrated in Fig. 2, which presents sample logit-hazard functions corresponding to the hazard plots in Fig. 1. The logit transformation has its largest effect on proportions near 0 (or 1), expanding the distance between these small values. In Fig. 2, because the hazard probabilities are small, the logit transformation widens the gap between the two functions, especially in the later years.

Inspection of the sample relationship between the predictor FEMALE and the entire logit-hazard profile in Fig. 2 motivates an appropriate format for population models of hazard as a function of predictors. When FEMALE=1 (for women), the logit-hazard function is higher relative to its location when FEMALE=0, indicating that in every year (except years 2 and 12) women are more likely to leave. So, ignoring any differences in the shapes of the profiles for the moment, the predictor FEMALE essentially displaces the logit-hazard profiles vertically, relative to each other.

Letting $h(t)$ represent the entire population hazard profile, a statistical model that relates the logit transform of $h(t)$ to the predictor FEMALE is:

$$logit\ h(t) = \beta_0(t) + \beta_1\ \text{FEMALE} \qquad (1)$$

The parameter $\beta_0(t)$ is the "baseline logit-hazard profile." It represents the value of the outcome (the entire logit-hazard profile) when FEMALE is zero (i.e., it specifies the profile for men). The baseline is written as $\beta_0(t)$, a function of time, and not as β_0, a single term unrelated to time (as in regression analysis), because the outcome $(logit\ h(t))$ is a temporal profile. The discrete-time hazard model specifies that differences in the value of the predictor "shift" the baseline logit-hazard profile up or down. The "slope" parameter, β_1, captures the magnitude of this shift; it represents the vertical shift in logit-hazard associated with a one unit difference in the predictor. Because the predictor here is a dichotomy, FEMALE, β_1 captures the differential

risk of leaving for women over men. If the model were fitted to the sample data in Fig. 1, the obtained estimate of β_1 would be positive because women are at a greater risk of leaving in every year.

The fitting of discrete-time hazard models provides a flexible approach to investigating educational transitions that attends to both censored and uncensored individuals. Although hazard models appear strange at first, they resemble the more familiar multiple regression models. Hazard models can incorporate several predictors simultaneously, permitting examination of one predictor's effect while controlling statistically for others'. To examine the effect of a teacher's age at hire (AGEHIRED) after controlling for sex, for example, it is necessary to add a second predictor to (1):

$$logit\ h(t) = \beta_0(t) + \beta_1 FEMALE + \beta_2 AGEHIRED \qquad (2)$$

The parameter β_2 assesses the difference in the elevation of the logit-hazard profile for two teachers whose ages are one year apart at hire, controlling for sex. If β_2 were negative, teachers who were older when hired would be less likely to leave in every year of their careers; if β_2 were positive, the reverse would hold.

It is also possible to examine the synergistic effect of several predictors by including statistical interactions in main-effects models, as in multiple regression analysis. Thus it is possible to explore whether the effect of a teacher's age at hire on their risk profile differs by gender by modifying (2):

$$\begin{aligned} logit\ h(t) = \beta_0(t) &+ \beta_1 FEMALE \\ &+ \beta_2 AGEHIRED + \beta_3 (FEMALE \times AGEHIRED) \end{aligned} \qquad (3)$$

and examining an estimate of β_3. By investigating such two-way interactions, Murnane et al. (1991) showed that women who were younger when hired were more likely to leave their teaching jobs than were either older women, or men of any age.

3.2 Including Time-varying Predictors in a Discrete-time Hazard Model

One advantage of hazard models is that they can include time-invariant and time-varying predictors. As befits their label, the former describe immutable characteristics of people, such as their sex or race, while the values of the latter, in contrast, may fluctuate with time, as might a teacher's salary, job assignment, marital status, or job conditions. Time-varying predictors are distinguished by a parenthetical "t" in the variable name.

The inclusion of time-varying salary (in thousands of dollars, corrected for inflation) in (3), for instance, permits asking whether teachers who are paid more are at a lesser risk of leaving teaching:

$$\begin{aligned} logit\ h(t) = \beta_1 FEMALE &+ \beta_2 AGEHIRED \\ &+ \beta_3 (FEMALE \times AGEHIRED) + \beta_4 SALARY(t) \end{aligned} \qquad (4)$$

In Eqn. 4, the logit-hazard profile depends on three

time-invariant, and one time-varying, predictors. In this model, although a teacher's salary fluctuates with time, its per-thousand dollar effect on the risk of leaving teaching is constant over time and is represented by the single parameter β_4. If β_4 is negative, more highly-paid teachers are less likely to leave their jobs. By including time-varying SALARY in their survival analyses, Murnane et al. (1991) show that better-paid teachers stay in the classroom longer.

The ease with which time-varying predictors can be incorporated into hazards models offers educational researchers an innovative analytic opportunity. Many important predictors of educational career paths fluctuate naturally with time. In traditional analyses, such temporal fluctuation has been well-nigh impossible to handle. With the advent of hazard modeling, this is no longer the case.

3.3 Interpreting Fitted Discrete-time Hazard Models

Discussion of methods for estimating the parameters of discrete-time hazard models, evaluating goodness-of-fit, and making inferences about the population is beyond the scope of this entry. In fact, all of these things are easily achieved using standard logistic regression analysis (Allison 1982, Efron 1988, Singer and Willett 1993). Once a hazard model has been fit, however, its parameters can be reported along with standard errors and goodness-of-fit statistics in the same way that the results of multiple regression analyses are reported.

Graphics are very useful for summarizing analytic findings. Just as fitted regression lines can be used to display the influence of important predictors so, too, can fitted survivor and hazard functions be displayed for prototypical people—people who share substantively important values of statistically significant predictors. This is illustrated in Fig. 3, which presents the results of fitting the model posited in (3) to the Michigan special educator data introduced in Fig. 1. In this model, there was a statistically significant interaction of gender and age-at-hire (preliminary analyses suggested that the latter predictor should be recoded as a dichotomy: 0 when teachers were 30 years old or younger when they began teaching, 1 if they were older than 30). Although the first years in teaching are riskiest for everyone, women under 30 are especially likely leave. Young women have an estimated median lifetime of just under 6 years, while the survivor functions for the other 3 groups remain above 50 percent even after 12 years, precluding estimation of precise median lifetimes.

Despite the roundabout path from question to finding, these graphic displays close the analytic circle. The data have been modeled appropriately, fitted hazard and survivor functions at prototypical values of important predictors summarize temporal fluctuations in risk, and the median lifetime statistic, estimated from the fitted survivor functions, summarizes the

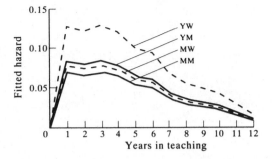

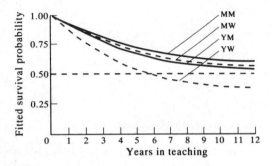

Figure 3
Fitted survivor and hazard functions plotted against years of teaching, for special educators in four demographic groups (young women, young men, mature women, and mature men)

careers of important subgroups in the intuitively meaningful metric of time.

3.4 What if the Effects of the Predictors Change over Time?

When processes evolve dynamically, the effects of both time-invariant and time-varying predictors may fluctuate over time. A predictor whose effect is constant over time has the same impact in all time-periods. A predictor whose effect varies over time can have a different impact on hazard in each time-period. Ironically, time-varying predictors can have time-invariant effects (and vice versa). Consider the effects of salary on the risk of leaving teaching. Salary is a time-varying predictor—its dollar value changes over time—but its *effect* on hazard may be constant over time. For instance, if the effect were time invariant, an extra US$1,000 per year would be an identical inducement whether the teacher were experienced or a novice. If the effect of salary varied over time, in contrast, an extra US$1,000 might have a bigger effect for novices, say.

The discrete-time hazard models posited so far have not permitted a predictor's effect to vary with time; they are called "proportional-odds models." Hazard profiles represented by such models have a special property: in every time-period ("t") under consideration, the effect of the predictor on logit-hazard is exactly the same. In Eqn. 1, for example, the vertical shift in the logit-hazard profile for women is always β_1 and, consequently, the logit-hazard profiles for men and women have identical "shapes" since their profiles are simply shifted versions of each other. Generally, in proportional-odds models, the entire family of logit-hazard profiles represented by all possible values of the predictors share a common shape and are mutually parallel, differing only in their relative elevations.

If the logit-hazard profiles are parallel and have the same shape, the corresponding "raw" hazard profiles are (approximate) magnifications and diminutions of each other—they are proportional. (For pedagogic reasons some mathematical liberties have been taken here. In discrete-time models, the proportionality of the raw hazard profile is only approximate because vertical shifts in logit-hazards correspond to magnifications and diminutions of the untransformed hazard profile only when the magnitude of the hazard probability is small (say, less than 0.15 or 0.20). In empirical research, discrete-time hazard is usually of about this magnitude, or less, and therefore the approximation tends to hold quite well in practice (see Singer and Willett 1993, for further discussion of the issues).) Because the model in (3) includes predictors with only time-constant effects, the four fitted hazard functions in Fig. 3 appear to have the required "proportionality."

But is it sensible to assume that the effects of all predictors are unilaterally time-constant and that all hazard profiles are proportional in practice? In reality, many predictors not only displace the logit-hazard profile, they also alter its shape. Even in Fig. 1, for example, the sample hazard profile for women differs in shape from that of men, suggesting that the effect of the predictor FEMALE fluctuates over time.

If the effect of a predictor varies over time, it is necessary to specify a "nonproportional model" that allows the shapes of the logit-hazard profiles to differ. When the effect of one predictor differs by the levels of another, it can be said that the two predictors "interact"; in this case, the predictor interacts with "time." In Figs.1 and 2, the sex differential in logit-hazard fluctuates from year to year suggesting that gender and time interact in the prediction of logit-hazard. To permit this effect in the model, the cross product of that predictor and time is included as an additional predictor (see Willett and Singer 1993).

4. Continuous-time Survival Analysis

So far in this entry, the focus has been on discrete-time survival analysis. In discrete-time, the fundamental quantity on which analyses are based—hazard—is intuitive and comprehensible; it is the conditional probability that the event of interest will occur in a particular time interval, given that it had not occurred in a prior interval. When time is measured continuously, in contrast, the exact instant at which the event of interest occurs is known. Therefore, hazard must be redefined because the probability that any event occurs at a single "infinitely-thin" instant of time tends to zero (by definition). In continuous-time, hazard is redefined as the instantaneous rate of event occurrence at each time (see Allison 1984), given that the event had not occurred up through the immediately prior instant. The new continuous-time hazard "rate" is less intuitive although, broadly speaking, it still describes the "risk" of event occurrence. It can, however, assume any value greater than, or equal to, zero.

Despite these fundamental changes in the definition of the central quantity, continuous-time survival analysis—like its discrete-time cousin—still proceeds in the same fashion. Again, the hazard profile is explicitly modeled. Now, however, the "outcome" is the "natural logarithm" of the continuous-time hazard rate but, as before, the hazard models can include main effects and interactions among multiple predictors, including time. When there are no interactions between any predictor and time, continuous-time hazard models are said to be "proportional-hazards" models—an assumption that can be rejected if necessary. Research findings are still displayed as fitted hazard and survivor functions in prototypical subgroups.

Allison's (1984) monograph provides excellent information on continuous-time survival analysis. Most mainframe computer packages currently contain software for conducting some form of continuous-time survival analysis, including BMDP, SAS and SPSS^x. Dedicated software designed for survival analysis on the personal computer is also widely available (Harrell and Goldstein 1994).

See also: Prediction in Educational Research

References

Allison P D 1982 Discrete-time methods for the analysis of event histories. In Leinhardt S (ed.) 1982 *Sociological Methodology*. San Francisco, California

Allison P D 1984 *Event History Analysis: Regression for Longitudinal Event Data*. Sage, Beverly Hills California

Cox D R 1972 Regression models and life tables. *Journal of Royal Statistical Society, Series B* 34: 187–202

Efron B 1988 Logistic regression, survival analysis, and the Kaplan–Meier curve. *Journal of American Statistical Association* 83(402): 414–25

Hanushek E A, Jackson J E 1977 *Statistical Methods for Social Scientists*. Academic Press, New York

Harrell F E, Goldstein R 1994 A survey of microcomputer survival analysis software: The need for an integrated framework. *The American Statistician*

Kalbfleisch J D, Prentice R L 1980 *The Statistical Analysis of Failure Time Data*. Wiley, New York

Murnane R J, Singer J D, Willett J B, Olsen R J, Kemple J J 1991 *Who Will Teach?: Policies that Matter*. Harvard University Press, Cambridge, Massachusetts

Singer J D 1992 Are special educators' career paths special? Results from a 13-year longitudinal study. *Exceptional Children* 59(3): 262–79

Singer J D, Willett J B 1991 Modeling the days of our lives: Using survival analysis when designing and analyzing longitudinal studies of duration and the timing of events. *Psych. Bull.* 110(2): 268–98

Singer J D, Willett J B 1993 It's about time: Using discrete-time survival analysis to study the duration and timing of events. *J. Educ. Stat.* 18: 155–95

Willett J B, Singer J D 1991 From whether to when: New methods for studying student dropout and teacher attrition. *Rev. Educ. Res.* 61(4): 407–50

Willett J B, Singer J D 1993 Investigating onset, cessation, relapse and recovery: Why you should, and how you can use discrete-time survival analysis to examine event occurence. *J. Consult. Clin. Psychol.* (Special issue on *Quantitative Methodology in the Measurement of Change*) 61(6): 952–965

Exploratory Data Analysis

G. Leinhardt and S. Leinhardt

Exploratory data analysis (EDA) is a collection of specialized tools and an approach to the analysis of numerical data which emphasizes the use of graphic displays and outlier resistant methods to detect and model patterns in data. Numerous researchers and statisticians have contributed to the development of EDA but the primary source of ideas is generally acknowledged to be John Tukey. Although many EDA tools have been known for some time, Tukey has created new procedures, improved older ones, and knitted them all together into a systematic method. Tukey's work, only partially described in his book, *Exploratory Data Analysis* (Tukey 1977), provides the data analyst with new capabilities for uncovering the information contained in numerical data and for constructing descriptive models.

Data exploration, as Tukey envisages it, is not simply an exercise in the application of novel tools. It is a phase of empirical research activity, one which follows data collection (or acquisition) and precedes the application of confirmatory or "classical" inferential procedures (Tukey 1973). It is, thus, part of that twilight zone which experienced researchers find so exciting and challenging, novice researchers fear and misunderstand, and few researchers ever report. The excitement of this phase of research derives in large measure from the prospect of discovering unforeseen or unexpected patterns in the data and, consequently, gaining new insights and understanding of natural phenomena. The fear that novices feel is partly a response to this uncertainty, but it is also partly due to traditional teaching which holds that "playing around" with data is not "good" science, not replicable, and, perhaps, fraudulent. Many experienced researchers pay lip service to this view, while surreptitiously employing ad hoc exploratory procedures that they have learned are essential to research. Exploratory data analysis, by making exploration routine and systematic, and by using theoretically justifiable procedures, opens the exploratory phase of research to public review, enhances its effectiveness, and allows for replicability.

Because Tukey's methods exploit the natural behavior of measurements, they allow researchers to rely on their intuitions. The simple logic of the methods helps clarify the process of modeling data and, consequently, makes it easier to detect errors in data or departures from underlying assumptions. Much of this is due to the graphical devices Tukey invented which are central to this approach because of their ability to portray a wide range of patterns that data can take. Well-designed graphics, such as those used in EDA, are useful for the guided searching that characterizes exploration and are also attractive mechanisms for communicating results to nontechnical audiences. As a consequence, EDA can serve in data analysis and for reporting the results of an analysis.

Many of the methods in EDA fall on the frontiers of applied statistics. Two important topics in statistics are the robustness and resistance of methods, terms which refer to the ability of a procedure to give reasonable results in the face of empirical deviations from underlying theoretical assumptions. Clearly, robust and resistant methods are particularly advantageous in social science research because empirical social science data are so often obtained in an ad hoc fashion, frequently under nonreplicable circumstances, on opportunistically defined variables whose relation to substantive theoretical constructs are vague at best. Exploratory data analysis is especially important in educational research, where many of the variables studied and data collected are brought into analyses not because well-verified, substantive theory demands their inclusion, but rather because investigators "feel" they ought to be, because they are "convenient" to use, or because measurements have been recorded in some assumed "reasonable" manner. Nor are the data typically produced as a consequence of a scientifically designed experiment. It is precisely in such research that EDA can be used to its greatest advantage because it is here that an open mind is an absolute necessity: the analyst rarely has the support of theoretically based expectations, and the real task confronting the data analyst is to explore—to search for ideas that make sense of the data (Simon 1977).

In the following brief description of EDA, only a few of the more usable techniques and the philosophical essence behind EDA are presented. Mathematical details are avoided but references to more extensive treatments are provided. The general objective of the procedures presented can be easily summarized. The procedures are tools for achieving resistant estimates of parameters for traditional additive and linear models. In this respect, they speak to a common empirical problem, the presence of outliers in data and the sensitivity of traditional methods of parameter estimation to highly deviant observations. Resistant analogs to three cases are presented: (a) a set of observations on a single factor at one level, (b) a set of observations on a single factor with multiple levels, and (c) a set of observations on two factors. In each case, the traditional approach to parameter estimation is mentioned first and then the EDA approach is detailed.

1. Organizing and Summarizing Individual Batches of Data

One of the first tangible products of a quantitative research project is a set of numbers, "data" that might contain information about the phenomenon or process under investigation. In many cases, the sheer amount of data to be analyzed can be overwhelming, leading an investigator to rely on summaries rather than dealing with all the values obtained. In addition to the impact that quantity can have, computer routines often present data values and summary statistics in a printed format which obscures rather than elucidates data properties. Automatically produced by routines designed to handle a wide variety of situations, output listings typically contain much that is distracting (e.g., decimal points, leading and trailing zeros, scientific notation) and little that is fundamental. In addition, such routines are usually designed to present values in what might be called an accounting framework, one that facilitates the location of identified values but provides little insight into the overall behavior of the data.

Even a small collection of data, for example, three variables for 50 cases, is extremely hard to visualize or to get a feel for. What is needed is a technique that preserves the detail of values but eliminates distracting noise and contributes to a first level of understanding. The stem-and-leaf display and the box plot are two such techniques.

2. Visual Organization: Stem-and-leaf Display

The stem-and-leaf display is an immensely useful and easily appreciated exploratory tool which can provide insightful first impressions. It combines the features of a sorting operation with those of a histogram. The basic procedure can be used to organize and provide information on a single batch of values in a wide variety of circumstances. (A batch is a collection of observations on a variable. The term is not meant to convey any notion of sampling from a population.)

Figure 1 presents a stem-and-leaf display of the number of 5-minute segments out of 40 in which each of 53 children was observed to be reading silently and is referred to as "direct silent" in the figure (Leinhardt et al. 1981). The arrows, words, and circles are for explanation only. To construct a stem-and-leaf display, each number in a batch is partitioned into a starting part (to the left of the bar) and a leaf (to the right of the bar). When single digits are used in leaves each starting part will be an order of magnitude larger than each leaf. A set of leaves for a given starting part is a stem. The unit of display records the scaled value.

To reconstruct a data value, juxtapose a starting part with a leaf and multiply by the unit. For example, consider the two leaves that form the first stem of Fig. 1: 6 and 9. To reconstruct the two data values that these leaves represent, simply juxtapose each leaf with the common starting part, 0, and multiply by 0.01, that is, $06 \times 0.01 = 0.06$; $09 \times 0.01 = 0.09$. As another example, consider the bottom-most stem in Fig. 1. It has only one leaf, 3. Juxtaposing the 3 with its starting part, 16, and multiplying by 0.01 yields 1.63. There are three starting parts 13, 14, and 15 that have no stems or leaves. This indicates that no observations have values between 1.27 and 1.63.

The display in Fig. 1 is actually the result of a two-step procedure (assuming the operation is carried out by hand). The first step normally yields a display in which the starting parts are ordered but the leaves on each stem are not. In the second step, each stem's leaves are ordered. This two-step procedure makes sorting a reasonably efficient operation.

Because all values in the display are represented by leaves occupying equal amounts of space, the length of a stem is proportional to the number of observations it contains. Thus, the display is like a histogram and provides information on shape and variation while also retaining information on individual values. This is true after the first step in construction. After the second step, the values are completely ordered and the display takes on the features of a sort. Because the display is like a histogram, anyone studying it can get the same kind of feeling for such elementary batch characteristics as overall pattern, bunching, hollows, outliers, and skewness that histograms provide. Those features that are akin to a sort allow the determination of maximum and minimum values quickly and, from them, the range of the values which can be used as a measure of overall variation.

Adding an inwardly cumulating count (depth) to the display greatly expands its utility. It facilitates

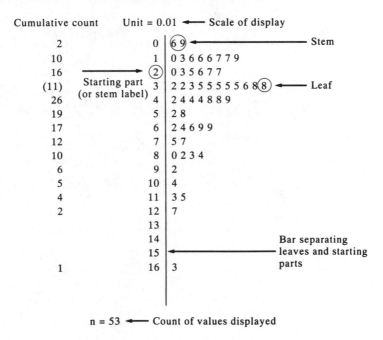

Cumulative count   Unit = 0.01 ◄── Scale of display

n = 53 ◄── Count of values displayed

Figure 1
A stem-and-leaf display of direct silent reading data

finding other order statistics besides the maximum and minimum, such as the overall median and the medians of the upper and lower halves of the batch, which Tukey calls the "hinges." To form such a count, the number of leaves on a stem are cumulated from both ends in toward the middle. The median is located (not its value) at a depth halfway into the batch from either end. The count of the number of leaves on the stem containing the median is given and put between parentheses because it is not cumulative.

To illustrate the use of this column of inwardly cumulating counts, the count column will be used to find the values of the median of the data in Fig. 1. The median will be located at depth $(n+1)/2$. Since there are 53 values, the median is at depth 27, that is, it is the 27th value in from either the high or low end of the sorted values. Counting into the batch from the low-value end (which happens to be at the top of this display), it can be seen that the 27th value is represented by a leaf on the fourth stem. The value of the median could just as easily have been determined by counting into the batch from the high-value end (at the bottom of the display).

While the stem-and-leaf display is useful for describing data, it can also be an effective exploratory tool. For example, looking at Fig. 1 an asymmetry can be seen skewing the values toward the high end. The clustering between 0.1 and 0.4 is obvious, as are the two groups at 0.6 and 0.8 and the modal group at 0.3. The minimum value, 0.06, and the maximum value, 1.63, are easily determined. There is a gap apparent

between 1.27 and 1.63. A researcher might be concerned, even at this point, with the question of why the maximum value seems to straggle out so much.

3. Numeric Summarization: Number Summaries and Letter-value Displays

While the stem-and-leaf display is a convenient and easily understood tool, it has its drawbacks. This is most evident when different batches of values are being compared. Although a simple comparison of the shapes of two batches can be achieved by placing the leaves of one batch on one side and the leaves of the second batch on the other side of a common set of starting parts, simultaneously comparing three or more batches using stem-and-leaf displays is obviously going to be difficult, possibly even confusing. While the visual quality of the stem-and-leaf display is a true asset in any first look at the behavior of a batch, it may be burdensome to continue to work with all the data values at once rather than a set of summary statistics.

The question is which summary statistics to use. The problem with choosing the mean and related statistics, such as the standard deviation, is their lack of resistance to the impact that one or a few deviant data values can have. Because the mean is a ratio of a sum to the number of values making up the sum, it can be made to equal anything by simply changing a single value in the sum. This is not a problem, of course, if the data are reasonably well-behaved. Empirical data,

521

however, often contain deviant values. Indeed, peculiar values are rather commonplace occurrences (recall the value of 1.63 in Fig. 1) and, regardless of their source, they can cause traditional summary statistics to misinform.

Other statistics exist which are less sensitive to deviant values than is the mean, and, while they may not yet be fully supported by the inference procedures available for the mean, they may still be preferable at the exploratory stage of an analysis, where inference is not yet a focal issue. Some of the more useful and commonly known resistant measures of location and variation can be derived from the median and other order statistics. Most order statistics are little affected by the presence of a few outliers in a batch. One common resistant order-statistic-based measure of variation is the interquartile range.

Tukey exploits the resistance of order statistics, especially the median, in EDA. His first step in the numerical summarization of a batch for exploratory purposes involves computing five order statistics: the median, the extremes (or maximum and minimum), and the medians of the upper and lower quartiles (i.e., the hinges). When these five numbers are grouped together, they are called a "five-number summary" and can be arrayed conveniently as LE(LH, M, UH)UE, for lower extreme, lower hinge, median, upper hinge, and upper extreme, respectively. Tukey has introduced a truncation rule to avoid the inconvenience of small fractional ranks when finding medians of segments of a batch. The rule is:

Depth of next median

$$= (1 + \lfloor \text{depth of prior median} \rfloor) / 2 \qquad (1)$$

The symbols $\lfloor$ and $\rfloor$ refer to the mathematical "floor" function which returns the largest integer not exceeding the number. That is, the fractional component of a value, in this case a fractional depth or rank, is discarded. This means that the only fractional depths used will be those that lie halfway between two consecutive values and, thus, will be easy to compute and understand. As a consequence of this truncation rule, exploratory summary statistics may not be exactly equal to analogous-order statistics whose computation is derived from more mathematically precise definitions.

The notion of a median is easily extended to provide a way of segmenting a batch resistantly. The hinges are themselves medians of segments, the upper and lower halves of the batch. Medians of the upper and lower quarters halve the quarter so that each segment bounds one-eighth of the values; medians of these segments bound 16ths, then 32nds, then 64ths, and so forth. In EDA, this process works outward from the center to the edges of a batch providing more and more detailed information on the behavior of the tails of an empirical distribution.

Although letter-value displays and five-number summaries (and extended number summaries in which medians of further foldings are recorded) provide useful, resistant information on location, their primary analytic use is in facilitating the computation of other features of batches. Differences of values provide information on spread or variation in a batch. For example, the range of silent reading data in Fig. 1 is computed by subtracting the lower extreme from the upper extreme: 1.63−0.06=1.57. The range, however, is not a very resistant measure of spread. Obviously, it is very sensitive to deviant values when these appear as extremes, a common occurrence. A more reasonable measure of spread is the range between the hinges. Analogous to the interquartile range, it is called a "hingespread." The hingespread (which is symbolized as dH) of the silent reading data is 0.69−0.26=0.43.

The hingespread is a statistic of central importance in elementary EDA. It is a useful tool in the search for values that deserve attention because they deviate from most values in a batch. This search can be started by computing another measure of spread, the "step," which is 1.5 times the hingespread. Using this quantity, one literally steps away from each hinge toward the extreme to establish another boundary around the central component of the data. These bounding values are called the "inner fences." Another step beyond these establishes the "outer fences." Note that the fences are not rank order statistics but are computed distances measured in the same scale as the values of the batch. Values that fall between the inner and outer fences are called "outside" values, and beyond these lie the "far outside" values. The two data values (or more if multiple observations occur at the same point) falling just inside the inner fences are called "adjacent values"; they are literally next to or adjacent to the inner fences.

It is useful to re-examine the stem-and-leaf display in Fig. 1 in light of the new information obtained on spread. In examining this display, it was noted that the data were evidently skewed out toward the high end. The numerical information on spread confirms this visual impression and suggests that one value at the high end deserves further attention. This value may be erroneous, or it may have been generated by a process different from that which generated the bulk of the values. Having identified a potential outlier, the problem of deciding what to do about it arises. If data are used which are made to appear highly asymmetric because of a few extreme observations, then it must be realized that many of the usual forms of inference, such as analysis of variance and least squares regression, will be strongly influenced by these few values. These procedures are not very resistant and, while removing values from empirical data should be done with utmost caution, the fact must be faced that unless omission of outliers is explored, fitted parameter values may describe the behavior of only a very small portion of the data. Replicability of findings in such situations is unlikely and generalizability is questionable.

Schematic plot	Number summary		Stem-and-leaf display Unit =10⁻²	
	LE	0.06	0	6 9
			1	0 3 6 6 6 7 7 9
	LH	0.26	2	0 3 5 6 7 7
	M	0.38	3	2 2 3 5 5 5 5 5 6 8 8
			4	2 4 4 4 8 8 9
			5	2 8
	UH	0.69	6	2 4 6 9 9
			7	5 7
			8	0 2 3 4
			9	2
			10	4
			11	3 5
			12	7
			13	
			14	
			15	
*	UE	1.63	16	3

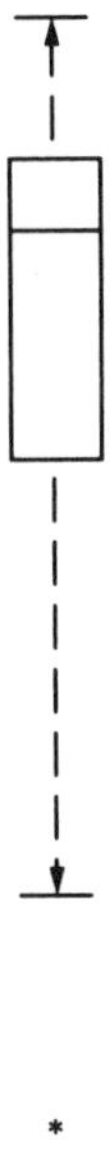

Figure 2
Schematic plot, five-number summary, and stem-and-leaf display for direct silent reading data

The theoretical rationale underlying this approach to identifying outliers is not explicitly developed in Tukey's book on EDA. Some implicit support is available, however, by examining the properties of a normally distributed population in terms of EDA order-statistic-based measures. In a Gaussian or normal population, 0.75 *dH* is approximately one standard deviation. Thus, 1.5 *dH*, a step, is approximately 2σ. Consequently, the inner fences, which are more than 2σ from the median, bound over 99 percent of the values of such populations. Observations drawn from a normal population that lie beyond the population's outer fences, which are an additional 2σ farther out, should indeed be rare.

4. Schematic Plots as Graphic Summaries

The quantities contained in number summaries and letter-value displays provide useful information on overall batch behavior. Most analysts, however, and certainly most nonspecialists, find that they can more easily appreciate the nuances of quantitative information when this information is displayed graphically. A schematic plot is an extremely useful graphic representation of the quantities contained in a number summary and, in fact, might well be considered a fundamental EDA summary device. It completely eliminates numbers (leaving them to a reference scale) and selectively obscures the data, drawing attention to some values and not others. Those values that are completely obscured are the values lying between the hinges, on the one hand, and those lying between the adjacent values and the hinges on the other. Attention is drawn by single marks to all values lying beyond the adjacent values. An example using the silent reading data appears in Fig. 2, which also shows the two other techniques that have been previously described.

Several points about schematic plots are worth noting. In the basic schematic plot, the width (or height, depending on orientation) of the box enclosing the central section of the data is arbitrary. However, this dimension can be used to represent information on other aspects of the data, such as batch size and significance of differences between medians (McGill et al. 1978). Whereas vertically oriented schematic plots are traditional and visually appealing, horizontal orientations are more effective for computerized printing operations because they permit a standard width to be used for any number of plots. Although the schematic plot is a visual device like the stem-and-leaf display, it is not as detailed and, indeed, is explicitly designed to reduce the amount of information being displayed. A related but even more elementary display, the box plot (so called because it consists of simply the box portion of a schematic plot and "whiskers" or lines extending to the extremes) obscures all except those in the five-number summary. Even though schematics speak to the issue of shape and spread, they can be somewhat misleading if gaps or multimodality occur between

Table 1
Summary of transformations: roles, procedures, and failures[a]

Data structure	Problem	Procedure	Failures
(a) Single batch	Asymmetry	Summary table (or equation)	Multimodality large gap
(b) One-way array	Spread heterogeneity	Diagnostic plot of log (dH_1) vs. log (x_1)	Inconsistency in dH_1
(c) Two-way array	Interaction	Diagnostic plot of comparison values	Idiosyncratic interactions
(d) Paired observations	Curvature	Slope ratios or equation	Nonmonotonocity
	Spread heterogeneity	(b above)	(b above)

a Sometimes the "correct" transformation is not well-approximated by kx^p for any "reasonable" choice of p

the adjacent values. Consequently, it is not advisable to use schematics as substitutes for stem-and-leaf displays, but rather as adjuncts.

5. Transformations

Frequently, naturally occurring data are modestly or extremely skewed, or exhibit some other property that make the data not normally distributed. Tukey emphasizes the need to consider the monotone transformation $y=kx^p$, where y is the transformed value, x is the original value, k is a constant set to -1 when p is less than zero and 1 otherwise. (The constant, k, retains order in the magnitude of the values when the transformation is a reciprocal.) The procedures for determining p are worked out and presented elsewhere and will not be described here (Leinhardt and Wasserman 1978). A summary of transformations is given in Table 1.

Thinking in terms of rescaled data values rather than raw data values is by no means straightforward and, given the central role that power transformations play in EDA, it is important that their rationale and validity are fully appreciated. There are several ways of thinking about transformations. One involves realizing that the well-grounded confirmatory tools of standard inferential statistics make specific assumptions concerning model structure and error properties. In many common procedures these include assumptions about normality of error distributions, additivity in parameters and variables, constancy of error variances, lack of functional dependence between error variance and variable location, and lack of interactions. When these assumptions are invalid, the procedures lose some of their appealing qualities. Their use in such problematic situations can be misleading. Unless procedures that deal directly with the known features of the data are used, one must resort to mathematical modification that adjusts the values so that their properties fit the assumptions of the model and/or estimation pro-

cedure. Transformations of scale can often provide the modifying mechanism.

An alternative view is more metatheoretical. In it the theoretical development of the social sciences is seen to trail that of the natural sciences in the sense of not yet having a well-developed, empirically verified, axiomatic and deductive body of theory from which the appropriate scale and dimension for representing a theoretical concept in terms of an empirical variable can be determined. Dimensional analysis in physics is an example of the power inherent in disciplines where such well-developed theory exists. In its absence, analysts must often use variables measured in arbitrary scales or variables defined in an ad hoc manner. Rarely is there any good reason to believe that such measures come in a form best suited to modeling relationships. In the absence of an a priori theory that could specify a model, EDA provides tools to determine whether rescaling a variable will lead to a better analysis.

6. Modeling Data

In EDA, models for data consist of two parts: a part that uses a mathematical statement to summarize a pattern in the data and a part that summarizes what is left over. Each observed value can be decomposed into a part that is typical of the pattern, the "fit," and a part that is not typical of the pattern, the "residual." Tukey constructs a verbal equation to represent a general class of models where the decomposition is additive:

$$\text{Data} = \text{Fit} + \text{Residual} \qquad (2)$$

Other models are not ruled out, but Tukey emphasizes the use of simple models because they are easily understood, are easily estimated, help reveal more complex features, and often provide a good first approximation to these complexities. Additionally, many other forms can be rendered in terms of Eqn. (2) through an appropriately chosen transformation. Consequently, Eqn. (2) plays a fundamental role in EDA.

The computational procedure is straightforward. The median is subtracted from each observed value. This yields a batch of residuals, that is, a batch of adjusted values indicating the amount by which each raw value deviates from the fitted central value. In terms of a horizontally formatted schematic plot, the computation of residuals is analogous to centering the raw data around their median and relocating the zero point on the horizontal axis so that this origin rests exactly on the median.

7. Model for Multiple Batches

Most research projects are not performed for the purpose of fitting single parameter models or obtaining a single summary statistic such as the mean or median. At the very least, the simplest objective involves comparing several batches in an attempt to determine whether one batch differs from another and by how much. A second-order question involves deciding whether an observed difference is important. These questions are traditionally approached through the analysis of variance (ANOVA) using ordinary least squares (OLS) estimation procedures. While OLS has estimable properties when special conditions hold (i.e., the parameter estimates are unbiased, consistent, and have minimal variance), some of these properties are lost when the conditions fail to hold. Such losses can result from the presence of a single outlier. An EDA-based approach which exploits graphical displays to detect data inadequacies is presented here which employs resistant measures in determining effects and provides a useful guide in obtaining a transformation that facilitates the use of classical procedures.

In classical ANOVA, the errors ε_{ij}, are assumed to be normally distributed random variables with zero mean and constant variance. Thus, the sum of squares for batch effects and the errors are multiples of χ^2 random variables. As a consequence, F ratios can be formed to test zero effect null hypotheses and symmetric confidence intervals can be constructed.

An analogous EDA procedure is presented here; one that is more resistant to outliers than ANOVA but lacking distributional assumptions and, consequently, lacking inferential tests. The purpose is to provide a resistant analysis that can be used in exploration. Furthermore, the EDA procedure provides a useful mechanism for studying the problem of inconsistency of variation in the errors, that is, heteroscedasticity.

The EDA modeling procedure is similar to that pursued in a classical analysis except that common effect and batch effect are estimated by medians and, consequently, involve different arithmetic computations.

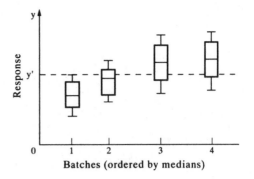

Figure 3
Box plots of multiple batches of hypothesis data

The model represented by the verbal Eqn. (2) yields a "fit" that is applicable to all batch values. For multiple batches, this model can be further elaborated so as to distinguish a general or common effect across all batches and a set of individual batch effects that are confined within their respective batches. Thus, the general model becomes:

$$\text{Data value}_{ij} = \underbrace{\text{Common effect} + \text{Batch}_j \text{ effect}}_{\text{Fit}} + \text{Residual}_{ij} \tag{3}$$

Conceptually, the model represents each observed data value as a conditional response determined in part by imprecision, noise, or error. No specific assumptions are made about this last ingredient except that, taken as a batch, the residuals are devoid of an easily described pattern. The information they contain relates solely to the overall quality of the model in terms of its ability to replicate the observed values.

The computational procedure is straightforward. First, consider the hypothetical multiple-batch data set represented by the box plots in Fig. 3. The median of the pooled batches is identified as the "common effect." Next, subtraction is used to "extract" this common effect from all data values. The result is simply a new centering of the adjusted batch values around a new grand median of zero. Second, the individual batch effects are obtained by subtracting the grand median from the individual batch medians. Finally, residuals are obtained by subtracting the batch effects from each adjusted value in the appropriate batch. The residuals are then examined as a whole and as batches. For the hypothetical example, the model is:

$$\text{Data value}_{ij} = \text{Common effect} + \begin{cases} \text{Batch effect}_1 \\ \text{Batch effect}_2 \\ \text{Batch effect}_3 \\ \text{Batch effect}_4 \end{cases}$$

$$+ \text{Residual}_{ij}. \tag{4}$$

The fitted value for the *i, j* th observation would simply be:

$$\text{Fit}_{ij} = \text{Common effect} + \begin{cases} \text{Batch effect}_1 \\ \text{Batch effect}_2 \\ \text{Batch effect}_3 \\ \text{Batch effect}_4 \end{cases} \quad (5)$$

8. Model for Two-way Classifications

A more complicated but quite common data structure arises when responses can be identified with the levels of two factors. The usual summary layout used to organize such data is the two-way table, an array of "responses" organized on the basis of row (*r*) and column (*c*) factors. Such two-dimensional arrays consist of *r*×*c* cells or entries. Each row or column of a factor is referred to as a factor level or factor version. Factors are usually ordinally or nominally scaled but may be interval scaled. Responses are usually ratio scaled. The data are conceived of as triples of values: two classifying variables and a response variable.

The usual approach to such data involves an elaboration of the one-way model. A model, additive in factor-level effects, is posited. The array of responses is decomposed into an overall level or common effect, row effects, column effects, and interaction effects. A two-way ANOVA using least squares is the traditional method employed to estimate the model's parameters and to test for significance. In ANOVA, the grand mean is used to estimate the common term, and row and column means of the adjusted data estimate the row and column effects.

Once again, the EDA approach is analogous. The differences lie in the lack of distributional assumptions for the errors and the use of medians to estimate model parameters. Because no distributional assumptions are made, the hypothesis tests that are possible with least squares cannot be done. However, the use of medians ensures a result that is more resistant to the impact of deviant values. Furthermore, the EDA procedure provides a useful way to detect interactions even when there is only one observation per cell. When certain kinds of interactions are present, the EDA procedure can lead to a choice of a power transformation of the data that eliminates the interactions, that is, yields a scale in which the additive model provides a reasonable summarization of the data.

The model is in many respects an extension of the one-factor, multiple-level model proposed earlier for multiple batches. Indeed, a two-way table of responses can be thought of as two interwoven sets of multiple batches. Considering the column factor as the only dimension, there is a set of *c* multiple batches, each containing a maximum of *r* values. Considering the row factor as the only dimension yields a set of *r* multiple batches, each

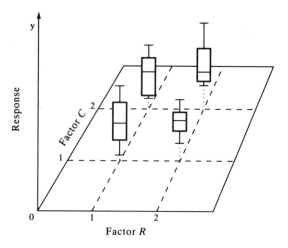

Figure 4

Graphical representation of hypothetical data for a two-way classification of responses (multiple unequal observations in each cell)

containing a maximum of *c* values.

Because the assumption is that each cell contains multiple observations, these data can be visualized as a two-way categorization of box plots as in Fig. 4. In the display, the vertical or *y*-axis is the scale on which the numeric response variable is measured. Factors *R* and *C* are categorical, so the distances between the levels, as well as their ordering, are arbitrary. The box plots of the multiply observed responses appear elevated above the origin plane by differing average positive amounts. The mathematical model represented involves a decomposition of the average elevation of each box plot into four parts: (a) an overall level; (b) a contribution from the column level (which occurs regardless of row level); (c) a contribution from the row level (which occurs regardless of column level); and (d) an error or residual. In verbal equation form this appears as:

$$\text{Data} = \overbrace{\begin{array}{c} \text{Common effect} + \text{Row effect} \\ + \text{Column effect} + \text{Residual} \end{array}}^{\text{Fit}} \quad (6)$$

Whether the grand mean or grand median is used to estimate the common term, the result is conceptually identical. Its removal by subtraction effectively translates the origin plane so that the data are distributed around the origin rather than above it as in the hypothetical example. It is thus analogous to removing the grand median from a set of multiple batches, or the median from a single batch, and using the adjusted values, that is, the raw values with the grand median subtracted out, in constructing a new display.

By assuming that row and column effects are consistent, the model asserts that there will be only one effect for a row level regardless of the number of column levels, their size, and their effects and vice versa. In other words, the effect of row level 1 will be to elevate (or depress) the values in cells (1,1) and (1,2) the same amount, say a_1. Similarly, the effect of column level 2, according to the model, will be to elevate (or depress) the values in cells (1,2) and (2,2) the same amount, say b_2. Thus, any process of fitting this model to data must be constrained to finding these amounts according to a criterion that ensures an additive result. Given some estimate of these effects, the extent to which the data fail to conform can be studied by examining the residuals.

Thinking in terms of multiple observations in each cell gives an opportunity to reflect on the occurrence of weird or deviant cell values in cases where there is only one observation per cell, a common situation. For example, analyses of previously reported data where access to raw values is not possible must usually proceed with cell values reported as averages. In many instances, even when raw values are available, only one observation per cell exists. Finally, in some cases it makes sense to think only in terms of single observations as in a longitudinal sampling frame, and, thus, the observed single cell entry, while drawn from a theoretical distribution of values, is the only observation that will ever be made.

In such cases, it is clear that when a single observation is drawn from the extremes of the cell distributions, a deviant cell results. Means of values, as was demonstrated earlier, provide little protection in such situations because they will be sensitive to any underlying asymmetries. The prospect of deviant observations in the cells as a consequence of poor initial measurement or erroneous data entry is obvious and remains a problem.

The traditional analytic procedure, using means and a least squares minimization criterion, will be highly sensitive to any instance of deviant cell values. As an alternative, Tukey suggests using "median polish." This procedure is relatively resistant and reasonably easy to perform. It involves the repeated (iterated) removal (subtraction) of medians. Several algorithms exist. The following procedure is relatively easy to perform by hand or to program for a computer.

First, the grand median is found and used to estimate the common effect. This term is removed (equivalent to a horizontal translation of the origin plane in Fig. 4) by subtracting the grand median from each cell value. The result of removing the common effect is a new array of positive and negative cell values centered around zero. Now a sweeping operation begins which alternately removes medians from the rows and then from the columns. There is no particular reason to start the steps on rows or on columns. However, because the solution provided by the algorithm is not exact, the results may differ slightly. The operation usually begins by sweeping rows.

In each sweep, each row or column median is found and subtracted out of its respective row and column of cell values. Usually, the process will quickly arrive at a point where row and column medians are zero or near zero. The values remaining in the table at this stage are the residuals. Row and column effects are calculated by adding the row and column medians obtained at each iteration. Individual fitted values can be found by using Eqn. (6) and the appropriate row and column effects. Row and column fits (i.e., estimated values) can be found by adding the common effect to the sum of each row effect and each column effect.

9. Conclusion

The tools and approaches that have been described comprise as much a philosophy of data analysis as a set of specific answers to a number of common data analysis problems. The philosophy is one in which the analyst's first task is viewed as discovery of evidence, not evaluation, and consequently the tools are designed to reveal unforeseen features rather than to create a decision-analytic framework for judging the importance of expected features. These evaluative tasks are left for another time and for different methods. Exploratory data analysis addresses the need for formulating models and developing hypotheses through the use of empirical data. Using data to test specific models and to determine the precision of parameter estimates remains the province of traditional inference.

There are many procedures associated with EDA which have not been discussed here. Some of these are considered in a number of articles and books. Several computer packages now contain EDA procedures. CMU-DAP is an especially versatile package of confirmatory and exploratory procedures. A system widely distributed by Pennsylvania State University, MINITAB, now also possesses some EDA capabilities.

Two features serve as continuous themes in the procedures that have been described. The first is the desire to use resistant procedures rather than to rely solely on traditional least square methods. The solution that Tukey provides in EDA is a set of fitting procedures that use medians instead of means. A good operational rule is to try both resistant and standard methods on a data set and to move cautiously when the two disagree. The second theme deals with deviations from simple models in the form of asymmetry, spread-by-level interaction, and curvilinearity. Tukey's solution here is a standard one, the use of transformations of scale so that in the new scale the data do not exhibit these patterns.

In conclusion, the belief should be reiterated that there is little in the philosophy of EDA that will be new to the experienced scientist. What is new, useful, and timely is the systematic and routine way in which Tukey's procedures allow this philosophy to be put into practice. Furthermore, while research scientists will appreciate these advantages, evidence indicates that EDA can be extremely helpful to students just commencing their education in statistical methods. Using EDA as an introduction to statistics and data analysis provides a refreshingly intuitive and intellectually appealing route to the development of quantitative analytic skills.

See also: Multivariate Analysis

References

Leinhardt S, Wasserman S S 1978 Quantitative methods of public management: An introductory course in statistics and data analysis. *Policy Analysis* Fall: 550–75

Leinhardt G, Zigmond N, Cooley W W 1981 Reading instruction and its effects. *Am. Educ. Res. J.* 18: 343–61

McGill R, Tukey J W, Larsen W A 1978 Variations of box plots. *Am. Stat.* 32: 12–16

Simon H S 1977 *Models of Discovery*. Reidel, Dordrecht

Tukey J W 1973 The zig-zagging climb from initial observation to successful improvement. In: Coffman W E (ed.) 1973 *Frontiers of Educational Measurement and Information Systems: 1973*. Houghton-Mifflin, Boston, Massachusetts

Tukey J W 1977 *Exploratory Data Analysis*. Addison-Wesley, Reading, Massachusetts

Further Reading

Erickson B H, Nosanchuk T A 1977 *Understanding Data*. McGraw-Hill Ryerson, Toronto, Ontario

Leinhardt G, Leinhardt S 1980 Exploratory data analysis: New tools for the analysis of empirical data. *Rev. Res. Educ.* 8: 85–157

McNeil D R 1977 *Interactive Data Analysis: A Practical Primer*. Wiley, New York

Mosteller F, Tukey J W 1977 *Data Analysis and Regression: A Second Course in Statistics*. Addison-Wesley, Reading, Massachusetts

Velleman P F, Hoaglin D C *Applications, Basics and Computing of Exploratory Data Analysis* (ABC of EDA). Duxbury, Boston, Massachusetts

Factor Analysis

D. Spearritt

Factor analysis is a technique for representing the relationships among a set of variables in terms of a smaller number of underlying hypothetical variables. It aims to describe the variation among a set of measures in terms of more basic explanatory constructs, and thus to provide a simpler and more easily grasped framework for understanding the network of relationships among those measures. Correlations might be computed, for example, among the scores of a group of students on measures of addition, subtraction, multiplication, division, vocabulary, and reading comprehension. A factor analysis of these correlations might show that the relationships among the tests could be almost completely explained in terms of two underlying variables, which might well be interpreted as computational ability and verbal ability.

1. Early Development of Factor Analysis

Although the technique of factor analysis is now applied in a wide variety of disciplines, it originated in the field of psychology. Toward the end of the nineteenth century, a number of psychologists turned their attention to experimental studies of intelligence and intellectual abilities. Spearman collected data to test his theory that mental activity could be explained in terms of a single central intellective function, "intelligence." Finding high correlations between estimates of intelligence and students' scores on tests of weight, light, and pitch discrimination, he concluded that

> all branches of intellectual activity have in common one fundamental function (or group of functions), whereas the remaining or specific elements of the activity seem in every case to be wholly different from that in all others. (Spearman 1904)

Subsequently, in his two-factor theory, the fundamental function was described as a general factor, "g," and the element specific to a particular activity as its specific factor, "s."

Spearman had noted that his matrices of correlations among intellectual abilities could be arranged hierarchically, showing a progressive decrease in value from left to right and from the upper to the lower rows of the table. He recognized that this would be the expected pattern of correlations if all mental processes reflected the operation of a single central intellective function, which operated at different levels of complexity. To test whether a set of correlations he had obtained among six variables conformed to this pattern, for instance, he computed the tetrad differences among the correlations, for example ($r_{13}r_{26} - r_{23}r_{16}$). Finding that they were approximately zero, he confirmed the hypothesis that the correlations could be explained by one general factor.

The two-factor theory was challenged by Thomson and other psychologists on both theoretical and empirical grounds. Working with larger batteries of tests and larger numbers of cases, Burt identified verbal, numerical, and practical group factors in school subjects in addition to a general factor; a "group factor" is one which is represented only in certain similar types of tests but not in others. Spearman later admitted the necessity of group factors, and British factorists adopted a factor model which incorporated both a general factor and group factors.

Hierarchical theories of mental structure had little

appeal for American psychologists. They preferred a multiple-factor approach in which several factors were extracted directly from a correlation matrix, without any initial assumption about the need for a general factor. In the early 1930s, Kelley and Hotelling sought a unique and exact mathematical solution to the problem of identifying the underlying factors in a correlation matrix, and developed the general method of principal components analysis put forward earlier by Karl Pearson. This method extracts successive uncorrelated components which account for as much of the variation among the scores of students on a set of variables as is possible at each stage.

Thurstone, the major American contributor to the development of factor analysis, noted that the addition of further tests to a battery could affect the factors identified by the principal components approach. He sought a method of analysis which would lead to the discovery of psychologically meaningful factors which were invariant, that is, supporting the same interpretation, over different test batteries.

In 1931, Thurstone accelerated the development of factor analysis by noting that Spearman's tetrad difference of

$$r_{13}r_{24} - r_{23}r_{14} = 0$$

was the equivalent of setting a second order minor or determinant to be equal to zero. In algebraic form,

$$\begin{vmatrix} r_{13}r_{14} \\ r_{23}r_{24} \end{vmatrix} = 0$$

He reasoned that "if the second-order minors must vanish in order to establish a single common factor, then must the third-order minors vanish in order to establish two common factors, and so on" (Thurstone 1947). This allowed him to use matrix algebra procedures to express the problem of determining the number of factors needed to account for an observed correlation matrix. He formulated the problem in terms of the fundamental factor theorem $\mathbf{FF'} = \mathbf{R}$, where $\mathbf{R}$ was the original correlation matrix and $\mathbf{F}$ was the factor matrix to be identified. $\mathbf{F}$ would consist of a matrix of coefficients or "loadings" of the original tests or variables on the "factors," and would usually be a rectangular matrix of lower rank than $\mathbf{R}$. His centroid method of analysis for solving this equation was superseded in the 1950s when computer technology made principal components and other solutions feasible.

Thurstone was also responsible for distinguishing two separate phases in the determination of factors—factor extraction and factor rotation. He recognized that the initial extraction of factors by the centroid method or by variants of the principal components method merely provided an arbitrary orthogonal set of reference axes—a set of axes at right angles to each other in two-dimensional, three-dimensional, or higher dimensional space depending upon the number of factors extracted—to represent the correlations among the tests or the relationships among the test vectors, and that any particular set of axes was only one of a very large number which would represent the correlations equally well. He claimed that the factor loadings determined at the factor extraction stage had no psychological meaning until they were rotated in the common factor space. Starting from the psychological assumption that there are some mental functions not involved in every intellectual task, Thurstone developed the criterion of simple structure to locate new positions for the reference axes. This required that the axes be placed so that each test would have significant loadings on only one or two factors and near-zero loadings on the remaining factors, and so that on each factor, a majority of the tests would have near-zero loadings. Unlike the British factorists, he made no initial assumption about the need for a general factor, but sought to determine "how many factors are indicated by the correlations without restriction as to whether they are general or group factors" (Thurstone 1947). It was left to the configuration of the test vectors to determine whether a general factor was needed in addition to other factors to explain the correlations among the tests.

Factor schools differed on the question of acceptable types of rotation. Most of the British factorists and a few of the American factorists insisted on orthogonal rotations; while a given axis could be rotated through any angle, the angle between that axis and other axes should remain at 90°. The factors therefore represented unrelated constructs. Thurstone, however, claimed that the restriction of unrelatedness or orthogonality of factors should not be imposed on the data. Application of the simple structure criterion would reveal whether the data could be represented by an orthogonal axis system. In most cases, however, the simple structure solution would require an oblique rotation of the initial axes, in which the angles between the rotated axes could be smaller or larger than a right angle. The factors emerging from an oblique rotation therefore tended to be themselves correlated. If the factors were correlated, the correlations among the factors could be further analyzed to yield second-order or higher order factors, which to the extent that they were represented in all tests in a battery, could be regarded as analogous to a general factor.

The most significant developments during this early period of factor analysis were: (a) Spearman's conceptualization of the two-factor theory; (b) its subsequent extension by British psychologists to a general plus group factor model, and a number of crucial contributions from L L Thurstone including (c) his generalization of the two-factor notion to a multiple factor analysis model; (d) his recognition of the need to rotate initially extracted factors to arrive at scientifically interpretable results; and (e) his development of the concept of oblique factors and of criteria for identifying factors. While the basic techniques of factor analysis were well-established by the 1950s, many problems remained. The initial extraction of factors still involved approximate methods, as did the estimation of test communalities, that is, that part of the variance of a test which it has in common with other tests in a battery. Criteria for determining the number of factors needed to explain the correlations were still approximate, and there was a substantial element of subjectivity in the graphical rotational procedures employed by factor analysts. In the ensuing years, many of these problems have been resolved or considerably refined, with theoretical advances being greatly facilitated by advances in computer technology.

2. The Basic Factor Model

The basic factor model assumes that a score on a variable can be expressed as a linear combination or as a weighted sum of scores on factors underlying performance in that variable. If three hypothetical factors F_1, F_2, F_3 were assumed to underlie performance in test j, scores (expressed in standardized form, that is, with a mean of zero and a standard deviation of 1) on test j could be represented by the equation

$$z_j = a_{j1}F_1 + a_{j2}F_2 + a_{j3}F_3 + U_j \tag{1}$$

where the a coefficients represent the loadings of test j on the respective common factors; F_1, F_2, and F_3 represent standard scores on these factors; and U_j represents scores on a factor unique to test j, including error of measurement. The standard scores of two persons on test j, for instance, might be expressed as follows:

$$\text{Person 1: } z_{j1} = a_{j1}F_{11} + a_{j2}F_{21} + a_{j3}F_{31} + U_{j1} \tag{2}$$

$$\text{Person 2: } z_{j2} = a_{j1}F_{12} + a_{j2}F_{22} + a_{j3}F_{32} + U_{j2} \tag{3}$$

Thus the loadings of test j on any one factor are the same for all persons, but the scores on a factor, whether common or unique, differ among persons.

Continuing with the above example, the standard score of Person 1 on test k would be given by

$$z_{k1} = a_{k1}F_{11} + a_{k2}F_{21} + a_{k3}F_{31} + U_{k1} \tag{4}$$

The product of the z scores of Person 1 on tests j and k, that is, $z_{j1}z_{k1}$ can be found by multiplying the expressions on the right-hand side of Eqns. (2) and (4). Summing the product of the standard scores on tests j and k over all N persons in the sample, and dividing the result by N gives

$$\frac{1}{N}\left(\sum_{i=1}^{N} z_{ji}z_{ki}\right) = a_{j1}a_{k1} + a_{j2}a_{k2} + a_{j3}a_{k3} \tag{5}$$

since the scores on the three factors are standard scores and the sum of the squares of standard scores is equal to N, and since product terms involving scores on different factors, whether common or unique, are equal

to zero, as the factors are by definition uncorrelated.

The expression on the left-hand side of Eqn. (5) defines the correlation between tests j and k, so that

$$r_{jk} = a_{j1}a_{k1} + a_{j2}a_{k2} + a_{j3}a_{k3} \tag{6}$$

That is, the correlation between any pair of variables can be expressed as the sum of the product of the loadings of those variables on each of the common factors. Using the vector terminology of matrix algebra, Eqn. (6) can be written as

$$r_{jk} = [a_j \ a_{j2} \ a_{j3}] \begin{bmatrix} a_{k1} \\ a_{k2} \\ a_{k3} \end{bmatrix} \tag{7}$$

Generalizing Eqn. (7) to represent the intercorrelations among n variables in terms of the three factors gives

Test

Test	1	2	.	j	k	.	n
1	r_{11}^{*}	r_{12}	.	r_{1j}	r_{1k}	.	r_{1n}
2	.		.	.	.		.
.		.	.	.	.	.	
j	r_{j1}	r_{j2}	.	r_{jj}^{*}	r_{jk}	.	r_{jn}	$=$
k	r_{k1}	r_{k2}	.	r_{kj}	r_{jk}	r_{kk}^{*}	r_{kn}
.		.	.	.	.	.	.
n	r_{n1}	r_{n2}	.	r_{nj}	r_{nk}	.	r_{nn}^{*}

Factors

Test	F_1	F_2	F_3
1	a_{11}	a_{12}	a_{13}
2	.	.	.
.	.	.	.
j	a_{j1}	a_{j2}	a_{j3}
k	a_{k1}	a_{k2}	a_{k3}
.	.	.	.
n	a_{n1}	a_{n2}	a_{n3}

$$\begin{bmatrix} a_{11} & . & . & a_{j1} & a_{k1} & . & a_{n1} \\ a_{12} & . & . & a_{j2} & a_{k2} & . & a_{n2} \\ a_{13} & . & . & a_{j3} & a_{k3} & . & a_{n3} \end{bmatrix} \tag{8}$$

which is conveniently represented by the matrix equation

$$\mathbf{R}_c = \mathbf{FF}' \tag{9}$$

where $\mathbf{R}_c$ is the matrix of correlations among the tests (which differs from the data-generated matrix $\mathbf{R}$ in that the asterisked diagonal entries consist of the correlation shared by the respective test with other tests in the battery and is less than unity), $\mathbf{F}$ is the matrix of test loadings on the factors, and $\mathbf{F}'$ is the transpose of the latter matrix. In

Eqn. (8), r_{jk} of Eqn. (7) appears as the product of the jth row of the $\mathbf{F}$ matrix and the kth column of the $\mathbf{F'}$ matrix. Equation (9) indicates that a given $\mathbf{F}$ matrix would yield a unique $\mathbf{R}_c$ matrix, but that a given $\mathbf{R}_c$ matrix could be analyzed to yield many different factor matrices.

Equation (9) represents the common factor model. The complete factor model also incorporates the variance (ψ_j) unique to each test, thus:

$$\mathbf{R} = \mathbf{R}_c + \psi = \mathbf{FF'} + \psi \tag{10}$$

where $\mathbf{R}$ is the correlation matrix with unities in the diagonal cells, and ψ is the diagonal matrix

$$\begin{bmatrix} \psi_1 & 0 & . & 0 & . & 0 \\ 0 & \psi_2 & . & 0 & . & 0 \\ . & . & . & . & . & . \\ 0 & 0 & . & \psi_j & . & 0 \\ . & . & . & . & . & . \\ 0 & 0 & . & 0 & . & \psi_n \end{bmatrix}$$

Each of the unique test variances (ψ_j) is regarded as consisting of a reliable component (specific variance, s_j^2) and an unreliable component (error variance, e_j^2). The common factor variance or communality for each test is represented by the symbol h_j^2. Thus in the factor model the variance of a test is expressed as the sum of several components:

$$\sigma_j^2 = 1 = \underbrace{(a_{j1}^2 + a_{j2}^2 + \ldots + a_{jm}^2)}_{h_j^2} + \underbrace{(s_j^2 + e_j^2)}_{\psi_j} \tag{11}$$

The reliability coefficient (r_{jj}) of a test is the sum of the reliable components of variance, $(h^2_j + s^2_j)$ or $(1 - e^2_j)$.

It was assumed in the derivation of Eqn. (5) that the factors in the $\mathbf{F}$ matrix were uncorrelated, and this assumption is also implicit in Eqn. (10). Regarding this assumption as unnecessarily restrictive, Thurstone advocated the acceptance of oblique or correlated factors if warranted by the configuration of the test vectors. When Eqn. (10) is expanded to accommodate correlated factors, the basic factor equation becomes

$$\mathbf{R} = \mathbf{R}_c + \psi = \mathbf{F}\phi\mathbf{F'} + \psi \tag{12}$$

where ϕ represents the matrix of correlations among the factors.

In the present example,

$$f = \begin{bmatrix} 1 & r_{F1F2} & r_{F1F3} \\ r_{F2F1} & 1 & r_{F2F3} \\ r_{F3F1} & r_{F3F2} & 1 \end{bmatrix} \tag{13}$$

If the data can be satisfactorily explained by a set of

uncorrelated factors, then ϕ reduces to an identity matrix,

$$\mathbf{I} = \begin{bmatrix} 1 & 0 & 0 \\ 0 & 1 & 0 \\ 0 & 0 & 1 \end{bmatrix}$$

and Eqn. (12) reduces to Eqn. (10).

3. Exploratory versus Confirmatory Factor Analysis

Usually, the first objective in carrying out a factor analysis of a correlation or covariance matrix is to arrive at an $\mathbf{F}$ matrix of the following form:

	Factors						
Variables	*I*	*II*	*III*	:	*p*	:	*m*
Test 1	a_{1I}	a_{1II}	a_{1III}	:	a_{1p}	:	a_{1m}
Test 2	a_{2I}	a_{2II}	a_{2III}	:	a_{2p}	:	a_{2m}
:	:	:	:	:	:	:	:
Test$_j$	a_{jI}	a_{jII}	a_{jIII}	:	a_{jp}	:	a_{jm}
:	:	:	:	:	:	:	:
Test$_n$	a_{nI}	a_{nII}	a_{nIII}	:	a_{np}	:	a_{nm}

$$\tag{14}$$

This is the matrix of the loadings (a_{jp}) of a set of tests or other variables on a set of m underlying common factors, $m < n$. It is also referred to as a "factor structure matrix," representing the correlations of each of the tests with each of the factors. As pointed out earlier, it is only one of a large number of matrices which would satisfy the relationship expressed in Eqn. (10), and some rotation of the axes represented by the factors would be required to arrive at a meaningful representation of the original data.

In its early development, the large majority of applications of factor analysis were exploratory, the purpose being to explore the underlying dimensions of a set of data. While there has been some indulgence in blind exploration among the uninitiated, in the sense of seeing what factors emerge from any ill-assorted set of variables, the use of factor analysis to explore the dimensions of an educational or psychological domain of interest has mostly been in the context of well-designed studies in which hypotheses have been carefully formulated and variables have been carefully selected. Exploratory factor analysis, however, does not place specific restrictions on the number of factors which should appear in the $\mathbf{F}$ matrix or the subsequent rotated matrix, or on whether particular entries in the factor matrices or factor correlation matrices should be zero or non-zero; it is an unrestricted factor model.

The idea of testing the hypothesis that the relationships among a set of variables might be accounted for in terms of a restricted factor model emerged in the mid-1950s, and following the work of such authors as Howe, Anderson, Rubin, Lawley (1940), Jöreskog, and Gruvaeus, had led to the development of procedures for confirmatory factor analysis. In contrast with exploratory factor analysis, confirmatory factor analysis sets out to test whether the original correlation or covariance matrix can be represented by an underlying factor matrix with a specific number of factors and/or specified zero or nonzero entries in factor matrices and/or factor correlation matrices. Instead of extracting an initial arbitrary **F** matrix and subsequently rotating that matrix, confirmatory factor analysis tests the specific hypothesis that the correlation or covariance matrix can be explained by an **F** matrix of a specified form, for example, by a matrix involving exactly three factors with a specified pattern of loadings as in (A) and of factor correlations as in (B) below:

		(A)				(B)		
	I	II	III			I	II	III
Test 1	*x*	*x*	0		I	1	*x*	*x*
Test 2	*x*	*x*	0		II	*x*	1	0
Test 3	*x*	*x*	0		III	*x*	0	1
Test 4	*x*	*x*	0					
Test 5	*x*	0	*x*					
Test 6	*x*	0	*x*					
Test 7	0	0	*x*					
Test 8	0	0	*x*					

Maximum likelihood methods are used to estimate the nonzero (x) elements in these matrices, given the original correlations or covariances among the variables. If a goodness-of-fit test then shows that the observed matrices do not deviate significantly ($p > 0.10$) from the hypothesized factor solutions, the specific theoretical hypothesis is held to be confirmed. Adequacy of "fit" is considered further in Sects. 4 and 6 below.

4. Initial Extraction of Factors

Many approaches to the determination of the initial **F** matrix have been developed since Thurstone proposed his centroid method of analysis, and many earlier methods have been superseded as a result of the development of computers. One set of reference axes and its associated **F** matrix have the important property that they enable a set of correlated variables to be described in terms of a set of orthogonal (uncorrelated) axes which account for the maximum amount of variance remaining among the variables as each axis in the new set is determined.

Equation (15) presents a correlation matrix for three tests: Vocabulary (V), Comprehension (C), and Arithmetic Problems (A).

$$\mathbf{R} = \begin{array}{c} (V) \\ (C) \\ (A) \end{array} \begin{bmatrix} 1.0 & 0.6 & 0.2 \\ 0.6 & 1.0 & 0.4 \\ 0.2 & 0.4 & 1.0 \end{bmatrix} \quad (15)$$

with columns (V) (C) (A)

This matrix can be represented by an ellipsoid of points in three-dimensional space, defined by three orthogonal axes X, Y, and Z. The ellipsoid would take the shape of an elongated football oriented from one corner of a room at floor level (the origin of the three-dimensional space) upwards toward the ceiling and outwards to the opposite walls. The first principal axis of the correlation matrix would be the major axis of the football; the second principal axis would pass through the centroid of the set of points and would be perpendicular to the first principal axis; the third principal axis would be perpendicular to both the first and second principal axes, representing the length of the line across the football if it had been flattened in one of its shorter dimensions. These three axes are called the "principal components" of the correlation matrix. The variances of the principal components are the latent roots or eigenvalues of **R** which are determined by solving the characteristic equation

$$|\mathbf{R} - \lambda\mathbf{I}| = 0 \quad (16)$$

These eigenvalues show the variance of the points along the first, second, and third principal axes of the football to be 1.823, 0.817, and 0.360 respectively.

The orientation of the principal axes with respect to the original axes is given by a set of eigenvectors corresponding to each eigenvalue; these are the direction cosines of each principal axis. By multiplying the elements of the eigenvectors by the square root of the corresponding eigenvalues, the loadings of the tests on the new axes would be found to be

	1st principal component	2nd principal component	3rd principal component
V	0.800	−0.475	0.366
C	0.888	−0.110	−0.446
A	0.627	0.762	0.164

(17)

Principal component analysis describes the relationships among the original n variables in terms of n new uncorrelated factors, rather than in terms of a reduced number of factors. Principal axes can be found, however, for the matrix $\mathbf{R}_c$ (see Eqn. [9]), in which the correlations in the diagonal cells represent the variance which each variable has in common with other variables in the set, not including the unique variance. This application of the principal axes method is referred to as "principal factor analysis."

The principal factor method will be illustrated with the aid of the fictitious matrix in Eqn. (18), which is based on the correlations among the scores of 200 15-year old secondary school students on examinations in English, French, Italian, physics, and chemistry, but in which the diagonal values of unity have been replaced by the communality, h^2_j, (see Eqn. [11]) of each variable. The communality is that part of the variance of each variable which it holds in common with one or more other variables in the set, or that part of the variable's self-correlation attributable to common factor variance in the set of variables. The squared multiple correlation of each variable with all of the other variables in the set is now usually accepted as the communality estimate, and has replaced the original values of unity in the diagonal cells of the matrix in Eqn. (18), which is therefore designated as R_c.

		(1)	(2)	(3)	(4)	(5)
		English	French	Italian	Physics	Chemistry
$R_c =$	(1)	(0.59)	0.63	0.65	0.31	0.20
	(2)	0.63	(0.41)	0.45	0.27	0.18
	(3)	0.65	0.45	(0.44)	0.10	0.05
	(4)	0.31	0.27	0.10	(0.36)	0.55
	(5)	0.20	0.18	0.05	0.55	(0.31)

(18)

The principal factors for R_c can be determined by finding the eigenvalues and eigenvectors of the above matrix. As the communality estimates are approximations, however, it is common practice to recompute them from the loadings determined for the principal factors, and to iterate this process until the communality estimates are stabilized. The iterated principal axis factor solution for the R_c matrix in Eqn. (18) is

Variables	Factors (p)					
(j)	I	II	III	IV	V	h²
F = English	0.880	−0.239	−0.009	−0.069	−0.017	0.837
French	0.684	−0.129	−0.204	0.068	0.005	0.531
Italian	0.642	−0.372	0.190	0.030	0.013	0.587
Physics	0.506	0.588	−0.021	−0.064	0.016	0.606
Chemistry	0.398	0.604	0.091	0.068	0.013	0.536
Eigenvalues	2.069	0.923	0.087	0.019	0.001	

(19)

In the **F** matrix in Eqn. (19), an $n \times m$ matrix, the values of the communalities are obtained by $\sum_{p=1}^{m}$ for each test, and the eigenvalues by $\sum_{j=1}^{n} a^2_{jp}$ for each factor. It

will be seen that the eigenvalues decrease in size from the first to later factors. The question arises as to how many of these factors are worth retaining for subsequent processing. The rank of the correlation matrix, that is, the order of the highest nonvanishing determinant of R_c, would indicate the minimum number of factors needed to describe the original set of relationships among the variables. If a matrix is of rank 2, the relationships among the set of variables can be expressed in two-dimensional space; if it is of rank 3, a three-dimensional space is required; and so on. However, clear-cut determination of the rank of a matrix is seldom possible with observed data in the social sciences because of the problem of estimating communalities, fluctuations due to the sampling of individuals, and errors of measurement in the variables.

The number of factors of the original **R** matrix with eigenvalues greater than or equal to 1 is often taken as an indication of the number of initially extracted factors to be retained for further processing; such factors account for at least the equivalent of the total variance of any of the variables being analyzed. In the **R** matrix on which Eqn. (18) is based, two eigenvalues are greater than 1. While this criterion is a useful starting point, it may underestimate the number of factors required to account for the correlational data, and may well be supplemented by other criteria. In Cattell's Scree test (1966), the eigenvalues are graphed from highest to lowest, and factors are accepted only for those eigenvalues above the point on the graph where the eigenvalues level off. With squared multiple correlations as communality estimates in the R_c matrix, the number of eigenvalues greater than the number of corresponding eigenvalues for a correlation matrix based on random data provides a further indication of the number of factors (Montanelli and Humphreys 1976). Subjective criteria, such as discarding factors which account for less than 5 percent, say, of the total variance, on the grounds of their lack of practical importance, may also be considered. A further useful guide is the number of factors built into a well-designed factor analytic study. A comprehensive and readily applicable set of criteria for determining the number of factors has been proposed by Carroll (1993).

The principal factor method is the most commonly used of the least squares approaches to the estimation of the initial **F** matrix; it is described as a "least squares approach," since extracting the maximum variance at each stage is equivalent to minimizing the unexplained variance or residual correlations between the variables.

The method of maximum likelihood, proposed in theoretical terms by Lawley in 1940, and made feasible by procedures developed in the 1960s (Jöreskog 1966, 1979, Jöreskog and Lawley 1968) is also widely used to determine the initial factor matrix, **F**. The method is more efficient than other procedures in the sense that the estimated factor loadings have a smaller sampling variance. It also provides a large sample test of significance for assessing the adequacy of different hypotheses about the number of common factors needed to account for the observed correlation or covariance matrix.

Under the principle of maximum likelihood, the parameter value(s) are sought which maximize the likelihood of a sample result. In its application to factor analysis, the parameter factor matrix **F** is estimated which would have the greatest likelihood, under a given hypothesis about the number of common factors, of generating the observed correlation or covariance matrix. This involves, in the case of uncorrelated factors, the minimization of a function $G(\mathbf{F}, \psi)$ where **F** represents the matrix of factor loadings, and ψ the diagonal matrix of unique variances. When the maximum likelihood estimates of **F** and ψ have been determined, the hypothesis that the n-variable observed matrix can be accounted for by the designated number of common factors (k) can be tested for moderately large N through the χ^2 statistic with $\frac{1}{2}$ degrees of freedom.

Application of the maximum likelihood factor analysis procedure to the correlation matrix in Eqn. (18) with unities in the diagonal cells showed that one factor was insufficient to account for the correlations ($\chi^2 = 69.487$, d.f. = 5, p = 0.000). Maximum likelihood loadings for an **F** matrix were then estimated on the assumption that the **R** matrix could be accounted for by two factors. This **F** matrix is

Factor

Variables (j)	I	II	
F = English	0.934	−0.136	
French	0.670	−0.033	
Italian	0.657	−0.257	(20)
Physics	0.440	0.739	
Chemistry	0.297	0.567	
Eigenvalues	2.037	0.953	

The probability that the observed correlation matrix **R** could have been generated from this **F** matrix is very high, namely 0.998 ($\chi^2 = 0$). The hypothesis that the observed correlation matrix can be accounted for by two underlying factors is therefore accepted.

When the procedure was first developed, the convention with empirically derived data was to accept the hypothesized number of factors as soon as the probability that the observed correlation matrix could be accounted for by that number of factors exceeded 0.10. Since χ^2 values varied with sample size, the significance test criterion in the maximum likelihood method tended to overestimate the number of factors when the sample size was large. It can be supplemented by other indexes of goodness-of-fit developed by Jöreskog and others (see Sect. 6), but most of these also vary with sample size. The appearance of singlet factors, on which only one variable has a substantial loading, may also indicate that too many factors have been extracted. Comparison of the two-dimensional plots based on Eqn. (20) and the first two columns of the matrix in Eqn. (19) shows that the configurations from the maximum likelihood and princi-

pal factor solutions are quite similar. Other approaches to the initial extraction of factors are indicated in Sect. 8.

In matrices with well-defined groupings of variables, as in the 5×5 correlation matrix in Eqn. (18), the various methods for the initial extraction of factors tend to identify the same factors even though factor loadings may differ from one solution to another. Most researchers will find that either the principal factor or maximum likelihood procedures will meet their needs, but it is often instructive to obtain both solutions.

5. Rotation of Factors

As outlined in Sect. 1, Thurstone argued that the initial factors needed to be rotated within the common factor space to arrive at a psychologically meaningful solution. He evolved the concept of simple structure to guide such rotations. As the principles of order implicit in simple structure are germane to a range of disciplines, the rotation of factors in exploratory factor analysis has continued to rely on this general concept.

In searching for new positions to which the original arbitrary orthogonal factor axes should be rotated to give substantive meaning to the factors, the investigator can choose to undertake an orthogonal or an oblique rotation. In the former case, the angles between all of the new factor axes remain at 90°, and the factors remain uncorrelated. In the latter case, the angles between the new axes can be smaller or larger than 90°, with the result that rotated factors may themselves be correlated. The difference between the two types of rotation is illustrated in Fig. 1 for the five-variable correlation problem in Eqn. (18), using as the initial factor plots the factor loadings from a two-factor principal factor solution for this matrix, since there were two eigenvalues greater than unity in the original **R** matrix. The principal factor matrix in this case is

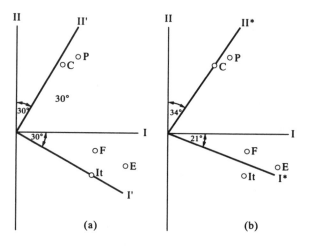

(a)   (b)

Figure 1
Orthogonal (a) and oblique (b) rotations of initial reference axes in Eqn. (21)

	I	II
F = English	0.905	−0.267
French	0.659	−0.128
Italian	0.615	−0.349
Physics	0.523	0.616
Chemistry	0.389	0.562

(21)

These loadings are plotted against the original factor axes I and II. The new positions of the axes after an orthogonal rotation are shown as I′ and II′ in Fig. 1(a). Figure 1(b) gives the new positions of the axes, I* and II*, after an oblique rotation.

In Fig. 1(a), the axes have been rotated clockwise through an angle of approximately 30°. Their placement could be subjectively determined, keeping in mind the need to have some variables with zero or near-zero loadings on each factor. The loadings of the variables on the new axes can be found from the formula **FT = B**, where **T** is the transformation matrix and **B** is the rotated factor matrix. In this particular rotation,

	I′	II′
T = I	cos(−29° 45′)	−sin(−29° 45′)
II	sin(−29° 45′)	cos(−29° 45′)

	I′	II′
= I	0.877	0.481
II	−0.481	0.877

(22)

	I′	II′
B = English	0.92	−0.20
French	0.64	−0.20
Italian	0.71	−0.01
Physics	0.16	0.79
Chemistry	0.07	0.68

(23)

The factor coefficients or factor loadings in Eqn. (23) could be read directly from Fig. 1(a) by measuring the orthogonal projections of the test points on axes I′ and II′ respectively. This matrix of orthogonal projections of the test points on the new axes is known as the "factor structure matrix"; the entries represent the correlations between the test vectors and the factors. The matrix of coordinates of the test points on the new axes, however, defines the "factor pattern matrix"; this is the matrix of coefficients which would be needed to estimate the standard scores of each person on the original variables, as set out in Eqn. (1). The factor pattern and factor structure are identical in an orthogonal factor solution but differ in an oblique solution.

In Fig. 1(b), the axes have been placed through the two distinct clusters of points, so that each cluster will have high loadings on one factor and zero or near-zero loadings on the other. Factor 1 has been rotated clockwise through 21°27′ to the new position I*, and Factor II through 34°28′ to the new position II*. Since the angle of 77° between the two new axes is not a right angle, the rotation is oblique. The orthogonal projection of the endpoints of the test vectors on the new axis system is given by **FΛ = S** where

	I*	II*
Λ = I	cos(−21° 27′)	cos(55° 32′)
II	sin(−21° 27′)	sin(55° 32′)

	I*	II*
= I	0.9307	0.5659
II	−0.3657	0.8245

is the matrix of direction cosines of the new axes with respect to the original axes. Post-multiplying **F** in Eqn. (21) by **Λ** gives the factor structure matrix

	I*	II*
S = English	0.94	−0.29
French	0.66	−0.27
Italian	0.70	−0.06
Physics	0.26	0.80
Chemistry	0.16	0.68

(24)

which represents the correlations of the tests with the factors. The correlation between the two rotated factors is given by the off-diagonal element in

$$\boldsymbol{\varphi} = \boldsymbol{\Lambda}'\boldsymbol{\Lambda} = \begin{bmatrix} 1.000 & 0.225 \\ 0.225 & 1.000 \end{bmatrix}$$

which represents a moderate degree of correlation. In representing the scores of persons in terms of a smaller number of factors, however, the coordinates of the test vectors with respect to the new oblique axes, which form the factor pattern matrix, are of more interest. These are given by **P = Sφ⁻¹**; in the present example, the factor pattern matrix is

	I*	II*
P = English	0.92	−0.08
French	0.63	−0.13
Italian	0.72	−0.10
Physics	0.08	0.78
Chemistry	0.01	0.68

(25)

The **S** matrix in Eqn. (24) could be read directly from Fig.1 (b) by finding the orthogonal projections of the test vectors on Factors I* and II*, and the **P** matrix in Eqn. (25) by finding their oblique projections on these two factors.

A comparison of the matrices in Eqns. (23) and (25) shows the advantages of oblique over orthogonal rotations if the factors are correlated. The factor definition is clearer in the oblique solution; zero or near-zero loadings indicate more clearly that physics and chemistry are not represented in Factor I* and that the three languages are not represented in Factor II*. Some knowledge of the nature of the variables is required to interpret the factors. Each factor must be inspected to determine what the variables with high loadings have in common which is not present in the variables with low loadings, and then named appropriately. The task is deceptively simple in the present example. Since the variables with high loadings on Factor I'/I* are language examinations, and the variables with low loadings are not, this factor can be interpreted as a "language ability factor." Similarly, Factor II'/II* can be interpreted as a "scientific ability/achievement factor." The task of interpretation can be much more demanding in studies involving many variables and several factors.

The new positions of the axes in Fig. 1 were obtained by analytic methods of rotation, which replaced the subjective graphical methods used prior to the 1950s, in which investigators inspected plots of each pair of factors from the **F** matrix. The first fully analytic procedures for rotation developed by Carroll (1953) and other factor analysts became known as "quartimax procedures." They tend to yield a general factor, and are not widely used.

The analytic criterion used to obtain the orthogonal factor solution in Fig. 1(a) was developed and subsequently refined by Kaiser (1958). It is known as the "varimax criterion," and aims to simplify the columns of the factor matrix by maximizing over all factors the variance of the squared factor loadings in each column, after first dividing each factor loading by the square root of the relevant variable's communality to give equal weight to the factors in the rotation. It requires the maximization of the function

$$V = n \sum_{p=1}^{m} \sum_{j=1}^{n} \left(\frac{a_{jp}}{h_j} \right)^4 - \sum_{p=1}^{m} \left(\sum_{j=1}^{n} \frac{a_{jp}^2}{h_j^2} \right)^2 \qquad (26)$$

The varimax criterion, which is designed to generate factors on which some variables have high loadings and others have low loadings, has been found to be highly satisfactory for orthogonal rotations, and is very widely used.

The placement of the new axes in Fig. 1(b) was determined with the aid of the most widely used oblique analytic rotation criterion, known as the "direct oblimin criterion" (Jennrich and Sampson 1966). Following the same principles as Carroll's earlier biquartimin criterion,

that is, the minimization over pairs of factors of the cross-products of squared factor loadings, the minimization of the covariances of these squared loadings, and the use of a coefficient to vary the relative weight given to these two components in order to control the degree of obliqueness of the factors, Jennrich and Sampson rotated the **F** matrix directly to the factor pattern matrix, **P**, by minimizing the function

$$G(\mathbf{P}) = \sum_{p<q=1}^{m} \left(\sum_{j=1}^{n} b_{jp}^2 b_{jp}^2 - \frac{\delta}{n} \sum_{j=1}^{n} b_{jp}^2 \sum_{j=1}^{n} b_{jp}^2 \right) \qquad (27)$$

where b_{jp} and b_{jq} are the elements of the matrix **P** and δ is the variable quantity which controls the degree of obliqueness of the factors. Computer packages usually allow the investigator to apply a range of values of δ to facilitate the selection of a solution which best conforms to simple structure. Factors tend to be too oblique when $\delta = 0$, and become less oblique as δ becomes more negative. DAPPRF (Direct Artificial Personal Probability Rotation Function), an oblique analytic rotational procedure proposed by Tucker and Finkbeiner (1981), was found by Carroll (1993) to yield clearly interpretable solutions in a large number of datasets.

6. Advances in Confirmatory Factor Analysis

The major advance in factor analysis since the late 1960s has been the development of confirmatory factor analytic procedures. In the course of developing maximum likelihood procedures for exploratory factor analysis, Jöreskog saw their possibilities for testing hypothesized matrices. Recognizing that factor analysts generally wished to specify only some of the parameters in a hypothesized matrix, and to allow others to vary, he reformulated the factor analysis model to incorporate fixed parameters, constrained parameters (unknown in value but equal to one or more other parameters), and free parameters. He expressed the model in terms of a variance-covariance or dispersion matrix which becomes a correlation matrix if the variables are in standardized form. That is,

$$\mathbf{\Sigma} = \mathbf{\Lambda} \, \boldsymbol{\phi} \, \mathbf{\Lambda}' + \mathbf{\psi} \qquad (28)$$

where Σ is the dispersion matrix of observed scores, Λ is an $n \times m$ matrix of factor loadings, φ is the factor correlation matrix, and ψ is the diagonal matrix of unique variances. In confirmatory factor analysis, the investigator is free to specify fixed values for particular parameters in Λ, φ, and ψ, given some restriction on the total number of fixed parameters. The matrix Σ is then estimated by maximum likelihood procedures under these conditions, and a χ^2 test applied to determine whether the observed dispersion matrix Σ differs from the estimated matrix $\hat{\Sigma}$.

The value of χ^2, however, varies with sample size so that its use as a test of goodness-of-fit is open to criticism.

Most of the many indexes of goodness-of-fit developed in the 1970s and 1980s have been shown to be affected by sample size (Marsh et al. 1988). Indexes which are independent of sample size, including one proposed by McDonald, have been discussed by McDonald and Marsh (1990). Along with Jöreskog (1979), they point out that decisions to accept or reject a hypothesized model will still need to take account of substantive and theoretical as well as statistical considerations.

Despite these problems of determining goodness-of-fit, the confirmatory factor analysis model has provided great flexibility for testing a wide variety of hypothesized factor patterns in which relationships among the factors may be orthogonal or oblique or a mixture of the two. It has been used, for example, to analyze data from multitrait, multimethod studies (Werts et al. 1972), to illuminate a long-standing controversy on the identification of reading comprehension skills (Spearritt 1972), and to test the simplex assumption underlying Bloom's taxonomy of educational objectives (Hill and McGaw 1981). It has facilitated the comparison of the factorial structure of a given set of variables in subpopulations varying, for example, in gender, age, ethnicity, or socioeconomic status (e.g., Byrne and Shavelson 1987).

The model set out in Eqn. (28) forms part of a more general model for the analysis of covariance structures, which was subsequently elaborated by Jöreskog to handle a wide range of statistical models for multivariate analysis. The LISREL computer program, which provides for the analysis of linear structural relationships by the method of maximum likelihood and various least squares procedures, has become a basic tool for studying not only exploratory and confirmatory factor analysis models, but also path analysis models and models relating to cross-sectional and longitudinal data (see *Path Analysis and Linear Structural Relations Analysis*). A multivariate data screening program called PRELIS was developed by Jöreskog and Sörbom (1988) as a preprocessor for LISREL, and has to be applied if the data include ordinal or "censored" (e.g., highly skewed) variables, in which case product–moment correlations would be inappropriate. Output from the PRELIS program can be used in the main LISREL program to give correct estimates of standard errors and χ^2 values when the distributions are non-normal. New features in the LISREL 7 version of the main program (Jöreskog and Sörbom 1989) include new types of least squares estimation procedures, the analysis of ordinal and other non-normal variables (including dichotomous variables which can be regarded as representing underlying continuous variables), and the consideration of differences in group means in simultaneous analysis of data in several groups. A similar program called EQS (Bentler 1985) avoids the assumption of multivariate normality of variables and is relatively easy to use. Microcomputer (PC) versions of PRELIS, LISREL 7, and EQS are also available.

7. Some Additional Methodological Aspects of Factor Analysis

7.1 Construction of Factor Scales

When factors are identified as a result of a factor analysis, it is possible to calculate a factor score for each person on the new factors, for example, a language score and a science score. With some exceptions, the calculation of factor scores has not been an important feature of educational and psychological studies in which the emphasis has been mainly on the identification rather than the measurement of factors. In some disciplines, however, the chief concern has been to create composite factor scales to facilitate further study of a topic.

The most widely used method of calculating a person's factor scores has been to regress the factor loadings on each factor in the factor structure matrix against the original set of variables. A matrix of factor-score coefficients or regression weights can be found from the formula

$$\mathbf{W} = \mathbf{S}'\mathbf{R}^{-1} \tag{29}$$

where $\mathbf{S}$ is the rotated factor structure matrix and $\mathbf{R}$ is the original correlation matrix. Factor scores are conventionally presented as standard scores, derived by applying the regression weights to a person's standard score on each of the original variables.

7.2 Hierarchical Factor Solutions

Hierarchical factor solutions were attractive to early British factorists because of their hierarchical theories of cognitive processes. Accordingly, a general factor was extracted from the correlation matrix as a first step group factors were then extracted from the residual correlations (Burt 1950, Vernon 1961). Even without the initial assumption of a general factor, the American oblique rotational methods could still yield an hierarchical factor solution. Provided the data yielded sufficient primary factors, the correlations among these factors could themselves be analyzed to arrive at second-order and higher order factors. If the matrix of primary-factor correlations were of unit rank, a second-order general factor would emerge. Schmid and Leiman (1957) showed how such hierarchical solutions could be made orthogonal; many examples of higher-order hierarchical solutions are presented by Carroll (1993). The testing of hierarchical factor models has become more feasible with LISREL confirmatory factor analysis programs; Marsh and Hocevar (1985) used these programs to compare first-order, second-order, and third-order factor models of the structure of self-concept.

7.3 Comparison of Factors

Coefficients of congruence designed to measure the degree of similarity between pairs of factors derived from different sets of variables in the same domain and the degree of similarity between loadings on pairs of corresponding factors derived when the same set of variables is applied to different subpopulations are summarized in Harman (1976) and Gorsuch (1983). Comparisons of factor matrices can be made through confirmatory factor analysis procedures.

7.4 Assumptions of Linearity

It is usually assumed in factor analysis (necessarily so with maximum likelihood procedures) that the variables have a multivariate normal distribution in the population which has been sampled, and this implies that the variables are linearly related. Where this is not the case, multivalued variables may be normalized as a first step. Factor analysis of dichotomously scored variables such as test items is feasible when the regressions of the items on the factors can be assumed to be linear (McDonald 1985) and LISREL 7 provides a program for such variables. Following his earlier work with dichotomous variables, Muthén together with Kaplan (1985) has shown that non-normal categorical variables such as Likert scales can also be factor analyzed. Factor analysis models in which factors are not linearly related to variables have been extensively investigated by McDonald (1967) with applications in item response theory in the 1980s.

8. Computer Programs

Widely available statistical packages such as SPSS, SAS, BMDP, and OSIRIS, and their PC versions where applicable, all contain factor analysis programs. For the initial extraction of factors, the researcher usually has the option of selecting the principal factor, maximum likelihood, Rao canonical, Alpha, or image method of factoring. Varimax and direct oblimin rotational solutions with nominated values of δ are available in most programs, along with other rotational methods such as, for instance, Quartimax and Equimax in SPSS and SAS, and Promax in SAS. Two-dimensional plots of the rotated factors, and the necessary matrix of coefficients for producing factor scores, are also usually obtainable.

9. Applications of Factor Analysis

Factor analysis has made its most direct contribution to education through its influence on the composition of test batteries used for educational or vocational guidance. Batteries of tests such as the SRA Primary Mental Abilities battery and the Psychological Corporation's Differential Aptitude Tests were designed to yield separate scores for students on aptitudes or abilities such as number computation, verbal reasoning, verbal comprehension, abstract reasoning, clerical speed and accuracy, mechanical reasoning, space relations, language usage, and word fluency. Factor analytic studies have also contributed to the selection of areas to be tested in achievement test batteries, such as reading comprehension, listening

comprehension, and comprehension and interpretation in mathematics, science, and social studies. Factor analysis has served to identify skills, abilities, and areas of achievement which are relatively independent, and has thus avoided unnecessary duplication of measurement in providing a profile of a student's performance. Factor studies have also often provided the framework for personality and interest inventories used in guidance and counseling.

The major impact of factor analysis has been in the area in which it was first employed, that is, in the study of intellectual or cognitive abilities. It has been used to map the broad areas of human abilities which are needed to account for the variation which occurs in the performance of subjects on a great variety of mental tasks. Factor studies of particular importance in this respect include many which made use of the Educational Testing Service's kit of cognitive abilities (French 1954) and its revisions in 1963 and 1976, and those leading to Guilford's Structure of Intellect model and the Cattell and Horn theory of "crystallized" and "fluid" intelligence. These have been supplemented by more recent testing of hierarchical models of intelligence by Gustafsson and others. Abilities isolated at one level, such as reasoning ability or memory, have also been subjected to detailed factor analyses of their infrastructure (see *Models of Intelligence*). These studies have produced a very considerable body of knowledge about the structure of human cognitive abilities, effectively epitomized by Carroll (1993) in terms of a three-level hierarchical factor model, based on his reanalyses of 461 datasets obtained in 19 countries for the period 1925 to 1987.

In applications in education, factor analytic studies have been undertaken in such diverse areas as prose style, administrative behavior, occupational classification, attitudes and belief systems, and the economics of education. The technique is still in extensive use in the exploration of abilities, in the refining of tests and scales, and in the development of composite variables for use in research studies. The educational implications of factors and factor models in the areas of profile assessments of students, teaching and learning, and educational policy have been discussed by Spearritt (1996).

Factor analysis will remain an important technique for reducing and classifying sets of variables as a means of improving theoretical understanding in various disciplines, and for testing hypotheses about structural relationships among sets of variables. Exploratory factor analysis procedures will continue to reveal the broad structure of educational and psychological domains, and to generate theories about this structure. Confirmatory factor analysis procedures should assist in formulating and testing more precise theories about structural relationships in these domains. In the search for explanations about how and why such structural relationships take the form they do, closer links can be expected to be developed between factor analysis and path analysis models. Further methodological developments might be expected in the application of factor analysis to non-normal variables, and in the development of nonlinear models where linear models prove to be inadequate. Considerable scope remains for research on the emergence of factors, involving neurological, general environmental, and schooling influences, while factor studies of the abilities tested in different school subjects would be highly relevant to the design of school curricula.

See also: Factorial Modeling; Models and Model Building; Multivariate Analysis; Q-Methodology

References

Bentler P M 1985 *Theory and Implementation of* EQS: A Structural Equations Program. BMDP Statistical Software, Los Angeles, California

Burt C 1950 Group factor analysis. *Br. J. Psychol. Stat. Sect.* 3: 40–75

Byrne B M, Shavelson R J 1987 Adolescent self-concept: Testing the assumption of equivalent structure across gender. *Am. Educ. Res. J.* 24: 365–85

Carroll J B 1953 An analytical solution for approximating simple structure in factor analysis. *Psychometrika* 18: 23–38

Carroll J B 1993 *Human Cognitive Abilities: A survey of factor-analytic studies.* Cambridge University Press, New York

Cattell R B 1966 The Scree test for the number of factors. *Mult. Behav. Res.* 1(2): 245–76

French J W (ed.) 1954 *Manual for Kit of Selected Tests for Reference Aptitude and Achievement Factors.* Educational Testing Service, Princeton, New Jersey

Gorsuch R L 1983 *Factor Analysis,* 2nd edn. Erlbaum, Hillside, New Jersey

Harman H H 1976 *Modern Factor Analysis,* 3rd edn. University of Chicago Press, Chicago, Illinois

Hill P W, McGaw B 1981 Testing the simplex assumption underlying Bloom's taxonomy. *Am. Educ. Res. J.* 18(1): 93–101

Jennrich R I, Sampson P F 1966 Rotation for simple loadings. *Psychometrika* 31(3): 313–23

Jöreskog K G 1966 Testing a simple structure hypothesis in factor analysis. *Psychometrika* 31(2): 165–78

Jöreskog K G 1979 A general approach to confirmatory maximum likelihood factor analysis. In: Jöreskog K G, Sörbom D (eds.) 1979 *Advances in Factor Analysis and Structural Equation Models.* Abt, Cambridge, Massachusetts

Jöreskog K G, Lawley D N 1968 New methods in maximum likelihood factor analysis. *Br. J. Math. Stat. Psychol.* 21(1): 85–96

Jöreskog K G, Sörbom D 1988 PRELIS: *A Program for Multivariate Data Screening and Data Summarization. A Preprocessor for* LISREL. *Scientific Software Inc., Mooresville, Indiana*

Jöreskog K G, Sörbom D 1989 LISREL 7: *A Guide to the Program and Applications.* Scientific Software Inc., Mooresville, Indiana

Kaiser H F 1958 The varimax criterion for analytic rotation in factor analysis. *Psychometrika* 23: 187–200

Lawley D N 1940 The estimation of factor loadings by the method of maximum likelihood. *Proc. Roy. Soc. Edin.* 60: 64–82

Marsh H W, Balla J R, McDonald R P 1988 Goodness-of-fit indexes in confirmatory factor analysis: The effect of sample size. *Psych. Bull.* 103(3): 391–410

Marsh H W, Hocevar D 1985 Application of confirmatory factor analysis to the study of self-concept: First- and higher order factor models and their invariance across groups. *Psych. Bull.* 97(3): 562–82

McDonald R P 1967 *Nonlinear Factor Analysis.* William Byrd, Richmond, Virginia

McDonald R P 1985 *Factor Analysis and Related Models.* Erlbaum, Hillsdale, New Jersey

McDonald R P. Marsh H W 1990 Choosing a multivariate model: Noncentrality and goodness-of-fit. *Psych. Bull.* 107(2): 247–55

Montanelli R G Jr, Humphreys L G 1976 Latent roots of random data correlation matrices with squared multiple correlations on the diagonal: A Monte Carlo study. *Psychometrika* 41: 341–8

Muthén B, Kaplan D 1985 A comparison of some methodologies for the factor analysis of non-normal Likert variables. *Br. J. Math. Stat. Psychol.* 38(2): 171–89

Schmid J, Leiman J M 1957 The development of hierarchical factor solutions. *Psychometrika.* 22: 53–61

Spearman C 1904 "General intelligence" objectively determined and measured. *Am. J. Psychol.* 15(2): 201–93

Spearritt D 1972 Identification of subskills of reading comprehension by maximum likelihood factor analysis. *Read. Res. Q.* 8(1): 92–111

Spearritt D 1996 Carroll's model of cognitive abilities: Educational implications. *Int. J. Educ. Res.* 25(2)

Thurstone L L 1947 *Multiple-factor Analysis: A Development and Expansion of the Vectors of the Mind.* University of Chicago Press, Chicago, Illinois

Tucker L R, Finkbeiner T C 1981 *Transformation of factors by artificial personal probability functions.* Research Report RR-81-58, Educational Testing Service, Princeton, New Jersey

Vernon P E 1961 *The Structure of Human Abilities,* 2nd edn. Methuen, London

Werts C E, Jöreskog K G, Linn R L 1972 A multitrait-multimethod model for studying growth. *Educ. Psychol. Meas.* 32(3): 655–78

Further Reading

Cattell R B 1971 *Abilities, Their Structure, Growth and Action.* Houghton Mifflin, Boston, Massachusetts

Comfrey A L, Lee H B 1992 *A First Course in Factor Analysis,* 2nd edn. Erlbaum, Hillsdale, New Jersey

Guilford J P 1967 *The Nature of Human Intelligence.* McGraw-Hill, New York

Kim J O, Mueller C W 1978 *Factor Analysis: Statistical Methods and Practical Issues.* Sage, Beverly Hills, California

Factorial Modeling

P. R. Lohnes

Factorial modeling (FaM) provides researchers with a simple method for constructing latent structural variables linking theory with correlational data. Structural variables emphasize construct validity rather than predictive power in the linear components fitted by data analysis to vector variables. At the research design stage, the researcher who is planning to use FaM is required to name the latent variables (hereafter called factors) and to specify each of them by means of an exclusive subset of the independent variates (i.e., the measurements). The researcher is also required to specify an order of extraction of the factors, because the mathematical simplicity and computational efficiency of FaM are purchased at the expense of order dependence of the factors. The FaM data analysis yields a structural equation for every observational variate and attributes all explained variance unambiguously among the factors. This is possible because the factors are constructed to be mutually uncorrelated. Partitioning of criterion variance into dependent contributions from uncorrelated factors is particularly useful in educational policy studies, where intervention decisions have to be justified by straightforward causal inferences.

The method was named factorial modeling to encourage comparison with factorial analysis of variance. In the design of experiments, a balanced sampling scheme creates uncorrelatedness of the causal factors to permit unambiguous causal inferences. In observational studies, FaM creates uncorrelated causal factors by analysis where they cannot be created by the sampling scheme. Causal inferences from FaM do not possess the high internal validity of inferences from a randomized factorial experiment, but if the data represent an important natural system in situ, the external validity of the factorial model may be much higher than that of any possible experiment. When the constructs of a theory represent interdependent attributes, the corresponding factors of a FaM model for data represent the partial contents of their constructs which are nonoverlapping with the contents of previously extracted factors. Thus FaM is a method which resembles multiple partial correlation.

Factorial modeling does not employ an algorithm derived by the differential calculus of linear systems. The method may appeal to researchers who fear that multivariate regression methods overpower many of the data collections available in education. The rationale for FaM is that using noncalculus multivariate mathematics on data will produce loose-fitting models that may be readily transferred to new situations.

1. Mathematics

Factorial modeling extracts ordered orthogonal factors by the method of matrix exhaustion. Each factor is specified by assignment to it of an exclusive subset of the independent variates. It is weighted by the covariances of those specifying variates with a selected dependent variate in the residual matrix prevailing at the start of the factoring step. For the first factor the weights are simply the bivariate correlations of the specifying variates with the selected criterion, or simple predictive validities. For all later factors, the weights are residual covariances representing residual predictive validities. It is not necessary that every independent variate be assigned to the specification of one of the factors, but it is highly desirable that at least two variates specify each factor. Otherwise, the total variance for a single variate specifying a factor will be swept out, resulting in $h^2 = 1$ for that variate and a degenerate structural equation for it. The object of modeling is to regress criteria on latent variables, not on observed variates.

Let an idempotent matrix containing ones on the main diagonal in the positions corresponding to the positions in the correlation matrix of the specifying variates for the kth factor, and zeros everywhere else, be identified as $\mathbf{I}_k$. Let

$$\mathbf{v}_k = \mathbf{I}_k \mathbf{r}_c \tag{1}$$

where $\mathbf{r}_c$ is the column of the residual matrix $\mathbf{C}_k$ which belongs to the selected criterion. Then $\mathbf{v}_k$ is a vector of the order of $\mathbf{R}$ (which may be designated p for the count of all the measurement variates, independent plus dependent), but the only nonzero elements of $\mathbf{v}_k$ are predictive validities of the specification variates for the kth factor. For the following equation

$$\mathbf{h}_k = (1/\sqrt{\mathbf{v}_k'\ \mathbf{C}_k \mathbf{v}_k})\mathbf{v}_k \tag{2}$$

when $k = 1$, $\mathbf{C}_1 = \mathbf{R}$, the correlation matrix for the measurements. When $k = 2$, $\mathbf{C}_2$ is the covariance matrix remaining after the first factor has been exhausted from $\mathbf{R}$. In general, $\mathbf{C}_k$ is the residual covariance matrix after $k - 1$ factors have been exhausted.

Then the structural coefficients for the kth factor are

$$\mathbf{s}_k = \mathbf{C}_k\ \mathbf{h}_k \tag{3}$$

and $\mathbf{C}_k$ is *exhausted of* $\mathbf{s}_k$.

$$\mathbf{C}_{k+1} = \mathbf{C}_k - \mathbf{s}_k\ \mathbf{s}_k' \tag{4}$$

When all n planned factors have been computed, their column vectors of structural coefficients are assembled in a $p \times n$ matrix $\mathbf{S}$. Now the theory plus error partition of $\mathbf{R}$ is given by

$$\mathbf{R} = \mathbf{S}\,\mathbf{S}' + \mathbf{C}_{n+1} \tag{5}$$

The elements of the main diagonal of the theory matrix $\mathbf{S}\,\mathbf{S}$ are the proportions of the variate variances explained by the theory for the data, called the communalities, h_j^2. The square roots of the elements of the main diagonal of $\mathbf{C}_{n+1}$ are the disturbance weights, d_j, which apply to the combined unknown sources of variance in each of the variates. From these results a structural equation can be written for each variate

$$z_j = s_{j1}f_1 + s_{j2}f_2 + \ldots + s_{jn}f_n + d_j\,u_j \tag{6}$$

In this equation the f_k are the factor scores and the u_j is a uniqueness score, that is, a score for the combination of all other sources of variance in z_j. Dropping the final addend gives the multiple regression equation

$$z_j s_{j1}f_1 + s_{j2}f_2 + \ldots + s_{jn}f_n \tag{7}$$

This shows that any structural coefficient s_{jk}, besides being a product–moment correlation between a variate and a factor, is also a standardized multiple regression weight for the regression of the kth variate on the kth factor, and its square, s_{jk}^2, is the contribution of the kth factor to the explanation of the variance in the jth variate. The squared multiple correlation coefficient is the communality

$$R_j^2 = h_j^2 = s_{j1}^2 + s_{j2}^2 + \ldots + s_{jn}^2 \tag{8}$$

Thus the canon of unambiguous attribution of variance is satisfied.

Two salient facts emerge from this mathematics. The exact definition achieved for each factor beyond the first is order dependent, in the sense that it depends in part on the order in which the factors are extracted. Also, as factoring continues, the degrees of freedom for arbitrary location of a factor are reduced and the disciplinary force of the uncorrelatedness requirement over the hypothetical location of the factor becomes stronger.

As originally proposed by Lohnes (1979) FaM required the designation of a key criterion toward which all the factors were oriented. Lohnes has modified the algorithm so that when there are multiple criteria, it searches the vectors of residual predictive validities of the specification variates for a factor to find the largest sum of squares of those validities, and orients the factor to that criterion for which it has, in this sum of squares sense, the largest predictive validity. The program provides for the user to override this feature by designating the criterion variate toward which each factor is to be oriented, and it is permissible to designate the same criterion for all the key factors, thus restoring the original emphasis on a key criterion.

The current program for FaM also incorporates an improved algebra for computing coefficients defining the latent variables as linear functions of some of the variates. The new algebra supplies true zero coefficients in every possible place. Only the specification variates for the first factor enter its operational definition. Only the specification variates for the first two factors enter the operational definition of the second factor. For any other factor, only the specification variates for it and the previously extracted factors enter the operational definition. Thus the minimum number of nonzero coefficients required to maintain the uncorrelatedness of the factors is employed. For $k = 1, 2,\ldots, n$, and letting s_k be the kth column of $\mathbf{S}$, and b_k be the kth column of the factor scoring coefficients matrix $\mathbf{B}$, the coefficients for the kth factor may be computed as

$$\mathbf{b}_k = \mathbf{h}_k - \mathbf{h}_k'\mathbf{s}_{k-1}\,\mathbf{b}_{k-1} - \mathbf{h}_k'\mathbf{s}_{k-2}\mathbf{b}_{k-2} - \ldots \tag{9}$$
$$- \mathbf{h}_k'\mathbf{s}_2\mathbf{b}_2 - \mathbf{h}_k'\mathbf{s}_1\mathbf{h}_1$$

For the first factor the results is

$$\mathbf{b}_1 = \mathbf{h}_1 \tag{10}$$

For the second factor

$$\mathbf{b}_2 = \mathbf{h}_2 - \mathbf{h}_2'\mathbf{s}_1\mathbf{b}_1 \tag{11}$$

Every $\mathbf{b}_k$ will contain true zeros in the positions of all the variates except those variates entering the specification of the first k factors.

In order to explore the possible consequences of an observed or manipulated change in a single independent variate, the algebra of the model may be read "backwards" (i.e., reversing the inferred paths of causal influence from the factors to the variates), computing the changes in factors that might be concomitant with a change in a given variate, and then the consequences of such changes in factors for changes in criterion variates. A table with w rows representing the criterion variates and q columns representing the independent variates (so that $w + q = p$), in which each element ∇_{jm} reports the possible change (in standard deviation) in the mth independent variate, contains elements

$$\nabla_{jm} = \sum_{k=1}^{n} s_{jk}\,b_{mk} \tag{12}$$

where $j = 1,2,\ldots, w$ and $m = 1,2,\ldots, q$.

If Δ_m is the fraction of a standard deviation change actually observed or produced in an independent variate, the corresponding possible change in a criterion may be computed as

$$\Delta_j = \Delta_m\,\nabla_{jm} \tag{13}$$

This is a highly tenuous interpretation of the model for the data, and the educational policymaker must be very cautious in using it. (The FORTRAN program for FaM should be requested from the author at 401 Baldy Hall, SUNYAB, Amherst, New York 14260, USA.)

There is no distribution theory for FaM, so it is not a statistical modeling procedure strictly speaking.

Table 1
Correlation matrix for informed condition (N=111)[a]

MF 1	1.00								
MF 2	0.74	1.00							
E 1	0.31	0.41	1.00						
E 2	0.31	0.40	0.80	1.00					
W 1	0.40	0.46	0.64	0.63	1.00				
W 2	0.40	0.50	0.56	0.57	0.82	1.00			
AA	−0.15	−0.18	−0.22	−0.16	−0.34	0.34	1.00		
G	−0.20	−0.24	−0.21	−0.18	−0.44	−0.38	0.67	1.00	
AP	−0.06	−0.11	−0.09	−0.06	−0.21	−0.20	0.59	0.64	1.00

a MF = motive to avoid failure; E = emotionality; W = worry; AA = arithmetic/algebra; G = geometry; AP = applied mathematics

However, Reeves (1990) demonstrates the use of both jack-knife and bootstrap methods for obtaining empirical resampling standard errors for the FaM path coefficients. A choice of one or the other of these methods should satisfy the user who requires *t*-tests or confidence intervals for the path coefficients.

2. Example

Hagtvet (1981), in an effort to challenge the conventional representation of test anxiety as a unitary construct, hypothesized a three-dimensional hierarchical set of test anxiety factors, which included a general factor (specified by "motive to avoid failure" scales) and two response factors ("emotionality," which refers to self-perceived affective–physiological arousal, and "worry," which refers to focusing of attention on irrelevant cognitions of shortcomings and risks). He also posited that the general factor would be the dominant source of text anxiety in situations where subjects were surprised with an unannounced test, whereas the response factors would be more psychoactive in situations where subjects had a period of time to prepare for an announced test.

Hagtvet made random assignments of ninth grade classes to the two situations. The criterion variates were three tests of the Norwegian national mathematics battery. Two questionnaire scales to specify each of the three anxiety factors were administered one month in advance of the mathematics tests. Sample sizes of 111 pupils in the informed group and 66 pupils in the uninformed group were available for analysis.

Factorial modeling models were computed for each group. Both models confirmed the three-factor theory well, and the hypothesis about the effects of the situations was sustained. The uninformed subjects model showed the general factor contributing moderately to variance on all three mathematics tests while the re-

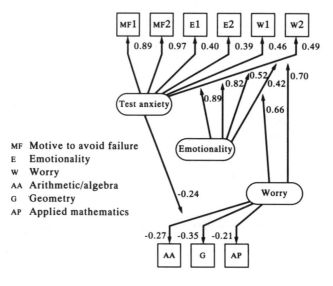

MF Motive to avoid failure
E Emotionality
W Worry
AA Arithmetic/algebra
G Geometry
AP Applied mathematics

Figure 1
FaM model for informed condition

Table 2
FaM model for informed condition[a]

| Variate | Factors | | | *d* | *h*[2] |
	General anxiety	Emotionality	Worry		
MF	0.89	−0.05	0.00	0.46	0.79
MF 2	0.97	0.03	0.00	0.24	0.94
E 1	0.40	0.89	−0.02	0.21	0.96
E 2	0.39	0.82	0.04	0.41	0.83
W 1	0.46	0.52	0.66	0.29	0.92
W 2	0.49	0.42	0.70	0.30	0.91
AA	−0.18	−0.15	−0.27	0.94	0.13
G	−0.24	−0.12	−0.35	0.90	0.20
AP	−0.09	−0.05	−0.21	0.97	0.05

a MF = motive to avoid failure; E = emotionality; W = worry; AA = arithmetic/ algebra; G = geometry; AP = applied mathematics; *d* = disturbance; *h*[2] = commun

Table 3
Factor scoring coefficients[a]

| Variate | Factors | | |
	General anxiety	Emotionality	Worry
MF 1	0.367	−0.168	−0.143
MF 2	0.696	−0.318	−0.270
E 1	0.000	0.759	−0.529
E 2	0.000	0.393	−0.274
W 1	0.000	0.000	0.758
W 2	0.000	0.000	0.719

a MF = motive to avoid failure; E = emotionality; W = worry

sponse factors contributed essentially nothing. In the informed subjects model (Tables 1, 2, 3, and Fig. 1) the general anxiety contribution to the mathematics tests was greatly reduced, whereas the "worry" factor contributed to the variance in all three criteria. The FaM analyses thus tested and supported both the factor structure and the situational effects aspects of Hagtvet's theory.

A further example of factorial modeling is provided in Lohnes (1986), where the results of analyses of data using FaM may be compared with those obtained through the use of alternative procedures.

See also: Factor Analysis; Latent Trait Measurement Models

References

Hagtvet K A 1981 Towards a three dimensional concept of test anxiety: A factorial modeling study. Unpublished paper available from Institute of Psychology, University of Bergen, Bergen

Lohnes P R 1979 Factorial modeling in support of causal inference. *Am. Educ. Res. J.* 16(4): 323–40

Lohnes P R 1986 Factorial modeling. *Int. J. Educ. Res.* 10(2): 181–89

Reeves D J 1990 A comparison of jack-knife and bootstrap methods in estimating standard errors for factorial modeling. Unpublished HD doctoral dissertation, State University of New York, Buffalo, New York

Further Reading

Ackerman W B, Lohnes P R 1981 *Research Methods for Nurses*, Chaps 10, 11, 12. McGraw-Hill, New York

Galois Lattices

C. Ander, A. Joó and L. Mérö

The Galois lattice (*G*-lattice) is a graphic method of representing knowledge structures. The nodes of *G*-lattices represent all the possible concepts in a given body of knowledge in the sense that a notion defines a set of individuals or properties with no exceptions or idiosyncrasies. A *G*-lattice provides a tool to represent all the possible developmental phases to reach a given total knowledge via different partial knowledge structures.

G-lattices are pure algebraic structures and may contain contingent features caused by irregular and random data. In this entry some algorithms are proposed to develop the *G*-lattice method so that statistical analyses can be incorporated. These algorithms are based on the possible omissions of individuals or properties from the data so that the resulting *G*-lattice

can be reduced as much as possible. The greatly simplified structure represented by the resulting *G*-lattice is still valid for a large percentage of individuals or properties. This is an alternative approach to statistical significance as this approach refers to strict logical relations.

1. On Binary Variables

Binary variables abound in educational research. Right or wrong answers, the presence or absence of certain properties, choices, and rejections in tests can be considered as sets of binary variables. However, there are only a few mathematical procedures that are developed exclusively for binary variables. Statisticians usually

Table 1
Model of results of 12 pupils on 12 tasks

Pupils Tasks	1	2	3	4	5	6	7	8	9	10	11	12
1	–	–	–	+	–	+	–	–	+	–	+	+
2	–	–	–	+	–	+	+	–	–	–	+	+
3	–	–	+	–	–	+	–	–	–	–	+	+
4	–	–	–	–	+	+	–	–	–	+	–	–
5	–	–	–	–	+	+	–	–	–	+	–	–
6	–	–	–	–	+	+	–	–	–	+	–	–
7	–	–	–	+	–	+	–	–	–	+	+	+
8	–	–	–	+	–	+	–	–	–	+	–	–
9	–	–	–	+	–	+	–	–	–	+	–	–
10	–	–	–	+	–	+	–	–	–	+	–	–
11	–	–	+	–	–	–	+	–	–	–	+	+
12	–	+	+	–	–	–	+	–	–	–	+	–

propose building up indices from binary variables and then apply common statistical procedures to analyze relationships between the indices.

In many cases, however, one may be interested in the interconnections of the binary variables themselves and when indices are built a great part of these interconnections may be lost. The strength of the connection between any two binary variables can, of course, be measured before composing indices of them. But how can one tell which connections are to be measured? In the case of only 20 binary variables there are more than one million possible connections if all the subsets of the binary variables are considered. Measuring only pairwise connections may be an unreasonable oversimplification.

The Rasch model has been proposed especially for evaluating test data and works well in many cases. A significant restriction of the Rasch model, however, is that it assumes homogeneity of items and, in connection with this homogeneity, that the test items should be ranked unequivocally according to their level of difficulty. The expectation of the test constructor may be different from this.

Task *b* may be easier than task *c* for those who were able to solve task *a*, while task *c* may be easier than task *b* for those who were not able to solve task *a*. This kind of connection may emerge when the solution of task *a* presupposes some kind of knowledge that renders the solution of task *b* obvious but obscures a commonsense solution for task *c*. This implies that the degree of difficulty of the tasks is a partial ordering relation rather than a full one. This means that a lattice model may characterize the connections between the difficulties of the tasks better than a linear model. In such a model it may happen that one task is easier or more difficult than another and it may happen that two tasks are incomparable. However, even two incomparable tasks may prove to be comparable when referenced to other tasks.

The method described in this entry is appropriate for these kinds of problems. It has been developed as a purely algebraic model and it will first be presented in its original form, and then developed into a statistical procedure. The procedure is also applicable to problems other than the one described above. It models the way of forming concepts and, therefore, it may be a useful tool in designing instructional materials.

2. The Galois Lattice

Let $I = \{i_1, i_2, \ldots, i_n\}$ denote the set of n individuals and $T = \{t_1, t_2, \ldots, t_k\}$ denote the set of k features. Let $R \subset I \times T$ denote a relation that is defined in the pair of one individual and one feature. The relation R assumes that $i_j\, R\, t_m$ is valid if the individual i_j has the feature t_m, and otherwise, the relation is not valid. The inverse of the relation R is denoted by R^{-1} and $t_m\, R^{-1}\, i_j$ is the same as $i_j\, R\, t_m$. Let I_1 be an arbitrary subset of I and let $R(I_1)$ denote the set of those features that are valid for all individuals in I_1. Similarly, a subset $R^{-1}(T_1)$ denotes the set of individuals showing all the features in T_1.

The subset of individuals I_1, shall be called a "closed set" of individuals if $I_1 = R^{-1}[R(I_1)$ is true. Similarly, the subset T_1 of features is called a "closed subset of features" if $T_1 = R[R^{-1}(T_1)$ is true. The sets I_1 and T_1 are said to be in "Galois connection" (or G-connection) if $R(I_1) = T_1$ and $R^{-1}(T_1) = I_1$ are true. Clearly if a set of individuals is in G-connection with a set of features then both sets are closed.

The principal aim is to investigate subsets that are in G-connection. To illustrate the meaning of a G-connection let the individuals be pupils and the features be a set of tasks. In this case a G-connection between a set of pupils I_1 and a set of tasks T_1 implies that all the following statements are valid:

(a) all pupils in I_1 have solved the tasks in T_1;

(b) there is no pupil outside I_1 who solved all the tasks in T_1;

(c) there is no task outside T_1 that was solved by all the pupils in I_1

It has been proved that the closed subsets of the set I of individuals constitute a lattice if the lattice operations are defined as follows (there are two operations in a lattice, the union and the intersection):

$$I_1 \cup I_2 \stackrel{\text{def}}{=} I_3 \quad \begin{array}{l} \text{If (a) } I_1 \subset I_3,\, I_2 \subset I_1 \text{ and} \\ \text{(b) } I_3 \text{ is the smallest among the closed} \\ \text{sets satisfying (a)} \end{array}$$

$$I_1 \cup I_2 \stackrel{\text{def}}{=} I_3 \quad \begin{array}{l} \text{If (c) } I_3 \subset I_1,\, I_3 \subset I_2 \text{ and} \\ \text{(d) } I_3 \text{ is the largest among the closed} \\ \text{sets satisfying (c)} \end{array}$$

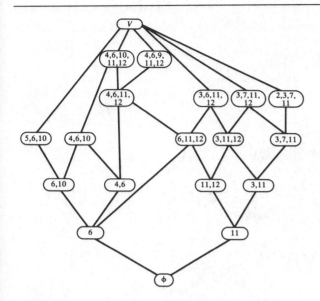

Figure 1
Representation of the Galois lattice

The closed subsets of T constitute a lattice in a similar way, only T is substituted for I everywhere in the previous definition. These two lattices are isomorphic and an isomorphism between them is defined by the G-connections. As a consequence of this fact, the two sets can be represented in the same drawing; the union of a pupil set corresponds to the intersection of a task set and vice versa.

Figure 1 presents an example illustrating these notions. Figure 1 is a Galois lattice representation of the data in Table 1. Table 1 contains the results of 12 pupils on 12 tasks; the rows of the matrix correspond to the pupils and the columns of the matrix correspond to the tasks; "+" represents a correct solution and "–" represents a wrong one. Table 2 presents the closed sets of pupils and also the closed sets of tasks. The correspondence between the closed pupil sets and the closed task sets is clear.

There are 19 closed sets in this example including the empty set (ϕ). Figure 1 shows the lattice of the closed sets of tasks. The set of all the tasks (which is obviously closed) is denoted by V and is at the top of the figure. Two elements in the lattice are connected by an edge if one of them includes the other and there is no third closed set which includes one of the two tasks and is included in the other.

The same diagram presents the lattice of the closed sets of pupils, too. In this case the task sets in Fig. 1 can be substituted with the appropriate pupil sets according to Table 2. Then V in Fig. 1 will denote the empty pupil set and ϕ in Fig. 1 will denote the set of all pupils. Moving upward in the graph of Fig. 1 one finds more and more narrow pupil sets and larger and larger task sets. Two closed sets of tasks in the lattice determine their union: the union of two sets in the lattice is the lowest point in the lattice from which a path of edges leads to both given sets. This is apparently not always the same as their set-theoretical union. A similar statement is valid for intersection. For example, the union of the closed sets {4,6,10} and {6,11,12} in the net or lattice structure is {4,6,10,11,12} and their intersection is {6}. In this case the union and the intersection coincide with the set-theoretical union and intersection. On the other hand, the union of the closed sets {4,6,10} and {5,6,10} in the lattice is the full task set, which is not the same as their set-theoretical union. Their set-theoretical union is the set {4,5,6,10} but this is not a closed set. These kinds of features allow interesting interpretations which will be shown later.

The lattice of closed sets as defined above is called a "Galois lattice" (or G-lattice). If the feature set is interpreted as properties, then a closed set of features can be interpreted as a notion. In this interpretation the concept of a notion is defined in a strict but very logical way: a notion should define a set of individuals with no exceptions and no idiosyncrasies; and conversely, if a set of individuals share a set of properties and no other individual has the same set of properties, then this set of individuals should correspond to a notion. Biologists, for example, narrow down their worlds to special properties of their interest and try to define the species as a notion in the previous sense. They might ask questions like "Is 'horse' a notion in this sense?"

Table 2
Table of closed sets

Set number	Closed sets of pupils	Closed sets of tasks
1	ϕ	1,2,3,4,5,6,7,8,9,10,11,12
2	1	4,6,9,11,12
3	3	3,6,11,12
4	7	4,6,10,11,12
5	11	3,7,11,12
6	12	2,3,7,11
7	3,11	3,11,12
8	11,12	3,7,11
9	1,2,7	4,6,11,12
10	3,11,12	3,11
11	4,5,6	5,6,10
12	1,2,3,7	6,11,12
13	7,8,9,10	4,6,10
14	1,2,3,7,11	11,12
15	1,2,3,7,11,12	11
16	1,2,7,8,9,10	4,6
17	4,5,6,7,8,9,10	6,10
18	1,2,3,4,5,6,7,8,9,10	6
19	1,2,3,4,5,6,7,8,9,10,11,12	ϕ

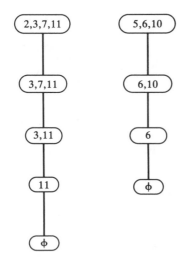

Figure 2
Subsets of the Galois lattice

This methodology for creating notions can be witnessed in archaic societies as described by Durkheim (1902), in modern phonetics (here individuals correspond to sounds and the properties correspond to their discriminative features), and this way of creating notions emerges in semantics (Katz and Fodor 1963) and in cybernetics (Fay and Takács 1975).

3. Applications in Education

Figure 1 will now be examined from an educational point of view. There are 12 tasks, so there are 2^{12}, or 4096 possibilities to investigate subsets of tasks and to measure the strength of connections in the subset. However, there is no need for that many measurement points because Fig. 1 includes all the significant information. It can be readily seen that anybody who solved task 3 also solved task 11, as all the closed subsets containing 3 also contain 11. No pupil solved both task 3 and task 4, because only V contains both of these tasks and V corresponds to the empty pupil set. There are pupils (at least one) who solved only task 6 and there are pupils who solved only task 11, because these single numbers are closed sets. On the other hand, if a pupil solved task 6 and also solved task 11 then he or she also solved task 12, because the union of {6} and {11} in the lattice is the set {6,11,12}. Some connections of this kind could also have been read from the matrix on Table 1. However, in Fig. 1 *all* connections of this kind can be read without any difficulty. The Galois lattice is a good tool for displaying connections and also for identifying them.

From a Galois lattice it can be immediately stated whether one task is easier or more difficult than an-

other, or whether they are incommensurable. In Fig. 1, for example, task 11 is clearly easier than task 3 or task 12. Task 3 and task 4 cannot be compared as to their difficulty because there was no pupil solving both of them.

The Rasch model aims at setting up an order of the tasks according to their difficulty. This would mean, in the strict sense, that for any two tasks *a* and *b* it should be true that either all the pupils who solved task *a* also solved task *b* (i.e., *b* was easier than *a*) or all the pupils who solved task *b* also solved task *a* (i.e., *a* was easier than *b*). This strict supposition is never fulfilled in large samples, and therefore it is accepted if these statements are true at a particular probability level (e.g., 0.95 or more). Before dealing with statistical matters, the situation in which the Rasch model can properly be applied should be examined. It is easy to see that a necessary and sufficient condition of the correct application of the Rasch model (in the strict sense) is that in the *G*-lattice of the task set only one path should lead from the bottom to the top. In other words, the *G*-lattice should look like that in Fig. 2. Figure 2 displays the *G*-lattice of two subsets of the original task set for which the easier/harder relation unequivocally holds between any two tasks.

It was stated above that the *G*-lattice contains all significant information. This raises the question as to how Fig. 2 can be derived from Fig. 1. There is a very simple way to find all the Rasch-type subsets in the *G*-lattice. One has only to search for all the paths from the top of the graph to the bottom which pass through points fulfilling the following condition: the passed point can be reached from any higher passed points in only one way in the lattice. It can be easily checked that the paths in Fig. 2 have this property.

A figure is always more than just its parts put together. Therefore one may ask what Fig. 1 *in toto* expresses. The claim is that the Galois lattice expresses the structure of knowledge and the possible ways of increasing that knowledge. In Fig. 1, if someone solves task 5, this implies that he or she

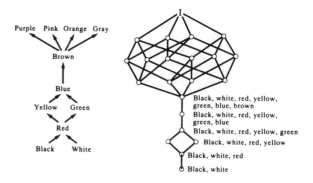

Figure 3
Evolution of color terminology and its Galois model

solves tasks 6 and 10 as well, since the only path to task 5 leads through these two tasks. The knowledge represented by task 4 can be reached in two ways: the shorter path leads immediately through task 6, but the longer path may lead through tasks 11 and 12 and only then through tasks 6 and 3. This longer path results in reaching the full knowledge represented in the tasks as a by-product. This kind of information is indispensable, for example, for the designer of instructional materials who wants to know which part of the target knowledge can be reached in several ways, what are the actual paths, what are their lengths, and so forth.

Finally the following theoretical question arises. We have started from a data matrix without any explicit or implicit time parameter. On the other hand, the *G*-lattice was interpreted as the possible paths of increasing knowledge in order to solve some tasks. When, however, the knowledge necessary for solving another task must have been previously acquired, the dimension of time immediately appears in the interpretation. The question is whether one may infer from the result of a process (i.e. the test results) the process itself. In the present case this kind of inference seems to be acceptable and is in accordance with the theory of multilinear evolution (Carneiro 1973). Berlin and Kay (1969) used a similar method for determining the order of appearance of the names of different colors in more than 100 languages. They treat the problem in a fashion analogous to the one followed in this entry. They state that in all languages the notion of red must have existed before the notion of blue appeared, but the notion of blue never appears immediately after red: either yellow or green (but never both) must exist before the notion of blue appears. These ideas are presented in Fig. 3.

4. Qualitative and Quantitative Methods

The method of *G*-connections can be used only for fairly small samples (e.g., for school classes) in its present form. If the number of individuals increases, the resulting *G*-lattice becomes immensely complex. For 1,000 pupils and 50 tasks the number of nodes in the *G*-lattice may be of the order of the number of neurons in the human brain. The *G*-lattice must be radically simplified, that is, the irrelevant closed sets should be discarded from the lattice. Set theory and abstract algebra in general do not provide any tool for this. Therefore one has to look for statistical methods.

There are two simple methods available. The first possibility is to discard individuals and/or features from the starting matrix according to some relevant point of view (criteria). The other possibility is to discard elements from the final result, from the *G*-lattice, independently from the starting matrix. Neither of these ways seems to lead to satisfactory results. It is almost impossible to define relevant criteria to discard elements without losing important connections.

A satisfactory compromise between the above possibilities is to discard elements from the starting matrix according to the effect of the discarded individual on the *G*-lattice. First of all, if two individuals have the same features, then discarding one of them will not affect the resulting *G*-lattice at all. The next step should result in reducing the *G*-lattice. The basic idea of the following algorithm is to discard as few individuals as possible so that it should result in as big a reduction in the *G*-lattice as possible.

The researcher has first to define a *c* threshold value. This *c* value should express the complexity of the *G*-lattice so that the researcher judges this complexity to be tolerable. The following algorithm results in a *G*-lattice with *c* nodes as a maximum at the price of possibly discarding a few individuals.

Step 1. Compute the number of nodes in the *G*-lattice as a result of discarding the i_1, i_2,..., i_n *individuals. Let k* be the index for which the resulting *G*-lattice is the smallest.

Step 2. Discard the *k*-th individual from the starting matrix.

Step 3. Check whether the *G*-lattice resulting from the present starting matrix consists of more than *c* nodes. If yes, continue with Step 1; if no, the procedure is finished.

The given procedure is very simple, but it takes a lot of computing time. However, if the number of individuals is about 1,000 to 2,000 and the number of features is fairly small (about 20), this algorithm can be performed on personal computers in a few hours. The asymmetry in the features and the individuals is quite logical because in educational research (as in other research areas) the features are stable elements and the individuals are incidental. On the other hand, the best algorithms for computing a *G*-lattice take a computing time in one variable which increases exponentially with the amount of data, while in the other variable the time increases only $N.\log N$ times, where *N* is the number of data in the variable. Thus, asymmetrical data are more favorable from a computing point of view.

One may interpret the above algorithm as if, in every step, the "most disturbing" individual were discarded, namely, the individual who contributed most to the complexity of the given *G*-lattice. In this sense, the pupil who fills out the test in a completely random way is extremely disturbing. This fact suggests the need to devise a tool for filtering out the "random" pupils from the matrix by trying to substitute a pupil by a random pupil, that is, with a test-sheet filled by a random generator. If the resulting *G*-lattice is not more complex than the original one, the pupil, most probably, filled out the test at random. Of course, several trials with different random substitutions will increase the reliability of this method.

A *G*-lattice computed from a random data matrix is usually very much larger than a lattice computed from real data. In the case of a 12 by 12 random starting matrix the resulting G-lattice, with a probability greater than 0.95, will consist of more than 100 points. The graph in Fig. 1 consists of only 19 nodes and this is typical for this matrix size. However, some unwanted random effects may also occur in real data. Coding error is a trivial example. A more subtle one is an unimportant computation error made by the pupil.

The proposed algorithm will initially discard those pupils whose results are either unreliable or very uncharacteristic. However, it can sometimes occur that about 30 percent of the pupils must be discarded before the lattice is reduced to the given threshold (e.g. 100-nodes). This is still satisfactory, because it means that 70 percent of the pupils can be described in a fairly simple way. Suppose, for example, that the lattice in Fig. 1 was not the result of Table 1 but represented the result of 1,000 pupils after discarding 300 of them. In this case it can be claimed that the statements read from the G-lattice are valid for at least 70 percent of the pupils. This would seem to be a fairly poor result since statisticians usually work with much higher significance levels. Nevertheless, these results refer to strict logical relations like "those who solved tasks 6 and 11 also solved tasks 12." This is a very different kind of statement from the one that "the correlation of the two variables is 0.68 ± 0.12 at a significance level of 5 percent." It cannot be stated, in general, which of the two statements is stronger.

The method of Galois lattices can be interpreted from both a qualitative and a quantitative point of view. The qualitative train of thought would be: discard the most disturbing individuals to eliminate random effects. Even the most apparent properties of a horse are not valid for all horses. Horses which are perissodactyls have an odd number of toes; but some of them may be injured and have an even number of toes on some legs. It would, however, not be reasonable to form a separate class of this latter type. Rather, it is more reasonable to discard these animals from the system. The described method presents the most stable categories and the aberrant cases should be compared with these stable categories, rather than included in them.

The quantitative approach starts from the fact that the size of the resulting G-lattice depends on an a priori decision about what degree of complexity is tolerable. If the structure of the knowledge in a certain domain is in fact more complex than the given threshold, simplifications may bias the result. If this is the case, then one must really work with the traditional statistical methods. However, the Galois method does not exclude statistical analyses; they can still be incorporated in the G-lattice. For example, the nodes of the G-lattice can be drawn to be proportional to the number of individuals corresponding to the closed set. Also, the edges of the G-lattice can be labeled with the probability of one pupil belonging to that edge. (In this case in any horizontal line the sum of the probabilities attached to the crossed edges is 1.) In this way, the

G-lattice is appropriate for deciding whether the test is in accordance with the Rasch model or not. It can also be decided that if the Rasch model can be fitted to 95 percent of pupils, then 5 percent are omitted. And if the test is very far from satisfying the criteria of the Rasch model there is still the possibility, by using the G-lattice, of creating a sub-test which is in accordance with the Rasch model at the 95 percent level.

5. *Complexity of a Relation*

The complexity of a G-lattice has been defined simply by the number of nodes in the lattice. However, it is not self-evident that a lattice with more nodes is really more complex than another lattice with a fewer number of nodes. In fact, it is not even true in the commonsense meaning of complexity. The discarding algorithm described above provides a way of comparing the complexity of two Galois lattices (and of two arbitrary relations) in a sense that is closer to the everyday meaning of complexity. An algorithm for this task is given in the following paragraphs.

Let M_1 and M_2 be two binary matrices both with n rows and k columns. Let the relations induced by the matrices be denoted R_1 and R_2. Let the G-lattices corresponding to the relations be denoted G_{1i} and G_{2i}. The index i means that this is the i-th iteration. Now perform the discarding algorithm on both lattices with the threshold chosen as $c = 1$. (This means that all individuals but one are discarded in the consecutive steps as 1 individual can only give 1 closed set.) The lattices obtained in the successive steps are denoted $G_{11}, G_{12}, \ldots, G_{1,n-1}$ and $G_{21}, G_{22}, \ldots, G_{2,n-1}$ respectively. Finally, let the number of nodes in a lattice L be denoted $|L|$. Thus, the relation R_1 is more complex than the relation R_2 if

$$\sum_{i=0}^{n-1} |G_{1i}| > \sum_{i=0}^{n-1} |G_{2i}|$$

holds. Thus the complexity of the original G_{10} and G_{20}

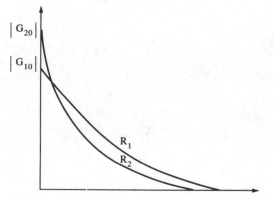

Figure 4

Measuring the complexity of the Galois lattice

lattices is compared by means of the number of nodes in the consecutive reductions.

This notion of complexity is really closer to the everyday notion of complexity because it also takes into consideration the effect of the individuals on the lattice. If the number of nodes in a lattice is very large only because of a few irregular individuals then the complexity measured in this way will be fairly low. An example of this effect is in Fig. 4 where in the case of relation R_1 the number of nodes decreases only slowly, while in the case of R_2 the number of nodes decreases fairly quickly. Thus, the relation R_1 proves to be more complex than R_2 even if the number of nodes in the starting lattice R_2 involves more nodes than R_1. This measuring algorithm expresses the heuristic that it is reasonable to consider a structure fairly simple if it seems very complex only because of a few irregular elements.

In a similar way one can check whether a relation is more or less complex than another referring to the features instead of the individuals. In this case, of course, the features should be consecutively discarded.

The proposed discarding algorithm discards the individuals one by one, which, theoretically, may result in fewer decreases than if one discards two or more individuals at once. Theoretically, a more "greedy" algorithm could produce a faster decrease of nodes, but this would be fairly hazardous in this case. Such an algorithm would involve the risk that a subset is discarded not because it is really irregular or random but because it is regular but in a different way from the majority, which might change the interpretation. This does not happen if the individuals are discarded one by one.

6. Conclusion

In a study of discourse reading, Kádár-Fülöp(1985) used the Galois lattice technique to carry out a detailed investigation of the errors made on a set of 5 test items by samples of approximately 1,700 Grade 4 and 1,650 Grade 8 students. By comparing the lattice structures for the Grade 4 students and the Grade 8 students, gains in reading skills during the four years of schooling could be examined. While this technique has not been widely used, it has the potential to assist in the teasing-out of learning hierarchies and the study of basic learning competencies in a manner that has not been possible with Guttman and Rasch scaling techniques.

See also: Cluster Analysis; Partial Order Scalogram Analysis

References

Berlin B, Kay P 1969 *Basic Color Terms, Their Universality and Evolution*. University of California Press, Berkeley, California

Carneiro R L 1973 The four faces of evolution. In: Honigmann J J (ed.) 1973 *Handbook of Social and Cultural Anthropology*. Rand McNally, Chicago, Illinois

Durkheim E 1902 De quelque formes primitives de classification. *L'Année sociologique*, 1901–1902. Presses Universitaires de France, Paris

Fay G, Takács D V 1975 Cell assemblies in cellular space. *J. Cybern.* 5(3): 65–86

Kádár-Fülöp J 1985 CTD reading study. *Eval. Educ.* 9(2): 117–64.

Katz J J, Fodor J A 1963 The structure of a semantic theory. *Language* 39: 170–210.

Hierarchical Linear Modeling

S. W. Raudenbush and A. S. Bryk

A prominent theme in methodological criticism of educational research during the 1980s was the failure of many quantitative studies to attend to the hierarchical, multilevel character of much educational field research data (Burstein 1980, Cooley et al. 1981, Cronbach 1976). The traditional linear models used by most researchers require the assumption that subjects respond independently to educational programs. In fact, students are commonly nested within classrooms, schools, districts, or program sites so that responses within groups are context dependent. When analysts ignore the nested structure of such data, problems of aggregation bias (Cronbach and Webb 1975, Robinson 1950) and misestimated precision (Aitkin et al. 1981, Walsh 1947) often result.

Perhaps more profound than such technical difficulties, however, is the impoverishment of conceptualization which single-level models encourage. Important educational effects operate within each level of the social organization of schooling, and these effects are undoubtedly interactive across levels. Researchers need to formulate explicit, multilevel models which enable the testing of hypotheses about effects occurring within each level and the interrelations among them (Burstein 1980, Cooley et al. 1981, Rogosa 1978).

During the 1980s, several methodologists working independently developed modeling and estimation procedures appropriate for hierarchical, multilevel data assumed normally distributed (Aitkin and Longford 1986, DeLeeuw and Kreft 1986, Goldstein 1987, Mason et al. 1983, Raudenbush and Bryk 1986). Despite some differences, these procedures share two core features. First, such methods enable researchers to formulate and test explicit statistical models for processes occurring within and between educational units. Under appropriate assumptions, multilevel modeling resolves the problem of aggregation bias. Such bias occurs in part because a variable can take on different meanings and have different effects at various levels of aggregation, and in part because estimation of such effects is prone to selection biases at each level (Burstein 1980).

Second, these methods enable specification of appropriate error structures, including random intercepts and random coefficients. Asymptotically efficient estimates of the variances and covariances of random effects are available for unbalanced designs. In most settings, appropriate specification of error components solves the problems of misestimated precision which have previously plagued hypothesis testing. Such misestimated precision arises when a conventional linear model analysis is used to analyze hierarchical data structures because standard error estimates fail to include components of variance and covariance arising from grouping effects.

Hierarchical linear models are also referred to in the literature as multilevel linear models (Mason et al. 1983, Goldstein 1987), random coefficient models (Rosenberg 1973), and complex covariance component models (Longford 1987). The term "hierarchical linear models," created by Lindley and Smith (1972) and abbreviated HLM for convenience, derives from the fact that data to which the models apply are hierarchically structured.

Four volumes focusing on educational application of these models are now available. Goldstein (1987) provides a broad overview of the methodology. Leading methodologists consider an array of statistical issues in Bock (1989). Raudenbush and Willms (1991) provide nonstatisticians with a conceptual introduction by collecting educational applications of the models from a number of countries. Bryk and Raudenbush (1992) give a comprehensive account of the models and estimation theory while focusing on strategies for data analysis illustrated by many detailed examples.

1. Basic Two-level Model

Although a hierarchical linear model may consist of any number of levels, all of the general properties of HLM are present in the two-level case. For clarity of exposition, the basic features of the two-level model are described in the context of research on how schools affect the social distribution of student achievement. In this case, the two-level HLM consists of a within-school and a between-school model. Other applications of two-level HLMs to educational research problems are reviewed later in this entry.

Formally, in the within-school equation, the achievement of student i in school j, Y_{ij} is represented as a function of student background characteristics, X_{ijk} and a random error, r_{ij}.

$$Y_{ij} = \beta_{j0} + \beta_{j1}X_{ij1} + \beta_{j2}X_{ij2} + ... + \beta_{jK}X_{ijK} + r_{ij} \quad (1)$$

where r_{ij} is assumed normally distributed with mean zero and some variance structure, Σ. In principle, Σ may take on a variety of forms within HLM (Goldstein 1987). In most applications, however, a homogenous error is assumed, that is, $Var(r_{ij}) = \sigma^2$, and the r_{ij} errors are mutually independent.

The parameters of this within-school model contain the following information:

(a) The intercept β_{j0} represents the base level of achievement in school j. If each of the X_{ijk} is deviated around its respective school mean, $\bar{X}_{ijk}$, then β_{j0} is the average achievement in school j, μ_j.

(b) Each regression coefficient, β_{jk}, indicates the strength of association between a student background characteristic, X_{ijk}, and achievement.

Equation (1) differs from a conventional multiple regression model in that the intercepts and the regression coefficients are allowed to vary over the population of schools. Taken together, the parameters of Eqn. (1) indicate how student achievement is distributed within school j. If the values of these parameters were known it would be possible to compare the distribution of achievement in different schools by comparing these coefficients. Of course, the parameters of Eqn. (1) are not known and must be estimated. In a sense Eqn. (1) may therefore be viewed as a measurement model, and estimation consists of using the available data to measure the distribution of achievement in each school.

Each β_{jk} represents some aspect of the social distribution of achievement. Variation among schools in these micro-level parameters (Mason et al. 1983) is represented through a set of between-school equations where each of the K regression coefficients, β_{jk}, is expressed as a function of school-level variables, W_{pj}, and a unique residual school effect, U_{jk}:

$$\beta_{jk} = \gamma_{0k} + \gamma_{ik}W_{1j} + \gamma_{2k}W_{2j} + ... + \gamma_{pk}W_{pj} + U_{jk} \quad (2)$$

distribution effects in schools j	effects of specific school characteristics on the distribution of achievement within schools	unique effect associated with school j

Since the unique effects associated with school j may covary, HLM applications typically assume that the U_{jk} are normally distributed with a mean of 0 and a full variance–covariance matrix, T.

Equation (2) models how features of schools affect the distribution of achievement within them. The γ_{pk} coefficients, sometimes referred to as macro-level parameters, represent the influence of school-level factors such as size, disciplinary climate, and academic organization on the distribution of effects among students within each school. For example, suppose that β_{j1} is the regression coefficient of mathematics achievement on students' social class. The size of this coefficient measures the extent to which initial differences among students' family background are related to subsequent achievement levels within a school. Does the strength of this relationship vary across schools? If yes, do certain school characteristics act to attenuate the effects of family background on student outcomes? These are illustrative of the kinds of hypotheses that can be formulated in the between-school model.

2. Statistical Estimation

An obvious difficulty with estimating hierarchical linear models is that the K outcome variables in the between-school equations, β_{jk}, are not directly observed. However, they can be estimated using standard regression techniques such as ordinary least squares, but these estimates, $\hat{\beta}_{jk}$, are estimated with error, that is

$$\hat{\beta}_{jk} = \beta_{jk} + \varepsilon_{jk} \tag{3}$$

Substituting from Eqn. (3) into Eqn. (2) for β_{jk} yields an equation in which the estimated relation $\hat{\beta}_{jk}$, varies as a function of measurable school characteristics and an error term equal to $U_{jk} + \varepsilon_{jk}$:

$$\hat{\beta}_{jk} = \gamma_{0k} + \gamma_{1k} W_{1j} + \gamma_{2k} W_{2j} + \ldots + \gamma_{pk} W_{pj} + U_{jk} \tag{4}$$

Equation 4 resembles a conventional linear model except that the structure of the error term is more complex. A consequence of this more complex error term is that neither the γ coefficients nor the covariance structure among the errors can be appropriately estimated with conventional linear model methods. Advances in statistical theory and computation, however, make this estimation possible (see Raudenbush 1988 for a full review).

From a technical point of view, estimation of the γ coefficients in Eqn. (4) can be viewed as a generalized or weighted least-squares regression problem where the weighting factor involves the covariance structure among the errors, $U_{jk} + \varepsilon_{jk}$. Maximum likelihood estimation of these covariance structures can be obtained using iterative computational techniques.

As a result, efficient estimates for the γs are also available.

2.1 Variance–Covariance Estimation

The statistical theory which forms the basis for estimation and inference in hierarchical linear models draws on Lindley and Smith (1972), Novick et al. (1972), and Smith (1973) who developed Bayesian estimation procedures for hierarchically structured data. The major obstacle to widespread use of their results has been the computational complexity of a full Bayes solution using numerical integration. A feasible alternative, termed empirical Bayes procedures (Morris 1983) consists of substituting maximum likelihood estimates for the variances and covariance components implied in Eqns. (1) and (2), and estimating values for β and γ conditional on these point estimates. Although closed-form analytic expressions for the variance–covariance components of an HLM are not available, developments in iterative approaches to maximum likelihood, especially the EM algorithm of Dempster et al. (1977), have made covariance components estimation accessible even for large databases. Some notable applications of the EM algorithm in random coefficients regression include Rubin (1981), Strenio et al. (1983), and Raudenbush and Bryk (1986). Other numerical approaches to maximum likelihood estimation of covariance components in HLM have also been developed including iterative generalized least squares (Goldstein 1987) and the Fisher scoring method (Longford 1987).

2.2 General Properties of HLM Estimators

The statistical estimators used in hierarchical linear models have several important properties. First, the precision of the $\hat{\beta}_{jk}$ coefficients will vary across schools because the amount of data available in each school will generally vary. In estimating the γ coefficients, HLM methods weight the contribution of the $\hat{\beta}_{jk}$ from each school proportional to its precision. This optimal weighting procedure minimizes the effects of unreliability in the $\hat{\beta}_{jk}$ on inferences about model parameters.

Second, the estimation procedures are fully multivariate since they take into account the covariation among the β coefficients. To the extent that these parameters covary, estimation will be more precise.

Third, HLM estimation enables the investigator to distinguish between variation in the true school effects, β_{jk}, and the sampling variation which arises because $\hat{\beta}_{jk}$ measures β_{jk} with error. That is, from Eqn. (3),

$$Var(\hat{\beta}_{jk}) = Var(\beta_{jk}) + Var(\varepsilon_{jk}) \tag{5}$$

or

total observed variance	parameter + variance	sampling variance

Knowledge of the amount of parameter variability is important in the process of formulating HLMs and in evaluating their results.

Fourth, the method enables estimation of the covariation among the β coefficients, that is, parameter covariance which can be of substantive interest. For example, in applications of HLM to measuring change, estimated parameter variances and covariances provide the basis for a maximum likelihood estimate of the correlation of change with initial status. This correlation, an important parameter in research on change, is routinely misestimated by conventional techniques.

Finally, the method enables improved estimates of the β coefficients in each school. Hierarchical linear models borrow strength from the fact that the estimation of β is being repeated across a number of schools. The usefulness of this particular feature of HLM in educational research is presented below.

3. Applications of Hierarchical Linear Models

Two conceptually different types of educational research problems can be investigated with these models. In the first type, interest focuses on the micro-parameters or random effects (i.e., the β coefficients in Eqn. 1). The within-unit model may be a regression equation for each school (as in Eqn. 1). In other HLM applications, the within-unit model might be a growth model for each individual, or a model of treatment effects in one of many studies. The research goal is to estimate a separate regression equation for each school, a growth trajectory for each person, or an effect size for each study, even when the data available for that school, child, or study are sparse. The HLM estimates for these micro-parameters, often called shrinkage estimators (Efron and Morris 1979), have smaller expected mean square error than do other alternatives such as ordinary least squares estimators computed separately from the data in each unit.

In the second type of application, attention is directed toward the macro-parameters, or fixed effects (i.e., the γ coefficients in Eqn. 2). The research now focuses on why some schools have smaller regression slopes than others, why some children grow faster than others, and why some studies report larger effects than others.

3.1 Improved Estimation of Individual Effects

One of the major uses of HLM is to estimate a separate linear model for each unit where strength can be borrowed from the fact that the estimation procedure is being replicated across the set of units. Rubin (1983) reviews several educational applications of this type.

To understand the concept of borrowing strength, it is necessary to return to Eqn. (1), which specifies a regression equation for each of many schools, and denotes the conventional ordinary least squares estimate of the regression coefficients β_j as $\hat{\beta}_j$. In general, $\hat{\beta}_j$ will be highly unstable if the sample size for school j is small or if there is little variation within school j on the independent variables.

The next step is to denote the average value of β_j across all schools as μ_β. The estimate of μ_β will be far more stable than the individual estimates $\hat{\beta}_j$. So the researcher might simply use $\hat{\mu}_\beta$ to estimate β_j rather than using the unstable estimate $\hat{\beta}_j$. However, the quantity μ_β will be an inaccurate estimate of β_j if the $\hat{\beta}_j$s vary markedly from school to school. Thus, the analyst confronts a dilemma: whether to use the unbiased but unstable estimate $\hat{\beta}_j$ of the stable but perhaps badly biased estimate μ_β.

The Empirical Bayes estimate for the micro-parameters enables the researcher to resolve this dilemma by employing a shrinkage estimator β_j^* which is a composite of $\hat{\beta}_j$ and μ. The improved estimator has the form

$$\beta_j^* = \Lambda_j \hat{\beta}_j + (1 - \Lambda_j) \hat{\mu}_\beta$$

The weight Λ_j accorded to $\hat{\beta}_j$ is the reliability of $\hat{\beta}_j$ as an estimate of β_j. The more reliable the within-group estimator, the more weight accorded to it in composing β_j^*. The weight accorded to μ_β is $1-\Lambda_j$ which is proportional to the degree of concentration of the β_js around the mean μ_β. The more concentrated the $\hat{\beta}_j$s around μ_β, the better μ_β is as an estimate of β_j, and so the more weight it is accorded. The estimate β_j^* is referred to as a shrinkage estimator since β^* is equivalent to the conventional estimator $\hat{\beta}_j$ shrunk toward its mean μ_β. The degree of shrinkage is proportional to $1-\Lambda$, which is a measure of the unreliability of $\hat{\beta}_j$.

A number of studies illustrate the value of shrinkage estimation in educational studies. Novick et al.(1971, 1972), Rubin (1980), and Braun et al. (1983) demonstrate how shrinkage improves predictive validity of admissions applications. Aitkin and Longford (1986) consider use of shrinkage estimators in identifying effective schools. Willms and Raudenbush (1989) use shrinkage to demonstrate that school effects over time may be far more stable than previously indicated in studies using standard regression methods. Shrinkage estimators also have significant application in the quantitative synthesis of research findings or "meta-analysis." Rubin (1981) used this approach to ask: "How large is the largest effect of coaching on the Scholastic Aptitude Test?" Raudenbush and Bryk (1985) productively re-evaluated the controversy over teacher expectance effects using these estimators.

3.2 Estimating Cross-level Effects

In the examples above, the goal was to obtain improved estimates of a set of relations occurring in individual units such as schools or studies. However, HLMs can also be used to relate these within-unit relations or micro-parameters to group characteristics. This permits investigation of questions such as: Why is the effect of pupil background on achievement stronger in some schools than others? Why do some experiments obtain larger effects than others? What is the effect of maternal speech on growth in vocabulary?

Previous attempts to answer such questions have confronted perplexing methodological difficulties: misestimated standard errors, aggregation bias, and inadequate methods for examining heterogeneity of regression. However, HLM methods largely resolve these problems (for an in-depth review of these difficulties and how they are largely resolved through hierarchical modeling, see Raudenbush and Bryk 1988). The major issues are summarized below.

3.3 Misestimated Standard Errors

This problem occurs in multilevel data when investigators fail to take into account the dependence among the outcome data within a particular unit such as a classroom or school. This dependence arises as a result of shared experiences among individuals within an organizational unit because of the ways individuals are either grouped together or individually select organizational membership. Hierarchical linear models enable investigators to resolve this problem by incorporating the unique effects associated with individual units (i.e., the U_{jk} in Eqn. 2) into the model. The resultant intraclass correlation is thus taken into account by HLM in the standard error estimates for the γ coefficients.

The consequences of misestimated precision in past analyses of educational data are clearly demonstrated by Aitkin et al. (1981) in their reanalysis of data from Bennett (1976) which had reported that formal teaching methods were associated with greater academic progress than were open classroom techniques. The Bennett study had used children as the unit of analysis, ignoring the clustering of students within classrooms. When the data were reanalyzed to include the random effects of classrooms, substantially larger standard errors resulted, and several key inferences in the original study were thrown into doubt.

3.4 Aggregation Bias

A large part of the difficulty with aggregation bias in educational settings is that a variable can take on different meanings and therefore have different effects at different levels of aggregation within an organizational hierarchy. The average social class of a school (a measure of normative environment of the collective), can have an effect on student achievement above and beyond the individual child's social class (a measure of the tangible and intellectual resources in a child's home environment). Hierarchical linear models resolve this problem by allowing a decomposition of any observed relationship between variables into separate components at each level.

Raudenbush and Bryk (1986) have illustrated this use of HLM in a reanalysis of data on the effects of public and private schooling. Their HLM analysis, which decomposed the relationship between social class and student achievement into within- and between-school components, found smaller sector effects than reported in earlier analyses (Coleman et al. 1982) which had analyzed the data solely at the student level.

3.5 Heterogeneity of Regression

Slope heterogeneity occurs when a relationship between an independent and dependent variable varies across units such as classrooms or schools. Although this phenomenon has often been viewed as a methodological nuisance, the causes of such heterogeneity of regression can be a central concern in educational research. For example, educational sociologists (Barr and Dreeben 1983, Bidwell and Kasarda 1980) argue that a major consequence of school organization is to differentiate the experiences of individuals within these organizations. Since the organization of schools and classrooms varies, heterogeneity of regression is likely, and should be a focus of investigation, not just another factor relegated to the error term.

Perhaps the most significant advantage of HLM is that it permits representation of random within-unit regression slopes and modeling variation in these slopes as a function of unit-level characteristics. The rationale for slopes-as-outcomes has been forcefully argued by Burstein (1980). Until the development of the estimation strategies discussed above, however, there was no efficient way to fit such models. With the emergence of these techniques, applied research using slopes as outcomes has begun to appear.

DeLeeuw and Kreft (1986) examined how the relationships between student background and teachers' expectations varied across schools as a function of the average IQ level of schools. Lee and Bryk (1989) formulated a within-school model for the distribution of academic achievement with regard to student social class, minority status, and academic background. They then examined how variations among schools in the social distribution of achievement depended on the normative environments and academic organization of schools. Mason et al. (1983) have used multilevel models in cross-national research on fertility. The within-unit model represents the effects of education and urban versus rural context on family fertility. Variation across countries in these regression parameters is explained as a function of the efficacy of family planning programs and level of economic development.

The modeling of slopes as outcomes also provides a powerful set of techniques for studying individual change (Bryk and Raudenbush 1987). In the micro-level model, individual status on some trait is represented as a function of individual growth trajectory plus random error. At the macro- or between-person level, the parameters of the individual growth trajectories are modeled as a function of differences among subjects in background characteristics, instructional experiences, and possibly experimental treatments. Bryk and Raudenbush (1987) demonstrate how this HLM formulation allows solution of several longstanding problems in the measurement of change, including assessment of the reliability of measures of status and rate of change, and correlation between initial status and rate of growth.

4. Three-level Applications

All of the examples mentioned above involve two-level HLMs. Some three-level applications have also begun to appear. Goldstein (1987) describes an example involving students nested within schools and schools within districts where each level—the student, the school, and the district—is formally represented in the model.

Willms and Raudenbush (1989) describe a three-level model for studying the stability of school effects over time. Schools were compared at each of several time points with an independent sample of students tested on each occasion. In the first level of the HLM, the achievement of each student at each time depends on the school average at that time plus the effect of student background. At the second level, the school's average is allowed to vary over time. At the third and final level, rate of change in each school's average achievement is represented as a function of changes in school organization, composition, and climate. This model permits efficient estimation of both mean effectiveness and change in effectiveness over time, and an assessment of the stability of the actual school effects rather than the stability of the estimated effects.

Bryk and Raudenbush (1988) present a three-level model for research on school effects which combines individual growth modeling with an explicit representation of the organizational structures of schooling. They use this model to study the effects of child poverty and school poverty concentration on children's growth in mathematics. The first level is an individual growth model for students' mathematics achievement over five occasions between Grades 1 and 3. Each of the parameters of the growth model are represented in the level 2 model as a function of student background characteristics such as child's poverty status. The effects of school characteristics including poverty concentration are introduced at level 3.

Three-level models have been utilized to incorporate information about measurement error into inferences about educational effects. Extending the results of Longford (1990a), Raudenbush et al. (1991) used a three-level model to assess the reliability of organizational measures. At the first level, each item for each person varied around a person mean. At level 2, the person means varied around the school mean, and at level 3, the school means varied around a grand mean. The approach elucidated the simple principles that determine reliability of measurement at the person and organizational levels. The analysis also produced estimates of the true score correlations at each level between responses of teachers within schools and between the school means. These correlations are corrected for measurement error. These estimated true-score correlations were, in every instance, higher than were the correlations among the observed scores, especially for those scales having few items.

5. Next Wave of Innovation

Three innovations under rapid development will add to the multilevel approaches now available to researchers. These are: (a) models for nonnormal errors, (b) crossed random effects models, and (c) models for structural relations.

5.1 Nonnormal Errors

Most of the published applications of multilevel analysis utilize models that assume normally distributed errors. This is not surprising, both because continuously distributed outcomes like test scores are common in educational research and because software development for normal error models has progressed very rapidly. However, nonnormal error models are not new. Aitkin and Anderson (1985) and Wong and Mason (1985) each developed and illustrated closely related approaches to multilevel logistic regression, appropriate for binary outcomes. Goldstein (1991) considers multilevel log-linear models and Longford's work (1990b) evaluates alternative approaches to estimation in nonnormal random effects models. Such models will enable researchers to examine dichotomous outcomes such as school dropout and retention in grade and behavioral counts such as absenteeism and instances of misbehavior from a multilevel approach. These analytical procedures are now available in the HLM4 computer program (Bryk et al. 1996).

5.2 Crossed Random Effects Models

The applications described above require that the data structure is a "pure hierarchy," for example with students nested in classrooms and classrooms in schools. However, a large class of potentially interesting multilevel analyses will have a crossclassified character. Raudenbush (1994) analyzes data representing two important examples. In the first case, it is necessary to estimate the effects of both schools and neighbourhoods on students' educational attainment. Because schools draw students from several neighborhoods and neighborhoods send students to multiple schools, the data have a "crossed" structure. In the second example, the goal is to estimate the effect of each primary-school teacher on the growth of the children as they pass through the primary grades. Each year the students are nested within classrooms; however, each year the students have a new teacher and a new collection of classmates. The analysis illustrates how to gauge the effect of a teacher on the growth trajectory of each student.

5.3 Structural Relations

All of the models discussed involve single endogenous outcome variables. In many cases, researchers will wish to study examples of the following type: students are nested within high schools, and information is available on multiple student-level endogenous variables (e.g., motivation and achievement) as well as exogenous variables measured at both the student and school levels. A standard linear structural relations analysis would be inapplicable in this case because of the nested structure of data. Goldstein and MacDonald (1988) suggested an estimation strategy that would allow the extension of the linear structural relations model to the multilevel setting. The model would also incorporate a measurement model for both latent predictors and outcomes. No software or illustrative examples were offered, however. Muthén (1990, 1991) showed how a similar estimation strategy could be implemented in special cases using conventional structural equation software, and provided several illustrative examples. Perhaps surprisingly, Schmidt (1969) suggested a solution to this problem in the case of balanced data, though variables were required to vary at each level.

6. Conclusion

The implications of the developments described in this entry are extensive for the design, conduct, and analysis of data in research studies in the fields of education, psychology, and sociology. Further developments in the area of hierarchical linear models and multilevel analysis must be expected during the 1990s, with widespread application to school and classroom research, to the analysis of longitudinal data, and to studies of student growth.

See also: Regression Analysis of Quantified Data

References

Aitkin M, Anderson D A, Hinde J 1981 Statistical modelling of data on teaching styles. *Journal of the Royal Statistical Society*, Series A 144(4): 419–61

Aitkin M, Anderson D A 1985 Variance component models with binary response: Interviewer variability. *Journal of the Royal Statistical Society*, Series B 47(2): 203–10

Aitkin M, Longford N 1986 Statistical modelling issues in school effectiveness studies. *Journal of the Royal Statistical Society*, Series A 149(1): 1–43

Barr R, Dreeben R 1983 *How Schools Work*. University of Chicago Press, Chicago, Illinois

Bennett N 1976 *Teaching Styles and Pupil Progress*. Open Books, London

Bidwell C E, Kasarda J D 1980 Conceptualizing and measuring the effects of school and schooling. *Am. J. Educ.* 88(4): 401–30

Bock R D (ed.) 1989 *Multilevel Analysis of Educational Data*. Academic Press, New York

Braun H I, Jones D H, Rubin D B, Thayer D T 1983 Empirical Bayes estimation of coefficients in the general linear model from data of deficient rank. *Psychometri.* 48(2): 171–81

Bryk A S, Raudenbush S W 1987 Application of hierarchical linear models to assessing change. *Psych. Bull.* 101(1): 147–58

Bryk A S, Raudenbush S W 1988 Toward a more appropriate conceptualization of research on school effects: A three-level linear model. *Am. J. Educ.* 97(1): 65–108

Bryk A S, Raudenbush S W 1992 *Hierarchical Linear Models: Applications and Data Analysis Methods*. Sage, Beverly Hills, California

Bryk A S, Raudenbush S W, Congdon R T 1996 HLM: *Hierarchical Linear and Nonlinear Modeling with the HLM/2L and HLM/3L Programs*. Scientific Software International, Chicago, Illinois

Burstein L 1980 The analysis of multi-level data in educational research and evaluation. *Rev. Res. Educ.* 8: 158–233

Coleman J S, Hoffer T, Kilgore S B 1982 *High School Achievement: Public, Catholic, and other Private Schools Compared*. Basic Books, New York

Cooley W W, Bond L, Mao B 1981 Analyzing multi-level data. In: Berk R A (ed.) 1981 *Educational Evaluation Methodology: The State of the Art*. Johns Hopkins University Press, Baltimore, Maryland

Cronbach L J 1976 *Research on classrooms and schools: Formulation of questions design and analysis*. Occasional paper of the Stanford Evaluation Consortium. Stanford University, Stanford, California

Cronbach L J, Webb N 1975 Between- and within-class effects in a reported aptitude-by-treatment interaction: Reanalysis of a study by G L Anderson. *J. Educ. Psychol.* 67(6): 717–24

DeLeeuw J, Kreft I 1986 Random coefficient models for multilevel analysis. *J. Ed. Stat.* 11(1): 57–85

Dempster A P, Laird N M, Rubin D B 1977 Maximum likelihood from incomplete data via the EM algorithm. *Journal of the Royal Statistical Society* Series B 39: 1–38

Efron B, Morris C 1979 Data analysis using Stein's estimator and its generalizations. *Journal of the American Statistics Association* 74: 311–19

Goldstein H 1987 *Multilevel Models in Educational and Social Research*. Oxford University Press, Oxford

Goldstein H 1991 Non linear multilevel models, with an application to discrete response data. *Biometrika* 78(1): 45–51

Goldstein H, McDonald R P 1988 A general model for the analysis of multilevel data. *Psychometri.* 53(4): 455–67

Lee V E, Bryk A S 1989 A multilevel model of the social distribution of high school achievement. *Sociol. Educ.* 62(3): 172–92

Lindley D V, Smith A F M 1972 Bayes estimates for the linear model. *Journal of the Royal Statistical Society* Series B 34: 1–41

Longford N T 1987 A fast scoring algorithm for maximum likelihood estimation in unbalanced mixed models with nested random effects. *Biometrika* 74(4): 817–27

Longford N T 1990a Multivariate variance component analysis: An application in test development. *J. Ed. Stat.* 15(2): 91–112

Longford N T 1990b Variance component models for observational data. In: van den Eiden P, Hox J, Hauer J (eds.) 1990 *Theory and Model in Multilevel Research: Convergence or Divergence?* SISWO Publication 351, Amsterdam

Mason W M, Wong G Y, Entwistle B 1983 Contextual analysis through the multilevel linear model. In: Leinhardt S (ed.) 1983 *Sociological Methodology 1983–1984*, Vol. 14. Jossey-Bass, San Francisco, California

Morris C 1983 Parametric empirical Bayes inference: Theory and applications. *Journal of the American Statistics Association* 78(381): 47–65

Muthén B 1990, 1991 Multilevel structural equation modeling. Papers presented at the annual meeting of the American Educational Research Association, Boston, Massachusetts and San Francisco, California

Novick M R, Jackson P H, Thayer D T 1971 Bayesian inference and the classical test theory model: Reliability and true scores. *Psychometri.* 36(3): 261–88

Novick M R, Jackson P H, Thayer D T, Cole N S 1972 Estimating multiple regression in m groups—A cross validation study. *Br. J. Math. S.* 25: 33–50

Raudenbush S W 1988 Educational applications of hierarchical linear models: A review. *J. Ed. Stat.* 13(2): 85–116

Raudenbush S W 1994 A crossed random effects model with applications in cross-sectional and longitudinal research. *J. Educ. Stat.*

Raudenbush S W, Bryk A S 1985 Empirical Bayes meta-analysis. *J. Ed. Stat.* 10(2): 75–98

Raudenbush S W, Bryk A S 1986 A hierarchical model for studying school effects. *Sociol. Educ.* 59(1): 1–17

Raudenbush S W, Bryk A S 1988 Methodological advances in analyzing the effects of schools and classrooms on student learning. *Review of Research in Education* 15: 423–75

Raudenbush S W, Rowan B, Kang S J 1991 A multilevel, multivariate model for studying school climate with estimation via the EM algorithm and application to US High School Data. *J. Ed. Stat.* 16: 295–330

Raudenbush S W, Willms J D 1991 *Schools, Classrooms, and Pupils: International Studies of Schooling from a Multilevel Perspective*. Academic Press, New York

Robinson W S 1950 Ecological correlations and the behavior of individuals. *Am. Sociol. Rev.* 15: 351–57

Rogosa D 1978 Politics, process, and pyramids. *J. Ed. Stat.* 3(1): 79–86

Rosenberg B 1973 Linear regression with randomly dispersed parameters. *Biometrika* 60(1): 65–72

Rubin D B 1980 Using empirical Bayes techniques in the Law School Validity Studies. *Journal of the American Statistics Association* 75(372): 801–27

Rubin D B 1981 Estimation in parallel randomized experiments. *J. Ed. Stat.* 6(4): 377–400

Rubin D B 1983 Some applications of Bayesian statistics to educational data. *Statistician* 32(1): 55–68

Schmidt W H 1969 Covariance structure analysis of the multivariate random effects model. (Unpublished doctoral dissertation, University of Chicago).

Smith A F M 1973 A general Bayesian linear model. *Journal of the Royal Statistical Society* Series B 35: 67–75

Strenio J L F, Weisberg H I, Bryk A S 1983 Empirical Bayes estimation of individual growth curve parameters and their relationship to covariates. *Biometrics* 39: 71–86

Walsh J E 1947 Concerning the effect of the intraclass correlation on certain significance tests. *Annals of Mathematical Statistics* 18: 88–96

Willms J D, Raudenbush S W 1989 A longitudinal hierarchical linear model for estimating school effects and their stability. *J. Educ. Meas.* 26(3): 209–32

Wong G Y, Mason W M 1985 The hierarchical logistic regression model for multilevel analysis. *Journal of the American Statistical Association* 80(391): 513–24

Further Reading

DerSimonian R, Laird N M 1983 Evaluating the effect of coaching on SAT scores: A meta-analysis. *Harv. Educ. Rev.* 53(1): 1–15

Huttenlocher J E, Haight W, Bryk A S, Seltzer M 1988 Parental speech and early vocabulary development. (Unpublished manuscript, University of Chicago)

Raudenbush S W, Bryk A S 1989 Quantitative models for estimating teacher and school effectiveness. In: Bock D (ed.) 1989 *Multi-level analysis of educational data*. Academic Press, New York

Shigemasu K 1976 Development and validation of a simplified m-group regression model. *J. Ed. Stat.* 1(2): 157–80

Stiratelli R, Laird N, Ware J H 1984 Random effects models for serial observations with binary response. *Biometrics* 40: 961–71

Willms J D, Raudenbush S W 1994 A longitudinal hierarchical linear model for estimating school effects and their stability. *J. Educ. Meas.*

Hypothesis Testing

J. D. Finn

The systematic formulation and testing of hypotheses is as essential to education and the social sciences as it is to other scientific disciplines. Although the hypothetico–deductive approach to educational research is often difficult to implement, it is particularly important for a field in which causal variables may be multifaceted and imperfectly measured, and rigorous experimental control can be attained only infrequently. This entry provides an overview of the ways in which hypotheses are generated, and the logic behind the statistical procedures commonly used to test them.

Hypotheses are informed propositions or speculations about values of two or more variables that may be observed concomitantly. In general, better informed hypotheses contribute more directly to models of social behavior, but it is not necessary that hypotheses derive from a great deal of prior knowledge or extensive theoretical reasoning. The simple observation that more boys than girls enroll in science courses may lead to speculation about a variety of precursors, including different aptitude levels, different interest levels, or various reward structures. Hypotheses may derive from previous empirical findings. For example, it has been noted for many years that greater amounts of "time-on-task" are generally associated with increased levels of learning among elementary and secondary school students (Atkinson 1968). Also, high-aptitude students are able to master school-related material at a faster rate than low-aptitude students (Denham and Lieberman 1980). These findings may lead to a further speculation that when instruction is limited to a fixed-time-period class, the achievement difference between high- and low-ability students will be greater than under variable time conditions.

Finally, hypotheses may be derived from a carefully formulated model that attempts to explain a class of outcomes. For example, according to the Getzels (1963) model of observed social behavior, school performance may be explained by an interaction of role expectations defined by the institution and values internalized by the individual. Harrison (1968) extrapolated a set of propositions from this model to explain the performance of children from advantaged home environments whose school performance is poor, and others from disadvantaged homes whose school performance is outstandingly high. These propositions derive entirely from the Getzels conceptualization, and as such were speculative. The empirical testing of the hypotheses contributed both to understanding school performance, and to the adequacy of the original model.

When empirical data are not available or seem contradictory, competing hypotheses may appear equally likely. For example, if there was concern about the effects of teachers' experience on their grading practices, it might be reasoned that as teachers accrue more years of experience, they become more accepting of average or poor performance; thus it would be hypothesized that years' teaching experience is directly related to grades (the more years, the higher the grades tend to be). An inverse but reasonable hypothesis is that more experienced teachers become more rigid and evaluative, and tend to give generally lower grades. These alternatives may be weighed against one another using a two-sided test (described below).

Much educational research is nonexperimental and involves a large number of possible variables, each of which may be an antecedent or an outcome of others. Hypotheses may be formulated to guide the data collection and analysis. As an alternative, an "empirical" approach may be taken in which data on many variables are collected and many different analyses are attempted once the data are in (Ellis 1952). In the absence of hypotheses to guide data collection and analysis, the findings that emerge may not be among the more meaningful that the study can provide, and the most important variables may not be given the extra attention they deserve. Complex relationships involving several variables may be overlooked in the attempt to seek out those that are obvious. Through the empirical approach, the relationships that are discovered may have arisen spuriously out of the many that were possible, and may not be replicable. On the other hand, the hypothetico–deductive approach does not preclude exploring a data set for other outcomes that were not anticipated.

Hypothesis formulation and testing are important for yet another reason. No matter how derived, hypotheses are informed propositions. Not only do they direct attention to particular relationships, but they anticipate through logic, theory, or from prior evidence what the nature of those relationships may be. When a hypothesis is confirmed through empirical observations, the outcome is supported not once but twice. Further discussion of the role and logic of hypothesis testing is found in Cohen (1960), Kerlinger (1986), Platt (1964), and Popper (1968).

1. Hypothesis Restatement

Before a hypothesis can be tested empirically, it must be restated in symbolic form. Consider several examples. A mathematics teacher believes that he or she is doing an effective job of teaching students to perform basic operations with fractions. The school principal is willing to grant a salary increment if students actually perform better on a test of fractions than if they were merely guessing the answers. If the test selected has 10 items each with 5 choices (1 choice correct) then the students could guess an average of 2 items correctly. The teacher, claiming to be effective, hypothesizes that the mean of all students subjected to instruction is higher than 2; symbolically the hypothesis is represented as $H_1: \mu > 2$. H_1 is the research hypothesis being forwarded, and μ is the mean score on the 10-item test.

One consequence of a mastery learning approach to instruction is that the average amount of material learned will be greater than with a nonmastery approach. If μ_1 is the mean achievement score of all Grade 8 students learning French as a foreign language through a mastery approach, and μ_2 is the mean of all Grade 8 students learning through a traditional lecture approach, then the research hypothesis can be stated as $H_1: \mu_1 > \mu_2$. Additionally, mastery learning is hypothesized to reduce the dispersion of performance scores. This is expected because students who are slow learners are given additional time and support, and thus are not as far behind the faster students when the unit is complete. If σ_1 is the standard deviation, a measure of dispersion of achievement scores in the mastery condition, and σ_2 is the standard deviation under a traditional approach, this hypothesis is symbolized as $H_2:\sigma_1 < \sigma_2$. Both H_1 and H_2 may be tested in a single investigation of mastery learning.

The hypothesis that more experienced teachers give higher grades asserts that there is a positive relationship between the two variables. If ρ is the correlation of years' experience with average grades given by a teacher, then the hypothesis is represented as $H_1:\rho>0$ (i.e., the correlation is greater than zero, or positive). The second possibility is that tenure and grades are inversely related, or that the correlation is negative, that is, $H_2:\rho<0$. Statisticians usually write these together, as $H_1:\rho \neq 0$, but it is important to keep in mind that two distinct possibilities are being tested.

2. Hypothesis Testing Procedures

Hypothesis testing begins with the supposition that the researcher's hypothesis is false. This counter-statement of the original proposition is the "null hypothesis," usually represented as H_0. For example, the null hypothesis regarding the mathematics teacher asserts that students attending his or her class perform at or below guessing level, that is, $H_0:\mu \leqslant 2$. If mastery learning does not raise mean performance, it may yield the same or lower average scores; this null hypothesis is $H_0:\mu_1 \leqslant \mu_2$. Both positive and negative correlations between experience and grades are hypothesized. Thus, the null hypothesis is that there is no association between the two variables, or $H_0:\rho=0$. In contrast to the null hypothesis, the statistical restatement of the researcher's original proposition (H_1) has come to be termed the "alternate" hypothesis, somewhat of a misnomer for the scientist's best informed judgment.

Systematic observations are made that bear directly on the hypothesis. This involves deciding on an appropriate sample of students, teachers, or other unit, and deciding on appropriate measurement instruments. The data are summarized into a numerical index that indicates the extent to which the null hypothesis is contradicted—the "test statistic." Finally the test statistic is assessed to determine whether the data contradict the null hypothesis to such a great extent that it is very unlikely the null hypothesis is true and thus the researcher's original hypothesis is supported.

2.1 Samples and Populations

Hypotheses describe relationships among variables for a particular "population" of persons (or groups, or institutions) defined by a specifiable set of characteristics. For example, the mathematics teacher claims effectiveness with all groups of children, say, whose ages are 7 through 12 years, who are of normal intelligence, have sound hearing, eyesight, and motor

control, and who may have other specific attributes. While certain factors limit the intended population, others, such as locale or time, do not. Thus the hypothesis pertains to last year's class and next year's as well as the present class. However, effectiveness may not be permanent and it may be necessary to reconsider the hypothesis at a later time, or test the original hypothesis by taking samples in each of several years. The population to which the global mastery learning hypothesis applies may be much broader, including children of a wide range of abilities and ages, but a single investigation testing these propositions would specify a number of limiting factors including the school subject area.

It is not necessary to examine the entire population to decide whether a study's hypotheses are supported. Instead an inference may be drawn based on a "representative sample" of observations—that is, a group of subjects that is usually far smaller than the entire population, but whose characteristics approximate those of the population as nearly as is feasible. Still, the hypothesis being tested remains sample free; it is a proposition regarding the population that usually extends far beyond the individuals actually observed. If this were not the case, teachers would have no confidence in the mastery learning approach the following semester or in an untested school, and schools might never invest in new materials "demonstrated" to be effective.

Two principles of sampling are essential: randomization and replication. Randomization is a method of drawing subjects from the larger population such that each subject is as likely to be selected as every other subject, and a particular combination of subjects comprising the entire sample is as likely to be chosen as any other combination of the same number of subjects. Randomization produces an "unbiased" sample in that members of the population with any particular characteristic (e.g., young, old, male, female) are not systematically overselected.

Replication—conducting the study with more rather than fewer subjects—is also necessary to obtain a representative sample. In general, the larger the sample, the more nearly its characteristics will approximate those of the population. However, other factors may be weighed in deciding how large a sample should be, including the amount of information gained by adding additional subjects to a sample. Also, if locating a subject, testing or interviewing, and recording and scoring responses requires extensive time and effort, a balance must be sought between the need for additional subjects and the costs involved.

2.2 Measures

The selection of appropriate measurement instruments is important both because inaccurate measures can produce erroneous decisions about a hypothesis and because measures that are defined too narrowly can limit the generality of the hypothesis test. In addition, a reasonable degree of "referent generality" (Snow 1974) is desirable; that is, the domain of responses should not be limited unduly. for example, in the mastery learning experiment, achievement might be represented by the total score on a test of French vocabulary. Even with a single score, greater generality is obtained by "item sampling"—that is, by choosing a representative sample of easy and difficult vocabulary items from the curriculum. Further, achievement may be defined more broadly to include vocabulary, comprehension, and pronunciation subtests, or both cognitive and attitudinal assessments. A "multivariate" approach to outcome measurement is particularly important when the response variable is somewhat ambiguously defined (e.g., personality traits, affective responses), and employing corresponding multivariate statistical procedures will increase both the replicability and referent generality of the investigation.

2.3 Summarizing the Data and Deciding

Once the subjects of an investigation have been observed or tested, the quantitative data are summarized through "descriptive statistics," that is, summary indexes that characterize the sample only. These often include simple measures such as the mean scores for the total sample and for each identified subsample, measures of dispersion such as the standard deviation, and measures of the relationships among variables (e.g., differences among means, correlations).

At least one of these statistics must provide direct information regarding the hypothesis being investigated. This statistic is converted to a standardized measure of the extent to which the research hypothesis is supported by the data (and the null hypothesis contradicted), and is called the "test statistic." For example, from a sample of N students taking the 10-item test of fractions, the sample mean $\bar{X}$ and the sample standard deviation S might be obtained. Since the hypothesis is that the population mean is greater than 2, the difference $\bar{X}-2$ is calculated, and becomes the basic element in the test statistic, $t=(\bar{X}-2)/(S/N^{1/2})$. The denominator $S/N^{1/2}$ is a scaling factor that puts the t statistic into a standard convenient metric. The more effective the instructor, the larger t will be.

Likewise the test statistics for the two mastery learning hypotheses are measures of the extent to which the hypotheses are supported by data from the sample. Suppose that a sample of N_1 students learn French through the mastery approach and have an average vocabulary score $\bar{X}_1$ and standard deviation S_1, and N_2 students learn by attending traditional lecture classes and have a mean vocabulary score $\bar{X}_2$ and standard deviation S_2. Then the test statistic for testing the difference between the two population means has the difference between the two samples means as its basic component, $D=\bar{X}_1-\bar{X}_2$. The test statistic is $t=D/S_D$ where S_D, a function of the standard deviations and the sample sizes, expresses the difference in a convenient

standard metric. The test is conducted by determining whether t is sufficiently greater than zero (i.e., $\bar{X}_1$ above $\bar{X}_2$) to convince us that μ_1 is above μ_2, and mastery learning is generally effective for French vocabulary. The test statistic for comparing the standard deviations is a direct comparison of the dispersions for the two samples, $F = S_1^2/S_2^2$ Since the hypothesis asserts that σ_1 is below σ_2, the F statistic is examined to see if it is enough below unity to be convincing that H_2 is supported for the populations generally.

A test statistic for the correlation of experience with grades is a t statistic that has the sample correlation r as its major component; this is $t= r [N-2)/(1-r^2)]^{1/2}$. A t value sufficiently above zero (positive correlation) or sufficiently below zero (negative correlation) will convince researchers that one of the research hypotheses is supported. This is termed a "two-sided" or "two-tail" test; the other tests, for which only evidence in one direction will convince researchers that the research hypothesis is supported, are termed "one-sided" or "one-tail" tests.

The decision is made by referring the test statistic to tables that are found in most basic statistics textbooks. The logic by which the tables are formed may be exemplified for the test that $\mu>2$. It should first be assumed that the null hypothesis is true and that $\mu=2$. If the study of teacher effectiveness is conducted many times with different samples (e.g., approaching an infinite number of times) a very large collection of $\bar{X}$'s would be obtained. Each sample mean would be a little different, and none would be exactly 2 because samples are not the entire population. Fortunately, it is possible to determine theoretically the point that separates the 1 percent of the $\bar{X}$'s the farthest above 2 from those closer to 2 or below 2. This value is called the "critical value" of $\bar{X}$. It may also be converted to a t statistic for convenience, and placed into a table of critical values of t that typically has the percentages (1 or 5) as its column heading, and different sample sizes as the row labels. The percentages (column headings) are usually referred to as α.

The t table described above is assembled from statistical theory based on the assumption that the null hypothesis is true. In reality, the experiment would be conducted only once, a single $\bar{X}$ and t statistic calculated. The test statistic is then compared with the critical value in the table. If it exceeds the critical value, then the sample mean is very unlikely to have arisen from a population in which the null hypothesis is true, and the null hypothesis is deemed false and the instructor effective. The conclusion is expressed by saying that "the null hypothesis is rejected" or "the sample mean is (statistically) significantly different from 2."

The same procedure is followed for the mastery learning hypotheses. In the case of 2 standard deviations, the critical value would be a fraction below 1, and the null hypothesis is rejected only if the F statistic is smaller than this value. For the 2-sided test of the correlation, 2 critical values would be necessary, 1 negative and 1 positive. If the test statistic is lower than the negative critical value or higher than the positive one, one of the research hypotheses is supported and the null hypothesis is rejected. Because of its central role in generalizing from the sample to the population, the test statistic is termed an "inferential statistic."

2.4 The Possibility of Being Wrong

It is likely, but not necessary, that a decision about the entire population based on a single sample is correct. Unfortunately, the actions based on hypothesis tests must often be taken even in the face of this uncertainty —for example, the principal must decide whether or not to award the mathematics teacher a salary increment; curriculum specialists must decide whether or not to invest in mastery learning procedures.

A test statistic that exceeds the respective critical value (e.g., a high mean score for students of the mathematics teacher) is unlikely to have been observed if the teacher were not effective. However, if the sample by coincidence contains only the most able students, then it may be concluded that the hypothesis of effectiveness is correct when in fact it is not. This is a "Type I error," that is, rejecting a true null hypothesis. Since the researcher never knows if this has occurred, random sampling and a relatively large sample are particularly important, and pilot testing an investigation an excellent idea. On the other hand, choosing a small α value, thus requiring a larger test statistic before concluding that the research hypothesis is supported, reduces the likelihood of such an error. Thus, when a supported research hypothesis implies an important finding or action (e.g., more money and lifelong employment for the teacher), the investigator may deliberately use a small α level. When the possible benefits of a supported hypothesis are so important that even weak evidence suggests that an action be taken (e.g., a new medication for a formerly incurable form of disease) a larger probability of making a Type I error may be acceptable.

If the sample data do not support the research hypothesis and it is concluded that the null hypothesis is true, this too may be erroneous—a "Type II error." The probability of a Type II error is controlled in practice by taking a sufficiently large number of subjects (Cohen 1988).

2.5 Power Analysis

The question must be addressed in any research study as to how many subjects should be involved in the investigation. A power analysis of a planned investigation seeks to provide the researcher with the number of subjects needed for a specific hypothesis to be given a reasonable chance of being proven correct.

The central issue may be stated in the following words.

On the assumption that a research hypothesis is true, for the parameter of interest, what is the minimal value by which the experimental group must differ from the control group or a reference value in order for the validity of the hypothesis to be established? (see Kraemer and Thiemann 1987 p. 10).

In order to answer this question the researcher needs to have conducted a preliminary study from which the parameter of interest is estimated, whether it is a mean, percentage, or correlation coefficient. A "critical effect size" is then calculated as the difference between the experimental mean and the control mean divided by a measure of variability. Then on the assumption that the research hypothesis is true, a probability must be set for the investigation yielding a significant result that involves rejecting the null hypothesis. This value is the power of the significance test, and thus together with other information enables an appropriate sample size to be determined. For a straightforward treatment of the analysis required Kraemer and Thiemann (1987) should be consulted, and for a more extensive treatment Cohen (1988) is available.

2.6 Multiple Tests of Significance

In education research it is not uncommon for an investigator to be faced with a situation in which tests of several hypotheses are needed, for example, to determine if the correlations among three or more variables are statistically significant or to see if there are differences among three or more population means. The probability of making one or more Type I error when conducting *one* test of significance is preset by the researcher to an acceptable small value (α). However, the probability of making one or more Type I errors when conducting *several* tests of significance— called the "familywise" or "experimentwise" Type I error rate—is greater than this. The familywise error rate must also be preset to a low value if the findings of the study are to be replicable.

One procedure for accomplishing this was recognized early in the twentieth century by R A Fisher and advanced by Ryan (1960). It is based on the *Bonferroni inequality* that states that the familywise Type I error rate for a set of m tests of significance is no greater than the sum of the α's used for the separate tests. On this basis the familywise error rate for a set of m statistical tests can be preset to a small value, e.g., .05. This is divided by m to establish the value of α and thus the critical value, to be used for each test. For example, if all pairwise comparisons are to be tested among three means (μ_1 with μ_2, μ_1 with μ_3, and μ_2 with μ_3) and the researcher wishes to maintain a familywise error rate of .05, the value of α for each comparison is .05/3 = .0167

Use of the Bonferroni inequality makes it more difficult to obtain statistical significance, especially as the number of tests increases. As an alternative a researcher might decide to conduct each test with a preset α and then decide if the familywise error rate is "acceptable." Thus, if four correlation coefficients are tested for significance, each with $\alpha = .02$, then the familywise rate is no greater than .08. Although larger than .05, this may not be so large that is seriously threatens the validity of the study's conclusions. More information about the Bonferroni approach can be found in all three textbooks listed in the Conclusion.

3. Conclusion

Hypothesis testing procedures constitute an important methodology for the advancement of the educational and social sciences. The technical formulation of hypothesis testing is detailed in a large number of textbooks including excellent introductions by Glass and Hopkins (1996), Ott (1993), and Anderson and Finn (1996). At the same time, hypothesis tests comprise only part of the results of an empirical investigation. It is also of the utmost importance to inspect as many descriptive data as is feasible to understand a study's major findings, to estimate important population characteristics, and to interpret the relationships that are or are not confirmed.

See also: Significance Testing; Multivariate Analysis; Research Paradigms in Education; Quasi-experimentation

References

Anderson T W Finn J D 1996 *The New Statistical Analysis of Data*. Springer-Verlag, New York
Atkinson R C 1968 Computer-based instruction in initial reading. *Proceedings of the 1967 Invitational Conference on Testing Problems*. Educational Testing Service, Princeton, New Jersey
Cohen J 1988 *Statistical Power Analysis for the Behavioral Sciences*, 2nd edn. Erlbaum, Hillsdale, New Jersey
Cohen M R 1960 *A Preface to Logic*. Meridian, New York
Denham C, Lieberman A 1980 *Time to Learn*. National Institute of Education, United States Department of Education, Washington, DC
Ellis A 1952 A critique of systematic theoretical foundations in clinical psychology. *J. Clin. Psychol.* 8: 11–15
Getzels J W 1963 Conflict and role behavior in the educational setting. In: Charters W W, Gage N L (eds.) 1963 *Readings in the Social Psychology of Education*, 1st edn. Allyn and Bacon, Boston, Massachusetts
Glass G V, Hopkins K D 1996 *Statistical Methods in Education and Psychology*, 3rd edn. Allyn and Bacon, Needham Heights, Massachusetts
Harrison F I 1968 Relationship between home background, school success, and adolescent attitudes. *Merrill-Palmer Q.* 14: 331–44
Kerlinger F N 1986 *Foundations of Behavioral Research*. Holt, Rinehart and Winston, New York
Kraemer H C, Thiemann S 1987 *How Many Subjects? Statistical Power Analysis in Research*. Sage, Newbury Park, California
Ott R L 1993 *An Introduction to Statistical Methods and Data Analysis*, 4th edn. Duxbury Press, Belmont, California
Platt J R 1964 Strong inference. *Science* 146: 347–53
Popper K R 1968 *Conjectures and Refutations: The Growth of Scientific Knowledge*, 2nd edn. Basic Books, New York
Ryan T A 1960 Statistical tests for multiple comparisons of proportions, variances and other statistics. *Psych. Bull.* 57: 318–28
Snow R E 1974 Representative and quasi-representative designs for research on teaching. *Rev. Educ. Res.* 44: 265–91

Interaction, Detection, and its Effects

K. Marjoribanks

In his analysis of experimental design, Fisher proposed that when research is undertaken "we are usually ignorant which, out of innumerable possible factors, may prove ultimately to be the most important, though we may have strong presuppositions that some few of them are particularly worthy of study. We have usually no knowledge that any one factor will exert its effects independently of all others that can be varied, or that its effects are particularly simply related to variations in these other factors" (Fisher 1966 pp. 94–95). Fisher suggested that if investigators confined their attention to any single factor, it might be inferred either that they were the unfortunate victims of a doctrinaire theory as to how experimentation should proceed, or that the

time, material, or equipment at their disposal was too limited to allow attention to be given to more than one narrow aspect of the problem. Fisher then challenged investigators to examine not only the possible influences of multiple factors but to design studies that analyzed the possible effects of interactions between multiple factors. He observed that such interactions might, or might not, be considerable in magnitude, and it would be of importance in practical cases to know whether they were considerable or not.

Similarly, Costner has claimed that "the lack of attention to nonadditive effects in our data analysis and the awkward implications of our attempts to include an exploration for such effects stands in sharp contrast to the frequency with which nonadditivity is implicitly assumed or explicitly stated in substantive discussions of social science (Costner 1988 p. 45). Costner has suggested:

> There are several possible reasons for this discrepancy between substantive claims and methodological procedures. Some might propose that it would be premature to explore more complex effects until the simpler additive effects have been established. That proposition seems to ignore the fact that it may be difficult to establish the simple effects if we ignore the nonadditive effects; we will be plagued repeatedly by contradictory findings as we explore the results of different studies. Others might suggest that the discrepancy occurs because of the division of labor in social science between methodologists, who prefer additive effects and assume that they suffice, and the substantive specialists, who may not realize that their ideas are inaccurately represented in data analysis. Still others may point to the difficulty of incorporating appropriate explorations for interaction effects in many of our commonly employed data analysis procedures. This is, perhaps, something of an illusion since nonadditive or interaction effects can always be explored by examining the relationships between two variables within subcategories of a third variable. (Costner 1988 p. 47)

Costner concluded that whatever the reason "the discrepancy between assumptions of nonadditivity in substantive claims and assumptions of additivity in data analysis strikes a jarring note in contemporary social science methodology. We need more satisfactory ways of exploring for nonadditivity in conjunction with our most commonly used data analysis procedures" (Costner 1988 pp. 47–48).

In this entry, some of the issues related to an understanding of interaction and the detection of interaction effects are examined and studies from educational research that illustrate the investigation of interactions are presented.

1. Ordinal, Disordinal, and Hybrid Interactions

It has been proposed (Pedhazur 1982 p. 350) that "when main effects are studied, each factor's independent effects are being considered separately. That is, a given combination of treatments (one from each factor) may be particularly effective because they enhance the effects of each other, or particularly ineffective because they operate at cross purposes, so to speak." Pedhazur suggests, for example, that:

> It is possible that a combination of a given teaching method with a certain type of reinforcement is particularly advantageous in producing achievement that is higher than what would be expected on the basis of their separate effects. Conversely, a combination of a teaching method and a type of reinforcement may be particularly disadvantageous in leading to achievement that is lower than would be expected on the basis of their separate effects. Or, to take another example, a specific teaching method may be particularly effective in a given region—say, urban—

whereas another teaching method may be particularly effective in another region—say, suburban. When no effects are observed over and above the separate effects of the various factors, it is said that the variables do not interact, or that they do not have joint effects. When, on the other hand, in addition to the separate effects of the factors they have joint effects as a consequence of specific treatment combination, it is said that the factors interact with each other. (Pedhazur 1982 p. 350)

If interactions are present in research then it has been proposed that they should be classified as being either ordinal or disordinal (Lindquist 1953). The distinction may be illustrated by considering the diagrams in Fig. 1, where each diagram is a representation of fictitious relationships between measures of aptitudes and achievement outcomes for students in two instructional treatment groups.

In Fig. 1a the parallel lines indicate that across the observed aptitude levels there is a constant difference in achievement outcome scores between the two treatment groups, A and B. Thus, in relation to the outcome measure there is no interaction between the aptitude and treatment variables. Ordinal interaction is represented in Fig. 1b. Although treatment A is relatively more effective at high ability levels, the achievement outcome scores for students in treatment A remain greater than the scores of treatment B students at all aptitude levels. Disordinal interaction is reflected in the diagram in Fig.1c. At aptitude levels below x_1 the outcome scores of treatment B students are higher than those of treatment A students. The two treatments appear to be equally effective at the aptitude level of x_1. Above the level x_1, however, students from treatment A have higher outcome scores than students from treatment B. It has been proposed that the decision as to whether an interaction is ordinal or disordinal is based on the point at which the regression lines in such figures cross each other. If this point is outside the range of interest, then the interaction is considered as being ordinal.

In a further classification, interaction effects have been labeled as being either pure ordinal, pure disordinal, or hybrid (Leigh and Kinnear 1980 pp. 842–43). It is suggested that some interactions may be ordinal with one factor as the abscissa and disordinal with the other. Pure ordinal interaction characterizes the situation in which, regardless of the factor used as the abscissa, a consistent rank order relationship exists for levels of a factor or factor combination between levels of the abscissa factor. Pure disordinal interaction occurs when regardless of the factor used as the abscissa, lines connecting treatment combinations for two levels of the other component(s) cross at least once. Hybrid interaction differs from pure ordinal interaction in that the rank order of treatment profiles is invariant between levels of one or more factors, and it varies between levels of one or more remaining factors. The slopes of two or more lines will vary

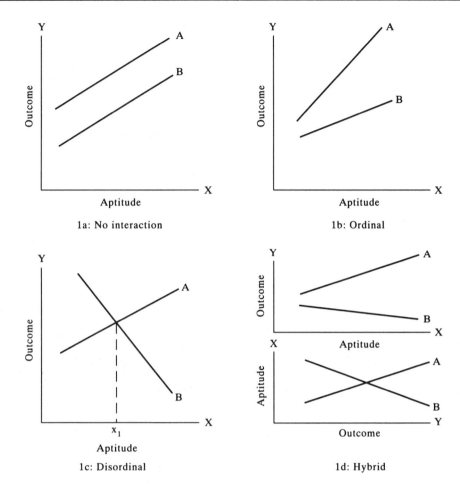

Figure 1
Graphical representation of interaction types

inversely between two or more levels of any of the possible factors, but they do not necessarily have to cross. Because this inverse relationship implies that in a two-factor interaction contrast, the largest and smallest mean values occur at the same abscissa level, the lines must also cross on the graph in which the other factor serves as the abscissa. A graphical representation of such a hybrid interaction is shown in Fig. 1d.

Cronbach and Snow (1977 p. 31) have suggested that often, researchers have stressed the value of disordinal interactions and have tended to dismiss ordinal interactions. The ordinal interaction was regarded as a mere artifact of the choice of measuring scales for the dependent variable. They have indicated, for example, that in many studies of aptitude–treatment interactions, students to the right of the crossover point were to be sent to one treatment and students to the left were assigned to the other treatment strategy. An ordinal interaction (no crossover) would imply the same treatment for all students. It is claimed

by Cronbach and Snow (1977) however, that such an argument about instructional decisions needs to be modified. They have proposed that if the treatment that yields the greater outcome is much costlier than the other, then the ordinal interaction effect on outcome becomes a disordinal effect on payoff. It is suggested that the more expensive method should be applied only to those who would find it so advantageous that its extra cost is likely to be repaid in benefits. Even if the cost-corrected interaction is ordinal, the differential assignment of students would be required when facilities available for one treatment are limited. The scarce treatment would be provided for those students most likely to profit from it; that is, students from the end of the range where the payoff differential is greatest. The graphs in Fig. 2 illustrate a change in ordinality when treatment costs are considered. In the example it is assumed that treatment A is much more expensive than treatment B. After outcome scores are adjusted for treatment costs, the ordinal interaction

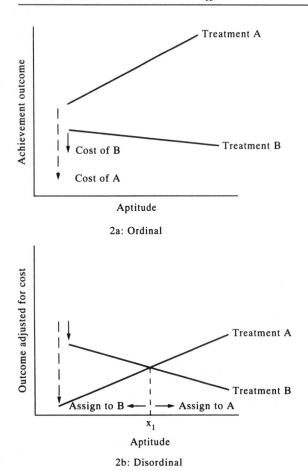

Figure 2
Ordinality alteration when expense of treatments is considered

that is represented in Fig.2a translates to a disordinal interaction as shown in Fig.2b. Rather than assigning all students to treatment A, as Fig. 2a would suggest, the adjusted interaction indicates that a more appropriate instructional decision might be to assign only those students with aptitude scores greater than x_1 to treatment A, and all other students to treatment B.

The analysis of ordinal, disordinal, and hybrid interactions indicates the sensitivity that needs to be adopted when interpreting interactions in educational research.

2. Detection of Interaction Effects

It has been suggested (O'Malley 1988 p. 625) that "There are two very different approaches to the detection of interaction: (a) an empirical search for interactions in a data set, and (b) the inclusion of an interaction effect in a statistical model and a test of its significance."

2.1 Searching for Interaction

O'Malley indicated that "The availability of high-speed computers has made it possible to search algorithmically through large data sets for interactions. One common automated search procedure is called AID, an acronym for Automatic Interaction Detection" (O'Malley 1988 p. 625). This technique subdivides persons into groups and subgroups, by successively splitting the total sample so that there is a maximum variation between groups and minimum variation within groups with respect to the criterion variable. The criterion variable must be either an interval-scaled variable or a dichotomous variable. Another detection technique that is similar to AID is labeled THAID. In this technique the criterion variable is associated with membership of one of a number of mutually exclusive groups. Again the sample is split into subgroups so that the number of correct predictions of membership of each group is maximized and the differences between the groups are also maximized with respect to the proportion of persons in each group category.

It is explained, however, that such search procedures are highly susceptible to error and that "there is considerable potential for detecting interactions which fail to replicate in new samples. This failure to replicate is because the interaction may be due to sample variability. The usual tests of statistical significance are not suitable in search procedures, and therefore are not very useful in determining significant interactions. Consequently, it is very important to use search procedures only with samples of large numbers of cases (as a rule of thumb, at least 1,000) in order to reduce sampling error. Further, it is advisable that the search procedure be conducted on one sample, and the validity of the resulting model be tested on another sample. However, if only one sample is available, the original can be split into separate search and validation groups" (O'Malley 1988 p. 626).

A more traditional technique for searching for interactions is the examination of residuals, "the difference between observed values of data and values predicted on the basis of some additive models. In the absence of interaction, there will be no systematic association between the residuals and the variables used in the prediction. While inspection of residuals can be very useful, it is also true, as with the automated search procedure, that results of searches can be misleading. It is usually preferable to have an interaction hypothesized, for which a test can be performed" (O'Malley 1988 p. 626).

2.2 Analysis and Testing of Interaction Effects

Interaction effects have typically come to the attention of behavioral and social scientists through the analysis of variance. In analysis of variance, which is used generally with nominally scaled research factors, interactions are functions of cell means, usually differences between differences of means. However, the idea of interaction is far more general than that represented by analysis of variance. Interactions are defined and may be studied using quantitative scales, or using combinations of qualitative and nominal scales. In fact, a single (independent) variable can be formed to carry the effect of the interaction of any aspect of any research factor (nominal or quantitative) with any aspect of another research factor (nominal or quantitative), and so on, for interactions of a higher order (see Lubinski and Humphreys 1990, MacCallum and Mar 1995). It is useful to point out that both analysis of variance and multiple regression or correlation analysis are realizations of the least-squares general linear model. However, multiple regression or correlation analysis is by far the more general procedure as it incorporates means of representing as sets of independent variables not only nominal scales but also straight-line and curvilinear (including polynomial) functions, variables with missing data, and interactions among variables of all kinds. Multiple regression or correlation analysis can be used to analyze the data of analysis of variance but the reverse does not hold. In fact, analysis of variance can be viewed as a special case of multiple regression or correlation analysis where the conditions are regular, that is, with equal cell sizes in factorial and split-plot designs and with equal sample sizes and intervals in trend analysis. Indeed it has been suggested (Tatsuoka 1988 p. 742) that a number of researchers "have done much to popularize, in the behavioral and social sciences, the use of multiple regression analysis in situations where analysis of variance has traditionally been the main if not the sole analytic tool. This has been hailed by many as a recent innovation, but in point of fact some early writings of R A Fisher indicate that he invented ANOVA as a computational tool to get around the intractable computational difficulties, in the precomputer era, that arose when multiple regression was applied to designed experiments—that is, when the independent variables were qualitative variables (such as different fertilizers, different varieties of corn, etc.) that were manipulated by the experimenter."

In defining what is meant by interaction when multiple regression models are used, two variables, u and v, are said to interact in accounting for variance in Y, when over and above any additive combination of their separate effects, they have a joint effect (see Cohen and Cohen 1975 for the development of this explanation). This is another way of saying that u and v operate jointly in relating to Y and they also operate conditionally. The relationship between u and Y depends on the value of v being stronger for some values of v than for others. Such a conditional relationship is symmetrical, the relationship between v and Y depending on the value of u. That is, to state the matter more precisely, a nonzero $u \times v$ interaction effect means that the regression of Y on v varies with changes in u. Whatever the nature of u and v, then the $u \times v$ interaction is carried in the $u \, v$ product and can be understood in terms of

joint, or conditional, or nonuniform relationships with Y. However, the $u \times v$ interaction "is carried by," not "is" the $u \, v$ product. This is because, in general, $u \, v$ will be linearly correlated with both u and v, often quite substantially. Only when u and v have been linearly partialed from $u \, v$ does it, in general, become the interaction (independent variable). That is,

$$u \times v = uv \cdot u, v$$

where the $u \times v$ notation is used to represent an interaction and $u \, v$ indicates a product that only becomes an interaction when its constituent parts are partialed.

Similarly, in a three-way interaction such as $u \times v \times w$, the interaction is carried by the product $u \, v \, w$ from which the constituent variables and two-way products are partialed. That is,

$$u \times v \times w = uvw \cdot u, v, w, uv, uw, vw$$

What is being claimed is that the product variable (say) $X \, Z$ contains the interaction together with variance that is linearly accounted for by X and Z. When this latter variance is removed from $X \, Z$ by partialing, it is precisely the $X \times Z$ interaction that remains; that is, $X \, Z \cdot X, Z$. The latter will have zero correlation with X and Z (by construction), and will be correlationally invariant over linear transformations of X and Z, and with an invariant t (or F) value.

The significance of interactions in regression models may most appropriately be examined by analyzing hierarchical regression equations in which independent variables are entered in a predetermined order so that prior variables are partialed from later ones. Consider, for example, the regression of Y on the variables X, Z, and their product $X \, Z$. Then:

$$Y = b_1 X + b_2 Z + b_3 XZ + a$$

where bs are the raw score regression weights and a the Y-intercept. The amount of variance associated with the addition of an independent variable (its unique contribution) is its squared semipartial r. It is a semipartial r because the other (independent) variables have been partialed from the (independent) variable in question but not from Y. In relation to the product variable, its squared multiple semipartial correlation with Y is:

$$r^2_{Y(XZ \cdot X, Z)} = R^2_{Y \cdot X, Z, XZ} - R^2_{Y \cdot X, Z}$$

which is the increment in Y variance accounted for when the product $X \, Z$ is added to its constituent variables, X and Z, as a third independent variable.

2.3 Analysis of Polynomials: Special Case of Interactions

If an $X \times Z$ interaction is interpreted in relation to Y as meaning that the slope of the Y on X regression line varies as Z varies, then it is possible to interpret a partialed power of X as an interaction. It is suggested (see Cohen and Cohen 1975 for the development of this explanation) that when the constituents of a product are linearly partialed there is an interaction; for example, $X \times Z = X Z \cdot X, Z$. Similarly, when the constituents of an integral power are linearly partialed, there is a curve component, for example, $X \times X = X X \cdot X = X^2 \cdot X$. Further, just as $X Z \cdot X, Z$ is necessarily orthogonal to X and Z, whatever the correlations among X, Z, and $X Z$, so, too, is $X^2 \cdot X$ necessarily orthogonal to X, whatever the correlation between X and X^2 (usually close to unity). Partialed variables (residuals) correlate zero precisely with the variables that have been partialed from them, by construction (or definition). That is, an $X \times X$ interaction ($X^2 \cdot X$) can be interpreted as meaning that the slope of the Y on X regression line varies as X varies. Polynomials may be analyzed in hierarchical regression equations with linear functions preceding quadratic, preceding cubic, and so on, and with main effects preceding two-way, preceding three-way interactions, and so forth, so that terms of lower order are partialed from those of higher order and not vice versa.

An illustration of using hierarchical regression models to detect interactions is presented in the following analysis of relationships between intellectual ability, attitudes toward school, and academic achievement for children from different family groups.

3. Ability and Attitude Correlates of Academic Achievement: Family–Group Differences

In psychological models of educational performance academic achievement is related typically to measures of intellectual ability and attitudes. In a review of such models, it was suggested (Haertel et al. 1983 p. 86) that the "presage conditions considered by the various theorists most often include cognitive and attitudinal attributes of individual learning." In contrast, sociological research of academic performance has tended to concentrate on examining relations between achievement and measures of social status and parent socialization.

It seemed appropriate, therefore, to examine a model of academic achievement that included intellectual ability, attitudes, and refined family environment measures. A study was generated (Marjoribanks 1987) from the proposition that for children from different family environments, relations among their ability, attitudes toward school, and academic achievement vary. For the investigation, children's family environments were defined conjointly by social status indicators and proximal social psychological variables. The definition of proximal family environments was based upon a seminal study (Kahl 1953 p. 193) of "common-man" boys. Kahl observed that in lower-middle social status groups it was possible to identify "getting-by" and "getting-ahead" families. In getting-by families,

boys were encouraged to enjoy themselves while they were young. The boys "were told to stay in high school because a diploma was pretty important in getting jobs nowadays, but they were allowed to pick their own curriculum according to taste" (Kahl 1953 p. 193). The possibility of pursuing a college education was rarely considered. In contrast, parents who believed in getting ahead started to apply pressure from the beginning of their sons' school careers. "They encouraged high marks, they paid attention to what was happening at school, they stressed that good performance was necessary for occupational success, and they suggested various occupations that would be good for their sons" (p. 201). For Marjoribanks's study, families were classified by social-status characteristics and by the family dimensions of getting-by or getting-ahead. In each of the four family groups, defined by the social status and environment dimensions, relations were examined between children's ability, attitudes toward school, and academic achievement.

Data were collected from 928 Australian families. Each family had an 11-year old child, and the analyses related to those children (472 boys, 456 girls). Family social status was measured by an equally weighted composite of parents' occupations and education. From interviews conducted in homes, parents' socialization was defined by the interrelated components of achievement training, independence training, achievement-value orientations, and aspirations. Families were classified as having a getting-ahead orientation if they stressed achievement training, encouraged independence, were individualistic, and had high aspirations for their children. In contrast, families were labeled as having a getting-by orientation if they expressed relatively low achievement training, encouraged dependence, were collectivistic, and had lower aspirations.

The children's intellectual ability was measured with Raven's Progressive Matrices. Academic achievement was assessed using the Class Achievement Test in Mathematics and the Primary Reading Survey Tests, devised by the Australian Council for Educational Research. A two-factor affective–cognitive model of attitudes was adopted for the construction of an attitude-to-school measure.

For the analysis, children were classified into four family groups which were defined by the median split of scores on the social status and parent-socialization measures. The family groups were labeled middle status/getting-ahead (146 boys, 141 girls), middle status/getting-by (59, 55), lower status/getting-ahead (81, 76), and lower status/getting-by (186 boys, 184 girls).

Relations among ability, attitudes, and academic achievement for children from the different family types were investigated by plotting regression surfaces generated from hierarchical regression models. In the models, product terms were included to test for possible interaction effects and squared terms were added to examine possible curvilinear relations. Prior investigations had indicated the possible presence of interaction and curvilinear associations between measures of children's individual attributes and their school-related outcomes. That is, the hierarchical regression models were of the form $Y = b_1 X + b_2 Z + b_3 X \times Z + b_4 X^2 + b_5 Z^2 + \text{constant}$, where Y, X, and Z represented measures of academic achievement, intellectual ability, and attitudes to school respectively.

In the following illustration only the relationships among ability, affective school attitudes, and children's mathematics achievement have been presented. For the analysis, each predictor variable was transformed by subtracting means from the raw scores of the relevant measures. Aiken and West have indicated, for example, that:

> The literature on regression with higher order terms contains many admonitions about the problems of multicollinearity. However, these problems are not the usual problems of multicollinearity in regression analysis in which two supposedly different predictors are highly correlated. The multicollinearity in the context of regression with higher order terms is due to scaling, and can be greatly lessened by centering variables. Uncentred X' and X'^{2} will be highly correlated. But if instead we use centered predictor X and it is normally distributed, then the covariance between centered predictor X and X^2 is zero. Even if X is not normally distributed, the correlation between X and X^2 will be much lower than the correlation between X' and X'^{2}. Uncentered X' and Z' will both be highly correlated with their crossproduct X'Z'. But if X and Z are bivariate normal, then the covariance between each centered variable X and Z and the product term XZ is zero. When X and Z are centered, the only remaining correlation between first order and product terms or between first order and second order terms is that due to nonnormality of the variables. (Aiken and West 1991 p. 35)

Aiken and West also examined the relationship between the centered raw score analysis with centered X, and Z, and their crossproduct XZ as predictors and a "standardized" solution. In this latter solution, z_x and z_z are initially calculated and then their product $z_x z_z$ is formed. These values are used as the predictors in regression analysis with z_y as the criterion. "The *unstandardized* solution from that analysis is the appropriate 'standardized' solution for use with multiplicative terms" (Aiken and West 1991 p. 44).

From the raw regression weights that were generated from the hierarchical analyses, regression surfaces were plotted. In Fig. 3 the surfaces show the regression-fitted relations among ability, affective attitudes, and mathematics achievement for boys and girls in each family group. In the surfaces, the horizontal axes represent the ability and affective-attitude variables while the vertical axis represents mathematics achievement. On each axis, the scores were standardized with means of 50 and standard deviations of 10.

The surfaces in the four family groups indicated that girls' affective attitudes toward school were not related to mathematics performance at different ability levels. At each attitude value, however, girls' ability had significant linear associations with mathematics achievement.

For boys, the variations in the surfaces were more complex. In the middle social-status groups, intellectual ability had a curvilinear association with mathematics achievement. Indeed, ability tended to act as a threshold variable. Until a certain ability level was reached, there was no significant association with mathematics scores. After that threshold value, however, further increases in ability were related to increasing changes in performance. In middle-status and getting-ahead families, for example, at an affective attitude value of 70, the fitted-mathematics scores were 47, 48, 51, and 58 at ability levels of 30, 40, 50, and 60, respectively. Also, for boys in middle-status and getting-ahead families, affective attitudes were not related significantly to mathematics scores at any ability level. In contrast, for boys in middle-status and getting-by families, increases in affective attitudes were actually related to decrements in mathematics performance. The shape of the boys' surface in lower-status and getting-by families indicated the presence of a significant interaction effect. At low ability levels, the boys' affective attitudes were not associated with mathematics achievement; at high ability levels, however, increments in affective attitudes were related to sizable increases in performance. That is, the surfaces in Fig. 3 indicated that when children were classified into family groups, there were family and gender differences in the complexity of the relations among ability, affective attitudes, and mathematics achievement. Indeed, the study suggests that an understanding of the variation in children's academic achievement is likely to be enhanced by examining models that test interaction and curvilinear relationships.

The study just described illustrates the potential value of including interaction and polynomials, the special case of interactions, in survey educational research. Some of the most interesting analyses of interaction, however, have involved investigations of possible aptitude–treatment interactions in experimental studies. Some developments in aptitude–treatment interaction research are examined in the following section.

4. Aptitude–Treatment Interactions

Much educational research has adopted either situation or trait models to examine students' school learning. In the situation model, relationships are examined between students' learning contexts and outcome measures. Whereas in the trait model, associations between students' individual attributes and measures of their performance and behavior are investigated. Increasingly, however, investigators are using interaction theoretical and methodological frameworks in

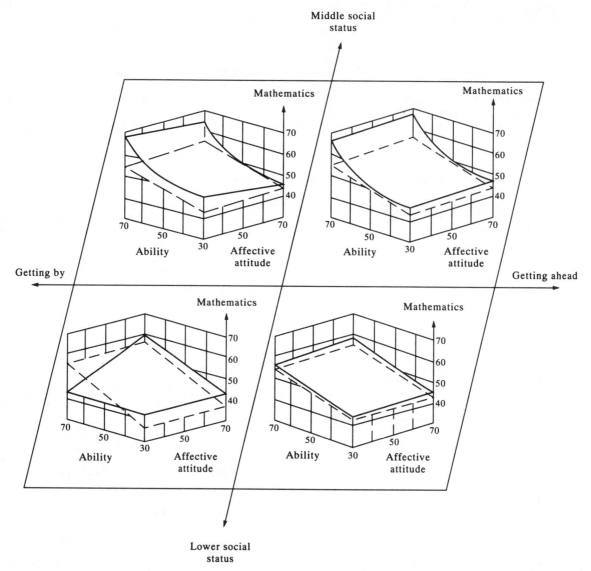

Figure 3
Fitted mathematics achievement scores in relation to ability and affective attitudes for children from different family groups[a]
a —— boys' surfaces, – – – girls' surfaces

which learning outcomes are related to students' individual characteristics, their learning contexts, and the interaction between individual attributes and situations.

A special case of the more general person–environment framework is the aptitude-treatment interaction model. It has been suggested (Snow 1991) that the investigation of aptitude–treatments attempts to increase an understanding of why and how different students benefit from various kinds of instruction. From such investigations it is hoped that adaptive instructional conditions can be created that will lead

to an improvement of learning situations to match the needs and characteristics of different students.

Corno (1979) has contended, however, that statistical analyses of aptitude–treatment interactions (ATIs) typically ignore the hierarchical (students nested within classes) character of classroom data. The concern is particularly important, given that research conclusions may be altered by reanalyses that take the hierarchical nature of the data into account. It has been suggested that in ATI research, analyses need to be conducted at three hierarchical levels: (a) between classes, (b) pooled within classes, and (c) overall individuals. For between-class investigations, students are assigned their class mean on each variable which weights each mean by the class size, and the analyses pose the question, "Do classes respond to treatments differently depending on the average level of aptitudes?" Pooled within-class studies adopt student and outcome scores deviated from the class mean and ask, "Does response to treatment depend on where the student is placed on aptitude relative to other students?" Analysis for overall students, which is characteristic of most ATI research, ignores class distinctions by regressing raw individual student outcomes onto similarly defined aptitudes to examine whether, "response to treatments depends on individual student aptitudes." That is, regressions and interactions divide—at least in principle—into group and individual components that have distinct substantive meanings. Recognition of these distinctions forces a radical change in thinking about ATI. Once two distinct interactions are conceived it becomes apparent that previous ATI studies have not asked as penetrating a set of questions as they might. Except for a few studies of teacher effects, investigators of ATIs have reported a single component ATI, calculated either between classes or on pooled classes.

In an investigation of self-appraisal data for students in two treatment groups, Corno et al. (1981) observed that between-class effects accounted for 62 to 81 percent of the variation in a number of affective outcome measures while pooled within-class effects were related to only 11 to 35 percent of the variation in scores. Although there were no significant ATIs in the individual overall or within-class pooled analyses there were three significant ATIs for the between-classes analyses. Classes with lower scores on general ability, for example, had more favorable attitudes if they were part of a treatment group in which parents instructed children in classroom strategies. In contrast, classes of higher ability had more favorable attitudes if they were part of a treatment group that received no special parent instruction in strategies. The exploration of between-group and within-group effects generates the possibility of new interpretations of much ATI research. Many analyses of ATI have been based on the assumption that all ATI effects occur independently in different students. However, while such an assumption is probably true for instruction administered to students singly, it may not be true when students work side by side, in classrooms.

However, such between-group analyses ignore the effects of aggregation bias. It has been proposed (Keeves and Sellin 1988 p. 695) that "The task facing educational research workers which is of vital importance in the study of classrooms, schools and school districts, as well as in cross-national studies of educational achievement, is the development of appropriate procedures for the analysis of multilevel data. The general framework for such procedures is that of multiple regression, with the outcome variables regressed on variables which measure student as well as teacher, classroom and school characteristics." Keeves and Sellin suggested that "The procedures must take into consideration the nesting of students within classrooms, and possibly classrooms within schools, and make full provision for the clustering or grouping effects of the micro units within the macro units ... The general class of models which have been developed for the analysis of multilevel data has become known as 'hierarchical linear models' (HLM)" (Keeves and Sellin 1988 p. 695).

It has been suggested (Raudenbush and Bryk 1986 p. 13) that "HLM is a powerful tool that permits a separation of within-school from between-school phenomena and allows simultaneous consideration of the effects of school factors not only on school means but also on structural relationships within schools." It has been further proposed (Lee and Bryk 1989 p. 173) that "By their very nature, questions about school effects require the exploration of hierarchical relationships. Such investigations involve a search of statistical associations between school factors, on the one hand, and student-level variables, on the other hand. Fortunately, recent developments in the statistical theory of hierarchical linear models (HLM) now provide appropriate tools for modeling within- and between-school phenomena." As they suggested, "Such a methodology allows direct representation of the influence of school factors on structural relations within schools. Specifically, HLM enables the investigator explicitly to represent a set of regression coefficients as multivariate outcomes to be simultaneously explained as a function of measured differences between schools. Hence, the variation among schools in regression slopes (for example, the relationship between social class and achievement) become dependent measures to be explained by school-level characteristics" (Lee and Bryk 1989 p. 174).

Such concerns as expressed by Corno and the later developments for the analysis of multilevel data have led to conclusions (Snow 1991) such that, from the research undertaken so far, no simple or general principles for matching students and teachers, teaching methods, or school environments have emerged. Snow has proposed that it is necessary to move beyond a reliance on isolated aptitude–treatment studies and develop programmatic research and development, if such research is to have a significant impact on classroom instruction. He also suggested (Snow 1989 p. 8) that "There are many new conceptions about the psychological structures and processes involved in learning and development in relation to instruction, and of individual differences in aptitude and achievement as well. These new constructs are reshaping and elaborating our view of instructional theory. Unfortunately, the new constructs have mostly been demonstrated piecemeal, in small-scale situations; their generality and relations to one another are thus not yet well investigated or understood." Conceptual, methodological, and statistical advances provide, however, the opportunity for a greater understanding of aptitude–treatment interactions.

5. Conclusion

Research findings provide support for the adoption of interactionist models in educational research. However, the models that have been used should be considered only as an initial approximation of the complexity of interrelationships among measures of person, situation, and outcome variables. In future research there is a need to measure with greater sensitivity contexts, person variables, and outcomes. All these characteristics are multivariate and it is likely to be found that situations and parts of situations will produce different effects on a variety of outcome measures and will produce different effects on different individual characteristics depending on the pattern of their initial stages. For subsequent research the following equation might be estimated:

$$I_{j,t_2} = \sum b_j I_{j,t_1}^* + \sum b_k E_{k,t_{1-2}}^* + \sum b_{jk}(I_{j,t_1}^*)(E_{k,t_{1-2}}^*)$$

where I_{j,t_2} is a given individual characteristic. The first term on the right hand side of the model is a weighted composite of a number of antecedent individual characteristics (the asterisk indicates that the characteristics are in an optimal mathematical form; for example, linear, quadratic, or logarithmic for prediction). The second term is a similar intervening context composite and the last term is a weighted composite of products of antecendent characteristics and situations.

Research based on the proposed generalized model, with appropriate measures and statistical techniques, would allow for the multiplicity of possible causes in the two domains, of persons and situations, and the possibility that initial characteristics interact with context measures, influencing later characteristics. Only by the adoption of such an analysis of interaction is it likely that our understanding of the complex nature of educational problems will be enriched.

See also: Regression Analysis of Quantified Data

References

Aiken L S, West S G 1991 *Multiple Regression: Testing and Interpreting Interactions*. Sage, Newbury Park, California

Cohen J, Cohen P 1975 *Applied Multiple Regression: Correlation Analysis for the Behavioral Sciences*. Erlbaum, Hillsdale, New Jersey

Corno L 1979 A hierarchical analysis of selected naturally occurring aptitude–treatment interactions in the third grade. *Am. Educ. Res. J.* 16(4): 391–409

Corno L, Mitman A, Hedges L V 1981 The influence of direct instruction on student self-appraisals: A hierarchical analysis of treatment and aptitude-treatment interaction effects. *Am. Educ. Res. J.* 18(1): 39–61

Costner H L 1988 Research methodogy in sociology. In: Borgatta E F, Cook K S (eds.) 1988 *The Future of Sociology*. Sage, Newbury Park, California

Cronbach L J, Snow R E 1977 *Aptitudes and Instructional Methods: A Handbook for Research on Interactions*. Irvington, New York

Fisher R A 1966 *The Design of Experiments*, 8th edn. Oliver and Boyd, Edinburgh

Haertel G D, Walberg H J, Weinstein T 1983 Psychological models of educational performance: A theoretical synthesis of constructs. *Rev. Educ. Res.* 53(1): 75–91

Kahl J A 1953 Educational and occupational aspirations of "common man" boys. *Harv. Educ. Rev.* 23: 186–203

Keeves J P, Sellin N 1988 Multilevel analysis. In: Keeves J P (ed.) 1988 *Educational Research, Methodology, and Measurement: An International Handbook*. Pergamon Press, Oxford

Lee V E, Bryk A S 1989 A multilevel model of the social distribution of high school achievement. *Sociol. Educ.* 62(3): 172–92

Leigh J H, Kinnear T C 1980 On interaction classification. *Educ. Psychol. Meas.* 40(4): 841–43

Lindquist E F 1953 *Design and Analysis of Experiments in Psychology and Education*. Houghton Mifflin, Boston, Massachusetts

Lubinski D, Humphreys L G 1990 Assessing spurious "moderator effects": Illustrated substantively with the hypothesized (synergistic) relation between spatial and mathematical ability. *Psychol. Bull.* 107: 385–93

MacCallum R C, Mar C M 1995 Distinguishing between moderator and quadratic effects in multiple regression. *Psychol. Bull.* 118: 415–21

Marjoribanks K 1987 Ability and attitude correlates of academic achievement: Family-group differences. *J. Educ. Psychol.* 79(2): 171–78

O'Malley P M 1988 Detection of interaction. In: Keeves J P (ed.) 1988 *Educational Research, Methodology, and Measurement: An International Handbook*. Pergamon Press, Oxford

Pedhazur E J 1982 *Multiple Regression in Behavioral Research: Explanation and Prediction*, 2nd edn. Holt, Rinehart and Winston, New York

Raudenbush S, Bryk A S 1986 A hierarchical model for studying school effects. *Sociol. Educ.* 59(1): 1–17

Snow R E 1989 Toward assessment of cognitive and conative structures in learning. *Educ. Researcher* 18(9): 8–14

Snow R E 1991 Aptitude–treatment interaction models of teaching. In: Marjoribanks K (ed.) 1991 *The Foundations of Students' Learning*. Pergamon Press, Oxford

Tatsuoka M M 1988 Regression analysis. In: Keeves J P (ed.) 1988 *Educational Research, Methodology, and Measurement: An International Handbook*. Pergamon Press, Oxford

Log–Linear Models

J. J. Kennedy and Hak Ping Tam

Log–linear models are used to analyze cross-tabular data. Specifically, they are used either to describe relationships or to document effects when data are frequencies presented within the context of contingency tables. Log–linear models are used to greatest advantage when cross-tabulations are presented in contingency tables of three or more dimensions. In this entry, an attempt will be made to illustrate the basic features of a log–linear analysis by subjecting educational data that are contained within a three-dimensional table to a particular application of log–linear modeling known as a "logit-model analysis."

1. A Brief Historical Perspective

Prior to 1970, for all practical purposes, comprehensive analyses of contingency tables were limited to tables of two dimensions. In typical, traditional, two-dimensional analyses, either the null hypothesis of "independence" or the hypothesis of "homogeneity of proportional response" are tested initially with the familiar chi-square statistic, developed in 1900 by Karl Pearson. The statistic is shown below.

$$\chi^2 = \sum_{all}^{cells} \frac{(f_0 - F_e)^2}{F_e} \tag{1}$$

where *observed* elementary cell frequencies (f_0) are compared to cell frequencies that are *expected* (F_e's) under the hypotheses above. If the fit between observed and expected frequencies exceeds chance expectation, as indicated by a significant χ^2 statistic, then either the independence hypothesis or the hypothesis of homogeneity of proportional response is rejected. In either case, for tables of only two dimensions, the Pearsonian chi-square given by Eqn. (1), along with the subsequent development of a number of measures of association for two-way tables (see Reynolds 1984), have served researchers well for seven decades.

However, researchers are often able to construct contingency tables of three, four, or more dimensions. It was not until the prominent introduction of log–linear models in the early 1970s, however, that methodology became available that would accommodate the analysis of tables of high dimensionality. Largely as a result of the pioneering work of Fienberg (1972), Haberman (1974), Bishop et al. (1975), Bock (1975), and most particularly, Goodman (1978), major advances in log–linear theory were made in the 1970s that enabled researchers to subject multidimensional tables to comprehensive analysis. These advances were followed in the 1980s by major improvements in the computational software (e.g., BMDP4F, SAS CATMOD, SPSS LOG–LINEAR, etc.). Also, during these two decades there appeared a number of didactic papers (Shaffer 1973, Marks 1975, Knoke and Burke 1980, Green 1988, Kennedy 1988) and books (Fienberg 1977, Upton 1978, Kennedy 1983) that were written to inform research practitioners of the existence of this relatively new system for the analysis of categorical data. As a result of the refinements in theory, software, and didactic publications, the use of log–linear models has become well established in fields such as sociology and biostatistics. Since categorical data are frequently collected in educational and psychological inquiry, a comparable increase in log–linear applications is likely to be seen in these fields in the future.

2. Preliminary Requirements and Considerations

Before a concrete example is introduced, the manner in which log–linear models are applied (i.e., modes of inquiry) and the requisite conditions associated with credible log–linear analyses will be reviewed.

2.1 Modes of Inquiry

There are two distinct orientations to the analysis of contingency tables. The first is a "symmetrical" orientation: statistical inquiry that seeks to identify relationships (or associations) between or among variables. For two-dimensional tables, a symmetrical orientation is operative when the hypothesis of variable independence is under test. For this test, no explicit attempt is made to cast one of the variables as an explanatory (independent) variable and the other variable as a response (dependent) variable. The second is an "asymmetrical" orientation: inquiry that seeks to document effects (i.e., differences between groups) with respect to the manner in which groups respond over levels of a designated response variable. For a table of two dimensions, one variable (say Variable *A*) is perceived as an explanatory variable while the other (Variable *B*) is designated as a response variable. When the null hypothesis is one of homogeneity of proportional response, asymmetrical inquiry is indicated.

When tables are of high dimensionality the distinction between inquiries that are symmetrical and those that are asymmetrical is of central importance. In addition to sampling considerations, the distinction is critical because it affects the choice of log–linear models that may be applied. Whereas the number of general log–linear models that may be specified in the symmetrical case is considerable, the number of models that may be assessed in the asymmetrical case is restricted. As will be shown, only a subset of general log–linear models qualify for use in an asymmetrical analysis.

2.2 Requisite Conditions

The underlying conditions and statistical assumptions for log–linear analyses are extensions of those associated with traditional analyses of two-dimensional contingency tables (see Hays 1988 pp. 780–81). Hence, all variables that define the table must be categorical. The variables may be dichotomies (e.g., females vs. males) or they may be polytomies (e.g., Africans, Americans, Asians, Europeans); they may be ordered (e.g., small, medium, large) or unordered (e.g., engineers, mathematicians, physicists) (see *522034*).

In all instances, however, members of the sample should be assigned to only one level of each categorical variable (mutual exclusivity) so that when the variables are crossed to form the multidimensional table, subjects appear in only one of the elementary cells of the table. If it should happen that subjects are counted more than once in the table, the underlying statistical assumption of response independence is likely to be violated, and the resulting chi-square statistics are likely to be positively biased.

In addition, if chi-square statistics are to serve as good approximations to the multinomial in symmetrical inquiry, or the product-multinomial for asymmetrical inquiry (see Kennedy 1992 Chap. 2), the size of samples should be sufficiently large. In practice, however, log–linear analysts are afforded a great deal of flexibility both with respect to analyzing sparse tables and tables that contain zero cell frequencies, especially when zero frequencies are not structural (e.g., pregnant males) but instead simply due to the small size of the sample (see Fienberg 1977 p. 108, Clogg and Eliason 1987, Agresti 1990 pp. 244–50).

3. An Illustrative Example: The Productivity of Teacher Educators

Data are those collected, but not analyzed, in doctoral research conducted by McCullough (1992) in the United States. McCullough sought to describe prospective teacher educators, that is, graduate students who were enrolled in advanced programs designed to prepare college teachers who, in turn, would prepare teachers of children in elementary and secondary schools. McCullough identified 668 prospective teacher educators enrolled in PhD or DEd programs in seven universities in the midwestern state of Ohio.

Of interest here are the usable self-reports of 489 prospective teacher educators ($n = 489$) with respect to three selected categorical variables: (a) grade point average (GPA) earned at the master's level prior to ad-

Table 1

Cross-classification of prospective teacher educators by masters-level GPA, completion of a master's thesis, and level of scholarly production

A_i: GPA	B_j: Thesis	C_1	C_2	C_3	C_4	[AB]
A_1 – Above	B_1 – Yes	29	34	15	14	92
	B_2 – No	80	44	27	28	179
A_2 – Below	B_1 – Yes	25	22	16	5	68
	B_2 – No	77	47	19	7	150
[C] Main Marginals		211	147	77	54	489

(header spanning C_1–C_4: C_k: Scholarly Production)

vanced training, (b) completion or noncompletion of a thesis at the master's level (thesis), and (c) the number of papers presented or articles published (scholarly production) as an advanced graduate student.

The first two variables, variables that may be regarded as indicators of scholarly productivity, will be treated as explanatory variables. In general, the first variable will be labeled Variable *A* and its constituent levels will be indicated with subscript "*i*" where ($i = 1,2, \ldots, a$). In particular, the first explanatory variable is:

Variable *A* – master's level GPA:
$A_1 = above$ 3.70
$A_2 = below$ 3.70

The second explanatory variable, labeled Variable *B* with subscript j ($j = 1,2 \ldots, b$) is:

Variable *B* – completion of a master's *thesis*:
$B_1 = yes$
$B_2 = no$

The third variable, "scholarly production," consisted of four categories based on subject responses to several questions pertaining to the number of conference papers and articles that students wrote or co-authored as part of their graduate experience. The third variable will be termed Variable *C* with subscript k ($k = 1,2, \ldots, c$) and it is:

Variable *C* – level of *scholarly production*
$C_1 = none$ no evidence of scholarly production
$C_2 = moderate$ 1–3 presentations or articles
$C_3 = high$ 4–5 presentations or articles
$C_4 = very\ high$ 6 or more presentations or articles

The 489 prospective teacher educators were cross-classified on the basis of their self-reported standing on the three variables and resultant tabulations are given in the $2 \times 2 \times 4$ contingency table presented as Table 1.

An examination of [C] in Table 1, that is, the main marginals for scholarly production, revealed that 211 sample members (43%) had not presented a paper or co-authored an article. A consideration of the marginals in the 2×2 [AB] revealed that only 160 students

(33%) had written a master's thesis, but 271 (55%) of students had earned a GPA of 3.70 or higher (a letter grade of A- or higher in most universities).

Having acknowledged differences in the marginal distributions of [C] and [AB], primary interest is directed toward the possible *effects* (group differences) of GPA and thesis on the variable of scholarly production. Since scholarly production will be regraded as a response variable, and since it comprises more than two categories, the log–linear analysis to be performed can be designated more specifically as a multinomial logit-model analysis.

4. An Overview of Major Operations

A log–linear analysis is a relatively complex process. It is based in the theory of exponential families (see Andersen 1990 Chap. 3) and, when implemented, consists of numerous orchestrated operations. An outline of major steps associated with typical symmetrical analyses will be found in Kennedy (1992 pp. 70–71). There follows below a reconstruction of major steps that are applicable when inquiry is asymmetrical, steps that will be illustrated when McCullough's (1992) data are analyzed.

4.1 Specification of Models

A log–linear analysis includes the specification, fitting, and assessment of multiple models, a task that is readily accomplished with the help of modern computer programs. The researcher's substantive intentions and mode of inquiry ultimately determine the number and nature of models that are analyzed. If inquiry is symmetrical and exploratory, a considerable number of general log–linear models are likely to be examined. If inquiry is asymmetrical, however, only a limited number of models, that is, those that can serve as logit models, are appropriate. A quick glance ahead to Table 2 will provide a preview of the logit models that will be specified in the analysis of McCullough's data.

4.2 Generation of Expected Cell Frequencies

For every specified model, a set of expected elementary cell frequencies, based on maximum-likelihood procedures, will be provided. Computer programs provide these expectancies by employing one of two iterative computational algorithms. BMDP4F, for example, uses the iterative proportional fitting algorithm developed in 1940 by W E Deming and F F Stephan (see Kennedy 1983 pp. 239–42), while SAS CATMOD and SPSS LOG–LINEAR use an alternative iterative procedure known as the Newton–Raphson (see Haberman 1978 pp. 10–15). For comparable models, identical expected cell frequencies, symbolized by F_{ijk}'s for three-dimensional tables, are produced by the two computational algorithms.

4.3 Assessing the Goodness-of-Fit of Models

For models specified, chi-square goodness-of-fit statistics are obtained and then used to assess the degree of agreement between F_{ijk}'s and the elementary cell frequencies actually observed (f_{ijk}'s). The preferred goodness-of-fit statistic in log–linear work is not the familiar Pearsonian chi-square given by Eqn. (1), however, but rather it is an alternative chi-square statistic developed 24 years later by R A Fisher. The preferred statistic is the *maximum-likelihood-ratio chi-square*, which for three-dimensional tables is

$$L^2 = 2 \sum_{all}^{cells} (f_{ijk}) \left(\ln \frac{f_{ijk}}{F_{ijk}} \right) \tag{2}$$

where ln denotes natural logarithms, that is, logs to the base $e = 2.718282$. Though χ^2 and L^2 are asymptotically equivalent, as will be shown there are decided advantages associated with the use of the L^2 in log–linear work.

4.4 Assessing the Importance of Model Parameters

For the most part, in an asymmetrical analysis, goodness-of-fit L^2's are obtained so that *component chi-squares* (or part chi-squares) can be calculated. Component chi-squares are then used to assess the importance of specific "interaction" terms that appear in log–linear models. It will become apparent that an assessment of the interactive λ^{ac} term that appears in Model (1), (2), and (3) will be important in the analysis to be performed (see Table 2). If, for example, it can be shown that the inclusion of λ^{ac} in a model has the effect contributing significantly to the fit of observed frequencies, a significant association between GPA (Variable A) and scholarly production (Variable C) is indicated, and consequently, from an asymmetrical perspective, significant differences (effects) between the two GPA subsamples, relative to their response to the scholarly production variable, will be indicated. In short, if λ^{ac} is found to be significant, logit-model main effects for GPA (Variable A) will be claimed.

Component chi-squares are calculated, therefore, to evaluate the importance of λ^{ac} and other interactive terms. The component for λ^{ac} may be obtained by subtracting the goodness-of-fit chi-square observed for Model (1) from the goodness-of-fit chi-square observed for Model (0), specifically

$$L^2_{(0-1)} = L^2_{(0)} - L^2_{(1)} \tag{3}$$

A quick glance at Table 2 will reveal that Model (0) contains all terms in Model (1) with the notable exception of the λ^{ac} term. Hence, the magnitude of component chi-square given by Eqn. (3) indicates the extent to which λ^{ac} contributes to explanation of observed data. The component chi-square reflects the strength of the association between Variables A and C, and hence reflects the strength of logit-model main effects associated with GPA. Moreover, the component chi-square can be tested for statistical significance.

The appropriate number of degrees of freedom (*df*) for the testing of component chi-squares is given by parallel subtraction. For example, the *df* that describe the sampling distribution of the component given by Eqn. (3) are

$$df_{(0-1)} = df_{(0)} - df_{(1)} \qquad (4)$$

In sum, the computation and testing of component chi-squares, along the lines suggested above, are critical steps in the performance of an asymmetrical analysis.

4.5 Summarizing and Advancing Omnibus Findings

Subsequent to testing relevant components—the components for λ^{ac}, λ^{bc}, and λ^{abc} in the example to follow—results are interpreted and then summarized in a fashion that is reminiscent of an analysis of variance (ANOVA). If, for example, the component given by Eqn. (3) is found to be statistically significant (and it will be), the omnibus finding will be that significant logit-model main effects have been detected between levels of the GPA variable with respect to their patterns of response to the scholarly production variable. If the component for λ^{bc} should be found to be significant (and it will be), then main effects due to the thesis variable are present. Finally, if the component for λ^{bc} is found to be significant (but it will not be), significant logit-model first-order interaction between GPA and thesis can be claimed.

4.6 Following up Omnibus Results

When response is polytomous, additional procedures are needed to explicate results. In the Goodman tradition, the majority of analysts attempt to follow up results by interpreting the lambda parameters that appear in log–linear models. This approach, however, is fraught with problems as is revealed by the numerous papers that have acknowledged many of these problems and have attempted further to offer partial remedies (Kaufman and Schervish 1986, Alba 1987, Clogg and Eliason 1987). The major problem with interpretation of lambda parameters is that comparisons are expressed ultimately in terms of odds or logged odds, a cumbrous expression of outcome that is not well understood by most researchers.

In response to lambda interpretation, alternative follow-up methodologies have been proposed that are analogous to the performance of *t*-test contrasts following an ANOVA. Bock (1975 pp. 531–35), for example, introduced contrasts based on the Newton–Raphson (see Marascuilo and Levin 1983 pp. 425–33), that are available to advanced users of SPSS LOG-LINEAR. More recent, and less complex, is a multiple comparison approach proposed by Kennedy and Bush (1988) that is based on the method of tabular reformulation. This approach, best illustrated in Kennedy (1992 Chap. 6), not only overcomes several of the problems associated with contrasts based on the

Newton–Raphson, but permits focused comparisons to be interpreted in terms of differences in proportional responses, a most attractive metric for most consumers of research. Later, a brief illustration of the Kennedy–Bush approach will be provided.

5. An Illustrative Multinomial Logit-Model Analysis

Having surveyed the six principal operations, they will now be implemented on data provided by McCullough (1992).

5.1 Specification of Legitimate Logit Models

The models that will be used on McCullough's data are specified in Table 2. In general, the four models displayed in the table are applicable for asymmetrical analyses of three-dimensional tables when (and only when) Variable *C* has been designated the response variable. Notice that each model generates elementary cell values that are the logs of expected cell frequencies. (Conversion of $\ln F_{ijk}$'s to F_{ijk}'s, however, is readily accomplished.) Notice too that models become systematically less *restrictive*—that is, fewer terms are set to zero—as models are viewed from Model (0) to unrestricted Model (3).

The most restrictive model, the base model, is Model (0): a model that contains a "point of departure" term (λ) common to all models, a lambda term for each of the main marginals (i.e., λ^a, λ^b, and λ^c), and a two-variable lambda term (λ^{ab}) which saturates the relationship between explanatory Variables *A* and *B*. Although limitations on space will not permit a thorough discussion of these lambda parameters, several basic points should be discussed.

It is important to know, for example, that the five terms in Model (0) indicate that five sources of observed information are used by this model to generate F_{ijk}'s. Used by Model (0) to generate F_{ijk}'s are: (a) the observed tabular *n* (e.g., *n* = 489); (b) observed

Table 2
Log-linear models for a logit-model analysis of three-dimensional tables

Model number	Log-Linear Models
(0)	$\ln F_{ijk} = \lambda + \lambda_i^a + \lambda_j^b + \lambda_k^c + \lambda_{ij}^{ab}$
(1)	$\ln F_{ijk} = \lambda + \lambda_i^a + \lambda_j^b + \lambda_k^c + \lambda_{ij}^{ab} + \lambda_{ik}^{ac}$
(2)	$\ln F_{ijk} = \lambda + \lambda_i^a + \lambda_j^b + \lambda_k^c + \lambda_{ij}^{ab} + \lambda_{ik}^{ac} + \lambda_{jk}^{bc}$
(3)	$\ln F_{ijk} = \lambda + \lambda_i^a + \lambda_j^b + \lambda_k^c + \lambda_{ij}^{ab} + \lambda_{ik}^{ac} + \lambda_{jk}^{bc} + \lambda_{ijk}^{abc}$

main marginals for [A], [B], and [C]; and (c) observed frequencies in the 2 × 2 configuration for [AB]. However, aside from the fact that the F_{ijk}'s produced by Model (0) are constrained to yield the observed frequencies in [A], [B], [C], and [AB], remaining cell frequencies are generated in a non-systematic, random fashion.

Hence, if the F_{ijk}'s given by Model (0) should be found to fit observed elementary cell frequencies extremely well, it follows that λ^{ac}, λ^{bc}, and λ^{abc} are not needed to explain observed data. And if λ^{ac} is not needed, main effects due to GPA (Variable A) are not indicated. By the same logic, if λ^{bc} is not needed, main effects associated with the thesis variable are not indicated; and finally, if λ^{abc} is not needed, interaction between GPA and thesis is not present. It should be no surprise that Model (0) is frequently called the "null-logit model."

However, if the null-logit model should *not* fit observed data well, as disclosed by a substantial goodness-of-fit chi-square, satisfactory explanation of data will necessitate the inclusion of additional terms that involve response Variable C. The need to incorporate these additional terms suggests that logit-model main effects, or interaction effects, are present.

Assume for the moment that Model (0) does not fit observed data well, but it is found that by fitting observed frequencies in the 2 × 4 [AC] configuration —by incorporating λ^{ac} in a model such as is seen in Model (1)—a significant improvement in explanation is realized. If this is the case, then it can be said that discernable differences exist between the two GPA<ox> groups with respect to their profiles of response to the scholarly production variable. Moreover, if the λ^{bc} term in Model (2) is needed to achieve an acceptable fit, main effects for the thesis variable are indicated. Finally, if λ^{abc} is needed to explain data, then interaction between GPA and thesis, analogous to first-order interaction in the ANOVA, is present.

Returning to the example, the models shown in Table 2 were specified in McCullough's data. On most computer programs, specification is accomplished by entering the observed marginals that are used by the model to generate elementary cell frequencies. To specify Model (3) on BMDP4F, SPSS LOG–LINEAR, or SAS CATMOD, for example, one requests a fit of [A], [B], [C], [AB], [AC], [BC], and [ABC]. In sum, Model (3) fits all observed frequencies in the 2 × 2 × 4 table and, accordingly, Model (3) is termed the "saturated model."

5.2 Generating Expected Cell Frequencies

By way of illustration, the F_{ijk}'s provided by Model (0) are displayed in Table 3.

The F_{ijk}'s for this particular model can be obtained from basic probability theory embodied in the following expression:

$$F_{ijk} = f_{ij}p_k \qquad (5)$$

where f_{ij}'s are observed frequencies in [AB], and p_k's are observed proportions for main marginal [C]. Using Eqn. (5) for F_{111}, for example, gives

$$F_{111} = (92)\left(\frac{211}{489}\right) = (92)\,(.4315) = 39.70$$

But realize that in actual practice, F_{ijk}'s are provided by either the Deming–Stephan or Newton–Raphson algorithms.

5.3 Assessing Models for Goodness-of-Fit

Consider first the adequacy of fit provided by the null-logit model which is accomplished by comparing the F_{ijk}'s produced by Model (0) (shown in Table 3) to corresponding f_{ijk}'s (shown in Table 1). Substituting into the likelihood-ratio chi-square given by Eqn. (2) yields

$$L^2_{(0)} = 2\left[(29)\ln\left(\frac{29}{3970}\right) + \ldots + (7)\ln\left(\frac{7}{1656}\right)\right]$$
$$= 2\,[(29)\,(-0.3141) + \ldots + (7)\,(-0.8611)]$$
$$= (2)\,[12.6333]$$
$$= 25.27$$

The number of degrees of freedom for $L^2_{(0)}$ is equivalent to the number of elementary cells that are free to vary subsequent to subtracting constraints imposed on the table by fitting observed marginals. For Model (0), subsequent to fitting [A], [B], [C], and [AB],

Table 3
Expected cell frequencies produced by Model (0), the Null-Logit Model

A_i: GPA	B_j: Thesis	C_1	C_k: Scholarly Production C_2	C_3	C_4	[AB]
A_1 – Above	B_1 – Yes	39.70	27.66	14.49	10.16	92
	B_2 – No	77.24	53.81	28.19	19.77	179
A_2 – Below	B_1 – Yes	29.34	20.44	10.71	7.51	68
	B_2 – No	64.72	45.09	23.62	16.56	150
[C] Main Marginals		211	147	77	54	489

independent estimates of only 9 of the original 16 cells are possible since seven cells must assume specific values to produce the fitted marginals. Hence, $L^2_{(0)}$ is tested with $df = 9$ which will be found to achieve statistical significance at the 0.003 level. Since Model (0) does *not* fit observed data well, significant effects associated with the two explanatory variables are suggested.

Table 4 provides a summary of goodness-of-fit statistics. For each model, Table 4 also presents an "Akaike's information criterion," or AIC statistic for short (see Sakamoto and Akaike 1978). One of several versions of the AIC statistic is given by

$$AIC = L^2 - 2(df) \qquad (6)$$

which when applied to Model (0) yields

$$AIC = 25.27 - (2)(9) = 25.27 - 18.00 = 7.27$$

Akaike's information criterion statistics are used to greatest advantage in symmetrical inquiry (see Kennedy 1992 p. 128) where the principal task is to select from among competing models a model that is deemed the most *acceptable* model: namely, a model that represents the optimal balance between simplicity (parsimony) and ability to explain observed data. In general, the lower the value of AIC, the more acceptable the model. Since Model (3) exhibits the smallest AIC statistic (AIC = −2.95), of models shown, it represents the *best* explanation of data. It should be noted that additional model selection criteria have been proposed. These include the BIC (Schwarz 1978) and Mallow's C_P-type statistic (Jolayemi and Brown 1984). A comparison of model selection techniques can be found in Clayton et al. (1986). It should be noted that present inquiry is asymmetrical where emphasis is placed on assessing the strength of components. Even so, the AIC or alternative selection statistics are useful when investigators are faced with the task of selecting the most appropriate logit model to use when explicating results.

5.4 Testing Component Chi-squares for Statistical Significance

As mentioned, the computation and testing of relevant component chi-squares are central in asymmetrical

Table 4
Residual chi-squares and AIC statistics associated with the fit of log-linear logit-models

Model	Marginals Fitted	L^2	df	p	AIC
(1)	[AB], [C]	25.27	9	0.003	7.27
(2)	[AB], [AC]	11.95	6	0.063	−0.05
(3)	[AB], [AC], [BC]	3.05	3	0.384	−2.95
(4)	[ABC]	0.00	0	1.000	0.00

Table 5
Summary of the logit-model analysis of scholarly production by master-level GPA and master's thesis[a]

Model/Source	L^2	df	p
(2) Due to GPA	13.32	3	0.004
(3) Due to Thesis | GPA	8.91	3	0.031
(4) Due to GPA × Thesis	3.05	3	0.384
(1) Null/Total	25.28	9	0.003

a The sum of reported effect components is not exactly equivalent to 25.27 due to rounding error

analyses. Since specific components are not typically provided by computer programs, they must be obtained by investigators by means illustrated in connection with Eqn. (3). To test obtained components, the appropriate number of df is determined by means of Eqn. (4). The results of component testing for the example are shown in Table 5.

Observe that Table 5 resembles a summary table for a two-way ANOVA and then recall that an important feature of an orthogonal (equal n) two-way ANOVA is that specific sums of squares are additive. Notice that additivity is also manifested in Table 5 in that the goodness-of-fit chi-square for the null-logit model ($L^2 = 25.27$) can be partitioned into three additive components:

(a) a *marginal* component ($L^2 = 13.32$, $p < 0.004$) that reflects the strength of the marginal association between Variables A and C and thus, in the asymmetrical case, reflects the strength of logit-model main effects associated with GPA;

(b) a *partial* component ($L^2 = 8.91$, $p < 0.031$) that reflects the strength of the association between Variables B and C subsequent to statistically removing the influence of Variable A, and thus reflects the strength of main effects for the thesis variable "given" effects due to GPA;

(c) a component ($L^2 = 3.05$, $p < 0.384$) that reflects the strength of the interaction between the two explanatory variables.

The additivity of specific components is a direct result of the use of likelihood-ratio chi-squares, not Pearsonian chi-squares, one of several desirable properties associated with L^2 in log–linear work.

5.5 Advancing Omnibus Findings

If the 0.05 level is adopted as the criterion for statistical significance, examination of Table 5 reveals that significance is associated with the main effects for GPA ($p < 0.004$) and the main effects for the thesis variable ($p < 0.031$), where the latter effects are independent of effects due to GPA. The fact that the component for the thesis variable exhibits partialed effects in this analysis is due to the fact that λ^{bc} has been assessed subsequent to λ^{ac} (see Kennedy 1992 pp. 122–23). (It would have been possible to obtain a partialed component for GPA by altering the order of entry of λ^{ac} and λ^{bc} in examined models.) Finally, evidence suggestive of interaction between GPA and the thesis variables is unquestionably absent ($p < 0.384$).

5.6 Following Up Omnibus Results

Having concluded to this point that response to the polytomous scholarly production variable differs for students with GPAs above and below 3.70, and that differences in response are also present between students who wrote or did not write a thesis, the remaining task is to elucidate these differences. The method chosen for brief demonstration is called the "method of focused comparisons."

Focused comparisons are single degree-of-freedom contrasts based on reformulated fourfold (2×2) tables. Comparisons are independent of order of performance, capable of affecting an exact partitioning of component chi-squares, and readily interpretable in terms of either differences in odds or, most importantly, differences in proportions. To satisfy diverse outcomes, four distinct types of comparisons have been proposed: marginal, partialed, compound, and interactive.

Chosen for brief mention here are *partialed* comparisons, that is, comparisons that are well suited to pursue the omnibus effects associated with the thesis variable (i.e., $L^2 = 8.91$, $p < 0.031$). Three focused comparisons were performed to compare thesis and nonthesis students on specific patterns of scholarly production. Because partialed comparisons were performed, potentially confounding effects associated with the GPA variable were removed, much like the comparison of adjusted groups means in the context of an analysis of covariance. The performed comparisons were:

(a) *Comparison (1)*. To implement this comparison, pseudo-numeric contrast coefficients that sum to zero were established on both the response variable and the sample factor. For the first comparison, coefficients on response were:

C_1	C_2	C_3	C_4
+1	−0.33	−0.33	−0.33

a contrast between no evidence of scholarly activity (C_1) and evidence of some scholarly activity, where the latter response is the aggregate of C_2, C_3, and C_4. For this and the remaining two comparisons, since the sample factor consists of only two levels (completion vs. noncompletion of a thesis), by default, coefficients on the sample were:

B_1	B_2
+1	−1

(b) *Comparison (2)*. The second comparison imposed the following coefficients on the response variable:

C_1	C_2	C_3	C_4
0	+1	−0.50	−0.50

As mentioned, the previously established default coefficients on the sample factor were used.

(c) *Comparison (3)*. The final comparison imposed the following coefficients on response:

C_1	C_2	C_3	C_4
0	0	+1	−1

Unfortunately, a detailed account of procedures used to perform these comparisons is beyond the scope of this entry. Procedures are described in detail, however, in Kennedy (1992 Chap. 6).

Before results are examined, it is important to note that the comparisons above were not designed primarily to accommodate substantive research questions that might be of interest, but rather they were designed so that the total set of three comparisons would be *mutually orthogonal*. (If the response coefficients for the three comparisons are studied, it will be seen that the sum of cross-products for all comparison pairs are zero, hence, the three focused comparisons can be said to be mutually independent.) This was done to demonstrate a most desirable property of focused comparisons; namely, that focused orthogonal comparisons are capable of affecting an *exact* partitioning of relevant component chi-squares, the component for thesis given GPA in the present case. With this capacity, the liberal use of nonorthogonal focused comparisons can be defended with greater conviction in actual practice.

During the performance of the comparisons, a number of steps were implemented that essentially led to the reformulation of the original $2 \times 2 \times 4$ contingency table such that for each comparison it was reduced to a simple fourfold (2×2) comparison table. The steps in question are not difficult to perform and do not require computer assistance. Suffice it to say that after

577

the identification of each fourfold table, conventional tests on the hypothesis of homogeneity of proportional response (or independence) were performed using the likelihood-ratio chi-square.

The single-*df* chi-square found for Comparison (1) turned out to be $L^2 = 8.483$, $p < 0.0004$. One of several precise conclusions that can be offered is that when students who completed and did not complete a thesis were compared, a significantly greater *proportion* ($p < 0.0004$) of students who completed a thesis reported some evidence of scholarly production, even after scholarly production attributed to GPA had been taken into account.

The ability of focused comparisons to capture relevant components is demonstrated in Table 6 where the results of the three orthogonal comparisons are summarized. Notice that comparison chi-squares sum to the composite chi-square for thesis given GPA. Also notice that Comparison (1) explained, almost in its entirety, main effects due to the thesis variable. (The component for the first comparison accounts for 8.48 out of 8.91 or 95% of the overall component.) As it turned out, efforts beyond an interpretation of Comparison (1) are neither needed nor warranted.

Parenthetically, parallel focused comparisons were implemented to follow up main effects due to the GPA variable. Here the principal finding was given by Comparison (3) where the scholarly production of high GPAs exceeded that of lower GPAs ($p < 0.005$) in the fourth category (C_4).

6. Recent Developments and Applications

Much progress has been made on the analysis of longitudinal data, ordered categorical data, and the development of new techniques that are often used in conjunction with log–linear models. A very readable account of the broad range of time dependent categorical data analysis, that includes discussion of log–linear models, has been proffered by Hagenaars (1990). Before several new supporting techniques are cited, a few words on ordered categorical variables will be offered.

6.1 The Analysis of Ordered Categories

Often classes of a categorical variable are amenable to ordinal scaling. Obvious educational examples are Grade Level (1st grade, 2nd grade, etc.) and responses on a five-point Likert-type attitude scale. If liberties are taken, McCullough's scholarly production variable could be perceived and treated as an ordered variable. In any event, it has long been recognized that when legitimate ordered variables are analyzed by traditional methods, information embedded in the order is ignored and potential inferential power is lost. For this reason, serious attention has been devoted to framing log–linear models that accommodate order. The basis for much of the work on ordered categories will be found in Goodman (1979), work that has been refined and reported well in a number of texts such as Agresti (1990 pp. 269–74).

To illustrate briefly the nature of this new work in a two-dimensional context, consider the 2×4 [*BC*] table that can be constructed with McCullough's data. Here, both the thesis and scholarly production variables will be considered ordered, a condition that lends itself to a type of log–linear modeling known as *linear-by-linear*. Logical rank values or scores are assigned to each variable, say u_j's to GPA that satisfy the condition that $u_1 \leqslant u_2$, and v_k's to the scholarly production variable such that $v_1 \leqslant v_2 \leqslant \ldots \leqslant v_4$. The log–linear model that can now be used on the [*BC*] is

$$\ln F_{jk} = \lambda + \lambda_j^b + \lambda_k^c + \beta(u_j - \bar{u})(v_k - \bar{v})$$
$$\text{where } \bar{u} = \frac{1}{b}\sum_{j=1}^{b} u_j \text{ and } \bar{v} = \frac{1}{c}\sum_{k=1}^{c} v_k.$$

Here the coefficient β can be regarded as a regression coefficient. If there is no association between GPA and scholarly production, the test on H$_0$: $\beta = 0$ will not result in significance. However, if β is significant, the variables are associated. Assuming an association, since the u_j's and v_k's are known, it is possible to fashion these values as an additional parameter and assess the fit of this linear-by-linear model by calculating a likelihood-ratio chi-square. This and other models

Table 6
Results of three orthogonal fully partialed focused comparison on scholarly production by completion versus noncompletion of a Master's Thesis

Comparison	Response Design C$_1$	C$_2$	C$_3$	Comparison Chi-Squares C$_4$	L^2	df	p
(1)	1	−0.33	−0.33	−0.33	8.483	1	0.000
(2)	0	1	−0.50	−0.50	0.014	1	0.906
(3)	0	0	1	−1	0.408	1	0.523
Overall:	Due to Thesis given GPA				8.905	3	0.031

have been extended for use with tables of higher dimensionality (see Agresti 1990 pp 274–81).

6.2 Further Reading On Related Developments

An approach that is frequently taken in conjunction with log–linear modeling is the "analysis of residuals." Historically, the most prominent treatments of this subject were provided by Haberman (1973) and Brown (1974). A more recent treatment is offered by Simonoff (1988.)

There are two relatively new methodologies that are being used with increasing frequency as complements to log–linear analyses. The first is a descriptive technique known as *correspondence analysis*. Helpful discussions have been provided by Goodman (1986), van der Heijden and de Leeuw (1985), and van der Heijden et al. (1989). The second is a taxonomical technique known as *configural frequency analysis*, a technique that initially fits log–linear models but then attempts to identify prominent clusters of subjects that share a common pattern of response to several categorical variables. An authoritative book on this subject has been written by von Eye (1990), and an introductory presentation by Kennedy (1992 Chap. 9) (see *Correspondence Analysis of Qualitative Data; Configural Frequency Analysis of Categorized Data*).

6.3 Further Educational Examples

Earlier it was implied that log–linear models have yet to be used extensively in educational settings. Examples of their use, however, include studies in graduate student retention (Ott et al. 1984) and test item bias (Baker and Subkoviak 1981, Mellenbergh 1982). It was also implied that an increase in the use of log–linear models and related techniques will likely occur in the decade of the 1990s. This prediction is predicated on the fact that categorical data are frequently encountered in educational and social science research.

See also: Factorial Modeling; Hierarchical Linear Models; Latent Trait Measurement Models

References

Agresti A 1990 *Categorical Data Analysis*. Wiley, New York
Alba R D 1987 Interpreting the parameters of log-linear models. *Sociol. Meth. Res.* 16(1): 45–77
Andersen E B 1990 *The Statistical Analysis of Categorical Data*. Springer-Verlag, London
Baker F B, Subkoviak M J 1981 Analysis of test results via log-linear models. *Appl. Psychol. Meas.* 5(4): 503–15
Bishop Y M M, Fienberg S E, Holland P W 1974 *Discrete Multivariate Analysis: Theory and Practice*. MIT Press, Cambridge, Massachusetts
Bock R D 1975 *Multivariate Statistical Methods in Behavioral Research*. McGraw-Hill, New York
Brown M B 1974 Identification of the sources of significance in two-way contingency tables. *Appl. Stat.* 23(3): 405–13

Clayton M K, Geisser S, Jennings D E 1986 A comparison of several model selection procedures. In: Goel P, Zellner A (eds.) 1986 *Bayesian Inference and Decision Techniques*. North Holland, Amsterdam
Clogg C C, Eliason S R 1987 Some common problems in log–linear analysis. *Sociol. Meth. Res.* 16(1): 8–44
Fienberg S E 1972 The analysis of incomplete multi-way contingency tables. *Biometrics* 28(1): 177–202
Fienberg S E 1977 *The Analysis of Cross-classified Categorical Data*. MIT Press, Cambridge, Massachusetts
Goodman L A 1978 *Analyzing Qualitative/Categorical Data: Log–linear Models and Latent-structure Analysis*. Addison-Wesley, London
Goodman L A 1979 Simple models for the analysis of association in cross-classifications having ordered categories. *J. Am. Stat. Assoc.* 74(367): 537–52
Goodman L A 1986 Some useful extension of the usual correspondence analysis approach and the usual log–linear models approach in the analysis of contingency tables. *Int. Stat. Rev.* 54(3): 243–70
Green J A 1988 Log–linear analysis of cross-classified ordinal data: Applications in developmental research. *Child Dev.* 59(1): 1–25
Haberman S J 1973 The analysis of residuals in cross-classified tables. *Biometrics* 29(1): 205–20
Haberman S J 1974 *The Analysis of Frequency Data*. University of Chicago Press, Chicago, Illinois
Haberman S J 1978 *Analysis of Qualitative Data. Vol. 1: Introductory Topics*. Academic Press, New York
Hagenaars J A 1990 *Categorical Longitudinal Data: Log–linear Panel, Trend, and Cohort Analysis*. Sage, Newbury Park, California
Hays W L 1988 *Statistics*, 4th edn. Holt, Rinehart and Winston, New York
Jolayemi E T, Brown M B 1984 The choice of a log–linear model using a C_P-type statistic. *Comp. Stat. Data Anal.* 2: 159–65
Kaufman R L Schervish P G 1986 Using adjusted cross-tabulations to interpret log-linear relationships. *Am. Sociol. Rev.* 51(5): 717–33
Kennedy J J 1983 *Analyzing Qualitative Data: Introductory Log–linear Analysis for Behavioral Research*. Praeger, New York
Kennedy J J 1988 Applying log–linear models in educational research. *Aust. J. Educ.* 32(1): 3–24
Kennedy J J 1992 *Analyzing Qualitative Data: Log–linear Analysis for Behavioral Research*, 2nd edn. Praeger, New York
Kennedy J J, Bush A J 1988 Focused comparisons in logit–model contingency table analysis. Paper presented at the meeting of the American Educational Research Association, New Orleans, Louisiana, April 1988
Knoke D, Burke P J 1980 *Log–linear Models*. Sage University Paper series on Quantitative Applications in the Social Sciences, Series No. 07–020. Sage, Beverly Hills, California
Marascuilo L A, Levin J R 1983 *Multivariate Statistics in the Social Sciences: A Researcher's Guide*. Brooks/Cole, Monterey, California
Marks E 1975 Methods for analyzing multidimensional contingency tables. *Res. Higher Educ.* 3(3): 217–31
McCullough J 1992 Demographic and biographic characteristics of prospective teacher educators and their motives for becoming teacher educators. Unpublished PhD dissertation, Ohio State University, Columbus, Ohio

Mellenbergh G J 1982 Contingency table models for assessing item bias. *J. Educ. Stat.* 7:105–18

Ott M D, Markewich T S, Ochsner N L 1984 Logit analysis of graduate student retention. *Res. Higher Educ.* 21(4): 439–60

Reynolds H T 1984 *Analysis of Nominal Data*, 2nd edn. Sage University Paper series on Quantitative Applications in the Social Sciences, Series No. 07–007. Sage, Beverly Hills, California

Sakamoto Y, Akaike H 1978 Analysis of cross-classified data by AIC. *Ann. Inst. Stat. Math.* 30 (Part B): 185–97

Schwarz G 1978 Estimating the dimension of a model. *Ann. Stats.* 6(2): 461–64

Shaffer J P 1973 Defining and testing hypotheses in multi-dimensional contingency tables. *Psych. Bull.* 79(2): 127–41

Simonoff J 1988 Detecting outlying cells in two–way contingency tables via backwards-stepping. *Technometric* 30(3): 339–45

Upton G J G 1978 *The Analysis of Cross-tabulated Data.* Wiley, New York

van der Heijden P G M, de Leeuw J 1985 Correspondence analysis: Used complementary to log–linear analysis. *Psychometrika* 50(4): 429–47

van der Heijden P G M, de Falguerolles A, de Leeuw J 1989 A combined approach to contingency table analysis using correspondence analysis and log–linear analysis. *Appl. Stats.* 38(2): 249–92

von Eye A 1990 *Introduction to Configural Frequency Analysis: The Search for Types and Anti-types in Cross-classifications.* Cambridge University Press, Cambridge

Measures of Variation

J. P. Keeves

Of major interest and concern to the educational research worker is the observed variation of naturally occurring events in human behavior and educational practice. Not only does variation occur naturally in human characteristics, but it also arises in response to different treatment conditions acting to influence learning and the consequent stability and change in those characteristics. In addition, variation arises as a result of what has come to be known appropriately as "error," which is associated with the random fluctuations of observations about an expected value. Such error occurs as a consequence of variability involving the observer, the variability in the procedures or the instruments used for observation, and variability in the object being measured.

Statistics has been referred to by Fisher (1970) as the study of the variation observed in the investigation of populations:

> The conception of statistics as the study of variation is the natural outcome of viewing the subject as the study of populations: for a population of individuals in all respects identical is completely described by a description of any one individual, together with the number in the group. The populations which are the object of statistical study always display variation in one or more respects. (p. 3)

Thus the educational research worker and statistician are necessarily concerned not only with the individual within the population under investigation, but also with the different conditions and circumstances that have contributed to the variation in the observations and measurements that are made.

This entry presents the different measures of variation that are widely used in educational research. First, consideration is given to measures that relate to variation about the mean value. Second, a less extensive treatment is provided regarding measures that refer to variation about the median value. The former set of measures are of greater interest in practical investigations since they are rigorously defined, easily calculated, and more readily amenable to algebraic treatment and to systematic analysis. Thus, the mean and its associated measures of variation are generally employed in situations where the variables may be considered to involve interval or ratio data. However, the use of the median and its measures of variation is preferred in some situations, where the data are essentially ordinal in nature or where outlying values may distort the location of the mean and spread of values recorded.

Since statistics is the study of variation, it is not surprising that reference should be made in other entries in this *Handbook* to the analysis of variance (see *Variance and Covariance, Analysis of*) and to the procedures by means of which the variation in a set of data can be partitioned into different components that can be ascribed to different factors (see *Multilevel Analysis*). These different factors may be associated with treatment conditions, naturally occurring variation, or different sources of error.

The analytic procedures employed in conventional statistical work generally involve one particular measure of variation that is obtained as the mean square of the deviations of individual observations about the population mean with which they are associated. This measure of variation, the "variance" has important properties that have enabled an extensive body of statistical theory to be developed around the analysis of variances and covariances and the partitioning of variance into separate components. However, the calculations involved in the analysis of variances are generally more complex than can be made by simple hand calculations with a data set obtained from observation and empirical research. As a consequence, it is very common for such sets of data to be systematically fed into a computer and only the summary statistics to be examined in detail. Nevertheless, it is generally rewarding to examine the raw data rather more thoroughly, and to tease out some simple relationships from an initial exploratory analysis of the data (see *Exploratory Data Analysis*).

One measure of variation that can be readily used in the initial examination of sets of data is the "range." Simple analytical procedures have been developed which involve the analysis of range values that can be readily applied to raw data and which involve nothing more than addition and subtraction. Because of a growing need for educational research workers to examine rather more carefully the raw data with which they are working, reference is made to some analytical procedures associated with range values. It is hoped these references may encourage not only their use, but also a thorough examination of raw data before it is subjected to more complex computer-based analyses.

In addition, consideration is given in this entry to the use of measures of variation to describe score distributions. Measures of "skewness" and "kurtosis" are also discussed and comments made on the use of these measures in analytical procedures that require a generally normal distribution. Furthermore, accounts are given both of the use of the "Lorenz curve" and the "Gini coefficient" as measures of the degree of equitable distribution of a characteristic and the use of the "intraclass correlation" and the "ratio of homogeneity" as measures of variation which are used with cluster samples.

1. Measures of Variation Associated with the Mean

Three measures of variation associated with the mean are widely used in statistics: the "mean deviation," the "standard deviation," and the "range." However, it is the standard deviation or its square, the "variance," that is most extensively used in statistical analysis in the field of education. Nevertheless, it may be of some guidance to list, following Guilford (1965), the considerations that apply when deciding which of these three measures of variability to use in any particular situation.

The *mean deviation* should be used when:

(a) there are extreme deviation values which would seriously bias the estimates of other measures of variation such as the standard deviation;

(b) a measure of variation is required without the additional labor of calculating squares and sums of squares; or

(c) the distribution of scores is nearly normal, and the mean deviation can be used to estimate the standard deviation using the relationship, standard deviation = 1.253 mean deviation.

The *standard deviation* should be used when:

(a) an accurate and dependable measure of variation is required and the shape of the distribution can be assumed (e.g., normal, rectangular);

(b) further analyses that depend upon the square of the standard deviation, namely, the variance, are likely to be carried out; or

(c) interpretation of the data set with respect to the normal distribution curve or other distributions, which is known to apply, is needed.

The *range* should be used when:

(a) a large body of data is available, that involves replication of measurement over many occasions;

(b) a quickly calculated measure of variation is needed; or

(c) information is needed about extreme scores which occur on some occasions and not on others.

Thus, with respect to ease of calculation, the three measures may be ranked in the order of the range, the mean deviation, and the standard deviation. However, with respect to the stability of the estimate and its constancy under replication or with repeated sampling, these three measures should be ranked in the reverse order: the standard deviation, the mean deviation, and the range.

1.1 Mean Deviation

The mean deviation is the arithmetic mean of the deviation scores of the observed scores about their mean value, disregarding the algebraic signs of the deviation scores.

$$d = \frac{\Sigma \mid x - \bar{x} \mid}{n} \qquad (1)$$

where $\mid x - \bar{x} \mid$ = the deviation score for the observed score x about the mean value $\bar{x}$; the modulus sign $\mid x \mid$ indicates disregard of the algebraic sign of the deviation scores; and n = number of score values. The deviation scores, using an analogy with concepts employed in physics, may be regarded as moments about the center of gravity, and the simple sum of the deviations, taking into consideration their algebraic signs, is equal to zero. The mean deviation is rarely used.

1.2 Standard Deviation

The most widely used measure of variation is the standard deviation. It is sometimes referred to as the "root mean square deviation" since computationally it involves calculating the deviation scores as for the mean deviation, squaring these scores to eliminate the problems associated with the algebraic sign of the deviation scores, summing the scores and dividing by the number of scores involved and taking the square root of the value so obtained. If a population of scores is involved, the population standard deviation (σ) is given by:

$$\sigma = \sqrt{\frac{\Sigma(x - \mu)^2}{n}} \tag{2}$$

where μ = the population mean.

If, however, a sample of scores is involved, the value based on Eqn. (2) is biased and the estimate of the population standard deviation (s) is given by

$$s = \sqrt{\frac{\Sigma(x - \bar{x})^2}{n - 1}}$$

where $\bar{x}$ = the estimate of the mean.

The estimate of the variance (σ^2) is given by the sample variance (s^2) where

$$s^2 = \frac{\Sigma(x - \bar{x})^2}{n - 1}$$

Several computational results are of interest since the standard deviation and the variance are so widely used in statistical analysis as measures of variation.

For the purposes of calculating the standard deviation for ungrouped sample data it is commonly more convenient to write the expression for the variance in a different form.

$$s^2 = \frac{\Sigma(x - \bar{x})^2}{n - 1}$$
$$= \frac{\Sigma(x^2 - 2x\bar{x} + \bar{x}^2)}{n - 1}$$
$$= \frac{[\Sigma x^2 + n\bar{x}^2 - 2n\bar{x}^2]}{n - 1}$$

since $\Sigma\bar{x}^2 = n\bar{x}^2$ and $\Sigma 2x\bar{x} = 2\bar{x}\Sigma x = 2n\bar{x}^2$, thus:

$$s^2 = \frac{\Sigma x^2 - n\bar{x}^2}{n - 1} \quad \text{and } s = \sqrt{\frac{\Sigma x^2 - n\bar{x}^2}{n - 1}}$$

An alternative formula for the standard deviation which does not require the calculation of the mean ($\bar{x}$) and which may be used directly in computation is:

$$s = \sqrt{\frac{n\Sigma x^2 - (\Sigma x)^2}{n(n - 1)}}$$

Before the availability of computers, it was common to group data in order to simplify computation. The formula for calculating the standard deviation (s)

from sample data grouped in the form of a frequency distribution is:

$$s = h \sqrt{\frac{1}{n - 1} \left[\Sigma fx'^2 - \frac{(\Sigma fx')^2}{n} \right]}$$

where h = group interval, f = group frequency, x' = value of coded score associated with each group. To use this formula, a standard statistical text (e.g., Ferguson 1966) should be consulted.

If a constant (c) is added to or subtracted from the values of all observations made in a sample, then the standard deviation remains unchanged. This can be readily seen if the deviation score is obtained for an observed score expressed as ($x + c$) where the mean value is also expressed as ($\bar{x} + c$).

$$d = (x + c) - (\bar{x} + c) = x - \bar{x}$$

Recognition of this result permits the rescaling of scores by the addition or subtraction of a constant without changing the standard deviation.

If all observations made on a sample are multiplied by a constant, then the standard deviation is also multiplied by the absolute value of that constant. This result can be seen readily if the observed score is expressed as (cx) and the mean score is expressed as ($c\bar{x}$). The deviation score is $cx - c\bar{x} = c(x - \bar{x})$. After squaring, sum over n observations and divide by $n - 1$ then:

$$\frac{\Sigma(cx - c\bar{x})^2}{n - 1} = \frac{c^2\Sigma(x - \bar{x})^2}{n - 1} = c^2 s^2$$

It should be noted that if c is negative, the positive square root would be taken as the multiplier of s, and the absolute value of the constant is used rather than the negative value associated with the multiplying constant. Recognition of this result permits the rescaling of scores, which may involve the multiplication or division of the scores by a constant value.

The use of computational procedures which involve the addition of a constant or multiplication by a constant, are of considerable importance in improving the accuracy with which calculations can be carried out using computers and calculating devices.

Of particular utility in educational research and practice are "standard scores." A standard score (z) is obtained by calculating the deviation from the mean and dividing this value by the standard deviation, namely:

$$z = \frac{x - \bar{x}}{s}$$

Standard scores have a mean of zero and a standard deviation of unity and are particularly useful in comparing scores across samples and populations that have different standard deviations. Many statistical formulations can be derived and expressed more conveniently using standard scores rather than raw scores or deviation scores. In addition, they sometimes enable computations to be carried out more accurately. It should be noted that the calculation of standard scores does not change the shape of a frequency distribution.

1.3 Pooled Estimates of Variance

A situation commonly occurs in practice where it is necessary to pool two estimates of variance obtained with samples of different sizes (n_1 and n_2). Several different computational procedures are used according to whether the situation is one where: (a) the population variance σ^2 is known; (b) the population variance is unknown and two variance estimates s_1^2 and s_2^2 are available and there is no difference between the means; and (c) the population variance is unknown and there are significant differences between the estimates of the means ($\bar{x}_1$ and $\bar{x}_2$). The formulas used in these three situations for combining variances are presented without proof but with reference to sources where further information on these formulas can be obtained.

(a) If the population variance is known to be the same for both samples the variance of the pooled mean is given by (Hays 1963 p. 209):

$$\sigma_m^2 = \frac{\sigma^2}{n_1 + n_2}$$

If the population variances (σ_1^2 and σ_2^2) are known to be different for the two samples which were drawn the pooled variance of the scores in the combined sample is:

$$\sigma_c^2 = \frac{(n_1\sigma_1^2 + n_2\sigma_2^2)}{n_1 + n_2}$$

The variance of the mean is given by:

$$\sigma_m^2 = \frac{\sigma_c^2}{n_1 + n_2}$$

(b) If the population variance is unknown and estimates for the variances of the two samples (s_1^2 and s_2^2) have been calculated and it is assumed that there are no significant differences between the two sample mean values, then the pooled estimate of the variance of the scores in the combined sample is (Hays 1963 p. 210):

$$s_c^2 = \frac{(n_1s_1^2 + n_2s_2^2)}{n_1 + n_2 - 2}$$

(c) If the variance is unknown, and the mean, variance, and number of cases for each group are $\bar{x}_1$, s_1^2, and n_1 and $\bar{x}_2$, s_2^2, and n_2 respectively, then the estimated variance of the combined group is (Ferguson 1966 p. 72):

$$s_c^2 = \frac{(n_1 - 1)s_1^2 + (n_2 - 1)s_2^2 + n_1d_1^2 + n_1d_2^2}{n_1 + n_2 - 1}$$

where $\bar{x}_1 - \bar{x} = d_1$ and $\bar{x}_2 - \bar{x} = d_2$ and

$$\bar{x} = \frac{n_1\bar{x}_1 + n_2\bar{x}_2}{n_1 + n_2}$$

In cases (b) and (c) it is assumed that the populations are sufficiently large that samples are drawn without replacement of the elements selected. If the population is small a finite population correction must be applied.

This correction involves multiplying the variance estimate by ([T − n] / n) where T is the number of elements in the population, and n the number of elements in the sample, drawn without replacement of elements.

1.4 Coefficient of Variation

It is commonly found in practice that the mean and the standard deviation increase or decrease together. This may be illustrated with data collected in the First Science Study conducted by the International Association for the Evaluation of Educational Achievement (IEA) (Comber and Keeves 1973). In Table 1 the standard deviations of science test scores are recorded, together with the mean scores on an 80-item test and the reliability estimates of the test using the Kuder–Richardson Formula 20 (KR-20) for the 18 countries that participated in the study at the 14-year old level. The rank order correlations between the standard deviation estimates and the mean scores and reliabilities are also presented. The correlations reported indicate strong relationships between the standard deviation and mean score, and between the standard deviation and reliability of the test. The latter relationship with the reliability of the test provides an indication of the source of the reported relationships with respect to the properties of the test. However, it is of greater interest to note the example of a strong relationship between the standard deviation and the mean.

The widespread occurrence of such a relationship where ratio scales are employed has led to the introduction of a measure of variation referred to as the "coefficient of variation" and defined as the ratio of the standard deviation to the mean:

$$c = \frac{s}{\bar{x}}$$

where c is the coefficient of variation, s = the sample standard deviation, $\bar{x}$ = the sample mean (Snedecor and Cochran 1967 pp. 62–64).

In Table 1, for each country sample the coefficient of variation is calculated. Except for the three developing countries, India, Chile, and Iran, the values of the coefficient show a high level of constancy across countries and the coefficient would appear to be a characteristic of the common test which was employed. It is clear that in the three developing countries named, the test behaves in a different manner when comparisons are made with the 15 more developed countries.

A knowledge of the relative variation is valuable in many situations where empirical evidence is being collected using a ratio scale or raw scores on a test. Differences in the magnitudes of this coefficient of

Table 1
Science total test standard deviations

Country	Standard deviations of scores	Mean science test score (80 items)	Reliability KR-20	Coefficient of variation $s/\bar{x}$
Japan	14.8	31.2	0.89	0.47
Scotland	14.2	21.4	0.89	0.66
England	14.1	21.3	0.89	0.66
Australia	13.3	24.6	0.87	0.54
New Zealand	12.9	24.2	0.86	0.53
Hungary	12.7	29.1	0.85	0.44
Sweden	11.7	21.7	0.83	0.54
United States	11.6	21.5	0.83	0.54
Federal Republic of Germany	11.5	23.7	0.84	0.49
Finland	10.6	20.5	0.80	0.52
Italy	10.2	18.5	0.81	0.55
Netherlands	10.0	17.8	0.85	0.56
Belgium (Flemish)	9.2	21.2	0.74	0.43
India	9.0	7.6	0.78	1.18
Chile	8.9	9.2	0.80	0.97
Belgium (French)	8.8	15.4	0.80	0.57
Thailand	8.1	15.6	0.65	0.52
Iran	6.1	7.8	0.57	0.78
Rank correlation with standard deviation	1.0	0.85	0.92	

Source: Comber and Keeves (1973 p. 164)

variation, across situations where parallel sets of such data are gathered, warrant attempts to discover the reason why these differences have been observed. It should be noted that since *c* is the ratio of two measures having the same unit of measurement it is, as a coefficient, independent of the unit employed. A word of warning is, however, necessary. Since this coefficient is such a convenient index to report, there is a tendency to overlook the information contained in the means and standard deviations for the original data from which values of the coefficient were obtained. Thus, in the example recorded, the values of the test mean, and the standard deviations across countries are shown to be related to the properties of the test itself, namely, the reliability. However, the relatively large values of the coefficient of variation for both England and Scotland warrant further examination as do the relatively small values for Hungary and Japan. Furthermore, it is necessary to caution that the coefficient of variation should only be used with ratio scale data or the equivalent.

1.5 Range

In situations where a considerable body of data is available for systematic examination, relatively simple routine statistical procedures are required. The range provides a measure of variation that is not only easy to compute but also can be readily explained to persons without a sophisticated knowledge of statistics. The range is the spread of measures from the highest to the lowest. It is defined as: Range = (maximum value–minimum value).

Where data are rounded to integer values, the range is sometimes calculated as:
Range = (maximum value–minimum value + 1).

The range has the valuable computational property that the estimates of its values can be added and averaged without bias being introduced. Thus it is common in working with the range, if less than 10 measures are available, to simply calculate the range as a measure of variation. However, if more than 10 measures are available, it is customary to divide the measures into subsamples in a random way, and calculate the range for each subsample and then to average the values across subsamples.

Values of the range can be used to obtain an estimate of the variance (σ^2) of a sample according to the formula (Snedecor and Cochran 1967 pp. 39–40).

$$\hat{\sigma} = \frac{\bar{R}}{d}$$

where $\bar{R}$ is the mean range, and *d* is the range factor.

In using the range to obtain an estimate of the standard deviation, the range factor (*d*) employed depends on the subsample size *n* and not on the number (*k*) subsamples taken with the ranges $R_1, R_2, \ldots R_k$

In Table 2, values of the range factor (d) for subsamples of different sizes are recorded.

It is of interest to note that for small samples the range is nearly as efficient as the standard deviation for

Table 2
Range factors for samples of different sizes

Subsample size (n)	Range factor (d)	Subsamplesize (n)	Range factor (d)
2	1.13	12	3.26
3	1.69	14	3.40
4	2.06	16	3.53
5	2.33	18	3.64
6	2.53	20	3.73
7	2.70	30	4.08
8	2.85	40	4.33
9	2.97	50	4.50
10	3.08	100	5.02

Source: Snedecor and Cochran (1967 p. 40) with modifications.

the estimation of the variance of these small samples. Moreover, in order to obtain rough estimates of the standard deviation of a small sample, it is convenient to remember approximate range factors of 2, 3, 4, and 5 for samples of 4, 10, 30, and 100 respectively. It is surprising that the range is not more widely used in educational research as a simply calculated measure of variation that can be readily employed to obtain rough estimates of variances or standard deviations.

1.6 Use of Range in Analysis

Since the range may be employed to provide a readily calculated estimate of the standard error of a mean, it may subsequently be used to test for significance differences between means or to test for interaction effects in two-way analyses of variance. For further discussion of the use of the range in the analysis of variation, articles by Hartley (1950), Patnaik (1950), and David (1951) should be consulted. In addition, the calculation of the sampling variability of large complex samples remains a major problem in educational research that, while commonly ignored, may be conveniently handled by the use of a subsample range procedure (see *Sampling Errors in Survey Research*). In this procedure the complex sample may be divided into four balanced subsamples, following fully the stratification of the sample design and without subdividing the primary sampling units. For each subsample the statistics of interest may be calculated, and their ranges across the subsamples obtained, from which their standard deviations may be estimated (Peaker 1965). The use of four subsamples rather than more avoids unnecessary work, while maintaining adequate accuracy. However, it is important that the four subsamples should be fully independent. If they are not, there is on the one hand a serious danger that the errors will be underestimated. On the other hand, if the subsamples do not balance approximately for size there is a danger that the errors will be overestimated.

2. Measures of Variation Associated with the Median

In investigations where a distribution of observed values is truncated or incomplete at either end, or where there is extreme skewing in one tail of the distribution, the median is commonly used as the descriptive measure of central tendency. In such situations where the median is employed, related measures of variation are required. The two traditional measures have been the interquartile range and the semi-interquartile range. These measures are commonly used in exploratory data analysis for the description of distributions of observed values, particularly in educational research for test score distributions, with the growing use of box and whisker plots.

2.1 The Interquartile Range (Q)

The interquartile range is the spread of the distribution between the first quartile, which has one quarter of the series of measures below it and the third quartile, which has three quarters of the series of measures below it. The interquartile range is the spread of the middle 50 percent of the measures in the series. The interquartile range (Q) is related to the variance of a normal distribution by the relationship $Q = 1.3490\sigma$ (see Guilford 1965).

2.2 The Semi-interquartile Range (q)

The semi-interquartile range (q) is, as its name suggests, half of the interquartile range and has the advantage that it can be shown diagrammatically on either side of the median. It is thus the measure of dispersion most commonly employed when the features of a distribution lead to the use of the median rather than the mean as a measure of central tendency. The semi-interquartile range (q) is related to the variance of a normal distribution by the relationship $q = 0.6754\sigma$.

2.3 Use of Quartiles to Indicate Skewness

If the value associated with the median is denoted as Q_2 and the values associated with the first and third quartiles are denoted as Q_1 and Q_3 respectively, then for a normal distribution, it would be expected that:

$Q_3 - Q_2 = Q_2 - Q_1 = q$ (the semi-interquartile range). If, however, this equality relationship does not hold, then the distribution is skewed.

Positive skewness is observed if $(Q_3 - Q_2) > (Q_2 - Q_1)$.

Negative skewness is observed if $(Q_3 - Q_2) < (Q_2 - Q_1)$.

The relative magnitudes of these distances give some indication of the extent of skewness present.

3. Measures of the Shapes of Distributions

Any set of measurements made may be represented by a frequency distribution. It is commonly possible to identify the theoretical frequency distribution

585

which underlies the measures recorded. Any theoretical frequency distribution can be represented by its moments, the two best known of which are the mean, or measure of central tendency, and the variance or measure of dispersion. The idea of moments is drawn by analogy from the field of mechanics where the first moment is the coordinate of the center of gravity, and the second moment is the radius of gyration. The first four moments of a set of measurements about the arithmetic mean are as follows:

$$m_1 = \frac{\Sigma(x - \bar{x})}{n} = 0$$

where $\bar{x}$ = the mean.

$$m_2 = \frac{\Sigma(x - \bar{x})^2}{n} = \frac{n - 1}{n} s^2$$

where s^2 = the sample variance.

$$m_3 = \frac{\Sigma(x - \bar{x})^3}{n}$$

$$m_4 = \frac{\Sigma(x - \bar{x})^4}{n}$$

In general, the rth moment about the mean is given by:

$$m_r = \frac{\Sigma(x - \bar{x})^r}{n}$$

The third and fourth moments are commonly used to test the shape of a frequency distribution.

3.1 Testing for the Normal Distribution

It is commonly assumed that the data are normally distributed or are drawn from an underlying normal distribution in the testing of estimated parameters for statistical significance. Moreover, conformity to a known distribution, commonly the normal distribution, is required for estimation using certain statistical procedures, which employ maximum likelihood methods, such as LISREL (see *Path Analysis and Linear Structural Relations Analysis*). The third (m_3) and fourth (m_4) moments are indicators of nonnormality of a distribution of measures.

The scale factor associated with m_3 and m_4 is eliminated by dividing the rth moment by $(\sqrt{m_2}) = m_2^{r/2} = \sigma^r$, since m_2 is an estimator of σ^2.

(a) Measures of skewness

The commonly used measure of *skewness* (g_1) is defined from the third moment m_3 adjusted by the corresponding scale factor $m_2^{r/2}$, namely:

$$g_1 = \frac{m_3}{m_2^{3/2}} = \frac{m_3}{\sigma^3}$$

When $g_1 = 0$, $m_3 = 0$ and the distribution is symmetrical.

If $g_1 > 0$, the distribution is positively skewed with a tail to the right.

If $g_1 < 0$, the distribution is negatively skewed with a tail to the left.

Commonly numerical values of g_1 greater than 2 are associated with a distribution that is too skewed to be considered to be normal.

(b) Measures of kurtosis

The commonly used measure of *kurtosis* (g_2) is defined from the second and fourth moments as:

$$g_2 = \frac{m_4 - 3m_2^2}{m_2^2} = \frac{m_4}{\sigma^4} - 3$$

When g_2 is zero, the distribution is normal.

If $g_2 < 0$, the distribution is flatter than normal, or platykurtic.

If $g_2 > 0$, the distribution is more peaked than normal, or leptokurtic.

Commonly, numerical values of g_2 greater than 2 are associated with a distribution that is either too platykurtic or too leptokurtic to be considered to be normal.

3.2 An Index of Inequality

One important representation of inequality is diagrammatic in nature, namely, the "Lorenz curve." It leads to the calculation of an index of inequality, the "Gini coefficient." This index is found to be useful as a measure of the variability or disparity in comparisons of the provision of education or the outcomes of

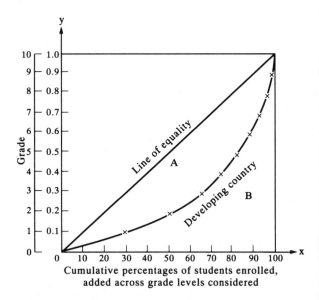

Figure 1
Lorenz curve for disparities across grades in levels of enrollment of students

education across different groups, such as schools, school districts, or countries. Lorenz curves are drawn by plotting the cumulative incidence of an appropriate criterion measure against the cumulative percentage incidence of the units of observation. An example is provided in Fig. 1, where the disparities across grades in levels of enrollment of students is under consideration. Along the y-axis grade levels of schooling to Year 10 are recorded and along the x-axis the cumulative percentages of students enrolled in successive grades are recorded.

In most school systems of developed countries there is an approximately equal distribution of students across grades, because the requirements of compulsory education prevent dropping out at higher grade levels to seek employment. However, in many developing countries there is a successive decline in enrollments across grades. The Lorenz curve for the developed countries approaches the line of equality shown in Fig. 1. However, in developing countries, the Lorenz curve for participation in schooling falls below the diagonal and is concave toward the diagonal. A single Lorenz curve can be assessed with respect to the diagonal line of equality, since the closer the curve is to the diagonal the greater the degree of equality, and the further the curve is from the diagonal, the greater the degree of disparity.

The units of observation could be individual students, schools, or districts, and the characteristic under consideration could be measures of financial provision, services supplied, or achievement of educational outcomes, such as the percentage achieving mastery on a literacy test.

The Gini coefficient is also used to express the relationship shown by the area between the Lorenz curve and the diagonal relative to the triangular area under the line of equality. In Fig. 1, the area between the curve and the diagonal is indicated by A, and the area between the curve and the bounding x-axis and the 100 percent ordinate is indicated by B.

The Gini coefficient is $G = A/(A + B)$. This coefficient approaches zero for high levels of equality and would have a value of 1.0 in cases of total inequality.

The Gini coefficient is calculated using the formula:

$$G = \sum_{i=1}^{n} (p_{i-1}q_i - p_iq_{i-1})$$

where p_i = cumulative proportion of the characteristic under investigation, and q_i = cumulative proportion of the criterion measure.

Johnstone (1981) warns that the coefficient is not invariant of the units of measurement employed. Hence, the Gini coefficient must relate the cumulative percentage or proportion of the characteristic to the cumulative percentage or proportion of the criterion if a meaningful and generalizable index is to be calculated. Thus, in the example given above in Fig. 1, the grade levels from 1 to 10 cumulate proportionally from 0.1 for Grade 1 to 1.0 for Grade 10.

Johnstone (1981 pp. 28–84) provides detailed information on the steps involved in the calculation of the Gini coefficient and presents an alternative formula advanced by Sen (1973 p. 31) where:

$$G = 1 + \frac{1}{n} - \frac{2}{n^2\bar{x}} [y_i + 2y_2 + \dots ny_n]$$

where n = number of units, $\bar{x}$ = average value of the characteristics across all units, y_i = proportion of the characteristic in unit i.

The use of this formula does not demand that the ranked proportions should be added together but does require that the proportions of the characteristic (y_i) have been ranked in descending order.

Johnstone (1981 pp. 94–96) also notes that the Gini coefficient does not indicate in any way the level of the characteristic being measured, but only the relative distribution of the characteristic across the population under consideration. Furthermore, the Gini coefficient does not indicate where the inequality is located within a system; it merely assesses the extent to which inequality is present. For a statistical treatment Kendall and Stuart (1958) should be consulted.

An example of the use of the Gini coefficient in the study of the extent of variation between schools in the proportion of students achieving mastery on reading and numeracy tests in the different Australian school systems is provided by Ross (1977). It was shown that in some school systems the proportion of students in a school not achieving mastery was evenly spread across the school system, while in other systems the majority of students who had not achieved mastery was located in relatively few schools. It was argued that these different situations required different strategies for the allocation of resources which would provide programs of remedial assistance to schools.

4. Measures of Clustering

Investigations in the field of education are almost inevitably required to collect data from students who are clustered together in classrooms, which are grouped together within schools, and from schools which are combined together to form a school system at the community, regional, or national level. It has been learnt from experience in education that members of any group are more like each other than they are like the members of any other group. Thus the students within one class in a school are commonly more like the other members of that class than they are like the members of other classes. This is a consequence both of the factors that operate to cluster individuals into a group and of the treatment conditions that apply within each group. The effects of this clustering of individual members within a group are observed in the measures of variation that are recorded in empirical investigations. As a result there is almost invariably a reduction in variance if the data obtained at the individual level are aggregated to a higher or group level.

Problems arise in the analysis of the variation between individuals and groups in three ways. First, there is considerable error involved if the parameters are estimated separately for each group and then examined between groups. Second, it is necessary to allow for the different effects of treatment conditions at different levels. Third, it is necessary to partition the sampling and measurement errors involved into components which operate at the different levels. The examination of these problems lies outside the scope of this entry (see *Multilevel Analysis; Hierarchical Linear Modeling*). However, here the concern is with the different indexes that have been advanced to measure the extent of clustering that occurs in situations where complex cluster samples are of necessity involved in investigations.

4.1 The Correlation Ratio (η)

The simplest index of clustering of individuals within groups is given by a correlation ratio, *eta*, (η). If y is the dependent variable and x the independent variable and if each group corresponds to one x_i value and $\bar{y}_i$ is the group mean of y and $\bar{\bar{y}}$ is the mean of the group means then the correlation ratio is given by:

$$\eta_{yx}^2 = \frac{\sum_{i=1}^{n} m_i (\bar{y}_i - \bar{\bar{y}})^2}{\sum_{i=1}^{n} \sum_{j=1}^{m_i} (y_{ij} - \bar{\bar{y}})^2}$$

This may also be expressed as
η^2 = Sum of Squares between groups/Total Sum of Squares.

Alternatively the correlation ratio may be expressed in terms of the F ratio

$$\eta_{yx}^2 = \frac{(n-1)F}{(n-1)F + (N-n)}$$

where n is the number of groups;
m_i is the number of individuals within each group; and
N is the total number of individuals

It should be noted that there is of course another correlation ratio (η_{xy}^2) which arises if y is regarded the independent variable and x is the dependent variable. The two correlation ratios arise from the existence of the two regression lines between variables x and y.

The standard error of a correlation ratio is given by:

$$se = \frac{1 - \eta^2}{\sqrt{N - 1}}$$

where N = total number of cases.

The correlation ratio can be tested for being significantly different from zero using the F ratio:

$$F = \frac{\eta^2(N - n)}{(n - 1)(1 - \eta^2)}$$

where n = number of groups, and N is the total number of individuals.

In addition, the correlation ratio (η) can be used to test for the significance of the departures of a regression line (y regressed on x) from linearity using the F ratio:

$$F = \frac{(\eta^2 - r^2)(N - n)}{(n - 2)(1 - \eta^2)}$$

where r = the product moment correlation coefficient. The value of the correlation ratio (η^2) is best obtained from a one-way analysis of variance to obtain the sum of squares between groups and the total sum of squares for the dependent variable.

4.2 Omega Squared

If x is an independent variable that provides the basis for the clustering of the dependent variable y, then a measure of the extent of clustering is given by the ratio *omega squared* (ω^2) which indicates the proportion of variance in y accounted for by x. Thus if σ_y^2 is the variance of y, and given groups clustered in terms of variable x, the conditional distribution of y given x has variance $\sigma_{y|x}^2$, then the reduction in the variance of y as a result of clustering is $\sigma_y^2 - \sigma_{y|x}^2$ and the proportional reduction ω^2 is given by:

$$\omega^2 = \frac{\sigma_y^2 - \sigma_{y|x}^2}{\sigma_y^2}$$

A further expression for ω^2 is given in terms of the F ratio

$$\hat{\omega}^2 = \frac{(n - 1)(F - 1)}{(n - 1)(F - 1) + N}$$

where n is the number of groups and N is the total number of individuals.

An alternative expression is given by

$$\hat{\omega}^2 = \frac{\text{Sum of Squares between Groups} - (n - 1)\,\text{Mean Square within Groups}}{\text{Total Sum of Squares} + \text{Mean Square within Groups}}$$

It should be noted that where η^2 is a descriptive statistic for a sample, $\hat{\omega}^2$ is an estimate of a population parameter ω^2. Furthermore, if F < 1, then $\hat{\omega}^2$ becomes negative, and is best taken to be zero.

The expression for omega squared (ω^2) is increasingly being used as a measure of the strength of an association between the independent and dependent variables. It replaces tests of statistical significance which are very dependent on the number of cases involved.

4.3 Intraclass Correlation

A further way of expressing the idea that clustering within groups accounts for variance of the dependent variable y was initially proposed through defining a population intraclass correlation coefficient (ρ_1)

$$\rho_1 = \frac{\sigma_g^2}{\sigma_g^2 + \sigma_w^2}$$

where σ_g^2 = the variance associated with groups,

σ_w^2 = error variance within groups,

$\sigma_g^2 + \sigma_w^2$ = total variance (σ_t^2).

In order to understand more fully just what the intraclass correlation coefficient is measuring, it is necessary to discuss its derivation and definition.

If from each of n schools a pair of students of the same age or grade is selected, one of whom is a boy and one a girl, it is possible to examine the correlation between these students in two different ways (Fisher 1970 pp. 213–49). First, they may be divided into two sets, the boys and the girls, and with matched pairs. It is then possible to proceed to calculate the product moment correlation coefficient between the two sets of measures in the normal way.

The correlation coefficient so calculated is termed the "interclass correlation coefficient". Second, it may not be possible or desirable to distinguish which measurements belong to boys or to girls in the matched pairs. The problem, however, arises as to which of the two students from each school should be considered in the first column. This difficulty is overcome by using a symmetric table in which each pair is entered twice in the correlation table, first as (x_{i1}, x_{i2}) and then as (x_{i2}, x_{i1}). There will now be $2n$ entries and the correlation coefficient is given as:

$$r_{xx} = \frac{1}{(2n-1)s^2} \left[\sum_{i=1}^{n} (x_{i1} - \bar{x})(x_{i2} - \bar{x}) \right.$$

$$\left. + \sum_{i=1}^{n} (x_{i2} - \bar{x})(x_{i1} - \bar{x}) \right]$$

$$= \frac{2}{(2n-1)s^2} \left[\sum_{i=1}^{n} (x_{i1} - \bar{x})(x_{i2} - \bar{x}) \right]$$

where

$$\bar{x} = \frac{1}{2n} \sum_{i=1}^{n} (x_{i1} + x_{i2})$$

and

$$s^2 = \frac{1}{2n-1} \left[\sum_{i=1}^{n} (x_{i1} - \bar{x})^2 + \sum_{i=1}^{n} (x_{i2} - \bar{x})^2 \right]$$

This correlation coefficient is called the "intraclass correlation coefficient."

The difference between the two correlation coefficients becomes clearer if the selection of three or more students from each school is considered. The intraclass correlation coefficient can still be calculated using all measures with each set of three students arranged into three pairs each having two entries in the symmetric table so that the three students give rise to six entries in the table. The interclass correlation coefficient is restricted to two equal subsets of students.

Now consider the case in which m students are selected from each of n schools and derive an expression for the intraclass correlation coefficient following Weatherburn (1946 pp. 97–99).

The symmetric table is constructed with $m(m-1)$ pairs of value for each of n schools.

The total number of entries N is given by:

$N = n.m(m-1)$.

If x_{ij} denotes the measure of the characteristic for the jth student in the i th school, then $i = 1, 2, \ldots n$ and $j = 1, 2, \ldots m$.

Each value of x_{ij} which occurs in one column of the correlation table will have a paired value in the other column for each of the other $(m-1)$ values from the same school. Thus each value of x_{ij} occurs $(m-1)$ times in each column.

The mean of this distribution which is the same in each column is:

$$\bar{x} = \frac{(m-1)\sum_{i=j}^{n} \sum_{j=1}^{m} (x_{ij})}{nm(m-1)} = \frac{\sum_{i=j}^{n} \sum_{j=1}^{m} (x_{ij})}{nm} \tag{3}$$

Likewise the variance of the distributions in each column which are the same is:

$$s^2 = \frac{1}{nm} \sum_{i=j}^{n} \sum_{j=i}^{m} (x_{ij} - \bar{x})^2 \tag{4}$$

The intraclass correlation coefficient (ρ) is given by an extension of the usual formula with $j \neq k$:

$$\rho = \frac{\sum_{i=1}^{n} \sum_{j=1}^{m} \sum_{k=1}^{m} (x_{ij} - \bar{x})(x_{ik} - \bar{x})}{nm(m-1)s^2} \tag{5}$$

The numerator may be summed first with respect to k, then to j and finally i and reduces to $m^2 n s_s^2 - nms^2$ where s_s^2 = variance of the school mean values. That is:

$$\rho = \frac{m^2 n s_s^2 - nms^2}{nm(m-1)s^2}$$

$$= \frac{ms_s^2 - s^2}{(m-1)s^2} \tag{6}$$

By rearranging, it can be shown that:

$\rho(m-1)s^2 = ms_s^2 - s^2$, and:

$$\frac{s_s^2}{s^2} = \frac{1 + \rho(m-1)}{m} \qquad (7)$$

If it is noted that:

mns_s^2 = Sum of squares between schools (SS_B)

and mns^2 = Total sum of squares (SS_T)

= Sum of squares between schools (SS_B) +
Sum of squares within schools (SS_W)

Then Eqn. (6) can be rewritten:

$$= \frac{mSS_B - (SS_B + SS_W)}{(m-1)(SS_B + SS_W)}$$

$$= \frac{(m-1)SS_B - SS_W}{(m-1)SS_B + (m-1)SS_W}$$

Dividing the numerator and denominator by $(n-1)$ $(m-1)$, the following is obtained:

$$\rho = \frac{\dfrac{SS_B}{n-1} - \dfrac{SS_W}{(n-1)(m-1)}}{\dfrac{SS_B}{n-1} + \dfrac{(m-1)SS_W}{(n-1)(m-1)}}$$

$$= \frac{MS_B - MS_W}{MS_B + (m-1)MS_W} \qquad (8)$$

where

MS_B = Mean square between schools, and
MS_W = Mean square within schools.

Since $F = MS_B/MS_W$ from a one-way analysis of variance,

$$\rho = \frac{F-1}{F + (m-1)} \qquad (9)$$

Equations (8) and (9) may be used with a one-way analysis of variance table given as Table 3 to obtain estimates of the intraclass correlation coefficient when there are unequal numbers of students (m_i) selected from within n schools, since it is unlikely in practice that the numbers of students sampled per school are equal.

When all values of m_i are equal, then from Table 3:
Expected (Between Schools Mean Square)

$= \sigma_w^2 + m\sigma_g^2$

Expected (Total Mean Square)

$= \sigma_w^2 + \left[\dfrac{N-m}{N-1}\right]\sigma_g^2$

If n, the number of schools in the sample is large compared to the number of students within each school (m), that is N is large compared with m, then

Expected (Total Mean Square) $= \sigma_w^2 + \sigma_g^2$

Thus $\sigma_t^2 = \mathrm{Var}\, x_{ig} = \sigma_w^2 + \sigma_g^2$

and $\sigma_s^2 = \mathrm{Var}\, \bar{x}_i$

$$= \frac{\text{Expected (Between Schools Mean Square)}}{m}$$

$= \sigma_g^2 + \sigma_w^2/m$

If s^2 is considered the estimate of σ_t^2 and s_s^2 the estimate of σ_s^2, assume a large sample of schools (n), and ignore the bias associated with a sample rather than a population, then by substituting in Eqn. (6)

$$\rho = \frac{m\sigma_s^2 - \sigma_t^2}{(m-1)\sigma_t^2}$$

Substituting $\sigma_s^2 = \sigma_g^2 + \sigma_w^2/m$ and $\sigma_t^2 = \sigma_w^2 + \sigma_g^2$ the following expression is obtained:

$$\rho = \frac{\sigma_g^2}{\sigma_g^2 + \sigma_w^2} \quad \text{or} \quad \frac{\sigma_g^2}{\sigma_t^2}$$

Thus, if certain assumptions are made as indicated above, the intraclass correlation can be regarded as a measure of the relative contributions of the between

Table 3
One-way analysis of variance for a random effects model

Item	Degree of freedom	Sum of squares	Mean squares	Expected mean square[a]
Between group	$n-1$	$\sum\limits_{i=1}^{n} m_i(\bar{x}_i - \bar{\bar{g}})^2$	$MS_B = \dfrac{SS_B}{n-1}$	$\sigma_w^2 + m\sigma_g^2$
Within group	$N-n$	$\sum\limits_{i=1}^{n}\sum\limits_{j=1}^{m_i} (x_{ij} - \bar{x}_i)^2$	$MS_W = \dfrac{SS_W}{N-n}$	σ_w^2
Total	$N-1$	$\sum\limits_{i=1}^{n}\sum\limits_{j=1}^{m_i} (x_{ij} - \bar{\bar{g}}_i)^2$	$MS_T = \dfrac{SS_T}{N-1}$	$\sigma_w^2 + \left[\dfrac{N-m}{N-1}\right]\sigma_g^2$

a All values of m_i are considered equal

group and the within group or error variances (see Fisher 1938 pp. 228–30). However, in practice estimates of the intraclass correlation are best made through a one-way analysis of variance, rather than through the ratio of the between group to the total variance. Moreover the significance of the intraclass correlation can be tested using the F-ratio from the one-way analysis of variance.

It should be noted that from Eqn. (7), namely,

$$\frac{s_s^2}{s^2} = \frac{1 + \rho(m - 1)}{m}$$

the limits of ρ are readily specified:

(a) when there is complete homogeneity within groups, that is when $s_s^2 = s^2$ then $\rho = 1$;

(b) when there is extreme heterogeneity within groups, that is, when $s_s^2 = 0$ then $\rho = -1/(m - 1)$; and

(c) when the homogeneity is equivalent to a random sorting into groups, then $\rho = 0$ and $s_s^2 = s^2/m$

4.4 Ratio of Homogeneity

In most situations which arise in educational research studies, not only are the samples which are drawn clustered as students within classrooms and classrooms within schools, but also classroom groups of students are randomly selected from within classrooms or schools. In addition, the sample of schools selected is commonly stratified and different sampling fractions are employed across different strata. Such variations in the complexity of the sample design, as well as losses in execution, tend to increase the variance of the measures. Consequently, it is necessary to allow for the effects of clustering through the use of a ratio of homogeneity (*roh*) rather than the intraclass correlation (see Kish 1965 pp. 161–62). This ratio is introduced by analogy with the intraclass correlation coefficient (ρ or *rho*). In addition, because of the complexity of the sample design, this ratio is best estimated not by analysis of variance procedures but by jackknife, balanced repeated replication, bootstrap, or subsampling procedures. Furthermore, an index of sample complexity, the design effect (*deff*) is introduced as the ratio of the estimated sample variance to the equivalent variance for a simple random sample of the same size.

One expression for *deff* is:

$$deff = \frac{var[t(c)]}{var[t(srs)]}$$

where var $[t(c)]$ = the estimated variance of the statistic t for the complex sample size N.

and var $[t(srs)]$ = the estimated variance of the statistic t for the simple equivalent sample of size N.

where $N = \bar{m}n$ and $\bar{m}$ is the average group size.

By analogy with Eqn. (7) above

where $\frac{ms_s^2}{s^2} = 1 + \rho(m - 1)$

deff may be expressed in the form

$$deff = 1 + roh(\bar{m} - 1) \tag{10}$$

Thus *roh* is estimated from *deff* and the sample variance of a complex sample. It should be noted that both *deff* and *roh* take into account not only the effects of clustering, but also the effects of stratification and differential losses across strata. Moreover, *roh* and *deff* are applicable to a wide range of statistics in addition to the sample mean.

4.5 Use of Intraclass Correlation and Ratio of Homogeneity

(a) *To Describe the Degree of Complexity of a Sample*
Both the intraclass correlation (*rho*) and the ratio of homogeneity (*roh*) may be used to describe the complexity of a sample associated with the estimation of a mean value or other statistic. However, with a large complex sample, the use of one-way analysis of variance procedures to estimate the intraclass correlation underestimates the effects of design on the mean value, since variability arises from sources other than the clustering of individuals within groups. As a consequence the ratio of homogeneity (*roh*) is employed and is estimated from the design effect after the variance of the mean for the complex sample has been estimated by the jackknife, balanced repeated replication, bootstrap, or subsampling procedures. For other statistics such as correlation coefficients and regression coefficients, only the ratio of homogeneity (*roh*) is applicable (see *Sampling Errors in Survey Research*).

(b) *To Estimate Reliability*
Analysis of variance procedures may be used to partition the components of variance which arise in measurement from different sources. From these variance components the different intraclass correlation coefficients (*rho*) which provide indexes of reliability associated with the different sources of error may be calculated (see *Reliability*).

(c) *To Estimate Similarity*
An important use of the intraclass correlation coefficient (*rho*) is as an index of similarity between different sets of measures. It is particularly useful in situations where there are more than two sets of measures being compared and where there are different numbers of cases in each set. It should be noted that *rho* calculated from a one-way analysis of variance takes into account the differences between the means of each set. Care, however, must be taken in setting up the one-way analysis of variance that the clusters form the treatments.

(d) *Comparison between the Intraclass and the Interclass Correlation Coefficients*
The interclass correlation coefficient (r) calculated as a product moment correlation, requires two matching sets of data with equal numbers of cases. It does not take into account the difference between the means of the two sets. However, the intraclass

591

correlation coefficient (*rho*) obtained with two matching sets of data does take into account the difference between the means of the two sets, if the coefficient is calculated from a one-way analysis of variance. Thus the difference between the two coefficients reflects the difference between the means of the two sets. The significance of the difference of the means between the two sets can be examined by carrying out a two-way analysis of variance.

5. Conclusion

Educational research has typically sought to estimate and examine mean values and the primary use of the examination and estimation of measures of variation has been for the estimation of error associated with the measurement of the mean. There is, however, a growing interest in the variability of other statistics and the factors influencing it. As a consequence, developmental work (see, e.g., Goldstein 1987) has been directed toward the estimation of variance components and the standard error of other statistics.

See also: Variance and Covariance, Analysis of

References

Comber L C, Keeves J P 1973 *Science Education in Nineteen Countries: An Empirical Study*. Wiley, New York
David H A 1951 Further applications of range to the analysis of variance. *Biometrika* 38: 393–09
Ferguson G A 1966 *Statistical Analysis in Psychology and Education*, 2nd edn. McGraw-Hill, New York
Fisher R A 1938 *Statistical Methods for Research Workers*, 7th edn. Oliver and Boyd, Edinburgh
Fisher R A 1970 *Statistical Methods for Research Workers*, 14th edn. Oliver and Boyd, Edinburgh
Goldstein H 1987 *Multilevel Models in Educational and Social Research*. Griffin, London
Guilford J P 1965 *Fundamental Statistics in Psychology and Education*, 4th edn. McGraw-Hill, New York
Hartley H O 1950 The use of range in analysis of variance. *Biometrika* 37: 271–80
Hays W L 1963 *Statistics for Psychologists*. Holt, Rinehart and Winston, New York
Johnstone J N 1981 *Indicators of Education Systems*. Kogan Page, London
Kendall M G, Stuart A 1958 *The Advanced Theory of Statistics*, 2nd edn. *Vol. 1: Distribution Theory*. Griffin, London
Kish L D 1965 *Survey Sampling*. Wiley, New York
Patnaik P B 1950 The use of mean range as an estimator of variance in statistical tests. *Biometrika* 37: 78–87
Peaker G F 1965 The Certificate of Secondary Education: School-based examinations. In: Schools Council 1965 *Examination Bulletin No. 5*. HMSO, London
Ross K N 1977 Some demographic influences on variation between schools. In: Bourke S F, Keeves J P (eds.) 1977 *The Mastery of Literacy and Numeracy. Australian Studies in School Performance*, Vol. 3. Australian Government Publishing Service, Canberra
Sen A 1973 *On Economic Inequality: The Radcliffe Lectures*. Clarendon, Oxford
Snedecor G W, Cochran W G 1967 *Statistical Methods*, 6th edn. Iowa State University Press, Ames, Iowa
Weatherburn C E 1946 *A First Course in Mathematical Statistics*. Cambridge University Press, Cambridge

Missing Data and Nonresponse

D. Holt

One of the purposes of survey design is to provide a sample which has a known relationship to the survey population so that the sample can be used to make estimates for the population parameters. Good design will provide efficient estimates which are unbiased or nearly so. It will take advantage of the population structure through techniques such as stratification and multistage sampling so as to yield a sample which will permit efficient estimation of the various population characteristics. One of the problems with survey research is that no matter how carefully the survey is designed, the actual outcome is imperfect. Problems occur because of nonresponse so that the sample which is actually achieved is deficient in comparison to what was intended. The reasons for nonresponse are complex and depend to some extent on the nature of the study, the survey procedures, and the relationship between the subjects and the researcher. How serious a problem this is and the effect on the survey objectives will depend on the level of nonresponse and how much respondents differ from nonrespondents in the variables of interest in the particular study.

This entry considers these problems and the procedures which can be adopted to reduce the effects of missing data and nonresponse in the estimates made from survey studies.

1. Problems Encountered in Survey Studies

In a survey of schools, for example, it may simply be the case that some selected subjects are unavailable on the day of the survey because of illness or absenteeism.

Alternatively it may be the conscious choice of some selected individuals or their parents not to respond. A third situation, which can affect not just one subject but many, occurs when a third party, a head teacher, for example, decides on behalf of a whole school, not to cooperate in a particular study. This creates a cluster of nonresponses from the selected subjects in that school. In the wider context of research studies which involve direct contact with individuals rather than via a school or similar institution, the situation is like other social surveys; nonresponse can result from direct refusal to cooperate, failure to contact the chosen subject or, more rarely, failure to collect the required information because of communication, language, or other similar problems. Failure to make contact is a broad category which includes a variety of situations. This failure may be due to prolonged absence of the subject or because the subject is simply unavailable on each occasion when contact is attempted. Alternatively, the subject may no longer be living at the last known address if the available information is out of date. The term "unit nonresponse" is used where no information is obtained for some selected individuals. In other cases, answers to some questions are not given in an otherwise complete response. These may, for example, be more sensitive or personal questions which the respondent chooses not to answer. This is known as "item or question nonresponse."

Thus no matter how carefully the original sample design was made to achieve a sample properly representative of the population of interest, the final data yielded will represent a loss of some of the originally chosen subjects. How much effect this will have depends heavily on the type of study, the means of data collection, the nature of the data required and the purposes of the study. At one extreme a well-designed study with carefully executed methodology and the full support of education authorities may achieve almost complete response. Here nonresponse could be such a small problem that it could be considered unlikely to effect significantly any of the conclusions drawn from the survey data. At the other extreme, poorly chosen methodology with poor follow-up using out-of-date information could result in a wholly inadequate response rate of 20 percent or less. It is the first responsibility of researchers to strive for as high a response rate as possible, but it is nevertheless common for well-designed social surveys with good methodology to achieve response rates of only 75 percent to 85 percent. Surveys based on schools or similar institutions are often carried out in favorable circumstances and might be expected to yield a higher response rate than this. It must be emphasized that the overall response rate, while important, is not a complete guide: it is quite possible that even when this is high, the level of response for particular subgroups may still be too low. Different ethnic groups, for example, may yield different response rates and if the research objectives call for separate statistical analyses for each ethnic group or a comparison between them, a low response rate in one group would still cause concern even though the response rate for all ethnic groups taken together was satisfactory.

Nonresponse may affect the survey results in two ways: first, there is the effect of reducing the achieved sample size below that intended. This alone will decrease the precision of estimates. If this were the only effect it could be overcome by enlarging the initial sample size and so allowing for a reduction in sample size due to nonresponse. The second and potentially more important and intransigent, effect is due to the fact that nonrespondents may differ systematically from respondents. The achieved sample is no longer fully representative of the original population and may result in biased population estimates. There is a substantial social survey literature showing that response rates differ with various factors such as age, social class, and urban/rural location. In particular, response rates are lower in inner city areas.

Consider the simple case of estimating the mean reading test score of a population of schoolchildren. Imagine that the population consists of two groups: (a) potential respondents (R) who if they happen to be selected into the sample would be available on the survey day and would respond; and (b) potential nonrespondents (NR), who if selected would be unavailable on survey day perhaps through illness or absenteeism or would refuse to respond. It is assumed that the two groups have mean reading test scores of μ_R and μ_{NR} respectively and that in the whole population the proportion of potential respondents is P_R. The proportion of potential nonrespondents is $P_{NR} = 1 - P_R$.

The mean reading age for the whole population is μ,

$$\mu = P_R\mu_R + P_{NR}\mu_{NR} \tag{1}$$

but the achieved sample will contain only respondents and, subject to sampling fluctuation, will have a mean reading age of μ_R. The bias in using only the respondents is B,

$$B = P_R\mu_R + P_{NR}\mu_{NR} - \mu_R \tag{2}$$
$$= P_{NR}(\mu_{NR} - \mu_R)$$

Thus the bias is proportional to the difference in mean reading age between respondents and nonrespondents and to the proportion of the population who are potential nonrespondents. It should be noted that this bias is not reduced simply by increasing the sample size. The hopeful dictum that a large enough sample solves all problems does not apply to this situation. Researchers sometimes try to overcome the nonresponse problem by replacing nonrespondents with extra sampled individuals. This will overcome the reduction in overall sample size but since replacements will be drawn from the respondent subpopulation the nonresponse bias will remain. The basic difficulty has been illustrated above in the simplest of all cases when trying to estimate the population mean. In more complex situations such as estimating a correlation coefficient the same principle applies although the systematic difference between respondents and nonrespondents is concerned with characteristics other than just the mean of each group. Under appropriate assumptions, the work of Pearson (1903) and Anderson (1957) on the effects of selection when estimating population characteristics is relevant.

2. Data Collection Methods to Reduce Nonresponse

It is generally held that the best way to attack the nonresponse problem is at source by achieving as high a response rate as possible. The methods used to do this are varied but all involve careful attention to procedures and a willingness to devote a disproportionate amount of the resources and effort available to potential nonrespondents. The basic data collection method may be crucial and it is usually the case that direct contact involving an interviewer will yield a higher response rate than a mail questionnaire although the latter is considerably cheaper in most situations. For interview surveys, refusals can be minimized by improved training for interviewers and sometimes a second contact by a more senior and experienced member of the field force. It is an obvious help if the objectives of the survey are clearly presented and may be seen to be of benefit. There is evidence from social surveys that some refusals represent a situational response from people for whom the particular moment of contact is inconvenient or who happen at that time to be less responsive than they might otherwise be. For such people a second contact on another occasion will often meet with success. It is the interviewer's task to minimize the influence of factors which might lead to refusal and so promote the likelihood of a successful outcome. For mail surveys, response rates are typically lower but reminder cards, repeat mailing, telephone or interview follow-up will often improve this although not so far as to compare with the response rate from interview surveys. In the usual situation in schools, the respondent is the student who is not initially approached directly to take part in the study. In this case the same principles apply to parents, administrators, and teachers who control access to the child. The level of cooperation achieved will greatly affect the quality of the survey. In other cases, such as higher education, it is more likely that the eventual respondent will be approached directly. Even in this case the active cooperation of authorities can minimize subsequent frame and response problems.

The question of noncontact is separate from refusal. The use of an accurate, up-to-date sampling frame is an important factor especially when home addresses are required. Clearly people who are completely unavailable at the time of the survey through prolonged absence may be contacted later if this is practicable. People who are simply difficult to contact need to be sought at a variety of times on different days both in the daytime and evenings in order to maximize the possibility of successful contact. Call-backs and finding out from others when a person is likely to be available are both important parts of good fieldwork. Mail questionnaires and telephone interviews often overcome this initial contact problem although for mail surveys at least the motivation to respond is not as strong which more than offsets the gain.

The case of movers is sometimes a particularly difficult problem. If each mover is followed to a new address which is distant from the original, the field organization needs to be exceptionally well-controlled. The cost of such follow-ups can be very great. For wide-scale surveys, the sample is often designed using multistage sampling techniques so that the chosen samples cluster into locations saving considerably on travel costs. If this clustering relies on outdated information then movers will be located outside of the selected clusters and heavy costs will be incurred for each respondent who is followed to a new address. For longitudinal studies, where the same subject is contacted repeatedly, the problem can be severe unless the telephone is used for contacts after the initial one. This will save the fieldwork travel costs if subjects have access to a telephone and the subject matter of the study lends itself to a telephone inquiry. For cross-sectional surveys the problem of movers is often overcome to a large degree by a conceptual change in the sampling unit so that it is not the individual but some other more stable unit, linked to individuals that is used. Thus the sampling unit might be addresses or schools which are located at fixed points and the final sample is taken from the *de facto* membership of each selected unit at the time of the study. In this way a sample is achieved which is still representative of the whole population (including recent movers, for example) without having to trace specific individuals who have moved. Such a method may be suitable for schoolchildren or general population surveys but will have limited use if the target population is only associated with a small proportion of the general population of units to be sampled. For example, if the survey is concerned with graduates then a sample of all addresses will yield relatively few university graduates. A sampling frame provided by the university of the last known address of each graduate, however outdated, may be the best information available (see *Sampling in Survey Research*).

3. Statistical Adjustment for Nonresponse

However good the fieldwork procedures are, and however great the effort made, a residual nonresponse problem will remain. Good survey methods are the first line of attack and will reduce the problem but not eliminate it. The second line of attack is concerned with statistical analysis techniques to correct for nonresponse bias. These sometimes require collection of additional data. The essential difficulty is that nonrespondents by their very nature are unobserved and the proposed methods all depend to a greater or lesser extent on assumptions which are difficult to verify directly. All of the methods assume that in some way respondents and nonrespondents are alike in the sense that data from respondents may be used in such a way as to make allowance for nonrespondents. The adjustment made can take various forms such as: (a) duplicating the survey data from a child with a similar attendance record to the nonrespondent's; (b) giving greater weight in the analysis to children with similar attendance records to nonrespondents; or (c) some more sophisticated form of statistical adjustment using the attendance record as a covariate. The exact form of this will depend upon the type of statistical analysis required and assumptions about the relationship between the survey variables and attendance. The duplication of an individual data record as described in (a) is known as "hot-decking" (Madow 1979). This is more widely used in large-scale surveys.

A variety of methods of adjustment for nonresponse fall under the heading of "reweighting." The population is divided into a set of mutually exclusive and exhaustive "weighting classes" with proportions {P_c} in each class c=1...C. Extending the framework described for equation (1) the proportion of respondents and nonrespondents in the cth class are P_{cR} and P_{cNR} with means μ_{cR} and μ_{cNR} respectively. The population mean μ may be expressed as

$$\mu = \sum_c P_c(P_{cr}\mu_{cR} + P_{cNR}\mu_{cNR}) \tag{3}$$

and the overall proportion of respondents in the population is given by:

$$P_R = \sum_c P_c P_{cR} \tag{4}$$

The bias of the mean of the sample respondents as an estimator for μ is

$$\text{bias } (\bar{y} R) = A + B$$

$$\text{where } A = \sum \frac{P_c \mu_{cR}(P_{cR} - P_R)}{P_R} \tag{5}$$

$$\text{and } B = \sum_c P_c P_{cNR}(\mu_{cR} - \mu_{cNR})$$

Component (A) is the component of bias related to the differences in response rates between weighting classes. If all weighting classes had the same response rate this component would be zero. Component (B) is that related to differences between respondent and nonrespondent means within each weighting class. If the means of respondents and nonrespondents are the same within each weighting class then this component will be zero. A number of reweighting methods eliminate component (A) and leave a residual, hopefully

smaller bias of component (B). The choice of weighting classes should be determined by the information available and the idea that within the weighting class μ_{cR} and μ_{cNR} are as similar as possible.

In a survey of schoolchildren, for example, basic demographic characteristics such as age and sex would be useful to define weighting classes. However, nonresponse may be caused by absenteeism on the survey day. If reading ability is the variable of interest then overall one might expect this to be correlated with absenteeism rates. If attendance records over a period are available for all children in the population then these together with age and sex could be used to define weighting classes. The essential assumption is that for children with the same age, sex, and attendance record the average reading ability of respondents and nonrespondents will be similar. In a sense, for two similar children it is a matter of chance which one happened to be absent from school on the survey day. If this is so then conditioning on attendance record will remove some of the nonresponse bias.

The poststratified estimator is given by

$$\bar{y}_{pst} = \sum_c P_c \bar{y}_{cR}$$

where $\bar{y}_{cR}$ is the sample mean for respondents in the cth weighting class. When a small number of characteristics are used to define weighting classes poststratification can be used. When the number of poststratification categories is too large a more robust method is "raking ratio estimation" (Brackstone and Rao 1976).

The essential requirement for poststratification and raking ratio estimation is that information about the proportion {P_c} of the entire population in each weighting class is available. In some situations this information is unavailable for the whole population but is available for the original selected sample (including nonrespondents). In this case a form of poststratification or raking ratio estimation can still be used to eliminate bias component (A). Now poststratification or raking ratio estimation can be used to make "estimates" for the original selected sample including nonrespondents and the estimation procedure from this point to the whole population is that which would have been used had there been no nonresponse at all. In practice, of course, the two stages of estimation are combined. Holt and Elliott (1991) provide details of this together with a description of raking ratio estimation.

Other methods of nonresponse adjustment may involve modeling the nonresponse mechanism in some way. For example, Bartholomew (1961) proposed a simple form of adjustment which is primarily concerned with failure to make contact in social surveys and requires a single recall. He argued that successful first calls were clearly biased since they favored people who spent much of their time at home. Bartholomew suggested that at the time of the first unsuccessful call, as much information as possible should be obtained from other members of the household, neighbors and so on, so as to yield as good a chance of success at the first recall as possible. He then suggested that successful interviews at the first recall could be weighted to represent also the failures at the first recall stage. The essential assumption is that the additional information collected at the first call helps in the assumption that successes and failures at the first recall are similar and to provide the link between respondents and nonrespondents.

Politz and Simmons (1949) were also concerned with noncontact and suggested that data be collected from respondents to allow adjustment for nonresponse without making any recalls. The essential idea is that contact is directly related to the availability of the subject during the survey period and people who are more often unavailable during the survey period will be underrepresented in the achieved survey data. Each respondent is asked about the periods when they were available for interview during the survey period and these data can be used to reweight the survey data. For example, someone who was at home on two days during the survey period is twice as likely to have been contacted as someone at home on only one day. The implicit assumption is that for any given level of availability, respondents can represent nonrespondents with whom no contact was made.

Algebraically, the Politz–Simmons method is a special case of the general situation when some auxiliary information is known which may be used to adjust estimation methods to allow for nonresponse. The special feature of the method is that unlike other reweighting methods such as poststratification and raking ratio estimation, the Politz–Simmons method does not require any auxiliary information for the whole population or the original sample including nonrespondents. However, the weights used vary considerably and this leads to a loss of efficiency for the estimation method.

Throughout it has been assumed that the auxiliary information, age group for example, is a categorical variable and this leads to adjustment through the reweighting. Conceptually there is no further difficulty if the auxiliary information is not grouped but is treated as a continuous variable. If age is known for each respondent and the average age for the entire population is known then the adjustment could take the form of a ratio or regression estimate but the basic principle is the same.

The cases described here represent relatively simple situations. Anderson (1957) investigated these issues for multivariate analyses. Little (1980) and Rubin (1976) and also both authors in Madow (1979) have developed a comprehensive framework describing the basis of statistical inference in the presence of nonresponse. In all the cases described here it has been assumed that the response mechanism is such that the distribution of data from respondents is the same as that for nonrespondents given the same value of the auxiliary variables. When this assumption cannot

be made, the situation becomes much more complex. Heckman (1979) has considered this situation in the context of econometric models. Related work is reported by DeMets and Halperin (1977) in epidemiology, and Nathan and Holt (1980) in sample survey theory.

For example, if auxiliary information is available as variable x and an estimate is required of the regression coefficient of variable y on variable z then a modification to the usual statistical formula would be

$$\beta_{yz} = \frac{s_{yz} + \dfrac{s_{yx}s_{zx}}{s_{xx}}\left(\dfrac{\sigma_{xx}}{s_{xx}} - 1\right)}{s_{zz} + \dfrac{s_{xx}^2}{s_{xx}}\left(\dfrac{\sigma_{xx}}{s_{xx}} - 1\right)}$$

Here s_{yz} is the sample covariance between variables y and z based on the data achieved from respondents and similarly for s_{xx}, s_{yx}, and so on. For the auxiliary variable x, σ_{xx} is the known population value of the variance. Thus if x were the attendance record for schoolchildren, s_{xx} would be the sample variance for respondent schoolchildren, and σ_{xx} would be the corresponding variance calculated from all the schoolchildren's attendance records whether they were in the sample or not.

Thompson and Siring (1979) have used the number of call-backs required for a successful interview to model response mechanism in terms of an auxiliary variable (household size). By using Norwegian data where the true responses are obtainable from other sources, they are able to investigate the success of their methods and the extent to which call-backs are needed. For their empirical studies they show that their attempts to remove nonresponse bias are an improvement and that a substantial number of call-backs are worthwhile.

4. Item Nonresponse

Almost all of this discussion has focused on the question of unit nonresponse when a complete record is missing from the desired sample data. In practice these cases tend to be dealt with by reweighting methods. The question of item or question nonresponse is important although in practice it often tends to be a much smaller issue than unit nonresponse. In general, reweighting techniques are not used so much for item nonresponse. This is because the existing data from other questions gives a much richer source of auxiliary information for the record with missing values. This is often used to "predict" or "impute" the missing values so that the record is "completed" with imputed values which are consistent with the original data in the record. Normal estimation methods are then applied to the completed data set. In this case imputation is regarded as a separate process from estimation.

There are difficulties about this approach which arise because at the estimation phase the imputed data are treated as if they were original data. This is described by Rubin (1987) who suggests techniques known as multiple imputation as a solution (see *Missing Scores in Survey Research*).

5. Conclusion

This entry has been focused on cross-sectional studies although many of the general principles apply to longitudinal studies where selected individuals are followed over time. In addition, such studies involve other methodological problems of nonresponse. Sample attrition over time and the increasing efforts which must be made to maintain contact are the most obvious. An account of these problems specifically related to longitudinal studies is given by Goldstein (1979).

See also: Survey Research Methods; Cross-sectional Research Methods; Longitudinal Research Methods; Sampling in Survey Research; Sampling Errors in Survey Research; Missing Scores in Survey Research

References

Anderson T W 1957 Maximum likelihood estimates for a multivariate normal distribution when some observations are missing. *J. Am. Stat. Assoc.* 52: 200–03
Bartholomew D H 1961 A method of allowing for "not-at-home" bias in sample surveys. *Appl. Stat.* 10: 52–59
Brackstone G J, Rao J N K 1976 Raking ratio estimators. *Survey Methodology* 2: 63–69
DeMets D, Halperin M 1977 Estimation on a simple regression coefficient in samples arising from a sub-sampling procedure. *Biometrics* 33: 47–56
Goldstein H 1979 *The Design and Analysis of Longitudinal Studies: Their Role in the Measurement of Change.* Academic Press, New York
Heckman J 1979 Sample selection bias as a specification error. *Econometrica* 47: 153–61
Holt D, Elliott D 1991 Methods of weighting for unit nonresponse. *The Statistician* 40: 333–42
Little R J A 1980 Models for non-response in sample surveys. Invited paper, European Conference of Statisticians, Brighton
Madow W G (ed.) 1979. *Symposium on Incomplete Data: Preliminary Proceedings.* United States Department of Health, Education and Welfare, Washington, DC
Nathan G, Holt D 1980 The effect of survey design on regression analysis. *J Royal Stat. Soc. Bull* 42: 377–86
Pearson K 1903 On the influence of natural selection on the variability and correlation of organs. *Phil. Trans. Royal Soc. Am.* 200: 1–66
Politz A, Simmons W 1949 I An attempt to get the "not at homes" into the sample without callbacks. II Further theoretical considerations regarding the plan for eliminating callbacks. *J. Am. Stat. Assoc.* 44: 9–31
Rubin D B 1976 Inference and missing data. *Biometrika* 63: 581–92
Rubin D B 1987. *Multiple Imputation for Nonresponse in Surveys.* Wiley, New York
Thompson I, Siring E 1979 On the causes and effects of non-response: Norwegian experiences. In: Madow W G (ed.) 1979

Further Reading

Cochran W G 1977 *Sampling Techniques*, 3rd ed. Wiley, New York.
Kalton G 1983 *Compensating for Missing Survey Data.* Survey Research Center, Institute for Social Research, University of Michigan, Ann Arbor, Michigan
Kish L 1965 *Survey Sampling.* Wiley, New York
Krewski D, Platek R, Rao J N K (eds.) 1981 *Current Topics in Survey Sampling.* Symposium, Carleton University, May 7–9, 1980. Academic Press, New York
Moser C A, Kalton G 1971 *Survey Methods in Social Investigation*, 2nd edn. Heinemann, London
Steeh C G 1981 Trends in non-response rates, 1952–79. *Public Opinion Quarterly* 45: 40–57
Yates F 1981 *Sampling Methods for Census and Surveys*, 4th edn. Griffin, London

Mobility Tables

R. Erikson

Mobility tables have long been the main device for the analysis of social mobility. A mobility table is basically a transition matrix, with social origins as row entries and social destinations as column entries. Origins and destinations refer to the social class or social status of the subject of enquiry at two different points in time and are usually measured by the same class schema or status scale, which results in mobility tables normally being square with the same entries in rows and columns. In a study of intergenerational mobility, origins usually refer to the class or status of the family of origination while destinations refer to the class or status at an adult age from the time of entry to the labor market and onward. In a study of intragenerational mobility, origins often refer to the individual's position at first job, while destinations again refer to his or her position at some later age.

1. Analyzing a Mobility Table

A mobility table, given a class schema with k classes, may most conveniently be written as in Table 1, where f_{ij} is the observed frequency of persons in class j with origin in class i.

Mobility tables have typically been analyzed with the help of percentages as in the first major treatise on social mobility (originally published in 1927) by Sorokin (1959). Thus, analyses have concerned inflows, studied by percentage distributions of origins for each destination ($f_{ij}/f\cdot j$), and outflows, represented by the distribution of destinations for each origin ($f_{ij}/f_i\cdot$). A natural measure of the total mobility implied by a mobility table is furthermore the proportion of cases located outside the main diagonal ($(n-\Sigma f_{ii})/n$). The application of these measures formed the principal mode of analysis in major studies published in the 1950s (Rogoff 1953, Glass 1954, Svalastoga 1959, Carlsson 1958) and the first comprehensive comparative studies of mobility (Lipset and Bendix 1959, Miller 1960).

It was clear at an early stage that the amount of mobility observed in a specific mobility table is to a large extent dependent upon the shapes of the marginal distributions, especially on how much the destination distribution of a table differs from the origin distribution. However, marginal distributions are normally assumed to be determined by forces external to the mobility process, mainly the level and pace of economic development. Comparisons between tables, say, referring to different points in time or to different nations, are thus difficult to interpret if the marginal distributions differ among the tables compared—which typically is the case—since the mobility measure will depend on both some "intrinsic" rate of mobility and on extrinsic effects from economic development. The total mobility suggested by a mobil-

Table 1
Example of a mobility table (abbreviated)

| Origin | Destination | | | |
	1 ... j		k ...	Σ
1	f_{11}	f_{1j}	f_{1k}	$f_1.$
⋮				
i	f_{i1}	f_{ij}	f_{ik}	$f_i.$
⋮				
k	f_{k1}	f_{kj}	f_{kk}	$f_k.$
Σ	$f._1$	$f._j$	$f._k$	n

ity table was therefore commonly separated into two parts—the assumed intrinsic rate, called "exchange" or "pure mobility," and the extrinsically determined rate, called "structural" or "forced mobility." Forced or structural mobility was then measured as the amount of mobility that—under varying assumptions—must appear, given the marginal distributions, and pure or exchange mobility was defined as the rest; that is, total mobility minus forced mobility. Attempts were also made to measure the association between origins and destinations in such a way that the measure of association would be independent of the origin and destination distributions. The measure most commonly used for this purpose was the association or mobility index ($f_{ij}n/f_i\cdot f\cdot j$) which for each cell of the mobility matrix was calculated as the observed frequency divided by the frequency expected under the assumption of independence between origins and destinations. However, neither this index nor the separation of total mobility into structural and exchange mobility solved the general problem, since neither solution is in fact independent of the marginal distributions. The problem of comparing mobility tables with differing marginals was actually not solved until the introduction of log–linear methods in the 1970s (see *Log-Linear Models*).

Another classic problem relates to the dimensionality of a mobility table. Many researchers have assumed that the classes or status groups defining the table could be ordered on some single hierarchical scale (cf. Glass 1954), but studies of the dimensionality of mobility tables have consistently shown that there are at least two dimensions involved (cf. Carlsson 1958, Blau and Duncan 1967, Domanski and Sawinski 1987). Since the assumption that classes or status groups form an ordered scale allows the use of more sophisticated methods of analysis, researchers have often been tempted to make, and have indeed made, this assumption, in spite of the overwhelming evidence that more than one dimension must be recognized. The rationale given has then often been that the scale chosen at all events accounts for most of the interaction in the table. In their study of social mobility in the United States, Blau and Duncan (1967) sought to go beyond the analysis of mobility tables as such for regression analyses, based on the assumption that the 17 status groups they distinguished could be placed on a vertical scale. Through this introduction of "status attainment" research, they had a remarkable impact on sociology in the years to follow, both in opening up this area of research and more generally in showing the strength and advantages of regression-based techniques, such as path analysis.

2. Log–Linear Methods

With the introduction of log–linear analysis in the 1970s, however, the study of mobility tables as such returned. The work of Goodman (1972, 1979) and

Hauser (1978, Featherman and Hauser 1978) laid the ground for an extensive use of these methods in the analysis of social mobility. Goodman introduced log–linear models generally and especially "association models," while Hauser introduced "levels models." Log–linear models had several advantages. They solved the old problem of comparing the strength of association between origins and destinations in tables with different marginal distributions and made it possible to test whether this association differs between tables. They also made it possible for researchers to formalize and test hypotheses about specific patterns of mobility and likewise to test for specific differences in mobility patterns between tables.

The problem of separating structural from exchange mobility was reformulated and turned into a distinction between two aspects of social mobility: —(a) absolute rates, that is, inflows, outflows, etc; (b) relative rates or social fluidity, that is, the association between origins and destinations considered independently of marginal distributions (Goldthorpe 1980, cf. Sobel 1983). The amount of social fluidity is determined by the interaction between origins and destinations in a log–linear model where the marginal distributions are fitted exactly. It is then easy to test whether social fluidity differs between nations or over time, provided that mobility tables based on the same class schema are available.

3. Topological Models

With levels or "topological models" the cells in a mobility table are separated into two or more levels where the interaction between origins and destinations may differ between cells on different levels while being set to the same among cells on the same level; that is, independence holds among these cells. This means that a levels model treats all the association in a mobility table as occurring between levels. The first levels models developed by Hauser (1978) and used by, for example, Goldthorpe (1980) introduced levels —often about as many as the number of classes defining the table—mostly on an ad hoc basis. One such model, which has been widely used—and sharply put into question—is the quasi-symmetry model (cf. Sobel et al. 1985), where each pair of cells symmetrically located around the main diagonal is placed on a separate level. In later applications the levels have been more structured, in that different levels have been connected to separate effects assumed to influence rates of mobility. Thus, Erikson and Goldthorpe (1992a, 1992b) introduced models in which hierarchical divisions, propensities for inheritance, distinctions between economic sectors, and affinities between classes in terms of, for example, blue collar or white collar status are entered as separate effects. Such models not only make it possible to study the effects of different aspects of class structure on the mobility process but also allow

for the testing of differences between tables in these respects (cf. Xie 1992).

4. Association Models

"Association models," again, are based on the assumption of a rank order between classes or status groups. Classes or status groups are assigned scores on a scale—most often of socioeconomic status—and the interaction between origins and destinations, that is, social fluidity, in a mobility table is then accounted for by a measure of association between these scores. With simpler association models the scores are taken from sources extrinsic to the table (e.g., occupational prestige ratings), but in log–multiplicative models (Goodman 1979) the scores are intrinsic to the table and chosen so as to account for as much association as possible. Models that are based on just one scale generally fail to achieve an acceptable fit, which should come as no surprise in view of the well-established multidimensionality of mobility tables. Some researchers have therefore combined association and levels models, most often by putting the cells on the main diagonal on several separate levels (cf. Ganzeboom et al. 1989). Attempts have also been made to account for the multidimensionality of mobility tables by entering several scales to account for the interaction between origins and destinations in mobility tables. Hout (1988) in his SAT-model thus entered scales for status, autonomy, and training to account for mobility in the United States and he included several separate levels as well as several scales to model social mobility in Ireland (Hout 1989; cf. Hout and Hauser 1992).

5. Multidimensional Tables

Another development, which relates to the path-analytical approach, concerns the simultaneous analysis of tables with more than two dimensions. The dimensions that are included in addition to origins and destinations are typically level of education or class of first full-time job. There are several examples of analyses of three-way tables (cf. Hout 1989 Chap. 9, Erikson and Goldthorpe 1992a Chap. 8) but so far models applied have been relatively primitive; that is, no major breakthrough in the analysis of multidimensional tables has taken place.

6. Prospects

In the 1980s the dramatic development of techniques for analyzing mobility tables underscored Hout's observation that "new findings and analytical developments come faster and more furiously in this field than in any other in sociology" (1983 p. 7). It must be expected that this development will continue in the late 1990s and that the methods and models will spread to other areas of educational and sociological research. However, the path of development may leave the analysis of mobility tables proper and turn to logistic regression where individual characteristics are entered as independent factors. Another area where advancements in mobility research may appear is event history analysis, but the actual application of this method may become hampered by the difficulty of collecting empirical data suitable for this approach. With growing interest in lifelong and recurrent education and in career development, longitudinal studies that trace the effects of social origins and education on qualifications attained and occupational advancement will become central to educational and social research. In the analyses of such studies the regression analysis of life-course data, log–linear and logit methods may all prove to be essential.

See also: Log-Linear Models

References

Blau P M, Duncan O D 1967 *The American Occupational Structure.* Wiley, New York

Carlsson G 1958 *Social Mobility and Class Structure.* Gleerups, Lund

Domanski H, Sawinski Z 1987 Dimensions of occupational mobility: The empirical invariance. *European Sociological Review* 3

Erikson R, Goldthorpe J H 1992a *The Constant Flux: A Study of Class Mobility in Industrial Societies.* Clarendon Press, Oxford

Erikson R, Goldthorpe J H 1992b The CASMIN project and the American dream. *European Sociological Review* 8

Featherman D L, Hauser R M 1978 *Opportunity and Change.* Academic Press, New York

Ganzeboom H, Luijkx R, Treiman D J 1989 Intergenerational class mobility in comparative perspective. *Research in Social Stratification and Mobility* 8

Glass D V (ed.) 1954 *Social Mobility in Britain.* Routledge, London

Goldthorpe J H 1980 *Social Mobility and Class Structure in Modern Britain,* 2nd edn. Clarendon Press, Oxford

Goodman L A 1972 A general model for the analysis of surveys. *Am. J. Sociol.* 77

Goodman L A 1979 Simple models for the analysis of association in cross-classifications having ordered categories. *Journal of the American Statistical Association* 74

Hauser R M 1978 A structural model of the mobility table. *Soc. Forces* 56

Hout M 1983 *Mobility Tables.* Sage, Beverly Hills, California

Hout M 1988 More universalism, less structural mobility: The American occupational structure in the 1980s: *Am. J. Sociol.* 93(6): 1358–1400

Hout M 1989 *Following in Father's Footsteps: Social Mobility in Ireland.* Harvard University Press, Cambridge, Massachusetts

Hout M, Hauser R M 1992 Symmetry and hierarchy in social mobility: A methodological analysis of the CASMIN model of class mobility. *Eur. Sociological Rev.* 8

Lipset S M, Bendix R 1959 *Social Mobility in Industrial Society.* University of California Press, Berkeley, California

Miller S M 1960 Comparative social mobility. *Current Sociology* 9

Rogoff N 1953 *Recent Trends in Occupational Mobility.* Free Press, Glencoe, Illinois

Sobel M E 1983 Structural mobility, circulation mobility and the analysis of occupational mobility: A conceptual mismatch. *Am. Sociol. Rev.* 48(5): 721–27

Sobel M E, Hout M, Duncan O D 1985 Exchange, structure and symmetry in occupational mobility. *Am. J. Sociol.* 91(2): 359–72

Sorokin P A 1959 *Social and Cultural Mobility,* 2nd edn. Free Press, Glencoe, Illinois

Svalastoga K 1959 *Prestige, Class and Mobility.* Gyldendal, Copenhagen

Xie Y 1992 The log–multiplicative layer effect model for comparing mobility tables. *Am. Sociological Rev.* 57(3): 380–95

Multitrait–Multimethod Analysis

H. W. Marsh and D. Grayson

In educational research there is a need to validate systematically constructs that are used. Campbell and Fiske (1959) argued that construct validation requires both convergent and discriminant validity (see *Validity*). They proposed the multitrait–multimethod (MTMM) design in which two or more traits are each assessed by two or more methods. Traits are attributes such as multiple abilities, attitudes, behaviors, or personality characteristics, whereas methods refer broadly to multiple test forms, methods of assessment, raters, or occasions. This entry summarizes briefly the MTMM design, the Campbell–Fiske guidelines for evaluating MTMM data, and subsequent latent variable models based on confirmatory factor analysis

1. The Campbell and Fiske Approach

Consider a MTMM matrix (see Table 1) based on three traits ($T1$, $T2$, $T3$) and three methods ($M1$,

Table 1
Multitrait—multimethod correlation matrix

Variables[a]	T1M1	T2M1	T3M1	T1M2	T2M2	T3M2	T1M3	T2M3	T3M3
Method 1									
T1M1	(0.89)[b]								
T2M1	0.384[c]	(0.79)[b]							
T3M1	0.441[c]	0.002[c]	(0.92)[b]						
Method 2									
T1M2	0.662[d]	0.368[e]	0.353[e]	(0.84)[b]					
T2M2	0.438[e]	0.703[d]	0.008[e]	0.441[c]	(0.89)[b]				
T3M2	0.465[e]	0.069[e]	0.871[d]	0.424[c]	0.136[c]	(0.95)[b]			
Method 3									
T1M3	0.678[d]	0.331[e]	0.478[e]	0.550[d]	0.380[e]	0.513[e]	(0.87)[b]		
T2M3	0.458[e]	0.541[d]	0.057[e]	0.381[e]	0.658[d]	0.096[e]	0.584[c]	(0.90)[b]	
T3M3	0.414[e]	0.027[e]	0.825[d]	0.372[e]	0.029[e]	0.810[d]	0.582[c]	0.135[c]	(0.94)[b]

Source: Byrne and Shavelson (1986)
a The nine MTMM variables are scale scores representing all combinations of the three traits ($T1$=School selfconcept, $T2$=Verbal self-concept, $T3$=Mathematical self-concept) and three methods ($M1$, $M2$, and $M3$ representing three different self-concept instruments). For $N=817$, correlations greater than 0.07 are statistically significant ($p < 0.05$) b Monotrait—monomethod coefficients (or reliability estimates) c Heterotrait—monomethod coeffecients d Monotrait—heteromethod coefficients (convergent validities) e Heterotrait—heteromethod coefficients

$M2$, $M3$) consisting of correlations among $M \times T = 9$ measures, each reflecting a combination of one trait and one method. The MTMM matrix is divided into triangular submatrices of correlations among different traits assessed with the same method (heterotrait–monomethods [HTMM]—the elements indicated by a superscript c in Table 1), square submatrices of relations among measures assessed with different methods (heterotrait–heteromethods [HTHM]—the elements indicated by a superscript e in Table 1), and relations among the same traits assessed with different methods (convergent validities—the elements indicated by a superscript d in Table 1).

In the Campbell–Fiske approach (1959), an evaluation of a MTMM matrix is used to infer convergent validity, discriminant validity, and method effects. "Convergent validity" refers to true score or common factor trait variance; it is inferred from large, statistically significant correlations between different measures of the same trait. "Discriminant validity" refers to the distinctiveness of the different traits; it is inferred when correlations among different traits are less than the convergent validities and reliabilities. "Method effect" refers to the influence of a particular method that inflates a correlation among the different traits measured with the same method; it is inferred when correlations among traits measured by the same method exceed correlations among the same traits measured by different methods. These inferences are embodied in 6 guidelines—guidelines 1–4 originally proposed by Campbell and Fiske and two others based on their recommendations—that are applied to the MTMM matrix in Table 1 ($TiMp$ is the combination of one of the multiple traits [Ti, Tj, Tk . . .] and one of the multiple methods [Mp, Mq, Mr . . .], and $r(TiMp$,

$TjMq$) is a correlation between two manifest scores):

(a) Convergent validities are substantial ($r[TiMp$, $TiMs] >> 0$). All nine convergent validities—indicated by superscript d in Table 1—are statistically significant, varying between 0.54 and 0.87 (mean $r = 0.70$), thus providing strong support for this guideline.

(b) Convergent validities are higher than HTHM correlations ($r[TiMp$, $TiMq] > r[TjMp$, $TiMq]$ and $r[TiMp$, $TiMq]r > [TjMq$, $TiMp]$). Because convergent validities (mean $r = 0.70$) are higher than the HTHM correlations—indicated by superscript e in Table 1—(mean $r = 0.31$) in all 36 comparisons, there is good support for this guideline of discriminant validity.

(c) Convergent validities are higher than HTMM correlations ($r[TiMp$, $TiMq] > r[TiMp$, $TjMp]$) and ($r[TiMp$, $TiMq] > r[TiMq$, $TjMj]$). Because the convergent validities (mean $r = 0.70$) are higher than the HTMM correlations—indicated by supercript c in Table 1—(mean $r = 0.35$) for 33 of 36 comparisons, there is reasonable support for this criterion of discriminant validity. All three failures involve $M3$ where correlations among the traits (mean $r = 0.44$) are higher than for $M1$ (0.28) or $M2$ (0.33).

(d) The pattern of correlations among different traits is similar for different methods ($r[TiMp$, $TjMq] > r[TkMp$, $TlMq]$) implies ($r[TiMr$, $TjMs] > r[TkMr$, $TlMs]$). All correlations between $T2$ and $T3$ are consistently small (mean $r = 0.06$) whereas $T1$ is substantially correlated with both $T2$ (mean

$r = 0.42$) and $T3$ (mean $r = 0.45$), thus providing support for this guideline.

(e) HTMM and HTHM correlations are all substantially less than their reliabilities ($r[TiMp, TjMp])/([r(TiMp, TiMp) r(TjMp, TjMp]^{1/2} \ll 1$). Campbell and Fiske (1959) specifically stated that a clear violation of discriminant validity occurred "where within a monomethod block, the heterotrait values are as high as the reliabilities" (p. 84) and that "the elevation of the reliabilities above the heterotrait–monomethod triangle is further evidence for discriminant validity" (p. 97). The formal inclusion of this guideline will encourage researchers to evaluate systematically the reliability of their measures, to focus more on the quality of measurement of each trait-method unit, and to evaluate the implicit assumption of equally reliable measures underlying all the guidelines. The coefficient alpha estimates of reliability—indicated by superscript b in Table 1—(0.79 to 0.95; mean = 0.89) are all substantial and none of the disattenuated correlations approaches 1.0, providing good support for this guideline of discriminant validity.

(f) Method effects—a typically undesirable source of bias—are inferred when HTMM correlations substantially exceed HTHM correlations ($r[TiMp, TjMp] > r[TiMp, TjMq]$). Campbell and Fiske (1959 p. 85) stated that "the presence of method variance is indicated by the difference in level of correlation between parallel values of the monomethod block and the heteromethod block, assuming comparable reliabilities among the tests" and Marsh (1988) operationalized this test of method effects. In Table 1 the mean HTMM correlation (0.35) is modestly larger than the mean HTHM correlation (0.29), although the mean HTMM correlations are larger for $M3$ (0.44), than for $M2$ (0.33) and $M1$ (0.28). This suggests modest method effects associated with at least $M3$.

Important problems with inferences based on these guidelines are well-known (Marsh 1988). Campbell and Fiske (1959) were aware of most of these limitations, specifically stating that their guidelines should be viewed as "common-sense desideratum" (p. 83). Their intent was to provide a systematic, formative evaluation of MTMM data at the level of the individual trait-method unit, qualified by the recognized limitations of their approach, not to provide summative, global summaries of convergent validity, discriminant validity, and method effects. It is recommended that these guidelines should be used as an initial formative evaluation of all MTMM data even when more sophisticated latent variable approaches are applied and that this formative orientation in the MTMM paradigm must not be lost in the development of mathematically more sophisticated approaches to MTMM data. More generally, Campbell and Fiske had a heuristic intention to encourage researchers to consider the concepts of convergent validity, discriminant validity, and method effects; in this intention they were remarkably successful.

2. Latent Variable Approaches, Proper Solutions, and Goodness of Fit

Limitations in the Campbell–Fiske approach led to the development of latent variable models (see *Path Analysis and Linear Structural Relations Analysis*) and an evaluation of their ability to fit MTMM data. Whereas there are no well-established guidelines for what minimal conditions constitute an adequate fit, a general approach is to: (a) show that the solution is well-defined by establishing that the model is identified, the iterative estimation procedure converges, parameter estimates are within the range of permissible values, and the size of the standard error of each parameter estimate is reasonable; (b) examine the parameter estimates in relation to the substantive, *a priori* model and common sense; (c) evaluate the X^2 and subjective indices of fit (e.g., Marsh et al. 1988, Marsh 1988) for each model and values obtained from alternative models. If a solution is ill-defined, then further interpretations must be made cautiously if at all. If the parameter estimates make no sense in relation to the substantive, *a priori* model, then fit may be irrelevant. An improper solution may not warrant serious consideration and if a model frequently results in improper solutions across a wide range of applications for which the model is intended, then the usefulness of the model is limited.

3. The Confirmatory Factor Analysis (CFA) Approach

MTMM matrices, like other correlation matrices, can be factor analyzed to infer the underlying dimensions. Factors defined by different measures of the same trait effects, whereas factors defined by measures assessed with the same method effects. With CFA the researcher can define models that posit *a priori* trait and method factors, and test the ability of such models to fit the data. In the general CFA model (see CFA–CTCM model in Fig. 1) adapted from Jöreskog (1974) (also see Marsh 1988, 1989; Widaman 1985): (a) there are at least three traits ($T = 3$) and 3 methods ($M = 3$); (b) $T \times M$ measured variables are used to infer $T + M$ *a priori* factors; (c) each measured variable loads on one trait factor and one method factor but is constrained so as not to load on any other factors; (d) trait/trait correlations and method/method correlations are freely estimated, but trait/method correlations are fixed to be zero; and

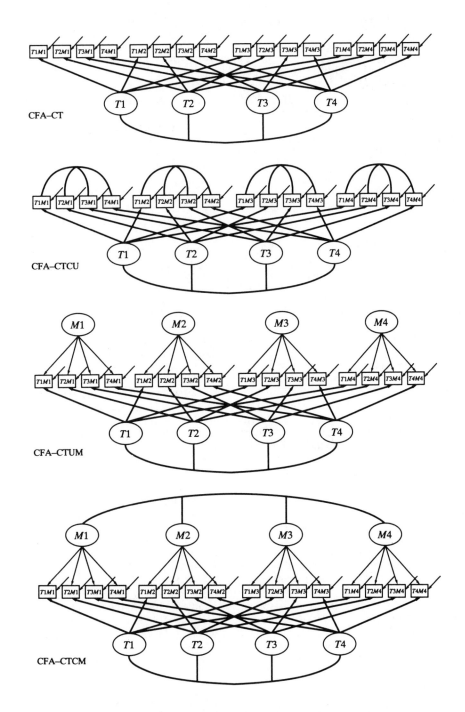

Figure 1
Four confirmatory factor analysis (CFA) models for a design with four traits (*T*) and four methods (*M*).
a Each of the $T \times M = 16$ measured variables (*T*1*M*1, *T*2*M*1, . . . *T*4*M*4) is represented by a single measured variable (the boxes) and the latent trait factors (*T*1, . . . *T*4) and latent method factors (*M*1, . . . *M*4) are represented as ovals. CT = correlated trait model. CTCU = correlated trait/correlated uniqueness model. CTUM = correlated trait/uncorrelated method model. CTCM = correlated trait/correlated method model. (Note: For $T > 3$, CT is nested under the remaining 3 models, and CTUM is nested under CTCM and CTCU. For $T = 3$, CTUM and CTCU are equivalent. There is no nesting relation for CTCM and CTCU.)

(e) the uniqueness of each scale is freely estimated but assumed to be uncorrelated with the uniqueness of other scales.

The CFA–CTCM parameters, so long as the solution is proper, provides unambiguous interpretations of convergent validity, discriminant validity, and method effects: large trait factor loadings support convergent validity, large method factor loadings indicate the existence of method effects, and large trait correlations—particularly those approaching 1.0—indicate a lack of discriminant validity. Also, in standardized form, the squared trait loading, the squared method factor loading, and the error component sum to 1.0 and can be interpreted as components of variance for each score. These effects are not the same as the convergent, discriminant, and method effects inferred from the Campbell–Fiske approach. Consistent with Kenny and Kashy's (1992) (also see Marsh and Grayson 1991) assertion, Campbell and Fiske's original guidelines (1959) (also see Campbell and O'Connell 1982) seemed to be implicitly based on the latent–variable approach embodied in the CFA models. From this perspective, the operationalizations of convergent validity, discriminant validity, and method effects in the CFA approach may better reflect Campbell and Fiske's (1959) original intentions than do their own guidelines.

Researchers have proposed many variations of the CFA–CTCM model and Widaman (1985) developed a taxonomy of models that was subsequently expanded by Marsh (1988, 1989). This taxonomy is designed to be appropriate for all MTMM studies, to provide a general framework for making inferences about the effects of trait and method factors, and to objectify the complicated task of formulating models and representing the MTMM data. Whereas detailed consideration of the taxonomy is beyond the scope of the present investigation (see Marsh 1989), four models (see Fig. 1) are considered that can be recommended as the minimum set of models that should be applied in all CFA/MTMM studies.

The trait-only model (CFA–CT) posits trait factors but no method effects, whereas the remaining models posit trait factors in combination with different representations of method effects. Because the trait-only model is nested under the other CFA models, the comparison of this model with the other models tests for the existence of method effects. Implicit in such tests is Jöreskog's contention that "method effects are what is left over after all trait factors have been eliminated" (1971 p. 128) (also see Marsh 1989).

The model with correlated trait factors but uncorrelated method factors (CFA–CTUM) differs from the CFA–CTCM model only in that correlations among the method factors are constrained to be zero. Hence the comparison of these models tests for correlated trait factors.

In the correlated uniqueness model (CFA–CTCU), method effects are inferred from correlated uniquenesses among measured variables based on the same method instead of being inferred from method factors (see Marsh 1989, Marsh and Bailey 1991, Kenny and Kashy 1992). Like the CFA–CTUM model, the CFA–CTCU model assumes that effects associated with one method are uncorrelated with those associated with different methods. The CFA–CTCU models differs from the CFA–CTCM and CFA–CTUM models in that the latter two models implicitly assume that the method effects associated with a given method can be explained by a single latent method factor (i.e., unidimensional method factors) whereas the correlated uniqueness model does not. This important distinction, however, is only testable when there are at least four traits. When there are three traits, the CFA–CTUM and the CFA–CTCU models are equivalent.

The juxtaposition of the CFA–CTCM, CFA–CTCM, and CFA–CTCU models is important. So long as all three models result in proper solutions, the comparison of CFA–CTUM and CFA–CTCU models tests whether the method effects associated with each method form a unidimensional method factor, whereas the comparison of the CFA–CTUM and CFA–CTCM models tests whether effects associated with different methods are correlated. Because the CFA–CTCU and CFA–CTCM models are not nested, their comparison is more complicated. For example, if both the CFA–CTCM and CFA–CTCU models fit the data substantially better than the CFA–CTUM model, all three models may be wrong: the CFA–CTUM model is wrong because it assumes unidimensional method factors and because it assumes uncorrelated method factors; the CFA–CTCM model is wrong because it assumes unidimensional method factors; the CFA–CTCU model is wrong because it assumes that the effects associated with each method are unrelated to the effects associated with other methods.

From a practical perspective, the most important distinction between the CFA–CTCM, CFA–CTUM and CFA–CTCU models is that the CFA–CTCM model typically results in improper solutions, the CFA–CTUM model often results in an improper solution, and the CFA–CTCU almost always results in proper solutions (Kenny and Kashy 1992, Marsh 1989, Marsh and Bailey 1991; also see Wothke 1987). For example, Marsh and Bailey (1991), using 435 MTMM matrices based on real and simulated data showed that the CFA–CTCM model typically resulted in improper solutions (77% of the time), whereas the CFA–CTCU model nearly always (98% of the time) resulted in well-defined solutions. When both solutions were proper, parameter estimates based on the CFA–CTCU model tended to be more accurate and precise in relation to known parameter values based on simulated data. Even for data specifically constructed to have correlated method effects as posited in the CFA–CTCM model but not the CFA–CTCU model, the CFA–CTCU model was more likely to converge to a proper solution and provided more accurate parameter estimates even though it was not able to fit the data completely, thus indicating that it was not a "true" model. Improper solutions for the CFA–CTUM and particularly the CFA–CTCM models were more likely when the MTMM design was small (i.e., $3T \times 3M$ vs. $5T \times 5M$), when the sample size was small, and when the assumption of unidimensional method effects was violated. From this practical perspective, the advantages in comparing the CFA–CTCM, CFA–CTUM and CFA–CTCU models may be of limited relevance because in many applications only the CFA–CTCU model results in a proper solution.

In conclusion, some recommendations can be offered about the design of CFA MTMM studies. The typical MTMM study is a $3T \times 3M$ design with a sample size of about 125. This design is apparently not adequate for the appropriate application of the CFA approach and may account for some of the problems typically encountered. The minimum sample size should be at least 250 and probably much larger given the apparent instability of CFA MTMM solutions. It may be unrealistic to estimate 6 latent factors from only 9 measured variables. The Marsh and Bailey study (1991) suggests that more stable solutions can be obtained when the number of traits and methods increased at least up to the $7T \times 4M$ and $6T \times 6M$ designs that they considered. Also, the differentiation of models in Fig. 1 requires $T > 3$. For these reasons it is recommended that a minimum of 4 traits and 3 methods be used, although it would preferable to have even more traits and methods. If these minimal recommendations of $T = 4$, $M = 3$, and $N > 250$ cannot be achieved, the CFA approach may not be appropriate and, if pursued anyway, should be interpreted cautiously.

4. Composite Direct Product Model

The CFA models implicitly assume that trait and method effects are additive, but Campbell and O'Connell (1982) suggested that the relation may be multiplicative. Both the additive and multiplicative models posit that correlations between traits measured with the same method will be higher than correlations between traits measured with different methods—a method effect. If this method effect is additive, then the increase in correlation due to this method effect is expected to be of a similar size for large and small correlations. In a multiplicative model, however, the method effects are systematically larger for traits that are more highly correlated, systematically smaller for traits that are less correlated, and zero for traits that are uncorrelated (i.e., the method effect multiplied by zero is zero) Browne (1984) proposed a multiplicative relation between latent trait and method factors in his composite direct product (CDP) model such that:

$$Pc = Pm \times Pt \qquad (1)$$

where Pm is the $(m \times m)$ correlation matrix of

relations among latent method factors with a typical element being $r(Mr, Ms)$, Pt is the $(t \times t)$ correlation matrix of relations among latent trait factors with a typical element being $r(Ti, Tj)$, Pc is the $(mt \times mt)$ correlation matrix of relations among latent variable scores with a typical element being $r(TiMr, TjMs) = r(Ti, Tj)\, r(Mr, Ms)$, and x is the Kronecker product.

Browne's CDP model can be fitted to a typical MTMM matrix and it provides parameter estimates that can be used to evaluate the Campbell–Fiske guidelines (Bagozzi and Yi 1990, Browne 1984, Marsh and Grayson 1991). The CDP model offers a mathematically elegant and parsimonious model of MTMM data. Whereas it has not been applied as widely as the CFA approach, existing research suggests that it typically results in proper solutions. Consistent with Browne's claim, the CDP model provides clear evidence about the Campbell–Fiske guidelines and about convergent and discriminant validity as embodied in these guidelines. The CDP model also provides parameter estimates that are typically consistent with patterns observed in the MTMM matrices. Due in part to its parsimony, it may be reasonable to fit the CDP model in problems that do not meet the minimum recommended standards ($T=4$, $M=3$, $N>250$) in the CFA approach. Therefore, subject to the continued demonstration of its success, the CDP model is recommended—but with some qualifications. In particular, its parsimony is achieved at the expense of implicit assumptions that may be worrisome such as: (a) the convergent validities for all the different traits are equal (i.e., $r[TiM1, TiM2] = r[M1, M2]$ for all values of i); (b) the size of method effects is the same for different traits (i.e., $r[TiMr, TjMs]/r[TiMr, TjMr] = r[Ti, Tj] \times r[Mr, Ms]/r[Ti, Tj] = r[Mr, Ms]$ for all values of i and j); and (c) the size of correlations among traits is the same for all methods (i.e., $r[TiMr, TjMr] = r[Ti, Tj]$ for all values of r). Pt correlations typically reflect the pattern of correlations among traits in the MTMM matrix, but only if this pattern is consistent across methods. Pm correlations typically reflect the extent of agreement between different methods, but only if the agreement is consistent across all traits. Whereas the overall fit of the model provides an indirect test of these assumptions, common sense suggests that they will typically be false so that a more detailed evaluation of the implications of violating these assumptions is needed. Also, because of these implicit invariance constraints, the CDP model does not provide a very useful formative evaluation of specific trait-method units that was the original basis of the MTMM paradigm.

There are also some broader, philosophical concerns about the CDP model. The model is apparently based on an uncritical acceptance of the original Campbell–Fiske guidelines. Thus, for example, Browne (1989) cited the general acceptance of the four Campbell–Fiske requirements for multitrait–multimethod correlation matrices and the CDP focuses specifically on these requriements. Whereas the heuristic value and intent of the Campbell–Fiske guidelines is widely endorsed, there is not widespread agreement that their literal translation as "requirements" as embodied in the CDP model is widely accepted. Whereas the application of the CDP approach certainly provides an objectivity to evaluating the Campbell–Fiske guidelines, it is not clear that the CDP model eliminates widely recognized ambiguities in the interpretation of the Campbell–Fiske guidelines. Furthermore, if the underlying assumption of a multiplicative relation between traits and methods is taken literally, then the logic bases of the Campbell–Fiske guidelines, the application of factor analysis, and even the classical approach to test theory appear to be problematic.

5. Other Considerations

Despite substantial new developments in MTMM analyses, it is not possible in the space available to cover some relevant considerations such as an evaluation of problems with the Campbell–Fiske guidelines, the ANOVA model and extensions presented by Wothke (1987) and Kenny and Kashy (1992), the use of more than one method variable, application of hierarchical CFA (Marsh and Hocevar 1988, Bagozzi and Phillips 1991), and the inclusion of external validity criteria in addition to the MTMM variables (Marsh 1989).

6. Summary and Implications

MTMM data has an inherently complicated structure that will not be fully described in all applications by any of the models or approaches considered here. There is, apparently, no "right" way to analyze MTMM data that works in all situations. Instead, it is recommended that researchers consider several alternative approaches to evaluating MTMM data—an initial inspection of the MTMM matrix using the Campbell–Fiske guidelines followed by fitting at least the subset of CFA models in Fig. 1 and the CDP model. The Campbell–Fiske guidelines should be used primarily for formative purposes, the CDP seems most appropriate as a summative tool, and the CFA models apparently serve both summative and formative purposes. It is, however, important that researchers understand the strengths and weaknesses of the different approaches. The appropriate interpretation of MTMM data requires an interplay between theory, measurement, and statistical methods. Despite the inherent complexity of MTMM data, the combination of common sense, a stronger theoretical emphasis on the design of MTMM studies, a stronger emphasis on the quality of measurement at the level of trait-method units, an appropriate arsenal of analytical tools such as these recommended here, and a growing understanding of these analytic

tools will allow researchers to use the MTMM design effectively.

See also: Validity; Exploratory Data Analysis)

References

Bagozzi R P, Yi L 1990 Assessing method variance in multitrait–multimethod matrices: The case of self-reported affect and perceptions at work. *J. Appl. Psychol.* 75: 547–60

Bagozzi R P, Phillips L 1991 Assessing construct validity in organizational research. *Adm. Sci. Q.* 36: 421–58

Browne M W 1984 The decomposition of multitrait–multimethod matrices. *Br. J. Math. S. Psychol.* 37: 1–21

Browne M W 1989 Relationships between an additive model and a multiplicative model for multitrait–multimethod matrices. In: Coppi R, Bolasco S (eds.) 1989 *Multiway Data Analysis.* North-Holland, Amsterdam

Byrne B M, Shavelson R J 1986 On the structure of adolescent self-concept. *J. Educ. Psychol.* 78: 474–81

Campbell D T, Fiske D W 1959 Convergent and discriminant validation by multitrait–multimethod matrix. *Psych. Bull.* 56(2): 81–105

Campbell D T, O'Connell E J 1982 Methods as diluting trait relationships rather than adding irrelevant systematic variance. In: Brinberg D, Kidder L H (eds.) 1982 *New Directions for Methodology of Social and Behavioral Science: Forms of Validity in Research.* Jossey-Bass, San Francisco, California

Jöreskog K G 1971 Statistical analyses of sets of congeneric tests. *Psychometrika* 36(2): 109–33

Jöreskog K G 1974 Analyzing psychological data by structural analysis of covariance matrices. In: Atkinson R C, Krantz D H, Luce R D, Suppes P (eds.) 1974 *Contemporary Developments in Mathematical Psychology,* Vol. 2. W H Freeman, San Francisco, California

Kenny D A, Kashy D A 1992 Analysis of the multitrait–multimethod matrix by confirmatory factor analysis. *Psych. Bull.* 112: 165–72

Marsh H W 1988 Multitrait–multimethod analyses. In: Keeves J P (ed.) 1988 *Educational Research Methodology, Measurement and Evaluation: An International Handbook.* Pergamon Press, Oxford

Marsh H W 1989 Confirmatory factor analyses of multitrait–multimethod data: Many problems and a few solutions. *App. Psychol. Meas.* 13(4): 335–61

Marsh H W, Balla J, McDonald R P 1988 Goodness-of-fit indices in confirmatory factor analysis: The effect of sample size. *Psych. Bull.* 103: 391–410

Marsh H W, Hocevar D 1988 A new, more powerful approach to multitrait–multimethod analyses: Application of second-order confirmatory factor analysis. *J. Appl. Psychol.* 73: 107–17

Marsh H W, Bailey M 1991 Confirmatory factor analysis of multitrait–multimethod data: A comparison of alternative models. *Appl. Psychol. Meas.* 15(1): 47–70

Marsh H W, Grayson D 1991 *Multitrait–Multimethod Data: An Evaluation of Five Analytic Approaches.* ERIC Document No. ED342 797, Washington, DC

Widaman K F 1985 Hierarchically nested covariance structure models for multitrait–multimethod data. *Appl. Psychol. Meas.* 9: 1–26

Wothke W 1987 *The Estimation of Trait and Method Components in Multitrait–Multimethod Measurement.* ERIC, Washington, DC

Further Reading

Alwin D F 1974 Approaches to the interpretation of relationships and the multitrait–multimethod matrix. In: Costner H L (ed.) 1974 *Sociological Methodology 1973–74.* Jossey-Bass, San Francisco, California

Browne M W, Cudeck R 1989 Single-sample cross-validation indices for covariance structures. *Multivariate Behavioral Research* 24: 445–55

Cudeck R 1988 Multiplicative models and MTMM matrices. *J. Educ. Stat.* 13: 131–47

Graham J W, Collins N L 1991 Controlling correlations bias via confirmatory factor analysis of MTMM data. *Multivariate Behavioral Research* 26(4): 607–29 ·

McDonald R P, Marsh H W 1990 Choosing a multivariate model: Noncentrality and goodness-of-fit. *Psych. Bull.* 107: 247–55

Millsap R E 1990 A cautionary note on the detection of method variance in multitrait–multimethod data. *J. Appl. Psychol.* 75: 350–53

Schmitt N, Stults D M 1986 Methodology review: Analysis of multitrait–multimethod matrices. *Appl. Psychol. Meas.* 10: 1–22

Sullivan J L, Feldman S 1979 *Multiple Indicators: An Introduction.* Sage, Beverly Hills, California

Wothke W, Browne M W 1990 The direct product model for the MTMM matrix parameterized as a second order factor analysis model. *Psychometrika* 55: 255–62

Nonparametric and Distribution-free Statistics

M. Cooper

Statistical inference methods most commonly taught and employed in educational research assume a knowledge of the nature of the probability distributions of variables in the populations from which samples are drawn. Tests of significance used when making statistical inferences very often depend on the assumption of an underlying normal distribution, although other underlying distributions, such as those of Student's *t* or Fisher's *F*, are sometimes assumed instead. In practice, however, situations often arise where little is really known about the nature of the distribution of a variable in the population, or where the distribution in the sample suggests that the usual assumption about the distribution in the population is untenable. Under these circumstances it may be desirable to use what is known as a "distribution-free" statistical procedure.

In educational research, distinctions should be made between variables according to the properties of the measurements that can be made on the variables. Measurement usually provides data in one of four classes: nominal, ordinal, interval, and ratio (see *Measurement in Research Education*). Nonparametric statistical procedures are appropriately used with nominal and ordinal data. Subject to certain assumptions, "classical" parametric statistical procedures are applicable to interval and ratio data. However, it has been shown that nonparametric procedures can sometimes be used very effectively in situations where parametric procedures would normally be applied. In such cases, the interval and ratio data are reduced to a form that is compatible with methods which are appropriate for nominal and ordinal data.

There are two major classes of nonparametric statistical procedures. The first class employs only the sign properties of the data, and all observations above a chosen fixed value are assigned a "plus" or a unit value (1) while all those at or below the fixed value are assigned a "minus" or a zero value (0). The second class of nonparametric techniques uses the rank properties of the data, and all observations are assigned a rank-order value. The subsequent statistical procedures involve the making of inferences based on the ranks assigned. It is evident that when nonparametric methods are applied to interval and ratio data, only part of the information available is used. Although it was initially believed that a heavy price would be paid for the loss of efficiency in the application of a statistical test under these conditions, there may be gains made in the robustness and validity of the test employed. This is particularly true where small samples are being used or where little is known about the underlying population distribution of the variable under investigation.

1. Methods

The terms "nonparametric" and "distribution-free" tend to be used interchangeably. A nonparametric test is, generally speaking, one in which no hypothesis is made about the value of a parameter in a statistical density function. In many so-called "nonparametric tests," the value of the test statistics is derived from ranks or frequencies, which are sample-dependent quantities that cannot be specified by a single observation. The distribution of the observation characteristic used in such a test thus tends to be discrete and specifiable exactly; this makes the test free of the distribution of the population from which the observations were drawn.

Because nonparametric tests use neither ratio nor interval data, they do not test directly for parameters calculated from magnitudes. Rather, tests using ranks and frequencies test for relationships between parameters such as medians and proportions. Many of the more common classical, parametric tests that are appropriately used with ratio or interval data have nonparametric analogues for use with ordinal or categorical data.

Most tests using ordinal data are based on expressions applicable to unbroken sequences of positive integers. Tied observations therefore render such tests somewhat inaccurate, and corrections have to be applied.

A number of nonparametric tests are based on discrete sampling distributions constructed by Fisher's method of randomization. In a typical two-sample test, the test statistic might be the sum S_i of the N_i ranks in sample i. In Fisher's technique, the value of S_i for each of the possible N $N_1 + N_{2}C_{Ni}$ combinations of the data is found, and the distribution of S_i is formed. Under the assumption of equal probability of occurrence of each such combination, the corresponding probability distribution is determined. The statistical test then involves finding the combined probability of occurrence of the rank-sum associated with the data and of any rank-sum that is equally or more extreme, and comparing this "exact probability" with the level of significance.

Since the distributions of many test statistics approach normality when samples are large, exact probability tests usually have associated large-sample tests based on the normal or chi-squared distributions.

The first application of a nonparametric technique appears to have been when Arbuthnott (1710) used the "sign test." This test is based on the binomial distribution developed by Bernoulli in 1713 which, as de Moivre showed in 1733, approaches the normal distribution when samples are large in size. Brief details of a number of nonparametric tests are presented below.

2. Correlation Coefficients

There are two general classes of correlation coefficient used in nonparametric statistics: those dealing with variables measured ordinally and those for use with categorical data (see *Correlational Procedures in Data Analysis*).

2.1 Ordinal Data

When two variables, X and Y, are measured by ranks, either Spearman's "correlation coefficient" or Kendall's "correlation index" may be used to indicate the intercorrelation of X and Y. Spearman's so-called "coefficient" is essentially the Pearson coefficient calculated on the basis of ranks instead of interval data. Assuming no tied observations, Spearman's formula provides a quick way of calculating the coefficient. If the difference of ranks for subject i is represented by d_i, Spearman's formula (ρ_s) is given (assuming no tied observations) by

$$\rho_s = 1 - 6\Sigma d_i / (N^3 - N) \tag{1}$$

where N is the size of the sample. The hypothesis of independence may be tested using Fisher's method of randomization, ρ_s being calculated for each pair of rank sets possible for the given N. For large samples, the standard normal deviate, z, may be used as the test statistic. This is given by

$$z = [1 - 6\Sigma d_i] / [N(N + 1) (N - 1)^{1/2}] \tag{2}$$

Kendall's index of rank correlation, τ, is based on his general theory of rank correlation. For subject i, an indicator variable a_i is assigned the value $+1$, 0, or -1 depending on whether performance on one variable is better, equal, or worse than that on the other. The formula for τ is

$$\tau = \Sigma a_i / N_{C2} \tag{3}$$

The sampling distribution of τ is constructed by Fisher's method of randomization. When samples are large, it approaches normality with zero mean and variance equal to $N(N - 1) (2N + 5) / 18$ (Kendall 1970).

2.2 Categorical Data

If both variables are dichotomies, the appropriate correlation index is either the phi coefficient, φ, or Goodman's 8 index. The absolute value of φ ranges from 0 to 1, and is essentially that of the Pearson coefficient calculated on the basis of nominal unit- and zero-values instead of interval data. When data are summarized in a 2×2 contingency table, φ is given by

$$\phi = (f_{00}f_{11} - f_{01}f_{10}) / (\text{product of marginals})^{1/2} \tag{4}$$

where f_{ij} is the frequency associated with category i of one variable and category j of the other. The ϕ statistic is related to discrete X^2 by the expression $\phi^2 = X^2/N$. The value of Goodman's 8 index, which is not restricted to the -1 to 1 range, is given by

$$8 = ln [(f_{00}f_{11}) / f_{01}f_{10}] \tag{5}$$

When either variable has more than two categories (say I categories in one variable and J in the other), correlation may be measured by the mean-squared contingency coefficient, M, or by Cramer's index, V. Both are related to X^2:

$$M^2 = X^2 / [X^2 + N]$$

$$\text{and } V^2 = X^2 / X^2 / [N \min(I - 1, J - 1)] \tag{6}$$

For those indexes related to X^2, this statistic may be used to test the hypothesis of independence with reference to the continuous chi-squared distribution, with $(I - 1)(J - 1)$ degrees of freedom. The general formula for X^2 is often replaced by a formula that is specific to the particular statistical design involved. In many cases, Yates's correction for continuity is applied so that discrete data may be tested by reference to the continuous chi-squared distribution.

2.3 Coefficient of Concordance

Kendall's coefficient of concordance (W) may be used with a single sample as an indicator of the relationship among many ordinally measured variables. For this procedure, each subject is ranked across all variables, a rank sum for each variable being obtained. W is the ratio of the sum of squares among the rank totals to the sum of squares that would be obtained if all subjects were to rank identically across all variables.

If the rank sum for variable j is T_j, a formula for W is

$$W = \{(12\Sigma T_j^2) / (N^2 K[K^2-1])\}-3(K+1) / (K-1) \tag{7}$$

where N subjects are ranked across K variables (Kendall 1970).

3. Two Independent Samples

Nonparametric analogues of Student's t test for independent samples include the Mann–Whitney (Wilcoxon) test, the normal scores tests, and Fisher's exact test.

3.1 Mann–Whitney (Wilcoxon) Test

For this test, all subjects are ranked across both samples, the rank sum for one sample being determined.

If this sample contains N_1 of N subjects, Fisher's method of randomization may be used to determine a value of the rank sum T_1 for each of the $^NC_{N_1}$ possible sets of N_1 ranks selected from the N ranks available. Under the assumption that all such sets have equal probability of occurrence, the probability distribution for T_1 may be determined.

The Mann–Whitney version of the test employs the statistic U, defined as $\min(U_1, U_2)$ where, for sample i,

$$U_i = T_i - \tfrac{1}{2}N_i(N_i + 1) \tag{8}$$

For large samples, a normal approximation is available, where

$$z = [U - \tfrac{1}{2}N_1 N_2] / [N_1 N_2(N_1 + N_2 + 1) / 12]^{1/2} \tag{9}$$

Where there are tied observations, a correction term may be applied (Hays 1973 p. 780).

3.2 Normal Scores Tests

Under certain conditions, greater power may be achieved by the substitution of normal scores for ranks (Marascuilo and McSweeney 1977).

The van der Waerden test replaces ranks with inverse normal scores. For rank i, the inverse normal score W_i is the value of z corresponding to the $100i/(N+1)$ centile point in the normal distribution, there being N subjects in both samples combined. The sum, s, of the W_i in one sample is the test statistic. Fisher's method of randomization may be used to construct a sampling distribution of s. Under the assumption of equal probability of occurrence of each set of normal scores, the probability distribution for s may be determined. For large N, a normal approximation is available, where

$$z = s / \{[N_1 N_2 / N(N - 1)]\Sigma W_i^2\}^{1/2} \tag{10}$$

The Terry–Hoeffding test uses the expected values of the corresponding normal-order statistic, usually referred to as expected normal scores, E_i. These have been likened (Marascuilo and McSweeney 1977) to the best guess as to the value of the original scores as reconstructed from the ranks. The sum, s, of the E_i in one sample is the test statistic. The sampling distribution of s is constructed as for the van der Waerden test. For large N, the normal deviate may be used, z being given by

$$z = s / \{[N_1 N_2 / N(N - 1)]\Sigma W_i^2\}^{1/2} \tag{11}$$

The Bell–Doksum test employs random normal scores and may be used with large samples only. N values of z are randomly selected from normal distribution tables, ordered, and matched with the ordered ranks 1 to N. In each sample, each rank is replaced by the corresponding random normal score. The test statistic is standardized from

$$z = [(S_1/N_1) + (S_2/N_2)]/[(1/N_1) + (1/N_2)]^{1/2} \tag{12}$$

3.3 Fisher's Exact Test

Fisher's exact test may be used when two independent populations are dichotomized on a particular characteristic. If X_i of the N_i subjects in sample i have the characteristic, the proportion having it in population i is estimated by $p_i = x_i/N_i$. The probability of occurrence of (x_1, x_2) given their sum, based on the hypergeometric distribution, is

$$P[(x_1,x_2) \mid x_1 + x_2]=\,^{N_1}C_{x_1}\,^{N_2}C_{x_2} / \,^{N_1+N_2}C_{x_1+x_2} \tag{13}$$

A probability distribution associated with the set of all $x_1 x_2$ possible pairs, given N_1 and N_2 and holding x_1+x_2 constant, is constructed and used for testing the hypothesis $p_1=p_2$, or $p_1-p_2 = 0$. Modifications to Fisher's exact test, that allow for the difference between the actual P-value and the level of significance (due to the discrete nature of the distribution), have been proposed by Overall (1980) and by Tochter (1950). For large samples, a normal approximation is available, where $z = (\hat{p}_1 - \hat{p}_2) / \{\hat{p}_0(1 - \hat{p}_0)[(1/N_1) + (1/N_2)]\}^{1/2}$, $\hat{p}_0$ being given by $\hat{p}_0 = (x_1 + x_2)/(N_1 + N_2)$.

The two-sample median test is an application of Fisher's exact test, in which lying above (or below) the median is the characteristic of interest. Observations lying at the median may be discarded, or assigned to cells so as to make the test more conservative, or less.

3.4 Other Tests

Included among two-sample tests is a number which will not be elaborated upon here. Examples are the Kolmogorov–Smirnov test for goodness of fit, the Wald–Wolfowitz runs test, and the Moses test of extreme reactions (Siegel 1956).

4. Matched-pairs Tests

If observation j in sample 1 is X_j, the match in sample 2 being Y_j, the difference is $d_j = X_j - Y_j$. The test statistic for the sign test, previously mentioned, $S = \Sigma(d_j \mid d_j > 0)$, has a binomial probability distribution.

The Cox–Stuart (1955) S_2 and S_3 tests for monotonic increase (or decrease) in a sequence of observations are an extension of the sign test, where corresponding observations in earlier and later sections of the sequence form the matched pairs.

For the Wilcoxon matched-pairs signed-ranks test, pair j is assigned a "signed rank" $r_j = a_j R_j$, where $a_j = 1$ if $d_j > 0$, $a_j = -1$ if $d_j \leqslant 0$, and R_j is the rank of $|d_j|$ in the set of absolute observation differences. The absolute sums of the positive and negative signed ranks are T_P and T_N (or T_+ and T_-), respectively. Either is used as the test statistic. The probability distribution of T_P or T_N is determined by Fisher's randomization method. For large numbers (N) of paired-observations, the test statistic for the normal approximation is

$$z = [T_P - \tfrac{1}{4}N(N+1)]/[N(N+1)(2N+1)/24]^{1/2} \qquad (14)$$

In a normal-scores version of the Wilcoxon test, positive normal scores are assigned to the unsigned ranks and re-signed according to the signs of the ranks. The test statistic is $T_P = \Sigma W_j \mid W_j > 0$, where W_j is the signed normal score for pair j. The exact test is based on Fisher's method of randomization, the normal approximation for large N uses

$$z = (2T_P - \Sigma W_j) / (\Sigma W_j^2)^{1/2} \qquad (15)$$

(Marascuilo and McSweeney 1977)

5. Tests for Many Independent Samples

Nonparametric analogues of the classical one-way analysis-of-variance F test include the Kruskal–Wallis test, normal scores versions, and a test for homogeneity of k proportions (Marascuilo and McSweeney 1977).

5.1 k-sample Normal-scores Tests

For the Kruskal–Wallis test, all N observations are ranked across all k samples. The test statistic, which is approximately distributed as chi-squared with $k-1$ degrees of freedom, is

$$H = [12\Sigma(S_j^2 / N_j)/N(N + 1)] - 3(N + 1) \qquad (16)$$

where S_j is the sum of the N_j ranks in sample j. Scheffé-like post hoc procedures are available, as are tests for polynomial trend. Tobach et al. (1967) have evolved a post hoc procedure for use with small samples. Steele (1960) has proposed post hoc procedures for pairwise comparisons, in which two-sample Wilcoxon tests may be used at the $2a/k(k-1)$ level of significance. Bradley (1968) has presented a method of collapsing data in a factorial design so that the Kruskal–Wallis test may be used to test for main and interaction effects.

5.2 Multi-sample Normal-scores Tests

The ranks in the Kruskal–Wallis design may be replaced by normal scores, the test statistic for this test being

$$W = (N - 1)\Sigma(S_j^2/N_j)T \qquad (17)$$

where S_j is the sum of the N_j normal scores in sample j and T is the sum of all N squared normal-scores. Scheffé-like post hoc procedures are available (Marascuilo and McSweeney 1977).

5.3 Homogeneity of Proportions

The design used for the two-sample Fisher exact test may be extended to k independent samples each dichotomized on a characteristic of interest. The hypothesis of homogeneity of proportions having the characteristic may be tested by use of chi-squared. The multi-population median test is an application. Post hoc procedures are available, as are tests for polynomial trend. When samples are small, an arcsine transformation may be applied to the proportions, the test statistics being

$$U_0 = \sum_j N_j \,[\hat{\phi} - (\Sigma N_j \hat{\phi}_j)/\Sigma N_j]^{1/2} \qquad (18)$$

where

$$\hat{\phi}_j = 2 \sin^{-1} \hat{p}_j^{\,1/2}[0 < \hat{p} < 1] \qquad (19)$$

$\hat{p}_j$ being the proportion of the N_j subjects in sample j having the characteristic (Marascuilo and McSweeney 1977).

5.4 Homogeneity of Vectors of Proportions/Frequencies

Vectors of proportions, each vetor deriving from a distinct population may be tested using the chi-squared test. When the frequencies relate to the same ordered categories of a dependent variable—such as measured by means of a Likert scale, Marascuilo and Dagenais (1982) have proposed post hoc procedures following a Kruskal-Wallis test of the hypothesis of homogeneity.

5.5 Multivariate Analysis of Variance

A nonparametric analogue of one-way multivariate analysis of variance has been proposed by Katz and McSweeney (1980). Two post hoc procedures are provided; one, the multivariate Scheffé-like technique, allows examination of as many contrasts as desired, the overall error rate being established at a specified value for the entire set. The other, the univariate Scheffé-like technique, limits examination to within-variable contrasts.

5.6 Analysis of Covariance

Techniques for the analysis of data in a k-sample design with p dependent variables and q covariates have been proposed by Quade (1967), Puri and Sen (1971), and McSweeney and Porter (see Marascuilo and McSweeney 1977). All use ranks; the second may also be based on normal scores.

In the Quade test, observations for each variable are ranked across all subjects, the ranks being subjected to linear regression techniques to generate errors of estimate, which are then subjected to conventional analysis of variance. The McSweeney–Porter test, which has approximately the same power as the Quade test, performs conventional analysis of covariance on the ranks.

6. Repeated Measures

6.1 The Friedman Model

The Friedman test may be used to test for homogeneity of mean ranks in a one-way design in which N subjects are each ranked over k occasions. The test statistic, which is associated with $k-1$ degrees of freedom, is

$$X^2 = [12\Sigma T_j^2 / Nk(k + 1)] - 3N(k + 1) \qquad (20)$$

where T_j is the rank-sum for occasion j. Scheffé-like post hoc procedures are available.

A normal-scores version (Marascuilo and McSweeney 1977) is also available. Marascuilo and McSweeney (1977 p.369) advocate a multiple matched-pair Wilcoxon test as being much superior to the Friedman test when only simple contrasts are to be examined.

6.2 Tests for Change

Among tests for change in behavior, in which a sample is measured on a categorical variable on two occasions, are the Bowker and McNemar tests. The former, used for dichotomous variables, is based on the binomial distribution; the latter uses a chi-squared statistic.

The Cochran Q test is an extension of the McNemar test in which N subjects are measured on k occasions on a dichotomous variable giving scores of 0 or 1. The test statistic is

$$Q = [k(k - 1) \Sigma (T_j - T/k)^2] / (k \Sigma S_i - \Sigma S_i^2) \qquad (21)$$

where T_j is the sum of observations for example j, S_i is the total score for subject i, and T is the total score for the sample. Scheffé-like post hoc procedures exist (Marascuilo and McSweeney 1977).

7. Nonparametric Tests in Blocking Designs

7.1 Two-sample Tests

In the Hodges–Lehmann test, scores are replaced by deviations from block means. These deviations are then ranked across all N subjects, thus "aligning" the observations. If S of the n_i subjects in block i are in sample A, the sum of their S_i ranks being W_i, the test statistic is $W = \Sigma W_i$. A sampling distribution of W may be formed by a tedious method of randomization, leading to an exact test. In block i, the expected value, E_i, and variance, V_i, of W_i are

$$E_i = S_i \Sigma (R_{ij} / N_i) \qquad (22)$$

and

$$V_i = [S_i(N_i - S_i)/(N_i - 1)]\{[\Sigma R_{ij}^2)/N_i] - [(\Sigma(R_{ij}^2)/N_i]^2\} \qquad (23)$$

For the normal approximation for large samples, therefore, the test statistic is

$$z = (W - \Sigma E_i) / \Sigma V_i \qquad (24)$$

A correction for continuity may be applied.

A test referred to by Marascuilo and McSweeney (1977) as a "multiple Wilcoxon test" may be used as an alternative. Here, observations are ranked within blocks, ranks for sample B being discarded. For this large-sample test, the expected value, E_i, and variance, V_i, are

$$E_i = \tfrac{1}{2}S_i(N_i + 1) \qquad (25)$$

and

$$V_i = S_i(N_i + 1) (N_i - S_i) / 12 \qquad (26)$$

7.2 Multi-sample Tests

For the k-sample design with b blocks, an extension of the Hodges–Lehmann test may be used. The test statistic, which is distributed approximately as chi-squared with k-1 degrees of freedom, is

$$W = b^2(N - 1) \Sigma[R_j - \tfrac{1}{2}(N + 1)]^2 /k\Sigma V_i \qquad (27)$$

where R_j is the mean rank for sample j, N is the total number of subjects, and V_i is the variance of the ranks in block i. Post hoc simultaneous confidence intervals may be constructed.

Alternatively, Marascuilo and McSweeney (1977) present a technique in which ranks in the above test are replaced by normal scores.

8. Nonparametric Tests for Interaction

8.1 Multi-sample Design with Two Dichotomous Variables

When subjects in a k-sample design are classified on two dichotomous variables, a series of k 2×2 tables results. If a proportion, $\hat{p}_{ij}$, of subjects in sample j are classified into the first category of the first variable and the ith category of the second, the difference of the proportions is $\hat{D}_j = \hat{p}_{1j} - \hat{p}_{2j}$. Homogeneity of the D_j, indicating no interaction, may be tested by means of a chi-squared test. Components of interaction in the populations may then be identified by means of post hoc procedures.

8.2 Second-order Interaction in a One-sample Design

Interaction involving a multicategory variable (A) and two dichotomies (B and C) on which a single sample is classified may be tested by means of a chi-squared test. If a proportion, $\hat{p}_{ijk}$ of the subjects in category k of A are classified into category i of B and category j of C, a measure of the association of B and C in A_k is Goodman's index of association (8), estimated by

$$\hat{8}_k = \ln(\hat{p}_{11k}\hat{p}_{22k}\hat{p}_{12k}\hat{p}_{21k}) \tag{28}$$

The hypothesis for the test of second-order interaction is that of homogeneity of 8 across all categories of A (Marascuilo and McSweeney 1977).

9. Relative Efficiency of Nonparametric Tests

Many of the nonparametric analogues of classical tests have high relative efficiency. The Mann–Whitney (Wilcoxon) test, the Wilcoxon signed-ranks test, and the Kruskal–Wallis test, for example, all have an asymptotic relative efficiency (ARE) of about 0.955 relative to their analogues when assumptions of normality and homogeneity of variance hold for the parametric test (Marascuilo and McSweeney 1977). When underlying distributions are non-normal, the efficiency is never below 0.864 and can exceed unity. Blair and Higgins (1980) report that the Wilcoxon rank-sum test generally holds "very large power advantages" over the t-test. The substitution of normal scores for ranks can boost the efficiency considerably.

10. Computer Packages

The NPAR TESTS subprogram of the *Statistical Package for the Social Sciences* (Nie et al. 1975) offers analysis for a number of the more common techniques. The program BMDP3S from the *Biomedical Computer Programs* (Dixon 1975) provides analysis for a few procedures. Perhaps the most comprehensive set of user-interactive nonparametric computer routines is available in EZSTAT (Cooper 1992).

See also: Significance Testing; Bayesian Statistics; Descriptive Data, Analysis of

References

Arbuthnott J 1710 An argument for Divine Providence, taken from the constant regularity observ'd in the births of both sexes. *Philosophical Transactions* 27:186–90

Blair R C, Higgins J J 1980 A comparison of the power of Wilcoxon's rank-sum statistic to that of Student's t statistic under various nonnormal distributions. *J. Educ. Stat.* 5:309–66

Bradley J V 1968 *Distribution-free Statistical Tests*. Prentice-Hall, Englewood Cliffs, New Jersey

Cooper M 1992 EZSTAT: *Nonparametric Section*. School of Education Studies, University of New South Wales, Sydney

Cox D R, Stuart A 1955 Some quick tests for trend in location and dispersion. *Biometrika* 42:80–95

Dixon W J (ed.) 1975 BMDP: *Biomedical Computer Programs*. University of California Press, Berkeley, California

Hays W L 1973 *Statistics for the Social Sciences*, 2nd edn. Holt, Rinehart and Winston, New York

Katz B M, McSweeney M 1980 A multivariate Kruskal–Wallis test with post hoc procedures. *Multivariate Behav. Res.* 15:281–97

Kendall M G 1970 *Rank Correlation Methods*, 4th edn. Griffin, London

Marascuilo L A, McSweeney M 1977 *Nonparametric and Distribution-free Methods for the Social Sciences*. Brooks-Cole, Monterey, California

Marascuilo L A, Dagenais F 1982 Planned and post hoc comparisons for tests of homogeneity where the dependent variable is categorical and ordered. *Educ. Psychol. Meas.* 42:777–81

Nie N H, Hull C H, Jenkins J G, Steinbrenner K, Bent D H 1975 *Statistical Package for the Social Sciences*. McGraw-Hill, New York

Overall J E 1980 Continuity correction for Fisher's exact probability test. *J. Educ. Stat.* 5:177–90

Puri M L, Sen P K 1971 *Nonparametric Methods in Multivariate Analysis*. Wiley, New York

Quade D 1967 Rank analysis of covariance. *J. Am. Stat. Ass.* 62:1187–200

Siegel S 1956 *Nonparametric Statistics for the Behavioral Sciences*. McGraw-Hill, New York

Steele R G D 1960 A rank-sum test comparing all pairs of treatments. *Technometrics* 2:197–207

Tobach E, Smith M, Rose G, Richter D 1967 A table for making rank and sum multiple paired comparisons. *Technometrics* 9:561–67

Tochter K D 1950 Extension of Neyman–Pearson theory of tests to discontinuous variates. *Biometrika* 37:130–44

Partial Order Scalogram Analysis

S. Shye

Partial order scalogram analysis (POSA) or the more specific partial order scalogram analysis by base coordinates (POSAC) is a multivariate data analytic technique for processing and graphically depicting nonmetric data. Specifically, POSAC is used for scaling individuals by the smallest number of scales logically consistent with the complexity of the data (Shye 1985). It is characterized by its focus on order relations that exist among objects, where the objects, in most usages, are the score profiles of individual subjects to be scaled. When analyzing a set of objects, the term "order relations" means that in some well-defined sense, any one of the following relations holds:

(a) Object A is comparable to object B (in symbols: A $\lesssim$ B); then further specification should tell whether:

   (i)   A is greater than B (A>B); or
   (ii) A is equal to B (A=B); or
   (iii) A is smaller than B (A<B).

(b) Object A is incomparable to object B (in symbols A $\nlessgtr$ B).

The POSAC technique is employed in order to scale individual subjects according to the smallest number of scales logically consistent with the complexity of the attribute (e.g., intelligence, social adaptability). Hence POSAC is an extension of the unidimensional scale known as the Guttman scale (Guttman 1950) to configurations of higher dimensionalities. Much of the mathematical development of POSAC and all of its published applications have been so far with respect to two-dimensional scalogram configurations.

The geometrical depiction afforded by POSAC yields the following desiderata for empirical data:

(a) a new profile, of shorter length (fewer scores) than the original one, is assigned to every individual;

(b) the possibility of abstracting fewer (and possibly more "fundamental") variables for the contents investigated.

Partial order scalogram analysis has been referred to as "nonmetric factor analysis" by Coombs and his associates in their works on partial order models (Coombs and Kao 1955, Coombs 1964). Guttman observed that POSA is a special case of his multi-dimensional scalogram analysis (Shye 1978, Zvulun 1978) and applied it to attitude research and content classification problems (Guttman 1954, 1959, 1972). Since then POSAC has been employed in various social studies (e.g., Shye and Elizur 1976). Mathematical studies of POSA and of its relationship to smallest space analysis (SSA) have been carried out by Shye (1976, 1985) (see *Smallest Space Analysis*). A specially developed computer program, POSAC/LSA, permits the processing of empirical data by computing the best two-dimensional configuration. Along with smallest space analysis and other nonmetric procedures, POSAC belongs to the family of intrinsic data analysis methods advocated by facet theory (Shye 1978, Shye et al. 1994).

This entry covers the following: (a) an illustration of the essential idea of POSAC; (b) a mathematical formulation of partial order scalograms; and (c) the uses of POSAC for scaling individuals and for interpreting derived scales.

1. The Essential Idea of POSA: An Illustration

Each individual in a particular population may be observed as to whether he or she possesses each of three traits, T_1, T_2, T_3. An individual receives a score $T_1 = 1$ if he or she possesses trait T_1 and $T_1 = 0$ if not, and similarly for T_2 and T_3. A profile 101, for example, would be assigned to an individual who is observed to possess traits T_1 and T_3 but not T_2. If the three specific traits conceptually represent a single general trait such as health (or sociability, or intelligence, or any other), then an individual with profile 011 may be said to be healthier (or more sociable, etc.) than the one with profile 010 because he or she has all the specific health traits of the latter ($T_2 = 1$) as well as additional one(s) ($T_3 = 1$). Hence 011 and 010 are comparable profiles. These relationships between the two profiles can be represented schematically by a directed graph thus:

$$010$$

$$\downarrow$$

$$011$$

If in a given set of profiles all profile pairs are comparable, the set constitutes a perfect scale or a Guttman scale. For example,

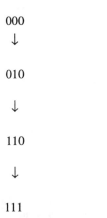

000

↓

010

↓

110

↓

111

However, two individuals with profiles 110 and 011 are incomparable with respect to their health because the specific health traits of each are different: the former exceeds the latter in one trait (T_1) but falls short of the latter in another trait (T_3). For the same reason, 110 and 001 are incomparable (even though 110 has two specific health traits and 001 only one). (In this analysis the specific traits are not assumed to be of equal weight; in fact their relative weights may be unknown or undefined.)

In a schematic representation, incomparability between profiles is characterized by the absence of a directed line between them. The relations among the four profiles 010, 011, 110, and 001 are representable thus:

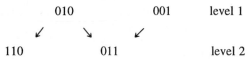

| 010 | | 001 | level 1 |
| 110 | 011 | | level 2 |

In such partial order diagrams it is customary and helpful to locate all profiles having a similar total score (i.e., the sum of the scores on all tests—here the number of traits possessed) on the same horizontal level of the

scalogram. This permits the omission of the arrowheads without causing misunderstanding: the line segments are assumed to point downwards.

In POSA the absence of profiles from the empirical data is presumed to reflect something about the structure of the investigated traits for the population in question. Such absence can often lead to a more economic representation of the data.

For example, in studying a particular population with respect to the three dichotomous traits T_1, T_2, and T_3 the following profiles have been observed:

	T_1	T_2	T_3
profile a	0	0	0
profile b	0	0	1
profile c	0	1	0
profile d	1	0	0
profile e	0	1	1
profile f	1	1	0
profile g	1	1	0

In this list the profile 101 is missing. Under appropriate experimental conditions and with certain assumptions, this may mean that this profile is impossible; in other words, that the mechanism investigated is such that the occurrence of $T_1 = 1$ and $T_3 = 1$ implies the occurrence of $T_2 = 1$. This structural interdependence among the three traits permits a simplification in the data representation in that the order relations among observed profiles can be represented in a two-dimensional space (see Fig. 1) instead of a three-dimensional space, which three traits are expected to produce when they are not interdependent.

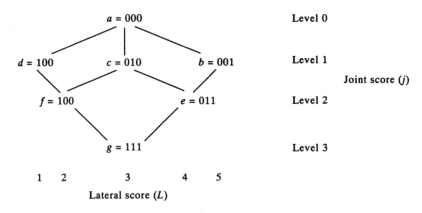

Figure 1

A two-dimensional partial order configuration of three dichotomous traits. Note that if the location of any two profiles (say, 100 and 010) were interchanged, lines would cross

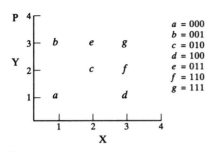

P

Y

X

a = 000
b = 001
c = 010
d = 100
e = 011
f = 110
g = 111

Figure 2
Minimum space diagram for profiles *a* through *g*

That the configuration is indeed two-dimensional is evidenced by the fact that the diagram could be drawn without crossings among the line-segments that represent comparability relations (if the missing profile 101 is added to the diagram, crossings are unavoidable).

Since the seven profiles (a–g) contain profiles that are incomparable, they do not form a perfect scale and so their dimensionality cannot be 1. Hence 2 is the minimum partial order dimensionality for that set of profiles.

Given the configuration of Fig. 1, two scores are sufficient to identify a profile (and reproduce all three original scores): one score, the joint score, specifies the level to which the profile belongs; the other, the lateral score, locates the profile within the level. Moreover, the two new scores are likely to have substantive meanings. The question of interpreting the joint and lateral axes will be examined below.

A more general way of thinking about (and determining) the partial order dimensionality of a given set of observed data is by answering the following question: what is the smallest coordinate space (i.e., the space with the minimum number of coordinates) into which observed profiles can be mapped (as points) such that all original order relations among profiles ("greater than," "smaller than," "incomparable to") are preserved by the assigned coordinate values? For example, the seven profiles, a–g, can be mapped into a space of just two coordinates X and Y as shown in the minimal space POSAC diagram in Fig. 2.

As may be verified, the mapping transforms the original three-variable profiles into new two-variable profiles in such a way that the relation between every pair of profiles remains the same after the transformation. For instance, the three-variable profiles c = 010 and e = 011 are transformed by the mapping (see Fig. 2) into the two-variable profiles 22 and 23 respectively (the xy coordinates of c and e); and indeed the relation between the original profiles (010 is less than 011) is preserved (22 is less than 23). Considering another pair, the profiles 011 and 110 are incomparable and indeed so are their transformations 23 and 32. The mapping similarly preserves all other order relations among profile pairs.

Although Fig. 1 is essentially ordinal (the exact profile locations are immaterial), it may be viewed as a rota-

tion of Fig. 2. In well-designed research or assessment exercises, the axes X and Y can be found to correspond to essential factors, or "fundamental variables," of the investigated contents.

The concepts discussed above (comparability, partial order dimensionality, etc.) apply to any number (n) of tests (variables) having any number of ordered categories. The partial order dimensionality m may be anywhere between 1 and n ($1 \leq m \leq n$). Since much of the experience with POSAC has been with m=2, this entry is confined to two-dimensional analysis. (Two is the lowest dimensionality that permits the representation of incomparability relations between profiles.)

When the number of profiles is small, a two-dimensional POSA can be carried out by hand. For a large number of profiles a computer program, the POSAC/LSA, is available. For a given set of profiles, the program seeks an optimal two-dimensional minimal space diagram as well as a spatial mapping of the analyzed variables in accordance with the role they play in structuring the scalogram (Shye and Amar 1985).

2. Partial Order Scalograms: A Mathematical Formulation

Each of N subjects $p_1, \ldots, p_N$ in a population P may receive a score in each of n tests $v_1, \ldots, v_n$ where the range of each test is $A_i = (1, 2, \ldots, \alpha_i)$, where i=1, \ldots, n; and $\alpha_i \geq 2$. A_i may be regarded as a set ordered by the relations $\alpha_i >, \ldots, > 2 > 1$ and one should consider the cartesian set $A = A_1 \ldots A_n$ ($n \geq 2$). Each component set A_i is called a facet and each element $a \varepsilon A$ ($a = a_1 a_2 \ldots a_n$, $a_i \varepsilon A_i$) is a profile in the n tests. $a' > a$ if $a'_j \geq a_j$ for all j = 1, \ldots, n and if there exists j', $1 \leq j' \leq n$ with $a'_{j'} > a_{j'}$ (where $a = a_1 \ldots a_n$ and $a' = a_1 \ldots a'_n$). a' and a are comparable ($a \lessgtr a'$) if $a' > a$, or $a > a'$, or $a' = a$, and otherwise are incomparable ($a \$ a$). The score $S(a)$ of a profile a is $S(a) = \Sigma^n_{j=1} a_j$.

A scalogram is a mapping of $P \rightarrow A$ from a population P to the cartesian set A. The subset A' of profiles of A onto which elements of P are mapped, is called the scalogram range, or briefly scalogram. The subset $A(s) \subset A'$ of all profiles having the score s is a level of the scalogram.

If every two profiles in the range A' of a scalogram are comparable, the scalogram is a Guttman scale.

A (and therefore also $A' \subset A$) is a partial order set with respect to the relation $\geq$.

The partial order dimensionality of a scalogram A' is the smallest m ($m \leq n$) for which there exists an m-faceted cartesian set $X = X_i \ldots X_m$, $X_i = 1, 2, \ldots \xi]_i$, i = 1 \ldots m and there exists a 1–1 mapping, $Q: X' \Leftrightarrow A'$ from a subset X' of X onto A' so that if $Q(x') = a'$ and $Q(x) = a$ then $a > a' \Leftrightarrow x > x'$.

The function Q is called a conversion and the cartesian set X is called the minimal space of A'. A function $Q^*: X \rightarrow A'$ from the entire cartesian set $X = X_1 X_2$ onto A' is a full conversion if it is an extension of a conversion and

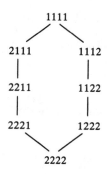

Figure 3
Partial order diagram of a double scale, for $n = 4$

if for every x, $x' \varepsilon X'^c$, $x > x' \Rightarrow a \geqslant a'$ whenever $Q^*(x) = a$ and $Q^*(x') = a'$.

Some elementary results are shown below.

THEOREM 1. Let $A' \subset A$ be any scalogram, and let $a' \varepsilon A'^c$. The dimensionality of the scalogram $A'' = A' \cup \{a'\}$ is no smaller than that of A'.

In certain senses (such as reproducibility of the original n scores from a smaller number of scores) the two-dimensional analogues of the one-dimensional Guttman scale are identifiable families of scalograms which can be determined for every given n.

A scalogram in n tests is a double scale if it is made up of exactly two complete scales. If the tests are all dichotomous ($\alpha_i = 2$, $i = 1, \ldots, n$), the scalogram can be characterized as follows: there exists a permutation of the tests which results in the profiles being all of at most two "runs" of digits (and the scalogram contains all such profiles). For example, if $n = 4$ the partial order diagram of a double scale is as shown in Fig. 3.

THEOREM 2. Double scales are two-dimensional for every n.

A scalogram in n dichotomous tests belongs to the family of diamond scalograms if it contains (after a suitable permutation of the tests) all profiles of n 1's and 2's with at most three runs of digits. For example, if $n =$

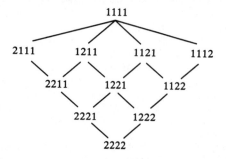

Figure 4
Partial order diagram of a diamond scalogram for $n = 4$

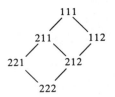

Figure 5
Two-dimensional dense, nonstandard scalogram

4 the partial order diagram of a diamond scalogram is as shown in Fig. 4.

THEOREM 3. Diamond scalograms are two-dimensional for every n.

Important notions in scalogram theory are those of dense scalograms and standard scalograms. A two-dimensional partial order scalogram is dense if each of its levels, s, can be uniquely ordered so that if two profiles, say $a = a_1 a_2 \ldots a_n$ and $a' = a'_1 a'_2 \ldots a'_n$ are adjacent in that order, then first the profile $a \cup a' \equiv \max(a_1, a'_1) \max(a_2, a'_2) \ldots \max(a_n, a'_n)$ and the profile $a \cap a' \equiv \min(a_1, a'_1) \min(a_2, a'_2) \ldots \min(a_n, a'_n)$ are of scores $s+1$ and $s-1$ respectively; and second, both $a \cup a'$ and $a \cap a'$ are in the scalogram. For example, double scales are not dense, but diamond scalograms are.

A two-dimensional partial order scalogram is a standard scalogram if it is dense and if every pair of its tests (out of the n tests) crosses (that is, forms a two-dimensional scalogram, or, in other words, no pair of its tests form a Guttman scale). The scalogram shown in Fig. 5, for example, is two-dimensional and dense but is not standard, because two of its tests (the first and second) form a scale.

In two-dimensional standard scalograms, exactly two tests—the polar tests—can be singled out as being, in a sense, the farthest apart among all test pairs. For instance, the correlation between them (if all profiles occur with equal frequency) is the smallest. This observation is the first step in the analysis of the structural relationship between the "profile (subject) space" (the partial order configuration), on the one hand, and the test space (the space obtained by the smallest space analysis [SSA]), on the other. The value of polar tests in research applications is that in contrasting their contents a "first approximation" of the meanings of the scalogram axes is afforded.

Mathematical analyses show (Shye 1976, 1985) that in standard scalograms the other (nonpolar) tests further refine the structure of the lateral axis (as well as the X, Y axes) of the scalogram with a corresponding refinement in the interpretability of these axes. The scalogram axes (J and L; or alternatively X and Y, of Sect. 1 above) are the factors of the contents analyzed, and in this sense scalogram analysis merits the name of "nonmetric factor analysis" proposed by Coombs and Kao (1955).

Partial order scalograms structure the observed profiles so that individual subjects may be classified and rated. A structural analysis of the scalogram tests (i.e., variables), however, can result in a test space that is merely a special version of the smallest space analysis of the tests. Smallest space analysis, that maps tests according to the roles these tests play in structuring partial order scalograms, is of particular value. Two such versions (termed lattice space analysis 1 and 2) have been proposed and applied through the use of the POSAC/LSA computer program.

2.1 Lattice Space Analysis 1

This procedure for mapping scalogram tests is based on the observation that in a standard scalogram considerable information concerning the structure of the interrelationships among scalogram tests is embodied in the two boundary scales of the scalogram, namely, the scales that envelop the scalogram's partial order diagram. The LSA 1 procedure maps the tests in a two-dimensional array so that the polar tests are relatively far apart while all other tests are located in the space according to the order in which they change their values on the boundary scales. This procedure, illustrated below, has been shown to be equivalent to a version of smallest space analysis in which the coefficient of similarity is a newly defined structural (not distributional) coefficient and the metric employed is the lattice ("city block") distance.

2.2 Lattice Space Analysis 2

This procedure is based on the observation that in the minimal space of a two-dimensional partial order scalogram, each test has a partitioning line (or lines) that divide the space into regions according to the values of that test. For instance, in the minimal space shown in Fig. 2, the vertical line that separates profiles a, b, c, and e from profiles d, f, and g pertains to Test T_1. It divides the space into a region where $T_1 = 0$ (profiles a, b, c, e) and another region where $T_1 = 1$ (d, g, f). Similarly, an L-shaped partitioning line separates the region where $T_2 = 0$ (profiles a, b, d) from the region where $T_2 = 1$ (profiles c, e, f, g). In the analyses of empirical data involving many variables and possibly some "noise," the partitioning lines do not usually have simple shapes. In LSA 2, each of the scalogram tests is characterized by its similarity (assessed by correlation coefficients) to each of four ideal-type tests. The latter are "pure content" tests which could conceivably be devised for the content universe. They are defined by the shapes of their partitioning lines in the scalogram minimal space diagram: vertical (representing one polar test), horizontal (representing another polar test), L-shaped (representing an attenuating test—one whose high values tend to concentrate in the middle of the lateral axis), and inverted L-shaped (representing an accentuating test—one whose high values tend to concentrate in the ends of the lateral axis).

The resemblance of each scalogram test to these four ideal types helps determine to what extent it plays the role of one or the other of the two polar tests, or of an attenuating or accentuating test.

3. The Uses of POSAC for Structuring Concepts and Scaling Individuals

Multiple scaling by POSAC is a valuable tool for tackling theoretical and practical problems of assessment. Perhaps more than other multivariate procedures it requires the researcher to formulate a clear definition of the concept involved (respect to which individuals are assessed) and to construct variables or tests that cover that concept reasonably well. If that concept (or a well-defined aspect of it) turns out to be two-dimensional in the sense of the partial order scalogram (or even nearly two-dimensional), the pay-off may be considerable: through LSA, variables making up the concept may be characterized according to their role in shaping the concept and in determining the meaning of the scalogram axes; and the partial order scalogram itself provides an efficient two-score scaling of the individual observed.

The POSAC/LSA computer program produces pictorially the best (two-dimensional) minimal space for the empirical data and, in addition, relates that diagram to external variables (variables that are not included in the scalogram itself). Lattice space analysis aids the investigator in interpreting the scalogram axes and in testing regional hypotheses (see *Smallest Space Analysis*).

To demonstrate the interplay between concept definition and scalogram structure, a hypothetical example will be considered.

A researcher is interested in assessing the educational level of individuals of a given population. One procedure might be to devise n tests that represent sufficiently well, in his or her opinion, the notion of education sufficiently well. The tests may be graduated with respect to their difficulty for the population in question and then a Guttman scale may be expected. If indeed one is empirically obtained, the structure of the concept, as represented by the tests, is the simplest: LSA identifies no polar tests, and exhibits no interpolar spread so the dimensionality of the test space is, in a sense, 0 and the concept is monolithic. This could occur perhaps if education is defined as general knowledge represented by a series of tests ordered by their difficulty, so that if an individual passes any one test he or she is sure to pass all easier tests (Elizur and Adler 1975).

However, a more structured definition of "education" may result in a selection of variables whose interdependence is neither so high nor so simple. For instance, the tests may be selected to represent a range of topics such as those taught in schools; and, moreover, the topics may be considered to be ordered by some substantive criterion, for example, from the sciences to the humanities (say, physics, biology, history of science, grammar, literature).

617

A possible hypothesis—and a possible result for such a test sampling—could be that pass-or-fail scoring of the tests would produce a diamond scalogram. The logic of such a scalogram is that if a person passes any two tests in the series he or she also passes all tests that are in between these two, in the order specified above. For n = 5 tests, the scalogram is given in Fig. 6. Figure 6(a) shows the partial order diagram with its joint (J) and lateral (L) axes; and Fig. 6(b) presents the minimal

space diagram with its X and Y axes. Note that here the figures facilitate a clear interpretation for each of the scalogram axes. These interpretations for the J and L axes, or alternatively the X and Y axes, are indeed more fundamental than the original tests and qualify as factors of "education" as this concept is conceived and represented by the tests.

Lattice space analysis for the above scalogram identifies the first and the last tests in the series as the

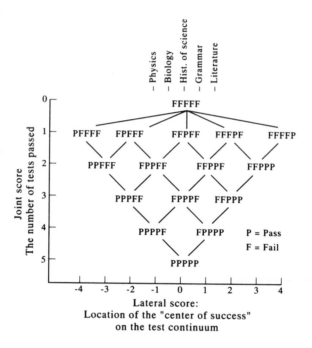

(a) Partial order diagram representation

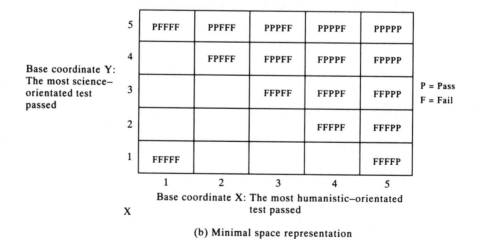

(b) Minimal space representation

Figure 6
The diamond scalogram hypothesis for passing a series of ordered tests

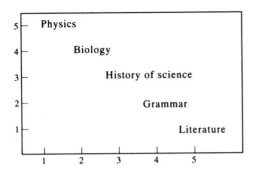

Figure 7
LSA of the diamond scalogram of Fig. 6, hypothesized for a series of tests

two scalogram poles and places all other tests in the expected order on a straight line between the two. The test space for the diamond scalogram is of dimensionality 1 (akin to Guttman's 1954 simplex) as shown in Fig. 7.

The diamond scalogram is characteristic of certain linear processes. It has been found empirically to accommodate data in a study of exposure to evening television programs (Levinsohn 1980) (the series of test questions was: "Do you watch television at 7.00 pm? at 7.30 pm? ... at 10.30?"), reflecting the fact that the population investigated tended to switch their television sets on just once, watch for varying lengths of time, and then switch off (and only few switch it on and off more than once).

A more complex definition of education can lead to a more structured scalogram. For instance, it may be desirable to define education to include not only tests of

knowledge but also a test of balanced exposure to areas of knowledge and perhaps also a test of the individual's tendency to study in depth whatever area in which he or she is knowledgeable. For simplicity, just four tests will be considered and it may be assumed that they are dichotomous pass/fail tests (each test in turn could be made up of many items having their own internal structures).

Test T_1: knowledge in the humanities	P/F
Test T_2: knowledge in the sciences	P/F
Test T_3: tendency to balance knowledge in the two areas	P/F
Test T_4: expertise in areas of knowledge	P/F

Given an appropriate design, it may be hypothesized that the profiles FFFP and FFPP in the test T_1 T_2 T_3 T_4 respectively would not be observed since lack of knowledge in both the humanities ($T_1 = F$) and the sciences ($T_2 = F$) could not go together with expertise ($T_4 = P$) in any of them. Also the profiles PPFF and PPFP are unlikely to be observed because knowledge in both the humanities and the sciences does indicate—let it be assumed—a balanced exposure to the two areas. A partial order scalogram of the remaining 12 profiles turns out to be two-dimensional. Figure 8 shows this and offers interpretations of the scalogram axes.

Passing T_1 (knowledge in humanities) characterizes the left-hand side of the partial order diagram while passing T_2 (knowledge in sciences) characterizes its right-hand side. Profiles with passing grades in T_3 (balanced knowledge) tend to occur in the middle range of the lateral axis and profiles with passing grades in T_4 (expertise) characterize the extreme ends of that axis. In the language of Sect. 2, T_1 and T_2 are the polar tests of the scalogram; T_3 is an attenuating test, and T_4 is an accentuating test. The LSA 1 diagram (Fig. 9) describes these roles graphically.

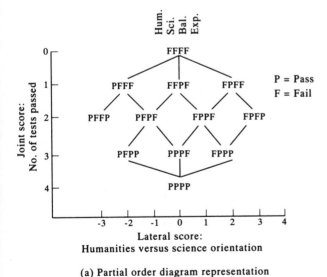

(a) Partial order diagram representation

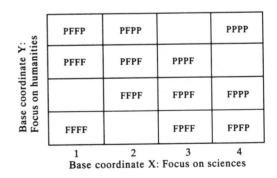

(b) Minimal space representation

Figure 8
A hypothesized four-test scalogram for "education"

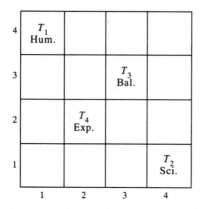

Figure 9
LSA of the scalogram of Fig. 8, hypothesized for four education indicators

This scalogram, made up of what may be called four ideal-type tests, has been found empirically—for example, in a study of job rewards, the loss of which was feared by a sample of government accounting unit workers, following the introduction of computerized procedures (Shye and Elizur 1976). Fear of job loss and of loss of interest in work constituted the two polar variables. Fear of encountering difficulties in performing the job and of being transferred to another unit constituted the attenuating and the accentuating variables, respectively.

In another application, Lewy and Shye (1990) decoded the structure of teachers' attitudes toward Higher Mental Function Curricular Objectives (HMCO)for disadvantaged pupils, and derived appropriate scales. Questionnaire items designed to cover various aspects of rote learning were processed by the POSAC/LSA computer program. POSAC joint axis (1st scale), provided an overall measure of support of rote learning versus insistence on HMCO for those pupils. The LSA 2 diagram (Fig. 10) helped in inferring the meaning of POSAC lateral axis (2nd scale). That meaning was found to be governed by two polar items: (a) focus on fact learning (for disadvantaged pupils) in itself; and (b) fact learning as leading to comprehension; hence a resignation versus instrumentality continuum was implied for the lateral POSAC axis. The item "experimentations in class take time from systematic coverage" was found to play an accentuating role; that is, disapproval of experimentation accentuates whatever pole (resignation or instrumentality) is dominant in teachers' attitudes.

See also: Smallest Space Analysis; Facet Theory; Scaling Methods; Multivariate Analysis; Factor Analysis

References

Coombs C H 1964 *A Theory of Data*. Wiley, New York
Coombs C H, Kao R C 1955 *Nonmetric Factor Analysis*. University of Michigan Press, Ann Arbor, Michigan
Elizur D, Adler I 1975 *Information Deprivation*. Israel Institute of Applied Social Research, Jerusalem

Guttman L 1950 The basis for scalogram analysis. In: Stouffer S A et al. (eds.) 1950 *Measurement and Prediction*, Vol. 4. Princeton University Press, Princeton, New Jersey
Guttman L 1954 A new approach to factor analysis: The radex. In: Lazarsfeld P F (ed.) 1954 *Mathematical Thinking in the Social Sciences*. Free Press, New York
Guttman L 1959 A structural theory for intergroup beliefs and action. *Am. Sociol. Rev.* 24: 318–28
Guttman L 1972 A partial-order scalogram classification of projective techniques. In: Hammer M, Salzinger K, Sutton S (eds.) 1972 *Psychopathology: Contributions from the Social, Behavioral, and Biological Sciences*. Wiley, New York
Levinsohn H 1980 *Patterns of TV Viewing and Radio Listening Among the Arab Population in Israel*. Israel Institute of Applied Social Research, Jerusalem
Lewy A, Shye S 1990 Dimensions of attitude toward higher mental function circular objectives (HMCO): A partial order scalogram analysis. *Quality and Quantity* 24: 231–44
Shye S 1976 *Partial Order Scalogram Analysis of Profiles and its Relationship to the Smallest Space Analysis of the Variables*. Israel Institute of Applied Social Research, Jerusalem
Shye S 1978 Partial order scalogram analysis. In: Shye S (ed.) 1978 *Theory Construction and Data Analysis in the Behavioral Sciences*. Jossey-Bass, San Francisco, California
Shye S 1985 *Multiple Scaling: The Theory and Application of Partial Order Scalogram Analysis*. North Holland, Amsterdam
Shye S, Elizur D 1976 Worries about deprivation of job rewards following computerization: A partial order scalogram analysis. *Hum. Relat.* 29: 63–71
Shye S, Amar R 1985 Partial order scalogram analysis by base coordinates and lattice mapping of the items by their scalogram roles. In: Canter D (ed.) 1985 *Facet Theory: Approaches to Social Research*. Springer-Verlag, New York
Shye S et al. 1994 *Introduction to Facet Theory*. Sage, Newbury Park, California
Zvulun E 1978 Multidimensional scalogram analysis: The method and its application. In Shye S (ed.) 1978

Figure 10
Attitude toward fact learning (vs. comprehension): LSA differentiating among types of such attitude

Path Analysis and Linear Structural Relations Analysis

A. C. Tuijnman and J. P. Keeves

Since the 1960s there have been major advances in educational research in the statistical procedures available for examining networks of causal relationships between observed variables and hypothesized latent variables. These procedures are considered in this entry using the related names of path analysis, causal modeling, and linear structural relations analysis. While the ideas underlying path analysis were first used in educational research by Burks (1928), these ideas lay largely dormant for over 40 years in this field until used by Peaker (1971) in England, largely because of the heavy computational work involved. The developments in education and the social and behavioral sciences have followed those advanced earlier in the field of genetics (Wright 1934). The techniques were introduced more generally into the social sciences by Duncan (1966) and articles by Land (1969), Heise (1969), and Duncan (1969) served to systematize the procedures being used and to clarify many of the issues involved. The approach employing these techniques enables the investigator to shift from verbal statements of a complex set of interrelationships between variables to more precise mathematical ones, which are commonly represented in diagrammatic form, and to estimate the magnitudes of the causal relationships involved. Stokes (1968, 1974) developed the procedures of path analysis from first principles, which emerged as equivalent to ordinary least squares regression analysis (see Keeves 1988).

A more general term for the analytical techniques involved, namely "structural equation modeling," is also used. As implied by this name a set of mathematical equations is employed to formulate the structural relations which are hypothesized to exist between a network of observed and latent variables, and the model is tested to determine the extent to which it accounts for the covariation between the observed measures. A variety of strategies is available for the examination of such models, and this entry considers the different approaches that are now widely employed in educational, behavioral, and social science research in the field of structural equation modeling.

This entry makes a distinction between path analysis, in which least squares regression procedures are used to maximize the variance explained, and procedures in which the model is estimated and the fit between the model and the data examined. The former is considered in greater depth (see *Path Analysis with Latent Variables*) and the latter in the discussion that is presented below.

1. Causal Explanation

It is rare in educational research for an investigator to proceed with an inquiry in which evidence is assembled without maintaining some theoretical perspectives, whether implicitly held or explicitly stated, that guide the design of the investigation and that influence the analyses carried out. In such analyses there is interest in examining the patterns in the covariation between measures and testing whether these patterns are consistent with the theoretical perspectives which are held. However, it is not possible to impute causal relationships from a study of the covariation between measures, and it is necessary to assume a scheme of causation derived from the theoretical perspectives which are maintained. Where these theoretical perspectives extend beyond simple description, they commonly involve ideas of causation which are probabilistic and stochastic in nature in so far as a time sequence is also involved. It is these ideas of causation that are examined in the analysis of data.

Thus hypotheses or sets of hypotheses in the form of structural equation models or path models are advanced, during the design stage of an investigation, and are subsequently available for examination after the data have been assembled. The results may lead to acceptance or rejection of a hypothesis or model. Alternatively, it may be possible to refine a model and resubmit it for further examination, or it may be necessary to abandon the model being advanced and at a later stage modify the theoretical perspectives which gave rise to the model.

It is important to note that the use of correlational data to reach causative conclusions is not acceptable under classical statistical inference (see *Significance Testing*). Thus if a causative model (M) predicts correlational relations (C) and the data observed (D) are such that C is *not* consistent with D, then the model (M) can legitimately be rejected. However, under classical statistical inference it cannot be affirmed that because the data (D) are consistent with the correlational relations (C) that they support the model (M) (Games 1990). Nevertheless, in educational research studies the researcher is rarely able to conduct an appropriate experiment, and it is necessary to develop models from theory and to examine systematically the models in order to advance theoretical understanding. This, however, does not mean that a causative relationship can be established.

1.1 Causation in Nonexperimental Research

In an experimental research study the investigator manipulates certain explanatory variables of interest and measures the effects of manipulation on an outcome variable. However, to ensure that the effects on the outcome are caused by the changes in the experimental conditions, it is necessary to control for other variables that might also influence the outcome and so confound the relationships observed. Unfortunately, in educational research it is rarely possible to randomize fully the subjects to whom different treatment conditions are administered by the manipulation of explanatory variables. Furthermore, many variables of interest to the educational researcher cannot be changed by manipulation, for ethical and operational reasons. As a consequence, a quasi- or nonexperimental study must be carried out. Under such circumstances the investigator must employ statistical controls in place of the controls that might have been achieved by randomization. However, the use of statistical controls demands an explanatory scheme that determines the nature of the analysis to be used in examining the covariation between variables in the data collected.

1.2 Role of Models and Theory

In the design of an empirical study, whether experimental, quasi-experimental, or nonexperimental, theory necessarily has a central place. From theory, hypotheses or models must first be advanced, since they determine, among other things, not only the manner in which the data are to be analyzed, but also the type of data to be collected. In general, the analyses are designed to make a decision on whether or not a hypothesis or model is consistent with the empirical evidence. If the hypothesis or model is not consistent with the data, then the model may need to be modified, or doubt may be cast on the theory that gave rise to the hypothesis or model. However, it is important to recognize that the consistency of a hypothesis or a model with the data collected does not furnish proof of theory, but it may provide support for theory. The role of models in relation to theory does not differ according to whether an investigation is experimental, with full randomization, quasi-experimental, or nonexperimental. What differs between the different types of studies is the extent to which randomization is used to control for variables that might confound the patterns of covariation observed between variables, and the extent to which statistical control must be exercised.

The function and purpose of the causal models which are used in path analysis and structural equation modeling are to specify as fully as possible the interrelations between variables so that appropriate statistical control might be employed. The use of a causal model has further advantages in so far as it makes explicit the interrelations between variables that are derived from theory. Moreover, it serves as a heuristic device in the development of theory and in the conduct of inquiry. Subsequently, it permits the teasing out of the complex network of effects, together with estimating the magnitudes of effects, that might be considered to

operate in a particular problem situation in educational inquiry.

1.3 Two Approaches to the Testing of Models

Two general strategies have evolved for the testing of models with empirical data, or more precisely stated, whether a model advanced from theory fits the data or is consistent with the observed data. In the least squares approach in which the residuals between the observed values and the predicted estimates are minimized (see *Regression Analysis of Quantified Data*) no assumptions need to be made about the form of the relationships between variables which exist in the population from which a sample is drawn. Thus it is not necessary to assume an underlying multivariate normal distribution in the population in order to estimate the magnitude of effects. However, in order to test for statistical significance such assumptions must commonly be made, and probability levels are generally calculated under the assumptions of: (a) a multivariate normal distribution in the population, and (b) that the sample is a simple random sample from the specified population. The former assumption is commonly investigated by an examination of each of the variables introduced into an analysis for normality. However, the latter which is difficult to achieve in educational research studies is commonly ignored with unfortunate consequences for the statement of the statistical significance of the findings recorded. Alternative techniques such as jackknifing (Tukey 1977) may be used to provide standard errors of the parameters being estimated, and these techniques neither assume knowledge of the nature of the underlying distribution in the population nor test estimates for statistical significance (see *Sampling Errors in Survey Research*).

In the use of maximum likelihood procedures of analysis, it is assumed that the general form of the population distribution from which the sample was drawn can be specified. Commonly, this is assumed to be the multivariate normal distribution. The PRELIS 2 computer program (Jöreskog and Sörbom 1993) provides a test of the multivariate normality of a set of variables. However, while the distribution of the population parameters can be assumed, the values of these parameters are not known. In the absence of such knowledge it is possible to take appropriate arbitrary values, and treat them as if they were the actual values and estimate the likelihood of observing particular values for the variables under consideration in a single observation drawn from such a population. With several variables, it is possible to estimate the joint likelihood for a single observation, and subsequently to estimate the population parameters that would enable the sample observations to have the greatest joint likelihood. As a consequence the values so calculated are the "maximum likelihood estimates" of the population parameters, using as the method of analysis the "maximum likelihood estimation" procedure. The further question which must be asked concerns how well the estimates made under these conditions for a particular model fit the observed data. A goodness of fit test is employed to compare the maximum likelihood estimates with the observed data. If the level of discrepancy in fit exceeds a particular level, usually taken to be less than the 10 percent level of significance for data involving a simple random sample of moderate size, of say 400 cases, drawn from a specified population, the estimated model is said not to fit the data and must be rejected. If the level of discrepancy does not exceed this specified level, and is greater than 10 percent, the model is accepted as a good fit to the data.

If the residuals obtained from the use of a least squares estimation procedure are normally distributed, then the least squares estimates and the maximum likelihood estimates of the parameters of a model are identical. However, the maximum likelihood approach and its tests of goodness of fit are very dependent on the use of significance levels associated with a simple random sample, which is rarely available in educational research. As a consequence the level of fit of a model to the data while very useful for refining a model and for comparing models has had limited value in providing evidence of the validity of a particular model. In addition to the maximum likelihood estimation procedure there is another function that has similar properties under the same assumptions, namely the generalized least squares estimator. Different estimation problems with different types of observed measures require different kinds of weight matrices in generalized least squares estimation (Hayduk 1987, Jöreskog and Sörbom 1989). Thus it has been possible to extend the use of the maximum likelihood approach by employing generalized least squares and weighted least squares estimation procedures.

One of the major developments in this field in the decade from 1980 to 1990 has involved estimation methods that were not dependent on the assumption of continuous multivariate normal distributions in the observed data. Browne (1984) advanced an asymptotic distribution free (ADF) estimation procedure in which information about the skewness and kurtosis of a distribution was incorporated. Muthén (1984) also developed an approach for estimating models that contained a mixture of different types of measurement scales and that employed polyserial and polychoric correlations for variables that were measured in terms of categories, but were associated with a continuous multinormal distribution. The calculation of these different types of correlation coefficients is provided for in PRELIS 2, a preliminary program that is used prior to analysis with LISREL 8 (Jöreskog and Sörbom 1993).

In the section that follows path analysis and the estimation of parameters using least squares procedures are discussed. In the subsequent section maximum likelihood and related techniques are considered in relation to linear structural equation modeling.

2. Path Analysis

Consider a simple causal model which contains four observed variables X_1, X_2, X_3, and X_4 that are, from theoretical considerations, regarded as being causally related as indicated in Fig. 1. The residual or disturbance variables, which represent those effects that are not considered in the causal model, are denoted R_u, R_v, and R_w.

The following conventions are employed in the path diagram:

(a) A causal relationship is indicated by a unidimensional arrow from the determining variable to the variable dependent on it.

(b) A noncausal correlation between variables that are not dependent on other variables in the system is represented by a bidirectional curved arrow; and the magnitude of a noncausal correlation is indicated by the zero-order correlation coefficient between the two variables (r_{ij}), but such a correlation is not present in the model shown in Fig. 1.

(c) Causal relationships which involve disturbance variables and represent forces outside the system, not correlated with the variables immediately determining the dependent variables, are indicated by unidirectional arrows from the disturbance variables under consideration.

(d) The magnitude of the relationship associated with an arrow, indicating one-way causation in the path diagram, is given by a path coefficient (p_{ij}), where i denotes the dependent variable and j denotes the independent or determining variable.

The system shown in Fig. 1 contains no noncausal relationships between the variables. Those variables that are not dependent on other variables in the model are known as "exogenous variables," and "residual variables" while the variables that are dependent on other variables are known as "endogenous variables."

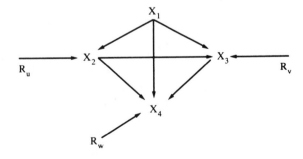

Figure 1

Path model for variables X_1, X_2, X_3, and X_4, with disturbance variables R_u, R_v, and R_w

In addition, in this system there are no variables that are linked by reciprocal causation or feedback. A model where there is a strictly ordered arrangement of variables, and where there is no reciprocal relationship is known as a "recursive" model; and a model which includes such a reciprocal relationship is a "nonrecursive" model.

2.1 Basic Theorem

The basic theorem of path analysis may be stated in the general form:

$$r_{ij} = \sum_k p_{ik} \cdot r_{jk} \tag{1}$$

which may be derived from the general Eqn.

$$X_i = \sum_k p_{ik} X_k \tag{2}$$

where the subscripts i and j denote two variables in the system and the subscript k denotes variables from which paths lead directly to X_i. This allows the mathematical relations between the variables to be expressed as a set of linear equations called the "path model":

$$r_{12} = p_{21} \tag{3}$$

$$r_{13} = p_{31} + p_{32}r_{12} \tag{4}$$

$$r_{23} = p_{32} + p_{31}r_{12} \tag{5}$$

$$r_{14} = p_{41} + p_{42}r_{12} + p_{43}r_{13} \tag{6}$$

$$r_{24} = p_{42} + p_{41}r_{12} + p_{43}r_{23} \tag{7}$$

$$r_{34} = p_{43} + p_{41}r_{13} + p_{42}r_{23} \tag{8}$$

These equations can be solved to obtain the six path coefficients ($p_{21}, p_{31}, p_{32}, p_{41}, p_{42}, p_{43}$) in terms of the six observed correlation coefficients ($r_{12}, r_{13}, r_{23}, r_{14}, r_{24}, r_{34}$).

An important extension of the theorem expressed in Eqn. (1) is when $i = j$, then

$$r_{ij} = 1 = \sum_k p_{ik} \cdot r_{ik} \tag{9}$$

This relationship allows the path coefficient of a disturbance variable to be calculated.

By the substitution of r_{12} from Eqn. (3), r_{13} from Eqn. (4), and r_{14} from Eqn. (6) in Eqns. (4) to (8) the following equations are produced to show the underlying processes responsible for the observed correlations.

$$r_{21} = p_{21} \tag{10}$$

$$r_{31} = p_{31} + p_{21}p_{32} \tag{11}$$

$$r_{32} = p_{21}p_{31} + p_{32} \tag{12}$$

$$r_{41} = p_{41} + p_{21}p_{42} + p_{21}p_{32}p_{43} + p_{31}\,p_{43} \tag{13}$$

$$r_{42} = p_{42} + p_{21}p_{41} + p_{21}p_{31}p_{43} + p_{32}p_{43} \tag{14}$$

$$r_{43} = p_{43} + p_{31}p_{41} + p_{32}p_{42} + p_{21}p_{32}p_{41} + p_{21}p_{31}p_{42} \tag{15}$$

Thus it can be seen from the mathematical equations that:

(a) r_{21} comes about because X_2 is influenced by X_1 (p_{21});

(b) r_{31} is observed because X_3 is directly influenced by X_1 (p_{31}) and X_1 also acts indirectly through X_2 to influence X_3 ($p_{21}\,p_{32}$).

2.2 Direct and Indirect Effects

Terms in Eqns. (10) to (15) like $p_{21}, p_{31}, p_{32}, p_{41}, p_{42}, p_{43}$ are referred to as direct effects, and, p_{43} for example, represents the effects of X_3 on X_4 after controlling for the effects of X_1 and X_2. Compound terms, for example $p_{21}\,p_{32}$, represent the indirect effects of X_1 on X_3 which operate through the mediating variable X_2 as is seen in Fig. 2(b).

2.3 Decomposition of Correlations

Equations (10) to (15) show that it is possible to decompose into different components the observed correlation between two variables, where one is exogenous and the other endogenous within a path model,

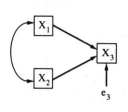
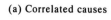

(a) Correlated causes

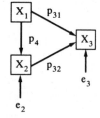

(b) Mediated causes

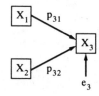

(c) Independent causes

Figure 2
Different types of causal relationships between three variables

or between two endogenous variables within a path model. For example, the correlation (r_{31}) between X_1 and X_3 where X_1 is exogenous and X_3 is endogenous, as is seen in Fig. 2(b), can be decomposed as shown in Eqn. (11) into two parts, namely: (a) a direct effect of X_1 on X_3, and (b) an indirect effect which is mediated through X_2 (p_{21} p_{32}). However, in a model as shown in Fig. 2(a) in which X_1 and X_2 are both exogenous variables operating on X_3, which is endogenous to both X_1 and X_2, then as seen from Eqn. (4), there is part of r_{31} which is left unanalyzed since it is due to correlated causes (r_{12} p_{32}). Furthermore, if as in Fig. 2(b), X_1 influences X_2 which in turn influences X_3, while X_1 also directly influences X_3, then from Eqn. (12) part of the correlation (r_{23}) between X_2 and X_3 arises from the direct influence of X_2 on X_3 (p_{32}), while a further part (p_{21} p_{31}) is spurious and arises because both X_2 and X_3 share a common cause, namely X_1. The spurious part of r_{23} is given by r_{23}-p_{32} which is equal to p_{31} p_{21}. It is also possible for variables X_1 and X_2, as shown in Fig. 2(c) to have independent effects on X_3. In such circumstances the correlation r_{13} between X_1 and X_3 is due solely to the direct effect of X_1 on X_3 (p_{31}), and the correlation between X_2 and X_3 is also due solely to the direct effect of X_2 on X_3 (p_{32}).

Thus a correlation coefficient can be decomposed into several different components: (a) a direct effect, (b) an indirect effect, (c) an unanalyzed effect due to correlated causes, and (d) a spurious effect due to common causes. The sum of a direct effect and an indirect effect is referred to as a "total effect," or is sometimes known as an "effect coefficient." However, not all correlations can be decomposed into all four components. Thus spurious effects are only observed for correlations between endogenous variables as seen in Fig. 2(b) while unanalyzed effects are only observed when the model includes correlated exogenous variables, as seen in Fig. 2(a) (see Hauser 1973a).

2.4 Model Specification

One of the essential requirements of any path model is that it should contain all the variables of consequence to the problem situation. Moreover, it is critical that the variables are placed in the logically and temporally correct structural sequence and in an appropriate functional form. With respect to the latter such models generally assume a linear relationship and a multivariate normal distribution, because it is the simplest and most robust functional form. However, if theory were to support the transformation of variables to provide for quadratic, cubic, or logarithmic functional relationships, appropriate modifications to a model are possible, but rarely employed. In general, the equations from which parameter estimates are made may be misspecified and the estimates made may be biased under certain circumstances. These occur if the model: (a) excludes important causal factors that may influence the variables included in the model; (b) specifies a linear relationship when a non-linear form is more appropriate; (c) assumes a causal relation when a reciprocal relation, or noncausal association, or a mediated causal effect would better apply; and (d) ignores the possibility of a moderating effect between two antecedent variables to influence an endogenous variable.

2.5 Identification

If the number of equations in a model is equal to the number of parameters to be estimated, and there is a unique value obtained for each parameter, and a unique solution for each equation, then the model is said to be "just identified." If, however, the number of equations in a model exceeds the number of parameters to be estimated, then the model is said to be "overidentified." Overidentification in models is generally a result of the imposition of constraints or restrictions which are required by theory, and a common such constraint is that certain path coefficients are logically assumed to be zero. A model is said to be *underidentified*, if it contains insufficient information for the estimation of all parameters in the model, because the number of parameters to be estimated exceeds the number of equations in the model. Such a model may not be testable, unless it is theoretically possible to impose restrictions that would eliminate certain parameters from inclusion in the equations of the model or that would add further equations to the model to permit complete estimation. Thus, while the issue of identification applies to a model, it is probably more profitable to consider the issue of identification as applying to the estimation of particular parameters. In conclusion, it is important to note that a fully recursive model in which all variables in the model are interconnected is a just identified model. More detailed discussions of the problem of identification are provided by Johnston (1972), Duncan (1975), and Heise (1975).

2.6 Model Testing

The validity of a causal model can be assessed in terms of its ability to reproduce the observed correlations between the variables. In a just identified model, where all parameters are estimated with unique solutions, the model will always be found to fit the data perfectly, and no test of validity can be applied to the model. Pedhazur (1982) discusses the two broad approaches that can be employed in the examination of models: (a) tests of overidentified models and (b) model trimming.

The testing of an overidentified model is undertaken by comparing the observed and the reproduced correlation matrices between the variables in the model. The determinants of these matrices are used to calculate a function involving the likelihood ratio with an approximate χ^2 distribution and with the number of degrees of freedom equal to the number of overidentifying restrictions. Fully recursive models which are just identified and have no overidentifying restrictions, can be fully reproduced, and if an attempt were made to calculate the value of χ^2, it would be zero, indicating a perfect fit. The larger the difference between the value of χ^2 obtained and the number of degrees of freedom the poorer the level of fit. If the level of fit has a probability of less than 10 percent, the model is generally rejected as being of poor fit. However, while the number of degrees of freedom employed in this test is independent of the number of cases, the calculated value of χ^2 is dependent on the number of cases involved in testing the model. Since large samples are necessary to obtain stable estimates of the parameters of a model, there is a high degree of probability that a particular model will be rejected on the grounds of poor fit to the data. Consequently, it would seem more appropriate to give attention to the size of a related goodness of fit index (Q) which may have values between zero and unity. The closer Q is to one, the better the fit. For further details of these procedures Pedhazur (1982 pp. 617–620) and Specht (1975) should be consulted.

Similar problems arise in model trimming and the refinement of a model by the removal of causal paths from the model, where an estimated parameter is close to zero. In the testing of the parameter estimates, t and F ratios are employed, both of which depend upon sample sizes. Thus, while it is commonly of value to engage in model trimming by the deletion of trivial paths for which the estimates of the path coefficients obtained are close to zero, tests of statistical significance *can be inaccurate* when large complex samples have been employed. Despite this flaw, standard error estimates are nevertheless used in assessing the levels of relative significance of path coefficients. Furthermore, some judgment level of the magnitude of such standardized path coefficients is sometimes employed, such as $|p| \geqslant 0.05$, to indicate those paths that should be retained. However, in well-developed fields of investigation some critics of research contend that such model trimming when applied post hoc, is exploratory in nature, and largely ignores consideration of the theoretical grounds for the inclusion of a particular parameter in a model.

Ultimately in the testing and refinement of models the principles of coherence and parsimony would seem the most appropriate to apply. The principle of coherence refers to the level of agreement between theoretical considerations and the inclusion of a path in a model on the basis of its magnitude estimated in the testing of the model. The principle of parsimony implies the deletion of a path and a parameter from a model, if there are only tenuous empirical and theoretical grounds for supporting its inclusion.

3. Parameter Estimation using Least Squares Procedures

A variety of procedures are available for obtaining estimates of the parameters of a model in which the principle of least squares is employed to minimize the difference between the observed and the estimated values.

3.1 Ordinary Least Squares Procedures

The most direct procedure for the estimation of the parameters of a model involves ordinary least squares estimation (see *Regression Analysis of Quantified Data*). A linear path equation, such as,

$$X_4 = p_{41}X_1 + p_{42}X_2 + p_{43}X_3 + p_{4w}X_w$$

may be expressed in standardized form:

$$X_4 = \beta_1 X_1 + \beta_2 X_2 + \beta_3 X_3 + \varepsilon$$

or in metric form

$$X_4 = a + b_1 X_1 + b_2 X_2 + b_3 X_3 + e$$

where β and b are the standardized and metric regression coefficients respectively and ε and e are the corresponding error terms. In metric form all variables retain their original units of measurement, while in standardized form all variables have been centered to their means ($\bar{X} = 0$) and to a variance of unity ($s^2 = 1$).

Metric coefficients lend themselves to more direct interpretation, and are comparable across different data sets. Standardized coefficients are only interpretable in terms of standard deviation units, but since within a model, all variables have the same metric, their effects may be meaningfully compared. In so far as the standardized measures have been standardized from different variances for different samples, the standardized path coefficients are not strictly comparable across different samples.

There is a range of ordinary least squares procedures that can be employed for the testing of specific path models. These procedures include multiple regression, factorial modeling, canonical analysis, and discriminant analysis. However, most path models are conceived in such ways that they can be tested and the parameters estimated using multiple regression procedures.

3.2 Nonrecursive Models

In a nonrecursive model, a reciprocal relationship between two variables is included in the model. This may lead to the underidentification of both the model and certain variables within the model. Two strategies of analysis which involve least squares principles are employed to estimate the parameters of such models, namely: (a) indirect regression and (b) two-stage least squares regression.

3.2.1 Indirect regression. The crucial feature of a reciprocal causal model which is necessary to permit the estimation of a reciprocal effect through a procedure

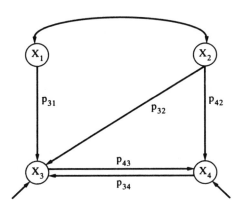

Figure 3a
An indirect regression model

called indirect or instrumental variable regression is that one variable in the model affects only indirectly one of the two variables involved in the reciprocal relationship. Such a variable is referred to as an instrumental variable, and the number of path coefficients to be estimated is equal to or less than the number of correlation coefficients available for substitution. Hauser (1973b) presents the elementary algebra required to calculate the values of all path coefficients in a simple nonrecursive model through the application of the basic theorem of path analysis.

In Fig. 3a, X_1 is the instrumental variable having an effect on variable X_3 but not directly on variable X_4, and only indirectly through variable X_3. The path equations are first solved for p_{42} and p_{43}. These values are then used to solve for p_{34}. Subsequently, this value is used to solve the path equations for p_{31} and p_{32} (see also Heise 1975).

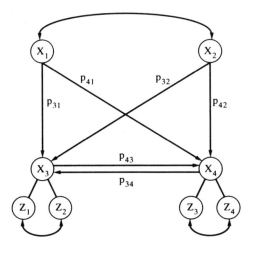

Figure 3b
A two-stage least squares model

However, unless a large sample is employed the estimates obtained using a single instrumental variable are likely to be unstable. An alternative procedure is provided by two-stage least squares regression (Cohen and Cohen 1983).

3.2.2 Two-stage least squares regression. In Fig. 3b an example of a model is shown where X_1 and X_2 both influence X_3 and X_4 which also reciprocally influence each other. However Z_1 and Z_2 act as instrumental variables for X_3, and Z_3 and Z_4 are instrumental variables for X_4. In the first stage X_1, X_2, Z_1 and Z_2 are used to estimate X_3, and X_1, X_2, Z_3 and Z_4 are used to estimate X_4. In the second stage these regression estimates of X_3 and X_4, each of which is independent of the causal influence of the other, are employed in the equations in the further estimation of X_3 and X_4 and the path coefficients p_{34} and p_{43} are obtained.

It is necessary to note that while there may not be significant multicollinearity between the original explanatory variables in a model, there may be high and damaging multicollinearity in the second stage regressions involving the values estimated at the first stage. A major consequence of high multicollinearity is large standard errors (Berry 1984). If the model is just identified, the two-stage least squares regression procedure yields an optimal solution. However, if the model is overidentified the method of generalized least squares regression provides a more robust set of parameter estimates together with standard errors that are not larger than and generally smaller than the two-stage least squares regression estimates. Tests which require the variables to be expressed in standardized form have been devised to examine whether one reciprocal effect is significantly larger than the other (James 1981).

3.3 Simple versus Latent Variable Models

The advantage of using ordinary least squares methods in the fitting of simple path models to directly observed variables is that such methods are readily applied and yield readily interpretable results. If the purpose of the data analysis is to indicate whether or not a certain relationship exists while other variables are being held constant; or if the aim is to rank order the explanatory capacity of antecedent variables in influencing a given dependent variable in terms of a few, broad categories of relationships, for example, strong, medium, and weak effects; then the use of simple path models can be defended on the grounds that the value added by employing more sophisticated estimation procedures would not balance the cost of the additional effort required.

The accuracy and hence usefulness of simple path models and least squares estimation procedures critically depend on the reliability of the variables and on whether the quality of the data is such that the use of maximum likelihood estimation procedures is justified. Simple path models do not allow the researcher to take into account that the variables on which the model is based are likely to be imperfectly measured. Yet it is certain that most variables commonly employed in social and educational research are beset by error (see *Reliability in Educational and Psychological Measurement*). Whereas one part of this error involves measurement error and is unique to the variable, a second component depends on certain characteristics of the study, such as the design and sampling procedures that were used in the data collection (see *Selection Bias in Educational Research; Sampling Errors in Survey Research*). The variables that are specified in a path model tend to have this second component of error in common; hence their residuals tend to correlate. Unique and common errors influence both the accuracy of parameter estimates and the stability of the path model as a whole.

If the purpose of the data analysis is to examine the causal relationship among a series of variables, or if the intention is to calculate precise estimates of the parameters in a model based on fallible indicators, then the use of multiple indicator modeling techniques is generally to be recommended. Where multiple observed variates are used to create a single variable that is a construct and not directly observable, the newly formed variable has come to be known as a latent variable. Such latent variables have greater reliability and validity than observable or manifest variates. Latent variable models, which are more powerful than simple path models but also much more demanding on the researcher, present an attractive means of estimating the strength of causal relationships among variables. They also overcome some of the problems of measurement error and correlated residuals that beset most psychological, sociological, and educational research studies in which use is made of indicators that are not directly observable, such as intelligence, gross domestic product, or the quality of teaching and learning in schools (see *Path Analysis with Latent Variables*).

4. Linear Structural Relations Analysis

One of the strategies employed for the analysis of path models that involve latent variables and a complex set of structural equations is known as "linear structural relations analysis."

Suppose that an investigator is interested in studying the stability of cognitive ability between the ages of 10 and 20 years, as well as the predictive capacity of home background and formal educational attainment in influencing cognitive ability. This research question, which is addressed in a study conducted by Husén and Tuijnman (1991), poses two basic problems of scientific inference. The first concerns the measurement of unobservable or latent variables, such as home background and educational attainment; the second involves that of estimating the causal relationships among these latent variables and their relative

explanatory capacity. As is explained below, linear structural relations analysis offers a means of solving both problems in a rigorous way. Several computer programs are available for the analysis of structural equation models, namely LISREL (Jöreskog and Sörbom 1989), EQS (Bentler 1985), and LISCOMP (Muthén 1987).

4.1 Measurement Model

Linear structural relations models generally consist of two components: a measurement model and a linear structural equation model. The key to overcoming the first problem is to estimate a measurement model in which each latent variable is identified on the basis of multiple observed indicators, so that the reliabilities of the latter and the validity of the former can be taken into account. For example, home background can be identified using indicators such as the level of education attained by the father and mother and the social prestige afforded by their occupations. The purpose of the measurement model is to extract the common dimension that underlies these four indicators. In this way an unobserved or latent variable—home background—is created, which is free of measurement error variances that are associated with the indicators. As in the case of commonality or factor analysis, the loadings can—after squaring—be interpreted as a lower bound estimate of the reliability of each of the four indicators in measuring the latent variable, home background. The variance which these indicators explain in the latent variable can moreover be interpreted as an estimate of construct validity (Heise and Bohrnstedt 1970).

In this example provided by Husén and Tuijnman's (1991) study the full measurement model would represent a factor analytic structure where each of the latent variables is measured by several high-loading indicators. A computer program can then be used to estimate the disattenuated (i.e., free of measurement error) correlation coefficients and the path coefficients among the latent variables in the structural model. The basic premise of factor analysis, namely, that a clear and stable factor structure is obtained if the indicators load strongly on only one latent construct and weakly on all the others, applies equally well in the case of a measurement model. If the indicators have significant factor loadings on more than one latent construct, then the stability of the structural model is in danger, and unbiased estimators of the disattenuated correlation coefficients generally cannot be obtained unless explicit allowance is made for this disturbance, something that can also be done in a structural model.

4.2 Structural Model

The method estimates not only the unknown reliability and validity coefficients in the measurement model, but also the structural parameters that are associated with the hypothesized, putative cause-and-effect relationships among the latent constructs. This is done in the linear structural relations model, which specifies the causal relationships among the latent variables as well as the random disturbance terms. As Jöreskog and Sörbom (1989) note:

> Because each equation in the model represents a causal link rather than a mere empirical association, the structural parameters do not, in general, coincide with coefficients of regressions among observed variables. Instead, the structural parameters represent relatively unmixed, invariant and autonomous features of the mechanism that generates the observed variables. (1989 p. 1)

In the example under consideration, this means that the estimates of the structural parameters among the four latent variables, for example, the stability of cognitive ability at 10 and 20 years of age, as well as estimates of the predictive capacity of home background and formal educational attainment in influencing cognitive ability, may be interpreted as relatively stable and unbiased path coefficients. Figure 4 presents the full structural model. Both the measurement and structural components of the model are easily recognized. It can be seen that the first latent variable, home background, is measured with three indicators. The reliability coefficients and related measurement errors are displayed, as well as the residual variances among the indicators. It can also be seen that the parameter showing the effect of home background on cognitive ability at age 10 years is statistically significant, whereas this is not the case with respect to the effect of this predictor on cognitive ability at age 20 years.

4.3 Model Specification and Assumptions

Jöreskog and Sörbom (1989 pp. 4–6) present the three equations that define a full structural model, the basic assumptions that guide model specification and the conventions used in modeling as follows:

Consider random vectors $\eta' = (\eta_1, \eta_2, \ldots, \eta_m)$ and $\xi' = (\xi_1, \xi_2, \ldots, \xi_n)$

of latent dependent and independent variables, respectively, and the following system of linear structural relations

$$\eta = B\eta + \Gamma\xi + \zeta. \tag{1.1}$$

where B $(m \times m)$ and Γ $(m \times n)$ are coefficient matrices and $\zeta' = (\zeta_1, \zeta_2, \ldots, \zeta_m)$ is a random vector of residuals (errors in equations, random disturbance terms). The elements of B represent direct effects of η-variables on other η-variables and the elements of Γ represent direct effects of ξ-variables on η-variables. It is assumed that ζ is uncorrelated with ξ and that Γ-B is nonsingular.

Vectors η and ξ are not observed, but instead vectors $y' = (y_1, y_2, \ldots, y_p)$ and $x' = (x_1, x_2, \ldots, x_q)$ are observed, such that

$$y = \Lambda_y\eta + \varepsilon, \tag{1.2}$$

and

$$x = \Lambda_x\xi + \delta, \tag{1.3}$$

where ε and δ are vectors of error terms (errors of

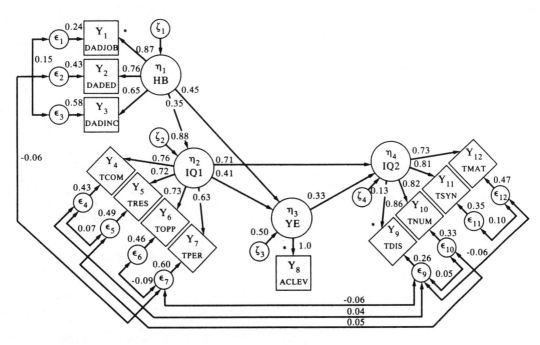

Figure 4
Parameter estimates in a model examining the effect of schooling on adult IQ test scores

measurement or measure-specific components). These equations represent the multivariate regressions of y on η and of x on ξ, respectively. It is convenient to refer to y and x as the observed variables and η and ξ as the latent variables. The errors ε and δ are assumed to be uncorrelated between sets but may be correlated within sets. The assumption that ε is uncorrelated with δ can be relaxed.

In summary, the full model is defined by the three equations,

Structural equation model: $\eta = B\eta + \Gamma\xi + \zeta$

Measurement model for y: $y = \Lambda_y\eta + \varepsilon$

Measurement model for x: $x = \Lambda_y\xi + \delta$

with the assumptions,

(a) ζ is uncorrelated with ξ;

(b) ε is uncorrelated with η;

(c) δ is uncorrelated with ξ;

(d) ζ, ε, and δ are mutually uncorrelated;

(e) Γ–B is nonsingular.

If certain rules are followed in the path diagram, it is possible to derive the model equations from the path diagram and to derive the LISREL parameter matrices. The following conventions for path diagrams are assumed:

(a)   Observed variables such as x- and y-variables are enclosed in squares or rectangles. Latent variables such as ξ- and η-variables are enclosed in circles or ellipses. Error variables such as δ-, ε- and ζ-variables are included in the path diagram and are enclosed in small circles.

(b)   A one-way arrow between two variables indicate a postulated direct influence of one variable on another. A two-way arrow between two variables indicates that these variables may be correlated without any assumed direct relationship.

(c)   There is a fundamental distinction between independent variables (ξ-variables) and dependent variables (η-variables). Variation and covariation in the dependent variables is to be accounted for or explained by the independent variables. In the path diagram this corresponds to the statements: (i) no one-way arrows can point to a ξ-variable; (ii) all one-way arrows pointing to an η-variable come from ξ- and η-variables.

(d)   All direct influences of one variable on another must be included in the path diagram. Hence the nonexistence of an arrow between two variables means that it is assumed that these two variables are not directly related. They may still be indirectly related.

If the above conventions for path diagrams are followed it is always possible to write the corresponding model equations by means of the following general rules:

(a)   For each variable which has a one-way arrow pointing to it there will be one equation in which this variable is a left-hand variable.

(b)   The right-hand side of each equation is the sum of a number of terms equal to the number of one-way arrows pointing to that variable and each term is the product of the coefficient associated with the arrow and the variable from which the arrow is coming.

4.4 Input Data, Moment Matrices, and Fit Functions

The LISREL computer program (Jöreskog and Sörbom 1993) can not only read a raw data matrix Z, but also a moment matrix M, a covariance matrix S, or a correlation matrix R, consisting of a combination of different types of correlation coefficients. PRELIS, the preprocessor for the LISREL program, is the appropriate tool for computing these matrices and assigning the desired input format.

PRELIS can handle a large number of problems with the distributional properties of the raw data, and can also compute an appropriate matrix for use by the LISREL program. Besides recoding and transforming raw data, PRELIS can be used to compute variance and covariance matrices based on either raw or normal scores, as well as moment matrices involving different correlation coefficients such as product moment, canonical, polychoric and tetrachoric, and bi- and polyserial coefficients. It is, moreover, possible to declare, before computing the desired matrix, which types of scales have been assigned to the variables —ordinal, continuous, or censored—so that optimal scores can be used in estimating the moment matrix.

The metric of the observed variables that are used in forming the latent variables can be retained or suppressed. As a first step in the analysis of structural equation models, the metric properties of one of the observed variables is normally assigned to the latent variable. The researcher then has the option of working with the latent variables in their unstandardized form, or the latent variables can be standardized in a second step. Because the transfer of the metric of one variable to another is beset with both conceptual and statistical problems the latter option is normally to be preferred.

Another advantage of the PRELIS program is that it can produce an estimate of the "asymptotic" (large sample) covariance matrix of the estimated correlation matrix (Browne 1982, Jöreskog and Sörbom 1993). This asymptotic matrix can be analyzed with the (generally or diagonally) weighted least squares method in the version of LISREL available in the early 1990s, thus allowing the relaxation of the otherwise often violated assumption of a multivariate normal distribution of data that binds the applicability of maximum likelihood estimation. This version of LISREL features four fit functions in addition to the three already mentioned—that is, maximum likelihood (ML), generally weighted least squares (WLS), and diagonally weighted least squares (DWLS). These additional methods for obtaining parameter estimates are: instrumental variables (IV), two-stage least squares (TSLS), unweighted least squares (ULS), and generalized least squares (GLS).

This variety of methods available for computing matrices and estimating parameters makes PRELIS and LISREL a very powerful model building tool. Some of the problems besetting the use of maximum likelihood estimation procedures in path analysis can be solved, for example, those associated with the use of ordinal, dichotomous and nonnormally distributed variables, through choosing from the range of methods available in the later versions of LISREL and PRELIS. However, certain problems remain in the testing for statistical significance of the specific parameters that are estimated.

4.5 Goodness of Fit and Testing the Model

The LISREL measurement model provides a number of statistics for checking whether the latent variables and their multiple indicators are adequately specified. It is rare for a LISREL measurement model to appear problem-free when specified for the first time. It is also much more common for the researcher to work on the improvement of the model through a repeated process of model specification, fit assessment, and diagnosis of the problem, followed by model respecification. Large measurement errors besetting some or all of the indicators, which negatively affect the validity of the constructs to be identified, is one of the most common problems at this stage in the model building process. If the measurement errors are large, then it is also likely that there are significant correlations among the residual variances or error terms. In this case the measurement model will often have to be modified; for example, by removing indicators, by allowing an indicator to be associated with more than one latent construct, or by explicitly allowing for correlations among the residuals.

The overall adequacy of a structural model is determined, first, on the basis of the interpretability of the parameter estimates; and second, on the basis of the consistency of the results compared with those obtained in contrast models computed with comparison data sets or, if such are not available, by crossvalidating the results on a split-half independent sample.

The following criteria, estimates for which are provided by the LISREL program, are often used in assessing the "overall goodness of fit" of a model to the data: the value of χ^2 relative to the degrees of freedom, the probability that the true χ^2 value is larger than the obtained value, the adjusted goodness

of fit index, the root mean square residual, root mean square error of approximation, and the number of fitted relative to unconstrained residuals. Users of LISREL are aware of the fact that the χ^2 statistic, which measures the discrepancy between the observed and the fitted covariance matrix, should actually be interpreted as a "badness-of-fit" measure, since a small chi-square value denotes good fit and a large χ^2 poor fit.

The following guidelines can be used in interpreting these overall goodness of fit criteria: the fit of a model may be judged acceptable if the χ^2 value is close to the number of degrees of freedom (a ratio of 2 or less is usually sufficient); a probability value P which is greater than the 0.10 level is commonly used as a threshold for statistical significance; a goodness of fit value which exceeds 0.90; and a value of the root mean square residual and the root mean square error of approximation (RMSEA) which should lie below 0.05. The RMSEA fit index would appear to be a key index in determining the fit of a model, since many of the other indexes are very dependent on sample size (Gustafsson and Stahl 1996). Furthermore, the fewer the number of unconstrained residuals with standardized values outside the range from −2.0 to 2.0, the better the fit of the model is judged to be.

Apart from the above criteria which are useful in examining the overall fit of a model to the data, there are also many ways of detecting lack of fit in parts of the model. The obvious statistics to be studied in this case are the values of the structural parameters themselves, their standard errors, the disattenuated correlations among latent variables, the squared multiple correlations associated with validity, and the coefficients of determination which are associated with prediction.

4.6 Refining the Model

As mentioned above, it is normally necessary to refine the measurement model, often even many times, before an adequate model is obtained. Since the way the measurement model is specified and its adequacy in terms of the properties of the resulting latent structure is decisive for the results that are eventually obtained, it is sound strategy to seek to crossvalidate the model building process using a split-half sample or some other means.

The LISREL computer program features two powerful tools for assessing detailed fit and diagnosing possible sources of the lack of fit in parts of the measurement or structural model: a facility for plotting standardized residuals and an option for computing modification indices. A Q-plot of standardized residuals offers an easy route for identifying outliers, which are indicative of problems such as nonlinearity, nonnormality or of a specification error in the model. Once a problem is detected in this way, the modification indices can be employed in order to look for a possible remedy. Such indices are measures of the predicted decrease in the χ^2 value if a single constraint in the model were to be relaxed and the model re-estimated. The improvement in fit is interpreted in terms of a χ^2 distribution with 1 degree of freedom. Although these modification indices make it easy to identify ill-fitting constraints, such parameters should only be freed if this can be justified on grounds of a plausible theoretical explanation. On balance, however, Q-plots and modification indices are an important innovation, since they greatly facilitate the process of detecting inadequacies in a model, and diagnosing and remedying their sources.

The refinement of the structural model follows a course similar to that used in simple path analysis. All structural parameters in a model are normally kept unconstrained until after the measurement model is judged adequate on grounds of both theory and the detailed assessment of goodness of fit statistics. After this, the estimates of the statistical significance of individual, structural parameters, such as the standard errors, are examined. Although the theory used in calculating the standard errors in LISREL normally requires a simple random sample, standard error estimates are usually examined even if this condition is not met. In models fitted to data collected with a stratified, complex sampling design, the threshold for accepting that a given structural parameter actually exists and is nonzero in the population is a t-value with magnitudes of 2.5 or higher. Structural parameters failing to achieve significance at this threshold level are removed from the model—not all at once but in several stages and in descending order of probability of statistical significance.

4.7 Additional Features

The LISREL computer program is very flexible and can handle both standard and nonstandard models and submodels, such as congeneric measurement models, factor analysis models, and recursive and nonrecursive path models. Nonstandard structural models include two-wave models which are much used in psychology and education, and simplex models, which are useful for time series analysis in econometric research, longitudinal models, and sample equivalent models. LISREL is a powerful tool especially for analyzing time series and longitudinal data, since it can handle the problem of highly correlated residuals in autoregression models in which similar variables that are measured for the same group over time are specified.

It is also possible to analyze simultaneously data from several independent samples according to models in which certain parameters are specified to be invariant. This is referred to as simultaneous factor analysis or multisample model building. This approach is especially useful if measurements on both an experiment and a control group are available, because the effect of an intervention can be evaluated in a simultaneous analysis of a model in which some or all variables except the treatment variables are constrained to be equal over the groups.

Jöreskog and Sörbom (1991) introduced a new language for path and structural equation modeling, SIMPLIS, which replaces the laborious program input that was previously required. The innovation makes it very easy to specify LISREL models, because all that is required of the user is to name the observed and latent variables and formulate the model as a simple path diagram. The LISREL 8 program, also introduced in the early 1990s, can accept both the traditional program input as well as SIMPLIS commands. In addition Windows versions of the program are now available and are relatively easy to operate. This program, which calculates the desired model can immediately display the results in a simple path diagram on the video monitor.

5. Structural Equation Models and the Problems of Multilevel Analysis

One of the most important problems in educational research to be tackled in the late 1980s has been the development of analytical methods for the examination of multilevel data (see *Multilevel Analysis*). The LISREL programs permit the simultaneous analysis of up to 10 different data sets (Tuijnman and Ten Brummelhuis 1992). However, this simultaneous procedure does not permit the modeling and estimation of fixed and random effects at the macro level. Muthén has developed an approach to categorical variable estimation that is available in the software program LISCOMP (Muthén 1987) and has subsequently extended the use of this approach both to the partial modeling of multilevel educational achievement data (Muthén 1989) and to the analysis of change (Muthén 1991). In the analysis of change data, the measures of individual performance which are obtained at different points in time form the micro level. More recently Muthén and his colleagues in Sweden have solved many further problems in the multilevel analysis of structural equation models, and the STREAMS program (Gustafsson and Stall 1996) is now available for the multilevel analysis of such models.

See also: Multivariate Analysis; Multilevel Analysis Regression of Quantified Data

References

Bentler P M 1985 *Theory and implementation of EQS: A Structural Equation Program.* BMDP Statistical Software, Los Angeles, California

Berry W D 1984 *Nonrecursive Causal Models.* Sage, Beverly Hills, California

Browne M W 1982 Covariance structures. In Hawkins E M (ed.) 1982 *Topics in Applied Multivariate Analysis.* Cambridge University Press, Cambridge

Browne M W 1984 Asymptotically distribution free methods for the analysis of covariance structures. *Brit. J. Math. S.* 37: 62–83

Burks B S 1928 *The Relative Influence of Nature and Nurture upon Mental Development: A Comparative Study of Parent–Foster Child Resemblance and True Parent–*

Child Resemblance. National Society for the Study of Education, Chicago, Illinois

Cohen J, Cohen P 1983 *Applied Multiple Regression/Correlation Analysis for the Behavioral Sciences*, 2nd edn. Erlbaum, Hillsdale, New Jersey

Duncan O D 1966 Path analysis: Societal examples. *Am. J. Sociol.* 72: 1–16

Duncan O D 1969 Contingencies in constructing causal models. In Borgatta E F (ed.) 1969 *Sociological Methodology 1969.* Jossey-Bass, San Francisco, California

Duncan O D 1975 *Introduction to Structural Equation Models.* Academic Press, New York

Games P A 1990 Correlation and causation: A logical snafu. *J. Exp. Educ.* 58(3): 239–46

Gustaffson J-E, Stall P A 1996 STREAMS *User's Guide Structural Equation Modeling Made Simple.* Goteborg University, Göteborg

Hauser R M 1973a Disaggregating a social-psychological model of educational attainment. In Goldberger A J, Duncan O D (eds.) 1973 *Structural Equation Models in the Social Sciences.* Seminar Press, New York

Hauser R M 1973b *Socioeconomic Background and Educational Performance.* American Sociological Association, Washington, DC

Hayduk L A 1987 *Structural Equation Modeling with LISREL: Essentials and Advances.* Johns Hopkins University Press, Baltimore, Maryland

Heise D R 1969 Problems in path analysis and causal inference. In Borgatta E F (ed.) 1969 *Sociological Methodology 1969.* Jossey-Bass, San Francisco, California

Heise D R 1975 *Causal Analysis.* Wiley, New York

Heise D R, Bohrnstedt G W 1970 Validity, invalidity and reliability. In Borgatta E F (ed.) 1970 *Sociological Methodology 1970.* Jossey-Bass, San Francisco, California

Husén T, Tuijnman A C 1991 The contribution of formal schooling to the increase in intellectual capital. *Educ. Researcher* 20(7): 17–25

James L R 1981 A test for asymmetric relationships between two reciprocally related variables. *Multivariate Behavioral Research* 16(1): 63–82

Johnston J 1972 *Econometric Methods*, 2nd edn. McGraw Hill, New York

Jöreskog K G, Sörbom D 1989 LISREL7. *A Guide to the Program and Applications*, 2nd edn. SPSS Publications, Chicago, Illinois

Jöreskog K G, Sörbom D 1991 SIMPLIS. *A New Command Language for LISREL Modeling.* Department of Statistics, University of Uppsala, Uppsala

Jöreskog K G, Sörbom D 1993 PRELIS 2. *A Program for Multivariate Data Screening and Data Summarization. A Prepocessor for LISREL,* 2nd edn. Scientific Software Inc., Mooresville, Indiana

Keeves J P 1988 Path analysis. In Keeves J P (ed.) 1988 *Educational Research, Methodology, and Measurement: An International Handbook.* Pergamon Press, Oxford

Land K C 1969 Principles of path analysis. In Borgatta E F (ed.) 1969 *Sociological Methodology 1969.* Jossey-Bass, San Francisco, California

Muthén B O 1984 A general structural equation model with dichotomous, ordered categorical and continuous latent variable indicators. *Psychometri.* 49: 115–32

Muthén B O 1987 LISCOMP: *Analysis of Linear Structural Relations using a Comprehensive Measurement Model.* Scientific Software, Mooresville, Indiana

Muthén B O 1989 Latent variable modeling in heterogeneous populations. *Psychometri.* 54: 557–85

Muthén B O 1991 Analysis of longitudinal data using latent variable models with varying parameters. In Collins L M, Horn J L (eds.) 1991 *Best Methods for the Analysis of Change.* American Psychological Association, Washington, DC

Peaker G F 1971 *The Plowden Children Four Years Later.* National Foundation for Educational Research, Slough

Pedhazur E J 1982 *Multiple Regression in Behavioral Research.* Holt, Rinehart and Winston, New York

Specht D A 1975 On the evaluation of causal models. *Social Science Research* 4(2): 113–33

Stokes D E 1968 Compound paths in political analyses. *Mathematical Applications in Political Science* 5

Stokes D E 1974 Compound paths: An explanatory note. *American Journal of Political Science* 18: 191–214

Tuijnman A C, Ten Brummelhuis A C A 1992 Predicting computer use in six education systems: Structural models of implementation indicators. In: Plomp T, Pelgrum H (eds.) 1993 *The IEA Study of Computers in Education.* Pergamon Press, Oxford

Tukey J W 1977 *Exploratory Data Analysis.* Addison Wesley, Reading, Massachusetts

Wright S 1934 The method of path coefficients. *Annals of Mathematical Statistics* 5: 161–215

Path Analysis with Latent Variables

N. Sellin and J. P. Keeves

Since the early 1970s path analysis and causal modeling have gained acceptance in educational research as well as in research in the social and behavioral sciences. The procedures employed have been developed to incorporate three main problems. First, in educational situations there are many outcomes as well as many explanatory factors to be considered. The analysis of the measures employed to represent these outcomes and explanatory constructs is confounded by problems of multicollinearity, measurement error, and validity. Measurements made on variables gain in strength and consistency if they are combined as related indicators of an underlying latent construct. Second, theory in educational research has advanced during the latter half of the twentieth century so that it is now possible to develop strong models that can be submitted to examination, and the estimation of the magnitude of the parameters of such models is of considerable theoretical interest and practical significance. Third, it is widely recognized that not only should the direct effects of explanatory variables be taken into consideration, but the mediating and moderating effects of such variables, as well as spurious and disturbance effects, should be examined. Those three issues have led to the development of latent variable path analysis and structural equation modeling (see *Path Analysis and Linear Structural Relations Analysis*).

Two general approaches have emerged in this field for the examination of models advanced from theoretical considerations. The first builds on the use of least squares regression analysis to predict and explain the effects of variables on one or more criteria. The emphasis in this approach is prediction and to maximize the amount of variance of the criteria explained by the predictors. The second approach builds upon maximum likelihood estimation procedures. This involves obtaining estimates of free parameters of a model, subject to specified constraints imposed by the fixed parameters, so that the covariance matrix derived from the estimations made is as close as possible to the covariance matrix based on the hypothesized model. Thus, the estimates obtained of the free parameters of the model are such that the difference between the covariance matrices of the observed data and the model are minimized. In this second approach the methods of parameter estimation employed distinguish between procedures that are dependent on the assumption of multivariate normality and those that are not. Normal theory estimation is associated primarily with the LISREL series of programs that employ both maximum likelihood estimation procedures and generalized and weighted least squares procedures (see *Path Analysis and Linear Structural Relations Analysis*) and the work of Jöreskog and Sörbom (1989). Asymptotic distribution free estimation is employed when the data are not multivariate normal and is associated with the work of Browne (1982, 1984) and Muthén (1984, 1987).

This entry restricts itself to consideration of the approach that employs partial least squares (PLS) regression analysis to maximize prediction and the explanation of variance which was developed by Wold (1977, 1982). This approach is less well-known than the other approaches outside of continental Europe, with the developmental work having been carried out in Sweden and Germany. It has the clear advantages that no assumptions need be made about the shape and nature of the underlying distributions of the observed and latent variables. This permits the analysis of data of dichotomous variables that are not associated with an underlying continuous distribution, which is a distinct advantage for a variable such as sex of student, or for the use of variables to represent countries in cross-national comparative studies. Furthermore, the approach recognizes that nearly all data employed

in educational research involve the use of complex cluster sample designs. As a consequence, procedures of statistical significance, that are heavily dependent on testing for statistical significance with assumptions of simple random sampling and multivariate normal distributions, are largely inappropriate. Least squares regression procedures are known from extensive experience to be robust. However, there is no proof, beyond very simple models which are equivalent to principal components analysis and canonical correlation analysis, that convergence in the iterative procedures employed is complete. There is the ever-present danger of a false minimum in the test for the iterative procedure, and thus an erroneous solution in the estimation process. Consequently, some form of testing by replication would appear to be essential to validate the solutions obtained with partial least squares analysis.

It should be noted, however, that partial least squares path analysis as a technique is quick in analysis, and convergence generally takes place rapidly; is flexible in use in the testing of complex models; and is relatively easy for a novice, but who has sound theoretical perspectives, to employ. Furthermore, while greater stability of the solution is attained with large samples, it does not demand large samples for effective operation, as is explained below. The maximum likelihood estimation approach is considered elsewhere (see *Path Analysis and Linear Structural Relations Analysis*).

1. Historical Developments of PLS

The development of partial least squares analysis has been heavily dependent on the partial least squares procedures advanced by Wold (1965, 1966) from work primarily in economics. Wold also recognized that principal components and canonical correlation analysis procedures could be presented as path diagrams (see *Multivariate Analysis*), and recognized the advantages of using latent variables formed by principal components and canonical correlation analysis in path analytic studies (Peaker 1971, Keeves 1972). In addition, Wold (1977) recognized that through the use of partial least squares regression procedures it would be possible in a single analysis, employing an iterative process, to form a latent variable with regression weights, as a "rosette" to carry the regression relationship through to path analysis with latent variables. Thus, he saw the merging of procedures employed in regression analysis by econometricians with principal components and factor analytic procedures employed primarily by psychometricians together with the developments in path analysis employed in sociological research (Noonan and Wold 1983). By the mid-1970s, a general algorithm for iterative PLS estimation of path models with latent variables was available and by the late 1970s the basic design for PLS estimation of path models with latent variables was established (Wold 1977).

At the beginning of the 1990s two versions of computer programs for latent variable path analysis, using partial least squares regression procedures and both having been prepared in Germany, were available for use on IBM mainframe computers and desktop computers. The LVPLS (Version 1.8) program is a data-analytic package containing six main programs together with a program manual, that was prepared by Löhmoller (1984) for use in the batch mode. Sellin (1990) prepared a related program PLSPATH (Version 3.01) for use primarily in an interactive mode, and with large data sets of up to 200 variables. The availability of these programs has extended the use of PLS more widely, and it is evident that further developmental work on these programs, which are written in Fortran 77, is urgently needed as the possibilities of the very flexible approach to data analysis becomes evident to educational research workers outside Continental Europe. The problems of multilevel analysis, and the fit of models to data obtained with complex sample designs remain to be resolved and introduced into the computer program.

2. Specification of Models

The use of partial least squares analysis demands the development from theory of a well-specified model for examination and estimation. Although the approach is flexible, it should not be seen to be exploratory and lacking in rigor, as are some other regression analysis procedures, such as stepwise regression analysis. A PLS model is formally defined by two sets of linear equations, called the inner model and the outer model. The inner model specifies the hypothesized relationships among latent variables (LVs), and the outer model specifies the relationships between LVs and observed or manifest variables (MVs). Without loss of generality, it can be assumed that LVs and MVs are scaled to zero means so that location parameters can be discarded in the equations that follow. The inner model equation can be written as:

$$\eta = B\eta + \Gamma\xi + \zeta \tag{1}$$

where η symbolizes a $(g \times n)$ matrix of variables that are dependent on other variables in the model, the endogenous LVs, and ξ a $(h \times n)$ matrix of exogenous LVs, those variables which are not dependent on other variables in the model, and with n denoting the number of cases. The matrices B and Γ denote $(g \times g)$ and $(g \times h)$ coefficient matrices, respectively, and ζ represents the $(g \times n)$ matrix of inner model residuals. The basic PLS design assumes a recursive inner structure. The endogenous LVs can then be arranged in such a way that B is lower triangular with zero diagonal elements. The inner model equation is subject to predictor specification:

$$E(\eta| \eta\xi) = B\eta + \Gamma\xi \tag{2}$$

which implies $(E\xi\zeta') = 0$ and $E(\eta\zeta') = \zeta\zeta'$, with $\zeta\zeta'$ being a $(g \times g)$ diagonal matrix. That is, the inner model is assumed to constitute a causal chain system with uncorrelated residuals.

The outer model equations are given by:

$$x = \Pi_x\xi + \varepsilon_x \tag{3}$$

$$y = \Pi_y\eta + \varepsilon_y \tag{4}$$

where x and y denote $(k \times n)$ and $(m \times n)$ matrices of MVs. Π_x and Π_y represent $(k \times h)$ and $(m \times g)$ coefficient matrices, while ε_x and ε_y symbolize the matrices containing outer model residuals. In the basic PLS design, the MVs are assumed to be grouped into disjoint blocks with each block representing one LV. That is, each MV is assumed to belong to just one LV and, hence, each row of Π_x and Π_y is assumed to contain just one nonzero entry. The nonzero elements of Π_x and Π_y are called loadings. Since the loadings and the LVs are unknown, some standardization is necessary to avoid both conceptual and statistical problems. As a general rule, all LVs are assumed to be standardized to unit variance; i.e. VAR (ξh) = VAR (ηg) = 1.0. Similar to the inner model, predictor specification is adopted for the outer model equations. For example, predictor specification applied to Eqn. (4) gives:

$$E(y|\eta) = \Pi y\eta \tag{5}$$

with $E(\eta\varepsilon_y') = E(\xi\varepsilon_y') = E(\zeta\varepsilon_y') = 0$. In words, the outer model residuals are assumed to be uncorrelated with the LVs and with the inner model residuals.

In addition to predictor specification applied to inner model and outer model equations, a fundamental principle of PLS modeling is the assumption that all information between observables is exclusively conveyed by latent constructs. This has two implications, namely: (a) that PLS models do not involve any direct relationships among MVs; and (b) that the outer residuals of one block are assumed to be uncorrelated with the outer residuals of all other blocks.

The formal specification of PLS models also includes relations for substitutive prediction of endogenous MVs. The corresponding relations are obtained when the inner model Eqn.(1) is used to substitute the endogenous LVs involved in the outer model Eqn.(4). This gives:

$$y = \Pi_y(B\eta + \Gamma\xi) + u \tag{6}$$

with $u = \Pi_y\zeta + \varepsilon_y$. Wold (1982) calls this substitutive elimination of latent variables or SELV. As can be seen from Eqn.(6) the SELV relation connects endogenous MVs with LVs that are indirectly connected (via the inner model) with the respective sets of MVs. The ensuing residuals are, by virtue of Eqns.(2) and (5) above, uncorrelated with the corresponding predictor LVs.

635

The basic model can also be extended so that a block may contain more than one latent variable. Moreover, the basic model can be modified so that the manifest variables are not disjoint between blocks, but are shared across more than one latent variable. These extensions provide for more complex models with a sizeable number of manifest and latent variables built into the model. It is also possible to combine categorical variables, such as type of school attended, into a latent variable, by the omission of one category as a dummy variable. The weights employed in combining the observed variables are estimated in the analysis and the omitted category merely receives a zero weight. Such a procedure would not seem to be appropriate with other latent variable estimation approaches. Furthermore, in common with other approaches, PLSPATH, but not LVPLS, through the incorporation of two-stage least squares regression into the computer program is able to estimate the parameters of a nonrecursive inner model, as is illustrated below.

3. Model Estimation

The key feature of PLS is the explicit estimation of latent variable scores by means of least squares methods. This has considerable advantages. Two points should be noted in addition to those mentioned above. First, no identification problems arise if the specified model is recursive. For nonrecursive models, the well-known classical conditions of identifiability (i.e. rank and order condition) can be applied so that identification is rarely a problem. Second, the PLS algorithm provides estimated case values of latent variables which can be used for testing purposes and case-oriented analyses. It is, for example, possible to employ distribution-free statistical methods, such as jackknifing, in order to evaluate PLS modeling results.

The above equations and the accompanying set of assumptions constitute the structural or the theoretical form of PLS models. The LVs, the inner model coefficients and the weights and loadings are, of course, unknown and must be estimated. It is beyond the scope of this entry to present the algorithm for PLS estimation in great detail. Reference is made to Wold (1982) for a comprehensive and thorough exposition of PLS.

The PLS parameter estimation proceeds in two steps. The first step involves the iterative estimation of LVs as linear composites of their associated MVs. The second step involves the noniterative estimation of inner model coefficients. The estimated LVs are defined as:

$$\text{est. } (\xi) = X = W_x x \tag{7}$$

$$\text{est. } (\eta) = Y = W_y y \tag{8}$$

where W_x and W_y represent $(h \times m)$ and $(g \times k)$ weight matrices, with nonzero weights corresponding to the grouping of MVs into $(h + g)$ disjoint blocks. The

matrices X and Y contain estimated LV scores which are standardized so as to give each LV unit variance.

The estimated LVs defined above are, in the second step of PLS estimation, used to estimate the inner model coefficients by means of standard least squares methods. Thus these inner model coefficients are estimated using standard path analytical procedures. That is, for recursive inner models, the respective coefficients are obtained by ordinary least squares (OLS) regression applied to each inner model equation separately.

The core of the PLS procedure is obviously the determination of the weights defining LV estimates. These weights are obtained iteratively by a series of either simple or multiple OLS regressions applied to each block of MVs. The investigator has the choice between two modes of weight estimation, called outward mode and inward mode. It may be noted that the distinction between the outward and inward blocks corresponds to the differentiation between reflective and formative indicators made by Hauser (1973). Reflective or outward indicators are assumed to "reflect" the corresponding latent construct. A typical example would be a set of attitude items assumed to reflect an underlying attitudinal dimension. Formative or inward indicators, on the other hand, are assumed to "form" or "produce" a latent construct. An example would be a set of teacher behaviors assumed to form a specific teaching style. Related to the outward mode are the further possibilities of employing principal components analysis noniteratively to form a LV from the cluster of MVs, or employing just one MV to reflect a particular LV.

The specification of the inner model, the block structure (i.e., the grouping of MVs into $(h + g)$ disjoint blocks), and the estimation mode to be applied to each block together constitute what can be called the PLS iteration model. The iteration model specifies the way in which the estimation of a given PLS model proceeds.

The estimation of outward blocks is based on an iterative sequence of simple OLS regressions where the respective MVs are considered as dependent variables. The estimation of inward blocks is based on multiple OLS regression where the MVs are used as independent variables. It should also be noted that the PLS algorithm incorporates, as special cases, principal components and canonical correlations. As shown by Wold, one-block PLS models estimated by the outward mode are numerically and analytically equivalent to the first principle component, while the first canonical correlation is obtained from the two-block PLS models when blocks are estimated by the inward mode. Since the general features of principle component and canonical correlation analysis can be expected to carry over to multiple-block PLS models, it is a general advice to use the inward mode for exogenous LVs and the outward mode for endogenous LVs in order to increase the predictive power of the corresponding inner model and outer model relations. Such statistical considerations should not generally overrule theoretical assumptions with regard to reflective and formative measurement relations. However, sometimes where the use of the inward mode is argued for an exogenous LV, a high degree of multicollinearity between the MVs, requires that the outward mode must be employed to get meaningful weights and loadings.

It is important to recognize that although both the weights and the loadings are available for the combination of MVs to derive LVs, it is the weights that are effective and should be reported where the inward or formative mode is used, and the loadings that should be reported where the outward mode is used. These loadings are the correlations between the LV and each of the related MVs.

It is also important to note that in the iterative procedure employed in the PLS estimation only a subset of the manifest variables is included in the analysis at any one time in the outer model estimations. Furthermore, once the latent variables have been estimated, only these latent variables are included in the inner model estimations. Thus the requirement of a sufficient number of cases for least squares estimation applies to only a subset of the variables at any stage and not to the total number of variables included in the analysis. As a consequence PLS analyses can be employed effectively with a much fewer number of cases than is generally required by other analytic procedures. Nevertheless, with a large number of cases greater stability in the estimates is ensured.

Because of the uncertainties with respect to whether a true minimum has been reached in the iterations, five criteria are employed to identify when it is appropriate to terminate the iterations, namely, (a) the greatest difference between weight estimates; (b) the mean of the squared multiple correlations of the LVs; (c) the root mean square of LV correlations; (d) the mean of the absolute LV correlations; and (e) the root mean square of loadings. Convergence is achieved when all these scalar quantities do not change by more than 0.00001 or a similar specified value.

4. Model Trimming

Sometimes problems are encountered in the estimation of a hypothesized model. Care must be taken in the refinement of a model in order to achieve convergence as well as to obtain a meaningful and well-fitting model. An important criterion is that of parsimony, in so far as it is of little value to include in a model variables and paths of the effects of one variable on another that do not contribute to prediction and the explanation of variance.

Partial least squares analysis programs do not place great reliance on tests of statistical significance, since the computation and use of standard errors in regression analysis necessarily assumes both a simple random sample and a multivariate normal distribution for the observed and the latent variables. Simple random samples are rare in educational research. Moreover, it seems likely that at least some of the variables in a model will violate the assumptions of normality. The problems of lack of normality in the estimation of standard errors can be largely overcome through the use of jackknifing, but the procedure is very tedious to employ with complex cluster samples and is considered below in a rare case where a simple random sample was drawn. As a consequence, in the use of PLS programs extensive reliance is placed on rules of thumb.

The first step in the refinement of a model is the trimming of the manifest variables (MVs) that are combined to obtain the latent variables (LVs). If the inward mode is employed, a weight of less than 0.1, associated with a correlation of approximately 0.1, contributes less than one percent to the explanation of a latent variable and the predictor variable must be regarded as having a trivial effect. If the outward mode is employed, a loading of less than 0.3 indicates that a LV contributes less than 10 percent to explaining an observed MV, and the relationship between the MV and the LV is slight. A more stringent rule of thumb may be used for a loading in the case of the outward mode of 0.55 which indicates that the LV has approximately 30 percent of variance in common with the observed MV. However, if the contributing MVs are theoretically and empirically homogeneous then a loading of 0.3 would seem acceptable.

The second step is the refinement of the inner model. Here path coefficients are generally trivial if they fall below 0.1 and the predictor latent variable contributes less than one percent to the explanation of an endogenous latent variable in a model. If, however, there is a strong theoretical case for the inclusion of a particular path in a model, then a path with a path coefficient in excess of 0.05 could remain in the model, provided a very large sample had been used.

In all cases where paths have been deleted and the effects of variables are under consideration, the matrices of residuals provide useful information of cases of lack of fit of variables to the model. Cases arise where a latent variable is clearly an orphan, being neither influenced by other latent variables in a model nor influencing other latent variables. Here the requirement of parsimony and overall model fit, imply the deletion of such a latent variable from a model.

5. Model Evaluation

The PLS procedure is characterized as a "prediction oriented" approach, because it basically aims at optimal least squares prediction of endogenous LVs and MVs. It will also be recalled that predictor specification as applied to inner and outer model relationships constitutes an integral part of the structural form of PLS models. Hence, in addition to the examination of point estimates (i.e., loadings, weights, and inner model coefficients), an important part of model evaluation is the examination of fit indices reflecting the predictive power of estimated inner and outer model relationships. Three descriptive fit indices can be derived from the inner and outer model equations given earlier. First, R^2 values can be computed for each inner model equation. Second, the squared correlations between MVs and their associated LV estimates can be used to assess the predictive power of outer model relations. Following factor-analytic terminology, these indices are commonly called communalities. Third, similar to the computation of communalities, squared correlations can also be calculated from relations derived by substitutive prediction. These indices are called redundancies and can be interpreted as indicating the joint predictive power of inner and outer model relations.

The statistics referred to above can be used in essentially the same way as the familiar R^2 computed for multiple regression equations. They reflect the relative amount of "explained" or "reproduced" variance of LVs and MVs. However, the researcher will usually wish to go beyond evaluating predictive relations in purely descriptive terms.

5.1 Stone–Geisser Test

Since PLS provides estimated case values of LVs and estimated case values of inner and outer residuals, as an alternative to conventional statistical tests Wold (1982) proposed the general use of the Stone–Geisser test (SG-test) of predictive relevance (Stone 1974, Geisser 1974). The SG-test basically produces jackknife estimates of residual variances while jackknife standard errors of point estimates can be obtained as a by-product (Tukey 1977). The general idea is to omit or "blindfold" one case at a time, to re-estimate the model parameters on the basis of the remaining cases, and to reconstruct or predict omitted case values on the basis of re-estimated parameters. An adaptation of Ball's (1963) Q^2 can then serve as the test criterion. As applied to $i = 1, 2, \ldots,$ n cases and to the familiar case of multiple OLS regression, Q^2 is defined as:

$$Q^2 = 1.0 - [\Sigma_n(Y_i - X_i b_{(i)})^2] / [\Sigma_n(Y_i - \bar{Y}_{(i)})^2] \quad (9)$$

where Y_i denotes the ith case value of the dependent variable and X_i the row vector of the ith case values of, say, k predictor variables. $\bar{Y}_{(i)}$ represents the jackknife mean of Y (i.e., the mean when the ith case is omitted), and $b_{(i)}$ is the ($k \times 1$) coefficient vector obtained when the ith ith case is exempted from estimation. From Eqn. (9) it can be seen that Q^2 is nothing other than a jackknife analogue of the familiar R^2. The tested model equation has more predictive relevance the higher Q^2 is, and model modifications, such as the deletion of predictor variables, can be evaluated by comparing Q^2 values. It should be noted that, contrary to R^2, Q^2 values may increase when predictors are deleted. This indicates, intuitively speaking, that "noise" emanating from irrelevant predictor or instability of parameter

estimation has been removed. Q^2 values may also turn out to be negative. The specified model is then said to be misleading because the trivial prediction in terms of sample means is superior to the prediction derived from the tested model relation.

The SG-test allows straightforward extension to PLS models (see Wold 1982). The corresponding procedures provide indices of the predictive relevance of inner and outer model relations as well as jackknife standard errors of PLS parameter estimates that can be used for testing purposes. However, jackknifing is a very tedious procedure to employ where complex cluster sample designs are used, and as a consequence has rarely been tried with complex samples in PLS analyses.

5.2 Reliability Coefficients

Another index of the fit of a model to the observed data has been developed from a strategy employed in the maximum likelihood approach. If O represents the null model, and T the model of interest, n is the number of independent parameters with k the number of manifest variables, and N is the number of cases, then Tucker and Lewis (1973) proposed a reliability index for the Model T compared to the null Model O:

$$r_{to} = \frac{L_t/f_t - L_o/f_o}{L_o/f_o - \frac{1}{N}} \quad (10)$$

where L is the maximum likelihood loss function, and the degrees of freedom are:

$$f = \frac{(k^2 + k)}{2} - n$$

Bentler and Bonett (1980) contended that the reliability index should be free of sample size and proposed a reliability coefficient given by:

$$r_{to} = \frac{L_t - L_o}{L_o}$$

However, Marsh et al. (1988) have shown that this and alternative indexes are not free from the effects of sample size, while the Tucker and Lewis coefficient is. For comparing the fit of PLS models this descriptive index would seem to have some utility.

5.3 Three other Indicators

For examining the overall strength of a PLS model, three further measures are available for use.

(a) Mean of squared multiple correlations of endogenous LVs—this is the arithmetic average of the multiple R^2 for the endogenous LVs. The larger the value of this index the greater the amount of variance explained by the model.

(b) RMS Cov (E, U)—this index is the root mean square of the covariances between the residuals of the MVs and the residuals of the LVs. Loosely, it is the average correlation of residuals of the LVs and MVs. The lower this coefficient the better the model.

(c) Redundancy coefficient—this index is an average of the amount of variance of the endogenous variables that is explained by the manifest variables in the model. A high or moderate value indicates good fit.

In the absence of a jackknife estimate of Q^2, it would seem of value to take a half sample, following the full design of the sample, to replicate the analysis on the half-sample, and then to compare the two solutions for the stability of the estimates. Alternatively, naturally occurring subgroups may provide opportunities for replication that would yield evidence of the stability of estimates.

6. An Example

Sellin (1986) provides an example of the analysis of a non-recursive model using PLSPATH and the two-stage least squares regression procedure (see *Path Analysis and Linear Structural Relations Analysis*). The data analyzed were obtained with simple random sampling (Keeves 1972). Through the use of a less than optimal routine it was possible to estimate jackknife standard errors. The results of the analysis are presented in the path diagram shown in Fig. 1. However, the standard errors shown in Fig. 1 must be interpreted with caution, as they tend to underestimate sampling variation.

The most interesting aspect of the model is the nonrecursive relation between Final Achievement and Final Attitude. In Fig. 1 it can be seen that the estimated effect of Final Attitude on Final Achievement turned out to be much smaller than the corresponding effect of Final Achievement on Final Attitude. The estimated effect of Final Attitude on Final Achievement (0.053) must, in fact be regarded as trivial, since the associated standard error (0.036) is an underestimate. Hence, the nonrecursive model formulation is not supported by the data. All other parameters shown in the model may be regarded as significant.

7. Limitations of PLS Analytical Procedures

While partial least squares path analysis procedures have many strengths when used with the data that are commonly available in educational research, they have several important shortcomings.

First, PLS procedures cannot model measurement error. Most variables of interest in educational research are measured with some degree of error. Measurement error in the exogenous variables can bias the estimates of parameters that are made. Measurement error in the endogenous variables reduces the variance explained and in so far as the standard errors of the estimates are taken into account, they are larger than would be expected. The formation of latent variables serves to

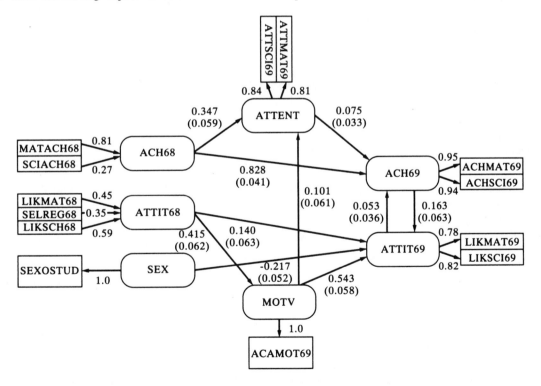

Figure 1
An example of a nonrecursive model

639

increase the reliability of such variables and to reduce the measurement error associated with them. However, LISREL permits the modeling of the measurement error associated with observed variables.

Second, in much measurement in educational research it is necessary to employ variables that are observed as censored or in discrete categories, but that have underlying continuous and normal distributions. Procedures were advanced by Muthén (1984) to estimate polyserial and polychoric correlations for such variables with stronger relationships being estimated and analyzed. The use of such procedures is now routine in LISREL analyses, but have not been employed or made available for PLS analyses.

Third, there are inevitably unmeasured correlations between the observed variables. Such correlations are not modeled in PLS analyses, although they can be in LISREL analyses, with general improvement in the fit of the model to the data.

Fourth, until very recently no path analytic procedures have sought to model the hierarchical or nested nature of the data widely used in educational research. Cheung and Keeves (1990) have employed principal components analysis together with hierarchical linear modeling in an attempt to overcome this weakness in current methods of analysis. However, their approach does not involve the simultaneous analysis of a multilevel path model, but rather the use of a series of separate steps.

Finally, it is not possible with PLS analyses to compare simultaneously the path models for separate data sets to test whether the path models may be considered highly similar or significantly different. Without such a test, for example, in the analyses of data for male and female students, it is necessary to assume that identical models are in operation for both sex groups. Such an assumption does, however, permit the estimation of the direct and indirect effects of Sex of Student on endogenous latent variables in PLS analyses.

In conclusion, it would seem unfortunate that the procedures made available for latent variable path analysis using partial least squares regression analysis is not more widely known outside continental Europe and that developmental work would appear to have ceased on this flexible and readily used analytic tool.

See also: Path Analysis and Linear Structural Relations Analysis; Multivariate Analysis

References

Ball R J 1963 The significance of simultaneous methods of parameter estimation in econometric models. *Appl. Stat.* 12: 14–25

Bentler P M, Bonett D G 1980 Significance tests and goodness of fit in the analysis of covariance structures. *Psych. Bull.* 88(3): 588–606.

Browne M W 1982 Covariance structures. In: Hawkins E M (ed.) 1982 *Topics in Applied Multivariate Analysis*. Cambridge University Press, Cambridge

Browne M W 1984 Asymptotically distribution free methods for the analysis of covariance structures. *British Journal of Mathematical and Statistical Psychology* 37(1): 62–83

Cheung K C, Keeves J P 1990 Testing multilevel product-process networks. *Int. J. Educ. Res.* 14(3): 307–15

Geisser S 1974 Contribution of the written discussion of the article by M. Stone. *Journal of the Royal Statistical Society* Series B 36: 134–47

Hauser R M 1973 Disaggregating a social–psychological model of educational attainment. In: Goldberger A J, Duncan O D (eds.) 1973 *Structural Equation Models in the Social Sciences*. Seminar Press, New York

Jöreskog K G, Sörbom D 1989 *LISREL 7. A Guide to the Program and Applications*, 2nd edn. SPSS Publications, Chicago, Illinois

Keeves J P 1972 *Educational Environment and Student Achievement*. Almqvist and Wiksell, Stockholm

Löhmoller J B 1983 *LVPLS Program Manual Version 1.6*. Zentralarchiv Universität Köln, Köln

Marsh H W, Balla J R, McDonald R P 1988 Goodness of fit indexes in confirmatory factor analysis: The effect of sample size. *Psych. Bull.* 103(3): 391–410

Muthén B O 1984 A general structural equation model with dichtomous ordered categorical and continuous latent variable indicators. *Psychometri.* 49(1): 115–32

Muthén B O 1987 *LISCOMP: Analysis of Linear Structural Relations using a Comprehensive Measurement Model*. Scientific Software, Mooresville, Indiana

Noonan R D, Wold H 1983 Evaluating school systems using partial least squares. In: Choppin B, Postlethwaite T N (eds.) 1983 *Evaluation in Education: An International Review Series*, Vol. 7. Pergamon Press, Oxford

Peaker G F 1971 *The Plowden Children Four years Later*. National Foundation for Educational Research, Slough

Sellin N 1986 Partial least squares analysis. *Int. J. Educ. Res.* 10(2): 189–200

Sellin N 1990 *PLSPATH Version 3.01. Program Manual*. Hamburg

Stone M 1974 Cross- validatory choice and assessment of statistical predictions. *Journal of the Royal Statistical Society* Series B 36, 111–47

Tucker L R, Lewis C 1973 A reliability coefficient for maximum likelihood factor analysis. *Psychometri.* 38: 1–10

Tukey J W 1977 *Exploratory Data Analysis*. Addison-Wesley, Reading, Massachusetts

Wold H 1965 A fix-point theorem with economic background. *Arkiv för Matematik* 6: 209–46

Wold D 1966 Non-linear estimation by iterative least squares procedures. In: David F N (ed.) 1966 *Research Papers in Statistics: Festschrift for. J. Neyman*. Wiley, New York

Wold H 1977 Open path models with latent variables. In: Albach H, Halstedt E, Henn R (eds.) 1977 Kuantative Wirtschaftsforschung: Wilhelm Krelle zum 60. Geburstag. Mohr, Tübingen

Wold H 1982 Soft modeling: The basic design and some extensions. In: Jöreskog K G, Wold H (eds.) 1982 *Systems under Indirect Observation. Part II*. North Holland Press, Amsterdam

Further Reading

Falk R R, Miller N B 1991 *A Primer for Soft Modeling*. University of Akron Press, Akron, Ohio

Löhmoller J B 1989 *Latent Variable Path Modeling with Partial Least Squares*. Springer-Verlag, New York

Muthén B O 1989 Latent variable modeling in heterogeneous populations. *Psychometri.* 54: 557–85

Profile Analysis

J. P. Keeves

During the latter decades of the twentieth century greatly increased use has been made of visual displays in the presentation of statistical and quantitative information. In part this is due to the ease and accuracy with which different types of graphs can be drawn using microcomputers in order to present such information. In part it is a consequence of increased dependence on television for obtaining information. But it is also in part a consequence of the ease with which quantitative data can be stored and subsequently accessed and with which complex analyses can be carried out. However, these developments also result in the need to present the findings of such analyses simply and in ways that can be readily understood.

These visual displays of information are commonly set out in the form of profiles. As a consequence, the use of profiles in practice and research has greatly increased, for the presentation of data on school performance regarding individual students to parents and teachers, regarding school and class groups to schools, principals, teachers, and administrators, and regarding major subgroups. This entry considers the use of profiles to present information. It is also concerned with the examination and analysis of profiles to extract meaning beyond what is immediately apparent in the visual display.

1. Definitions of "Profile" and "Profile Analysis"

In analyzing and recording the findings of many investigations in the field of education, comparisons are made between persons or groups of persons in terms of a set of measurements on specific related characteristics. For each person or group of persons a "profile" is obtained on a set of variables. Thus a profile may be defined as "a set of different measures of an individual or a group, each of which is expressed in the same unit of measure" (Kerlinger 1964 p. 614). The comparison between profiles for persons or groups on the same set of variables is known by the generic term "profile analysis." The term "profile" is derived from the common practice of plotting, as a graph or delineation, the scores of a person or a group on a battery of tests. The investigator who wishes to make comparisons between persons or between groups should pay particular attention to the choice of variables to be used in the set making up the profile. In addition, the investigator should take care to ensure that the scale used for recording data for the different measures is the same or metrically equivalent. Frequently standard score scales are employed where the measures have been standardized on the defined target population or on a sample drawn from that population.

2. Characteristics of Profiles

Nunnally (1967) has drawn attention to the fact that there are three major features of a score profile for any person or group of persons: level, dispersion, and shape. "Level" is defined as the mean score of the person or group over the set of variables in the profile. The concept of level can be employed only if the variables are concerned with similar properties of an individual or group and it is appropriate to add together the scores on the variables and calculate a mean. "Dispersion" of a score profile is related to the scatter or spread of the scores and indicates the extent to which the scores of the profile diverge from the average. A measure of dispersion is the standard deviation of the scores on the variables for each person or group from the mean score or level. The third characteristic of a profile is its "shape." An indicator of shape is the rank order of scores on the variables for each person or group. Thus it would be possible for two persons or groups to have profiles at the same level and with the same dispersion, but to differ markedly in shape.

3. Visual Display of Profiles

The most common form of visual display of a profile is a line graph for each individual or group across a set of scores. However, sometimes a profile compares the performance on two or more occasions, or on two scores for a set of individuals or a set of groups. Either Cartesian (rectangular) coordinates may be employed with a horizontal or vertical profile or polar (circular) coordinates may be used. Cartesian coordinates serve to emphasize a difference in shape, while polar coordinates serve to emphasize a difference in level (see Keeves 1992).

Where there is interest in the error of measurement for an individual or in the variability of scores for a group of individuals, which is related to the error of measurement of the mean of the group, then a confidence interval is commonly used to present the accuracy or spread (Gronlund 1976). Shading is also used to suggest the probability or confidence that can be ascribed to scores within the confidence interval (Masters 1990). It is particularly important to show the likely error of measurement when reporting information of an ipsative or intraindividual nature in order to prevent the impression being given that performance has been recorded with a high level of precision, without error, and is fixed and unchangeable over time. The widespread use of profiles in the presentation of information in counseling and guidance demands that such data are shown in an accurate way.

4. Comparisons of Profiles

Studies in which profiles have been compared have used a large number of techniques for assessing profile similarity (Cronbach and Gleser 1953). A common approach to the assessment of profile similarity is to consider the measurements that have been made on the set of variables as coordinates, and the scores of a group or a person on the variables as a point in the space defined by ordinates or dimensions associated with the variables. The distance between any two points, given k variables, may be calculated by the generalized Pythagorean formula:

$$\mathrm{D}^2_{12} = \sum_{i=1}^{k} (x_{i1} - x_{i2})^2 \text{ or } D_{12} = \sqrt{\sum_{i=1}^{k} (x_{i1} - x_{i2})^2}$$

for variables $i=1 \ldots k$

Either D or D^2 can be used as a measure of similarity. The use of D is generally preferred to other possible measures because it gives less weight to larger differences, although the measure of similarity D is not normally distributed. D as an index of profile similarity considers level, dispersion, and shape, and it has the advantage of being the basis for other more powerful techniques of profile analysis. Such procedures may involve cluster analysis and multidimensional scaling (see *Cluster Analysis; Scaling Methods*).

A second commonly used index of profile similarity is the Pearson product–moment correlation coefficient. It should be noted that the product–moment correlation coefficient based on raw scores provides the same result as that obtained using scores standardized within profiles. The product–moment correlation coefficient used in this way is a special case of the D measure, which ignores the differences in level and dispersion between the two sets of measure. It follows that the product–moment correlation coefficient is only sensitive to differences in shape between the two profiles. Cronbach and Gleser (1953) have also provided a weighted similarity index which can be used when the sets of scores on the variables do not have a strong first principal component.

5. Reliability of Comparison of Two Measures within Profiles

It is common when examining profiles of individual students to make comparisons between standard scores on individual subjects; for example, that the student is better in mathematics than in a foreign language. The reliability of the two tests and their intercorrelation needs to be taken into account when such statements are made, since the reliability of the difference score is given by:

$$r_{dd} = \frac{r_{xx} + r_{yy} - 2r_{xy}}{2 - 2r_{xy}}$$

where r_{dd} =the reliability of the difference score, $(x_i - y_i = d)$
r_{xx} and r_{yy} =the reliabilities of the two tests, and r_{xy} =the intercorrelation between the tests.

For example, if the reliabilities of a mathematics test and a foreign language test are 0.8, and their intercorrelation is 0.7, then the reliability of the difference is approximately 0.33. If differences in a profile are to be considered then the measures compared need to: (a) be highly reliable, (b) have low intercorrelations, and (c) be independent of one another if the differences are to have clear meaning (Cooley 1971).

6. Profiles and Moderator Effects

In the examination of moderator or interaction effects it is important to draw the profiles for subgroups that are hypothesized to be associated with a moderator variable. If the profiles diverge or converge to a significant extent a test should be applied for an interaction effect. If the profiles are parallel for the groups under consideration, no moderator effect is present (see *Interaction and Detection of its Effects in Educational Research*).

7. Conclusion

It is important that before using the techniques of profile analysis, consideration should be given to the strength, assumptions, and limitations associated with the indexes of similarity that are available, because different indexes will lead to different conclusions. If correctly used, profiles can be examined through multivariate analysis, as well as through the simple comparison of the profiles obtained from two persons or groups. Where the groups are known in advance of the analysis, the multivariate technique of discriminant analysis may be used to compare the groups. However, when the grouping of persons is not known in advance of the analysis, the function and purpose of the analysis are to cluster persons in terms of their profiles on the set of variables. Here the multivariate techniques of cluster analysis, multidimensional scaling, and smallest space analysis may be applied to cluster the persons into groups.

See also: Multivariate Analysis; Discriminant Analysis; Cluster Analysis; Scaling Methods; Smallest Space Analysis

References

Cooley W W 1971 Techniques for considering multiple measurements. In: Thorndike R L (ed.) 1971 *Educational Measurement*, 2nd edn. American Council on Education, Washington, DC
Cronbach L J, Gleser G C 1953 Assessing similarity between profiles. *Psych. Bull.* 50: 456–73
Gronlund N E 1976 *Measurement and Evaluation in Teaching*, 3rd edn. Macmillan Inc., New York

Keeves J P (ed.) 1992 *The IEA Study of Science III: Changes in Science Education and Achievement: 1970–1984.* Pergamon Press, Oxford

Kerlinger F N 1964 *Foundations of Behavioral Research.* Holt, Rinehart and Winston, London

Masters G et al. 1990 *Profiles of Learning: The Basic Skills Testing Program in New South Wales.* ACER, Hawthorn

Nunnally J C 1967 *Psychometric Theory.* McGraw-Hill, New York

Projections of Educational Statistics

D. E. Gerald and W. J. Hussar

Each nation has designated a center or unit that is responsible for collecting, analyzing, and disseminating information related to the status and progress of education in that country. An important aspect of this work includes the development of projections of enrollment, of high school graduates, and of classroom teachers, as well as producing projections on expenditure and average annual teacher salaries in public elementary and secondary schools. These projections are used by individuals and organizations in business, industry, government, the media, and education whose work requires information on projected developments and trends affecting education in that country. This entry is concerned with the techniques employed in the making of such projections and their use in planning and policy-making.

1. Use of Projections in Planning and Policy-making

In all countries it is necessary to make projections of key education statistics to facilitate planning and legislation. Moreover, in conjunction with socioeconomic and demographic data, educational projections provide the information needed to assess and monitor the progress of education in each country. Because projections can be constructed under different scenarios —low, middle, and high alternatives—alternative projections provide a range of possible outcomes to prepare decision-makers and planners for contingencies. Such contingencies have important budgetary implications for a country because expenditure on education is a significant part of the national budget of most countries.

Projections can be persuasive and, therefore, are commonly needed to lend credibility to long-term plans and proposed policies. In many instances, projections are developed in relation to the formulation of policies (United Nations 1984, Hopkins 1983). Projections, which are used to provide the best estimates about the future, given certain assumptions, indirectly contribute to developing policy. Furthermore, projections, which are used as warnings of where present trends are heading in the future, shape a policy to reverse, maintain, or promote such trends. Another use of projections is to determine the effects of a proposed policy.

The use of projections to develop long-term plans and make decisions is evident within the education system itself. This is because a considerable time lag exists between implementing plans for educational reforms and realizing the effects of such reforms (Hemler 1983). At a minimum, a planning horizon of 10 years is required to respond and to meet educational needs in a timely manner.

Projections also provide data about the future, and strengthen the quality of decisions made (Ascher and Overholt 1983). As such, forecasting is not an end in itself, but is the beginning of a process that leads to planning, decision, and action. For example, educational administrators need enrollment projections for long-range planning (Weldon et al. 1989). Projections of the number and ages of children to be served by a school district are required to analyze and reach decisions affecting facility requirements, staffing, and budgets.

Members of the business and industrial communities use educational projections as part of their information base for long-term strategic planning. With planning horizons of one, five, and ten years, projections are inputs into planning models to project demand for products such as graduation caps and gowns and cafeteria services. Book publishers use grade-specific enrollment projections to calculate the number of textbooks to print. Businesses and industry also use projections to determine the supply of high school graduates and college-educated personnel to staff companies. Another use in some countries is illustrated by leading institutions that make student loans for college attendance. High school graduate projections are used in such countries as inputs into models for projecting college enrollments. Accurate projections of college enrollments help these institutions to determine the loan volume needed for student aid.

2. Projecting Education Statistics

Beginning with current survey data and demographic age-specific data and projections derived from

643

a national census, public elementary and secondary enrollment is projected using expected grade retention and enrollment rates. Projections of high school graduates are based primarily on enrollment projections, while those for classroom teachers, school expenditure, and teacher salaries are based on enrollment projections and relevant economic variables. In the sections that follow the projection of each of these different statistics is considered in turn.

2.1 Public Elementary and Secondary Enrollment

This section provides a discussion of the data, methodology, and assumptions that may be used to develop projections of public elementary and secondary enrollment. The general approach to projection is that employed in the United States, and as a consequence the examples provided reflect the manner in which education is organized in that country. The general principles described would, however, apply to the projections made in other countries.

First, an education census or a survey is needed to collect data on current enrollment in kindergarten, individual Grades 1 through 12, ungraded classes, and adult classes. In addition, population estimates for the past two decades and population projections for the decade ahead are needed to develop the projections for these education statistics.

The grade retention or cohort-survival method is widely used to project public elementary and secondary school enrollment. The grade retention rate method starts with 6-year olds entering first grade and follows their progress through public elementary and secondary schools. Using the historical series of enrollment statistics by grade, the method computes the rate for the number of children who "survive" the year and enroll in the next grade the following year. This procedure is used to calculate retention rates for Grades 2 through 12. These rates are projected using exponential smoothing and are then applied to the current enrollment levels to yield grade-by-grade projections for future years. To obtain projections of enrollments for kindergarten, first grade, ungraded elementary, ungraded secondary, and adult levels, enrollment rates are computed. The various enrollments are expressed as percentages of the respective populations for the past two decades. These percentages are projected and applied to corresponding population projections for the decade ahead. Projections of kindergarten enrollment are thus based on population projections of 5-year olds, first grade on 6-year olds, ungraded elementary on 5- to 13-year olds, ungraded secondary on 14- to 17-year olds, and adult on 18-year olds. Grade retention and enrollment rates are projected and held constant throughout the projection period at levels consistent with the most recent rates.

A single exponential smoothing technique is used to project the grade retention and enrollment rates. This technique produces a constant projection and is suitable for historical data that do not vary drastically from year to year. This smoothing technique places more weight on recent observations than on earlier ones. The weights for observations decrease exponentially for data from those years further in the past. As a result, the older data have less influence on projections. The rate at which the weights of older observations decrease is determined by the smoothing constant selected.

The smoothing equation commonly employed is as follows:

$$P = aX_i + a(1 - a)X_{t-1} + a(1-a)^2X_{t-2} \qquad (1)$$
$$+ a(1 - a)^3X_{t-3} + \ldots$$

where: P = projected constant (e.g., retention rate); a = smoothing constant ($0<a<1$); and X_t = observation for time t (e.g., the actual retention rate at year t).

This equation illustrates that the projection is a weighted average based on exponentially decreasing weights. For a high smoothing constant, weights for earlier observations decrease rapidly. For a low smoothing constant, decreases are more moderate. A smoothing constant of 0.4 is commonly used to derive a rate at which the weights of earlier observations are decreased.

To obtain projections of elementary enrollment (kindergarten through Grade 8), kindergarten enrollment, ungraded elementary enrollment, and enrollment in Grades 1 through 8 are summed.

A public elementary enrollment projection model may be stated as follows:

$$EG_t = K_t + E_t + \sum_{j=1}^{8} G_{jt} \qquad (2)$$

where: t = subscript denoting time; j = subscript denoting grade; EG_t = total enrollment in elementary Grades K–8; K_t = enrollment at the nursery and kindergarten level; E_t = enrollment in elementary special and ungraded programs; and G_{jt} = enrollment in Grade j. To obtain projections of secondary enrollment Grades 9 through 12, ungraded secondary enrollment, adult enrollment, and enrollment in Grades 9 through 12 are summed.

The public secondary enrollment projection model is as follows:

$$SG_t = S_t + PG_t + \sum_{j=1}^{12} G_{jt} \qquad (3)$$

where: t = subscript denoting time; j = subscript denoting grade; SG_t = total enrollment in secondary Grades 9–12; S_t = enrollment in secondary special and ungraded programs; PG_t = enrollment in adult programs; and G_{jt} = enrollment in Grade j.

Data estimated in population projections must assume a changing fertility rate (e.g., 2.2 births per woman) and a changing net immigration rate expressed in terms of people per year. High and low estimates of these parameters provide alternative high and low projections of education statistics. These

644

assumptions affect enrollment projections in kindergarten and elementary grades. The grade retention rate method assumes that past trends in factors affecting public school enrollments will continue over the projection period. This assumption implies that all factors influencing enrollments will display future patterns consistent with past patterns. Therefore, the method has limitations when there are unusual changes in the data. This method implicitly includes the net effects of such factors such as dropouts, deaths, nonpromotion, and transfers to and from different types of schools.

Where major fluctuations are observed, it is necessary to ascribe these to clearly identifiable causes, such as in some countries the decline in fertility rates which occurred in the late 1960s and early 1970s.

2.2 High School Graduates

This section describes the data, methodology, and assumptions which may be used to develop projections of high school graduates. Census or survey data from the past two decades on the number of high school graduates provide the initial information. In addition, Grade 12 enrollments over the same period are required.

Projections of high school graduates may be developed in the following manner. For each major administrative region the number of school graduates is expressed as a percentage of Grade 12 enrollment in public schools for the past two decades. This percentage is projected using single exponential smoothing and applied to projections of Grade 12 enrollment to yield projections of high school graduates for the decade ahead.

By using single exponential smoothing, the number of high school graduates as a percentage of Grade 12 enrollment is assumed to remain constant at levels consistent with most recent rates. This method assumes that past trends in factors affecting high school graduates will continue over the projection period. It may, however, be necessary in some situations to make the estimates separately for males and females because of sex differences in both enrollment rates at Grade 12 and graduation rates.

2.3 Classroom Teachers

This section describes the data, methodology, and assumptions used to develop projections of the number of classroom teachers. The basic data on classroom teachers used to develop the projections may be obtained from a census of schools or from surveys over the past three decades. To estimate the number of teachers by organizational level (elementary and secondary), the proportion of teachers by organizational level is also required if separate projections are being made by educational level. In addition, local educational receipts per capita from central sources and disposable income, obtained from an economic forecasting organization, may be employed to increase the accuracy of the projections.

The number of school teachers is projected separately for the elementary and secondary levels. The elementary teachers are modeled as a function of per capita income, educational receipts per capita from central sources, and elementary enrollment. Secondary teachers are also modeled as a function of per capita income, educational receipts per capita from central sources, but lagged by three years, and secondary enrollment. Both per capita income and educational receipts per capita from central sources are expressed in constant dollars.

The particular equations shown were selected on the basis of their statistical properties, such as coefficients of determination (R^2), the t-statistics of the coefficients, the Durbin–Watson statistic, and residual plots. The elementary classroom teacher model is:

$$ELTCH + b_0 + b_1PCI + b_2SGRANT \qquad (4)$$
$$+ b_3ELENR$$

where: ELTCH = number of elementary classroom teachers; *PCI* = income per capita in constant dollars; *SGRANT* = educational receipts per capita from central sources in constant dollars; and *ELENR* = number of students enrolled in elementary schools. Each variable affects the number of teachers in the expected way. As people receive more income, the system spends more money on education, and as enrollment increases, the number of elementary teachers hired increases.

The secondary classroom teacher model is:

$$SCTCH = b_0 + b_1PCI + b_2SGRANT3 \qquad (5)$$
$$+ b_3SCENR$$

where: *SCTCH* = number of secondary classroom teachers; *SGRANT3* = educational receipts per capita from central sources in constant dollars, lagged by three years; and *SCENR* = number of students enrolled in secondary schools. Again, each variable affects the number of teachers in the expected way.

Three alternative projections of classroom teachers are commonly developed to indicate a range of possible outcomes. These alternatives vary assumptions about the growth paths for two of the key variables in the teacher model, namely, disposable personal income per capita, and local educational receipts from central sources per capita. Under the middle alternative it may be assumed that the economy will decline and then recover. The low alternative assumes that the economy will continue to grow over the projection period, but at a slower rate than the middle alternative. The high alternative assumes that the economy will grow more rapidly than the middle alternative. The third variable in the teacher model, enrollment by organizational level, is the same for all three alternatives, or it may be varied to take into account the possible perturbations in the enrollment estimates.

2.4 Current Expenditures of Public Elementary and Secondary Schools

The current expenditures of elementary and secondary schools are projected for the 1990s. Several alternative sets of projections may be developed. Data used to produce the current expenditure projections are based on information of expenditure over a sample period of suitable length.

There has been an extensive amount of research, both theoretical and empirical, concerning the demand for public goods such as education expenditures. The most theoretically developed and empirically tested model is the median voter model. According to this model, the demand for education in a community reflects the median voter's preference for the commodity (Inman 1979). The median voter model is used as a basis for the model employed to produce the current expenditure projections.

In the standard median voter model, education expenditures are a function of four types of independent variables: (a) income variables, (b) intergovernmental aid variables, (c) price variables, and (d) other variables believed to be related to the public's educational preferences. The model used to produce the projections contains a variable from each of the first three categories of variables. The current expenditure per pupil projection model is:

$$\ln(CUREXP) = b_0 + b_1\ln(PCI) \qquad (6)$$

$$+ b_2\ln(SGRANT) + b_3\ln(ADAPOP)$$

where: $\ln$ = natural logarithm; $CUREXP$ = current expenditures of public elementary and secondary schools per pupil in average daily attendance, in constant dollars; PCI = disposable personal income per capita, in constant dollars; $\ln$ = natural logarithm $SGRANT$ = educational receipts from central sources per capita in constant dollars; and $ADAPOP$ = ratio of average daily attendance to the population.

Alternative sets of projections for revenue receipts may be employed. To produce the projections of educational receipts from central sources per capita in constant dollars, a model containing four independent variables may be employed. An appropriate educational receipts projection model is:

$$\ln(SGRANT) = b_0 + b_1\ln(PERTAX1) \qquad (7)$$

$$+ b_2\ln(BUSTAX1) + b_3\ln(ADAPOP)$$

$$+ b_4\ln(RCPIANN/RCPIANN1)$$

where: $\ln$ = natural logarithm; $SGRANT$ = educational receipts from central sources per capita in constant dollars; $PERTAX1$ = personal taxes and nontax receipts in constant dollars, lagged one period; $BUSTAX1$ = indirect business taxes and tax accruals, excluding property taxes per capita, in constant dol-

lars, lagged one period; $ADAPOP$ = ratio of average daily attendance to the population; and $RCPIANN$ equals the inflation rate measured by the Consumer Price Index; and $RCPIANN1$ equals the inflation rate measured by the Consumer Price Index lagged one period.

The bases for the four projection alternatives for current expenditures were three sets of projections for disposable personal income and three sets of projections for educational receipts from central sources. For example, the middle–high alternative projections were produced using the middle projections for both variables.

2.5 Average Annual Salaries of Teachers in Public Elementary and Secondary Schools

The average annual salaries of teachers in public elementary and secondary schools may be projected for the decade ahead. Four alternative sets of projections may be developed.

The average annual salaries of teachers may be calculated as the arithmetic mean of the total amount regularly paid to teachers, before deductions. Historical data on teacher salaries are required.

A teacher salary model includes three variables which measure the demand for teachers and is:

$$\ln(SALARY) = b_0 + b_1\ln(CUREXP)$$

$$+ b_2\ln(ADAPOP) + b_3(ADA_1/ADA_2) \qquad (8)$$

where: $\ln$ = natural logarithm; $SALARY$ = average annual salaries of teachers in constant dollars; $CUREXP$ = current expenditures of schools per pupil in average daily attendance, in constant dollars; $ADAPOP$ = ratio of average daily attendance to the population; ADA_1 = average daily attendance lagged one period and ADA_2 = average daily attendance lagged two periods.

A sample period of the previous three decades is used to estimate the model. The model is estimated using a technique to correct for autocorrelation.

Four alternative scenarios are developed for teacher salaries. Each is based on one of the four alternative scenarios of current expenditures per pupil.

3. Accuracy and Limitations of Projections

3.1 Accuracy of Projections

The accuracy of projections largely depends on the reliability of the data sources, the validity of techniques used to construct the projections, and, for some techniques, the assumptions concerning the independent variables. These limitations are discussed in the following section. This section reviews the reliability of projections in terms of their errors.

The mean absolute percentage error (MAPE) may be used to measure the accuracy of the projection. The MAPE is the average value of the absolute value of errors expressed in percentage terms. To compute the MAPE, the values appearing in the projections are compared to the recorded values appearing in the previous versions of the projections. The absolute differences are then grouped by lead time of projections (i.e., one year into the future, two years into the future) to calculate the average of errors. The resultant MAPEs indicate the likely average percent of deviation between the projection and the actual value for specific numbers of years into the future.

For shorter lead times of one to two years, the projections of enrollment, high school graduates, and classroom teachers in the public schools have smaller errors than those for longer lead times. The current expenditure and teacher salaries projections have relatively larger errors, even for short lead times, due to changes in the economy.

3.2 Limitations of Projections

Any projection is limited by the data sources, the projection techniques, and the assumptions used to produce the projections (Ascher 1978). The limitations of projections affect their reliability in providing information about the future and in their usefulness in various applications. An understanding of the limitations allows for a more careful use and interpretation of the projections.

One difficulty about data sources is that projections frequently must be constructed for statistics for which there are very little historical data. In those instances, the number of possible projection techniques is limited. A second potential problem is that data in a time series may not be consistent due to changes in survey or census forms. Such changes make it more difficult to estimate the model and more difficult to evaluate its performance.

In this entry the use of exponential smoothing and regression techniques in the projection models has been discussed. The exponential smoothing technique is appropriate for statistics, such as enrollment and high school graduate projections, where the variation between historical data points is generally not large. This smoothing technique is suitable for historical data that do not vary drastically from year to year. The weights for observations decrease exponentially as movement is made further into the past. As a result, the older data have less influence on projections. The rate at which the weights of older observations decrease is determined by the smoothing constant selected. Proper selection of the smoothing constant allows the user to place more or less weight on the most recent data.

The regression technique is appropriate to estimate the models for classroom teachers and current expenditure. This technique is used when a strong causal relationship exists between the variable being projected and the independent variables.

These two estimation techniques use historical data to estimate the projection models. With these techniques, it is assumed that the future trend will be the same as in the past. With the ordinary least squares regression technique, it is assumed that the relationships between dependent and independent variables will continue to hold throughout the projection period.

Projections of education statistics frequently rely on projections of other statistics. For example, the projection of elementary and secondary enrollment relies on age-specific population projections produced by a national census. The projections of teachers, current expenditures, and teacher salaries rely on projections of economic variables. These educational projections are limited by the accuracy of these other population and economic projections.

Frequently, several sets of projections are presented which are based on alternative sets of demographic and/or economic assumptions. These alternatives represent best judgments of reasonable upper and lower bounds for each projected series. Users are able to choose the set of assumptions which they think are most likely and to contrast the impact of the differing sets of assumptions.

4. Future Developments

It is necessary to upgrade projection methodologies through ongoing model development. While enrollment and graduate projections are primarily based on demographic data, efforts are necessary to continue to improve the econometric models for classroom teachers, current expenditures, and teacher salaries. Work on estimating several different models using simultaneous equations is clearly a promising line of development.

References

Ascher W 1978 *Forecasting: An Appraisal for Policy-Makers and Planners.* Johns Hopkins University Press, Baltimore, Maryland.

Ascher W, Overholt W 1983 *Strategic Planning and Forecasting: Political Risk and Economic Opportunity.* Wiley, New York

Helmer O 1983 *Looking Forward: A Guide to Futures Research.* Sage, Beverly Hills, California

Hopkins F S 1983 The planning mission before us. In: Fowles J (ed.) 1983 *Handbook of Futures Research.* Greenwood Press, Westport, Connecticut

Inman R P 1979 The fiscal performance of local governments: An interpretative review. In: Mieszkowski B, Straszheim M (eds.) 1979 *Current Issues in Urban Economics.* Johns Hopkins University Press, Baltimore, Maryland

United Nations Ad Hoc Expert Group on Demographic Projections 1984 *Population Projections: Methodology of the United Nations.* United Nations, Department of International Economic and Social Affairs, Population Studies, No. 83, New York

Weldon W, Hurwitz E, Menacker J 1989 Enrollment projections: Techniques and financial implications. *School Business Affairs* 55(10): 28–31

Further Reading

Abraham B, Ledolter J 1983 *Statistical Methods for Fore-*

casting. Wiley, New York

Gerald D, Hussar W 1996 *Projections of Education Statistics to 2006.* US Department of Education, National Center for Education Statistics, Washington, DC

Holden K, Peel D A, Thompson J L 1990 *Economic Forecasting: An Introduction.* Cambridge University Press, Cambridge

Regression Analysis of Quantified Data

M. M. Tatsuoka

Regression analysis refers to a broad class of statistical techniques that are designed to study the relationship between a criterion (or dependent) variable, Y, and one or more predictor (or independent) variables, $X_1, X_2, \ldots, X_p$. The means by which such study is effected is a regression equation, which is an equation of the general form

$$\hat{Y} = (X_1, X_2, \ldots, X_p) \tag{1}$$

where the circumflex on the Y denotes that what is represented by the function of the X's is a "predicted" or "modeled" Y-value rather than one that is actually observed.

The function $f(\ )$ may, at one extreme, be a simple linear function of a single predictor (i.e., $b_0 + b_1 x$). At the other extreme it may be a complicated weighted sum of several predictors raised to various powers and include also products of two or more predictors (e.g., $b_0 + b_1 X_1 + b_2 X_2 + b_3 X_1^2 + b_4 X_1 X_2 + b_5 X_1 X_2^2$). The terms may even include transcendental functions such as $\log X_j, e^{x_j}$, and so forth. However, such a term may be defined as a separate predictor, and the task of determining the combining weights (or regression coefficients) will become more involved but no new principle will have to be invoked.

What is the general principle involved in determining the regression coefficients? It is desirable that the modeled Y-values, $\hat{Y}_i$ (where i represents the i-th individual in the sample), should "be as close as possible" to their actually observed counterparts Y_i. More specifically, "closeness" can be defined so as to mean small total (or average) squared discrepancies between Y_i and $\hat{Y}_i$. That is, the quantity

$$Q = \sum_{i=1}^{N} (Y_i - \hat{Y}_i)^2 \equiv \sum_{i=1}^{N} e_i^2 \tag{2}$$

can be defined as the "loss function," which is to be minimized by appropriate choice of the regression-coefficient values. (Here N is the sample size, and e_i is simply another symbol for $Y_i - \hat{Y}_i$, known as "error" or "lack of fit" of the i-th observation to the model.) This is the famous least squares principle.

Of course, invoking the least squares principle, by itself, does not completely solve the problem of determining the regression coefficients. Before that, a decision must be made on what particular functional form to adopt for $f(\ )$; that is, the regression model must be chosen. Until this choice is made, the very task of minimizing the loss function is ill-defined. For instance, the minimum Q attainable by adopting the class of linear functions $f(X) = b_0 + b_1 X$ as the regression model and determining the optimal b_0 and b_1 values will, in general, be "undercut" if one allows a quadratic function $f(X) = b_0' + b_1' X + b_2' X^2$ as a candidate and determines the optimal values of b_0', b_1', and b_2. Thus, the choice of a type of regression model is the crucial first step before one can even apply the least squares principle.

Ideally, there should be some theoretical grounds for making this choice. A substantive theory in the field of research should dictate whether to adopt, say, a linear, quadratic, or exponential regression model. Unfortunately, it is seldom the case in behavioral science that there is a substantive theory precise enough to specify a particular type of regression model. It is thus frequently necessary to proceed by trial-and-error. In this case, the decision is guided by another principle of scientific endeavor: the canon of parsimony, which holds that a more complicated model should not be used when a simpler one will suffice.

In the context of choosing a regression model, this usually means that a linear model should be tried first, and only if this proves not to yield an "adequate" fit should a sequence of more complicated models be tried successively. A crucial point here is how to decide whether the fit offered by a given regression model is adequate or not. One way is to test whether or not a significant decrease would be obtained in the loss function Q if one were to go from the simpler to the more complicated model. Only if the decrease $Q_1 - Q_2$ (say) is significantly greater than zero would there be justification for using the second model. To ignore this and jump suddenly to a complicated, well-fitting model would be to commit the error of "overfitting" the sample at hand. An excellent fit may be obtained to the current dataset, but this would more likely than not incur a drastic drop in the extent of fit in a future sample from the same population, when an attempt is made to replicate (cross-validate) the finding or utilize the regression equation.

What was said above concerning the choice of a class of regression models holds equally well with regard to the number of predictor variables to include. Even when the mathematical form of a model is fixed, say to a multiple linear regression form, the fit can generally be improved by adding more and more predictor variables. But the more that is added, the less likely it will be that the extent of fit achieved in the sample at hand will hold up in future samples. Hence, a predictor variable should not be added to an existing multiple regression equation unless the addition results in a significant decrease in the loss function Q—or, as is shown below—a significant increase in the squared multiple correlation coefficient.

In the forgoing, nothing was said about the purposes of regression analysis, since it was assumed that the reader was familiar with at least the simplest (or most practical) of the purposes served; namely the prediction of such things as college or job performance for the screening or guidance of candidates. However, regression analysis is coming more and more to be used for a purpose that has traditionally been served by analysis of variance (ANOVA) and analysis of covariance (ANCOVA). This usage will be discussed below after a description of several models, their properties, and some problems inherent in regression analysis.

It should also be pointed out here that a regression model, properly speaking, requires the values of the independent variable(s) to be fixed by the researcher. Examples would be ages of the subjects to be used, dosages of a drug to be administered, and so on. This is in counterdistinction to the correlation model, in which dependent and independent variables alike are random variables, whose values are "brought along" by the subjects sampled—for example, course grades and pretest scores; height and weight. Most of the techniques of regression analysis are applicable equally to the regression and correlation situation, although some differences in significance tests and so on do exist. This entry will speak for the most part in the language of the regression model; this allows one to refer to groups defined by values of the independent variable(s), and hence to subgroup means of Y.

1. Models, Properties, and Problems

1.1 Simple Linear Regression

The simplest regression model takes the form of a single-predictor linear equation,

$$\hat{Y} = b_o + b_1 X \tag{3}$$

where the constants are determined, as mentioned

earlier, so as to minimize the loss function $Q = \Sigma(Y - \hat{Y})^2$. The results turn out to be

$$b_1 = \Sigma x_i y_i / \Sigma x_i^2 \tag{4}$$

and

$$b = \hat{Y} - b_1 \hat{X} \tag{5}$$

(Here $x_i = X_i - \bar{X}$ and $y_i = Y_i - \bar{Y}$ are deviations from the means.) b_1 is called the coefficient of regression of Y on X—or, simply, the "regression coefficient" —while b_o *is the* Y-intercept. These constants are unbiased estimates of the corresponding population constants β and β_0.

When b_1 and b_0 as defined by Eqns. (4) and (5) are substituted back into the expression for Q with $\hat{Y}$ replaced by $b_0 + b_1 x$, after doing some algebra, the following is obtained:

$$Q_{min} = \Sigma y^2 - (\Sigma xy)^2 / \Sigma x^2 \tag{6}$$

This is called the residual sum of squares of Y, denoted SS_{res}. Factoring out Σy^2 in the right-hand expression yields

$$SS_{res} = (\Sigma y^2)[1 - (\Sigma xy)^2 / (\Sigma x^2 \Sigma y^2)] \tag{7}$$

The reader may recognize the fraction in the brackets to be equal to the square of the product–moment correlation coefficient r_{xy}. Thus,

$$SS_{res} = (\Sigma y^2)(1 - r_{xy}^2) \tag{8}$$

Recalling that SS_{res} is another symbol for Q_{min}, the minimum value of the loss function that can be achieved for the given regression model by using the optimal b_0 and b_1, it can be seen that the larger r_{xy} is in absolute value, the smaller Q_{min} is. (Of course $0 \leqslant r_{xy} \leqslant 1$, as the reader probably knows.)

Equation (8) may also be written as $SS_{res} = \Sigma y^2 - r_{xy}^2 \Sigma y^2$, and it may further be shown that

$$r_{xy}^2 \Sigma y^2 = \sum_{i=1}^{N} (y_i - \hat{Y})^2 \tag{9}$$

which is called the sum of squares due to linear regression, symbolized $SS_{lin.reg.}$. It therefore follows that

$$r_{xy}^2 = SS_{lin.\,reg.} / SS_{tot} \tag{10}$$

where SS_{tot} has been written for Σy^2 (since this is the total sum of squares of ANOVA). This is the mathematical formulation of the well-known statement that "the squared correlation is the proportion of the variability of the dependent variable that is associated with its linear regression on the independent variable."

The reader may recall that the t statistic for testing the significance of a correlation coefficient is $t = r(N-2)^{1/2}/(1-r^2)^{1/2}$, which follows a t distribution with $N-2$ degrees of freedom when the null hypothesis is true. The square of this statistic, which may be rearranged slightly to read

$$F = \frac{r^2/1}{(1-r^2)/N-2)} \tag{11}$$

follows an F distribution with 1 and $N-2$ degrees of freedom. Substituting for r^2 and $1 - r^2$ from Eqns. (10) a9 11 13nd (8), respectively, the following is obtained:

$$F = \frac{SS_{\text{lin. reg.}}/1}{SS_{\text{res}}/(N-2)} \tag{12}$$

or, upon rewriting the numerator and denominator as mean squares,

$$F = \frac{MS_{\text{lin. reg.}}}{MS_{\text{res}}} \tag{13}$$

which bears an obvious resemblance with the customary F ratio in one-way ANOVA: $F=MS_b/MS_w$.

1.2 Multiple Linear Regression

One way in which the simple linear regression Eqn. (3) can be complexified by one step is to add a second predictor variable to get

$$\hat{Y} = b_o + b_1 X_1 + b_2 X_2 \tag{14}$$

The constants b_o, b_1, and b_2 are again determined by minimizing $Q = \Sigma(Y - \hat{Y})^2$ with $\hat{Y}$ replaced by the second member of Eqn. (14). Setting the appropriate partial derivatives equal to zero results in the equations:

$$(\Sigma x_1^2)b_1 + (\Sigma x_1 x_2)b_2 = \Sigma x_1 y \tag{15}$$

$$(\Sigma x_2 x_1)b_1 + (\Sigma x_2^2)b_2 = \Sigma x_2 y \tag{16}$$

and

$$b_0 = \bar{Y} - b_1 \bar{X}_1 - b_2 \bar{X}_2 \tag{17}$$

The first two of these equations, called the normal equations, may be written in a compact form by defining the sum-of-squares-and-cross-products (SSCP) matrix of the predictor variables,

$$S_{xx} = \begin{bmatrix} \Sigma x_1^2 & \Sigma x_1 x_2 \\ \Sigma x_2 x_1 & \Sigma x_2^2 \end{bmatrix} \tag{18}$$

the vector of regression coefficients (more precisely, partial regression coefficients),

$$b = \begin{bmatrix} b_1 \\ b_2 \end{bmatrix} \tag{19}$$

and the vector of sums of cross products (SCP) between predictors and criterion,

$$S_{xy} = \begin{bmatrix} \Sigma x_1 y \\ \Sigma x_2 y \end{bmatrix}. \tag{20}$$

The normal equations then become

$$S_{xx}b = S_{xy} \tag{21}$$

which may be solved to yield

$$b = S_{xx}^{-1} S_{xy} \tag{22}$$

(provided that S_{xx} is nonsingular). The similarity between this and Eqn. (4) for the one-predictor case is evident—especially if the latter is deliberately rewritten in the form

$$b_1 = (\Sigma x^2)^{-1}(\Sigma xy) \tag{23}$$

Those who are not familiar with matrix algebra may either simply follow the formal analogy with the one-predictor situation described in the previous subsection or refer to a reference such as Green (1976) or to the matrix-algebra chapter in any of several multivariate analysis texts (e.g., Tatsuoka 1988).

If Eqn. (14) is generalized to

$$\hat{Y} = b_0 + b_1 X_1 + b_2 X_2 + \ldots + b_p X_p \tag{24}$$

one has only to define a larger SSCP matrix (with p rows and p columns) S_{xx} and larger (p-dimensioned) vectors b and S_{xy} to go into Eqn. (21). The equation for the Y-intercept b_0 is not worth rewriting in matrix notation. The general case can be simply written as

$$b_0 = \bar{Y} - b_1 \bar{X}_1 - b_2 \bar{X}_2 - \ldots - b_p \bar{X}_p \tag{25}$$

The index which measures how well (or poorly) a multiple linear regression model fits a given set of observations—that is, how small the minimum value of Q can be made by choosing regression coefficients and intercepts that satisfy Eqns. (21) and (25)—is defined as the product–moment correlation coefficient $r_{Y\hat{Y}}$ between the observed and modeled criterion scores Y and $\hat{Y}$. This is called the "multiple correlation coefficient" and is symbolized as R _y.123. . .p_ (or simply R if the context makes it clear what the criterion and predictor variables are). R may be computed by actually determining each person's "predicted" (i.e., modeled) Y score, $\hat{Y}_i$, from Eqn. (24) and correlating it with the observed Y score, Y_i. This, however, would be extremely tedious to do, and in practice one of several algebraically equivalent formulas is used that gives the same result. One of these is $R^2 = S'_{xy} b / \Sigma y^2$, where S'_{xy} (or S_{yx}) is the transpose of S_{xy}—that is, a row vector with the same elements as the S_{xy} defined before. Nevertheless, it is important to keep in mind that $R=r_{\hat{Y}Y}$.

A test of the null hypothesis that the population multiple correlation coefficient is zero may be carried out by using an F statistic that is a direct generalization of that displayed in Eqn. (11) for the one-predictor case:

$$F = \frac{R^2/p}{(1-R)/(N-p-1)} \tag{26}$$

which follows an F distribution with p and $N - p - 1$ degrees of freedom under the null hypothesis.

A more important test, in view of the earlier admonition against proceeding to a more complicated regression model than warranted by the data, is one that allows a test to be carried out to determine whether the addition of a new predictor results in a significant decrease of the loss function. This may now be restated in terms of an increase in the squared correlation coefficient, by using the relation between Q_{min} (i.e., SS_{res}) and r^2 given by Eqn. (8) and its multiple-predictor extension. For if the residual SS using one predictor X_1 is denoted by $SS_{res(1)}$ and that using two predictors, X_1 and X_2, by $SS_{res(2)}$ then the decrease in Q, $SS_{res(1)} - SS_{res(2)}$, is, by Eqn. (8) and its two-predictor extension, equivalent to $(\Sigma y^2)(R^2 - r^2)$. Hence, the F statistic for testing the significance of the increase from r^2 to R^2 is

$$F = \frac{(R^2 - r^2)/1}{(1 - R^2)/(N - 3)} \tag{27}$$

The divisor, 1, in the numerator is the difference, 2−1, between the numbers of predictors; the $N-3$ dividing the denominator is $N-p-1$ with $p=2$. The degrees of freedom of this F statistic are 1 and $N-3$. More generally, the statistic for testing the significance of the increase in R^2 (or the "incremental R^2" as it is often called) in going from a p-predictor model to a $(p+1)$-predictor model is

$$F = \frac{(R_{p+1}^2 - R_p^2)/1}{(1 - R_{p+1}^2)/(N - p - 2)} \tag{28}$$

which has an F distribution (under the null hypothesis) with 1 and $N-p-2$ degrees of freedom.

The incremental R^2 is sometimes used in the reverse (then called the decremental R^2) as a measure of how much the predictability of the criterion decreases when a particular predictor variable is removed from a multiple regression equation. This was called the "usefulness" of that predictor by Darlington (1968) in an article that compares the advantages and disadvantages of several measures of the relative importance of each predictor variable in predicting or "expanding" the criterion. The best known of such measures is, of course, the standardized regression weight b_j^* (or "beta weight") associated with each variable, which is related to the corresponding raw-score regression weight b_j by the equation $b_j^* = (s_j/s_y)b_j$ where s_j and s_y are the standard deviations of X_j and Y, respectively. However, Darlington points out several drawbacks of the beta weight as a measure of each variable's contribution to the predictability of the criterion.

1.3 Polynomial Regression

Another way in which the simple linear Eqn. (3) may be complexified is to add, successively, a term in X^2, X^3, and so on, while holding the number of actual predictor variables to one. Such a regression equation is called a polynomial regression equation of degree m, when X^m is the highest degree term involved. The effect of adding higher degree terms is to enable the modeling of datasets in which the Y means corresponding to the distinct values of X trace curves of more and more complicated forms.

Once again, it cannot be overemphasized that the mistake should never be made of overfitting the data at hand by using a polynomial equation of a degree higher than warranted. In fact, it can be seen without too much difficulty that, if there are K distinct values of X in the dataset (and hence at most K distinct Y-means), the subgroup Y-means $\bar{Y}_1, \bar{Y}_2, \ldots, \bar{Y}_K$ can be fitted perfectly by a polynomial regression equation of degree $K-1$. (This is because the number of constants whose values can be chosen in a polynomial equation of degree $K-1$ is K, which is the number of Y-means to be fitted.) Clearly such a fit is spurious and would never begin to hold up in a subsequent sample.

The determination of the regression coefficients and the successive significance testing may be done by precisely the same methods that were described for multiple linear regression in the preceding subsection. This should not be difficult to see, because in a cubic regression equation (for instance) the successive powers X, X^2, and X^3 may be regarded as three different predictor variables, X_1, X_2, and X_3, respectively. Thus, the SSCP matrix for the normal equations may be written by the simple device of starting out with the SSCP matrix appropriate to the three-predictor linear model case, then moving the subscripts upwards to the position of exponents, and finally using the rule of exponents ($x^m x^n = x^{m+n}$). The SSCP matrix then becomes

$$S_{xx} = \begin{bmatrix} \Sigma x^2 & \Sigma x^3 & \Sigma x^4 \\ \Sigma x^3 & \Sigma x^4 & \Sigma x^5 \\ \Sigma x^4 & \Sigma x^5 & \Sigma x^6 \end{bmatrix} \tag{29}$$

Similarly, the predictor-criterion SCP vector S_{xy} becomes

$$S_{xy} = \begin{bmatrix} \Sigma xy \\ \Sigma x^2 y \\ \Sigma x^3 y \end{bmatrix} \tag{30}$$

With S_{xx} and S_{xy} thus, constructed, the normal equations [Eqn. (21)] are written and solved in exactly the same way as before.

The multiple correlation coefficient, defined as $R = r_{\hat{Y}Y}$ in the context of multiple linear regression, can be used in conjunction with polynomial regression equations just as well. Hence, it can be computed as $R^2 = S'_{xy} b/\Sigma y^2$ with the newly defined S_{xy} and b solved from the redefined normal equations.

The significance tests, both for a given multiple correlation coefficient itself and for the residual from the polynomial regression equation of a given degree, can likewise be conducted in the ways described in the previous subsection. For the former the F statistic given in Eqn. (26) is used, where the p used for the number of predictors may be replaced by m to denote the degree of the polynomial. Similarly, for testing, if it is warranted to go from an m-th degree equation to an $(m+1)$-th, Eqn. (28) may be used, again with p replaced by m.

Although the foregoing significance tests are generally adequate and commonly used, there is one troublesome thing about them. This is that, in using these formulas, it is tacitly being assumed that the residual sum of squares, $(1 - R^2)\Sigma y^2$ or $(R^2_{m+1})\Sigma y^2$ as the case may be, is attributable to "pure sampling error." This would be true if it was known that the degree of the regression equation entertained at any given stage is indeed the correct population model (in which case there would be no need to conduct a significance test). Otherwise, SS_{res} would be an overestimate of pure sampling error, since it would include also a portion due to regression of Y on a higher degree term of X. For this and other reasons, it is often advisable to use an alternative approach to constructing and testing polynomial regression equations, which is known as the method of orthogonal polynomials. Very briefly, this approach uses a sequence of polynomials $P_1(X), P_2(X), P_3(X)$, and so on, instead of pure powers of X as the terms of the regression equation. Thus, for example, a cubic regression equation would be written as $\hat{Y} = a_0 + a_1 P_1(X) + a_2 P_2(X) + a_3 P_3(X)$.

For situations when the values that X can take are equally spaced (and hence can, by a suitable linear transformation, be transformed into 1, 2,..., K) and each of these X values is taken by the same number of cases, there is a specific sequence of orthogonal polynomials $P_1(X), P_2(X),..., P_{K-1}(X)$ for each K. These were originally derived by R A Fisher, and tables of their values are available in many textbooks on experimental design (see, e.g., Winer 1971). As explained in these books, orthogonal polynomials have the important property that, for each K their values for $X=1, 2,..., K$ sum to 0. Hence, the polynomial values may be used as coefficients of a contrast among the subgroup means of Y. For example, with $K=5$ and $j=1$,

$$\hat{\psi}_1 = P_1(1)\bar{Y}_1 + P_1(2)\bar{Y}_2 + \ldots + P_1(5)\bar{Y}_5 \qquad (31)$$

is a contrast of the five subgroup means of Y "attributable" to the first-degree polynomial, $P_1(X)$.

A further important property is that, associated with each contrast $\hat{\psi}$ for any given K, there is a sum of squares $SS(\hat{\psi}_j)$, with one degree of freedom, that constitutes an additive component of the between-groups sum of squares in the following sense:

$$SS(\hat{\psi}_1) + SS(\hat{\psi}_2) + \ldots + SS(\hat{\psi}_{K-1}) = SS_b \qquad (32)$$

Moreover, the partial sums of these $SS(\hat{\psi}_j)$'s are related to the SS due to regressions of successive degrees:

$$SS(\hat{\psi}_1) = r^2\Sigma y^2 = SS_{lin. reg.} \qquad (33)$$

$$SS(\hat{\psi}_1) + SS(\hat{\psi}_2) = R^2_2\Sigma y^2 = SS_{quad. reg.} \qquad (34)$$

$$SS(\hat{\psi}_1) + SS(\hat{\psi}_2) + SS(\hat{\psi}_3 = R^2_3\Sigma y^2 = SS_{cubic reg.} \qquad (35)$$

and so forth. (Here each $R_m = r_{\hat{Y}Y_m}$ is the correlation of Y with the m-th degree regression.)

Consequently, the question of whether or not the m-th degree regression equation is "adequate" for modeling the K subgroup means of Y may be tested by

$$F = \frac{\left[SS_b - \sum_{j=1}^{m} SS(\hat{\psi}_j)\right] / (K - 1 - m)}{MS_w} \qquad (36)$$

With $K-1-m$ and $N-K$ degrees of freedom. If this is significant, it is possible to proceed to the $(m+1)$-th degree equation; if not, it can be concluded that the m-th degree equation is adequate.

1.4 Multiple Nonlinear Regression

This combines the complexities of multiple-linear and polynomial regression models. That is, higher degree terms of each of several predictors, and possibly products among two or more predictors, constitute the terms of the regression equation. Geometrically, this would represent a curved surface or "hypersurface." Such an equation can again be treated like a multiple linear regression, with each term regarded as a separate predictor. Hence, nothing new in the way of determining the regression coefficients, computing multiple correlation coefficients, and conducting significance tests needs to be added.

However, the presence of product terms (which could go beyond the simple $X_1 X_2$ type and include such monstrosities as $X_1^2 X_2 X_3$) does introduce a considerable difference in interpretation. To illustrate the point, the simplest case will be examined:

$$\hat{Y} = b_0 + b_1 X_1 + b_2 X_2 + b_3 X_1 X_2 \qquad (37)$$

By collecting the last two terms, this may be rewritten as

$$\hat{Y} = b_0 + b_1 X_1 + (b_2 + b_3 X_1)X_2 \qquad (38)$$

which somewhat resembles a multiple linear regression equation with two predictors X_1 and X_2, except that the coefficient of X_2 is not a constant but is itself a linear function of X_1. What this means is that the effect of X_2 on the criterion Y depends on the value of X_1. Assuming $b_3<0$, it can be seen that the larger X_1 is, the larger the coefficient $b_2 + b_3 X_1$ of X_2 becomes, hence the greater the effect of X_2 on Y. This, as the reader may have recognized, is what is known as interaction in ANOVA. The effects of the two independent variables are not simply additive, but are exerted jointly—each enhancing the effect of the other.

2. ANOVA and Multiple Regression

Since the mid-1960s or so, the writings of Darlington (1968), Kerlinger and Pedhazur (1973), Cohen and Cohen (1975), and others, have done much to popularize, in the behavioral and social sciences, the use of multiple regression analysis in situations where analysis of variance has traditionally been the main if not the sole analytic tool. This has been hailed by many as a recent innovation, but in point of fact some early writings of R A Fisher indicate that he invented ANOVA as a computational tool to get around the intractable computational difficulties, in the precomputer era, that arose when multiple regression was applied to designed experiments—that is, when the independent variables were qualitative variables (such as different fertilizers, different varieties of corn, etc.) that were manipulated by the experimenter.

The nature of the difficulty is not hard to see even in the case of one-way designs with qualitative independent variables having a large number of "levels"—for example, five or six different instructional methods for teaching some subject matter. Since there is no a priori ordering to the different teaching methods, it will not do to define a variable called "method," denoted X, give it the values 1, 2, 3, . . ., 6 (say), and use it as the independent variable in a simple linear regression analysis. Rather a technique has to be used known as "coding," of which there are several varieties.

Perhaps the most widely used type is that known as "dummy variable coding." Suppose there are K categories (K different teaching methods, K different religions, etc.) to the independent variable. $K - 1$ dummy variables $X_1, X_2, . . ., X_{K-1}$ are then introduced and values assigned to members of the different categories as follows:

$X_1 = 1$ and $X_2 = X_3 = . . . = X_{k-1} = 0$
for Category 1 members;

$X_2 = 1$ and $X_1 = X_3 = . . . = X_{K-1} = 0$
for Category 2 members:

.

.

.

$X_{K-1} = 1$ and $X_1 = X_2 = . . . = X_{K-2} = 0$
    for Category $K - 1$ members;

$X_1 = X_2 = X_3 = . . . = X_{K-1} =$
    for Category K members.

A multiple (linear) regression analysis of the criterion variable Y (a suitable measure of achievement in the subject matter, observed on the entire sample) is then carried out. The test of significance of the multiple correlation coefficient thus obtained gives results identical to those given by the familiar F = test of ANOVA;

$$F = \frac{R^2/(K-1)}{(1-R^2)/(N-K)} = \frac{MS_b}{MS_w} \qquad (39)$$

where the first ratio comes from Eqn. (26) with p replaced by $K - 1$. The curious reader will no doubt wonder why this should be so. Why do two techniques so seemingly different as multiple regression and ANOVA yield identical results?

Before answering this question, it is useful to look at how the technique of coding is extended to designs involving two or more factors. For specificity, suppose it is desirable to handle a 3×4 factorial-design ANOVA by the multiple regression approach via dummy-variable coding. Two dummy variables U_1 and U_2 (say) would be used for coding the three categories of factor A, and three dummy variables X_1, X_2 and X_3 for the four levels of B. How is the interaction A $\times$ B expressed? The reasoning introduced in Sect. 1.4 has simply to be applied so that the product of two variables represents an interaction between them. It is thus necessary to form all possible products between one of the U's and one of the X's—that is, U_1X_1, U_1X_2, U_1X_3, . . ., U_2X_3 and treat these as six additional predictor variables. There would therefore be a total of $2 + 3 + 6 = 11$ "dummy" predictor variables in the multiple-regression version of the 3×4 ANOVA problem. It is easy to see that the number of predictor variables increases rapidly with the complexity of the design; so it is not surprising that Fisher should have striven, and succeeded, in inventing the alternative computational routines of ANOVA. Without the benefit of a computer, the solution of the normal equations (21) is a formidable task even when $p = 4$ or 5.

Returning now to the question of identity of the results obtained by the usual ANOVA method and the multiple-regression approach, just outlined, it can be recalled that a set of K group means of Y, $\bar{Y}_1$, $\bar{Y}_2$, . . ., $\bar{Y}_k$ can be perfectly fitted by a polynomial regression equation of degree $K - 1$. Hence, as pointed out earlier, the sum of squares $R_{k-1}^2 \Sigma y^2$ due to the regression equation of degree $K - 1$ is equal to SS_b, since $\Sigma n_k(\hat{Y} - \bar{Y})^2 = \Sigma n_k(\bar{Y}_k - \bar{Y})^2$ when $\hat{Y} = \bar{Y}_k$ for each group. It therefore follows that $(1 - R_{k-1}^2) \Sigma y^2 = SS_w$, and hence that Eqn. (26) becomes

$$F = \frac{R^2/(K-1)}{(1-R^2)/(N-K)} = \frac{MS^b}{MS^w} \qquad (40)$$

which is the customary F-test of ANOVA.

Consequently, in order to show that the same holds for the multiple correlation of Y with the $K - 1$ dummy variables X_1, X_2, X_{K-1} introduced above, it need only be shown that

$$R_{Y \cdot X_1 X_2 . . . X_{K-1}} = R_{Y \cdot XX^2X^3 . . . X^{K-1}} \qquad (41)$$

Although a general proof of this relation requires some background in linear algebra, it is a simple matter to verify that it holds for, say, $K = 3$.

It stands to reason (and it can be proved both algebraically and geometrically) that the criterion variable Y has the same multiple correlation with X_1 and X_2 as it does with X and X^2. This reasoning can be extended to the general case of $K - 1$ dummy variables for K groups. Each dummy variable may be shown to be a linear function of X, X^2, . . ., X^{K-1} where X may be given the values 0, 1, . . ., $K-1$ (or 1, 2, . . ., K or any K distinct values for that matter) for members of the K groups, respectively. Hence Y has the same multiple correlation with X_1, X_2, . . ., X_{K-1} as it does with X, X_2, . . ., X^{K-1}, and since it is already known that r^2_{Y} $_{\hat{Y}_{K-1}}$ $\Sigma y^2 = SS_b$, it follows that the significance test of $R_{YX_1X_2...X_{K-1}}$ is equivalent to the F test MS_b/MS_w of ANOVA.

Two other coding systems that are often used are effect coding and contrast coding. In the former, which is a special case of the latter, all members of a particular group (usually the Kth) are given the value -1 in all the $K-1$ coding variables, while members of one and only one of the other groups are given a $+1$ on each coding variable in turn, members of all other groups getting 0's. Thus, for instance, with $K = 4$:

1	0	0	for Group-1 members
0	1	0	for Group-2 members
0	0	1	for Group-3 members
−1	−1	−1	for Group-4 members.

Note that the columns here constitute the coding variables. This system has the advantage that the resulting regression coefficients b_1, b_2, . . ., b_{K-1} represent the successive treatment effects $\bar{Y}_1 - \bar{Y}$, $\bar{Y}_2 - \bar{Y}$, . . ., $\bar{Y}_{K-1} - \bar{Y}$ (assuming that members of Group j got the 1 on the j-th coding variable).

In the more general contrast coding system, it is usual to use—as the values of each coding variable for the several groups—any set of numbers that add up to zero, with the further condition that no column (listing the values for one coding variable) be a linear combination of the other columns. Thus, the first three columns below qualify as values for a set of contrast coding variables, but the last three columns do not, because VI = IV + V.

	I	II	III	IV	V	VI
Group I:	3	0	0	1	0	1
Group 2:	−1	2	0	−1	1	0
Group 3:	−1	−1	1	−1	0	−1
Group 4:	−1	−1	−1	1	−1	0

Each contrast coding variable asks a specific question. For example, I above asks whether $\bar{Y}_1$ differs significantly from the average of $\bar{Y}_2$, $\bar{Y}_3$, and $\bar{Y}_4$; II asks whether $\bar{Y}_2$ differs significantly from the average of $\bar{Y}_3$ and $\bar{Y}_4$. When the contrasts further satisfy the condition of orthogonality—that is, when the products of corresponding values of any pair of coding variables sum to zero (as do those in the set I, II, III)—the resulting analysis has an interesting property. Namely, the coding variables are then uncorrelated among

themselves, and hence the squared multiple R is the sum of the squares of the zero-order r's of the several coding variables with the criterion: $R^2_{Y \cdot 12...(K-1)} = r^2_{Y1} + r^2_{Y2} + . . . + r^2_{Y, K-1}$

2.1 Advantages of the Multiple Regression Approach

The advantages of the multiple regression approach to ANOVA are implicit in the above discussions. The main advantage is that, with a judicious choice of coding variables, it is possible to dispense with the two-stage procedure of carrying out "global" significance tests and then going on to more specific, "fine-grained" significance tests that address specific issues, and go directly to the latter.

Another advantage is that a mixture of quantitative and categorical variables can be used as the independent variables in multiple regression whereas in ANOVA the independent variables must all be categorical or deliberately categorized (e.g., "high," "medium," "low" in mechanical aptitude), thus resulting in a loss of information.

Also, there is a greater flexibility available to the researcher in the order in which the independent variables are entered into the analysis. Since, at each stage, the significance of the increase in R^2 is tested, this corresponds to asking whether or not the later entered variable affects the criterion over and above the effects associated with the earlier entered variables.

Finally, and somewhat ironically, the "simplified" computational routines that Fisher developed in the precomputer days for ANOVA are mixed blessings at best in the computer age. Multiple regression offers a unified approach that dispenses with having to use specific formulas for specific designs.

An approach that further formalizes, generalizes, and routinizes the multiple regression approach is called the general linear model approach. This avoids (at least initially) an explicit coding of members of different subclasses by using coding variables and, instead, utilizes what is called the design matrix to specify the structural equation of the design being used. The interested reader is referred to treatises by Bock (1975), Finn (1974), and to a brief, introductory booklet by Tatsuoka (1975).

3. Concluding Remarks

Space limitations have precluded the discussion of several ancillary but nevertheless noteworthy topics in the forgoing. Cursory mention will therefore be made of some of them here, and the reader will be referred to suitable sources.

3.1 Correction for Shrinkage

One consequence of using the least squares principle in determining the regression coefficients (more precisely, estimating the population regression coefficients) and the multiple correlation coefficient is that the latter is necessarily "inflated" for what can reasonably be expected as the correlation $r_{Y\hat{Y}}$ when the equation is used in a subsequent sample. A correction is therefore called for, and one that is commonly used is Wherry's shrinkage formula,

$$R_w^2 = 1 - \frac{N-1}{N-p}(1-R^2) \qquad (42)$$

where N is the sample size, p. the number of predictor variables, and R and R_w are the observed and "corrected" (or deflated) multiple-R, respectively.

This formula, however, is not the most appropriate one, for it is actually an estimate of what the population R^2 would be if the regression coefficients were optimized in the population as a whole. A better shrinkage formula is that developed by Stein (1960), which reads

$$R_s^2 = 1 - \frac{N-1}{N-p-1}\frac{N-2}{N-p-2}\frac{N+1}{N}(1-R^2) \qquad (43)$$

What this equation gives is an estimate of the cross-validated $r_{Y\hat{Y}}^2$ in the population, using the sample-based regression equation. It therefore is closer to what is being looked for, that is the $r_{Y\hat{Y}}^2$ in a subsequent sample, using the current regression equation.

3.2 Alternative Predictor-weighting Schemes

By the same token as the sample R^2 is an overestimate of the population R^2 and the cross-validated $r_{Y\hat{Y}}^2$ in the population, the observed regression coefficients b_j or b_j^*, as the case may be, are extremely unstable from one sample to the next. Several authors have therefore proposed alternative weighting schemes, the most recent of which is Wainer's (1976) unit-weight system, which holds that not much predictive power is lost by simply giving every standardized predictor a weight of one. While this has considerable intuitive appeal, some cautions against uncritical acceptance of the proposal are given by Laughlin (1978) and by Pruzek and Frederick (1978), to which Wainer (1978) responds in defence.

3.3 Ridge Regression

A different problem occurs when one predictor has a high multiple correlation with some of the others. In this situation the sample SSCP matrix $\mathbf{S}_{xx}$—or correlation matrix $\mathbf{R}_{xx}$ of the standardized predictors are being used—becomes close to singular, and the solution of the normal equations for $\mathbf{b}$ or $\mathbf{b}^*$ becomes extremely inaccurate. One method designed to cope with this problem (often called the problem of multicollinearity) is known as ridge regression, and it consists essentially of modifying the correlation matrix by subtracting a suitable constant from the diagonal elements. Marquardt and Snee (1975) present a good exposition of this method.

3.4 Applications

Applications of multiple regression analysis in educational research—especially those of the "technological" variety designed for practical prediction purposes

—are too numerous even to think of reviewing in the limited space available. A highly selective, minuscule set of abstracts of some of the more innovative and research-oriented applications is given here, and the reader is referred to other sources of research examples.

An often cited and early example of the "ANOVA qua multiple regression" type of research of Cronbach's (1968) reanalysis of Wallach and Kogan's (1965) study of creativity in young children. The original researchers did a 2×2 ANOVA for each sex separately, using dichotomies on indexes labeled "intelligence" and "creativity" as the independent variables and measures of social interaction and confidence in schoolwork as the criteria. Cronbach used the sequential multiple regression approach entering intelligence [renamed "achievement" (A) to avoid "surplus connotations"]and creativity [likewise renamed "flexibility" (F)]first and then adding sex (S), AS, FS, and AFS, testing the incremental R^2 each time. Outcomes that contradicted Wallach and Kogan's original results were that a significant $A \times F$ interaction was found on several dependent variables while the $A \times S$, $F \times S$, and $A \times F \times S$ interactions were in general nonsignificant.

In a study of the effects of classroom social climate on learning, Anderson (1970) included quadratic and product terms of the predictors, using samples at random from about 110 high-school physics classes. The criteria were post-test–pretest gain scores on a physics achievement test, a test on understanding science, and two other tests. Treating males and females separately, a total of eight multiple regression equations were constructed, entering IQ, LEI (learning environment inventory), IQ $\times$ LEI, (IQ)^2 and (LEI)^2 sequentially as predictors in each case. Not surprisingly, the IQ $\times$ LEI interaction was found significant in many cases, but the detailed graphical presentations of the resulting response surfaces are well worth careful study.

Another ingenious study relating environmental forces to cognitive development was that by Marjoribanks (1972), who was interested also in the possible effects of ethnic background (Canadian Indians, French Canadians, Jews, southern Italians, and WASPs). Specifically, eight "environmental variables" (P) (press for achievement, press for intellectuality, press for independence, etc.) plus ethnicity (E) served as the independent variables, and four subtests (verbal, number, spatial, and reasoning) of the SRA Primary Mental Abilities Test constituted the dependent variables. The main results for the verbal subtest (which was the most highly affected by the independent variables) was that $R^2_{V \cdot P_1P_2\ldots P_8E_1E_2\ldots E_4} = 0.61$ while $R^2_{V \cdot P_1P_2\ldots P_8} = 0.50$ and $R^2_{V \cdot E_1E_2\ldots E_4} = 0.45$ (Note that there are eight variables in the environmental press set, since each is a quantitative variable in its own right, while there are four coding variables for the five ethnic groups.) From these three R^2 values, it may be inferred that the proportion of variability in verbal ability attributable to environmental press alone is $0.61 - 0.45 = 0.16$, while that attributable to ethnicity alone is $0.61 - 0.50 = 0.11$. This subtraction of squared multiple R's is in the same spirit as that of incremental (or decremental) R^2 s, described above. Note, however, that the differencing is here done for sets of variables (the eight environmental variables as a set, and the four ethnic variables as a set) rather than individual variables. The systematic study of the separate effects of single sets of independent variables and the joint effects of two or more sets, when the independent variables fall into natural clusters as they do here, was called commonality analysis by Mayeske et al. (1969) who used it as a prominent tool in a reanalysis of the well-known Coleman et al. (1966) Report *Equality of Educational Opportunity*.

More than one study in the area of detection and correction of salary inequalities (between the sexes, among ethnic groups, etc.) have used multiple regression as their main analytic tool.

Birnbaum (1979), however, argues that it is fallacious to conclude, on the basis of a regression analysis of salary on merit (as measured by the typical indices of number of journal articles and other publications, ratings of teaching, years of experience, etc.), that discrimination exists whenever the actual salaries (Y) for a minority group fall short of the predicted salaries ($\hat{Y}$) based on the regression equation for the majority group (e.g., white males). He contends that the opposite regression—that of merit on salary—should also be considered. Group bias should be inferred only if a particular group is shown to have a lower mean salary holding merit constant and to have higher mean merit holding salary constant. An equitable system is proposed in which part of the salary increase is based on merit alone while another part is based on both merit and current salary in a compensatory manner (i.e., with current salary fixed, a person with greater merit gets a larger raise, whereas with merit fixed, a person with lower current salary gets a larger raise).

Besides Kerlinger and Pedhazur (1973) and Cohen and Cohen (1975), the following are excellent sources for discussions of illustrative research studies using regression analysis—and, in the second case, related techniques such as canonical correlation, covariance structure analysis, factor analysis, and path analysis: Pedhazur (1982) and Kerlinger (1977).

3.5 Computer Programs

No account of regression analysis would be complete without some mention of the available computer programs. Briefly, all the well-known computer packages such as BMD, BMDP, OSIRIS, SAS, and SPSS include one or more multiple regression and/or general linear model programs. A package that is not typically implemented at a computer center but requires one's own typing in the FORTRAN file is the package included in Cooley and Lohnes's (1971) textbook. In addition, a stand-alone program for the general linear model, called MULTIVARIANCE, is available from International Educational Resources, Inc.

Each of these programs has its advantages and disadvantages, so it is not feasible to rate them from "best" to "least desirable." One thing that all these programs have in common is the stepwise multiple regression (Draper and Smith 1966) capability—something that was implicit through all the foregoing discussions but never explicitly mentioned; that is, adding predictors one at a time so that the incremental R^2 at each step is as large as possible and terminates the adding when the resulting incremental R^2 is not significant at a prescribed level. A related procedure is that of adding the independent variables successively in a predetermined order—not necessarily that which will maximize the incremental R^2—having to do with some sort of priority ordering either chronological or theoretical. It will be recalled that all the research examples alluded to, utilized this procedure.

Finally, it is almost trite to say that, with the increasing availability and popularity of microcomputers, one should become cognizant of the availability and efficiency of software capable of carrying out multiple regression and other statistical analysis that is proper to or compatible with each machine. A short-range economy may prove to be a long-term waste unless a brand is carefully selected to match its capabilities with a person's needs and plans.

See also: Multivariate Analysis; Models and Model Building

References

Anderson G J 1970 Effects of classroom social climate on individual learning. *Am. Educ. Res. J.* 7: 135–52

Birnbaum M H 1979 Procedures for the detection and correction of salary inequities. In: Pezzullo T R, Brittingham B F (eds.) 1979 *Salary Equity: Detecting Sex Bias in Salaries Among College and University Professors.* Lexington Books, Lexington, Massachusetts

Bock R D 1975 *Multivariate Statistical Methods in Behavioral Research.* McGraw-Hill, New York

Cohen J, Cohen P 1975 *Applied Multiple Regression/Correlation Analysis for the Behavioral Sciences.* Erlbaum, Hillsdale, New Jersey

Coleman J S et al. 1966 *Equality of Educational Opportunity.* United States Government Printing Office, Washington, DC

Cooley W W, Lohnes P R 1971 *Multivariate Data Analysis.* Wiley, New York

Cronbach L J 1968 Intelligence? Creativity? A parsimonious reinterpretation of the Wallach-Kogan data. *Am. Educ. Res. J.* 5(4): 491–511

Darlington R B 1968 Multiple regression in psychological research and practice. *Psych. Bull.* 69: 161–82

Draper N R, Smith H 1966 *Applied Regression Analysis.* Wiley, New York

Finn J D 1974 *A General Model for Multivariate Analysis.* Holt, Rinehart and Winston, New York

Fisher R A *Statistical Methods for Research Workers*, 10th edn. Oliver and Boyd, Edinburgh

Green P E 1976 *Mathematical Tools for Applied Multivariate Analysis*. Academic Press, New York

Kerlinger F N 1977 *Behavioral Research: A Conceptual Approach*. Holt, Rinehart and Winston, New York

Kerlinger F N, Pedhazur E J 1973 *Multiple Regression in Behavioral Research*. Holt, Rinehart and Winston, New York

Laughlin J E 1978 Comments on "Estimating coefficients in linear models: It don't make no nevermind". *Psychol. Bull.* 85: 247–53

Marjoribanks K 1972 Ethnic and environmental influences on mental abilities. *Am. J. Sociol.* 78: 323–37

Marquardt D W, Snee R D 1975 Ridge regression in practice. *Am. Statistician* 29: 3–20

Mayeske G W et al. 1969 *A Study of Our Nation's Schools*. United States Office of Education, Washington, DC

Pedhazur E J 1982 *Multiple Regression in Behavioral Research: Explanation and Prediction*, 2nd edn. Holt, Rinehart and Winston, New York

Pruzek R M, Frederick B C 1978 Weighting predictors in linear models: Alternatives to least squares and limitations of equal weights. *Psych. Bull.* 85: 254–66

Stein C 1960 Multiple regression. In: Olkin I, Ghurye S G, Hoeffding W, Madow W G, Mann H B (eds.) 1960 *Contributions to Probability and Statistics: Essays in Honor of Harold Hotelling*. Stanford University Press, Palo Alto, California

Tatsuoka M M 1975 *The General Linear Model: A "New" Trend in Analysis of Variance*. Institute for Personality and Ability Testing, Champaign, Illinois

Tatsuoka M M 1988 *Multivariate Analysis: Techniques for Educational and Psychological Research*, 2nd edn. Macmillan, New York

Wainer H 1976 Estimating coefficients in linear models: It don't make no nevermind. *Psych. Bull.* 83: 213–17

Wainer H 1978 On the sensitivity of regression and regressors. *Psych. Bull.* 85: 267–73

Wallach M, Kogan N 1965 *Modes of Thinking in Young Children: A Study of the Creativity-Intelligence Distinction*. Holt, Rinehart and Winston, New York

Winer B J 1971 *Statistical Principles in Experimental Design*, 2nd edn. McGraw-Hill, New York

Further Reading

Aitken L S, West S G 1991 *Multiple Regression: Testing and Interpreting Interactions*. Sage, Newbury Park, California

Darlington R B 1990 *Regression and Linear Models*. McGraw-Hill, New York

Robust Statistical Procedures

H. Huynh

In this entry, a review is made of some well-known robust/resistant statistical procedures useful in analysis of large data sets. These techniques are most suitable in the presence of outlying observations. Details are provided for robust estimation of means and regression coefficients in the linear model, and for robust approaches to analysis of variance and covariance.

1. Effect of Outliers on Traditional Statistical Procedures

Statistical inference based on commonly used procedures such as the t test, multiple regression, and analysis of variance and covariance are part of the least squares (LS) method.

1.1 Least-Square Estimates

In general, LS estimates are obtained by minimizing the sum of squares of appropriate deviations or residuals. When the data satisfy the condition of normality, LS estimates are known to fulfill important optimization criteria in terms of efficiency and minimum variance. In addition, these estimates have well-established sampling distributions which allow important statistical inference to be carried out in a straightforward manner.

1.2 Data Transformation

When normality does not hold, efforts may be made to transform the data to an approximate normal distribution so that LS procedures can be used efficiently. For a positively skewed variable such as family income, family size, or Scholastic Aptitude Test (SAT) score among low-achieving students, a logarithmic or square-root transform would bring the distribution closer to a normal distribution. On the other hand, for a negatively skewed variable such as raw score on an easy test, vacation expense among affluent families, or parental income of students attending private universities, an exponential or square transformation might be sufficient. If the attempt to normalize the distribution succeeds, then the data analysis may be carried out through the use of traditional LS methods and conveniently available software. Otherwise, a suitable nonparametric procedure may be employed.

1.3 Outliers

Large data sets in education (and in other fields) often contain an unknown proportion of outlying observations ("outliers," "wild shots"). Somehow these observations seem to be out of touch with the mainstream of the data set. In general, outliers may constitute a natural part of the data or they may be caused by errors in making or recording the observations.

In the first case, outliers are the results of a contaminated distribution in which the majority of data follow a specified distribution (such as a normal distribution) and only a small percentage (the wild shots) follow another distribution with considerably heavier tails (Tukey 1960, 1962). Here, the wild shots may not be inherently wrong observations. Rather, they constitute the part of the data which simply cannot be described by the model postulated for the remaining majority. As a consequence, they are a very important part of the data which needs to be detected and carefully studied.

Outliers may also be bad data points caused by errors in making or recording observations. These errors may be corrected in a small study. In most large-scale projects, however, financial and time constraints may render such corrections unfeasible.

1.4 Difficulty in Detecting Outliers

Statistical literature is rich with procedures for detecting outliers in very general situations such as multiple regression (Barnett and Lewis 1978). In general, a LS analysis is first conducted and the residuals are obtained for all observations. Each residual will then be examined to determine whether it is unexpectedly large for the situation under consideration. However, because of their large squared contribution to the sum of squares which needs to be minimized, outliers tend to distort the LS regression line and may push the otherwise "good" observations away from this line. Not only will this disturbance make it difficult to sort out the outlying ("bad") observations, but it may also create the impression that some "good" observations are candidates for outliers (see Fig. 1 of Wu 1985 p. 319).

2. M-Estimation

Alternative approaches to LS procedures have been described in the literature (see Hogg 1979, Wu 1985). Typically, these procedures are designed to lessen the impact of suspected outliers by giving them small or even zero weights in the estimation process. By doing so, the estimates are mostly determined by the main body of the data and are only marginally influenced by the small portion of the data suspected to be outliers.

Among the many alternatives to LS, the robust *M*-estimation advanced by Huber (1973, 1981) has received considerable attention because it appears to be a natural extension of the LS process.

2.1 Overall Framework

M-estimation was first introduced for the central location μ (mean or median) of a symmetric distribution. Let $x_1, \ldots, x_n$ be the data from a random sample and let $\hat{\mu}$ be an estimate for the parameter (population value)

μ. The residuals (or deviations) are $r_i = x_i - \hat{\mu}$ where $i = 1, \ldots, n$. To obtain the LS estimate, the sum of squares $SS = \Sigma r_i^2$ needs to be minimized. Now let the function ψ (r_i) be equal to r_i for all observations. The LS estimate may then be obtained by solving the equation $\Sigma \psi (r_i) = 0$, a process which yields the sample mean $\bar{x}$. From this equation, it may be seen that the LS estimate is very susceptible to any observation with a large absolute residual. Hence the LS estimate is not a robust/resistant estimate.

Another commonly used estimate for the population mean is the sample median (Md). If n is an odd number and when the central observations are not equal, the median is the $(n+1)$-th ordered value of the sample data. This estimate minimizes the sum $\Sigma |r_i|$ of the absolute deviations, a process which bears names such as "least absolute residual (LAR)," "least absolute deviation (LAD)," or "L1." Now let the function $\psi (r_i)$ be equal to -1, 0, and 1 if r_i is negative, zero, and positive respectively. Then the median satisfies the equation $\Sigma \psi (r_i) = 0$. With most extreme observations entering this equation through either -1 or 1, it appears obvious that the median is very robust/resistant to outliers.

For various theoretical reasons, Huber proposed that a "compromised" *M*-estimate be obtained by taking a following process of combining the LS and LAR estimates. With d as an acceptable measure of scale (or variability) for the data, let $z = r_i/d$, $i = 1, \ldots, n$, be the rescaled residuals. Now let the function $\psi (z_i)$ be equal to z_i when $|z_i| \leq a$, to $-a$ when $z_i < -a$, and to $+a$ when $z_i > a$, where a is a suitably chosen positive constant (the "tuning constant"). In other words, the function $\psi (z_i)$ takes the LS-estimation form when z_i is close to zero and the LAR-form when z_i is far from zero. Then the *M*-estimate is obtained by solving the equation $\Sigma \psi (z_i) = 0$. The process is equivalent to minimizing the sum $\Sigma \rho (z_i)$ where the function $\rho (z_i)$ is equal to z_i^2 (as in LS) when z_i is close to zero and is proportional to $|z_i|$ (as in LAR) when z_i is far from zero.

2.2 Scale Measure and Tuning Constant

Some commonly used measures of scale are $d_1 = $ median $(x_i - Md)/0.6745$ and $d_2 = (Q_3 - Q_1)/1.1349$ where Q_1 and Q_3 are the first and third quartiles.

When the sample comes from a normal distribution, use of the *M*-estimate instead of the more efficient LS estimate $\bar{x}$ would result in a loss of efficiency. Using the *M*-estimate, however, would protect the estimate from being adversely influenced by a few outlying observations. When the tuning constant is set at $a = 1.5$, the loss in efficiency is roughly at 5 percent when the normality condition holds.

2.3 Other ψ Functions

The Huber *M*-estimate takes into account all observations, and gives outliers the equal contributions of $\psi = a$ or $+a$. In some situations it may be wise to down play observations as they turn more and more extreme and to be able to delete observations altogether if they do not seem to belong to the main body of the data. This may be accomplished by letting the function ψ (z_i) come back to 0 as z_i moves farther from 0 and settles finally at 0 at some point. These ψ functions are referred to as "redescending ψ functions."

The commonly mentioned redescending ψ functions are those proposed by Hampel, Andrews (the sine estimate), and Tukey (the bigweight estimate) (see Hogg 1979). The Andrews and Tukey functions are very similar in shape and, due to their continuity, are easier to manipulate than the Hampel function. The Andrews function ψ (z_i) is set at $a \sin (z_i/a)$ for $|z_i| \leqslant a\pi$, π being 3.1416, and at 0 elsewhere. At the 5 percent loss of efficiency, the tuning constant a stands at roughly 2.1. For small z_i, ψ (z_i) is approximately z_i.

2.4 Asymptotic Standard Error

Let $\hat{\mu}$ be a robust estimate for the parameter μ based on a sample of n observations. Then $\hat{\mu}$ follows asymptotically (i.e., when n is large) a normal distribution with a mean equal to μ and a variance equal to $d^2 \Sigma \psi^2$ $(z_i)/[\Sigma \psi' (z_i)]^2$ where ψ' is the derivative of ψ.

2.5 Numerical Example 1

For the 17 sample observations: 5, 6, 7, 7, 8, 8, 8, 9, 10, 10, 10, 10, 11, 15, 17, 59, and 99, the mean is 17.59. As can be seen, the sample mean is strongly affected by the two obvious outliers 59 and 99. Without these outliers, the mean would be 9.40. The Huber process yields an estimate of 9.78 based on all 17 observations. Starting with all 17 observations, the final stage of the Andrews process assigns a zero weight to the outliers and provides a robust estimate of 8.26. Both the Huber and Andrews estimates are very close to the mean 9.40 of the reduced data set.

3. Regression

By carrying out the M-estimation to the residuals in linear regression, robust estimates for the regression coefficients may be found.

3.1 General Framework

Let the dependent variable y be predicted by a linear combination of p predictors $x_1, \ldots, x_p$. For the j-th subject in the sample, the residual takes the form $r_j = y_j - \hat{y}_j = y_j - \Sigma_i \beta_i x_{ij}$, in which the β_i are the regression coefficients. The LS estimates for these coefficients minimize the sum of squares $SS = \Sigma r_j^2$ and satisfy the system of p (linear) equations resulting from the equalities $\underset{j}{\Sigma} r_j x_{ij} = 0$, $i = 1, \ldots, p$. It may be seen that outliers, with their large (absolute) residuals, have strong impact on the LS estimates.

To reduce the impact of large residuals, the LAR estimates may be found by minimizing the sum of the absolute residuals $\Sigma |r_j|$ (Gentle 1977). M-estimates may also be found by use of a function ψ which reduces the contribution of large residuals. To do this, let d be a spread measure for the residuals, $z_j = r_j/d$, and $\psi (z_j)$ be a function chosen from those defined in Sect. 2.1 and 2.3. Then robust estimates for the regression coefficients satisfy the p (nonlinear) equations of the form $\underset{j}{\Sigma} \psi (z_j) x_{ij} = 0$, $i = 1, \ldots, p$. It has been proposed that d be found by taking the median of all the non-zero residuals and dividing this by 0.6745.

3.2 Computations and Software

Unlike the LS method, there is no closed-form procedure (e.g., without iterations) to compute the spread measure d and the robust regression coefficients. There are at least three ways to iterate the estimates, namely the Newton–Raphson procedure, the H-algorithm, and the weighted least square (WLS) solution. All are fully described in Huber (1973). However, with WLS regression already programmed in large-scale software such as SAS (1982, 1986), the WLS iterations have been more fully described and studied.

To implement the WLS iterations, let the weight w_j be equal to 1 when $z_j = 0$ and to $\psi (z_j)/z_j$ when $z_j \neq 0$, $j = 1, \ldots, n$. Starting with some initial estimates for the regression coefficients such as the LAR (or even the LS), the weight w_j can be computed for each subject. Then new values for the regression coefficients, the spread measure d, and the residuals can be obtained by carrying out the WLS regression of y on the predictors $x_1, \ldots, x_p$ with w_j as the weight function. Using the updated residuals, another iteration may be carried out in the same manner, and so on until convergence is achieved in the estimates. An illustration of SAS codes for WLS iterations is provided in Huynh (1994).

The following provides a partial list of computer software for robust regression.

(a) Minitab Macros: listed in Staudte and Sheather (1990).

(b) LINWDR: developed by R Dutter.

(c) ROBETH: written at ETH, Zurich, and continuously updated at the University of Lausanne.

(d) TROLL: developed at MIT and extended at the United States National Bureau of Economic Research's Computer Research Center.

(e) PROGRESS: developed at the University of Brussels and the University of Delft.

Details regarding Items (b)–(e) are given in Hampel et al. (1986).

3.3 Numerical Example 2

The left part of Table 1 lists a modified form of a data set previously analyzed by Daniel and Wood

Table 1
Data and residuals for Numerical Example 2

Obs. No.	x_1	x_2	x_3	y	LS	Huber	Andrews
1	80	27	89	182	70.3	141.4	146.2
2	80	27	88	37	−76.0	−3.8	1.1
3	75	25	90	157	69.7	123.0	127.0
6	62	24	87	78	30.3	55.7	58.2
5	62	22	87	18	−21.8	−2.1	−0.7
6	62	23	87	18	−25.8	−3.2	−1.2
7	62	24	93	19	−21.2	−2.4	−0.4
8	62	24	93	20	−20.2	−1.4	0.6
9	58	23	87	15	−16.6	−2.8	−1.0
10	58	18	80	14	−6.5	0.5	0.3
11	58	18	89	14	4.8	1.9	0.9
12	58	17	88	13	6.6	1.9	0.4
13	58	18	82	11	−6.9	−2.2	−2.6
14	58	19	93	12	3.8	−0.5	-1.4
15	50	18	89	8	23.0	2.8	1.3
16	50	18	86	7	18.3	1.3	0.1
17	50	19	72	8	−2.2	−1.0	−0.4
18	50	19	79	8	6.5	0.1	0.1
19	50	20	80	9	4.8	0.1	0.6
20	56	20	82	15	−4.9	1.4	1.9
21	70	20	91	15	−36.0	−9.2	−8.7

(1971), and later reanalyzed by Andrews (1974). The modified data set will be used to compare the results of the LS, Huber, and Andrews regression coefficients. The original data contain 21 observations ("subjects"), each with one dependent variable (y) and three predictors x_1, x_2, and x_3. (Including the predictor $x_4 = 1$ assigned to the constant in the equation for multiple regression, there are actually $p = 4$ independent variables.) The data represent 21 days of operation of a plant which oxidizes ammonia to nitric acid. Four of these y-values were judged to be in error due to their unusual behavior (see Daniel and Wood 1971), and were assigned a weight of zero in the sine regression analysis (Andrews 1974). All values of the independent variables are retained in the modified data set. In addition, all y-values except those of Nos. 1, 3, and 4 are also kept intact; the y-values for these are changed drastically so that the effects of outliers (or bad data points) can be vividly displayed in the LS and robust regressions.

The right part of Table 1 reports the residuals computed from the LS and robust regression equations. The data clearly point out the undue influence of the altered observations on the LS regression line. Although observation No. 2 is identified by its LS residual as the least fitted to the regression line, it is not considered as unusual in the analysis by Daniel and Wood, and in the reanalysis by Andrews. The Huber and Andrews procedures successfully point out the unusually large residuals associated with observations Nos. 1, 3, 4, and 21. All of them are given a zero weight by the Andrews process.

The successful performance of the robust alternatives for regression is again documented in Table 2. This table reports the LS and robust regression results based on the entire 21 data points and the LS regression coefficients based on the reduced set of data of the 17 "good" observations. The Huber and Andrews estimates based on the entire 21 points are in close agreement with the LS estimate based on 17 "good" observations.

3.4 Some Observations

Numerical Example 2 along with others documented in Huynh (1982, 1994) lead to the following observations:

(a) For data sets which contain no apparent outliers, the LS and robust estimates for the regression coefficients do not appear to differ substantially from each other.

(b) For "messy" data (with suspected or obvious outliers), the LS estimates may vary considerably from those provided by the robust procedures.

(c) Observations considered as outliers by the LS procedure may not be outliers at all under robust regressions.

(d) A robust regression procedure, such as the one proposed by Andrews, may be able to detect outliers automatically by giving them weights that are zero or close to zero.

4. Robust Analysis of Variance

Analysis of variance (ANOVA) pertains to the process of partitioning the variation of the dependent variable into several components which are relevant to the situation. By use of appropriate dummy (0/1) variables, ANOVA problems may be treated as special cases

Table 2
Results of LS and robust regression

No. of Obs.	Procedure	Constant	β_1	β_2	β_3
21	LS	−126.82	3.03	3.99	−1.25
	Huber	−42.79	0.85	1.08	−0.16
	Andrews	−37.46	0.81	0.56	−0.07
17	LS	−37.65	0.80	0.58	−0.07
	Huber	−37.03	0.82	0.53	−0.07
	Andrews	−37.22	0.82	0.53	−0.07

Table 3
Data set used in Numerical Example 3[a]

Region	Education of father (in years)				
	≤8	9-11	12	13-15	≥16
Northeast	25.3 (1)	25.3 (5)	18.2 (9)	18.3 (13)	16.3 (17)
North Central	32.1 (2)	29.0 (6)	18.8 (10)	24.3 (14)	19.0 (18)
South	38.8 (3)[b]	31.0 (7)	19.3 (11)	15.7 (15)	16.8 (19)
West	25.4 (4)	21.1 (8)[c]	20.3 (12)	24.0 (16)	17.5 (20)

Source: US Department of Health, Education and Welfare ([1992] Department of Health and Human Services) 1972, *Infant Mortality Rates: Socioeconomic Factors, United States*. Vital and Health Statistics Series 22, No. 14. National Center for Health Statistics, Rockville, Maryland (DHEW publication number [HSM] 72-1045). Data from Table 8, p. 21
a Enclosed within parentheses is the sequence of the observation   b changed to 99.9   c changed to 0.1

of the linear model. This has led to the development of robust procedures for ANOVA as an application of robust regression.

Works on robust ANOVA include papers by Schrader and McKean (1977), Schrader and Hettmansperger (1980), Braun and McNeil (1981), and Huynh (1994).

4.1 General Framework

Ruppert (1985) discusses the use of pseudo-observations and existing LS software to perform a robust ANOVA. Let K be the bias correction factor discussed in Huber (1981) (which may be taken as 1 when p/n is small) and $\lambda = Kd [\Sigma \psi'(z_j)]/n$, where ψ' is the derivative of the weight function ψ. The pseudo-observation for the j-th subject is defined as $y_j^* = \hat{y}_j + \lambda \psi(z_j)$ where $\hat{y}_j$ is the predicted value of the dependent variable based on the robust regression. A robust ANOVA may then be carried out by replacing each observed y_j by the pseudo y_j^* and then partitioning the sum of squares of the y_j^* via a LS software.

4.2 Numerical Example 3

This example is based on the data in Table 3 which lists the infant mortality data in the United States, classified by father's education (Factor A) and region (Factor B), for the period 1964–6. (For purposes of identification, the observations are numbered according to the numerals enclosed within the parentheses.) The data was used by Godfrey (1985) to illustrate the process of fitting by organized comparisons. This process provides residuals which indicate the potential outlying nature of the observations 38.8 (No. 3) and 21.1 (No. 8).

To magnify the effect of outliers in a robust ANOVA for a two-way design, the observation 38.8 of Table 3 is increased to 99.9 and the observation 21.1 is reduced to 0.1. (The remaining 18 observations are kept intact.)

A traditional (LS) two-way ANOVA is first carried out for all the 20 observations of the altered table under the model without interaction between the two factors A and B: $y_{ij} = \mu + \alpha_i + \beta_j + e_{ij}$. The results reported on the top of Table 4 indicate a nonsignificant contribution of the A and B factors. The LS residuals (not reported here) point to five potential outliers: Nos. 3 and 8 (the altered observations), and Nos. 1, 2, and 15 (original observations).

To carry out the robust Andrews analysis, seven dummy variables are created, four for Factor A and

Table 4
Results of LS and robust ANOVA based on pseudo-observations for Numerical Example 3

Procedure	Data	Source	DF	MS	*F*-ratio	*P*-value
LS	20 obs.	A	4	552.20	1.85	0.18
		B	3	347.83	1.16	0.36
		Error	12	299.93		
Andrews Robust	20 obs.	A	4	80.00	12.92	<0.01
		B	3	12.96	2.19	0.16
		Error	10	6.04		
LS	17 obs.	A|μ	4	83.17	21.67	<0.01
		B|μ, A	3	13.98	3.64	0.06
		Error	9	3.84		

and three for Factor B. In the final iteration, the two altered observations are assigned WLS weights of zero and are thus effectively deleted in the robust analysis. Except for No. 15, all other observations are weighted about fully; hence they may be considered as "good" observations of the data set.

To illustrate the effectiveness of the robust ANOVA in the presence of outliers, outlying observations Nos. 3, 8, and 15 are deleted and the reduced table is analyzed using a LS ANOVA for a two-way table with incomplete data.

The results of the Andrews robust analysis and of the LS analysis for the reduced table are also reported in Table 4. This table shows that these two analyses provide very similar results and that the variance due to Factor A is statistically significant.

5. Other Robust Estimation Procedures

There are other families of ψ functions (see Wu 1985, Staudte and Sheather 1990). In addition, there are other robust estimation procedures such as those based on order statistics (*L*-estimation) and normal scores (*R*-estimation), ridge regression, and adaptive estimation (Hogg 1979).

6. Conclusion

In regression analysis (and in ANOVA), a couple of "wild shots" or outliers might exert undue influence on the LS results. Therefore it is prudent to be cognizant of observations which somehow are not right or should not be part of the current data set, and to try either to eliminate them or to reduce their influence in the data analysis. Robust procedures, especially those with a redescending ψ, would provide a regression line which is reasonably free of the "real" outliers; in the process, they would be able to identify the "real" outliers with an acceptable level of accuracy.

Not much is gained by conducting a robust analysis on a set of data with no apparent outliers. For data with outliers, however, robust estimates may depart substantially from the LS results. These observations reinforce the recommendations made by Hogg (1979) regarding a sensible regression analysis: that is, to perform the usual LS analysis along with a robust procedure such as that used by Andrews. If the two sets of results are close to each other, the (traditional) LS estimates and relevant statistics should be reported. On the other hand, if substantial discrepancies occur, the observations with unexpectedly large residuals should be carefully looked at and checked to determine whether they contain errors of any type or if they represent significant situations under which the postulated regression model is not applicable.

See also: Scaling Methods; Regression Analysis of Quantified Data; Multivariate Analysis

References

Andrews D F 1974 A robust method for multiple regression. *Technometrics* 16(4): 523–31

Barnett V, Lewis T 1978 *Outliers in Statistical Data*. Wiley, New York

Braun H I, McNeil D R 1981 Testing in robust ANOVA. *Communications in Statistics* A10(2): 149–65

Daniel C, Wood S F 1971 *Fitting Equations to Data*, 2nd edn. Wiley, New York

Gentle J E 1977 Least absolute values estimation: An introduction. *Communications in Statistics* B6(6): 313–28

Godfrey K 1985 Fitting by organized comparisons: The square combining table. In: Hoaglin D C, Mosteller F, Tukey J (eds.) 1985

Hampel F R, Ronchetti E M, Rousseeuw P J, Stahel W A 1986 *Robust Statistics: The Approach Based on Influence Functions*. Wiley, New York

Hogg R V 1979 Statistical robustness: One view of its use in applications today. *The American Statistician* 33(3): 108–15

Huber P J 1973 Robust regression: Asymptotic, conjecture, and Monte Carlo. *Annals of Statistics* 1(5): 799–821

Huber P J 1981 *Robust Statistics*. Wiley, New York

Huynh H 1982 A comparison of four approaches to robust regression. *Psych. Bull.* 92(2): 505–12

Huynh H 1994. Robust procedures for multiple regression and analysis of variance. In: Thompson B (ed.) 1994 *Advances in Social Science Methodology*. JAI Press, Greenwich, Connecticut

Ruppert D 1985 M-estimator. In: Kotz S, Johnson N L (eds.) 1985 *Encyclopedia of Statistical Sciences*. Wiley, New York

SAS 1982 *SAS User's Guide: Statistics*. SAS Institute, Cary, North Carolina

SAS 1986 *SAS System for Regression*. SAS Institute, Cary, North Carolina

Schrader R M, Hettmansperger T P 1980 Robust analysis of variance based upon a likelihood ratio criterion. *Biometrika* 67(1): 93–101

Schrader R M, McKean J W 1977 Robust analysis of variance. *Communications in Statistics* A6(9): 879–94

Staudte R G, Sheather S J 1990 *Robust Estimation and Testing*. Wiley, New York

Tukey J W 1960 A survey of sampling from contaminated distributions. In: Olkin I (ed.) 1960 *Contributions to Probability and Statistics*. Stanford University Press, Stanford, California

Tukey J W 1962 The future of data analysis. *Annals of Mathematical Statistics* 33: 1–67

Wu L L 1985 Robust estimation of location and regression. In: Tuma N B (ed.) 1985 *Sociological Methodology*. Jossey-Bass, San Francisco, California

Further Reading

Hoaglin D C, Mosteller F, Tukey J W (eds.) 1985 *Exploring Data, Tables, Trends, and Shapes*. Wiley, New York

Mosteller F, Tukey J W 1977 *Data Analysis and Regression*. Addison-Wesley, Reading, Massachusetts

Sampling Errors in Survey Research

K. N. Ross and M. Wilson

The difference between a sample estimate for a particular statistic and the population parameter obtained from a complete analysis of all members of the defined target population is called the "sampling error" for that sample. In most practical situations the value of the population parameter is unknown, and therefore it is not possible to calculate the sampling error for a particular sample. Instead, through a knowledge of the behavior of estimates derived from all possible samples, it is sometimes possible to estimate the average, or expected, sampling error, even though the value of the population parameter is unknown.

The notion of an average, or expected, sampling error is usually summarized in terms of the mean square error. The mean square error, MSE, is the expected value of the squared difference between a sample value; for example, the sample mean $\bar{x}$, and the population parameter, μ, taken over all possible samples. Denoting the expected value of the sampling distribution of sample means by $E(\bar{x})$, the mean square error of the sample mean may be written as:

$$MSE(\bar{x}) = E(\bar{x} - \mu)^2$$

$$= E[\bar{x} - E(\bar{x})]^2 + [E(\bar{x}) - \mu]^2 \qquad (1)$$

$$= \text{Variance of } \bar{x} + (\text{Bias of } \bar{x})^2.$$

In most well-designed samples the bias of a sample estimate is either zero or small, tending toward zero with increasing sample size. Therefore, the mean square error is usually described in terms of the variance.

This entry considers the issues involved in the estimation of sampling errors and variance, the empirical procedures employed in their estimation, and the developments that occurred in the 1980s, to model the structure of complex sample designs and improve the estimation of variance components (see *Sampling in Survey Research*).

1. Estimation of Sampling Errors

1.1 Simple Random Samples

The educational researcher is usually dealing with a single random sample of data rather than all possible samples from a population. The variance of a sample estimate therefore cannot be calculated exactly. Instead, by using formulas derived by statisticians, estimates are made of the variance from the internal evidence of a single sample of data.

For a simple random sample of n elements drawn without replacement from a large population, the variance of the sample mean may be estimated from a single sample by using the following formula (Kish 1965 p. 41):

$$\text{var}(\bar{x}) = \frac{s^2}{n} \qquad (2)$$

where var $(\bar{x})$ refers to the sample estimate of the variance of $\bar{x}$, and s^2 is the unbiased estimate of the variance of the element values. A factor called the "finite population correction" has been left out of the formula because the population is assumed to be large.

In many practical survey research situations the sampling distribution of the sample mean, and many other sample estimators, is approximately normally distributed. The approximation improves with increasing sample size, even though the population of element values is far from normal (Kish 1965). Consequently, by taking the square root of the estimated variance it is possible to obtain an estimate of the standard error of the sampling distribution and thereby calculate confidence limits for the corresponding parameter.

In the case of the sample mean, the estimate of the standard error would be:

$$SE(\bar{x}) = \sqrt{\text{var}(\bar{x})} = \frac{s}{\sqrt{n}} \qquad (3)$$

Although there is general agreement among statistical authors concerning the formula for estimating the standard error of the sample mean for a simple random sample of elements, there are sometimes differences of opinion about the appropriate formulas for calculating the variance of more complex statistics. These differences generally become insignificant for the typically large population and sample sizes that are associated with educational survey research. In Table 1 the formulas for calculating the standard error of several commonly used statistics have been listed. The formulas were selected from one source (Guilford and Fruchter 1978).

The formulas in Table 1 are based on a simple random sample of n elements which are measured on m variables. The symbol s refers to the standard deviation and the symbol $R_{i.jkl}$ refers to the multiple correlation coefficient associated with a regression equation which uses i as the criterion variable and j, k, and l as predictor variables.

1.2 Complex Samples

Educational research is generally conducted by using data obtained from complex sample designs which

Table 1
Formulas for estimation of sampling error when data are gathered by using a simple random sample design

Sample Statistic	Estimator of standard error
Mean	$\dfrac{s}{\sqrt{n}}$
Correlation coefficient	$\dfrac{1}{\sqrt{n}}$
Standardized regression coefficient	$\sqrt{\dfrac{1-R^2_{1.234\ldots m}}{(1-R^2_{2.345\ldots m})(n-m)}}$
Multiple regression coefficient	$\dfrac{1}{\sqrt{n-m}}$

employ techniques such as stratification, clustering, and varying probabilities of selection. Computational formulas are available to provide estimates of the standard errors of descriptive statistics such as the sample mean for a wide range of these sample designs. Unfortunately, the computational formulas required for estimating the standard errors for analytical statistics such as correlation coefficients, standardized regression coefficients, and multiple correlation coefficients are not readily available for sample designs that depart from the model of simple random sampling. These formulas are either enormously complicated or, ultimately, they prove to be resistant to mathematical analysis (Frankel 1971). Reviews of

this area by Wolter (1985), Skinner et al. (1989), and Lee et al. (1990) provide detailed descriptions of the mathematical foundations of this complex area.

As a result of the lack of suitable sampling error formulas for many analytical statistics estimated from complex sample designs, researchers have tended to accept estimates based on formulas which assume that data have been gathered by using simple random sampling procedures. While overestimates of sampling errors may lead to errors of a conservative kind, underestimates have the potential to misrepresent the stability of sample statistics in a fashion that might lead to erroneous conclusions concerning the importance of research findings.

The research evidence available concerning the magnitude of sampling errors for statistics such as means, correlation coefficients, regression coefficients, and multiple correlation coefficients suggests that the use of formulas based on the assumption of simple random often results in gross underestimation of sampling errors for many sample designs commonly used in educational research (Peaker 1975, Ross 1978, Ross 1991). The degree of underestimation may be summarized by the "design effect" or "Deff" value. In Table 2 some values of $\sqrt{\text{Deff}}$ have been presented for a two-stage sample design employed in seven countries during a cross-national research study carried out by the International Association for the Evaluation of Educational Achievement (IEA) (Peaker 1975). For each country, the number of schools selected at the first stage, m, and the number of students selected within the sample schools, $\bar{n}$, has been presented.

The value of $\sqrt{\text{Deff}}$ represents the factor by which sampling errors, obtained from formulas based on simple random sampling assumptions, must be multi-

Table 2
Mean values of $\sqrt{\text{Deff}}$

obtained for seven countries participating in the First IEA Science Study Project at the 14-year old level

Country	Cluster size			Value of $\sqrt{\text{Def}}$	
	Schools m	$\bar{n}$	Means	Corr. coeff.	Regn. coeff.
Australia	225	24	2.4	1.7	1.3
Chile	103	13	2.6	1.6	1.6
Finland	77	30	2.2	1.7	1.3
Hungary	210	33	3.2	1.9	1.5
New Zealand	74	27	1.9	1.4	1.4
Scotland	70	28	2.4	1.5	1.2
Sweden	95	26	1.8	1.2	1.3
Mean $\sqrt{\text{Deff}}$	—	—	2.3	1.6	1.4

plied in order to obtain estimates of the actual value of the sampling error for the complex sample design. For example, from the data presented in Table 2, the standard error of a correlation coefficient for Australia based on the complex two-stage sample of $n_c = m\,\bar{n}$ elements would be:

$$SE(r_c) = \sqrt{\text{Deff}}\; SE(r_{srs}) = \frac{1.7}{\sqrt{n_c}} \qquad (4)$$

where $SE(r_c)$ is the standard error of a correlation coefficient for the complex two-stage sample design of n_c elements, and $SE(r_{srs})$ is the standard error which would be estimated from the appropriate formula in Table 1, which is based on the assumption that there was a simple random sample of n_c elements.

In Table 2 the values of $\sqrt{\text{Deff}}$ for means are higher than for correlation coefficients and regression coefficients. This result has occurred consistently for other types of sample design in a range of studies (Kish and Frankel 1970, Ross 1987).

2. Empirical Techniques for the Estimation of Sampling Errors

The calculation of the $\sqrt{\text{Deff}}$ adjustment factor requires that the researcher be able to estimate the sampling errors of statistics derived from complex sample designs. In the absence of suitable formulas based on distribution theory for many analytical statistics, a variety of empirical techniques have emerged which provide "approximate variances that appear satisfactory for practical purposes" (Kish 1978 p. 20).

These techniques may be divided into two broad groups: (a) random subsample replication, and (b) Taylor's series approximations.

2.1 Random Subsample Replication

In random subsample replication, a total sample of data is divided into two or more independent subsamples, each subsample following the overall sample design except for the sampling fraction and sample size. Finifter (1972) has described the procedure that is then employed in the following terms: "A distribution of outcomes for a parameter being estimated is generated by each subsample. The differences observed among the subsample results are then analyzed to obtain an improved estimate of the parameter, as well as a confidence assessment for that estimate" (Finifter 1972 p. 114). The main approaches to this technique have been independent replication (Mahalanobis 1946, Deming 1960), jackknifing (Tukey 1958), balanced repeated replication (McCarthy 1966), and the bootstrap (Efron 1979).

The use of "independent replication" to estimate errors in surveys was first introduced by Mahalanobis

(1946) for agricultural surveys carried out in India. Deming (1960) refined this technique as "replicated sampling" and demonstrated that it was useful for estimating the sampling errors of a wide range of statistics. In replicated sampling, several subsamples, rather than one full sample, are selected from the population. Each of these subsamples follows the same sample design. Sample estimates, y_i, of the statistic y are then calculated for each subsample. The variation between these independent estimates provides a means of assessing the sampling error associated with the overall estimate.

For k subsamples the statistic y may be estimated from the mean of the k subsample estimates, $\bar{y}$, and then the variance of y is approximated by the variance of the mean of the subsample estimates:

$$\text{Var}(y) \approx \frac{\Sigma(y_i - \bar{y})^2}{k(k-1)}. \qquad (5)$$

The independent replication technique considers the overall estimate as the mean of an unrestricted random sample of k subsample estimates. Therefore, provided the subsamples represent independent replications of each other, the technique may be used with any complex sample design.

The independent replication technique was used by the IEA in a study of mathematics achievement of students in 12 countries (Peaker 1967). An important feature of this technique is that sophisticated computer programs are not required for the estimation of sampling errors because the analyses required for the overall dataset are simply repeated on each of the subsamples.

Kish (1965) presented a variety of arguments that may be advanced in favor of employing either large or small numbers of independent replications. Kish favored at least 20 replications, Deming (1960) recommended 10, and Peaker (1967) employed 4 to estimate errors in the IEA studies. The use of 10 replications provides an appealing result in terms of computational simplicity (Kish 1965). In this case, due to the relationship between the range and the variance of elements in a sample, the variance of the statistic y may be estimated as:

$$\text{Var}(y) \approx \left[\frac{\text{Range }(y_i)}{10}\right]. \qquad (6)$$

The development of the "jackknife" procedure may be traced back to an earlier method used by Quenouille (1956) to reduce the bias of estimates. Further refinement of the method (Tukey 1958, Mosteller and Tukey 1968, 1977) has led to its application in a range of social science situations where formulas are not readily available for the calculation of sampling errors. The application of the jackknife procedure requires that estimates of statistics be made on the total sample of data, and then, after dividing the data

665

into groups, the calculations are made for each of the slightly reduced bodies of data which are obtained by omitting a subgroup in turn. These subgroups should be constructed according to the same approach used in Deming's technique.

Let y_i be an estimate of a statistic y based on the data that remain after omitting the ith subgroup and let y_{all} be the estimate based on the total sample data. k pseudovalues y_i^* $(i = 1, \ldots, k)$ can be defined based on the k complements:

$$y_i^* = ky_{all} - (k - 1)y_i. \tag{7}$$

The jackknife value is defined as:

$$y^* = \frac{1}{k} \sum_{i=1}^{k} y_i^*. \tag{8}$$

The variance of the statistic y may be estimated from the variance of the jackknife value:

$$\text{Var}(y) \approx \left[\sum_{i=1}^{k} y_i^{*2} - \frac{1}{k} \left(\sum_{i=1}^{k} y_i^* \right)^2 \right] \Big/ k(k-1) \tag{9}$$

Tukey (1958) advanced the proposals that the pseudovalues could be treated as if they were approximately independent observations and that Student's t distribution could be applied to these estimates in order to construct approximate confidence intervals for y^* or y_{all}. Later empirical work by Frankel (1971) provided firm support for these proposals when the jackknife technique was applied to complex sample designs and a variety of regression-related statistics.

Substituting for y_i^* in the expression for $\text{var}(y^*)$ permits the variance of y^* to be estimated from the k subsample estimates, y_i, and their mean, $\bar{y}_i$, without the need to calculate pseudovalues.

$$\text{var}(y^*) = (k - 1)/k \sum_{i=1}^{k} (y_i - \bar{y}_i)^2 \tag{10}$$

Wolter (1985 p.156) has shown that replacing y^* by y_{all} in the right hand side of the first expression for $\text{var}(y^*)$ will provide a conservative estimate of (y^*)— the overestimate being equal to $(y_{all} - y^*)^2/(k - 1)$. In practice, these expressions for $\text{var}(y^*)$ have also been used to estimate the variance not only of Quenouille's estimator y^*, but also of y_{all} (Wolter 1985 pp. 155, 172). That is,

$$\text{var}(y_{all}) = 1/k(k - 1) \sum_{i=1}^{k} (y_i^* - y_{all})^2 \tag{11}$$

Or, after substituting for y_i^*,

$$\text{var}(y_{all}) = (k - 1)/k \sum_{i=1}^{k} (y_i - y_{all})^2 \tag{12}$$

Wolter (1985) and Rust (1985) have presented an extension of these formulae for complex stratified sample designs in which there are k_h primary sampling units in the *hth* stratum (where $h = 1, 2, \ldots, H$). In this case, the formula for the variance of y_{all} employs y_{hi} to denote the estimator derived from the same functional

form as y_{all}—calculated after deleting the *ith* primary sampling unit from the *hth* stratum:

$$\text{var}(y_{all}) = \sum_{i=1}^{H} (k_h - 1)/k_h \sum_{h=1}^{k_h} (y_{hi} - y_{all})^2 \tag{13}$$

Where $K = \sum_{i=1}^{H} k_h$ is the total number of samples to be formed.

The majority of sample designs used in educational research employ schools as primary sampling units. For these sample designs, the K estimates of y_{hi} are obtained by removing one school at a time from the total sample and then applying the same functional form used to estimate y_{all} for each reduced sample. Where geographical areas are used as the primary sampling unit, followed by the selection of more than one school per area, the estimates of y_{hi} are commonly based on reduced samples formed by omitting one geographical area at a time from the total sample.

The jackknife procedure has been extensively used in the large-scale educational evaluation studies carried out by the IEA (Peaker 1975). Rust (1986) found that for typical sample designs the best estimates are obtained when one primary sampling unit is omitted for each jackknife replication.

A computer program within the OSIRIS statistical software system (Survey Research Center 1981) has been designed to carry out jackknife calculations for regression-related statistics. However, even for large samples, provided there are only a few statistics and only a few subsamples it is feasible to carry out the necessary calculations by hand following the preparation of pseudovalues on the computer. A number of user-written SAS procedures have become available to carry out the jackknife procedure for complex samples. These include: PROC JACKREG (Hobbs and Chilko 1983), PROC JRR (Rochan and Kalsbeek 1983), and WESVAR (Westat Inc. 1989).

A PC version of WESVAR (Brick 1996) has been released that computes estimates and replicate variance estimates from survey data collected using complex sampling and estimation procedures. Sampling errors can be estimated for different types of survey statistics and for a whole range of complex sample designs, including multistage, stratified, and unequal probability samples. WesVarPC computes parameter estimates for linear and logistic regression models, and provides a test for the overall fit of the regression model as well as tests for the significance of linear combinations of variables included in the model, using the replication for variance estimation of jackknifing and balanced repeated replication.

The "balanced repeated replication" technique was developed by McCarthy (1966) in order to permit variance estimates to be made from sample designs which featured the maximum amount of stratification possible (two primary selections per stratum) and yet still permitted variance estimates to be made from a single sample of data.

Consider a population divided into h strata and the primary sampling units within each of these strata are allocated to two random halves of equal size. A primary sampling unit is then selected from each half stratum. A half-sample replicate is formed by randomly choosing one of these primary sampling units for each stratum. The number of possible half samples which can be drawn from the data is 2^h. Variance estimates are then computed from the squared difference between the total sample estimate and the half-sample replicate estimate.

Thus, if y_{all} is an estimate of a statistic y based on the total sample of data, then the variance of this statistic may be estimated by $(y_i - y_{all})^2$, where y_i is the estimate based on a half sample (Kish and Frankel 1970).

In order to increase the precision of the variance estimate the researcher may select k repeated replications and then the variance of the statistic y may be estimated from the mean of the k computed variances:

$$\text{Var}(y) \approx \sum_{i=1}^{k} (y_i - y_{\text{all}})^2 / k \qquad (14)$$

McCarthy's (1966) main contribution in this area was to develop a method for choosing a specific subset of half samples which contained all of the information available in the total set of half samples. Frankel (1971) carried out extensive tests of this technique and showed that it was suitable for generating sampling errors for a variety of statistics employed in multiple regression analysis. A computer program, based on Frankel's research, has been distributed within the OSIRIS statistical software system (Survey Research Center 1981). An important feature of this software is that it is capable of producing estimates of sampling errors for both the balanced repeated replication and the jackknife techniques. Several user-written SAS procedures have been produced to carry out balanced repeated replication. These include: PROC BRRVAR (Wise 1983) and WESVAR (Westat Inc. 1989).

A PC version of WESVAR (Brick et al. 1996) has been released that computes estimates and replicates variance estimates from survey data collected using complex sampling and estimation procedures. Sampling errors can be estimated for different types of survey statistics and for a whole range of complex sample designs, including multistage, stratified, and unequal probability samples. WESVARPC computes parameter estimates for linear and logistic regression models, and provides a test for the overall fit of the regression model as well as tests for the significance of linear combinations of variables included in the model, using the replication for variance estimation of jackknifing and balanced repeated replication.

2.2 The Bootstrap Technique

Put very generally, the "bootstrap" technique (Efron 1979) is as follows (see Fig. 1). The statistician interested in estimating the distribution of a statistic $R(y,$ F) based on some data y and a probability distribution F: R must be well-defined given F; y is, of course, known; and F is unknown, or, at best, known up to some parameter set. For example, R might be the mean $\bar{y}$, and the aspect of its distribution that is of interest might be the standard error; there are n data points in y (for sampling situations, these might be the primary sampling units). The bootstrap solution is to base an empirical distribution F^* on y, then to resample y^* from F^*. The distribution of $R(y^*, F^*)$, in which all elements are known, is considered an estimator of $R(y, F)$, and it can be used to investigate the distributional properties of R, such as its standard error.

In the example of the mean, a large number of samples, say 500 to 2,000, would be drawn from y using simple random sampling of primary sampling units or data points with replacement, each sample being of size n (i.e., F^* is a distribution with mass $1/n$ on each data point in y). The mean is calculated for each of these bootstrap samples, and the standard deviation of the bootstrap samples is used to estimate the sampling error of the mean. Note that no parametric assumptions about the distribution F of y have been made: the empirical distribution of y has been used as a surrogate for such assumptions. A general introduction to the topic is given in Efron and Tibshurani (1986) (see *Simulation as a Research Technique*).

Straightforward application of the technique to complex sample survey data (referred to as the "naive bootstrap" by Rao and Wu [1988]) results in inconsistent estimators. Fortunately Rao and Wu have provided corrected formulas that reduce this problem. Although the technique has some advantages when a normality assumption is not valid, it has been found to be less stable than the jackknife and Taylor's series approaches (Rao and Wu 1988). Interest in the preparation of software that will apply the bootstrap to survey research data has grown—and programs such as BOJA, distributed by the Progamma organization in the Netherlands have come onto the market in the early 1990s.

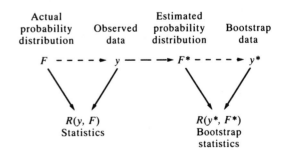

Figure 1
Schematic illustration of the bootstrap process
Source: Efron and Tibshurani 1986 (adapted)

2.3 Taylor's Series Approximations

The use of Taylor's series approximations was initially suggested by Kendall and Stuart (1969) and is often described as a more direct method of variance estimation than the "replication" approaches. In the absence of an exact sampling variance formula, the Taylor's series is used to approximate a numerical value of the first few terms of a series expansion of the variance formula. The majority of applications in social science research have been limited to the use of Taylor's series terms up to the first partial derivatives (Kish and Frankel 1970).

Kendall and Stuart (1969 pp. 231–32) showed that if $g(y)$ is a function of the k variates $y_1, y_2, \ldots, y_k$, which have means $\theta_1, \theta_2, \ldots, \theta_k$, then providing $g(y)$ is differentiable, the Taylor's series for $g(y_1, y_2, \ldots, y_k)$ may be written as:

$$g(y) = g(y_1, y_2, \ldots, y_k)$$

$$= g(\theta_1, \theta_2, \ldots, \theta_k) + \sum_{i=1}^{k} \frac{\partial g}{\partial y_i} (y_i - \theta_i) \qquad (15)$$

$$+ \text{ terms of order } n^{-1} \text{ or less.}$$

The partial derivatives in the above expression are calculated at the appropriate expected values.

For large sample sizes, that is, large n values, the approximation is made that $g(y)$ may be expressed as a sum of the first two terms on the right hand side of the above equation.

Then, with this assumption in mind, the sampling variance of $g(y)$ is approximately equal to the sampling variance of the first degree terms of the Taylor's series approximation. That is,

$$\text{Var}[g(y)] \approx \text{Var} \left[\sum_{i=1}^{k} \frac{\partial g}{\partial y_i} y_i \right]. \qquad (16)$$

since $g(\theta_1, \theta_2, \ldots, \theta_k)$ and $\sum_{i=1}^{k} (\partial g / \partial y_i) \theta_i$ are both constants (Frankel 1971 pp. 27–28).

The application of this estimator of the sampling variance of $g(y)$ requires that values for the partial derivatives can be obtained, and that the values of these, when they are evaluated for the sample data, are reasonable approximations to their true values.

In the relatively simple situation where $g(y)$ is a ratio mean, y/x, based on two variables, x and y, measured for a simple random sample of intact but unequal sized clusters, the partial derivatives may be obtained readily. Kish (1965 p. 207) showed that:

$$\text{Var}\left(\frac{y}{k}\right) \approx \frac{1}{x^2} \left[\text{var}(y) + \left(\frac{y}{x}\right)^2 \text{var}(x) \right.$$

$$\left. - 2\left(\frac{y}{x}\right) \text{cov}(x, y)\right].$$

The evaluation of partial derivatives when estimates of the sampling variances of correlation or regression coefficients are required becomes a much more unwieldy exercise (Frankel 1971, Mellor 1973, Rust 1985). Beyond these elementary analytical statistics, it would appear that very few attempts have been made to tackle the extensive algebra required to make series approximations for more complicated multivariate statistics obtained from complex samples.

A number of computer programs have been produced that employ Taylor's series approximations for the estimation of sampling errors associated with means and proportions (Shah 1981a), ratio means (Shah 1981b, Survey Research Center 1981), and regression coefficients (Hidiroglou et al. 1979, Holt 1979). All of these programs are based on subroutines which describe formulas for the partial derivatives of the appropriate statistics. Woodruff and Causey (1976) have produced a more generalized approach in which the partial derivatives of many complicated statistics may be estimated by means of a numerical approximation technique. Wilson (1989) has presented a detailed study of the Woodruff–Causey approach when it is applied to a variety of sample designs that are commonly employed in educational survey research.

In the late 1980s efforts were made to extend the availability of this computer software to the users of personal computers. Reviews of this and related work have been presented by Cohen et al. (1986, 1988) and Carlson et al. (1990). In particular, Fuller et al. (1989) and Ogden and Liebman (1991) have produced personal computer programs that utilize Taylor's series approximations.

3. Modeling the Structure of Complex Sample Designs

Several related techniques were introduced during the 1980s that can be considered as ways to model the structure of complex sample designs of the kinds that are employed in educational research. Advances in the application of numerical estimation techniques to the problem of covariance component estimation in unbalanced nested designs (Dempster et al. 1977, Goldstein 1987, Longford 1987), based on the groundbreaking work of Lindley and Smith (1972), led to the application of covariance component models in various applied fields. They are variously known as "multilevel linear models," "mixed effects or random effects models," "random coefficient regression models," and "hierarchical linear models," with the labels reflecting mainly the field of application, but also (less often) differences in formulation. The standard (educational) application of a (two-level) covariance component model could be applied to a situation where students were sampled within schools as well as being sampled from a school population. More complex possibilities include the modeling of repeated measures within individual students, and other levels of nesting. These models can be applied to a number of types of problems in educational research, among them, improved estimation of individual effects, the modeling of cross-level effects, and the partitioning of covariance components. It is this last that is most relevant to the estimation of sampling errors, although the major emphasis of many researchers appears to be the first and second (e.g., Bryk and Raudenbush 1992). Thus, although there is a burgeoning list of applications of these models in educational research, and although many of the applications are to survey sample data, the formal use of the techniques to address the issue of sampling errors has received little attention. For example, this is reflected in the fact that what is probably the most popular program in the field, HLM (Bryk et al. 1988), was not available in a version that correctly processed weighted data until 1992. It will be some time before these developments match the complexity present in many educational survey samples (e.g., combinations of clustering and stratification), and it will be somewhat longer before numerical techniques such as jackknifing and the bootstrap can be used to free them from the strict assumptions of multivariate normality which currently characterize their application. But it is a development well worth watching out for.

4. Conclusion

This entry has mainly concentrated on describing the steps that might be taken to cope with the problems of sample error estimation in educational surveys. It is well worth reiterating the importance of such efforts. It is not just an esoteric game for sampling statisticians. Almost all research in education based on quantitative data is founded on some sort of survey design. Every such analysis, from the most modest comparison of means up to the sophisticated analyses possible within computer packages such as LISREL (Jöreskog and Sörbom 1989), is subject to distortion of its results of an order of magnitude similar to those exemplified in Table 2. Application of the methods described above is as yet not very common, but a computer program STREAMS (Gustafsson and Stahl 1996) has now been released for analysis of data, using structural equation modeling and the LISREL approach, that provides for the partitioning of covariance components at two levels (but not for the modeling of cross-level effects) and thus for the appropriate estimation of effects and their errors in multilevel sample designs. There is a great need for research on the development and application of these techniques in the diverse contexts that characterize educational research today.

See also: Hierarchical Linear Models; Multivariate Analysis; Path Analysis and Linear Structural Relations Anlaysis; Path Analysis with Latent Variables; Measures of Variation; Survey Research Methods; Sampling in Survey Research

References

Brick J M, P James P, Severynse J 1996 *A User's Guide to WesVarPC*. Westat Inc, Rockville, Maryland

Bryk A S, Raudenbush S W 1992 *Hierarchical Linear Models: Applications and Data Analysis Methods*. Sage, Newbury Park, California

Bryk A S, Raudenbush S W, Seltzer M, Congdon R 1988 *An Introduction to HLM: Computer Program and User's Guide*. Scientific Software, Mooresville, Indiana

Carlson B L, Johnson A E, Cohen S B 1990 An evaluation of the use of personal computers for variance estimation for complex survey data. *Proceedings of the Survey Research Methods Section of the American Statistical Association* 724–6

Cohen S B, Burt V L, Jones G K 1986 Efficiencies in variance estimation for complex survey data. *The American Statistician* 40(2): 157–60

Cohen S B, Xanthopoulos J A, Jones G K 1988 An evaluation of statistical software procedures appropriate for regression analysis of complex survey data. *J. Off. Stat.* 4(1): 17–34

Deming W E 1960 *Sample Design in Business Research*. Wiley, London

Dempster A P, Laird N M, Rubin D B 1977 Maximum likelihood from incomplete data via the EM algorithm. *J. Roy. Stat. Soc. (Series B)* 39(1): 1–38

Efron B 1979 Bootstrap methods: Another look at the jackknife. *Annals of Statistics* 41(1): 1–26

Efron B, Tibshurani R 1986 Bootstrap methods for standard errors, confidence intervals, and other methods of statistical accuracy. *Stat. Sci.* 1(1): 54–77

Finifter B M 1972 The generation of confidence: Evaluating research findings by random subsample replication. In: Coster H I (ed.) 1972 *Sociological Methodology: 1972* Jossey-Bass, London

Frankel M R 1971 *Inference from Survey Samples: An Empirical Investigation*. Institute for Social Research, University of Michigan, Ann Arbor, Michigan

Fuller W A, Kennedy W, Schnell D, Sullivan G, Park H J 1989 *PC Carp Manual*. Statistical Laboratory, Iowa State University, Ames, Iowa

Goldstein H I 1987 *Multilevel Models in Educational and Social Research*. Oxford University Press, Oxford

Guilford J P, Fruchter B 1978 *Fundamental Statistics in Psychology and Education*, 6th edn. McGraw-Hill, New York

Gustafsson J-E, Stahl P A 1996 *STREAMS User's Guide Structural Equation Modeling Made Simple*. Göteborg University, Göteborg

Hidiroglou M A, Fuller W A, Hickman R D 1979 *Super Carp*, 4th edn. Survey Section, Iowa State University, Ames, Iowa

Hobbs G, Chilko D M 1983 Robust regression and PROC JACKREG. *Proceedings of the Survey Research Methods Section of the American Statistical Association*, 729–37

Holt M M 1979 *Standard Errors of Regression Coefficients from Sample Survey Data*. Research Triangle Institute, Research Triangle Park, North Carolina

Jöreskog K G, Sörbom D 1989 *LISREL 7 User's Reference Guide*. Scientific Software, Mooresville, Indiana

Kendall M G, Stuart A 1969 *The Advanced Theory of Statistics*, 3rd edn, Vol. 1. Griffin, London

Kish L 1965 *Survey Sampling*. Wiley, New York

Kish L 1978 On the future of survey sampling. In: Krishnan

Namboodiri N (ed.) 1978 *Survey Sampling and Measurement*. Academic Press, New York

Kish L, Frankel M R 1970 Balanced repeated replications for standard errors. *J. Am. Stat. Assoc.* 65(331): 1071–94

Lee E S, Forthofer R N, Lorrimer R J 1990 *Analyzing Complex Survey Data*. Sage, Newbury Park, California

Lindley D V, Smith A F M 1972 Bayes estimates for the linear model. *J. Roy. Stat. Soc. (Series B)* 34(1): 1–41

Longford N T 1987 A fast scoring algorithm for maximum likelihood estimation in unbalanced mixed models with nested random effects. *Biometrika* 74(4): 817–27

Mahalanobis P C 1946 Recent experiments in statistical sampling in the Indian Statistical Institute. *J. Roy. Stat. Soc.* 109(4): 326–78

McCarthy P J 1966 *Replication: An Approach to the Analysis of Data from Complex Surveys: Development and Evaluation of a Replication Technique for Estimating Variance*. DHEW, Washington, DC

Mellor R W 1973 Subsample replication variance estimators. (Doctoral dissertation, Harvard University)

Mosteller F, Tukey J W 1968 Data analysis including statistics. In: Lindzey G, Aronson E (eds.) 1968 *The Handbook of Social Psychology*, 2nd edn. *Vol. 2: Research Methods*. Addison-Wesley, Reading, Massachusetts

Mosteller F, Tukey J W 1977 *Data Analysis and Regression: A Second Course in Statistics*. Addison-Wesley, Reading, Massachusetts

Ogden C, Liebman E 1991 *PC STRATTAB: A Tabulation Program Using Taylor Series Approximations for Estimating Standard Errors*. MPR Associates, Berkeley, California

Peaker G F 1967 Sampling. In: Husén T (ed.) 1967 *International Study of Achievement in Mathematics: A Comparison of Twelve Countries*, Vol. 1. Wiley, New York

Peaker G F 1975 *An Empirical Study of Education in Twenty-one Countries: A Technical Report*. Wiley, New York

Quenouille M H 1956 Notes on bias in estimation. *Biometrika* 43: 353–60

Rao J N K, Wu C F J 1988 Resampling inference with complex survey data. *J. Am. Stat. Assoc.* 83(401): 231–41

Rochon J, Kalsbeek W D 1988 Variance estimation from multistage sample survey data: The Jackknife repeated replicate approach. *Proceedings of the Survey Research Methods Section of the American Statistical Association* 848–53

Ross K N 1978 Sample design for educational survey research. *Eval. Educ.* 2(2): 105–95

Ross K N 1987 Sample design. *Int. J. Educ. Res.* 11(1):57–75

Ross K N 1991 *Sampling Manual for the IEA International Study of Reading Literacy*. IEA Reading Literacy Study Coordinating Center, University of Hamburg, Hamburg

Rust K 1985 Variance estimation for complex estimators in sample surveys. *J. Off. Stat.* 1(4):381–97

Rust K 1986 Efficient replicate variance estimation. *Proceedings of the Survey Research Methods Section of the American Statistical Association*

Shah B V 1981a *Standard Errors Program for Computing of Standardized Rates from Survey Data*. Research Triangle Institute, Research Triangle Park, North Carolina

Shah B V 1981b *Standard Errors Program for Computing of Ratio Estimates from Sample Survey Data*. Research Triangle Institute, Research Triangle Park, North Carolina

Skinner C J, Holt D, Smith T M F (eds.) 1989 *Analysis of Complex Surveys*. Wiley, Chichester

Survey Research Center 1981 *OSIRIS IV User's Manual*, 7th edn. Survey Research Center, Ann Arbor, Michigan

Tukey J W 1958 Bias and confidence in not-quite large samples: Presented at Ames, Iowa. *Ann. Maths. Stat.* 29: 614

Westat Inc. 1989 *The WESVAR Procedure*. Westat Inc., Rockville, Maryland

Wilson M 1989 An evaluation of Woodruff's technique for variance estimation in educational surveys. *J. Ed. Stat.* 14(1): 81–101

Wise L L 1983 *The PROC BRRVAR procedure: Documentation*. American Institute for Research, Palo Alto, California

Wolter K M 1985 *Introduction to Variance Estimation*. Springer, New York

Woodruff R A, Causey B D 1976 Computerized method for approximating the variance of a complicated estimate. *J. Am. Stat. Assoc.* 71(354): 315–21

Significance Testing

J. K. Lindsey

Scientific research, in education as elsewhere, involves the construction of models to represent observable reality. When a research worker studies some phenomenon, he or she will often have in mind some well-specified hypothesis about these models. Significance testing deals with the checking of such hypotheses. Since a hypothesis can never be verified by any finite amount of data and since someone may subsequently observe data that contradict it, it is necessary to specify hypotheses of interest that can be rejected. In order to be useful, such an approach must be formalized. (For a more detailed discussion, see Lindsey 1996.)

This entry considers the three alternative approaches that have been advanced to address these issues. Because of the controversy that exists, a rigorous treatment is required; otherwise, the material presented is likely to be misleading and to add to the confusion that has arisen in the area.

In the statistical context, there will be a "family of models," $f(y; \psi)$, which can be considered as possible candidate mechanisms which could have generated the data, y. A capital letter will represent as yet unobserved data, a random variable, while the corresponding small letter signifies that actually observed. The unknown "parameters," ψ, distinguish among the different members of the family. For any given, fixed value of the parameters, the probability of any possible observation can be calculated from this function.

Thus, a model is meant to describe certain aspects of some population under study. Relationships among variables are given by specific parameters in the model. Both these and the overall validity of the model may be tested. The testability of causality depends uniquely on the way data are collected: whether it is experimental or not. Nothing in the model-building and testing process can change this. See, for example, Cox (1992), and the concluding discussion below. If measurement error is important, it must be explicitly incorporated as part of the model. If simple random sampling is not used, the more complex sampling scheme should also be included in the model (Holt et al. 1980). For example, with cluster sampling, intraclass correlation will be required. As long as the sample plan does not depend on the response variable being observed, it will have no influence on modeling, or on the resulting testing (Hoem 1985). This is called "noninformative" sampling. The most common example of informative sampling is a retrospective study: people are selected, for example, according to their profession, and their education level ascertained. However, those who have died or migrated cannot be interviewed. These are the same criteria as apply for missing observations to be noninformative.

Once the data have been actually observed, it is possible to look at the family of models in a different light. It is now called the "likelihood function," written $L(\psi;y)$, although it is still mathematically identical to the model function given above. By looking at different values of the parameters, it is possible to calculate, each time, the probability of the observed data. Those that make the data more probable are said to be more likely. The one parameter value that makes the data most probable is called the "maximum likelihood estimate" (MLE).

The likelihood function is the basis of modern statistics. The elaboration of hypotheses and their testing will be developed in this context. In a short entry such as this, it is not possible to give specific techniques for all situations; for that, the reader may consult a reliable introductory statistical text. In this entry, the idea is to outline the general theory of significance testing, using a rather arbitrary selection of common simple techniques as examples. However, statistical theory is not a unified field; it is subject to certain controversies. As will be seen, this is reflected in the ways significance testing may be handled.

1. Fisherian Tests

Suppose that a specific, completely defined, statistical model, with $\psi = \psi_0$, a known fixed value, is under consideration as an hypothesis. Then, if the observed value of some suitable "test statistic" such as a mean,

calculated from the data, is rare or improbable as compared to other possible, but unobserved, values of the statistic, the hypothesis might be considered to be questionable, and, in extreme cases, rejected. Exactly how this process can be carried out will be elaborated in what follows; much of this section is generally applicable to all three approaches to significance testing.

The reasoning behind this procedure is that *any* observed data set always has small probability, even if it is the most probable one for a given model. This is especially so as the number of observations increases. Thus, such a probability has no absolute meaning. Instead, it is necessary to look at the total probability of the set of all possible observations, under the model, which are at least as rare. This probability is called the "P-value." *This is a probability about the data, not about the parameters.* If it is small, there are only two possibilities: either a rare event has happened or the hypothesis, is false. This is known as a "pure" or "Fisherian test of significance" (Fisher 1954). The close relationship to Popperian theory of falsification of scientific hypotheses is evident. However, Fisher had already developed his approach to testing before Popper published his philosophy of science.

Consider the following three sets of binomial observations with their MLE of the probability of success, π:

n	y	$\hat{\pi}$
20	13	0.750
200	115	0.575
2000	1046	0.523

For each set, the P-value is about $\alpha = 0.021$ under the model, $\pi_0 = 0.5$, indicating rather rare events. This shows how, as the sample size, n, increases, an MLE ever closer to its hypothesized value will nevertheless be rejected.

In a simple (monotone) case, suppose that $T(\mathbf{Y})$, with $t(\mathbf{y})$ its observed value, is a test statistic, such that

$$Pr(T(\mathbf{Y}) \geq t(\mathbf{y}); \psi_0) = \alpha$$

so that large values are rare. If a fixed probability value, α, say 0.05, is chosen as indicating rarity, what has been done, in effect, is to replace the full data set by a single binary value indicating whether the data are in the rare set or not. However, with modern statistical software, it is no longer necessary to adopt such a fixed value, like the traditional 5 percent. P-values are always provided by statistical software and they should be reported. Fixing the significance level is only applicable in a one-shot decision context, where a clear choice must be made based on the available information. Such a situation is found, for example, in industry or in medical drug testing, but rarely in educational research.

In a Fisherian test, there is only concern for what has happened, as compared to what might have occurred. No long-run frequency arguments, concerning what might happen in the future, are involved. The aim is to maximize the chance of the conclusions being correct given only what has actually been observed. The appeal of this significance test is that it allows making an absolute statement about one model, in the light of the data, without comparing it to any other. The drawback is that it involves a drastic loss of information by the data reduction process just mentioned. As well, there is obviously no wish to reject a hypothesis if no alternative model is available to replace it. But, in such a situation, would a significance test be performed in the first place?

1.1 Exact Tests

In certain simple cases, it is possible to calculate the exact probabilities for test statistics. For normal distribution models, such as standard multiple regression and analysis of variance, the well-known tests based on the Chi-squared, t, and F distributions are exact. Tables of probabilities are widely available and computer statistical packages all provide them.

Another famous illustration is "Fisher's exact test" for independence in a 2×2 contingency table. This is the most fundamental case of testing an hypothesis about the relationship between variables.

Suppose that X and Y are two variables, each only taking two possible values, zero and one, giving a table of frequencies n_{ij} with $n_{i \cdot}$ and $n_{\cdot j}$ the marginal totals. Then, $t_0 = n_{\cdot 2}$ is the total number of times that Y is observed to be one in a sample, and $t_1 = n_{22}$ the number of times Y and X are simultaneously one. This can be modeled by a logistic regression:

$$\log \left(\frac{\pi_i}{1 - \pi_i} \right) = \beta_0 + \beta_1 x_i$$

where π_i is the probability of Y_i being 1 when $X = x_i$. For the hypothesis that X and Y are independent, or that $\beta_1 = 0$, the exact P-value is given by:

$$\Pr(T_1 \geqslant t_1) = \frac{\displaystyle\sum_{i = t_1}^{min\,(t_0, n_1)} \binom{n_{\cdot 1}}{i} \binom{n_{\cdot 2}}{t_0 - i}}{\binom{n_{\cdot \cdot}}{t_0}}$$

For the table,

	$y = 0$	$y = 1$
$x = 0$	0	4
$x = 1$	3	2

the P-value is 0.167, so that, for the model with no relationship between X and Y, the results are not a rare event. However, in the second table,

	$y = 0$	$y = 1$
$x = 0$	19	4
$x = 1$	14	12

the P-value is 0.039, indicating that this would be a rather improbable result for the independence model.

This exact test can easily be generalized to larger tables. It is very important when the frequencies in a table are small, so important that specialized commercial software is available just for this type of problem!

1.2 Asymptotic Tests

Since exact tests of significance are only feasible in special cases, it is important to have available approximate tests, usually asymptotic, when the number of observations is sufficiently large. Since all the information in the observations is contained in the likelihood function, it is natural to use (minus two times) its logarithm, the deviance, with an asymptotic Chi-squared distribution, called a "likelihood ratio test." Large values indicate a rare event, under a given fixed model. The "degrees of freedom" (DF) is the number of parameters fixed by hypothesis.

Consider again the contingency table problem. For large tables, calculation of the exact P-value is complex. An asymptotic approximation may be based on the deviance

$$D = 2 \left[n_{\cdot \cdot} \log (n_{\cdot \cdot}) + \sum_{i=1}^{I} \sum_{i=1}^{J} n_{ij} \log(n_{ij}) \right.$$

$$\left. - \sum_{i=1}^{I} n_{i \cdot} \log (n_{i \cdot}) - \sum_{i=1}^{J} n_{\cdot j} \log (n_{\cdot j}) \right]$$

This is often called G^2, with $(I - 1)(J - 1)$ DF in the context of log–linear and logistic models.

For the first table above this gives a value of 4.727, with 1 DF. The probability of a Chi-squared value as large as this is about 0.030. Here, the total number of observations is too small for the approximation to be very good. For the second table, a deviance of 4.763 is obtained, with P-value 0.029. With more observations this time, the approximation is better.

Approximations to the log likelihood ratio test are sometimes used: the asymptotic normal distribution of the MLE (of β_1) gives a "Wald test" and the score statistic a "Rao score" or "Lagrange multiplier test."

1.2.1 Example of an asymptotic test.
In the second table above, the MLE is $\beta_1 = 1.404$ with standard error (s.e.) 0.676, in the logistic model. Because of the zero in the first table, an estimate of β_1 cannot be made there. Thus, the Wald statistic is $1.404/0.676 = 2.076$ with a P-value from the normal distribution of 0.038.

The Rao score approximation to the likelihood ratio test for a 2×2 contingency table is

$$\sum_i \sum_j \frac{\left(n_{ij} - \frac{n_i \cdot n_{\cdot j}}{n_{\cdot\cdot}} \right)^2}{\frac{n_i \cdot n_{\cdot j}}{n_{\cdot\cdot}}}$$

which is the well-known Pearson Chi-squared statistic. For the first table, this gives a value of 3.600 with P-value, 0.058, and, for the second table, 4.591 with P-value 0.032.

1.2.2 Another example. Exactly the same procedures can be used when a probability distribution is hypothesized to describe population frequencies. A Poisson distribution might be chosen for the number of times a student is sick during the year. Then, this hypothesis can be checked with a *"goodness of fit test."*

The Wald and Rao score tests have certain advantages, especially when the model of interest sets certain parameters to zero. The Wald test is simple to apply, since, if the s.e. of an estimate is available, a rough rule of thumb is that a value of the MLE at least twice as large as the s.e. will only occur with about probability 0.05 if the true value is zero. However, this test is particularly sensitive to transformations of the parameters and can give poor results in many situations. The other two tests are both parametrization invariant. The Rao score test has the advantage that it can be obtained from the simpler model, with the parameters set to zero, without calculating the MLE of those parameters. In complex cases, only the deviance may give sensible answers. Thus, generally, it should be preferred to the others, which are approximations to it, even although they are all asymptotically equivalent.

2. Neyman–Pearson Tests

In certain circumstances, it is desirable to reduce the long-term risk of making mistakes in repeated applications of an inference procedure, instead of maximizing the possibility of being correct in the particular observed situation. Various criteria have been developed to accomplish this, in what is known as the Neyman–Pearson school of statistical inference (see Cox and Hinkley 1974).

2.1 Simple Null Hypothesis

Suppose, as before, that there is a family of parametric statistical models and some hypothesis, H, about the "correct" model. A "null hypothesis," usually denoted by H_0, is that (family of) model(s) of special interest, which is under test. However, there is also an "alternative hypothesis," denoted by H_A, that (family of) model(s) which is taken to be competing with H_0.

An hypothesis is said to be "simple" if it completely specifies the model, so that the family contains only one member and the probability of any possible outcome can be calculated. Otherwise, it is "composite." Two examples will follow.

A simple null hypothesis would be that the observations have a normal distribution, with mean $\mu = 0$ and variance $\sigma^2 = 1$. A composite alternative could be that $\mu > 0$ and $\sigma^2 = 1$.

A composite null hypothesis would be that the observations have a normal distribution, with $\mu = 0$ and unknown σ^2. A composite alternative could be that $\mu \neq 0$ with unknown σ^2.

2.1.1 Simple alternative hypothesis. For any value, α, with $0 < \alpha < 1$, let $\mathcal{Y}_\alpha$ be the corresponding set of possible observations which are taken to contradict H_0 at the "significance level" α. Then, $\mathcal{Y}_\alpha$ is called a "critical region" of size α. A significance test is defined by a set of such regions such that

- $\mathcal{Y}_{\alpha 1} \subset \mathcal{Y}_{\alpha 2}$ if $\alpha_1 < \alpha_2$
- $\Pr(\mathbf{Y} \in \mathcal{Y}_\alpha; H_0) = \alpha$ for all α
- the significance level of observation, y, is $p_y = \min(\alpha; y \in \mathcal{Y}_\alpha)$

Up to this point, the approach is just a reformulation of the Fisherian significance test of the previous section, with the same reduction in information. Thus, the P-value of that approach is now called the significance level.

However, since $\mathcal{Y}_\alpha$ may not be unique, some criteria are now required, based on the long run principle, for choosing it appropriately. First, look at the simplest case, where null and alternative hypotheses are both simple. In other words, compare two completely specified models.

Consider the probability, called the "power" (see below for further discussion), that an observation is in the critical region under the alternative hypothesis; that is, when the null hypothesis is false. Now, suppose that more than one possible critical region, $\mathcal{Y}^*_\alpha$, of size α exists. If

$$\Pr(\mathbf{Y} \in \mathcal{Y}_\alpha; H_A) > \Pr(\mathbf{Y} \in \mathcal{Y}^*_\alpha; H_A)$$

for all $\mathcal{Y}^*_\alpha \neq \mathcal{Y}_\alpha$

the critical region, $\mathcal{Y}_\alpha$ is called the "best critical region" of size α.

For the comparison of the two hypotheses, all of the information in the data is contained in the likelihood ratio comparing the two hypotheses:

$$\text{LR}(H_A, H_0; \mathbf{y}) = \frac{\text{L}(H_A; \mathbf{y})}{\text{L}(H_0; \mathbf{y})}$$

The larger is the ratio, the more evidence there is in the data against H_0. Since the two models are fixed, $\text{LR}(H_A, H_0; \mathbf{Y})$ is a test statistic, calculable from the data, with a probability distribution, so that there exists some unique value, c_α (which is what is traditionally looked up in the appropriate table for Chi-square, t, or F-tests), such that

$$\Pr(\text{LR}(H_A, H_0; \mathbf{Y}) \geqslant c_\alpha; H_0) = \alpha$$

The region defined by values LR(H_A, H_0; Y) $\geqslant c_\alpha$ is the size α "likelihood ratio critical region." According to the "Neyman–Pearson fundamental lemma," for any given size α, this is the best critical region. Two examples will follow.

First, consider a normal distribution with known variance, where two values of the mean are to be compared, such that $\mu_A > \mu_0$. The deviance is

$$D = \frac{(\mu_A^2 - \mu_0^2) - 2n\bar{y} \cdot (\mu_A - \mu_0)}{\sigma^2}$$

where $\hat{\mu} = \bar{y}.$ is the MLE of the mean. A critical region of the form LR $\geqslant c_\alpha$ is equivalent to one of the form $\bar{y}. \geqslant c_\alpha^*$ for the estimate of the mean.

Now, choose c_α^* to satisfy the size condition that the probability of the likelihood ratio being larger than this constant is α:

$$c_\alpha^* = \mu_0 + \frac{k_\alpha \sigma}{\sqrt{n}}$$

where k_α can be obtained from the appropriate software or table for the normal distribution. This does not depend on the value of μ_A chosen as alternative.

Second, and more generally, it can be shown that such tests exist for models based on what is known as the exponential family of distributions. This is important, since this family includes such models as logistic and log linear regression for discrete data, as well as certain duration or survival distributions for event histories, in addition to all normal theory models like that just given.

For discrete distributions, critical regions only change by discrete steps, so that it will usually be impossible to find a region with exactly a given size α. Consider a Poisson distribution, with the hypotheses, $\mu_0 = 1$ and $\mu_A = 10$.
The deviance for one observation is

$$D = 2(\mu_A - \mu_0) - 2y[\log(\mu_A) - \log(\mu_0)]$$

with possible critical regions

c_α^*	$\alpha = \text{Pr}(Y \geqslant c_\alpha^*; H_0)$
0	1.0000
1	0.6321
2	0.2642
3	0.0803
4	0.0190
5	0.0037
6	0.0006
7	0.0001
:	:
:	:

In hypothesis testing, the null and the alternative are not treated in the same way. The idea is that H_0 must be clearly specified and is the model of interest; the alternative only serves to indicate directions of departure from the null. Thus, in constructing critical regions, the two models are not treated symmetrically and there is no concern with which fits the observations better!

For the Poisson example, suppose that it is observed that $\Sigma y_i = 35$ for $n = 10$, giving MLE of the mean, $\hat{\mu} = 3.5$. Then, $D = -2 \log(\text{LR}) = 18.82$, indicating preference for μ_0, since it makes the data more probable (the likelihood ratio is less than one).

Under the null hypothesis, the MLE, $\hat{\mu}$, has an asymptotic normal distribution with mean and variance both μ_0. An asymptotic best critical region will be defined by

$$\frac{\hat{\mu} - \mu_0}{\sqrt{\mu_0}} \geqslant k_\alpha$$

where k_α is obtained from the normal distribution, as above, and the left hand side has a value of $(3.5-1)/1 = 2.5$. The probability of observing a value as extreme as this is 0.0062 so that the null hypothesis is rejected. Since the only alternative in the present situation is $\mu_A = 10$, this would imply accepting the latter, which goes against the evidence.

Similar examples can easily be constructed with the mean of a normal distribution. In all such cases, if the null and alternative hypotheses are interchanged, the new null is also rejected, even more strongly, however now being in agreement with the result obtained from examining the likelihood ratio.

2.1.2 Power. As has been seen, the probability, Pr($Y \in \mathcal{Y}_\alpha$; H_A), that the observations fall in the critical region if the (simple) alternative hypothesis is true (and, hence, the null hypothesis false), is called the power of the test against that alternative. Power is used to choose among possible tests, before the observations are made, one with higher power being preferred. Generally, a test with fewer degrees of freedom will have higher power.

The size, α, is sometimes known as the probability of Type I error since it is the long run frequency of rejecting the null hypothesis when it is true. One minus the power is sometimes known as the probability of Type II error since it is the long run frequency of "accepting" the null hypothesis when it is false. However, these terms are disappearing from statistical usage, both because of the loss of information the reduction to one fixed α level implies and because of the implication that either the null or alternative hypothesis must be accepted.

Instead, the power, taken as a function of possible hypotheses, can be examined. This is called the "power function"

$$\text{pow}(\,\psi_A\,;\,\mathcal{Y}_\alpha) = \text{Pr}(\mathbf{Y} \in \mathcal{Y}_\alpha;\,\psi_A\,)$$

Note that $\text{pow}(\psi_0;\,\mathcal{Y}_\alpha) = \alpha$.

2.1.3 Composite alternative hypothesis. The usual situation is that there is a collection of alternative hypotheses. Thus, evidence is required against all of that collection, something that may be difficult both to define and to attain.

One simple case can be handled immediately. If the same size α best critical region is obtained for all of these alternatives, the results of the previous section still apply. The test is called "uniformly most powerful" (UMP).

For example, for the one parameter exponential family, mentioned above, tests based on

$$t \geqslant c_\alpha^*$$

if $\psi_A > \psi_0$, where t is the appropriate test statistic, are UMP. On the other hand, if alternatives in both directions from the null hypothesis are of interest, no UMP test can exist.

If no UMP test exists, some rather arbitrary further criterion is needed to make the choice among possible tests. For example, it is possible

(a) to choose one of the H_A as "typical" and use the most powerful test for that alternative;

(b) to maximize the power locally, by taking H_A close to H_0;

(c) to maximize some weighted average of power for the different alternatives.

One solution is mathematically attractive and widely used, but statistically unsatisfactory: a critical region of size α is said to be *unbiased* if the power under all alternatives is greater than the size of the test. Then, among the unbiased regions, that one with the greatest power would be chosen. Otherwise, the test is said to be biased. This has the drawbacks that biased tests may nevertheless, be preferable for most alternatives, and that it does not take into account the direction of departure, so that evidence that $\psi > \psi_0$ could be used to conclude that $\psi < \psi_0$.

A more satisfactory, solution is to admit that two tests are really required, one for each direction, each with its own power function. Each region is usually taken to have size, $\frac{1}{2}\alpha$. This is called a "two-tailed test."

2.2 Composite Null Hypothesis

In all but very simple problems, the null hypothesis is composite. Three common cases are:

(a) a single parametric family of models, with a null hypothesis that the parameters take some subset of all possible values, the alternative being the others;

(b) a single parametric family of models, but where there are two types of parameters, those of interest, say, λ, and others which must be in the model, but are not studied in detail, say φ; the latter are called nuisance parameters;

(c) two different parametric families of models which are to be compared, one being the null hypothesis.

Here, only the most common case, the second, is considered.

In order to test that the mean is μ_0 in a normal distribution with unknown variance, the nuisance parameter, one approach would be to fix the nuisance parameter at some value, and then test the null hypothesis as previously. The significance level so obtained will change according to the fixed nuisance parameter value chosen. If the level does not vary very much in this way, the appropriate conclusion can be drawn about the null hypothesis. The drawback of this method is that the nuisance parameter is being allowed to take any possible value, when, in fact, there is unused information about it.

A second approach is to make the test at the MLE of the nuisance parameter. This, now, has the opposite effect, of assuming that the value of the nuisance parameter is known exactly. It will lead to the true significance level exceeding the size α when the null hypothesis is true.

2.2.1 Similar regions. Consider only one way of resolving the problem, that most commonly used. In this approach, what is sought is that

$$\text{Pr}(\mathbf{Y} \in \mathcal{Y}_\alpha;\,\lambda_0,\,\varphi) = \alpha \qquad \text{for all } \varphi$$

A region satisfying this criterion is called a "similar region" of size α, with the corresponding "similar test."

The general procedure is to condition on what is called a sufficient statistic for φ, so that the resulting conditional distribution will not depend on φ when H_0 is true. A sufficient statistic is a summary of the data which contains all of the information in it about the parameter. For any particular simple alternative, apply the Neyman–Pearson lemma to the conditional distribution to obtain the best critical region of size α. If this applies to all possible alternatives a "uniformly most powerful similar" (UMPS) region is obtained. Three examples will follow.

First, consider n observations from a normal distribution with unknown mean and variance, where μ is the parameter of interest. For fixed $\mu = \mu_0$, the sufficient statistic for σ^2 is $S = \Sigma(Y_i - \mu_0)^2$. The conditional distribution, given the observed value, s, is a Student t-distribution. The "Student t-statistic" is

$$t = \frac{(\bar{y}. - \mu_0)\sqrt{n(n-1)}}{\sqrt{\Sigma(y_i - \bar{y}.)^2}}$$

If the alternative is $\mu > \mu_0$, the critical region will be given by sufficiently large values of t, i.e.

$$\frac{t}{\sqrt{t^2 + n - 1}} \geqslant c_\alpha$$

which yields a UMPS test. In more complex situations, this Student t-test is applied to differences between means and to linear regression coefficients, all in the context of normal distributions models with nuisance parameter the unknown variance.

Second, consider n independent binary observations, Y_i, having possible values zero and one, each with corresponding fixed and known explanatory value, x_i. In a logistic regression, the sufficient statistics are $\mathbf{T} = (\Sigma\ Y_i, \Sigma\ x_i Y_i)$.

Let β_1 be the parameter of interest, with null value β_{10}. For this fixed value, t_0, the total number of ones, is sufficient for β_0 and the conditional probability is

$$\text{PR}\ (t_1 \mid t_0; \beta_1) = \frac{c(t_0, t_1)\,e^{\beta_1 t_1}}{\Sigma_u\ c(t_0, u)\,e^{\beta_1 u}}$$

where $c(t_0, t_1)$ is a complex function to be calculated. From this, Fisher's exact test, given above, can be derived. As in the previous example, if the alternative to β_{10} is $\beta_1 > \beta_{10}$, the UMPS test is obtained by summing the upper tail probabilities.

Third, consider two independent observations from Poisson distributions with means μ_i, where $\mu_1 = \lambda\mu_2$ and use the parameters, λ and $\varphi = \mu_2$, so that the joint distribution is

$$f(y_1, y_2; \lambda, \varphi) = \frac{e^{-\varphi(1+\lambda)}\varphi^{y_1 + y_2}\lambda^{y_1}}{y_1!\ y_2!}$$

For fixed $\lambda = \lambda_0$, the sufficient statistic for φ is $T_2 = Y_1 + Y_2$. Since this has a Poisson distribution with mean $\mu_1 + \mu_2 = \varphi(1 + \lambda)$, the conditional distribution is

$$f(y_1, y_2 \mid t_2; \lambda, \varphi) = \binom{t_2}{y_1}\frac{\lambda^{y_1}}{(1 + \lambda)^{t_2}}$$

a binomial distribution. If the alternative to λ_0 is $\lambda > \lambda_0$, the UMPS test rejects H_0 for large y_1, with a significance level obtained by summing the conditional distribution, at λ_0, over values of y_1 greater than or equal to that observed, for fixed total, t_2.

2.2.2 Likelihood ratio tests. The Neyman Pearson lemma can be extended in cases where similar regions are not available. The likelihood function can be maximized under the null and alternative hypotheses:

$$R = \frac{\max_{\psi_0} L(\psi; y)}{\max_\psi L(\psi; y)}$$

Small values are significant. When this quantity is transformed by taking minus two times its logarithm, the resulting "deviance" has an asymptotic Chi-squared distribution. Now, large values are significant. However, the optimum properties of likelihood ratios for simple hypotheses, in general, no longer apply.

3. Bayesian Tests

A third approach to statistical inference takes yet another tack. Since all information from the data is contained in the likelihood function, Bayesian statisticians hold, as a first principle, that identical likelihood functions must give the same inference. They then consider the parameters to have a probability distribution, whereas, up until now, only the data did. This distribution, before making the observations, will be based on prior knowledge and/or belief. The data are used to update it to give a posterior distribution, using Bayes' formula (see Berger and Wolpert 1988).

Most Bayesians affirm that classical significance tests necessarily give misleading or wrong answers (see Shafer 1982), because they violate the likelihood principle by using not only the observed but also less probable (unobserved) data. However, some admit that they must be accepted simply because they are so widely used.

Suppose that the "prior distribution" for the parameter is $p(\psi)$. This is combined with the likelihood function to give the required "posterior distribution":

$$p(\psi \mid y) \propto L(\psi; y)p(\psi)$$

It can be seen that the likelihood function is being weighted by the prior information. In contrast to the previous approaches, this gives a probability statement about the parameters, not just about the data.

If two simple hypotheses are to be compared, a posterior odds ratio is obtained:

$$\frac{p(\psi_A \mid y)}{p(\psi_0 \mid y)} = \frac{L(\psi_A; y)}{L(\psi_0; y)} \times \frac{p(\psi_A)}{p(\psi_0)}$$

If this is sufficiently large, the null hypothesis will be rejected.

When the hypotheses are composite, the functions must be integrated over the relevant set of parameters. Although this is simple in principle, it rapidly becomes mathematically intractable in all but very special cases. Thus, the Bayesian approach is, formally, very attractive, if it can be accepted that prior information and belief can be formulated mathematically as probability distributions. But, in most practical situations, it is beyond the power of existing computational facilities to perform the required calculations, although rapid progress is currently being made in this area (see *Bayesian Statistics in the Analysis of Data*).

4. Conclusion

Anyone preparing to use significance testing should be wary of pitfalls.

(a) The power of a test should not be overemphasized. Testing for independence between two variables by the hypothesis that the slope of a linear regression is zero may miss a nonlinear form of dependence. Yet it is more powerful than testing that all coefficients of a polynomial regression are zero. Similar examples may be given for testing independence in contingency tables with assumed linear ordering of the categories.

(b) A significant difference does not mean a scientifically important effect. With a sufficiently large sample, the most minute difference can be found significant, but this does not imply that it has any meaning in the field under study (see, e.g., Healy 1990). Likelihood, confidence, or posterior probability "interval estimation" of parameters is more reliable.

(c) Causality is present if dynamically modifying one variable necessarily induces a change in (the distribution of) another variable. If, in a (static) study, the exact reason why the first variable was modified is not known, a causal model can always be constructed, but never tested. An untestable hypothesis that "spurious correlation" is not present must be made. An approach, such as LISREL, attempts to include the interrelationships among as many such variables as possible. This cannot eliminate the problem, since the data are still essentially static. Thus, care must be taken in hypothesis-testing with such models, as Jöreskog (1981) has emphasized. However, this does not imply that causality cannot or should not be studied, only that it is a difficult problem (Cox 1992). Data, statistical and other, must be collected on all aspects of such relationships and combined in any suitable way in order to draw conclusions.

(d) Suppose that people at a number of different sites are testing some hypothesis, which in fact relates to a noneffect. At a 5 percent level, by chance, one institution in 20 will find a significant result —and will publish it!

More space has been given above to the Neyman–Pearson approach, not necessarily because it is superior, but because the school has placed more emphasis on testing and has spent more energy refining its methods. When only the current data are to be used to judge a hypothesis, the Fisherian approach seems preferable. If a series of concrete decisions is to be made on the basis of tests, it is preferable to choose the Neyman–Pearson procedures. If prior information, formulated as probabilities, is available, Bayesian methods will be applied. Thus, in certain circumstances, a test can be selected by objective criteria. However, the final choice of a general approach to significance testing may primarily be a matter of personal philosophical inclination (see Efron 1986 and the ensuing debate).

See also: Simulation as a Research Technique; Variance and Covariance, Analysis of; Bayesian Statistics in the Analysis of Data

References

Berger J O, Wolpert R L 1988 *The Likelihood Principle*, 2nd edn. Institute of Mathematical Statistics, Hayward California

Cox D R 1992 Causality: Some statistical aspects. *Journal of the Royal Statistical Society* A155: 291–301

Cox D R, Hinkley D V 1974 *Theoretical Statistics*. Chapman and Hall, London

Efron B 1986 Why isn't everyone a Bayesian? *American Statistician* 40: 1–11, 330–31

Fisher R A 1954 *Statistical Methods for Research Workers*, 12th edn. Oliver and Boyd, Edinburgh

Healy M J R 1990 Measuring importance. *Statistics in Medicine* 9(6): 633–37

Hoem J M 1985 Weighting, misclassification, and other issues in the analysis of survey samples of life histories. In: Heckmann J J, Singer B (eds.) 1985 *Longitudinal Analysis of Labour Market Data*. Cambridge University Press, Cambridge

Holt D, Smith T M F, Winter P D 1980 Regression analysis of data from complex surveys. *Journal of the Royal Statistical Society* A143: 474–87

Jöreskog K G 1981 Analysis of covariance structures. *Scandinavian Journal of Statistics* 8: 65–92

Lindsey J K 1996 *Parametric Statistical Inference*. Oxford University Press, Oxford

Shafer G 1982 Lindley paradox. *Journal of the American Statistical Association* 77(378): 325–51

Smallest Space Analysis

S. Shye

Smallest space analysis (SSA) is a multivariate data analytic technique which represents geometrically pairwise similarities existing within a set of observed items. For example, the items may be observed variables and the similarities may be the correlation coefficients computed between them. As such, SSA belongs to the class of paired comparisons techniques, including factor analysis (see *Factor Annalysis*), which, in a sense, constitutes a special case of SSA and is, historically, its ancestor. The term "smallest space analysis" (SSA) was coined by Guttman (1968) to indicate that a solution of smallest dimensionality to the geometrical representation problem is sought. When the given information about the pairwise similarities is treated as nonmetric, that is, only the relative degrees of similarity are represented, the dimensionality attained can be smaller than would otherwise be the case. Guttman (1968) presented computational procedures (algorithms) for solving a family of SSA problems within a unified mathematical formulation. These procedures have been computer programmed, originally by Lingoes (1973). Smallest space analysis, then, often refers to any of these programs (most often SSA-I and its modifications).

Along with similar procedures, such as Kruskal's (1964a, 1964b) multidimensional scaling and M-D-SCAL computer program, SSA is sometimes referred to as a multidimensional scaling (MDS) technique. Indeed, whenever some correlation coefficient (calculated on a population of individuals) is used as the similarity criterion between observed variables, a central issue of these techniques is that of ranking or scaling the individuals (see *Partial Order Scalogram Analysis of Nonmetric Data; Scaling Method*). The scaling is done with respect to a number of derived variables (factors) and hence is multidimensional. But it is anticipated that these derived variables will be fewer (and have more fundamental meanings) than the original set of observed variables. "Multiple Scaling," the study of relationships between the SSA of the variables on the one hand and the space in which individuals are scaled on the other, is of theoretical and practical importance (Shye 1985b; see *Partial Order Scalogram Analysis of Nonmetric Data*).

The full power of SSA is in formulating and testing theories, especially in complex (multivariate) systems typical of the behavioral sciences. In the application of SSA to theory construction, the variables to be mapped by SSA are selected so as to represent one general concept, or "content universe," definitionally equivalent to the set of variables that measure it. Typically, that set is infinitely large so that the observed variables constitute but a sample from the content universe. The insight that enabled SSA's application to theory construction may be coined by the following "continuity principle" (Shye 1972, 1978b; Shye et al. 1994):

> In the spatial representation of a content universe, not only every (actually) observed variable from that content universe is mapped into a point, but every point represents a (potentially) observable variable from that content universe (Shye 1972, Shye et al. 1994).

With the continuity principle, SSA is often referred to as Faceted SSA (FSSA) (Shye 1991). Faceted SSA suggests a strategy for theory construction, one that hinges on identifying correspondences between conceptual constructs—content subuniverses—and subregions in the representation space. Common patterns of space partitioning into regions are: axial (generalized simplex), angular (circumplex), and radial (radex). These patterns give rise to testable regional hypotheses whose confirmation has implications for scientific lawfulness and for scaling individuals (see *Facet Theory*). Faceted SSA computer program (Shye 1991) provides optimal partitioning of SSA solution by facets (content–classifications) supplied by the researcher.

1. Representation of Similarity Data by SSA

Suppose A, B, C, ... are objects such as variables, people, social groups, ideas, or countries. And suppose that for each pair of objects there are empirical data about how similar (or dissimilar) the pair is. The similarity may be expressed in the form of correlation coefficients, preference indicators, conditional probabilities, panel judgment scores, or any other quantified measure. It is desirable to represent these data in a geometrical space in such a way that each object is represented by a point in that space, and the empirical similarity within each pair of objects is represented by the geometrical proximity of their respective points: the more similar two objects are, the closer the points representing them in the geometrical space (see *Cluster Analysis*). It is sought to attain such a representation simultaneously for all object pairs, within a space whose dimensionality is the smallest possible. In practice, however, the problem is this: given a particular dimensionality m, (m = 1, 2, 3, etc.) what distribution of the points (each representing an object) in an m-dimensional space would best fit the similarity data?

A solution to this complex problem requires, first, its mathematical formulation, specifying the loss function to be minimized; the treatment of ties in the similarity data; and the distance function to be used in the geometrical space. Following contributions by Guttman and by Shepard (1962) a solution was found by Kruskal (1964a, 1964b) and in a rather general way by Guttman (1968) who proposed loss functions (Kruskal's stress or Guttman–Lingoes' alienation coefficient) and computational procedures were developed for solving the problem.

1.1 The Essential Idea: An Illustration

Suppose the pairwise similarities between three objects, A, B, and C have been found to be as shown in Table 1. A, B, and C could be, for example, three different schools and similarity could be assessed and scored (e.g., with respect to their educational philosophies) by a panel of judges.

An empirical procedure for scoring the degrees of similarity between objects might produce the numerical scores shown in Table 1, which are commonly written in a matrix form, as shown in Table 2.

Table 1
Pairwise similarities between three objects, A, B, and C

Object pairs	Similarity	Possible similarity score range (0-100)
A and B	Not similar	5
A and C	Very similar	85
B and C	Somewhat similar	30

Table 2
Matrix form of degrees of similarity between objects from numerical scores given in Table 1

	A	B	C
A	100	05	85
B	05	100	30
C	85	30	100

The essential information used in SSA is simply the ranking of similarities: thus the similarity scores 85, 30, and 5 are ranked 1, 2, and 3 respectively. Ignoring the diagonal values, the matrix of similarity ranks between A, B, and C is shown in Table 3. This matrix is the effective input of the SSA algorithm in its common versions, SSA-I and FSSA, for symmetric matrices.

In a two-dimensional Euclidean space with the familiar Euclidean distance function, A, B, and C can be easily mapped so that the similarity between any two of them is reflected by their proximity in the space, as shown in Fig. 1. The largest distance, between A and B, represents the fact that they are the least similar pair; B and C, being somewhat similar, are a little closer in the diagram; and the most similar pair, A and C, are the closest in the diagram. Thus, the rank order of the pairwise similarities is correctly represented by the (inverse) rank order of the representative pairwise distances. That this could be done on the flat page means that a two-dimensional space two is sufficient. But is it necessary? Could one-dimensional space

Table 3
Matrix of similarity ranks between A, B, and C from Table 2 data

	A	B	C
A	–		
B	3	–	
C	1	2	–

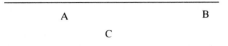

Figure 1
A two-dimensional mapping representing similarity relationships between the three objects

suffice? As Fig. 2 shows, the three objects can be placed on a straight line (a Euclidean, one-dimensional space) and yet all relative similarities are still correctly represented. This is, indeed, a solution of smallest dimensionality for the given similarity matrix.

In the above simple illustration it was easy to find a perfect geometrical representation for the matrix since it contained only three similarity coefficients. But in general, the task of constructing a geometrical representation of a similarity matrix becomes increasingly more difficult when the number of objects, n, increases. Then the number $n(n-1)/2$, of coefficients to be ranked and represented by ranked distances, is much larger (e.g., if n = 10, it is 45; if n = 50, it is 1,225). Hence the need for computer programs.

In general, the larger the number of objects, n, the larger the dimensionality required for a perfectly faithful representation. But a dimensionality m = n−2 (the number of objects minus 2) will always suffice (provided the untying in the output of ties in the input is permitted). Often, however, empirical interdependencies among objects (schools, variables, etc.) produce a pattern of similarities that can be represented fairly faithfully within a space of much lower dimensionality, thus facilitating a parsimonious interpretation of the space, linking it with predefined research contents and, ultimately, theories.

2. Versions of SSA

Versions of SSA differ both with regard to the kind of input they take (i.e., the matrix to be analyzed) and with regard to the specifications of the analysis itself (the treatment of tied values in the similarity matrix, and the choice of distance function for representing the similarity data). Some of the possibilities are reviewed briefly here.

2.1 Input Matrix

The similarity (or dissimilarity) matrix can be symmet-

A   C   B

Figure 2
A one-dimensional mapping representing similarity relationships between the three objects

ric, corresponding to the situation where the similarity of A to B (A and B being any two of the analyzed objects) is by definition equal to the similarity of B to A. Examples of symmetrical similarity relations include: product–moment correlation coefficients between two variables; judgmental scores directly assessing the (symmetrical) similarity of two objects, A and B. This is the case illustrated above, where in fact only half of the (off-diagonal) matrix entries are considered. This is the most popular version nowadays and is often referred to as SSA-I, the name given to the corresponding computer program in the Guttman–Lingoes series (Lingoes 1973).

Often, however, similarity is neither defined nor observed as a symmetrical relation: The similarity of A to B may differ from that of B to A. (Recall that similarity in this entry is a generic, umbrella concept for any relation that connotes affinity of any kind and that needs to be defined and quantified in any particular application.) Examples of asymmetrical relations are: conditional probabilities or conditional relative frequencies (probability of A given B does not equal probability of B given A; or, if A and B are social groups, say, the rich and the smart, respectively, then the relative frequency of A in B is not that of B in A); preference of association (if A and B are students, the extent to which A prefers to associate with B does not necessarily equal the extent to which B prefers to associate with A). Such data sets can be analyzed by SSA with the interpoint distances reflecting similarities based on either the matrix columns or the matrix rows. In the above illustration these choices would correspond to the ranking by active preference (preferring) vs. ranking by passive preference (being preferred). This version of SSA, too, has a corresponding computer program, SSA-II.

For further varieties of input matrices there are further versions of SSA including SSAR for analyzing rectangular matrices and others (Lingoes 1973).

2.2 Treatment of Ties

In SSA the mapping of objects into a geometrical space is done subject to (or accommodating as best as possible) the condition that the greater the similarity between two objects the smaller the distance between their point-images in the space.

In symbols, this condition for SSA-I is:

if $v_{ij} < v_{kl}$ then $d_{ij} > d_{kl}$

where v_{ij} and v_{kl} are the coefficients of similarity between objects (e.g., variables) i and j, and between objects k and l, respectively, as provided by the empirical data. d_{ij} and d_{kl} are the distances in the geometrical space between the points representing objects i, j and objects k, l respectively. This condition, however, does not specify what representation should be attempted if $v_{ij} = v_{kl}$. Two main possibilities may be considered:

(a) The first is to insist on representing equal similarities by equal distances, that is, if $v_{ij} = v_{kl}$, then d_{ij}

$= d_{jk}$. That is, equality in similarity coefficients is represented by equality in distance relations. In conjunction with the first condition stated above, this is the strong monotonicity condition. The strong monotonicity condition is appropriate when importance is attributed to the equality in similarities as such, and hence it is desirable to preserve the information about equality in the spatial representation. This is the case in the lattice space analysis (LSA) version which emphasizes structural aspects of the data and association with the individual profile space (see *Partial Order Scalogram Analysis of Nonmetric Data*).

(b) The second possibility is to allow equality in similarity coefficients to be represented freely with any of the two distances being larger than the other ("untying of ties"). Solutions of SSA based on this weaker condition of so-called semistrong monotonicity could be of lower dimensionality which is consistent with the general aim of the analysis. Indeed, this semistrong monotonicity condition is the choice made in the most current applications of the SSA program series.

2.3 Distance Functions

A variety of distance functions that may be used in SSA include Minkowsky, Euclidean, or other and even semimetrics (functions that do not obey the triangle inequality); the exact functional form for the common SSA versions is given in Guttman's (1968) original paper. So far, however, the familiar Euclidean distance function has been the most widely used.

A further version of SSA, the lattice space analysis (LSA), has been proposed (Shye 1976, 1985b) in which the lattice ("city block") distance function is employed. This version seems appropriate when the concern is with structural issues such as the connection between SSA and partial order scalograms for scaling the individual subjects.

3. Comparison with Other Techniques

Several writers have reviewed multidimensional scaling (MDS) techniques. Carroll and Arabie (1980), taking Coombs (1964) *Theory of Data* as a point of departure, have developed a general taxonomy for the numerous MDS models and methods advanced in recent years. Others compare MDS computational procedures for their technical merits (e.g., Lingoes and Roskam 1973). Here only a brief comparison of SSA with the more traditional technique, factor analysis, will be made, based on Guttman (1982).

Both SSA and factor analysis are used to represent correlation matrices in a geometrical space for the purpose of formulating the essential concepts (dimensions) of the contents sampled by the observed variables. Both represent each variable as a point and vary the distances d_{ij} between the points inversely with the correlation variables i, j. In factor analysis, as in SSA-III output, the points are the termini of vectors extending from a common origin and the distances are the scalar products of these vectors. In that, SSA-III is the SSA version closest to factor analysis.

However, in factor analysis, the distances are related to correlations by an exact function, and if the vectors are all corrected to be of unit length, that inverse relation is $d_{ij} = \sqrt{2(1 - r_{ij})}$. In SSA, distances can be related to correlations by any monotone decreasing function. The exact relation is determined by the data and is provided in the SSA programs by a graphical plot ("Shepard diagram"). This a priori restriction to a particular function in factor analysis constitutes a strong constraint in the analysis and in this sense factor analysis is a specialized case of SSA. The result is that for a given set of data the dimensionality of the SSA solution cannot be larger, and often is smaller than that of the factor analytic solution (see Schlesinger and Guttman 1969 for an empirical example). A dramatic parsimony is achieved by SSA, for example, in the case of the simplex, a one-dimensional configuration in SSA, which, in factor analysis, may require n−1 factors (n = number of variables).

Another important difference is that factor analysis requires the r_{ij} to be product–moment coefficients. This is because it uses regression analysis for relating the individual factor scores to their variable scores. In this exercise, however, the analysis suffers from the indeterminacy of the relation of the desired score space to the calculated space for the variables. For a review of the indeterminacy problem see Steiger and Schonemann (1978).

In SSA, any real numbers, interpretable as similarity coefficients, can be used for r_{ij}. The space of individuals is left to be treated in its own right according to any relevant theoretical or technical consideration. This, of course, does not preclude attempts to relate the two spaces mathematically or substantively (see below).

SSA-I with the Euclidean distance function is further contrasted with factor analysis by its coordinate-free representation which is conducive to the discovery of patterns of regional contiguity, for example, simplex, circumplex, radex (Shye 1978c, 1988).

4. Relating the Space of Variables to the Space of Individual Profiles

Since SSA is concerned directly with similarity among objects (which could, as a specialized case, be correlation among variables) it is not based on, nor does it assume, the existence of individuals' scores. Nevertheless, in cases where SSA is carried out with reference to some statistical coefficient computed on a population of individuals, it is of interest to characterize relationships between structural and interpretational features of the SSA space of the variables, on the one hand, and the associated space of the individuals' space (ordering them by their score profiles), on the other. In relating the two spaces there are a number of specifications that need to be made concerning the principles of structuring the two spaces: the exact nature of the statistical coefficients to be employed (whether product moment or any other); the version of SSA employed; the technique for ordering individuals; and so on. Mathematical results on this question have been obtained by Shye (1976, 1985b, Shye and Amar 1985) with reference to partial order scalograms of individuals' scores (a multidimensional generalization of the unidimensional Guttman scale) and a special version of SSA, lattice space analysis, LSA (see *Partial Order Scalogram Analysis of Nonmetric Data*).

5. Uses of SSA for Theory Construction

Beyond being a mere device for visually displaying the multiple similarity relationships among objects, SSA can help in exploratory and confirmatory studies and aid in theory construction. Several examples from reported research illustrate that the utility of SSA hinges on the identification of reliable correspondences between clearly defined objects and interobject similarities, on the one hand, and patterns of partitioning the SSA space into regions, on the other hand.

5.1 Uses of SSA: Some Examples

5.1.1 Sociogram of a community elite. Some 50 members of a community elite of a small city in Germany played the role of objects in an SSA carried out by Laumann and Pappi (1973). In one of the analyses, reproduced in Fig. 3, the similarity criterion was interpersonal professional or business contact. It was found that "integrative centrality" of the leaders, as measured by an independent index, corresponded to leaders' proximity to the center of the SSA map (in facet theoretic terms: integrative centrality constituted a radial facet); and that leaders' institutional sector (education, economic, religious, or science sector) corresponded to circularly ordered sections in the SSA map (i.e., "institutional sectors" constituted an angular facet). The resulting business/professional network helped structure the community influence system and contributed to the theory of community decision-making.

That interest or professional sectors are circularly ordered in SSA has also been found in a sociogram of experts, mapped by the proximity of their values (Shye 1982).

Sociograms based on SSA have also been used to depict the structure of social relations in school classes.

5.1.2 Testing a hypothesis on the structure of achievement motive. Smallest space analysis was used by

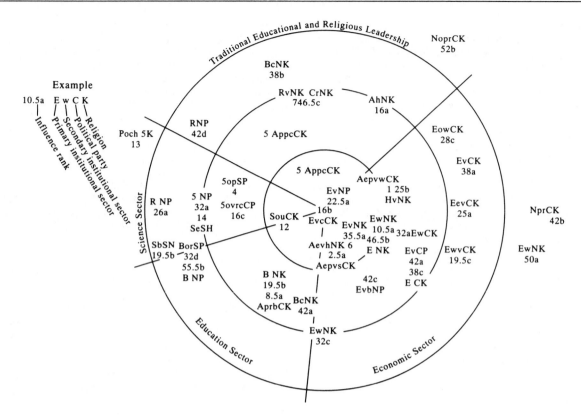

Figure 3
Business/professional network (Guttman–Lingoes coefficient of alienation = 0.148)
Source: Laumann and Pappi (1973)

Shye (1978a) to confirm the hypothesized structure of the concept of achievement motive. On the basis

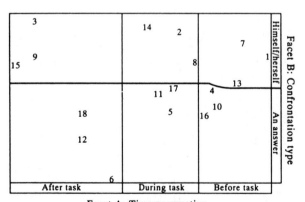

Facet A: Time perspective

Figure 4
The empirical structure of achievement motive depicted as a "duplex" (the product of two axial facets). Space diagram of intercorrelations among 18 variables. Two-dimensional SSA: coefficient of alienation = 0.17

of a content analysis using the facet technique (see *Facet Theory*), the concept of achievement motive was derived. A hypothesis concerning the structure of achievement motive was also formulated. The hypothesis stated how the conceived structure of the concept would be manifested in an empirical SSA in terms of prespecified regions, spatial arrangement of the regions, and the dimensionality of the arrangement. Subsequently, the 18 variables were observed on a sample of executive managers and the intercorrelations among them were taken as the similarity measure for SSA. The resulting SSA (see Fig. 4) confirmed the anticipated structure by exhibiting regions that correspond to the preconceived aspects of achievement motive and arranged these aspects in space according to rationalized criteria. An analogous picture was also obtained in a study of the wider concept of achievement orientation among school children (Shye 1980).

5.1.3 The structure of visual and audio stimuli
Reviewing many studies by himself and others, Shepard (1978) found that when certain sets of stimuli are spatially represented according to the perceived similarity between them, they form a circle (circumplex). This is true, in particular, of colors

differing in hue, and of musical sounds differing in chroma. This is especially noteworthy because from the purely physical point of view the stimuli are linearly ordered by their wavelengths. Hence the observed circularity could well be an instructive indication of the way in which the human mind tends to structure these sets of stimuli.

Circularity can be often regarded as the outcome of two (or more) polarities. This is illustrated in the nonmetric modeling of behavioral systems.

5.1.4 The structure of intelligence. An important contribution of SSA to solving a theoretical problem is its application to the field of intelligence testing theory. Since Alfred Binet (1857–1911) introduced the notion of individual intelligence scores, the need to define intelligence has led to theories about its structure. Among these, Spearman's TFT (two-factor theory) with its general factor ("g") of intelligence, and Thurstone's multiple factor generalization of Spearman's theory are especially noteworthy. By employing SSA (together with an appropriate definition of intelligence items) Schlesinger and Guttman (1969) confirmed the radex as the pattern that best structures intelligence tests, thereby not only identifying factors of intelligence but also depicting meaningful relationships among them, through their spatial arrangement.

In the intelligence radex one partitioning, into concentric rings, corresponds to the nature of the task required by the intelligence item: whether rule-inferring (center), rule-applying (ring around center), or achievement (outer ring). The other partitioning, into circularly ordered wedge-like sectors, is according to the "language," or "material," of the intelligence items: whether figural, numerical, or verbal (see

Fig. 5). Since then, the radex theory of intelligence has been confirmed in many studies (e.g., Snow et al. 1984, Shye 1988), and has been further refined (Guttman and Levy 1991, Klauer and Shye 1991).

5.2 Generalizations for Research and Theory Construction

The above examples as well as numerous applications of SSA in the study of intelligence, attitudes, personality, and social organization, illustrate that SSA focuses on stable aspects of data and hence can assist in scientific research and theory construction. In working with SSA it is useful to identify recurring patterns of regional contiguity and spatial arrangements by labeling them. "Simplex" denotes a linear arrangement of the analyzed objects; in the "circumplex," objects are circularly ordered (see Sect. 5.1.3 above). "Radex" denotes a double partitioning of a two-dimensional SSA space (a) into rings by concentric circles and (b) into sections by radii emanating from the center (see Sect. 5.1.1 above). Duplex is a double partitioning of two-dimensional SSA by two sets of parallel lines (see Sect. 5.1.2). The question of comparing empirical structures, specifically in the context of educational research, is discussed by Shye (1981).

See also: Facet Theory; Partial Order Scalogram Analysis Of Nonmetric Data; Scaling Methods; Multilevel Analysis; Multivariate Analysis; Models of Intelligence

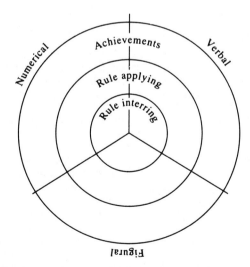

Figure 5
The radex of intelligence (schematic diagram)

References

Carroll J D, Arabie P 1980 Multidimensional scaling. *Annu. Rev. Psychol.* 331: 607–49

Coombs C H 1964 *A Theory of Data.* Wiley, New York

Guttman L 1968 A general nonmetric technique for finding the smallest coordinate space for a configuration of points. *Psychometri.* 33: 469–506

Guttman L 1982 Facet theory, smallest space analysis and factor analysis. *Percept. Mot. Skills.* 54(2): 491–93

Guttman L, Levy S 1991 Two structural laws for intelligence tests. *Intelligence* 15: 79–103

Klauer K J, Shye S 1991 *Formalization of Inductive Reasoning.* Israel Institute for Applied Social Research and Aachem, Jerusalem

Kruskal J B 1964a Multidimensional scaling by optimizing goodness to fit to a nonmetric hypothesis. *Psychometri.* 29: 1–27

Kruskal J B 1964b Nonmetric multidimensional scaling: A numerical method. *Psychometri.* 29: 115–29

Laumann E O, Pappi F U 1973 New directions into the study of community elites. *Am. Sociol. Rev.* 38: 212–30

Lingoes J C 1973 *The Guttman–Lingoes Nonmetric Program Series.* Mathesis, Ann Arbor, Michigan

Lingoes J C, Roskam E E 1973 A mathematical and empirical analysis of two multidimensional scaling algorithms. *Psychometri.* 38(4 Pt. 2): 93

Schlesinger I M, Guttman L 1969 Smallest space analysis of intelligence and achievement tests. *Psych. Bull.* 71: 95–100

Shepard R N 1962 The analysis of proximities: Multidimensional scaling with an unknown distance function (Parts I and II). *Psychometri.* 27: 125–40, 219–46

Shepard R N 1978 The circumplex and related topological manifolds in the study of perception. In: Shye S (ed.) 1978 *Theory Construction and Data Analysis in the Behavioral Sciences.* Jossey-Bass, San Francisco, California

Shye S 1972 *On Mapping Sentences and their Deviation through the Use of SSA.* Israel Institute of Applied Social Research, Jerusalem

Shye S 1976 *Partial Order Scalogram Analysis of Profiles and Relationship to Smallest Space Analysis of the Variables.* Israel Institute of Applied Social Research, Jerusalem

Shye S 1978a Achievement motive: A faceted definition and structural analysis. *Multivariate Behavioral Research* 13(3): 327–46

Shye S 1978b On the search for laws in the behavioral sciences. In: Shye S (ed.) 1978 *Theory Construction and Data Analysis in the Behavioral Sciences.* Jossey-Bass, San Francisco, California

Shye S 1978c Facet analysis and regional hypotheses. In: Shye S (ed.) 1978 *Theory Construction and Data Analysis in the Behavioral Sciences.* Jossey-Bass, San Francisco, California

Shye S 1980 A structural analysis of achievement orientation derived from a longitudinal study of students in Israeli schools. *Am. Educ. Res. J.* 17(3): 281–90

Shye S 1981 Comparing structures of multidimensional scaling (SSA). *Stud. Educ. Eval.* 7(1): 105–09

Shye S 1982 Compiling expert opinion on the impact of environmental quality of a nuclear power plant: An application of a systemic life quality model. *Int. Rev. Appl. Psychol.* 31(2): 285–302

Shye S 1985 *Multiple Scaling: The Theory and Application of Partial Order Scalogram Analysis.* North Holland, Amsterdam

Shye S 1988 Inductive and deductive reasoning: A structural reanalysis of Ability Tests. *J. Appl. Psychol.* 73(2): 308–11

Shye S 1991 Faceted smallest space analysis (FSSA): A computer program for the PC. Israel Institute of Applied Social Research, Jerusalem

Shye S, Amar R 1985 Partial order scalogram analysis by base coordinates and a lattice mapping of the items by their scalogram roles. In: Canter D (ed.) 1985 *Facet Theory Approaches to Social Research.* Springer-Verlag, New York

Shye S et al. 1994 *Introduction to Facet Theory.* Sage, Newbury Park, California

Snow R E et al. 1984 The topography of ability and learning correlations. In: Sternberg R J (ed.) 1984 *Advances in the Psychology of Human Intelligence*, Vol. 2. Erlbaum, Hillsdale, New Jersey

Steiger J H, Schonemann P H 1978 A history of factor indeterminancy. In: Shye S (ed.) 1978 *Theory Construction and Data Analysis in the Behavioral Sciences.* Jossey-Bass, San Francisco, California

Social Network Analysis

A. S. Klovdahl

A social network is a set of nodes connected by relationships of one kind or another. The usefulness of the concept of a network stems from its relevance across a range of social phenomena, its ability to move beyond explanations made solely in terms of characteristics of individuals, and its capacity to link different levels of analysis. Social network analysis provides fruitful concepts and powerful methods (see Coleman 1958, Mitchell, 1969, Barnes 1972). A brief introduction to these ideas is presented here focusing on the concepts employed, graph theory, the inferences drawn and analyses of networks, observation of networks, and the computer programs available for network analysis. In conclusion, some caveats and challenges are discussed.

1. Conceptual Considerations

Early students of sociometric methods helped to lay the foundations of social network analysis, and anyone wishing to study social networks would do well to begin with a review of the sociometric literature (see *Sociometric Methods*). As one example, Moreno (1953 pp. 153–61) provided a series of sociometric diagrams showing same-sex/different-sex contacts among students in Grades K (Kindergarten) to 8. These data can give rise to fruitful hypotheses about the effects of changing gender relationships among adults on patterns of contact among schoolchildren (see Eder and Hallinan 1978). Similarly, the classic work of Coleman (1961) on sociometric networks in high schools remains a worthwhile starting point for anyone studying adolescents in modern society.

The concepts and tools employed to study networks of persons can be used to study networks in which the nodes are other kinds of units (e.g., organizations) but the emphasis here is on networks in which the nodes are persons and the links are social relationships. Even allowing for this restriction the term "social network" has been used in a variety of ways, so additional conceptual distinctions are needed.

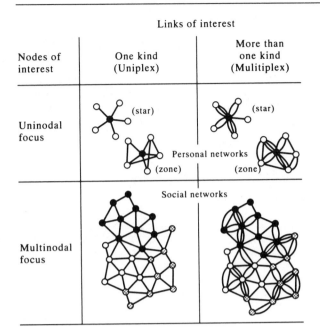

Links of interest

Nodes of interest	One kind (Uniplex)	More than one kind (Mulitiplex)

Uninodal focus

Multinodal focus

Figure 1
The concept of a network

The focus of network research may be on one node (or kind of node) or more than one. Similarly, the focus may be on one type of relationship or more than one. In other words, in any network study, in terms of nodes, the focus may be uninodal or multinodal; in terms of relationships, on uniplex (single-stranded) or on multiplex (multistranded) relationships. When these two basic dimensions are cross-classified a useful categorization of the "objects" of network research results.

Social network studies may examine uniplex relationships or multiplex relationships (column headings in Fig. 1). When studying schoolchildren, for example, the focus may be restricted to friendship relationships. Or, studies may focus on the extent children (or teachers or administrators) are connected by multistranded relationships, for example, as a consequence of living in the same neighborhood, attending the same church, and associating with each other during school (or work) hours.

Similarly, some studies may emphasize single nodes; others, multiple nodes (row labels in Fig. 1). As, by definition, a social network consists of a set of nodes, a uninodal focus means concern with how the network in which an individual is embedded affects the focal individual or is affected by the individual. For example, how much encouragement to study or to smoke reaches an individual from the others (e.g., friends) to whom he or she is directly linked? Does the focal person influence definitions of normative behavior in the network? In contrast, with a multinodal

focus the concern is with the whole set of nodes. For example, is the network as a whole structured into one or two large cliques or into many dyads, triads, or other small clusters? And, of course, what are the consequences of this?

Most network studies observe more than one kind of social relationship, though individual analyses may concentrate on only one kind. In practice, then, network research can often be categorized according to whether the focus is uninodal or multinodal. Put simply, most network research looks at either personal networks or social networks. A personal network consists of a focal individual and the other persons (associates) linked directly to this individual by various kinds of social relationships. The personal networks actually observed may be (first-order) "stars" or (first-order) "zones," depending on whether links among the associates (independent of the focal person) are considered (see Fig. 1). In any population, there are as many personal members as there are members of the population. A social network, in contrast, consists of a whole set of nodes and the social relationships connecting them. Depending on the kinds of nodes and relationships of interest, a large social network may consist of distinguishable regions. Everyone in these regions may be connected together; all of the regions may be connected together. In other words, in any population everyone may be connected together to form a single social network (see Srinivas and Beteille 1964, Barnes 1972).

Sociometric diagrams, sociograms, and other visual representations of networks (e.g., Fig. 1) can be useful for stimulating insights and for making complex ideas more clear (Klovdahl 1981, 1986), but these are most powerful when tied closely to mathematical models. Accordingly, any fruitful foray into social network analysis requires an understanding of some basic mathematical ideas.

2. Graph Theory

At the most elementary level, a social network can be seen as a realization of a " *graph*," or " *digraph*," as conceptualized in mathematical graph theory (Flament 1963, Ore 1963, Harary et al. 1965, Wilson 1979). Simply defined, a graph consists of a finite nonempty set $V = V(G)$ of p nodes together with a set $E(G)$ of q unordered pairs of distinct nodes of V. A digraph (directed graph) consists of a finite non-empty set of nodes together with a set A of ordered pairs of distinct nodes in V. Paired nodes represent links (edges/arcs/lines) between nodes (vertices/points). In a graph the links between nodes are nondirectional; in a digraph they have direction. Visual representations of a social network viewed as a graph and as a digraph are provided (see Fig. 2).

The three basic matrices relevant for describing graphs and digraphs are the adjacency matrix, the

(a) Visual representations

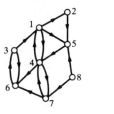

(i) A digraph (D)

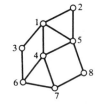

(ii) A graph (G)

(b) Relevant matrices

Adjacency, A(D) =

	1	2	3	4	5	6	7	8
1	0	1	0	1	1	1	0	0
2	0	0	0	0	1	0	0	0
3	1	0	0	0	0	1	0	0
4	1	0	0	0	0	1	1	0
5	0	0	0	1	0	0	0	0
6	0	0	1	0	0	0	0	0
7	0	0	0	1	0	1	0	0
8	0	0	0	0	1	0	1	0

Adjacency, A(G) =

	1	2	3	4	5	6	7	8
1	0	1	1	1	1	0	0	0
2	1	0	0	0	1	0	0	0
3	1	0	0	0	0	1	0	0
4	1	0	0	0	1	1	1	0
5	1	1	0	1	0	0	0	1
6	0	0	1	1	0	0	1	0
7	0	0	0	1	0	1	0	1
8	0	0	0	0	1	0	1	0

Reachability, R(D) =

	1	2	3	4	5	6	7	8
1	1	1	1	1	1	1	1	0
2	1	1	1	1	1	1	1	0
3	1	1	1	1	1	1	1	0
4	1	1	1	1	1	1	1	0
5	1	1	1	1	1	1	1	0
6	1	1	1	1	1	1	1	0
7	1	1	1	1	1	1	1	0
8	1	1	1	1	1	1	1	1

Reachability, R(G) =

	1	2	3	4	5	6	7	8
1	1	1	1	1	1	1	1	1
2	1	1	1	1	1	1	1	1
3	1	1	1	1	1	1	1	1
4	1	1	1	1	1	1	1	1
5	1	1	1	1	1	1	1	1
6	1	1	1	1	1	1	1	1
7	1	1	1	1	1	1	1	1
8	1	1	1	1	1	1	1	1

Distance, N(D) =

	1	2	3	4	5	6	7	8
1	0	1	3	1	1	2	2	∞
2	3	0	4	2	1	3	3	∞
3	1	2	0	2	2	1	3	∞
4	1	2	2	0	2	1	1	∞
5	2	3	3	1	0	2	2	∞
6	2	3	1	3	3	0	4	∞
7	2	3	2	1	3	1	0	∞
8	3	4	3	2	1	2	1	0

Distance, N(G) =

	1	2	3	4	5	6	7	8
1	0	1	1	1	1	2	2	2
2	1	0	2	2	1	3	3	2
3	1	2	0	2	2	1	2	3
4	1	2	2	0	1	1	1	2
5	1	1	2	1	0	2	2	1
6	2	3	1	1	2	0	1	2
7	2	3	2	1	2	1	0	1
8	2	2	3	2	1	2	1	0

Figure 2
A digraph and a graph

reachability matrix and the distance matrix (see Fig. 2). The cell entries (a_{ij}) in an adjacency matrix indicate direct (one-step) links between pairs of nodes. For example, in the digraph shown (Fig. 2) the links between nodes #1 and #4, in both directions, are represented by a *1* in cell 1–4 and a *1* in cell 4–1. The two nodes are *adjacent* ($a_{14}=1$ and $a_{41}=1$) to each other; each is *reachable* from the other in one step. The link from #2 to #5 is represented by a *1* in cell 2–5 and the absence of a (direct, one-step) link from #5 to #2 by a *0* in cell 5–2. For the graph the link between #2 and #5 is represented by a *1* in cell 2–5 and a *1* in cell 5–2, and the absence of a link between #4 and #8 is represented by *zeros* in cells 4–8 and 8–4. The adjacency matrix for a graph is always symmetric; for a digraph it may be symmetric or asymmetric.

The cell entries (r_{ij}) in a reachability matrix indicate whether particular pairs of nodes are connected in any number of steps. For example, in both the digraph and the graph (Fig. 2) nodes #1 and #4 are each reachable from the other, in one step, as evident from the adjacency matrix ($a_{14}=a_{41}=1$) and reflected in the values $r_{14}=r_{41}=1$ in the reachability matrix. However, despite $a_{34}=a_{43}=0$ in both adjacency matrixes, $r_{34}=r_{43}=1$ in each case because, although not connected directly, the two nodes are indirectly connected. In both, #3 can reach #4 in two steps, and vice versa. By convention $r_{ii}=1$—each node is considered reachable from itself.

The cell entries (d_{ij}) in a distance matrix give the number of steps along the shortest path (sequence of connected links) between each pair of nodes (Buckley and Harary 1990). For example, in the digraph (Fig. 2) the shortest path from node #1 to node #3 is 3 steps ($d_{13}=3$); in the graph it is 1 step. In the digraph, the shortest path from #1 and #5 is 1 step; from #5 to #1 it is 2; in the graph, it is 1 in either direction. In the digraph, #8 can reach all other nodes by a path of some length, but none of the other nodes can reach #8—the distance between each and #8 is "infinity" (∞). In both, from #8 to #4 there are two shortest paths, one via #5 and one via #7.

The information in these basic matrixes leads to other relevant concepts, such as connectedness. In a graph or digraph, if each pair of nodes is reachable from the other it is said to be (strongly) connected. Thus, a population represented in graph–theoretic terms would be connected if each individual can *reach* all others. Alternatively it might consist of a number of connected components, with individuals connected within each component but no connections (bridges) between different components.

In theory both graphs and digraphs can be used to represent the structure, in social network terms, of any population. In practice the nature of the observations possible is constraining. For example, some students may experiment with injectable drugs, and in the process share needles with more experienced users. A person who shares needles may shoot *upstream* or *downstream* from someone else, and information about the direction of the link, the direction of the sharing, may be useful for evaluating risks of infection (e.g., with the human immunodeficiency virus, HIV). Ideally, then, this network of experimenting students and experienced drug-users would be represented as a digraph. In reality, it may be difficult to observe the *direction* of needle sharing accurately enough to justify a digraph rather than a graph representation. Thus, it may be necessary to make simplifying assumptions about social relationships, and the social networks connecting individuals in the relevant population(s) represented as graphs.

3. Observation

In order to study networks it is necessary to observe them. Two key issues that arise here concern name generators and designs for observing networks.

3.1 Name Generators

A primary issue in any network research involves deciding the social relationships to be studied and determining how to observe these. In research involving participant observation, a social relationship may be observed directly, or at least a sequence of behaviors taken to indicate a social relationship may be observed. In observation based on questionnaires or interviews more indirect indicators of social relationships must be elicited. For example, a respondent may be asked to name his or her friends. The response, the naming of individuals, is taken to indicate that the specified kind of relationship exists between the respondent and the person(s) named. A number of questions naturally

arise in this context. What does the researcher mean by the term "friend" (or any other concept referring to a social relationship) and is this shared by respondents? What are the relative merits of open-ended name generators as compared to, if available, complete lists of others in the population(s) of interest? What is the relative validity/reliability of different kinds of name generators? These kinds of questions have been addressed in the network literature (see Marsden, 1990) but must be considered in the context of any particular study design.

3.2 Designs for Observing Networks

There are three basic kinds of designs for making observations on networks: nodes designs, sequences designs and populations designs. In a nodes design (Fig. 3), individual nodes are selected independently of each other. In other words, some of the same kinds of designs used to select individuals in traditional social research can be used to select individuals who are nodes in a network. For example, students may be selected randomly from a master list and asked about their links to others. Nodes designs typically are used to study personal networks (as "stars" or "zones"—see Fig. 1). In principle, a nodes design could be used to study social networks (Fig. 1); in practice, the size of the sample required to observe a connected region of a large social network may be too large to be feasible (Klovdahl 1989).

In a sequences design (Fig. 3) an initial node is

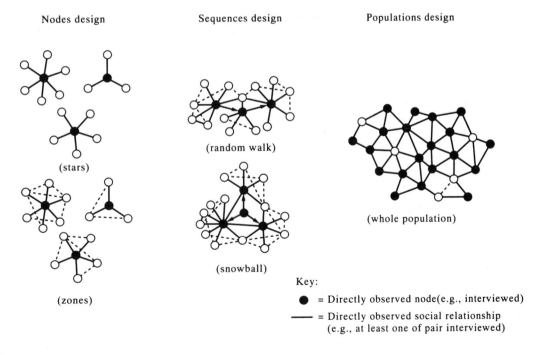

Nodes design   Sequences design   Populations design

(stars)

(zones)

(random walk)

(snowball)

(whole population)

Key:

● = Directly observed node(e.g., interviewed)

── = Directly observed social relationship (e.g., at least one of pair interviewed)

Figure 3
Designs for network observations

selected independently but the selection of the subsequent nodes is from the list provided by a previous (e.g., initial) respondent. The selection of the initial nodes is independent; the selection of sequential nodes is dependent. A snowball sampling design is the classic example of a sequences design (Goodman 1961). A random walk design is another example (Klovdahl 1989). These kinds of designs can make feasible observations of social networks not otherwise possible. For example, snowball designs have been used to obtain information of the social networks of young drug-users, as a basis for developing effective disease prevention programs (e.g., for HIV, hepatitis B). Similarly, random walk designs have been used to determine how urban residents in contemporary cities are connected together to form large social networks (Klovdahl 1989, Liebow 1989).

In a populations design (Fig. 3) an attempt is made to observe all members of a population. Ideally, studies using a populations design focus on more than one population to permit comparison and population (social network) level inference (Stinchcombe 1968). When all, or even most, of the members of a population provide information on their network connections, a vast array of procedures for analysis is available.

4. Inference and Analysis

In network studies, as elsewhere, research design determines possible and legitimate forms of inference and analysis. Accordingly, inference and analysis are most easily considered by reference to the data from different designs for making network observations (Fig. 3).

4.1 Nodes Data

If a nodes design has been used to make network observations, employing one of the probability sampling procedures often found in research on individuals (e.g., simple random sampling, stratified cluster sampling), the tools available for making inferences in traditional social research for inference and analysis are available. For example, network data obtained in this manner can serve as the basis for inferences about the characteristics of the individuals in the network, the number of ties they maintain with others, the kinds of social relationships they have, and so on (Marsden 1987). Similarly, the individuals selected and the associates to whom they are linked may be considered as clusters, and (after correcting for any overlap) the tools for estimation based on cluster sampling used to describe the personal networks of these individuals (Sudman 1978). In addition, tools for making inferences about the pairs or dyads in which individuals are involved can also be employed, for example, using well-known tests for differences between paired individuals. Beyond these, there is

a growing body of tools developed for the purpose of making inferences about characteristics of larger social networks (e.g., density of ties) on the basis of data from randomly selected individual nodes (Frank 1981). And, observations of individual nodes can also serve as the basis for analyzing the role/position structure of the relevant populations (Burt 1980, Marsden 1989). Here, the idea is that the patterns of social ties maintained by individuals (taking into account ties which do not exist as well) are the building blocks from which larger social structures are constructed (Knoke and Kuklinski 1982, Scott 1991). In other words, using this approach it is not seen as necessary to observe connected regions of larger social networks to begin to describe how a population is structured by its pattern of social relationships.

4.2 Sequences Data

When network observations are made with a sequences design the initial nodes, if selected with a probability sampling procedure, can serve as the basis for inferences about individuals and personal networks, as with a nodes design. The precision of the estimates made using data from the initial nodes in a sequences design, in general, depends on the number of initial nodes observed in a particular study. For example, given 300 possible interviews, if a design called for one-step (two-node) sequences, 150 initial nodes would be available for estimation (of characteristics of individuals) purposes ($300 = 150 \times 2$); if two-step (three-node) sequences, 100 would be available; if three-step (four-node) sequences, 75 independently selected initials would be available; and so on. Clearly, more precise estimates of characteristics of individuals in a population would be obtained with designs calling for more, shorter sequences. However, usually a major aim of sequences designs (whether snowball or random walk) is to learn more about connected regions of large social networks, and as longer sequences are more likely to provide this kind of information, sequences designs may permit only rough estimates of characteristics of individuals. Clearly, if the purpose of a study is to estimate characteristics of individuals, this can be done more efficiently using the kinds of sampling designs employed by census organizations.

Although the initial nodes in a sequences design are selected independently of each other, the other nodes are not independently selected, and this has implications for inference and analysis. In essence, the selection is of sequences of linked observations from the population of all possible sequences, not individuals from a population of individuals.

4.2.1 Markov models.
Markov methods provide the simplest and most well-known procedures for making inferences from sequential-dependent data (Kemeny and Snell 1960, Howard 1971, Gottman and Roy 1990). Using Markov models, a number of useful properties of social networks may be estimated, such

as transition probabilities, order of dependency for the model best representing the underlying structure, and so on (Anderson and Goodman 1957). A related problem is to find the most suitable clusterings (or "lumps") of connected individuals (Kemeny and Snell 1960). Flows (e.g., of information, influence, and infectious agents) through a social network can be estimated, for example, using mean first passage times (Beshers and Laumann 1967). The complexity and power of possible models of social structure developed from observed sequences are virtually unlimited, and can provide significant new insights into social phenomena.

4.3 Population Data

When all (or most) individuals in a population, and their network ties, have been observed, many tools are available for analysis. The characteristics that may be examined, ideally in relation to other independent and dependent variables, include characteristics of the individuals in the population(s) studied, of their social relationships, of their personal networks, of the cliques, clustering, or regions in which their personal networks are embedded, and of the large social networks that connect the individuals together. The density of social ties in the network as a whole may be of interest, that is, the total number of social relationships (perhaps of a particular kind) relative to the number possible (see Edwards and Monge 1977), along with the reachability of individuals, as well as the reachability of the network as a whole. Distance may also be of interest—that is, how many individuals can be reached by a focal individual in a particular number of steps, and the average distance between individuals in a large (connected) social network. The centrality of individuals and the extent to which social networks are centralized are important properties as well (Freeman 1978). That is, some individuals in networks occupy positions that put them astride more paths between others, and hence their structural position alone makes it possible to exert control over flows (e.g., information) through a network. In addition, a variety of methods for discovering cliques or clusters in social networks are available, for modeling the role/position structure of populations, in terms of algebraic topology, lattices, and so on (Burt 1980, Knoke and Kuklinski 1982, Scott 1991).

5. Network Analysis Packages

Computer programs/packages are essential for analyses of complex relational data and many relevant computer tools are now available. The most versatile are two major social network analysis packages (for personal computers): GRADAP (Stokman and Sprenger 1989), and UCINET (Borgatti et al. 1992).

GRADAP (graph definition and analysis package) assumes that networks are represented as mathematical graphs (or digraphs) and provides a powerful set of tools for manipulating networks and analyzing them (Stokman and Sprenger 1989). GRADAP (version 2.0) can handle networks of up to 6,000 nodes and 60,000 social relationships. The main strength of GRADAP is its close link to mathematical graph theory. The package includes the data used for illustrative purposes in the manual.

UCINET is an integrated set of procedures for network analysis (Borgatti et al. 1992). Network data may be input in a variety of formats, for example, as adjacency matrixes, or as linked lists. There are a variety of procedures for manipulating data. With UCINET it is possible to calculate various graph/digraph measures (e.g., reachability, density), to compute a number of centrality measures (e.g., degree, betweenness, and Bonacich power), to detect cliques and clans (e.g., n-clique, k-plex), to identify structural equivalence, to carry out multidimensional scaling on network data, and so on. Depending on hardware configuration and specific procedure used, UCINET (version IV) can handle networks from as large as 180 nodes to over 500 nodes. Also provided with the package are a number of network datasets from previous studies and a Monte Carlo procedure for generating random networks. The main strength of UCINET is the diversity of procedures it provides.

These packages are complementary: no single network analysis package is likely to meet every need. Moreover, specialized programs for particular purposes (e.g., for lattice analysis (Duquenne 1992)) can usually be located without great difficulty.

6. Caveats and Challenges

The main caveats when contemplating network research are the possible sensitivity of some of the information that may be sought and the complexity of the resulting data. In some cases—in different cultures, in particular arenas, for some topics—persons readily provide (to bona fide researchers) the nominative data (e.g., names and addresses) usually required to reconstruct the social networks in which they are enmeshed. In other cases, obtaining even data on unnamed individuals in someone's personal network may be difficult. Pretests are essential. In addition, except when relatively small populations are involved, the process of transforming raw data from individuals into network data is likely to be more time-consuming than necessary if not anticipated and planned from the start of a study.

The easiest designs to implement are nodes designs, as information on personal networks can be obtained with little modification to traditional sample survey designs. Populations designs, where feasible, typically provide the greatest range of opportunities for analyses. Sequences designs provide the greatest challenges, as well as enticing opportunities for studying the large social networks that connect individuals in modern societies.

Despite the challenges, social network analysis provides a unique opportunity to move beyond attempts to explain educational and other social phenomena solely in terms of characteristics of individuals; to begin to explore how the patterns of social relationships in which individuals are embedded, and how their locations in the larger interpersonal networks affect them; and how in turn these individuals affect other individuals, the organizations, the communities, and the societies in which they are involved. Some of the earliest studies of social network phenomena were carried out in schools, and one of the most promising areas for future research on social networks is in the sphere of education.

See also: Sociometric Methods

References

Anderson T W, Goodman L A 1957 Statistical inference about Markov Chains. *Annals of Mathematical Statistics* 28: 89–110

Barnes J A 1972 *Social Networks: Module in Anthropology* Addison-Wesley, Reading, Massachusetts

Beshers J M, Laumann E O 1967 Social distance: A network approach. *Am. Sociol. Rev.* 32: 225–36

Borgatti S P, Everett M G, Freeman L C 1992 UCINET IV, Version 1.0. Analytic Technologies, Columbia, South Carolina

Buckley F, Harary F 1990 *Distance in Graphs.* Addison-Wesley, Redwood City, California

Burt R S 1980 Models of network structure. *Ann. Rev. Sociol.* 6: 79–141

Coleman J S 1958 Relations analysis. *Human Organization* 17: 28–36

Coleman J S 1961 *The Adolescent Society: The Social Life of the Teenager and its Impact on Education.* Free Press, New York.

Duquenne V 1992 GLAD: *A Program for Lattice Analysis.* Centre National de la Recherche Scientifique, Paris

Eder D, Hallinan M T 1978 Sex differences in children's friendships. *Am. Sociol. Rev.* 43(2): 237–50

Edwards J A, Monge P R 1977 The validation of mathematical indices of communication structure. In: Ruben B D (ed.) 1977 *Communication Yearbook I.* Transaction Books, New Brunswick, New Jersey

Flament C 1963 *Applications of Graph Theory to Group Structure.* Prentice-Hall, Englewood Cliffs, New Jersey

Frank O 1981 A survey of statistical methods for graph analysis. In: Leinhardt S L (ed.) 1981 *Sociological Methodology.* Jossey-Bass, San Francisco, California

Freeman L C 1978 Centrality in social networks: Conceptual clarification. *Social Networks* 1: 215–39

Goodman L A 1961 Snowball sampling. *Annals of Mathematical Statistics* 32: 148–70

Gottman J M, Roy A K 1990 *Sequential Analysis: A Guide for Behavioral Researchers.* Cambridge University Press, Cambridge

Harary F, Norman R Z, Cartwright D 1965 *Structural Models: An Introduction to the Theory of Directed Graphs.* Wiley, New York

Howard R A 1971 *Dynamic Probabilistic Systems: Vol. I: Markov Models.* Wiley, New York

Kemeny J G, Snell J L 1960 *Finite Markov Chains.* Van Nostrand, Princeton, New Jersey

Klovdahl A S 1981 A note on images of networks. *Social Networks* 3: 197–214

Klovdahl A S 1986 VIEW-NET: A new tool for network analysis. *Social Networks* 8: 313–42

Klovdahl A S 1989 Urban social networks: Some methodological problems and possibilities. In: Kochen M (ed.) 1989 *The Small World.* ABLEX, Norwood, New Jersey

Knoke D, Kuklinski J H 1982 *Network Analysis.* Sage, Beverly Hills, California

Liebow E B 1989 Category or community: Measuring urban Indian social cohesion with network sampling. *Journal of Ethnic Studies* 16(4): 67–100

Marsden P V 1987 Core discussion networks of Americans. *Am. Sociol. Rev.* 52(1): 122–31

Marsden P V 1989 Methods for the characterization of role structures in network analysis. In: Freeman L C, White D R, Romney A K (eds.) 1989 *Research Methods in Social Network Analysis.* George Mason University Press, Fairfax, Virginia

Marsden P V 1990 Network data and measurement. *Annual Review of Sociology* 16: 435–63

Mitchell J C 1969 The concept and use of social networks. In: Mitchell J C (ed.) 1969 *Social Networks in Urban Situations: Analyses of Personal Relationships in Central African Towns.* Manchester University Press, Manchester

Moreno J L 1953 *Who Shall Survive? Foundations of Sociometry, Group Psychotherapy and Sociodrama.* Beacon House Inc., Beacon, New York

Ore O 1963 *Graphs and their Uses.* Random House, New York

Scott J 1991 *Social Network Analysis: A Handbook.* Sage, Newbury Park, California

Srinivas M N, Beteille A 1964 Networks in Indian social structure. *Man* 54: 165–68

Stinchcombe A L 1968 *Constructing Social Theories.* Harcourt, Brace and World, New York

Stokman F N, Sprenger C J A 1989 GRADAP: Graph Definition and Analysis Package. Iec ProGAMMA, Groningen

Sudman S 1978 *Applied Sampling.* Academic Press, New York

Wilson R J 1979 *Introduction to Graph Theory*, 2nd edn. Academic Press, New York

Sociometric Methods

L. J. Saha

Sociometry and sociometric methods are concerned with the study of the ways people interact with one another. Knowledge about how people in groups choose one another for friendship, work, and other activities tells us much about group structures and the ways they change. This knowledge also tells us about the ways that individuals in groups behave, and why. It also provides us with guidelines for the development and implementation of intervention strategies to change group interaction and structures.

The origins and development of sociometry are inextricably linked with educational research. Moreno, the originator of sociometry and the sociometric method, based many of his early observations on studies of student classroom structure and the evolution of groups (Moreno 1934). He clearly documented the structures of groups from kindergarten to the eighth grade. The analysis of group properties is facilitated by the sociometric test which requires an individual to choose his or her associates for any group of which he or she is or might become a member. The individual is expected to make the choices without restraints and is not limited to members of his or her own group. In order to be sociometric, the test must determine, according to specified criteria (e.g., sitting or working together), the feelings of individuals toward each other (attraction or rejection). The representation of these choices in two-dimensional space is known as a "sociogram," which portrays in graphic form the sociometric "stars," the "isolates," the "cliques," and other patterns of group structure.

Virtually no aspect of the educational process has been unexplored by sociometric research, including cognitive development, creativity and innovativeness, school success, and teacher effectiveness. Sociometric measures have also been used to study educational processes at all levels, from kindergarten (Wasik et al. 1993) to university (Guldner and Stone-Winestock 1995).

1. Early and Recent Uses of Sociometric Methods

Both the techniques of designing a sociometric test, as well as the statistical procedures for analyzing the results, have undergone considerable change over the years.

In its original form, the sociometric test was deceptively simple. Northway (1967) suggests that in any test, three or four criteria should be used as the basis for choices, the choices should be limited in number, and the choice questions should be stated in the conditional mood. Hence, the appropriate question

is not "With whom do you associate," but "If all things were possible and you could associate with anyone you liked, with whom would you choose to associate?" Although Northway argued that three criteria and three choices for each individual were desirable, others have contended that an unspecified number of choices is necessary to locate the full range of choice patterns (Lindzey and Byrne 1968). Furthermore, Remer (1995) argues that in its original form envisaged by Moreno, sociometric research included an action orientation and a warming process prior to the choice or rating exercise. Participants in sociometric research would also consider the results of the research and explain them. These elements were integral to Moreno's sociometric research. He calls the original Moreno form "strong sociometry" and the derivatives, which are more common today and which usually focus on the choice or rating process only, "weak sociometry".

There have been many variations on the standard sociometric question. One has been the "self-rating method" whereby the subject predicts by whom he or she will be chosen and how all members of the group will relate to each other through their choices. Other methods include "scaling instruments" which are designed to elicit ratings of members of groups in terms of their capacity to meet certain needs, such as affiliation and recognition. More complex approaches have combined sociometric data with other information to portray the group structure more accurately, while the time spent with individuals on certain tasks and interpersonal attractiveness have also found their way into sociometric tests.

In fact, it has been found that different approaches can produce different sociometric results. Schwarzwald et al. (1986) found that "nomination" and "rating" methods resulted in different patterns of sex and ethnic group cleavages in the classroom. In terms of willingness to participate in activities of low, medium, or high intimacy, junior high school students were asked to identify three classmates most desired as partners for each activity (the nomination approach), and also to rate students in terms of a positive desire for each classmate (the rating approach). The researchers found that the nomination technique produced a heightened picture of sex and ethnic cleavage relative to the rating approach, and also that the former was insensitive to the level of intimacy of the sociometric content.

1.1 Quantitative Methods in Sociometric Analysis

The earliest approach to the quantification and organization of sociometric data was the matrix whereby all choices are recorded and then summed. The names of individuals are listed along the vertical and horizontal axes and the choices are recorded in the cells for each criterion which is being tested. According to Northway (1967) the total number of choices for all criteria provides a social acceptance score or an indication of sociometric status. The actual number of persons choosing the subject gives a social receptiveness score, while the number of individuals chosen by the subject gives a social expansion score. It is also possible to identify groups of individuals for whom choices are or are not reciprocated, as well as the social isolates who neither choose nor are chosen.

Other methods have been applied to sociometric data. Of considerable use has been the probability model which identifies individuals who receive greater or fewer choices than they would ordinarily receive by chance. More complex matrix approaches consist of reordering rows and columns, by trial and error, until the clique structure of the group is located. Likewise, factor analysis has been used to identify and isolate underlying dimensions of group structure (Proctor and Loomis 1951, Lindzey and Byrne 1968, Hallinan 1974).

1.2 Graphic Presentation of Sociometric Data

The sociogram provides a graphic portrayal of sociometric information. It is constructed on the principle that choices between individuals may be symmetric (reciprocated), asymmetric (not reciprocated), or nonexistent. The major limitation of the sociogram is that it cannot deal adequately with large groups. Some researchers have argued, for example, that 20 persons is

the ideal size for sociometric analysis, although more have been used.

In its original form, group members were designated by symbols with lines and arrows to indicate the direction of choice (Moreno 1934 pp. 33–44). Northway (1967) introduced the notion of the "target sociogram" which contained four concentric circles similar to an archery target. Each circle represented four quartiles or the four levels of probability: significantly above chance, above chance, below chance, and significantly below chance—from the center outward. The "stars" were placed in the center circle and the "isolates" in the outside circle. A vertical line through the center of the diagram was used to separate males and females, and the choice levels for each circle were usually indicated below each circle line (Northway 1967, Gronlund 1959).

Recent usage of the sociogram has tended to focus on cliques rather than individuals. An early example of this clique-oriented structure is found in Coleman's (1961) analysis of adolescent friendship groups and their value systems. Hargreaves (1967) focused his attention on the clique structure of groups rather than individual "stars" or "isolates." Figure 1 reproduces a sociogram from Hargreaves's analysis of Form 4A boys in Lumley Secondary Modern School for Boys in England. Here it can be seen that Clique A dominates the group structure but with Cliques B and C also prevalent. The "star" of Clique A is Adrian (No. 29) who is also school captain.

The sociogram can display some of the main features of group sociometric structure, and also some of

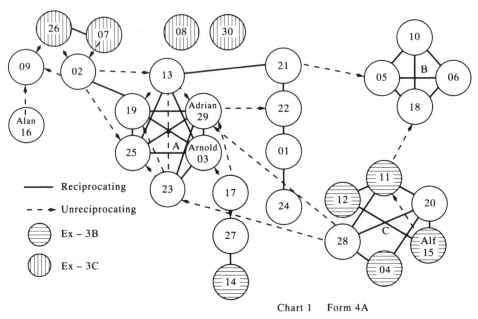

Chart 1   Form 4A

Figure 1
Sociogram depicting group structure of Form 4A (hatched circles represent students not in form 3A the previous year)

the variations in structure within different organizational environments. For example, Ford (1969) studied friendship choice in three English secondary schools (grammar, comprehensive, and modern secondary) to test the hypothesis that the comprehensive school students would manifest more sociometric mixing than students in the other two types of schools because of its more heterogeneous student population. In the event, she found that sex differentiation in sociometric choices prevailed in all schools and in all streams. Furthermore she found that differentiation by social class in all schools and streams also prevailed, except for the top three streams in the elite grammar school. Students in the comprehensive school, although in heterogeneous social environments, tended to choose friends from their own social class and from within their stream. These patterns are clearly visible in the sociograms which Ford constructed (see Ford 1969 pp. 86–99).

Ford concluded that the exceptional case of the upper streams in the grammar school could be explained in terms of the dominance of the high aspirations of all students in these streams, irrespective of class background, and thus indicates the greater importance of "class of aspiration" over "class of origin" in sociometric choices.

1.3 Limitations of Sociometric Data

The sociogram can sometimes be misused or misinterpreted. Gronlund (1959) has identified four common errors: (a) the sociogram usually depicts a graphic picture of desired associations, not actual associations; (b) the sociogram depicts the internal structure of the group, and therefore provides an incomplete depiction of group structure; (c) the choice patterns are sometimes seen as representing a fixed group structure rather than a changing social process; and (d) the sociometric structure will appear different when constructed by different individuals.

There is a further problem related to that previously noted by Schwarzwald et al. (1986) above. The findings of sociometric research sometimes appear to contradict findings using other methods. This was the case with Denscombe et al. (1986) who found that the ethnic bias resulting from a sociometric study of British primary school students did not agree with the perceptions of teachers, who reported a high level of student integration and inter-racial mixing. A study using fieldwork observations of the same students supported the teachers' perceptions rather than that resulting from the sociometric research. It would appear that the sociometric research design produces a particular description, and sometimes explanation, of social reality using a specific measurement, but that other designs and measurements may result in other descriptions or explanations. Finally Carlson-Sabell et al. (1992) argue that conventional sociometric instruments do not provide for the measurement of negative preference as well as positive preference, that is both

attraction and repulsion. They provide evidence which suggests that contradictory preferences may underlie choice, and that positive and negative preferences may not be linearly related. Given these limitations the interpretations and generalizations based on conventional sociomenric methods must be made with care.

2. Sociometrics and Educational Research

The importance of sociometry for educational research rests on the recognition that individual behavior is profoundly influenced by the group of which the individual is a member. Within the classroom, motivation, achievement, conduct, pupil–pupil and pupil–teacher relations are affected by group social composition and particularly informal group structure. A selective discussion of the findings of educational research using sociometric techniques points to some patterns of classroom behavior resulting from the sociometric context.

2.1 Intelligence and Achievement

There are distinct sociometric differences between students with extremely high or low intelligence (Gronlund 1959). Low intelligence may interfere with social acceptance by a person's peers, but high intelligence is not sufficient for high sociometric status. Pupils tend to choose those who are similar in intelligence, and a high deviation from group norms results in low peer acceptance. Gronlund (1959) identifies many studies which suggest that high levels of achievement are related to high social acceptance, but the direction of causality is not clear. However, the relationship is strongest where achievement is most highly valued by the group. The same pattern seems to hold for other skills which are highly valued, for example, in sport, playing a musical instrument, or social skills.

2.2 Social Factors

Social factors influence sociometric choice. Hollingshead's (1949) study pointed to high class homophily with regard to adolescent friendship patterns: two-thirds of all girls' clique relations and more than half the boys' were between members of the same social class. A reanalysis of recent data from Elmtown showed less choice between class equals, which suggests that over time the class structure in Elmtown had become more open and flexible, and hence less a criterion for sociometric choice (Cohen 1979).

Similar patterns have been found regarding other social factors, such as family status, residential proximity and even child-rearing strategies. Hart et al. (1990) report a study of mothers and their first-to-fourth grade children, using home interviews with the mothers before the beginning of the school year, and subsequent studies of the pupils after the school

year began. They found that children of power assertive mothers also practiced assertive techniques, and
they expected successful outcomes for these assertive
methods. However, these assertive pupils were less
accepted by their peers in terms of sociometric choice.

2.3 Classroom Interaction

It is generally recognized that greater involvement
in group activity and satisfactory social relationships
leads to less emotional tension and thus provides a better environment for classroom learning. Shared group
activities tend to promote greater affective ties, and
teachers can manipulate the classroom situation to promote greater interaction and thus more interpersonal
relationships. Classroom organization, both controlled
and uncontrolled by the teacher, has a pronounced
effect on the social development of students.

2.4 Educationaly Handicapped

Sociometric measures have been used to assess the
social acceptance or rejection of children with learning
difficulties, and to provide the basis for intervention
strategies. Hagborg (1994), for example, used sociometric measures to investigate the social relations of
a number of handicapped children and adolescents in
different educational settings. This sociometric data,
combined with additional information from other sources, provided the basis for the development of intervention strategies designed to improve the integration
of the handicapped. However, as noted above, sociometric data indicate the extent to which an individual
is accepted or rejected, but do not always indicate why.
Nevertheless, as Ochoa and Olivarez (1995) conclude,
it is clear that sociometric measures can identify the
link between behavior patterns and low sociometric
status, and the risk this poses for later life difficulties.

3. Applicability of Sociometrics to the Improvement of Social and Cognitive Development

The knowledge derived from sociometric research is
directly applicable to the improvement of social and
cognitive development. Sociometric grouping whereby each individual is best placed for his or her
own social and cognitive development is fundamental. Sociodrama and the use of roleplaying have also
received attention for promoting beneficial classroom
structures. Finally, a recognition of the importance of
power and influence, leadership and headship, both
between students and between teacher and student,
facilitates the utilization of group structures already
present in the classroom setting.

4. Future Directions in Sociometric Research

There has been much renewed interest in the development and use of sociometric measures in recent years

in a range of contexts, including education (see Blake
and McCanse 1989).

New developments in sociogram construction include three-dimensional models based on a number
of variables. Klovdahl (1982) has used computer
programs to create and manipulate visual, including
stereoscopic, representations of sociometric data and
has suggested that the increasing availability of sophisticated interactive computer graphics promises to
stimulate the development of theory about complex
relational data. Many of these developments are taking
place in the broader field of social network research,
which includes the study of communities and organizations, as well as schools and other educational
institutions. Johnson et al. (1994) provide a useful discussion of the use of sociometric status with network
analysis.

Hallinan (1974) finds the traditional quantitative
techniques of sociometric analysis too weak for an adequate analysis of the complexity of group sentiment
and structure, and argues that there is more promise
in the use of powerful mathematical theories and
methods, such as Markov chains, matrix algebra, abstract algebra, game theory, and differential equations.
Similarly Gazda and Mobley (1994) argue that the use
of multidimensional scaling (MDS) "has great promise
for expanding sociometric applications" (p. 94). More
recently Maasen et al. (1996) have demonstrated the
two-dimensional structure of sociometric status using
rating data.

With respect to schooling, greater attention to the
process of group formation, its development and decline, is required to understand better the dynamics of
classroom interaction and their consequences. Finally,
there is need to utilize what is now known about socio-
metrics in educational practice, particularly classroom
pedagogy, to improve further classroom learning and
general school effectiveness.

References

Blake R R, McCanse A A 1989 The rediscovery of sociometry. *Journal of Group Psychotherapy, Psychodrama
and Sociometry* 42(3): 148–65
Carlson-Sabelli L, Sabelli H C, Patel M, Holm K 1992 The
union of opposites in sociometry. *Journal of Group Psychotherapy, Psychodrama and Sociometry* 44(4): 147–71
Cohen J 1979 Socioeconomic status and high school friendship choice: Elmtown's youth revisited. *Social Networks*
2(1): 65–74
Coleman J S 1961 *The Adolescent Society: The Social Life
of the Teenager and its Impact on Education*. Free Press,
New York
Denscombe M, Szulc H, Patrick C, Wood A 1986 Ethnicity and friendship: The contrast between sociometric
research and fieldwork observation in primary school
classrooms. *Brit. Educ. Res. J.* 12(3): 221–35
Ford J B 1969 *Social Class and the Comprehensive School*.
Routledge and Kegan Paul, London
Gazda G M, Mobley J A 1994 Multidimensional scaling:

high-tech sociometry for the 21st century. *Journal of Group Psychotherapy, Psychodrama and Sociometry* 47(2): 77–96

Gronlund N E 1959 *Sociometry in the Classroom*. Harper and Row, New York

Guldner C A, Stone-Winestock P 1995 The use of sociometry in teaching at the university level. *Journal of Group Psychotherapy, Psychodrama and Sociometry* 47(4): 177–85

Hagborg W J 1994 Sociometry and educationally handicapped children. *Journal of Group Psychotherapy, Psychodrama and Sociometry* 47(1): 4–14

Hallinan M T 1974 *The Structure of Positive Sentiment*. Elsevier, New York

Hargreaves D H 1967 *Social Relations in a Secondary School*. Routledge and Kegan Paul, London

Hart C H, Ladd G W, Burleson B R 1990 Children's expectations of the outcomes of social strategies: Relations with sociometric status and maternal disciplinary styles. *Child Dev.* 61(1): 127–37

Hollingshead A B 1949 *Elmtown's Youth: The Impact of Social Classes on Adolescents*. Wiley, New York

Johnson J, Ironsmith M, Poteat G M 1994 Assessing children's sociometric status: issues and the application of social network analysis. *Journal of Group Psychotherapy, Psychodrama and Sociometry* 47(1): 36–48

Klovdahl A S 1982 A note on images of networks. *Social Networks* 3(3): 197–214

Lindzey G, Byrne D 1968 Measurement of social choice and interpersonal attractiveness. In: Lindzey G, Aronson E (eds.) 1968 *The Handbook of Social Psychology. Vol. 2: Research Methods*, 2nd edn. Addison-Wesley, Reading, Massachusetts

Maasen G H, Akkermans W, Van Der Linden J L 1996 Two-dimensional sociometric status determination with rating scales. *Small Group Research* 27(1): 56–78

Moreno J L 1934 *Who Shall Survive? A New Approach to the Problem of Human Interrelations*. Nervous and Mental Disease, Washington, DC

Northway M L 1967 *A Primer of Sociometry*. University of Toronto Press, Toronto

Ochoa S H, Olivarez A 1995 A meta-analysis of peer rating sociometric studies of pupils with learning disabilities. *J. Spec. Educ.* 29(1): 1–19

Proctor C H, Loomis C P 1951 Analysis of sociometric data. In: Jahoda M, Deutsch M, Cook S W (eds.) 1951 *Research Methods in Social Relations: With Special Reference to Prejudice, Part. 2: Selected Techniques*. Dryden, New York

Remer R 1995 Strong sociometry: a definition. *Journal of Group Psychotherapy, Psychodrama and Sociometry* 48(2): 69–74

Schwarzwald J, Laor T, Hoffman M 1986 Impact of sociometric method and activity content on assessment of intergroup relations in the classroom. *Brit. J. Educ. Psychol.* 56(1): 24–31

Wasik B H, Wasik J L, Frank R 1993 Sociometric characteristics of kindergarten children at risk for school failure. *Journal of School Psychology* 31: 241–57

Further Reading

Sociometry: A Journal of Interpersonal Relations 1937–78 (since 1978 known as *Social Psychology*)

Suppressor Variables

J. P. Keeves

A special problem that has arisen in both studies of prediction and of explanation in educational research is associated with the presence of suppressor variables. The presence of suppression effects can be observed both with partial correlation coefficients and partial regression coefficients. An example of a suppression effect is where the partial correlation coefficient between a predictor variable and a criterion variable after controlling for a second predictor variable is larger than the corresponding zero-order correlation coefficient. It should be noted that the effect may be an interrelated one and the second predictor variable may also exhibit a substantial change in its partial correlation with the criterion.

Horst (1966) has reported an example of the phenomenon of a suppression effect from a study of the prediction of success in the primary training of pilots during the Second World War. It was found that mechanical, numerical, and spatial ability tests had significant positive correlations with the criterion,

success as a pilot. However, while verbal ability had relatively high positive correlations with these three predictor variables, it had a very low positive correlation with the criterion. It is perhaps not surprising that verbal ability should correlate highly with the other predictors which were measured by pencil and paper tests, and should act as a suppressor variable, with a negative weight, in the combined prediction equation. In this case the verbal ability test was used to partial out reading factors which were serving to attenuate the relationships associated with the mechanical, numerical, and spatial ability tests.

Conger has developed a definition of suppression effects:

> A suppressor variable is defined to be a variable which increases the predictive validity of another variable (or set of variables) by its inclusion in a regression equation. This variable is a suppressor only for those variables whose regression weights are increased. (Conger 1974 pp. 36–37)

In addition, Conger (1974) and Cohen and Cohen (1975) have identified three kinds of suppression effects that can occur in regression analyses between two predictor variables and a criterion variable.

(a) *Classical suppression*. This occurs when one predictor has a correlation with the criterion of zero but has a significant regression coefficient when the criterion is regressed on both predictors. The regression coefficient of the other predictor variable will also be increased by the inclusion of the suppressor variable in the regression equation.

(b) *Negative suppression*. This effect was identified by Darlington (1968) and occurs when both predictor variables are correlated positively with the criterion variable and are correlated positively with each other. However, when the criterion variable is regressed on both predictors the suppressor variable has a negative regression coefficient. Thus the direction of the relationship between the predictor and the criterion has changed as a consequence of the suppression effect.

(c) *Reciprocal suppression*. This effect was identified by Conger (1974) and occurs when both predictor variables are correlated positively with the criterion variable and are correlated negatively with each other. Alternatively, it occurs when one predictor is correlated positively with the criterion variable and the other predictor is correlated negatively with the criterion, but the two predictors are correlated positively with each other. When the criterion variable is regressed on both predictor variables, the suppression effect operates to increase the magnitude of the regression coefficients of both predictor variables.

Tzelgov and Stern (1978) and Tzelgov and Herick (1991) have examined the range of possible relationships which exist between the three variables and have identified the mathematical conditions existing between the three variables that give rise to the three different types of suppression effects as well as the situation under which no suppression effects occur.

Cooley and Lohnes (1976 p. 160) have drawn attention to a phenomenon which all who have used multiple-regression analysis extensively, whether for the estimation of path coefficients in path analysis, or for studies of explanation, through the use of stepwise regression analysis, or for the purposes of prediction with a theoretically based prediction model, are well-aware. They refer to the phenomenon as one of "bouncing betas". The "bouncing" of standardized partial regression coefficients can arise in several ways. First, through the inclusion of an additional variable in the regression analysis that acts as a suppressor variable, and it should be noted that under certain circumstances a regression coefficient will exceed 1.0 when a suppression effect is present. Second, the "bouncing" can occur in a replicated study, where sampling variations change the interrelationships between the variables. Third, "bouncing" can occur in a study where measurement error can distort the interrelations between the variables. The results of "bouncing" can be of considerable significance not only where suppression effects are operating but also where there is a substantial degree of multicollinearity between the predictor variables.

In developing a prediction equation many have argued that suppressor variables should be used to refine the prediction model. Cronbach (1950) was among the first to suggest that response sets in achievement testing could be allowed for by the use of a suppressor variable measuring a tendency to answer "true" to objective test items. In the same way it has been proposed that in personality assessment, scores on personality inventories could be corrected by the inclusion of a measure of response style for socially desirable responses as a suppressor variable in the prediction equation. However, the evidence available over a long period with respect to the predictive effectiveness of suppressor variables in personality assessment (Thorndike 1949, Wiggins 1973) is not impressive and suppressor variables that operate consistently to improve prediction are rare. In practice it would seem wise not to include a suppressor variable in a prediction equation unless the inclusion of the variable was strongly supported on theoretical and rational grounds. Nevertheless, the idea of using a suppressor variable in prediction models must remain an interesting possibility.

In explanation studies, the research worker must be extremely wary that suppressor variables are not being introduced into the analyses without a sound theoretical basis. The dangers are particularly great when stepwise regression analysis is employed, and where a suppressor variable is introduced with a marginal increase in the variance accounted for, but with a marked influence on the partial regression coefficients arising from the inclusion of the variable.

See also: Regression Analysis; Validity; Prediction in Research; Multivariate Analysis

References

Cohen J. Cohen P 1975 *Applied Multiple Regression/Correlation Analysis for the Behavioral Sciences*. Erlbaum, Hillsdale, New Jersey.

Conger A J 1974 A revised definition for suppressor variables: A guide to their identification and interpretation. *Educ. Psychol. Meas.* 34: 35–46

Cooley W W, Lohnes P R 1976 *Evaluation Research in Education*. Irvington, New York

Cronbach L J 1950 Further evidence on response sets and test design. *Educ. Psychol. Meas.* 10: 3–31

Darlington R B 1968 Multiple regression in psychological research and practice. *Psychol. Bull.* 69: 161–82

Horst P 1966 *Psychological Measurement and Prediction*. Wadsworth, Belmont, California

Thorndike R L 1949 *Personal Selection: Test and Measure-*

ment Techniques. Wiley, New York

Tzelgov J, Stern I 1978 Relationships between variables in three variable linear regression and the concept of suppressor. *Educ. Psychol. Meas.* 38: 325–35

Tzelgov J, Herick A 1991 Suppression situations in psycho-

logical research: definitions, implications and applications. *Psych. Bull.* 109(3): 524–36

Wiggins J S 1973 *Personality and Prediction: Principles of Personality Assessment*. Addison-Wesley, Reading, Massachusetts

Variance and Covariance, Analysis of

J. D. Finn

The analysis of variance, introduced by Sir Ronald Fisher near the beginning of the twentieth century, is widely used by behavioral and social scientists. As a class of statistical models, "ANOVA" provides a means for analyzing data that is both rigorous logically and mathematically, and sufficiently broad to address questions posed in a wide spectrum of investigations. This entry describes the range of different analysis of variance models, the questions they address, the types of data for which they are appropriate, and the logic by which they operate. Several newer developments and recent thinking about ANOVA procedures are described and demonstrated in an investigation of students' motivation.

The main function performed by ANOVA is to compare systematically the mean response levels of two or more independent groups of observations, or of a set of observations measured at two or more points in time. Analysis of variance techniques are validly applied in each of three types of investigations (Bock 1975): (a) experiments, in which subjects are assigned at random to treatments determined by the investigator: (b) comparative studies, whose purpose is to describe differences among naturally occurring populations; and (c) surveys, in which the responses of subgroups of a single population are to be compared.

Consider several examples. First, an experiment might be conducted in which one randomly assigned group of students receives no formal spelling instruction, a second group receives 15 minutes of spelling instruction per day, and a third group 30 minutes per day. At the end of the experiment, the effectiveness of spelling instruction is assessed by comparing the mean scores of the three groups on a common spelling test. Second, a recent large-scale comparative study examined differences among the achievement levels of students attending American public schools, private schools with religious affiliation, and other private schools. Although many different analyses were employed, ANOVA provides the most direct comparison of mean achievement across the three types of institutions. Third, the International Association for the Evaluation of Educational Achievement (IEA) international surveys sampled children in such a way

that the final sample represented the entire age cohort attending school within each participating country. Subjects within a country may be subclassified by their responses even after the data are collected, to examine differences in mean response level among subgroups of interest. In an example described below, Swedish 13-year olds are classified according to their fathers' occupations, and average levels of achievement motivation are compared using ANOVA. In a survey, unlike other types of investigations, removing the researcher-defined subclassifications still yields an intact population (all Swedish 13-year olds). Nevertheless, whenever mean comparisons are of concern, ANOVA remains an appropriate and powerful analytic tool.

The examples above are described as having one measured response variable. Studies that yield two or more interrelated response measures (i.e., multiple dependent variables) require multivariate analysis of variance ("MANOVA") tests and estimates. For example, the spelling experiment might have included a subtest covering words that were explicitly part of the curriculum and another covering words of similar difficulty that were not taught. Achievement in three types of American schools may have been measured in terms of multiple subject areas (mathematics, reading, social studies, etc.) or in terms of both cognitive and affective outcomes. In each case, summing the measures will obscure important differences among the subscales, while separate analyses of each scale may give contradictory or confusing results and limit the replicability of the investigation. Appropriate MANOVA procedures maintain the integrity of the original measures while providing tests and estimates that pertain to the set of responses jointly.

Repeated measures analysis is employed in investigations in which the same subjects are observed at two or more points in time or under two or more experimental conditions. These include pretest-posttest studies or educational or social interventions, longitudinal studies in which data are collected on the same scale repeatedly, and within-subject experiments in which subjects are measured on the same response variable under several experimental conditions. Both univariate and multivariate analysis of variance models may be used with repeated measures data, depending on the distribution of the multiple measurements. The two types of analyses are described and compared in Bock (1975 Chap. 7).

1. Analysis of Variance Models

Analysis of variance procedures are based on linear models that depict the partition of scores on a measured dependent variable into prespecified components. Consider hypothetical scores of subjects in the spelling experiment who have been exposed to 0, 15, or 30 minutes of instruction per day. The design would be described as a one-way or one-factor design with three "levels"—that is, three different treatment conditions. The ANOVA model describes a typical score as the sum of three components: a response level common to all subjects in the total population of potential subjects (μ); a deviation from μ common to all subjects who receive treatment one (no instruction), treatment two (15 minutes), or treatment three (30 minutes)—α_1, α_2, or α_3, respectively; and a deviation from the average response under a particular treatment unique to the individual subject, ε_{ij}. Thus if Y_{ij} represents the response for typical subject i in treatment group one, two, or three (j), the ANOVA model is:

$$Y_{ij} = \mu + \alpha_j + \varepsilon_{ij} \tag{1}$$

For example, if the final test has 20 spelling words, the average score for all Grade 5 students might be 8. Further, the average spelling score of all Grade 5 students who receive 15 minutes of instruction per day might be 10, and one student in this group might obtain a score of 13. Then α_2 is the systematic advantage or "effect" of receiving this instructional treatment, $10 - 8 = 2$, and the unique term for the individual scoring 13 is $13 - 10 = 3$.

Fitting the ANOVA model to empirical data consists of performing two general statistical functions: tests of significance and the estimation of effects. In the spelling experiment, the null hypothesis asserts that the means of the three groups are equal, or equivalently that the three α's are equal; that is,

$$H_0 : \alpha_1 = \alpha_2 = \alpha_3 \tag{2}$$

The test of significance provides a sample-based decision as to whether this hypothesis is supported or refuted. If the test reveals that the groups have different means, the researcher may estimate the α's or the differences among them (see Sect. 1.2).

As a more complex example, consider that students are classified by sex and exposed to mastery or nonmastery instruction in simple operations with fractions. The experimental design is pictured in Fig. 1, together with hypothetical mean scores on a test of fractions given at the end of the experiment. The

	Mastery	Nonmastery	All
Males	42	38	40
Females	30	32	31
All	36	35.5	

Figure 1
Mean scores for hypothetical mastery learning equipment

design is a two-way or two-factor design (sex and method) with two levels of sex (M and F) and two levels of method (mastery and nonmastery). There is a total of four "cells" in this design. The ANOVA model for a typical subject in the experiment is:

$$Y_{ijk} = \mu + \alpha_j + \beta_k + \gamma_{jk} + \varepsilon_{ijk} \tag{3}$$

Again, μ is the mean response common to all subjects in all cells, or 35.5 in the example. The effects of being a male or female are α_1 and α_2, respectively; for example, males enjoy an average advantage of $\alpha_1 = 40 - 35.5 = 4.5$ points on the test. Also, β_1 and β_2 are the effects of being exposed to the mastery or nonmastery approach, respectively; for example, mastery students enjoy an average of $\beta_1 = 36 - 35.5 = 0.5$ points. The term γ_{jk}, unlike any in the one-factor model is the "interaction" or average effect attributable to a particular combination of sex and method. For example, males' 4.5 point advantage and mastery students' 0.5 advantage might lead to the belief that males learning by mastery would have an average score of 40.5 (35.5 + 4.5 + 0.5 points). Instead the actual mean is 42, and the interaction for the cell is $\gamma_{11} = 42 - 40.5 = 1.5$. Factors uniquely associated with males learning by this approach appear to elevate the scores further; if the interactions are large, the investigator may wish to explore further what these may be. Finally, an individual subject with a score of 38 would have a unique component (ε) of $38 - 42 = -4$.

Three general tests of significance are obtained under this model: tests of whether the means for males and females are different, whether the means for mastery and nonmastery approaches are different, and whether there is any significant interaction. These are represented symbolically as:

$$H_0(1) : \alpha_1 = \alpha_2 \tag{4}$$
$$H_0(2) : \beta_1 = \beta_2 \tag{5}$$
$$H_0(3) : \text{All } \gamma_{ik} = 0 \tag{6}$$

If a statistical significance is found, further analysis might include estimating the magnitude and direction of the differences. If significant interaction is found [i.e., $H_0(3)$ rejected], then the mastery-nonmastery difference is not as large (or small) for males as it is for females, and separate differences for males and females must be inspected.

The concept of interaction is all that is necessary to generalize to models with more than two classification factors. Thus most textbooks give limited attention to higher order designs, and are usually restricted to studies with equal numbers of subjects in the cells. With this (artificial) simplification, tests of significance are easily computed using ordinary scalar algebra and estimated effects are simple differences of the marginal means. Unequal-N designs, although arising frequently in practice, require matrix algebra to obtain the appropriate sums of squares for significance testing and proper estimates of effects and their differences. The study described in the following sections has unequal Ns, and exemplifies the information provided by the more general and realistic application of ANOVA.

1.1 Tests of Significance

The terms μ, α_j, β_k, and γ_{jk} in Eqns. (1, 3) in classical statistical theory represent fixed population constants, while Y and ε are random variables whose distribution may be inferred from the characteristics of the measurement scale (see Sect. 3). The basic ANOVA hypotheses assert that the population constants have particular values or that the means are equal to one another. An inference concerning whether a hypothesis is supported or contradicted may be made from a representative sample of observations.

For example, assume that N subjects are randomly and independently assigned to $J = 3$ different instructional conditions with N_1 students in the no spelling group, N_2 in group 2 (15 minutes), and N_3 in group 3 (30 minutes). At the end of two weeks, a 20-word spelling test is administered and the mean scores for the three groups are found to be some values $\bar{Y}_1$, $\bar{Y}_2$, and $\bar{Y}_3$, respectively. The mean of all subjects is $\bar{Y} = \Sigma N_j \bar{Y}_j / N$.

Two measures are obtained from these descriptive data for the test of significance: an index of how different the three means (or the three α's) are from one another in the sample, and a measure of how variable individuals' scores are within the experimental groups. If differences among the group means are large in comparison to differences among individuals, then the groups are clearly distinguishable and it is likely that the null hypothesis [Eqn. (4)] is false. If differences among individuals are relatively large instead, then groups vary no more than random differences among subjects, and the null hypothesis is considered supported.

The measure of differences among means is the "mean square between groups,"

$$MS_B = \frac{\Sigma N_j (\bar{Y}_j - \bar{Y})^2}{J - 1} \tag{7}$$

The basic component in MS_B is $(\bar{Y}_j - \bar{Y})$, a sample value that estimates the population α_j. The difference between the mean of each group and the mean of all observations, calculated from the sample, is large if the subgroup means are very different from one another and small if they are close in value. Thus MS_B, a summary of these differences, is generally larger when group means are far from one another and smaller if the subgroup means are close together.

The measure of differences among individual subjects within the groups is "mean square within groups,"

$$MS_W = \frac{\sum_j \sum_i (Y_{ij} - \bar{Y}_j)^2}{\sum_i (N_j - 1)} \tag{8}$$

The basic component is a sample value for ε_{ij}, that is, the difference of the individual score (Y_{ij}) from the mean in the particular group ($\bar{Y}_j$). These differences are squared and summed across all subjects in all groups, and then divided by $\Sigma (N_j - 1)$. The greater the variation among individuals within the groups, the greater MS_W will be.

The test statistic is the ratio F= MS_B/MS_W—the F test, and is referred to in tables of the F distribution found in most statistics textbooks. The parameters needed to look up the F value are the probability of a Type I number of error acceptable to the researcher and the "degrees of freedom" between groups ($J - 1$) and within groups [$\Sigma(N_j - 1)$]. If F exceeds the tabled critical value, MS_B is sufficiently larger than MS_W to conclude that group differences predominate, and H_0 is rejected. If the critical F value is not exceeded, the null hypothesis of no difference is maintained. In the two-way design, in addition to mean square within groups, there is a separate mean square between, and an F statistic for each hypothesis (Eqns. 4, 5, and 6).

1.2 Estimation of Effects

In addition to tests of significance, it is important to determine the magnitude and direction of differences among the means, and to locate groups that may not differ from one another even if the overall null hypothesis is rejected. The most straightforward approach is to estimate preselected contrasts among the parameters in the model. In the spelling experiment, if H_0 is rejected, the difference between the no spelling condition and the average of the two instructional conditions [$\alpha_1 - (\alpha_2 + \alpha_3)/2$] might be examined. Also, the difference between 15 and 30 minutes of instruction, $\alpha_2 - \alpha_3$, could be estimated. Common statistical methods allow the determination of these differences in raw-score units and in standard deviation units ("effectsizes"), and to draw confidence intervals on the contrasts, or to re-express them in t-statistic form. Any contrasts that are required may be estimated. When there is a physical metric underlying the group differences (e.g., time in the spelling experiment) "orthogonal polynomial" contrasts may be particularly useful. These reveal the extent to which a unit increase in time is accompanied by an additional unit increase on the spelling test, and thus results for amounts of time not studied may be predicted. Additional interpretive devices include plots of the estimated differences and "predicted means" obtained by eliminating nonsignificant effects from the ANOVA model.

1.3 An Example of Two-way ANOVA

A random sample of 102 13-year old Swedish students whose total school performance placed them among the top 5 percent or lowest 5 percent of students of their age was drawn from the data bank of the IEA international survey of science achievement. The subjects were further subclassified according to their father's occupation, into four levels: professional, manager, skilled laborer, or unskilled laborer. The resulting design had two factors—two levels of school performance and four occupational levels. The investigation focused on differences among the groups in children's achievement motivation. The IEA "need achievement" measure was used for this purpose, obtained by administering a paper-and-pencil attitude questionnaire to each student in the survey. Mean scores and the number of students in each subgroup of the sample are given in Fig. 2. While motivation levels tend to be lower among children of less skilled parents, the difference between the best and poorest students is clearer. A summary of the ANOVA computations is presented in typical "source table" form in Table 1.

The F-ratio for performance differences (14.89) exceeds the 0.05 critical value of 3.96; there is a significant difference between the means of the best and poorest students in need achievement, and $H_0(1)$ [Eqn. (4)] is rejected. The F-ratio for occupational differences does not exceed the tabled critical value of 2.72; there is not a significant difference among the four means and $H_0(2)$ [Eqn. (5)] is maintained. Finally, the F-ratio for interaction does not exceed its critical value and $H_0(3)$ [Eqn. (6)] is maintained.

Table 1

Analysis of variance source table for need achievement scores

Hypothesis	Degrees of freedom	Mean square	F ratio
Performance [Eqn. (4)]	1	149.73	14.89
Occupation [Eqn. (5)]	3	23.60	2.35
Interaction [Eqn. (6)]	3	1.98	0.20
Subjects within groups	94	10.06	

a Significant at $p < 0.05$

The direction of the performance difference is obvious from Fig. 2. Since the marginal means for occupational groups decrease monotonically, for purposes of extending the example particular contrasts on that dimension may be examined. Specifically, one may estimate contrasts between the achievement motivation of children whose fathers are in particular occupational groups and the achievement motivation of children whose fathers are in an occupational group requiring less skill development. That is, the children of professional fathers may be compared with the average of the children of all the other occupational groups; the children of managers may be compared with the children of skilled and unskilled laborers; and the children of skilled laborers may be compared with the children of unskilled laborers, on the basis of achievement motivation. The estimates of these contrasts are summarized in Table 2, obtained by employing a general estimation algorithm for unequal-N designs.

The average need achievement of children of professionals is estimated to be 1.12 points above that of other children of fathers in other occupational

		Father's occupation			
	Professional	Manager	Skilled laborer	Unskilled laborer	All
Best 5%	22 13.23	6 13.67	25 11.28	4 12.25	12.35
Poorest 5%	6 10.67	7 10.29	20 9.10	12 8.83	9.42
Bath	12.68	11.85	10.31	9.69	11.06

Figure 2

Mean need achievement scores of 13-year old Swedish students (sample sizes in upper left inserts)

groups. This is about one-third of a pooled within-group standard deviation ($S = 3.17$). The average need achievement of children of managers is 1.69 points above that of laborers, or slightly over half a standard deviation. The standard error of this difference is 0.99 points so that the difference is 1.70 standard errors in magnitude. This result may be referred to the t-distribution with 94 degrees of freedom and exceeds the 0.05 critical value in one tail. The data would support a hypothesis that this particular difference is positive. Thus, while there are no overall differences in need achievement among children whose fathers differ by occupation, the data indicate that children of managers have higher average motivation levels than children of laborers; further research to confirm this finding may be warranted.

2. Analysis of Covariance Models

Many studies obtain data on additional antecedent variables that have numerical scales. For example, the study to compare three types of American schools may reasonably obtain parents' income, a concomitant of the type of school children attend, as well as individual schooling outcomes. Income need not be subdivided into discrete categories but may be included in the analysis as a "covariate." Likewise, the investigation of spelling performance might include a measure of children's spatial visualization to test whether it partially explains spelling outcomes.

Analysis of covariance is an extension of ANOVA procedures to incorporate one or more measured scales as additional antecedent variables. The "ANCOVA" model is:

$$Y_{ij} = \mu + \alpha_j + \beta(X_{ij} - \bar{X}) + \varepsilon_{ij} \qquad (9)$$

X_{ij} is the score for the individual on the covariate, and $\bar{X}$ is the mean of all observations. β is the regression coefficient reflecting the extent to which scores on the criterion Y are dependent on the covariate X. Three hypotheses are tested through this model. First, are there differences among the subgroups on response variable Y, eliminating ("holding constant") differences attributable to the covariate? The null hypothesis is identical to Eqn. (2), although adjustments are made to the within and between mean squares for the influence of the covariate. Second, is there a significant correlation of X and Y among individuals within the subgroups, eliminating (holding constant) group mean differences? The null hypothesis is:

$$H_0(2) : \beta = 0 \qquad (10)$$

Finally, is the relationship of X and Y as strong among individuals in one subgroup as it is in the others? The null hypothesis is:

$$H_0(3) : \beta_1 = \beta_2 = \beta_3 \qquad (11)$$

where β_1, β_2, β_3 are separate regression coefficients for each of the three spelling groups. The equivalence of regression coefficients is a necessary condition for the rest of the analysis to be valid, since only one common value of β is included in Eqn. (9). Also, the test may have substantive importance. In the spelling experiment, for example, it may be important to know if more instructional time can lower the dependence of performance on spatial aptitude.

ANCOVA was developed originally for use in experiments. In this application, measurement of the covariate must precede the experimental manipulation. Since groups are assigned at random, their averages on the covariate will not differ. On the other hand, the covariate may be related to differences among individuals within the groups and the residuals (ε_{ij}) are reduced by including X in the model. Thus, mean square within groups will tend to be smaller than in the corresponding ANOVA model, and the sensitivity of the statistical test is increased.

In nonexperimental studies, ANCOVA is a general procedure whenever some antecedent variables define discrete groups of observations and others have well-measured scales. In this context, the covariate(s) may be measured simultaneously with the dependent variables. The availability of general computer programs for ANCOVA obviates the need for such poor data analytic practices as dichotomizing well-measured scales to adapt them to an analysis of variance model, or dummy coding categorical variables to force them into a regression analysis framework.

3. Assumptions Underlying ANOVA and ANCOVA

Four major properties of the distribution of the dependent variable (Y) are important to the validity of the procedures described in this article. First, the units of scale must be well-defined and small relative to the range of the variable, so that a continuous probability function (i.e., the normal distribution) is a reasonable approximation; the scale should have at least ordinal properties and should have nearly equal or equal appearing intervals. Second, the distribution of the response variable should approach normality in the population, although not necessarily in the sample. This is assured by the central limit theorem for the majority of educational and psychological measures, but should be examined whenever departure from normality may become extreme. Third, the variance or standard deviation of the dependent variable should be equal in the populations represented by all of the subgroups in the design (although not necessarily in the samples).

ANOVA is moderately robust to violations of the normality and equal variance requirements and a program of research summarized in Glass and Hopkins (1996) demonstrates the impact of departure from these conditions. On the other hand, the fourth requirement

Table 2
Contrasts among occupational groups in children's achievement motivation

Contrast	Average difference	Standard error	Difference in standard deviations
Professionals-others $\beta_1-(\beta_2+\beta_3+\beta_4)/3$	1.12	0.77	0.35
Managers-laborers $\beta_2-(\beta_3+\beta_4)/2$	1.69	0.99	0.53
Skilled-unskilled $\beta_3-\beta_4$	−0.17	0.95	−0.05

is the *sine qua non* of valid statistical tests with ANOVA models: the observations must be sampled and respond independently of one another. If dependencies arise because the same subjects or groups are measured repeatedly, then multivariate models should be employed. Otherwise, independent observations are essential to all aspects of the analysis, including both sample calculations and theoretical underpinnings, and cannot be compromised.

4. Multiple Comparisons

Multiple comparisons which involve testing of pairwise differences between subgroup means and other contrasts among subgroup means are frequently conducted after the initial analysis is completed. These "post hoc" comparisons have become common practice, and are recommended as a follow-up to a significant ANOVA. In testing multiple comparisons some correction should be made to the significance level for the fact that several contrasts are being made on the same data set. Many different approaches have been proposed, but one based on the *Bonferroni inequality* is probably the most convenient to employ. This principle states that the probability of making at least one Type I error out of a set of m tests of significance is no greater than the sum of the Type I error rates (α's) used for the separate tests. On this basis an error rate for a set of m comparisons can be preset to a small value, e.g., .05. This is divided by m to establish the value of α to be used for each comparison.

For example, if all pairwise comparisons are to be tested among three means (μ^1 with μ^2, μ^1 with μ^3, and μ^2 with μ^3) and the Type I error rate for the set of comparisons is .05, the value of α to be used for each comparison is .05/3 = /0167. Alternatively the researcher might decide to conduct each test with a predetermined α and then decide if the error rate for the entire set is "acceptable." Thus, if four comparisons are tested, each with $\alpha = .02$, then the error rate for the set of comparisons is no greater than .08. This may not be so large that it would seriously threaten the validity of the study. Extensive information about other approaches to multiple comparisons is given in Glass and Hopkins (1996) and Ott (1993).

5. Texts and Computer Programs

Textbooks by Glass and Hopkins (1996), Ott (1993), and Anderson and Finn (1996) give particularly clear introductions to ANOVA with examples from the social sciences and education. The text by Scheffé (1959) remains the classic introduction to a wide range of issues related to ANOVA at a more mathematical level. An introduction to MANOVA with real-data examples is given in Bock (1975) and Stevens (1996). ANOVA for unequal-N designs is discussed at length in these multivariate compendia. Good introductions to ANCOVA are given by Gourlay (1953) and Elashoff (1969) although there is generally a paucity of good textbook coverage.

The computations for any but the simplest ANOVA design require the use of a computer. Several programs will accurately perform the calculations for the widest range of models, including equal and unequal N's, univariate and multivariate responses, analysis of variance and covariance, and complex as well as simple designs. These include subprograms that are part of general purpose packages such as SPSS (distributed by SPSS, Inc., in Chicago, Illinois) and SAS (distributed by the SAS Institute in Raleigh-Durham, North Carolina) and MULTIVARIANCE (Finn and Bock 1988), a specialized program that is very powerful for simple and complex ANOVA and MANOVA designs. All are available for personsl computers as well as the mainframe and all are relatively user-friendly.

See also: Significance Testing; Hypothesis Testing; Regression Analyses of Quantified Data

References

Anderson T W, Finn J D 1996 *The New Statistical Analysis of Data.* Springer-Verlag, New York
Bock R D 1975 *Multivariate Statistical Methods in Behavioral Research.* Scientific Software, Chicago, Illinois
Elashoff J D 1969 Analysis of convariance: A delicate instrument. *Am. Educ. Res. J.* 6: 383–401
Finn J D, Bock R D 1988 *MULTIVARIANCE PC (Version 7.3).* Scientific Software, Chicago, Illinois
Glass G V, Hopkins K D 1996 *Statistical Methods in Education and Psychology,* 3rd edn. Prentice-Hall, Englewood Cliffs, New Jersey

Gourlay N 1953 Covariance analysis and its applications in psychological research. *Br. J. Stat. Psychol.* 6: 25–33

Ott R L 1993 *An Introduction to Statistical Methods and Data Analysis*, 4th edn. Duxbury Press, Belmont, California

Scheffé H 1959 *The Analysis of Variance*. Wiley, New York

Stevens J 1996 *Applied Multivariate Statistics for the Social Sciences*, 3rd edn. Lawrence Erlbaum, Mahwah, New Jersey

Measurement in Educational Research

Introduction: Advances in Measurement in Education

J.P. Keeves

Educational research commonly involves the investigation of stability and change in the characteristics of individuals and social groups. In order to examine stability and change it is necessary to make measurements on the characteristics that are of interest. Moreover the making of measurements on the chosen characteristics requires the abstraction and refinement of constructs and the devising and development of observable characteristics associated with those constructs. These constructs, observable characteristics and measurements are not only required for research activity, but are also useful in educational practice, including: (a) the appraisal of student learning, (b) the certification of student performance, (c) the diagnosis of problems in learning, (d) the selection of individuals and groups for the provision of learning experiences, (e) the guidance of individuals in their future learning, (f) the evaluation of learning programs, and (g) the design of curricula.

The major problems associated with measurement for both educational research and educational practice involve the meaningfulness, accuracy and the consistency with which measurements are made. In more technical terms, these are the validity, precision and reliability of the measurements respectively. Over the past 100 years, since Sir Francis Galton published *Inquiry into Human Faculty and its Development*, and Stanley Hall published *The Study of Children* both in 1883, the science of educational measurement has progressed towards more explicit and precise ways of specifying and appraising the constructs and observables that are of relevance to education. These advances have been made through the use of appropriate statistical, mathematical and psychological theories to support the identification and quantification of constructs and observable characteristics. Both the progress made in the development of theory in education and psychology, and in the ease with which computations can now be carried out through the use of electronic computers have led to marked advances in the field of educational measurement during the latter decades of the twentieth century. The challenge to educational researchers and to practitioners is not only to keep abreast of these developments but also to learn to use them in ways that would facilitate both the conduct of inquiry and the improvement of educational practice. Nevertheless, there has been, at the same time as developments have occurred, a turning away by many in education from the use of measurement both in research and practice in education.

1. Concerning the Nature of Measurement

1.1 The Quantitative or Qualitative Debate

It is frequently claimed that there are two different modes of inquiry in education which lead to the quantitative and qualitative approaches to research. However, this simple dichotomy involves a serious failure to understand the nature of both quantities and qualities. Kaplan in *Scientific Methods in Educational Research*, argues that it is necessary to emphasize that measurement is not an end in itself, it merely performs an instrumental function in inquiry. He also argues that there is a danger of assuming that measures have an inherent value, without regard for the nature of the object being measured, and the intrusion of the observer into the measurement process. Furthermore, there is a tendency to disregard how the number assigned in measurement should be used in analysis. The treatment of measurement as if it had intrinsic scientific value is referred to by Kaplan (1964) as the *Mystique of Quantity*. There is, however, a more pervasive *Mystique of Quality*, which considers that any attempt that is made to measure in educational research is a gross distortion and obfuscation of both objects and events. Those who adhere to this perspective regard qualitative methods as the only meaningful way to investigate an educational problem.

If these two views are considered as alternatives or even as opposites that are complementary then a serious misunderstanding of the nature of both quantities and qualities has occurred. Kaplan (1964, p. 207) has clarified the point at issue in the following terms:

> Quantities are *of* qualities, and a measured quality *has* just the magnitude expressed in its measure.

Every measurement demands some degree of abstraction. The assigning of a number to an observable characteristic or relationship requires the refinement of that characteristic or relation before measurements can be made. This is not an assumption of measurement; it is a *requirement* that the characteristic or relation should be accurately specified and should be unidimensional before measurement is attempted.

1.2 Single or Multiple Observations

A general distinction must be drawn between measurements that are made through a single observation or judgment and measurements that are made by combining in an appropriate way multiple observations or judgments. Errors of measurement arise from three distinct sources: (a) variability in the making of the observation or judgment by the observer, (b) variability in the making of the observation or judgment due to the instrument being employed, and (c) variability in the characteristic being measured. Errors arising from the third source demand the making of multiple measurements by the sampling of behaviors or observable phenomena associated with the characteristic or relationship under survey. It is, however, not uncommon to make multiple observations in order to estimate and allow for observer errors and instrumental errors. Such procedures necessarily lead to the combining of the multiple observations in an appropriate way.

Consequently reliance on a single observation or judgment is relatively rare in measurement in educational research and practice, and the use of multiple observations is widespread. Substantial problems arise because the multiple observations must be combined. Cronbach (1960), using an analogy with the recording of music, draws attention to the distinction made between bandwidth and fidelity. Thus in measurement with multiple observations it is necessary that the range of observations employed is sufficiently wide to provide a meaningful indicator of the variability in the characteristic or relationship under investigation. The range of observations is associated with the bandwidth of the recording. However, it is also necessary with multiple observations to ensure that the range of observations employed is sufficiently narrow to provide a high degree of fidelity. Only thus is it possible to ensure that the measurements are unidimensional and that it is meaningful to combine observations. This balance between bandwidth and fidelity becomes increasingly important as advances occur in educational measurement where multiple observations are made.

The same issues must be considered when multiple observations are made because of random variability that arises from the instrument employed. Thus most observations involve error. However, the word "error" implies not a mistake, but like the "knights errant" of old, a wandering about a central position. Where random error is associated with measurement, then statistical procedures can be employed which, according to established conventions, enable greater precision of measurement to be obtained. It is, however, the issues of bandwidth and fidelity that must be tackled in the improvement of measurement in educational research.

1.3 Bandwidth and Fidelity

The terms, bandwidth and fidelity, have some overlap in meaning with the more technical terms of validity and reliability, but they are not synonymous, with these more familiar terms. Moreover, they are increasingly being used in situations where validity and reliability do not suffice, since they are more directly related to the combining of observations and judgments in the making of measurements.

Fidelity demands that not only should a characteristic or relationship be accurately defined, but the measurements should satisfy the requirement of unidimensionality. The development of procedures for confirmatory factor analysis (see *Factor Analysis*) provide a rigorous test of unidimensionality, that is based on the variability in the items and in the sample employed. Bejar (1983 p. 31) has, however, drawn attention to the fact that unidimensionality as tested under these conditions does not imply that only a single characteristic is involved in responding or that a single process operates. If several characteristics or processes were to operate in unison, then unidimensionality would also hold. However, if the characteristics or processes did not operate together then it would not be meaningful to assign numbers to any combination of the items employed, unless another operation such as that of prediction, were to provide the rule for combination. If a set of measurements lacked this necessary fidelity, and if several identifiable dimensions were involved, then each dimension would need to be considered separately and a profile of measures recorded.

The power of measurement is that once a characteristic or relationship has been specified in detail and in a meaningful way with sufficient bandwidth, then the quantities that are obtained as measures of two objects or events can be compared. Where measurement is made through a single observation, the issues of bandwidth and fidelity do not apply; consequently, there is a heavy burden placed on the single observation.

The idea of bandwidth is employed to ensure that there is a sufficient range of manifestations of the characteristic being measured for meaningful representation of that characteristic. If variability exists in the characteristic, a range of instances is required to represent adequately that characteristic. Consequently under some circumstances observations can be said to supply redundant information and serve no useful purpose and must be rejected. Observations can also supply information that can be shown not to relate to the specified characteristic and they must also be rejected. Thus decisions need to be made prior to the undertaking of measurement on the bandwidth of acceptable observations when variability exists in the characteristic being measured.

1.4 Precision

In education it is common to make measurements in the form of graded responses or ratings. It is also common in the use of rating scales to assign numbers to response categories that assume equal spacing, and to assume that the error involved in rating is the same across response categories. It is also generally assumed that greater precision is obtained through the use of a greater number of response categories that have each been carefully specified. In more advanced treatments of measurement in education (Andrich 1995a, 1995b) it is assumed that categories do not have equal spacing, that errors of assignment to response categories can not be ignored, and that the response categories employed are meaningful and have been carefully specified. In general, the larger the number of response categories the more precise the measurement. However, there may be a limit to the number of response categories that can be employed effectively in measurement by the observers making the measurement or by respondents to a rating scale.

1.5 Using Numbers in Measurement

The great advantage of using numbers to specify the degree or extent of a characteristic or relationship is that mathematics has provided the rules and procedures for working with numbers and matrices in order to examine relationships. In addition, statistics has provided the rules and procedures for examining the probabilities with which results might be observed and the levels of magnitude and importance of such results. It is here through the development of mathematical and statistical procedures that great advances have occurred. Computers have made extensive computation possible, so that computations that could not a few decades ago be contemplated, can now be done almost instantaneously. These mathematical and statistical procedures are necessary, not only because the interrelations between variables in educational research are complex, but also because measurements made in educational research often involve considerable error and require large samples of observations or persons for a hypothesized relationship to be detected. The rules and procedures provided by mathematics and statistics permit both the hypothesizing of relationships between measured variables and the subsequent testing of these hypothesized relationships, together with the estimation of the magnitude of the effects.

Since the mid-1990s the computers available in the office, the classroom and the home have become so ubiquitous that they have had the capacity to transform much research in education as well as the processes of instruction and learning. However, the full benefit of the computation that can be carried out by these powerful computers is not achievable without advances in the theory of measurement. Consequently, it is of interest to examine the major developments that have occurred in recent decades in educational measurement. It is also of value to emphasize the simplicity of the ideas involved, and the ease with which computers can be employed to carry out the necessary computation. In addition, it is important to indicate the potential that these developments in both educational measurement and computer analysis of data have for further advances in both educational research and practice.

Nevertheless, there is also sometimes a marked distrust of the use of computers and the application of measurement theory. The alternative of merely employing a verbal description has greater inherent dangers, since the same words mean different things to different people. Consequently, it is important to remember that while measurement and the computer analysis of data are not ends in themselves, there are many issues that can now be addressed as a result of the emergence of new measurement procedures and computer processing techniques.

Perhaps the most significant problem in education involves learning itself. That learning occurs in schools and homes is beyond doubt. However, so little is known about the factors that actually have been proved to influence learning, beyond the power of time as a variable, that a major issue of concern in educational research and practice, involves the study and advancement of learning. Progress in this field demands the more accurate measurement of learning over longer periods of time.

2. Advances in the Theories of Measurement

Nearly 100 years ago in 1905, Binet and Simon published the report of their initial scale for the assessment of intelligence. At approximately the same time Spearman published his model for test scores that laid the foundations of classical test theory. This theory, with its concepts of *true score, measurement error* and the index of *test reliability* dominated the field of educational and psychological measurement for approximately 50 years. In time a substantial body of statistical theory and related computational techniques was assembled, and entries on *Classical Test Theory, Measurement in Educational Research, Reliability, Scaling Methods* and *Validity* provide an account of current knowledge and understanding of educational measurement from this perspective. Nevertheless, two major issues emerged over time as significant problems. The first involved the estimation of the contribution of different sources of error to the total error variance associated with the use of a test. The second was related to the selection of items or tasks that were included in a particular version of a test, since most tests employed in education were formed as a combination of items or tasks. Although parallel forms could be developed for tests, in general, the selection of items was left to the judgment of test constructors or research workers who developed a particular instrument.

Gradually, two other competing theoretical approaches to educational and psychological measurement evolved. The theories involved have become known as *generalizability theory* which uses what might be referred to as a random sampling model, and *item response theory* for which a range of statistical models has been developed commonly based on the use of the logistic transformation. Generalizability theory remains relatively close to classical test theory, and is clearly oriented towards the obtaining of a total score. However, it differs from classical test theory in so far as the items employed are, in general, selected randomly from a pool of items. This enables the different components of variance to be calculated which are associated with variability between items and between persons, and enables reliabilities to be estimated for these different facets of error.

Item response theory is primarily concerned with the probabilities associated with the level of performance of an individual relative to a particular item. This leads to major differences between the two theories in the specification of the content being tested. In generalizability theory there is a pool of homogeneous items from which a sample of items can be drawn. Alternatively, it is possible to stratify items by type and content into a hierarchy of levels of difficulty from which sampling can occur. In item response theory, it is necessary to ensure that the items are located along a latent trait continuum, that is invariant across the groups of students to whom the test is given. However, provided the items satisfy this condition of unidimensionality the specific items employed in a test need not be randomly selected.

A further important difference between generalizability theory and item response theory, is that in generalizability theory the estimates of errors of measurement and the reliability of a test apply to the test as a whole. However, in item response theory it is possible to assign an estimate of error to each person and each item at each level of the continuum.

In classical test theory a correction for guessing on multiple choice items may be applied. However, this correction is likely either to underestimate or overestimate the extent to which guessing might have occurred on particular items, although it does not make allowance for the extent to which individuals might differ in their tendency to guess. In generalizability theory an adjustment could be made both for guessing and for carelessness using Bayesian procedures, but this necessarily applies to the test as a whole and not to individual items (Morgan 1979). However, in the three-parameter logistic model in item response theory an allowance is made for guessing with respect to each individual item, with the assumption that guessing is

a characteristic of items and not persons (see *Multiple Choice Tests, Guessing in*).

Criterion-referenced measurement (see *Criterion Referenced Measurement*) involves another theory of test construction and use which permits the interpretation of the performance of a person taking a test to be related to well-defined objectives (Popham 1978). There is, in addition, a type of criterion-referenced test referred to as a mastery test which is based on models of school learning (Carroll 1963, Block 1971, Bloom 1974). However, both of these approaches to test development encounter problems in the selection of items and the determination of an appropriate standard across all items in a test for the assignment of mastery, or for achieving a criterion level of performance.

Classical test theory has been employed, traditionally, in the construction of achievement tests. It may be referred to as 'weak true score' theory since it merely involves two assumptions that: (a) the observed raw scores can be decomposed into two additive components, namely, true score and error; and (b) repeated estimates of true scores for a person are not linearly correlated with the error scores for that person. The entry on *Classical Test Theory* argues that 'strong true score theory' which employs an appropriate statistical model awaits development, and when such development has occurred it could well replace existing procedures. However, towards the end of the twentieth century it is 'weak true score theory' that remains the most widely used approach for the construction and scoring of tests, as well as for other types of instrumentation in educational research and practice. Nevertheless, 'weak true score theory' presents many problems for the user including the dependence of the reliability estimate on the variability in the sample that was tested, as well as the deviation of the scale of scores from an interval scale, although with a large number of items the scale would seem to approximate satisfactorily to an interval scale. The main problem associated with the use of generalizability theory is that rarely is there a large pool of appropriate test items from which sampling could occur in the construction of a test (see *Item Banking*).

3. Conjoint Measurement and Item Response Theory

One of the major problems in measurement in education and in the social and behavioral sciences is that there is an interaction between the person being measured and the instrument involved in measurement at the time measurements are made. As a consequence the performance of a person is not independent of the measuring instrument employed. This uncertainty or confounding that arises between the person and the instrument is to some degree removed by the procedures of conjoint measurement proposed by Rasch in 1960. In conjoint measurement it is always the performance of a person relative to a particular item that is being considered in terms of probabilities. Thus a person's ability is set at the same level as the difficulty of an item if that person has a specified probability, commonly 50 percent, of responding correctly to the item.

Furthermore, clear benefits would be gained in educational measurement if the students measured by an instrument and the items in that instrument were located on a common scale. In this way the idea of a criterion level of performance could be replaced by the location of a student's level of performance with respect to particular items. Specific levels or standards of performance on a scale of this type could also be stated and shown in terms of either the characteristics of the items or the characteristics of the students or alternatively by a defined level on the scale, once a fixed point had been set to anchor the scale with respect to items or to students.

Rasch (1960) also proposed that the logistic function could be employed to construct an interval scale that would relate the position of an item on a scale, which was associated with the characteristic being measured, to a student's probability of success on that item. In the scale of conjoint measurement, when the level of performance of a student just matches the difficulty level of an item then the student would have a one to one chance or a 50 percent probability of answering the item correctly or incorrectly. The Rasch model is then constructed as a logistic function of the odds associated with the performance level of a person with respect to the difficulty level of an item.

The logistic transformation of the response odds enables the item and person parameters and their estimated values to be expressed as separate components on the conjoint scale. Conditional probabilities are then used to separate the person parameters from the item calibration, and the item parameters from the estimation of the person parameters. The requirement for this estimation procedure to provide meaningful results would be that both the items and the persons must fit a unidimensional model and behave in a consistent way across different samples. This requirement simply imposes a restriction, similar but not completely identical to that used in classical test theory, that should be satisfied before it is considered appropriate to add together item responses to obtain a total score.

In achievement testing using classical test theory such a restriction is sometimes applied through item analysis and item selection, although a sufficiently large number of items is commonly employed to prevent nonconforming items from having a damaging effect on a total score. In attitude and descriptive scale construction it has been an accepted practice for items to be eliminated from a scale if they did not satisfy this requirement (see *Attitudes, Measurement of; Descriptive Scales*) for the additivity of scores, which is similar to that of unidimensionality. The more restrictive requirements for Rasch scaling is a small price to pay for the advantages of measurement that are gained by using the logistic function to construct a scale of performance.

It should be noted that the Rasch scale is not only an interval scale, but also has its own natural metric, with the scale unit referred to as a logit. All that is required is that a fixed point should be specified in order to determine the location of the scale. In addition, the errors involved in the estimation of both the item difficulty parameters and the person performance parameters are obtained for each individual item and person, rather than for the instrument as a whole, provided conditions of independence of observation of items and persons are maintained. This scaling procedure eliminates the dependence of the item parameters on the sample of persons used in calibration, and the dependence of the person parameters on the sample of items used. Under these circumstances, the scale so formed has some properties of an absolute scale, but fails to have an absolute zero, being an interval, but not a ratio scale. Such a scale has substantial advantages in educational and psychological measurement, with the only requirement that the items and the persons used in the calibration of the scale must satisfy the condition of unidimensionality (see *Rasch Measurement Theory*).

3.1 Advantages of Rasch Measurement

Some of the immediately obvious advantages of the Rasch scale in educational measurement can be listed. First, in the equating of different instruments that are known to measure the same student trait or the same underlying dimension of performance, all that is required is the appropriate location of the zero points of the two scales in terms of the relative average difficulty levels of the items. The ease with which the equating of instruments (see *Equating of Tests*) on the same scale can be carried out, and the ease with which it is possible to test whether two instruments measure the same dimension, is of great advantage in the investigation of learning.

Second, when two subgroups drawn from a common population are administered the same calibrated instrument, they may differ considerably in their mean level of performance. However, the relative positions of the difficulty parameters of particular items on the calibrated scale would only change if items were biased with respect to the two groups (see *Item Bias*). The detection of biased items provides information of value in education, because the existence of bias reflects either differences in the learning experiences involved for providing a correct response to the item, or deficiencies in the construction of an item so that it would favor one particular group to the disadvantage of the other group.

Third, the location of persons on the same scale as items permits the ready identification of the inconsistent behavior of persons. A particular person might be expected to respond correctly to those items whose difficulty level was well below that person's performance level. This permits the accurate diagnosis of problems in student learning since items can be readily identified that a particular person is expected to get correct.

Fourth, while the tendency for a student to guess responses could have damaging consequences for the unidimensionality of a scale, if students were advised not to guess at random in responding to test items, then their scores could be accurately calculated using the information available on the set of items to which they responded. There would, however, be the need for the items to be calibrated on a scale using a sample of persons who had responded to all items. Furthermore, there would be the need for a student not to have omitted a subset of items that reflected a particular content bias. If these restrictions were satisfied, then the problem of guessing would be largely avoided.

Finally, in the estimation of a person's performance on a specific characteristic, it would be possible to select from a pool of calibrated items a subset of items which were close to that person's level of performance and to use a sufficient number of items in that subset to estimate that person's performance to a specified degree of accuracy. A computerized testing procedure, referred to as adaptive testing, (see *Adaptive Testing*) has been developed to facilitate the estimation of a person's performance without subjecting that person to a lengthy test containing a very large number of items that added little to the accuracy of estimation.

Some of these advantages of the Rasch model are shared with the two- and three-parameter item response models (see *Item Response Theory*) which introduce an item discrimination parameter and guessing parameter respectively to the model. The use of these alternative models requires large samples of persons for calibration and the estimation of these parameters of the model is no longer independent of the sample of persons or the items employed. The requirement that all items and persons involved in scale calibration should conform to the Rasch model has the benefits of simplicity and generality that are lost when the two and three parameter models are used. However, a price is paid for the use of the Rasch model, that involves the exclusion from calibration of nonfitting items and persons. However, estimates of person performance may nevertheless be made for those persons excluded, and considerable advantages are gained through improved measurement.

3.2 Extensions of the Rasch Model in Educational Measurement

Many variations of the simple Rasch model considered above have been developed by scholars in Australia, Europe and at the University of Chicago in the United States.

3.2.1 Rating Scale Analysis. Andrich (1978) developed a variation of the unidimensional Rasch model that allowed for polychotomous response categories and specified that the particular threshold parameter for each category was the same across all items contained in the scale. This model is of particular value in the analysis of performance ratings on a set of related characteristics, for attitude scales of the Likert type and for view or descriptive scales (see *Rating Scale Analysis; Descriptive Scales*).

3.2.2 Partial Credit Model. The partial credit model was formulated by Masters (1982) to provide a further extension of the unidimensional Rasch Model in order to include a different threshold parameter for each item and for each response category of a polychotomous response item. This model allows a different number of response categories for each item and this type of analysis is of particular value in the scaling of examination questions involving constructed responses, which are scored in the range from O to 9. Furthermore, the partial credit model can be used for the scaling of ratings and attitudinal and descriptive questionnaires in circumstances where the response categories differ across items (see *Partial Credit Model*).

3.2.3 Essay Scoring Model. Andrich has extended these procedures to the scoring of essay type questions, where marks are assigned in a range from 0 to 25, or more, and where it is extravagant and unnecessary to estimate all possible parameters. In this model the rating scale analysis model has been redefined so that the spread, skewness and kurtosis of a set of scores on several essays are taken into consideration. This model has considerable potential for use in the scaling of essay type examinations and other performance assessment tasks (see *Essays, Equating of Marks*).

3.2.4 Facet Model. In addition to the calibration of items and persons on a common scale, it is also possible to extend the Rasch model to include raters, markers, or judges, so that the performance of different raters can be measured on the same common scale beside items and persons. The only requirement for the employment of this model besides that of unidimensionality is that raters should be randomly assigned to items or should jointly rate all items. Likewise persons could be required to select without bias the items to which they wished to respond, if they did not respond to all items (see *Judgements, Measurement of*).

3.2.5 Saltus Model. In the investigation of developmental levels it may be assumed that there is not an underlying continuity between levels and that the levels involve a discrete transition, break in continuity or saltus. Wilson (1984) has proposed a variation of the Rasch model, the Saltus model, to allow for such systematic jumps in responding to achievement test items that are assumed to be related to different developmental levels (see *Developmental Levels, Measurement of*).

3.3 Multidimensional Models

It must be recognized that not all items might be measuring along same dimension, but it is a requirement for the use of the simple Rasch model that the items, their score categories and the persons must be located along a unidimensional scale. However, if it is meaningful to assign items to a restricted number of dimensions, then multidimensional analysis procedures could be employed in order to scale responses on more than one dimension, with the several scaled cores being measured with a common metric (Wilson and Adams 1993) (see *Latent Trait Measurement Models*).

The strengths of the Rasch model lie in the simplicity of the algebra involved as well as in the extension of the model to cover a range of situations. No longer is unidimensionality a restriction, provided a limited number of dimensions have been hypothesized, and the items and persons are constrained to those dimensions. There is no place for noise or for items and persons that do not conform to the dimensions specified in a model. If the necessary requirements of the model are satisfied, the benefits are substantial for the shift from deterministic approaches to measurement in education, to probabilistic and stochastic models in order to advance the accuracy of measurement. There remain some limitations associated with a ceiling or floor for a particular instrument when respondents answer correctly all items or no items respectively. However, the ceilings or floors are false in so far as the use of further items that conform to the unidimensional scale involved would permit the accurate estimation of performance. Thus unlike classical test theory, where the test or instrument is the scale, in Rasch scaling the scale is independent of the items in the test and the sample employed in calibration.

It must be recognized that problems are encountered if a latent trait scale does not remain invariant over the population being investigated. However, the capability exists to develop a scale that has the property of invariance, as well as to construct multidimensional scales. Insufficient work has been carried out into the use of multidimensional scales to determine the limitations imposed on the research questions that can be meaningfully investigated. In addition, further research is required into the robustness of scales measuring educational achievement in contrast to tightly defined cognitive abilities, as well as the validity of the results obtained under different circumstances.

4. Assessment, Evaluation and Measurement

The ideas of assessment, evaluation and measurement permeate much discussion in education. It is important to recognize that these three terms need to be interpreted separately and differently. However, in the minds of many researchers and practitioners these terms together with the topic of testing, would seem to be used interchangeably. What assessment, evaluation and measurement have in common is testing. Each frequently, but not always, makes use of tests. Nevertheless, none of these terms is synonymous with testing, and the types of tests required for each of the three processes may be very different. The three processes are considered below in reverse order.

4.1 Measurement

The regular dictionary definition of 'assigning a numerical quantity to . . .' serves well in most applications of educational measurement. While instruments such as rulers and stopwatches can be used directly to measure height and speed, many characteristics of educational interest must be measured indirectly. Thus ability tests are typically used to measure such characteristics as intelligence, and achievement tests are used to measure the amount of knowledge learned or forgotten. The items employed in these tests are manifestations of a latent variable. They are not the characteristic itself. Latent trait test theory, or as it is now known, item response theory, recognizes this separation and seeks to estimate performance on the underlying latent characteristic. Likewise, classical test theory also considers a *true score* as distinct from a *raw score*. However, classical test theory can only estimate a true score by using the group properties of a test, the reliability and standard error of measurement, unless multiple measures are obtained. Item response theory does not need to employ such concepts as reliability and standard error of measurement in the measurement of individual performance, since errors of estimation are calculated for each person separately. It is, nevertheless, apparent that measurement is not undertaken as an end in itself. It is a useful operation in the processes of evaluation, or for research where characteristics must be measured, or as part of the tasks of assessment of student performance.

4.2 Evaluation

In general, the use of the term "evaluation" is reserved for application to abstract entities such as programs, curricula and organizational situations. Its use implies a general weighing of the value or worth of something. Evaluation commonly involves making comparisons with a standard, or against criteria derived from stated objectives, or with other programs, curricula or organizational situations. Evaluation is primarily an activity involved in research and development. It may require the measurement of educational outcomes, and it may involve the testing of both individuals and groups. Its potential importance in the improvement of educational practice is widely recognized, but fierce controversy surrounds the issue of the methods that should be used and the part that measurement should play in the conduct of an evaluation. Indeed it is possible for an evaluation to be conducted that does not involve any measurement of observable characteristics and that makes judgements against specified criteria in a holistic way which involves an ethnographic approach to evaluation. Most judgements of an evaluative kind that are made in education would seem to be holistic in nature and to be based on a global examination of a situation.

4.3 Assessment

In general, the term "assessment" should be reserved for use with reference to people. It may include the administration of tests, or it may simply involve activities of grading or classifying according to some specified criteria. Student achievement in a particular course might be assessed, or students' attitudes towards particular aspects of their schooling might be examined. Such assessments are commonly based on an informal synthesis of a wide variety of evidence, although they might include the use of test results, or responses to attitude scales and questionnaires.

Attention is increasingly being given to improving the quality of assessment, through the systematic specification of levels in performance assessment. However, such assessments can be converted to a scale of measurement through the use of the partial credit model (see *Partial Credit Model*), or the scaling of essay marks (see *Essays, Equating of Marks*), and there is little need to view assessment as a process that does not involve measurement. It is, nevertheless, unfortunate that the term "student evaluation" is now being widely used as a consequence of the growing emphasis on the evaluation of educational programs and the financial support made available for such work. The use of the term student evaluation implies making a value judgment on the performance of a student that involves a consideration of the student's worth relative to other students. This is unnecessary and undesirable, because the development of a scale of achievement permits student learning to be examined, and learning is a responsibility which is shared by the student, the school, and the home. No longer is it necessary to consider a student's worth relative to other students, if the emphasis in education is on the facilitation of student learning and the attainment of standards of performance. Such an approach to the assessment of student performance would radically change the traditional procedures based on selection and competition.

4.4 Concerning the Entries in this Section

The entries in this section are subdivided into three parts. In the first part in an **Introduction to Measurement** entries are presented that relate to *Classical Test Theory and Generalizability Theory*, . The measurement issues and procedures considered in the entries involve those widely used procedures that have been traditionally employed in educational and psychological measurement.

In the second part on **Item Response Theory Measurement** entries are included that relate to item response theory which has been developed during the period since the early 1960s in order to advance the accuracy and strength of measurement in education and psychology. Many of the issues involved in item response theory have been raised in the earlier pages of this introduction. It is, however, necessary to comment that greater emphasis has been placed on Rasch measurement in this discussion than on the two-parameter and three-parameter models that are presented in the entry on *Item Response Theory*. This greater emphasis is a consequence of the stronger measurement properties that are seen to be associated with the Rasch model, and the greater range of problem situations in which it can be seen to be employed.

The third part on **Applications of Measurement in Research** presents entries that involve both classical test theory, and item response theory and are concerned with the uses of measurement in a wide range of problem situations. The entries, in general, consider the issues involved and the procedures adopted to confront these issues in order to make meaningful measurements. Research requires the careful design and construction of instruments to serve the purposes of inquiry and to establish relationships that represent in a coherent way phenomena in the real world.

References

Andrich D 1978 A rating formulation for ordered response categories. *Psychometri.* 43: 561–73

Andrich D 1995a Models for measurement, precision and the non-dichotomization of graded responses. *Psychometri.* 60: 7–26

Andrich D 1995b Further remarks on the non-dichotomization of graded responses *Psychometri.* 60: 37–46

Bejar I I 1983 *Achievement Testing: Recent Advances.* Sage, Beverly Hills, California

Block J H 1971 *Mastery Learning, Theory and Practice* Holt, Rinehart and Winston, New York

Bloom B S 1974 Time and Learning. *Am. Psychol.* 29: 682–88

Carroll J B 1963 A model of school learning. *Teach. Coll. Rec.* 64: 723–33

Cronbach L J 1960 *Essentials of Psychological Testing.* Harper and Row, New York

Kaplan A 1964 *The Conduct of Inquiry.* Chandler, San Francisco, California

Masters G N 1982 The Rasch model for partial credit scoring. *Psychometri.* 47: 149–74

Morgan G 1979 *A Criterion-referenced Measurement Model with Corrections for Guessing and Carelessness.* Australian Council for Educational Research, Hawthorn

Popham W J 1978 The case for criterion referenced measurements. *Educ. Researcher* 7 (11): 6–10

Rasch G 1960 *Probabilistic Models for Some Intelligence and Attainment Tests.* University of Chicago Press, Chicago, Illinois

Wilson M 1984 *Measuring Stages of Growth. A Psychometric Model of Hierarchical Development.* Australian Council for Educational Research, Hawthorn

Wilson M, Adams R J 1983 Marginal maximum likelihood estimation for the ordered partition model. *J. Ed. Stat.* 18 (1): 69–90

(a) Introduction to Measurement

Classical Test Theory

J. A. Keats

After a brief statement about measurement theory, this entry describes "weak true score theory," its implications and difficulties in practice. This section is followed by short statements on guessing in multiple choice tests, item homogeneity and "ordinal true score theory." The problems of weak true score theory gave rise to the development of "strong true score theory", which is described in detail. Finally there is a short section on the future of true score theory.

Although measurements of different kinds, such as educational and psychological, have been used for many centuries in different cultures, it is only in this century that theories of measurement have been developed. This fact raises the question of the role of theory when so much practical application has existed without it. One answer could be that although theory had not been enunciated it was implicit in practice: for example, the need for accurate standards of measurement became evident when subjective methods of marking essay examinations were found to be unreliable.

In mathematics, the need for an axiomatic approach became widely recognized in the late nineteenth century, and was also prevalent in the sciences in relation to physical measurement. Campbell's influential book on the theory of measurement was a result of this movement (see Campbell 1957). The practices of measurement could now be evaluated in terms of this theory.

Twenty-three years after the first publication of Campbell's book in 1917, a committee of the British Association for the Advancement of Science concluded that measurement in education and psychology was not of the same kind as physical measurement, in that the combining condition for physical measurement had no parallel in those disciplines (see Ferguson et al. 1940). In the early 1960s extensions of physical measurement to conjoint measurement axioms and theory were explicitly stated by Luce and Tukey (1964) and implicit in the work of Rasch (1980). Whereas physical measurement theory refers to a common attribute, say weight, of a certain class of objects, "conjoint measurement" refers to two classes of objects for which the interaction between one member of each class can be quantified in some way so that certain axioms are satisfied. Conjoint measurement could apply to educational and psychological measurement (see *Measurement in Educational Research*).

Weak true score theory can be seen as an application of the theory of errors in physical measurement without consideration of the question of whether or not this theory is applicable to test data. The most complete statement of weak true score theory was given by Gulliksen (1950). Strong true score theory is based on axioms which have been shown empirically to be more applicable to objective tests than those of weak true score theory. This stronger theory was published by Keats and Lord (1962), Keats (1964a, 1964b), and Lord (1965).

1. Weak True Score Theory

The assumptions of weak true score theory include the assumption of linear independence and the assumption that the observed quantity, the raw score, can be decomposed into two additive components: the true score and the error score. The assumption of linear independence asserts that repeated estimates of true score for the same person are not linearly correlated, which implies that true score and error score are not linearly correlated. From these assumptions it is possible to show that: (a) the variance of raw scores is equal to the variance of true scores plus the variance of error scores; (b) the correlation between two sets of raw scores from parallel tests, or the reliability of the tests over the population, is equal to the ratio of the variance of true scores to the variance of raw scores; and (c) if a test of reliability R is increased or decreased in length by a proportion k of its original number of items, the reliability of the new test will equal kR / which is known as the Spearman–Brown formula.

In order to estimate a true score range from a raw score it is necessary to assume that error variance is constant over raw score and that the regression of true score on raw score is linear. The first of these assumptions has been shown to be untrue in practice by Keats (1957), among others, while the latter assumption has broad implications, as will be shown below, and also may not be true in practice. Given these two assumptions, the formula proposed by Kelley (1947) would appear to be the most appropriate. This formula may be written as:

$$Est[T] = R_{x \cdot x} X + [1 - R_{x \cdot x}]M(X)$$
$$= M(X) + R_{x \cdot x}[X - M[X]$$

where $Est[T]$ is the estimate of true score; $R_{x \cdot x}$ is the reliability of the raw score, X; and $M(X)$ is the mean of X, which is of course equal to $M(T)$, the mean of T, since it is assumed that the mean of the error scores is zero.

The "reliability" of the raw score may be estimated in several different ways. It has been defined as the ratio of true score variance to raw score variance, which may be shown to be equal to the correlation between two tests of the same length and measuring the same characteristic. Thus, the correlation between scores on parallel tests provides a direct measure, but there is the problem of defining parallel tests. This problem may be tackled by matching tests item by item in terms of the difficulty and discriminating power of corresponding items. If the results of only one testing are available, two parallel tests of half the length can be formed by matching items and randomly allocating one of each pair to each of the parallel halves. The correlation between the two halves (r) is not a measure of the reliability of the total test (R), which is twice as long, but the Spearman–Brown formula $R = 2r/(1 + r)$ relates these two quantities. This formula generalizes to the formula $R = kr/([1 + k − 1]r)$ given above (see *Reliability*).

Other estimates of reliability may be obtained using the Kuder–Richardson formula 20 (KR20) and:

$$KR20 = \frac{n}{n-1}\left\{ 1 - \frac{nM(p)M(q) - n\,\text{Var}(p)}{\text{Var}(x)} \right\}$$

where n is the number of items, $M(p)$ is the mean of the item difficulties, $M(q) = 1 − M(p)$, $\text{Var}(p)$ is the variance of p, and $\text{Var}(X)$ is the variance of raw scores. In addition: $Alpha = n[1 − Sum\,\text{Var}(i)/\text{Var}(X)]/(n − 1)$ where $\text{Var}(i)$, $i = 1. . . . . .n$, is the variance within each of the n components. With only two possible scores within each component, *Alpha* is equal to *KR20*. However, *Alpha* assumes that the three or more item scores form an equal interval scale and this assumption is unlikely to be true in practice. Keats (1951) showed that *KR20* is uniquely related to the "concordance coefficient w" (Kendall and Gibbons 1990) and is thus a measure of the extent to which items order subjects in the same way. This relationship suggests a different method of scoring polytomous items using the mean rank of subjects giving each of the alternatives. With dichotomous items this leads to a linear transformation of the sum of item scores (Keats 1951) but this is not the case with three or more alternatives in each item. With three or more alternatives scored in the way suggested here, the coefficient W can be calculated and transformed into a generalization of *KR20*, which is different from coefficient alpha as usually calculated.

The other important concept arising from weak true score theory is that of "validity." In its simplest and most practical form this concept refers to the extent to which a test predicts future performance in a given situation. This is known as "predictive validity." Other types of validity include "face validity," which relates to the validity of the test as perceived by the person tested, and could therefore affect the motivation of that person.

"Construct validity" is usually defined by factor-analytic methods and relates to the extent to which the test measures a more general construct defined by a group of similar tests. "Content validity" is based on expert opinion. For practical purposes, predictive validity is the most important but should be determined for each applied situation. In this sense, tests are not generally valid but may be valid for a number of different situations (see *Validity*).

When it is proposed to use tests to replace complicated and expensive physiological examinations it is also important to show that the tests have "concurrent validity" in that they agree with the results of physiological examinations carried out at the same time. Because many forms of validity are based on correlation coefficients it is important to remember that the value obtained depends upon the variance of the group on the measures used to establish this validity. In general, validity also depends on reliability and can be shown to increase as reliability is increased, which is achieved by adding to the test further items measuring the same attribute.

One of the embarrassments of weak true score theory arises from the paradox that the more internally consistent a test is beyond a certain point, the lower is the correlation between raw score and true score. The paradox arises because the relationship between raw score and true score can become nonlinear at high levels of internal consistency.

This kind of embarrassment has led to the seeking of more satisfactory theories. The concept of reliability itself has been criticized on the grounds that its value is affected by restricting or expanding the range of true scores in the sample. What has less often been noted is that average error variance, and so the reliability measure, is also affected by the skewness of the raw score distribution. Thus the usefulness of the reliability coefficient can be questioned unless steps are taken to control these two factors. The concept of reliability has also been criticized on the grounds that it is an index that is applied to the whole test. Under "Item Response Theory" it is claimed that the information function for a test or even an item should be used instead of a single reliability coefficient (see *Item Response Theory*).

Weak true score theory leads naturally to the adoption of "standard scores" with a prescribed mean and standard deviation as the derived score to be used in practice. This approach, although widely followed, has some disadvantages. First, the standard score is often interpreted in terms of the normal distribution, so that a standard score of one standard deviation above the mean is taken to correspond to the 84th percentile of the population. The fact that test scores are not necessarily normally distributed (Keats 1951) shows that this interpretation is not valid.

To overcome this difficulty some test constructors proceed from the percentiles in the standardization sample directly to "normalized scores" with fixed mean and standard deviation, usually taken as 100 and

15 respectively. It would seem preferable to proceed from the estimated population percentiles to the normalized scores, but this practice is rarely followed (see ACER 1951 for an example of this method). Population percentiles can be estimated under the conditions of strong true score theory described below.

Another disadvantage of the approach of using standard scores for an age group as the derived score is that it precludes the possibility of measuring growth. This applies whether or not the derived scores have been normalized. The overall growth of ability within a population has been ironed out by setting the mean of each age group at 100. Bayley (1955) discussed this problem and attempted to solve it by ad hoc methods. This problem can be overcome by defining a latent ability variable which is on the same scale at all age levels.

A procedure which also derives readily from weak true score theory with the assumption of linear regression of true score on raw score is that of "linear equating." There are various methods of collecting and analyzing data with a view to equating the derived scores on two parallel tests. These methods are summarized by Angoff (1988).

It should be noted that if derived scores are obtained by normalizing through percentiles, then the appropriate method of equating is through estimates of population percentiles obtained by using methods described below under strong true score theory.

Another way of defining a derived score or "intelligence quotient" (IQ) stems from Binet and Simon (1916). A mean score by chronological age (CA) curve is defined empirically for the age range over which the test can be used. A person's score can be converted to a "mental age" (MA) by means of the graph, and thence to an IQ from the formula IQ = 100MA/CA. Mental age can also be estimated by defining a basal age in terms of items appropriate for each age level as the highest age at which a person succeeds on all of the items plus two months for each item passed beyond this age.

This approach, using the concept of mental age, has been questioned by Thurstone (1926) on the grounds that it can not be applied to people whose ability is above the adult average, and that the wrong regression line is used. The correct regression would be that of age on score rather than score on age. For these and other reasons this method has become less frequently used in practice. However, there are ways of meeting these criticisms and so preserving this approach, which has proved to be very useful for studying cognitive growth.

2. Guessing in Multiple Choice Questions

While true score theory can be applied to various types of testing and examination, the applications have been mainly in the area of objective testing of the multiple choice kind. In this type of testing the question arises as to the extent to which the subject can give the correct response by randomly guessing from a small number of alternatives—usually four or five, but sometimes as few as two, as in true-false questions.

The first suggestion for adjusting the number correct score (X) for guessing was referred to as formula scoring, which produced an adjusted score (X') by means of the formula:

$$X' = X - W/(N - 1)$$

where W is the number of wrong answers given and N is the number of alternatives. However, the assumptions of formula scoring have been found to be untenable (Hutchinson 1986) (see *Multiple Choice Tests, Guessing in*).

The guessing phenomenon was studied by Brownless and Keats (1958) using a method of repeated testing in which subjects were given a test in the standard way and then, without notice, were given the same test one week later. From data for two tests with five alternatives they found that the effective number of alternatives was 3.6 and 3.5.

Thus, to use five as the basis for inferring the probability of a correct response by guessing for all subjects would not be valid. The extent of guessing was much smaller on the verbal test than on the nonverbal test, but there was evidence that learning was greater on the nonverbal test while memory effects were smaller for that test.

In the case of three-parameter item response theories, a pseudo-guessing parameter (c) is introduced, which may be different for different items but is assumed to be the same for all subjects independent of their abilities. Using the model of Brownless and Keats (1958), which Wilcox (1982) has described as the first "state"—as opposed to trait—model of cognitive performance, it is possible to test the assumption that the effective number of alternatives is the same for all subjects, independent of their ability as measured by raw score. Keats and Munro (1992) report a study using this procedure with 755 subjects. The correlation between the average effective number of alternatives for each subject and score on the first testing was −0.53 and −0.43 for space rotations and mechanical reasoning tests respectively. The conclusion is that the effective number of alternatives, and so the probability of success by guessing, is significantly correlated to the ability of the subject.

To conclude this discussion of guessing, it should be noted that the inclusion of a term for guessing in the Rasch model as proposed by Keats (1974) destroys the consistency property of that model as shown by Colonius (1977).

Finally, de Gruijter and van der Kamp (1984 p. 177) have reported results that show that including the pseudo-guessing parameter in three-parameter models makes the difficulty and discriminating power parameters not comparable between items, and so makes them meaningless. Furthermore, although the pseudo-guessing parameter should theoretically always be greater than $1/N$, in practice estimates of this parameter are mostly less than this value. Keats and Munro (1992) provide a possible explanation for this finding.

In short, the problem of guessing has never been solved in either true score theory or item response theory. In the latter case the admission of such a phenomenon is contrary to the assumption that correct responses are due solely to the ability parameter. There is a strong argument for using only constructed response questions in situations such as tailored testing in which some form of latent trait or item response theory is essential.

3. Item Homogeneity

Before proceeding to the discussion of strong true score theory it is important to note a concept which was variously called unidimensionality, "item homogeneity", "local independence," and factorial purity, and was also variously quantified. Factor analysis was suggested by McDonald (1985) as a satisfactory method of testing for homogeneity.

Lord (1952) showed that such analysis could also be a test for local independence on the assumption that ability was normally distributed and that the item response curve was the cumulative normal distribution which implied the use of tetrachoric correlations. Local independence can be tested directly by considering the relationship between pairs of items for subjects at the same score level.

Item homogeneity can be thought of as an important adjunct to weak true score theory in that it provides a way of testing whether or not a collection of items constitutes a measure of a single homogeneous variable. However, it is assumed by strong true score theory based on the binomial error model, and is an essential assumption in latent trait theory and item response theory. A minor variation of the assumption is also used by Cliff (1989) in his "ordinal true score theory" discussed below.

4. Ordinal True Score Theory

Keats (1951) showed that raw score was linearly related to the sum of the orderings of subjects by each of the items and, as such, could form the basis for obtaining a best estimate of the true order in a sense associated with least squares (Kendall and Gibbons 1990).

These observations have suggested an ordinal true score theory of the kind proposed by Cliff (1989). He defined local independence of rankings by any pair of items in terms of the probability of their being in agreement on the ordering of subjects, and this is independent of whether or not either is in agreement with the true ordering. He showed that this was equivalent to requiring that the partial rank order correlation between the two items, given the true ordering, was zero, as measured by Kendall's partial tau (Kendall and Gibbons 1990). The similarity between this definition and the usual one for local independence is evident. He defined a true rank order without ties and, in addition to assuming local independence as defined for rankings, he also assumed the proportional distribution of subjects tied on one item

between those correctly and incorrectly ordered on the other. He then showed that many of the characteristics of reliability coefficients found in weak true score theory could be demonstrated in ordinal true score theory without having to assume interval scale properties, or define them in terms of conjoint measurement.

While Cliff's criticism of two- and three-parameter item response theory—that neither can form the basis of an interval scale—is sound, his only objection to the Rasch theory is on practical grounds, which may well apply in some form to ordinal true score theory. However, applications which require only an ordinal scale could well be based on this ordinal theory.

The major contribution of this work is to show that it is not necessary to assume interval scale properties to derive a theory which both yields many of the results of weak true score theory and does not seem to have some of the embarrassing paradoxes of weak true score theory.

5. Strong True Score Theory

The weaknesses of weak true score theory arise from the fact that estimates of true score cannot be obtained without making further assumptions about the constancy of error variance at different raw score levels and the linearity of the regression of true score on raw score. The variation of error variance with raw score was reported by Keats (1957) who suggested the formula:

$$\text{Error Variance} = x(n - x)/(n - 1)$$

where x represents raw score and n the number of items in the test. Thus error variance is equal to the estimated variance of a binomial distribution.

This model became known as the binomial error model, because the distribution of errors was binomial. It fitted published data relating error variance to raw score values. The binomial error model forms the basis of the only strong true score theory that has been thoroughly explored (see Keats and Lord 1962, Keats 1964a, 1964b). The general form of the theory may be stated as:

$$g(x) = \int_{-\infty}^{\infty} (^n_x) p^x (1 - p)^{(n - x)} f(p) \, dp$$

where $g(x)$ represents the frequency distribution of raw scores, p represents the probability of a correct response or relative true score ranging from 0 to 1, and $f(p)$ represents the frequency distribution of relative true scores. Keats and Lord (1962) showed that:

$$g(x + 1) [1 - \text{Mean}(p/x + 1)]$$
$$= (n - x) \, \text{Mean}(p/x) g(x)/(x + 1)$$

which related terms in the frequency distribution of raw scores to the regression of relative true score on raw score, which may or may not be linear.

In the case of linear regression of true score on raw score Keats and Lord (1962) have shown that the frequency distribution of raw scores is the negative hypergeometric distribution. Keats (1951) as well as Keats and Lord (1962) showed that this distribution gave a good representation of observed raw score distributions. In this special case the relative true scores are distributed according to the Beta function as the simplest possible case.

However, it is not necessary to assume linearity, as Keats (1964a) has shown that nonlinear regressions represented by orthogonal polynomials leads to natural generalizations of the hypergeometric distribution. From the bivariate distribution of raw score and relative true score, which can be generated numerically by methods described by Keats (1964a) and Keats and Lord (1962), the range of true scores corresponding to a given raw score can be estimated. Thus strong true score theory meets the two criticisms raised against weak true score theory if the generalized form of the hypergeometric distribution is used. This generalized form may be written as:

$$g(x) = [(-n)_x (a_1)_x (a_z) \, x. \ldots] / [(b_1)_x (b_z)_x \ldots x!]$$

where

$$(a_1)_x = a_1(a_1 + 1)(a_1 + 2) \ldots \ldots \ldots (a_1 + x - 1)$$

and a_1 and b_1 are constants of the linear regression of relative true score on raw score, and a_2 and b_2 are constants from the orthogonal parabolic component of regression and so on for cubic, quartic, and so forth, orthogonal components.

Another form of generalization of the beta binomial model which depends on linear regression of true score on raw score was proposed by Lord (1965). Instead of relaxing the linear regression assumption as in the case of generalized hypergeometric distribution, this proposal approximates the generalized binomial distribution and adds parameters a and b to the beta distribution such that $o < a < p < b < 1$, so that relative true score has a reduced range.

The first of these is introduced to take some account of differences in item difficulty and the second is to allow for guessing and fatigue, reducing the possible range of true score. While this form of strong true score theory produces a reduced chi-square value when fitting the raw score distribution, even to the extent of producing chi-square values which are significantly too small, it does not account for nonlinear regression of true score on raw score.

Although the complete form of the strong true score theory has been in the literature since 1964 it has never been included in standard texts, which seem to prefer the special form of the beta-binomial model which assumes linear regression of true score on raw score (see Lord and Novick 1968, de Gruijter and van der Kamp 1984). They do not provide methods for testing this assumption and, if significant curvilinearity is found, incorporating the degree of this curvilinearity into the model. In this respect the beta-binomial model, whether defined by two or up to six parameters, is not an improvement on weak true score theory but the "generalized negative hypergeometric model" is.

Given that the generalized hypergeometric distribution can produce theoretical frequencies which, when compared with observed frequencies at each score level, yield a total chi-square value close to the degrees of freedom, it is possible to generate percentiles that estimate the population percentiles. The aim is not to reduce the chi-square value to as low a figure as possible by adding further parameters because, if successful, this will simply preserve the sampling fluctuations in the data, and one might just as well use the sample percentiles. The estimates of the population percentiles can be used to produce normalized derived scores or to equate tests through percentiles.

Other ways of producing normalized derived scores have been suggested. In view of the binomial error model it is tempting to use the arc–sin transformation to stabilize the approximate error variance at each score level and produce a more nearly normal distribution, and this has been suggested with or without minor changes. Ikeda (1989), among others, has suggested the logit transformation, or a variation of this, as a means of obtaining a normalized derived score with constant error variance at each level. He was interested in producing a method which teachers could use without major calculations, and produced some impressive results.

Perhaps the most remarkable characteristic of the strong true score theory is its robustness. Keats (1964b) reported that, of eleven tests and data from samples ranging from 1,000 to 11,000 cases, two tests showed nonsignificant chi-square values for linear regression and three showed nonsignificant values for quadratic regression. Of the remaining six, four showed significance at the 5 percent level and only two showed significance beyond the 1 percent level. Cubic and higher order curvilinear regressions were not examined. Ikeda (1989) reported even more remarkable data for seven samples in the range 320,000–350,000 cases. Using only the assumption of linear regression of true score on raw score, four of the seven samples yielded chi-square values close to the degrees of freedom. Unfortunately the remaining three samples were not checked for quadratic or higher order regression. It should be noted that with such large samples, cluster sampling methods would have to be used and these would have the effect of reducing the effective number of degrees of freedom.

What makes this robustness of strong true score theory so remarkable is the fact that the theory leads to a representation of the frequency distribution of raw scores without taking into account the difficulties of the individual items. In other words, the theory assumes that the difficulties of items are equal, a possibility discussed by Keats (1967) in terms of combining individuals' performances.

On the other hand Lord (1965), in his presentation of a form of strong true score theory, weakened the assumption of equal item difficulty slightly and incorporated further parameters restricting the range of true scores. With these changes he was able to improve the goodness of fit to the observed frequency distribution to the extent that the chi-square value became significantly too small, and sampling fluctuations in the observed distribution were incorporated in the theoretical distribution. Such a result can hardly be thought of as desirable in practice or theory.

The concept of "item difficulty" used in most test theories is an average across subjects, and as such does not necessarily apply to any particular person. If a person gives the incorrect response to a question, it can be concluded that the question was too difficult for the person, without any implication as to its difficulty for a group of people. The difficulty of the test for the person is reflected in the person's score, which may be compared to another person's score to decide which has the greater ability in the field tested. In item response theories that use two or more item parameters, one item may appear more difficult than another for low scorers but easier than the same item for high scorers. This incongruity is avoided by the Rasch theorists who insist that items should be equal in discriminating power.

As stated earlier the binomial error aspect of strong true score theory shows that error variance is related to raw score by the formula:

$$\text{error variance} = x(n - x)/(n - 1).$$

Thus error variance depends only on the raw score and number of items in the test. If this quantity is averaged over a given sample of subjects it is possible to derive the formula for $KR21$ from the average error variance.

Once again the model behaves as if all items are of the same difficulty, but in this case there is a simple correction that can be made by defining $k = (1 - KR20)/(1 - KR21)$, where $0 < k \leqslant 1$ and:

$$\text{error variance} = kx(n - x)/(n - 1).$$

Keats (1957) showed that this formula gives a good representation of the graph of error variance against raw score for tests with moderate spread of item difficulty. Thus error variance is defined independently of reliability apart from the correction term, which should remain fairly constant across samples. However, average error variance and reliability will depend on the distribution of scores in the sample and so can hardly be considered as constant characteristics of the test.

In summary it can be said that strong true score theory based on generalized hypergeometric distributions derived from the binomial error model as shown here is complete in that the regression of true score on raw score, linear or nonlinear, leads to estimates of true scores for each raw score. Furthermore the bivariate distribution of true scores and raw scores can be estimated, and leads to confidence limits for the estimates of true score.

The assumptions of weak true score theory needed to obtain estimates of true score and confidence intervals for these include the assumption of linear regression of true score on raw score and constancy of error variance over raw scores, and normal distribution of true scores has been shown to be untenable in empirical data as well as in theory. As a consequence of these findings the concept of reliability as usually defined is practically useless as a basis for estimating true score and its confidence limits (de Gruijter and van der Kamp 1984 pp. 53–57).

A further criticism of weak true score theory in general arises from the factor analytic approach to test theory developed by McDonald (1985). He makes the point that raw score could be composed of general factor score, specific factor score, and error score, and shows that from this point of view certain formulas for reliability such as alpha and $KR(20)$ are biased downwards, unless the variance of specific factor scores is zero.

However, this approach usually assumes linear relationships between factor scores and raw scores and homoscedasticity which are assumed by weak true score theory, and have been shown to be untenable. Moreover, there seems to be no empirical evidence of the extent to which specific score variance is important. As McDonald (1985 pp. 215–16) concedes, and has been noted above, the reliability coefficient is of doubtful value. Whether it would be possible to develop a form of factor analysis which would be compatible with strong true score theory has yet to be established.

6. *Future Use of the Strong True Score Theory*

At the practical level, an atheoretical approach to testing will undoubtedly continue (with all its inefficiencies) as will weak true score theory, with its emphasis on item selection in terms of difficulty and discriminating power and on reliability coefficients which are often meaningless figures. As far as strong true score theory is concerned, it will be noted that this was formulated in the early 1960s at a time when the theory of conjoint measurement was also developing.

The practicability of using latent trait theory was increasing because of the availability of computers of greater speed and capacity. Thus, developments in latent trait theory, or item response theory as it has been called more recently, have been very rapid in the past 25 years. However, with its problems of unmet assumptions and uninterpretable parameters, as well as estimation difficulties noted above, the three- and two-parameter models may become less popular in future. This could well lead to a resurgence of interest in strong true score theory and an extension of its use in practice. The development of computers makes solving for the parameters of strong true score theory easy, and so its use in estimating true score and its confidence range, establishing norms, and equating tests is likely to increase.

See also: Measurement in Educational Research; Rasch Measurement, Theory of; Multiple Choice Tests, Guessing in; Scaling Methods

References

Angoff W H 1988 *Scales, Norms and Equivalent Scores.* Educational Testing Service, Princeton, New Jersey

Australian Council for Educational Research (ACER) 1951 *ACER Intermediate Test D.* Australian Council for Educational Research, Melbourne

Bayley N 1955 On the growth of intelligence. *Am. Psychol.* 10: 805–18

Binet A, Simon T 1916 *The Development of Intelligence in Children.* Loyd M Dunn, Honolulu

Brownless V, Keats J A 1958 A re-test method of studying partial knowledge and other factors influencing item response. *Psychometri.* 23(1): 67–73

Campbell N R 1957 *Foundations of Science* (formerly *Physics: The Elements*). Dover Publications, New York

Cliff N 1989 Ordinal consistency and ordinal true scores. *Psychometri.* 54(1): 75–91

Colonius H 1977 On Keats' generalization of the Rasch model. *Psychometri.* 42: 443–45

De Gruijter D N M, van der Kamp L J T 1984 *Statistical Models in Psychological and Educational Testing.* Publication Service, Amsterdam

Ferguson A, Meyers C S, Bartlett R J 1940 Quantitative estimation of sensory events. Final report. *Advancement of Science* 2: 331–49

Gulliksen H 1950 *Theory of Mental Tests.* Wiley, New York

Hutchinson T P 1986 Evidence about partial information from an answer-until-correct administration of a test of spatial reasoning. *Contemp. Educ. Psychol.* 11: 264–75

Ikeda H 1989 Applicability of logit transformation to test score. In: Keats J A, Taft R, Heath R A, Lovibond S H (eds.) 1989 *Mathematical and Theoretical Systems.* Proc. 24th Int. Congress of Psychology of the International Union of Psychological Science. North Holland, Amsterdam

Keats J A 1951 *A Statistical Theory of Objective Test Scores.* Australian Council for Educational Research, Melbourne

Keats J A 1957 Estimation of error variances of test scores. *Psychometri.* 22: 29–41

Keats J A 1964a Some generalizations of a theoretical distribution of mental test scores. *Psychometri.* 29: 215–31

Keats J A 1964b Survey of test score data with respect to curvilinear relationships. *Psychol. Rep.* 15: 871–74

Keats J A 1967 Test theory. *Annu. Rev. Psychol.* 18: 217–38

Keats J A 1974 Applications of projective transformations to test theory. *Psychometri.* 39(3): 359–60

Keats J A, Lord F M 1962 A theoretical distribution of mental test scores. *Psychometrika* 27: 59–72

Keats J A, Munro D 1992 The use of the test-retest method to study guessing, partial knowledge, learning and memory in performance on multiple choice tests. *Bulletin of the International Test Commission*

Kelley T L 1947 *Fundamentals of Statistics.* Cambridge University Press, Cambridge

Kendall M G, Gibbons J D 1990 *Rank Correlation Methods,* 5th edn. Edwin Arnold, London

Lord F M 1952 *A Theory of Test Scores.* Psychometric Monographs No. 7. University of Chicago Press, Chicago, Illinois

Lord F M 1965 A strong true score theory, with applications. *Psychometri.* 30: 239–70

Lord F M, Novick M R 1968 *Statistical Theories of Mental Test Scores.* Addison-Wesley, Reading, Massachusetts

Luce R D, Tukey J W 1964 Simultaneous conjoint measurement: A new type of fundamental measurement. *J. Math. Psy.* 1: 1–27

McDonald R P 1985 *Factor Analysis and Related Methods.* Erlbaum, Hillsdale, New Jersey

Rasch G 1980 *Probabilistic Models for Some Intelligence and Attainment Tests.* University of Chicago Press, Chicago, Illinois

Thurstone L L 1926 The mental age concept. *Psychol. Rev.* 33: 268–78

Wilcox R R 1982 Some empirical and theoretical results on an answer-until-correct scoring procedure. *Br. J. Math. S.* 35: 57–70

Criterion-referenced Measurement

R. K. Hambleton

Criterion-referenced tests are constructed to permit the interpretation of examinee test performance in relation to well-defined objectives (Popham 1978). There are three common uses for criterion-referenced test scores: (a) to describe the level of examinee performance, (b) to assign examinees to mastery states (e.g., "masters" and "nonmasters"), and (c) to describe the performance of groups of examinees in program evaluation studies. Criterion-referenced tests are receiving extensive use in schools, industry, and the military because they provide information which is valued by instructors and policy-makers and is different from the information provided by norm-referenced tests. This entry will describe: (a) basic criterion-referenced testing concepts; (b) norm-referenced versus criterion-referenced tests; (c) content specifications; (d) criterion-referenced test development; (e) measurement models, reliability, and standard setting; (f) applications of criterion-referenced tests; and (g) emerging trends and research.

1. Basic Concepts

The first article on the topic of criterion-referenced testing appeared in the *American Psychologist* (Glaser 1963). Over 1,000 papers on the topic have been published since then, and the scope and direction of educational testing has been changed dramatically. Glaser was interested in assessment methods that would provide information for making a number of individual and programmatic decisions arising in connection with specific objectives or competencies. Norm-referenced tests were seen as limited in terms of providing the desired kinds of information.

At least 57 definitions of criterion-referenced measurement have been offered in the literature. Popham's (1978) definition (see above) is the most widely used. Five points about the definition are important. First, terms such as "objectives," "competencies," and "skills" are used interchangeably in the field. Second, the objectives measured by a criterion-referenced test must be well-defined. Well-defined objectives make the process of item writing easier and more valid, and improve the quality of test score interpretations. The quality of score interpretations is improved because of the clarity of the content or behavior domains to which test scores are referenced. There is no limit to the breadth or complexity of a domain of content or behaviors defining an objective. The intended purpose of the test will influence the appropriate breadth and complexity of domains. Diagnostic tests are typically organized around narrowly defined objectives. End-of-year assessments would normally be carried out with more broadly defined objectives. Third, when more than one objective is measured in the test, examinee performance can be reported on each objective or group of objectives of interest. Fourth, Popham's criterion-referenced test definition does not include a reference to a cutoff score or standard. It is common to set a minimum standard of performance for each objective measured in a criterion-referenced test and to interpret examinee performance in relation to it. The use of criterion-referenced test scores for describing examinee performance is common (e.g., the best estimate of student A's performance in relation to the domain of content defined by the objective is 70 percent) and standards are not needed for this type of score use.

The fact that a standard (or standards) may not be needed with a criterion-referenced test may surprise some persons who have assumed (mistakenly) that the word "criterion" in "criterion-referenced test" refers to a "standard" or "cutoff score." In fact, the word "criterion" was used by Glaser (1963) and, later, by Popham and Husek (1969) to refer to a domain of content or behavior to which test scores are referenced. Finally, criterion-referenced testing is not synonymous with assessing low-level basic skills with multiple-choice items. All important educational outcomes can be assessed within a criterion-referenced framework, and the mode of assessment should be based on valid testing methods. Objective item formats, performance assessments, portfolios, as well as other formats which lead to valid information about examinee proficiency may be used in test development.

It is common to see terms like "criterion-referenced tests," "domain-referenced tests," and "objectives-referenced tests" in the psychometric literature. Popham's definition of a criterion-referenced test is similar to one that Millman and others proposed for a domain-referenced test. There are no essential differences between the two if Popham's definition

for a criterion-referenced test is adopted. The term "domain-referenced test" is a descriptive one and therefore it is less likely to be misunderstood than the term "criterion-referenced test." One reason for continuing to use the term "criterion-referenced test," even though it is less descriptive and its definition has become muddled in the psychometric literature, is that there is considerable public support for "criterion-referenced tests."

Objectives-referenced tests consist of items that are matched to objectives. The principal difference between criterion-referenced tests and objectives-referenced tests is that, in a criterion-referenced test, items are organized into clusters with each cluster serving (usually) as a representative set of items from a clearly defined content domain measuring an objective, while, with an objectives-referenced test, no clear domain of content is specified for an objective, and items are not considered to be representative of any content domain. Therefore, interpretations of examinee performance on objectives-referenced tests should be limited to the particular items on the test.

2. Norm-referenced versus Criterion-referenced Tests

Proponents of norm-referenced and criterion-referenced tests waged a battle in the 1970s for supremacy of the achievement testing world. A third group argued that there was only one kind of achievement test from which both criterion-referenced and norm-referenced score interpretations could be made when needed. It is clear that there was no winner, although the uses of criterion-referenced tests have increased substantially around the world. Also, a reduction in the amount of norm-referenced testing has taken place.

There was no winner in the debate because it is clear that it is meaningful to distinguish between two kinds of achievement tests, and both kinds of tests should have important roles to play in providing information for test users. Norm-referenced achievement tests are needed to provide reliable and valid normative scores for comparing examinees. Criterion-referenced achievement tests are needed to facilitate the interpretation of examinee performance in relation to well-defined objectives, and the uses of these tests extend well beyond schools to include the whole area of credentialing.

Although the differences between norm-referenced tests and criterion-referenced tests are substantial, the two kinds of tests share many features. In fact, it would be a rare individual who could distinguish between them from looking at the test booklets alone. They often use the same item formats; test directions are similar, and both kinds of tests can be standardized.

There are, however, a number of important differences between them. The first difference is test purpose. A norm-referenced test is constructed specifically to facilitate comparisons among examinees in the content area measured by the test. It is common to use age-, percentile-, and standard-score norms to accomplish the test's purpose. Since test items are (or can be) referenced to objectives, criterion-referenced score interpretations (or, more correctly, objectives-referenced score interpretations) are possible but they are typically limited in value because of the (usually) small number of test items measuring any one objective in the test. Criterion-referenced tests, on the other hand, are constructed to assess examinee performance in relation to a set of objectives. Scores may be used (a) to describe examinee performance, (b) to make mastery–nonmastery decisions, and (c) to evaluate program effectiveness. Scores can be used to compare examinees but comparisons may have relatively low reliability if score distributions are homogeneous.

The second difference is in the area of content specificity. It is common for designers of both test types to prepare test blueprints or tables of specifications. It is even possible that norm-referenced test designers will prepare behavioral objectives. But criterion-referenced test designers should prepare considerably more detailed content specifications than provided by behavioral objectives to ensure that criterion-referenced test scores can be interpreted in the intended way. This point will be considered further in the next section. Thus, with respect to content specifications, the difference between the two types is in the degree to which test content should be specified.

The third difference is in the area of test development. With norm-referenced tests, item statistics (difficulty and discrimination indices) serve an important role in item selection. In general, items of moderate difficulty (p-values in the range 0.30 to 0.70) and high discriminating power (point biserial correlations over 0.30) are most likely to be selected for a test because they contribute substantially to test score variance. Test reliability and validity will generally be higher when test score variance is increased. In contrast, criterion-referenced test items are only deleted from the pools of test items measuring objectives when it is determined that they are not consistent with the content specifications, violate standard principles of item writing, or if the available item statistics reveal serious noncorrectable flaws. Item statistics can be used to construct parallel forms of a criterion-referenced test or to produce a test to discriminate optimally between masters and nonmasters in the region of a standard of performance on the test score scale.

The fourth and final major area of difference between criterion-referenced tests and norm-referenced tests is test score generalizability. Seldom is there interest in making generalizations from norm-referenced achievement test scores. The basis for score interpretations is the performance of some reference group. In contrast, score generalizability is usually of interest with criterion-referenced tests. Seldom is there interest in the performance of examinees on specific sets of test items. When clearly specified objective statements are available, and assuming test items are representative of the content domains from which they are drawn, examinee test performance can be generalized to performance in the larger domains of content defining the objectives. It is this type of interpretation which is (usually) of interest to criterion-referenced test users.

3. Content Specifications

Behavioral objectives had a highly significant impact on instruction and testing in the 1960s and 1970s. But, while behavioral objectives are relatively easy to write and have contributed substantially to the specification of curricula, they do not lead to clearly defined content descriptions defining objectives. Popham (1974) described tests built from behavioral objectives as "cloud-referenced tests." Several suggestions have been made for addressing the deficiency in behavioral objectives and thereby making it possible to construct valid criterion-referenced tests. These suggestions include the use of item transformations, item forms, algorithms, and structural facet theory.

Possibly the most versatile and practical of the suggestions was introduced by Popham (1978) and is called "domain specifications," or sometimes "item specifications," or "expanded objectives." Domain specifications serve four purposes: (a) to provide item writers with content and technical guidelines for preparing assessment material; (b) to provide content and measurement specialists with a clear description of the content and/or behaviors which are to be covered by each objective, so that they can assess whether the assessment materials are valid; (c) to aid in interpreting examinee performance; and (d) to provide users with clear specifications of the breadth and scope of objectives. Some educational measurement specialists have even gone so far as to suggest that the emphasis on content specifications has been the most important contribution of criterion-referenced testing to measurement practice (Berk 1984).

Building on the work of Popham (1978), Hambleton (1990) suggested that a domain specification could be divided into four parts:

(a) *Description.* A short, concise statement of the content and/or behaviors covered by the objective.

(b) *Sample directions and test item/assessment task.* An example of the test directions and a model test item/assessment task to measure the objective.

(c) *Content limits.* A detailed description of both the content and/or behaviors covered by the objec-

The student will identify the tones or emotions expressed in paragraphs.

Sample directions and test item
Directions: Read the paragraph below. Then answer the question and circle the letter beside your answer.

Jimmy had been playing and swimming at the beach all day. Now it was time to go home. Jimmy sat down in the back seat of his father's car. He could hardly keep his eyes open.

How did Jimmy feel?

A. Afraid   B. Friendly   C. Tired   D. Kind

Content limits
1. Paragraphs will describe situations which are familiar to Grade 3 students.
2. Paragraphs should contain between three and six sentences. Readability levels should be at the third grade (using the Dale-Chall formula).
3. Tones or emotions expressed in the passages should be selected from the list below:

sad	mad	angry	kind
tired	scared	friendly	excited
happy	lucky	smart	proud

Response limits
1. Answer choices should be one word in length.
2. Four answer choices should be used with each test item.
3. Incorrect answer choices may be selected from the list above.
4. Incorrect answer choices should be tones or emotions which are familiar to students in Grade 3 and which are commonly confused with the correct answer.

Figure 1
A typical domain specification in the reading area

tive, as well as the structure and content of the item pool. (This section should be clear enough so that items/assessment tasks may be divided by reviewers into those items/assessment tasks that meet the specifications and those items/assessment tasks that do not.) Sometimes clarity is enhanced by also specifying areas which are not included in the content domain description.

(d) *Response limits.* if objective item formats are used, a description of the kind of incorrect answer choices which should be prepared is provided. The structure and content of the incorrect answers should be stated in as much detail as possible. If performance tasks are used as the assessment mode, this section should describe the details for scoring the examinee's work.

An example of a domain specification using multiple-choice test items as the assessment mode is shown in Fig. 1. Once properly prepared domain specifications are available, the remaining steps in the test development process can be carried out.

4. Criterion-referenced Test Development

It is essential to specify clearly the domain of content or behaviors defining each objective which is to be measured in the test. The mechanism through which the objectives are identified will vary from one situation to the next. For high school graduation exams, the process might involve district educational leaders meeting to review school curricula and identifying a relatively small set of important broad objectives (e.g., reading comprehension, mathematics computations). When criterion-referenced tests are needed in an objectives-based instructional program, it is common to define a curriculum in broad areas (and sometimes into a two-dimensional grid). Then, within the cells of the grid, the sets of relevant objectives, often stated in behavioral form, are specified, reviewed, revised, and finalized. With certification exams, it is common to first conduct a "role delineation study" with individuals working in the area to identify the responsibilities and activities which serve to define a role. Next, the knowledge and skills which are needed to carry out the role are identified.

A set of 12 steps for preparing criterion-referenced tests adapted from Hambleton (1990) is suggested in Table 1.

5. Measurement Models, Reliability, and Standard Setting

Throughout the 1970s and early 1980s, numerous statistical models were advanced to provide criterion-referenced measurement with a solid technical foundation. The special issue of *Applied Psychological Measurement* published in the fall of 1980 still remains in 1993 as one of the most useful single references on criterion-referenced measurement models and reliability assessment (Hambleton 1980).

The binomial test model and (less frequently) the compound binomial test model have been used as a basis for estimating examinee proficiency, determining test length, assessing reliability, and setting standards (see Hambleton et al. 1978). Other researchers have applied decision theoretic models, latent class models, random sampling models, and item response models to various technical topics (van der Linden 1980).

The major breakthrough in criterion-referenced test reliability was the recognition that, when mastery–nonmastery decisions are the focus of attention, reliability of decisions (over parallel-forms or a retest

Table 1
Steps for constructing criterion-referenced tests

Steps	Comments

1. Preliminary considerations:
  (a) Specify test purposes.
  (b) Specify groups to be measured and (any) special testing requirements (due to examinee age, race, sex, socioeconomic status, handicaps, etc.).
  (c) Determine the time and money available to produce the test.
  (d) Identify qualified staff.
  (e) Specify an initial estimate of test length.
	This step is essential to ensure that a test development project is well-organized, and that important factors which might have an impact on test quality are identified early.

2. Review of objective statements; write domain specifications:
  (a) Review the descriptions of the objectives to determine their acceptability.
  (b) Make necessary objective statement revisions to improve their clarity.
  (c) Write and review the domain specifications.
	Domain specifications are invaluable to assessment material writers when they are well-done. Considerable time and money can be saved later in revising assessment materials if the writers are clear on what it is that is expected of them.

3. Item writing:
  (a) Draft a sufficient amount of assessment material for pilot testing.
  (b) Carry out editing.
	Some training of assessment material writers in the importance and use of domain specifications, and in the principles of assessment material writing is often essential.

4. Assessment of content validity:
  (a) Identify a sufficient pool of judges and measurement specialists.
  (b) Review the test material to determine their match to the objectives, their representativeness, and their freedom from bias and stereotyping.
  (c) Review the test materials to determine their technical adequacy.
	This step is essential. Assessment materials are evaluated by reviewers to assess their match to the objectives, their technical quality, and their freedom from bias and stereotyping.

5. Revisions to test materials:
  (a) Based upon data from 4(b) and 4(c), revise test materials (when possible) or delete them.
  (b) Write additional test material (if needed) and repeat step 4.
	Any necessary revisions to test material should be made at this step and, when additional test materials are needed, they should be written, and step 4 carried out again.

6. Field test administration:
  (a) Organize the test material into forms for pilot testing.
  (b) Administer the test forms to appropriately chosen groups of examinees.
  (c) Conduct item analyses, and validity and bias studies.
	The test material is organized into booklets and administered to appropriate numbers of examinees. That number should reflect the importance of the test under construction. Appropriate revisions to test material can be made here. Item statistics are used to identify items which may be in need of revision: (a) items/tasks which may be substantially easier or harder than other items/tasks measuring the same objectives, and (b) items/tasks with negative or low positive discriminating power.

7. Revisions to test material: (a) Revise test materials when necessary or delete them using the results from 6(c).	Whenever possible, malfunctioning test material should be revised and added to the pools of acceptable test material. When revisions to test material are substantial, they should be returned to step 4.

8. Test assembly:
  (a) Determine the test length, and the number of forms needed and the number of items/tasks per objective.
  (b) Select test items/tasks from the available pool of valid test material.
  (c) Prepare test directions, practice questions, test booklet layout, scoring keys, answer sheets, etc.
	Test booklets are compiled at this step. When parallel forms are required, and especially if the tests are short, item/task statistics should be used to ensure matched forms are produced.

Table 1 (continued)
Steps for constructing criterion-referenced tests

Steps	Comments
9. Selection of a standard: (a) Initiate a process to determine the standard to separate "masters" and "nonmasters."	A standard-setting procedure must be selected and implemented. Care should be taken to document the selection process.
10. Pilot test administration: (a) Design the administration to collect score reliability and validity information. (b) Administer the test form(s) to appropriately chosen groups of examinees. (c) Evaluate the test administration procedures, test items/tasks, and score reliability and validity. (d) Make final revisions based on data from 10(c).	At this step, test directions can be evaluated, scoring keys/guides can be checked, and reliability and validity of scores and decisions can be assessed.
11. Preparation of manuals: (a) Prepare a test administrator's manual. (b) Prepare a technical manual.	For important tests, a test administration manual and a technical manual should be prepared.
12. Additional technical data collection: (a) Conduct reliability and validity investigations.	No matter how carefully a test is constructed or evaluated, reliability and validity studies should be carried out on an ongoing basis.

administration) is more important than test score reliability (as reflected in the myriad of norm-referenced test score reliability indices). Various single and double test administration decision consistency indices have entered the measurement literature since 1973 (see Hambleton and Novick 1973, Traub and Rowley 1980, Berk 1984).

Standard setting (see *Standard Setting in Criterion-referenced Testing*) is the most controversial aspect of criterion-referenced measurement and is central to many applications. Numerous methods currently exist for standard setting. The most popular of the judgmental methods is the "Angoff method" which involves a group of judges determining how minimally competent examinees (i.e., borderline examinees) will (or should) perform on the items/tasks in the test. The most popular of the empirical methods is the "contrasting groups method" which involves identifying groups of "masters" and "nonmasters" and then considering their actual performance on the test. The standard is set to minimize some function of the false-positive and false-negative errors. For example, it is common in testing practice to choose a standard which minimizes the sum of false-positive and false-negative errors. False-positive errors result when "nonmasters" pass the test; false-negative errors result when "masters" fail the test. When the sum of these errors is used as the function to minimize in standard setting, both errors are being considered equally important. Other loss functions may be chosen to weight the two types of errors differently.

6. Applications of Criterion-referenced Tests

Criterion-referenced tests (or domain-referenced tests, mastery tests, competency tests, basic skills tests, or certification exams, as they are alternatively called) are being used in a large number of settings. Criterion-referenced tests are finding substantial use in schools. Classroom teachers use criterion-referenced test score results to locate students correctly in school programs, to monitor student progress, and to identify student deficiencies. Special education teachers are finding criterion-referenced test scores especially helpful in diagnosing student learning deficiencies and monitoring the progress of their students. Criterion-referenced test results are also being used to evaluate school programs. While it is less common, criterion-referenced tests are finding some use in higher educational programs as well (e.g., those programs based upon the mastery learning concept). Also, criterion-referenced tests are in common use in military and industrial training programs.

It has become common for departments of education and (sometimes) school districts to define sets of skills (or objectives) which students must achieve in order to be promoted from one grade to the next, or, in some states, to receive high school diplomas. The nature of these criterion-referenced testing programs varies dramatically from one place to another. For example, in some places, students are held responsible for mastering a specified set of skills at each grade level. In other places, skills which must be acquired are specified at selected grade levels, and in still other places, only a set of skills which must be mastered for high school graduation is specified.

One of the most important applications of criterion-referenced tests is to the areas of professional certification and licensure. It is common, for example, for professional organizations to establish entry-level examinations which must be passed by candidates before they are allowed to practice in their chosen professions. In fact, many of these professional organizations have also established recertification exams. A typical examination will measure the competencies which define the professional role and candidate test performance is interpreted in relation to minimum standards which are established. Hundreds of professional organizations, including most groups in the medical and allied health fields, have instituted certification and recertification exams.

7. Emerging Trends and Research

Without a doubt, the most important trends in criterion-referenced measurement in the early 1990s involve: (a) the assessment of higher level cognitive objectives such as critical thinking, reasoning, problem-solving, and writing; and (b) more use of performance assessments such as constructed response questions, projects, and portfolios (Hambleton 1993). Both trends are being stimulated by massive school reform movements, advances in cognitive psychology, and shortcomings with the multiple-choice test item format. But, with both trends, substantial research is needed in defining these higher level objectives and assessing them with appropriate levels of reliability and validity. Standard-setting methods, which can be applied to performance task data, is an especially important topic for additional research.

See also: Measurement in Educational Research Evaluation Models and Approaches

References

Berk R A (ed.) 1984 *A Guide to Criterion-Referenced Test Construction.* Johns Hopkins University Press, Baltimore, Maryland

Glaser R 1963 Instructional technology and the measurement of learning outcomes. *Am. Psychol.* 18: 519–21

Hambleton R K (ed.) 1980 Contributions to criterion-referenced testing technology. *Appl. Psychol. Meas.* 4: 421–581

Hambleton R K 1990 Criterion-referenced testing methods and practices. In: Gutkin T, Reynolds C (eds.) 1990 *The Handbook of School Psychology*, 2nd edn. Wiley, New York

Hambleton R K 1993 The rise and fall of criterion-referenced measurement? Paper presented at the joint meeting of AERA and NCME, Atlanta, Georgia

Hambleton R K, Novick M R 1973 Toward an integration of theory and method for criterion-referenced tests. *J. Educ. Meas.* 10: 159–70

Hambleton R K, Swaminathan H, Algina J, Coulson D B 1978 Criterion-referenced testing and measurement: A review of technical issues and developments. *Rev. Educ. Res.* 48: 1–47

Popham W J 1974 An approaching peril: Cloud-referenced tests. *Phi Del. Kap.* 55: 614–15

Popham W J 1978 *Criterion-Referenced Measurement.* Prentice-Hall, Englewood Cliffs, New Jersey

Popham W J, Husek T R 1969 Implications of criterion-referenced measurement. *J. Educ. Meas.* 6: 1–9

Traub R E, Rowley G R 1980 Reliability of test scores and decisions. *Appl. Psychol. Meas.* 4: 517–46

van der Linden W J 1980 Decision models for use with criterion-referenced tests. *Appl. Psychol. Meas.* 4: 469–92

Decision Theory in Educational Testing

W. J. van der Linden

In most educational situations, tests are used for decision-making rather than measurement purposes. The ultimate purpose in these cases is to use test scores not as quantitative ability estimates but merely as data on which qualitative decisions can be based. Examples of such decisions are admissions to training programs, pass–fail decisions, certification, treatment assignment in individualized instructional systems, and the identification of optimal vocational alternatives in guidance situations. In all of these examples, decisions are ordinarily based on cutting scores carefully selected in order to optimize the actions to be taken.

In spite of the fact that tests are used mostly for decision-making, much psychometric research has been aimed at improving the use of educational and psychological tests as means for estimating ability scores from test performances. The first to recognize this paradox were Cronbach and Glaser (1965) in their classical monograph *Psychological Tests and Personnel Decisions*. At first their plea for a more decision–theoretical approach to testing had more impact on (personnel) psychologists than on educators. During the 1970s, however, the situation changed dramatically, and in the mid 1990s the use of decision theory in educational testing is one of the main research topics. The major impetus for this has come from the introduction of novel testing procedures in individualized instructional systems, and from such politically controversial issues as culture-fair selection for schools.

This entry describes the various decision problems that can be met in the practice of educational testing and shows how (Bayesian) decision theory can be applied to optimize the use of tests for decision-making.

1. A Typology of Test-based Decision-making

Test-based decisions can be classified in many ways. A simple typology is the following, which is based on the use of flowcharts to define different types of decision-making. In each decision problem, three common elements can be identified: (a) the test that provides the information the decision is based on, (b) the treatment with respect to which the decision is made, and (c) the criterion by which the success of the treatment is measured. "Treatment" is a generic term here, standing for any manipulation aimed at improving the condition of individuals. Examples include training programs, the use of special instructional materials, therapeutic measures, and the like. The criterion may be any type of success measure, but is often a test itself. With the aid of these elements, four basic flowcharts can be formed, each defining a different type of decision-making.

1.1 Selection Decisions

In selection problems, the decision is whether or not to accept individuals for a treatment. The test is administered before the treatment takes place and only individuals promising satisfactory results on the criterion are accepted. Selection decisions may imply that individuals who are rejected are not admitted to the institute providing the treatment, or have to leave the institute if they were already in it. Figure 1 shows the flowchart of a selection problem. Examples of selection decisions are admission examinations to schools, hiring of personnel in industry, or the intake of students for a remedial program.

The selection problem is the oldest decision problem in the history of educational testing. Traditionally, the problem has been approached as a prediction problem in which regression lines or expectancy tables are employed to predict whether the criterion scores of individuals exceed a certain value. Only individuals with criterion scores above the threshold are accepted. Selection decisions with quota restrictions (see below) have long been evaluated with the aid of Taylor–Russell (1939) tables, which give success ratios for a number of parameters characterizing the selection situation (see *Regression of Quantified Data*).

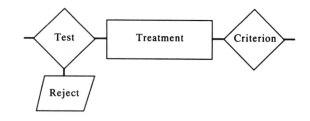

Figure 1
Flowchart of a selection decision

1.2 Mastery Decisions

Mastery decisions are made for individuals who have already undergone a treatment. Unlike selection decisions, the question is not whether individuals are qualified for admittance to a treatment, but whether they have profited enough from a treatment to be dismissed. Figure 2 shows the flowchart of a mastery decision. For this type of decision problem the test and the criterion coincide. More particularly, the test is an unreliable representation of the criterion, or, equivalently, the criterion can be considered the true score underlying the test. As the test is unreliable, erroneous decisions are possible and a mastery decision problem exists.

Mastery decisions usually imply that individuals may leave the institute providing the treatment, or proceed with another treatment. Examples of mastery decisions are pass–fail decisions, certification decisions, and decisions with respect to therapeutic success.

Interest in mastery decisions has grown because of the introduction of such modern instructional systems as individualized instruction, mastery learning, and computer-aided instruction. In the past the main concern has been for issues related to standard setting procedures; that is, to procedures for selecting threshold values on the (true-score) criterion separating "masters" from "nonmasters." The influence of measurement error on decision-making was simply ignored. That this may lead to serious decision errors was clearly demonstrated by Hambleton and Novick (1973).

1.3 Placement Decisions

This type of decision problem differs from the preceding two in that alternative treatments are available.

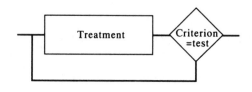

Figure 2
Flowchart of a mastery decision

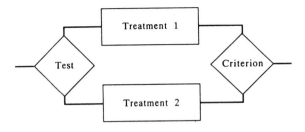

Figure 3
Flowchart of a placement decision (case of two treatments)

The success of each treatment is measured by the same criterion. All individuals are administered the same test, and the task is to assign them to the most promising treatment on the basis of their test scores. Unlike the selection problem, each individual is assigned to a treatment. The case of placement decisions with two treatments is represented in Fig. 3. Examples of placement decisions can be found in individualized instruction, where students typically are assigned to different routes through an instructional unit or are offered alternative instructional materials.

Interest in placement decisions has emanated from aptitude-treatment interaction (ATI) research, which was motivated by the finding that individuals may react differentially to treatments and that above average treatments may be worse in individual cases. The placement decision problem has mostly been approached as a prediction problem to be tackled using linear-regression techniques. For each treatment there is a regression line of the criterion on the test score, and individuals are assigned to the treatment with the largest predicted criterion score. The methodology needed for detecting ATIs is reviewed in Cronbach and Snow (1977).

1.4 Classification Decisions

In classification decisions, the problem also consists of a choice among a number of different treatments. As opposed to placement decisions, however, each treatment has a different criterion. The situation is as shown in Fig. 4. In order to be able to compare criterion performances across different treatments, it is necessary to transform each criterion to a common utility scale. Examples of classification decisions can be found in vocational guidance situations in which most promising schools or careers must be identified or in testing for military service.

The most popular approach to classification decisions has been the use of linear-regression techniques again. For each treatment, the regression line of its utility (which equals transformed criterion) scores on the test scores is estimated and individuals are assigned to the treatment with the largest predicted utility score. Usually, as more than one criterion is present, there is not a single test, but a battery of tests covering the various aspects of all of the criteria. If so, the use of multiple- rather than bivariate-regression techniques has been the traditional choice.

1.5 Combinations of Elementary Decisions

In practice, the decisions in the above typology are mostly met in combination. A simple example is a decision problem in which more than one treatment is available, but not all individuals are accepted for a treatment. These features create a combination of a selection and a placement problem. Another example is a selection decision, where after the treatment a mastery test is administered to assess its success. However, all such combinations of decisions can be mapped on flowcharts built up of Figs. 1–4 as elements.

A new development is to simultaneously optimize decision rules for systems of combinations of decisions rather than to optimize the individual decisions one at a time (Vos 1990, 1991, Vos and van der Linden 1987). The advantage of a simultaneous approach is that more realistic utility structures can be adopted; for example, structures in which the utilities involved the separate decisions are modeled as a function of an individual's position on the last criterion in the system. Also, test scores on one test automatically provide collateral information for decisions based on scores on other tests. A practical application of simultaneous optimization of decision rules is individualized instruction, for example, as implemented in CAI systems. In such systems, at various points of time small sets of items are used to make a selection, mastery, or placement decision.

1.6 Possible Constraints and Extensions

For each type of decision-making, one or more of the following constraints or extensions may be in force:

(a) Quota restrictions. In some cases, the number of vacancies per treatment is constrained by a quota. Such quotas usually simplify the derivation of optimal rules for selection decisions (accept individuals with the highest test scores until the quota is filled), but complicate placement or classification decisions.

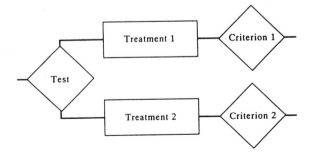

Figure 4
Flowchart of a classification decision (case of two treatments)

(b) Multiple criteria. More than one criterion can be necessary to measure success of treatments. In decision theory such cases are known as multiple-objective or multiattribute decision-making. Methodology to analyze cases with multiple criteria is given in Louviere (1988).

(c) Multiple tests. The presence of multiple criteria may also be a reason to replace a single test by a full battery of tests. As a consequence, the decision must be made on the basis of multivariate information, which complicates the decision rule.

(d) Multiple populations. In some applications, populations varying on a socially relevant attribute can be distinguished. If the test is biased against one of the populations, the problem of fair decision-making arises (Gross & Su 1975, Novick and Petersen 1976).

(e) Adaptative testing. Tests may be administered adaptively, selecting consecutive items to match the current estimate of the individual's ability. In this case, decision rules have to be modified accordingly, for example, using the framework of sequential Bayesian decision-making (Lindgren 1976).

2. Optimizing Decisions Based on Tests

Decision theory is a branch of statistics addressing the use of data as an aid in decision-making. More specifically, it is concerned with how random data on "true" or future states of nature and utilities associated with the possible outcomes of the decision process can be combined to design optimal decision rules. In the above decision problems, the data are provided by a test. Since a test may not produce reliable data, it has to be considered a random indicator of an individual's performance. For a population of individuals, test and criterion scores relate to each other in a way that is fully specified by their joint probability distribution. In some decision problems, a psychometric model is needed to specify this distribution.

Several approaches to optimizing decisions can be taken, one of which is Bayesian decision theory. It is indicated below how (empirical) Bayesian theory tackles the four decision problems and provides optimal decision rules (called Bayes rules). First, the Bayesian solution to a classification problem is described. This problem, in a formal sense, is the most complicated decision problem. Then, it will be indicated how solutions to the other decision problems can be obtained by imposing certain restrictions and modifications on the classification model. To enhance understanding, however, in treating these topics some mathematical precision will be sacrificed (see *Bayesian Statistics in the Analysis of Data*).

The classification problem is formalized as follows.

Suppose a series of individuals, who can be considered as being randomly drawn from a population, must be classified into $t + 1$ treatments indexed by $j = 0, \ldots, t$. The observed test scores are denoted by a random variable X with discrete values $x = 0, \ldots, n$. Each treatment leads to a certain performance on its corresponding criterion, which is denoted by a continuous random variable Y_j with range R_j. It is assumed that the joint distributions of X and Y_j are given by probability functions $\eta_i(x, y_i)$. Since all individuals are administered the same test, it holds for the marginal probability function $\lambda_i(x)$ of X that:

$$\lambda_j(x) = \lambda(x) \tag{1}$$

for all values of j.

Generally, a decision rule is a function that indicates for each possible observation which of the possible actions is to be taken. In the present problem the observations take the form $X = x$, and the possible actions are the assignments to one of the treatments $0, \ldots, t$. It is assumed that the optimal rule takes a monotone form; that is, it can be defined using a series of cutting scores $0 = c_0 \leqslant c_1 \ldots \leqslant c_j \leqslant \ldots \leqslant c_{t+1} = n$ $(t \leqslant n)$, where treatment j is assigned to individuals whose scores satisfy $c_j \leqslant X < c_{j+1}$. For an optimal rule to be monotone, some conditions must be met (Ferguson 1967), which are not unrealistic for the present problems.

Suppose that, for individuals assigned to treatment j, the decision-maker is able to express his or her preferences for the outcomes $Y_j = y_j$ on a numerical scale. Technically, such an evaluation is known as a utility function. If utility functions can be established for all treatment–criterion combinations, all possible outcomes of the decision have been made comparable on a common scale. To express its dependency on both the criterion and the chosen treatment, utility functions will be denoted as $u = u_j(y_j)$. Figure 5 shows some examples of utility functions that have received some interest in the literature. The threshold function represents the case where a critical value on the criterion discriminates between successful and unsuccessful performances. The other two functions increase more gradually with the criterion performance. The choice of a utility function may be facilitated by varying its form and studying the robustness of the optimal decision rule to these variations (e.g., Vijn and Molenaar 1981).

For each possible series of cutting scores $(c_1, \ldots, c_t)$ the expected utility of the decision procedure can be calculated as:

$$B(c_1, \ldots, c_t) \equiv \sum_{j=0}^{t} \sum_{i=1}^{c_{j+1}} \int_{R_j} u_j(y_j) \, \eta_j(x, y_j) dy_j \tag{2}$$

The set of optimal cutting scores in the Bayesian sense is the choice of values for $(c_1, \ldots, c_t)$ maximizing the expected utility. A simple procedure to find these values is as follows. Using Eqn. (1) the expected utility can be written as:

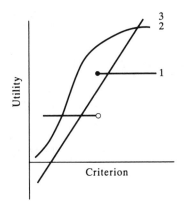

Figure 5
Examples of utility functions: (1) threshold; (2) normal ogive;
(3) linear

$$B(c_1, \ldots, c_t) \equiv \sum_{j=0}^{t} \sum_{i=1}^{c_j+1-1} \lambda(x) \int_{R_j} u_j(y_j)\, \omega_j(y_j | x) dy_j$$

(3)

where $\omega_j(y_j|x)$ is the conditional probability function of y_j given $X = x$. For known utility and probability functions, the integral in this expression only depends on x and j. As $\lambda(x) \geq 0$, the double sum in Eqn. (3) is maximized if for each possible value of x the value of j is selected for which the integral is maximal. The monotone character of the problem, assumed here, guarantees that the optimal value of j changes at a series of cutting scores on x. More theory on Bayes rules for classification decisions and its application to the problem of choosing optimal programs in secondary education is given in van der Linden (1987).

The placement problem differs from the classification problem in that all treatments lead to the same criterion. Therefore, it holds that:

$$Y_j = Y \tag{4}$$

$$\omega_j(y_j | x) = \omega_j(y | x) \tag{5}$$

$$u_j(y_j) = u_j(y) \tag{6}$$

for all values of j. Differences between the utility functions now arise only from their treatment dependency, for instance, because each treatment involves a different amount of costs. The restrictions in Eqns. (4–6) only simplify the expected utility expression in Eqn. (3); Bayes rules for the placement problem are found in the same way as for the classification problem. Solutions to the placement problem for some intuitively appealing utility functions are given in Cronbach and Glaser (1965) and van der Linden (1981).

In the mastery decision problem, the true score variable τ underlying the test score is considered as the criterion. All individuals have followed the same treatment, so there is no treatment variable modifying

the relation of test scores to criterion scores. Hence, the subscript j in $\omega_j(y | x)$ can be dropped. Usually two true states are defined—the mastery ($\tau \geq \tau_c$) and the nonmastery state ($\tau < \tau_c$), where t_c is a standard chosen for instructional reasons. Different utility functions for the mastery and the nonmastery decision are distinguished. Generally, the former increases in the criterion τ, because the utility of a mastery decision tends to be larger for students with higher true scores. Analogously, the utility of a nonmastery decision decreases in the true score. The mastery decision model follows if, in addition to Eqns. (4–6), the following restrictions are imposed:

$$y_i = \tau_i \equiv EX_i \tag{7}$$

$$\omega_j(y | x) = \omega(y | x) \tag{8}$$

with $u_0(y)$ decreasing in y, $u_{1(y)}$ increasing in y, and where $j = 0, 1$ denotes the nonmastery and mastery decision respectively. Cutting scores maximizing the expected utility under these restrictions have been examined for threshold (Huynh 1976), linear (van der Linden and Mellenbergh 1977), and normal-ogive utility functions (Novick and Lindley 1978, van der Linden 1980).

As in mastery decisions, selection decisions involve only one treatment for which individuals are either accepted or rejected. When an individual is rejected, he or she is of no value to the institute making the selection decisions. This is formalized by putting the utility for the rejection decision equal to zero. Further, the criterion is always an external variable and not a true score underlying the test. In summary, optimal selection decisions follow from maximizing the expected utility in Eqn. (3), if in addition to the restrictions in Eqns. (4–6) the following restrictions are imposed:

$$\omega_j(y | x) = \omega(y | x) \tag{9}$$

$$u_0(y) = 0 \tag{10}$$

where $j = 0, 1$ denotes the rejection and acceptance decision, respectively.

3. Miscellaneous Results

As indicated above, in practice the four types of decisions discussed in this entry are not always met in their pure form. Further constraints and extensions may apply. Optimal rules for selection and placement decisions under quota restrictions are given in Chuang et al. (1981) and van der Linden (1990) respectively. If multiple populations must be distinguished, as is the case, for example, in culture-fair selection, each population may entail its own utility and probability functions, and cutting scores must be selected for each population separately. Optimal rules for culture-fair selection are given in Gross and Su (1975), Mellenbergh and van der Linden (1981), and Petersen (1976). Reckase (1983) discusses the use of Wald's probability ratio test with mastery decisions based on adaptive testing procedures. If the decision rule has to be based on multiple tests, the posterior distributions in Eqn. (3) are conditional on multivariate data. The derivation of optimal rules is still possible, but numerically more involved than in the case of univariate data.

References

Chuang D T, Cheng J J, Novick M R 1981 Theory and practice for the use of cut-scores for personnel decisions. *J. Educ. Stat.* 6(2): 107–28

Cronbach L J, Glaser G C 1965 *Psychological Tests and Personnel Decisions*, 2nd edn. University of Illinois Press, Urbana, Illinois

Cronbach L J, Snow R F 1977 *Aptitudes and Instructional Methods: A Handbook for Research on Interactions.* Irvington, New York

Ferguson T S 1967 *Mathematical Statistics: A Decision–Theoretic Approach.* Academic Press, New York

Gross A L, Su W H 1975 Defining a "fair" or "unbiased" selection model: A question of utilities. *J. Appl. Psychol.* 60(3): 345–51

Hambleton R K, Novick M R 1973 Toward an integration of theory and method for criterion-referenced tests. *J. Educ. Meas.* 10(3): 159–70

Huynh H 1976 Statistical consideration of mastery scores. *Psychometri.* 41(1): 65–79

Lindgren B W 1976 *Statistical Theory*, 3rd edn. Macmillan, New York

Louviere J J 1988 *Analyzing Decision Making: Metric Conjoint Analysis.* Sage Publications, Newbury Park, California

Mellenbergh G J, van der Linden W J 1981 The linear utility model for optimal selection. *Psychometri.* 46(3): 283–93

Novick M R, Lindley D V 1978 The use of more realistic utility functions in educational applications. *J. Educ. Meas.* 15(3): 181–91

Novick M R, Petersen N S 1976 Towards equalizing educational and employment opportunity. *J. Educ. Meas.* 13(1): 77–88

Petersen N S 1976 An expected utility model for "optimal" selection. *J. Educ. Stat.* 1(4): 333–58

Reckase M D 1983 A procedure for decision making using tailored testing. In: Weiss D J (ed.) 1983 *New Horizons in Testing: Latent Trait Theory and Computerized Adaptive Testing.* Academic Press, New York

Taylor H C, Russell J T 1939 The relationship of validity coefficients to the practical effectiveness of tests in selection: Discussion and tables. *J. Appl. Psychol.* 23: 565–78

van der Linden W J 1980 Decision models for use with criterion-referenced tests. *Appl. Psychol. Meas.* 4(4): 469–92

van der Linden W J 1981 Using aptitude measurements for the optimal assignment of subjects to treatments with and without mastery scores. *Psychometri.* 46(3): 257–74

van der Linden W J 1987 The use of test scores for classification decisions with threshold utility. *J. Educ. Stat.* 12(1): 62–75

van der Linden W J 1990 Applications of decision theory to test-based decision making. In: Hambleton R K, Zaal J N (eds.) 1990 *Advances in Educational and Psychological Testing: Theory of Applications.* Kluwer, Boston, Messachusetts

van der Linden W J, Mellenbergh G J 1977 Optimal cutting scores using a linear loss function. *Appl. Psychol. Meas.* 1(4): 593–99

Vijn P, Molenaar I W 1981 Robustness regions for dichotomous decisions. *J. Educ. Stat.* 6(3): 205–35

Vos H J 1990 Simultaneous optimization of decisions using a linear utility function. *J. Educ. Stat.* 15(4): 309–40

Vos H J 1991 Simultaneous optimization of the aptitude treatment interaction decision problem with mastery scores. In: Wilson M (ed.) 1991 *Objective Measurement: Theory into Practice.* Ablex Publishing Corporation, Norwood, New Jersey

Vos H J, van der Linden W J 1987 Designing optimal rules for instructional decision making in CAI systems. In: Moonen J, Plomp T (eds.) 1987 *Developments in Educational Software and Courseware.* Pergamon Press, Oxford

Equating of Tests

M. J. Kolen

Multiple forms of educational tests contain different items, but are built to the same specifications. The forms typically differ somewhat in difficulty. Test form equating often adjusts scores on the multiple forms to account for these difficulty differences. This entry considers the procedures employed for the equating of tests.

1. Purpose and Context

Multiple forms of a test built to the same content and statistical specifications, but containing different items, are often needed for test security purposes and for comparing examinee performance over time. Test forms typically differ somewhat in difficulty, even though test developers attempt to construct test forms to be as similar as possible to one another. Equating is often used when multiple forms of a test exist and examinees taking different forms are compared with one another. Equating makes adjustments for difficulty differences, thus allowing forms to be used interchangeably. After successful equating, examinees are expected to earn the same score regardless of the test form administered.

Equating has become a prominent topic in the United States for at least two reasons. First, there has been a growth of the type of testing that requires multiple forms. Second, test developers have had to make reference to equating in order to address issues raised by testing critics and test legislation. This increased visibility has led to various publications on equating. Before 1980, Angoff (1971) was the primary comprehensive source on equating. Since 1980, the Holland and Rubin (1982) book, the chapter by Petersen et al. (1989), and the Kolen and Brennan (1995) book have been published. In addition, introductory treatments of traditional equating methods by Kolen (1988) and item response theory methods by Cook and Eignor (1991) have been published. Also, there have been many journal articles, presentations of papers at meetings, and research reports. Papers by Cook and Petersen (1987), Skaggs and Lissitz (1986), a special issue of *Applied Psychological Measurement* (Brennan 1987), and a special issue of *Applied Measurement in Education* (Dorans 1990) provide an introduction to this literature. Because equating has been used predominantly with multiple-choice tests, the focus of this entry is on equating multiple-choice tests. The equating of other types of tests is discussed briefly.

Processes similar to equating exist that are better referred to as scaling to achieve comparability (Petersen et al. 1989). One of these processes is vertical scaling (frequently referred to as vertical "equating"), which is used with elementary achievement test batteries. In these batteries, students are typically administered test questions matched to their current educational level (e.g., grade level). Vertical scaling allows the scores of examinees at different levels to be compared and allows for the assessment of an individual's growth over time.

Another example of scaling to achieve comparability is converting scores on one test to the score scale of another test, where both tests are measuring similar constructs, such as reading tests from two different publishers. As with vertical scaling, solutions to these problems do not allow the tests to be used interchangeably because the content of the tests is different. In addition, the development of these tests typically is not coordinated, so there are often differences in what the tests are measuring.

Although similar statistical procedures are often used in scaling and equating, their purposes are distinct. Whereas scaling is used to make scores comparable on tests that are purposefully built to be different, equating is used to make scores interchangeable on multiple forms that are built to be as similar as possible.

Scale scores are typically used in testing programs that use multiple forms. In these programs, a score scale is established based on the initial form of the test. The score scale is chosen to enhance the interpretability of scores by incorporating useful information into the score scale. The scale is maintained through an equating process that places scores from subsequent forms on the score scale that was established initially.

2. Properties of Equating Relationships

Define Form X as a new form and Form Y as an old form. Assume that a conversion of Form Y raw scores to scale scores was previously constructed, and that the purpose of equating is to be able to convert Form X raw scores first to Form Y raw scores and then to scale scores.

There are various desirable properties for equating relationships. For the "symmetry property" to hold, the function used to transform a score on Form X to the Form Y scale must be the inverse of the function used to transform a score on Form Y to the Form X scale. This symmetry property rules out regression as an equating method, because the regression of y on x is, in general, different from the regression of x on y. The "same-specifications property" requires that forms be built to the same content and statistical specifications. Symmetry and same-specifications are two properties that need to be achieved in order that scores across multiple test forms can be used interchangeably.

There are other properties of equating that are desirable, but that might not always be achievable such as "Group invariance." Ideally, the equating relationship should be the same regardless of the group of examinees used to conduct the equating. Because this property cannot be expected to hold precisely for all populations of examinees, the population of examinees used to develop an equating relationship needs to be clearly stated.

The property of "equal distributions" states that score distributions should be the same across equated multiple forms for a given population. Define x as score on Form X and y as score on Form Y. Also, define F as the distribution function of equated x and G as the distribution function of y. If e is the function used to equate scores on Form X to the Form Y scale, then the equal distribution property is achieved if

$$F[e(x)] = G(y). \tag{1}$$

When the equal distribution property holds, the same proportion of examinees in the population would score below any particular cut score on any equated form.

The "equity" property, as described by Lord (1980), states that, after equating, examinees should be indifferent to which form they are administered. Precise specification of this definition of equity requires the consideration of a test theory model. Define $F[e(x)|\tau]$ as the cumulative distribution of converted scores for examinees with a particular true score, and $G(y|\tau)$ as the cumulative distribution on Form Y for examinees with a particular true score. Equity holds if

$$F[e(x)|\tau] = G(y|\tau) \text{ for all } \tau. \tag{2}$$

This definition implies that examinees with a given true score have identical observed score means, standard deviations, and distributional shapes of converted scores on Form X and scores on Form Y. Note that identical standard deviations implies that the standard error of measurement at any true score needs to be equal on the two forms. Lord (1980) showed that, under fairly general conditions, the equity property holds only if Form X and Form Y are essentially identical.

Morris (1982) suggested a less restrictive version of equity, referred to as "first-order equity." If first-order equity holds, examinees with a given true score have the same mean converted score on Form X as they have on Form Y. Defining E as the expectation operator, an equating achieves first-order equity if

$$E[e(x)|\tau] = E(y|\tau) \text{ for all } \tau. \tag{3}$$

The achievement of all the desirable properties is most likely impossible, although they might be closely approximated in actual equating situations. Typically, one or more of these properties are made the focus of a particular equating.

3. Equating Designs

A variety of designs (Angoff 1971) is used for collecting data for equating. The group of examinees included in the equating study should be reasonably representative of the group of examinees that will be given the test under typical test administration conditions. The choice of a design involves considering both practical and statistical issues. Three of the most commonly used designs that involve equating one intact test form with another such form are considered here. Pre-equating designs (Petersen et al. 1989), in which the new form is constructed from items or parts of previously administered tests, are not considered here.

3.1 Random Groups Design

A spiraling process is typically used to implement the random groups design, where alternate examinees in a test center are administered the forms to be equated. In one method for spiraling, Form X and Form Y are alternated when the test booklets are packaged. When the booklets are handed out, the first examinee receives Form X, the second examinee Form Y, the third examinee Form X, and so on. If large groups of examinees are used that are representative of the group of examinees that will be given the test under typical test administration conditions, then the difference between group-level performance on the two forms is a direct indication of the difference in difficulty between the forms.

In the random groups design, each examinee takes only one form of the test, thus minimizing testing time. However, the random groups design requires the forms to be available and administered at the same time, which might be difficult in some situations. Also, because different examinees take the forms to be equated, larger sample sizes are needed than in some other designs.

3.2 Single Group with Counterbalancing Design

In the single group with counterbalancing design the same examinees are administered both Form Y and Form X. To deal with order effects, the order of administration of the two forms is counterbalanced. In one method for counterbalancing, one half of the test booklets are printed with Form X following Form Y, and the other half are printed with Form Y following Form X. In packaging, booklets having Form X first are alternated with booklets having Form Y first. When the booklets are handed out, the first examinee gets Form X first, the second examinee Form Y first, the third examinee Form X first, and so on. When the tests are administered, each test form is separately timed.

In the single group equating design with counterbalancing, the data from the form administered second are useful only if the order effects are constant across forms. For this reason, order effects need to be studied empirically. If order effects are not constant across forms, then the data from the form administered second might need to be disregarded.

Also, because two forms must be administered to the same students, testing time needs to be doubled, which often is not practically feasible. If fatigue and practice are effectively controlled by counterbalancing, then the single group design with counterbalancing has relatively small sample size requirements because, by taking both of the forms, each examinee serves as his or her own control.

3.3 Common-item Nonequivalent Groups Design

The common-item nonequivalent groups design is used when more than one form per test date cannot be administered because of test security or other practical concerns. In this design, Form X and Form Y have a set of items in common, and different groups of examinees are administered the two forms. There are two variations of this design. When the score on the set of common items contributes to the examinee's score on the test, the set of common items is referred to as internal. Typically, internal common items are interspersed among the other items in the test. When the score on the set of common items does not contribute to the examinee's score on the test, the set of common items is referred to as external. Typically, external common items are administered as a separately timed section.

In this design, test score summary statistics are influenced by a combination of examinee group differences and test form differences. A major task in equating using this design is to disentangle these group and form differences.

The common-item nonequivalent groups design is widely used in practice. A major reason for its popularity is that this design requires that only one test form be administered per test date. The administrative flexibility offered by nonequivalent groups is gained at some cost. Strong statistical assumptions are required to disconfound group and form differences.

A variety of practical approaches were described by Brennan and Kolen (1987) to deal with the problems associated with this design. One important consideration is that the set of common items should be proportionally representative of the total test forms in content and statistical characteristics, as illustrated by Klein and Jarjoura (1985). That is, the common-item set should be a miniature version of the total test form, and needs to be a large proportion (say, at least 20 percent) of the total test. The common items also need to behave similarly on the old and new forms, as illustrated by Zwick (1991). To help ensure similar behavior, each common item should occupy a similar location on the two forms. Also, the common items should be exactly the same (e.g., no wording changes or rearranging of alternatives) in the old and new forms. A large number of common items should be used, as this usually allows for better content representativeness and greater stability. In addition, the groups administered the two forms should be reasonably similar, because extreme dissimilarities in groups have been found to cause problems in equating, as illustrated by Cook et al. (1988).

4. Equating Relationships and Estimation

To conduct equating, the relationship between alternate forms needs to be specified and estimated. The focus in traditional observed score equating methods is on the scores that are observed, although sometimes test theory models are used to estimate observed score equating relationships. Item response theory (IRT) and true score equating methods exist that make heavy use of test theory models.

4.1 Traditional Equating Methods

In traditional observed score equating methods, score correspondence is found by setting certain characteristics of the score distributions equal for a specified population of examinees. For example, in equipercentile equating, a score on Form X is considered to be equal to a score on Form Y if the two scores have identical percentile ranks in a population. Thus, x is equivalent to y if in the population of examinees.

$$F[e(x)] = G(y) \tag{4}$$

The goal of equipercentile equating is for the distribution of converted scores on Form X to be the same as the distribution of scores on Form Y. This goal is the equal distribution property stated in Eqn. 1.

Linear equating is another observed score method of equating. The goal of linear equating is for the mean and standard deviation of converted scores to be equal on the two forms. The linear equating function in the population is

$$l(x) = \sigma(y) \left[\frac{x - \mu(x)}{\sigma(x)} \right] + \mu(y) \tag{5}$$

where μ is a population mean and σ is a population standard deviation.

The estimation of equating relationships in the random groups design involves substituting statistics for the parameters in Eqns. 4 and 5. In equipercentile equating, the resulting equating relationship is typically irregular and subject to a considerable sampling error at those points where few examinees score. For this reason, smoothing methods are used. Methods for smoothing the score distributions are referred to as presmoothing methods (see Kolen 1991 for a review) and methods for smoothing the equipercentile relationship as postsmoothing methods (e.g., Kolen 1984). Either type of method, used analytically, can improve equating precision.

If the shapes of the score distributions for Form X and Form Y differ, which often occurs when the forms differ in difficulty, then equipercentile and linear relationships differ. However, even in these situations, the linear and equipercentile relationships are similar near the mean score. When interest is primarily in scores near the mean, such as when a cutting score is used that is near the mean score, then linear methods are sufficient. When interest is in scores all along the score scale and sample size is large, then equipercentile equating is often preferable to linear equating. A common rule of thumb is that a minimum of 1,000–2,000 examinees per form are needed for equipercentile equating, whereas fewer examinees are needed for linear equating.

The estimation of observed score equivalents in the common-item nonequivalent groups design requires that strong statistical assumptions be made. Define score on the common items as v. In the Tucker linear method, the linear regression of x on v is assumed to be equal for the examinees taking Form X and the examinees taking Form Y. A similar assumption is made about the linear regression of y on v. In the Levine linear observed score method, similar assumptions are made about true scores rather than observed scores. No method exists to directly test these assumptions using the data that are collected for equating, because examinees take only one form. An equipercentile counterpart of the Tucker method exists that is referred to as frequency estimation (Angoff 1971).

Linear methods have been developed for equating true scores on test forms. The Levine true score method is based on assumptions that are similar to the Levine observed score method, but equates true scores. Hanson (1991) showed that applying the Levine true score equating relationship to observed scores results in the property of first-order equity when the test forms meet congeneric test theory model assumptions. Linear true score methods are likely to be most useful when tests differ in length, and therefore in reliability. For this reason, linear true score methods are often referred to as methods for unequally reliable tests. Curvilinear methods for equating true scores exist that make use of strong true score models (see Lord 1980 Chap. 17).

4.2 IRT Methods

Item response theory (IRT) models assume that examinee ability (θ) can be described by a single latent variable and that items can be described by a set of item parameters (Lord 1980). For multiple-choice tests, the probability that examinees of ability θ correctly answer item g is symbolized $P_g(\theta)$. Item response theory models are based on strong statistical assumptions that need to be checked before the methods are applied. The θ-scale has an indeterminate location and spread. For this reason, one θ-scale sometimes needs to be converted to another linearly related θ-scale. If scores are to be reported on the number-correct scale, then there are two steps in IRT equating. First, the θ-scales for the two forms are considered to be equal or set equal. Then number-correct score equivalents on the two forms are found.

In many situations, the parameter estimates for the two forms are on the same θ-scale without further transformation. In general, no transformation of the θ-scales is needed in the following situations: (a) in the random groups design or the single group design when the parameters for Form X and Form Y are estimated separately using ability scales with the same mean and standard deviation; (b) in the single group design when parameters for the two forms are estimated together; and (c) in the common-item nonequivalent groups design when Form X and Form Y parameters are estimated simultaneously. The typical situation in which a transformation of the θ-scale is required is in the common-item nonequivalent groups design when the Form X and Form Y parameters are estimated separately. In this situation, the parameters for one form are linearly transformed to the θ-scale of the other form. In one procedure for equating, the mean and standard deviation of the estimated θ-values are set equal. Additional methods of equating the θ-scales also exist (see Haebara 1980, Stocking and Lord 1983).

After the parameter estimates are on the same scale, IRT true score equating can be used to relate number-correct scores on Form X and Form Y for score reporting purposes. In this procedure, the true score on one form associated with a given θ is considered to be equivalent to the true score on another form associated with that θ. In IRT the true score on Form X for an examinee of ability θ is defined as

$$\tau_X(\theta) = \sum_{g:X} P_g(\theta) \qquad (6)$$

where the summation $g:X$ is over items on Form X. True score on Form Y for an examinee of ability θ is defined as

$$\tau_Y(\theta) = \sum_{g:Y} P_g(\theta) \qquad (7)$$

where the summation $g:Y$ is over items on Form Y. Given a θ, the score on Form X, $\tau_X(\theta)$, is considered to be equivalent to the score on Form Y, $\tau_Y(\theta)$. In practice, estimates of the parameters are used in Eqns. 6 and 7.

As a practical procedure the estimated true score relationship is applied to observed scores. However, no theoretical reason exists for treating scores in this way. Rather, doing so has been justified in item response theory by showing that the resulting true score conversions are similar to observed score conversions (Lord and Wingersky 1984). Procedures exist for using IRT methods to conduct equipercentile equating (Lord 1980), although these methods have not been used much in practice.

Any application of unidimensional IRT methods requires that the test forms be unidimensional and that the relationship between ability and probability of correct response follow a specified model. These requirements are difficult to justify for many educational achievement tests, although the methodology might be robust to violations in some circumstances. Item response theory methods also have substantial sample size requirements, although the sample sizes for the Rasch model (Wright and Stone 1979) are considerably less than those for the three parameter logistic model (Lord 1980). In any application of IRT to equating, the fit of the models needs to be carefully analyzed.

5. Equating Issues

Minimizing equating error is a major goal when deciding whether or not to equate forms, when designing equating studies, and when conducting equating. Random equating error is present whenever samples from populations of examinees are employed to estimate parameters (e.g., means and standard deviations) that are used to estimate an equating relationship. Random error diminishes as sample size increases. Random error is typically indexed by the standard error of equating.

Systematic equating error results from violations of the assumptions of the particular equating methodology used. For example, in the common-item nonequivalent groups design, systematic error results if the assumptions of statistical methods used to disconfound form and group differences are not met. Systematic error might also be present if the group of examinees used to conduct the equating differs substantially from the group of examinees who are administered the test operationally. Systematic equating error typically cannot be quantified in actual equating situations.

Equating error of both types needs to be controlled because it can propagate over-equatings and result in scores on later forms not being comparable to scores on earlier forms. In testing programs that use many test forms, the selection of the previously equated form or forms influences equating error. For example, in the common-item nonequivalent groups design a new test form is often equated to two previously equated forms by including two sets of common items. The results from each of the two equatings could be compared for consistency, and this provides a check on the adequacy of the equating. The results could be averaged, which might provide more stable equating.

Many testing programs, because of practical constraints, cannot use equating for comparing examinee scores and assessing score trends over time. For example, sometimes security issues prevent test items from being administered more than once, such as when all items administered are released after the test is given. All equating designs require more than one administration of at least some items. In other practical situations the amount of equating error might be so large that equating would add more error into the scores than if no equating had been done. For example, suppose that the common items behave differently from one testing to the next because of changes in item position. In such a case, no equating might be preferable to equating, using the common items. Equating with small sample sizes might also introduce more error than it would remove. In these situations, no equating might be preferable to equating. Even without equating, scores of examinees who are given the same form can be compared with one another. If most decisions are made among examinees tested with the same form, then not conducting equating might have minimal consequences. However, not equating would make it difficult to chart trends over time and to compare examinees who were given different forms.

In some circumstances, equating can be used with nonmultiple-choice tests. To equate such tests with observed-score methods, equating proceeds in the same way as it does with multiple-choice tests. With IRT, if the test items are not dichotomously scored, then generalizations of the standard IRT models must be used, such as the model developed by Masters (1982). One practical problem often occurs when equating tests that are not multiple-choice with the common-item nonequivalent groups design. In this situation, it can be very difficult to develop a set of common items that is representative of the entire test, because there are so few items on the test. This problem is especially severe with essay tests, where a test form might contain only one or two essay items (see *Essays: Equating of Marks; Partial Credit Models; Rating Scale Analysis*). Recently there has also been considerable interest in developing comparable scores between computerized tests and paper-and-pencil tests, and

between alternate forms of computerized tests. Kolen and Brennan (1995) review many of the related issues.

6. *Equating and Related Procedures In Testing Programs*

To provide an indication of the variety of equating procedures that are in use, some examples of equating methods are presented. In the United States, the ACT (American College Testing 1989) and the SAT (Scholastic Aptitude Test) (Donlon 1984) are the two major tests used for college admissions purposes. Different forms of the tests are given multiple times during any year. Examinees who test on different dates are compared to one another, so there is a need to conduct equating.

The ACT tests are equated using a random groups design. Forms are spiraled in test centers in a special operational equating administration. The forms are equated using equipercentile methods with postsmoothing. The equated forms are used in subsequent administrations.

The SAT is equated on each test date using a common-item nonequivalent groups design with external common items. Typically, a single form is administered along with an equating section that is not part of the score of the examinee, but the examinees do not know which section is not scored. The use of the external common-item section allows the scored items of the examination to be released to examinees while still allowing for equating in the future. The forms are equated to two previously administered forms using two common-item sections. When the SAT is equated, IRT, linear, and equipercentile methods are all examined.

The Iowa Tests of Basic Skills (Hieronymus and Hoover 1986) are vertically scaled using a scaling test method, in which a scaling test is constructed to span various levels of educational development. The scaling test is spiraled with the tests that are typically used at each educational level. Equipercentile procedures are used to scale each test to the scaling test. The California Achievement Tests are vertically scaled by using IRT methods. Yen (1983) provided a detailed discussion of these methods. Petersen et al. (1989) discussed issues in vertical scaling.

The National Assessment of Educational Progress (NAEP) in the United States uses common-item methods with item response theory methods to conduct equating (Zwick 1991). This program also uses item sampling to estimate group-level achievement rather than achievement at the individual level. Intriguing scaling issues in NAEP arise from changes in specifications over time.

In a study to examine the feasibility of using the Rasch latent trait measurement model in the equating of the Australian Scholastic Aptitude Test, Morgan (1982) found that all items used in the test needed to fit a unidimensional latent trait model at the test development stage. On two occasions, in 1970–71 and 1983–84, Keeves and Schlerdren (1992) also used the Rasch model to equate and scale science achievement tests employed at the 10-year-old, 14-year-old, and secondary school levels in 10 different countries through the use of different sets of bridging items.

7. Conclusion

The equating methods outlined in this entry have been shown to produce adequate equating results for the random groups design when the following conditions are met:

(a) Test forms are built to the same carefully defined content and statistical specifications.

(b) The examinee groups are reasonably representative of the group of examinees who are going to be administered the test operationally.

In addition to (a) and (b), the common-item nonequivalent groups design requires additional conditions:

(c) The groups taking the two forms are similar to one another.

(d) The common items are representative of the full test in content and statistical characteristics, and are at least 20 percent of the full test.

(e) The common items behave similarly in the forms that are equated.

Item response theory methods also require that the test forms are at least close enough to being unidimensional for practical purposes. Linear methods also require either that the score distributions be similar in shape or that interest is only in scores near the mean score. Equipercentile and IRT methods require large sample sizes.

The adequacy of scaling to achieve comparability and vertical scaling depends on the purpose of the scaling and how the results are to be used. Scaling to achieve comparability is probably much more dependent on the groups sampled and on the design used to collect the data, than is equating.

See also: Item Response Theory; Latent Trait Measurement Models; Classical Test Theory; Scaling Methods

References

American College Testing 1989 *Preliminary Technical Manual for the Enhanced* ACT *Assessment.* American College Testing, Iowa City, Iowa

Angoff W A 1971 Scales, norms, and equivalent scores. In: Thorndike R L (ed.) 1971 *Educational Measurement*, 2nd edn. American Council on Education, Washington, DC

Brennan R L (ed.) 1987 Problems, perspectives and practical issues in equating. *Appl. Psychol. Meas.* 11(3): 221–306

Brennan R L, Kolen M J 1987 Some practical issues in equating. *Appl. Psychol. Meas.* 11(3): 279–90

Cook L L, Eignor D R 1991 NCME instructional module: IRT equating methods. *Educational Measurement: Issues and Practice* 10(3): 37–45

Cook L L, Eignor D R, Taft H L 1988 A comparative study of the effects of recency of instruction on the stability of IRT and conventional item parameter estimates. *J. Educ. Meas.* 25(1): 31–45

Cook L L, Petersen N S 1987 Problems related to the use of conventional and item response theory equating methods in less than optimal circumstances. *Appl. Psychol. Meas.* 11(3): 225–44

Donlon T F (ed.) 1984 *The College Board Technical Handbook for the Scholastic Aptitude Test and Achievement Tests.* College Entrance Examination Board, New York

Dorans N J 1990 Equating methods and sampling designs. *Applied Measurement in Education* 3(1): 3–17

Hanson B A 1991 A note on Levine's formula for equating unequally reliable tests using data from the common item nonequivalent groups design. *J. Ed. Stat.* 16(2): 93–100

Haebara T 1980 Equating logistic ability scales by a weighted least squares method. *Japanese Psychological Research* 22(3): 144–49

Holland P W, Rubin D B (eds.) 1982 *Test Equating.* Academic Press, New York

Hieronymus A N, Hoover H D 1986 *Iowa Tests of Basic Skills Manual for School Administrators Levels 5–14 ITBS Forms G/H.* Riverside Publishing Co., Chicago, Illinois

Keeves J P, Schlerdren A 1992 Changes in science achievement: 1970–1984. In: Keeves J P (ed.) *The IEA study in Science III. Changes in Science Education and Achievement: 1970–1984.* Pergamon Press, Oxford

Klein L W, Jarjoura D 1985 The importance of content representation for common-item equating with nonrandom groups. *J. Educ. Meas.* 22(3): 197–206

Kolen M J 1984 Effectiveness of analytic smoothing in equipercentile equating. *J. Ed. Stat.* 9(1): 25–44

Kolen M J 1988 An NCME instructional module on traditional equating methodology. *Educational Measurement: Issues and Practice* 7(4): 29–36

Kolen M J 1991 Smoothing methods for estimating test score distributions. *J. Educ. Meas.* 28(3): 257–82

Kolen M J, Brennan R L 1995 *Test Equating. Methods and Practices.* Springer-Verlag, New York

Lord F M 1980 *Applications of Item Response Theory to Practical Testing Problems.* Erlbaum, Hillsdale, New Jersey

Lord F M, Wingersky M S 1984 Comparison of IRT true-score and equipercentile observed-score "equatings." *Appl. Psychol. Meas.* 8(4): 453–61

Masters G N 1982 A Rasch model for partial credit scoring. *Psychometrika* 47(2): 149–74

Morgan G 1982 The use of the Rasch latent trait measurement model in the equating of Scholastic Aptitude Tests. In: Spearritt D (ed.) 1982 *The Improvement of Measurement in Education and Psychology.* ACER, Hawthorn

Morris C N 1982 On the foundations of test equating. In:

Holland P W, Rubin D B (eds.) 1982

Petersen N S, Kolen M J, Hoover H D 1989 Scaling, norming, and equating. In: Linn R L (ed.) 1989 *Educational Measurement*, 3rd edn. American Council on Education and Macmillan, New York

Skaggs G, Lissitz R W 1986 IRT test equating: Relevant issues and a review of recent research. *Rev. Educ. Res.* 56(4): 495–529

Stocking M L, Lord F M 1983 Developing a common metric in item response theory. *Appl. Psychol. Meas.* 7(2): 201–10

Wright B D, Stone M H 1979 *Best Test Design*. Mesa Press, Chicago, Illinois

Yen W 1983 Use of the three-parameter model in the development of a standardized test. In: Hambleton R L (ed.) 1983 *Applications of Item Response Theory*. Educational Research Institute of British Columbia, Vancouver

Zwick R 1991 Effects of item order and context on estimation of NAEP reading proficiency. *Educational Measurement: Issues and Practice* 10(3): 10–16

Generalizability Theory

L. Allal and J. Cardinet

Generalizability theory provides a conceptual framework for estimating the reliability of behavioral measurements obtained by virtually any kind of procedure: test, rating scale, observation form. It helps educational researchers and decision-makers to determine whether it is possible to interpret the observed differences between objects of study, given the random fluctuations that affect the measurement instruments. It also provides theoretical and methodological guidelines for the construction of more precise and/or less costly measurement procedures.

Historically, within the context of classical test theory, a variety of procedures were developed for estimating different aspects of reliability: (a) calculation of test–retest correlations to estimate the stability of measurements over different testing occasions; (b) correlation of scores obtained from parallel forms of a test to estimate the equivalence of measurements based on different sets of items; and (c) application of various formulas to estimate the internal consistency, or homogeneity, of a pool of test items. Generalizability theory offers a comprehensive set of concepts and estimation procedures for treating any one or, simultaneously, all of these aspects of reliability. It is applicable, moreover, to complex measurement designs not considered in classical theory.

1. Basic Concepts

Behavioral measurements used in educational research and decision-making are almost always based on procedures involving one or more sources of potential error due to fluctuations in the conditions of measurement. In generalizability theory, the design of a measurement procedure implies the specification of the admissible variations that can occur along one or several facets, for instance, items, occasions, correctors, or observers. Any given observed score is considered to be a sample from the universe of scores that would exist if measurements were obtained under all admissible conditions. The classical concept of "true" score is replaced in generalizability theory by the concept of universe score, which Cronbach et al. (1972) define as follows:

> The ideal datum on which to base the decision would be something like the person's mean score over all acceptable observations, which we shall call his "universe score." The investigator uses the observed score or some function of it as if it were the universe score. That is, he generalizes from sample to universe. *The question of "reliability" thus resolves into a question of accuracy of generalization, or generalizability* (p. 15).

In conducting a generalizability study, it is necessary to include all relevant facets of the universe of admissible observations in the factorial design used for data collection. The design must include at least one facet formed by random sampling of measurement conditions, and may entail any number of other facets constituted by random or fixed modes of sampling. For example, if data are collected by a design in which persons are crossed with a random sample of items, the facet "items" could be nested within the levels of a fixed facet such as "instructional objectives," or it could be crossed with levels of a random facet such as "occasions." It would also be possible to construct a design in which items are nested within objectives and crossed with occasions.

Once the data have been collected, the standard procedures of analysis of variance (ANOVA) are applied to determine the mean squares and to estimate the variance components corresponding to all sources of variation in the design. The choice of the appropriate ANOVA model is determined by the mode of sampling (random, finite random, or fixed) of the levels of each facet.

For a simple design in which persons are crossed with items, variance components can be estimated by the random effects model for three sources of variation: persons (σ_p^2), items (σ_i^2 and error ($\sigma_{pi,e}^2$) For a more complex design in which items are nested in fixed objectives, the appropriate mixed effects model would be used to estimate the variance components for five sources of variation: persons (*P*), items (*I:O*), objectives (*O*), and the interactions $P \times (I:O)$ and $P \times O$.

Once the variance components have been estimated, the principles of generalizability theory are used to determine the allocation of the components for the estimation of three major parameters.

(a) *Universe score variance.* This parameter, symbolized by $\sigma^2(\mu)$, is defined as the variance of the expected values of the scores belonging to the universe of admissible observations. It reflects the systematic variations due to differences among the objects of measurement. For the $p \times i$ design described above, it is estimated by the variance component estimate due to persons $\hat{\sigma}_p^2$

(b) *Relative error variance.* Observed scores are frequently interpreted by comparing the relative positions of the objects of measurement within the score distribution. In this case, the sources of error are limited to the interactions of the objects of measurement with the facet(s) formed by random sampling of the conditions of measurement. The relative error variance, symbolized by $\sigma^2(\delta)$, is estimated by the sum of the weighted variance component estimates corresponding to the sources of relative error. Each component is weighted inversely to the number of times its effect is sampled when calculating the average score of one of the objects of measurement. For the $p \times i$ design, the estimate of relative error variance is based on a single variance component estimate $\hat{\sigma}^2(\delta) = \hat{\sigma}_{pi,e}^2 / n_i$, where n_i is the number of levels of the facet items.

(c) *Absolute error variance.* For some situations, particularly in the areas of criterion-referenced and domain-referenced measurement, the observed scores are used as estimates of universe scores. In crossed designs, if decisions are based on the absolute rather than the relative values of the observed scores, additional sources of error must be considered. The absolute error variance, symbolized by $\sigma^2(\Delta)$, includes the components of relative error plus the components that are due specifically to the facet(s) formed by random sampling of the conditions of measurement. Thus, for the $p \times i$ design, the estimate of absolute error variance is based on two variance component estimates $\hat{\sigma}^2(\Delta) = \hat{\sigma}_{pi,e}^2 / n_i + \hat{\sigma}_i^2 / n_i$.

The precision of measurement provided by a given design is assessed by a generalizability coefficient, defined as the ratio of the universe-score variance to the expected observed-score variance. For the case of relative comparisons of observed scores, the expected observed-score variance is composed of the universe-score variance plus the relative error variance. The corresponding generalizability coefficient for the $p \times i$ design is defined as $E\rho_\delta^2 = \sigma_p^2 / (\sigma_p^2 + \sigma^2(\delta))$.

If decisions are based on the absolute values of the observed scores, the estimate of absolute error variance, $\hat{\sigma}^2(\Delta)$, would be used in place of $\hat{\sigma}^2(\delta)$, and a corresponding coefficient would be estimated by $\hat{\sigma}_p^2 / (\hat{\sigma}_p^2 + \sigma^2(\delta))$.

The interpretation of these coefficients is analogous to that of classical reliability coefficients. Values approaching 1.0 indicate that the scores of interest can be differentiated with a high degree of accuracy, despite the random fluctuations of the measurement conditions.

Cronbach et al. (1972) distinguish two stages in the application of generalizability theory. The first is the generalizability (G) study carried out by the developer of the measurement procedure. Its aim is to furnish estimates of the variance components for all sources of variation of potential interest to future users. On the basis of this information, various modifications of the initial G-study design can be analyzed in the context of decision (D) studies. The purpose of a D-study is to determine the most appropriate measurement procedure for a particular situation in which the information will be used. Certain modifications may be required because of practical constraints; for instance, a limitation on the availability of training supervisors could lead to a reduction in the number of observations per trainee. Other design modifications may be considered in order to improve the precision of measurement. The most obvious example is the reduction of measurement error by increasing the number of levels of the random facets which, as shown in the G-study, make the largest contributions to the error variance. For example, in the case of the $p \times i$ design, an increase in the number of items (n_i) would lead to a decrease in the estimates of both relative and absolute error, as defined by the formulas presented above.

An accessible introduction to the basic principles of generalizability theory, including clearly presented illustrations and practice exercises, is provided by Shavelson and Webb (1991).

2. Extensions of Generalizability Theory

Among the contributions to generalizability theory since the initial 1972 publication by Cronbach et al., five areas of development will be mentioned.

The first is the work on problems associated with the underlying statistical models used in generalizability analysis. Brennan (1992) has proposed a formal presentation of the theory that includes useful clarifications with respect to the definition and estimation of generalizability parameters based on variance components estimated by mixed models of ANOVA.

Smith (1981) has analyzed a second problem of

estimation: the instability of variance component estimates when small samples are used in complex G-study designs. He shows that more accurate estimates of variance components can be obtained by combining the results of multiple small-scale G-studies.

Efforts to develop multivariate extensions of the theory constitute a third area of investigation. In addition to the proposals of Cronbach et al. (1972) for the generalizability analysis of profiles of scores, work has been carried out on multivariate methods for estimating the components of variance and covariance associated with composite scores defined by canonical coefficients or other weighting schemes. Having compared generalizability coefficients for multivariate composites based on different weighting schemes, Shavelson et al. (1989) suggest that the most adequate approach may be to use weights derived from a confirmatory factor analysis fitted to a conceptual model of the composite.

A fourth area of development is based on the principle of symmetry which, as proposed by Cardinet et al. (1981 p. 184), affirms "that each factor of a design can be selected as an object of study, and generalizability theory operations defined for one factor can be transposed in the study of other factors." This principle has led Cardinet and his colleagues to develop a framework for generalizability analysis that is applicable to a wide range of situations in educational measurement, including situations where the objects of measurement (whether persons or other factors) are formed by the crossing and/or nesting of several factors (fixed or random). Generalizability theory is thus extended to the analysis of the sources of error and bias that occur when multifaceted measurement procedures are applied to multifaceted populations.

A further advantage of the proposed framework is its usefulness in situations where the data are collected in order to carry out comparisons along each of several facets which are of interest to educational decision-makers. In multipurpose educational surveys, for example, school administrators may wish to compare achievement levels of classes or of school districts, whereas curriculum developers may be interested in comparisons of achievement levels for different items or sets of items. To deal with these multiple measurement aims, Cardinet et al. (1981) propose a clear separation between the initial phases of analysis, based on analysis of variance (leading to estimation of variance components without reference to any particular aim of measurement), and the subsequent phases, based on the principles of generalizability theory, in which several alternative measurement designs can be defined and analyzed. In each design, two types of facets are distinguished: the facets of differentiation (corresponding to the objects of measurement) and the facets of instrumentation (corresponding to the conditions or instruments of measurement). It is then possible to determine the allocation of the variance component estimates for the estimation of the variance of differentiation (universe–score variance) and the error variances associated with a design. In the final phase of the framework, various modifications of the initial design are considered in order to optimize the measurements needed for different decision-making or research purposes.

A fifth area of development concerns the optimization of the decision-study design. Cardinet and Tourneur (1985) have developed a procedure called "facet analysis" used to estimate contributions of facet levels to error variance; atypical levels ("outliers") are thus detected and, as far as possible, excluded from the universe of observations and/or population under study, thereby reducing the error variance. Marcoulides and Goldstein (1990) have dealt with the question of determining the optimal number of observations when resource constraints are imposed on the investigator. Sanders et al. (1989) propose a more general method, using a "branch-and-bound algorithm," to determine the minimum number of observations per subject needed to achieve a specified generalizability coefficient (or threshold). The advantage of this method is that it takes into account various mathematical constraints defined by the user, and can provide exact integer optimization solutions.

3. An Illustration of Generalizability Analysis

In this illustration, the principles of generalizability analysis are applied to a design that typifies several aspects of data collection in the field of education measurement. In many instances, rather than simple random sampling of persons from a homogeneous population, persons are randomly sampled within levels of one or more fixed stratification variables. The data collection design thus entails the nesting of the facet persons within other facets. For example, pupils may be nested within facets such as age, sex, grade, and instructional treatment; or in the case of a study of teaching behavior, teachers may be nested within facets such as type of training, years of experience, and sector of employment. In a similar manner, measurement procedures (e.g., tests and rating scales) are often constructed by the generation of randomly equivalent items nested within levels of one or more fixed classification variables (e.g., objectives, content chapters, and tasks) corresponding to the dimensions of a predetermined table of specifications.

To illustrate the application of generalizability theory for designs of this type, the following example is used. A 30-item multiple-choice test has been administered to a sample of 100 eighth-grade pupils—50 boys and 50 girls. The test has been constructed to measure pupil achievement with respect to three instructional objectives, and is composed of 10 items per objective.

The data collection design for this example is formed by four facets. The random facet pupils (*P*) is nested within the fixed facet sex (S). Items (I) constitute a second random facet nested within the fixed facet objectives (O). The facets $P{:}S$ and S are crossed with the facets $I{:}O$ and O.

For this design, variance components can be estimated for eight sources of variation, the four sources corresponding to the main effects of the facets (S, $P{:}S$, O, $I{:}O$), and the four sources corresponding to the interactions among facets $S \times O$, $S \times (I{:}O)$, $(P{:}S) \times O$, $(P{:}S) \times (I{:}O)$. Since two facets of the design, S and O, are fixed, the variance components would be estimated using the appropriate mixed model of ANOVA.

Once the variance components have been estimated, several directions of generalizability analysis could be considered, depending on the aim of measurement. For illustrative purposes, two contrasting cases are described using the terminology proposed by Cardinet et al. (1981). The description of each case is limited to the definition of the measurement design and the corresponding allocation of the variance component estimates for the estimation of the generalizability parameters (see Table 1).

The first, and more conventional, case is the use of the test scores to compare pupil achievement levels in the context of school certification or placement decisions. In this situation, the aim of measurement is to differentiate pupils while generalizing over items based on a fixed set of objectives. If decisions pertain to individual pupil scores regardless of sex, the measurement design is defined by two facets of differentiation ($P{:}S$ and S) and two facets of instrumentation ($I{:}O$ and O).

The estimation of the differentiation (i.e., universe–score) variance is based on the variance component estimates for the two facets of differentiation, $P{:}S$ and S. The relative error variance is estimated on the basis of the variance component estimates due to the interactions of the differentiation facets with the random instrumentation facets. For this design, the sources of relative error correspond to the following interactions $(P{:}S) \times (I{:}O)$, $S \times (I{:}O)$. The estimate of absolute error variance includes the above interaction components plus the variance component estimate due to the effect of the random instrumentation facet $I{:}O$.

The second case to be considered is the comparison of the achievement levels attained for different instructional objectives, as might be required in the context of curriculum evaluation or in a survey monitoring educational outcomes of the school system. In this case, the aim of measurement is to differentiate objectives, while generalizing over random sampling of items and of pupils nested within sex. The measurement design therefore includes a single differentiation facet (O) and three instrumentation facets ($I{:}O$, $P{:}S$, S).

The corresponding allocation of the variance component estimates differs in several respects from that of the previous design (see Table 1). The estimation of the differentiation variance is based on the variance component estimate for the facet O. The estimate of the relative error variance includes the estimated variance components for the random facet $I{:}O$, and for the interactions of $I{:}O$ and O with the random instrumentation facet $P{:}S$. The absolute error variance is estimated on the basis of the above components plus the component due to the random instrumentation facet $P{:}S$.

In examining the indications in Table 1, it can be seen that the allocation of the variance components is quite different depending on the aim of measurement. Only one source of relative error, $(P{:}S) \times (I{:}O)$, is allocated in the same way for the two cases under consideration. It should be noted, moreover, that in computing the estimates of the generalizability parameters for these designs, different coefficients would be used for the weighting of the components entering into the formulas.

4. Areas of Application

In addition to applications of generalizability theory in the classical field of norm-referenced measurement of individual differences, other areas of application have been developed. In the brief description that follows, selected references are given for five areas.

4.1 Accuracy of Large Scale Performance Assessments

In mandated assessment programs that concern statewide populations or large stratified samples, reports present performance summaries at several levels—schools, districts, the state as a whole—in order to determine whether the results meet accepted standards. Generalizability analysis can estimate the degree of uncertainty associated with the summary scores (Cronbach et al. 1995).

Table 1
Allocation of the variance component estimates for the estimation of generalizability parameters associated with two contrasting aims of measurement

	Aim of measurement	
Generalizability parameters	Differentiation of pupils	Differentiation of objectives
Differentiation variance	$P : S$ S	O
Relative error variance	$(P : S) \times (I : O)$ $S \times (I : O)$	$I : O$ $(P : S) \times (I : O)$ $O \times (P : S)$
Absolute error variance	Components of relative error, plus: $I : O$	Components of relative error, plus: $P : S$

740

4.2 Multifaceted Ratings and Observations

Generalizability theory has been frequently applied to investigate multiple sources of error affecting ratings, such as ratings of instruction (Gillmore et al. 1978), or of job requirements (Webb and Shavelson 1981). The theory has also been used to conduct G-studies based on observational data pertaining to teacher behavior, and to teacher–student interactions (Erlich and Borich 1979).

4.3 Assessment of Individual Learning

The universe of admissible observations, as postulated by generalizability theory, constitutes a useful basis for domain-referenced interpretation of diagnostic test scores (Webb et al. 1987). Estimates of absolute error variance are appropriate for setting confidence intervals around scores provided by domain-referenced or criterion-referenced tests. Brennan and Kane (1977) have developed an "index of dependability" for mastery testing in which observed scores are used to estimate the positions of universe scores with respect to a specified criterion. When measuring individual progress, or the variation of an individual's performance for several instructional objectives, applications of generalizability theory can be based on techniques developed by Cardinet (1994).

4.4 Multipurpose Surveys of Educational Outcomes

The flexibility of generalizability theory, as enlarged by the principle of symmetry, is particularly useful for dealing with multiple problems of reliability in large-scale surveys involving multifaceted measurement procedures applied to multifaceted populations. Tourneur and Cardinet (1981) present the analyses carried out in a mathematics curriculum evaluation to determine the precision of differentiation for content domains and test series, as well as for performance levels of different student subpopulations (i.e., classes, grades, and regions).

4.5 Analysis of Instrument Bias

In order to identify possible sources of bias, as reflected in the interactions of test items with facets such as sex, social class, ethnic group, it is possible to carry out a facet analysis (Bertrand 1988) or, more broadly, to use ANOVA-based techniques in conjunction with other approaches (Osterlind 1983). Generalizability theory has also been applied to improve grade comparability in the context of cross-moderation of secondary school examinations (Johnson and Cohen 1983).

Review articles by Shavelson and Webb (1981) and by Shavelson et al. (1989) provide further information on the developments that have given generalizability theory an ever increasing range of application as a framework for measurement design and analysis in education.

See also: Reliability in Educational and Psychological Measurement; Variance and Covariance, Analysis of; Sampling in Survey Research; Criterion-referenced Measurement; Rating Scales; Test Bias; Measurement in Educational Research

References

Bertrand R 1988 Pourquoi de nouvelles théories de la mesure? *Mes. Eval. Educ.* 11(2): 5–21

Brennan R L 1992 *Elements of Generalizability Theory*, 2nd edn. American College Testing Program, Iowa City, Iowa

Brennan R L, Kane M T 1977 An index of dependability for mastery tests. *J. Educ. Meas.* 14(3): 277–89

Cardinet J 1994 Control of the value of an intra-subject measurement design. In: Laveault D, Zumbo B, Gessaroli M, Boss M (eds.) 1994 *Modern Theories of Measurement: Problems and Issues* . Faculty of Education, University of Ottawa, Ottawa

Cardinet J, Tourneur Y, Allal L 1981 Extension of generalizability theory and its applications in educational measurement. *J. Educ. Meas.* 18(4): 183–204

Cardinet J, Tourneur Y 1985 *Assurer la Mesure*. Peter Lang, Berne

Cronbach L J, Gleser G C, Nanda H, Rajaratnam N 1972 *The Dependability of Behavioral Measurements: Theory of Generalizability for Scores and Profiles*. Wiley, New York

Cronbach L J, Linn R L, Brennan R L, Haertel E 1995 Generalizability analysis for educational assessments. *Evaluation Comments*, Summer: 1–29

Erlich O, Borich G 1979 Occurrence and generalizability of scores on a classroom interaction instrument. *J. Educ. Meas.* 16(1): 11–18

Gilmore G M, Kane M T, Naccarato R W 1978 The generalizability of student ratings of instruction: Estimation of the teacher and the course components. *J. Educ. Meas.* 15(1): 1–13

Johnson S, Cohen L 1983 *Investigating Grade Comparability Through Cross-Moderation*. Schools Council, London

Marcoulides G, Goldstein Z 1990 The optimization of generalizability studies with resource constraints. *Educ. Psychol. Meas.* 50(4): 761–68

Osterlind S J 1983 *Test Item Bias*. Sage, Newbury Park, California

Sanders P F, Theunissen T J J M, Baas S M 1989 Minimizing the number of observations: A generalization of the Spearman–Brown formula. *Psychometri.* 54(4): 587–98

Shavelson R J, Webb N M 1981 Generalizability theory: 1973–1980. *Br. J. Math. Stat. Psychol.* 34(2): 133–66

Shavelson R J, Webb N M 1991 *Generalizability Theory: A Primer*. Sage, London

Shavelson R J, Webb N M, Rowley G L 1989 Generalizability theory. *Am. Psychol.* 44(6): 922–32

Smith P L 1981 Gaining accuracy in generalizability theory: Using multiple designs. *J. Educ. Meas.* 18(3): 147–54

Tourneur Y, Cardinet J 1981 L'étude de la généralisabilité d'un survey. *Educ. Rech.* 3(1): 33–50

Webb N M, Shavelson R J 1981 Multivariate generalizability of general educational development ratings. *J. Educ. Meas.* 18(1): 13–22

Webb N M, Herman J L, Cabello B 1987 A domain-referenced approach to diagnostic testing using generalizability theory. *J. Educ. Meas.* 24(2): 119–30

Item Bias

J. D. Scheuneman and C. A. Bleistein

Item bias procedures are used to determine whether the individual items on an examination function in the same way for two groups of examinees, usually defined by racial and ethnic background, sex, age and experience, or condition of handicap. These procedures would be applied when the examinee groups of interest appear to differ in their mean level of the ability, knowledge, or skill being measured, making a direct comparison of their performance on the items inappropriate. In most instances these methods are applied when no criteria of the abilities, knowledges, or skills being measured are available outside of the examination in question.

Although the test performance of various population subgroups has long been of interest, the issue of the fairness of the use of tests with these subgroups came into prominence in the measurement literature in the late 1960s and early 1970s. A number of procedures were proposed and evaluated (see *Test Bias*), but all required some criterion of performance in the college or job setting, the two situations in which these methods were most frequently applied.

At the same time, test publishers became interested in instituting procedures to identify problematic items, which could then be revised or eliminated before the test forms were finalized. Criterion measures could not be obtained until tests were in use, however, making the existing procedures inapplicable. Consequently, a number of procedures were devised which were useful where external criteria were unavailable.

Although not all of the procedures that have been suggested have stood the test of time, a number of methods are now generally accepted as useful in isolating items that appear to function differently for two groups. Such methods are now included as part of the test development process of a number of tests (Berk 1982, Diamond and Elmore 1986). Notice, however, that, just as the test bias procedures are inapplicable in this setting, the item bias procedures are not appropriate for evaluating bias or fairness in test use.

For the purpose of this entry, the various methods for detecting item bias are divided into two categories. In the first of these categories are methods based on observed item responses and test scores that use classical measurement methods. The second category contains those approaches based on "true" abilities, as in item response theory models and methods. Throughout the entry, the term "item bias" has been replaced by "differential item functioning" (DIF). This term is coming to be preferred by many researchers because of its focus on what is actually observed rather than suggesting inferences about the nature of the effect. (See Scheuneman 1982 for a discussion of this point.)

1. Classical Approaches

1.1 Transformed Item Difficulty Methods

Essentially these methods of detecting DIF involve calculating percent correct item difficulties (p-values) for two groups of examinees, and transforming the p-values to another metric in order to make the relationship between the respective difficulty values linear. The most widely used of these procedures is the delta plot method (Angoff and Ford 1973). In this procedure, p-values are converted to deltas; that is normal deviates with a mean of 13 and a standard deviation of 4. Typically, a plot on a bivariate chart of the deltas for two groups of equivalent ability will form an ellipse along the 45-degree line through the origin which would represent equal difficulty of the items. When the groups being compared differ in ability, the points will be displaced from this line and the ellipse may be rotated somewhat from 45 degrees. See Fig. 1 for an example of a delta plot.

The major axis of the ellipse is defined in terms of the points representing the item difficulties for the two groups. Using X and Y to represent the respective item difficulties for the two groups being compared, the major axis is given by:

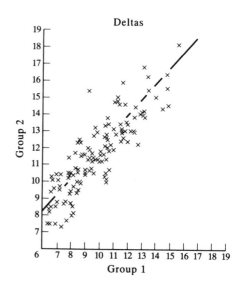

Figure 1

Example of transformed item difficulties (deltas) plotted for two groups

$$Y = aX + b \tag{1}$$

where:

$$a = \frac{(S_y^2 - S_x^2) \pm \sqrt{(S_y^2 - S_x^2) + 4r_{xy}^2 S_x^2 S_y^2}}{2r_{xy}S_xS_y}, \tag{2}$$

and

$$b = M_y - aM_x \tag{3}$$

The distance of each item from the major axis is measured by:

$$d_i = (ax_i - y_i + b)/a^2 + 1 \tag{4}$$

Other indices used with the delta plot method include the standard deviation of d_i and the correlation between the delta values of the two groups, the magnitude of which reflects the degree to which items rank in the same order of difficulty in both subgroups. The method may also be generalized to the investigation of several groups simultaneously (Angoff 1975). Modifications have been proposed by Sinnott (1980) and Rudner et al. (1980a).

Advantages of the delta plot method are that it is simple, inexpensive, easily explained, and does not require large numbers of examinees, although a reasonably large set of items is required to assure that the major axis is well-defined. A principle disadvantage is that when two groups differ in their mean ability, an item that is unusually discriminating will result in larger item difficulty differences, while an item that has particularly low discrimination will show smaller differences than the other items on the test even when the items are not functioning differentially. Angoff (1982) suggested using groups matched on ability to circumvent this problem. The method is sample dependent, as is the case for all the classical procedures, and the delta values for different-sized samples are not equally reliable. This latter difficulty can be overcome by using an arcsin transformation rather than the inverse normal transformation used by the delta plots (Cardall and Coffman 1964, Plake and Hoover 1979–80).

1.2 Item Discrimination Procedures

Pairs of item discrimination indices (point-biserials) for different ethnic or gender groups have been plotted in the manner described for transformed item difficulties and the plots examined for outliers in an attempt to identify differentially functioning items. Green and Draper (1972) used point-biserial correlations to separate the items in a test into "best half" and "worst half" and defined differentially functioning items as those chosen as best for one group and worst for another. These methods have the same advantages as the transformed item difficulty methods. Unfortunately, studies of these procedures have suggested that these methods lack validity for identifying items that

function differentially (Ironson and Subkoviak 1979, Rudner 1977, Shepard et al. 1981).

1.3 Contingency Table Approaches

The contingency table methods were first suggested by Scheuneman (1979) based on a definition stating that for an item that does not function differentially, persons of equal ability have equal probability of a correct response regardless of their group membership. This definition was operationalized in a contingency table made up of group membership and ability, which was defined by score ranges on the test or subtest on which the item appeared (see *Contingency Tables*). A number of variations of this technique have since been suggested and are discussed below. All of these methods assume that the test score, which is used as the ability measure, is valid and reliable and that the test is essentially unidimensional. Without unidimensionality, it cannot be assumed that two people with the same score have equivalent ability.

1.3.1 Chi-square methods. Scheuneman's (1979) contingency table method and variations which use a chi-square value as an index are collectively referred to as chi-square methods. After collapsing the score scale into J intervals (typically 3 to 5), an index value is computed. Scheuneman's original index, C2, which is based only on correct responses, is calculated as follows:

$$C2 = \sum_{j=1}^{j} \frac{(E_{j1} - O_{j1})^2}{E_{j1}} + \sum_{j=1}^{j} \frac{(E_{j2} - O_{j2})^2}{E_{j2}} \tag{5}$$

where:

O_{jk} = the observed frequency of correct responses for score interval j and group k;
$E_{jk} = P_{j.} N_{jk}$ = the expected frequency of correct responses for score interval j and group k;
$P_{j.}$ = proportion correct across all groups within score interval j;
N_{jk} = the number of examinees in score interval j and group k.

The procedure may be readily extended to evaluate item functioning for several groups simultaneously. Not only does this provide computational efficiency, but the results provide information on the relative standings of the groups that is not available from pairwise comparisons. For example, if four groups are being compared and the item with a high index value is functioning similarly for three of them, it is clear for which group the item is functioning differentially and whether this group is favored or disfavored by the item.

Scheuneman's method has been criticized because the associated index is not distributed as the chi-square, although it has a chi-squarelike appearance. Hence it does not have an associated sampling distribution and significance tests cannot properly be employed. The modification that has most commonly been suggested includes the incorrect responses in the contingency table, a variation often attributed to Camilli (1979). It is possible to derive a formula including this information which permits the chi-square index to be obtained without actually having to compute the expected values for the incorrect responses (Scheuneman 1981). This formula is as follows:

$$\chi^2_{full} = \sum_{j=1}^{j} \frac{(E_{j1} - O_{j1})^2}{E_j(1 - P_{j0})} + \sum_{j=1}^{j} \frac{(E_{j2} - O_{j2})^2}{E_{j2}(1 - P_{j0})} \qquad (6)$$

The chi-square methods have several important advantages: notably their intuitive appeal due to the use of groups matched on ability, simplicity, and appropriateness for small sample sizes. They are also inexpensive to obtain. The C2 and the full chi-square index tend to produce very similar results (Scheuneman 1986), but can be contrasted on a number of points. When sample sizes are large, the full chi-square has tended to perform somewhat better in research studies, but minimum samples are probably about 300 in contrast to about 100 for the C2 index. The full chi-square does better in evaluating difficult items; the C2 does better for easy items. Both methods have been criticized because groups may not be equivalent in ability within the broad score intervals used.

1.3.2 Log–linear methods. General log–linear models provide a means of analyzing qualitative data through their relationship to the elements of contingency tables (see *Log-Linear Models*). The application of these models to the evaluation of DIF involves: (a) the construction of a three-way contingency table (ability level by group by item response) for each item similar to that used with the chi-square methods; (b) specification and fitting of the models of interest; (c) calculation of a residual goodness-of-fit measure, such as the chi-square likelihood ratio (G2); and (d) testing for significant differences between models; that is the difference between the G2 obtained for the two models.

Three hierarchical models are typically used in the study of DIF. The first tests for a main effect of ability level; in the second, a term is added for a main effect of group; and the last requires a term for the interaction of ability with group. If Model 1 adequately fits the data, no DIF exists. If Model 2 provides a significantly better fit, the item is exhibiting DIF that is uniform across ability levels; and if Model 3 is needed to explain the data, the DIF is nonuniform in nature (see Mellenbergh 1982).

Examples of research applying this methodology to the detection of DIF include the work of Alderman and Holland (1981), Mellenberg (1982), and van der Flier et al. (1984). An advantage of log–linear models over the other contingency table methods is that they provide added information by distinguishing between uniform effects, resulting where the differential functioning is with regard to difficulty only, and nonuniform effects, resulting where differences

in item discrimination also exist. They may also be used with relatively small sample sizes. The major disadvantage is that the available software uses an iterative algorithm to process the data so the method is more expensive than the other classical procedures and requires more expertise to use.

1.3.3 Mantel–Haenszel procedure. This procedure, developed by Mantel and Haenszel (1959), is closely related to log–linear procedures for detecting first-order interactions, and has been used extensively in biomedical research. Its application to the study of DIF was introduced by Holland (Holland and Thayer 1988). As with the other contingency table methods, performance is compared for group members of comparable ability, with total test score as the matching criterion. The Mantel–Haenszel (MH) estimate (α_{MH}) is a weighted average of the odds ratio at each of j scores, and may be interpreted as the average factor by which the likelihood that a member of one group answers the item correctly exceeds the corresponding likelihood for a member of the other group. The equation for the MH estimate is:

$$\alpha_{MH} = \left(\sum_j A_j D_j / T_j \right) \Big/ \left(\sum_j B_j C_j / T_j \right) \qquad (7)$$

where:

A_j = the number of group 1 members responding correctly;
B_j = the number of group 1 members responding incorrectly;
C_j = the number of group 2 members responding correctly;
D_j = the number of group 2 members responding incorrectly;
$T_j = A_j + B_j + C_j + D_j$ = the total number of examinees with score j who responded to the item.

An α_{MH} value of 1.00 indicates that a correct response is equally likely for both groups. If α_{MH} is greater than 1.00, group 1 members are more likely to respond correctly, and if less than 1.00, group 2 members have the advantage. To test the hypothesis of independence of response and group membership, a one-degree of freedom chi-square test is associated with the MH estimator and is calculated as:

$$\chi^2_{MH} = \frac{\left(\left| \sum_j A_j - E(A_j) \right| \frac{1}{2} \right)^2}{\sum_j S(A_j)^2} \qquad (8)$$

where:

$$E(A_j) = [(A_j + B_j)(A_j + C_j)] / T_j, \qquad (9)$$

and:

$$S(A_j)^2 = \frac{(A_j + B_j)(C_j + D_j)(A_j + C_j)(B_j + D_j)}{T^2_j(T_j - 1)} \qquad (10)$$

A major difference between the MH procedure and the contingency table methods discussed so far is that it matches on total test score by unit intervals, thus avoiding the problems associated with collapsing the score scale into categories. Sample sizes required are therefore greater than those required for the previously discussed methods (about 500 per group), but smaller than those for the three-parameter item response theory models to be discussed below. In addition, the MH procedure does not require computer programs using expensive iterations as do log–linear and item response theory models. If nonuniform DIF is of concern, MH may not be the best choice of method since it may fail to detect instances of this type of DIF.

1.4 Standardization Procedure

The standardization procedure, developed by Dorans and Kulick (1986), is based on an empirical item response function where the probability of a correct response to an item is estimated by the observed proportion correct at each ability level (typically measured in unit intervals of total test score). Estimates of the conditional probability of success at each score level are developed on the "reference group," the group that forms the performance reference for the "focal group" (the group of interest, which is typically the lower scoring group). The reference group is usually the larger sample and provides the most stable estimates across the score range.

The DIF index provided by the standardization method uses a weighting function supplied by the standardization group. In practice, the weight chosen has been the number of focal group examinees at a given score level (K_j) because this weights the differences between the probabilities of a correct response for the reference and focal groups most heavily at score levels most often achieved by the focal group members. However, other options are available for the weighting function. The item discrepancy index is the standardized p-difference (D_{STD}), defined as:

$$D_{STD} = \sum_j K_j (P_{jf} - P_{jr}) / \sum_j K_j \qquad (11)$$

where:

$(K_j / \sum K_j)$ = the weighting factor;
P_{jf} = the probability that a focal group member at a given score level will answer the item correctly;
P_{jr} = the corresponding probability for the reference group.

An advantage of the standardization procedure is that visual aids have been developed to assist in interpretation. Graphical displays of the conditional probabilities of successful performance and the difference between these probabilities for focal and base groups for each item are shown in Figs. 2a and 2b. Typically, these plots are produced only for items flagged for high values of D_{STD}.

Computationally the standardization and Mantel–Haenszel approaches are very similar, with the primary difference being in the weights used, although the standardization estimates tend to be more stable. The principle disadvantage of both methods is

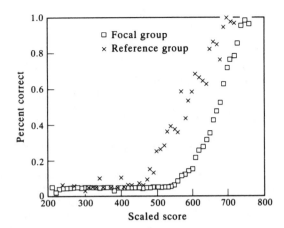

Figure 2a
Conditional probabilities of successful performance for reference and focal groups

that large samples are required for stable estimation. (See Dorans 1989 for a comparison of these two procedures.)

1.5 Logistic Regression Method

Conceptually related to the contingency table methods, particularly the log–linear method, the logistic regression method is designed to detect both uniform and nonuniform DIF (Swaminathan and Rogers 1990). Rather than treating the ability dimension as a set of unordered categories, however, this procedure retains ability as a continuum. In the model, the probability of a correct response is a function of z, where:

$$Z_i = \tau_0 + \tau_1 \theta + \tau_2 g + \tau_3 (\theta g) \qquad (12)$$

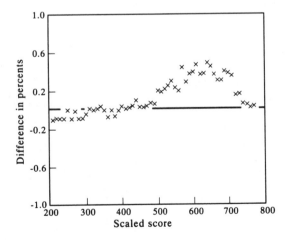

Figure 2b
Difference in conditional probabilities of successful performance between reference and focal groups

745

and $\tau_0 \tau_1$ = intercept and slope of the logistic function;
θ = examinee ability;
g = 1 for examinees belonging to group 1 and 0 for examinees belonging to group 2;
θg = the product of g and θ.

The parameter τ_2 corresponds to the group difference in performance and τ_3 to the interaction between group and ability. An item shows uniform DIF if $\tau_2 \neq 0$ and τ_3 = 0, and nonuniform DIF if $\tau_3 \neq 0$, whether or not τ_2 = 0. The values of τ_1, τ_2, τ_3, and τ_4 are estimated using maximum likelihood methods. Significance tests are available.

This method has not yet been widely evaluated but appears to compare well with the Mantel–Haenszel procedure for simulated instances of uniform bias, and will detect instances of nonuniform bias that the MH procedure misses. It is more difficult to compute, however, and, because it uses iterative procedures, is more expensive than MH and many of the other classical procedures.

1.6 Distractor Analysis

In addition to flagging items for DIF, distractor analysis may be used to help provide an explanation of the result. Scheuneman (1982) described three methods for analysis of distractors: (a) her comparison of mean-scaled scores of individuals responding to each option, (b) Veale and Foreman's (1983) chi-square based on the incorrect options only, and (c) Frary and Giles's (1980) Rasch model method. Green et al. (1989) propose the use of log–linear models to examine the possibility of a subgroup-by-option interaction when ability is held constant. They advocate analyzing DIF through incorrect responses and describe their method as the study of differential distractor functioning. Any of the contingency tables methods can also be used to analyze distractors, where sample sizes are large enough, by repeating the procedures on one or more of the distractors rather than on the keyed response.

2. Item Response Theory Approaches

The DIF procedures using item response theory (also known as latent trait theory) are often considered preferable to the classical approaches discussed above because of their theoretical underpinnings. The assumption of item response theory (IRT), that makes it useful for investigating DIF, is that the estimated parameters of the item response function (IRF) are invariant for different samples drawn from the same population (see *Item Response Theory*). Hence, if parameters are estimated separately for two groups, the resulting IRFs of an item which is functioning equivalently for those groups should be the same (apart from a linear transformation of scale). This means that the probability of a correct response for persons at a given ability level is the same for both groups, a statement equivalent to the definition given for the contingency

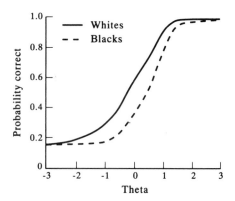

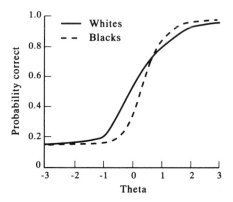

Figure 3
IRFS obtained for two items that demonstrate DIF for Black and White examinees

table methods except that the true ability scale is used rather than observed test scores. Where there is DIF, however, the IRFs will be displaced from each other somewhat. Fig. 3 shows the IRFs for two such items.

2.1 Three-parameter Methods

Although all of the IRT methods agree that an item for which the IRFs are different for two groups is functioning differentially for those groups, a number of procedures for distinguishing such differences from error of parameter estimation have been suggested. As yet, no clear preference for any one of these procedures has emerged.

In the method proposed by Rudner (1977), the items are calibrated separately for each of the two groups being compared and equated for scale. The area between the two obtained curves is then approximated by summing the difference between the probability of a correct response at small increments of ability. The formula for the area is expressed by:

$$\varphi_k = \sum_{-4.0}^{4.0} | P_1(u_k = 1 | \theta_j) - P_2(u_k = 1 | \theta_j) | \Delta\theta \quad (13)$$

where $P(u_k=1)$ = the logistic function with the parameter values that were obtained when calibrating the item for group k, and $\Delta\theta = .005$.

Once the item calibrations have been done, this statistic can be calculated readily with a simple computer program. Perhaps for this reason it is the method used in most of the research comparing the three-parameter IRT methods to other DIF procedures. Raju (1990) has developed significance tests for both signed and unsigned area measures, thus enhancing the usefulness of this method.

For the procedure suggested by Lord (1980), items are first calibrated with all examinees together in order to get better estimates of the c parameters. These are then held constant and the a and b parameters are re-estimated for the two groups separately and equated for scale. Lord then suggests a chi-square test which permits simultaneous comparison of the a and the b parameters in the two separate calibrations. The significance test is asymptotic; it assumes that the abilities are known, rather than estimated; and can be applied only to maximum likelihood estimates of a and b. The primary disadvantage of this method is that it requires a complex computer program to obtain the chi-square values, although this is not particularly expensive to run once the parameter estimates have been obtained.

Linn and Harnish (1981) suggested a procedure that compares the actual performance of focal group members with that predicted by the model. The items are first calibrated on the total group and estimates of ability are obtained for the focal group. Fit is then assessed with a standardized difference score using the following formula:

$$Z_i = \frac{1}{N_f} \sum_{ef} \frac{U_{ij} - P_{ij}}{P_{ij}(1 - P_{ij})} \quad (14)$$

where:

$U_{ij} = 1$ if item i is answered correctly by person j, and 0 otherwise;

N_f = the number in group f;

P_{ij} = estimated probability that person j would answer item i correctly, based on the fitted model from combined groups.

This method permits the use of IRT methods in instances where the total sample is large enough for IRT-item calibration, but the focal group of interest is not. This is a common situation for practical applications of DIF methods. As with the area method, the statistics are easy to compute once the calibrations have been done. If the model does not fit the data for that item, either for the focal or reference group, however, DIF may be identified where it does not in fact exist.

In those instances where the IRT model can be shown to fit the data, these procedures offer a strong theoretical basis and the advantages of true ability estimates

rather than observed scores. Research suggests that these methods are superior to the classical approaches for the identification of DIF (Ironson and Subkoviak 1979, Rudner et al. 1980b, Shepard et al. 1981). In general, however, the three-parameter methods will be more expensive than either the classical methods or the Rasch model methods. LOGIST, one of the more frequently used computer programs for parameter estimation, is an iterative program and is consequently very expensive to run. Large samples are required (at least 1,000 people per group and 40 items), and the c parameters often fail to converge. Robustness of the estimation techniques to violation of the IRT model assumptions is unknown. (See Hills 1989 for a summary of the advantages and disadvantages of the different IRT indices as well as several of the classical indices.)

2.2 The Rasch Model

In the Rasch model, the discrimination of the items is assumed to be constant and the lower asymptote of the IRF is assumed to be zero (see *Rasch Measurement, Theory of*). Hence, if the IRFs for two groups differ, the difference must be in the location parameter, d, representing item difficulty. The two most common procedures used for evaluating DIF with the Rasch model examine either the differences in difficulty between groups (the difficulty shift), or the fit of each item to the model in each group (Draba 1977, Durovic 1975, Wright et al. 1976).

To analyze a difficulty shift, the d parameters are estimated for each group separately and placed on the same scale. A t statistic may then be used to evaluate the difference in d parameters for the two groups for each item, where:

$$t_i = (d_{i1} - d_{i2})/(SE_{i1}^2 + SE_{i2}^2) \quad (15)$$

and SE represents the standard error of d. If t is large, the item is functioning differentially in the two groups.

Analysis of the fit of each item to the model assumes that a non-DIF item will have a similar fit in each group. Again, statistics are generated for each group separately and a chi-square with one degree of freedom is computed for each item in each group as:

$$\chi^2 = Z_{ij}^2 = \frac{[x_{ij} - E(x_{ij})]^2}{S^2(x_{ij})} \quad (16)$$

where:

x_{ij} = an individual's score ($i = 1$ or 0) on item j;

$E(x_{ij})$ = the expected response predicted by the model;

$S^2(x_{ij})$ = the variance of the expected value.

The overall fit of an item is given by the mean square:

$$MS_i = \sum_{j}^{n} Z_{ij}^2 [L/(n-1)(L-1)] \quad (17)$$

where: L = test length and n = the number of individuals in the sample.

MS has an expected value of 1 and a standard error of $2L/(n-1)(L-1)$. Fit of each item to the model for different groups has also been assessed by the difference in mean square residuals (Wright et al. 1976).

In their evaluation of DIF, Rudner et al. (1980b) found the difficulty shift analysis to be better than the fit statistic. Shepard et al. (1981) found a near perfect correlation of results between the difficulty shift statistic and a delta plot distance measure. Both studies found that the Rasch model methods worked less well than the chi square procedures.

The major advantages of the Rasch model are the theoretical parameter invariance and the availability of the computer programs to process the data inexpensively. There is disagreement regarding the minimum sample required. Some have argued that as few as 100 are adequate to obtain good estimates of the *d* parameter (Wright 1977). The crucial problem for these techniques is whether the Rasch model provides an adequate fit to the data.

3. Prospects and Challenges for Research

Work will continue into the future on statistical or procedural refinements of the methods described above. New statistical methods may also emerge in the coming years. Two major challenges will need to be met in future research that go beyond the methodologies used in the early 1990s. First is the challenge set by modes of assessment other than multiple choice where items may not be dichotomously scored. Further, some of these assessment modes may not have an internal criterion measure of ability, such as a total score used with multiple-choice tests, that is adequate for the use of the DIF procedures as they are conceptualized. Second is the challenge raised by the frequent inability of researchers to move beyond the statistical results to an understanding of why these differences occur and what corrective actions—if any—might be taken.

See also: Measurement in Educational Research

References

Alderman D L, Holland P W 1981 *Item Performance Across Native Language Groups on the Test of English as a Foreign Language*. Educational Testing Service, Princeton, New Jersey

Angoff W H 1975 The investigation of test bias in the absence of an outside criterion. Paper presented at the National Institute of Education Conference on Test Bias, Annapolis, Maryland

Angoff W H 1982 The use of difficulty and discrimination indices in the identification of biased test items. In: Berk R A (ed.) 1982

Angoff W H, Ford S F 1973 Item–race interaction on a test

of scholastic aptitude. *J. Educ. Meas.* 10: 95–106

Berk R A (ed.) 1982 *Handbook of Methods for Detecting Test Bias*. Johns Hopkins University Press, Baltimore, Maryland

Camilli G 1979 A critique of the chi square method for assessing item bias. Unpublished paper, Laboratory of Educational Research, University of Colorado, Boulder, Colorado

Cardall C, Coffman W E 1964 *A Method for Comparing the Performance of Different Groups on the Items in a Test*. Educational Testing Service, Princeton, New Jersey

Diamond E E, Elmore P B 1986 Bias in achievement testing: Follow-up report of the AMECD Commission on Bias in Measurement. *Meas. Eval. Couns. Dev.* 19: 102–12

Dorans N J 1989 Two new approaches to assessing differential item functioning: Standardization and the Mantel–Haenszel method. *Applied Measurement in Education* 2: 217–33

Dorans N J, Kulick E 1986 Demonstrating the utility of the standardization approach to assessing unexpected differential item performance on the Scholastic Aptitude Test. *J. Educ. Meas.* 23: 355–68

Draba R E 1977 *The Identification and Interpretation of Item Bias*. Statistical Laboratory, Department of Education, University of Chicago, Chicago, Illinois

Durovic J J 1975 Test bias: An objective definition for test items. ERIC Document Reproduction Service No. ED 128 381, Washington, DC

Frary R B, Giles M B 1980 Multiple choice test bias as reflected by examinee selection of inappropriate answers. Report submitted to the National Institute of Education under grant No. NIE-G-79–0140

Green B F, Crone C R, Folk V G 1989 A method for studying differential distractor functioning. *J. Educ. Meas.* 26: 147–60

Green D R, Draper J F 1972 Exploratory studies of bias in achievement tests. ERIC Document Reproduction Service No. ED 070 794, Washington, DC

Hills J R 1989 Screening for potentially biased items in testing programs. *Educational Measurement: Issues and Practice* 8(4): 5–11

Holland P W, Thayer D T 1988 Differential item performance and the Mantel–Haenszel procedure. In: Wainer H, Braun H I (eds.) 1988 *Test Validity*. Erlbaum, Hillsdale, New Jersey

Ironson G H, Subkoviak M J 1979 A comparison of several methods of assessing item bias. *J. Educ. Meas.* 16: 209–25

Linn R L, Harnish D 1981 Interactions between item content and group membership in achievement test items. *J. Educ. Meas.* 18: 109–18

Lord F M 1980 *Application of Item Response Theory to Practical Testing Problems*. Erlbaum, Hillsdale, New Jersey

Mantel N, Haenszel W 1959 Statistical aspects of the analysis of data from retrospective studies of disease. *Journal of the National Cancer Institute* 22: 719–48

Mellenbergh G 1982 Contingency table models for assessing item bias. *J. Ed. Stat.* 7: 105–18

Plake B S, Hoover H D 1979–80 An analytical method of identifying biased test items. *J. Exp. Educ.* 48: 153–54

Raju N 1990 Determining the significance of estimated

signed and unsigned areas between two item characteristic curves. *Appl. Psychol. Meas.* 14: 197–207

Rudner L M 1977 An evaluation of select approaches for biased item identification. (Doctoral dissertation, Catholic University of America)

Rudner L M, Getson P R, Knight D L 1980a Biased item detection techniques. *J. Ed. Stat.* 5: 213–33

Rudner L M, Geston P R, Knight D L 1980b A Monte Carlo comparison of seven biased item detection techniques. *J. Educ. Meas.* 17: 1–10

Scheuneman J D 1979 A method of assessing bias in test items. *J. Educ. Meas.* 16: 143–52

Scheuneman J D 1981 A response to Baker's criticism. *J. Educ. Meas.* 18: 63–66

Scheuneman J D 1982 A posteriori analyses of biased items. In: Berk R A (ed.) 1982

Scheuneman J D 1986 Differential item performance: Use of computer simulation to evaluate indices. In Angoff W H (ed.) 1986 *Differential Item Performance: Methodological and Measurement Issues.* American Educational Research Association, San Francisco, California

Shepard L A, Camilli G, Averill M 1981 Comparison of procedures for detecting test-item bias using both internal and external ability criteria. *J. Educ. Stat.* 6: 317–75

Sinnott L T 1980 *Differences in Item Performance Across Groups.* Educational Testing Service, Princeton, New Jersey

Swaminathan H, Rogers H J 1990 Detecting differential item functioning using logistic regression procedures. *J. Educ. Meas.* 27: 361–70

Van der Flier H, Mellenbergh G, Ader H J, Wijn M 1984 An iterative item bias detection method. *J. Educ. Meas.* 21: 131–45

Veale J R, Foreman D I 1983 Assessing cultural bias using foil response data: Cultural variation. *J. Educ. Meas.* 20: 249–58

Wright B D 1977 Solving measurement problems with the Rasch model. *J. Educ. Meas.* 14: 97–115

Wright B D, Mead R J, Draba R 1976 *Detecting and Correcting Test Item Bias with a Logistic Response Model.* Statistical Laboratory, Department of Education, University of Chicago, Chicago, Illinois

Item Writing Techniques

J. L. Herman

Item writing techniques provide rules and prescriptions for constructing sound test items, items that measure what they are intended to measure. Until relatively recently, these rules have incorporated the conventional wisdom of test writers and have provided only general guidance on how to devise test items that do not clue or unnecessarily confuse an examinee's response. Since the 1960s, however, in tandem with the growth of criterion-referenced testing, item writing techniques increasingly have focused attention on the nature and structure of test content and ways to define and operationalize what is being measured. The match between the intended content of a test and that of test items is no longer left to the implicit understanding of the item writer; rather, newer item writing technologies provide explicit, specific rules to help insure that test items measure particular domains of knowledge, skills, and/or abilities. This entry provides an overview to a range of current item writing techniques. It is limited to techniques for measuring academic achievement and focuses principally on selected response or "objective" measures.

1. Conventional Guidelines

Conventional item construction guidelines help inhibit the inclusion of extraneous factors in test items that confound an examinee's response. They concentrate on factors such as linguistic, semantic, and grammatical features that may enable an unknowing examinee to give a correct response or that may prevent a knowing examinee from responding correctly.

Typical rules for multiple-choice items, short answer and completion items, and true–false response items are given in Fig. 1 (Gronlund 1971, Conoley and O'Neil 1979).

2. Techniques for Constructing Replicable Test Items

While general guidelines of the sort listed in Fig. 1 are useful for constructing sound test items, they represent necessary but not sufficient criteria. Left open is the issue of how to construct items that capture and validly reflect intended test content. A number of approaches to this problem have evolved over the years; these approaches differ in the degree of specificity, amount of discretion left in the hands of the item writer, and replicability of the items generated.

Content–process matrices represent the loosely structured end of the continuum, where item writers are accorded a great deal of discretion in devising individual items. Derived from a curriculum general scheme described by the work of Tyler and Bloom, broad subject domains are partitioned into two dimensions of content and process. Content includes the key concepts of the subject field and process the levels of reasoning specified by Bloom's taxonomy. Subject area experts write items they consider appropriate for each cell of the matrix, guided only by the simple content-process designation.

Criterion-referenced approaches, exemplified first by objectives-based techniques and later by domain

---

Typical rules for multiple-choice items:

1. The stem of the item should be meaningful by itself and should present a clear problem.
2. The stem should be free from irrelevant material.
3. The stem should include as much of the item as possible except where an inclusion would clue. Repetitive phrases should be included in the stem rather than being restated in each alternative.
4. All alternatives should be grammatically consistent with the item stem and of similar length, so not as to provide a clue to the answer.
5. An item should include only one correct or clearly best answer.
6. Items used to measure understanding should contain some novelty and not merely repeat verbatim materials or problems presented in instruction.
7. All distractors should be plausible and related to the body of knowledge and learning experiences measured.
8. Verbal associations between the stem and correct answer or stereotyped phrases should be avoided.
9. The correct answer should appear in each of the alternative positions with approximatley equal frequency and in random order.
10. Special alternatives such as "none," "all of the above" should be used sparingly.
11. Avoid items that contain inclusive terms (e.g., "never," "always," "all") in the wrong answer.
12. Negatively stated item stems should be used sparingly.
13. Avoid alternatives that are opposite in meaning or that are paraphrases of each other.
14. Avoid items which ask for opinions.
15. Avoid items that contain irrelevant sources of difficulty, such as vocabulary, or sentence structure.
16. Avoid interlocking items, items whose answers clue responses to subsequent items.
17. Don't use multiple choice items where other item formats are more appropriate.

Typical rules for short answer and completion items:

1. A direct question is generally better than an incomplete statement.
2. Word the item so that the required answer is both brief and unambiguous.
3. Where an answer is to be expressed in numerical units, indicate the type of units wanted.
4. Blanks for answers should be equal in length. Scoring is facilitated if the blanks are provided in a column to the right of the question.
5. Where completion items are used, do not leave many blanks.
6. For completion items, leave blank only those things that are important to remember.
7. In composing items, don't take statements verbatim from students' textbook or instruction.

Typical rules for true-false or alternative response items:

1. Avoid broad general statements for true-false items.
2. Avoid trivial statements.
3. Avoid negative statements and especially double negatives.
4. Avoid long complex sentences.
5. Avoid including two ideas in a single statement unless cause-effect relationships are being measured.
6. Include opinion statements only if they are attributed to particular sources.
7. True statements and false statements should be approximately the same length.
8. The number of true statements and of false statements should be approxiamtely equal.
9. Avoid taking statements verbatim from students' text or instruction.

Figure 1
General guidelines for item writing

referencing, provide more direction for item writers' efforts. Objectives specify observable stimulus and response conditions that describe the nature of the task that is expected of the learner and conditions under which the task is to be performed. The objective becomes the target of assessment, and test items are generated to match the conditions specified, for example, "Given a short story, the student will select, from among four given alternatives, the main idea."

The probability that items produced by two writers will be parallel is higher for objectives-based approaches than for content–process schemes; however, significant discretion and areas of item writer variability still exist. For example, different writers may vary in their definitions of "short story," in the extent to which main ideas are stated or implied, in the amount of supporting detail, and so on.

More fine-grained specifications of the intended test content have been developed to control this variability and to define more precisely the domain of behavior to be assessed—descriptions that serve to prescribe test item development. The goal of these more elaborate specifications is to define a pool of items that represents an important universe of knowledge or skill domain—such that student performance on one set of items drawn from the domain would generalize to a second set of items and to the entire defined domain. In its most highly prescribed form, domain specifications provide an exhaustive set of rules for generating a set of related test items. For example, item forms developed by Hively et al. (1973) include:

(a) general description of what the item form is about;

(b) item form shell, which provides a sample item as it would be administered to examinees and the common unvarying elements of each item generated;

(c) stimulus and response characteristics, which describe the theoretical characteristics of the item generation scheme and the dimensions which are varied to comprise the replacement sets;

(d) replacement schemes and replacement sets, which detail the exact mechanics of generating item pools for the given domain;

(e) scoring specifications, which describe the properties to be used to distinguish between a correct and an incorrect response (see Fig. 2).

Similarly, Osburn has described item forms which (a)

generate items with a fixed syntactical structure; (b) contain one or more variable elements; (c) define a class of item sentences by specifying the replacement sets for the variable elements. Facet design, originated by Guttman, likewise specifies a universe of content in terms of a mapping sentence that contains variable facets—the latter operates like replacement sets in Hively's item forms.

The most highly specific item forms and mapping sentence approaches permit computerized test item writing. Using author languages such as COURSEWRITER, PLANIT, and TUTOR, a series of computer commands define the wording of an item form and the way the variable elements are chosen or computed.

The applicability of highly specific item forms has been questioned for content areas which are not highly structured; their cost feasibility and widespread practical utility are also a concern. Popham and Baker have both suggested a compromise strategy to optimize descriptive rigor and feasibility. Derived from

---

Producing a number satisfying a given order relation to specified number(s) (spoken form).

General description

The child is asked to say the name of a number that bears a specified order relation ("greater than" or "less than") to a given number of numbers in the range 0 through 20. Given numbers are presented in spoken form and response is spoken.

Stimulus and response characteristics

Constant for all cells

The presentation is completely spoken: a spoken response is required

Distinguishing among cells

Three scripts are used asking respectively for a number greater than a given number, for a number less than a given number, and for a number greater than one given number and less than another.
Within the third script, three conditions are allowed:
(1) first given numeral greater than second with required number possibly an integer; (2) first given numeral greater than second with required number necessarily not an integer; and (3) first given numeral less than second so that the solution to the problem is the empty set.

Varying within cells

Within each cell, the given numbers are integers from the range 0 through 20 chosen so that the correct response (when it is not the empty set) can be a real number from the range 0 through 20.

Item form shell

Materials None	
Directions to examiner Read script to child Write down child's exact words	Script Tell me a number that is _____

Replacement scheme

(a) Script
Cell 1: "less than b_1" "greater than b_1"
Cells 3, 4, 5: "greater than b_1 but less than b_2"

(b) Numerals with script
Cell 1: Choose b_1 from R.S. 9.1
Cell 2: Choose b_1 from R.S. 9.2
Cell 3: Choose two numbers from R.S. 9.3
Cell 3: Choose two numbers from R.S. 9.3
    Let b_1 = smaller number; b_2 = larger number
    Reject if $b_2 - b_1 \leqslant 1$
Cell 4: Choose b_1 from R.S. 9.3
    Let $b_2 = b_1 + 1$
Cell 5: Choose two numbers from R.S. 9.3
    Let b_1 = larger number; b_2 = smaller number
    Reject if $b_1 = b_2$

Replacement sets

R.S. 9.1: Whole numbers 0, 1, 2....., 19
R.S. 9.2: Whole numbers 1, 2, 3....., 20
R.S. 9.3: Whole numbers 0, 1, 2....., 20

Scoring specifications

Cell 1: Any real number X where $X > b_1$
Cell 2: Any real number X where $X < b_1$
Cell 3: Any real number X where $b_1 < X < b_2$
Cell 4: Any real number X where $b_1 < X < b_2$
Cell 5: Any response equivalent to saying that there are no numbers which can fulfill the conditions.

Cell matrix

Script (a)	"greater than b_1"	"less than b_1"	"greater than b_1 but less than b_2"		
Numerals (b)	$0 \leqslant b_1 \leqslant 19$	$1 \leqslant b_1 \leqslant 20$	$0 \leqslant b_1 \leqslant 18$ $b_1 + 2 \leqslant b_2 \leqslant 20$	$0 \leqslant b_1 \leqslant 19$ $b_2 = b_1 + 1$	$1 \leqslant b_1 \leqslant 20$ $0 \leqslant b_2 < b_1$
	(1)	(2)	(3)	(4)	(5)

Figure 2
Sample Item form

Hively's work, their approach features an expanded objective which delimits the nature of the intended content and response and provides explicit rules for generating test items. First known as amplified objectives and in their more recent refinement, domain specifications, these statements detail (a) a general description of the knowledge, skill, or attitude being measured; (b) content limits, which describe the range of eligible content for constructing the item stem; (c) response limits, which describe the nature of the correct response, including specific criteria for judging the adequacy of a constructed response, or rules for generating distractors for multiple-choice items; and (d) sample items and directions for administration. Figure 3 provides a sample domain specification.

3. Item Writing Algorithms

Domain specifications provide rules for generating test items, and the source of such rules has received modest attention. Hively has indicated the curriculum as a source, and has described inductive and deductive approaches to generating item generation rules

---

Grade level:	Grade 3
Subject:	Reading comprehension
Domain description:	Students will select from among written alternatives the stated main idea of a given short paragraph
Content limits:	1. For each item, student will be presented with a 4-5 sentence expository paragraph. Each paragraph will have a stated main idea and 3-4 supporting statements.
	2. The main idea will be stated in either the first or the last sentence of the paragraph. The main idea will associate the subject of the paragraph (person, object, action) with a general statement of action, or general descriptive statement of action, or general descriptive statement. For example, "Smoking is dangerous to your health," "Kenny worked hard to become a doctor," "There are many kinds of seals."
	3. Supporting statements will give details, examples, or evidence supporting the main idea.
	4. Paragraphs will be written at no higher than a third grade reading level.
Response limits:	1. Students will select an answer from among four written alternatives. Each alternative will be a complete sentence.
	2. The correct answer will consist of a paraphrase of the stated main idea. Paraphrased sentences may be accomplished by employing synonyms and /or by changing the word order.
	3. Distractors will be constructed from the following:

(a) One distractor will be a paraphrase of one supporting statement given in the paragraph (e.g., alternative "a" in the sample item).

(b) One or two distractors will be generalizations that can be drawn from two of the supporting statements, but do not include the entire main idea (e.g., alternative "d" in the sample item).

(c) One distractor may be a statement about the subject of the paragraph that is more general than the main idea (e.g., alternative "b" in the sample item).

Format:	Each question will be multiple choice with four possible responses.
Directions:	Read each paragraph. Circle the letter that tells the main idea.
Sample item:	Indians had many kinds of homes. Plains Indians lived in teepees which were made from skins. The Hopi Indians used bushes to make round houses, called hogans. The Mohawks made longhouses out of wood. Some Northeast Indians built smaller wooden cabins.

What is the main idea of this story?

a. Some Indians used skins to make houses.
b. There were different Indian tribes.
c. Indians built different types of houses.
d. Indian houses were made of wood.

Figure 3
Sample domain specifications

and schemes. Others have attempted to describe rules for item generation which are applicable across curricula and content areas, for instance, assessing prose learning and comprehension and concept learning.

3.1 Linguistic-based Approaches to Item Writing

Bormuth (1970) was among the first to stress the need for an item writing technology, and pioneered linguistic-based approaches to assess prose learning and assure a logical connection between test items and instructional materials. Bormuth proposed a detailed set of rules for transforming segments of prose instruction into test items, using his "wh-transformation." He described transformations for two types of items: those derived from a single sentence, and those derived from the relationship between sentences. For example, a sentence is selected from the instructional materials, a substantive word is deleted and replaced with the appropriate *wh* word (*who, what, when, where*, etc.), and the item is constructed by transforming the sentence into a question.

Anderson emphasized the use of paraphrasing in constructing such test items. He pointed out that verbatim questions do not require comprehension, but merely recall. To assess whether an examinee has comprehended the original information, it must be paraphrased and then transformed. He outlined two requirements for paraphrased statements: (a) they have no substantive words in common; (b) they are equivalent in meaning. In addition to assessing comprehension of prose materials, Anderson also outlined a method for testing concepts and principles by substituting particular terms for superordinate ones and replacing with synonyms all remaining substantive words, a process further operationalized by Conoley and O'Neil.

Bormuth's transformational approaches were further refined by Finn (1975) who used case grammar to develop an 82-step algorithm for selecting sentences and for transforming them into questions. Finn's procedures were subsequently streamlined into three major steps:

(a) analyzing the text and selecting the sentences, including procedures for screening tests and selecting the most instructionally relevant and significant sentences, for writing summary sentences, and for using word frequency analyses to identify keywords;
(b) transformation of sentences into questions, by clarifying referents and simplifying the selected sentences, replacing the keyword noun, and rewriting the sentences and a question;
(c) construction of distractors, from learner-free responses, from a fixed list of keywords, or from other similar function words in the instructional passage.

3.2 Concept Learning Approaches to Item Writing

Tiemann and Markle's (1978) research on concept learning provides guidance on how to circumscribe and define valid domains for teaching and assessment. A concept represents a class of objects, events, ideas, or relations which vary among themselves, but are nonetheless classified as the same. For example, the concept "dog" includes dobermans, spaniels, poodles, mutts; "democracy" subsumes parliamentary and congressional varieties; "reinforcer" includes endless specific instances. Concept testing basically involves assessing generalization to *new* examples and discrimination of nonexamples of a particular concept.

Systematic analyses of the critical and variable attributes of a concept are central to both teaching and testing. Critical attributes are those which are common to all members of the class, while variable attributes are those which may differ among members; these attributes define and differentiate the concept domain. For example, all dogs have four legs and a tail, but vary in size, color, length of hair, and so on. Examples and nonexamples of the concept, embodying the presence and/or absence of these various attributes, are constructed for teaching, and new, previously unencountered examples of both types are used to test students' understanding. Novel examples are essential —otherwise simple recall rather than higher levels of thinking are being assessed. Further, examples and nonexamples representing systematic variation of critical and variable attributes can heighten the diagnostic value of resultant test items.

3.3 Other Approaches to Higher Levels of Learning

Williams and Haladyna's (1982) typology is also concerned with constructing higher level test items and provides rules for matching syntactical forms with objectives at various cognitive levels. They define a three-dimensional matrix for classifying objectives and test items: content (including facts, concepts, and principles); task (including reiteration, summarization, illustration, prediction, evaluation, application); and response mode (selected and constructed). Generic objectives for each cell describe the type of situation to which the examinee must respond, the nature of the information or stimulus presented, and the type of response required, for instance, "name," "identify," "define." After selecting the content and task to be tested, the item writer can then use the matrix to determine how to construct an appropriate test item. The Instructional Quality Inventory, developed for use in United States military training, relies on a similar content by task matrix and is particularly concerned with objective/test consistency and adequacy.

4. Summary and Conclusion

In summary, a range of item writing strategies has been advanced since the 1970s. These strategies have been aimed predominantly at defining a universe or domain of knowledge to be tested and at assuring a match between test items and significant instructional content; they seek to maximize instructional and content validity.

Unfortunately, however, there appears to be conflict between features which maximize such validity and those which affect feasibility. For example, the approaches which offer the greatest descriptive rigor are least likely to be implemented by teachers because of time, cost, and technical sophistication requirements. These more elaborate approaches may be more feasible for large-scale national, state, and province assessments, and for creating item banks which are maximally useful for instructional planning and certification—situations where greater resources are available, and resultant items are intended for widespread use.

Item writing is but one step in the test development process. Sound procedures must be used at all steps to assure test validity.

See also: Item Response Theory

References

Bormuth J R 1970 *On the Theory of Achievement Test Items.* University of Chicago Press, Chicago, Illinois

Conoley J, O'Neil H F 1979 A primer for developing tests items. In: O'Neil H F (ed.) 1979 *Procedures for Instructional Systems Development.* Academic Press, New York

Finn P J 1975 A question-writing algorithm. *J. Read. Behav.* 4: 341–67

Gronlund N E 1971 *Measurement and Evaluation in Teaching,* 2nd edn. Macmillan, New York

Hively W, Maxwell G, Rabehl G, Sension D, Lundin S 1973 *Domain-referenced Curriculum Evaluation: A Technical Handbook and a Case Study from the Minnemast Project.* CSE Monograph Series in Evaluation No. 1. Center for the Study of Evaluation, University of California, Los Angeles, California

Tiemann P W, Markle S M 1978 *Analyzing Instructional Content: A Guide to Instruction and Evaluation.* Stipes, Champaign, Illinois

Williams R G, Haladyna T 1982 Logical operations for generating intended questions (LOGIQ): A typology for higher level test items. In: Roid G, Haladyna T (eds.) 1982

Further Reading

Anderson R C 1972 How to construct achievement tests to assess comprehension. *Rev. Educ. Res.* 42: 145–70

Millman J 1980 Computer-based item generation. In: Berk R (ed.) 1980 *Criterion-referenced Measurement.* Johns Hopkins University Press, Baltimore, Maryland

Roid G, Haladyna T 1980 The emergence of an item writing technology. *Rev. Educ. Res.* 50: 293–314

Roid G, Haladyna T 1982 *A Technology for Test-item Writing.* Academic Press, New York

Measurement in Educational Research

J. A. Keats

In describing the application of measurement principles to educational research, it is impossible to separate the contributions that have come from numerous disciplines—education, psychology, sociology, physical sciences, and mathematical statistics. There is little to be gained from making such separations, but certain approaches tend to be known by the name of their principal protagonist and this reference tends to imply that a particular person's discipline is the one making the contribution. No such implication is intended in the present account when techniques are referred to by their customary name.

Measurement in education has been practiced for more than a millennium in China and for centuries elsewhere. However, it was not until the beginning of the twentieth century that research workers studying educational problems became concerned about measurement methods. This situation also existed in the physical sciences where Campbell's (1917) account of physical measurement was the first to be widely recognized and adopted. It was not until educational measurement methods had developed considerably that it was possible to compare them with physical measurement and this was done by a committee of the British Association for the Advancement of Science in 1938 (Ferguson et al. 1940).

In the first four decades of the twentieth century two quite different educational measurement techniques were developed for quantifying individual differences. The first of these was developed by Alfred Binet in the context of an educational problem associated with compulsory education. Binet not only constructed an instrument for deciding whether or not a child could benefit from formal education as it was in those days, but also established the criteria of item difficulty and discriminating power that are still currently used for the selection of items, tasks, and so on to be used in educational and psychological tests.

While Binet was constructing a psychological instrument to solve an educational problem, others such as Sir Francis Galton and Spearman (1904) were developing and applying statistical methods suitable for the study of individual differences. Binet's criteria of difficulty and discriminating power which he defined graphically were soon converted to statistical indices which in the case of discriminating power was sometimes associated with a test of statistical significance. However, Binet's developmental measure, the mental age, was severely criticized by those with a more statistical approach as being ambiguous in definition and lacking generality (Thurstone 1926). Thurstone recommended measures based on the standard score at particular age levels.

It was only pointed out in the 1980s (Keats 1982a) that the differences between the approaches of Binet and Thurstone were not only those of the convenience of one measure as opposed to another but went much deeper. Both approaches implied that cognitive growth could be described by a single number. However, Binet's approach implied that individual differences at any age level could be accounted for by differences in rate of growth, whereas Thurstone's approach implied that individual differences at all ages arose from differences in the value approached at intellectual maturity, but that rate of approach to the ultimate level is the same in percentage terms. According to Thurstone's implicit assumption, everyone reaches a given fraction —for example, one-half of his or her ultimate level at a particular age level. In the case of physical height this assumption is very nearly correct. With Binet's assumption, all human beings are approaching the same ultimate level but at quite different rates. Both Binet's and Thurstone's implicit assumptions have been shown to be seriously in error (Keats 1982a).

While these arguments were proceeding, a third criterion for selecting items, that of item homogeneity, was being ignored. Spearman (1904) had established conditions that would lead to the conclusion that the relationships between a given set of measures could be accounted for by a single variable or factor. Spearman used these techniques known as "factor analysis" to try to establish a single general ability underlying all tests of cognitive performance (see *Factor Analysis*). While Spearman's thesis was proved incorrect empirically, his methods could have been used to establish criteria for concluding that a given set of cognitive tasks or items all measured the same underlying variable, that is, were homogeneous. This condition for educational and psychological measurement was not stressed until the middle of the twentieth century. Thus the three criteria for incorporating cognitive tasks into a single instrument with a single score are difficulty, discriminating power, and homogeneity.

1. The Relationship between Educational Measurement and Physical Measurement

The conditions for physical measurement stated by Campbell (1917) involved two basic operations each requiring a condition to be satisfied. The first of these is an operation of ordering whereby two objects can be compared with respect to (say) weight and a decision made as to which is heavier. In this case the condition to be met is that of "transitivity", so that if object A is judged to be heavier than object B and object B heavier than object C then object A *must* be judged to be heavier than object C. Failure to meet this condition could be due to unreliability in the comparing instrument or to a confusion in the dimensionality on which the objects are being compared.

Given that the ordering condition can be met with consistency, a second operation must be possible, that of combining; that is, two or more objects can be combined with respect to the dimension being measured in such a way that the combination can be compared on that dimension with any other object or combination of objects. With a consistent ordering operation and a combining operation it is possible to associate a number with any object by combining standard units and subunits. The combining or "additivity" condition is that the number associated with object A plus that associated with object B must equal the number associated with the combination of A and B. If the additivity condition holds for all pairs of objects then the set of numbers associated with these operations and objects is unique apart from a multiplying constant to convert, for example, pounds to kilograms.

With the development of educational measurement using objective testing methods, rating scales, attitude scales, and so on, the question of the extent to which these methods can be made to satisfy Campbell's conditions naturally arose. A Committee of the British Association for the Advancement of Science (BAAS) in 1938 examined this question in the context of psychological applications of these techniques and concluded that they did not do so completely (Ferguson et al. 1940). The ordering operation and condition could be met by a number of methods with allowance for unreliability of comparisons, but a suitable combining operation could not be identified and so the additivity condition could not be checked.

Following the BAAS report, Gulliksen (1946) pointed out that, in the case of the method of paired comparisons, a combining of differences operation was in fact defined and additivity of differences could be checked. This observation led naturally to the definition of interval scales; that is, scales for which differences between objects could be measured but for which no zero point could be defined from the data obtained by the method of measurement used. Stevens (1951) proposed a fourfold classification of measurement methods:

(a) nominal scales, which are really unordered classifications of objects;

(b) ordinal scales, which have an operation of ordering which exhibits transitivity;

(c) interval scales, which have ordering and combining operations for *differences* and which meet the consistency conditions of transitivity and additivity;

(d)   ratio scales, which satisfy Campbell's criteria for fundamental measurement of individual objects.

Stevens' classification has been widely adopted in the literature reporting educational and psychological research since the early 1950s. However, his conclusion that certain types of statistical procedures are applicable or inapplicable to one or more types of scale has caused considerable controversy. This conclusion has not been substantiated in terms of the assumptions underlying the various statistical techniques and so should not be taken seriously.

2. Conjoint Measurement

The general lack of a combining operation in educational and psychological research was finally overcome by research workers in Denmark and the United States, who apparently developed conjoint measurement independently at approximately the same time. Technical accounts of this theory are contained in Luce and Tukey (1964) and Ross (1964). The latter account is marred by a general "theorem" which is not only incorrectly proved but is in fact untrue. Rasch (1960), working at the Danish Institute for Educational Research, published what amounts to an application of conjoint measurement to the preparation of objective tests and analysis of data obtained from their application. His method has been developed and widely applied in recent years (see *Rasch Measurement, Theory of*).

The simple account given here follows Coombs et al. (1970) using objective testing as an example. The measurement method is based on a matrix or table

in which rows correspond to groups of subjects who have each attempted all of the items which define the columns. The entries in the cells of the table, for example P_{gi} *are the proportions of subjects in group g who give the correct response to item i.* Table 1 displays such a table. If the letters a, b, c denote the measures corresponding to any three of the groups of subjects and p, q, and r to the measures corresponding to any three of the items then it must be possible to define three functions, φ, f and h such that:

(a) $\varphi(a,p)=f(a)+h(p)$, that is, the function is decomposable into two additive components which are separately functions of a and p;

(b) $\varphi(a,p) \geqslant \varphi(b,q)$ if and only if $P_{ap} \geqslant P_{bq}$.

The following axioms are sufficient for the existence of functions satisfying the above conditions:

(a)   the cancellation axiom: if $P_{ap} \geqslant P_{bq}$ and $P_{br} \geqslant P_{cq}$ then $P_{ar} \geqslant P_{cp}$;

(b)   the solvability axiom: if $P_{ap} \geqslant t \geqslant P_{ap}$ for some real t then there exists a p such that $P_{ap} = t$ and the corresponding condition for the individual differences subscripts.

All measures of the type a, b, c and p, q, r satisfy the conditions for an interval scale which may under certain circumstances be transformed to a ratio scale. In the 30 years following the first formulation of the theory of conjoint measurement there have been relatively few attempts to apply the theory to research in either education or psychology. The next section describes attempts to apply the theory to educational and psychological testing.

3. Latent Trait Theory

Rasch (1960) proposed a transformation of the proportions obtained in tables such as those in Table 1. He observed that if

$$\frac{P_{gi}}{1 - P_{gi}} = \frac{A_g}{D_i} \tag{1}$$

where A_g is now used to denote the ability of group g and D_i the difficulty of item i then:

$$\text{Logit}(P_{gi}) = \log \frac{P_{gi}}{1 - P_{gi}} = \log A_g - \log D_i \tag{2}$$

which meets the order-preserving and additivity conditions. The values of $\log A_g$ satisfy interval-scale conditions and the values of A_g thus satisfy ratio-scale conditions. Similarly, the values of D_i satisfy the conditions for a ratio scale. Rasch presents examples

Table 1
Proportions of subjects in groups giving the "correct" responses to items

		1	2	3	...	Items i	...	j	...	N
Groups	1	P_{11}	P_{12}	P_{13}	...	P_{1i}	...	P_{1j}	...	P_{1N}
of	2	P_{21}	P_{22}	P_{22}	...	P_{2i}	...	P_{2j}	...	P_{2N}
Subjects										
	g	P_{g1}	P_{g2}	P_{g2}	...	P_{gi}	...	P_{gj}	...	P_{gN}
	n	P_{n1}	P_{n2}	P_{n3}	...	P_{ni}	...	P_{nj}	...	P_{nN}

of test data that satisfy the conditions of this model and some that do not. Other workers have made empirical investigations of the applicability of the model to tests that were not constructed in accordance with the model, and often report satisfactory fits of the data by the model.

Many years before Rasch's publication, Lord (1952) had developed the theory of the normal ogive latent ability model. The methods of estimating ability values for the normal model are very complex and certainly require computer assistance. It is thus not surprising that latent ability models and measures were not used in educational and psychological research until after Rasch's logit model had appeared with its much greater simplicity.

From the time that advances in electronic computers made the normal ogive model a viable alternative to the logit model (sometimes called the "one-parameter logistic model," a title that is somewhat misleading) there has been considerable discussion as to which model should be used. Before summarizing the points made in this controversy it is as well to remember that the advantages of using latent ability measures are not questioned. The most efficient way of obtaining estimates of these measures, however, is the subject of considerable current debate.

One of the reasons for the greater simplicity of the Rasch logit model lies in the fact that the model assumes that, although the test items have different difficulties, they all have the same discriminating power. This restriction is necessary if the axioms of conjoint measurement are to be satisfied, and places an added restraint on selecting items for a test: they must not only have significant discriminating power, but also, at least approximately *equal* discriminating power. The advantage claimed for such instruments is that the simple, number correct score is a sufficient statistic for estimating ability. It is also a consistent estimate. There are other consequential advantages related to chaining or equating tests.

The disadvantages of the logit model are argued in terms of the fact that, given (say) 200 trial items, a test of 80 items chosen with tight restriction on discriminating power will in general have lower reliability than one also of 80 items in which the highly discriminating as well as the moderately discriminating items are included. However, to utilize this to produce greater reliability for the estimation of latent ability, it would not be possible to use the simple, number correct score as the basis of estimation. Some kind of weighted score would be required. These matters are demonstrated by Birnbaum (1968).

Birnbaum suggested what is usually taken to be the inclusion of an item discrimination parameter in the logit model but what is really a different model: the two- (or more correctly three-) parameter logistic model. In terms of the logit model, Birnbaum's model would be:

$$\frac{P_{gi}}{1 - P_{gi}} = \left(\frac{A_g}{D_i}\right)^{C_i} \tag{3}$$

where C_i is the index of discriminating power of the item. In terms of dimensional analysis this equation is unbalanced unless C_i is dimensionless for all items which it is not. Thus the Rasch form is the only logit model that is dimensionally balanced.

However, Birnbaum and others write the alternative model by transforming A_g into a_g and D_i into d_i where $A_g = e^{a_g}$ and $D_i = e^{d_i}$, from which

$$\frac{P_{gi}}{1 - P_{gi}} \quad \frac{e^{c_i a_g}}{e^{c_i d_i}} \quad \text{or logit } (P_{gi}) = c_i (a_g - d_i) \tag{4}$$

or

$$P_{gi} = \frac{e^{c_i a_g}}{e^{c_i a_g} + e^{c_i d_i}} \quad \text{or} \quad \frac{e^{c_i(a_g - d_i)}}{e^{c_i(a_g - d_i)} + 1} \tag{5}$$

This logistic model is dimensionally balanced if c_i is taken to be of dimensionality (ability)$^{-1}$ which is defensible. Similar definitions are used in the normal ogive model (Lord 1952). The sacrifices made for this additional parameter are, first, that the number correct score is no longer a sufficient statistic for the estimate of ability, and the ability estimates obtained are not on a ratio or even an interval scale. However, the additional care needed to construct tests to meet the conjoint measurement conditions in the way Rasch suggests is worthwhile. The further application of latent ability measures to the measurement of cognitive growth will be discussed later.

4. Frequency Distributions of Educational and Psychological Measurements

A further problem associated with measurement of individual differences relates to the frequency distribution of scores on objective tests obtained from administration to large random samples. This problem has practical significance because of the use of percentile ranks and normalized percentile scores as derived scores. Keats (1951) was the first to suggest on general theoretical grounds that the negative hypergeometric distribution should give a reasonable representation of score distributions. Because of computational problems he followed Pearson (1930) in using the Beta function to estimate the theoretical frequencies. Keats demonstrated that this method gave good representations of most frequency distributions found in practice, and was useful not only in providing stable estimates of percentile points but also in revealing bias in samples.

At approximately the same time Mollenkopf (1949) showed that the error variance of an objective test was greatest for the middle range of scores and least for extreme scores. Keats (1957) showed that a binomial error distribution accounted for this phenomenon and

Lord (1965) gave a general account of the binomial error model. Keats and Lord (1962) showed that the binomial error model together with linear regression of true score on raw score leads to a derivation of the negative hypergeometric distribution. This finding stimulated considerable further research into representations of data obtained from objective tests. Lord (1965) looked into possible additional forms of the distribution of true scores while Keats (1964) examined some of the effects of nonlinear regressions of true scores on raw scores. Many of these results and some additional ones were brought together in Lord and Novick (1968).

The practical usefulness of theoretically based frequency distributions in defining percentile values on objective tests for carefully defined populations has seldom been applied in practice, despite the obvious advantages in standardizing and equating tests. More recently Huynh (1976) has confirmed the robustness of the negative hypergeometric distribution and suggests its use when criterion-referenced as opposed to normatively based tests are being developed (see below).

5. Parameters of Persons

Gulliksen (1950) based his theory of mental tests essentially on the notion that a raw score on the test could be thought of as consisting of a true score and an error score that were additive and uncorrelated. He showed that much of the existing test theory could be derived in these terms. There were, however, problems of strict definition and of estimation which were not developed. Lord and Novick (1968) attempted to solve these problems by means of axioms they claimed to be not inconsistent with conjoint measurement. However, Lumsden (1976) severely criticized true score theory on the grounds that any set of axioms that had been proposed for the definition of true score was unlikely to be satisfied in any domain so far explored.

Rasch (1960) also implicitly criticized true score theory when he complained that, as a student, he was always being assessed on an arbitrarily difficult set of tasks and relative to an undefined population. He argued strongly for ability measures that did not have these relativities associated with them but were "person parameters" in an absolute sense. Criticism of a similar kind was being expressed by Bayley (1955) who pointed out that it was impossible to develop a quantitative theory of cognitive development unless such an absolute measure could be developed. She did not seem to accept the notion that latent trait measures of the Rasch type could meet these requirements. Subsequently two extensive longitudinal studies, those reported by McCall et al. (1973) and by Hindley and Owen (1979), have been carried out without using such measures.

More recently Lumsden (1978) has proposed that in addition to a level parameter of the latent trait kind one could also distinguish between subjects in terms of the extent to which their performance varies with the difficulty of the task. Some subjects obtain most of their score on what are usually called "easy" items and fail on "difficult" items whereas others perform almost as well on the difficult items as they do on the easy ones. This concept is the person's equivalent of the concept of discriminating power of an item; that is, the extent to which a low-scoring subject gives the right answer much less often on more difficult items than less difficult items. Attempts to establish this as a reliable and valid dimension for persons have not so far been very successful. A possibility-related measure of a subject's tendency to guess (Miles 1973) has also not been developed to a stage where it can be regarded as an established dimension.

Keats (1982a) criticized the term "person parameter," which has been commonly used following Rasch (1960), on the grounds that in the cognitive area subjects continue to develop up to an age of approximately 20 years. Thus an estimate of this parameter at age 10 years will be consistently different from one at 15 years. Such a variable quantity hardly deserves to be called a parameter. He proposed a more basic parameter which determines the greatest level the subject will approach with age, and raised the question as to whether this was the basic person parameter or whether a rate of development parameter might be required as well as or even instead of a greatest level parameter.

By assuming that cognitive development could be represented in terms of a latent ability being projectively related to time, Keats (1982a) showed that Binet's mental-age measure was only a consistent measure if all subjects were approaching the same adult value at quite different rates. The deviation measure advocated by Thurstone (1926) and Wechsler (1939) among others is, on this assumption, stable only if rate of development is approximately the same for each subject, but that the adult value approached varies from person to person. Using longitudinal data reported by Skodak and Skeels (1949), Keats was able to show that both a rate parameter and adult level parameter seemed to be important. In a subsequent paper Keats (1982b) considered mechanisms that could be thought of as underlying cognitive development and thus gave these parameters a theoretical significance independent of their mensurational significance.

Even though current evidence suggests that in the quantification of general ability an independent rate and asymptote parameter are required to represent development, this must not be taken to mean that purely rate of development models are not applicable in educational research. If minimal skills in reading and number work are considered, which almost all can master, it is still significant to measure how quickly they are mastered by subjects of different ability and in different settings. There is much more research to be done investigating personal parameters in these areas.

The question of discontinuities in the development

of ability or in mastering minimal skills was investigated by Keats (1989). Such discontinuities could be caused by commencing formal education or by head injury of a severe kind. His earlier model (Keats 1982a) was expanded to take into account these types of discontinuity.

6. Criterion-reference Testing

This form of educational measurement arose in part as a reaction to normative testing, which relates a person's performance to that of a particular norming group; for example, an age group or a grade group. The objective of this form of testing is to relate the person's performance to some kind of standard or level of mastery, but the problem arises of attempting to define such a standard in terms of a test performance. This problem exists whether or not the score on the test has been converted to some kind of derived score such as a standard score or even to an estimate of some underlying latent trait.

Various ways of solving the basic problem of setting a mastery level in terms of a test score have been suggested. These range from the exercising of a value judgment by curriculum experts through decision theory approaches which assume knowledge of true mastery score to utilizing the ratio of the two costs of misclassification (i.e., false positives and false negatives) and alternatively the use of an independent criterion such as degree of success in a referral task. Huynh (1976) suggested that mastery classification should imply a high probability of success in training to which only persons classed as masters at the lower level are admitted. He explored the statistical implications of this approach in terms of the beta-binomial model (Keats and Lord 1962) with constant losses and pass–fail referral performance.

There are very few areas of knowledge for which content criteria can be specified precisely. Mechanical arithmetic could be considered as one such area and a criterion of (say) 90 percent accuracy could be required in adding and/or multiplying two, digit numbers by two-digit numbers. However, such criterion referencing ignores the fact that some combinations are more likely to produce errors than others, and also the fact that some students make systematic errors due to inappropriate strategies. Thus the problems of developing criterion-referenced instruments touch on the very core of the educational process. Until more of the theoretical problems of education are solved the possibility of developing useful criterion-referenced instruments seems to be unattainable.

In this context the development of computer-administered tests is proceeding rapidly. The further goal of adapting items to the level of performance of the student is also being approached in some areas. It should also be possible to develop programs to explore the patterns of errors made by a particular student, to determine deficient strategies that can be corrected. The interaction between measurement and diagnosis and treatment of weaknesses in performance must be studied in detail before criterion referencing can be successful. The wide use of computers should facilitate this work (see *Criterion referenced Measurement*).

7. Measurement of Attitudes

Attitude measurement began as a result of Thurstone's development of scale values for stimuli on dimensions for which there is no corresponding physical measure. Using the method of paired comparison, Thurstone and Chave (1929) showed that it was possible to find scale values for statements reflecting positive and negative attitudes and that subjects could be measured in terms of the scale values for statements they agreed with. Shortly after Thurstone's contribution Likert (1932) suggested that the methods that had been developed for constructing objective tests of cognitive abilities could be applied to the construction and use of scales for measuring attitudes. Later still Guttman (1947) proposed criteria that could be used to select statements that formed a scale (see *Thurstone Scales; Attitudes, Measurement of*).

A valuable collection of scales for the quantification of attitudes has been provided by Shaw and Wright (1967). Their publication corresponds in many ways to the *Mental Measurements Yearbooks* published by the Buros Institute (e.g., Conoley and Kramer 1989) in the field of psychological testing, but is more immediately useful because the scales are presented in full along with the evaluative material. As a means of organizing their material Shaw and Wright classified scales according to the quantified attitudes. The classes of attitudes that are distinguished are attitudes toward social practices, social issues and problems, international issues, abstract concepts, political and religious issues, ethnic and national groups, "significant others," and social institutions. A revised edition of this volume is urgently needed.

The three methods—Thurstone's, Likert's, and Guttman's—use different models as the basis of their quantification methods, and all have some current use. Allport and Vernon (1931), among others, have used essentially ranking methods to obtain measures that are then interpreted as if they corresponded to Likert's scales. This confusion of models by Allport and Vernon is quite unscientific, as it can lead to unjustified interpretations of data and the neglect of other possible interpretations. Models for ordinal data are relatively recent.

The Likert method of constructing and applying attitude scales is by far the most common, as it resembles most closely the objective test approach. The major difference arises from the fact that, whereas items in cognitive tests are usually scored as either +1 (correct) or zero (incorrect), the Likert items often have alternatives of the kind "strongly agree, agree, undecided,

759

disagree, strongly disagree" which are scored 2, 1, 0, −1, and −2 respectively. However the inclusion of the alternative "undecided" has been shown to lead to anomalous results and so should possibly not be used. In any case the use of integers such as 2, 1, 0, −1, and so on tends to destroy the ordinal characteristics of items when the item scores are added to produce a total score.

There was little practical or theoretical development of this method from the 1930s until the 1980s. Andrich (1989) applied the Rasch approach to model building to the analysis of attitudinal data collected by either the Likert or the Thurstone method. In particular, he indicated ways in which data could be collected and analyzed to test the assumptions of these two methods.

The Thurstone method depends on the possibility of reliably scaling statements in terms of the attitude level of persons who would endorse the statement. He suggested the method of paired comparisons as a way of determining these scale values, but because of the experimental time required by this method he developed other, quicker procedures. Thurstone emphasized that the scale values obtained by one of these methods should be independent (up to a linear transformation) of the attitudes of the judges scaling the statements. This condition has rarely been checked in practice and is similar to the requirement of the Rasch model that the estimates of the difficulties of items should be independent of the abilities of the subjects used to obtain them.

Given that sufficient numbers of appropriately scaled statements are available, a subject's attitude can be measured by averaging the scale values of those items he or she endorses. Again, the second requirement for the Rasch model should apply in that the measurement obtained for a subject should not depend on the particular set of statements with which the subject is presented. This condition is harder to check because available Thurstone scales tend to have a relatively small number of items, so that any sampling of these statements would tend to give unreliable as well as coarse measures.

Guttman scales can be best thought of as Likert scales with items of infinite discriminability. If the Likert scale items meet the requirements of the Rasch model then the Guttman scale property, that a person's score indicates precisely which items he or she endorsed, is weakened to the extent that, for each score, the probability of it being obtained with each of the possible patterns can be calculated. If the items in the scale have a wide range of item parameter values and high discrimination there will be a most probable pattern for each score. In the rarely obtained case of a perfect Guttman scale these most probable patterns will, of course, have a probability of unity.

The unifying effect of applying the Rasch model to methods of measuring attitudes should be clear from the above discussion. Only with the restrictions of this model is it possible to justify giving unique interpretation to the usual raw score, whether from an ability test, an attainment test, or an attitude scale. If more general models that allow for variation in the discriminating power of items are used then the value of the measure differs from one pattern of responding to another. Even for an instrument of only 20 items, there are at least one million patterns of responding but only 21 possible raw scores. Thus the data reduction possibilities obtained by using the Rasch model are enormous.

8. Multivariate Approaches to Measurement in Education

Spearman (1904) proposed that measures of cognitive achievement, including sensory judgments, could be accounted for by an underlying single factor or general ability. Much of the data he used came from school achievement measures and the balance from the psychophysical laboratory. This approach was developed and explored for almost 30 years before Thurstone (1931) proposed multivariate factor analysis.

Both methods were directed toward the problem of representing human cognitive performance in terms of a relatively small number of cognitive factors. The technical problems of factor analysis have been actively investigated for more than 50 years and, although they cannot be said to have been completely solved, many least squares and maximum likelihood methods are now available for exploring and testing data. Most, if not all, are available in the form of computer programs. However, there is still debate as to which method is the most appropriate in a given situation and the various methods do not produce the same results (see *Factor Analysis*).

On the substantive side, many attempts have been made to define the significant factors by means of which individual differences in cognitive behavior can be represented. Thurstone proposed a set of primary mental abilities and provided research instruments to measure these. More recently, groups working with J W French (Ekstrom et al. 1976) have proposed, after a great deal of empirical research, 23 cognitive ability factors and have provided at least three tests measuring each of these. The tests are referred to as cognitive factor reference tests and are intended for use in identifying factors rather than for direct use in assessment or selection situations.

The predominant tendency today is to use a large number of group factors, rather than to retain Spearman's concept of a general factor, and to supplement this with well-established group factors. However, this practice tends to obscure the one most pervasive and substantiated result from cognitive achievement studies: namely, that measures of cognitive performance with quite different content are almost always positively related. It is probably true to assert that if the general-plus-group factor approach were adopted the number of cognitive factors to be referenced would be reduced from 23 to perhaps as few as 15 uncorrelated measures.

In the case of personality or temperament factors, the group led by French (Dermen et al. 1978) has had a much more difficult task as there is far less agreement about which factors have been clearly and reliably defined. The manual of reference tests for temperament factors reflects this uncertainty by the fact that only 18 of the 28 factors listed could be confirmed by the group. The remainder, however, have often been reported in the literature. A further problem with temperament scales is that they are far more susceptible to the effects of response styles than are cognitive tests.

While the French group has provided a valuable service to educational research by investigating both cognitive and personality factors in this almost exhaustive fashion, it should be noted that almost all of their work has been carried out on adults. There is still the task of determining to what extent they also apply to children in primary and secondary schools. For at least some factors this question has some urgency for educators who wish to obtain a concise way of recording children's cognitive performance.

Factor analytic methods can also be regarded as ways of accounting for patterns or structures in correlations between variables by postulating more fundamental variables underlying the manifest observations. Two other ways of accounting for such patterns in correlation are also of concern when considering measurement in educational research. The first concerns the special patterns that arise in developmental studies when measures are administered on several different occasions to the same group of subjects. The second seeks to interpret patterns in terms of causal relationships and is called "path analysis" (see *Path Analysis and Linear Structural Relations Analysis*).

Anderson (1940) was the first to propose an explanation for the particular pattern of correlations obtained in developmental studies when performance on a particular measure, at a given age level, is correlated with performance on the same measure at other age levels. When all such correlations are tabulated the table obtained usually exhibits a distinctive pattern, sometimes called a "simplex pattern" (Anderson 1940). Anderson demonstrated that such a pattern could be generated by means of cumulations of random numbers. Thus the first measure would be a random number and the second measure would consist of the first measure plus a second random number, and so on. In due course there would be considerable overlap between one measure in the series and the next, and so high correlation. Thus development could be thought of as random cumulations of the products of experience without any individual differences parameters (Humphreys 1960)

This possible explanation of development was repeated by many writers without any great amplification until Drösler (1978) demonstrated, using time series methods, that it was possible to distinguish graphically between simplex patterns that could have arisen in this fashion and those that could not. From published data Drösler showed that educational achievement tests provided correlation patterns that were *not* inconsistent with Anderson's proposed explanation over most of the compulsory education period. However, general ability or aptitude tests reject the Anderson proposal for age levels above approximately five years. This finding has been confirmed for other sets of published data. Thus educational measures can be classified into those that do and those that do not conform to the random cumulation model. Factor analysis is not an appropriate method in the case of developmental data.

A second situation in which the factor analytic model is not an appropriate one for analyzing tables of correlations between measures obtained in educational research is one in which relationships are asymmetric, in that A can influence B but B cannot influence A. An example would be where a social class measure is related to school achievement. It is most unlikely that a child's school achievement could affect his or her parents' social class whereas social class could influence school achievement. A method that accounts for patterns of correlations under these circumstances is path analysis, and both least squares and maximum likelihood programs are available for estimating the weightings of causal paths (see *Path Analysis and Linear Structural Relations Analysis*).

A related form of studying correlations between educational measures is the method of Herbst (1970), which he termed "cyclic network analysis." In that publication Herbst illustrated application of this method using measures of pupil's work effort, boredom, and anxiety in relation to work expected by the teacher as perceived by the pupil. Later developments in factor analysis include the methods of Goldstein and McDonald (1988), which enable the researcher to analyze data from two-level hierarchical populations such as teachers and pupils nested under teachers. Applications of these methods should lead to the identification of classroom and school factors in addition to individual differences factors.

See also: Scaling Methods; Latent Trait Measurement Models; Factor Analysis; Rasch Measurement, Theory of

References

Allport G W, Vernon P E 1931 *A Study of Values: A Scale for Measuring the Dominant Interests in Personality: Manual of Directions*. Houghton Mifflin, Boston, Massachusetts

Anderson J E 1940 *The Prediction of Terminal Intelligence from Infant and Preschool Tests*. Thirty-ninth Yearbook, National Society for the Study of Education. American Educational Research Association, Chicago, Illinois

Andrich D 1989 Distinctions between assumptions and requirements in measurement in the social sciences. In:

Keats J A, Taft R, Heath R A, Lovibond S H (eds.) 1989 *Mathematical and Theoretical Systems*. Elsevier Science Publications, Amsterdam

Bayley N 1955 On the growth of intelligence. *Am. Psychol.* 10: 805–18

Birnbaum A 1968 Some latent trait models and their use in inferring an examinee's ability. In: Lord F M, Novlick M R (eds.) 1968 *Statistical Theories of Mental Test Scores*. Addison Wesley, Reading, Massachusetts

Campbell N R 1917 *Foundation of Science: The Philosophy of Theory and Experiment*. Dover Publications, New York

Conoley J C, Kramer J J 1989 *The Tenth Mental Measurement Yearbook*. Buros Institute, Nebraska

Coombs C H, Dawes R M, Tversky A 1970 *Mathematical Psychology: An Elementary Introduction*. Prentice Hall, Englewood Cliffs, New Jersey

Dermen D, French J W, Haran H H 1978 *Guide to Factor Reference Temperament Scales 1978*. Educational Testing Service, Princeton, New Jersey

Drösler J 1978 Extending the temporal range of psychometric prediction by optimal linear filtering of mental test scores. *Psychometri.* 43: 533–49

Ekstrom R B, French J W, Harman H H 1976 *Manual for Kit of Factor-referenced Cognitive Tests, 1976*. Educational Testing Service, Princeton, New Jersey

Ferguson A et al. 1940 Quantitative estimation of sensory events: Final report. *Advancement of Science* 2: 331–49

Goldstein H, McDonald R P 1988 A general model for the analysis of multilevel data. *Psychometri.* 53: 455–67

Gulliksen H 1946 Paired comparisons and the logic of measurement. *Psychol. Rev.* 53: 199–213

Gulliksen H 1950 *Theory of Mental Tests*. Wiley, New York

Guttman L 1947 The Cornell technique for scale and intensity analysis. *Educ. Psychol. Meas.* 7: 247–79

Herbst P G 1970 *Behavioural Worlds: The Study of Single Cases*. Tavistock, London

Hindley C B, Owen C F 1979 An analysis of individual patterns of DQ and IQ curves from 6 months to 17 years. *Br. J. Psychol.* 70: 273–93

Humphreys L G 1960 Investigations of the simplex. *Psychometri.* 25: 313–23

Huynh H 1976 Statistical consideration of mastery scores. *Psychometri.* 41: 65–78

Keats J A 1951 *A Statistical Theory of Objective Test Scores*. Australian Council for Educational Research, Hawthorne

Keats J A 1957 Estimation of error variances of test scores. *Psychometri.* 22: 29–41

Keats J A 1964 Some generalizations of a theoretical distribution of mental test scores. *Psychometri.* 29: 215–31

Keats J A 1982a Comparing latent trait with classical measurement models in the practice of educational and psychological measurement. In: Spearritt D S (ed.) 1982 *The Improvement of Measurement in Education and Psychology: Contributions of Latent Trait Theories*. Australian Council for Educational Research, Hawthorne

Keats J A 1982b Ability measures and theories of cognitive development. In: Messick S (ed.) 1982 *Festschrift*

for F M Lord. Educational Testing Service, Princeton, New Jersey

Keats J A 1989 Formulation of a mathematical theory of intelligence. In: Heath R A (ed.) 1989 *Current Issues in Cognitive Development and Mathematical Psychology*. University of Newcastle, Shortland

Keats J A, Lord F M 1962 A theoretical distribution of mental test scores. *Psychometri.* 27: 59–72

Likert R 1932 A technique for the measurement of attitudes. *Arch. Psychol.* 140

Lord F M 1952 A theory of test scores. *Psychometric Monogr.* 7

Lord F M 1965 A strong true-score theory, with applications. *Psychometri.* 30: 239–70

Lord F M, Novick M R 1968 *Statistical Theories of Mental Test Scores*. Addison-Wesley, Reading, Massachusetts

Luce R D, Tukey J W 1964 Simultaneous conjoint measurement: A new type of fundamental measurement. *J. Math. Psy.* 1: 1–27

Lumsden J 1976 Test Theory. *Annu. Rev. Psychol.* 21: 251–80

Lumsden J 1978 Tests are perfectly reliable. *Br. J. Math. S.* 31: 19–26

McCall R B, Appelbaum M I, Hogarty P S 1973 Developmental changes in mental performance. *Monogr. Soc. Res. Child Dev.* 38 (3, No. 150)

Miles J 1973 Eliminating the guessing factor in the multiple choice test. *Educ. Psychol. Meas.* 33: 637–51

Mollenkopf W G 1949 Variation of the standard error of measurement. *Psychometri.* 14: 189–230

Pearson K (ed.) 1930 *Tables for Statisticians and Biometricians*, 3rd edn. Cambridge University Press, Cambridge

Rasch G 1960 *Probabilistic Models for some Intelligence and Attainment Tests*. Danish Institute for Educational Research, Copenhagen

Ross S 1964 *Logical Foundations of Psychological Measurement: A Study in the Philosophy of Science*. Munksgaard, Copenhagen

Shaw M E, Wright J M 1967 *Scales for the Measurement of Attitudes*. McGraw-Hill, New York

Skodak M, Skeels H M 1949 A final follow-up study of one hundred adopted children. *J. Genet. Psychol.* 75: 85–125

Spearman C 1904 "General intelligence," objectively determined and measured. *Am. J. Psychol.* 15: 201–93

Stevens S S (ed.) 1951 *Handbook of Experimental Psychology*. Wiley, New York

Thurstone L L 1926 The mental age concept. *Psychol. Rev.* 33: 268–78

Thurstone L L 1931 Multiple factor analysis. *Psychol. Rev.* 38: 406–27

Thurstone L L, Chave E J 1929 *The Measurement of Attitude: A Psychophysical Method and Some Experiments with a Scale for Measuring Attitude toward the Church*. University of Chicago Press, Chicago, Illinois

Wechsler D 1939 *The Measurement of Adult Intelligence*. Williams and Williams, Baltimore, Maryland

Missing Scores in Survey Research

A. E. Beaton

In survey research and educational assessment, the problem of missing scores is widespread. The respondents in a sample may refuse to cooperate despite the surveyors' urging and the offering of rewards. In educational settings, a school principal may refuse to allow an infringement on student time for participating in an assessment or survey. Even with school cooperation, students may be absent or unavailable at the necessary time, and special sessions to accommodate them may not be feasible. Finally, a student may not complete all parts of a test nor all items in a questionnaire. Despite extensive efforts to avoid missing scores, some are inevitable in large surveys or assessments.

Missing scores may result in a serious problem for data analysis and interpretation. If the missing scores are few and can be considered missing at random, the problem may not be severe, and there are a number of statistical techniques such as listwise deletion or multiple imputations, which are discussed below, that are available for data analysis and interpretation. On the other hand, if the scores are not missing at random, if the reasons for missing scores are related to the topic being surveyed, then the survey results may be biased in unknown and inestimable ways, perhaps seriously. For example, if schools with low-scoring students tend to refuse to participate in an assessment, then the distribution of scores derived solely from the students in participating schools will be not representative of the entire population. If absentee students tend to have lower scores, then the average for schools with many absentees will be artificially high. Small percentages of missing scores are often ignored, but large percentages may result in large estimation biases and improper interpretations of the results.

There is no really good way to handle scores that are not missing at random. It should be stressed that the best procedure is to avoid or minimize missing scores through strong efforts to encourage the subjects to participate. Some ideas about how to improve participation in mail surveys are presented by Dillman (1983). Details of the efforts to encourage participation and assure good operations that were used in a United States educational assessment are discussed by Caldwell et al. (1992).

In this entry several common ways are considered for handling missing scores of the sort often encountered in educational research, surveys, and assessments. More particularly, the discussion is restricted to continuous variables of the type that are used in regression and multivariate analysis. A more general review of missing data techniques is presented by Anderson et al. (1983). Two outstanding recent books in this area are *Multiple Imputation for Nonresponse in Surveys* (Rubin 1987) and *Statistical Analysis with Missing Data* (Little and Rubin 1987).

1. Commonly Available Techniques

For linear statistics such as regression, analysis of variance, and multivariate analysis of variance, two approaches to missing scores are commonly used and incorporated in statistical systems such as SPSS (Norusis 1990).

1.1 Listwise Deletion

The listwise deletion method involves removing from an analysis any observations (i.e., subjects or cases) that have any missing data at all. Programs incorporating this feature require that a list of all variables, whether dependent, independent, or concomitant, be submitted before the accumulation of summary statistics. Every observation is examined for data completeness; if any datum is missing in an observation, then it is excluded from all accumulations. If an accumulation such as a cross-product matrix is used for several different analyses, then the entire observation will be excluded from all analyses, even though it might be complete for some analyses, because of missing scores for others.

This method produces unbiased estimators of population parameters if the data are missing at random. However, the method may substantially reduce the sample size if a few scores are missing from many observations; in some cases, such as a balanced incomplete block spiraling, the sample size will be reduced to zero since by design there will be no observations with complete data. In some cases, the data loss can be reduced by removing one or a few scores on which there is a substantial amount of missing data, although, of course, at the loss of the available scores and at the risk of model misspecifications in pursuant data analyses.

A technical advantage of this method is that it produces a positive definite or semidefinite cross-products matrix whether or not the data are missing at random, and estimated or predicted values and their residuals for the observations with complete data can be produced. A serious disadvantage is that this method ignores the potential bias introduced when scores are not missing at random; the resultant estimates are, therefore, biased to an unknown degree.

1.2 Pairwise deletion

The pairwise deletion method involves computing each cross-product or correlation using all observations for which the pair of scores are available. In accumulating cross-products, each pair of variables is examined for each observation and, if both variables are present, then they are included in the accumulations. An observation may, therefore, be included in some cross-products and correlations but not in others in the same matrix. The accumulation of data separately for different pairs of variables increases the computing time and storage requirements of the computer.

This method produces consistent estimators of population parameters if the scores are missing at random. An advantage of this method is that it uses all available scores for estimating a cross-product or correlation. A serious technical disadvantage is that this method does not guarantee that the resultant matrices will be positive definite or semidefinite, and experience has shown that this irregularity will commonly occur in practice. A regression analysis using a cross-product or correlation matrix produced in this way may have a negative determinant and, if allowed to proceed, may produce multiple correlations greater than unity. A cross-product, covariance, or correlation matrix with a negative determinant is inconsistent with any conceivable set of real numbers, indicating that the pairwise correlations cannot be a good estimate of the correlation matrix if the missing scores were known. Consequently, inexperienced or nontechnical users may not know how to deal with the problems and may misinterpret their results. Furthermore, the production of estimated or predicted values and their residuals is not clearly defined, since data for producing them are not available. It is also a serious disadvantage that this method ignores the potential bias introduced when scores are not missing at random.

2. Imputation methods

Another approach to missing scores involves filling in the blanks or imputing missing values. Several different methods have been used, including filling in means, estimated values, estimated values plus error, the hot deck, and multiple imputations, which are discussed below. Since all missing scores are replaced by real numbers, all of these methods result in cross-product, covariance, and correlation matrices that are at least positive semidefinite, and it is possible to compute estimated values and residuals.

It is important to realize that all of the imputation methods imply a model for estimating the missing score through knowledge of the available data. If the knowledge of other variables is accurate and the model is exact, then the missing scores can be imputed exactly, although this is unlikely to be the case. In most cases, the models will involve uncertainty; thus the missing score will not be known exactly, and a distribution of possible scores can be estimated, as in the plausible value method discussed below. This factor is important in understanding the concept of missing at random as used in imputation models. In this section, missing at random will mean missing at random conditional on the available data and the accuracy of the model for the missing scores. Instead of assuming that the missing scores are simply randomly missing from the entire population, it is assumed that something is known about the missing observations and that there is an assumed model for estimating their values. For example, if a boy from a professional family is absent, and the model suggests some homogeneity of scores among gender and socioeconomic groups, then it is assumed that the missing score was randomly missing from the population of boys from professional families. The accuracy of this assumption will, of course, affect the results.

2.1 Filling in Means

Filling in means is an imputation method that will seldom be an adequate approach to the missing score problem, although it is occasionally used. This method involves simply replacing missing scores with the mean value of that score from the available data on other observations. This method takes no advantage of data on other variables and is equivalent to assuming that the missing scores are all from students who are exactly at the average, which is very unlikely to be true. This method places the mean of the data with some filled-in scores at the same place as the mean of the available scores. However, this method results in a peaked distribution with a smaller variance than the distribution of the available scores. Correlation of scores with filled-in means with other variables will be distorted.

2.2 Filling in Estimated Values

Filling in estimated values is somewhat less problematic than filling in means but still inadequate. The general idea is to fill in the blanks with an estimate of missing scores from available data on other variables which are available. This may be done, for example, by using a single, highly correlated variable that is available for an observation or by using a set of available estimation variables and multiple regression. These methods imply that the missing scores are linearly related to the available variables that are used for imputation, and that a missing score is at the point estimated from the available data, that is, at the middle of the distribution of those observations with the same values for the scores used for imputation. If several estimation variables are employed, the process can become quite complicated, because the estimator variables may themselves be missing, thus requiring searching for a pattern of existing scores for each observation to estimate the value of its missing score. Filling in estimated values will usually result in a score distribution with a smaller variance than that of the nonmissing scores, since the variance of the predicted values will generally be less than the available values if the (multiple) correlation is less than unity. The correlations among such filled-in values will generally be increased because exact linear relationships are built in.

2.3 Filling in Estimated Values plus Error

Filling in estimated values plus error responds to the fact that filling in the estimated value alone tends to reduce the variance of the filled-in vector of scores from that of the observed data. To correct for this situation, a random error may be added to the estimated value, thus increasing its variance. In a regression situation assuming normally distributed error, the error would be randomly selected from a normal distribution with a mean of zero and a standard deviation equal to the standard error of estimate in estimating the missing score from the available data. This procedure is, therefore, similar to filling in estimated values, except that the uncertainty introduced by imputation is also incorporated in the model. In the case of randomly missing data from a multivariate normal distribution, this procedure will properly estimate the variances of the individual variables, but not in general the correlations among them.

2.4 Hot Decking

The hot deck procedure is another way of filling in the blanks (Rockwell 1975). Originally, the hot deck procedure was used in census computations to impute missing values. The technique replaces a missing value with the value of the last observation with similar known characteristics. For example, if the score of a rural eighth-grade girl were missing, it would be replaced by the score of the last rural eighth-grade girl who did have a score. This method can clearly be improved by replacing the value with a random draw from all available observations with similar characteristics. This method is somewhat analogous to the fill in the blank with estimated values plus error when the predictors are categorical.

2.5 Multiple Imputation

The multiple imputation approach involves imputing more than one, perhaps many, values for each missing score. For background, Dempster et al. (1977) showed that the EM algorithm produced maximum likelihood estimates from incomplete data under very general conditions. In the case of regression analysis with the assumption of a multivariate normal distribution, estimation of the covariance matrix was iterative, estimating the missing scores and then their covariance matrix repeatedly. The process was computer intensive but ultimately convergent. The original results did not produce a data matrix with imputed values that would generate the covariance matrix directly; this was the result of a separate calculation in the EM algorithm. Multiple imputations as a direct approach to missing values in survey data were first proposed by Rubin (1977, 1978)

Multiple imputations work as follows. With the available data and one or more models for imputation, several equally likely values are imputed for each missing score. This can be thought of as developing several equivalent data sets with filled in values; each data set is as likely to be accurate as any other, as far as the surveyor knows. Data analyses are then done several times, once for each imputed data set. The parameter estimates from the several data analyses are then averaged to produce a single parameter estimate. The variance of the several parameter estimates is added to the usual sampling error, so that the error due to imputation is acknowledged and included in the total error variance associated with the parameter estimate. If the model and assumptions are true, then Rubin has shown that the method produces maximum likelihood estimates. The multiple imputation method is described in detail in Rubin (1987) and Little and Rubin (1987).

2.6 Plausible Values Imputation

The multiple imputation technique has been developed and elaborated by Mislevy (1991) under the name of "plausible values." This method has been used extensively in the National Assessment of Educational Progress (NAEP) (Beaton and Zwick 1992, Johnson 1992). The technology is described in detail by Mislevy, Beaton, Kaplan and Sheehan (1992), by Mislevy, Johnson and Muraki (1992), and by Mislevy (1992).

The general idea is to impute several "plausible" values for each missing score, each value selected at random from the estimated posterior distribution of the missing score given the available data and a model for nonresponse. These plausible values, therefore, incorporate the uncertainty into both the imputation and analysis processes. In this application, no student receives all assessment questions and thus all scores are missing by design, although partial information is available. Students are randomly assigned booklets and so the scores may be considered missing at random. Five plausible values are drawn for each missing score, and each data analysis is run five times, once for each set of plausible values. The results of the five analyses are averaged. The variance of the results from one set of imputations to another is added to the sampling variance to make a total estimate of the uncertainty of the results. Mislevy (1991) has developed this theory in general and in particular for item response models, and Beaton and Johnson (1990) have developed the methodology for linear models.

The multiple imputation approach has the advantage, like other imputation methods, of allowing analyses to be done with standard statistical systems. A disadvantage is that the computations are more extensive, since the analyses must be repeated for each plausible value and then summarized after completion. A strong advantage of this approach is that it recognizes and estimates the error introduced by imputation.

3. Comment on Nonrandom Missing Scores

From consideration of the methods of handling nonrandomly missing scores as if they were randomly missing, it can be seen that the bias introduced is ignored, despite the fact that this bias may be large. Rubin (1987) has noted that the surveyor usually does know something about the reason for missing scores, and that this knowledge can be incorporated into data analyses. As noted above, the imputation models do imply a belief about the missing scores, although they do not usually check the adequacy of the model. Rubin has suggested that the uncertainty about different possible imputation models can be investigated by trying several different imputation models using different assumptions about the relationship between the missing scores and the available data. Summarizing across the results using different models would give a measure of the sensitivity of the imputations to the models as well as the uncertainty within a single model.

The methods of Rubin directly face the many issues of missing scores thoughtfully and thoroughly. This is seemingly the best technology for missing scores that is available. It is better, however, to avoid or minimize the missing scores so that their imputation is not necessary or has little effect on the interpretation of results.

See also: Missing Data and Nonresponse in Survey Research; Survey Research Methods; Sampling in Survey Research; Sampling Errors in Survey Research

References

Anderson A B, Basilevsky A, Hum D P J 1983 Missing Data. In: Rossi P H, Wright J D, Anderson B (eds.) 1983 *Handbook of Survey Research*. Academic Press, New York

Beaton A E, Johnson E 1990 The average response method of scaling. *J. Ed. Stat.* 15(1):9–38

Beaton A E, Zwick R 1992 Overview of the National Assessment of Educational Progress. *J. Ed. Stat.* 17(2): 95–109

Caldwell N, Slobasky R, Moore D, Ter Maat J 1992 Field operations and data collection. In: Johnson E G, Allen (eds.) 1992 *The NAEP 1990 Technical Report*. National Center for Education Statistics, Washington, DC

Dempster A P, Laird N, Rubin D B 1977 Maximum likelihood from incomplete data via the EM algorithm. *Journal of the Royal Statistical Society* B39: 1–38

Dillman D A 1983 Mail and other self-administered questionnaires. In: Rossi P H, Wright J D, Anderson A B (eds.) 1983 *Handbook of Survey Research*. Academic Press, New York

Johnson E G. 1992 The design of the National Assessment of Educational Progress. *J. Educ. Meas.* 29(2): 95–110

Little R J A, Rubin D B 1987 *Statistical Analysis with Missing Data*. Wiley, New York

Mislevy R J 1991 Randomization-based inferences about latent variables from complex samples. *Psychometri* 56(2), 177–96

Mislevy R J 1992 Scaling procedures. In: Johnson E G, Allen (eds.) 1992 *The NAEP 1990 Technical Report*. National Center for Education Statistics, Washington, DC

Mislevy R J, Beaton A E, Kaplan B, Sheehan K M 1992 Estimating population characteristics from sparse matrix samples of item responses. *J. Educ. Meas.* 29(2): 133–61

Mislevy R J, Johnson E G, Muraki E 1992 scaling procedures in NAEP. *J. Ed. Stat.* 17(2): 131–54

Norusis M J 1990 *SPSS/PC + 4.0 Base Manual*. SPSS, Chicago, Illinois

Rockwell R C 1975 An investigation of imputation and differential quality of data in the 1970 census. *Journal of the American Statistical Association* 70(1): 39–42

Rubin D B 1977 The design of a general and flexible system for handling non-response in sample surveys. Manuscript prepared for the US Social Security Administration

Rubin D B 1978 Multiple imputations in sample surveys—a phenomenological Baysean approach to non-response. *Proceedings of the Survey Research Methods Section of the American Statistical Association*

Rubin D B 1987 *Multiple Imputation for Nonresponse in Surveys*. Wiley, New York

Multiple Choice Tests, Guessing in

H. J. Rogers

Generally defined, guessing on test items occurs whenever an examinee responds to an item with less than perfect confidence in the answer. As such, guessing may be "blind," "cued," or "informed." Blind guessing occurs when an examinee has no idea of the correct answer and responds randomly. Cued guessing occurs on selection-type test items when an examinee does not know the answer and responds to some stimulus in the item such as an unintended clue or intentional mislead. Informed guessing occurs when the examinee's response is based on partial knowledge about the question.

Guessing of one form or another can occur on any type of test item, whether multiple choice or free response. However, it is generally considered to be a serious problem only on multiple choice tests, because of the greater likelihood of a correct answer through guessing. The primary psychometric problem arising from guessing on test items is that it increases the error variance of test scores, thereby reducing their reliability and validity. Since the 1920s, when multiple choice tests came into widespread use, there has been considerable research on ways to reduce the effects of guessing on test scores. This entry considers the many different approaches that have been proposed, reviews the research carried out to examine these approaches, and assesses the gains and losses associated with each approach.

1. Corrections for Guessing

1.1 Formula Scoring

Much of the research on corrections for guessing has focused on correction formulas applied to the scores after testing. The most widely used correction formula is based on the assumption that an examinee either knows the correct answer and chooses it, or does not know the answer and omits or responds randomly. From this perspective, wrong answers are the result of unlucky guessing; if this is so, the number of wrong answers can be used to predict the number of lucky guesses, which can then be deducted from the examinee's score. For example, on a four-option multiple choice test, a randomly guessing examinee will average one right answer (lucky guess) for every three wrong answers (unlucky guesses); thus, a third of the number of wrong answers should be deducted from the examinee's score.

The standard correction for guessing is given by the formula

$$F = R - \frac{W}{(A - 1)}$$

where R is the number of right answers, W is the number of wrong answers, and A is the number of response options per item. Associated with the use of the correction formula are test directions that instruct examinees to omit items rather than guess randomly, as wrong answers will be penalized. Omits are not counted as wrong answers in this formulation.

A corresponding correction can be applied to the item difficulty index or p-value (the proportion of examinees answering the item correctly). The corrected p-value is given by the formula (Thorndike 1982)

$$p_c = p - \frac{p_w}{(A - 1)}$$

where p is the proportion of examinees answering the item correctly and p_w is the proportion of examinees attempting the item who answered it incorrectly. A problem with this correction is that when the propor-

tion of correct answers falls below the chance level (due to particularly attractive distractors), it is possible to obtain a corrected item difficulty index less than zero (Thorndike 1982).

Argument about the appropriateness and effectiveness of formula scoring and the associated test directions continues in the early 1990s. Lord (1975) remarked that formula scoring is an area "where two informed people often hold opposing views with great assurance" (p. 7). Critics of formula scoring claim that: (a) it is based on false assumptions about examinee behavior, and (b) it penalizes examinees with certain personality traits.

With respect to the first point, critics argue that examinees who do not know the answer to a test item rarely respond randomly. If this were so, the distractors for an item would be chosen with approximately equal frequency. This is rarely the case, as can easily be shown. Thorndike (1982) illustrated this point with the example of a set of verbal analogy items from a published test, where the most popular distractor was, on average, chosen by about 20 percent of examinees and the least popular by about 4 percent of examinees.

Another criticism of the formula-scoring assumption is that it ignores the possibility that an examinee has either misinformation or partial knowledge (Rowley and Traub 1977). If examinees respond on the basis of misinformation, the formula overcorrects, since examinees lose not only the point for the question but an additional fraction of a point for behavior that cannot be considered to be guessing. If informed guessing based on partial knowledge is held to be undesirable, then the formula undercorrects, since examinees are more likely to get an item right in this case than if they had been randomly guessing.

Whether informed guessing should be penalized at all is another issue. It has been argued that informed guessing increases true score variance rather than error variance and hence enhances the validity of scores (Mehrens and Lehman 1986). Moreover, when examinees respond on the basis of partial knowledge, their test scores are based on a greater sample of content than if they omit, as instructed under formula-scoring directions, and hence may have greater validity. If examinees with partial knowledge are not to be penalized, the test directions should instruct examinees to omit only if they cannot eliminate any of the answer choices.

In answer to criticisms of the formula-scoring assumption, Lord (1975) described an alternative assumption which provides a more defensible basis for formula scoring. Lord's assumption is that the difference between an answer sheet obtained under formula-scoring directions and the same answer sheet obtained under number-rights directions is that omits, if any, on the former, are replaced by random guesses on the latter. Under this assumption, it can be shown that while the number-right and formula scores are unbiased estimators of the same quantity, the formula score has smaller error variance and is therefore preferable. Rowley and Traub (1977) pointed out that Lord's assumption is tenable only if examinees are able to distinguish informed guesses from random guesses. Some studies (e.g., Sheriffs and Boomer 1954, Slakter 1968, Votaw 1936) have shown, however, that under formula-scoring directions, examinees omit items which they have a greater-than-chance probability of answering correctly. Lord (1975) criticized these studies on methodological grounds.

With respect to the argument that formula-scoring confounds personality traits with test scores, there is a considerable body of research which shows that the extent to which examinees comply with the instructions associated with formula scoring (i.e., the instruction to omit rather than to guess randomly) reflects a personality trait which may disadvantage some examinees (see Diamond and Evans 1973, Rowley and Traub 1977 for reviews of this research). Examinees who are unwilling to take risks may omit rather than answer a question they feel uncertain about even if they have partial knowledge, and consequently lose more points than they would have by answering. Examinees who are more willing to take risks will not be penalized on average, since at most they will lose the points gained by randomly guessing. The research in this area indicates that the tendency to omit under formula-scoring directions is a personality trait which is more reliably measured by multiple choice tests than the cognitive trait of interest.

The primary argument in favor of formula scoring is that it increases the reliability and validity of scores (Mattson 1965, Lord 1975). While the argument has theoretical merit (under the assumptions of formula scoring), empirical studies have not yielded unequivocal support (Diamond and Evans 1973, Rowley and Traub 1977). Increases in reliability and validity, where obtained, are generally small (for a review, see Diamond and Evans 1973). Rowley and Traub (1977) suggested that even when increases in reliability are obtained, the increase may reflect the reliability of measurement of the personality trait rather than a reduction in the error variance of the true scores on the cognitive component.

A second argument in favor of formula scoring is based on empirical studies that show that formula scoring tends to equalize the mean scores of randomly equivalent groups of examinees who have been given different instructions regarding guessing. Angoff and Schrader (1984) compared the mean number-right and formula scores of groups of examinees who were given either number-right or formula-scoring directions and found that while there was a significant difference in the mean number-right scores of the two groups, there was almost no difference in the mean formula scores. The authors concluded that the difference in number-right scores was due largely to chance responding. Angoff and Schrader (1986), using the same data,

drew the additional conclusion that partial knowledge is often misinformation: that is, low-ability examinees with misinformation are deterred from responding under formula-scoring directions (and hence lose fewer points than they would have under number-right scoring) as often as higher-ability examinees with partial knowledge (who lose more points than they would have otherwise), with the result that there is no net effect on formula scores. This conclusion, however, does more to support the argument that the mean scores of the groups are an inappropriate basis for comparison of the effects of test directions than it does to support the argument in favor of formula scoring.

An alternative formula score used by Traub et al. (1969) is given by

$$F = R + \frac{O}{A}$$

where O is the number of omits. Under this procedure, examinees gain a chance score on items they omit, rather than a penalty for wrong answers. This formula scoring procedure may be less disadvantageous to the timid examinee (Mehrens and Lehman 1986), but on the other hand, may disadvantage better students who have partial knowledge but who prefer to accept the omit reward rather than attempt the question (Wood 1976). Hence, personality factors may once again be confounded with scores obtained under formula-scoring directions.

Lord (1975) noted that the omit-reward formula produces scores which are perfectly correlated with standard formula scores. This is true, however, only if the scores are obtained under the same testing conditions. The scores will not be perfectly correlated when each is obtained under directions appropriate to the procedure, since the directions will differentially affect omitting behavior.

1.2 Item Response Theory Approaches

Item response theory (IRT) is a test theory which has come into wide use only since the early 1970s. Item response theory provides an alternative approach to the problem of guessing. Under IRT, an examinee's observed performance on a test item is assumed to depend on the examinee's underlying and unobservable ability or trait level and characteristics of the test item. The relationship is expressed in the form of a mathematical function, or item characteristic curve, which gives the probability of a correct response to an item as a function of the person and item parameters. Under item response theory, the examinee ability estimate is not a simple transformation of number-correct test score; it is estimated in the presence of parameters describing the test item, and hence takes into account the characteristics of the item (see *Item Response Theory*).

The most general of the commonly used item response models, referred to as the "three-parameter model," assumes that examinee performance on a test item is affected by three characteristics of the item: its difficulty, discrimination, and a factor which reflects the probability that a very low ability examinee will answer the item correctly. This parameter of the item is denoted the *c*-parameter and is sometimes referred to as a "pseudoguessing" parameter. Items differ in their *c*-parameters according to their difficulty and the attractiveness of the distractors. The three-parameter item response model is given by the equation

$$P(u = 1 \mid \theta) = c + (1 - c) \; \frac{e^{a(\theta - b)}}{1 + e^{a(\theta - b)}}$$

where *u* is the examinee's response to the item (taking the value 1 for a correct response), θ is the examinee's ability, *a* is the item discrimination parameter, *b* is the item difficulty parameter, and *c* is the pseudoguessing parameter. Examples of three-parameter item characteristic curves are shown in Fig. 1.

While the *c*-parameter does indicate that there is a nonzero probability of a correct answer even for the lowest ability examinees, it does not indicate the probability of a correct answer through random guessing. The *c*-parameter for multiple choice items is often lower than the chance probability of a correct answer because of the attractiveness of the distractors.

Although the *c*-parameter is considered to be a characteristic of the item rather than the examinee, its effect does depend on the ability level of the examinee. Hence, it does take into account the individual examinees' differential probabilities of guessing and its incorporation in the model allows for the adjustment of the ability estimate to take into account the possibility of guessing. However, whenever the *c*-parameter is nonzero, the precision of estimation of ability is reduced. Hence, as in the case where test score is used as the trait estimate, the occurrence of guessing increases error variance and is therefore undesirable.

In practice, satisfactory parameter estimation in the three-parameter model requires large samples of examinees and long tests. The *c*-parameter is often poorly estimated, even when data are abundant. For this reason, many practitioners choose more restrictive models, incorporating only one or two item parameters. These models are easier to fit to test data. However, one- and two-parameter models assume that very low ability examinees have zero probability of obtaining a correct answer, and therefore make no allowance for guessing behavior. If guessing is a factor in examinee performance, the ability of the examinee will be overestimated and the estimate will contain greater error.

Waller (1989) suggested a modification of the one- and two-parameter models which would yield an ability estimate corrected for guessing without including a lower asymptote parameter. Waller suggested that at each stage of the estimation process, an examinee's ability estimate be based only on the items for which the examinee has a greater-than-chance probability of answering correctly. Waller's initial evaluation of this model indicated that it does not fit real data as well as the three-parameter model. Waller concluded that the three-parameter model is better able to model partial-knowledge guessing, since the *c*-parameter has an effect throughout the ability range, whereas Waller's model only considers random guessing, which is most likely to occur among low ability examinees. There appears to have been no follow-up research with respect to this model.

1.3 Other Approaches

Two other testing procedures designed to circumvent the problem of guessing in multiple choice tests and allow for assessment of partial knowledge are confidence testing and elimination testing procedures.

Confidence testing requires examinees to indicate their degree of confidence in each of the response options for an item or simply in the option they choose; guessing and partial knowledge can thus be identified. Various schemes for allotting confidence points have been proposed. Echternacht (1972) provided a review of confidence testing procedures. Studies of confidence testing procedures have produced mixed results with respect to improvements in reliability and validity of scores. For example, Hambleton et al. (1970) found that confidence testing produced more valid but less reliable scores; Hakstian and Kansup (1975) concluded that confidence testing procedures do not result in any increase in reliability or validity. An obvious disadvantage of confidence testing procedures is that they require increased testing time and are more difficult for examinees. In addition, there is some evidence (Jacobs 1971, Hansen 1971) that the personality factor of "general confidence" contaminates scores obtained under confidence testing procedures.

Elimination testing requires examinees to eliminate the answer choices they believe to be incorrect, with points awarded for each incorrect option eliminated and points deducted if the correct answer is elimi-

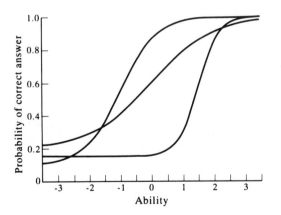

Figure 1

Three-parameter item characteristic curves

nated. There are many variants on the basic procedure. As with confidence testing procedures, research has shown no clear advantage to elimination procedures. Hakstian and Kansup (1975) summarized the research in this area and observed that there was no evidence of an increase in reliability and, at best, provisional evidence for an increase in validity. These authors concluded on the basis of their own study that there was no empirical support for elimination testing procedures.

Because of the lack of empirical evidence supporting the use of these procedures, neither is widely used and there has been little research in this area since the 1970s.

2. Detection of Guessing in Multiple Choice Tests

Apart from procedures for correcting for guessing in multiple choice tests, a number of procedures exist for detecting "aberrant" test-taking behavior such as guessing. These procedures are known generally as "appropriateness measures."

Perhaps the simplest appropriateness measure is the personal biserial correlation (Donlon and Fischer 1968). The personal biserial correlation coefficient is a measure of the relationship between the examinee's response pattern and the item difficulties (p-values). When the examinee responds in a consistent manner, he or she should answer easier items correctly more often than difficult items, hence the correlation should be high; if the examinee is randomly guessing, then he or she will obtain a correct answer on more difficult items than expected, leading to a lower correlation coefficient.

Other appropriateness measures are based on a comparison of the examinee's observed response pattern with that expected under certain assumptions. One such measure is Sato's Caution Index (Sato 1975), which is obtained by first computing the covariance between the item difficulties and the examinee response pattern; this covariance is then compared with the covariance between item difficulty and the perfect Guttman response pattern for an examinee with that total score. The ratio of these quantities will be close to one when the examinee responds in a consistent manner and close to zero when the response pattern is extremely aberrant.

A number of appropriateness measures are based on item response theory. An example of an appropriateness measure based on IRT is the person-fit statistic, which can take a variety of forms. A general person-fit statistic is the mean squared standardized residual, given by

$$f = \frac{1}{n} \sum_{i=1}^{n} \frac{[u_i - P(\theta)]^2}{P(\theta)[1 - P(\theta)]}$$

where n is the number of items, u_i is the response of the examinee to item i, and $P(\theta)$ is the probability that an

examinee with ability θ will answer the item correctly. The probability of a correct answer is obtained using the parameter estimates obtained under the chosen item response model.

Other non-IRT and IRT-based appropriateness measures are described and evaluated in Harnisch and Linn (1981) and Drasgow et al. (1987). These appropriateness measures are designed to detect aberrant response patterns, but not to correct test scores or ability estimates for the aberrant responses. If an examinee's appropriateness measure indicates an aberrant response pattern, the examinee must be retested to obtain a more valid and reliable estimate of ability or achievement.

3. Conclusion

Despite over 50 years of research, there appears to be no generally accepted and satisfactory way of correcting for guessing in multiple choice test scores. While arguments have been made for and against formula scoring, there is no conclusive empirical evidence that formula scores are more reliable and valid than number-right scores, but some evidence suggests that formula-scoring test directions lead to the confounding of a personality factor with test score. Item response theory offers an alternative approach, but the practical problems of implementing IRT procedures may preclude the use of such procedures in some testing situations. Indices for detecting aberrant response patterns are available, but these measures offer no aid in correcting for the guessing observed.

Practical steps that can be taken to ameliorate the problem of guessing include ensuring that power tests are not administered under speeded conditions, that directions about guessing and scoring are clearly stated, that the test is of sufficient length so that guessing cannot substantially influence scores, and that the test is of appropriate difficulty for the examinees being tested.

See also: Validity; Measurement in Educational Research

References

Angoff W H, Schrader W B 1984 A study of hypotheses basic to the use of rights and formula scores. *J. Educ. Meas.* 21(1): 1–17
Angoff W H, Schrader W B 1986 A rejoinder to Albanese, "The correction for guessing: A further analysis of Angoff and Schrader." *J. Educ. Meas.* 23(3): 237–43
Diamond J, Evans W 1973 The correction for guessing. *Rev. Educ. Res.* 43(2): 181–91
Donlon T F, Fischer F E 1968 An index of an individual's agreement with group determined item difficulties. *Educ. Psychol. Meas.* 28: 105–13
Drasgow F, Levine M V, McLaughlin M E 1987 Detecting inappropriate test scores with optimal and practical appropriateness indices. *Appl. Psychol. Meas.* 11(1): 59–79

Echternacht G J 1972 The use of confidence testing in objective tests. *Rev. Educ. Res.* 42(2): 217–36

Hakstian A R, Kansup W 1975 A comparison of several methods of assessing partial knowledge in multiple-choice tests: II. Testing procedures. *J. Educ. Meas.* 12(4): 231–39

Hambleton R K, Roberts D M, Traub R E 1970 A comparison of the reliability and validity of two methods for assessing partial knowledge on a multiple-choice test. *J. Educ. Meas.* 7(2): 75–82.

Hansen R 1971 The influence of variables other than knowledge on probabilistic tests. *J. Educ. Meas.* 8(1): 9–14

Harnisch D L, Linn R L 1981 Analysis of item response patterns: Questionable test data and dissimilar curriculum practices. *J. Educ. Meas.* 18: 133–46

Jacobs S S 1971 Correlates of unwarranted confidence in responses to objective test items. *J. Educ. Meas.* 8(1): 15–19

Lord F M 1975 Formula scoring and number-right scoring. *J. Educ. Meas.* 12(1): 7–11

Mattson D 1965 The effects of guessing on the standard error of measurement and the reliability of test scores. *Educ. Psychol. Meas.* 25(3): 727–30

Mehrens W A, Lehman I I 1986 *Using Standardized Tests in Education*, 4th edn. Longman, New York

Rowley G L, Traub R E 1977 Formula scoring, number-right scoring, and test taking strategy. *J. Educ. Meas.* 14(1): 15–22

Sato T 1975 *The Construction and Interpretation of S-P Tables*. Meiji Tosho, Tokyo

Sheriffs A C, Boomer D S 1954 Who is penalized by the penalty for guessing? *J. Educ. Psychol.* 45: 81–90

Slakter M J 1968 The effect of guessing strategy on objective test scores. *J. Educ. Meas.* 5(3): 217–22

Thorndike R L 1982 *Applied Psychometrics*. Houghton Mifflin Co, Boston, Massachusetts

Traub R E, Hambleton R K, Singh B 1969 Effects of promised reward and threatened penalty on performance on a multiple-choice vocabulary test. *Educ. Psychol. Meas.* 29(4): 847–61

Votaw D F 1936 The effect of do-not-guess directions upon the validity of true-false or multiple-choice tests. *J. Educ. Psychol.* 27: 698–703

Waller M I 1989 Modeling guessing behavior: A comparison of two IRT models. *Appl. Psychol. Meas.* 13(3): 233–43

Wood R 1976 Inhibiting blind guessing: The effect of instruction. *J. Educ. Meas.* 13(4): 297–308

Further Reading

Hambleton R K, Swaminathan H, Rogers H J 1991 *Fundamentals of Item Response Theory*. Sage, Newbury Park, California

Objective Tests

† B. H. Choppin

Objective methods of observation are those in which any observer who follows the prescribed rules will assign the same values or categories to the events being observed as would another observer. Similarly, an objective test is one for which the rules for scoring it are so specific and comprehensive that anyone who marks a test script in accordance with these rules will arrive at the same test score. Most objective tests used in education are composed of a sequence of individual "objective" test items (sometimes called "structured-response items") in which the testees must choose their answers from a specified list of alternatives rather than by creating them for themselves. It is important to remember, however, that the definition relates to the method of scoring the test and not to the format of its constituent items as such. Not all objective tests require the student to select from a presented list. Items which require the student to write down a phrase, a word, or a number, and in the scoring of which there are clear and unequivocal rules for deciding whether the response is right or wrong, also qualify as "objective."

Objective tests stand in clear contrast to essay examinations and other forms of open-ended tests in which few constraints are put on the testee. Such tests are characterized by the very great variation in the responses that are produced even among students of similar ability or attainment, and their scoring requires the examiner to weigh a variety of evidence, a task which calls for substantial amounts of personal judgment. As a result, different examiners usually arrive at different scores for the same essay, and hence this type of assessment is not regarded as objective.

Objective tests may also be distinguished from short-answer (or restricted-response) tests in which, although the testee must produce his or her own answers, the constraints imposed by the formulation of the question are such as to make the scoring more objective. For example, students might be asked to draw a diagram of a terrestrial telescope paying particular attention to the characteristics and positioning of the lenses. The scoring instructions might dictate that the student's response be accepted as correct if and only if the objective lens has a longer focal length than the eye-piece. Tests of this last type are sometimes referred to as "semiobjective tests."

1. Areas of Application

Objective tests are widely used to measure intelligence, aptitude, and achievement (or attainment). Almost all tests of aptitude and intelligence are of the objective type because of the uses to which such measures are put. Raw scores of intelligence or aptitude have little meaning in themselves, and need to be translated to well-established scales before they can be used. In consequence, reliability of the scores is a major consideration and using objective test formats is one way to maximize this.

However, the appropriateness of objective tests for the measurement of achievement is much more controversial. Essay tests are still preferred to objective tests for most educational purposes in many countries. Where the teacher scores the tests for a single class, objectivity as such is less important, and the advantages of getting the students to express themselves fully and openly tend to outweigh the demands for a reliable score. For example, although the typical American high-school teacher will use objective tests (self-developed) for routine assessment of students on a weekly or monthly basis, the teacher in England or Wales will almost always prefer to use nonobjective tests for this purpose. The system of public examinations in England and Wales, which certify levels of attainment for secondary school leavers, are largely nonobjective despite the need for reliability (given the importance of the results to the future careers of individual students). However, it should be noted that the proportion of objective test material in these examinations has been increasing in recent years.

2. Item Formats

Most objective test items appear in one of four alternative formats. These will be considered in turn below, and examples of each type appear in Fig. 1.

2.1 Supply Items

Unlike the other types in which the student is selecting from a list of alternative responses presented to him or her, the supply type of item requires a student to construct a response. However, the question is so structured as to limit the scope of the student's response so that (ideally) there will be one, and only one, acceptable answer. Demanding that the student construct rather than recognize the response avoids some of the common criticisms of objective tests described below. However, it does give up some of the convenience (such as automated scoring) that selection-type items offer. The format's most frequent area of application is in mathematics on questions which call for a specific quantitative answer. However, Fig. 1 demonstrates that it can be used effectively in other areas.

Specification of the acceptable answers is an essential part of the item construction process, but there is always the danger that certain students will invent unforeseen answers that could arguably be accepted as correct. For example, on item 1(b) in Fig. 1 the student might respond "N_2." It is advisable with supply items to compile a comprehensive list of answers that give appropriate evidence of achievement before scoring begins. Note that the criterion is not grammatical correctness nor even truth. The answer "invisible" to question 1(b) makes the statement true, but does not demonstrate that the student has achieved the objective being tested.

2.2 The True/False Item Format

The true/false item presents a declarative statement and requires the examinee to indicate whether he or she judges it to be true or false. (Some generally similar items have other dichotomous response options such as yes/no or appropriate/inappropriate.) Although such items are easy to construct, this is not a format to be generally recommended. Tests composed of true/false items tend to be rather unreliable, and are particularly susceptible to contamination by guessing. Ebel (1970) argues that this is not serious and that true/false tests may be very efficient, but few other writers support this view. True/false items can be quite effective for assessing factual knowledge (especially if great precision is not required), but are usually inappropriate for testing more complex skills.

2.3 Multiple-choice Item Format

The multiple-choice item is by far the most frequently used in educational achievement testing. The number of alternative answers offered varies but is usually four or five. As a rule only one of the alternatives is correct, the others (the distractors) being constructed so as to provide plausible examples of common errors. If the distractors are carefully written a wrong-answer analysis can yield valuable diagnostic information about the types of error being made by students. Many variations of the basic format have been developed (Wood 1977) mainly to increase the amount of information elicited by an item or to improve its applicability to the testing of higher mental processes.

The chief difficulty in constructing good multiple-choice questions is to find appropriate distractors. To be effective they must be plausible at least to a substantial minority of students, yet they must be clear and unambiguously wrong in the judgment of experts. Distractors should not give inadvertent clues which permit testwise students to eliminate them irrespective of their ability to solve correctly the question. The multiple-choice questions given in Fig. 1 may be regarded as exemplars of the type.

Although they too may effectively be used to assess specific knowledge, multiple-choice items are readily

1. *Supply-type items*
    (a) A new school building has 12 classrooms. The school ordered 30 desks for each classroom. Only 280 desks were delivered. How many more are needed?

    _____

    (Scoring key: 80)

    (b) The gas which is most abundant in the atmosphere is:

    _____

    (Scoring key: Nitrogen)

    (c) Through which country does the canal that links the Mediterranean Sea to the Red Sea pass?

    _____

    (Scoring key: Egypt or UAR)

    (d) A solid element x forms two oxides which contain respectively 71.1% and 62.3% of x. Calculate the equivalent weight of x in each oxide. The specific heat of x is 0.084. Given that the product of the atomic weight and specific heat of a solid element is approximately 6.4, write down the formulae for the two oxides of x.

    _____ and _____

    (Scoring key: XO_2 and XO_3)

2. *True/false items*
    (e) The capital city of Sweden is Stockholm.   True : False
    (f) The rate of juvenile delinquency is usually higher in the older parts of a city.   True : False
    (g) The oceans are deepest at the center and shallowest near the edges.   True : False
    (h) Light rays always travel in straight lines.   True : False

3. *Multiple-choice items*
    (i) The amount of heat required to raise the temperature of one gram of a substance by one degree (°C) is called:
    (i)   its thermal conductivity;
    (ii) its specific heat;
    (iii) its thermal capacity;
    (iv) its thermal expansion.

    (j) John brought the skull of an animal to school. His teacher said she did not know what the animal was but she was sure that it was one that preyed on other animals for its food. Which clue, do you think, led her to this conclusion?
    (i)   The eye sockets faced sideways.
    (ii) The skull was much longer than it was wide.
    (iii) There was a projecting ridge along the top of the skull.
    (iv) Four of the teeth were long and pointed.
    (v)   The jaws could work sideways as well as up and down.

4. *Matching item format*
    For each piece of apparatus listed below, identify the scientist who invented it, and enter the appropriate code letter on the answer sheet.

	Apparatus		*Inventor*
(k)	X-ray spectrometer	(i)	Angstrom
(l)	Reflection grating	(ii)	Bragg
(m)	Interferometer	(iii)	Helmholtz
(n)	Ophthalmoscope	(iv)	Michelson
		(v)	Newton
		(vi)	Rowland
		(vii)	Thomson

Figure 1
Examples of objective test items

adaptable to measure more complex skills involving reasoning and analysis. It has been found to be relatively straightforward to construct an achievement test, all of whose items are in the multiple-choice format which assesses student performance on a wide range of objectives involving different skill levels.

2.4 Matching Items

The fourth widely used item format to be considered is the matching exercise. This is a logical extension of the multiple-choice item in which the same list of alternative responses is used for several items in sequence. An example of this format is included in Fig. 1.

The most obvious advantage of the matching item format is one of economy. More responses are obtained from the student for the same amount of reading. The format can be effectively employed to test knowledge of specific facts, but is generally unsuitable for more complex objectives. However, it has been suggested (Thorndike and Hagen 1969) that a variation of the format, the classification task, can be used to appraise comprehension and application-type objectives.

3. Disadvantages of Objective Tests

Many critics of the multiple-choice format have pointed out that it required students only to recognize the correct answer rather than to recall and/or construct it for themselves. It is suggested that recognition is a fundamentally lower form of behavior, and that many students who are able to recognize the correct answers on a test are unable to apply what they have learned in practice. In general, the research evidence does not support this. Students who are good recallers of knowledge are also good recognizers. Several studies (e.g. Godshalk et al. 1966, Choppin and Purves 1969) which compared objective tests with free-response essays written by the same students showed that the objective tests predicted overall performance on the essay about as well as the limited reliability of the essay scoring would permit.

Associated with this criticism is the complaint that objective tests place an undue emphasis on reading rather than writing skills, so that the latter tend to become devalued. Wood (1977) comments that although this may have some validity in the United States, elsewhere (e.g., in the United Kingdom) traditional testing practices have paid far too much attention to the ability of the testees to express themselves in writing.

A third form of criticism is that the multiple-choice test item typically presents the student with three or four times as many false answers as correct ones. As a rule the distractors are written so as to be quite plausible, and thus the opportunities for the student to "learn" incorrect information during the test session are substantial. Thorndike and Hagen (1969) note that little research had been done on this point.

Two other disadvantages of objective tests deserve mention. The first is that it is, in general, much easier to write objective test questions to test comparatively low-level skills (e.g., factual knowledge) than the more complex skills of analysis and synthesis. As a result, many existing objective tests are overloaded with items focusing on pieces of specific knowledge. Objective test items (particularly in the multiple-choice format) can be constructed to assess higher mental processes, but in general this is rather more difficult to do, and too often professional test constructors have not paid sufficient attention to this problem.

The other criticism is that objective tests encourage guessing behavior. Although a minority of critics (e.g., Hoffmann 1962) appear to regard guessing itself as an immoral activity on a par with betting on horses or using illegal drugs, most feel it is an appropriate behavior for the student, in a restricted choice situation, who lacks sufficient information to solve the test item directly. The problem arises from the number of correct guesses that occur. They can lead to an overestimate of an individual student's level of achievement, and tend to lower the measurement reliability for a whole group. Various countermeasures have been proposed.

4. Advantages of Objective Tests

Against these real or imagined disadvantages, there are clearly a number of benefits ensuing from the use of objective tests of achievement. The first is that by focusing the attention of the student, it is possible to gather information rapidly on particular parts of his or her learning—a feature especially important in diagnostic work and in formative evaluation. This focusing of individual items allows the test maker to control the scope of what is being assessed by the complete test, so that items may be sampled from across a very broad domain or from only a very narrow part of it. In contrast, responses on an essay-type examination are less subject to control by the examiner, and it is often difficult to persuade all students to provide evidence about their mastery of particular skills.

Minute by minute, an objective test is probably the most efficient basis for obtaining information about an individual's learning. Because of its structure, the instrument is relatively easy to score, is reliable, and its data are amenable to a wide range of statistical analyses. Automated scoring procedures have played a major part in making the multiple-choice item format so popular. These have ranged from a simple template (which when placed over a test or answer sheet allows the scorer to observe quickly how many correct responses have been selected), to computer-controlled electronic scanning machines which can "read" the pattern of pencil marks made on an answer sheet very rapidly. The use of such methods whether on a large or small scale substantially reduces the time and cost of achievement testing. However, it should be noted that some of the time saved in scoring may be used up by the additional time required for test preparation. Constructing clear, unambiguous, and valid objective test items is not an easy task.

Since each objective test item is usually short,

many of them can be included in a single test, and this contributes to the higher reliability that is usually achieved. The items can be spread more evenly over the topics to be covered, so that a more representative sampling of performance is obtained. Another way of stating this is to note that the score from a well-made objective test is likely to be more accurate than that from a comparable essay test. Two separate objective tests, based on the same content area, will rank an individual at more nearly the same place in his or her group, than would two free-response measures.

5. Summary

Objective tests have been found to be efficient and effective instruments for obtaining measures of learning as well as of general mental ability and aptitude. They yield scores that are more dependable than those from comparable open-ended tests, and their quality can be readily assessed through statistical item analysis.

Nevertheless, their full advantages are only realized when considerable care is exercised in their construction. Writers of objective items for achievement tests have an unfortunate tendency to concentrate on factual, and often trivial, information, and to produce tests which seem to distort the full range of educational goals. It is possible, however, to create objective test items which assess abilities to comprehend, interpret, and apply knowledge, to analyze and to synthesize ideas. The extra effort needed to write such items is justified when valid and reliable measures of achievement are desired.

See also: Item Writing Techniques; Measurement in Educational Research

References

Choppin B H, Purves A C 1969 Comparison of open-ended and multiple-choice items dealing with literary understanding. *Res. Teach. Eng.* 3: 15–24

Ebel R L 1970 The case for true–false test items. *Sch. Rev.* 78: 373–89

Godshalk F I, Swineford F, Coffman W E 1966 *The Measurement of Writing Ability.* College Entrance Examinations Board, New York

Thorndike R L, Hagen E 1969 *Measurement and Evaluation in Psychology and Education*, 3rd edn. Wiley, New York

Wood R 1977 Multiple-choice: A state of the art report. *Eval. Educ.* 1: 191–280

Further Reading

Ebel R L 1979 *Essentials of Educational Measurement*, 3rd edn. Prentice-Hall, Englewood Cliffs, New Jersey

Hoffmann B 1962 *The Tyranny of Testing.* Collier Macmillan, New York

Roid G H, Haladyna T M 1982 *A Technology for Test-item Writing.* Academic Press, New York

Reliability

† R. L. Thorndike and R. M. Thorndike

Any measurement presents a set of observations taken from some universe of responses by the examinee. The universe corresponds, it is hoped, to the latent attribute in which one is interested. In evaluating a measurement procedure, two broad questions are encountered that are different but overlapping. The first question is how accurately the observation sample represents the broader universe of responses from which it is drawn; the second is how faithfully that universe corresponds to the latent attribute in which there is interest. The first relates to what is commonly called the "reliability" of the measure, the second to its "validity." Collectively, they have been spoken of by Cronbach et al. (1972) as the "generalizability of the score"—the range of inferences that can be made from it. (While the discussion here is couched in terms of test scores, the concepts apply equally to all types of measurement.)

There are typically three sides to the issue of reliability: the basic rationale, the procedures for data collection, and the statistical procedures for data analysis. These facets interact in that certain empirical data sets are appropriate for certain conceptions of the universe to which inference is desired, and the possible types of statistical analysis depend on the data at hand. Ideally, the rational analysis of the universe to which generalization was desired should be primary and data collection and statistical treatment should flow from this analysis. Realistically, however, practical considerations may limit the data that it is possible to collect, and these limitations may set boundaries on the universe to which inferences can logically be made and on the statistical analyses that can be carried out.

This entry starts with a consideration of "classical" reliability theory. This is the true-score-and-error model of a test score that was presented by Spearman in 1904 and that provided the accepted theoretical model for discussions of reliability for the next 50 years. There follows an analysis of the multifacet model of reliability presented by Lindquist (1953) and elaborated by Cronbach et al. (1972). Then the discussion returns to the practical issues involved in data collection and analysis. Finally, the meaning of reliability in the context of domain mastery or criterion-referenced testing is briefly considered.

1. The Classical Reliability Model

The classical reliability model views a test score as having two additive components, the "true" score and a random "error." The error is defined as unrelated to the true score and as unrelated to the error that would occur in another measurement of the same attribute. The true score is defined as the value that the average of repeated measurements with the identical measure approaches as the number of measurements which is increased without limit. The term "identical" implies that it is possible to measure an individual repeatedly without changing that individual—a condition that obviously cannot be achieved in the real world. Though the model is in this respect, and some others, an oversimplification and not a representation of reality, development of the model brings out a number of relationships that are instructive and useful in the design and construction of tests and in the evaluation of test scores.

1.1 Basic Assumptions, Definitions, and Resulting Relationships

The basic assumptions of the model are as follows:

(a)   The obtained score is the sum of true score plus a random error; $X_{obt} = X_{true} + X_{error}$. The subscripts o, t, and e will be used for observed score, true score, and error respectively. The subscript x is used for the variance (S_x^2) of X_o.

(b)   Over the population, error is independent of true score; that is, $r_{te} = 0$.

(c)   In pairs of measures, the error in one measure is independent of the error in the other; that is, $r_{ee'} = 0$.

(d)   Two tests are parallel (or alternate or equivalent) forms if they are "constructed to the same specifications, give rise to identical distributions of observed scores . . ., covary equally with each other, and covary equally with any measure (Z) that is not one of the parallel forms" (Feldt and Brennan 1989 p. 108). Parallel forms are denoted by x and x'.

Given these assumptions, as the number of persons

or the number of measurements increases, the mean error approaches 0 as a limit. That is $\bar{X}_e \cong 0$ when the number of measures increases without limit. This follows from the definition of errors as random deviations from the true score that are equally likely to be positive or negative. Any consistent direction to "error" would be indistinguishable from, and hence assimilated as part of, the operational "true" score.

It follows that, in the limit, the mean of observed scores is equal to the mean of true scores; that is:

$$\bar{X}_o \cong \bar{X}_t \tag{1}$$

This relationship holds both for repeated measures of an individual and for the mean of a group. That is, as the number of observations increases, the observed mean approaches the mean of true scores and is an unbiased estimate of the true-score mean.

The variance of observed scores equals the true-score variance plus the error variance. Most of the development from here on will work with scores that are expressed as deviations from the mean; that is, $x = X - \bar{X}$. By definition

$$S_x^2 = \frac{1}{N} \sum (X_t + X_e)^2$$

Squaring, distributing terms and simplifying, and noting that $r_{te} = 0$ yields

$$S_x^2 = S_t^2 + S_e^2 \tag{2}$$

It can also be shown that the correlation between two parallel tests is equal to the true-score variance divided by the observed variance, that is:

$$r_{xx'} = S_t^2 / S_x^2 \tag{3}$$

Thus the alternate-forms reliability of a test equals true-score variance divided by observed variance. From this it follows that $S_t^2 = S_x^2 r_{xx'}$ and $S_t = S_x (r_{xx'})^{1/2}$.

Returning to Eqn. (2) and transposing, gives $S_e^2 = S_x^2 - S_t^2$.

But since $S_t^2 = S_x^2 r_{xx'}$, then $S_e^2 = S_x^2 - S_x^2 r_{xx'}$, or:

$$S_e = S_x (1 - r_{xx'})^{1/2}. \tag{4}$$

Thus the standard error of measurement, S_e, is estimated from the observed standard deviation and the alternate-forms reliability coefficient.

Next the correlation between observed score and true score, and the correlation between observed score and measurement error can be derived. Remembering that $x_o = x_t + x_e$,

$$r_{x_o x_t} = \cfrac{\frac{1}{N} \sum (x_t + x_e) x_t}{S_x S_t} = \cfrac{\frac{1}{N} \sum x_t^2 + \frac{1}{N} \sum x_t x_e}{S_x S_t}$$

But the second term in the numerator approaches

zero because of the independence of true score and error. Hence

$$r_{x_o}x_t = S_t^2/S_xS_t = S_t/S_x \qquad (5)$$

Referring to Eqn. (3), it was found that $r_{xx'} = S_t^2/S_x^2$, so $r_{x_oxt} = (r_{xx'})^{1/2}$. The correlation of an observed measure with the underlying true score is equal to the square root of the alternate-forms reliability coefficient.

Turning to observed score and error,

$$r_{x_o}x_e = \frac{\frac{1}{N} \sum (x_t + x_e)x_e}{S_xS_e} = \frac{\frac{1}{N} \sum x_tx_e + \frac{1}{N} \sum x_e^2}{S_xS_e}$$

Once again referring to the independence of true score and error, it can be seen that the first term of the numerator approaches 0, and

$$r_{x_o}x_e = S_e^2/S_xS_e = S_e/S_x$$

But from Eqn. (4), $S_e/S_x = [1 - r_{xx'}$ and, so $r_{x_o}x_e = (1 - r_{xx'})^{1/2}$. This correlation of observed score with error is a specific example of the more general expression $(1 - r_{xy})^{1/2}$, which has been called the coefficient of alienation when predicting y from x.

1.2 Effects of Increasing or Decreasing Test Length

In this section, the discussion turns now to the effects of increasing (or decreasing) the length of a test, considering *en route* the general expressions for the correlations of sums.

The equation for the mean of the unweighted sum of two or more variables is simply:

$$\text{Mean } (X_1 + X_2 + ... + X_k) = \bar{X}_1 + \bar{X}_2 + ... + \bar{X}_k$$

For two variables,

$$\bar{X}_{(1+2)} = \frac{1}{N} \sum (X_1 + X_2)$$

$$= \frac{1}{N} \sum X_1 + \frac{1}{N} \sum X_2$$

$$= \bar{X}_1 + \bar{X}_2$$

If X_1 and X_2 are equivalent forms of the same test, each will have the same mean, so one can write $\text{Mean}_{2X} = 2(\text{Mean } X)$. When the length of a test is doubled by adding equivalent items, the mean can be expected to double. More generally:

$$\text{Mean}_{kX} = k(\text{Mean } X)$$

If the variables are combined with different weights, then

$$\text{Mean}_{wtd\,sum} = \sum W_i\bar{X}_i \qquad (6)$$

Turning now to the variance of a sum:

$$S_{(X_1 + X_2)}^2 = \frac{1}{N} \sum (X_1 + X_2)^2$$

$$= S_1^2 + S_2^2 + 2r_{12}S_1S_2,$$

where the last term is twice the covariance of X_1 and X_2. When the two variables are equivalent forms of the same test, the effect of summing two tests is to double the length of the test, and:

$$S_{(X + X')}^2 = S_X^2 + S_{X'}^2 + 2r_{XX'}S_XS_{X'} \qquad (7)$$

But because the test forms are equivalent, and so have the same standard deviation, this can be expressed as:

$$S_{2X}^2 = 2S_X^2 + 2r_{XX'}S_X^2 = S_X^2(2 + 2r_{XX'})$$

and

$$S_{2X} = S_X(2 + 2r_{XX'})^{1/2} \qquad (8)$$

In general terms, when the length of a test is increased by a factor of k, the variance can be expected to increase by a factor of $k + k(k - 1)r_{XX'}$, in which case $S_{kx} = S_X[k + k(k - 1)r_{XX'}]^{1/2}$. The rate at which the standard deviation increases as the length is increased depends on the correlation between unit-length tests. At one limit, as the correlation approaches 0.00, the increase is proportional to $k^{1/2}$. At the other, as the correlation approaches 1.00, the increase is proportional to k.

Though covariances and correlations between tests have been applied here, average interim covariances and correlations could also be applied. The relationships developed between unit-length tests and longer tests also apply at the limit where the unit is a single item, and the k-length test is a test composed of k items.

What happens to the variance of true scores and to the variance of errors when the length of the test is doubled? Using Eqn. (8) and remembering that the correlation of true scores on alternate forms is 1.00, it can be seen that:

$$S_{(2t)}^2 = 2S_t^2 + 2r_{tt'}S_tS_{t'} = 4S_t^2$$

$$S_{(2t)} = 2S_t$$

To obtain the variance of errors, remembering that the correlation of errors on alternate forms is by definition 0, it follows that:

$$S_{(2e)}^2 = 2S_e^2 + 2r_{ee'}S_eS_{e'} = 2S_e^2$$

$$S_{(2e)} = S_e(2^{1/2})$$

In the general case of increasing test length by a factor k,

$$S_{kt}^2 = k^2S_t^2, \quad S_{kt} = kS_t$$

and $\qquad\qquad\qquad\qquad\qquad\qquad (9)$

$$S_{ke}^2 = kS_e^2, \quad S_{ke} = S_e(k)^{1/2}$$

Thus it can be seen that true-score variance increases as the square of change in test length, whereas error variance increases only as a linear function of test length, which accounts for the progressively greater reliability of a test as its length is increased.

A variety of interesting relationships can be derived when the sum of variables $X_1 + X_2 + \ldots + X_m$ is correlated with the sum of variables $Y_1 + Y_2 + \ldots + Y_n$. Consider first the case in which there is the same number of elements in each sum and in which all of both the X's and the Y's represent equivalent forms of the same test. Then, if the tests are in fact equivalent, all the covariances will be equal, except for sampling fluctuations, and the same will be true of all the variances. It can be shown that:

$$r_{(1 \text{ to } m)(1 \text{ to } m)} = \frac{m\bar{r}_{ii'}}{1 + (m-1)\bar{r}_{ii'}} \quad (10)$$

This is the general form of the Spearman–Brown Prophecy Formula to estimate the reliability of a test the length of which has been increased by a factor of m. When $m = 2$, then

$$r_{2X} = 2r_{XX'}/(1 + r_{XX'}) \quad (11)$$

This is the specific form for a double-length test. It is most frequently encountered in adjusting a split-half reliability coefficient obtained by correlating score on odd-numbered items with score on even-numbered items to estimate the reliability of the complete test.

When all the X's are to be considered equivalent forms of one test and all the Y's are equivalent forms of a different test, the correlation when one or both of the two tests are lengthened can be estimated. If both are lengthened, it can be shown that:

$$r_{(X_1 + \ldots + X_m)(Y_1 + \ldots + Y_n)}$$
$$= \frac{\bar{r}_{XY}}{(1/m + [\{m-1\}/m]\bar{r}_{XX'})^{1/2}(1/n + [\{n-1\}/n]\bar{r}_{YY'})^{1/2}} \quad (12)$$

For proofs of these relationships see Thorndike (1982).

This equation makes it possible to estimate what the effect would be on the correlation between any two variables, say a predictor test and some type of criterion measure, if more (or less) data were gathered for either or both. Suppose, for example, it had been found that the correlation between two forms of an aptitude test was 0.80, the correlation between two independently obtained supervisory ratings was 0.60, and the correlation of a single test with a single rating was 0.25. One might ask what the correlation would be between a test twice as long and the average of five ratings. As an estimate it would be found that:

$$r_{(2X)(5Y)} = \frac{0.25}{[1/2 + 1/2(0.80)]^{1/2}[1/5 + 4/5(0.6)]^{1/2}}$$
$$= 0.25/[(0.90)(0.68)]^{1/2} = 0.25/0.78 = 0.32$$

If one of the tests, say X, remains of unit length while the length of the other is changed, then:

$$r_{X(Y_i + \ldots + Y_n)} = \bar{r}_{XY}/(1/n + [\{n-1\}/n]\bar{r}_{YY'})^{1/2} \quad (13)$$

If the length of Y is now increased without limit, giving in effect the correlation between X and Y_t, the true score on Y, then:

$$r_{XY_x} = r_{XY_t} = r_{XY}/(r_{YY'})^{1/2} \quad (14)$$

If the length of both tests is allowed to increase without limit:

$$r_{X_xY_x} = r_{X_tY_t} = r_{XY}/[(r_{XX'})(r_{YY'})]^{1/2} \quad (15)$$

This is the general form of the correction for attenuation. It provides an estimate of the correlation between true scores on x and y, or measures that are of such a length that measurement errors are negligible. Taking the values from the previous illustration would give:

$$r_{XY} = 0.25/[(0.8)(0.6)]^{1/2} = 0.25/0.693 = 0.36$$

1.3 Problems in Defining True Score and Error

True score and error, of course, are not observables. Behavior samples are observed, and from these observations inferences about the constructs of "true score" and "error" are made. The inferences that can legitimately be made depend on the nature of the samples of behavior that are observed.

A universe of behavior samples for an individual has a dimension of content (items) as well as one of trials or occasions and possibly one of judges or appraisers. Variation in performance arises in part from the extent of variation in the specific content in terms of which the universe is assessed and in part from the context (time and appraiser) in which the performance is observed. The dimensions over which generalizations can be made depend on which dimensions have been allowed to vary. Any facet which is constant across all conditions of observation will appear as true score. For example, if different judges would evaluate a performance differently, but only one judge was used, scores will show a higher consistency than if judges had varied.

Content may be defined quite narrowly, as when all the words in a vocabulary test are drawn from a single area of knowledge such as biology, or broadly to cover the whole of a field. The universe may be defined solely in terms of content, or it may also be limited in terms of format—as when the measure of vocabulary consists only of words out of context presented in pairs, with the examinee to judge whether the members are synonyms or antonyms. As the definition of the universe is broadened, any single task or narrow sampling of tasks becomes less adequate to represent that universe. Thus, any estimate of reliability for a testing procedure appropriately refers to its precision as estimating some particular universe score, and it will depend as much on the definition of the universe as on the instrument.

2. Reliability Estimates and Variance Components

2.1 Error Variance

The classical definition of reliability (expressed in the notation of population parameters) was framed in terms of true score and error variance and took the form:

$$r_{XX'} = \sigma_t^2/\sigma_X^2 = \sigma_t^2/(\sigma_t^2 + \sigma_e^2)$$

What is included under the heading "error variance" depends on how the universe that the test score is presumed to represent is defined, with certain sources of variance being treated as error under one definition of the universe and as true score under another definition. In theory, at least, an ideal set of data and an ideal analysis would be those that allowed estimation of the magnitude of each possible component of variance, so that estimates could be made of the reliability of an instrument as representing universes defined in various ways, and so that the effectiveness of various alternative strategies for increasing the reliability of generalization to a particular universe score could be compared. If the different facets that are likely to be sources of variation in the resulting score have been identified, the theoretically ideal data-gathering and data-analysis design for getting information about the sources of error in an instrument or procedure would seem to be that of a completely crossed multidimensional analysis of variance.

A two-dimensional illustration is shown in Fig. 1. Suppose that each of N examinees has written answers to m test questions. Each answer has been evaluated by the same single reader. The $N \times m$ data matrix can be represented by the entries in the box. The border entries represent summations, where a subscript of a dot (.) indicates summation over the facet. In this matrix, each row represents a person and $X_{i.}$ is the sum over questions for person i, whereas each column represents a question and $X_{.j}$ represents the sum over all persons for question j.

The usual computations for analysis of variance (see, e.g., Winer et al. 1991) are:

Total sum of squares (SS_T) =
$$\sum_1^N \sum_1^m (X_{ij})^2 - (1/mN)(X_{..})^2$$

Persons sum of squares (SS_p) =
$$1/m \sum_1^N (X_{i.})^2 - (1/mN)(X_{..})^2$$

Questions sum of squares (SS_Q) =
$$1/N \sum_1^m (X_{.j})^2 - (1/mN)(X_{..})^2$$

Residual sum of squares (SS_{Res}) =
$$SS_T - SS_p - SS_Q \qquad (16)$$

and then

Persons mean square = $SS_p/(N-1)$ (17)
Questions mean square = $SS_Q/(m-1)$
Residual mean square = $SS_{Res}/[(N-1)(m-1)]$

A numerical illustration is shown in Table 1, in which each of a group of six examinees responded to the same set of four questions. All were evaluated by one examination reader.

The precision of the scores that result from a test composed of a set of m questions can now be investi-

Table 1
A numerical illustration of six examinees responding to a set of four questions

Examinees	Questions 1	2	3	4	Sum
1	9	6	6	2	23
2	9	5	4	0	18
3	8	9	5	8	30
4	7	6	5	4	22
5	7	3	2	3	15
6	10	8	7	7	32
Sum	50	37	29	24	140

$\Sigma(X_{ij})^2 = 972$ $\Sigma(X_i)^2 = 3486$
$\Sigma(X_j)^2 = 5286$ $(X_{..})^2 = 19{,}600$

    Total SS = $972 - 19{,}600/24 = 155.3$
Examinees SS = $3486/4 - 19{,}600/24 = 54.8$
Questions SS = $5286/6 - 19{,}600/24 = 64.3$
  Residual SS = $155.3 - 54.8 - 64.3 = 36.2$
Examinees MS = $54.8/5 = 10.96$
Questions MS = $64.3/3 = 21.43$
   Residual MS = $36.2/(3 \times 5) = 2.41$

X_{11} $\cdots$ X_{1j} $\cdots$ X_{1j}	$X_{1.}$
$\vdots$ $\vdots$ $\vdots$	$\vdots$
X_{i1} $\cdots$ X_{ij} $\cdots$ X_{im}	$X_{i.}$
$\vdots$ $\vdots$ $\vdots$	$\vdots$
X_{N1} $\cdots$ X_{Nj} $\cdots$ X_{Nm}	$X_{N.}$

$X_{.1}$ $\cdots$ $X_{.j}$ $\cdots$ $X_{.m}$ $X_{..}$

Figure 1
Two-dimensional matrix representing N examinees answering m questions

gated. Note that the only facet of the domain that can be studied is that of questions rated by the single rater. There is no evidence on the variability that would be introduced if the examinees were tested on different occasions or if the questions were rated by different judges. To obtain evidence on these facets, they would have to be systematically allowed to vary in the data-gathering and data-analysis design.

In this context, the usual situation is that all examinees respond to the same questions. When that is the case, "questions" becomes a fixed condition, does not vary, and consequently introduces no variance. Then the only source of error variance is the residual term: the interaction between persons and questions—that is the fact that each examinee does better on some questions and worse on others than would be expected in the light of that person's average performance and the difficulty of a given question for all examinees. The observed variance among persons includes both "true" between-persons variance and error, so it is necessary to subtract the error, to get an estimate of σ_t^2. Thus, σ_t^2 = Persons MS − Residual MS, and hence:

$$\text{Reliability} = \frac{\text{Persons } MS - \text{Residual } MS}{\text{Persons } MS} \quad (18)$$

In the illustrative example presented in Table 1, this becomes:

$$\text{Reliability} = \frac{1096 - 241}{1096} = 0.78$$

and the standard error of measurement is $(2.41)^{1/2}$ = 1.55.

The foregoing estimate applies to the total score; in this example the score is based on four questions. It is also possible to estimate the average error variance and the average reliability of a single element, in this illustration the response to a single question. The relationships are as follows:

$$\sigma_E^2 = \text{Residual } MS/m$$

$$\text{Reliability} = \frac{\text{Persons } MS - \text{Residual } MS}{\text{Persons } MS + (m - 1) \text{ Residual } MS} \quad (19)$$

For the example being considered, the values come out:

$$\sigma_E^2 = 2.41/4 = 0.60$$

$$\text{Reliability} = \frac{1096 - 241}{1096 + 3(241)} = 0.47$$

and the standard error of measurement equals $(0.60)^{1/2}$ = 0.77. Naturally, a score based on just a single question provides a much less accurate estimate of the universe score than one based on the pooling of a number of questions.

It is possible, of course, that questions are not uniform across examinees, and that it is not known which, from a pool of possible questions, a given examinee

is going to encounter. If that is so, and the questions vary from examinee to examinee, "questions" variance becomes part of error and must be so treated. There are then only two distinguishable components, examinees and residual, in which case:

$$\text{Total } SS = \Sigma\Sigma(X_{ij})^2 - (X_{..})^2/mN$$
$$\text{Persons } SS = 1/m \, \Sigma(X_{i.})^2 - (X_{..})^2/mN$$
$$\text{Residual } SS = \text{Total } SS - \text{Persons } SS$$
$$\text{Persons } MS = \text{Persons } SS/(N - 1)$$
$$\text{Residual } MS = \text{Residual } SS/[N(m - 1)]$$

Applying these relationships to the illustrative example considered here, gives

$$\text{Persons } SS = 54.8$$
$$\text{Residual } SS = 100.5$$
$$\text{Persons } MS = 54.8/5 = 10.96$$
$$\text{Residual } MS = 100.5/18 = 5.58$$

Reliability of total score = $(10.96 - 5.58)/10.96$ = 0.49

$$\text{Reliability of single item} = \frac{(1096 - 558)}{1096 + 3(558)} = 0.19$$

The reduction in reliability is quite dramatic in this example—and rightly so, because the questions obviously differed widely in their mean score for this group of examinees. If questions were allowed to vary among examinees, a substantial part of the differences among persons would be due to differences in question difficulty rather than differences in true score.

The approach to reliability through analysis of the facets of variance can be quite instructive, as the example brings out. It indicates in this case that a great deal of precision will be lost if different examinees are given different questions. However, for this conclusion to be dependable, it is important that the sample of questions be representative of the universe of admissible questions. Of course, if the estimate of examinee variance is to be meaningful, it is also important that the sample of examinees be representative of the population of examinees to which generalization is sought. Research workers in general and test-makers in particular are used to worrying about their sample of persons. However, if estimates are to be made about the size of effects from varying any other facet of the situation, equal attention must be devoted to sampling from the other facet. It may be desirable to have as large a sample from the facet of questions, or of raters, or of observation periods, as from the facet of persons.

2.2 The General Multifacet Model

In the illustration considered so far only one facet of the domain was varied—the facet represented by questions. Table 2 illustrates a two-facet problem. Suppose that each of the questions had also been read by a second reader and that this reader had assigned scores as shown on the right of the table. (The scores

Table 2
A two-facet problem representing six examinees responding to a set of four questions evaluated by two readers

Question: examinee	First reader				Second reader				Sum		
	1	2	3	4	1	2	3	4	First reader	Second reader	Both readers
1	9	6	6	2	8	2	8	1	23	19	42
2	9	5	4	0	7	5	9	5	18	26	44
3	8	9	5	8	10	6	9	10	30	35	65
4	7	6	5	4	9	8	9	4	22	30	52
5	7	3	2	3	7	4	5	1	15	17	32
6	10	8	7	7	7	7	10	9	32	33	65
Sum	50	37	29	24	48	32	50	30	140	160	300

Item sums for both readers 98 69 79 54

assigned by the first reader are repeated on the left.) The sums over questions and over questions and readers are shown at the right. The sums over examinees and over examinees and readers are shown at the foot of the table.

Table 2 presents the raw material for a three-way analysis of variance and allows the possibility of obtaining estimates of seven distinct components of variance. If the facet representing raters is designated k, the sums are as follows:

$$\sum_i \sum_j \sum_k (X_{ijk})^2 = 2{,}214 \text{ squares of single observations}$$

$$\sum_j \sum_k (X_{.jk})^2 = 12{,}014 \text{ squares of sums over persons}$$

$$\sum_i \sum_k (X_{i.k})^2 = 8{,}026 \text{ squares of sums over questions}$$

$$\sum_i \sum_j (X_{ij.})^2 = 4{,}258 \text{ squares of sums over readers}$$

$$\sum_j (X_{.j.})^2 = 23{,}522 \text{ squares of sums over both persons and readers}$$

$$\sum_k (X_{..k})^2 = 45{,}200 \text{ squares of sums over both persons and questions}$$

$$\sum_i (X_{i..})^2 = 15{,}878 \text{ squares of sums over both questions and readers}$$

$$(X_{...})^2 = 90{,}000 \text{ square of grand sum}$$

From these sums, the sum of squares associated with each component can be derived.

Total $SS = 2214 - 90{,}000/48 = 2214 - 1875.0 = 339.0$
Persons $SS = 15{,}878/8 - 1875.0 = 109.8$
Questions $SS = 23{,}522/12 - 1875.0 = 85.2$
Readers $SS = 45{,}200/24 - 1875.0 = 8.3$
$P \times Q = 4528/2 - 1875.0 - 109.8 - 85.2 = 59.0$
$P \times R = 8026/4 - 1875.0 - 109.8 - 8.3 = 13.4$
$Q \times R = 12{,}014/6 - 1875.0 - 85.2 - 8.3 = 33.8$
$P \times Q \times R = 339.0 - (109.8 + 85.2 + 8.3 + 59.0 + 13.4 + 33.8) = 29.5$

The seven mean squares can now be obtained by dividing the SS terms by their degrees of freedom, as shown in Table 3.

To estimate the seven variance components, it must be noted that each mean square at a given level already includes, within itself, variance represented in the higher levels of interaction. That is the persons-by-questions mean square includes a contribution from persons $\times$ questions $\times$ readers, and the persons mean square includes contributions from persons $\times$ questions and from persons $\times$ readers (each of which includes the three-way interaction). It must also be noted that the mean squares represent the values that attach to a sum of several observations. For example, the mean square for persons is a sum over four questions each read by two readers. If the variance component for a single observation is wanted, the given value must be divided by the number of observations on which it is based.

Taking these two points into account gives the following set of equations from which the variance components can be determined:

$$\sigma^2_{pqr} = MS_{pqr}$$

$$\sigma^2_{pq} = 1/n_r \, (MS_{pq} - MS_{pqr})$$

$$\sigma^2_{pr} = 1/n_q \, (MS_{pr} - MS_{pqr})$$

Table 3
Data matrix of mean squares for data in Table 2

Source	Sum of squares	Degrees of freedom	Mean square
Persons	109.8	5	21.96
Questions	85.2	3	28.40
Readers	8.3	1	8.30
$P \times Q$	59.0	15	3.93
$P \times R$	13.4	5	2.68
$Q \times R$	33.8	3	11.27
$P \times Q \times R$	29.5	15	1.97

$$\sigma^2_{qr} = 1/n_p \, (MS_{qr} - MS_{pqr})$$

$$\sigma^2_p = 1/n_q n_r \, (MS_p - MS_{pq} - MS_{pr} + MS_{pqr})$$

$$\sigma^2_q = 1/n_p n_r \, (MS_q - MS_{pq} - MS_{qr} + MS_{pqr})$$

$$\sigma^2_r = 1/n_p n_q \, (MS_r - MS_{pr} - MS_{qr} + MS_{pqr}) \quad (20)$$

Thus, σ^2_p is the average variance among persons for a single question scored by a single rater; σ^2_{qr} is the average interaction of questions with raters for a single person, and so forth. In this problem the values become:

$$\sigma^2_{pqr} = 1.97$$

$$\sigma^2_{pq} = 1/2 \, (3.93 - 1.97) = 0.98$$

$$\sigma^2_{pr} = 1/4 \, (2.68 - 1.97) = 0.18$$

$$\sigma^2_{qr} = 1/6 \, (11.27 - 1.97) = 1.55$$

$$\sigma^2_p = 1/8 \, (21.96 - 3.93 - 2.68 + 1.97) = 2.16$$

$$\sigma^2_q = 1/12 \, (28.40 - 3.93 - 11.27 + 1.97) = 1.26$$

$$\sigma^2_r = 1/24 \, (8.30 - 2.68 - 11.27 + 1.97) < 0$$

The values for the seven components of variance provide estimates of how important the various facets will be in producing variation in the estimates of a given examinee's ability. These values are worth examining with some care.

First, note that the estimate for readers is less than zero. Of course, variation less than zero is meaningless. What this value points out is that the values are estimates. Estimates may in some cases fall above the universe value and in some cases below. Furthermore, the estimates are often (and certainly in the data given in this example) based on a small number of degrees of freedom and are correspondingly unstable. There

were only two readers. It happened that these two were similar in the overall severity of their grading standards (though they differed rather markedly in their severity on specific questions), and given the interactions of readers with questions and with examinees, the residual contribution of readers per se is nil.

The result on readers points out the need, in studies of the importance of different variance components, to sample adequately from each of the facets—in this case examinees, questions, and readers. Practical realities often make it difficult to get as large or as well-designed a sample from such facets as test tasks, evaluators, and occasions as the sample of examinees, but the need is as great in the one case as in the other.

Returning to the list of variance components, it should be noted with satisfaction that the largest single component is that for persons (or examinees). This is the component that represents "true score" or "universe score" and is of primary interest in this assessment. The next largest component is that designated σ^2_{pqr}. This should more accurately be labeled $\sigma^2_{pqr} + \sigma^2_e$, because it incorporates both the second-order interaction of person $\times$ question $\times$ reader and the random "error" in its purest form. With only one observation in each $p \times q \times r$ cell of Table 3, it is impossible to separate these two elements. In most instances it will happen that at the highest level of interaction there will be only a single observation, so that "error" and this highest interaction will be confounded.

The next three components, in order of size, are question-by-reader interaction (1.55), questions (1.26), and person-by-question interaction (0.98). All these involve the sampling of questions, and collectively they indicate that the particular set of questions included in the test is a very potent determiner of the score that a given examinee will achieve. From the viewpoint of a strategy for accurate measurement, the size of these components indicates that it will be important (a) for all examinees to answer the same questions, and (b) for the number of questions to be large.

The importance of the different variance components can be seen more clearly if the "coefficient of reproducibility" (the ratio of expected true or universe score variance to expected observed variance) is calculated. Universe variance for a score that is the sum of observations on n_q questions, each rated by n_r readers, is given by:

$$\sigma^2_{\text{true}} = (n_q n_r)^2 \, \sigma^2_p$$

where σ^2_p is the estimate of the persons variance component. This follows from Eqn. 9, because to add questions and readers is in effect to increase the length of the behavior sample. The expected observed variance is given by:

$$\sigma^2_{\text{obs}} = (n_q n_r)(n_q n_r \sigma^2_p + n_q \sigma^2_r + n_r \sigma^2_q$$
$$+ n_q \sigma^2_{pr} + n_r \sigma^2_{pq} + \sigma^2_{qr} + \sigma^2_{pqr} \quad (21)$$

With appropriate divisions in both numerator and denominator, the coefficient of generalizability becomes:

$$\frac{\sigma^2_{\text{true}}}{\sigma^2_{\text{obs}}} = \frac{\sigma^2_p}{\sigma^2_p + \dfrac{\sigma^2_q}{n_q} + \dfrac{\sigma^2_r}{n_r} + \dfrac{\sigma^2_{pq}}{n_q} + \dfrac{\sigma^2_{pr}}{n_r} + \dfrac{\sigma^2_{qr}}{n_q n_r} + \dfrac{\sigma^2_{pqr}}{n_q n_r}} \quad (22)$$

Using the data derived from Table 3, this gives:

$$\frac{\sigma^2_{\text{true}}}{\sigma^2_{\text{obs}}} =$$

$$\frac{2.16}{2.16 + \dfrac{1.26}{4} + \dfrac{0}{2} + \dfrac{0.98}{4} + \dfrac{0.18}{2} + \dfrac{1.55}{8} + \dfrac{1.97}{8}}$$

$$r_{XX'} = 2.16/3.25 = 0.66$$

This coefficient is an estimate of the correlation that would be obtained between two sets of scores for a group of examinees, when each examinee is tested with a random set of four questions chosen independently for that examinee and rated by a random two readers also chosen independently for each examinee.

Looking only at the denominator, the source of most of the "error variance" becomes evident. Thus:

$$\sigma^2_{\text{obs}} =$$

$$\begin{array}{ccccccc} 2.16 + (0.32 & + 0 & + 0.24 & + 0.09 & + 0.19 & + 0.25) \\ p & q & r & pq & pr & qr & pqr \end{array}$$

The largest components of the error variance, in order of size, are questions (0.32); the interaction of

persons, questions, and readers (0.25); and the interaction of persons and questions (0.24). The strategy for reducing all these would be to increase the number of questions. This would increase the divisors in the largest terms of the denominator of Eqn. (22)—and hence would reduce those largest terms and increase the precision of the resulting score. If the number of questions were doubled, this would give

$$\sigma^2_{\text{obs}} = 2.16 + (0.16 + 0 + 0.12 + 0.09 + 0.10 + 0.12)$$
$$= 2.75$$
$$r_{XX'} = 2.16/2.75 = 0.79$$

By contrast, if the number of readers were doubled without any change in the number of questions, this would give:

$$\sigma^2_{\text{obs}} = 2.16 + (0.32 + 0 + 0.24 + 0.04 + 0.10 + 0.12)$$
$$= 2.98$$
$$r_{XX'} = 2.16/2.98 = 0.72$$

and the gain in precision would be a good deal less.

2.3 Nonrandom Questions and Readers

Up to this point, it has been assumed that both the questions facet and the readers facet have been sampled at random, such that a given examinee could have any four questions drawn from the universe of admissible questions rated by any two readers drawn from the universe of admissible readers. It is a good deal more common for the set of questions (and possibly the readers) to be the same for all examinees. If the set of questions will be uniform for all examinees, the variance component associated with questions (σ^2_q) disappears, which gives:

$$\sigma^2_{\text{obs}} = 2.16 +$$
$$(0 + 0.24 + 0.09 + 0.19 + 0.25) = 2.93$$
$$r_{XX'} = 2.16/2.93 = 0.74$$

Naturally enough, an estimate of a person's standing in the group is appreciably more precise when it is known that all members of the group will take the same test. If it is also known that the readers will be the same for all examinees, two other variance components (σ^2_r and σ^2_{qr}) drop out of the observed variance, leaving:

$$\sigma^2_{\text{obs}} = \sigma^2_p + \frac{\sigma^2_{pq}}{n_q} + \frac{\sigma^2_{pr}}{n_r} + \frac{\sigma^2_{pqr}}{n_q n_r}$$

For the data given this becomes:

$$\sigma^2_{\text{obs}} = 2.16 + (0.24 + 0.09 + 0.25) = 2.74$$
$$r_{XX'} = 2.16/2.74 = 0.79$$

Thus, in the example considered here, keeping the

questions and readers uniform for all examinees raises the true-score variance, as a percentage of the total, from 0.66 to 0.79.

It is also possible that there is interest only in a specific set of test questions, considering these to be the universe to which it is wished to generalize. The questions facet then becomes a fixed facet, rather than one that is sampled randomly from some larger universe. Considering a certain facet to be fixed has two effects: (a) the interaction between persons and that fixed facet, σ^2_{pq} in this illustration, is treated as a component of true score rather than error; and (b) the component associated with that fixed facet (σ^2_q) disappears. Thus

$$\sigma^2_{true} = \sigma^2_p + \sigma^2_{pq}/n_q$$

$$\sigma^2_{obs} = \sigma^2_p + \frac{\sigma^2_{pq}}{n_q} + \frac{\sigma^2_r}{n_r} + \frac{\sigma^2_{pr}}{n_r} + \frac{\sigma^2_{qr}}{n_q n_r} + \frac{\sigma^2_{pqr}}{n_q n_r}$$

$$\sigma^2_{true} = 2.16 + 0.24 = 2.40$$

$$\sigma^2_{obs} = 2.40 + (0 + 0.09 + 0.19 + 0.25) = 2.93$$

$$r_{XX'} = 2.40/2.93 = 0.82$$

If there were interest in generalizing only to this set of questions as appraised by these specific readers, this could be shown by:

$$\sigma^2_{true} = 2.16 + 0.24 + 0.09 \qquad = 2.49$$

$$\sigma^2_{obs} = 2.49 \qquad\qquad + 0.25 = 2.74$$

$$r_{XX'} = 2.49/2.74 = 0.91$$

2.4 Confounding of Variance Components

In all of these analyses, the situation has been one in which the design for collection of the original data was completely "crossed"—that is every examinee answered every question and every response was evaluated by every rater. Collection of the original data in this format has very real advantages in that it allows for the generation of estimates (though somewhat fragile ones because of small n's for some of the facets) of all the variance components. However, it may not always be possible to gather such data. Thus the readers might vary from one examinee to another

and it might not be known which reader had read a particular examinee's paper. It might only be known that two from a sizable universe of readers had read a given paper. In this case, the reader is said to be "nested within persons." When it is not known which readers have read a given examinee's paper, certain of the variance components become confounded and cannot be separated from one another. Specifically, reader variance (σ^2_r) cannot be separated from the interaction between reader and examinee (σ^2_{pr}), because information for a particular pair of readers can be identified only within the data for a single examinee. Similarly, σ^2_{qr} and σ^2_{pqr} cannot be separated. Thus the only identifiable variance components are, σ^2_p σ^2_q, σ^2_{pq} (σ^2_r, σ^2_{pr}) and (σ^2_{qr}, σ^2_{pqr}). Table 4 shows how the data for our illustrative problem would be analyzed. It should be noted that both the sum of squares and the degrees of freedom collapse for the two components that are confounded.

The analysis of variance components also reduces to just the five that can be isolated. Thus:

$$\sigma^2_{qr,pqr} = MS\,(Q \times R,\ P \times Q \times R)$$

$$\sigma^2_{pq} =$$

$$1/n_r\,[MS(P \times Q) - MS(Q \times R,\ P \times Q \times R)]$$

$$\sigma^2_{r,pr} =$$

$$1/n_q\,[MS(R,\ P \times R) - MS(Q \times R,\ P \times Q \times R)]$$

$$\sigma^2_q = 1/n_p n_r\,[MS(Q) - MS(P \times Q)] \qquad (23)$$

$$\sigma^2_p = 1/n_q n_r\,[MS(P) - MS(P \times Q) -$$

$$MS(R,\ P \times R) + MS(Q \times R,\ P \times Q \times R)]$$

For the data of the example shown in Table 4, this becomes:

$$\sigma^2_{qr,\,pqr} = 3.52$$

$$\sigma^2_{pq} = 1/2\,(3.93 - 3.52) = 0.20$$

$$\sigma^2_{r,\,qr} = 1/4\,(3.62 - 3.52) = 0.02$$

$$\sigma^2_q = 1/12\,(28.40 - 3.93) = 2.04$$

Table 4
Analysis of variance components when readers are nested within persons

Component	Sum of squares	Number of degrees of freedom	Mean square
P	109.8	5	21.96
Q	85.2	3	28.40
$(R, P \times R)$	8.3 + 13.4	6	3.62
$P \times Q$	59.0	15	3.93
$(Q \times R, P \times Q \times R)$	33.8 + 29.5	18	3.52

$$\sigma_p^2 = 1/8\ (21.96 - 3.93 - 3.62 + 3.52) = 2.24$$

The analyses of true score and observed variances parallel the development previously given, except that the confounding prevents the testing of some of the models. Thus, for generalization to a situation in which each examinee is tested with a random set of four questions drawn from the universe of admissible questions:

$$\sigma_{true}^2 = 2.24$$
$$\sigma_{obs}^2 = 2.24 + (2.04/4 + 0.02/2 + 0.20/4 + 3.52/8)$$
$$= 2.24 + (0.51 + 0.01 + 0.05 + 0.44) = 3.25$$
$$r_{XX'} = 2.24/3.25 = 0.69$$

If it were known that all examinees would have the same questions, then:

$$\sigma_{obs}^2 = 2.24 + (0.01 + 0.05 + 0.44) = 2.74$$
$$r_{XX'} = 2.24/2.74 = 0.82$$

If, however, there were interest only in generalizing to a universe of scores on these specific questions, then the following would apply:

$$\sigma_{true}^2 = 2.24 + 0.05 = 2.29$$
$$r_{XX'} = 2.29/2.74 = 0.84$$

The effects of uniform readers or a universe of only specified readers cannot be analyzed because the required variance components involving readers are confounded.

It is even conceivable that both questions and readers could be confounded with person (though it is unlikely that data would be gathered in this form). This would occur if all that was known was that, in the original analysis of the test, each examinee had taken some form of a test composed of four questions and that each person's paper had been read by some pair of readers. Confounding then becomes complete, and all that can be isolated are between-persons and within-persons components of variance, as shown in Table 5.

$$\sigma_p^2 = 1/n_q n_r\ [MS(p) - MS(\text{within})]$$
$$= 1/8\ (16.50) = 2.06$$
$$\sigma_{obs}^2 = 2.06 + 5.46/8 = 2.06 + 0.68 = 2.74$$
$$r_{XX'} = 2.06/2.74 = 0.74$$

The estimate indicates that, for a randomly chosen four-question test read by two randomly chosen readers, 74 percent of the variance is true-score or universe

variance of persons and the other 26 percent is contributed by the composite of all other components. No further analysis of the situation is possible. This value may be compared with the 66 percent found in Sect. 2.2, which results from the variance components of the completely crossed data. That the agreement is not better than this must be attributed to the small number of degrees of freedom underlying several of the specific variance components.

This two-facet illustration of the variance-components approach to analysis of reliability and the precision of measurement has been discussed in some detail, because it serves to exhibit both the logic and the empirical possibilities of the method. The same type of approach is possible with three or more varied facets, but the number of variance components approximately doubles each time a facet is added. In such multifacet studies, obtaining the full set of completely crossed data becomes quite an undertaking. Furthermore, obtaining samples of adequate size and of suitable randomness for each facet can present serious practical difficulties.

The variance-components model is one into which practically all the conventional procedures for gathering data on reliability can be fitted, and understanding any procedure is enhanced by seeing how it handles the several components of variance. The simplest procedure is to test each examinee with two forms of a test, giving everyone form A followed by form B—either immediately or at some later date. It has then been the usual procedure to compute the correlation between form A and form B. This is a single-facet problem, but the facet is a compound one that could be designated test-form-confounded-with-order. Thus there are three variance components: (a) persons, (b) test-form-and-order, and (c) the interaction of components (a) and (b). Component (b) shows up as a difference between mean scores on the two forms and does not influence the correlation, because product–moment correlations are based on deviations from the respective group means. Thus,

$$r_{AB} = \frac{\sigma_{persons}^2}{\sigma_{persons}^2 + [\sigma_{(persons \times forms)}^2]/2}$$

It is necessary to divide by 2 because the persons-by-forms component is based on two forms.

Coefficient alpha (α) (Cronbach 1951) and its spe-

Table 5
Analysis of completely confounded variance components

Component	Sum of squares	Number of degrees of freedom	Mean square
p	109.8	5	21.96
Within p	229.2	42	5.46

cial case, Kuder–Richardson Formula 20 (Kuder and Richardson 1937), are also single-facet approaches in which analysis is carried out at the item level. Thus, in the case under consideration there is: (a) a between-persons variance component, (b) a between-items component, and (c) an interaction-of-persons-with-items component. Once again, items are considered to be a fixed effect. The results from this analysis can be shown to be algebraically equivalent to coefficient alpha, computed by the equation:

$$\alpha = [n/(n - 1)] \, [1 - \sum_{i=1}^{n} S_i^2 / S_X^2] \qquad (24)$$

where S_i^2 is the variance of item i and S_X^2 is the variance of test X.

If a test is appreciably speeded and there are a number of students who do not have time to attempt a number of items then coefficient alpha tends to become meaningless because there are a number of empty cells in the persons-by-items data matrix. In effect, a value of zero is assigned to each of these empty cells, but it is done in the absence of data. The series of zeros for a given examinee produces a kind of spurious consistency in his or her scores on the later items and consequently inflates to some degree the estimate of the reliability coefficient.

3. Reliability with Conventional Data-collection Strategies

Carrying out a systematic analysis of variance components is the most instructive way to obtain a complete understanding of the sources of error in a measurement procedure. However, collecting the data for such a complete analysis is rarely practical and perhaps not really necessary. The circumstances of life usually do make it possible (a) to give two presumably equivalent forms of a test and study the correlation between the resulting two sets of scores, (b) to give the same test form on two separate occasions and study the correlation between the results from the two testings, or (c) to give a single test form consisting of several sections or a number of items and study the consistency of performance over the sections or items. Much of the evidence on test reliability stems from one or other of these procedures.

The foregoing procedures permit the allocation to error of only certain components of variance (see Thorndike 1951). Consequently, each provides a somewhat different and limited definition of the universe being sampled by the test. However, each offers some information about the generalizability from a testing procedure. Anastasi (1988) gives examples of how to estimate the effects of item and time variance from combinations of these approaches.

3.1 Reliability Estimated from Equivalent Forms

If two equivalent forms of a test are administered, the correlation between them serves as an estimate of the reliability coefficient (see Eqns. 2 and 3). The value obtained for this coefficient is critically dependent on the heterogeneity of the group to which the two forms are administered—that is on the size of σ_{true}^2. For this reason, an estimate of the error variance or of its square root, the standard error of measurement (Eqn. 4), is often a more serviceable statistic than the reliability coefficient. It is a good deal less sensitive to the range of talent in the sample on which the reliability estimate is based.

So far the error variance has been treated as though it kept the same value at all levels of the latent attribute. Of course, this is not necessarily the case. A test often measures more accurately within certain limits on the latent attribute than it does at other points; the location of higher accuracy depends on the way in which the items that compose the final test were chosen. For example, it is common for test producers to include more items of moderate than extreme difficulty on a test. This practice focuses the test's ability to make accurate discriminations near the center of the score range and results in the highest precision for the greatest number of examinees. Precision, as indicated by S_e, will suffer at the extremes of the distribution because each observation is, in effect, based on a smaller sample of behavior. The standard error of measurement, estimated from the correlation between two forms of a test, is a pooled overall estimate of precision, an estimate that is often better replaced by estimates at each of a number of different score levels. A procedure for obtaining those estimates is provided by Thorndike (1982).

3.2 Reliability Estimated from Retesting

As indicated above, an alternative data-gathering strategy is to use one specific measure of a latent attribute and to repeat the identical measure after an interval. This is a reasonable strategy if (a) all test exercises are so similar in content or function that any one sample of exercises is equivalent to any other, and (b) the exercises are sufficiently numerous or nondescript that, at the second testing, there will be little or no memory of the responses given on the initial testing. Specific memory will, of course, become a less serious problem as the interval between the two testings is lengthened. However, as the time interval is lengthened, the impact of intervening experiences or of differential growth rates on the variation from one testing to the other increases. The variation then becomes, in increasing proportion, an indicator of instability of the underlying attribute over time, rather than of lack of precision in the measuring instrument.

The standard error of measurement at each score level can appropriately be obtained from retesting with the identical test. It now provides information about the consistency with which persons at different ability levels respond to the test tasks. The difference in mean score between the first and second testing constitutes a variance component reflecting some mixture of practice effect and growth between the two testings. The two are not separable, but the relative importance of each can be inferred at least crudely from the length of the interval between testings.

3.3 Reliability Estimated from Internal Consistency

The third data-collecting strategy relies on the internal analysis of a single test administration. This has very great practical advantages because (a) it requires development of only a single form of the test, and (b) cooperation of examinees is required for only a single period of testing. These practical advantages have led test-makers and research workers to use procedures of internal analysis frequently, in spite of their fairly severe theoretical limitations. One limitation is, of course, that all testing is done within a single brief period, so no evidence can be obtained on changes in individual performance from one occasion to the next. Another limitation is that the estimates of reliability become more and more inflated as the test is speeded. This issue will be discussed further after the basic procedures have been set forth.

The early procedure for extracting reliability estimates from a single administration of a test form was to divide the test items into equivalent fractions, usually two equivalent halves, and obtain two separate scores —one for each fraction. The correlation between the two half-test scores was corrected by Eqn. 11 to give an estimate of the reliability coefficient for the full-length test.

When items are numerous and arranged either by subarea or in order of gradually increasing difficulty (or by increasing difficulty within subareas), putting alternate items into alternate test forms has often seemed a sound strategy for achieving equivalence: hence the odd–even correlations often reported. An investigator or test-maker must decide in each case whether this or some other procedure is the most reasonable way to define equivalent halves for the instrument she or he is studying.

Those extracting reliability estimates from a single test administration have tended increasingly to base the estimates on analysis of variance approaches, in which single items constitute the units on which the analysis is based. The analysis is built on the assumption that all items are measures of the same underlying attribute—that is that the test is homogeneous in content. For this reason, when a test score is based on items from two or more diverse content/process domains, it is usually necessary to apply the analysis to the items from each domain separately and then to use a formula for the correlation of sums to estimate the reliability of the total score. Analysis of variance procedures do not depend on any particular choice in subdividing the items, and they approximate an average of all the possible correlations that might have been obtained by different ways of assigning items to alternate forms. When the assumption of homogeneity

of function measured is justified, this would appear to be the most objective way to determine consistency across the items of the test (see *Measures of Variation*).

The most general form of the analysis of item variance is provided by Cronbach's coefficient alpha (Eqn. 24). This expression is quite general in its application. It will handle test exercises in which scores can take a range of values, as in essay tests or in inventories that provide multiple levels of response. It can even be applied when the "items" are themselves groups of test exercises.

When all n items are scored either 0 or 1, coefficient alpha reduces to the form reported earlier by Kuder and Richardson (1937) and known as "Kuder–Richardson Formula 20." It is:

$$KR_{20} = \left(\frac{n}{n-1}\right)\left(1 - \frac{\Sigma p_i q_i}{S_X^2}\right) \tag{25}$$

where p_i and q_i are the proportion of examinees passing and failing, respectively, item i. A lower-bound estimate of this value, which is exact if all items are of the same difficulty, is provided by Kuder-Richardson Formula 21, which takes the form:

$$KR_{21} = \left(\frac{n}{n-1}\right)\left(1 - \frac{\Sigma n\bar{p}\bar{q}}{S_X^2}\right)$$

where $\bar{p}$ is the mean percent of correct responses, and $\bar{q}$ the mean percent of incorrect responses. KR_{21} can also be expressed as:

$$KR_{21} = \left(\frac{n}{n-1}\right)\left(1 - \frac{\bar{X} - (\bar{X}^2)/n}{S_X^2}\right) \tag{26}$$

This formula provides a convenient way to get a quick, conservative estimate of coefficient alpha, because it requires information only on the mean, standard deviation, and number of items in the test. It differs from the full formula by the amount nS_p^2 / S_X^2 where S_p^2

is the variance of the item difficulty indices, p. For a test of 50 or more items, this element is likely to be no greater than 0.02 or 0.03. For example, if the items have a range of p-values from 0.30 to 0.90 with a standard deviation of 0.10, and the test's standard deviation is 6 points (a realistic figure) for a 50-item test, this gives:

$$\frac{50(010)^2}{6^2} = \frac{050}{36} = 0.014$$

Thus, with tests of a length commonly encountered in practice, Eqn. (26) provides a very serviceable approximation.

It was indicated earlier that coefficient alpha in its standard form is applicable only to homogeneous tests in which all items are designed to measure the same common latent attribute. When test items are not designed to be measures of a single homogeneous attribute, a test may often be divided into subtests each of which is designed to be homogeneous in what it measures. Then Eqns. (24), (25), or (26) can be applied to each subtest separately to estimate the reliability (in the internal-consistency sense) of the subtest. Thorndike (1982) illustrates how an index of total test reliability can be thus obtained.

4. Reliability of Domain Mastery or Criterion-referenced Tests

In discussing reliability up to this point, the main concern has been the precision with which an individual can be located on the scale of a latent attribute through the administration of a test. Within limits, this conception can still be applied to a domain mastery test. The adaptation that may be required is to think of the attribute as having a limited range, because the tasks that fall within a precisely defined domain may have a limited range of difficulty. Within that range, correlations may be attenuated because of the presence of substantial numbers of perfect (or zero) scores. Such scores indicate individuals who fall at the boundaries of the difficulty range of the domain and who are in a sense not fully measured. The presence of such scores acts to attenuate correlation coefficients by reducing test score variance. The location of these extreme cases on a continuous scale representing the domain is in a sense indeterminate, so it is difficult to estimate a meaningful standard error of measurement for them.

Within the domain mastery model, interest usually focuses on some one level of performance—often 80 or 90 percent correct answers—that has been defined as constituting "mastery" of the domain. When this is the case, the critical issue so far as reproducibility of results is concerned would appear to be whether another sample from the domain would lead to the same decision (mastery or nonmastery, as the case may be) for each individual.

The most direct approach to answering the question of consistency in the critical decision is to obtain two test scores for each individual by administering two equivalent test forms—equivalent in that each sampled by the same rules from the defined domain. The two could be given concurrently or with a lapse of time, depending on the nature of the universe to which generalization is sought. From the test results, a 2 × 2 table such as the one shown in Fig. 2 can be produced.

Figure 2 would present the basic data on consistency, but finding a statistic that adequately evaluates the test is not easy. The simple percentage of cases with consistent decisions depends on the range and level of talent in the group. In the extreme case, for example with a group for whom the domain is completely new and untaught (no-one approaches mastery), an appearance of a very accurate test is obtained, because all cases will fall in the upper left-hand cell. Of course, consistency of performance could also appear if the

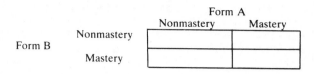

Figure 2
Structure of results from a domain mastery test

test were extremely easy for all members of the group. Furthermore, if the group were extremely varied in competence (including a number for whom the test was very hard, a number of others for whom it was very easy, and very few who were just about at the threshold of mastery), high consistency of placement would be the rule. In all of these cases, consistency in placement reflects properties of the groups tested rather than excellence of the test. Furthermore, in the intermediate range of excellence of examinees, both percentage of agreement and the point correlation represented in the phi coefficient are sensitive to the proportional split between the two groups.

If the two forms of the test have been equated for difficulty and if it is reasonable to assume that, within the domain as defined, competence shows a normal distribution, then it is possible to postulate a normal bivariate distribution of competence underlying the score distribution on the tests, and a tetrachoric correlation for the fourfold table can be appropriately calculated. This should be relatively independent of the average level of ability in the group tested, though it would be sensitive to the variability in the ability being studied and would be higher for a group that is more heterogeneous in ability. However, the tetrachoric correlation coefficient will not be sensitive to differences in the proportion achieving the criterion score level on form A and form B. If these differences appear to be due to something in the forms themselves, rather than to the sequence of testing, the tetrachoric correlation will yield an overestimate of the test's reliability.

Various measures that have been proposed for use with criterion-referenced tests depend in some way on the average of squared deviations of test scores from the established "mastery" level, developed as formulas analogous to those for error variance. However, these formulas are substantially (perhaps even primarily) dependent on level of competence within the group of examinees, and they reveal little about the properties of the test as a testing instrument. They seem to be going off in an unproductive direction.

If there is dissatisfaction with the conventional reliability coefficient when a test is being used for mastery decisions, perhaps the best alternative is the standard error of measurement for scores within a range of a few percentage points above and below the critical percentage that is defined as "mastery." This is one index that does not depend to any substantial degree on the range or level of talent within the group, but solely on consistency of performance from trial to trial. Though this statistic might be difficult to interpret in terms of proportion of cases receiving the same decision on two testings (that does depend on the nature of the group), the standard error would permit comparison of one test with another.

The procedures for calculating a standard error of measurement directly from score discrepancies are described in Thorndike (1982), and these procedures can be applied in the present case. The form that the results might take can be illustrated for a triad of tests (unfortunately not designed to be mastery tests) for which standard errors by score level happen to be available. Consider the Cognitive Ability Tests at Level A. Standard errors of measurement based on a sample of 500 and expressed as percentage of correct items were as follows for examinees with an average score of from approximately 70 to 90 percent of correct answers:

(a) verbal test—3.96 percent;

(b) quantitative test—3.99 percent;

(c) nonverbal test—3.15 percent.

Within the limits of the data, these results would be interpreted as showing that the verbal test and the quantitative test are quite comparable in the precision with which a judgment can be made that a person has achieved "mastery" of their domain, but that the nonverbal test permits this decision to be made with appreciably greater precision.

5. Special Issues in Reliability

5.1 Attenuation of Correlations Due to Unreliability

The effect on the correlation between measures of increasing the reliability of a test by increasing its length was described in Sect. 1.2. One of the implications of this development is that it makes clear there is no single correlation between two traits. Since all measures have less than perfect reliability and, by assumption, errors of measurement are uncorrelated either within or between tests, the observed correlation must be less than the correlation between true scores. This fact is known as "attenuation", and Eqn. (14) and (15) provide estimates of what the correlation between perfect measures of two traits would be, that is, the "disattenuated correlations."

Disattenuated correlations are useful for two purposes. First, they can be used to determine whether substantial gain in predictive validity is possible by making either the predictor or the criterion measure more reliable. If Eqn. (14) shows a substantial gain in the correlation between the observed predictor and a perfect criterion but not between a perfect predictor and an observed criterion, for example, then a gain in

predictive validity can be expected if the reliability of the criterion measure is improved, but little gain would accrue from improving the predictor.

The second major use of disattenuated correlations is to indicate the maximum correlation that could be expected between two variables, or, conversely, whether two variables are really distinct. If two tests correlate 0.70, and each has a reliability of 0.80, then $r_{tt} = 0.88$ and it can be asked whether it is scientifically useful to consider them to measure separate concepts.

In applying the correction for attenuation, the type of reliability estimate used is important. Lower reliabilities will occur when items are sampled (parallel forms) than when they are fixed (test–retest) and when times are sampled (delayed retest) rather than fixed (immediate retest or internal consistency). For a given level of correlation between the variables, lower reliability estimates will produce higher disattenuated correlations. Therefore, a reliability estimate that is appropriate to the use to be made of the test is important.

5.2 Reliability of Differences and Discrepancies

It is common practice for educators and clinicians to examine the pattern of scores from a multiscore test or battery and to interpret score differences as indicating areas of relative strength or weakness. This practice, while inviting, poses some serious problems. Referring to Eqn. (7) for the variance of sums, the variance of differences is $S^2_{(X + X')} = S^2_X - S^2_{X'} + 2r_{XX'}S_XS_{X'}$. Thus, if two tests are uncorrelated, the variance of their sum is equal to the variance of their difference, but if they are positively correlated the variance of the difference will be less than the variance of the sum by an amount proportional to the correlation between the two tests. This reduction in variance has important consequences for the reliability of the difference score defined as diff = $X-Y$. The reliability of such a score is

$$r_{\text{diff}} = \frac{1/2(r_{XX'} + r_{YY'}) - r_{XY}}{1 - r_{XY}} \qquad (27)$$

where $r_{XX'}$ and $r_{YY'}$ are the reliabilities of the two tests and r_{XY} is the observed correlation between the tests (see Thorndike 1997 pp. 111–14 for a discussion of this).

Closely related to the problem of difference scores is the problem of errors in prediction. Research on test bias, learning disabilities, and underachievement often depends on the discrepancy between a predicted score on some criterion and actual score on that variable to identify the individuals of interest. The standard error of estimate (see *Correlational Procedures in Data Analysis*) is given by $S_{Y.X} = S_Y (1 - r_{YX})^{1/2}$. It can be shown (see Thorndike 1963) that the reliability of the discrepancy between predicted and actual performance is given by

$$r_{\text{disc}} = \frac{r_{YY'} + r_{X^2Y}r_{XX'} - 2r_{XY}^2}{1 - r_{XY}^2} \qquad (28)$$

Combining Eqns. (27) and (28), the standard error of measurement of a discrepancy score is

$$S_{\text{disc}} = S_Y(1 + r_{XY}^2 - r_{YY'} - r_{XX'}r_{X^2Y})^{1/2}$$

Using the very reasonable values of $r_{XX'} = 0.90$, $r_{YY'} = 0.80$, and $r_{XY} = 0.50$, the reliability of discrepancy scores on Y would be 0.71, and S_{disc} would be $0.47S_Y$.

5.3 Clinical Reliability

One potential source of error variance in testing is examiner/scorer inconsistency. For machine-scored tests this source is limited to errors in test administration and should be essentially zero, but for essay tests, product ratings, and many of the assessments made in educational practice, the potential for errors arising from this source is very real. The reliability of a test score depends on the context in which that particular measurement was made, not on procedures used during standardization research. For example, a test publisher may base reliability estimates on test protocols that have been scored by two or more carefully trained raters who are also monitored for consistency, thus eliminating most scorer error. When the test is used in practice, the real or clinical reliability of the scores will be lower than that estimated in standardization to an unknown degree, because practitioners may not be as highly trained and certainly are not subject to the same level of scoring verification. Consequently, the standard error of measurement will be higher, and some clinical applications such as the analysis of subtest specificity will be based on inflated values.

There is no single value that represents the correct reliability of a test. The most appropriate value depends on how the test scores will be used. The design for data collection should allow for all the sources of error variation that will occur in the application of the test to be present in the reliability study. Only then can the test user know how much confidence to place in the test scores.

See also: Measurement in Educational Reasearch; Scaling Methods

References

Anastasi A 1988 *Psychological Testing*, 6th edn. Macmillan, New York

Cronbach L J 1951 Coefficient alpha and the internal structure of tests. *Psychometri.* 16: 297–334

Cronbach L J, Gleser G, Nanda H, Rajaratnam N 1972 *The Dependability of Behavioral Measurements: Theories of Generalizability for Scores and Profiles.* Wiley, New York.

Feldt L S, Brennan R L 1989 Reliability In: Linn R L (ed.) 1989 *Educational Measurement*, 3rd edn. Macmillan, New York

Kuder G F, Richardson M W 1937 The theory of the estimation of test reliability. *Psychometri.* 2: 151–60

Lindquist E F 1953 *Design and Analysis of Experiments in Psychology and Education.* Houghton Mifflin, Boston, Massachusetts

Thorndike R L 1951 Reliability In: Lindquist E F (ed.) 1951 *Educational Measurement.* American Council on Education, Washington, DC

Thorndike R L 1963 *The Concepts of Over- and Underachievement.* Teachers College, New York

Thorndike R L 1982 *Applied Psychometrics.* Houghton Mifflin, Boston, Massachusetts.

Thorndike R M 1997 *Measurement and Evaluation in Psychology and Education*, 6th edn. Macmillan, New York

Winer B J, Brown D R, Michels K M 1991 *Statistical Principles in Experimental Design*, 3rd edn. McGraw-Hill, New York

Scaling Methods

P. Dunn-Rankin and Shuqiang Zhang

Scaling refers to a group of statistical methods that measure the relationships among psychological objects by arranging them in one or more dimensions. It is concerned with objects about which people can manifest some attitude or perception. Usually the experimenter wishes to know the relationship among a set of objects; that is, how far apart they are and in what relative directions they may lie. As a visual metaphor, the configuration reveals the mental organization of psychological objects. This entry discusses several of the most useful scaling tasks and methods. The educational researcher should become aware of the extensive number and diversity of other scaling methods that exist by consulting the references.

1. Psychological Objects

Psychological objects can be tangible, such as chairs, stools and sofas, but they can also be non-physical, such as concepts, impressions, propositions, beliefs or tendencies. Psychological objects are most often presented as sentences or statements such as "There will

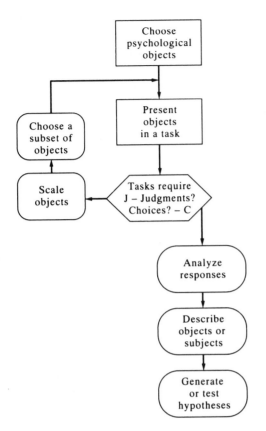

Figure 1
Diagrammatic representation of attitudinal measurement

always be wars" or "I hate war." With young children, the objects are often pictures.

2. Judgments or Choices

The two major responses that subjects can make to a set of psychological objects are (a) similarity judgments and (b) choices (preferences). The type of response is determined by the measurement objectives of a particular study or experiment. If a psychological scale is to be constructed, then the responses to the objects should initially be judgments of similarity. Once the scale values have been created the preferences of a group of subjects can be determined.

Figure 1 presents a diagrammatic outline for attitudinal measurement. First the psychological objects are chosen, dictated by the interests of the experimenter. Once the objects have been created or obtained they are presented in a task. If the task elicits judgment of similarities, the objects can be initially scaled. From such an analysis, a subset of them may be chosen

and formulated into a more sensitive scaling instrument. The revised instrument can then be presented to the target group(s). Should preferences instead of judgments be obtained, a direct descriptive analysis is made. Such analyses can generate or test hypotheses.

3. Tasks

The great variety of scaling methodologies, which were initiated in the 1960s, have been "tried out" for three decades. Educators and researchers find that a limited number of established tasks and analyses appear to be most functional. The tasks can be divided into four areas. These include: (a) ordinal tasks, (b) ordered category ratings, (c) similarity judgments, and (d) free clustering (see Table 1).

Differences in these primary tasks create differences in the direction and kind of analyses that can be performed on the resulting data. Generally, however, a similarity or dissimilarity matrix of some kind forms the interim data amenable to subsequent analysis. Similarities, sometimes expressed as correlations, show how closely one object resembles the other. Dissimilarities, typically expressed as Euclidian distances, are the opposite of similarities. The larger the distance between two objects, the less similar they are.

4. Ordinal Tasks (Ranking)

Ordinal tasks involve ranking psychological objects in some way to produce what Shepard et al. (1972) labeled "dominance data." Ranking can be accomplished directly or derived from pairing the objects and counting the votes for each pair. The votes are inversely related to a ranking and can be called "rank values." For example, three statements: (a) "Teacher gives you an A," (b) "Friends ask you to sit with them," and (c) "Be the first to finish your work," are paired in

Table 1
Tasks for assessing people's judgments or choices about psychological objects

Types of Tasks	Examples
Ordering	"Who or what is best, next best, etc.?"
Ordered Categories	"Onions," are they: Good—: —: —: —Bad
Similarity Judgments	"How similar are fish and chicken?"
Clustering	"Put the similar words together."

all possible ways as shown below:

* (a) Teacher gives you an A.
  (b) Friends ask you to sit with them.

* (a) Teacher gives you an A.
  (c) Be the first to finish your work.

* (b) Friends ask you to sit with them.
  (c) Be the first to finish your work.

In this example the (*) represents the vote for a particular statement in each of the pairs. By counting the votes for each statement (those with the *), one finds that (a) gets 2 votes, (b) 1 vote, and (c) no votes, and the rank order for these statements has been established.

4.1 Circular Triads

It is possible for the votes to be circular. That is, a subject may like (a) better than (b), (b) better than (c), but (c) better than (a). This results in circular trial and tied votes. The analysis of circular triads is an interesting sidelight to the mental organization of psychological objects through pairwise comparisons. Circulatory cannot be identified from the commonly adopted method of direct ranking, which does not allow subjects to reveal their inconsistencies. Therefore, data collected through direct ranking may oversimplify psychological reality. A Fortran program for circular triad analysis TRICIR is available from *Scaling Methods* by Dunn-Rankin (1983).

4.2 Balanced Incomplete Block Designs

When the number of objects becomes larger than 20 (20 objects involve $K(K-1)/2 = (20)(19)/2$ or 190 pairs) then the time needed for a subject to vote on all the pairs becomes increasingly tedious. Balanced incomplete block (BIB) designs then are useful alternatives to complete pairing (Cochran and Cox 1957). In BIB designs, small subsets of the objects or statements are ranked in such a way that all possible paired comparisons can be inferred (Gulliksen and Tucker 1961).

One of the simplest of the BIB designs involves seven groups of three objects. This design, sometimes called a "Youden Square," looks as follows:

a b d
b c e
c d f
d e g
e f a
f g b
g a c

The task is to rank order just three objects at a time. The objects are related to the letters in each block or "row" of the design. Suppose the objects were adjectives and a subject ranked the adjectives in each "row" as follows:

(a) powerful_3_   rich_1_   good-looking_2_
(b) rich_2_   honest_1_   generous_3_
(c) honest_1_   good-looking_3_   famous_2_
(d) good-looking_2_   generous_3_   intelligent_1_
(e) generous_2_   famous_1_   powerful_3_
(f) famous_2_   intelligent_1_   rich_3_
(g) intelligent_1_   powerful_3_   honest_2_

Then rank values are derived by establishing a matrix in which 1 is inserted if the column object (adjective) is judged or preferred over the row object.

	a	b	c	d	e	f	g
a		1	1	1			1
b			1			1	1
c							1
d	1	1				1	1
e	1	1	1			1	1
f		1					1
g				1	1		
votes	0	3	5	2	1	4	6

The votes can then be utilized as a profile of dominance or ordered data for a given subject. The following values are given to the seven adjectives derived from the example above: (g) intelligent = 6, (c) honest = 5, (f) famous = 4, (b) rich = 3, (d) good-looking = 2, (e) generous = 1, and (a) powerful = 0.

While this simple illustration can be analyzed by hand, a computer program is needed to convert the data for larger designs. BIB, a Fortran program that converts various BIB designs to rank values, is available from Dunn-Rankin (1983).

5. Ordered Category Ratings

"Ordered category" subsumes many of the most frequently utilized unidimensional scaling methodologies. An example is provided in Fig. 2. These measures are commonly referred to as "summated ratings," "Likert scales," or "successive categories." Such titles, however, refer to different assumptions and different analyses about the data derived from ordered categories rather than the task itself.

5.1 Likert Scales.

Likert (1932) suggested that statements (psychological objects) should be written so that people with different points of view will respond differently. He recommended that statements of similar content represent one single dimension and vary widely in emphasis. For example, the statements "I would recommend this course to a friend," and "This is the worst course I have ever taken" will evoke different responses but are generally evaluative in nature or dimensionality.

Most common in the behavioral and social sciences

For the following statements A = Agree, TA = Tend to Agree, TD = Tend to Disagree, and D = Disagree.

	A	TA	TD	D
1. I will be lucky to make a B in this class	:___:	___:	___:	___:
2. This class has a tough professor.	:___:	___:	___:	___:
3. This is the kind of class I like.	:___:	___:	___:	___:
4. I would not take this class if it wasn't required.	:___:	___:	___:	___:
5. The demands for this class will *not* be high.	:___:	___:	___:	___:

Figure 2
The general form for an ordered category task

are survey instruments of the type shown in Fig. 2. The arithmetic average of the integers 1 to J (where J = the number of categories) assigned to responses in the categories is often immediately utilized as the value of a variable. Such analyses assume that category widths are of equal value.

The immediate use of summed scores may conflict with Likert's recommendation for unidimensionality and a unit value for each category. Efforts should be made to judge the similarities among the statements to see if the statements are, in fact, unidimensional. Green's (1954) successive interval scaling can then be used to eliminate redundant or non-discriminating statements and accommodate unequal intervals. TSCALE, a Fortran program to accomplish Green's successive interval scaling, is available from Veldman (1967).

Because similarities are likely to be multidimensional in character, subsets of items representing latent traits, factors, or dimensions should be established. Subsets of items generally are more reliable and valid than single items, because a specific construct or domain is better represented by several items rather than just one.

5.2 The Semantic Differential Scale

The semantic differential scale (Osgood et al. 1957) is anchored by a pair of antonyms related to a central psychological object or concept. For example:

POETRY

valuable	_:_:_:_:_:_:_	worthless
good	_:_:_:_:_:_:_	bad
interesting	_:_:_:_:_:_:_	boring
easy	_:_:_:_:_:_:_	hard
light	_:_:_:_:_:_:_	heavy
simple	_:_:_:_:_:_:_	complex

In this case, a single object or concept is evaluated on a number of bipolar semantic dimensions consisting of ordered categories. This is contrasted with many objects or statements evaluated on a single set of ordered categories. It is the dimensional structure of the adjective pairs in the semantic differential scale that is utilized to define the concept. This is accomplished by using "sets" of bipolar adjectives. An analysis might reveal, for example, that "valuable," "good," and "interesting" all belong to the same set or factor whereas "easy," "light," and "simple" belong to another.

6. Free Clustering

Free clustering is valuable because the underlying structure of the objects is not predetermined. In this task, the psychological objects (usually words, statements, or concepts) are individually listed on slips of paper or cards. The subjects are asked to put objects they feel are similar into the same group (even a single object may be a group). The subjects can constitute as many or as few groups as they consider to be necessary.

On the back of each card is written a different number (consecutive integers from 1 to k for K objects used). When the groups have been formed a new set of numbers is assigned to each group. Each different object in a particular group then receives the same particular group number.

The basic data might look as follows:

	Letters						
Subjects	a	b	c	d	e	f	
A	1	2	1	2	1	3	
B	2	1	2	1	2	1	
C	1	3	2	3	1	2	Group numbers
D	1	1	2	1	1	3	
E	1	1	2	1	2	2	

The integers in the data matrix represent group numbers.

Table 2
Similarities between lowercase English letters

	Percent Overlap Matrix					
	a	b	c	d	e	f
a	—					
b	0.40	—				
c	0.40	0.00	—			
d	0.40	1.00	0.00	—		
e	0.80	0.20	0.60	0.20	—	
f	0.00	0.20	0.40	0.20	0.20	—

Table 3
Distances between judges

Judges					
1	—				
2	2	—			
3	3	5	—		
4	6	8	5	—	
5	6	8	5	6	—

By calculating the percent overlap between each pair of letters, a matrix of similarity can be determined for these six lowercase English letters (see Table 2). This is accomplished by finding the number of times any two letters are found with the same group numbers and then dividing this sum by the number of subjects. A quick perusal of the similarity matrix indicates that "b" and "d" are seen as most alike for these subjects.

It is also possible to analyze the distances or dissimilarity between the judges. The interjudge similarities for the English letter data are presented in Table 3. PEROVER and JUDGED, two expandable Fortran programs to compute interobject and interjudge similarities respectively using pairwise comparisons, are available from Dunn-Rankin (1983).

Free clustering can also be done by listing the objects in the same consecutive sets (perhaps ten or more). Judges are then asked to mark or circle those objects that they would group together for a particular reason and to indicate, next to the grouping, a reason for the judged similarity. The reasons are sought by the experimenter and are an important adjunct to the analysis. In this task, an object can appear in more than one group and overlapping clusters may result from the analysis of the similarity matrices. Table 4, for example, reveals the responses of one subject through the clustering of eleven words.

In this example, the subject regroups each column of

words and a percent overlap matrix can be constructed for a single subject or a group of subjects.

7. Similarity Judgments

Judgments can be determined initially by (a) creating category designations as degrees of judgment as opposed to degrees of preference, (b) by pairing the objects and asking for similarity judgments, or (c) by a free clustering used to create groups of similar statements.

For example, a survey might initially ask special education teachers to "judge" the severity of behaviors in an ordered category task that runs from (N) Normal to (VA) Very Abnormal. Or the behaviors could be paired and a measure of judged similarity assigned to each pair. Or, finally, the stated behaviors could be clustered into groups based on the judges' estimates of their similarity. Each of these methods results in a matrix of similarities which is then analyzed to determine its dimensional characteristics. Once this is accomplished, a reduced set of statements are reframed into a single scale or into subsets of statements calling for subjects' preferences or perceptions or both.

8. Analysis of Ordered Preferences

8.1 Variance Stable Rank Sum Scaling

For psychological objects that are ordered there are a limited number of analyses that can be applied. The data consist of a subject by object matrix of correlated ranks or rank values. Rank scaling (Dunn-Rankin and King 1969) in which the scale values are proportional to the rank sums is quickly and easily applied. For example, a group of second grade children were asked what they most preferred as a reward following a job well done; an "A" grade, a score of "100", a gold star ("GS"), or the word *Excellent* ("Ex"). For these children, the objects were formed into the six possible pairs as shown in Fig. 3.

The circled objects in Fig. 3 indicate the preferred choice in each pairing for subject 1. The figure also

Table 4
Clusters in similarity matrices[a]

<u>shallot</u>	shallot	shallot	shallot	<u>shallot</u>	shallot	shallot
fool	<u>fool</u>	fool	fool	fool	fool	fool
demon	demon	<u>demon</u>	demon	demon	demon	demon
<u>shallow</u>	shallow	shallow	shallow	shallow	shallow	<u>shallow</u>
I'll	I'll	I'll	<u>I'll</u>	I'll	I'll	I'll
lemon	lemon	<u>lemon</u>	lemon	lemon	lemon	lemon
<u>fellow</u>	<u>fellow</u>	fellow	fellow	fellow	fellow	fellow
leek	leek	leek	leek	<u>leek</u>	<u>leek</u>	leek
isle	isle	isle	<u>isle</u>	isle	isle	<u>isle</u>
look	look	look	look	look	<u>look</u>	look
aisle	aisle	aisle	<u>aisle</u>	aisle	aisle	aisle

a Underlined words by the same subject in each set represent separate groups or clusters

Reward pairings

(Circled object was preferred in each pairing)

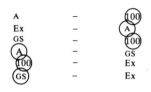

Sum of the choices

Ex	GS	A	100
0	1	2	3

Figure 3

Subject l's preference for the objects is shown and the rank values obtained by counting the choices for each object

shows the preference values for each subject by summing the votes for each object. Table 5 illustrates the rank values obtained for 24 subjects over the same objects. After obtaining the rank totals (R_j), the scale values are obtained (SV) by dividing each rank total by the maximum

rank possible and multiplying by 100. These values are presented in Table 5.

It is also possible to treat this problem as the Friedman two-way analysis of variance by ranks, which may entail various procedures for multiple comparisons among the scaled objects (Marascuilo and McSweeney 1977, Siegel and Castellan 1988, Wilcoxon and Wilcox 1964).

8.2 *MDPREF Analysis*

Multidimensional Preference Analysis (MDPREF) (Carroll and Chang 1970) can be accomplished through the MDS procedure in SAS (SAS Institute 1992). However, an earlier program MDPREF by Chang (1968) is much easier to use. MDPREF is an analysis of both subjects and objects. The subject (m) by object (n) matrix illustrated in Table 5, for example, can be decomposed into the product of an ($n \times g$) matrix = A and a ($g \times m$) matrix = B. A principal component analysis, the Eckart-Young decomposition (1936) performed on both matrices, attempts to capture the original data effectively. The objects are generally plotted in two dimensions with the subjects' preference vectors superimposed. The plot of objects reveals what common dimensions account for the different preferences

Table 5

Calculation of scale values (SV) from sum of the rank values

Subjects	Min	Ex	GS	A	100	Max
1	0	0	1	2	3	3
2	0	0	1	3	2	3
3	0	0	1	2	3	3
4	0	1	1	1	3	3
5	0	3	2	0	1	3
6	0	0	1	2	3	3
7	0	1	0	3	2	3
8	0	0	3	2	1	3
9	0	0	1	3	2	3
10	0	2	0	2	2	3
11	0	1	0	2	3	3
12	0	1	0	3	2	3
13	0	0	1	3	2	3
14	0	3	2	0	1	3
15	0	1	0	2	3	3
16	0	0	1	3	2	3
17	0	3	0	2	1	3
18	0	0	1	2	3	3
19	0	0	3	2	1	3
20	0	0	3	1	2	3
21	0	2	0	2	2	3
22	0	0	1	3	2	3
23	0	0	1	2	3	3
24	0	0	1	2	3	3
Sums (R_k)	0	18	25	49	52	72[$N(K$-l$)$]
SV ($100\ R_k/R_{max}$)	0	25	34.7	68.1	72.2	100

for the objects where as the preference rector of each subject shows how the person uses the identified dimensions to make choices.

Figure 4 provides an MDPREF analysis of the preference data shown in Table 5. The objects are plotted in two dimensions and the subjects are shown as preference vectors that have been fitted in the space of the objects in such a way as to best preserve the original scale values given by each subject (when the objects are projected perpendicularly onto the vectors). This analysis reveals that the choices between a "Gold Star" and "Excellent" are different for a few subjects while most of the subjects prefer "100" or an "A". Other preference directions are easily seen.

9. Analysis of Categorized Ratings

For categorized ratings, analyses are related to the average ratings for a specific group of judges or respondents. Most often Multidimensional Scaling (MDS), factor analysis, or clustering is employed to validate or establish the structure or dimensionality of the similarity or dissimilarity matrix of the objects or items.

The technique of "factor analysis," traditionally developed and used with tests of ability and achievement, has also been extensively applied to the reduction of similarity matrices of psychological objects.

The restrictive assumptions underlying factor analysis, e.g., normal distribution, linearity of relationship, and homogeneity of variance make the simpler assumptions underlying MDS attractive to researchers. Multidimensional scaling can also be employed to handle similarity matrices other than correlations such as matrices of Euclidian distances resulting from ranking or judging similarities of pairs and percent overlap matrices resulting from free clusterings.

9.1 Multidimensional Scaling

Multidimensional scaling is the name for a number of methods which attempt to represent spatially the distances within a set of stimuli. Most often similarity data are converted to Euclidian distances to determine a parsimonious spatial representation of the original data. This can be accomplished with only ordinal assumptions about the data.

Shepard and Kruskal's Nonmetric Monotonic MDS proceeds as follows:

(a) There is a given set of n objects.
(b) For every pair of objects (i and j) some measure of proximity is obtained. These measures are most often similarity data (Sij) such as correlations, associations, or judged similarities. When similarities are obtained, they are converted to theoretical distances ($\hat{d}_{ij}$) by subtracting from a constant.
(c) Several dimensions (t) are selected which may fit the data. As a first step, the n objects are randomly or selectively placed within the dimensional space selected.

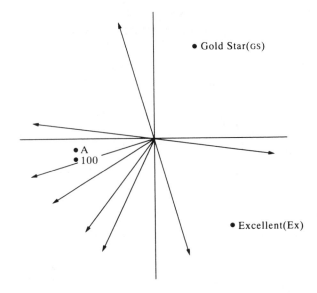

Figure 4

An MDPREF analysis of 24 students' responses to 4 reinforcers. The majority of the preference vectors point toward (A) and (100) and away from Gold Star (GS) and Excellent (Ex). Similar profiles lie on the same vector

(d) MDS searches for a replotting of the n objects so that the recalculated distances ($\hat{d}_{ij}$) are best related to the distances initially derived from the similarity data.

The process of arriving at the best spatial configuration to represent the original similarities has been presented effectively by Kruskal (1964). In this method, a resolution is made in steps (iterations). At each step, the objects are moved from their initial placement in the dimensional space and the physical distances between all pairs of objects are recalculated. The distances between pairs of objects in the new placement are ordered and then compared with the original theoretical distances between the same pairs of objects which have also been ordered. If the relationship is increasingly monotonic, that is, if the order of the new distances is similar to the order of the original distances, the objects continue to move in the same direction at the next step. If the relationship is not effectively monotonic, changes in direction or step length are made.

The object is to make the sum of the squared deviations between (d_{ij}) and ($\hat{d}_{ij}$) as small as possible. That is to make

$$\Sigma (d_{ij} - \hat{d}_{ij})^2$$

a minimum.

Kruskal averages the sum of squares of the differences by dividing by $\Sigma_{ij} d_{ij}^2$.

He then gets the formula back into the original linear units by taking the square root of this average. He calls this index "stress (S)." Kruskal uses numerical analysis (the

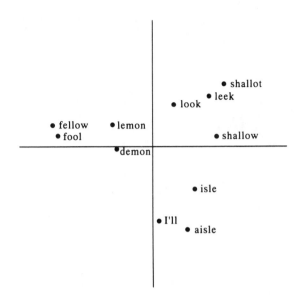

Figure 5
An MDS (KYST) analysis of a single subject's repeated clustering of 11 words. Phonetic, graphic, and semantic patterns are shown

method of steepest descent) to find the minimum stress. In general, the smaller the stress the better the fit.

The data of Table 4 (data for a single subject) was converted to a percent overlap matrix and analyzed using KYST (Kruskal-Young-Shepard-Torgerson MDS). The results are presented in Fig. 5. It is also possible to superimpose the results of cluster analysis (Aldenderfer and Blashfield 1991) on top of this configuration for an even better view of the data.

10. Analysis of Similarities

10.1 Individual Differences Scaling

The development of methodologies which relate differences between individuals to the dimensional aspects of the objects promises to have wide applications in the behavioral sciences. In factor analysis and MDS a parsimonious description of the objects is the primary purpose. In those methods, an "average" measure of similarity between pairs of objects is utilized as the primary data.

To measure individual differences, similarity or preference information between the objects must be obtained for each subject. Each subject responds to the same set of stimuli, for example, "color names" paired in all possible ways. Each subject has therefore a matrix of similarity representing all pairs of stimuli. LOMAT, a Fortran program that generates one similarity matrix for each subject based on similarity judgments of all possible pairs, is available from Dunn-Rankin (1983).

The most useful and popular representation of individual differences are the models of weighted Euclidean

space elucidated by Carroll and Chang (1970) (INDSCAL and MDPREF) and Young et al. (1976) (ALSCAL).

The INDSCAL (INdividual Differences SCALing) model assumes that different subjects perceive stimuli on a common set of dimensions. The authors assume that some dimensions may be more important for one individual than another. A color blind individual might weight the red–green dimension differently than subjects with normal vision. A weight of zero can occur for an individual who fails to use a dimension in making decisions of similarity, for example.

Individual Differences Scaling (for a detailed description, see Arabie et al. 1990) seeks to represent a large body of information in a more parsimonious way. The analysis seeks a small-dimensional solution for the objects and an individual weighting for each subject on these few (t) dimensions. Once a solution (a set of weights or loadings for each object and subject) is determined, calculated distances $(\hat{d}_{ij})$ between the objects are compared with the original distances (d_{ij}) between the objects provided by the proximity data. R squared (R^2) is used as a criterion in the comparison. INDSCAL or its improved alternative ALSCAL (Alternating Least Squares Scaling) (Young, Lewyckyj and Takane 1986) can be accomplished through the MDS procedure in SAS Version 6. But ALSCAL, existing in SAS Version 5 SUGI Supplementary Library, is easier to use. Another updated program SINDSCAL (Symmetric Individual Differences Scaling) is available from Bell Telephone Laboratories. Bell Telephone Laboratories can provide KYST, INDSCAL, MDPREF (along with PREFMAP), and about 20 other programs.

See also: Attitudes; Partial Credit Model; Rating Scale Analysis; Rating Scales; Factor Analysis

References

Aldenderfer M S, Blashfield R K 1991 *Cluster Analysis.* Sage, Newbury Park, California
Arabie P, Carroll J D, Desarbo W 1990 *Three-Way Scaling and Clustering.* Sage, Newbury Park, California
Carroll J D, Chang J-J 1970 Analysis of individual differences in multidimensional scaling via an n-way generalization of "Eckart–Young" decomposition. *Psychometrika* 35: 283–319
Chang J-J 1968 *Preference Mapping Program.* Bell Telephone Laboratories, Murray Hill, New Jersey
Cochran W G, Cox G M 1957 *Experimental Designs*, 2nd edn. Wiley, New York
Dunn-Rankin P 1983 *Scaling Methods.* Erlbaum, Hillsdale, New Jersey
Dunn-Rankin P, King F J 1969 Multiple comparisons in a simplified rank method of scaling. *Educ. Psychol. Meas.* 29: 315–29
Eckart C, Young G 1936 The approximation of one matrix by another of lower rank. *Psychometrika* 1: 211–18
Green B F 1954 Attitude measurement. In Lindsey G. (ed.) 1954 *Handbook of Social Psychology.* Addison–Wesley, Reading, Massachusetts
Gulliksen H, Tucker L R 1961 A general procedure for obtaining paired comparisons from multiple rank orders.

Psychometrika 26: 173–84

Kruskal J B 1964 Multidimensional scaling by optimizing goodness of fit to a nonmetric hypothesis. *Psychometrika* 29: 1–27

Likert R A 1932 A technique for the measurement of attitudes. *Arch. of Psy.* 140: 52–53

Marascuilo L A, McSweeny M 1977 *Nonparametric and Distribution-free Methods for the Social Sciences.* Brooks/Cole, Monterey, California

Osgood C E, Suci G J, Tannenbaum P H 1957 *The Measurement of Meaning.* University of Illinois Press, Urbana, Illinois

SAS Institute Inc. 1992 *SAS Technical Report P-222, Changes and Enhancements to Base SAS Software, Release 6.07.* SAS Institute Inc. Cary, North Carolina

Shepard R N, Romney A K, Nerlove S B (eds.) 1972 *Multi-dimensional Scaling: Theory and Applications in the Behavioral Sciences, Vol 1: Theory.* Seminars Press, New York

Siegel S, Castellan Jr N J 1988 *Nonparametric Statistics for the Behavioral Sciences*, 2nd edn. McGraw-Hill, New York

Veldman D J 1967 *Fortran Programming for the Behavioral Sciences.* Holt, Rinehart and Winston, New York

Wilcoxon F, Wilcox R A 1964 *Some Rapid Approximate Statistical Procedures.* Lederle, New York

Young F W, de Leeuw J, Takane Y 1976 Regression with qualitative and quantitative variables: An alternating least squares method with optimal scaling features. *Psychometrika* 41: 505–29

Young F W, Lewyckyj R, Takane Y 1986 The ALSCAL Procedure. In: *SUGI Supplementary Library User's Guide, Version 5.* SAS Institute, Cary, North Carolina

Standard Setting in Criterion-referenced Tests

R. K. Hambleton

One of the primary purposes of criterion-referenced tests is to make mastery decisions about examinees in relation to well-defined domains of content. This requires a standard or cutoff score on the test score scale to separate examinees into two performance categories, often labeled mastery and nonmastery. Sometimes multiple standards are set to separate examinees into more than two performance categories. For example, three standards may be set to separate examinees into four mastery categories: novice, apprentice, proficient, and advanced. For the purposes of this entry, discussion will center on setting one standard, though the extension to multiple standards on the same test score scale is straightforward.

All standard-setting methods in use in the early 1990s involve judgment and are arbitrary. Some researchers have argued that arbitrary standards are not defensible in education (Glass 1978). Popham (1978) countered with this response:

> Unable to avoid reliance on human judgment as the chief ingredient in standard-setting, some individuals have thrown up their hands in dismay and cast aside all efforts to set performance standards as arbitrary, hence unacceptable.
>
> But *Webster's Dictionary* offers us two definitions of arbitrary. The first of these is positive, describing arbitrary as an adjective reflecting choice or discretion, that is, "Determinable by a judge or tribunal." The second definition, pejorative in nature, describes arbitrary as an adjective denoting capriciousness, that is, "selected at random and without reason." In my estimate, when people start knocking the standard-setting game as arbitrary, they are clearly employing Webster's second, negatively loaded definition.
>
> But the first definition is more accurately reflective of

serious standard-setting efforts. They represent genuine attempts to do a good job in deciding what kinds of standards ought to be employed. That they are judgmental is inescapable. But to malign all judgmental operations as capricious is absurd. (Popham 1978 p. 168)

Many of the standards that are set by society to regulate behavior are set arbitrarily, but in the positive sense of the word. For example, fire, health, environmental, and highway safety standards are common and they are set arbitrarily. Professional judgment provides the basis for setting these standards. Criterion-referenced test standards are set arbitrarily too, but the process used in arriving at the standards is carefully planned and carried out by persons identified as suitable for setting the standards. Presumably sometimes standards are set too high or too low. Through experience and carefully designed validity studies of the test scores and decisions that are made, standards that are not "in line" can be identified and revised. The consequences of assigning: (a) a nonmaster to a mastery state (known as a false–positive error), or (b) a master to a nonmastery state (known as a false–negative error) on a credentialing examination, however, are considerably more serious than errors made on (say) a classroom test. Therefore, more attention should be given to the setting of standards on the more important testing programs.

Many of the available standard-setting methods have been described, compared, and critiqued in the measurement literature (Berk 1986, Glass 1978, Hambleton and Powell 1983, Shepard 1984). The methods can be organized into three categories: "judgmental," "empirical," and "combination." The judgmental methods require data from judges for setting standards, or require judgments to be made about the presence of variables (e.g., guessing) that influence the setting of a standard. Empirical methods are based on the analysis of actual criterion-referenced test results from two groups formed on the basis of a criterion variable. For example, the criterion variable would be a measure of success on a variable related to the contents of the criterion-referenced test. Also, empirical methods involve decision-theoretic concepts and procedures. Combination methods use both judgmental data and empirical data in the standard-setting process. Livingston and Zieky (1982) and Hambleton and Powell (1983) have developed guidelines for applying several of the methods.

Several of the popular judgmental, empirical, and combination methods are described next. Then some practical guidelines for setting standards are offered, along with a brief discussion of emerging trends and current research.

1. Judgmental Methods

With the judgmental methods, individual items are studied in order to judge how well a minimally competent examinee will perform on the test items. The minimally competent examinee is someone who has a proficiency score located right at the standard. Judges are asked to assess how or to what degree an examinee who could be described as minimally competent would perform on each item.

1.1 Nedelsky Method

With the Nedelsky (1954) method, judges are asked to identify distractors in multiple-choice test items that they feel the minimally competent student will be able to identify as incorrect. The assumption is then made that the minimally competent examinee would be indifferent to the remaining answer choices, and therefore he or she would choose one of the remaining choices at random. The minimum passing level for that item then becomes the reciprocal of the number of remaining answer choices. For example, suppose a judge reviews a test item and feels that a minimally competent examinee would recognize that two of the available five choices are incorrect. The expected score for the minimally competent examinee then is 0.33, since the assumption is made that all remaining choices (three remain) are equally plausible to the minimally competent examinee.

The judges proceed with each test item in a similar fashion, and, on completion of the judging process, each judge sums the minimum passing levels across the test items to obtain a standard. A judge's standard is the expected score on the test for the minimally competent examinee. Individual judges' standards are averaged to obtain a standard that is considered to be the best estimate of the standard.

Often a discussion of the judges' ratings will then take place, and judges have the opportunity to revise their ratings if they feel revisions are appropriate. And often judges do make revisions, since misreading of test items, overlooking of important features of test items, and even some carelessness in making the ratings are common in the item rating process. After judges provide a second set of ratings, again, each judge's item ratings are summed to obtain a standard on the test, and then the judges' standards are averaged to obtain a standard based upon the ratings of all of the judges.

The standard deviation of the judges' standards is often used as an indicator of the consensus among the judges (the lower the standard deviation, the more consensus there is among the judges on the placement of the standard). When the variability is large, confidence in the standard produced by the judges is lessened. Very often the goal in standard-setting is to achieve a consensus among the judges.

1.2 Ebel's Method

With the Ebel (1972) method, judges rate test items along two dimensions: relevance and difficulty. There are four levels of relevance in Ebel's method: essential, important, acceptable, and questionable. These levels of relevance are often edited or collapsed into two or three levels when the method is used in practice. Ebel used three levels of item difficulty: easy, medium, and hard. These levels of relevance and difficulty can be used to form a 4×3 grid for sorting the test items. The judges are asked to do two things:

(a) Locate each of the test items in the proper cell, based on their perceived relevance and difficulty.

(b) Assign a percentage to each cell representing the percentage of items in the cell that the minimally competent examinees should be able to answer.

The number of test items in each cell is multiplied by the percentage assigned by the judge, and the sum of these products, when divided by the total number of test items, yields the standard. As with all of the judgmental methods, the standards set by the individual judges are averaged to obtain a final standard.

1.3 Angoff's Method

When using Angoff's method (Angoff 1971), judges are asked to assign a probability to each test item directly, thus circumventing the analysis of a grid or the analysis of answer choices. Each probability is to be an estimate of the minimally competent examinee answering the test item correctly. Individual judges' assigned probabilities for items in the test can be summed to obtain a standard, and then the judges' standards can be averaged to obtain a final standard.

As with the other judgmental methods, it is common

practice to repeat the probability assignment process following discussions among the judges about their assigned probabilities. Sometimes, too, judges are provided with item statistics, or information which addresses the consequences (i.e., passing and failing rates) of various standards to aid them in the standard-setting process.

The method has been applied successfully to multiple-choice test items, and in a modified form to performance data. For example, suppose a standard for separating masters and nonmasters on a performance task is the goal. Judges, using a variation on the Angoff method, might be asked to specify the expected number of score points on the performance task (i.e., the standard) for the minimally competent examinee. Various standards from the judges can be averaged to obtain a final standard that would be used for classifying examinees as masters and nonmasters on the performance task.

2. Empirical Methods

Two of the typical methods in this category depend upon the availability of an outside criterion, performance measure, or true ability distribution. The test itself, and the possible standards, are observed in relation to these criterion scores. An "optimal" standard is then selected. For instance, Livingston's (1975) utility-based approach leads to the selection of a standard that optimizes a particular utility function. Livingston suggested the use of a set of linear or semilinear utility functions in viewing the effects of decision-making accuracy based upon a particular standard. A standard is selected to maximize the utility function.

A second method, by van der Linden and Mellenbergh (1977), leads to the selection of a standard that minimizes "expected losses." Scores from the criterion-referenced test of interest are used with an arbitrary standard to classify examinees into two categories: masters and nonmasters. Also, an external criterion, specified in advance, is used to dichotomize the examinee population into "successes" and "failures." Then an expected loss function (the quantity to be minimized) is specified. One simple possibility is the sum of false–positive and false–negative errors. A more interesting option is to weight the two types of errors by their importance. The standard on the test is then varied to find the one that minimizes expected losses over the sample of examinees. The standard that minimizes the chosen loss function is the one that is used with the test. Essentially, expected losses occur when examinees who score high on the external criterion (successes) fail the test, or when low-scoring examinees (failures) on the external criterion pass the test. The goal is to choose a standard to minimize the expected losses, which is accomplished by locating the standard on the test so that essentially the maximum

number of successful persons on the criterion pass the test and unsuccessful persons on the criterion fail the test.

Decision-oriented approaches, such as those developed by Livingston (1975), van der Linden and Mellenbergh (1977), and Hambleton and Novick (1973), are conceptually and technically appealing, but unfortunately the difficulty of obtaining criterion data, let alone suitable criterion data in most standard-setting studies, limits the applicability of the approaches. As a result, they are rarely used in practice.

3. Combination Methods

With these methods, judgments are made about the mastery status of a sample group of examinees from the population of interest. In a school context, these judgments would come from the teachers. The choice of combination method determines the nature of the required judgments. Next, one or more groups for whom mastery determinations have been made are administered the test. Details are offered next for analyzing the judgmental data and the test scores.

3.1 Borderline-group Method

This method requires that a definition be prepared of minimally acceptable performance in the content area being assessed. For example, here is the definition of the minimally proficient Grade 4 student in mathematics on the 1992 National Assessment of Educational Progress (NAEP) in the United States: fourth-grade students performing at the proficient level should consistently apply integrated procedural knowledge and conceptual understanding to problem-solving in the five NAEP content areas.

The judges (in practice, teachers who are familiar with the academic accomplishments of the examinees) are asked to submit a list of examinees whose performances would be so close to the standard or borderline that they could not be reliably classified as masters or nonmasters. The test is administered to this "borderline" group, and the median test score for the group may be taken as the standard. Alternatively, it may be decided to pass more or less than 50 percent of those examinees judged to be minimally competent examinees.

3.2 Contrasting Groups Method

Once judges have defined minimally acceptable performance in the domain of content of interest (or perhaps, they may be provided with a definition), the judges are asked to identify those examinees they are certain are either masters or nonmasters in relation to the domain of content of interest (Berk 1976). The test is administered to the two groups, and the score distributions for the two groups are compared. The point of intersection is often taken as the initial standard. An example is given in Fig. 1. The standard can be moved up to reduce the number of false–positive errors (examinees identified as masters by the test, but who were not in the masters group formed by the judges) or down to reduce the number of false–negative errors (examinees identified as nonmasters by the test, but who were in the masters group formed by the judges). The direction in which to move the standard will depend on the relative seriousness of the false–positive and false–negative errors. If the score distributions overlap completely, no mastery–nonmastery decisions can be made reliably. The ideal situation would be one in which the two distributions did not overlap at all. Then, the standard can be positioned between the two distributions, and the assignment of examinees to mastery states would be in complete agreement with the judges.

The validity of this approach to standard setting depends, in part, on the appropriateness of the judges' classifications of examinees. If the judges tend to err in their classifications by assigning examinees to the mastery group who do not belong, the result is that standards from the contrasting groups method are lower than they should be. On the other hand, the standards tend to be higher if judges err by assigning some masters to the nonmastery group who do not belong. Like the Angoff method, or modified Angoff method, the contrasting groups method can also be applied to performance assessment data.

4. Some Practical Guidelines for Setting Standards

A number of researchers have suggested guidelines to follow in setting standards (Hambleton and Powell 1983, Livingston and Zieky 1982). An updated list of guidelines for setting standards via judgmental methods is as follows:

(a) The importance of the resulting mastery–nonmastery decisions should impact substantially on the effort that is committed to the standard-setting process. With important tests, such as those used in awarding high school diplomas, and professional licenses and certificates, substantial effort should be committed to producing defensible standards and this effort would include compiling evidence to support the validity of the standards.

(b) The design of the standard-setting process should be influenced by the judges (and their backgrounds), test length, and test-item formats. For example, inexperienced judges may require substantial amounts of training, long tests may require that subgroups of judges be formed with each group assigned a different portion of the test, and some formats such as performance measures will require modifications to the common methods for setting standards.

(c) With important standard-setting initiatives, the full process should be field-tested prior to using it operationally. Serious errors can often be avoided with carefully conducted and evaluated field tests of the standard-setting process.

(d) The selection and number of judges should be given considerable attention. Can the judges represent the main constituencies, and are there enough judges to produce stable standards? The defensibility of the resulting standards depends very much on how this question is answered.

(e) The judges should take the test (or a part) under test-like conditions. This familiarity with the test and its administration will enhance the validity of the resulting standards. This reduces the common problem of judges underestimating the difficulty of the test and setting unreasonably high expectations for examinee performance.

(f) The judges should be thoroughly trained in the standard-setting process and be given practice exercises. The judges' understanding of the process is critical to their confidence in the process and the acceptability of the standards that are produced.

(g) It is desirable to provide an opportunity for judges to discuss their first set of ratings with each other prior to providing a final set of ratings. The second set of ratings will often be more informed and lead to more defensible standards because many sources of error due to misunderstandings, carelessness, inconsistencies, and mistakes can be removed. It has also become common to provide judges with item statistics and passing rates associated with different standards so that they have a meaningful frame of reference for providing their ratings.

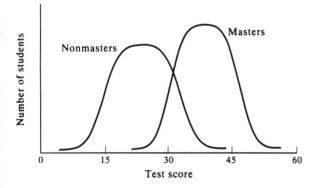

Figure 1
Contrasting groups method for standard setting

(h) The full process of standard-setting should be documented so that it is available if challenges to the standards arise. Every detail, from who selected the judges to the choice of method, and the resolution of differences among the judges should be documented for possible use later.

5. Emerging Trends and Research

Many researchers are still not comfortable with standard-setting methods in the 1990s. Criticisms center on both the logic of the methods and the ways in which the methods are being implemented. Clearly, there is a need for new ideas and more research. Both new methods and improved implementation of existing methods are needed. With respect to new methods, "policy-capturing" methods are now being developed for use with performance-based assessments (Hobson and Gibson 1983, Jaeger et al. 1993). The methods require judgments about the acceptability or nonacceptability of profiles of examinee scores across a number of performance tasks. These methods seemed to have potential with performance assessments, which are becoming popular, but the relative advantages and disadvantages of these new methods compared to modified Angoff methods are unknown. With respect to improved implementation, considerable attention is being focused on the implementation of the modified-Angoff method. Every aspect of it, from the initial definition of minimally competent examinees to the selection and training of judges, and the resolving of interjudge and intrajudge differences is being researched (Jaeger 1991, Mills et al. 1991)

6. Summary

The most controversial problem in criterion-referenced testing concerns setting standards on the test score scale to separate examinees into masters and nonmasters, or certifiable and noncertifiable. It is recognized by workers in the educational testing field that there are no true standards waiting to be discovered by well-designed psychometric research studies. Rather, setting standards is ultimately a judgmental process that is best done by appropriate individuals who: (a) are familiar with the test content and knowledgeable about the standard-setting method they will be expected to use; (b) have access to item performance and test score distribution data in the standard-setting process; and (c) understand the social and political context in which the tests will be used.

See also: Criterion-referenced Measurement

References

Angoff W H 1971 Scales, norms, and equivalent scores. In: Thorndike R L (ed.) 1971 *Educational Measurement*, 2nd edn. American Council on Education, Washington, DC

Berk R A 1976 Determination of optimal cutting scores in criterion-referenced measurement. *J. Exp. Educ.* 45: 4–9

Berk R A 1986 A consumer's guide to setting performance standards on criterion-referenced tests. *Rev. Educ. Res.* 56: 137–72

Ebel R L 1972 *Essentials of Educational Measurement.* Prentice-Hall, Englewood Cliffs, New Jersey

Glass G V 1978 Standards and criteria. *J. Educ. Meas.* 15: 277–90

Hambleton R K, Novick M R 1973 Toward an integration of theory and method for criterion-referenced tests. *J. Educ. Meas.* 10: 159–71

Hambleton R K, Powell S 1983 A framework for viewing the process of standard-setting. *Evaluation and the Health Professions* 6: 3–24

Hobson C J, Gibson F W 1983 Policy capturing as an approach to understanding and improving performance appraisal: A review of the literature. *Academy of Management Review* 8: 640–49

Jaeger R M 1991 Selection of judges for standard setting. *Educational Measurement: Issues and Practice* 10: 3–6, 10

Jaeger R M, Plake B S, Hambleton R K 1993 Integrating multidimensional performances and setting performance standards. Paper presented at the meeting of the American Educational Research Association, Atlanta, Georgia

Livingston S A 1975 *A Utility-based Approach to the Evaluation of Pass/Fail Testing Decision Procedures.* Report No. COPA-75-01, Center for Occupational and Professional Assessment, Educational Testing Service, Princeton, New Jersey

Livingston S A, Zieky M J 1982 *Passing Scores: A Manual for Setting Standards of Performance on Educational and Occupational Tests.* Educational Testing Service, Princeton, New Jersey

Mills C N, Melican G, Ahluwalia N T 1991 Defining minimal competence. *Educational Measurement: Issues and Practice* 10: 15–16, 22, 25–26

Nedelsky L 1954 Absolute grading standards for objective tests. *Educ. Psychol. Meas.* 14: 3–19

Popham W J 1978 *Criterion-referenced Measurement.* Prentice-Hall, Englewood Cliffs, New Jersey

Shepard L A 1984 Setting performance standards. In: Berk R A (ed.) 1984 *A Guide to Criterion-referenced Test Construction.* Johns Hopkins University Press, Baltimore, Maryland

van der Linden W J, Mellenbergh G J 1977 Optimal cutting scores using a linear loss function. *Appl. Psychol. Meas.* 2: 593–99

Taxonomies of Educational Objectives

V. De Landsheere

Originally, the term taxonomy (or systematics) was understood as the science of the classification laws of life forms. By extension, the word taxonomy means the science of classification in general and any specific classification respecting its rules, that is, the taxonomy of educational objectives.

A taxonomy related to the social sciences cannot have the rigor or the perfect branching structure of taxonomies in the natural sciences. In education, a taxonomy is a classification constructed according to one or several explicit principles.

The term "taxonomy of educational objectives" is closely associated with the name of B.S. Bloom. This is explained by the extraordinary worldwide impact of the *Taxonomy of Educational Objectives* first edited by Bloom in 1956. This taxonomy was enthusiastically received by teachers, educationists, and test developers because it offered easily understandable guidelines for systematic evaluation covering the whole range of cognitive processes (and not only the lower mental processes, as was too often the case in the past). This taxonomy had also a definite influence on curriculum development and teaching methods for the same reason: it emphasized processes rather than content matter, and helped determine a proper balance between lower and higher cognitive processes.

Bloom's Taxonomy of cognitive objectives was soon followed by taxonomies for the affective and psychomotor domains. Within two decades, several taxonomies were developed by other authors and a great number of philosophical and empirical studies appeared on this topic.

A presentation of the main taxonomies so far published follows.

1. The Cognitive Domain

1.1 Bloom's Taxonomy

This taxonomy, which has inspired the majority of the other taxonomies, uses four basic principles: (a) the major distinction should reflect the ways teachers state educational objectives (methodological principle); (b) the taxonomy should be consistent with our present understanding of psychological phenomena (psychological principle); (c) the taxonomy should be logically developed and internally consistent (logical principle); and (d) the hierarchy of objectives does not correspond to the hierarchy of values (objective principle).

The taxonomy itself comprises six cognitive levels:

(a) Knowledge: recall or recognition of specific elements in a subject area. The information possessed by the individual consists of specifics (terminology, facts), ways and means of dealing with specifics (conventions, trends, sequences, classifications, categories, criteria, universals), and abstractions in a field (principles, generalizations, theories, and structures).

(b) Comprehension:
  (i) Translation: the known concept or message is put in different words or changed from one kind of symbol to another.
  (ii) Interpretation: a student can go beyond recognizing the separate parts of a communication and see the interrelations among the parts.
  (iii) Extrapolation: the receiver of a communication is expected to go beyond the literal communication itself and make inferences about consequences or perceptibly extend the time dimensions, the sample, or the topic.

(c) Application: use of abstractions in particular and concrete situations. The abstractions may be in the form of general ideas, rules of procedure, or generalized methods. The abstractions may also be technical principles, ideas, and theories which must be remembered and applied.

(d) Analysis: breakdown of a communication into its constituent elements or parts such that the relative hierarchy of ideas is made clear and/or the relations between the ideas expressed are made explicit. One can analyze elements, relationships, organizational principles.

(e) Synthesis: the putting together of elements and parts so as to form a whole. This involves arranging and combining in such a way as to constitute a pattern of structure not clearly there before.

(f) Evaluation: evaluation is defined as the making of judgments about the value of ideas, works, solutions, methods, material, and so on. Judgments can be in terms of internal evidence (logical accuracy and consistency) or external criteria (comparison with standards, rules. . .).

The content validity of the taxonomy is not considered as perfect by any author but, in general they are satisfied with it: taken as a whole, it allows nearly all the cognitive objectives of education to be classified. Nevertheless, the taxonomical hierarchy is questionable and the category system is heterogeneous. De Corte (1973) has pointed out that the subcategories used are not always based on the same classification principle. He writes: "For knowledge, analysis and synthesis, the sub-categories correspond to a difficulty scale of products resulting from cognitive operations. For comprehension, the subdivisions are specifications of operations and not of their products. For evaluation, the subcategories depend on the nature of the criteria chosen to formulate a judgment."

Gagné (1964) has also pointed out that some categories or subcategories only differ in their content and not by formal characteristics which affect their conditions of learning.

According to Cox (De Corte 1973), the agreement on classification among the users of the taxonomy ranges from 0.63 to 0.85. The lack of reliability must come from the vagueness of the concepts for which the authors of the taxonomy propose essential rather than operational definitions.

The taxonomy has been elaborated for evaluation purposes. It has also been very useful in developing blueprints for curriculum development. It helped in identifying and formulating objectives, and, as a consequence, in structuring the material and specifying assessment procedures.

When developing a test for a particular curriculum, the curriculum often only presents a theme (Bacher 1973). No indication is given about which behaviors of the theme are to be tested. The test constructor is left to guess about which behaviors are to be tested. Furthermore, the taxonomy of objectives movement could signal a renaissance of nineteenth-century faculty psychology. Instead of training separate mental faculties such as memory, imagination, etc., one could artificially cultivate memory (knowledge in Bloom), application, analysis, synthesis, judgment, aptitudes.

Several authors are of the opinion that the taxonomy pays too much attention to knowledge, and not enough to higher mental processes.

It is not possible to use the taxonomy without reference to the behavioral background of the individual. There is an obvious difference between the individual who solves a specific problem for the first time and the individual who has met the same problem before. In both cases, however, the answer can be the same.

To test the validity of the hierarchical structure of the taxonomy, Madaus and his associates developed a quantitative causal model (see Fig. 1) to reveal not only the proportion of variance at each level explained directly by the preceding adjacent level, but also any proportion of variance explained indirectly by nonadjacent levels. The statistical techniques used were principle components analysis to identify the role of a factor of general ability g, and multiple regression analysis to measure the links between taxonomic levels. Hill (1984) has employed maximum likelihood estimation procedures, using LISREL, to list the hierarchical assumptions of the Bloom taxonomy, and has provided important evidence to support a hierarchical structure between the five higher-order categories.

In a pure hierarchy, there must be a direct link between adjacent levels and only between these two.

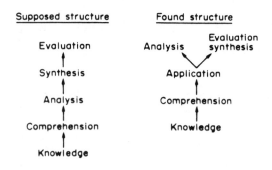

Figure 1

Schematic representation of an hypothesized perfect hierarchy and of the hierarchical structure found by Madaus et al. (1973)

As one proceeds from the lower to the higher levels in Bloom's taxonomy, the strength of the direct links between adjacent levels decreases and many links between nonadjacent levels appear. Knowledge, comprehension, and application are well-hierarchized. Higher up in the hierarchy, a branching takes place. On one side, analysis is found (even if the g factor is taken into account, analysis entertains an indirect link with comprehension). It is what Ebel (1973) calls the stage of content mastery. On the other side, synthesis and evaluation are found; they are differentiated clearly from the rest in that they are highly saturated in the g factor. This dependence increases if the material is not well-known to the students, or is very difficult, or if the lower processes have not been sufficiently mastered to contribute significantly to the production of higher level behaviors.

Horn (1972) suggested an algorithm to classify objectives along Bloom's taxonomy. He notes that in lower mental processes, objectives content and problem cannot be separated. For instance, for the objective: "The student will be able to list the parts of a plant", there is no problem. The answer will be possible only if the student has it "ready made" in his or her memory. For higher mental processes, the problem is general, and can be formulated without reference to a specific content.

To quasioperationalize Bloom's taxonomy, Horn takes the level of complexity of the problem posed as a classification criterion. At each level, he considers the formal aspect and content. Figure 2 presents Horn's algorithm.

Using Horn's algorithm, well-trained judges can reach a high interreliability in their classification of objectives.

Bloom's taxonomy is formulated in an abstract way. To help the users apply the taxonomy properly, Metfessel et al (1970) suggested a list of verbs and a list of objects which, appropriately combined, give the framework for an operational objective at the different taxonomic levels.

Bloom is aware of the limits of the instrument to

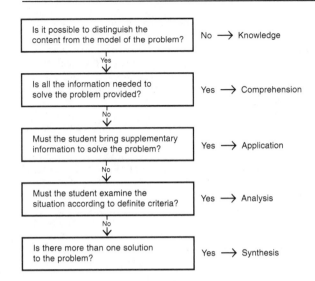

Figure 2
Horns algorithm

whose development he has contributed. What really matters to Bloom is that educators question as often as possible whether they have varied the cognitive level of the tasks, exercises, and examinations they propose, whether they stimulate their students sufficiently, and whether they really help them develop.

1.2 Guilford's Structure of Intellect Model

To organise intellectual factors, identified by factor analysis or simply hypothesized, Guildford (1967) designed a structure of intellect (SI) model (see Fig.3). This model was essentially conceived to serve the heuristic function of generating hypotheses regarding new factors of intelligence. The placement of any intellectual factor within this nonhierarchical model is

Figure 3
Guildford's Structure of Intellect Model

determined by its three unique properties: its operation, its content, and its product.

Content categories are:

(a) Figural: figural information covers visual, auditive, and kinesthesic sense.

(b) Symbolic: signs that can be used to stand for something else.

(c) Sematic: the verbal factor.

(d) Behavioral: behavioral content is defined as information, essentially nonverbal, involved in human interactions, where awareness or attention, perceptions, thoughts, desires, feelings, moods, emotions, intentions, and actions of other persons and of ourselves are important.

Operation categories are:

(a) Cognition: awareness, immediate discovery or rediscovery, or recognition of information in various forms; comprehension or understanding.

(b) Memory: retention or storage, with some degree of availability, of information in the same form in which it was committed to storage, and in connection with the same cues with which it was learned.

(c) Divergent production: the generation of information from given information where the emphasis is upon variety and quantity of output from the same source; this category is likely to involve transfer.

(d) Convergent production: the area of logical productions or at least the area of compelling inferences. The input information is sufficient to determine a unique answer.

(e) Evaluation: the process of comparing a product of information with known information according to logical criteria, and reaching a decision concerning criterion satisfaction.

Product categories are:

(a) Units: relatively segregated or circumscribed items of information having "thing" character.

(b) Classes: recognized sets of items grouped by virtue of their common properties.

(c) Relations: recognized connections between two items of information based upon variables or upon points of contact that apply to them.

(d) Systems; organized or structured aggregates of items of information, a complex of interrelated or interacting parts.

(e) Transformations: changes of various kinds, of existing or known information in its attributes, meaning, role, or use.

(f) Implications: expectancies, anticipations, and predictions, the fact that one item of information leads naturally to another.

Each cell of Guilford's model represents a factor that is a unique combination of operation, content, and product. For instance, cell 1 (see Fig. 3) represents cognition of figural units.

Can Guilford's model be utilized to formulate or at least to generate objectives? First of all, it can be noted that the three dimensions of the model are hierarchical at least to a certain extent. Furthermore, Guilford has discussed the implications of his model for education. He thinks that it indicates clearly the kinds of exercises that must be applied to develop intellectual abilities. He remarks, in particular, that school, in general, overemphasizes cognition and the memorization of semantic units. It is important, says Guilford, to apply oneself much more to the exercise of the other products: classes, relations, systems, transformations, and implications.

The fact that Guilford compares his model to Bloom's taxonomy and acknowledges important similarities between both of them seems to confirm that Guilford does not exclude the possibility that his model may be used to generate and classify objectives.

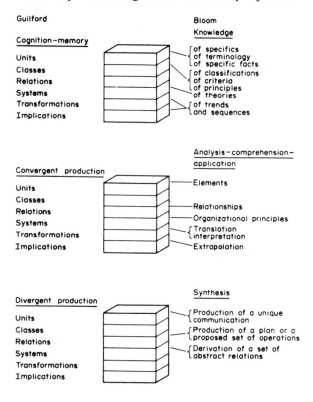

Figure 4
Parallelism between Guilford's model and Bloom's cognitive taxonomy

Guilford's model can absorb Bloom's whole cognitive taxonomy (see Fig. 4). By its greater precision, the SI model may allow easier operationalization and, more generally, may offer greater taxonomic possibilities.

De Corte (1973) has adapted and transformed Guilford's model. The four dimensions of De Corte's general model of classification are: (a) the subject matter of specific content of a given universe of objectives; (b) the domain of information to which the subject matter belongs (content in Guilford's model); (c) the produce: the objectives are classified with respect to the formal aspect of the information they produce (products in Guilford's model); (d) the operation is defined as in Guilford's model.

De Corte focuses on this fourth category and develops Guilford's five operations into a seven category system. Cognition comprises receiving-reproducing operations: (a) perception of information; (b) recall of information; (c) reproduction of information and productive operations; (d) interpretative production of information; (e) convergent production of information; (f) evaluative production of information; (g) divergent production of information.

De Corte's system is of interest in that it develops Guilford's model in such a manner that it becomes a practical tool for the definition of the cognitive objectives of education. It seems to indicate how Bloom and Guilford's contributions could be integrated and be of use to education.

1.3 The Gagné-Merrill Taxonomy

Gagné proposes a hierarchy of processes needed to achieve the learning tasks assigned by objectives. Merrill designates the behavior and psychological condition under which learning can be observed.

With Gagné's learning conditions, the push-down principle constitutes the basis of the Gagné-Merrill taxonomy. In the process of development, a person acquires behavior at the lower levels before acquiring behavior at the higher levels. Later, the conscious cognitive demand on the learner increases. Learners have an innate tendency to reduce the cognitive load as much as possible; consequently, a learner will attempt to perform a given response at the lowest possible level. The push-down principle states that a behavior acquired at one level will be pushed down to a lower level as soon as conditions have changed sufficiently so that the learner is able to respond to the stimulus using lower level behavior. It is rather surprising that this important principle is often neglected or even ignored in the literature related to the taxonomies of educational objectives.

The Gagné-Merrill taxonomy is an original formulation integrating the affective, psychomotor, and cognitive domains.

The following is a condensed version of Merrill's presentation:

(a) *Emotional behavior (signal learning)*. In the

presence of every stimulus situation, students involuntarily react with physiological changes which they perceive as feelings. The direction (positive or negative) and the relative magnitude of this emotional behavior can be inferred by observing the students' approach/avoidance responses in unrestrained choice situations.

(b) *Psychomotor behavior.* A student is able to execute rapidly, without external prompting, a specified neuromuscular reaction in the presence of a specific stimulus situation. The observable behavior is an overt skeletal-muscular response which occurs in entirety without hesitation. Psychological conditions of importance are the presence of a specific cue and the absence of prompts. Psychomotor behavior may be further broken down into three constituent behaviors.

First, topographic behavior (stimulus response) is where a student is able to execute rapidly without external prompting, a single new neuromuscular reaction in the presence of a particular stimulus cue. This can be observed as a muscular movement or combination of movements not previously in the student's repertoire. The important psychological conditions are the presence of a specific cue and the absence of prompts.

Secondly, chaining behavior where a student is able to execute, without external prompting, a coordinated series of reactions which occur in rapid succession in the presence of a particular stimulus cue, is observed as a series of responses, and occurs in the presence of a specified cue and in the absence of prompts.

Thirdly, skilled behavior is where a student is able to execute sequentially, without external prompting, complex combinations of coordinated psychomotor chains, each initiated in the presence of a particular cue when a large set of such cues are presented. In some skills, cue presentation is externally paced while in other skills cue presentation is self-paced. This is seen as a set of coordinated chains, and occurs when there is a paced or unpaced presentation of a set of cues and an absence of prompts prior to or during the performance.

(c) *Memorization behavior.* A student immediately reproduces or recognizes, without prompting, a specific symbolic response when presented with a specific stimulus situation. The observable behavior always involves either reproduction or recognition of a symbolic response, and occurs under psychological conditions similar to those of psychomotor behavior. Memorization behavior can be broken into naming behavior where a student reproduces or recognizes, without prompts, a single symbolic response in the presence of a particular stimulus cue; serial memorization behavior (verbal association) which occurs in the presence of a particular stimulus cue, so that a student reproduces, without prompting, a series of symbolic responses in a prespecified sequence; and discrete element memorization behavior (multiple discrimination) where a student reproduces or recognizes, without

prompting, a unique symbolic response to each of a set of stimulus cues.

(d) *Complex cognitive behavior.* The student makes an appropriate response to a previously unencountered instance of some class of stimulus objects, events, or situations. This can further be broken into classification behavior, analysis behavior, and problem-solving behavior.

Classification behavior (concept learning) is where a student is able to identify correctly the class membership of a previously unencountered object or event, or a previously unencountered representation of some object or event. It occurs when the student must make some kind of class identification, the important psychological conditions being the presentation of unencountered instances or non-instances.

Analysis behavior (principle learning) is when a student is able to show the relationship between the component concepts of an unencountered situation in which a given principle is specified as relevant. The student must first identify the instances of the several classes involved in the situation and then show the relationship between these classes. The psychological condition of importance is presentation of a situation which the student has not previously analyzed or seen analyzed.

Problem-solving behavior is when a student is able to select relevant principles and sequence them into an unencountered problem situation for which the relevant principles are not specified. Creativity and/or divergent thinking occurs when some of the relevant principles are unknown to the student and the strategy developed represents a new higher order principle. It can be observed when the student must synthesize a product which results from analyzing several principles in some appropriate sequence and generalize new relationships not previously learned or analyzed. The psychological conditions of importance are: an unencountered problem for which the relevant principles are not specified, and which in some cases may require principles not previously analyzed by the student or perhaps even by the instructor.

Without any doubt, Gagné-Merrill's taxonomy provides some order in the field of fundamental learning processes. However, it does not claim exhaustivity, and certain categories such as "process learning" and "problem solving" are rather vague.

D'Hainaut (1970) believes that Gagné does not give enough emphasis to the creative processes. Divergent thinking can be categorized under the heading "problem solving", but this category is perhaps too large.

Merrill and Gagné have made two important contributions to the definition of objectives. Their categories are expressed in terms of definite behavior and the psychological conditions are considered, although these conditions are still to be integrated into an operational definition of objectives.

1.4 Gerlach and Sullivan's Taxonomy

Sullivan in association with Gerlach (1967) attempted to replace a description of mental processes in general terms (as in Bloom's taxonomy) by classes of observable learner behaviors which could be used in task description and analysis. Their model is empirical. After listing hundreds of learning behaviors, Sullivan has progressively grouped them into six categories, each headed by a typical verb. The six categories are ordered according to the increasing complexity of behaviors they represent, but the whole does not constitute a rigorous hierarchy and, for that reason, cannot be considered as a true taxonomy.

(a) Identify: the learner indicates membership or non membership of specified objects or events in a class when the name of the class is given.

(b) Name: the learner supplies the correct verbal label (in speech or writing) for a referent or set of referents when the name of the referent is not given.

(c) Describe: the learner reports the necessary categories of object properties, events, event properties, and/or relationships relevant to a designated referent.

(d) Construct: the learner produces a product which meets specifications given either in class or in the test item itself.

(e) Order: the learner arranges two or more referents in a specified order.

(f) Demonstrate: the learner performs the behaviors essential to the accomplishment of a designated task according to pre-established or given specifications.

Gerlach and Sullivan consider their "taxonomy" as a check list helping to ensure that no important behavior is forgotten when planning school activities. This may succeed, as long as "mastery objectives" (i.e. objectives concerning a fully defined behavior universe) are kept in sight. However, the six categories suggested do not cover creative productions and do not even make a clear place for transfer.

1.5 De Block's Taxonomy

De Block (1975) suggests a model of teaching objectives (see Fig. 5). He thinks that teaching pursues objectives in three directions: (a) from partial to more integral learning. Comprehension seems more desirable than rote learning (knowledge); in this perspective, mastery and integration are final objectives; (b) from limited to fundamental learning. Facts gradually become background data; concepts and methods come to the fore; (c) from special to general learning. The objective is thinking in a productive rather than in a reproductive way, taking initiatives, and being able to adapt oneself to a great variety of situations.

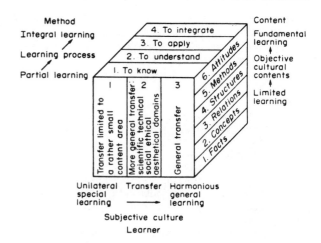

Figure 5
De Block's model of instruction

The combination of all subcategories yields 72 classes of objectives. De Block's system does not deal sufficiently with the criteria by which it is recognized whether an objective has been achieved or not. However, it can certainly help teachers to reconsider their activities, and to make their students work at higher cognitive or affective levels.

1.6 Conclusion to the Cognitive Domain

Not one of these taxonomies can be considered as entirely satisfying. Looking at highly nuanced classifications, only moderate reliability can be hoped for. If the system is reduced to a few operationalized categories, content validity decreases.

The taxonomy of Bloom and his associates has already been used successfully by hundreds of curriculum and test developers throughout the world. Furthermore, it has stimulated fruitful discussion and reflection on the problem of objectives. The several taxonomies that appeared after Bloom are useful to curriculum developers, to test constructors, and to teachers planning their next lesson and preparing mastery tests for their pupils.

2. The Affective Domain

According to Bloom, the affective domain includes objectives which describe changes in interest, attitudes, and values, and the development of appreciations and adequate adjustment.

What are the main difficulties in the pursuit of affective objectives? Imprecision of concepts, overlap of the affective and the cognitive domains, cultural bias (Western culture still tends to consider feelings as the most secret part of personality), ignorance about affective learning processes, and poor evaluation instruments.

So far, the only significant taxonomy for the affective domain is the one published by Krathwohl et al. (1964), hence the brevity of this section when compared to the first.

2.1 *Krathwohl's Taxonomy*

The main organizing principles for the cognitive domain were "from simple to complex" and "from concrete to abstract". It soon appeared that these could not be used for the affective domain which dealt with attitudes, interests, values, and so on. After a long search, the authors discovered an ordering principle that was precisely characteristic of affective development: the degree of internalization, that is, the degree of incorporation of the affects within the personality. When the process of internalization is completed, the person feels as if the interests, values, attitudes, etc. were his or her own and lives by them. In Krathwohl's taxonomic terms, the continuum goes from merely being aware that a given phenomenon exists, and giving it a minimum attention, to its becoming one's basic outlook on life. The main organizing principles in Krathwohl's taxonomy are receiving, responding, valuing, organization, and characteristics.

(a)   Receiving: "Sensitivity to the existence of certain phenomena and stimuli, that is, the willingness to receive or attend to them." Receiving consists of three subcategories that represent a continuum: (i) awareness; (ii) willingness to receive; and (iii) controlled or selected attention.

(b)   Responding: "Behavior which goes beyond merely attending to the phenomena; it implies active attending, doing something with or about the phenomena, and not merely perceiving them." Subcategories of responding are: (i) acquiescence in responding; (ii) willingness to respond; and (iii) satisfaction in response.

(c)   Valuing: "It implies perceiving phenomena as having worth and consequently revealing consistency in behaviour related to these phenomena." The individual is motivated to behave in the line of definite values. Subcategories: (i) acceptance of a value; (ii) preference for a value; and (iii) commitment.

(d)   Organization: "For situations where more than one value is relevant, the necessity arises for (i) the organization of the values into a system; (ii) the determination of the interrelationships among them; and (iii) the establishment of the dominant and pervasive one." Subcategories are: (i) conceptualization of a value and (ii) organization of a value system.

(e)   Characteristics by a value or value complex: "The values already have a place in the individual's value hierarchy, are organized into some kind of internally consistent system, have controlled the behaviour of the individual for a sufficient time that he has adapted to behaving in this way."

Subcategories are: (i) generalized set and (ii) characterization.

The most striking feature of this taxonomy is its abstract, general character. Krathwohl is aware of the problem. The taxonomy deals with objectives at the curriculum construction level. This means that objectives as defined in the taxonomy are approximately midway between very broad and very general objectives of education and the specific ones which provide guidance for the development of step-by-step learning experiences.

For a short presentation of Krathwohl's taxonomy, G. De Landsheere (1982) tried to find a classification principle that would be easier to formulate in behavioral terms than internalization. He suggested a continuum of activity, or of personal engagement. De Landsheere's frame of reference was developmental psychology. He wrote: "An individual has really reached the adult stage if his behaviour has found its coherence, its logic and stability; he has developed at the same time a sound tolerance to change, contradiction, frustration; he is cognitively and affectively independent; he is, at the same time, able to abide by his engagement and feelings." Education is a long process leading to this ultimate balance.

De Landsheere suggests the following taxonomy:

(a)   *The individual responds to external stimulation.*

(i)   The individual receives: this is a rather amorphous stage. The individual encounters, for instance, beauty or ugliness without any reaction, like a mirror that would not reflect any image. This behaviour is hard to distinguish from the cognition (in Guilford's sense) that takes place before memorization. Only some manifestation of attention is observable.

(ii)   The individual receives and responds to the stimulus: an observable reaction takes place. The individual obeys, manifests pleasure by his or her words or attitudes. At this stage, there is not yet explicit acceptance or rejection that would reflect a deliberate choice.

(iii)   The individual receives and reacts by accepting or refusing: now the individual knows what he or she wants or likes, provided things or events are presented.

(b) *The individual takes initiatives.*   The individual tries spontaneously to understand, to feel, and then act according to the options available. Here the adult stage is reached. For instance, the individual lives a life in accordance with his or her values, feelings, beliefs, likings, but is also able to change his or her mind if convincing proofs or arguments are offered. This stage is parallel to evaluation in the cognitive domain.

The classification suggested by De Landsheere seems clearer than Krathwohl's taxonomy, but more limited. Objectives can be more easily operationalized, but the criticism of Krathwohl's work also applies here.

2.2 Conclusion to the Affective Domain

The situation in the affective domain remains unsatisfactory. Why does it appear that so much work is still to be undertaken in the field? Krathwohl has not succeeded in filling completely the gap in the theoretical framework and the methodology of educational evaluation in the affective domain. A more systematic attack on the problem of affective objectives is required, and, in particular, an inventory of existing studies, experiments, and evaluation instruments in the field should be undertaken. Indubitably, the affective domain will constitute a priority area in the field of educational research in the decades to come.

3. The Psychomotor Domain

Why is the psychomotor domain important? First of all motion is a necessary condition of survival and of independence. Life sometimes depends on physical strength correctly applied, on agility, and on rapidity. Locomotor behavior is needed to explore the environment and sensory-motor activities are essential for the development of intelligence. Some Psychomotor behaviors such as walking and grasping, are also necessary for physical and mental health to be maintained. Dexterity is crucial for the worker, and also in civilizations giving a lot of time to leisure, corporal ability plays a considerable role in artistic and athletic activities.

Numerous taxonomies have been developed for the psychomotor domain. Some of them tend to be comprehensive, a strict parallelism with the taxonomies inspired by Bloom and Krathwohl for the cognitive and affective domains. Others have been developed for specialized fields and have, in many cases, a very technical character. Only six taxonomies which fall in the first category are presented in this article.

Ragsdale, Guilford, Dave, and Kibler's taxonomies are summarized very briefly for they are mainly of historical interest.

3.1 Ragsdale's Taxonomy

As early as in 1950, Ragsdale published a classification for "motor types of activities" learned by children. He worked with three categories only: (a) object motor activities (speed, precision): manipulation or acting with direct reference to an object; (b) language motor activities: movement of speech, sight, handwriting; (c) feeling motor activities: movements communicating feelings and attitudes.

These categories are so general that they are of little help in the definition of educational objectives.

3.2 Guilford's Taxonomy

Guilford (1958) suggested a simple classification in seven categories that is not hierarchical, and also does not seem of great utility for generating objectives. The seven categories are: power, pressure, speed, static precision, dynamic precision, coordination, and flexibility.

3.3 Dave's Taxonomy

Dave's classification (1969), although also rather schematic, can be considered as an embryo of a taxonomy. The categories are: initiation, manipulation, precision, articulation, naturalization (mechanization and internalization). The meaning of the first three categories is clear. Articulation emphasizes the coordination of a series of acts which are performed with appropriate articulation in terms of time, speed, and other relevant variables. As for naturalization, it refers to the highest level of proficiency of an act that has become routine.

3.4 Kibler's Classification

Kibler and his associates suggest a classification (1970) more developed than that of previous authors. The main frame of reference is developmental child psychology.

(a) Gross movements: movements of entire limbs in isolation or in conjunction with other parts of the body (movements involving the upper limbs, the lower limbs, two or more bodily units).

(b) Finely coordinated movements: coordinated movements of the extremities, used in conjunction with the eye or ear (hand-finger movements, hand-eye coordination, hand-ear coordination, hand-eye-foot coordination, other combinations of hand-foot-eye-ear movements).

(c) Nonverbal communication behaviours: facial expression, gestures (use of hands and arms to communicate specific messages), bodily movements (total bodily movements whose primary purposes are the communication of a message or series of messages).

(d) Speech behaviours: sound production (ability to produce meaningful sounds), sound-word formation (ability to coordinate sounds in meaningful words and messages), sound projection (ability to project sounds across the air waves at a level adequate for reception and decoding by the listener), sound-gesture coordination (ability to coordinate facial expression, movement, and gestures with verbal messages).

3.5 Simpson's Taxonomy (1966)

Simpson's taxonomy can be divided into five main categories.

(a) *Perception.* This is the process of becoming aware of objects, qualities, or relations by way of the sense organs.

  (i) Sensory stimulation: impingement of a stimulus upon one or more of the sense organs (auditory, visual, tactile, taste, smell, kinesthesic).
  (ii) Cue-selection: deciding to what cues one must respond in order to satisfy the particular requirements of task performance, for example, recognition of operating difficulties with machinery through the sound of the machine in operation.
  (iii) Translation: relation of perception of action in performing a motor act. This is the mental process of determining the meaning of the cues received for action, for example, the ability to relate music to dance form.

(b) *Set.* Preparatory adjustment of readiness for a particular kind of action or experience.

  (i) Mental set: readiness, in the mental sense, to perform a certain motor act.
  (ii) Physical set: readiness in the sense of having made the anatomical adjustments necessary for a motor act to be performed.
  (iii) Emotional set: readiness in terms of attitudes favourable to the motor act's taking place.

(c) *Guided response.* Overt behavioral act of an individual under the guidance of the instructor (imitation, trial and error).

(d) *Mechanism.* Learned response has become habitual.

(e) *Complex overt response.* The individual can perform a motor act that is considered complex because of the movement pattern required. A high degree of skill has been attained. The act can be carried out smoothly and efficiently.

  (i) Resolution of uncertainty: the act is performed without hesitation.
  (ii) Automatic performance: the individual can perform a finely coordinated motor skill with a great deal of ease and muscle control.

Simpson suggests that there is perhaps a sixth major category: adapting and originating. "At the level, the individual might originate new patterns of actions in solving a specific problem."

The weakness of this taxonomy is to be found again in its very abstract and general formulation.

3.6 Harrow's Taxonomy

As operationally defined by Harrow (1972), the term "psychomotor" covers any human voluntary observable movement that belongs to the domain of learning.

Harrow's taxonomy is the best available for the psychomotor domain, although some of the category descriptives are unsatisfactory:

(a) Reflex movements: segmental, intersegmental, suprasegmental reflexes.

(b) Basic-fundamental movements: locomotor, non-locomotor, manipulative movements

(c) Perceptual abilities:

  Kinesthetic discrimination: body awareness (bilaterality, laterality, sidedness, balance), body relationship of surrounding objects in space.
  Visual discrimination: visual acuity, visual tracking, visual memory, figure-ground differentiation, perceptual consistency.
  Auditory discrimination: auditory acuity, tracking, memory.
  Tactile discrimination: coordinated abilities: eye-hand and eye-foot coordination.

(d) Physical abilities: endurance (muscular and cardiovascular endurance), strength, flexibility, agility (change direction, stops and starts, reaction-response time, dexterity).

(e) Skilled movements: simple adaptive skill (beginner, intermediate, advanced, highly skilled), compound adaptive skill (beginner, intermediate, advanced, highly skilled), complex adaptive skill (beginner, intermediate, advanced, highly skilled).

(f) Nondiscursive communication: expressive movement (posture and carriage, gestures, facial expression), interpretative movement (aesthetic movement, creative movement).

In fact, Harrow does not describe her model in relation to a general, unique criterion (i.e., coordination), but simply looks for a critical order; mastery at an inferior level is absolutely necessary to achieve the immediate higher level in the hierarchy of movements.

This taxonomy has great qualities. First, it seems complete, not only in its description of the major categories of psychomotor behavior, but also in terms of the subcategories within the different taxonomic levels. Furthermore, the author defines the different levels clearly. For each subcategory, she proposes a clear definition of the concept and indicates, where necessary, the differences from other authors who have written in this field. She also presents concrete examples.

Harrow's taxonomy seems to be of direct use to teachers in physical education. Level (c) is specially interesting for preschool and for elementary-school teachers. It contains a good example of a battery for testing the perceptive abilities of pupils, diagnosing difficulties, and proposing appropriate remedial exercises. The author underlines the dependence between the cognitive and psychomotor domains at the level of perceptual abilities. Several examples also show the great inter-relation between the three domains. However, Harrow's hierarchy is not governed by a specified criterion, such as internalization or coordination. Moreover, the sub-categories are not mutually exclusive.

3.7 Conclusion to the Psychomotor Domain

It seems that taxonomies in the psychomotor domain have not yet been given the attention they deserve. They should be tried in many varied situations and their relations with the other two domains should be carefully investigated.

4. Conclusion

The cognitive domain is the best developed. First, it is by nature favourable to the construction of logical models. Secondly, schools have traditionally been interested in cognitive learning, especially in the acquisition of factual knowledge which in turn leads to easy evaluation.

Compared with the cognitive domain, the affective domain is less developed. Only since about 1970 has the educational world been trying to change the situation (in the past, affectivity has sometimes been intensively cultivated, but nearly always in terms of indoctrination processes). Affects seem less observable than cognitive activities and in most cases are less susceptible to rigorous measurement.

One would think that the psychomotor domain would present fewer difficulties, but little systematic work has been undertaken. In most Western educational systems, physical and artistic education is comparatively neglected in the curriculum.

Despite certain weaknesses, the two taxonomies with which Bloom is associated, and Harrow's taxonomy dominate the field. The others should, however, not be neglected, since they supply further clarifications and suggestions.

At present, the taxonomy movement in education is of great value. Even though the instruments are so far imperfect, they stimulate educators to fruitful reflection. Half-way between the great ideological options and the micro-objectives, the taxonomies seem to relate philosophy and educational technology and practice. It is one of their great merits.

References

Bacher F 1973 La docimologie. In: Reuchlin M (ed.) 1973 *Traité de psychologie appliquée*. Presses Universitaires de France (PUF), Paris

Bloom B S (ed.) 1956 *Taxonomy of Educational Objectives: The Classification of Educational Goals*, Handbook 1: *Cognitive Domain*. McKay, New York

Dave R H 1969 *Taxonomy of Educational Objectives and Achievement Testing. Developments in Education Objectives and Achievement Testing. Developments in Educational Testing*, Vol. 1 University of London Press, London

De Block A 1975 *Taxonomie van Leerdoelen*. Standard Wetenschappelijke Uitgererij, Amsterdam

De Corte E 1973 *Onderwijsdoelstellingen*. Universitaire Pers, Louvain

De Landsheere G 1982 *Introduction à la recherche en éducation*. Thone, Liège; Armand Colin, Paris

D'Hainaut L 1970 Un modèle pour la détermination et la sélection des objectifs pédagogiques du domaine cognitif. *Enseignement Programmé* 11: 21–38

Ebel R L 1973 Evaluation and educational objectives. *J. Educ. Meas.* 10: 273–79

Gagné R M 1964 The implications of instructional objectives for learning. In: Lindvall C M (ed.) 1964 *Defining Educational Objectives*. University of Pittsburgh Press, Pittsburgh, Pennsylvania

Gerlach V, Sullivan A 1967 *Constructing Statements of Outcomes*. Southwest Regional Laboratory for Educational Research and Development, Inglewood, California

Guilford J P 1958 A system of psychomotor abilities. *Am. J. Psychol* 71: 164–74

Guilford J P 1967 *The Nature of Human Intelligence*. McKay, New York

Harrow A J 1972 *A Taxonomy of the Psychomotor Domain: A Guide for Developing Behavioral Objectives*. McKay, New York

Hill P W 1984 Testing hierarchy in educational taxonomies: A theoretical and empirical investigation. *Eval. Educ.* 8: 181–278

Horn R 1972 *Lernziele und Schülerleistung: Die Evaluation von den Lernzielen im kgnitiven Bereich*, 2nd edn. Beltz, Weinheim

Kibler R J, Barker L L, Miles D T 1970 *Behavioral Objectives and Instruction*. Allyn and Bacon, Boston, Massachusetts

Krathwohl D R, Bloom B S, Masia B B 1964 *Taxonomy of Educational Objectives: The Classification of Educational Goals*, Handbook 2: *Affective Domain*. McKay, New York

Madaus G F, Woods E N, Nuttal R L 1973 A causal model analysis of Bloom's taxonomy. *Am Educ. Res. J.* 10: 253–62

Metfessel N S, Michael W B, Kirsner D A 1970 Instrumentation of Bloom's and Krathwohl's taxonomies for the writing of educational objectives. In: Kibler R J, Barker L L, Miles D J (eds.) 1970

Simpson E J 1966 *The Classification of Educational Objectives, Psychomotor Domain*. University of Illinois, Urbana, Illinois

Further Reading

De Landsheere V, De Landsheere G 1992 7th revised edn. *Definir les objectifs de l'education*. Presses Universitaires de France (PUF), Paris

Merrill M D 1971 Necessary psychological conditions for defining instructional outcomes. In: Merrill M D (ed.) 1971 *Instructional Design: Readings*. Prentice-Hall, Englewood Cliffs, New Jersey

Ragsdale C E 1950 How children learn motor types of activities. *Learning and Instruction* 49th Yearbook of the National Society for the Study of Education, Washington, DC

Test Bias

C. K. Tittle

Bias is defined as prejudice or having a particular bent or direction. To say a test is biased is to charge that it is prejudiced or unfair to groups or individuals characterized as different from the majority of test takers. These groups may include ethnic minorities, women or men, individuals whose first language is not English, and persons with handicapping conditions. Charges of test bias have been based on examination of the content and format of individual test items, group differences in average performance, and the use of tests. As multiple choice testing has had increased use for teacher certification and licensure, there have been charges that these tests are biased against minority teachers.

A trend has developed toward testing formats other than multiple choice and essay examinations. There is the likelihood that bias concerns will arise for these alternative forms of assessments of both students and teachers. Assessments may now include observations, videotapes, interviews, science experiments, and so on. As these methods indicate, there will be less standardization in the future in both the context and scoring (rating) of assessments (Linn et al. 1991), as well as fewer samples of examinee performance. The procedures to examine bias will be broadened to include studies of components of score variance not just due to characteristics of the assessee, but also to the context (task/stimulus) and the characteristics of the rater or judge. Thus, the term "test" bias encompasses "assessment" bias.

Detailed reviews of test and item bias methods can be found in Berk (1982), Cole and Moss (1989), and Camilli and Shepard (1994).

1. Investigating Between-group Differences

Test bias, from a broader, construct-oriented perspective, has been examined in studies of tests used in crosscultural research and in earlier attempts to develop tests that are culture free or culture fair. Early research in the 1900s on intelligence measures recognized the problems of testing children in different groups; for instance, those whose native language was not English. With the development of group mental tests and the first large-scale use of tests, the Army Alpha in the First World War, these measures came into wider use and to the attention of the public. By the 1920s crosscultural test results were being used to counter deterministic interpretations of mental test scores. In the 1930s there were studies of the effect of language and culture on test scores. During the 1940s and 1950s, there were again studies of racial differences in intelligence measures. Havighurst and Davis studied the relation of social class and test performance, and Eells, with others, attempted to develop culture-fair mental tests.

No one in the late 1990s would claim that a test can be culture free or culture fair, nor is there consensus on a set of procedures that would establish that a test measures the same construct for groups with different social and cultural environments (Poortinga and van de Vijver 1991). However, there has been a series of studies since the early 1970s giving renewed attention to the theory underlying tests, the test development process, and a broader view of the validity evidence appropriate for the justification of tests used in educational settings. While there are arguments to be made for a purely technical definition of bias and validity (Cole and Moss 1989), there are strong arguments to be made for the inclusion of politics, values, and consequences in considering the full context of test interpretation and test use in which issues of test bias arise (Cronbach 1988, Messick 1989, Shepard 1993).

A theory-oriented perspective on test bias seeks to provide an understanding of the observed group differences based on characteristics on which individuals in any group may differ. The goal is to develop explanatory models in which gender or ethnic group membership does not directly predict the test scores or outcomes of interest (Eccles et al. 1983). In such explanatory models, group membership is related to educational and psychological characteristics that in turn are directly related to the achievement score or educational outcome of interest. Test or assessment bias concerns are likely to arise in situations where psychological and educational variables are not used in explanatory models of observed group differences. For example, in labeling group differences as due to fixed attributes of the group (boys or girls, their gender) or to genetic differences (e.g., females cannot do mathematics, males have greater variability in scores), there is a foreclosure of understandings on which educators can make appropriate inferences and use assessment information for educational goals. Thus, some research on test bias now seeks a greater understanding of the influences on test scores of educational experiences, psychological characteristics, culture, and language. For a broadly related review, see Gipps and Murphy (1994).

Other research seeking explanatory models of between-group performance on test scores uses cognitive psychology theory within a (mostly multiple choice format) measurement framework (Scheuneman and Gerritz 1990, Scheuneman et al. 1991) to examine cognitive process and linguistic influences on item and test performance. Yet other research uses alternative models for assessment of learners and teachers that seeks to build on cognitive constructivist theories and uses more complex forms of assessment tasks (Shulman 1989, Snow 1989) and scoring rubrics and training of raters (Lane et at. 1996).

2. Settings for Test Use

The fundamental role of validity, validation arguments, and the ruling out of plausible alternative interpretations in questions of test bias are made clear in describing the settings for test use. Validity of a test or, more accurately, the validity of inferences and actions based on test scores has been established typically through the strategies of: (a) criterion-related or predictive studies for validity evidence; (b) content analyses for validity evidence; and (c) construct studies for validity evidence. More broadly, validation procedures can also encompass evidence based on response processes, relations to other variables, internal structure, relevant literature, logical analyses, and so on.

Criterion-related studies provide evidence on the accuracy with which a test predicts a criterion, such as the use of a test of developed abilities to predict a criterion of college grades in an admissions setting.

Content-related validity evidence depends upon the definition of a domain of achievement to be sampled, the classification of test tasks in terms of this domain of reference, and expert judgment that the content of the test tasks sample or represent accurately the achievement domain, and includes administration and scoring procedures. An example is the application of conceptual and procedural knowledge in a measure of science achievement, along with the definitions or rubrics that are the scoring codes used by raters (teachers or other raters).

The construct strategy encompasses both the criterion and content analyses, as well as providing a more theory-based evaluation of the logical and empirical bases of determining how well a score represents a construct such as literacy or anxiety.

Several authors (e.g., Messick 1989) have suggested a more unified view of validity in which the role of construct validity is fundamental. The accuracy of an inference that a pupil cannot read based on the results of a single test score labeled as a measure of reading comprehension is dependent on more than expert classification or judgment of the test items in relation to instruction. The inference that an individual child cannot read assumes that motivation in the testing situation is optimal, that anxiety or unfamiliarity with the testing format does not interfere with performance, that questions can be answered only within the context of the reading passage, that the vocabulary is appropriate (e.g., within the child's experience or readily inferred from the context), that the child has had

opportunities to read genres similar to that of the text, and so on.

Further, from a theory-oriented perspective, there may be important variables to add to the assessment so that the reading comprehension score can be placed in the context of a theoretical model of the reading process. Examples from state testing programs in Illinois and Michigan (Tittle 1991) indicate that models may include items designed to measure students' ability to construct meaning from selected texts that are "mapped" for structure and content prior to item writing, there may be questions on topic familiarity (prior knowledge), and questions on knowledge about reading and reading strategies. Assessments may include self-reports of effort and interest in the reading tasks. Items to assess constructing meaning from text may have one, two, or three right answers, and literacy experiences may also be surveyed.

In these state assessment programs, reading is represented as an interactive process, between the reader, the text, and the context of the reading situation. Other examples of a theory-orientated perspective in test development and use are Baker's (1994) application of a cognitive information processing and expert–novice approach for history assessments. Lane et al. (1996) based the development of mathematics assessments on a cognitive constructivist perspective. Such theory-oriented perspectives in assessment should assist in gaining meaning from the test score and suggest areas on which classroom instruction can focus. There are, therefore, questions of an educational and psychological nature that should be examined when group differences in average test performance are observed. Construct-related validity evidence will provide the means to examine alternative, theory-related explanations for group differences in test performance.

Test bias in educational settings has another dimension. If evidence on the accuracy of interpretations is provided from a scientific perspective and it is satisfactory, there remain questions of the logical and empirical consequences of test use in a particular instance. These include the interpretations (meaning) and use (actions) of students and teachers, for example, based on the complete assessment process and resulting information (Tittle 1994). If an assessment is intended to encourage changes in teaching and learning in classrooms, then evidence for this intended use is needed. If in an admissions testing program proportionally fewer (in terms of the applicant pool) minority students are selected at elite institutions, what is the social value of this outcome? Similarly, if a career interest inventory used in counseling suggests fewer science and technological occupations to women than to men, what is the social value of this outcome? Whether one incorporates the social value and interpretive perspectives within an expanded conception of validity or considers values as a matter for public policy and hence separate from a technical definition of validity, these concerns are a part of the study of test bias in educational settings.

2.1 Admissions Testing

In the use of tests for admission to postsecondary education, a test is assumed to have prediction-related validity evidence to the extent that students scoring well on the test also do well on a criterion such as college grades. When there are differences between mean scores for groups such as men and women or majority–minority ethnic groups, the question arises as to whether the group differences are also reflected in criterion differences or whether they represent bias.

In defining selection bias, within-group regression equations are examined for differences in correlations and predictor reliabilities and differences in slopes, intercepts, or standard errors of estimate. The comparison of these statistics for different groups has shown few differences, with the exception of intercept differences. Typical findings in the United States with the Scholastic Aptitude Test (SAT) are that women's college grades are underpredicted, with the extent of underprediction varying from study to study; for White–Black comparisons, Black scores tend to be somewhat overpredicted and Whites underpredicted, with a common regression line. Results vary for other ethnic groups.

Since use of a single regression line leads to over- or underprediction of the criterion in some instances, several models were proposed in the 1970s as fair procedures for selecting students for an educational institution. In these models a criterion score (grades) and a predictor (test score) are available and a cut score on the test needs to be found for each group such that the definition of fair selection in a particular model is satisfied. The models allow for explicit consideration of values and effects of different types of selection decisions. Although the models were useful in identifying different policies that could be followed, in practice they have not been used. Thus there remains considerable argument about the issue of the bias or fairness in the use of a test such as the SAT, and the test typically is used with an overall group, single selection, or placement formula, often with no other predictors. Since the test is also used for course placement, to award scholarships, and to select precollege-age children for gifted programs, the underprediction of female criterion scores is of great concern.

Studies of SAT bias have examined factors such as speededness, item formats, test preparation or coaching (Bond 1989), test-taking strategies, and characteristics such as anxiety. These variables have not accounted for gender differences, especially on the mathematics test of the SAT. Wainer and Steinberg (1992) used large databases (47,000) of first-year college students who enrolled in and completed a mathematics course in their first semester. They examined average SAT mathematics scores for men and women within five specific types of first-year mathematics courses and at each academic grade (A, B, C, etc.) achieved in the course types.

When women and men were matched on each criterion grade achieved within each of the five courses (e.g., calculus) and their SAT scores examined, women's scores were about 33 SAT points lower. Prediction of college grades using SAT and sex found somewhat larger sex effects (women's course grades were underpredicted). The authors concluded: "There is evidence of differential validity by sex on the SAT-M; women score lower on average than men of comparable academic performance" (Wainer and Steinberg 1992). Since possible unfairness in the use of the SAT-M for selection, course placement, and scholarships involves social and political values, the authors propose that models of fairness of the 1970s be re-examined and alternatives to the SAT considered.

For selection of minorities the data are harder to examine, and with the general trend toward overprediction of grades (at least in the United States), explicit consideration of models of fairness are essential for the consideration of social and political goals. Novick (1980) suggested defining disadvantage operationally (e.g., family income) for each individual. A further refinement of this approach would be to identify the educational and psychological variables for which "disadvantage" is proxy, and link these to educational selection and placement within the postsecondary setting. Paradoxically, as the issue of test bias in selection has been clarified into its technical and social value components, there is a trend toward less selectivity on the part of many institutions in the United States. This trend should reinforce the use of tests specifically designed for placement and instruction, resulting in less use of traditional predictors such as the SAT.

2.2 Special Education Placement

The use of educational and psychological tests in placing students into special classes, as for the mildly retarded, has been the subject of controversy and court litigation. Two main issues are the overrepresentation of minorities in special education classes and bias in tests (including IQ tests) used for placements. Shepard (1989) provided a thorough analysis of definitions, the use of assessment in the identification of mild handicaps, and school placement issues. She identified a trend toward assessment measures and procedures that are more directly related to school placement and instructional decisions. As with the use of standardized tests, including IQ tests, the study of bias or fairness in school placement procedures has to be concerned with the potential adverse impact of the procedures (disproportionate classification of groups into special classes), and studies of effects—evidence that the classification into "treatments" is of educational benefit to children. Special issues in the testing of linguistic minorities and cultural minorities are also relevant, including language dominance and a child's understanding of any assessment procedures (Duran 1989).

2.3 Competency and Achievement Testing

In the United States, minimum competency testing (MCT) programs have been started by the majority of local school districts and states to assess basic academic skills. The tests are typically objective in form and measure reading and mathematics, sometimes language and writing skills. A passing score or standard for acceptable levels of student performance is established. The main uses of the test results are to certify students for grade promotion, graduation, or a diploma, and to classify or place students in remedial or other special service programs. A trend is toward assessment of problem-solving and "higher order thinking," and assessments that provide understanding of student conceptual knowledge, processes, and procedures used in problem-solving (Tittle 1991). Also, in North America and the United Kingdom, among other nations, concern with minimum competency is being replaced with programs to define national and state-level goals, standards, and alternative or performance assessment procedures. These assessment procedures are also beginning to be examined for bias in content, group differences, and adequacy of scoring procedures, as well as rater consistency and accuracy.

Although test bias issues have been raised in connection with the adverse impact of MCT on minority students, the courts have only supported a procedural fairness argument in delaying implementation of MCT for graduation or certification purposes. The argument was sustained that adequate educational opportunity to learn the skills and content of such tests must be provided to students. Programs of MCT typically use test bias procedures (see Sect. 3). Arguments about educational opportunity also arise in the context of developing national standards and assessments. That is, where high stakes national assessments may be implemented, questions can be asked: do students have equality of opportunity to learn, and how do we document the allocation of resources, including those of classroom processes or learning activities?

2.4 Evaluating Educational Programs

Issues of test bias in evaluation have been raised primarily in studies of compensatory education programs. The debates over the standardized achievement tests used in evaluation focus on group differences in test scores and individual items that are identified as biased—items that may represent life-styles or experiences more typical of middle socioeconomic White groups in United States culture. Major test publishers now routinely use item and test bias review procedures, with representatives of concerned groups included on judgmental review panels. As a result, the major tests are less subject to these criticisms. A

second focus is on the interpretation of scores and use of the tests. Bias in this context has involved concerns about (the inappropriate) inferences that some groups do not have the ability to learn what the tests are assessing. Increasing use of alternative assessments (portfolios, classroom tasks) are not likely to eliminate bias concerns in program evaluation.

2.5 Career Counseling

Career interest inventories and aptitude batteries are examined for bias against women and minorities. In the 1960s and 1970s there were efforts to define aspects of interest measurement and outcomes of career counseling that were likely to contribute to the uneven distribution of women and minorities in occupations. For women, sex bias was examined in stereotyping of female and male roles, in the development of new scales, and in providing the same range of occupations for men and women, as well as gender-neutral language; all were recommendations made in the 1974 *Guidelines for Assessment of Sex Bias and Sex Fairness in Career Interest Inventories*. Related issues are discussed in a series of papers edited by Tittle and Zytowski (1978), and in Harmon (1989). Cronbach (1988) demonstrated the severe problems for women and girls with an aptitude battery (Armed Services Vocational Aptitude Battery) used for classification/career counseling in high schools in the United States.

What little evidence is available suggests that the validity of interest inventories may be the same for minority and White groups. Because interest measures are frequently used within a program of career guidance in schools, studies of the effects or outcomes of using interest measures and vocational aptitude measures are critical. Outcome measures can provide evidence on bias or lack of fairness in measures employed in career counseling by using student ratings, the number of occupations considered by females and males and minorities, and the number of nontraditional occupations considered.

3. Test Bias Methodology

The study of test bias includes methods that use internal and, more rarely, external criteria. Current procedures to provide evidence to support the claim that an achievement test or minimum competency test (MCT) is unbiased or fair to women and minorities emphasize judgmental reviews and statistical studies of item bias. Judgmental reviews used in the test development process and in selecting achievement tests for use in large school districts and state programs are described by Tittle (in Berk 1982). Test planning, item writing and review, item tryout, selection of final items, and development of norms and scaling are all stages in the test development process where judgments are made that affect perceptions of test bias. Procedures include review forms and directions to judges to identify stereotyping of women, minorities, and the handicapped; whether content may be less familiar to particular groups; and whether students have had an opportunity to learn the test (item) content.

Studies carried out for large-scale testing programs and by publishers of achievement tests routinely examine test items for evidence of group differences in performance. Typically, these methodological studies examine the characteristics of item statistics based on the assumption that the test, over all items, is not biased. The methods rely upon detecting items that are by some definition aberrant from the majority of items in the test. Such statistical procedures look for examples of differential item functioning for groups of interest by means of the comparison of item difficulties (empirically-based procedures) or item characteristics curves (model-based procedures) (Cole and Moss 1989; Holland and Wainer 1993). Another method is to examine the internal structure of the test items or subtests by means of factor analyses compared across groups.

Although experimental studies have examined the "effect" of using test content more familiar to women and minorities than men and majority White groups (content thought to favor one group or another), they have yielded mixed results. Potentially more fruitful are studies that use theories of cognitive processing to characterize test items and to study item difficulty or differential item functioning indices for different groups (Scheuneman and Garritz 1990, Scheuneman et al. 1991). Other promising studies are in theory-based assessment programs (described above). The examples of state programs in reading assessment provide opportunities for examining whether group differences in text comprehension can be explained by psychological process variables as opposed to group ethnic variables. The comprehensive assessment model proposed by Snow (1989), as well as the work of Eccles et al. (1983), should also be valuable in providing explanatory models for studying test bias in a variety of subject matters.

4. Bias Considerations for Alternative Assessments

The majority of bias studies have been carried out using tests with multiple choice item formats. Alternative assessment formats include essays or written responses, carrying out experiments, performing problem-solving in group settings, putting together a portfolio of work (the arts, writing, or other subject areas). These assessments yield written products, observational ratings, and video- or audiotapes for evaluation. "Scores" on a task are typically sets of ordered categories (polytomous) rather than dichotomous. A method used with polytomously scored tasks in performance assessments is logistic discriminant

function analysis (Miller and Spray 1993, Wang and Lane 1996) or extensions of procedures for dichotomously scored items.

Cole and Moss (1989) identified studies of grading or judging writing and essay examinations that have examined the effects on raters of poor handwriting, labeling of groups as "honors" or "regular" students, and other variables irrelevant to the achievement construct of interest. Comparisons of compositions of writers from different countries have found differences in such variables as organization and style. In a study in Ireland, Bolger and Kellaghan (1990) compared the performance of boys and girls on multiple choice and short written response tests of mathematics, Irish, and English achievement. There was an effect of measurement format across all three achievement areas (males performed higher than females on multiple choice tests). Bridgeman and Lewis (1994) found gender differences on history multiple choice scores but not on essays or course grades for the Advanced Placement test (male scores one-half SD higher on multiple choice test). Studies in England and Australia (e.g., Adams 1983) have found supporting and nonsupporting results.

The change in format of the tasks to the use of complex stimuli combining print, audio, and visual components is likely to introduce other sources of possible bias. Tests of listening involve speech patterns and intonation that may vary for different linguistic communities. Tasks presented by videotape add the visual cues of discourse and patterns of social interactions that vary for sociocultural communities. Thus assessment of constructs of student learning or teacher performance will be in the context of stimuli that will be more variable for groups of concern. As another example of task fairness, consider science assessments. It is known that girls have different interests and experiences in science topics than boys, and the same may hold true for some minority groups.

Similarly, as the "product" or achievement outcome to be evaluated is presented for rating in different media (written, real-time or live performance, audio- or videotape), bias concerns will be evident. This time the bias concerns are with the characteristics of raters or observers and their experience in relation to the examinee's. There is little evidence that scoring by well-trained administrators of highly structured individually administered cognitive tasks (e.g., IQ measures) is biased by ethnic group or sex of the rater or examinee. (This is not to say that particular assessment instruments are appropriately used with examinees of different groups of concern.) Analogously, procedures are now being developed to detect and adjust for rater leniency and stringency (Englehard 1996, Raymond and Houston 1990). From an explanatory perspective, one think-aloud process study identified raters applying questionable reasoning processes while scoring complex portfolio assessments (Thomas et al. 1995).

However, there are studies of employment assessment centers that suggest the need for investigation of sources of score variance due to sex and ethnic characteristics of the rater and the individual being rated. Rater age and physical attractiveness of the examinee have been related to score variance. These are studies in which the rater has a complex task, since the examinee may be observed in the context of a group setting. Further, the examinee's performance may vary as a function of the group task and other aspects of the context for observing the task. Particularly where raters and examinees have different cultural and linguistic experiences such as those associated with gender and minority status, the possibility of bias or irrelevant score variance can be investigated.

Studies of bias will need to develop additional sets of procedures to provide evidence that scores based on ratings of student or teacher performance on more complex tasks are fair. This is likely to require more detailed specification of the characteristics of linguistic and cultural minorities that could influence ratings and performance and which are irrelevant to the assessment construct of interest. Studies in employment centers and in educational assessments suggest that rater bias is lessened if there is extensive development of the rating measure, careful selection of raters, lengthy rater training, and continued contact with raters during the rating period (Pulakos et al. 1989, Lane et al. 1996).

5. Summary and Conclusion

Examining a test or complex performance assessment for bias or fairness to groups and individuals is an important part of the development, tryout, administration, and evaluation of such instruments. In brief, it is an aspect of the validation and evaluation of the assessment system—from development to interpretations and limitations of scores, to score use, to consequences and values for individuals, groups, institutions, and society. Bias and fairness to groups need to be considered an integral part of the evaluation of educational assessments. The most frequently used procedures by test developers and publishers include attention to the specifications, reviews by judges of test content for bias, and use of statistical item bias analyses. Judgments and content reviews provide information that the statistical methods cannot, and the reverse is also true. Test bias studies for complex performance tasks and raters require additional procedures.

Group differences on test scores are leading toward two areas of research that hold promise for educationally relevant explanatory studies. One area of research arises within the measurement framework and applies theories from cognitive psychology. The second area of research arises from cognitive and constructivist theories. This research provides explanatory models of teaching and learning in which educational and psychological characteristics of individuals replace group membership in direct relationships to desired outcomes. Both areas of research hold promise for integrating psychological and measurement theory and for bringing testing closer to educational practice.

See also: Item Bias

References

Adams R J 1983 *Sex Bias in ASAT?* ACER, Hawthorn
Baker E L 1994 Learning-based assessments of history understanding. *Educational Psychologist* 29(2): 97–106
Berk R (ed.) 1982 *Handbook of Methods for Detecting Test Bias.* Johns Hopkins University Press, Baltimore, Maryland
Bolger N, Kellaghan T 1990 Method of measurement and gender differences in scholastic achievement. *J. Educ. Meas.* 27(2): 165–74
Bond L 1989 The effects of special preparation on measures of scholastic ability. In: Linn R L (ed.) 1989 *Educational Measurement*, 3rd edn. Macmillan, New York
Bridgeman B, Lewis C 1994 The relationship of essay and multiple-choice scores with grades in college courses. *J. Educ. Meas.* 31(1): 37–50
Camilli G, Shepard L A 1994 *Methods for identifying biased test items.* Sage, Thousand Oaks, California
Cole N S, Moss P A 1989 Bias in test use. In: Linn R L (ed.) 1989 *Educational Measurement*, 3rd edn. Macmillan, New York
Cronbach L J 1988 Five perspectives on the validity argument. In: Wainer H, Braun H I (eds.) 1988 *Test Validity.* Erlbaum, Hillsdale, New Jersey
Duran R P 1989 Testing of linguistic minorities. In: Linn R L (ed.) 1989 *Educational Measurement*, 3rd edn. Macmillan, New York
Eccles J S et al. 1983 Expectancies, values and academic behavior. In: Spence J T (ed.) 1983 *Achievement and Achievement Motives: Psychological and Sociological Approaches.* Freeman, San Francisco, California
Englehard G Jr 1996 Evaluating rater accuracy in performance assessments. *J. Educ. Meas.* 33(1): 56–70
Gipps C, Murphy P I 1994 *A fair test? Assessment, achievement and equity.* Open University Press, Buckingham
Harmon L W 1989 Counseling. In: Linn R L (ed.) 1989 *Educational Measurement*, 3rd edn. Macmillan, New York
Holland P W, Wainer H (eds.) 1993 *Differential item functioning.* Erlbaum, Hillsdale, New Jersey
Lane S et al. 1996 Generalizability and validity of a mathematics performance assessment. *J. Educ. Meas.* 33(1): 71–92
Linn R L, Baker E L, Dunbar S B 1991 Complex performance-based assessment: Expectations and validation criteria. *Educ. Researcher* 20: 15–21
Messick S 1989 Validity. In: Linn R L (ed.) 1989 *Educational Measurement*, 3rd edn. Macmillan, New York
Miller T R, Spray J A 1993 Logistic discriminant function analysis for DIF identification of polytomously scored items. *J. Educ. Meas.* 30(2): 107–22
Novick M R 1980 Policy issues of fairness in testing. In: van der Kamp L J T et al. (eds.) 1980 *Psychometrics for Educational Debates.* Wiley, New York
Poortinga Y H, van de Vijer F J R 1991 Culture-free measurement in the history of cross-cultural psychology. *Bulletin of the International Test Commission* 18: 72–87

Pulakos E D, White L A, Oppler S H, Borman W C 1989 Examination of race and sex effects on performance ratings. *J. Appl. Psychol.* 74: 770–80

Raymond M R, Houston W M 1990 *Detecting and correcting for rater effects in performance assessment.* ERIC Document Reproduction Service ED 361 369. (ACT RR 90–14)

Scheuneman J, Gerritz K 1990 Using differential item functioning procedures to explore sources of item difficulty and group performance characteristics. *J. Educ. Meas.* 27(2): 109–31

Scheuneman J, Gerritz K, Embretson S 1991 *Effects of Prose Complexity on Achievement Test Item Difficulty.* Educational Testing Service, Princeton, New Jersey

Shepard L A 1989 Identification of mild handicaps. In: Linn R L (ed.) 1989 *Educational Measurement*, 3rd edn. Macmillan, New York

Shepard L 1993 Evaluating test validity. *Review of Research in Educ.* 19: 405–50

Shulman L S 1989 The paradox of teacher assessment. In: 1989 *New Directions for Teacher Assessment. Proceedings of the ETS Invitational Conference.* Educational Testing Service, Princeton, New Jersey

Snow R E 1989 Toward assessment of cognitive and conative structures in learning. *Educ. Researcher* 18(9): 8–14

Thomas W H et al. 1995 *California Learning Assessment System portfolio assessment research and development project.* ETS Center for Performance Assessment, Princetown, New Jersey

Tittle C K 1991 Changing models of student and teacher assessment. *Educ. Psychol.* 26: 157–67

Tittle C K 1994 Toward an educational psychology of assessment for teaching and learning: Theories, context, and validation arguments. *Educ. Psychologist* 29(3): 149–62

Tittle C K, Zytowski D G (eds.) 1978 *Sex-fair Interest Measurement: Research and Implications.* National Institute of Education, Washington, DC

Wainer H, Steinberg L S 1992 Sex differences in performance on the mathematics section of the Scholastic Aptitude Test: A bidirectional validity study. *Harv. Educ. Rev.* 62: 323–36

Wang N, Lane S 1996 Detection of gender-related differential item functioning in a mathematics performance assessment. *Applied Meas. in Educ.* 9(2): 175–99

Thurstone Scales

D. Andrich

Thurstone's work in the 1920s and 1930s on constructing scales for measuring social variables, shows great care in formalizing the foundations of measurement and reflects a concern for the very foundations of scientific enquiry. He explicitly avoided the use of correlations, using instead linearity as a rationalizing principle, which means that if the value of object A is greater than that of object B by an amount a_1, and if the value of object B is greater than that of object C by an amount of a_2, then the value of object A should be greater than that of object C by an amount close to the sum $a_1 + a_2$. This entry considers his work and papers on scaling, which were written in the 1920s and 1930s, and republished in Thurstone (1959).

1. Unidimensionality

With the idea of linearity is the notion of unidimensionality. Thurstone appreciated that this is a relative concept and is constructed either to understand complex phenomena or to facilitate decision-making. Attitudes of people are clear examples of complex phenomena; yet Thurstone argued convincingly that there was a sense to placing them on a single continuum.

The various opinions cannot be completely described merely as "more" or "less." They scatter in many dimensions, but the very idea of measurement implies a linear continuum of some sort, such as length, price, volume, weight, age. When the idea of measurement is applied to scholastic achievement, for example, it is necessary to force the qualitative variations into a scholastic linear scale of some kind. (Thurstone 1959 pp. 218–19)

2. Defining a Continuum

Whatever the property to be measured, it is necessary to operationalize the continuum. This is done by formalizing the locations and spacings of the questions on the continuum. In principle, tests of achievement or attitude could be constructed in the same way in the sense that the test questions in one, and the statements in the other, can both be located on a continuum. In the former, the differences in location reflect differences in difficulty; in the latter, they reflect differences in what Thurstone called "affective values."

3. Statistical Formulations

Thurstone's mathematical–statistical formulations for his scales arise from the psychophysical methods and models of Fechner and Weber in which the basic data collection design is that of pair-comparisons. In such a design, each of a group of persons compares objects with respect to some physical property, such as weight or brightness, and declares which of the pair has more of the property. Thurstone contributed to the logic of psychophysics, and in the process, liberated the construction of scales for subjective values from the need of any physical continuum.

> One of the main requirements of a truly subjective metric is that it shall be entirely independent of all physical measurement. In freeing ourselves completely from physical measurement, we are also free to experiment with aesthetic objects and with many other types of stimuli to which there does not correspond any known physical measurement. (Thurstone 1959 pp. 182–83)

3.1 The Law of Comparative Judgment

The basis for this liberation was Thurstone's law of comparative judgment (Thurstone 1959 p. 39), which may be summarized as follows:

(a) When person n reacts to object i, the person perceives a value d_{ni} of the property in question. This value is assumed to be a continuous random variable defined by

$$d_{ij} = \alpha_i + \varepsilon_{ni} \tag{1}$$

where α_i is the scale value of object i and is constant with respect to all persons in a specified population, and ε_{ni} is the error component associated with person n. Over the population of persons, d_{ni} is defined to be normally distributed with mean α_i and variance σ_i^2.

(b) When person n compares two objects i and j then the person judges that object i has more of the property if the difference $d_{ni} - d_{nj} > 0$. In the population, this difference,

$$d_{ij} = d_{nj} - d_{nj} = (\alpha_i - \alpha_j) + (\varepsilon_i - \varepsilon_j), \tag{2}$$

is a continuous random variable normally distributed with mean value $\alpha_{ij} = \alpha_i - \alpha_j$ and variance $\sigma_{ij}^2 = \sigma_i^2 + \sigma_j^2 - 2\rho_{ij}\sigma_i\sigma_j$

This difference process for a fixed α_{ij}, is shown in Fig. 1 in which the shaded region represents the probability that $d_{ij} > 0$.

In empirical data, the proportion of persons who

judge that object i has more of the property than object j is an estimate of this probability. The associated estimate of $\alpha_i - \alpha_j$ then is the corresponding normal deviate. The step of transforming a proportion, taken as an estimate of a probability in a normal distribution, was, in fact, the key step in Thurstone's linearization of his scales.

The expression for σ_{ij}^2 was further modified by Thurstone (1959 p. 39) into special cases. One special case is to assume that the correlation ρ_{ij} is zero. A further specialization is to let $\sigma_i^2 = \sigma_j^2 = \sigma^2$. This produces Thurstone's Case V of the law of comparative judgment, and is the easiest case to apply. Torgerson (1958) and Bock and Jones (1968) elaborate on the law of comparative judgment and develop more advanced techniques for estimating the scale values. Edwards (1957) provides an excellent elementary treatment.

The central role of this model, which has not been properly understood, was to act as a "criterion" to which responses should conform rather than as a description of the responses—only if data conformed to the model could it be said that measurement had taken place. The model was *not* a statistical assumption about the data.

3.2 Attitude and Mental Testing

For constructing attitude scales, statements reflecting different intensities of attitude may be scaled through the pair-comparison design in which persons compare the affective values of statements and declare which has the greater value. By a simple redefinition of one of the variables, Thurstone applied the principles of the law of comparative judgment to mental testing. Effectively, the ability of each person replaced the value of one of the two entities which were compared. Thus the ability of a person was compared with the difficulty of a question.

A common classification of persons taken by Thurstone was an age group. Then the proportion of any age group which succeeded on any question was transformed to a normal deviate and used as a basis for scaling. This principle is described in detail in Thurstone (1925).

3.3 The Methods of Equal Appearing Intervals and Successive Intervals

The disadvantage of the pair comparison design is that it is time consuming. As a result, the much simpler method of rank ordering was adapted to the law of comparative judgment (Thurstone 1959) and models for incomplete pair comparison designs have been developed (Bock and Jones 1968).

Another adaptation for constructing an attitude scale was the design of "equal appearing intervals" and its extension to the method of successive intervals. After creating a list of some 100 statements, based on a literature search of the topic in question and opinions of experts, the statements are placed by 200 or 300

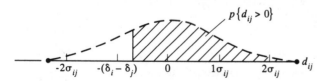

Figure 1
Probability that $d_{ij} > 0$ for fixed $(\delta_i - \delta_j)$ in a pair comparison design

judges into 11 intervals. These intervals are to be considered equally spaced in intensity on the affective continuum. Scale values for the statements are then computed on the assumption that the equal appearing intervals actually operate as if they were equal. For the method of successive intervals, the data collection design is essentially the same, except that estimates of scale values of intervals are calculated.

The model for computing the scale values is a direct extension of the model in Fig 1. If there are m boundaries or thresholds between the $m + 1$ successive intervals on the affective continuum designated by τ_1, $\tau_2, \ldots, \tau_k, \ldots, \tau_m$, the response corresponds to the interval in which the value of the random variable falls.

The estimate of the appropriate model probabilities is again given by a proportion; this time by the proportion of persons who classify the statement to be *in or below* a given category. By transforming these probability estimates to corresponding normal deviates, the scale values of both the statements and the category boundaries can be estimated.

The approach and modeling associated with the method of successive intervals has been used as a basis for analyzing data in which three or more categories have some order, and the mathematical statistical and computing techniques have been advanced considerably (Bock 1975). A contrasting approach to dealing with ordered categories is presented in Andrich (1978a).

4. Checks on the Scales

Once a set of statements or questions has been placed on a continuum, checks on the scales must be made. Because Thurstone was concerned that measurement be scientifically defensible, he stressed that the scales must be checked for validity, and that it must be possible for the data not to accord with the theory underlying the scale construction. The first check is that the ordering and spacing of the questions or statements is consistent with a theoretical appreciation of the continuum. Perhaps only some questions or statements need to be eliminated. Alternatively, it may be that the effects of dimensions other than the one intended have played too great a role. Finally, it may be that the scale construction is sound, and that a new understanding about the continuum has been revealed.

4.1 Statistical Tests

Formal statistical checks are also usually applied, which take advantage of the feature that the location estimates are a summary of the data. From this summary, and the model, an attempt is then made to "recover" the observed details of the data, usually the relevant proportions. To the degree that the detail is recovered, the scale is confirmed to be internally consistent. Such statistical checks on the model are

generally called "tests of fit": they test the fit between the data and the model.

Finally, it is possible to test directly the degree to which the differences among scale values of questions, taken in threes, satisfy the requirement of additivity mentioned in sect. 1 above. It should be appreciated that no test of fit is necessary and sufficient for the models, and the results of the different tests of fit are not mutually exclusive. Bock and Jones (1968) elaborate on the statistical tests of fit.

4.2 Principles of Invariance

Another requirement which can be applied to check the validity of a scale is that of invariance of scale values of statements across populations of persons who may have different attitudes.

> If the scale is to be regarded as valid, the scale values of the statements should not be affected by the opinions of the people who help to construct it. This may turn out to be a severe test in practice, but the scaling method must stand such a test before it can be accepted as being more than a description of the people who construct the scale. (Thurstone 1959 p. 228)

To the degree that the invariance is demonstrated across different groups of persons, including those with known differences on the trait under investigation, the scale is applicable across those groups. The scale is deliberately constructed both to capture the trait in question and to exhibit the desired properties of a measuring instrument.

4.3 Person Measurement

Thurstone also appreciated the complementary requirement that a person's measure should not depend on the actual questions used in a scale.

> It should be possible to omit several test questions at different levels of the scale without affecting the individual score. (Thurstone 1926 p. 446)

Interestingly, however, Thurstone never seemed to formalize a person parameter in his mathematical statistical models. And despite the specifications of invariance, both in the scaling of questions or statements and in the measurement of persons, he seemed to be constrained by considering persons always to be sampled from some specified population. Furthermore, the procedure for attitude measurement of individuals is essentially ad hoc: a person responds to an attitude scale, which consists of statements approximately equally spaced on the continuum, by either agreeing or disagreeing with each statement, and then the person's measure of attitude is taken as the median of the scale values of the statements endorsed. The implied mechanism when the person responds directly to a statement is that a person would endorse the statements in a given range on the scale which represented his or her attitude, and would tend not to endorse statements more extreme in either direction. This mechanism is that of unfolding (maximum probability), which was developed subsequently by Coombs (1964), a student of Thurstone's. The other type of scale, subsequently elaborated by Guttman (1950), implies that if a person endorses a statement of a particular scale value, then the person will tend to endorse all statements with smaller scale values and tend not to endorse all statements with greater scale values. This implied second mechanism is said to be cumulative (increasing probability), and Thurstone became aware of the possibility of using this mechanism directly.

> In a small 1929 monograph I described two types of attitude scales. These were called the *maximum probability type* and the *increasing probability type*. All our work was with the first type. Recently, there has been interest in the second type of scaling, which lends itself to certain types of attitude problems. The scaling of attitude statements can be accomplished directly from the records of acceptance and rejection for a group of subjects without the sorting procedure that we used, but as far as I know, such a scaling procedure has not yet been developed. (Thurstone 1959 p. 214)

In contrast to Thurstone's models, those of Coombs and Guttman implied a person parameter, but their models were deterministic, and did not apply the powerful statistical properties Thurstone introduced for the pair-comparison design to estimate the location of statements or test questions. A probabilistic model for the unfolding response mechanism was derived by analogy to Thurstone's law of comparative judgment by Andrich (1988), and the model which (a) is a probabilistic version of the Guttman-type scale; (b) permits measurements of persons and the scaling of statements from the direct endorsement or otherwise of the persons; and (c) which also captures all the properties of linearity articulated by Thurstone, is the simple logistic model known as the Rasch model

(Rasch 1960) (see *Rasch Measurement, Theory of*). The formal relationship between Thurstone's law of comparative judgment and the Rasch model is provided in Andrich (1978b).

See also: Latent Trait Measurement Models; Scaling Methods; Attidudes; Rasch Measurement, Theory of

References

Andrich D 1978a A rating formulation for ordered response categories. *Psychometrika* 43(4): 561–73
Andrich D 1978b Relationships between the Thurstone and Rasch approaches to item scaling. *Appl. Psychol. Meas.* 2(3): 451–62
Andrich D 1988 The application of an unfolding model of the PIRT type for the measurement of attitude. *Appl. Psychol. Meas.* 12(1): 33–51
Bock R D 1975 *Multivariate Statistical Methods in Behavioral Research*. McGraw-Hill, New York
Bock R D, Jones L V 1968 *The Measurement and Prediction of Judgment and Choice*. Holden-Day, San Francisco, California
Coombs C H 1964 *A Theory of Data*. Wiley, New York
Edwards A L 1957 *Techniques of Attitude Scale Construction*. Appleton–Century–Crofts, New York
Guttman L 1950 The problem of attitude and opinion measurement. In: Stouffer A et al. (eds.) 1950 *Measurement and Prediction: Studies in Social Psychology in World War II*, Vol. 4. Princeton Unversity Press, Princeton, New Jersey
Rasch G 1960 (reprinted 1980) *Probabilistic Models for Some Intelligence and Attainment Tests*. University of Chicago Press, Chicago, Illinois
Thurstone L L 1925 A method of scaling psychological and educational tests. *J. Educ. Psychol.* 16: 433–51
Thurstone L L 1926 The scoring of individual performance. *J. Educ. Psychol.* 17: 446–57
Thurstone L L 1959 *The Measurement of Values*. University of Chicago Press, Chicago, Illinois
Togerson W S 1958 *Theory and Methods of Scaling*. Wiley, New York

Validity

R. A. Zeller

That validity is essential to successful scientific activity is widely accepted among science methodologists, theoreticians, researchers, and philosophers. However, the reaction of most scientists to the question of validity has been one of the recitation of abstract ritualistic dogma of validity's importance, rather than a serious investigation of the place of validity in scientific research. In this entry, validity is first defined and contrasted with its companion concept in the measure-

ment process, reliability; the various types of validity are then described; and finally, a new definition of validity is offered.

1. The Definition of Validity

A "valid" research finding is one in which there is isomorphism between the reality that exists in the world and the description of that reality. A measure is valid if it measures what it is intended to measure. In other words, an indicator of some abstract concept is valid to the extent that it measures what it purports to measure. In science, indicators "purport" to measure concepts. Statements about relationships among concepts proceed in an orderly fashion only when indicators provide accurate representations of their respective concepts. When indicators are not valid, statements about the relationships among concepts become distorted.

There is widespread agreement that valid measurement is crucial to the success of scientific endeavors. For example, Hauser (1969 pp. 127–29) remarks: 'I should like to venture the judgment that it is inadequate measurement, more than inadequate concept or hypothesis, that has plagued social researchers and prevented fuller explanations of the variances with which they are confounded.' In a similar vein, Greer (1989) states:

> The link between observation and formulation is one of the most difficult and crucial of the scientific enterprises. It is the process of interpreting our theory or, as some say, of "operationalizing our concepts." Our creations in the world of possibility must be fitted to the world of probability; in Kant's epigram, "Concepts without percepts are empty." It is also the process of relating our observations to theory; to finish the epigram, "Percepts without concepts are blind." (p. 160)

Why, however, when it is so crucial to the success of scientific endeavors, does valid measurement receive ritualistic recitations instead of serious investigation? There are two important interrelated answers to this question. First, theoretical considerations (and hence, considerations of validity) were excluded from an early, important definition of "measurement." Second, it is immensely difficult to provide compelling evidence of validity. Each of these impediments to a vigorous and rigorous investigation of validity are discussed below.

1.1 An Inadequate Definition of Measurement

Stevens (1951 p. 22) defines measurement as " . . . the assignment of numbers to objects or events according to rules." While this definition takes into account the empirical activities associated with the measurement process, it ignores the theoretical ones. For example, suppose a researcher wanted to measure the concept "self-esteem." According to Stevens, the researcher would have accomplished that task by constructing a set of rules for the assignment of a number to each individual. Presumably, that number would empirically represent that individual's level of self-esteem. One possible "rule for assigning numbers" is: height divided by weight. Thus, someone who was 175 centimeters tall and weighed 70 kilograms would be assigned the number 2.5 (175/70 = 2.5). Another person who was 120 centimeters tall and weighed 60 kilograms would be assigned the number 2 (120/60 = 2).

However, height and weight do not provide a "valid" representation of an individual's self-esteem. The problem is that this rule fully satisfied Stevens's definition of measurement. More generally, any definition of measurement that considers only the world of sense experience is inadequate. An adequate definition of measurement must also include consideration of abstract theoretical concepts. In scientific discourse, when indicators are invalid, scientific statements about relationships among variables are distorted.

While Stevens allegedly defined measurement, he actually provided a context for assessing reliability. Reliability focuses on the extent to which a measurement procedure consistently yields the same result on repeated observations. Put in another way, reliability is the degree of repeatability or consistency of empirical measurements. In scientific discourse, when indicators are unreliable, scientific statements about relationships among the variables are obscured. Thus, the appropriate epigram concerning reliability and validity is:

Unreliability obscures; invalidity distorts

Stevens's definition lays the groundwork for reliability assessment; it focuses on the empirical. His definition is not relevant for validity assessment; it ignores the theoretical. Because it focuses exclusively on the empirical, reliability is much easier to assess than validity. Reliability assessment requires no more than manipulation of observations, whereas validity assessment requires consideration of both observations and concepts (see *Reliability*).

1.2 An Adequate Definition of Measurement

In this regard, Blalock (1968 p. 12) observes that "theorists often use concepts that are formulated at rather high levels of abstraction. These are quite different from the variables that are the stock-in-trade of empirical sociologists." In this tradition, measurement can be defined as the process of linking concepts to indicants. To illustrate the measurement process, the situation where a researcher wants to measure the concept "self-esteem" can again be used. According to Blalock, the research must engage in a variety of tasks to provide a valid measure of this concept. These tasks include: (a) defining the concept "self-esteem"; (b) selecting indicants that will provide empirical representations of the concept "self-esteem"; (c) obtaining empirical information for those indicants; and (d) evaluating the degree to which those indicants did, in fact, provide a valid representation of the concept "self-esteem." These four tasks can be outlined as follows:

(a) Defining the concept "self-esteem"—Rosenberg (1979 p. 54) defines self-esteem as a positive or negative orientation toward oneself. An individual of low self-esteem "lacks respect for himself, considers himself unworthy, inadequate, or otherwise seriously deficient as a person." On the other hand, a person of high self-esteem consider themself to be person of worth. High self-esteem carries no connotations of "feelings of superiority, arrogance, conceit, contempt for others, overweening pride." This, then constitutes a widely used theoretical definition of the concept "self-esteem."

(b) Selecting measures of self-esteem—Having defined self-esteem theoretically, Rosenberg then constructs indicants that he considers as measuring the concept (Rosenberg 1979 p. 291). The indicants are statements about oneself; subjects respond to these indicants by expressing strong agreement, agreement, disagreement, or strong disagreement. Some indicants are written with a positive description of self; examples include: "On the whole, I am satisfied with myself," and "I feel that I'm a person of worth, at least on an equal plane with others." Other indicants are written with a negative description of self; examples include: "I feel I do not have much to be proud of," and "I wish I could have more respect for myself." Rosenberg constructed five positive and five negative indicants of self-esteem.

(c) Obtaining empirical information for indicants— Rosenberg then obtains data for these indicants by asking adolescents to respond to each indicant in terms of the response categories.

(d) Evaluating the validity of the indicants—To what degree do the indicants represent the concept "self-esteem" empirically? The answer to this question is a major challenge in scientific discourse. There are a variety of approaches to this problem.

2. Types of Validity in Concept Measurement

Validation occurs within the context of a measurement situation. Thus, it is not the indicant itself that is being validated, but rather, it is the purpose for which the indicant is being used that is submitted to validation procedures. In Cronbach's words (1971 p. 447): "One validates, not a test, but an *interpretation of data arising from a specified procedure*."

2.1 Content Validity

Fundamentally, content validity focuses on the extent to which the content of an indicant corresponds to the content of the concept it is designed to measure. Rosenberg's self-esteem indicants focused on the same content as the conceptual definition of self-esteem. Thus, these items were judged to be content valid.

Establishing content validity involves specifying a domain of content for a concept and constructing or selecting indicants that represent that domain. Neither of these tasks can be done unequivocally. First, is Rosenberg's definition of self-esteem adequate? This question cannot be answered with certainty because of the

fundamental openness of meaning that is characteristic of concepts. As Kaplan (1964 p. 63) asserts: "As the theory is used—for scientific as well as practical purposes—its meaning is progressively more fixed; but some degree of openness always remains." Thus, in content validation, "acceptance of the universe of content as defining the variable to be measured is essential" (Cronbach and Meehl 1955 p. 282). Obtaining this acceptance has proved to be exceedingly difficult for many of the concepts in the social and behavioral sciences.

Second, do Rosenberg's indicants represent the domain of content? This question cannot be answered with certainty either, because of the fundamental nature of indicants. Specifically, indicants are designed to be as specific, as exact, and as bounded as the conceptual definitions and the research settings will allow. Hence, indicants never duplicate nor fully exhaust the meaning of the respective concept. Consequently, there are no commonly agreed criteria for evaluating whether content validity has or has not been established. Thus, while it is important to make a reasonable effort to establish the content validity of a set of indicants, these two liabilities prevent content validation from being sufficient for establishing the validity of indicants as measures of their respective concepts.

2.2 Criterion-related Validity

Criterion-related validity focuses on the correlation between an indicant and some criterion variable of interest. Within this context, the criterion-related validity of college board exam scores may be established by the degree to which they are correlated with performance in college. If this correlation is high, the indicant is considered to be criterion-related valid *for that criterion*.

There are two types of criterion-related validity: concurrent and predictive. *Concurrent validity* describes a criterion-related validity situation where the criterion variable exists in the present. For example, a researcher might wish to establish the awareness of students about their performance in school during the past year. In this situation, each student could be asked the question: "What was your grade point average last year?" This response could then be concurrent criterion validated by correlating it with the grade point average obtained from the school's records office.

Predictive validity describes a criterion-related validity situation where the criterion variable will not exist until later. For example, a researcher might wish to have students anticipate their performance in school during the next year. In this situation, each student could be asked the question: "What do you think your grade point average will be next year?" This response could then be predictive criterion validated by correlating it with the grade point average obtained from the school's records office after the elapse of a year.

Most tests used to screen applications for various occupational and educational opportunities are, by nature, concerned with predictive validity. The purpose of the test is to differentiate between those who will and will not be successful. Ordinarily, one cannot fully establish the predictive validity of such an instrument. This is because the instrument is actually used to choose who will and who will not be allowed into the respective positions. For example, suppose that a university entrance examination is administered to 2,400 applicants. The university establishes a minimum score for admission and admits those who surpass this score. The university then wishes to discover whether the entrance examination is effective in predicting who will and will not succeed in the program. It embarks upon "an evaluation research project" to assess the predictive validity of the entrance examination. The following discussion summarizes the practical and conceptual difficulties that such a research team would face.

In order to explore this situation, it is necessary to make some reasonable assumptions about the setting. First, there is a positive and relatively strong correlation between the score on the entrance examination and performance in the program. Second, the university will only admit half of the applicants. Third, the university uses performance on the entrance examination as the only criterion for admission. Fourth, only those students who exhibit a certain level of performance or better "succeed" in the program. Figure 1 provides a scatterplot of the behavior that would occur if these assumptions were, in fact, the case. In Fig. 1, the horizontal axis represents the score on the entrance exam (1 = lowest score; 6 = highest score). The vertical axis represents performance in the program (1 = lowest performance; 6 = highest performance). There are 100 observations at each of the 24 locations designated by the letters A, B, C, and D; these represent the 2,400 applicants to the program. The correlation between exam score and program performance is positive and, by social science standards, relatively strong ($r = 0.64$).

However, the university can only admit half of the applications to the program. The university admits those with a score of 4 or more on the admissions test (As and Cs in Fig. 1). A score of 4 or more is needed in order to "succeed" in the program. Hence, As are admitted and succeed; Bs are not admitted, but would have succeeded if they had been admitted; Cs are admitted but fail; and Ds are not admitted but would have failed in the program if they had been admitted.

After the program is over, the research team correlates entrance exam scores and performance in program ratings. This correlation is calculated on only the 1,200 who were admitted to the program (the As and the Cs). There was no "performance" score for those who were not admitted to the program (the Bs and the Ds). Hence, they are "phantom" observations. If they had been admitted to the program, 25 percent of them (the Bs) would have succeeded while 75 percent of them (the Ds) would have failed.

The correlation between entrance exam and program performance is positive and, by social science standards, relatively weak ($r = 0.32$). This delights the critics of the entrance exam who infer that the entrance exam provides little useful information about the potential for success in the program. Further examination of Fig. 1, however, shows that 75 percent of those admitted to the program succeeded. This success rate is substantially higher than the 50 percent success rate if applicants were admitted randomly. The correlation was weak because those who scored low on the entrance exam (and who probably would have failed the program) were not admitted to the program. Thus, the entrance examination is a more valuable tool than it appears in deciding which applicants are most likely to succeed by examining the performances of those who were admitted.

This illustrates a fundamental difficulty in the use of predictive validity in social research. When a predictor is used to choose which subset of applicants from a larger pool will be provided with an opportunity to succeed in a program, later attempts to assess the effectiveness of the predictor variable are undermined by the fact that the predictor was used as the admissions criterion.

Another difficulty in the use of criterion-related validity is that, for many concepts, no appropriate criterion measure exists. For example, there is no known criterion variable for self-esteem. The more abstract the concept, the more difficult it is to establish the viability of a potential criterion variable. Thus, while criterion-related validity appears to be an attractive method for establishing measurement validity, its value is largely an illusion.

2.3 Construct Validity

Construct validity focuses on the assessment of whether a particular measure relates to other measures consistent with a theoretically anticipated way. As Cronbach and Meehl (1955 p. 290) observe: "Construct validation takes place when an investigator believes his instrument reflects a particular construct, to which are attached certain meanings. The proposed interpretation generates specific testable hypotheses, which are a means of confirming

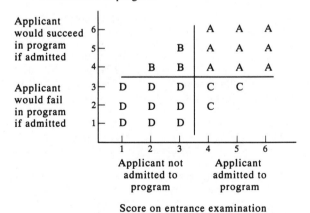

Figure 1
Relationship between entrance examination and performance in program

or disconfirming the claim." Thus, construct validity is established within a given theoretical context.

Establishing construct validity involves the following steps:

(a) defining concepts and anticipating relationships among them;

(b) selecting indicants to represent each concept;

(c) establishing the dimensionality of the indicants;

(d) constructing scales of indicants;

(e) calculating correlations among these scales; and

(f) comparing the observed correlations with the anticipated ones.

These steps are examined in turn below.

(a) Defining concepts and anticipating relationships among them—This step involves construction of a theory by defining concepts and anticipating relationships among them. For example, a theory might assert that social background factors cause self-esteem which, in turn, causes social and political knowledge, attitudes, and behavior. Specifically, a positive social background will cause a positive self-esteem which, in turn, will cause greater social and political knowledge and more positive social and political attitudes and behaviors.

(b) Selecting indicants to represent each concept—This step involves selection of indicants that represent each concept contained within the theory. For the purpose of this example, a researcher might wish to select the following indicants to represent each concept. Social background may be represented by years of father's formal education and years of mother's formal education. Self-esteem may be represented by the indicants that Rosenberg (1979 p. 291) used. Social and political knowledge, attitudes, and behavior may be represented by items measuring understanding of democratic principles, knowledge of government services, knowledge of political authorities, political efficacy, participation in community activities, and participation in school activities. An item measuring political cynicism may be used as a negative measure of this concept.

(c) Establishing the dimensionality of the indicants— The indicants designed to measure self-esteem may or may not represent the concept "self-esteem" well. If the indicants do represent the concept well, these indicants should intercorrelate positively and strongly. A common statistical procedure to evaluate the degree to which indicants intercorrelate positively and strongly is factor analysis. If a factor analysis reveals that the items correlate strongly and positively with one factor and do not correlate in a systematic fashion with any other factor, the dimensionality of those items as measures of their respective concept is established. When this does not occur, the construct validity of the items as measures of the concept is suspect. For a discussion of what is occurring when the dimensionality of the indicants is not established, see Zeller and Carmines (1980).

(d) Constructing scales of indicants—Once the dimensionality of the indicants is established, scales must be constructed so that a single measure of each concept may be used. A common way to construct such a scale from Likert items (such as those used in Rosenberg's self-esteem scale) is first to reverse score the items that measure the concept negatively. Then sum the scores of all items such that the higher the scale for an individual, the higher that individual's self-esteem is measured to be. An alternative procedure involves standardization of the items prior to implementing the above procedures.

(e) Calculating correlations among these scales—Once the scales have been constructed, they can be correlated with one another.

(f) Comparing the observed correlations with the anticipated ones—A pattern of correlations among the scales that is consistent with the pattern of correlations predicted by the theory provides both confirmation of the theory and construct validation for the scales designed to measure each of the concepts.

The usefulness of these techniques does not always lead to unambiguous inferences about the theoretical dimensionality of concepts. Therefore, factor analysis cannot be used as the sole criterion for establishing the adequacy of the concept-indicant linkage. On the contrary, naive and simplistic interpretation of factor structures (such as the automatic use of the default 1.0 eigenvalue cutoff for inclusion of factors and the varimax rotation) can be misleading in terms of the theoretical nature of the empirical indicants. Specifically, respondents may answer items without regard to their content. Some respondents engage in "response set" where they will agree (or disagree) with every item. This method artifact and others can systematically alter the pattern of intercorrelations among the indicants which, in turn, leads to a faulty inference about content validity.

Thus, the process of construct validation is, by necessity, theory laden. Indeed, it is impossible to "validate" a measure of a concept unless there exists a theoretical network that surrounds the concept. At the same time, this "theoretical network" need not be formal and fully developed to guide construct validity efforts. As Cronbach and Meehl (1955 p. 284) note: "The logic of construct validation is involved whether the construct is highly systematized or loose, used in ramified theory or a few simple propositions, used in absolute propositions or probability statements." What is required is that it is possible to state several theoretically derived hypotheses involving the particular concept. For a more complete discussion of the procedures for handling external associations with sets of indicants, see Curtis and Jackson (1962), and Sullivan and Feldman (1979).

However, what would the appropriate inference have been if the construct validity evidence had been negative? What should a researcher conclude if the empirically observed relationships are inconsistent with those that were theoretically anticipated? Four different interpretations are possible (Cronbach and Meehl 1955 p. 295). One possible interpretation is that the indicants of the concept lack construct validity; that is, that the indicants do not measure the concept that they purport to measure. Unfortunately, negative construct validity evidence is also consistent with three other interpretations: (a) the theoretical arrangement of the concepts was incorrect; and/or (b) the procedures for deriving hypotheses from the theory were incorrect; and/or (c) the indicants of the other concepts in the theory lack construct validity.

There is no foolproof procedure for determining which of these interpretations of negative evidence is correct in any given instance. Bits of evidence can be accrued from additional data analysis that may support one or more of these interpretations. However, it is important to acknowledge that the process of construct validation is more analogous to a detective searching for clues than it is analogous to an accountant proving out a balance. A researcher does not establish validity once and for all; instead, a researcher obtains bits of information that are consistent or inconsistent with a construct validity interpretation. The more systematic the pattern of such bits of information with construct validity, the more confidence can be placed in that interpretation.

3. Toward a New Definition of Validity

Each of the above procedures is useful in establishing the validity of scientific measurement. At the same time, all of the above procedures designed to establish measurement validity leave the researcher unsatisfied. Indeed, a researcher can fulfill all of the above criteria for validity and still be led to erroneous inferences about what is occurring. This happens because all of the above procedures assume a quantitative, survey research approach to social knowledge. However, such an approach used in isolation from other approaches runs the risk of missing important aspects of the situation and missing opportunities to provide even more compelling evidence of the causal linkages contained within the theory. The purpose of this section is to address how a researcher may wish to validate results by employing nonquantitative methods.

Qualitative researchers define validity in terms of "deeper knowledge of social phenomena . . . developed in intimate relationship with data" (Strauss 1987 p. 6). Validity from the qualitative perspective can be characterized as "pressing the flesh." Survey researchers search for statistical relationships among variables (Zeller and Carmines 1980). Validity from the survey research perspective can be characterized as "chasing the decimal

point." Experimentalists answer the validity question by appealing to the truth or falsity of causal propositions (Cook and Campbell 1979 p. 37). Validity from the experimental perspective can be characterized as "producing the effect." None of these approaches to validity, taken in isolation from the others, satisfy the quest for isomorphism between reality and observation. Therefore, it is necessary to offer a new definition of validity. This definition could be the criterion that social research would employ:

> A valid phenomenon has been established when pressing the flesh, chasing the decimal point, and producing the effect all provide the same messages about the nature of the phenomenon.

These criteria for establishing validity are both simple and awesome. According to this definition, validity is as much a process as a product. In this view, validity requires method diversity rather than method specialization; it requires both theoretical insight and attention to detail. Validity demands a virtual obsession with the identification of argumentation and observational flaws and establishing ways that those flaws can be handled convincingly. Under these conditions, it is not surprising that efforts to conduct valid research from the perspective of a single methodological approach are unsatisfying.

Strauss does an admirable job of pressing the flesh, but his refusal to chase the decimal point or produce the effect make his work uncompelling. His strength in providing insight through rich description is not matched by an effort to explore the limits of generalizability through parameter estimation of demonstrable causation. He therefore fails the validity test outlined above.

Jöreskog (1973), although an extremely clever and creative data analyst, does not appear to have any appreciation of the challenges to validity presented by data collection situations. Moreover, despite the insightfulness, elegance, and creativity of their work, it is naive for Heise and Bohrnstedt (1970) to claim to have identified a formula which differentiates reliability from validity when their formula does no more than differentiate between two kinds of reliability. They also fail the test of validity.

Few experimentalists are as gifted and creative as Aronson (1980), yet the application of his work to certain situations is unconvincing and unsatisfying. His causal propositions are demonstrated well and he is to be commended for his noble attempt to bridge the gap between qualitative and experimental work. However, he generalizes his results well beyond reasonable bounds, and the gap between his intuitive form of qualitative work and his laboratory experiments strains credulity. Thus, Aronson has clearly moved in a productive direction. At the same time, there remains an uncomfortable sense that much is left to be done.

3.1 Establishing Isomorphism between Reality and Observation

In order for research data to speak most powerfully to the

question being raised by the researcher, the above techniques should be used in concert. It is more difficult to be misled by the results that triangulate multiple techniques with compatible strengths than it is to be misled by a single technique which suffers from inherent weaknesses.

Hence, the general strategy of combining qualitative, survey, and experimental observation is that the methods be used interactively. While such a position is easy to articulate, it is difficult to implement. This implementation challenge is due in part to the fact that most researchers have a research method loyalty. Researchers are comfortable operating in their own area of methodological expertise, but are vulnerable outside that area. Moreover, the academic reward structure provides disincentives for such methodological diversity. In addition, those who are true believers in any technique look with skepticism upon someone who alleges expertise not only in that area but in other areas as well.

At the same time, one method used in isolation does not provide compelling answers to many research problems. The reason for this is clear. Different techniques differ dramatically in their purposes, goals, objectives, tactics, strategies, strengths, and weaknesses. The original questions that prompt the research and the new questions that emerge from its results require a blending of methods. As a result, while many scholars endorse the idea of combining various research techniques, few actually do it. The purpose of this section is to explore ways that alternative research techniques can be blended into a coherent research strategy.

The general strategy for establishing the isomorphism between reality and observation focuses on the definition of the problem. What is known and what needs to be known about the phenomenon? This phenomenon can be illustrated by the concept of "political correctness." Leo (1990 p. 22) defines political correctness in the popular press as "the narrow orthodoxy now ascendant on American campuses large and small . . . Affirmative action, bussing, gay rights, women's studies, the PLO, animal rights, bilingualism, the self-segregation of blacks on campus and censorship in the pursuit of tolerance are all politically correct." These causes have been championed by American political liberals. Critics of this concept argue that "political correctness" is a shorthand for conservative resistance to changes that are sweeping modern society.

In order to make valid observations about political correctness, a researcher may wish to employ qualitative techniques first. The researcher may wish to observe classroom discussions, talk to students, look at the content of papers, conduct focused interviews, and so on. In this way, the researcher can obtain a sense of whether allegedly prescribed ideas dominate discourse and whether proscribed ideas, when articulated, are negatively sanctioned. By "pressing the flesh," it is possible to obtain a sense of the degree to which students perceive a need to bring their own opinions into agreement with the opinions of their instructors.

The researcher may wish to conduct surveys to dis-

cover the percentage of students who hold one view or another. That percentage can then be compared to the percentage who articulate these views in student term papers. By "chasing the decimal point," one can establish whether a shift in opinion between the students' articulation of their own ideas and what they write in term papers occurs.

Experimental and quasi-experimental data may also address this question by establishing the conditions under which the ideas expressed in interaction do and do not coincide with the ideas written for evaluated term papers. By "producing the effect," one can establish what behaviors will and will not produce a classroom environment characterized by "political correctness".

If the messages received from each of these three approaches to the question provide similar "messages" about the pressure toward ideational conformity, a "valid" conclusion about the concept and its operation is warranted. For example, suppose an observer notes that some ideas are clearly prescribed while others are proscribed; a survey researcher shows that the percentage of students who articulate an idea on an anonymous questionnaire is higher than the percentage who articulate that idea in term papers, and an experimenter shows that an instructor can eliminate that change in percentage by including certain instructions, which are not currently in use, about the writing of term papers. All of these messages consistently demonstrate the operation of political correctness validly.

The messages received could consistently challenge the operation of the concept of political correctness. For example, suppose a wide variety of ideas are voiced without proscription, the percentages who articulate ideas anonymously and on term papers is equal, and no change in instructions alters this percentage. In this situation, all of the messages consistently demonstrate the operation of political fairness validly.

When the messages are in conflict, no valid conclusion can be drawn. For example, what is the researcher to conclude about the validity of political correctness if some ideas are clearly prescribed while others are proscribed, but the percentage who articulate ideas anonymously equals the percentage who write those ideas on a term paper? What should be concluded if a wide variety of ideas are voiced without proscription but the percentage of students who articulate an idea on an anonymous questionnaire is higher than the percentage who articulate that idea in term papers. These situations do not warrant an unambiguous judgment about the validity of the concept.

4. Conclusion

Validity has been considered in this entry. An indicator is valid to the degree that it empirically represents the concept it purports to measure. As such, valid measurement becomes the *sine qua non* of science. There are several strategies for establishing valid measurement including content, criterion-related, and construct validity. Though useful, each of these approaches is beset by difficulties that make an unambiguous inference about validity unwarranted. Specifically, inferences about validity do not lend themselves to solely quantitative or statistical solutions. On the contrary, an interactive research strategy combining quantitative and qualitative is advocated. A valid inference occurs when there is no conflict between messages received as a result of the use of a variety of different methodological procedures.

See also: Scientific Methods in Educational Research; Triangulation in Educational Research

References

Aronson E 1980 *The Social Animal*, 3rd edn. W H Freeman, San Francisco, California.

Blalock H M 1968 The measurement problem: a gap between the languages of theory and research In: Blalock H M, Blalock A B (eds.) 1968 *Methodology in Social Research*. McGraw-Hill, New York

Cook T D, Campbell D T 1979 *Quasi-Experimentation: Design & Analysis Issues for Field Settings*. Rand McNally, Chicago, Illinois

Cronbach L J 1971 Test validation. In: Thorndike R L (ed.) 1971 *Educational Measurement*, 2nd edn. American Council on Education, Washington, DC

Cronbach L J, Meehl P E 1955 Construct validity in psychological tests. *Psychol. Bull.* 52(4): 281–302

Curtis R F, Jackson E F 1962 Multiple indicators in survey research. *Am. J. Sociol.* 68: 195–204

Greer S 1989 *The Logic of Social Inquiry*, 2nd edn. Transaction, New Brunswick, New Jersey

Hauser P 1969 Comments on Coleman's paper. In: Bierstedt R (ed.) 1969 *A Design for Sociology: Scope, Objectives, and Methods*. American Academy of Political and Social Science, Philadelphia, Pennsylvania

Heise D R, Bohrnstedt G W 1970 Validity, invalidity, and reliability. In: Borgatta E F, Bohrnstedt G W (eds.) 1970 *Sociological Methodology 1970*, Jossey-Bass, San Francisco, California

Jöreskog K G 1970 A general method for analysis of covariance structures. *Biometrika* 57(2): 239–51

Kaplan A 1964 *The Conduct of Inquiry: Methodology for Behavioral Science*. Chandler, Scranton, Pennsylvania

Leo J 1990 The academy's new ayatollahs. US *News and World Report* December 10, p. 22

Rosenberg M 1979 *Conceiving the Self*. Basic Books, New York

Stevens S S 1951 Mathematics, measurement and psychophysics. In: Stevens S S (ed.) 1951 *Handbook of Experimental Psychology*. Wiley, New York

Strauss A L 1987 *Qualitative Analysis for Social Scientists*. Cambridge University Press, New York

Sullivan J A, Feldman S 1979 *Multiple Indicators: An Introduction*. Sage, Beverly Hills, California

Zeller R A, Carmines E G 1980 *Measurement in the Social Sciences: The Link Between Theory and Data*. Cambridge University Press, New York

(b) Item Response Theory Measurement

Essays: Equating of Marks

D. Andrich

The science of educational measurement has developed in order to enhance the validity and reliability of tests. Unfortunately, reliability can be attained readily at the expense of validity, which is illustrated by the use of tests composed of multiple-choice items compared to those that require extended responses. The multiple-choice item was developed because of its reliability in scoring, and has been accompanied by a voluminous amount of methodological research according to classical test theory (CTT), generalizability test theory (GTT), and latent trait theory (LTT). One feature of LTT is that it uses a response function with the item as the unit of analysis, making it possible to use different items for different persons, yet still estimate the location of all persons and all items on the same continuum (Weiss 1983, Kubinger 1988, Julian and Wright 1988).

Despite this theoretical and practical work on multiple-choice items, schools, colleges, and universities continue to require students to provide extended responses, often in the form of essays. Essays are considered a more valid means for assessing the higher levels of knowledge associated with analyzing, synthesizing, and evaluating information (e.g., Bloom et al. 1956).

Before proceeding, an important point of nomenclature must be clarified. It is common in LTT to refer to the location of a person or a trait as the person's "*ability*." This term can sometimes be interpreted as some ability determined entirely genetically. However, that is not the intention in LTT: instead, it is intended that a latent or underlying ability to produce a set of related manifest performances is inferred from the manifest performances. This latent ability to perform arises from the sum of all the person's relevant learning experiences. To avoid misinterpretation, the term "*ability/performance*" will be used throughout for the location on the latent trait.

Surprisingly, relatively little research on LTT has been applied to essays where the scores may range beyond single digit integers even though many features are directly analogous. First, more than one question is usually to be answered, which has the same purpose as having many multiple-choice questions—to sample a greater variety of content and to have a more precise estimate of each person's ability/performance. Second, often there is a choice, which acknowledges that it

is not necessary to answer only one set of questions to be able to provide evidence of appropriate knowledge in a certain field. Traditional text books (e.g., Chase 1978) consider that choice should not be permitted because scores obtained on different combinations of questions cannot be compared properly. Nevertheless, choice is provided in essay-type examinations, in part because of time constraints, but in part because it is considered more valid to provide students with some choice. The task then is to account for the difficulties of the questions, which is again analogous to the multiple-choice context–items are invariably of different difficulty, and using LTT it is possible to locate persons on the same continuum even though they have answered different questions. This entry applies a latent trait model to equate questions of an examination which was composed of four questions, where the maximum mark for each question was 25, and where the students were to answer any two of the four questions.

1. The Model

The model applied is an extension of Rasch's (1980) simple logistic model (SLM) for dichotomously scored items (Andrich 1988, Wright and Stone 1979). This model was derived theoretically by Rasch (1968), Andersen (1977), and Andrich (1978), and has been studied further (Wright and Masters 1982, Andrich 1985, Jansen and Roskam 1986), usually where the number of graded responses has been limited to single digit values. However, this procedure has had very restricted application in practice.

The SLM specifies a location parameter (ability/performance β) of the person and a location parameter (difficulty δ) of the item and takes the form:

$$\Pr\{X_{ni} = x; \beta_n, \delta_i\} = [\exp\{x\beta_n - x\delta_i\}]/\gamma_{ni} \quad (1)$$

where $\gamma_{ni} = 1 + \exp\{\beta_n - \delta_i\}$ is the normalizing factor that ensures that $\Pr\{X_{ni} = 0\} + \Pr\{X_{ni} = 1\} = 1$.

The extended logistic model (ELM) for ordered categories takes the form

$$\Pr\{x; \beta_n, \delta_i, \tau_i\} = [\exp\{x(\beta_n - \delta_i)$$

$$- \tau_{1i} - \tau_{2i} \ldots - \tau_{xi}\}]/\gamma_{ni} \quad (2)$$

where (a) τ_{xi} is the threshold between the (x-1)th and the xth response categories, there being m thresholds with $\tau_0 \equiv 0$; (b) $x \in \{0,1,2, \ldots, x, \ldots, m\}$ corresponds to the ordered category of the response; and (c)

$$\gamma_{ni} = \sum_{k=1}^{m} \exp\left[k(\beta_n - \delta_i) - \left(\sum_{y=1}^{k} \tau_{yi} \right) \right]$$

again is the normalizing factor. With m thresholds, a constraint such as $\Sigma_{x=1}^{m} \hat{\tau}_{xi} = 0$ is necessary within each item and $\Sigma_{i=1}^{1} \hat{\delta}_i = 0$ across items.

The curve of the rate of change of the expected value (EVC) with respect to β is given by

$$E[X_i; \beta, \delta_i, \tau_i] = \sum_{x=1}^{m} xPr\{x; \beta, \delta_i, \tau_i\}. \qquad (3)$$

These curves are shown in Fig. 1 for each question of the example. It can be seen that they have different locations (difficulties) and slopes. Different slopes result from different distances between the thresholds among questions and they correspond to the traditional

notion of discrimination—the closer the thresholds the greater the discrimination.

It is possible to estimate all thresholds for each question. However, where the maximum score is large, for example m = 25 as in the data set in this entry, it is extravagant to estimate all parameters. Here, the thresholds are reparameterized so that their spread, skew, and kurtosis are summarized: specifically,

$$- \sum_{k=1}^{x} \tau_{ki} = x_i(m_i - x_i)\theta_i.$$
$$+ x_i(m_i - x_i)(2x_i - m_i)\eta_i$$
$$+ x_i(m_i - x_i)(5x_i^2 - 5x_im_i + m_i^2 + 1)\psi_i$$

where θ_i is the average equal half-distance between thresholds, and where η_i and ψ_i indicate the asymmetric deviation (skewness) and symmetric deviation (kurtosis) from equidistance respectively. Pedler (1987) has derived the general expression for generating the successive polynomials for the category coefficients.

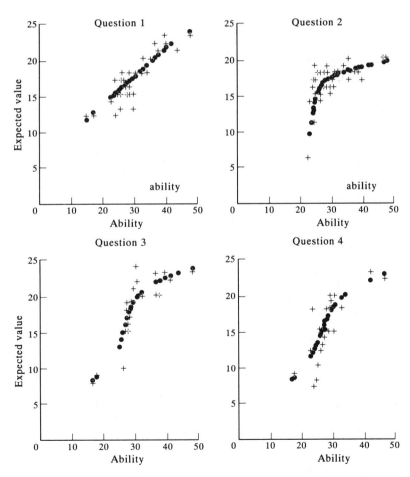

Figure 1
Points on the expected value curve (•) and observed scores (+) for each question

The following definitions further simplify the expressions: let

$$g_{1i} = g_1(x_i) = -x_i/m_i, \qquad\qquad \varphi(m_i) = \varphi_{1i};$$

$$g_{2i} = g_2(x_i) = x_i(m_i - x_i)/m_i^2, \qquad \varphi(m_i^2\theta_i) = \varphi_{2i};$$

$$g_{3i} = g_3(x_i) = x_i(m_i - x_i)(2x_i - m_i)/m_i^3, \qquad \varphi(m_i^3\eta_i) = \varphi_{3i};$$

$$g_{4i} = g_4(x_i) = x_i(m_i - x_i)(5x_i^2 - 5x_im_i + m_i^2 + 1)/m_i^4, \qquad \varphi(m_i^4\psi_i) = \varphi_{4i}.$$

The division of successive coefficients by m_i, m^2_i, etc, is used to account for the large value of m_i, and the consequent extremely small values of the parameters. Accordingly, the parameters δ_i, θ_i, and η_i are rescaled so that $\delta_i \to m_i\delta_i$, $\theta_i \to m_i^2\theta_i$, $\eta \to m_i^3\eta_i$, and $\psi \to m_i^4\psi$. In the subsequent presentation and in the results section these rescaled parameters are assumed. Using vector notation, the final probability is given by the simple equation:

$$\Pr\{x_{ni};\ \boldsymbol{\varphi},\ \beta_n\{ = [\exp\{g_i'\boldsymbol{\varphi}_i + x_{ni}\beta_n\}]/\gamma_{ni}. \qquad (4)$$

The basis for estimating the item parameter is the probability of the response pair (x_{ni}, x_{nj}) of each person n to a pair of questions i and j conditional on the total score $r_{nij} = x_{ni} + x_{nj}$. This is given by

$$\Pr\{(x_{ni}, x_{nj}) \mid r_{nij};\ \boldsymbol{\varphi}_i,\ \boldsymbol{\varphi}_j\} \qquad (5)$$

$$= \frac{\exp[g_i'\varphi_i + g_i'\varphi_j]}{\displaystyle\sum_{(x_{ni},x_{nj})\mid r_{nij}} \exp[g_i'\varphi_i + g_j'\varphi_j]}$$

in which the terms $\dfrac{1}{\gamma_{ni}\gamma_{nj}}$ and $\exp[_{nij}\beta_n]$ are eliminated.

This equation may be generalized across all pairs of items for each person, and then across all persons in deriving estimation equations for the item parameter estimates. Three points need to be noted in Eqn. (5). First, the person parameter β_n does not appear in the equation. Thus the estimates of the item parameters are independent of the distribution of abilities performances. Equally importantly, the equation implies that for a given total score of a person on two items which are intended to reflect the same latent trait, the differences in the responses to these two items is a function of the properties of the items, and not of the person. These properties include the relative difficulties of the items as in the dichotomous case, and in addition, the tendency for the items to spread, skew and flatten responses of each person, independently of the abilities performances of the different persons involved.

Second, when a person has a minimum total score of 0 on both items or a maximum score of $m_i + m_j$, the pair of responses are not included in the solution equations. Likewise, when a person has no response

to an item, that item is not paired with any other item. Thus missing data are handled routinely. Third, the generalization of Eqn. (5) across persons and items in the form of a continued product provides maximum likelihood-type estimates. However, because the same responses are used across different pairs of items, dependencies are created, and therefore the tests of fit and standard errors cannot be derived directly. The parameter estimates themselves are not affected unduly because the dependencies simply provide redundant, not contradictory, information. Nevertheless, further research, both analytic and through simulation studies following on from the work of van der Linden and Eggen (1986) in the dichotomous case, is required, and this is currently being carried out. This pairwise algorithm was studied extensively by Choppin (1983).

Given the estimates of the item parameters, and treating them as fixed, the ability/performance of each person is estimated by a direct maximum likelihood equation which takes the simple form

$$r_n = \sum_i x_{ni}\Pr\{x_{ni};\ \hat{\beta}_n,\ \hat{\varphi}\}, \qquad (6)$$

where $r_n = \sum_i x_{ni}$, with the summations carried over the items to which person n has responded.

Various tests of fit can be devised to help check the degree to which the data conform to the model. In this case one test of fit used is a graphical one in which the observed value of each person on each of the questions is compared with its expected value given the estimate of ability/performance of each person and the estimate of the item parameters. A second one considers the standardized residuals for each person. These are illustrated in the context of the example.

2. The Example

The example (see Table 1) involved a unit of study in social research methods at Murdoch University (Australia), and part of the assessment involved an examination in which students had to answer two of the four questions set. The possible range of marks for each question was 0 to 25. The examiners were experienced lecturers in the course, and they were all involved in the construction of the four questions. In addition, they discussed their marking schedules and agreed on them before they began. From a statistical point of view, the example involves a very small data set—only 72 persons responding to only two of four questions. However, its advantages are that it is a real example (already mentioned), and in being small, it permits the complete data set to be studied in detail to illustrate the significant features of the model, the analysis, and the interpretation. It also shows that large samples are not required to carry out a specific analysis.

In the assessment of the responses of the students,

Table 1
Data from four exam questions, each with a maximum score of 25, in which only two questions needed to be answered: persons ordered by total score

Item			1	2	3	4	Item			1	2	3	4
Person	Total Score	Ability Performance	Q1 25a	Q2 25	Q3 25	Q4 25	Person	Total Score	Ability Performance	Q1 25	Q2 25	Q3 25	Q4 25
1	17	16.77			9	8	37	35	29.22	15	20		
2	20	15.12	12			8	38	35	29.22	16	19		
3	21	17.48	12		9		39	35	29.22	15	20		
4	22	23.49		15		7	40	35	30.06	17			18
5	24	24.01		6		18	41	36	28.29		18	18	
6	26	23.07	14			12	42	36	28.29		17	19	
7	26	24.55		18		8	43	36	29.23	15		21	
8	27	24.84		14		13	44	36	30.08		17		19
9	28	23.99	15		13		45	36	30.08		16		20
10	28	24.81		15	13		46	36	30.90	18	18		
11	28	25.15		18		10	47	37	30.20	13		24	
12	28	25.15		15		13	48	37	30.20	15		22	
13	29	24.66	17	12			49	37	31.32		17		20
14	29	24.66	12	17			50	37	32.71	18	19		
15	30	25.39		20	10		51	38	30.61			20	18
16	30	26.11	15			15	52	38	33.42	20			18
17	31	26.35		19		12	53	38	34.57	18	20		
18	31	25.48	15	16			54	38	34.57	19	19		
19	31	26.35		19		12	55	39	31.71		19	20	
20	32	26.04	13	19			56	39	34.82		19		20
21	32	26.40	17		15		57	39	36.47	20	19		
22	32	26.88		19		13	58	40	38.42	21	19		
23	32	27.56	17			15	59	40	38.42	21	19		
24	32	27.56	17			15	60	41	36.22		18	23	
25	33	26.77	17	16			61	41	36.22		21	20	
26	33	27.01	18		15		62	41	40.46	23	18		
27	33	27.01	17		16		63	42	37.22	22		20	
28	33	27.49		19		14	64	42	37.22	20		22	
29	33	28.33	15			18	65	42	39.41		19	23	
30	34	27.03		15	19		66	42	42.67	22	20		
31	34	27.03		16	18		67	43	43.30		20	23	
32	34	27.67	17		17		68	43	47.66		21		22
33	34	28.21		19		15	69	44	40.83	22		22	
34	35	28.40	16		19		70	44	43.09	21			23
35	35	29.06		17		18	71	44	48.02		21	23	
36	35	29.22	18	17			72	44	48.44	23	21		

a Maximum score for each question is 25.0

a different examiner graded each question. Thus it is impossible from this design to distinguish between the effects of examiners and the properties of the questions. However, the same analysis, with corresponding changes to the interpretation, could be carried out if the data had been generated by one grader who graded all questions, or if the data came from one question having been graded by four different graders.

It is clear that calculating the mean and other statistics for each question makes it impossible to compare them—the students chose the questions, the questions were not assigned at random to the students, and so it cannot be assumed that random variation would ensure that the average ability/performance of students answering each question was the same. Table 2 shows the estimates of the parameters obtained for each question. It is evident from this Table that there are some differences in location (difficulty) among the questions, with question 2 (Q2) being the most difficult and question 3 (Q3) the easiest. However, in the presence of different discriminations of the questions it is not straightforward to interpret differences in difficulty.

Figure 1 shows the expected value curves (EVCs), defined in Eqn. (3) for each question. In order to make the abilities have more customary values, the

Table 2
Parameter estimates for each question: constraint on the location parameter only

	Location δ_i	(SE)	Scale θ_i	(SE)	Skew η_i	(SE)	Kurtosis ψ_i	(SE)
Q1	0.61	(1.82)	49.84	(4.05)	13.35	(5.61)	−10.56	(5.90)
Q2	25.75	(1.15)	69.94	(4.74)	50.24	(3.59)	75.98	(5.74)
Q3	−20.50	(1.64)	102.82	(4.19)	−66.96	(5.09)	64.85	(6.37)
Q4	−5.86	(1.54)	86.59	(5.41)	−35.50	(4.22)	53.13	(6.33)
	0.00							

estimated abilities performances were transformed linearly by multiplying them by 0.5 and adding 20: they are notated by $\hat{\beta}^* = 0.5\,\hat{\beta} + 20$. These figures show that the observed values tend to congregate around the EVCs. In addition, the curves for Questions 2 and 3 are somewhat similar: the other two are different from these and from each other. In traditional terms, Question 2 has not operated as effectively in discriminating among the students as the other questions. However, it is important to appreciate that unlike the typical situation with many multiple-choice items, this question cannot be eliminated. This point is elaborated in the discussion.

The six test characteristic curves (TCC) for each combination of two questions, are of major interest. Fig. 2 shows these curves. It will be recalled that for each combination of questions, the total score is sufficient for estimating the ability/performance; therefore, each total score for each combination transforms to a single ability/performance. As expected from the EVCs, the TCCs are also different from each other, so that the same total score on different combinations leads to different

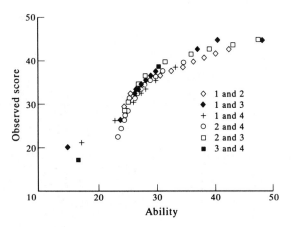

Figure 2
Points on the test characteristic curves for each of the combinations of questions mapped on to the same ability continuum

abilities. Interestingly, also, is that only two persons answered the combination of Questions 3 and 4, yet these total raw scores are mapped onto the same scale as are those of the other persons.

3. Further Issues, Interpretation, and Generalizations

So far, analogous features between tests composed of multiple-choice items and essay questions have been emphasized. There are, however, some important differences between the two, which rest primarily on the likely substantive applications of the procedure.

First, in university or college examinations it is unlikely that an examiner would wish to identify parameters of a question and use them again. Clearly, the questions may be retained or improved, but with the effect of the grader, the teaching, and so on it is more likely that the analysis would be repeated. Second, the transformed scores give a different ranking of students from the raw scores, even though the correlation in this case is high (0.92). This can have implications for who receives prizes, grades, or places in highly selective programs of study. Third, many of the usual aspects of the test of fit do not apply. For example, even though Question 2 did not operate as well as it might have and as well as the others, there was no opportunity to discard the question—given time, a remarking of all answers to that question might have been possible, but, as usual, there was no time in this case, and the original data had to be used. However, if for some reason the usual formal test of fit between the data and the model, which focuses on the questions, was required then the usual chi-square and likelihood ratio tests, which check specific violations of the model, can be used (Wright and Masters 1982).

Fourth, therefore, the important test of fit is at the level of the individual. Recall that because the total score on the questions answered is sufficient for the ability/performance estimate, all persons with the *same total score on the same questions* will have the same ability/performance estimate. This implies that the pattern or profile of scores is immaterial, and that

Table 3
Analysis of profiles of two persons who have answered the same two questions

Person	Questions	Ability/Performance estimate	Observed score	Expected score	Standardized residual z	Σz^2
17	2	26.350	19	16.563	0.683	0.923
	4		12	14.435	−0.676	
5	2	24.010	6	11.901	−0.974	4.026
	4		18	12.099	1.754	

there is no further information in the profile. This indeed is the case, provided that the data of the profile accord with the model. However, if the profile does not accord with the model, then the total score cannot be interpreted as sufficient, and therefore there is information in the profile. The key index for further information compares the observed and expected values for each question given the parameter estimates. If these are similar, then the profile has been recovered from the total score. Of course, the recovery will not be perfect, and the decision as to the adequacy of the recovery will be the usual combination of statistical inference and an understanding of what might be an important substantive difference.

For example, consider the information on the two profiles in Table 3. It is clear from the size of the standardized residuals that the profile of person 17 is recovered better than that of persons. Therefore, if there were the resources to remark some scripts, and if the choice were between reassessing the scripts of person 17 and person 5, the script of person 5 would be the one reassessed.

A single index for comparing consistency of profiles is given by the sum of the squared residuals, $\sum_{i} z^2_{ni}$, also shown in Table 3. Further research on the statistical properties of such an index is required, and while that research is important, the index can be used as it is in situations such as the one described. Already, many examining panels look for inconsistencies in marks awarded, and the procedure outlined systematizes this procedure by ordering the magnitude of the discrepancies. Then the number of profiles re-examined is as much a function of the expectations of examiners who have a substantive knowledge of the field, and the availability of resources, as it is a function of any statistical distribution.

See also: Rasch Measurement, Theory of; Rating Scale Analysis

References

Andersen E B 1977 Sufficient statistics and latent trait models. *Psychometri.* 42: 69–81
Andrich D 1978 A rating formulation for ordered response categories. *Psychometri.* 43: 561–73
Andrich D 1985 An elaboration of Guttman scaling with Rasch models for measurement. In: Brandon-Tuma N (ed.) 1985 *Sociological Methodology.* Jossey-Bass, San Francisco, California
Andrich D 1988 *Rasch Models for Measurement.* Sage, Beverly Hills, California
Bloom B S, Krathwohl D, Madaus G 1956 *Taxonomy of Educational Objectives.* McKay, New York
Chase C L 1978 *Measurement for Educational Evaluation,* 2nd edn. Addison-Wesley Reading Massachusetts
Choppin B 1983 *A Fully Conditional Estimation Procedure for Rasch Model Parameters.* Centre for the Study of Evaluation, Graduate School of Education, University of California, Los Angeles, California
Jansen P G W, Roskam E E 1986 Latent trait models and dichotomization of graded responses. *Psychometri.* 51: 149–74
Julian E R, Wright B D 1988 Using computerised patient simulations to measure the clinical competence of physicians. *Applied Measurement in Education* 1: 299–318
Kubinger K D 1988 On a Rash-model based test for noncomputerised adaptive testing. In: Langeheine R, Rost J (ed.) 1988 *Latent Trait and Latent Class Analysis.* Plenum, New York
Pedler P 1987 Accounting for psychometric dependence with a class of latent trait models. (Doctoral dissertation, University of Western Australia)
Rasch G 1968 A mathematical theory of objectivity and its consequence for model construction. European Meeting on Statistics, Econometrics and Management Science, Amsterdam.
Rasch G 1980 *Probabilistic Models for Some Intelligence and Attainment Tests,* 2nd edn. University of Chicago Press, Chicago, Illinois
van der Linden W J, Eggen T J H M 1986 An empirical Bayesian approach to item banking. *Appl. Psychol. Meas.* 10: 345–54
Weiss D (ed.) 1983 *New Horizons in Testing.* Academic Press, New York
Wright B D, Masters G N 1982 *Rating Scale Analysis.* MESA Press, Chicago, Illinois
Wright B D, Stone M H 1979 *Best Test Design.* MESA Press, Chicago, Illinois

Item Response Theory

M. L. Stocking

Item response theory (IRT) models the relationship between a person's level on the trait being measured by a test and the person's response to a test item or question (Lord 1980). Because trait levels are inherently unobservable, item response theory falls into the general class of latent trait models (see *Latent Trait Measurement Models*).

In contrast to classical test theory, item response theory makes strong assumptions about a person's behavior when responding to items. Many advantages accrue from these strong assumptions, for example: (a) it is possible to characterize or describe an item, independently of any sample of people who might respond to the item; (b) it is possible to characterize a person independently of any sample of items administered to the person; and (c) it is possible to predict properties of a test in advance of test administration.

Item response theory has some disadvantages. For some models it is currently not possible to check completely the accuracy with which the assumptions are met by the data. For data that appear to meet the assumptions, however, it is reassuring that predictions made from item response theory can often be independently verified. Applications of item response theory are generally more expensive than similar applications of classical test theory, and many applications of item response theory require the use of a computer.

1. Basic Concepts of Item Response Theory

1.1 Assumptions

Most item response theory models assume that only a single latent trait underlies performance on an item. This is often a reasonable assumption: most tests are constructed to measure a single trait—for example, verbal ability. Models that incorporate more than one latent trait are currently beyond the state of the art.

Item response theory assumes that it is possible to describe mathematically the relationship between a person's trait level and performance on an item. This mathematical description is called an "item response function," an "item characteristic curve," or a "trace line."

1.2 Item Response Functions

For dichotomously scored items (items that are scored right or wrong), the item response function (IRF) states mathematically the probability of a correct response for a given level of trait. This conditional probability is a function of the item characteristics or parameters. Usually, the mathematical function chosen to represent this conditional probability is from the logistic

ogive family or the normal ogive family of functions. There is little difference between the two. More practical work has been done using the logistic family, because of its mathematical simplicity.

If u_i stands for a response to item i (0 for incorrect and 1 for correct) and θ stands for the trait being measured, then the logistic item response function is:

$$P(u_i = 1|\theta) = c_i + (1 - c_i)/(1 + e^{-1.702a_i(\theta-b_i)}) \qquad (1)$$

The normal ogive item response function is:

$$P(u_i = 1 \mid \theta) = c_i + (1 - c_i)\Phi[a_i(\theta - b_i)] \qquad (2)$$

where $\Phi[]$ is the normal cumulative distribution function. In these equations a_i, b_i, and c_i are parameters that describe characteristics of item i. The pseudoguessing parameter c_i is the probability that an examinee with very low θ will respond correctly to the item. The item discrimination parameter a_i is related to the steepness of the curve at the point of inflection. The item difficulty b_i is the θ-level at the point of inflection.

Not all items require three parameters to characterize them adequately. Some work has been done with two-parameter models ($c_i = 0$). A great deal of work has been done with one-parameter models in which the items vary only in difficulty ($a_i = $ constant, $c_i = 0$). If this latter model is logistic, it is called the Rasch model (see *Rasch Measurement, Theory of*). Note that the three-parameter model in Eqn. (1) and Eqn. (2) subsumes models with fewer parameters.

Item response functions from different (logistic) models are displayed in Fig. 1. Two three-parameter IRFs are displayed in the bottom panel. It should be noted that both IRFs have nonzero pseudoguessing parameters and the discriminations and difficulties differ. The middle panel displays IRFs from the two-parameters family. Note that both IRFs have zero pseudoguessing parameters and the discriminations and difficulties differ. The top panel displays IRFs from the one-parameter family. They are parallel to each other and differ only by a shift in difficulty or location.

Item response models have also been developed for items with more complex scoring procedures. Consider a multiple-choice item for which it is informative to know which incorrect option was selected by a person. Item response theory applicable to this type of scoring has been developed by Samejima (1969), Bock (1972), and Masters (1982).

1.3 Information Functions

Information functions (Birnbaum 1968) are used to describe the measurement effectiveness of a test or an item at each level of the trait being measured. In

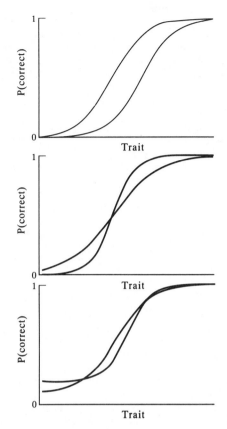

Figure 1
Two one-parameter IRFs (top), two two-parameter IRFs (middle), and two three-parameter IRFs (bottom)

$1 \mid \theta)$ is the item response function, $Q_i(\theta) = 1 - P_i(\theta)$; and $P_r^{'}(\theta)$ is the derivative of the item response function with respect to θ. The test information function $I(\theta)$ is defined as the maximum information available from a test, regardless of the scoring method. The test information function is the simple sum of the item information functions: $I(\theta) = \Sigma_{i=1}^{n} I(\theta, u_i)$, where n is the number of items in the test. For conventional tests $I(\theta)$ is typically a bell-shaped curve. Each item contributes to $I(\theta)$ independently of all other items in the test. In classical item and test analysis, the contribution of each item to test reliability and test validity depends upon what other items are in the test.

Information functions are useful when the metric established for measuring θ is not subject to challenge. However, slight changes in this metric can drastically alter the shape of an information function and hence the conclusions drawn.

1.4 Relative Efficiency Functions

If it is supposed that there are two tests, x and y, both measuring the same trait θ, then the relative efficiency (RE) function of test y versus test x, RE (y, x), is the ratio of their information functions at corresponding values of θ: RE $(y, x) = I(\theta, y)/I(\theta, x)$ (Birnbaum 1968). Most practical applications of item response theory will rely on relative efficiency functions since, unlike information functions, relative efficiency is invariant under any monotonic transformation of the metric used to measure θ.

If RE $(y, x) > 1$ for a particular θ, then test y gives more information than test x at that θ. Relative efficiency functions are useful tools for redesigning existing tests and for investigating novel tests, without actually administering them.

2. Choice of Models and Estimation Methods

The first steps in any application of item response theory to practical problems are to choose a mathematical model for the item response function and to obtain estimates of item parameters and perhaps the θs.

2.1 Choosing a Model

The choice of the appropriate model depends predominantly on the types of test questions and the scoring of the test questions.

Consider items that will be scored either correct or incorrect. If such an item is multiple-choice, that is, if it can be correctly answered by guessing, then an item response function containing a pseudoguessing parameter is desirable. If such an item is free-response, that is, if an examinee must produce a response rather than select one from a list of possible responses, then it is less likely to be correctly answered by guessing, and a two-parameter model with no pseudoguessing parameter is appropriate. If free-response items vary in difficulty but not in discrimination, then the one-parameter model is most appropriate.

contrast, classical test theory usually provides only one measure of effectiveness, which is applied to all people regardless of their θ.

The test information function for a particular scoring method has two equivalent definitions, both of which are useful. By the first definition, the information function for test score y, $I(\theta, y)$, is inversely proportional to the square of the length of the asymptotic confidence interval for estimating trait θ from score y. A high level of information at a particular θ means that this θ can be more precisely estimated from score y than a θ for which the level of information is relatively low.

The second definition states that the information function for test score y is the square of the ratio of (the slope of the regression of y on θ) to (the standard error of measurement of y for fixed θ). In this context, $I(\theta, y)$ can be viewed as a signal-to-noise ratio. The signal is the change in mean y due to a change in θ. The noise is measured by the standard error of measurement of y for fixed θ.

An item information function $I(\theta, u_i)$ is defined as $I(\theta, u_i) = [P_i^{'}(\theta)]^2 / [P_i(\theta)Q_i(\theta)]$, where $P_i(\theta) \equiv P(u_i =$

Similar kinds of considerations affect the choice of the appropriate model when test questions are scored by more complex methods.

In practice, the choice of the appropriate model is not independent of the amount of data available for estimating parameters of that model. In general, the larger the number of parameters in a model, the more data (in the form of examinee responses to items) are required to obtain good estimates of model parameters. In some cases, in the absence of adequate data, estimation errors will be reduced by choosing a less appropriate model with fewer parameters (see Lord 1983).

2.2 Choosing an Estimation Method

The process of obtaining estimates of model parameters is frequently referred to as "calibration." It is difficult for most models—and impossible for some—to obtain such estimates by hand. Many available computer programs, implementing a variety of statistical approaches to the estimation of parameters of many different models, have been developed over the past 20 years. LOGIST (Wingersky 1983) implements a joint maximum likelihood approach to estimating item parameters and θs for the one-, two-, and three-parameter logistic item response model. BILOG (Mislevy and Bock 1983) employs a marginal maximum likelihood approach to the estimation of item parameters for the same models, and a Bayesian approach to the estimation of θs. ASCAL (Vale 1985) employs a joint maximum likelihood approach with prior distributions imposed for the same models.

These programs are quite general in the sense of handling more than one model, therefore they may be less efficient and informative for a single model than computer programs designed to exploit aspects of that single model. BIGSTEPS (Wright and Linacre 1991) fully exploits features of the one-parameter model, along with extensions to partial credit models based on the one-parameter model.

3. Illustrative Applications

Parameter estimates are fallible approximations to true parameter values. To the extent that the approximations are close to the true parameter values, or appropriate methodology has been employed to take account of the uncertainty in the estimates (see Mislevy et al. 1993 and Tsutakawa and Soltys 1988), item response theory provides for many powerful applications to measurement problems.

3.1 Test Construction

Tests with prespecified measurement properties can be constructed from a pool of calibrated items. The first step is to specify a target information function for the new test. The shape of this target indicates the θ levels at which the test should provide the most precise measurement. Second, select items for the new test that will fill in areas under the target that might be difficult to fill, for example, areas where relatively few items are available. Third, compute the test information function for this part test. Fourth, add items that contribute information in areas that are far from meeting the target. Continue to choose items, always comparing the information function of the part test to the target, until a satisfactory approximation to the target has been reached.

Much work has been done to facilitate the solution of IRT-based test design problems using computerized item banks and more complex procedures for selecting test items. Methods of eliciting target information functions and incorporating content and other nonstatistical constraints on item selection have been developed which cast the test design problem as a mathematical programming problem (van der Linden and Boekkooi-Timminga 1989).

3.2 Redesigning an Existing Test

Relative efficiency functions provide a convenient way of investigating various design changes in a test and comparing them with the original test. Fig. 2 illustrates this.

The curves in Fig. 2 are relative efficiency functions for three different tests designed from an original 60-item test. Curve 1 is a test containing only the 30 harder items. This half-length test is less efficient for all test scores. The loss of efficiency is small, however, for high scores. Curve 2 is a test containing only the 30 easier items. This half-length test is less efficient at high scores but is actually more efficient than the full-length test at low scores. This is so because guessing on hard items by low-scoring people destroys information. Better measurement is obtained for these people by discarding the harder items. Curve 3 is a 60-item test with all b_i changed to a middle value. This "peaked" test measures very much better for the middle range of scores.

3.3 Equating

Equating is a measurement topic of interest to test publishers who produce many different forms of a test

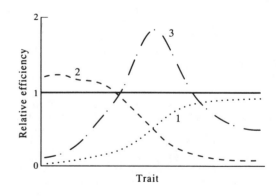

Figure 2
Relative efficiency functions of three modified tests

but wish to report scores on a single scale. The process of finding corresponding scores on different forms of a test is called "equating." In general, observed scores on two different forms of a test cannot be equated except under conditions that make the equating unnecessary (Lord 1980). However, true scores (see *Classical Test Theory*) can be equated under a wide variety of conditions, and item response theory facilitates true-score equating.

Suppose there are two tests, x and y, both measuring the same trait. The items in both tests are calibrated on the same scale. A person's (number-right) true score T_x, on test x is a transformation of the person's θ: $T_x = \sum_{i=1}^{n} P_i(\theta)$, where $P_i(\theta)$ is the item response function for item i evaluated at θ, and n is the number of items in test x. Similarly, the true score on test y is T_x, on test x is a transformation of the person's θ: $T_y = \sum_{i=1}^{m} P_i(\theta)$, where the sum is taken over the m items in test y. These two expressions imply that for any particular θ, a true score on test x and a corresponding true score on test y can be computed. These two true scores are equated because they represent the same trait level on two different measuring scales.

In practice, estimated item parameters are substituted into the two expressions, and equated pairs of true scores are computed for arbitrary values of θ. Even though only observed scores are known, the process continues as if the true-score equating holds for observed scores as well.

3.4 Item Bias

Items in a test that measures a single trait should measure the same trait in all subgroups of the population to which the test is administered. Items that fail to do so are biased for or against a particular subgroup. Since item response functions in theory do not depend upon the group used for item calibration, item response theory provides a natural method for detecting item bias.

Suppose a test is administered to two different groups and the item response functions are estimated separately for each group. If, for a particular item, the item response function for one group is uniformly higher than for the other group, then a person in the first group has a higher probability of a correct response for the same θ. This item is clearly biased in favor of the first group. Typical instances of item bias are not this clear. Usually item response functions will cross, rather than lie all above or all below each other. This means that the item is differentially biased at different θ levels.

3.5 Mastery Testing

Mastery tests are designed to determine if a person has reached a specified level of achievement, in which case the person is a "master." Item response theory can be used to construct optimal mastery tests.

If a pool of calibrated items is supposed, for which subject-matter experts have defined the mastery level, the test construction specialist then selects items from the pool that have the highest item information functions at that level. The test constructed in this way will measure most precisely at the mastery level, thus minimizing errors in classifying people. In addition, item response theory can aid in the determination of the optimal item difficulty, item weights, and cutting score, as well as in the necessary test length. Various test designs may be compared in relative efficiency.

3.6 Tailored Testing

Conventional tests are usually designed to measure best near the middle of the θ range for some group. A tailored test is one in which every person is administered items that measure that person's θ best. The general testing algorithm is as follows: (a) obtain an estimate of a person's θ; (b) from a pool of calibrated items, select an item that measures best at that θ; (c) administer and score the item and revise the estimated θ; and (d) if the estimate is precise enough, stop; otherwise, return to step (b). Many tailored testing designs are possible, most of which require a computer for item administration.

Information functions for tailored tests are generally higher than for conventional tests over a broad range of θ. Much work has been done in this field, investigating and implementing various designs (Dorans et al. 1990).

Item response theory is essential for many aspects of tailored testing. For example, conventional scoring does not apply, since every person may take a different test. In contrast, item response theory provides estimates of θ that are independent of the particular items administered. With item response theory, many different designs can be examined and evaluated using relative efficiency functions.

See also: Adaptive Testing; Latent Trait Measurement Models

References

Birnbaum A 1968 Some latent trait models and their use in inferring an examinee's ability. In: Lord F M, Novick M R (eds.) 1968 *Statistical Theories of Mental Test Scores.* Addison-Wesley, Reading, Massachusetts

Bock R D 1972 Estimating item parameters and latent ability when responses are scored in two or more nominal categories. *Psychometri.* 37(1): 29–51

Dorans et al. 1990. *Computerized Adaptive Testing: A primer.* Erlbaum, Hillsdale, New Jersey

Lord F M 1980 *Applications of Item Response Theory to Practical Testing Problems.* Erlbaum, Hillsdale, New Jersey

Lord F M 1983 Small N justifies Rasch methods. In: Weiss D (ed.) 1983 *New Horizons in Testing.* Academic Press, New York

Masters G N 1982 A Rasch model for partial credit scoring. *Psychometr* 47(2): 149–74

Mislevy R J, Bock R D 1983 BILOG: Item analysis and test scoring with binary logistic models (computer program). Scientific Software Inc., Mooresville, Indiana

Mislevy R J, Sheehan K M, Wingersky M S 1993 How to equate tests with little or no data. *J. Educ. Meas.* 30(1)

Samejima F 1969 Estimation of ability using a response pattern of graded scores. *Psychometr. Monogr.* No. 17, Vol. 34, Part 2

Tsutakawa R K, Soltys M J 1988 Approximation for Bayesian ability estimation. *J. Educ. Stat.* 13(2): 117–30

Vale C D 1985 ASCAL: Item parameter estimation program (computer program). Assessment Systems Inc., St Paul, Minnesota

van der Linden W J, Boekkooi-Timminga E 1989 A maximin model for test design with practical constraints. *Psychometri.* 54(2): 237–48

Wingersky M S 1983 LOGIST: A program for computing maximum likelihood procedures for logistic test models. In: Hambleton R K (ed.) 1983 *Applications of Item Response Theory*. Educational Research Institute of British Columbia, Vancouver

Wright B, Linacre M (1991) *A User's Guide to BIGSTEPS. MESA Press, Chicago, Illinois*

Further Reading

Hambleton R K, Swaminathan H 1984 *Item Response Theory: Principles and Applications*. Kluwer Nijhoff, Boston, Massachusetts

Hulin C L, Drasgow F, Parsons C K 1983 *Item Response Theory: Application to Psychological Measurement*. Dow Jones-Irwin, Homewood, Illinois

Item Sampling

A. E. Beaton

Item sampling is a fundamental concept in educational and psychological measurement. Educational and psychological attributes are often considered latent, that is, not directly observable, and thus must be measured indirectly. For example, a student's reading proficiency may not be measured directly if it is meant to encompass all of the language that a student can read, but it is possible to administer to a student a series of reading passages and to estimate the student's reading proficiency from the student's performance on the assigned passages. The accuracy of the estimate will depend on the properties of the construct being measured (e.g., reading), the selection of exercises, the estimation procedures, the student's willingness to be measured, the setting in which the passages were assigned, and a host of other factors. Item sampling is concerned with the selection of items in the test or assessment instrument being used in measurement. This entry considers the topics of matrix sampling, multiple matrix sampling, balanced incomplete block sampling, rotated sampling, the duplex design and incidence sampling.

1. General Sampling Theory in Educational Measurement

Item sampling is a special application of general sampling theory, which is well-documented in such texts as Hansen et al. (1953) and Kish (1965). However, most general sampling theory has been developed around the issues involved in estimating the parameters of the distribution of a variable in a population of objects, as when estimating the number of employed persons in a nation. In most such examples, the variable is assumed to be measured without error in each unit in the realized sample. In educational and psychological measurement, it is seldom reasonable to assume that the measurement of an attribute is without error, thus the general sampling theory has to be adapted appropriately.

In educational and psychological measurement, the items selected for administration are considered to be a sample from a population of items, that is, a sample from all of the possible items that measure the construct. For example, the items in a reading test may be considered a sample from the population of all relevant reading items. An item sample is often considered to be a simple random sample from an infinite population of items, although this is never literally true. As in sampling theory in general, the purpose of the item sample is to estimate population parameters. For a simple example, consider that a simple random sample of reading items has been administered to a single student, and that the student responded correctly to p of the items. Then, from sampling theory alone, it can be concluded that p is an unbiased estimator of π, the percentage of items that the student would have answered correctly if all items in the entire population of items had been administered. Using general sampling theory, the formula for estimating the standard error of p is $se_p = \sqrt{p(1-p)}/m$ where m is the number of items in the sample. If the sample of items is administered to a group of N students, then the proportion of items answered correctly for student i ($i=1,2,\ldots,N$), p_i, is an unbiased estimate of the parameter π_i, the proportion of items in the population of items that the particular student would have answered correctly. An example of a type of latent variable is π_i, which varies from student to student.

The simple random sampling of items is not necessarily either efficient or sufficient for many testing purposes, since the randomly selected items might not cover all the levels or the total breadth of possible performance. In cases where the test scores are to be used to compare students, the random selection of items might not produce a set of items that discriminates among students reliably enough for purposes of the test. In cases where the item population is large and diverse, the simple random sample might not tap all of the important facets of performance, in which case stratified sampling might be appropriate to ensure that some items are sampled from each important item subpopulation. Furthermore, the sampling errors associated with estimates of the latent variables may be reduced in situations where the item responses are related, that is, when information about whether or not a student answered one item correctly can improve the estimated probability that other items are answered correctly.

Selecting a unique sample of items for each individual student is rare in most testing situations. For example, in computer adaptive testing Wainer et al. (1990), the items that are administered to a student are tailored to a student's estimated proficiency. Items are drawn in a systematic, nonrandom way from a precalibrated, finite population of items. Item calibration processes require that the items have been previously administered to a fairly large population of students.

In educational and psychological measurement, it is often convenient to conceive of the population of examinees and the population of items together in matrix form, that is, considered as a very large (perhaps infinite) matrix with rows representing subjects and columns representing items. Matrix sampling usually involves selection of a sample of both subjects and items, with a selected sample taking the form of a smaller matrix. The concept of matrix sampling has evolved to include a number of more elaborate sampling designs, including multiple matrix sampling, balanced incomplete block sampling, rotated sampling, and the duplex design, which will be discussed below. Extensive discussion of the sampling properties of matrix sampling has been given by Wilks (1962), and Sirotnik and Wellington (1977).

2. Matrix Sampling

Matrix sampling involves the joint sampling of subjects and items from their respective populations. One example of matrix sampling would be a norming study that is designed to estimate the distribution of ability for a population of students so that, at a later time, the performance of individual students, or groups of students, can be compared to that population. In many wide-ranging student sampling plans, a stratified probability sample of students is selected in order to assure that major student groupings in the population are adequately represented in the sample for administrative efficiency. In selecting test items, there is an implicit or explicit sampling plan to assure that the major components or objectives of the test are covered. The data, representing student responses to a set of items, constitute a matrix sample.

The score of subject i ($i=1,2,\ldots,n$) on item j ($j=1,2,\ldots,m$) may be written as

$$x_{ij} = \mu + \alpha_i + \beta_j + \gamma_{ij}$$

where n is the size of the sample of students from the population of N students and m is the size of an independent random sample of items from the population of M items. The definition of μ is the expected value of x_{ij}, the grand mean over the entire population of students and items, $\alpha_i = \mu_i - \mu$, where μ_i is the average value of student i over the population of items, $\beta_j = \mu_j - \mu$, where μ_j is the average of item j over the population of students, and $\gamma_{ij} = x_{ij} - \mu - \alpha_i - \beta_j$, α_i, β_j, and γ_{ij} have average values of zero. Wilks (1962) shows that the expected value of the variance of the mean over all samples of n subjects and m items is

$$\sigma_x^2 = (n^{-1} - N^{-1})\,\sigma_\alpha^2 + (m^{-1} - M^{-1})\,\sigma_\beta^2 + $$
$$(n^{-1} - N^{-1})\,(m^{-1} - M^{-1})\,\sigma_\gamma^2$$

where

$$\sigma_\alpha^2 = \sum_i \alpha_i^2 / (N-1), \ \sigma_\beta^2 = \sum_j \beta_j^2 / (M-1), \text{ and}$$
$$\sigma_\gamma^2 = \sum_i \sum_j \gamma_{ij}^2 / (N-1)(M-1)$$

This decomposition is instructive in showing that the variance of the mean is composed of a component associated with sampling subjects, a component associated with sampling items, and a component associated with their interaction. If the test is considered fixed, that is, that the items are not a sample of items from a larger population, then $m = M$ and the variance of the mean is $(n^{-1} - N^{-1})\sigma_\alpha^2$. In addition, if the subject sample is assumed to be infinitely large, then $\sigma_x^2 = \sigma_\alpha^2 / n$, the standard definition of the sampling variance of a mean taken from a simple random sample of size n when the observations are measured without error.

A single matrix sample can be used for inferences about either the subject population, the item population, or both. If the aim of a norming study is to estimate the average percentage of correct answers to the particular sample of items on the test, then sampling theory indicates that the percentage of correct responses in a probability sample from that population is an unbiased estimator of the population value (using sampling weights if the students were selected with unequal probabilities). If the items can be considered a probability sample from a population of items, then the distribution of the correct scores for a student in the sample is also an unbiased estimate of the percentage of correct scores to any similarly sized sample of items from the item population (using item-sampling weights if the items were not selected with equal probability).

The error variance due to the sampling of subjects is usually called the sampling variance (and its square root is called the standard error). If simple random sampling were used, inferences to the population of students can be made using simple statistical formulas, but if stratified or cluster sampling were used, then other procedures for estimating sampling error such as the jackknife (Mosteller and Tukey 1968, Wolter 1985) should be used instead (see *Sampling Errors in Survey Research*).

Assuming that the item sample can be considered a random sample from the item population, the logic of classical test theory applies (Gulliksen 1987). A person's true score on an m item test is $\tau_i = m(\alpha_i + \mu) = m\mu_i$, that is, m times the proportion of items in the item population that would be answered correctly by that person. Let x_{ik} be the observed score for subject i on the kth ($k=1,2,...,k$) equally likely random sample of m items from the population of M items. The number of possible random samples of size m is $K = M! / [m!(M-m)!]$. Then, $\varepsilon_{ik} = X_{ik} - \tau_i$ is the error of measurement for individual i, the difference between the observed score on the k th possible test and the true score for subject i. The average error for subject i across all possible item samples of size m is $\sum_k \varepsilon_{ik} / K = 0$. The measurement variance across all subjects and possible samples of size m is $\sigma_e^2 = \sum_{ik} \varepsilon_{ik}^2 / NK$. The square root of the measurement variance is known as the (population) standard error of measurement.

Since an individual's score on a particular item, x_{ij}, is assumed to be selected from one of the K possible random samples of m items from the item population for that individual, $\Sigma_j x_{ij}$ is an unbiased estimate of τ_i, the true score for that subject. The estimated average value of τ_i across the population of subjects is therefore $\Sigma_{ij} x_{ij}/n$. An unbiased estimate of the item sampling variance of the true score $_i$ for subject i is $s_{\tau_i}^2 = m^2(1 - m/M)s_i^2$ where $s_i^2 = \Sigma_m(x_{ij} - x_i)^2/(m-1)$.

In educational and psychological measurement, it has been traditional to estimate the measurement variance using the concept of parallel tests. With a single matrix sample, there is only one "test," and so the sample of m items is considered to be two randomly equivalent samples of $m/2$ items; in practice, this is often done by considering the odd numbered and even numbered items as separate half-length tests. If the items are ordered in difficulty, the equivalence of the split halves can be improved by randomly assigning one of each pair of odd and even items to each split half. For simplicity, only tests with a total even number of items is discussed here.

Since the half tests were randomly selected from the overall item pool, the correlation between these split halves is an estimate of the population correlation

among samples of size $m/2$ from the item population. The correlation among tests of m items, that is, full-length tests, can be estimated using the Spearman Brown "prophecy" formula

$$\rho = 2\rho_{xx'} / (1 + \rho_{xx'})$$

where ρ is the estimated reliability of a test of length m and $\rho_{xx'}$ is the correlation between the two half-tests, each of length $m/2$ (Lord and Novick 1968) (see *Reliability*).

The decomposition of a score on a test into components attributable to subject sampling, item sampling, and their interaction or error is an example of the widely used statistical technique known as the analysis of variance (see *Variance and Covariance, Analysis of*). Indeed, Cronbach et al. (1972) have developed extensively the analysis of variance approach to analyzing test data in their important book *The Dependability of Behavioral Measurements: Theory of Generalizability for Scores and Profiles* (1972). They argue that many of the concepts of classical test theory can be reproduced and that test theory can be further developed by using the random and mixed effects models that are now widely used in the analysis of variance. Under basic assumptions about the nature of the phenomenon being measured and consideration of the design through which the data were collected, it may be possible to estimate many different components of variation and thereby estimate the uncertainty in the sample statistics as estimators of the corresponding population parameters. Therefore, consideration of the components of variance leads to statements about the "generalizability" of the properties of the test or assessment instrument. The Cronbach et al. generalizability approach is broadly applicable in educational and psychological measurement, beyond its applicability to matrix samples.

Item response theory, as generally practiced, is a different way of analyzing data from matrix samples. In most applications, IRT assumes that a single parameter, usually called θ_i, characterizes an individual's ability to answer the items in an item sample, and it further assumes that each item has one or more parameters that describe the relationship between the θ_i of all individuals and the observed item responses. Thus, IRT assumes that an individual's probability of answering an item correctly is a function of some properties of the item, the individual's ability, and the stochastic relationship between the ability and the item. The stochastic relationship is usually assumed to be nonlinear. Given a model for the stochastic relationship, IRT computer programs typically estimate the individual parameters, θ_i, and the parameters associated with each item. Item response theory is covered in detail by Lord (1980) (see *Item Response Theory*).

There are many special cases of matrix sampling which are of practical interest. For example, a norming study in which the only goal is to estimate how a population of students would do on a test containing only a particular set of items would involve only sampling error, not measurement error. A computer-assisted test that sampled from a pool of items to measure a particular student's ability to some pre-scribed degree of accuracy would have measurement error, but no sampling error. Although in many cases, a specific, measurable group of students is of interest and thus sampling error is not at issue, measurement error is of interest in almost all educational situations, since a hypothetical population of possible items is of concern, not the specific items on the test.

Matrix sampling is limited in practice by the matrix form of the sample, which implies that all students respond to the same items. The number of items that can be sampled is therefore limited to the number of items that can be responded to in the available time for each student. The following designs allow more extensive probes into the item population.

3. Multiple Matrix Sampling

Multiple matrix sampling is the selection of several matrix samples by selecting several distinct samples of students and administering to them different samples of items. The purpose of multiple matrix sampling may be to enlarge the sample of items from the item population without increasing the burden on individual students, or to reduce the burden on individual students without reducing the number of items, or both. In most matrix sampling, the sampling of both students and items is done without replacement so that the samples are nonoverlapping. As Lord (1962) noted, sampling with replacement would be somewhat more efficient; however, practical considerations may make administering a particular item to a student more than once unacceptable. Certain types of samples in which subsets of items are administered as parts of several tests are discussed in the following sections.

Multiple matrix sampling has been used widely in educational testing for some time. Any test with two or more parallel forms that was normed using a probability sample of students may be considered a multiple matrix sample. In his influential 1962 paper, Lord addressed the bias introduced in test norms by refusals of schools to cooperate, and he proposed estimating norms by item sampling as a way to reduce the burden on schools and students, thereby enhancing cooperation. To demonstrate his point he used multiple matrix samples from an available population. The National Assessment of Educational Progress (NAEP) in the United States used multiple matrix sampling in its assessments from 1969–82 in order to assess student competencies in a large population of assessment exercises.

Multiple matrix sampling forces a test designer to address the trade-offs in the allocation of resources. Increasing the sample of subjects while keeping the item pool fixed, reduces the sampling error but does

not reduce the measurement error. Increasing the sample of items while keeping the number of students responding to each item fixed, increases the total sample size and allows more precise estimation of the properties of the item population, but does not reduce the sampling error. Increasing either subject or item coverage involves some cost. Considerations of the size of sampling and measurement errors, as well as the cost of reducing them, are important in reaching an efficient sampling design. Methods for optimizing the efficiency of the sampling design are discussed by van der Linden (1987), van der Linden and Adema (1988), van der Linden (1988), and Berger (1989).

Multiple matrix sampling does allow estimating the joint distribution of items within a test but does not allow the estimation of the joint distributions of items in different item samples since typically no student takes more than one test. Parallel form reliability coefficients are, therefore, not computable. However, if the items are randomly selected for each test, the reliability coefficient of each test can be computed and the Spearman-Brown formula used to estimate the correlation between each test and a similarly sized random sample of items, that is, the other forms of the test. The several estimated correlations can be combined for an overall reliability estimate.

3.1 Balanced Incomplete Block (BIB) Sampling
Balanced incomplete block (BIB) spiraling is a complex form of multiple matrix sampling in which different students are given different samples of items but in a controlled way so that the item samples overlap. Its purpose is to keep the testing burden on each subject modest while sampling a large pool of items in such a way that the joint distribution of each pair of items is estimable.

The notion of controlled item overlap has been used in testing for some time as, for example, in the experimental section of the Scholastic Aptitude Test which has been used, among other things, to anchor the scales of different forms of the test (Angoff 1988). Some sampling properties of balance incomplete block matrix sampling are in Wilks (1962) and using these designs for efficient testing was proposed by Knapp (1968). Spiraling (defined below) was added to the BIB designs by Messick et al. (1983) and has been used extensively by the National Assessment of Educational Progress since 1983 (Beaton 1987).

The general strategy is as follows: instead of selecting item samples of the size that a student can respond to in the time available, item subsamples, that take a fraction of the student time, are selected. It is important that the various subsamples all require the same amount of time and use the same administrative procedures, since examinees in a testing session will be responding to different items. Each item subsample is paired with each other subsample and placed in some booklet using a balanced incomplete block design. The booklets are then spiraled, that is, placed in a random sequence and administered to the subjects in that random sequence.

An example of BIB spiraling may clarify the concept. If it is assumed that an hour of student time is available but that it is necessary to gather information about items that would require a student two hours to complete, then the two-hour item sample could be divided randomly into four half-hour subsamples which are denoted S1, S2, S3, and S4. For a completely balanced design, six booklets would be developed, containing subsamples {S1,S2}, {S1,S3}, {S1,S4}, {S2,S3}, {S2,S4}, and {S3,S4}. The correlations among all subsamples of items are therefore estimable. The NAEP has employed another design that uses item samples that require one-third of the available student time. A sample of items that would require two hours and 20 minutes of subject's time is selected and divided into seven subsamples. The subsamples are randomized and then assigned to seven booklets in a cyclic rectangle as follows:

Block

Booklet	1st	2nd	3rd
1	1	2	4
2	2	3	5
3	3	4	6
4	4	5	7
5	5	6	1
6	6	7	2
7	7	1	3

Each booklet contains three subsamples of items. Each item subsample is in three booklets, in each case paired with two different subsamples, and is in the first, second, and third position in a booklet exactly once. The booklets are then placed in a random sequence and then packaged in conveniently sized bundles such that each booklet appears an equal number of times in each position of a package.

There are many balanced incomplete designs that could be used in BIB spiraling. An excellent overview of such designs is in Cochran and Cox (1957). Note, however, that a balanced incomplete design is not necessarily available for a particular number of blocks with a given number of blocks to be placed in each booklet.

The advantages of BIB spiraling are several. Since every block of items is paired with every other block, each item is paired with each other item for some subsample of students, and thus the joint distribution of any pair of items can be estimated. Estimating the joint distribution of items is essential for studying the dimensionality of the item population. If administra-

tive procedures allow, it is possible to spiral together items from different subject areas (e.g., mathematics and science) and estimate the correlations among them. Parallel form reliability coefficients are computable among the subsamples scores. The spiraling improves the sampling errors by spreading the sample over more schools and thus reducing the clustering effect in the sample. The cost, however, is that more different forms of the test must be printed; in fact, if the number of item blocks is large, the number of different booklets needed to complete the design may be so large as to be impractical. The item subsamples must be strictly timed so that each booklet requires the same amount of testing time, and the test instructions are restricted to generalities since subjects in the same testing session will be administered different tests.

3.2 Rotated Sampling

Rotated sampling addresses some of the same concerns as balanced incomplete block spiraling, but in a simpler way. Rotated sampling allows the test developer to expand the number of items that are sampled but does not guarantee that each item is paired with each other item in some booklet, thus the relationships among some items are not directly observed. The unobserved relationships may be estimated indirectly from the observed data if sufficient assumptions are made. The test booklets may be spiraled together for administration if they have common timing and instructions.

Rotated designs have been used extensively by the International Association for the Evaluation of Educational Achievement (IEA) to allow a common block of items to be administered to all countries for international comparisons and to allow different countries to have additional items tailored to their own curricula, as well as to increase the range of items sampled in a testing program.

Using the same example as for BIB spiraling, a rotated design might be as follows:

Block

Booklet	1st	2nd	3rd
1	1	2	3
2	2	3	4
3	3	4	5
4	4	5	6
5	5	6	7

This design places the seven item blocks into five booklets, instead of seven as in the BIB design, but is unbalanced, in that blocks three, four, and five are in more booklets than the other blocks. Note that the joint distributions of the items in following combinations of blocks are not directly estimable: {1,4}, {1,5}, {1,6}, {1,7}, {2,5}, {2,6}, {2,7}, {3,6}, {3,7}, {4,7}.

There are many ways to form a rotated design. For example, if it is assumed that a seven-block item pool has a particularly important set of items that must be administered to all students, then the following design would suffice:

	Block		
Booklet	1st	2nd	3rd
1	1	2	3
2	1	3	4
3	1	4	5
4	1	5	6
5	1	6	7
6	1	7	2

All students are administered item block one as well as two of the six remaining blocks. The design is still unbalanced, since block one is administered more often than the others, but balanced among the remaining six blocks. Note, however, that some interblock relationships are not directly estimable since, for example, blocks two and five are not together in any booklet.

3.3 The Duplex Design

The duplex design (Bock and Mislevy 1988) can be considered as a stratified form of multiple matrix sampling. An item population can be stratified into a number of different categories such as items that measure various categories of educational objectives. A test which is administered to a subject consists of one randomly selected item from each item category. Many forms of the test are developed by sampling without replacement from the item strata. If the test timing and administration procedures permit, the various forms of the test may be spiraled together and administered to different students within a testing session.

The resulting data from the tests may be analyzed either by item category or by student. Analysis by item results in estimates of the adequacy of coverage of each category or educational objective in a population of students. The population of students may be small, such as a school, or large, such as a nation. Sampling efficiency is achieved by administering only one item in each category to an individual student. Analysis by student results in the estimate of the student's proficiency on a carefully constructed, multiobjective test. Under the random sampling assumption, the different tests are parallel. For information about the analysis of data collected using the duplex design, see Mislevy and Bock (1989).

Although the duplex design uses data quite efficiently, it assumes that the item population can be stratified into a fairly large number of categories; for example, if an hour of student time is available, then the design may allow 60 to 100 item categories. This level of detail is not usually achieved in practice. Furthermore, the design does not allow the study of the dimensionality of each category since only one item of each type is administered to a student and thus the joint distribution of performance is not directly estimable from the data.

4. Incidence Sampling

While developing the work of Hooke (1956a, 1956b), Sirotnik and Wellington (1977), proposed a general design for item sampling which they call incidence sampling. Incidence sampling generalizes item sampling by allowing the arbitrary sampling of subjects and of items. Unlike multiple matrix sampling which requires that the samples be in matrix form (i.e., the same items assigned to all subjects in a sample), incidence sampling allows for any sampling scheme. The sampling scheme is described by an incidence matrix of the same form as the population subject by item matrix. In the incidence matrix, an indicator variable is given the value of one if the item is selected for a subject and zero otherwise. Under this very general scheme, all of the various item sampling designs can be described as special cases of incidence sampling.

Sirotnik and Wellington use the "generalized symmetric means" approach of Hooke in order to establish the properties of incidence samples. This general approach can be used to estimate not only the average but also the higher order moments of the distributions from which the samples are selected. Sirotnik and Wellington's method also presents a method of computing the standard errors of the various moments.

The advantage of incidence sampling is that Sirotnik and Wellington (1977) have presented a general approach to computing estimates of the moments and standard errors from various item by subject samples. This fact is of substantial theoretical interest. However, the notation and algorithms are very complex and laborious, with the result that the methodology will be difficult to apply in practical survey work. (See *Item Banking in Testing and Assessment; Item Response Theory; Sampling in Survey Research; Sampling Errors in Survey Research; National Assessment of Educational Program*)

See also: Item Banking in Testing and Assessment; Item Writing Techniques

References

Angoff W H 1988 *Scales, Norms, and Equivalent Scores*. Educational Testing Service, Princeton, New Jersey

Beaton A E 1987 *Implementing The New Design: The NAEP 1983–84 Technical Report*. Educational Testing Service. Princeton, New Jersey

Berger M P F 1989 *On the Efficiency of IRT Models When Applied to Different Sampling Designs*. Research Report 89–4. University of Twente, Department of Education, Enschede

Bock R D, Mislevy R M 1988 Comprehensive educational assessment for the states: The duplex design. *Educ. Eval. Policy Anal.* 10(2): 89–102

Cochran W G, Cox G M 1957 *Experimental Designs*. 2nd edn. Wiley, New York

Cronbach L J, Gleser G C, Nanda H, Rajaratnam N 1972 *The Dependability of Behavioral Measurements: Theory of Generalizability for Scores and Profiles*. Wiley, New York

Gulliksen H 1987 *Theory of Mental Tests*, rev. edn. Erlbaum, Hillsdale, New Jersey

Hansen M H, Hurwitz W N, Madow W G 1953 *Sample Survey Methods and Theory*, Vols. 1 and 2. Wiley, New York

Hooke R 1956a Symmetric functions of a two-way array. *Ann. Math. Stat.* 27(1): 80–98

Hooke R 1956b Some applications of bipolykays to the estimation of variance components and their moments. *Ann. Math. Stat.* 27: 55–79

Kish L 1965 *Survey Sampling*. Wiley, New York

Knapp T 1968 An application of balanced incomplete block designs to the estimation of test norms. *Educ. Psychol. Meas.* 28(2): 265–72

Lord F M 1962 Estimating norms by item-sampling. *Educ. Psychol. Meas.* 22(2): 259–67

Lord F M 1980 *Applications of Item Response Theory to Practical Testing Problems*. Erlbaum, Hillsdale, New Jersey

Lord F M, Novick M R 1968 *Statistical Theories of Mental Test Scores*. Addison-Wesley, Reading, Massachusetts

Messick S M, Beaton A E, Lord F M 1983 NAEP Reconsidered: A New Design for a New Era. Educational Testing Service, Princeton, New Jersey

Mislevy R J, Bock R D 1989 A hierarchical item-response model for educational testing In: Bock R D (ed.) 1989 *Multilevel Analysis of Educational Data*. Academic Press, San Diego

Mosteller F M, Tukey J W 1968 Data analysis, including statistics. In Lindzey G, Aronson E (eds.) 1969 *Handbook of Social Psychology*, 2nd edn. Addison-Wesley, Reading, Massachusetts

Sirotnik, Wellington 1977 Incidence sampling: An integrated theory for "matrix sampling." *J. Educ. Meas.* 14: 343–99

van der Linden W J (ed.) 1987 IRT-based Test Construction. Research Report 87–2. University of Twente, Department of Education, Enschede

van der Linden W J 1988 *Optimizing Incomplete Sample Designs for Item Response Model Parameters*. Research Report 88–5. University of Twente, Department of Education, Enschede

van der Linden W J, Adema J J 1988 *Algorithmic Test Design Using Classical Item Parameters*. Research Report 88–2. University of Twente, Department of Education, Enschede

Wainer H et al. 1990 *Computerized Adaptive Testing: A Primer*. Erlbaum, Hillsdale, New Jersey

Wilks S S 1962 *Mathematical Statistics*. Wiley, New York

Wolter K H 1985 *Introduction to Variance Estimation*. Springer-Verlag, New York

Judgments, Measurement of

J. M. Linacre

The use of judges to rate examinee performance on test items is often necessary, but can cause a severe measurement problem. The Spearman true score model solution assumes a linear rating scale used by judges to rate each examinee at a true score with some error. True scores are the resultant measures but they are sample-dependent numerations, linear by assertion, but not in construction. Inter-rater reliability, the usual statistic of judge agreement, is of doubtful value, particularly when the intention is to measure individual examinee performances. Nevertheless, when the empirical departures from linearity are small and some components underlying the observations can be held to be interchangeable, generalizability theory—an elaboration of the true-score model—provides some useful information. In contrast, a Rasch model analysis capitalizes on the inevitable judge disagreement to construct a sample-free, objective, and linear measurement continuum. Models for both rating scales and rank orderings can be implemented. When true-score models are used, then equating of judged-tests is, at best, norm-referenced and hence sample-dependent. When Rasch models are used, the equating is criterion-referenced and hence sample-free.

1. Judgment and Measurement in Education

Expert judgment is required to rate the level of performance in many fields of education: written composition, music, drama, spoken language. The purpose of judging is to determine the best performances in a competition or what level of competence has been reached in a skill. The tasks, skills, or behaviors on which the examinees are rated will be called "items." All judges may rate all examinees on all items, or individual judges may be assigned to rate examinees on different items according to some judging plan. In practice, the optimum judging plan minimizes the number of judgments necessary to measure performances with the required precision.

Judgment is usually recorded by a judge making an independent ordinal rating of an examinee's performance on an item. The numeration of the discrete ratings on the scale is chosen for convenience in recording and ordering the categories. The situation may be as simple as each judge rating each examinee with 1 for success or 0 for failure on the only item, or as complex as each examinee performance involving several items, each with its own rating scale. The possible responses on the rating scales are categories defined in ascending order in terms of the performance level they represent (see *Rating Scales*).

The aim of the analysis is to derive from the ordinal, discrete ratings given by the judges final linear measures of performance for each examinee that are as fair and accurate as possible. This means that the measure given to an examinee must be estimated from, but be made statistically independent of, the particular judge or judges who rated that examinee. That is, the measure must be judge-free. In many situations, the measure must also be item-free; that is, independent of the particular items on which ratings were made. If the measure is also made independent of consideration of other examinees (i.e., person-free or sample-free) the measure can be termed "objective." Measures are usually subjected to further statistical analysis, such as means and standard deviations, that require measure linearity, not merely ordinal numeration over a finite interval, for meaningful interpretation (Stevens 1959).

When judging is repeated at a later time, but standards are to be maintained, or examinee performances are to be compared across sessions, there is also the requirement that examinee measures be independent not only of the composition of the judging panel, and of the particular items chosen for recording competence, but also of the local levels of performance of the examinees at any session. Consequently, the most effective measurement model is not one that most completely describes any particular judging situation, but rather one that yields the most stable basis for inference—that is, the most objective measures.

2. Measuring by True Scores

The perfect judging situation is often proposed to be that in which the ideal judge rates each examinee performance exactly at its "true score." The ratings given by empirical judges, however, rarely show complete agreement, and are therefore regarded as combining this fictitious "true score" with consistent judge differences and random error. This is analogous to the true-score model for objective testing and suffers from all its shortcomings (see *Classical Test Theory*).

Studies of judge behavior have identified numerous reasons for consistent differences between judges' ratings: leniency (severity) level, halo effect, and central tendency (Guilford 1954). Consistent differences are also found in interactions of judges with other aspects of the situation. A judge may be consistently lenient on one item, but consistently severe on another. Whatever part of each rating cannot be accounted for as a sum of the factors specified in the true-score model is treated as judge-generated random error (see *Rating Scales*).

Numerous studies have attempted to recover examinees' true scores from empirically observed ratings. The means of performing this is to construct a linear model in the rating metric of the form (Saal et al. 1980):

Observed Rating = True score + Judge effect + Interaction + Error $\qquad$ (1)

In spite of the effort expended on this model, the resultant true scores have proved deficient. Specifications of rating scales have been arbitrary and, despite the numerical labeling, nonlinear in function. Thus, on a rating scale labeled from 1 to 5, the difference in performance between 1 and 2 is unlikely to be the same as that between 2 and 3. Consequently, an estimated true score of 1.7 has no clear quantitative meaning.

For most applications of these models, true scores are only estimable when every judge rates every examinee on every item or when a sophisticated judging plan, such as a balanced incomplete block design (Braun 1988), is followed scrupulously. These constraints are impractical for large-scale test administration and so are seldom used.

The introduction into the measurement model of interaction effects, such as each judge's personal degree of bias against individual examinees, further limits the objectivity of the resultant measures. This is because interactions are local to the specific judging session. Better judge training is often proposed as the way to reduce interaction effects and error variance. Though judge training is beneficial, there is no example in the literature where it has eliminated judge differences.

3. Inter-rater Reliability

An inter-rater (inter-judge) reliability coefficient, analogous to the reliability coefficient of objective tests, is often reported as a measure of judge agreement. This coefficient ranges from 0 to 1 with higher values regarded as better. Even though the reliability coefficient is manifestly insensitive to differences in judge severities, a high value is treated as evidence that the sums of examinee ratings accurately reflect examinee performance.

In general, the greater the ratio of true score variance to error variance in Eqn. (1), the higher the reliability. This reliability is dominated by the range of examinee ability, the range of judge severity, and the range of item difficulty. Since these ranges are local to the judging situation, any particular reliability lacks general significance. Some research even reports the paradoxical result that "examiners who agree are likely to be wrong" (Harper and Misra 1976 p. 260).

4. Generalizability Theory

Generalizability theory, an elaboration of true-score theory, also mistakes ratings as linear. It specifies judging designs which, with additional assumptions, are intended to lead to estimates of measurement error. An implementation of this approach is the GENOVA computer program (Crick and Brennan 1982).

In a typical study, ratings are awarded by judges to examinees on items of performance according to a judging plan. The analyst specifies which aspect (examinees, judges, or items of performance) is the one to be measured. The other aspects, called "facets," are then sources of error. Error variances are calculated according to the judging plan and whether each facet is a random sample from a normally distributed admissible universe (e.g., of similar judges) or is the entire universe (e.g., all of a standardized test). These error variances are used to estimate a measurement error for the measure of interest (see *Reliability*).

If further, similar ratings are to be collected, a decision study can be performed to predict the error variances produced by revised judging plans. In particular, the decision study predicts what alterations to the previous judging plan would most reduce measurement error.

Generalizability theory is more successful when judges are in close numerical agreement, the test items are of similar difficulty, and the ratings are around the central, close to linear, part of the ordinal rating scale. In practice, the success of a generalizability study is actually evaluated only by the size of the error variances. Fit analysis and investigation of unexpected residuals is not undertaken (see *Generalizability Theory*).

5. Many-facet Rasch Measurement

Many-facet Rasch models address the inevitable error in the ordinal ratings by specifying that each examinee has an estimable probability of being awarded any possible rating on any item by any judge (see *Rasch Measurement, Theory of*). The data are evaluated as potential realizations of these probabilities. Each observation is modeled as an ordinal rating stochastically governed by a log-linear combination of the measures of one element from each facet (e.g., an examinee ability or performance from the examinees' facet, a judge severity from the judges' facet, and an item difficulty from the items' facet). These measures are estimated so that they are statistically independent of the particular observations comprising the data, but they are realized through the data. The measures estimated for the elements maximize the likelihood of the observed

ratings. An asymptotic standard error for each measure is provided. An implementation of this model is the *Facets* computer program (Linacre 1988).

These measures constitute a linear measurement system that locates all elements of all facets on a common interval continuum of infinite range. The item measures on this continuum define the underlying variable (see *Item Response Theory*). The depiction of all measures as points along a line has the familiar visual interpretation of equal distances that is so productive in physical science and engineering.

The residual differences between the data and their measure-based expected values become the basis of detailed quality-control fit statistics and rating diagnoses. Significant misfit associated with particular elements and unexpectedly large residuals for particular observations identifies and diagnoses anomalies. Remedial action can be taken and errant (highly improbable) observations can be evaluated for re-rating or omission prior to reporting.

5.1 Rasch Judging Plans

The only constraint on the judging plan is that the ratings must form a network of connections such that separate but comparable measures can be obtained for each examinee, judge, and item. This does not require that every examinee be rated by every judge or even that any single observation be replicated, that is, rated more than once. The requirement is only that a chain of observations connects every judge, item, and examinee directly or indirectly. This has proved usefully robust in practice even with idiosyncratic judging plans. Since only recorded observations are used to estimate measures, missing data or even mistakes in implementing the judging plan do not threaten the analysis or require remedial maneuvers. Missing data have no practical consequence so long as the available ratings form one connected network of the type discussed by Luce and Perry (1949).

Judging plans have succeeded in which each examinee is rated by only one judge on any particular item. The judges rotate across items and examinees so that every examinee is rated by more than one judge, although on different items. Each judge rates more than one item, but for different examinees (Lunz et al. 1990). There is considerable flexibility because there is no requirement that each judge rate the same number of examinees or use the same number of items.

Defective plans are those in which judges are specialists who rate only items in their own specialties. Then it becomes impossible to determine how much of the challenge to the examinee is due to the difficulty of the specialty and how much is due to the severity of the specialty judges. Other defective plans are those in which one panel of judges rates one group of examinees, while another independent panel rates another independent group. Then it is impossible to determine whether mean differences between the groups are due to a mean ability difference among examinees or a mean severity difference among judges. Even these defective plans can be used if reasonable assertions beyond the data can be made, such as the equal severity of randomly assigned judging panels or the equal ability of randomly sampled examinee groups.

5.2 Dichotomously Judged Items

Dichotomous items produce observations in one of two categories, usually labeled 0 and 1, and generally coded so that 1 means success on the item and 0 means failure. A relevant many-facet Rasch model is:

$$\log(P_{nij1} / P_{nij0}) = B_n - D_i - C_j \tag{2}$$

where

P_{aijl} = the probability that person n will earn a 1 on item i from judge j;
B_n = ability of person n;
D_i = difficulty of item i;
C_j = severity of judge j.

Person abilities are not expressed in nonlinear raw scores on the particular test, but rather in linear log-odds units (logits) that measure examinees' levels of success on whatever items they performed, but in a general measurement system. The other facets are also calibrated in logits on the same continuum.

Solving Eqn. (2) for P_{nij1}, since $P_{nij0} = 1 - P_{nij1}$,

$$P_{nij1} = \frac{exp(B_n - D_i - C_j)}{1 + exp(B_n - D_i - C_j)} \tag{3}$$

brings out the exponential form of the model. If an examinee of ability 1 logit is rated by a judge of severity 0 logits on a dichotomous item of difficulty 0 logits, the probability of the rating being a 1 is exp(1)/(1 + exp(1)) = 73%.

5.3 Rating Scales with Discrete Categories

When examinees are rated by judges on several items, each of which has its own ordinal rating scale, a relevant many-facet Rasch model is:

$$\log(P_{nijk}/P_{nijk-1}) = B_n - D_i - C_j - F_{ik} \tag{4}$$
$$k = 1, K_i$$

where

P_{nijk} = the probability that person n will earn a rating of category k on item i from judge j;
B_n, D_i, C_j are defined as above;
F_{ik} = additional difficulty of being rated in category k beyond that of being rated in category k-1 for item i;
K_i = the highest rating scale category, after ordinally renumbering of categories from 0.

The empirically observed rating scale is analyzed as ordinal categories representing increasing increments of performance. This redefinition replaces the arbitrary numeration of the original scale with a scale labeled in successive integers from 0 to K_i, in which each category label becomes the count of observed increments in performance above the lowest observed performance level.

Item difficulty, D_i, is usually defined such that the sum of all F_{ik} is set at 0. Thus the item difficulty, D_i, is calibrated at that point on the logit continuum at which the highest and lowest rating categories have equal probabilities of being awarded.

Zero or perfect scores are empirically inestimable. If there is a relevant context in which they can be embedded, they can be forced into the estimation procedure by means of simple Bayesian techniques (see *Bayesian Statistics in the Analysis of Data*).

5.4 Rating Scales with Unobserved Categories

The many-facet model for discrete intervals renumbers the observed ratings into an ordinally ascending rating scale. Each category of this new rating scale represents a count of increments of performance and has associated with it a difficulty measure. In practice, not all categories may be observed. When the unobserved categories are an artifact of sampling, a simple computational device suffices to maintain estimability (Wilson 1991). If, however, categories are unobserved because there are too many (e.g., a 0–100 rating scale), then representing the rating scale by a continuous rather than a discrete function can be useful.

A model for a continuous 0–100 rating scale, parallel to the discrete example above, is:

$$P_{nijk} = \frac{exp(k(B_n - D_i - C_j) - G_{ik})}{\int_{m=0}^{100} (exp(m(B_n - D_i - C_j) - G_{im})dm)} \tag{5}$$

where

P_{nijk} = the probability density that person n will earn a rating in category k on item i from judge j;
B_n, D_i, C_j are defined as above;
G_{ik} is a continuous function of k defining the rating scale structure for item i such that $G_{i0} = G_{i100} = 0$.

The function, G_{ik}, models the observed and unobserved parts of the rating scale. Since it is incompletely observed in the empirical data, its form must be specified by the analyst. Since the aim of the measurement model is to assist in interpretation and inference, it follows that the useful functions, G_{ik}, are ones with a few, readily interpretable parameters, such as polynomial or Fourier series (Andrich 1982, Muller 1987).

6. Measuring by Rank Ordering

Difficulties experienced in defining and using rating scales have led some analysts to prefer ranking examinees. Even when competent judges cannot agree on the category into which to place a performance, they may agree on which performance is better. This approach is attractive when the purpose is to find the best of a small number of examinees. When there is a criterion performance standard, this criterion performance can be ranked along with examinees to identify a pass–fail point.

The extent of agreement among judges ranking examinees depends on the variance in examinee performance. If several examinees have similar abilities, there can be little agreement among judges' rank-orderings (Harper and Misra 1976). Thus the reliability of rank-ordering is also sample-dependent. Nevertheless, summing rankings is often satisfactory for the purpose at hand.

6.1 Rasch Models for Rank Ordering

Lack of agreement between rank-orderings from different judges can be evaluated with a Rasch measurement model, and so used to obtain linear measures of the distances between examinees. The model for the simplest case, paired comparisons, is:

$$\log(P_{nmij} / (1 - P_{nmij})) = B_n - B_m \qquad (6)$$

where

P_{nmij} is the probability that person n is preferred to person m on item i by judge j;
B_n = ability of person n;
B_m = ability of person m.

This model enables measures, standard errors, and fit statistics to be obtained for each person. Though the judges and items are not parameterized explicitly, data partitioning enables quality-control fit statistics to be obtained for each judge and item. Thus idiosyncratic judging and uneven examinee performance across items can be detected.

Rank-ordering of more than two examinees introduces interexaminee observation dependency not present in ratings. Though this can be modeled explicitly, empirical studies indicate that modeling the rankings as ratings provides a practical approximation. Such a model, allowing tied and partial rankings, is:

$$\log(P_{nijk} / P_{nijk + 1}) = B_n - F_{ijk} \qquad k = 1, K_{ij} - 1$$
$$(7)$$

where

P_{nijk} = the probability that person n will be ranked k on item i by judge j;
B_n is defined as above;
F_{ijk} = additional difficulty of being ranked k beyond that of being ranked lower at k+1 in the rank-ordering on item i by judge j;
K_{ij} = the number of different rankings made by judge j on item i. The highest ranking is 1.

7. The Equating of Judged Tests

Equating judges from one testing session to another using true-score models remains intractable. Generalizability theory provides a mathematical solution provided that no variation in overall judge behavior or item or judge sampling occurs. Many examination boards attempt a solution by assuming that their distributions of examinee performances are the same from testing session to testing session. They then apply an arbitrary norm-referenced rule, say, that 80 percent of examinees shall always be said to succeed, whatever the actual level of competence.

Rasch measurement models yield individual judge severity estimates and individual item difficulty estimates. When the data fit the measurement model, these measures are statistically sample-free for judge, item, and examinee populations similar to those used to estimate these measures. Consequently, when there has been no substantive change in the corresponding judge or item, each measure can be used as maintaining its numerical value. The relative stability of measures can be verified by comparing the measures of common elements across testing sessions.

The characteristics of judges do change between, and even within, judging sessions. The characteristics of items change more slowly. Research indicates, however, that panels of experienced judges can maintain their overall group level of severity over time. Consequently, so long as each facet except one (usually examinees) of each new test has some components in common with the corresponding facets of the old test, the Rasch continua constructed for the two tests can be aligned, that is, equated. This enables the maintenance of criterion levels of performance (such as pass–fail points) from judging session to judging session despite the introduction of new judges and new items and the inevitable variations in distributions of examinee ability on the different occasions (see *Criterion-referenced Measurement*).

8. Unidimensionality

Both true-score and Rasch models specify that the variable to be measured is unidimensional. General lack of fit of data to model is an indication that the facets of the model do not add up to realize one variable in which greater competence by the examinees is expressed in terms of higher ratings awarded by the judges on the items. Such lack of fit is not unusual in practical examinations in which conflicting requirements such as speed, accuracy, and neatness are confounded. Under these circumstances, any decision based on a cumulative score involves an arbitrary weighting of the various nonhomogeneous components. Unlike truescore models, which tend to hide the underlying ambiguity, Rasch fit statistics point it out to the examination board, on whom policy decisions concerning the relative importance of the different components depend.

See also: Rating Scale Analysis; Partial Credit Model; Attitudes, Measurement of; Rasch Measurement, Theory of; Rating Scales

References

Andrich D 1982 An extension of the Rasch model for ratings providing both location and dispersion parameters. *Psychometri.* 47(1): 105–13

Braun H I 1988 Understanding scoring reliability: Experiments in calibrating essay readers. *J. Ed. Stat.* 13(1): 1–18

Crick J E, Brennan R L 1982 GENOVA: Generalized Analysis of Variance. Computer program. University of Massachusetts at Boston Computer Facilities, Dorchester, Massachusetts

Guilford J P 1954 *Psychometric Methods*, 2nd edn. McGraw Hill, London

Harper A E, Misra V S 1976 *Research on Examinations in India*. National Council of Educational Research and Training, New Delhi

Linacre J M 1988 Facets: Many-facet Rasch Measurement. Computer program. MESA Press, Chicago, Illinois

Luce R D, Perry A D 1949 A method of matrix analysis of group structure. *Psychometri.* 14(1): 95–116

Lunz M E, Wright B D, Linacre J M 1990 Measuring the impact of judge severity on examination scores. *Applied Measurement in Education* 3(4): 331–45

Muller H 1987 A Rasch model for continuous ratings. *Psychometri.* 52(2): 165–81

Saal F E, Downey R G, Lahey M A 1980 Rating the ratings: Assessing the Psychometric quality of rating data. *Psych. Bull.* 88(2): 413–28

Stevens S S 1959 Measurement, psychophysics and utility. In: Churchman C W, Ratoosh P (eds.) 1959 *Measurement: Definitions and Theories*. Wiley, New York

Wilson M 1991 Unobserved categories. *Rasch Measurement* 5(1): 128

Further Reading

Brennan R L 1992 *Elements of Generalizability Theory* Rev. edn. American College Testing Program, Iowa City, Iowa

Cardinet J, Tourneur Y 1985 *Assurer la mesure*. Lang, New York

Engelhard G 1992 The measurement of writing ability with a many-faceted Rasch model. *Applied Measurement in Education* 5(3): 171–91

Engelhard G, Wilson M (eds.) 1996 The Many Facet Rasch (Facets) Model. In *Objective Measurement: Theory Into Practice*. Vol. 3. Ablex, Norwood, New Jersey

Heller J, Sheingold K, Nunez A, Myford C 1996 Examining the Quality of Rater Reasoning: Confronting Barriers to Valid and Reliable Portfolio Assessment. Educational Testing Service, Princeton, New Jersey

Linacre J M 1989 *Many-facet Rasch Measurement*. MESA Press, Chicago, Illinois

Shavelson R J, Webb N M 1991 *Generalizability Theory*. Sage, Newbury Park, California

Latent Trait Measurement Models

H. Swaminathan

Latent trait theory, in general terms, is concerned with the identification of traits such as aptitudes, interests, cognitive abilities, and personality variables that give rise to observed behavior. These latent traits are unobserved but it is assumed that the values the subject has on them influences, or predicts, in a stochastic sense, the observed response(s) of the subject. The goal of latent trait measurement theory is to infer, based on the observed responses, the subject's values on these latent traits. In order to accomplish this goal, a statistical model which specifies the relationship between the observed responses and the set of latent traits is postulated. Once the statistical model is specified, the values the subject has on the latent traits is estimated using standard statistical procedures.

The statistical model that is used to specify the relationship between the observed response and the latent traits could take many forms; it could be linear, curvilinear, or nonlinear. The choice of model depends upon the nature of the observed response, the nature of the latent trait, and finally, the mathematical form that is deemed appropriate. The model may be taken as unidimensional if only one trait is believed to influence the observed responses, or multidimensional if more than one trait is invoked.

1. Linear Latent Trait Measurement Models

While the term "latent trait" appears to have been first introduced by Paul Lazarsfeld in 1950, the concept goes back to Spearman in the early years of the twentieth century. Spearman (1904), postulated that the observed score y_{ji} of examinee i on test j is related to the examinee's unobservable or latent ability, θ_i, according to the linear model

$$y_{ji} = \mu_j + f_j \theta_i + e_{ji} \tag{1.1}$$

where f_j is, in factor analysis terms, the "factor loading," and e_{ji} is the error or "unique score." The term μ_j is an additive constant which has no effect on the correlation between the observed score and the trait. It is included here for the sake of completeness.

The unifactor theory of Spearman was rejected by Thurstone who postulated that the correlations among

851

scores on a battery of tests can be more reasonably explained by a set of traits, which he termed "common factors." The factor model postulated by Thurstone takes the form

$$y_{ji} = \mu_j + f_{ji}\theta_{li} + f_{j2}\theta_{2i} + \dots + f_{jk}\theta_{ki} + e_{ji} \qquad (1.2)$$

where $f_{j1}, f_{j2}, \dots f_{jk}$ are the factor loadings associated with the k latent traits $\theta_1, \theta_2, \dots, \theta_k$. As with the unifactor model, the purpose of the multifactor model was to provide an explanation of the correlations among the observed test scores (see *Factor Analysis*).

The primary objective in measurement is to determine, through observations, the scores an examinee has on a set of latent traits that give rise to the observations. While the factor models proposed by Spearman and Thurstone were designed to provide an explanation of the observed correlations among the test scores in terms of the underlying latent trait, they also serve as measurement models through which the values the examinee has on the latent traits can be determined. The Spearman model can be thought of as a unidimensional measurement model and the Thurstone model as its multidimensional extension.

In principle, the factor models given by Eqns. (1.1) or (1.2) can serve as latent trait measurement models and have been used as such, albeit in a limited sense, in personality assessment and vocational classifications. In achievement and aptitude testing factor analytic methods have been used primarily in test construction, particularly for item selection and validity assessment, and not as a framework for measurement.

Classical test theory (Lord and Novick 1968), on the other hand, has provided the framework for measurement during the past few decades. The foundation of classical test theory lies in the decomposition of the observed score in terms of true score and error score that is

$$y_{ji} = \tau_{ij} + e_{ij} \qquad (1.3)$$

where τ_{ij} is the true score of examinee i on test j and e_{ij} is the error score. In comparing Eqn. (1.3) with the Spearman model given in Eqn. (1.1), it can be seen that τ_{ij} is further decomposed. While the classical test theory decomposition is a tautology (Lord and Novick 1968), the decomposition given by the factor model by Eqn. (1.1) is falsifiable, i.e., the Spearman model is a statistical model which may or may not fit the data (see *Classical Test Theory*).

The simplicity of classical test theory and the fact that the classical test theory "model" is not subject to model-data fit, makes it appealing. However, it has serious drawbacks in that the indices that characterize an item, that is, item difficulty and item discrimination, and that which characterize the test, that is, reliability, are not invariant across examinee subpopulations. Similarly, the score that is assigned to an examinee is dependent on the particular set of items administered to the examinee; consequently, the concept of parallel test forms is needed for comparing performance of examinees and for the definition of the reliability of the test. In addition, the standard error of measurement associated with the score assigned to the examinee is assumed to be the same for all examinees. As a result, the standard error of measurement is an average value across the score range of the examinees, and in one sense, not appropriate for any examinee. Finally, classical test theory does not provide a framework for assembling items in a test to meet a certain objective, e.g., assembling a set of items to yield a desired precision of measurement at a specified trait value (for more detail and further discussion on these issues see Lord 1980, Hambleton and Swaminathan 1985) (see *Item Response Theory*).

The need for a better framework for measurement than that provided by classical test theory has prompted measurement theorists to consider model based measurement procedures. The simplest model for measurement is the Spearman model, given by Eqn. (1.1). Since in this model the observed score of an examinee on a test is a function of the characteristic of the test and the trait level of the examinee, this model provides a framework for taking into account the interaction between the trait level of the examinee and the characteristic of the item. While this linear latent trait model is appropriate for relating test scores to underlying traits, it is not appropriate for relating an examinee's trait to his/her performance on a dichotomously scored item. Equation (1.1) represents the regression of the score y_{ji} on the latent trait θ_i and hence is the expected value of y_{ji} conditional on the value of θ_i. When y_{ji} is dichotomous, this expected value is the probability that $y_{ji} = 1$. Since the probability is bounded by zero and unity, the regression curve cannot be linear. Thus when items are scored dichotomously, non-linear models that relate the probability of a correct response to the underlying trait are required.

2. Nonlinear Latent Trait Measurement Models

2.1 Dichotomous Item Response Models

The problem of predicting a dichotomous dependent variable from an observed regressor variable was first addressed by Finney in the early 1930s in the context of bioassay. Finney chose the cumulative normal probability function (the area under the normal curve) to model the relationship between the probability of "success" and an observed regressor. This normal ogive model, or the probit model was extended by Lawley (1943) to the situation where the regressor was a latent variable. Lord (1952, 1953), in extending the work of Lawley, formalized latent trait theory, by introducing the "assumption of local independence."

The assumption of local independence, according to Lord and Novick (1968), " . . . is the foundation of latent trait theory." The assumption of local independence or conditional independence states that once all the latent traits that contribute to performance on a set of items are determined, the responses to the items are statistically independent. This assumption is similar to that found in factor analysis; when the factors that contribute to the correlations among observed variables are partialed out, the observed variables will cease to be correlated. While the assumption of local independence may seem obvious or trivial when stated in this manner, the implications are profound. The assumption of local independence is equivalent to the assumption that all the traits that are relevant are included in the latent trait model; that is, the complete latent space is specified.

The major issue with the assumption of local independence revolves around the assumed dimensionality of the latent space. If the assumed dimensionality is correct, then local independence holds. However, for convenience and for mathematical reasons a unidimensional latent trait model is usually assumed. If the complete latent space is not unidimensional, the assumption of local independence will not hold. Up until the mid-1990s no foolproof method exists for examining the dimensionality of the latent space. Factor analysis is an obvious choice for examining the dimensionality of the latent space. However, as noted earlier, factor analysis was considered inadequate to model the relationship between a dichotomous observed variable and a continuous latent variable. Given this, it does not make much sense to use the model that was deemed inappropriate to check the assumptions underlying a model that replaced it.

Like the factor model, "item response theory" (a term coined by Lord in the late 1970s to replace the more general term, "latent trait theory") is based on the assumption that an examinee's response to an item is a function of the examinee's trait level (also known as ability level or proficiency level) and the characteristics of the item. In contrast to the model in Eqn. (1.1), in item response theory it is the probability of a correct response that is modeled. The higher the proficiency level, the higher the probability of responding correctly to the item. This probability is also affected by the characteristics of the item; if the item is very "difficult" relative to the examinee's proficiency level, the probability of a correct response will be low (see *Item Response Theory*).

An item may be characterized by a number of parameters; if the item is characterized by only one parameter, the "difficulty" parameter, the item response model is called a "one-parameter" model. If the item is characterized by the difficulty parameter and the "discrimination" parameter, the item response model is termed a "two-parameter" model. A three-parameter model is one which specifies that examinees with very low proficiency level will have a nonzero probability of responding correctly to the item.

The two-parameter normal ogive model that relates the probability of correct response to an examinee's latent trait and the characteristics of the item is given below:

$$P[\,y_{ji} = 1 \mid \theta_i\,] = \int_{-x}^{a_j(\theta_i - b_j)} e^{-\frac{1}{2}z^2}\, dz \equiv \Phi[a_j\,(\theta_i - b_j\,)]$$

(2.1)

In the expression given above, y_{ji} is the response of examinee i on item j, a_j and b_j are the parameters that characterize the item, and θ_i is the latent trait of examinee i. The function $\varphi(x)$ yields a notational simplification of the normal ogive model.

It is easily seen that in this model, the probability is bounded between zero and one. When $\theta_i = b_j$, the probability of a correct response is 0.5. The higher the value of b_j, the higher the value of θ_i that is needed to have a 50 percent chance of passing the item. It is in this sense that this parameter is called the "difficulty parameter." Curves 1, 5, and 6 (corresponding to items 1, 5, and 6) in Fig. 1, follow two-parameter item response models. By examining the θ corresponding to $P = 0.5$, it can be seen that Item 1 has the lowest b value; Items 5 and 6 have higher but the same b value.

The slope of the curve given by Eqn. (2.1) at the point where the probability is 0.5 corresponds to the value of the parameter a_j. The parameter a_j is called the discrimination parameter since as this value increases, the curve rises sharply at the point $\theta_i = b_j$. This implies that examinees with trait values higher than b_j will have a markedly higher probability of responding correctly to the item than examinees who have trait values lower than b_j. The curves corresponding to Items 1 and 5 in Fig. 1 have the same discrimination parameter value. The curve corresponding to Item 6 rises less sharply then these two curves and hence Item 6 is less discriminating than either Item 1 or 5.

The similarity between the item response model

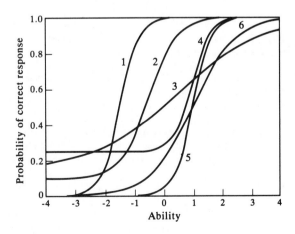

Figure 1

Six item response models

given by Eqn. (2.1) and the Spearman model given by Eqn. (1.4) is noteworthy. Clearly Eqn. (2.1) is the nonlinear analogue of the model given in Eqn. (1.4). Thus the item response models presented above are nonlinear factor models. To the extent that the item response function approximates a linear function, the results obtained using item response theory and linear factor model will be in agreement.

Curves corresponding to Items 2, 3, and 4 in Fig. 1 have nonzero probability of a correct response as θ_i approaches negative infinity. These curves are given by the equation

$$P[y_{ji} = 1 | \theta_i] = c_j + (1 - c_j)\Phi[a_j(\theta_i - b_j)] \quad (2.2)$$

The parameter c_j corresponds to the lower asymptote; Item 4 has the largest value for the c-parameter; and Item 2 has the lowest c-parameter value of the three items. Obviously, Items 1, 5, and 6 have the lowest possible values for the c-parameter, zero.

2.1.1 Logistic item response model. The normal ogive models are mathematically cumbersome. Berkson (1953) introduced the logistic cumulative distribution function to model the probability of success in the context of bio-assay. Birnbaum (1968) introduced these models in the mental measurement context.

The logistic function is given by the expression

$$P[y_{ji} = 1 | \theta_i] = c_j + (1 - c_j)\frac{e^{1.7a_j(\theta_i - b_j)}}{1 + e^{1.7a_j(\theta_i - b_j)}} \quad (2.3)$$

where the parameters have the same significance as in the normal ogive model. The scaling factor of 1.7 is introduced in the model to make the function as similar as possible to the normal ogive function. In almost all item response theory applications, the logistic model is the model of choice. The two-parameter model is obtained by setting $c_j = 0$ in Eqn. (2.3).

2.1.2 The invariance property. The items parameters in an item response model are parameters that characterize a curve. The values of these parameters must necessarily be the same along the points on the trait continuum. The parameters are therefore the same across subpopulations of examinees. It should be noted that the parameters obtained using the linear model given by Eqn. (1.4) will also be invariant when covariances rather than correlations are analyzed.

The parameter that characterizes an examinee's proficiency level is also invariant across different subsets of items as long as the dimensionality of the latent space remains the same. This invariance property distinguishes item response theory from classical test theory and serves as a powerful tool in test construction and trait assessment.

2.1.3 The Rasch model. When $c_j = 0$, and when the

item response models do not differ in discrimination, that is the item response functions have the same slope, the one-parameter model results. In Fig. 1 Items 1 and 5 have the same discrimination parameter values. These two items taken together follow the one-parameter model. The one-parameter model is usually written as

$$P[y_{ji} = 1 | \theta_i] = \frac{e^{(\theta_i - b_j)}}{1 + e^{(\theta_i - b_j)}} \quad (2.4)$$

While it is convenient to think of the one-parameter model as a special case of the two- and the three-parameter models, the one-parameter model was developed independently by Rasch (1960) using a totally different approach. Rasch was concerned with the principle of "objective measurement"—he felt that that the measurement of an examinee's proficiency level should in no way depend on the items used in the test. Similarly, two items should be comparable without any reference to the group of examinees to whom the item is administered. Using these two criteria he arrived at the one-parameter logistic model, or the Rasch Model (see *Rasch Measurement, Theory of*).

In the Rasch Model, it can be shown that the number right score contains all the information regarding an examinee's proficiency level, that is, two examinees who have the same number correct score have the same proficiency level. By conditioning the likelihood function (loosely speaking, the joint probability of the observations) on the number right score, it is possible to estimate the parameters that characterize the items without any reference to the examinees. In theory, it is also possible to estimate an examinee's proficiency level independently of the items administered by conditioning the likelihood function on the number of examinees who respond correctly to each item. This procedure, however, cannot be implemented in practice because of the excessive number of combinations that will result. The conditional estimation procedure described above is not possible with the multiparameter models; the invariance property has to be invoked with these models.

2.1.4 Features of the item response theory framework. When the item response model fits the data, the advantages afforded by the theory can be realized. For a complete discussion see Hambleton and Swaminathan (1985), Lord (1980). A few of the advantages are listed below.

(a) Item parameters are invariant across examinee subpopulations.

(b) Trait ability, or proficiency level parameters are independent of the set of items administered to the examinees.

(c) Precision of the trait estimates, or the standard error of measurement, can be determined at each trait level. This obviates the concept of reliability.

(d) The concept of information (inverse of the square of the standard error of measurement) provides a framework for test construction; the information provided by each item can be aggregated. Thus the contribution of each item to the precision of measurement can be assessed and this provides a basis for item selection.

(e) The invariance property of the trait parameters permits the administration of different items to different examinees. Testing can be "adapted" to an individual's trait level. This adaptive testing procedure has been shown to reduce testing time by at least 50 percent.

2.2 Models for Polytomously Scored Items

The models considered in the above sections are appropriate when the item is scored dichotomously. There are many situations where the items may be scored non-dichotomously, that is, polytomously. Ratings on a Likert scale, attitude measurement, and essay scoring are all examples where the items are polytomously scored. In addition in these situations the score categories are ordered. Scoring where the categories are unordered also occur as when the choice of distractors in multiple choice items is considered. Models for these types of scoring can be classified as nominal response models and ordinal response models (see *Attitudes, Measurement of; Rating Scales*).

2.2.1 The nominal response model.
The nominal response model where the response categories are unordered was first considered by Bock (1972). This model can be considered as an extension of the dichotomous model by considering the probability of choosing one category over another. Since the categories are unordered, the probability of choosing a category over the first category may be modeled. If π_i and π_0 are the probabilities of falling in categories j and 0 respectively, ($j = 1, 2, \ldots, k$), then, for an examinee with trait level θ (subscripts for the item and examinee are dropped for notational simplicity),

$$\frac{\pi_j}{\pi_j + \pi_{j-1}} = \frac{e^{a(\theta - b_j)}}{1 + e^{a_j(\theta - b_j)}} \tag{2.5}$$

where a_j and b_j are the parameters corresponding to the difference between category j and 0. It follows then that

$$\pi_j = \pi_0 e^{a_j(\theta - b_j)} \tag{2.6}$$

Since $\pi_0 + \pi_1 + \ldots + \pi_k = 1$, π_0 can be eliminated from the model to yield the probability of failing or choosing category j:

$$\pi_j = \frac{e^{a_j(\theta - b_j)}}{1 + \sum_{j=1}^{k} e^{a_j(\theta - b_j)}} \tag{2.7}$$

In this model, the examinee's trait value along with the category parameters determine which category the examinee chooses. A Rasch Model formulation is obtained by specifying a common a parameter value across the categories and across the items.

2.2.2 The ordinal response model.
In the ordinal response model the categories are ordered. In developing the model for this situation, the probability of choosing one category over the "preceding" category must be considered. Thus

$$\frac{\pi_j}{\pi_j + \pi_{j-1}} = \frac{e^{a(\theta - b_j)}}{1 + e^{a(\theta - b_j)}} \tag{2.8}$$

The important distinction between this model and the model in Eqn. (2.7) is that the discrimination parameter is not allowed to vary across the categories since otherwise the order will not be meaningful. The discrimination parameter, however, is permitted to vary across items. It follows that

$$\pi_j = \pi_{j-1} e^{a(\theta - b_j)} \tag{2.9}$$

This model yields the probability of choosing category 1, 2, 3, . . ., k in terms of the probability of choosing category 0:

$$\pi_j = \frac{e^{z_j}}{1 + \sum_{r=1}^{k} e^{z_r}},$$

where

$$z_t = \sum_{m=1}^{t} a(\theta - b_m). \tag{2.10}$$

The model given in Eqn. (2.10) is essentially that developed first by Andrich (1978, 1982) in the analysis of rating scales and by Masters (1982) in the context of partial credit scoring. These authors used a Rasch formulation of the model. Andrich (1978), by decomposing the parameter b_j into components specific to the item and to the response category, i.e., $b_j = b + t_j$, was able to provide a more finely tuned analysis of the choice process. The partial credit models of Andrich and Masters, and their generalization have important applications in performance assessment and essay scoring (see *Rating Score Analysis; Partial Credit Model*).

Samejima (1969) introduced an alternative model, the graded response model, for ordered responses. This model considers the probability that an examinee will respond *at or above* category j. In this model the probability that an examinee will choose a particular category is not easily determined. Comparisons between the partial credit and the graded response models are provided by Masters (1982).

3. Multidimensional Item Response Models

The item response models that were in use in the early 1990s were unidimensional models. The assumption that the latent space is unidimensional has been a source of concern for many practitioners and psychometricians. Unlike the factor analysis situation where a multidimensional extension of the Spearman model has been operationalized and developed fully, the multidimensional extension of the item response model is still in its infancy. While multidimensional models have been formulated by several researchers (see McDonald 1982; Bock et al. 1985; McKinley and Reckase 1982; Reckase and McKinley 1982; Sympson 1978) the models and procedures are not in operation.

Multidimensional item response models can be classified into compensatory models and noncompensatory models. In the compensatory model an examinee's trait value on one dimension compensates for the trait in another dimension, that is in a mathematics item, an examinee's mathematical knowledge may compensate for his/her lack of language skills. In the noncompensatory model an examinee is required to have a minimum value on all the relevant dimensions in order to respond correctly to the item. The mathematical form of the compensatory model (Reckase and McKinley 1982) is:

$$P[u = 1 | \theta_1, \theta_2] = \frac{e^{a_1(\theta_1 - b_1) + a_2(\theta_2 - b_2)}}{1 + e^{a_1(\theta_1 - b_1) + a_2(\theta_2 - b_2)}}$$

(3.1)

where θ_1, θ_2 are the trait values of the examinee on two dimensions, a_1, a_2 are the discrimination parameters on the two dimensions, and b_1, and b_2 are the difficulties on these dimensions. Reckase and McKinley (1983) have provided interpretations of the item parameters. The noncompensatory model was formulated by Sympson (1978). The two-dimensional model is given as a product of two unidimensional item response models, that is,

$$P[u = 1 | \theta_1 \; \theta_2] = \frac{e^{a_1(\theta_1 - b_1)}}{1 + e^{a_1(\theta_1 - b_1)}} \times \frac{e^{a_2(\theta_2 - b_2)}}{1 + e^{a_2(\theta_2 - b_2)}}.$$

(3.2)

Figures 2a and 2b provide illustrations of the compensatory and noncompensatory two-dimensional item response models. Despite the formulation of these models little is known about their utility and applicability to practical testing problems.

4. Conclusion

Latent trait measurement theory is a model based measurement theory that provides a general framework for testing and measurement. While linear latent trait models are appropriate when the observed responses are continuous, they are inappropriate when responses to items are dichotomously or polytomously scored. Item response models, which are non-linear latent trait models, are appropriate in the latter situation. Consequently, item response theory has emerged as the modern measurement theory. Procedures based on item response theory are the procedures of choice for test construction, trait estimation, and equating of tests. However, current interest in performance assessment and the possible move away from multiple choice items have resulted in an increased interest in models for nondichotomously scored items. While

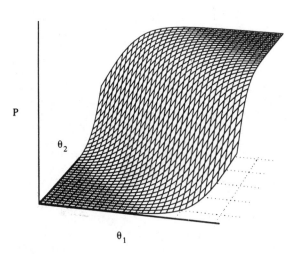

Figure 2a
A compensatory model

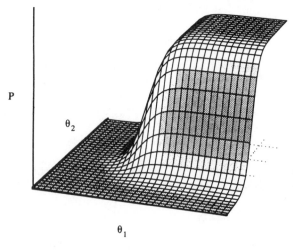

Figure 2b
A noncompensatory model

these models are in place, considerable research is needed before the models can be fully operationalized and used by practitioners. A major area of concern is with the unidimensional nature of the item response models. While research in multidimensional item response models is continuing, little progress has been made to date in the estimation of parameters and in understanding how the models could be applied. Considerable research efforts can be expected in this direction in the 1990s and beyond.

See also: Scaling Methods; Item Response Theory

References

Andrich D 1978 A rating formulation for ordered response categories. *Psychometri.* 43:561–73
Andrich D 1982 An extension of the Rasch model for ratings providing both location and dispersion parameters. *Psychometri.* 47: 105–13
Berkson J 1953 A statistically precise and relatively simple method of estimating the bio-assay with quantal response, based on the logistic function. *J. Am. Stat. Assoc.* 48: 565–99
Birnbaum A 1968 Some latent trait models and their use in inferring an examinee's ability. In: Lord F M, Novick M R 1968 *Statistical Theories of Mental Test Scores.* Addison-Wesley, Reading
Bock R D 1972 Estimating item parameters and latent ability when responses are scored in two or more nominal categories. *Psychometri.* 37: 29–51
Bock R D, Gibbons R, Muraki E 1985 *Full Information Factor Analysis.* MRC Report 85–1. Nat. Opinion Res. Ct. Chicago, Illinois

Hambleton R K, Swaminathan H 1985 *Item Response Theory: Principles and Applications.* Kluwer-Nijhoff, Boston, Massachusetts
Lawley D N 1943 On problems connected with item selection and test construction. *Proc. Royal Soc. Edin.* 61: 273–87
Lord F M 1952 A theory of test scores. *Psychometric Monograph* 7
Lord F M 1953 The application of confidence intervals and maximum likelihood to the estimation of an examinee's ability. *Psychometri.* 18: 57–75
Lord F M 1980 *Applications of item response theory to practical testing*
Lord F M, Novick M R 1968 *Statistical theories of mental test scores.* Addison-Wesley, Reading
McDonald R P 1982 Linear versus nonlinear models in item response theory. *App. Psych. Meas.* 4: 379–96
McKinley R L, Reckase M D 1982 *An extension of the two-parameter logistic model to the multidimensional latent space.* Res. Rep. ONR 83–2. The American College Testing Program, Iowa City, Iowa
Masters G N 1982 A rasch model for partial credit scoring. *Psychometri.* 47: 149–74
Reckase M D, McKinley R L 1982 The feasibility of multidimensional latent trait model. Paper presented at the meeting of the Am. Psych. Assoc., Washington, DC
Rasch G 1960 *Probabilistic models for some intelligence and attainment tests.* Danish Institute of Educational Research, Copenhagen
Samejima F 1969 Estimation of ability using a response pattern of graded scores. *Psychometriic Monograph*, 7
Spearman C 1904 General intelligence, objectively determined and measured. *Am. J. Psych.* 15: 201–33
Sympson J B 1978 A model for testing with multidimensional items. In: Weiss D (ed.) 1978 *Proceedings of the 1977 Computerized Adaptive Testing Conference.* University of Minnesota, Minneapolis, Minnesota

Partial Credit Model

G. N. Masters

The partial credit model is an extension of the Rasch model for dichotomously scored test data to outcomes recorded in more than two ordered response categories. One approach to the analysis of polychotomously scored data is to group the ordered response categories and to carry out multiple dichotomous analyses. A preferable approach is to implement a model for ordered response categories directly. The partial credit model is a general polychotomous item response model belonging to the Rasch family of measurement models.

1. A Mathematics Example

There are many situations in educational research in which students' attempts at a task can be categorized into several ordered levels of outcome. The use of multiple outcome categories is common practice when scoring performances on complex tasks like essay writing and problem-solving. But even in situations in which it is usual to score students' performances dichotomously (right/wrong), it is often possible to identify among students' "incorrect" answers varying degrees of partial understanding and so to define more than two levels of outcome on an item. This can be illustrated with the following item from a test of basic mathematics:

A calculator shows the figure 25.634817
Express this correct to two decimal places.

Students give a variety of answers to this item, but by far the most common are 25.63, 25.64, 2563.4817, and 0.25634817.

The usual dichotomous scoring of this item would give full credit for the first of these answers and no credit for any other. However, the second answer, 25.64, shows partial understanding: students who give this answer understand that correcting a number to two decimal places involves reducing to two the number of digits after the decimal point. These students appear to believe that because the original number is greater than 25.63 it must be rounded *up* to 25.64. The last two answers indicate no understanding of rounding and result from moving the decimal point two places (as in multiplication and division by 100). The most that can be said for these two answers is that they show some understanding of "two decimal places." This is more than can be said for the other answers that students give to this item (e.g., "25.634.817").

The answers given to this mathematics item by a group of 570-ninth grade students are summarized in Fig. 1. Students' answers have been grouped to form four ordered outcome categories: 25.63; 25.64; either 2563.4817 or 0.25634817; and some other answer. The 570 students have been divided into 10 equal-sized groups on the basis of their total mathematics test scores. Students with the lowest test scores are at the bottom of Fig. 1. Students with the highest test scores are at the top. Figure 1 shows the proportion of students in each test score group in each of the four outcome categories.

Among the lowest-scoring group of students (at the bottom of Fig. 1), only about 20 percent of students gave the correct answer, 25.63, to this item. The most common answer given by this group was either 2563.4817 or 0.25634817. More than 60 percent of incorrect answers given by this low-scoring group were of this type. Among the highest-scoring group (at the top of Fig. 1), about 80 percent of students gave the correct answer. Ninety percent of high-scoring students who gave incorrect answers to this item gave the answer 25.64. Figure 1 shows that the types of errors made on this item change with increasing mathematics test score. Very few of the incorrect answers given by students with low test scores show any understanding of rounding. In fact, about 20 percent of low-scoring students give "other" answers like 25.634.817, suggesting that these students may not even understand "two decimal places." In contrast, the incorrect answers given by high-scoring students display some understanding of rounding but reveal confusion about when to round up or down. In an instructional setting, it would be inappropriate to treat every student giving an "incorrect" answer to this mathematics item in the same way. The type of instruction in rounding decimal numbers required by most low-scoring students in Fig. 1 is likely to be very different from the instruction required by most high-scoring students.

The partial credit model is a statistical model for the analysis of test and questionnaire items for which two or more ordered levels of outcome are defined. Its purpose is to model changes in the distribution of

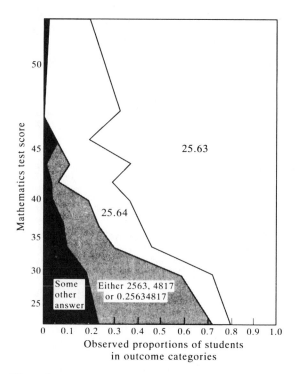

Figure 1
Observed proportions in outcome categories

students' answers over the available outcome categories with increasing competence. For the mathematics item described above, the four outcome regions as modeled by the partial credit model are shown in Fig. 2. The four regions of this map correspond to the four regions in Fig. 1. The difference is that these regions no longer show the observed proportions of students in each category, but show *modeled* proportions. The basic shapes of the smooth curves in Fig. 2 are fixed by the algebra of the partial credit model. The locations of these curves were estimated from the answers this group of 570 students gave to this item.

When students' answers to an item approximate the partial credit model (i.e., Fig. 1 resembles Fig. 2), that item can be used to help estimate students' locations on the path of developing competence that runs up the left edge of these figures. It is in this sense that the partial credit model is a "measurement" model: it provides a probabilistic connection between the categories of observed outcome on an item and locations on a latent path of developing competence. This probabilistic connection provides a basis for constructing measures of competence from students' performances on a set of items with multiple outcome categories.

2. Algebra of the Model

In common with all latent trait models, the partial credit model represents each student's level of competence

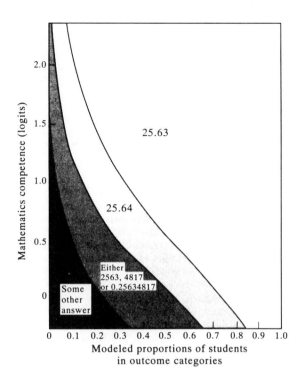

Modeled proportions of students
in outcome categories

Figure 2
Modeled proportions in outcome categories

or achievement as a location on a continuum of increasing competence. In Figs. 1 and 2, this continuum runs up the left edge of the figure. The location β_n of student n on this continuum is estimated from that student's answers to a set of appropriate items. Answers to each item are classified into a set of ordered outcome categories labeled 0, 1, 2, . . . m_i for that item. Under the partial credit model, the probability of student n's answer being in outcome category x of item i is given by

$$P_{nix} = \frac{1}{1 + \sum_{k=1}^{mi} \exp \sum_{j=1}^{k} (\beta_n - \delta_{ij})} \quad \text{for } x = 0$$

$$\text{and } P_{nix} = \frac{\exp \sum_{j=1}^{x} (\beta_n - \delta_{ij})}{1 + \sum_{k=1}^{mi} \exp \sum_{j=1}^{k} (\beta_n - \delta_{ij})} \quad (1)$$
$$\text{for } x = 1, 2, . . . m_i$$

where the parameters $\delta_{i1}, \delta_{i2}, \ldots, \delta_{im_i}$ are a set of parameters associated with item i which jointly locate the model probability curves for that item (see Fig. 2). There are m_i item parameters for an item with $m_i + 1$ outcome categories.

For the mathematics item described above, four outcome categories were defined meaning that 4−1=3 parameters $\delta_{i1}, \delta_{i2},$ and δ_{i3} were estimated for this item. These three estimates and the algebra of the model provide the modeled outcome regions in Fig. 2. At any estimated level of competence β_n, the partial credit model provides the widths $P_{ni0}, P_{ni1}, P_{ni2},$ and P_{ni3} of the four outcome regions at that level. These widths can be interpreted either as the estimated probabilities of a student at that level of competence responding in outcome categories 0, 1, 2, and 3, or as the expected proportions of students at that level of competence responding in these four categories. For values of β_n near the bottom of Fig. 2, P_{ni0} and P_{ni1} are larger than P_{ni2} and P_{ni3}. For values of β_n near the top of Fig. 2, P_{ni3} is large, and all other probabilities are small. A more complete discussion of the algebra of the partial credit model is provided by Masters (1982, 1988), Wright and Masters (1982), and Masters and Wright (1984).

3. Ordered Outcome Categories

The partial credit model could be applied to any set of test or questionnaire data collected for the purposes of measuring students' abilities, achievements, or attitudes provided that responses to each test or questionnaire item are scored in two or more ordered categories. There are many different ways in which a set of ordered outcome categories might be defined for a task. Some of these are considered below.

3.1 Levels of Partial Understanding

The four outcome categories defined for the mathematics item above were the product of a careful study of all answers given by students to this item. This approach to developing a set of outcome categories is described in some detail by Dahlgren (1984). For some tasks, the types of misconceptions and errors that are likely to occur will be well understood, making it possible to construct a set of outcome categories before the task is given to a group of students. For most tasks, however, the construction of a set of categories which capture levels of partial understanding will probably require a close study of students' responses. These might then be grouped according to the levels of understanding that they reflect.

> Starting with a comparatively large number of categories the researcher will gradually refine these, arriving at a smaller set of categories that may finally be difficult or impossible to collapse further. (Dahlgren 1984 p. 26)

Dahlgren describes this approach to constructing a set of outcome categories as the partitioning of the "outcome space" associated with a task. The final set of categories is then used in future applications of the task.

3.2 Multistep Problems

For complex problems which require the completion of a number of steps, it is usual to identify several intermediate stages in the solution of each problem and to award partial credit on the basis of the number of steps a student completes. This scoring procedure is common in subject areas like mathematics and the physical sciences where students must first identify the problem type, select an appropriate solution strategy, and then apply this strategy which may itself involve a number of steps. By awarding credit for the steps a student has successfully completed, a set of ordered outcome categories can be defined for each multistep problem.

4. Rating Scales

Another common method for recording performances on an item is to rate students' attempts at the item on a scale (e.g., 1 to 5). This scoring procedure is popular for recording performances on tasks like building a model, assembling a piece of apparatus, carrying out a procedure, and writing an essay. To ensure a degree of comparability across raters and over time, the criteria to be applied in rating performances on a task might be made explicit and accompanied by samples of student attempts at that task to illustrate the available score points.

Rating scales are also common methods of measuring attitudes and personalities. In these contexts, respondents are usually provided with a fixed set of response alternatives like "never," "sometimes," "often," "always," or "strongly disagree," "disagree," "agree," "strongly agree" to be used with all items on the questionnaire. Questionnaires of this form can be analyzed with the partial credit model. However, the fact that the response alternatives are defined in the same way for all items introduces the possibility of simplifying the partial credit model by assuming that, in questionnaires of this type, the pattern of modeled outcome regions (Fig. 2) will be the same for all items on the questionnaire and that the only difference between items will be a difference in location on the measurement variable (e.g., difficulty of endorsement). This assumption yields the rating scale model (see *Rating Scale Analysis; Attitudes, Measurement of*).

4.1 Question Clusters

Occasionally, test and questionnaire items come in clusters with all items in a cluster relating to the same piece of introductory text. Each item in a cluster could be treated as an independent item to be scored right or wrong. However, if items of this type are to be treated as independent dichotomously-scored items, then the assumption of local independence must be made. Each student's response to any one item must be assumed to be without the influence of his or her responses to the other items in that cluster. In most dichotomously scored tests, this is a reasonable assumption. But in an item cluster, items have a shared dependence on a common stem and so are less likely to be locally independent. In this context, it is often more appropriate to treat a cluster as a single "item" on which students' scores are counts of the questions in that cluster answered correctly and to take values between 0 and m_i *(where m_i is the number of questions in the cluster)*. In this way, m_i+1 ordered levels of outcome are defined for each cluster (Andrich 1982, Masters and Evans 1986).

4.2 Interactive Items

Finally, ordered outcome categories can be constructed from students' performances on computer-administered items which provide feedback to students during a test. The feedback given during a test may simply inform students of their success or failure on an item and offer a second attempt if the item is failed. Failure on a second attempt might be followed by a third or fourth attempt and credit awarded on the basis of the number of attempts required to provide the correct answer. This procedure is usually referred to as "answer-until-correct" scoring. Alternatively, students failing on their first attempt at an item might be given a "hint" and offered an opportunity to try again (Trismen 1981). Failure after a hint might be followed by further assistance and each student's score based on the number of hints required to arrive at the correct answer. This format not only defines several ordered levels of outcome for each item but also, through the careful construction of hints, might be used to trace students' misunderstandings to their source.

5. Related Models

The partial credit model is a latent trait (or item response) model and, in particular, is a member of the Rasch family of latent trait models. The relationship of the partial credit model to a number of other members of this family (e.g., Poisson counts model, binomial trials model) is described by Masters and Wright (1984). Several of these related models are considered briefly below.

5.1 Dichotomous Rasch Model

The dichotomous model (see *Rasch Measurement, Theory of*) is designed for the analysis of test items for which only two levels of outcome are defined (x=0 and x=1). The dichotomous model is obtained by setting $m_i=1$ in Eqn (1). This provides the model probabilities

$$P_{nix} = \frac{1}{1 + \exp(\beta_n - \delta_{i1})} \qquad \text{for } x = 0$$

$$= \frac{\exp(\beta_n - \delta_{i1})}{1 + \exp(\beta_n - \delta_{i1})} \qquad \text{for } x = 1$$

The resulting outcome map (Fig. 2) contains only two regions ("fail" and "pass") and the single parameter estimate δ_{i1} locates the modeled boundary between these two regions. This model is the best known of the item response models and is widely used for the analysis of educational tests.

5.2 Rating Scale Model

The rating scale model (see *Rating Scale Analysis*) can be used to analyze questionnaires in which a fixed set of response alternatives like "strongly disagree," "disagree," "agree," and "strongly agree" is used with every item on the questionnaire. The rating scale model is obtained by resolving the general item parameter δ_{ij} in Eqn (1) into two components: one for item i, and one associated with the transition between response alternatives $j-1$ and j:

$$\delta_{ij} = \delta_i + \tau_j$$

The rating scale model is obtained by substituting $(\delta_i + \tau_j)$ for δ_{ij} in Eqn (1):

$$P_{nix} = \cfrac{1}{1 + \sum_{k=1}^{m} \exp \sum_{j=1}^{k} (\beta_n - \delta_i - \tau_j)} \quad \text{for } x = 0$$

$$= \cfrac{\sum_{j=1}^{x} (\beta_n - \delta_i - \tau_j)}{1 + \sum_{k=1}^{m} \exp \sum_{j=1}^{k} (\beta_n - \delta_i - \tau_j)} \quad \text{for } x = 1, 2, \dots, m$$

When this model is applied, a single location δ_i is estimated for each item and m parameters $\tau_1, \tau_2, \dots, \tau_m$ are estimated for the $m+1$ response alternatives provided with the questionnaire.

5.3 Ordered Partition Model

The ordered partition model (Wilson 1993) can be applied when responses to an item are recorded in K_i categories, but some of these K_i categories, while qualitatively different, represent the same *level* of performance (i.e., the number of distinguishable levels of performance on item i, L_i, is less than the total number of response categories K_i). When $L_i = K_i$, the ordered partition model is simply the partial credit model.

The ordered partition model is obtained by introducing a vector B_i which indicates the level to which each response category belongs. If, for item i, response category k is to be assigned to level j, then $B_i(k) = j$ where j is an integer between 0 and L_i. Under the ordered partition model, the probability of person n responding in category k of item i is

$$P_{nik} = \frac{\exp(\beta_n B_i(k) + \xi_{ik})}{\sum_{h=1}^{ki} \exp(\beta_n B_i(h) + \xi_{ik})} \quad k = 1, 2, \dots K_i$$

where ξ_{i1} is defined as 0 and the item parameters in the partial credit model $((\delta))$ can be expressed in terms of the item parameters in the ordered partition model $((\xi))$. The estimation of the parameters in the model is described by Wilson and Adams (1993).

5.4 Other Constraints

Other cases of the partial credit model can be generated by imposing constraints on the values of the item parameters $\delta_{i1}, \delta_{i2}, \dots, \delta_{imi}$ for each item. One simple constraint is to restrict these parameters to a uniform spacing such that $(\delta_{i2} - \delta_{i1}) = (\delta_{i3} - \delta_{i2}) = \dots = (\delta_{im} - \delta_{im-1}) = \sigma_i$.

Under this constraint (Andrich 1982), only the mean item parameter δ_i and the uniform spacing σ_i are estimated for each item i. If there is a reason to expect that the outcome categories for every item on a test will be uniformly spaced, and the data conform to this expectation, this case of the partial credit model offers a more parsimonious representation than the full-rank model in that it requires the estimation of fewer parameters. This constrained version of the model may also be useful with small data sets which provide insufficient data to reliably estimate all parameters for an item.

Further cases of the partial credit model have been proposed by introducing other constraints on the item parameters (e.g., steadily increasing or steadily decreasing differences $(\delta_{i2} - \delta_{i1}) < (\delta_{i3} - \delta_{i2}) < \dots < (\delta_{im} - \delta_{im-1})$. In general, constraints such as these are only likely to be of value if they have a basis in theory (i.e., if they follow from the way in which the ordered categories have been defined).

6. Applications

Estimation algorithms for the partial credit model are described by Masters (1982), Wright and Masters (1982), Glas and Verhelst (1989), and Wilson and Adams (1993). Computer programs to implement these algorithms have been developed by Adams and Khoo (1993) and Wright and Linacre (1992).

In 1989 a special issue of *Applied Measurement in Education* described a range of applications of the partial credit model. Some areas of application are summarized briefly below.

6.1 Variable Definition

Figures 1 and 2 illustrate how, by classifying "incorrect" answers to an item into a number of ordered levels of understanding or completion, it is possible to build a more detailed picture of how competence in a subject area develops. This is an important general application of the partial credit model. The probabilistic connection between categories of observed outcome on an item and the latent continuum that these items are constructed to measure, enables each level of competence on the measurement variable to be interpreted in terms of the types of misconceptions or processing errors that are likely to be found among students at that level. Students with estimated locations near the top of Fig. 2, for example, are likely to have very different misunderstandings from students with estimated locations near the bottom of this figure.

Adams et al. (1987) have used this method to build a detailed picture of a path of developing competence in second language learning. The items in their instrument were questions posed to second language learners in face-to-face interviews. Each learner's response to a question was rated using a set of ordered outcome categories specific to that question.

The Ministry of Education in Western Australia has taken a similar approach to analyzing students' performances on written expression tasks. They have identified a number of aspects of writing competence and have developed a set of rating points for each of these aspects of writing. Each set of ordered rating points is illustrated using samples of student writing. In this way, a number of "ladders" of developing competence corresponding to different aspects of writing ability have been constructed and calibrated. These are used as a framework for scoring students' performances on writing tasks and provide a detailed picture of the development of writing competence.

Other examples of the use of partial credit analysis in variable construction are provided by Adams et al. (1990), Julian and Wright (1988), and Wright and Masters (1982).

6.2 Item Banking

Calibrated item banks are usually limited to dichotomously-scored test items. This is a serious limitation if the bank is to be used as part of a program of educational assessment. A large proportion of what is taught in schools is not adequately assessed with items that can be scored either right or wrong. If an item bank is to be useful as an assessment resource, it must be capable of incorporating calibrated tasks like essay-writing, problem-solving, and model-building.

The partial credit model provides a basis for the calibration of a range of tasks which cannot adequately be scored dichotomously. If these tasks are to be calibrated and included in an item bank, then it will usually be necessary to provide explicit guides to the scoring of individual tasks, possibly with samples of student responses to illustrate the score points to be used with each task. Some experimental work on the construction of banks of nondichotomously scored items is described by Masters (1984) and Masters and Evans (1986) (see *Item Banking in Testing and Assessment*).

6.3 Computer Adaptive Testing

The availability of a bank of calibrated items introduces the possibility of selecting items to suit an individual's current level of competence. If items are administered by computer, then the items to be presented to a student can be selected automatically during the course of a test. After each item is answered, the student's level of competence is re-estimated and the bank is searched for the most appropriate remaining item. (This is the item that provides most information at the student's current estimate.)

Computer adaptive testing can be generalized to items which use systems of partial credit scoring, thereby enabling the construction of tailored tests based on more complex outcome spaces than right and wrong answers. The simplest adaptive testing algorithm for the partial credit model uses the statistical "information" I_{ni} available from bank item i at competence level β_n. This can be calculated as

$$I_{ni} = \sum_{k=1}^{m_i} (k^2 P_{nik}) - \left(\sum_{k=1}^{m_i} k P_{nik} \right)^2$$

where $P_{nik}(k=1,2,\ldots,m_i)$ is the model probability of person n with an estimated level of competence β_n giving an answer in outcome category k of item i. The value of this information might be calculated for each item in a bank, given student n's current estimate, and the item with the largest value of I_{ni} chosen as the next item to be administered to person n.

Important foundational work on the extension of computer adaptive testing procedures to items which use systems of partial credit scoring has been done by Koch and Dodd (1986, 1989) and Dodd and Koch (1986, 1987). They describe a number of potential applications of this methodology, including the possibility of constructing computer adaptive questionnaires in which items designed to measure attitudes or opinions might be calibrated and selected to maximize the information available from a questionnaire. Another very promising application of this method is the construction of computer adaptive tests in which feedback is provided and multiple attempts are permitted at individual computer-administered test items (see *Adaptive Testing*).

See also: Rasch Measurement, Theory of; Latent Trait Measurement Models

References

Adams R J, Doig B A, Rosier M 1990 *Science Learning in Victorian Schools.* Australian Council for Educational Research, Melbourne

Adams R J, Griffin P E, Martin L 1987 A latent trait method for measuring a dimension in second language proficiency. *Language Testing* 4(1): 9–27

Adams R J, Khoo S T 1993 QUEST: *The Interactive Test Analysis System.* Australian Council for Educational Research, Melbourne

Andrich D 1982 An extension of the Rasch model for ratings providing both location and dispersion parameters. *Psychometri.* 47(1): 105–13

Dahlgren L O 1984 Outcomes of learning. In: Marton F, Hounsell D, Entwistle N (eds.) 1984 *The Experience of Learning.* Scottish Academic Press, Edinburgh

Dodd B, Koch W 1986 Relative efficiency analyses for the partial credit model. Paper presented at the annual meeting of the American Educational Research Association, San Francisco, California

Dodd B G, Koch W R 1987 Effects of variation in item step values on item and test information in the partial credit model. *Appl. Psych. Meas.* 11: 371–84

Glas C A W, Verhelst N D 1989 Extensions of the partial credit model. *Psychometri.* 54(4): 635–59

Julian E R, Wright B D 1988 Using computerized patient simulations to measure the clinical competence of physicians. *Appl. Meas. Ed.* 1(4): 299–318

Koch W R, Dodd B G 1986 Operational characteristics of adaptive testing procedures using partial credit scoring. Paper presented at the annual meeting of the American Educational Research Association, San Francisco, California

Koch W R, Dodd B G 1989 An investigation of procedures for computerized adaptive testing using the partial credit scoring. *Appl. Meas. Ed.* 2(4): 335–57

Masters G N 1982 A Rasch model for partial credit scoring. *Psychometri.* 47(2): 149–74

Masters G N 1984 Constructing an item bank using partial credit scoring. *J. Ed. Meas.* 21(1): 19–32

Masters G N 1988 The analysis of partial credit scoring. *Appl. Meas. Ed.* 1(4): 279–98

Masters G N, Evans J 1986 Banking non-dichotomously scored items. *Appl. Psychol. Meas.* 10(4): 355–67

Masters G N, Wright B D 1984 The essential process in a family of measurement models. *Psychometri.* 49(4): 529–44

Trismen D M 1981 The development and administration of a set of mathematics items with hints (ETS-RB-81-5). Educational Testing Service, Princeton, New Jersey

Wilson M R 1993 The ordered partition model: An extension of the partial credit model. *Appl. Psych. Meas.*

Wilson M R, Adams R J 1993 Marginal maximum likelihood estimation for the ordered partition model. *J. Ed. Stat.* 18(1):69–90

Wright B D, Linacre J M 1992 FACETS computer program. MESA Psychometrics Laboratory, University of Chicago, Chicago, Illinois

Wright B D, Masters G N 1982 *Rating Scale Analysis.* MESA Press, Chicago, Illinois

Further Reading

Adams R J 1988 Applying the partial credit model to educational diagnosis. *Appl. Meas. Ed.* 1(4): 347–62

Adams R J, Griffin P E 1986 *Scaling Tests of Spoken Language with the Rasch Partial Credit Model.* Victorian Ministry of Education, Melbourne

Harris J, Laan S, Mossenson L 1988 Applying partial credit analysis to the construction of narrative writing tests. *Appl. Meas. Ed.* 1(4): 335–46

Masters G N, Mislevy R J 1993 New views of student learning: Implications for educational measurement. In: Fredericksen N, Mislevy R J, Bejar I I (eds.) 1993 *Test Theory for a New Generation of Tests.* Erlbaum, Hillsdale, New Jersey

Muraki E 1992 A generalized partial credit model: Application of an EM algorithm. *Appl. Psych. Meas.* 16(2): 159–76

Pollitt A, Hutchinson C 1987 Calibrating graded assessments: Rasch partial credit analysis of performance in writing. *Language Testing* 4(1):72–92

Wilson M, Iventosch L 1988 Using the partial credit model to investigate responses to structured subtests. *Appl. Meas. Ed.* 1(4):319–34

Wilson M R, Masters G N 1993 The partial credit model and null categories. *Psychometri.*

Rasch Measurement Theory

P. Allerup

This entry is concerned with the use of the Rasch model as a diagnostic tool in the development of tests in order to identify items and persons that do not conform to the measurement model. It emphasizes the unique properties of the dichotomous Rasch model, and the problems encountered when items do not discriminate at the same level between individuals. This entry is of a technical nature and provides a mathematical and statistical treatment of the issues. This approach has been adopted because although the Rasch models are used increasingly in many parts of the world, texts that raise and address these issues are not readily available. Other entries in this *Encyclopedia* consider the applications of the Rasch model in a wide range of measurement problems (see *Adaptive Testing; Es-*

says: Equating of Marks; Item Banking; Partial Credit Model; Rating Acale Analysis).

1. Introduction to the Rasch Model

When the name "Rasch model" appears in connection with statistical analyses, it will often mean the so-called "dichotomous Rasch model" (Rasch 1960) or the "one-parameter logistic model," namely, the basic statistical model, used when analyzing a set of observations, $a_{vi}=0$ or $a_{vi}=1$, obtained from a study, where n students ($v=1, \ldots, n$) respond (correctly or incorrectly) to k ($i=1, \ldots, k$) test items. When Georg Rasch (1901–80) was still alive, he strongly opposed the use of "Rasch" as a label for the model—or rather models, since, in fact, the dichotomous model is only one model among a group of statistical models. Rasch himself referred to "models for measurement" or "measurement models."

Among the more prominent members of this group is the "general M-category model" (Rasch 1968), in which the responses a_{vi} take M different values (e.g., M=3: "agree"/"do not agree"/"do not know"). The general M-category model is, like the basic Rasch model, a statistical model for analyzing categorical information a_{vi} but the fact that the basic model summarizes the number of correct responses tends to suppress this aspect of the model. Although the multiplicative Poisson model was used as an illustrative example before 1960 by Rao (1952), it was Rasch (1960) who extensively used the multiplicative structure of the expected values $E(a_{vi})=\lambda_{vi}=\varepsilon_i\xi_v$ (λ is the expected value of a Poisson variable, splitting multiplicatively into ε and ξ characterizing row and column effects) in his working with the concept of specific objectivity (Rasch 1966a, 1966b, 1966c) and exploited the statistical properties of this class of models in practical statistical analysis. The general M-category model attained a position as a thoroughly investigated model when Andersen (1973) solved the problems of conditional estimation routines for the parameters and gave proofs for the statistical distributions in large samples of the statistics in a conditional framework. Later, it seems that a particular version of the general model, the so-called "one-dimensional general model," in which the item and individual parameters (originally being arrays containing as many parameters as the number of response categories but now reduced to a set of one-dimensional category and item parameters) (Andrich 1978, Allerup 1985, 1986, 1987) has been used at the cost of the general model.

The Rasch model with dichotomous responses $a_{vi}=0,1$ quickly became the model attracting most attention, and very soon Fischer (1974) published a comprehensive treatment of the mathematics of this model and the classical statistical methods. However, it seems that some of the powerful properties of this model have been disregarded in the way the model is used in practical data analysis. This occurs in two quite different situations that employ the model. The first is when the model is tested as a theoretical description of data (i.e., the model is tested for fit) but the model is rejected; in this case substantial knowledge is still available from the very way in which the model was rejected. The other situation is where the model is accepted as an adequate description but not all consequences of this acceptance are taken properly into consideration.

The aim of this entry is therefore twofold: to illustrate through examples that (a) rejection of the Rasch model can in itself represent valuable "end point" information, ready for important conclusive statements; and (b) that when data are further analyzed acceptance of the Rasch model implies the existence of a set of restrictions on the statistical hypotheses and analyses.

2. Uniqueness of the Dichotomous Rasch Model

In the examples below it is advocated that fitting data by the Rasch model is, in fact, a one-to-one correspondence between accepting a certain mathematical structure in the data and having available a definite set of practical tools—or interpretations—for the further analysis of data. A standard test of fit of a statistical model is always conducted by means of a (limited) set of test statistics derived under the model hypothesis; and considering the conventional problems of Type-I and II errors the analyst is led to accept or reject the model. Since test statistics are derived mathematical consequences under the model hypothesis they, by nature, can be "strong" consequences; that is, unambiguously derived consequences. Alternatively they can be "weak" in the sense that this particular test statistic is but one out of several other, important consequences of the model hypothesis. This is the problem of specificity of the statistics used for testing the statistical model; that is, how much can be inferred about the model from the test statistics? In order to make the position of the Rasch model clear it is necessary to reproduce briefly the proof of specificity of the test statistics, using the original terminology, since Rasch gave this proof only as a note in 1971.

Assume that the set of responses $a_{vi}=1$ ("correct") or $a_{vi}=0$ ("noncorrect") are organized in the well-known scheme (see Table 1) with $\xi_1, \ldots, \xi_n$ indicating the individual (latent) parameters and $\varepsilon_1, \ldots, \varepsilon_k$ indicating the item parameters.

The Rasch model, then, assigns the following probability in Eqn. (1) for obtaining the response a_{vi}

$$P(a_{vi}) = \frac{(\varepsilon_i\xi_v)^{a_{vi}}}{1 + \varepsilon_i\xi_v} \tag{1}$$

$i = 1, \ldots, k; \; v = 1, \ldots, n.$

From Eqn. (1) the probability of any matrix $((a_{vi}))$, conditional upon the marginals, is calculated

$$\sum_{i=1}^{k} a_{vi} = r_v \sum_{v=1}^{n} a_{vi} = s_i. \tag{2}$$

$r_v \; v=1, \ldots, n$ are the individual scores, $s_i \; i=1, \ldots, k$ are item totals, and show that this probability is independent of all of the parameters ξ_v, ε_i.

In fact, $\begin{bmatrix}(r_v)\\(s_i)\end{bmatrix}$ denoting the number of zero–one matrices with the marginals in Eqn. (2), it is possible to obtain, readily the conditional probability

$$p(((a_{vi})) \mid (r_v), (s_i)) = \frac{1}{\begin{bmatrix} (r_v) \\ (s_i) \end{bmatrix}}. \tag{3}$$

Since Eqn. (3) is dependent on the marginals (r_v) and (s_i) only, it shows, furthermore, that all such matrices are equally probable.

That Eqn. (3) proves true, then, is a necessary condition for the model to be true; thus, by means of the statistics (r_v) and (s_i) it offers an opportunity for test of fit of the model for an actual set of data.

However, in the following it can be proved that Eqn. (3) is also a sufficient condition for the model in Eqn. (1), provided the a_{vi}'s are stochastically independent.

No assumptions are required to write

$$p(a_{vi} = 1) = \frac{\lambda_{vi}}{1 + \lambda_{vi}}$$

$$p(a_{vi} = 0) = \frac{1}{1 + \lambda_{vi}} \qquad \lambda_{vi} > 0 \tag{4}$$

and it can be concluded from the independence of the a_{vi}'s that the probability generating function with the associated variables $((X_{vi}))=x$, for $a=((a_{vi}))$ is

$$\Pi \begin{bmatrix} a \\ x \end{bmatrix} \lambda = \Pi \left[\left(\begin{pmatrix} a_{vi} \\ x_{vi} \end{pmatrix} \right) \mid ((\lambda_{vi})) \right]$$

$$= \frac{\Pi \ \Pi}{(v) \ (i)} \frac{1 + \lambda_{vi} X_{vi}}{1 + \lambda_{vi}}. \tag{5}$$

If the associated variables $x_{vi} = x'_{vi} \cdot y_v z_i$ are factorized, and using the notation

$$y^r = y^{r_1} \cdot \ldots \cdot y^{r_n} \qquad x^a = \frac{\Pi \ \Pi}{(v) \ (i)} x_{vi}^{a_{vi}}$$

$$z^s = z^{s_1} \cdot \ldots \cdot z^{s_k} \qquad \lambda^a = \frac{\Pi \ \Pi}{(v) \ (i)} \lambda_{vi}^{a_{vi}} \tag{6}$$

$$r = (r_1, \ldots, r_n) \qquad s = (s_1, \ldots, s_k)$$

the generating function in Eqn. (5) can be written

$$\pi \begin{bmatrix} a \\ x \end{bmatrix} \lambda = \sum_{(r,s)} \Pi \begin{bmatrix} a \\ x \end{bmatrix} r, \ s, \ \lambda \cdot p(r, \ s|\lambda) y^r z^s. \tag{7}$$

Now, each factor in the generating function in Eqn. (5) may be transformed into one, with the parameter $\lambda=((1))$. In fact,

$$\Pi \begin{bmatrix} a_{vi} \\ x_{vi} \end{bmatrix} \lambda_{vi} = \frac{1 + \lambda_{vi} x_{vi} \cdot 1}{1 + 1} \cdot \frac{2}{1 + \lambda_{vi}}$$

$$= \Pi \begin{bmatrix} a_{vi} \\ \lambda_{vi} x_{vi} \end{bmatrix} 1 \cdot \frac{2}{1 + \lambda_{vi}}. \tag{8}$$

Thus, using the notation $u \circ v=((u_{vi} \ v_{vi}))$, which is valid for any two response matrices of the same order $(n, \ k)$, and

$$((x'_{vi} \ y_v z_i)) = x' \circ (y^*z)$$

$$((\lambda_{vi} x'_{vi} y_v z_i)) = \lambda \circ x' \circ (y^*z) \tag{9}$$

then, Eqn. (8) applied to Eqn. (5) leads to the identity

$$\Pi \begin{bmatrix} a \\ x \circ (y^*z) \end{bmatrix} |\lambda| =$$

$$\frac{\Pi \ \Pi}{(v) \ (i)} \cdot \frac{2}{1 + \lambda_{vi}} \cdot \Pi \begin{bmatrix} a \\ \lambda \circ x' \circ (y^*z) \end{bmatrix} |((1))| \tag{10}$$

Using the conditional approach in Eqn. (7), with powers of y and z for both sides of Eqn. (10) and identifying corresponding terms, the following general relation is obtained

$$\Pi \begin{bmatrix} a \\ x' \end{bmatrix} r, \ s, \ \lambda \ p(r, \ s|\lambda) =$$

$$\frac{\Pi \ \Pi}{(v) \ (i)} \cdot \frac{2}{1 + \lambda_{vi}} \cdot \Pi \begin{bmatrix} a \\ \lambda \circ x \end{bmatrix} r, \ s, \ ((1)) \cdot p(r, \ s|((1))). \tag{11}$$

For the particular pairs of observed marginals $(r, \ s)$ Eqn. (11) can, through the development of Eqn. (5) to Eqn. (7), be written as

$$\frac{\varphi(\lambda \circ x'|r, \ s)}{\varphi(x'|r, \ s)} = \frac{\Pi \ \Pi}{(v) \ (i)} \frac{1 + \lambda_{vi}}{2} \cdot \frac{p(r, \ s|\lambda)}{p(r, \ s|((1)))} \tag{12}$$

using that

$$\varphi(x'|r, \ s) = \sum x'^a \tag{13}$$

the summation being extended over all a_{vi}'s with fixed $(r, \ s)$.

Since the right-hand term of Eqn. (12) is independent of x', the left-hand term, for any x', is identical with what is obtained by putting $x'=((1))$. Consequently, the function φ satisfies the following functional equation

$$\varphi(\lambda \circ x'|r, \ s) = \frac{\varphi(\lambda|r, \ s)}{\begin{bmatrix} r \\ s \end{bmatrix}} \cdot \varphi(x'|r, \ s). \tag{14}$$

If Eqn. (13) is applied on both sides of Eqn. (14), using that $(\lambda \circ x')^a = \lambda^a \circ x'^a$, the following can be obtained immediately

$$\lambda^a = \frac{\varphi(\lambda|r, \ s)}{\begin{bmatrix} r \\ s \end{bmatrix}} \tag{15}$$

This is valid for any response matrix $((a_{vi}))$ with the marginals $(r, \ s)$. It follows, that for any two response matrices a and a', yielding the given marginals $(r, \ s)$:

$$\lambda^a = \lambda^{a'} \Leftrightarrow \sum_{(v)} \sum_{(i)} a_{vi} \kappa_{vi1} = \sum_{(v)} \sum_{(i)} a_{vi} \kappa_{vi1} \quad \kappa_{vi} = \log \lambda_{vi}$$

$$(16)$$

For any two admissible matrices a and a', being equal for all (v, i), except for a so-called "switch" in an intersection between two columns (i, j) and two rows (u, v):

a		a'	
1	0	0	1
0	1	1	0

Eqn. (16) requires that

$$\kappa_{ui} + \kappa_{vj} = \kappa_{uj} + \kappa_{vi} \qquad (17)$$

A final averaging in Eqn. (17) over the indices v and j leads to

$$\kappa_{ui} = \kappa_{u.} + \kappa_{.i} - \kappa_{..} \qquad (18)$$

which means that $\lambda_{ui} = \log \kappa_{vi}$ splits into a u-factor (row) and an i-factor (column). Inserting this factorization of λ into Eqn. (4), completes the proof that (3) is also a sufficient condition.

2.1 Consequences of the Uniqueness

The proof states that the Rasch model in Eqn. (1) is true if—and only if—the conditional distribution of the responses $((a_{vi}))$ given the marginals (r_v) and (s_i) is independent of the parameters $\varepsilon_1, \ldots, \varepsilon_k$ and $\xi_1, \ldots, \xi_n$ —briefly denoted as joint sufficiency of the marginals (r_v) and (s_i).

Before the conclusions from the proof of uniqueness of the Rasch model are fully drawn, it is necessary to consider another aspect of the model's uniqueness in terms of specific objective comparisons. In fact, Rasch (1966a, 1966b, 1966c) along with the development of statistical properties of the model, like the theorem of specificity shown above, was deeply attached to the problem of defining the general conditions under which individuals in Table 1 can be compared—or measured. The question to be solved was essentially the following: What are the formal requirements for being able to compare any two individuals v and u— through the parameters ξ_v and ξ_u—using any subset of the items—namely the item parameters—and end up with (stochastically) the same result? This formulation is, of course, an abbreviated form of Rasch's original request for objectiveness when comparing individuals. In one of his last papers Rasch (1977) summarized his work with specific objective comparisons and stressed that general objectivity seems to be an ambiguous concept, and hence objectivity needs a frame of reference—like the one given by Table 1—in order to be defined distinctly. Therefore, "specified" or "specific objective comparisons" among individuals (and among items) are the terms used by Rasch in order to

Table 1
Responses $a_{vi} = 0,1$ from n individuals to k items with individual parameters ξ_v $v=1, \ldots, n$ and item parameters ε_i $i=1, \ldots, k$

		Item No. 1 .... i .... k	Scores (r_v)
Individuals	1	1 0 1	1	$a_{1.}$
	2	1 1 0 .	0	$a_{2.}$
	.		.
	v	.... a_{vi}	$a_{v.}$
	.		.
	n		.
Item totals (s_i)		$a_{.1}$ ...... $a_{.i}$ .... $a_{.k}$	$a_{..}$

restrict, or specify, the comparisons to be undertaken in such frameworks as Table 1.

It turns out (Rasch 1968, 1977) that the request for specific objective comparisons is, in fact, in one-to-one correspondence with the Rasch model in Eqn. (1)—if response matrices $((a_{vi}))$ with $a_{vi}=0,1$ like the Table 1 data are considered.

Now, combining the conclusions from the proof of uniqueness and the properties of objectivity it is seen that:

{The Rasch model (1) is true}
if, and only if
{The marginals (r_v) and (s_i) are jointly sufficient statistics}
if, and only if
{Individuals (items) can be compared (specific) objectively}

The mutual characterization of (a) the statistical model, (b) the sufficiency of marginals, and (c) specific objective comparisons have a series of implications for the practical work. In fact, (b) enables the analyst —in principle by applying the test statistic in Eqn. (3) above—to carry out a test of fit of the model that is independent of all parameters; and to do it specifically. If the model is rejected, the individual total scores (r_v) are no longer sufficient statistics, and information about the ξ's is not exhausted by the r_v's. In other words, information is needed about which items have been answered correctly instead of knowing only the number of correct responses across all items. The way the test statistic rejects the model indicates the "direction" of misfit and, taking into account the specificity of the test statistic, "exactly" what is wrong is now known. Usually, the items are so-called nonhomogeneous, and proper use of the test statistics may point to, for example, the existence of two homogeneous subscales of the items rather than one. Rejection of the model is also equivalent to the fact that individuals— in terms of the ξ's—cannot be compared, irrespective of which items are used. That is, of course, not the same as claiming that individuals cannot be compared at all, but in this case, any statement concerning two individuals will be nonobjective in the sense that the result of the comparison will depend on something less "general" than what is covered by the whole range of items (e.g., the concept of "difficulty" valid for the items in many test forms).

3. Detecting Gender Differences

When test forms are analyzed, frequently a sample of boys and girls have answered a series of tasks, or items, which can be classified as correct ($a_{vi}=1$) or incorrect ($a_{vi}=0$). The complete set of observations is then gathered in a scheme like Table 1. In the Reading Literacy Study conducted by the International Association for the Study of Educational Achievements (IEA) (Elley 1992) the items were *a priori* collected in three subgroups, dealing with the reading of three different text types, but still the items could be more or less "difficult" within each reading domain. The caption applied to all items (viz., the ε's) is, therefore, a concept of difficulty and, consequently, "reading comprehension" or "reading ability" is the derived concept assigned to the ξ's of the individuals.

Part of the international calibration exercise, where one unique set of items acts as an international ruler, or Reading Scale, for comparing all students, is a test of fit of the Rasch model in Eqn. (1), in which special attention is given to test statistics revealing possible inhomogeneities between girls and boys. The issues are not that of investigating differences in the level of achievement—which can be studied after acceptance of the model by comparing the ξ's for the girls and the ξ's for the boys; rather, the question is raised whether the items are equally difficult for the girls and for the boys—irrespective of the general level of ability for the two sexes. In other words, are the item parameters $\varepsilon_1, \ldots, \varepsilon_k$ consistent across all students? Only in this case, of course, can the levels of achievement be compared properly without giving free score points to either of the gender groups because of inhomogeneity. Classical statistical analyses mix up these two aspects of measuring differences, since it is outside their mathematical formalization to distinguish between ability and difficulty in the way the Rasch model does. In order to demonstrate how test of fit of the Rasch model also brings about conclusive statements concerning gender differences, it is necessary, first of all, to take advantage of the sufficient reduction of the basic observations ((a_{vi})) conducted by the r_v's.

This is done in Table 2, where the individuals are classified according to their score values $r_v, v= 1, \ldots, n$. If the conditional approach is employed with the test statistic in Eqn. (3), the conditional probability can be calculated to achieve a correct response to Item No. i both for the boys and for the girls. Imagine that Table

Table 2
The number of $a_{.i}(r)$ of correct responses to Item No. i given by n_r individuals in score group = r[a]

Score r	Item No. 1	. . .	i	. . .	k	Number of individuals in score group n_r
0	0	. . .	0	. . .	0	n_0
.			.			.
r		. . .	$a_{.i(r)}$	. . .		n_r
.						.
$k-1$						n_{k-1}
k	n_k	. . .	n_k	. . .	n_k	n_k
Total	s_1	. . .	s_i	. . .	s_k	$n = \Sigma n_r$

a The total number of correct responses to Item No. i is $s_i, i = 1, \ldots, k$

2 summarizes data for the boys and the girls separately —$a_{.i}(r)$'s and $b_{.i}(r)$'s, referring to the boys and the girls respectively; and, further, n_r and m_r indicate the number of boys and girls in score group: r correct responses.

From the Rasch model in Eqn. (1) the distribution of $a_{.i}(r)$ and $b_{.i}(r)$ are derived as two binomials:

$$a_{.i}(r) \sim b(n_r, \theta_{ri}) \quad \theta_{ri} = \varepsilon_i^b[\gamma^{(i)}_{r-1}/\gamma_r]_b$$

$$b_{.i}(r) \sim b(m_r, \eta_{ri}) \quad \eta_{ri} = \varepsilon_i^g[\gamma^{(i)}_{r-1}/\gamma_r]_g$$

ε_i^b and ε_i^g are the difficulties for Item No. i for boys and girls respectively, and γ_r is the elementary symmetric function of $\varepsilon_1, \ldots, \varepsilon_k$ of order r (Rasch 1960, Fischer 1974)—$\gamma^{(i)}_{r-1}$ calculated without ε_i and suffixes b and g set to indicate that the γ's are calculated for the boys' and for the girls' ε's respectively. Notice that the individual parameters ξ's are eliminated! From Eqn. (19) the extended Hypergeometric probability in Eqn. (20) of $a_{.i}(r)=x$, conditional on $a_{.i}(r)+b_{.i}(r) = c_{.i}(r)$ is derived for each score level r:

$$p(a_{.i}(r) = x|c_{.i}(r) = c, n_r, m_r) =$$

$$\frac{\binom{n_r}{x}\binom{m_r}{c-x}\kappa_{ri}^x}{\sum_{j=0}^{c}\binom{n_r}{j}\binom{m_r}{c-j}\kappa_{ri}^j} \tag{20}$$

$$\kappa_{ri} = \frac{\theta_{ri}}{1-\theta_{ri}} \bigg/ \frac{\eta_{ri}}{1-\eta_{ri}} = \varepsilon_i^b/\varepsilon_i^g.$$

Under the hypothesis that Item No. i is equally difficult for boys and girls, H:$\varepsilon_i^b=\varepsilon_i^g$, it is observed that $\kappa_{ri}=1$ for each score value $r=1, \ldots, k-1$.

Evaluation of the test statistics $a_{.i}(r)$ in Eqn. (20) for $r=1, \ldots, k-1$ gives information on possible deviations from the hypothesis H and—using approximate $\chi^2(1)=u_r^2$ for the standardized $u_r=[a_{.i}(r)-E(a_{.i}(r)|H)]/\sigma(a_{.i}(r))$ at each level of the score=r—a summary test, $\chi^2(df)=\Sigma u_r^2$ $df=k-1$ across all score groups is obtained as an overall test for no gender differences—or sex bias—on item No. i.

As an example, Table 3 shows data from Items A and B. In Item A the hypothesis H is rejected, $p=0.02$ and the patterns of $a_{.i}(r)$ and $E(a_{.i}(r))$ clearly demonstrate an interaction between sex and ability, since the sign of the differences $a_{.i}(r)-E(a_{.i}(r)|H)$ shifts for low r's to high r's. For Item B the hypothesis H is also rejected ($p=0.00$), but here the situation is different, as a general sex bias is observed across all score groups, and in this case the degree of sex bias can be assessed, simply from the estimated value of K_r in (20), or $\log(\kappa_{ri}) = \log(\varepsilon_i^b) - \log(\varepsilon_i^b) \approx 0.14$, if a logarithmic interval scale is used for the difficulties.

4. Analysis of Item Discrimination

Another area of interest when applying Item Response Theory (IRT) models, is covered by the so-called "two-parameter logistic model" (Lord and Novick 1968) which is often cited as a generalization of the basic Rasch model in Eqn. (1). The practical need for formally extending the mathematical structure of the Rasch model appears when the statistical analysis of actual data fails to accept the Rasch model in Eqn. (1), and various indications as to why the model does not fit lead to the proposal of the two-parameter model in Eqn. (21):

$$P(a_{vi}) = \frac{e^{[\delta_i \theta_i + \sigma_v]a_{vi}}}{1 + e^{\sigma_i(\delta_i + \sigma_v)}} \qquad (a_{vi} = 0, 1)$$

$$(21)$$

$$\theta_i = \log(\varepsilon_i)$$

$$\sigma_v = \log(\xi_v)$$

In Eqn. (21) logarithmic scaling is applied with θ's as item parameters and σ's as individual parameters. To many users of classical test theory the concept of item discrimination—and therefore a model as in Eqn. (21)—is connected with evaluation of biserial correlations between responses to an Item a_{vi} and the total scores $r_v.=\Sigma a_{vi}$ ($v=1, \ldots, n$). To users of IRT models, the Item Response Functions or Item Characteristic Curves (ICC) with varying slope values interpreted as varying item discriminations, have for a long time (Lord 1980) been a natural part of the model construction. From this point of view the model in Eqn. (21) is, indeed, an evident, general framework for analyzing response data.

Obviously, when setting the item discrimination parameters $\delta_i=1$ $i=1, \ldots, k$ the Rasch model is obtained, formally, as a special case of the model in Eqn. (21). But what is really generalized from the Rasch model in Eqn. (1) to the model in Eqn. (21) beyond the mathematics? And what is not? First, it is impossible to give independent interpretations of the item and discrimination parameters; this can be seen by considering the mathematical structure of the model in Eqn. (21) and trying to identify the components δ_i, θ_i and σ_v —which control the probability completely. Since θ_i and σ_v interact additively, a constrained form, using $\theta_i+\sigma_v+\rho$ with $\theta.=\sigma.=0$ (i.e., average=zero), determines these two sets of parameters, but still the combined term $\theta_i+\sigma_v+\rho$ interacts multiplicatively with the δ_i. Hence, by "shrinking"—that is, dividing the term by some constant—the combined scale of difficulty and ability $\theta_i+\sigma_v+\rho$, it is possible to "compensate" by multiplying the δ_i's by the same constant in order to maintain the status quo, as regards the final value of the probability $p(a_{vi})$. Second, the discrimination parameters $\delta_1, \ldots, \delta_k$ are always unknown, and since this brings the model in Eqn. (21) outside the class of exponential distributions, it implies severe estimation problems of the parameters, including the δ's. Third,

Table 3
Observed $a_{.i}(r)$ and expected $E(a_{.i}(r)|H)$ responses under the hypothesis H of equal item difficulties for boys and girls on two items A and B[a]

r	n_r	m_r	Item A $a_{.i}(r)$	$E(a_{.i}(r)|H)$	u_r	Item B $a_{.i}(r)$	$E(a_{.i}(r)|H)$	u_r
0	0	0	0	0.00	.	0	0.00	.
1	4	8	0	0.00	.	0	0.00	.
2	16	32	4	4.00	0.00	10	5.00	3.27
3	69	86	22	17.81	1.40	33	27.15	1.93
4	121	159	40	51.86	−2.88	83	76.06	1.73
5	193	118	91	101.15	−2.37	176	168.80	2.54
6	89	57	89	89.00	.	89	89.00	.

$$\chi^2(4) = 15.87 \qquad\qquad \chi^2(4) = 23.86$$
$$\chi^2(p = 0.00) \qquad\qquad \chi^2(p = 0.02)$$

a n_r, m_r = the number of boys and girls respectively in score group = r u_r = approximate normal test statistic for each score level how can individuals be compared under the model in Eqn. (21)?

In Fig. 1 two ICC's with different slopes are displayed, and on the scale of ability (*x*-axis) two individuals with different levels of ability σ_1, σ_2 judge the difficulties of the two items from their chances of solving the two items correctly. It can be seen directly from the figure that their ranking of difficulties depends on the positions σ_1, σ_2 of the two individuals; the low-achieving σ_2 disagrees with the high-achieving σ_1. In other words, these two items cannot be compared objectively in terms of level of difficulty!

However, if the model in Eqn. (21) is not used as a formal basis for investigating the data, because of the drawbacks described, the question arises as to how to make inferences about the phenomenon brought about by varying the slopes of the ICCs. The varying slopes are usually observed already in the initial phase of the testing of the model (Allerup 1994), when the sufficiency of the r_v's is investigated and the empirically observed chances (estimated conditional ICC) of getting a correct response $a_{.i}(r)/n_r \approx \Theta_{ri}$ (compare Eqn. (19)) is studied as a function of r, $r= 1, \ldots, k-1$.

Since the probability of a correct response to Item No. *i*, conditional on the individual score $a_{vi}=r$, is given by

$$p(a_{vi} = 1|a_{v.} = r) = \varepsilon_i \frac{\gamma_{r-1}^{(i)}}{\gamma_r} = \frac{e^{\theta_i + \log(\gamma_{r-1}^{(i)}/\gamma_r^{(i)})}}{1 + e^{\theta_i + \log(\gamma_{r-1}^{(i)}/\gamma_r^{(i)})}}$$

$$\theta_i = \log(\varepsilon_i) \qquad\qquad (22)$$

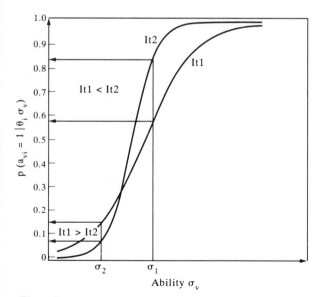

Figure 1
Item characteristic curves (ICC) for items It1 and It2 under the two-parameter model. Item difficulties evaluated ($a > b \Leftrightarrow$ "*a* easier than *b*") at two points σ_1 σ_2 on the scale of ability

it can be identified with the unconditional probability of the Rasch model Eqn. (1), using logarithmic scaling $\theta_i=\log\varepsilon_i$ $\sigma_v=\log\xi_v$

$$p(a_{vi}) = \frac{e^{(\theta_i + \sigma_{vi})a_{vi}}}{1 + e^{\theta_i + \sigma_v}} \qquad (a_{vi} = 0, 1) \qquad (23)$$

and the two-parameter extension of Eqn. (23) in Eqn. (21) can be captured directly from Eqn. (22) by the following model proposal

$$p(a_{vi}|v. = r) = \frac{e^{(\theta_i + \delta_i\lambda_{ri})a_{vi}}}{1 + e^{\theta_i + \delta_i\lambda_{ri}}} \qquad (a_{vi} = 0, 1) \qquad (24)$$

$$\lambda_{ri} = \log(\gamma_{r-1}^{(i)}/\gamma_r^{(i)})$$

The reason for suggesting (a) $\theta_i+\delta_i\lambda_{ri}$ rather than (b) $\delta_i(\theta_i+\lambda_{ri})$—which would otherwise make the equivalence to the two-parameter model in Eqn. (21) clearer—is that Eqn. (24) immediately represents a simple one-dimensional logistic regression (LR) of a_{vi} on the λ's for fixed Item No. *i* ($r=1, \ldots, k-1$) with slope=δ_i and intercept=θ_i. Considering $\lambda_{ri}=\lambda_{ri}(\theta_1, \ldots, \theta_k)$ as known by the estimated θ's, the λ's being by-products of the conditional maximum likelihood equations for $\theta_1, \ldots, \theta_k$ (Andersen 1973), tests of fit of LR can be conducted. Besides the usual likelihood ratio test (χ^2) for the shape of the conditional ICC (CICC) modeled by Eqn. (24), the hypothesis H:$\delta_i=1$ attracts attention, since $\delta_i=1$ $i=1, \ldots, k$ brings the model (24) back to the basic Rasch model in Eqn. (1). Furthermore, the "locally" LR-estimated intercept values θ_i can be compared with the "global" $\theta_i=\log(\varepsilon_i)$ from the initial estimation of the item difficulties (Allerup 1994). Notice, that Form (b) can be obtained from Form (a) by the transformation $\theta_i \to \theta+r_i=\theta_i/\delta_i$ (compare the remarks concerning independent interpretations of item difficulty and item discrimination in the two-parameter model). It is also worthy of note that the definition of item discrimination δ_i takes place in the model in Eqn. (24), which—like the basic model in Eqn. (22)—is conditional on the sufficient statistics $a_{v.}=r$ for the individual parameters $\sigma_1, \ldots, \sigma_n$ under the original Rasch model. This avoids the mathematical confusion caused by the use of $T_v=\Sigma_{(i)}\delta_i a_{vi}$ which, on known δ's, is sufficient for the individual parameter σ_v in the two-parameter model in Eqn. (21). An example with two items showing the results of analyzing the conditional ICCs by means of the logistic regression technique is displayed in Table 4.

It is seen from Table 4 that for Item No. B the test of fit rejects the hypothesized structure in Eqn. (24) ($p=0.002<0.05$) and, consequently, the ICC for this item not only falls outside what is predicted by the Rasch model, it also fails to conform with simple linear transformations of the basic logistic "S"-shape. For this reason no additional estimation of slope and intercept values takes place. From inspecting the dif-

Table 4

The frequency of correct responses $h_{ri} = a_{.i}(r)/n_r$ within score group=r out of n_r individuals in score group=r [a]

r	n_r	$a_{.i}(r)/n_r$	Item no. i = A $E(h_{ri}|LR)$	λ_{ri}	$a_{.i}(r)/n_r$	Item no. i = B $E(h_{ri}|LR)$	λ_{ri}
1	2	0.00	0.10	−2.85	0.00	0.07	−2.88
2	5	0.20	0.18	−1.96	0.20	0.25	−2.00
3	12	0.30	0.45	−1.36	0.08	0.19	−1.40
4	6	0.33	0.27	−0.86	0.00	0.13	−0.91
5	33	0.43	0.54	−0.41	0.21	0.31	−0.48
6	46	0.58	0.62	0.01	0.39	0.45	−0.07
7	91	0.67	0.36	0.43	0.32	0.38	0.34
8	183	0.69	0.70	0.86	0.54	0.52	0.77
9	376	0.82	0.78	1.34	0.65	0.61	1.24
10	588	0.86	0.85	1.91	0.75	0.70	1.82
11	915	0.91	0.92	2.76	0.77	0.81	2.67

Test of fit: $\chi^2(9) = 16.15$ (p = 0.06)　　　　　　　　　$\chi^2(9) = 26.50$ (p = 0.002)

LR-estimates: $\delta_A \approx 0.83$ 　　$\theta_A \approx 0.14$

Approx t: 　$t = -2.75$ 　　$t = 0.10$

　　　　　(p = 0.02) 　(p = 0.92)

a $E(a_{.i}(r)|n_r/LR)$ the expected frequency of correct responses under logistic regression (LR) and $\lambda_{ri}=\log(\gamma^{(i)}_{r-1} / \gamma^{(i)}_r)$ the independent variable in logistic regression; two items, Nos. A and B are studied

ferences between observed and expected frequencies no clear picture emerges of the reason for nonfit; frequently, for the low-scoring individuals, an overweight of observed corrects, namely, the $a_{.i}(r)$'s, is a sign of guessing. In Item No. A the situation is different, since test of fit of the item characteristic curve for this item does not reject the structure in Eqn. (24). The estimated item discrimination $\delta_A \approx 0.83$ and the approximate t-test for the hypothesis $\delta_A=1$ ($t=-2.75$, $p=0.02$) indicate that the ICC for Item No. A also does not fit the Rasch ICC. However, considering the acceptance of fit to a linear transformation of the basic Rasch ICC, namely, the model in Eqn. (24), it is desirable to look for other items that enjoy similar δ values. In fact, collecting a series of items of this type, it is possible to build up a subscale now fitting the basic Rasch model in Eqn. (1)—since the common δ_i value, then, would be absorbed into the difficulty parameter θ_i.

If, for various reasons, items satisfying the model in Eqn. (24) are employed with varying δ_i values—some of which are significantly different from unity—it should then be realized that the estimate of ability=σ_v is based upon the statistic $T_v=\Sigma_{(i)} \delta_i a_{vi}(a_{vi}=0,1)$ which submits the sum of item discriminations across those items answered correctly. Increasing T_v values—and ability σ_v estimates—are therefore a consequence of either responding correctly to items with high δ's, possibly being easy items with low θ_i's, or responding correctly to an increasing number of items. This again illustrates the confusion in the two-parameter model Eqn. (21) about the interpretation of the ability σ_v which, in the basic Rasch model, is unambiguously combined with the number of correct answers a_v.

5. Comparing the Results of Two Tests

In Sect. 3 it was demonstrated how the Rasch model can be used both to detect sex bias on a single item and to assess, quantitatively, the difference by means of the parameters of the model. Here, principally the same issue is addressed, but this time the point of departure lies in the data usually available to users after testing sessions: two sets of individual score values (i.e., the number of correct responses, a_v and b_v $v=1, \ldots, n$)—one from Test (I) and one from Test (II), displayed in Table 5. It is assumed that the two-test sessions are parallel, so that each individual has match-paired scores from the two tests. Furthermore, it is assumed that the Rasch model proves true for data within each of Tests I and II. This can be done either as a result of performing two separate tests of fit of the Rasch model, conducted at the single-item level, or, in the absence of single-item data, because of the underlying theorem of uniqueness of the model and the sufficiency of the item and individual scores.

In the light of this design a general question is considered: What kind of calculations can be undertaken using the scores a_v., b_v. in order to reveal the difference between Test I and Test II? One point of view could be that, having accepted the fit of the Rasch model and, consequently, being in a position where all information concerning the individual parameters σ_v, η_v are kept in the scores a_v., b_v., there is freedom to choose any kind of subsequent calculations based on a_v. and b_v. . In experimental psychology, for instance, Tests I and II (comprising words and nonwords) are used to identify certain reading literacy problems by taking notice of the magnitude of the

Table 5
Data from two parallel Tests I and II

Individual No. v	Test I Items 1 $\qquad$ $k1$	Score $a_{v.}$	Ability ξ_v	Test II Items 1 $\qquad$ $k2$	Score $b_{v.}$	Ability η_v
1	1 0 1 1 0 0	12	1.23	1 1 0 0 1 1	15	1.32
2	0 1 1 0 1 1	13	1.27	1 1 1 0 1 1	18	1.36
.	. . . . . .	.	.	. . . . . .	.	.
v	$((a_{vi}))$			$((b_{vi}))$		
.	. . . . . .	.	.	. . . . . .	.	.
n	1 1 0 1 0 0	9	0.98	1 0 1 1 0 0	8	0.95

a Single item responses a_{vi} (Test I) and b_{vi} (Test II) and individual abilities ξ_v, η_v $v=1, \ldots, n$ under the basic Rasch model Eqn. (1)

difference between Test I and II—the greater the difference, the more distinct is the impression of reading problems; and the more confident is the psychologist about using the difference between Test I and Test II outcomes for diagnostic purpose. The aim of analysis is therefore, in a way, "opposite" to the usual focus, since the statistical analysis is now directed toward identification of those individuals having the greatest deviation from—or rejection of—the hypothesis $H: \sigma_v = \eta_v$.

Numerous suggestions have been published as to how the difference between the two tests can be assessed. The simple algebraic difference (Mitterer 1982) $a_{v.} - b_{v.}$ between the number of correct responses, a simple quotient $a_{v.}/b_{v.}$ (Bryant and Impey 1986), a difference between standardized z-scores (i.e., $(a_{v.} - a_{..})/\sigma(a_{v.})$ considering all n individuals) have been proposed (Olson 1985) and even the so-called d, of signal detection theory (Snowling 1980), which is the distance (scaled in σ-units) between two mean values from normal distributions by means of cut-off points equal to the percentage of correct responses for Tests I and II. It is, however, easy to show that if these four ways of evaluating the difference between Tests I and II are used, it is possible to end up with incompatible results, leading to a contradictory rank order of the individuals.

There is also the problem of which method to choose. Is one method "better" or more "correct" than the other? The point is that, in fact, none of the methods mentioned is "correct," since none of the methods has properly taken care of the initial assumptions that tacitly lie behind all the methods. These are the use of individual scores as measures of ability and—although not explicit here—the use of item totals as measures of item difficulty. In other words the statistical sufficiency of item and individual scores, according to the theorem of uniqueness, inevitably leads to the Rasch model in Eqn. (1). What needs to be done, consequently, is to make explicit the use of the Rasch model in Eqn. (1), apply it to data available from the two tests, and attempt to develop a model-derived statistic,

which can be used to assess the individual differences between Tests I and II.

Let a distinction be made between two cases: (a) where all single-item responses $((a_{vi}))$ and $((b_{vi}))$ (and hence by calculation the individual scores $a_{v.}$, $b_{v.}$ $v=1, \ldots, n$) are known; and (b) where only the individual scores $a_{v.}$, $b_{v.}$ are known.

In both cases (a) and (b) the distribution of individual score values $a_{v.}$ and $b_{v.}$ can be obtained readily from the basic Rasch model in Eqn. (1)

$$p(a_{v.} = x) = \frac{\xi_v^x \gamma_x(\underline{\varepsilon})}{\sum_{j=0}^{k1} \xi_v^j \gamma_j(\underline{\varepsilon})}$$

$$p(b_{v.} = y) = \frac{\eta_v^y \gamma_j(\underline{\eta})}{\sum_{j=0}^{k2} \eta_v^j \gamma(\underline{\eta})} \tag{25}$$

$$\gamma_x(\underline{\varepsilon}) = \gamma_x(\varepsilon 1, \ldots, \varepsilon k1)$$

$$\gamma_y(\underline{\eta}) = \gamma_y(\eta 1, \ldots, \eta k2).$$

In Eqn. (25) the γ's are the elementary symmetric functions of item difficulties $\varepsilon_1, \ldots, \varepsilon_{k1}$ and $\eta_1, \ldots, \eta_{k2}$ in the two Tests I and II respectively.

For each individual from Eqn. (25) the distribution can be derived of $a_{v.} = x$ conditional on the sum of scores across both tests $a_{v.} + b_{v.} = c_{v.} = c$.

$$p(a_{v.} = x | c_{v.} = c) = \frac{\gamma_x(\underline{\varepsilon}) \gamma_{c-x}(\underline{\eta}) \kappa_k^x}{\sum_{j=0}^{k1} \gamma_j(\underline{\varepsilon}) \gamma_{c-j}(\underline{\eta}) \kappa_v^j} \tag{26}$$

$$\kappa_v = \xi_v / \eta_v$$

Note that the abilities ξ_v and η_v (cf. Table 5) enter this distribution by their ratios $\kappa_v = \xi_v / \eta_v$. Hence, if the objective was to test for consistent abilities $H_0: \xi_v = \eta_v$ across the two Tests I and II, the test distribution in Eqn. (26), being a kind of generalized

871

hypergeometric Fisher-exact-test, will serve as the basis with $\kappa_v=1$ $v=1, \ldots, n$ (Allerup 1986). Even the more relaxed hypothesis of a general "shift," Δ, in the level of abilities from Test I to Test II (viz., $H_1:\xi_v=\Delta\eta_v$) is captured by Eqn. (26) by testing $\kappa_v=\Delta$ $v=1, \ldots, n$. For these statistical tests to be carried out on real data it is necessary in case (a) to obtain access to the values of the difficulties ε_i and η_i of the two Tests I and II, either as known values from previous studies of the two reading tests, or as a result of estimating the parameters based on single-item data $((a_{vi}))$ and $((b_{vi}))$. In any case it turns out to be simple χ^2's adding up along the conditioning "c_v.-diagonals" in the $k1 \times k2$ cross tabulation of $(a_v., b_v.)$, using multinomials $p(a_v. \,|c_v.=c)$ on each $c_v.$-diagonal (Allerup 1986).

If, on the other hand, H_0 and H_1 are both rejected, the alternative hypothesis remains that the subjects do have different abilities in Tests I and II. In response to the question initially raised, it is necessary, therefore to measure the magnitude of span in ability between the two tests by simply estimating the κ_v's (e.g., as $\kappa_v \approx \hat{\xi}_v / \hat{\eta}_v$—the ratio of estimated abilities obtained from each of the Tests I and II).

At the same time, it can be seen that this "correct"

model-derived estimator for κ_v is not a function of the scores $a_v.$ and $b_v.$ that is comparable to the specifications in the four methods mentioned above. In fact, the usual maximum likelihood estimates (e.g., of $\xi_1, \ldots, \xi_n$) are obtained from solving the equations

$$r = \sum_{j=0}^{k1} \frac{\varepsilon_i \xi}{1 + \varepsilon_i \xi} \tag{27}$$

$$r = 1, \ldots, k1$$

with $\varepsilon_1, \ldots, \varepsilon_{k1}$ replaced by their conditional maximum likelihood estimates; it makes only little difference if the conditional maximum likelihood estimates are applied for the ξ's (Holst 1993).

An idea of the mathematical structure of the estimator for κ_v is available, however, when trying to solve the problem of estimating the difference between Tests I and II, κ_v, in case (b), where only the scores $a_v.$ and $b_v.$ are known. Under these circumstances it is impossible, of course, to conduct proper statistical tests of H_0 or H_1, since the item difficulties $\varepsilon_1, \ldots, \varepsilon_{k1}$ and $\eta_1, \ldots, \eta_{k2}$ are all unknown, and it is necessary to rely on appropriate approximate methods.

These are, like the development from Eqn. (22)

Table 6
Hypothetical item difficulties $\varepsilon_{i,i}$, $i=1, \ldots, 10$ in Tests I and II

	Item No.									
	1	2	3	4	5	6	7	8	9	10
Test I	0.67	1.79	2.01	0.22	0.67	1.12	1.56	0.45	1.79	2.01
Test II	0.27	2.72	0.54	0.82	2.45	0.54	1.90	1.09	1.36	0.82

Table 7
True, theoretical log κ_r-values for any combination of scores, r, s, on Tests, I and II, with item difficulties ε_i, i given in Table 6

Test I $s1$	Test II (Total score $r =$)							
	2	3	4	5	6	7	8	9
1	−0.01	−0.81	−1.37	−1.83	−2.26	−2.68	−3.13	−3.65	−4.34
2	0.79	−0.01	−0.57	−1.03	−1.46	−1.89	−2.35	−2.89	−3.67
3	1.34	0.53	−0.02	−0.49	−0.92	−1.35	−1.81	−2.37	−3.17
4	1.79	0.99	0.44	−0.03	−0.46	−0.89	−1.36	−1.92	−2.73
5	2.22	1.42	0.87	0.41	−0.03	−0.46	−0.93	−1.49	−2.31
6	2.65	1.85	1.31	0.84	0.41	−0.02	−0.49	−1.06	−1.88
7	3.10	2.32	1.78	1.32	0.89	0.45	−0.01	−0.58	−1.40
8	3.63	2.87	2.34	1.89	1.46	1.03	0.56	0.00	−0.82
9	4.34	3.66	3.16	2.71	2.29	1.86	1.39	0.83	0.01

to Eqn. (24), at hand if the unconditional probability $p(a_{vi}=1)$ of a correct response is identified with the conditional probability $p(a_{vi}=1|a_{v.}=r)$ given the score $a_{v.}=r$

$$p(a_{vi} = 1) = \frac{\varepsilon_i \xi_v}{1 + \varepsilon_i \xi_v} \approx p(a_{vi} = 1|a_{v.} = r)$$

$$= \frac{\varepsilon_i \dfrac{\gamma^{(i)}_{r-1}}{\gamma^{(i)}_r}}{\varepsilon_i \dfrac{\gamma^{(i)}_{r-1}}{\gamma^{(i)}_r}}. \qquad (28)$$

For score value$=r$, this leads to the identification of the ability $\xi(r)$, for individuals with $a_{v.}=r$

$$\xi(r) \approx \frac{\gamma^{(i)}_{r-1}}{\gamma^{(i)}_r}. \qquad (29)$$

If all ε's are equal $\varepsilon_1= \ldots =\varepsilon_{k1}=1$ (ε's constrained by $\pi\varepsilon_i=1$) the γ's are binominal coefficients

$$\gamma_r(\underline{\in}) = \binom{k1}{r} \qquad (30)$$

and the ratio in Eqn. (29) reduces to

$$\xi(r) \approx \frac{r}{k1 - r}. \qquad (31)$$

Even if the log difficulties $\theta_i=log(\varepsilon_i)$ $i=1, \ldots, k1$ are uniformly spread in the normally used interval $[-2.0, 2.0]$, Eqn. (31) represents a good mathematical approximation to the ratio of γ's in Eqn. (29). Together with a similar approximation for the η's

$$\eta(r) \approx \frac{r}{k2 - r} \qquad (32)$$

it is possible to obtain the final approximation for $\kappa_v=\xi_v/\eta_v$. In fact, observing score value $a_{v.}= r$ in Test I and score value $b_{v.}=s$ in Test II Eqns. (31) and (32) provides the following approximate estimate of $\kappa(r)$ (i.e., κ_v values for individuals with score $= a_{v.} = r$)

$$\kappa(r, s) \approx \frac{r/(k1 - r)}{s/(k2 - s)} \qquad (33)$$

$$r = 1, \ldots, k1 - 1$$

$$s = 1, \ldots, k2 - 1.$$

By Eqn. (33) a solution to the initial problem has been reached, and it can be seen that the mathematical structure of the estimate of κ_v is that of a ratio between two odd values (i.e., an "odd's ratio" of the number of correct responses for Tests I and II). The individual measure κ_v of discrepancy between Test I and Test II abilities is obtained under the Rasch model and it is, although mathematically simple in structure, incompatible with simple differences, z-scores, etc. mentioned above. Note, that under the condition $\varepsilon_1=\ldots=\varepsilon_{k1}=1$ Eqn. (26) becomes a simple, extended hypergeometric distribution, known from analysis of 2×2 contingency tables, and the "natural" estimate of κ_v (Johnson and Kotz 1969) is exactly the odd's ratio estimate listed in Eqn. (33).

The power of the $\kappa(r, s)$ approximation in Eqn. (33) can be illustrated by an example. Taking items in Tests I and II with assumed item difficulties ε_i, η_i $i=1, \ldots,$ 10 ($k=10$) listed in Table 6, the maximum likelihood estimates $\xi(r), \eta(r)$ $r=1, \ldots, 9$ corresponding to the nine score levels ($r=1, \ldots, k-1$) can be calculated from Eqn. (27) and, finally the true theoretical $\kappa(r,$

Table 8
Log odds values based on total scores r, s as approximative $\kappa(r, s)$ values in Eqn. (33)

Test I	Test II (Total score $r =$)								
s	1	2	3	4	5	6	7	8	9
1	−0.00	−0.81	−1.35	−1.79	−2.20	−2.60	−3.04	−3.58	−4.39
2	0.81	0.00	−0.54	−0.98	−1.39	−1.79	−2.23	−2.77	−3.58
3	1.35	0.54	0.00	−0.44	−0.85	−1.25	−1.69	−2.23	−3.04
4	1.79	0.98	0.44	0.00	−0.41	−0.81	−1.25	−1.79	−2.60
5	2.20	1.39	0.85	0.41	0.00	−0.41	−0.85	−1.39	−2.20
6	2.60	1.79	1.25	0.81	0.41	0.00	−0.44	−0.98	−1.79
7	3.04	2.23	1.69	1.25	0.85	0.44	0.00	−0.54	−1.35
8	3.58	2.77	2.23	1.79	1.39	0.98	0.54	0.00	−0.81
9	4.39	3.58	3.04	2.60	2.20	1.79	1.35	0.81	0.00

s) $=\xi(r)/\eta(r)$ $r=1,\ldots,9$ can be determined. These values, listed in Table 7, can be compared with the approximate $\kappa(r,s)$ values listed in Table 8.

It is seen that not only does Eqn. (33) approximate the true, Rasch-model-derived measure κ of individual distance between Tests I and II, mathematically a structure similar to well-known terms from contingency table analysis, but it also enjoys the property of being easy to calculate by means of the test scores r, s only.

See also: Adaptive Testing; Measurement in Educational Research

References

Allerup P 1985 *Why I Like to Read: Statistical Analysis of Questionnaire Data*. Danish Institute for Educational Research, Copenhagen
Allerup P 1986 *Statistical Analysis of MADRS: A Rating Scale*. Danish Institute for Educational Research, Copenhagen
Allerup P 1987 *Raschmodeller—Principper og Anvendelse*. Danish Institute for Educational Research, Copenhagen
Allerup P 1994 Development of the reading scales. In: Beaton A E (ed.) 1993 *IEA Reading Literacy Study; Technical Report*. International Association for the Evaluation of Educational Research, The Hague
Andersen E B 1973 *Conditional Inference and Models for Measuring*. Mentalhygiejnisk Forlag, Copenhagen
Andrich D 1978 A rating formulation for ordered response categories. *Psychometrika*. 43(4): 561–73
Bryant P, Impey L 1986 The similarities between normal readers and developmental and acquired dyslexics. *Cog.* 24: 121–37
Elley W B 1992 *How in the World do Students Read? IEA Study of Reading Literacy*. International Association for the Evaluation of Educational Research, The Hague
Fischer G 1974 *Einführung in die Theorie Psychologischer Tests*. Huber, Bern
Holst C 1993 *Item Response Theory*. Danish Institute for Educational Research, Copenhagen
Johnson N L, Kotz S 1969 *Discrete Distributions*. Wiley, New York
Lord F M 1980 *Applications of Item Response Theory to Practical Testing Problems*. Erlbaum, Hillsdale, New Jersey
Lord F M, Novick M R 1968 *Statistical Theories of Mental Test Scores*. Addison-Wesley, Reading, Massachusetts
Mitterer J O 1982 There are at least two kinds of poor readers: Whole-word poor readers and recoding poor readers. *Canadian Journal of Psychology* 36(3): 445–61
Olson R K 1985 Individual and developmental differences in reading disability. In: Mackinnon G E, Waller T G (eds.) 1985 *Reading Research: Advances in Theory and Practice*. Academic Press, London
Rao C R 1952 *Advanced Statistical Methods in Biometric Research*. Wiley, New York
Rasch G 1960 *Probabilistic Models for some Intelligence and Attainment Tests*. Danish Institute for Educational Research, Copenhagen
Rasch G 1966a An informal report on a theory of objectivity in comparisons. *Proc. of the NUFFIC Int. Summer Session in Science at "Het Oude Hof," The Hague*
Rasch G 1966b An individualistic approach to item analysis. In: Lazarsfeld P F, Henry N W (eds.) 1966 *Readings in Mathematical Social Science*. MIT Press, Chicago, Illinois
Rasch G 1966c An item analysis which takes individual differences into account. *Br. J. Math. S. Psych.* 19(1): 49–57
Rasch G 1968 A mathematical theory of objectivity and its consequences for model construction. Paper presented at the European Meeting on Statistics, Econometrics and Management Science, Amsterdam
Rasch G 1977 On specific objectivity—an attempt at formalizing the request for generality and validity of scientific statements. In: *Danish Yearbook of Philosophy*. Munksgaard, Copenhagen
Snowling M J 1980 The development of grapheme–phoneme correspondance in normal and dyslexic readers. *Journal of Experimental Child Psychology* 29(2): 294–305

Rating Scale Analysis

D. Andrich

Rating scales are used to help identify the degrees of a *property* or *trait* of an object or person when no instrument for measuring the trait is available. Dawes (1972) estimated that some 60 percent of social science studies have rated variables as the only form of dependent variable. Rating scales are used in attitude questionnaires where responses to statements take the form Strongly Disagree, Disagree, Neutral or Undecided, Agree and Strongly Agree, and in performance ratings where judges classify performances in categories like Poor, Fair, Good, and Excellent. The former, with semantically opposite extremes, is a bipolar scale, while the latter is a unipolar scale. Many variants on these formats exist. In some cases, descriptions of the two extreme categories are given, with the central categories denoted by cutoff points; in others, such as judgment of performance, operational examples at each level are provided. This entry considers the procedures employed in the analysis of rating scale data.

1. Contingency Tables

In many contexts individuals who belong to defined

Table 1
Format for ratings in contingency tables[a]
Please respond to the following statement in one of the categories provided:
There should be publicly defined standards which all students should pass before leaving high school

	Response score	Strongly disagree (0)−	Disagree (1)	Agree (2)	Strongly agree (3)	Total No
Teaching level	Elementary	f_{10}	f_{11}	f_{12}	f_{13}	N_1
	Secondary	f_{20}	f_{21}	f_{22}	f_{23}	N_2
	Tertiary	f_{30}	f_{31}	f_{32}	f_{33}	N_3

a f denotes frequency

classes are rated into categories. For example, educators involved with different aspects of education may provide an opinion on public examinations or competency testing. Table 1 shows the kind of format, called a contingency table, in which responses would be presented. A topic such as public examinations may prompt responses to more than one statement. Results are then often reported statement by statement and inferences are drawn regarding the level of support enjoyed by each issue.

2. Individual Classifications

Often classifications more refined than contingency tables are required. First, the performance of each person rated, or providing an opinion, may need to be considered individually rather than as a member of some population. Second, it may be necessary to obtain more precise information about that person than can be obtained from one statement or rating. Therefore, more than one statement on a related topic, or more than one task, is required. In situations with two or more statements or two or more tasks, the information is collapsed into a single value for each person. Table 2 shows the kind of format in which the responses would be presented.

Where many statements or tasks are provided, whether in opinion, attitude, performance, or achievement ratings, the statements or tasks have the same role as they do in Thurstone Scales to which dichotomous responses rather than ratings are required (see Thurstone 1927). That is, they serve to define a continuum, and the ratings can be seen as extensions and refinements to dichotomous responses such as Disagree or Agree and Correct or Incorrect. Viewed from this perspective, the increase in the number of categories beyond two helps to increase the precision. The greater the number of categories, and to the degree that the categories can be used meaningfully, the greater the precision.

Unlike performance ratings, where a rater rates a performance explicitly, the rater in attitude testing is the person whose attitude is to be assessed. Attitude questionnaires requiring such ratings are said to be of the Likert style, following the work by Likert (1932) on attitude measurement (see *Attitudes, Measurement of*).

3. Scoring the Response Categories

The scoring of the ordered response categories in rating scales has received a great deal of attention. The most elementary approach follows closely the measurement analogy.

With a formalized measuring instrument, any object can be placed between the two cutoff points or thresholds on a continuum mapped onto a real line. On a typical measuring instrument the thresholds are represented by line segments of equal width which cut the real line at equal intervals. The measure then is the number of thresholds the object is seen to pass

Table 2
Format for ratings of individuals Statements or tasks

Rating Score x		1 0 1 2	2 0 1 2	i 0 1 2	J 0 1 2
Person (ratee)	1	x_{11}	x_{12}	x_{1i}	x_{1J}
	2	x_{21}	x_{22}	x_{2i}	x_{2J}
	3	x_{31}	x_{32}	x_{3i}	x_{3J}
	.	.	.	.	.
	.	.	.	.	.
	n	x_{n1}	x_{n2}	x_{ni}	x_{nJ}
	.	.	.	.	.
	.	.	.	.	.
	N	x_{N1}	x_{N2}	x_{Ni}	x_{NJ}

number of thresholds the object is seen to pass and this measure may be refined by having smaller intervals between thresholds and by having thresholds represented by finer lines. Often, measurement errors are considered sufficiently small relative to the variation of the measured property that they are ignored and the measures are then treated as continuous variables.

By analogy, in the rating scale the thresholds are placed so that they indicate equal spacing, and the raters are supposed to place their response between two thresholds. Elementary quantification and analysis extend this measurement analogy. Thus the successive categories are scored with successive integers, and the resultant numbers are again treated as continuous variables. The integers may start with either 0 or 1. For convenience here, they will be taken to commence with 0 and to have a maximum of m, where there are m thresholds and therefore m+1 categories.

In the contingency table context, the relative status of each *group* g is calculated then simply by $r_g = \sum_{x=0}^{m} x f_{gx}$ while in the assessment of individuals on statements or tasks i, i=1, . . . k, the status of each *individual* n is calculated simply by $r_n = \sum_i x_{ni}$. That is, the integer ratings are simply summed. Standard analyses based on these summary statistics, and following the true score model of traditional test theory, have been developed. Guildford (1954, Chap. 11) provides a comprehensive discussion of the construction of rating scales and on the analyses using the above scoring. However, the assumption of equality of intervals, on which the integer scoring is supposed to be based, has been questioned often. This has led to more formal representations of the rating process.

4. Mathematical Response Models

Two qualifications to the elementary analogy to a measuring instrument are made. First, it is accepted that there is uncertainty in the classification, second that the distances between thresholds may not be equal and require estimating.

4.1 The Traditional Threshold Model

The traditional model, originating with Thurstone (1927), assumes a single response process centered at the location μ (of a group or individual). This process may be either the cumulative normal or the logistic distribution, but because the two are indistinguishable numerically after a linear scaling, and because the latter is more tractable, it is now usually preferred. Then the probability of a response above each threshold is the area beyond the threshold in the distribution, Fig. 1 shows the process for the logistic function, where the probability p_x^* of a response *above* threshold $\tau_x, x = 1, m$, is given by

$$p_x^* = \int_{\tau_x}^{\infty} \frac{\exp(x - \mu)/\sigma}{\{1 + \exp(x - \mu)/\sigma\}^2} dx = \frac{1}{\gamma} \exp\{(\mu - \tau_x)/\sigma\}$$

$$= \frac{1}{\gamma} \exp\{\alpha(\mu - \tau_x)\} \tag{1}$$

where (i) $\alpha=1/\sigma$ is termed the discrimination and (ii) $\gamma = 1 + \exp\{\alpha(\mu - \tau_x)\}$ which ensures that p_x^* and its complement, the probability of a response below threshold x, sum to 1. The probability p_x of a response in category x, x=0, 1, 2 . . ., m is given simply by the difference between successive cumulative probabilities: $p_x = p_{x-1}^* - p_x^*$ with $p_0^* \equiv 1$. Note that the ratio of p_x^* and $1 - p_x^*$ gives $p_x^*/(1 - p_x^*) = \exp\{\alpha(\mu - \tau_x)\}$ of which the natural logarithm $\log p_x^*/(1 - p_x^*) = \alpha(\mu - \tau_x)$ is called the *logit*.

The parameters α, μ, and τ_x may be qualified according to the context. For example, in a contingency table, the logit in Eqn. (1) may take the form $(\mu_g - \tau_x)$ where only the location of the groups vary, or $\alpha_g(\mu_g - \tau_x)$,

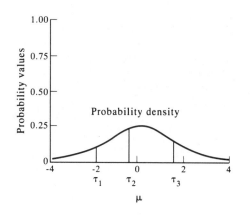

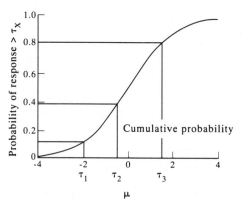

Figure 1
Probability of the response process with the Thurstone cumulative probability model

where the discrimination among groups also varies, or $\alpha_g(\mu_g - \tau_{xg})$ where the thresholds also vary among groups.

In the case for the assessment of individual n across more than one task or statement i, μ is resolved according to $\mu_{ni} = \beta_n - \delta_i$. Then if each task or statement is assumed to have the same discrimination and equal thresholds, the logit in (1) may take the form ($\beta_n - \delta_i - \tau_{xi}$).

The estimation of the parameters may be carried out in various ways. In the early work, and in the case where ratings are associated with a group or population, the proportions of responses in the respective categories were taken as a direct estimate $\hat{p}_x$ of the corresponding probabilities p_x. Then the estimates of $\mu - \tau_x$ were given simply by either the corresponding standard normal deviate, or the logit given by log $(\hat{p}_x^* / (1 - \hat{p}_x^*))$ for each group. More recent techniques involve the maximum likelihood estimation (MLE) procedure. This requires identifying the values of the parameters of the chosen model which maximize the probability for the data observed.

Likert originally correlated the estimates of locations using weights for categories in the manner described above, with those obtained by simply summing the integer scores. These correlations were generally very close to 1.00. As a result, and for simplicity, Likert and the majority of users of rating scales since then have used the simple integer scoring. That is, they have continued with the original measurement analogy.

While the characterization or measurement of individuals is often the main task, understanding and controlling the rating mechanism is also important. Therefore, researchers have continued to show concern about the assumption of equal intervals on the rating scales. The traditional threshold model and its mathematical formulation described above is one attempt to accommodate these concerns, for which Bock (1975 Chap. 8) provides the mathematics for contingency tables and Samejima (1969) for the assessment of individuals.

4.2 The Rasch Rating Model

A more recent formulation of a mathematical model for ratings (Andersen 1977, Andrich 1978) accommodates not only the features of a random response process and the estimation of thresholds, but also the simple integer scoring of the successive categories and the simple summing among tasks or statements. In addition, it has major epistemological differences with Thurstone's formulation referred to later. If p_x is again the probability that a rating, governed by a true value μ, is in category x, the model takes the form

$$p_x = \frac{1}{\gamma}\exp\{x\mu - \sum_{k=1}^{x} \tau_k\} \qquad (2)$$

where $\gamma = \sum_{k=0}^{x} \exp\{k\mu - \sum_{j=1}^{k}\tau_j\}$ is a normalizing factor

ensuring that $\sum_{x=0}^{m} p_x = 1$, and where $\tau_x, = 1, 2 \ldots, m$ are again m thresholds on the continuum. This model has been called the Rasch Rating Model because it has all the distinguishing properties of the Rasch model for dichotomously scored responses (see *Rasch Theory, Measurement of*). That is, the structural parameters of thresholds (and items) can be separated from the distributions of the groups (and persons). Fig. 2 shows the response probability curves for three ordered categories. As with Eqn (1), the exponent of Eqn (2) can be modified to suit the particular data collection format. Thus for contingency tables, the exponent may take the form $x\mu_g - \sum_{k=1} \tau_k$. Alternatively, if the thresholds are considered differently spaced from group to group, it may be modified to $x\mu_g - \sum \tau_{kg}$.

It is important to note one similarity and three differences between Eqns (1) and (2). First, they both take the logistic form. Second, in Eqn (1) the logit is given by the ratio of cumulative probabilities while in Eqn (2) it is given by the ratio of probabilities of *adjacent* categories: $(p_x / p_{x-1}) = \exp\{\mu - \tau_x\}$ from which $\ln(p_x / p_{x-1}) = \mu - \tau_x$. Third, the exponent in Eqn (2) has parameters that are additive, there being no general discrimination α as in the exponent of Eqn (1). Fourth, while the same term "threshold" is used in both models, because they are defined differently, they have different values.

When the MLE is used, the *sufficient statistics* for the estimate of μ_g is $r_g = \sum_{x=1} x f_{gx}$ and the sufficient statistic for the estimate of τ_x is $t_x = \sum_{i=1} f_{gx}$

Further, the solution equations for μ_g and τ_x respectively are

$$r_g = \frac{1}{\gamma} N_g \Sigma \exp\{x\hat{\mu}_g - \sum_{k=1}^{x} \hat{\tau}_k\}, \; g = 1, G,$$

$$t_x = \frac{1}{\gamma} \sum_g \exp\{x\hat{\mu}_g - \sum_{k=1}^{x} \hat{\tau}_k\}, \; x = 1, m.$$

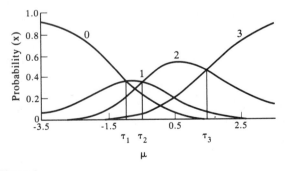

Figure 2
Probability of the response process with the Rasch cumulative threshold model

These equations with the imposed constraints $\sum_g \hat{\mu}_g = 0$ and $\sum_x \hat{\tau} = 0$ must be solved iteratively because they are implicit, and not explicit, equations in the parameters.

The existence of sufficient statistics shows that they contain all the information about the parameters that is available in the responses. In addition, these statistics are the simple sums of the integers, which is exactly the ones used in the elementary measurement analogy. Through Eqn (2), the constrained qualitative responses are mapped onto an additive or linear scale, which also estimates the thresholds. The simple total score r_g is then not seen as the sum of equally spaced thresholds as in the full measurement analogy, but as a count of the number of thresholds that have been passed. The weighting of the categories is taken account of by the threshold estimates. Andrich (1979) discussed the application of this model to contingency tables.

In the case of assessment of individuals, the location μ in the exponent of Eqn (2) is again modified to include a person parameter β_n and a difficulty or affective value parameter δ_i so that $\mu_{ni} = \beta_n - \delta_i$ giving the logit $(\beta_n - \delta_i) - \sum_{k=1}^{x} \tau_k$. Then the sufficient statistic for the person parameter β_n is $r_n = \sum_i x_{ni}$, for the task or statement parameter δ_i it is $s_i = \sum_n x_{ni}$, and for the threshold parameter τ_x it is $\tau_x = \sum_n \sum_i I_{nix}$ where $I_{nix} = 1$ if the response is in category x, and 0 otherwise. That is, t_x is simply the total number of responses in category x across all tasks or statements and across all persons.

Again, the statistic r_n for estimating the person parameter is identical to that used in the elementary measurement analogy and shown by Likert (1932) to be satisfactory for the measurement of persons. In fact, because $\hat{\beta}_n$ and r_n are monotonically related, their correlation is nearly perfect. The transformation of r_n to $\hat{\beta}_n$ again maps or transforms the qualitative responses onto a linear scale.

If it is assumed that the threshold spacings, whatever they are, are not equal across tasks or statements, then the exponent of Eqn (2) may be qualified further to $x\beta_n - \sum_{k=1}^{x} \tau_{ki}$, (Wright and Masters 1982). The total score $r_n = \sum_i x_{ni}$ remains the sufficient statistic for the person parameter β_n, thus indicating the appropriateness of scoring successive categories with successive integers while taking account of variations in spacing between the thresholds.

5. Connecting Ratings to Measurements

Because the Rasch Rating Model does not require that the distances between thresholds are equal, the integer score on each rating is not itself a measure. However, the parameter estimates are on a linear scale and are measures up to an interval level. With respect to a conformable set of statements or tasks, the only difference between usual measures and those estimated through the Rasch model for ratings is one of degree. The precision can be increased by increasing the number of tasks or statements. Thus the Rasch Rating Model formally completes the measurement analogy.

A related aspect of the Rasch Rating Model is that it formalizes the popular and simple, yet theoretically weak, Likert approach to the attitude measurement of individuals. Likert had originally proposed his approach to circumvent the time-consuming requirement of scaling statements required by the approaches of Thurstone. The formalization permits the Likert approach to subscribe to all the rigorous requirements of Thurstone for scales (see Thurstone 1927 Scale P), including the scaling of tasks or statements. In particular, and with respect to a conformable set of tasks or statements, any subset will lead to the same measure of a person. Similarly, the scale values of the statements and thresholds will be invariant across the abilities or attitudes of the persons measured. The linearity and this form of invariance are key aspects of Thurstone Scales. Andrich (1982) presented a full discussion of the way in which the Rasch Rating Model unifies the Thurstone and Likert approaches to scaling and measurement.

6. Quality Control

It is stressed that these invariance properties hold in data only if they conform to the Rasch Model; whether or not they do so conform, is an empirical question.

There are two related advantages in using the above explicit measurement model for analyzing ratings. The obvious one is that the measures—not simply ratings—become available. Second, and equally important, is that in the very process of attempting to obtain formal measurements, a greater understanding of the variable or trait in question should follow. A close examination of response patterns that do not conform to the rating model may be as informative in understanding the variable as when they do conform, and the Rasch Rating Model permits a refined analysis that detects lack of conformity in various ways.

6.1 The Response Pattern

One important and necessary feature for measurement, which can be checked, is whether the response pattern is internally consistent. According to the rating model, every person is expected to score higher on an easier question in achievement testing, or a smaller affective value in attitude measurement. If the ratings do not conform satisfactorily to this pattern, then a single measure to represent the responses cannot be justified.

This perspective leads naturally to the analysis of profiles.

6.2 The "Halo" Effect

There can be many sources of inconsistency, as in all measurement data. When judges rate performances, a judge may gain an overall impression that affects all his or her ratings of the performance, even if these ratings are supposed to reflect different criteria. This is called the "halo" effect. The ratings in this case are "too consistent" as a result of the artificial dependence among them.

6.3 Rater Leniency

In performance ratings, some raters may be more lenient or more harsh than others. If more than one rater rates with respect to a single task, then the rating model accounts for this effect. In particular, when δ is made to characterize the rater, it represents rater harshness. Alternatively, if more than one rater and more than one task are involved, then the logit in Eqn (2) may be further modified to include the rater effect. For example, it may take the form $x(\beta_v - \delta_i - \eta_j) - \sum_{k=1} \tau_k$ where η_j is the harshness of rater j. Other qualifications are also possible.

6.4 Response Sets

Another possible systematic source of inconsistency occurs when different individuals use the categories differently. For example, some raters may use the extreme categories, while others may use the central categories, relatively too often. Both types of response patterns, reflecting what are known as response sets, which can threaten valid measurement, can be identified by the relative location of the thresholds.

6.5 Number of Categories and the Neutral Category

In constructing rating response formats that will minimize the above problems, two further issues need to be considered. First, the number of categories should be large enough to take advantage of the judge's capacity to discriminate, but not greater. Guildford (1954) gave empirical evidence to guide the choice of the number of categories. Usually four or five are used for unipolar scales and five to nine for bipolar scales. Second, in bipolar scales, the Neutral or Undecided category has been the subject of much study. It seems not to attract responses consistent with those found on either side of it, it being a "catch-all" category in which people who do not understand the question, as well as people who are genuinely undecided, or neutral, respond. It seems best to construct statements that would attract few responses in this category, and then to exclude the category when the statements are used to obtain measures. Linacre (1989) covered these issues in greater detail.

7. Distinctions between the Rasch and Thurstone Models

While the models of Rasch and Thurstone can be used for the same purpose, there are some major conceptual differences between the two, and in a well-defined sense they are incompatible specifications. First, as indicated already, the Rasch Model permits a separation of the person and item parameters in the estimation, and therefore no assumptions about the distribution of the person parameters is necessary in any estimation. Such a separation is not possible in the Thurstone Model. Second, because the thresholds are determined by the cumulative probabilities in the Thurstone Model, the ordering of the estimates of the thresholds must be in the a priori order designated by the investigator. Therefore, any problem in the operation of the rating scale on this feature cannot be identified by the model, and all data, no matter how poorly collected, will always show the a priori ordering. In contrast, the threshold estimates in the Rasch Model may be disordered relative to the intended ordering of the categories, indicating that something has gone wrong in the specification or operation of the categories. The reversal of the threshold estimates does not in itself indicate exactly what has gone wrong.

However, one example seems consistent: when a *neutral* category is inserted in a bipolar scale, the Rasch Model consistently shows reversed threshold estimates, confirming other well-established evidence that this category does not operate on the same dimension as the other categories. Third, and most profound, is that in the Thurstone Model it is possible to collapse adjacent categories after the data are collected, and the estimates of the thresholds between other categories will not be affected. In contrast, in the Rasch Model, if the data collected with a particular set of categories conform to the model, then if a pair of adjacent categories are collapsed, the data will no longer conform to the Rasch Model with one fewer category. The implication of this result is that the specification of the categories, and the collection of data in these categories, is an integral part of the construction of the variable, and that if the separation of the person and item parameters is to be retained, these cannot be tampered with after the data are collected. The full implications of this result have not been explored.

See also: Rating Scales; Contingency Tables; Scaling Methods

References

Andersen E B 1977 Sufficient statistics and latent trait models. *Psychometri.* 42(1): 69–81

Andrich D 1978 A rating formulation for ordered response categories. *Psychometri.* 43(4): 561–73

Andrich D 1979 A model for contingency tables having an ordered response classification. *Biometrics* 35(2): 403–15

Andrich D 1982 Using latent trait measurement models to analyse attitudinal data: A synthesis of viewpoints. In: Spearritt D (ed.) 1982 *The Improvement of Measurement in Education and Psychology.* ACER, Melbourne

Bock R D 1975 *Multivariate Satistical Methods in Behavioral Research.* McGraw-Hill, New York

Dawes R M 1972 *Fundamentals of Attitude Measurement.* Wiley, New York

Guildford J P 1954 *Psychometric Methods,* 2nd edn. McGraw-Hill, New York

Likert R 1932 A technique for the measurement of attitudes. *Archives of Psychology* 140: 52

Linacre J M 1989 *Many-faceted Rasch Measurement* MESA Press, Chicago, Illinois

Samejima F 1969 Estimation of latent ability using a response pattern of graded scores. *Psychometric Monographs,* 134 (2, No. 17)

Thurstone L L 1927 Psychological analysis. *American Journal of Psychology* 38: 368–89

Wright B D, Masters G N 1982 *Rating Scale Analysis.* MESA Press, Chicago, Illinois

(c) Applications of Measurement in Research

Adaptive Testing

D. J. Weiss and J. L. Schleisman

An adaptive test is an educational or psychological test in which the questions/items to be administered to an examinee are selected based on the examinee's responses to previously administered items (Wainer 1990, Weiss 1985, Weiss and Betz 1973). This approach to test administration contrasts with a conventional test (e.g., a typical paper-and-pencil test) in which all examinees receive the same fixed set of items. Adaptive testing has also been called tailored (Lord 1971), response-contingent, programmed, computerized, automated, individualized, and branched testing. Adaptive testing can be differentiated from sequential testing. In a sequential test (Kingsbury and Weiss 1983), test items are administered either in a fixed order or are randomly selected from an item bank; in an adaptive test, items are selected from an item bank based on a prespecified item selection rule. Sequential and adaptive tests are similar in that the number of items administered to an examinee can vary, although they are based on different termination rules.

A variety of approaches have been developed for administering adaptive tests. In some approaches, a new item is selected after a single item is administered and scored. In others, a new block of items—sometimes called a "testlet" (Wainer and Kiely 1987)—is administered based on an examinee's performance on a previously administered set of items. An examinee's response to an item (or set of items) is scored and the next item(s) administered is based on the examinee's response to the previous item(s). If the response is correct, the next item administered will be a more difficult item; if the response is incorrect, the next item will be less difficult. Items are selected from an item bank that contains items with predetermined difficulties (and perhaps discriminations and other item characteristics).

An individual taking an adaptive test will receive a set of items that is most appropriate for his or her performance level within the limitations of the item bank —the items selected are adapted to the characteristics of the examinee during testing. Adaptive tests are designed to improve measurement over conventional tests by improving the efficiency of test administration —by administering the minimum number of items necessary to measure each examinee—and by controlling the precision of measurement. Some adaptive tests have been designed for individual administration by a trained psychometrist (e.g., the Stanford–Binet) while others have been proposed for paper-and-pencil administration, for example, Lord's (1971) flexilevel test. Computerized adaptive testing (CAT), in which test items are administered by an interactive computer, takes full advantage of the capabilities of adaptive testing.

In this entry the basic principles of adaptive testing are summarized and adaptive item selection procedures based on prestructured or unstructured item banks are described. In self-adapted testing, the examinee selects the difficulty of the next item based on feedback received from performance on previous items. Adaptive testing has been shown to increase measurement efficiency and precision. Adaptive testing has also been applied to personality assessment. Potential problems with adaptive testing and future research areas are also discussed.

1. Principles of Adaptive Testing

An adaptive test requires: (a) a precalibrated item bank, (b) a procedure for initial item selection, (c) a procedure for item selection during test administration, (d) a method for scoring the test, and (e) a procedure for terminating the test.

1.1 Initial and Adaptive Item Selection

If the first item is allowed to vary for each examinee, the test has a variable entry point; if all examinees begin testing with the same item, the test has a fixed entry. Prior information from a teacher, the examinee, demographic data, or previous test data can be used to determine the initial item selection for a variable entry test. Any information that is known to be correlated with the performance or trait estimates derived from the adaptive test will reduce test length or improve performance or trait estimation.

The item selection rule differs depending on the type of adaptive test being used. Adaptive item selection procedures are based either on prestructured item banks, which typically implement fixed-branching procedures, or unstructured item banks which implement variable-branching procedures. Scoring methods and termination rules are generally implemented in the context of the prestructured and unstructured item bank dichotomy.

1.2 Prestructured Item Selection/Fixed Branching

Early approaches to adaptive testing were based primarily on fixed-branching procedures, such as the individually administered Stanford–Binet intelligence test (Terman and Merrill 1960), originally developed by Alfred Binet in the early 1900s. Based on the examinee's responses to items at a given "mental age," items at another "mental age" are selected and administered to the examinee. Other types of adaptive tests that use prestructured item selection rules include two-stage (Lord 1971), pyramidal (Hansen 1969), flexilevel (Lord 1971), and stratified adaptive (stradaptive) tests (Weiss 1973).

Wainer and Kiely (1987) proposed a "multistage fixed-branching CAT model that substitutes multi-item 'testlets' for single items as the unit for test development and administration . . . . A testlet is a group of items related to a single content area that is developed as a unit and contains a fixed number of predetermined paths that an examinee may follow" (p. 190). Testlets (see also Kingsbury and Zara 1989, Thissen et al. 1989) can use a linear or hierarchical branching scheme. In a linear testlet, all examinees receive all items; in a hierarchical testlet, branching is based on previous responses. Testlets are combined to form a larger test. Similar to a two-stage test, an examinee who performed well on a previous testlet would be administered a testlet of higher difficulty; an examinee who responded poorly on items in the previous testlet would be administered a testlet of lower difficulty.

Although two-stage tests have minimal adaptive capability, Adema (1990) proposed mixed-integer linear programming models for constructing two-stage tests. Adaptive tests based on "testlets" are an implementation of the concepts underlying two-stage tests and are an extension of tests based on blocks of items with more than two stages and therefore have many of the limitations of the two-stage tests, even though they are implemented with more sophisticated models.

The fixed-branching item selection procedures have several limitations: (a) they do not use all information available from the items (i.e., they generally only make use of item difficulty and ignore other item characteristics such as discriminations and susceptibility to guessing); (b) they are based on arbitrary scoring methods; (c) with the exception of the stradaptive tests, they are based on a fixed termination criterion (i.e., all examinees receive the same number of items); and (d) the amount of adaptation for each examinee is limited.

1.3 Unstructured Item Banks/IRT-based Adaptive Testing

Variable-branching strategies based on item response theory (IRT), latent trait test theory, and item charac-

teristic curve theory which operate from unstructured but precalibrated item banks, have been developed and represent the state of the art in adaptive testing. IRT is a family of mathematical models that describe the probability of a correct response as a function of item characteristics and examinee characteristics. The three-parameter IRT model (Hambleton and Swaminathan 1985, Lord 1980) characterizes items by the three parameters: difficulty, discrimination, and pseudo-guessing; and examinees by using their performance or trait level. The Rasch (1960) or one-parameter (logistic) model describes items using only difficulty. The three item parameters can be combined into a single index called the "item information function," which describes how precisely an item measures at different performance or trait levels.

Item information is a primary criterion for selecting items in IRT-based adaptive testing. Two item selection procedures are commonly used: maximum information (Weiss and Kingsbury 1984) and Bayesian (Owen 1975). In maximum information adaptive testing, items are selected that provide maximum levels of item information at the examinee's currently estimated performance/trait level. The item is administered, and the examinee's performance/trait estimate is based on the responses to all previously answered test items using maximum likelihood estimation. The new performance or trait estimate is then used to select the next item to be administered to that examinee. This process is repeated until a termination criterion is reached.

Bayesian-based item selection uses Bayes's theorem to select the one item from all unadministered items that will minimize the Bayesian posterior variance of the performance/trait estimate after it is answered. Performance or trait level is then re-estimated using Bayesian estimation procedures, and the item bank is again searched to identify the unadministered item that minimizes the posterior variance. The procedure is repeated until some predetermined level of the Bayesian posterior variance is reached. This procedure permits more explicit use of prior information to determine starting points than does maximum information item selection. However, the use of prior information introduces biases into the scoring procedure that reduce levels of measurement precision for individuals whose performance or trait levels are not near the prior estimate (e.g., Weiss and McBride 1984).

IRT-based adaptive testing addresses the limitations of and offers advantages over non-IRT-based adaptive testing. The item's difficulty, discrimination, and guessing parameters can all be taken into account; scoring methods are not arbitrary; and item banks can be used efficiently because there is no predetermined branching structure.

A final advantage of IRT-based adaptive tests is that the termination criterion can be tailored to the purpose of testing. IRT scoring procedures allow for both performance or trait estimation and the estimation of individualized errors of measurement. Consequently, in situations where it is important to test all examinees to a given level of precision, the termination criterion can be based on precision of measurement; given an adequate item bank, testing can be continued for each examinee until the desired level of precision is reached. In other testing applications (e.g., selection of individuals against some predetermined criterion level of performance, such as in job or educational admissions testing or mastery testing), it is necessary to test an individual only long enough to determine whether she or he is above or below the cutoff value (e.g., Weiss and Kingsbury 1984).

The implementation of IRT-based adaptive testing involves substantial amounts of numerical calculation after each item is administered. Typically, calculations involve estimating the performance or trait level and its standard error, and the amount of information provided by each item at the current performance or trait estimate. Because of these computational requirements, IRT-based adaptive testing must be computer-administered and is the basis for most implementations of CAT.

1.4 Self-adapted Testing

Self-adapted testing (SAT) (Kingsbury and Zara 1989, Rocklin and O'Donnell 1987) has been proposed as a method to reduce test anxiety, which, it is believed, will maximize an examinee's performance. This is accomplished by allowing the examinee to choose the difficulty level of the items administered. For example, after answering an item, an examinee would be informed immediately whether the answer was correct or incorrect. The examinee would then choose the next item. The items in SAT are prestructured by difficulty into levels or strata, therefore, it is very similar to the stradaptive testing procedure, except that the examinee selects the difficulty of the next item. An obvious problem with this procedure is that an examinee may select only items that she or he can answer correctly (i.e., the examinee may never select an item from a stratum containing items of higher difficulty). Although this might result in reduced test anxiety, it might not yield much psychometric information about the examinee.

2. Improved Measurement Efficiency and Precision with Adaptive Testing

Research comparing conventional tests and adaptive tests has demonstrated that a major advantage of adaptive tests over conventional tests is increased measurement efficiency. Improved measurement efficiency occurs when test length is reduced, but measurements of comparable or superior quality are obtained. For example, McBride and Martin (1983), compared computer-administered conventional tests

and CATs and found that for any given test length the adaptive tests had higher reliabilities than the conventional tests. A 10-item CAT had a slightly higher reliability than a 25-item conventional test (0.87 vs. 0.86). McBride and Martin also determined how many items a conventional test would need to reach a reliability equal to that of a CAT. For a 5-item adaptive test, the conventional test would need to be 2.57 times as long or 12.85 items in length to attain the same level of reliability as the CAT.

Adaptive tests not only provide increases in measurement efficiency, but also improved measurement precision. Adaptive tests provide measurements of equal or greater precision than conventional tests of the same length (Wise and Plake 1989). McBride and Martin (1983) found that the alternate forms reliability of a 9-item adaptive test (0.800) was equal to that of a 17-item conventional test (0.798). Others (Olsen et al. 1989, Weiss 1982, Weiss and Vale 1987, Wise and Plake 1989) reported similar findings concerning measurement efficiency and precision. The decreases in test length of adaptive tests do not negatively affect validity; McBride and Martin found that scores on a 10-item adaptive test correlated 0.80 with a 50-item criterion test, but it took 30 items on a conventional test to reach the same level of validity.

3. Potential Problems with CAT

Perhaps the most commonly cited potential problem with CAT is context effects (Bunderson et al. 1989, Kingsbury and Zara 1989, Wainer and Kiely 1987). The effects of prior items in a test on succeeding items are known as "context effects." In conventional testing, each examinee receives the same items in the same order and, therefore, any context effects would exist for every examinee and should not differentially impact any particular examinee. In CAT, each examinee potentially receives different items and/or items in different orders. "Cross-information" (information that one item may inadvertently contribute about the answer to another) is a context effect. If Item 3 provided information that would help an examinee answer Item 5, then every examinee would have access to that information in a conventional test. However, in an adaptive test, only an examinee who received both Items 3 and 5 consecutively would have access to that information.

Another context effect is "unbalanced content," which refers to the situation in which there is repeated emphasis on a particular content area. For example, in an adaptive mathematics test designed to test the four basic mathematics skills (addition, subtraction, multiplication, and division), an examinee may only be administered items which require subtraction and addition. This unbalanced sampling of the different content areas can occur if item selection is based solely on psychometric criteria, particularly in nonhomogeneous content domains.

Another potential problem with adaptive testing, termed "lack of robustness," results from the fact that adaptive tests are often shorter than conventional tests and thus lack redundancy (Bunderson et al. 1989, Wainer and Kiely 1987). An item that is functioning poorly in an adaptive test might have a greater impact on test results than a poorly functioning item would have in a longer conventional test. This problem may be mitigated, however, by the fact that IRT-based CATs typically use item banks that consist primarily of items of high psychometric quality and are carefully analyzed before the tests are administered.

In a conventional test, items are usually presented in order of increasing difficulty. This procedure may give many examinees confidence by allowing them to experience success at the beginning of a test. In an adaptive test, the initial item administered is usually one of average difficulty. For a high-ability examinee, the items would increase in difficulty from the initial item administered; examinees of lower ability would probably experience failure on the initial items because they would be too difficult, and the subsequent items administered would decrease rather than increase in difficulty. This might cause frustration, anxiety, and lower performance in the lower ability group. This problem can be mitigated by the use of informed entry points based on appropriate prior information. Also, in a good adaptive test, all examinees will receive a set of items on which they will experience 50 percent success; therefore adaptive tests may have the beneficial effect of equalizing the psychological test-taking environment for both high and low ability examinees.

Another potential problem is the effect that reviewing items and changing responses might have on performance or trait estimates. Wise and Plake (1989) concluded that unless denying examinees the opportunity to review items and to change responses "adversely affects the test scores of a meaningful proportion of examinees . . . they should probably not be provided" (p. 7). Lunz et al. (1992) studied the effect of allowing examinees to review items and to alter responses. They examined what the ability estimates (and standard errors) of those who were allowed to review would have been if they had not been allowed to review. They found that the ability estimates correlated 0.98, which suggests that being able to review did not significantly alter the ability estimates of examinees and that the standard errors of measurement were not affected by review.

4. Application of Adaptive Testing to Personality Assessment

Although the majority of adaptive testing research has occurred with ability and achievement measurement, the principles and procedures apply equally well to the measurement of personality variables (Butcher

1987). For example, Waller and Reise (1989) compared two IRT-based adaptive testing strategies to a paper-and-pencil version of a personality scale. Their procedure involved "real-data simulation," namely, post-hoc simulation of adaptive tests using responses of examinees to a previously administered conventional personality scale. They found that the adaptive procedure resulted in a reduction in test length of as much as 50 percent without any loss in measurement precision. Using a decision-based adaptive testing strategy, they obtained a perfect success rate (i.e., no incorrect classifications) even though only 25 percent of the items, on average, were administered.

Roper et al. (1991) administered paper-and-pencil and CAT versions of the MMPI-2 to college students. They were interested in determining whether score comparability was compromised because fewer items were administered in the CAT version. No significant differences were found across modalities even though fewer items were administered in the CAT version.

5. Future Directions of Adaptive Testing

Adaptive testing, particularly CAT, moved from the research to the implementation stage during the early 1990s. Flexible microcomputer software for adaptive testing—the MicroCAT Testing System (Assessment Systems Corporation 1988) which is capable of administering almost any type of adaptive test—has been developed and upgraded. Several major testing programs in the United States have converted large testing programs to CAT administration, including the Educational Testing Service's Graduate Record Examination and Scholastic Aptitude Test. The National Council of State Boards of Nursing began nationwide CAT administration of its nursing licensing examinations in 1994 and the public school system in Portland, Oregon has converted many of its achievement tests to CAT administration (Kingsbury 1990).

Further research is needed to resolve the aforementioned potential problems described. New algorithms must also be developed and evaluated to integrate psychometric item selection criteria with content and other considerations, and research is needed on entry points and termination criteria for different testing applications.

Almost all CAT developments are based on power tests, yet speed is an important component of ability. There is a need to develop CAT models that will allow adaptation of examinee response latency or time of response presentation. In addition, almost all adaptive testing research has been based on multiple-choice items. However, both computer presentation of tests and the trend toward performance evaluation allow for a much richer and varied kind of test item than is possible with paper-and-pencil tests (e.g., Bunderson et al. 1989). These new kinds of test items will pose new challenges for the development of CAT.

See also: Item Response Theory; Item Sampling; Rasch Measurement, Theory of

References

Adema J J 1990 The construction of customized two-stage tests. *J. Educ. Meas.* 27(3): 241–39
Assessment Systems Corporation 1988 *MicroCAT 3.0* (Computer program). Assessment Systems Corporation, St Paul, Minnesota
Bunderson C V, Inouye D K, Olsen J B 1989 The four generations of computerized educational measurement. In: Linn R L (ed.) 1989 *Educational Measurement*, 3rd edn. Macmillan, New York
Butcher J N 1987 *Computerized Psychological Assessment: A Practitioner's Guide.* Basic Books, New York
Hambleton R K, Swaminathan H 1985 *Item Response Theory: Principles and Applications.* Kluwer-Nijhoff, Boston, Massachusetts
Hansen D N 1969 An investigation of computer-based science testing. In: Atkinson R C, Wilson H A (eds.) 1969 *Computer-assisted Instruction: A Book of Readings.* Academic Press, New York
Kingsbury G G 1990 Adapting adaptive testing: Using the MicroCAT testing system in a local school district. *Educational Measurement* 9(2): 3–6, 29
Kingsbury G G, Weiss D J 1983 A comparison of IRT-based adaptive mastery testing and a sequential mastery testing procedure. In: Weiss D J (ed.) 1983 *New Horizons in Testing: Latent Trait Test Theory and Computerized Adaptive Testing.* Academic Press, New York
Kingsbury G G, Zara A R 1989 Procedures for selecting items for computerized adaptive tests. *Applied Measurement in Education* 2(4): 359–75
Lord F M 1971 The self-scoring flexilevel test. *J. Educ. Meas.* 8(3): 147–51
Lord F M 1980 *Applications of Item Response Theory to Practical Testing Problems*, Erlbaum, Hillsdale, New Jersey
Lunz M E, Bergstrom B A, Wright B D 1992 The effect of review on student ability and test efficiency for computerized adaptive tests. *Appl. Psychol. Meas.* 16(1): 33–40
McBride J R, Martin J T 1983 Reliability and validity of adaptive ability tests in a military setting. In: Weiss D J (ed.) 1983 *New Horizons in Testing: Latent Trait Test Theory and Computerized Adaptive Testing.* Academic Press, New York
Olsen J B, Maynes D D, Slawson D, Ho K 1989 Comparisons of paper-administered, computer-administered and computerized adaptive achievement tests. *Journal of Educational Computing Research* 5(3): 311–26
Owen R J 1975 A Bayesian sequential procedure for quantal response in the context of adaptive mental testing. *Journal of the American Statistical Association* 70: 351–56
Rasch G 1960 *Probabilistic Models for Some Intelligence and Attainment Tests.* Danmarks Paedagogiske Institut, Copenhagen
Rocklin T, O'Donnell A M 1987 Self-adapted testing: A performance-improving variant of computerized adaptive testing. *J. Educ. Psychol.* 79(3): 315–19
Roper B L, Ben-Porath Y S, Butcher J N 1991 Comparability of computerized adaptive and conventional testing with the MMPI-2. *Journal of Personality Assessment* 57(2): 278–90
Terman L M, Merrill M A 1960 *Stanford–Binet Intelligence Scale.* Houghton Mifflin, Boston, Massachusetts
Thissen D, Steinberg L, Mooney J A 1989 Trace lines for testlets: A use of multiple-categorical response models. *J. Educ. Meas.* 26(3): 247–60
Wainer H 1990 *Computerized Adaptive Testing: A Primer.* Erlbaum, Hillsdale, New Jersey
Wainer H, Kiely G L 1987 Item clusters and computerized adaptive testing: A case for testlets. *J. Educ. Meas.* 24(3): 185–201
Waller N G, Reise S P 1989 Computerized adaptive personality assessment: An illustration with the absorption scale. *J. Pers. Soc. Psychol.* 57(6): 1051–58
Weiss D J 1973 *The Stratified Adaptive Computerized Ability Test.* Research Report No. 73–3. University of Minnesota, Minneapolis Department of Psychology, Minnesota
Weiss D J 1982 Improving measurement quality and efficiency with adaptive testing. *Appl. Psychol. Meas.* 6(4): 473–92
Weiss D J 1985 Adaptive testing by computer. *J. Consult. Clin. Psychol.* 53(6): 774–89
Weiss D J, Betz N E 1973 *Ability Measurement: Conventional or Adaptive?* Research Report No. 73–1. University of Minnesota, Department of Psychology, Psychometric Methods Program, Minneapolis, Minnesota
Weiss D J, Kingsbury G G 1984 Application of computerized adaptive testing to educational problems. *J. Educ. Meas.* 21(4): 361–75
Weiss D J, McBride J R 1984 Bias and information of Bayesian adaptive testing. *Appl. Psychol. Meas.* 8(3): 273–85
Weiss D J, Vale C D 1987 Adaptive testing. *Appl. Psychol.* 36(3/4): 249–62 (Special Issue: Computerized Psychological Testing)
Wise S L, Plake B S 1989 Research on the effects of administering tests via computers. *Educational Measurement* 8(3): 5–10

Attitudes, Measurement of

L. W. Anderson

Attitudes, interests, and values are central to the educative process both as ends and as means. Depending on whether they are positively or negatively directed towards a particular object they are considered to promote or inhibit student behavior in the classroom, the home, and the peer group and ultimately learning and the choice of a career. Furthermore, they are considered to influence choices to attend, respond, value, participate, and make a commitment to educational activities. Thus the development of favorable attitudes, interests, and values toward particular objects is a stated goal of most educational programs. Even when not stated as a goal, such programs influence the attitudes, interests, and values of the students who take part, again either positively or negatively. Many informal sources, for example, the mass media, also have an influence on attitude formation. The purpose of this entry is to examine this field, broadly regarded as attitudes and values, the methods used to measure such attitudes and values, and the quality of measurement these methods produce, as well as the practical problems involved in attitude measurement. It also considers the current status of attitude measurement and speculates on the future of attitude measurement in educational and psychological research. In addition, while the discussion in this entry refers primarily to attitudes, the boundary between attitudes and values is indistinct and the discussion applies equally well to the measurement of values.

1. Definitions of Attitude

Attitudes, relevant to education, are a subdomain of a wider field of attitudes toward a very broad range of objects that are investigated in the discipline of Social Psychology.

The term "attitude" has been defined in many different ways over the years. Fisher (1977) stated that the concept of attitude has had more definitions than any other concept in social psychology. Fishbein and Ajzen (1975) asserted that the term is "characterized by an embarrassing degree of ambiguity and confusion" (p. 1). As early as 1935, at least 16 definitions of attitude existed (Allport 1935). Despite the myriad of definitions, they share a set of common features.

Krathwohl et al. (1964) sought to order this field for the purposes of instruction and assessment by developing a taxonomy of educational objectives for what they termed the "affective domain". The basis of their classification is "internalization," which refers to the inner growth that takes place through "Acceptance by the individual of the attitudes, codes, principles, or sanctions that become part of himself in forming value judgments or in determining his conduct" (quoted by Krathwohl et al. 1964 from Good 1959 p. 296). While this approach to the ordering of this complex field has not gained widespread acceptance among psychologists, it would appear to be of considerable relevance and utility for educational practice.

In reviewing these definitions, Anderson (1981) identified five common features of attitudes: emotion, target, direction, intensity, and consistency.

1.1 The Emotional Component of Attitude

All who have attempted to define attitude agree that the concept involves feelings. This statement is not to suggest that attitudes only involve feelings. Attitudes may include cognitive and behavioral components as well (Cook and Selltiz 1964, Bagozzi and Burnkrant 1979). However, it is evident that attitude is an affective characteristic, and that emotions are involved. The feelings can be positive, negative, or somewhere in between. Thus, many attitudes exist along a continuum which ranges from negative to positive and passes through a point at which people simply do not care or do not know how they feel.

1.2 The Target of Attitudes

Despite the belief among some teachers that a particular student simply has a "bad attitude", attitudes are not general feelings. Rather, these feelings are directed toward or away from some target, that may often be an abstract idea. The most common targets in educational research and evaluation involve objectives that are associated with the school and specific curricula or subject areas within the school (e.g., reading, mathematics) (Anderson et al. 1989, Mortimore et al. 1988).

1.3 Direction of Attitudes

As implied in the two previous sections, attitudes are feelings which are directed toward or away from some target. When attitudes are favorably directed toward the target, they are said to be positive. Likewise, when they are directed unfavorably toward the target, they are said to be negative. It is not surprising, then, that the measurement of attitudes typically begins with the identification and specification of opposite (or bipolar) statements and adjectives, which involve the ideas of favorable or unfavorable, like or dislike, satisfied or dissatisfied.

1.4 Intensity of Attitudes

Not only do the emotional components of attitudes differ in their direction, but they also differ in their intensity. Some people experience and express more intense feelings than do others. Similarly, some feelings are more intense than others. For example, hate is more intense than dislike. Conversely, ecstasy is more intense than pleasure. Practically speaking, students who cannot wait until they get to school are different in terms of the intensity of their attitudes from those who enjoy school once there.

1.5 Consistency of Attitudes

The consistency of an attitude relates to the strength of an individual's feelings toward a particular object in different settings or situations. It differs both from the stability of attitudes over time, and the interrelatedness of kindred attitudes, which may involve a more deeply internalized world view.

Consistency differentiates attitudes generally held by an individual from the individual's emotional reactions to particular settings or situations. There is a difference between a student who likes school and one who likes school sometimes or who likes certain aspects of school. Separating the attitudes of an individual from that individual's reaction to a particular situation is not an easy problem to solve. Nonetheless, virtually all who have attempted to define attitude suggest that consistency is an important feature (Allport 1935, Fishbein and Ajzen 1975).

The third and fourth characteristics listed above permit the visual representation of an attitudinal response toward a particular object by an individual along a number line using a subjective self-rating from a totally unfavorable response (scaled as −1) to a totally favorable response (scaled as +1) and with a neutral response indicated by zero. It is instructive to note that the semantic differential method of measuring attitudes (Osgood et al. 1957) employs this visual representation of the attitude continuum, although commonly on a number line from 1 to 9, which conceals the bipolar nature of a response.

2. Attitudes and Attitude Change

Tesser and Shaffer (1990) have reviewed developments in the theoretical issues associated with the investigation of attitudes and attitude change. McGuire (1986) contended that the study of attitudes has "held hegemony" in the field of social psychology during three periods, namely the 1920s and 1930s, the 1950s and 1960s, and the 1980s and 1990s. During all three periods there has been concern for both issues of measurement and of attitude change. However, according to McGuire (1986), in the most recent period there is an additional concern for attitude structure. The same would also appear to be true in educational research. At the time of writing, research into attitude measurement would appear to be thriving and Oppenheim (1992) is testimony to this research activity as are the reports of the Second IEA Science Study (Postlethwaite and Wiley 1992, Keeves 1992).

Tesser and Shaffer (1990) strongly challenge the traditional definitions of attitudes in terms of affect, cognition, and behavior and advance the view that attitudes should be considered as if they were structures in memory, which is consistent with recent research in cognitive science and into brain functioning. Furthermore, Tesser and Shaffer (1990 p. 481) argue that "attitudes are evaluations based on beliefs, feelings and/or past behavior," and quoting Zarma and Rempel (1988) they distinguish between evaluation and affect. These arguments are based on the view that attitudes involve networks in memory that are retrieved as required. Such networks have characteristics of integrative complexity of structure and attitude extremity. These perspectives would appear consistent with the ordering dimension advanced by Krathwohl et al. (1964) of internalization. Moreover, they would seem

to support the existence of a reciprocal relationship between attitudes and behavior, by which attitudes influence behavior and behavior influences attitudes. Thus Tesser and Shaffer (1990 p. 497) argue that "the primary purpose of holding an attitude is object appraisal, i.e., making evaluative judgments about an attitude object that will have clear behavioral implications." Consequently, attitudes are seen to be dynamic in nature and under constant change as they interact with behavior and must be viewed in probabilistic rather than deterministic terms because of the complexity of structure of an attitudinal network. These distinctions between evaluation and affect and between direction and intensity have important consequences for the measurement of attitudes which has customarily involved self-report or the observation of behavior.

Attitudes cannot be observed directly; rather they have in the past been inferred from what a person *says* or *does*. Thus, attitude measurement has traditionally relied on either responses made to a set of statements or a series of adjectives or behaviors exhibited in a specific situation or a variety of situations. However, the relationship between self-report and behavioral measures of attitudes has generally been weak (Fishbein and Ajzen 1975). Kiesler et al. (1969) provide a critical analysis of theoretical approaches to attitude change and examine the factors affecting the relationship between attitudes and behavior.

3. Self-report Measures

A self-report measure consists of a series of sentences or adjectives (hereafter termed "items") to which those persons whose attitude is being measured are expected to respond. To measure attitude, these items must be: (a) related to the target of the attitude; (b) located somewhere on or along the attitudinal continuum; and (c) capable of being understood as intended by those who are expected to respond to the items.

In an attempt to construct self-report measures which meet these three criteria, four types of scaling techniques have been widely employed. Three of these techniques are named after the individuals who developed them—Thurstone (1928), Likert (1932), and Guttman (1950). The fourth, developed by Osgood et al. (1957), is referred to as the "semantic differential" technique.

The first three scaling techniques rely on sentences, while the fourth relies on adjectives to measure the strength and direction of the attitude. In addition, however, they differ in two other important respects: (a) the position of the items on the attitudinal continuum, and (b) the nature of the response required to indicate position along the continuum (see *Thurstone Scales*).

3.1 Position of Items Along the Attitudinal Continuum

The Thurstone and Guttman techniques require that the items be hierarchically ordered *along* the attitudinal continuum. That is, there should be some very negative items, some fairly negative items, some neutral items, some fairly positive items, and some very positive items. In contrast, the semantic differential technique requires that the items which involve two contrasting adjectives are placed at the two *ends* of the attitudinal continuum. Those responding to the items in fact are asked to place themselves along a number line by indicating their intensity of response. In a similar but not identical way, the Likert technique employs a range of items or statements, to which subjects are required to respond. These persons are also asked to respond with different degrees of affect along a continuum ranging from very unfavorable to very favorable or very negative to very positive.

3.2 The Nature of a Response

The Thurstone technique requires respondents by agreeing or disagreeing with statements to reveal their location along the attitudinal continuum. Their agreeing responses will tend to cluster around a particular position on the scale which is used to indicate their level of attitude. Thus their responses are noncumulative but focused. The Guttman technique requires respondents by agreeing or disagreeing with statements which are hierarchically ordered to identify a turning point above which they will agree with all statements and below which they will disagree with all statements. Thus their responses are cumulative and the turning point determines level of attitude. The Likert and semantic differential scale responses are both additive, in so far as the statements or adjectives represent a judgment sampling from a domain of stimuli, and the position of a response to a particular statement on the response scale provides a score that can be combined with the scores obtained in response to other statements to indicate level of attitude. Thus while the Thurstone and Guttman techniques require the "attitudinal statements" to be located at hierarchically ordered positions along the attitude continuum, neither the Likert nor the semantic differential techniques require this. However, the Likert and semantic differential techniques require the "responses" to be hierarchically ordered along an attitude continuum, which, like the continuum for the Thurstone and Guttman scales, must be bipolar.

3.3 The Construction of Attitudinal Items

Once the attitudinal object and the type of attitude scale has been determined, the next step is to develop an item pool, or collection of attitude statements from which a scale can be constructed. One way of preparing attitude statements, that will be meaningful and interesting to respondents, is to discuss attitudes toward the chosen object with individuals who are representative of the group to whom the scale will be administered and to record their comments as a basis for the writing of statements. Another procedure is

to ask a sample of respondents to complete a set of open-ended statements which relate to the attitudinal object. The responses to both approaches will include statements that, after careful editing, can be used as items in the pool. The statements should be submitted to field trials and refinement until an effective set of statements is obtained. The nature of the statistical procedures used in refinement are considered below and depend on the type of scaling procedure employed.

Self-report measures require, at a minimum, that those responding should find the items included in a scale meaningful and interesting. Edwards (1957) developed a set of 14 "informal criteria" for writing statements for inclusion on attitude scales. Furthermore, Thorndike (1982 p.50) has identified five suggestions for writing clear and unambiguous items. They are listed below.

(a) Ensure that each item involves feeling and affect and not belief or a statement of fact.

(b) Keep the language of the statements simple, clear, and direct.

(c) Each statement should contain only one complete thought.

(d) Avoid the use of statements that involve double negatives.

(e) Avoid the use of words that are vague modifiers or words that may not be understood by those who are asked to respond to the scale.

Recommendation (e) also pertains to the selection of adjectives for inclusion on semantic differential scales.

Shaw and Wright (1967) have provided a valuable collection of scales, and Anderson (1981) has identified a list of adjectives that are familiar to students in the elementary school grades for use in semantic differential scales. Oppenheim (1992 p.187–88) provides further excellent advice on designing attitude statements.

However, it should be recognized from the outset that as in any writing task much depends on the skill in the use of words and the expression of ideas of the person responsible for writing the attitudinal items.

3.4 Measurement Principles Employed in Attitude Scale Construction

A linear scaling model is the simplest available for attitude scale construction and implies the use of the number line proposed above. This model has the following requirements (Oppenheim 1992):

(a) *Homogeneity* or *unidimensionality* implies that the scale measures only one thing and that the items are internally cohesive.

(b) *Reliability* implies internal consistency which unfortunately is partly dependent upon the variability in the sample employed to estimate this characteristic.

(c) *Validity* implies the degree to which the scale measures what it purports to measure.

(d) *Linearity* implies that the intervals along the scale are equal or proportional.

(e) *Reproducibility* implies the extent to which hierarchically ordered items are involved in the scale, although this requirement is not essential for all types of scales.

4. Testing the Properties of Attitude Scales

These requirements of the linear scaling model are generally examined through the use of analytical procedures that test the properties of the scale by means of evidence that is based on relationships between the items in the scale or the internal characteristics of the scale, rather than being related to external criteria. Several different analytical procedures are now widely used and each warrants some consideration.

4.1 Item Analysis Procedures

If a unidimensional set of items has been identified and a decision has been made to combine items together with unit or equal weights, item analysis procedures such as those provided in SPSS (Norusis 1990) are available not only to identify items that do not conform to the requirements of unidimensionality, but also to calculate an index of reliability, Cronbach α (Cronbach 1951), for the attitude scale so formed.

$$\text{Coefficient } \alpha = \frac{n}{n-1}\left(1 - \frac{\sum_{i=1}^{n} s_i^2}{s_x^2}\right)$$

where n is the number of items, s_i^2 is the variance of item i, and s_x^2 is the variance of test x (see *Reliability in Educational and Psychological Measurement*).

4.2 Exploratory Factor Analytic Procedures

The simplest factor analytic procedure that is used to examine the properties and dimensionality of a set of attitude scale items is principal components analysis (see *Factor Analysis*). If the items are strongly homogeneous there will be only one principal component with an *eigen* value greater than unity. Even where this occurs there may be items that do not cohere with the remaining items in a scale, and generally items with a factor loading of less than 0.3 (i.e., items which do not correlate with the underlying latent dimension formed by the scale to the degree of 0.30 or have, in general terms, less than 10 percent of their variance in common with the latent dimension) are rejected. The reliability

of such a scale is given by the Kaiser and Caffrey (1965) formula

$$r_{tt} = \frac{n}{n-1}\left(\frac{\lambda - 1}{\lambda}\right)$$

where
r_{tt} = scale reliability
n = number of items
λ = the first *eigen* value from the principal components analysis.
Where a principal components analysis indicates only one factor, an optimally reliable scale with reliability given by r_{tt} can be constructed by weighting the items according to their factor weights. Otherwise unit or equal weights with consequent robustness are commonly employed.

Where a principal components analysis indicates more than one factor with an *eigen* value significantly greater than unity, the evidence indicates that there is more than one dimension being measured by the set of attitudinal statements. Oppenheim (1992) describes the use of varimax rotation procedures to identify the items associated with two or more orthogonal scales. However, where once it was considered essential that such attitude scales should be orthogonal to avoid the problems of multicollinearity in subsequent explanatory analyses, analytical techniques of latent variable construction (see *Latent Trait Measurement Models; Path Analysis and Linear Structural Relations Analysis*) do not demand that attitude scales be orthogonal. Carroll (1983) provides a detailed account of how oblique rotation procedures can be employed to form two or more unidimensional sets of items.

4.3 Confirmatory Factory Analysis Procedures

If a set of items is hypothesized to form a unidimensional scale then a rigorous test may be applied to confirm that such a scale exists. The unidimensionality of each scale with a multiscale instrument can be assessed using a congeneric test model approach (Jöreskog 1971). Each subscale is fitted to a one factor LISREL model (Jöreskog and Sörbom 1989). Heise and Bohrnstedt (1970) have provided a procedure for estimating the validity of a unidimensional scale from a confirmatory factor analysis. This index of validity is defined as the correlation between the measures and the true underlying variable. It does not indicate that the items measure what they were intended to measure, but that whatever the items are measuring, the index estimates the degree to which the composite that is constructed is correlated to the measures employed (see *Factor Analysis*).

4.4 Scalogram Analysis Procedures

The major issues addressed by scalogram analysis are those of the unidimensionality and reproducibility involved in the construction of a Guttman scale. The items in a Guttman (1944) scale must have the properties of being both ordinal and, as previously explained, cumulative. The confirmation that a scale is a Guttman scale is made on the basis of two coefficients: the "coefficient of reproducibility" and the "coefficient of scalability." The items on the scale postulated to be a Guttman scale are administered to a sizable sample, and the responses submitted to a Guttman scalogram analysis typically carried out by a standard computer program or by hand. The procedures in scalogram analysis assess whether and the degree to which the items and the responses to those items by the members of a sample deviate from an ideal scale response pattern.

Consider, for example, a scale in which five statements are ordered from negative to positive. If an "agree" response is indicated by "1" and a disagree response by "0", then a response pattern indicated by 11100 is consistent, since the three least positive statements are endorsed and the two most positive statements are not endorsed. However, a response pattern for the same five items of 11010 is clearly not consistent, with responses three and four being inappropriate. If an error is recorded every time a 1 appears to the right of a 0, then one error is seen in this simple example. The coefficient of reproducibility R is given by

$$R = 1 - \frac{\text{no of errors}}{\text{no of responses}}$$

If the coefficient of reproducibility for a scale is below 0.9 then that scale is considered to be unsatisfactory as a Guttman scale. However, this is not a sufficient condition for a Guttman scale, since it is also necessary to know the coefficient of scalability, which is the minimum marginal reproducibility index that could occur by chance given the number of respondents obtaining various total scores and the number of respondents endorsing each statement. Several computations are required to calculate this coefficient of scalability which indicates the extent to which the coefficient of reproducibility exceeds that which could be expected by chance. Guttman proposed that this coefficient should exceed 0.60 (Guttman 1950). Scalogram analysis can yield useful measures of attitudes, but such scales are difficult to construct unless they are relatively short. It must be recognized that Guttman scales are essentially deterministic in nature and failure to conform to the rigid structure of a Guttman scale is considered to involve error rather than reflecting the probabilistic nature of an attitudinally based response (see *Partial Order Scalogram Analyses of Nonmetric Data*).

4.5 Rasch Scaling Procedures

Thurstone (1959) recognized that maximum probability measurement formed an alternative mode of scaling to that type of scale that currently bears his name,

which he referred to as "increasing probability measurement." Moreover, such an alternative differs from the deterministic Guttman-type scale. Rasch scaling procedures permit statements and levels of responses to those statements as in a Likert-type scale to be placed along an attitude continuum, provided the statements and response categories associated with the statements fit the requirement of equal discrimination.

Two approaches are available for the Rasch scaling of polychotomous response categories to attitudinal statements. First, there is a "rating scale" model, as advanced by Andrich (1978), that assumes equal intervals across all statements for the distances along the scale between corresponding response categories (see *Rating Scale Analysis*). Second, there is the "partial credit" model, as proposed by Masters (1982), that permits the intervals to vary both for each response category and for each statement (see *Partial Credit Model*). Experience is being gained with these two models in the scoring of essay type questions and constructed response questions in achievement tests, but very little work has been undertaken in the construction and analysis of attitude scales. However, some important developmental work has been done by Andrich (1989) and Wilson (1991).

The potential advantages of the use of Rasch scaling procedures are both the testing for unidimensionality and the construction of an interval scale with both items and response categories as well as persons located on the same scale (see *Measurement in Educational Research*). The location of a person on the scale is determined as that scale value for which the person might be expected to respond to statements at that level with a 50 percent probability of providing a favorable or positive response. Furthermore, the location of an item on a scale is determined as that scale value for which a person located at that level might be expected, with a 50 percent probability, to provide a favorable or positive response to that item.

The advantages of an interval scale and of conjoint measurement, namely persons and items being located jointly on the scale, are substantial for measuring change over time. Likewise, the accurate equating of scales associated with parallel instruments (or sets of items) and of different groups of people are required for the analysis of attitude change, where several measurements at specified points of time are involved, and this can be readily done with Rasch scaled instruments.

4.6 Smallest Space Analysis

Alternative procedures to factor analysis that indicate the relationship between attitudinal statements and attitude scales in a one-, two-, or multidimensional space are provided by smallest space analysis. Smallest space analysis includes a range of techniques for representing geometrically pairwise similarities within a set of correlation coefficients (or other paired comparison measures) computed between observed variables. Smallest space analysis is also referred to as a multidimensional scaling technique, in which scaling is carried out with respect to more than one derived variable and hence is multidimensional. The analysis provides a solution of smallest dimensionality to the problem of the geometrical representation of the data (Guttman 1968). These procedures are of particular utility in examining a set of attitudinal statements that are known not to be unidimensional in an alternative way to that provided by factor analysis (see *Smallest Space Analysis; Scaling Methods*).

5. Behavioral Measures

Behaviors can be observed in two settings: natural and contrived. Natural settings are those in which people typically find themselves and are unaware that they are being observed. In contrast, contrived settings are those which are unfamiliar and/or those in which people are aware they are being observed.

Both settings have problems associated with them. While natural settings may have greater face validity, the behavior being investigated may occur very infrequently, thus making data collection time-consuming and costly. Unfortunately, while contrived situations may be less time-consuming and costly, the external validity (that is, the generalizability of the data across persons, settings, and times) may be suspect.

Regardless of the setting or occasion, it is important that multiple observations of the behavior(s) be made. The reliability of ratings made on the basis of one behavioral observation is no stronger than the reliability of inferences which are based on one item (see *Rating Scales*).

Sechrest (1969) contends that inferences about attitudes should be made on observations and ratings of people's behavior. Sechrest's advocacy of this position arises from concerns for the validity of attitude scales. However, consideration must be given to the extent to which attitudes can be inferred from overt behavior. Wicker (1969) summarized his review of relevant studies as follows:

> Taken as a whole, these studies suggest that it is considerably more likely that attitudes will be unrelated or only slightly related to overt behaviors than that attitudes will be closely related to actions. Product-moment correlation coefficients relating the two kinds of responses are rarely above .30 and often are near zero. Only rarely can as much as 10% of the variance of overt behavioral measures be accounted for by attitudinal data. (p. 65)

Much of the lack of relationship can probably be attributed to the use of a single behavioral indicator in the research. The reliability of behavioral measures could be increased by combining multiple indicators of behavior and by multiple observations. Some such attempts have been made in the measurement of self-esteem of students (Coopersmith 1967) using a checklist of behaviors believed to be related to the self-esteem of students.

6. Physiological Response Measures

Many of Sechrest's (1969) concerns could also be alleviated if an appropriate physiological measure of attitude could be found. To date a number of such measures have been proposed: the galvanic skin response (GSR), pupillary dilation and constriction, respiration rate, and heart rate are among them. While such measures do detect arousal or intensity, the information they provide is not specific enough for the measurement of an identified attitude. In particular, the evaluation dimension of the attitude concerned with the direction and target of the arousal remains unknown and possibly unknowable. As Fishbein and Ajzen (1975) conclude in their discussion of physiological measures: "it would definitely be desirable to have a non-verbal measure of attitude not under the subject's control, but it appears unlikely that any known physiological reaction will serve this purpose (Fishbein and Ajzen 1975 p. 94).

7. Projective Techniques

The effectiveness of attitude scales depends on both the frankness and the cooperation of the person responding. Projective techniques may be used to investigate attitudinal responses in order to overcome some of the barriers that prevent respondents from providing valid responses. Oppenheim (1992 p.211–12) lists such barriers.

(a) *Awareness.* Respondents are frequently unaware of their own attitudes and motives.

(b) *Irrationality.* Respondents tend to rationalize their attitudes and beliefs because society places a premium on rational and logical behavior.

(c) *Inadmissibility.* Since society sets norms and expectations, respondents are commonly reluctant to admit to holding negative or unfavorable attitudes.

(d) *Self-incrimination.* Respondents are reluctant to indicate a lower self-esteem or negative attitudes in order to maintain a high self-image.

(e) *Politeness.* Respondents prefer not to say negative, unpleasant, or critical things, unless they have specific complaints.

Oppenheim (1992 p.212) also identifies four commonly used approaches to the use of projective techniques.

(a) *Association*. Respondents are required to employ an approach which involves saying the first thing that comes to mind in anticipation that this will reveal an underlying or latent attitude or motive.

(b) *Fantasy*. Respondents are required to tell a story, to discuss a picture in imaginary terms or to guess, on the assumption that their attitudes rather than knowledge will be employed and such attitudes may be inferred from their responses.

(c) *Ambiguous stimuli*. Where the stimulus is indefinite or ambiguous, the respondent is required to project and interpret by employing latent attitudes.

(d) *Conceptualization*. Respondents' attitudes can be probed by requiring them to name, order, or group things.

All four approaches have much in common in so far as they all rely on spontaneity or interpretation, provided the respondent does not know the purpose lying behind the task or question. Thus, in the use of projective techniques the investigator should be as nondirective as possible. However, as with the inference of attitudes from behavior, issues of unreliability arise from the use of a single indicator or from a single interview session. As a consequence multiple indicators or several interview sessions should be used. While depth of understanding is achieved and the direction of a response is readily assessed, the target of the aroused response remains nonspecific (see *Projective Testing Techniques*).

8. Technical Quality of Attitude Measurement

Once attitude measures have been developed and administered, the technical quality of the resulting data must be examined. The predominant aspects of the technical quality of these measures are: (a) reliability, (b) validity, (c) distribution of scores.

8.1 Reliability of Attitude Measures

Reliability refers to the extent to which the responses or behaviors made by individuals are consistent across items, settings, raters and/or time. Consistency across items or settings is referred to as "internal consistency," while consistency across time is commonly labeled "stability," and across raters is called "interrater reliability."

Both the Thurstone and Guttman scales have estimates of internal consistency built into the techniques used to develop them. For Thurstone scales, internal consistency is estimated for each respondent by a mean error statistic which considers the range of scale values associated with the statements endorsed by the respondent or respondents. The smaller the range, the more consistent the responses. For Guttman scales, the estimate of internal consistency is based on the coefficients of reproducibility and scalability. For Likert and semantic differential scales, the traditional internal consistency estimate is the reliability coefficient α (Cronbach 1951). Rasch scaling methods have tended to employ inappropriately the alpha reliability coefficient, but a mean square error statistic would seem a more appropriate index of internal consistency (Andrich 1978, Masters 1982).

In general, the more items or settings used in making the measurement, the greater the internal consistency reliability. With respect to the Likert and semantic differential and ratings measures, a second factor, the number of response options employed, also influences the internal consistency reliability. In general, the more response options that are provided, the higher the reliability. An important caveat must be placed on this latter generalization, however. Osgood (1941) reported that in a 7-point scale, some respondents used only the extremes 1 and 7; others used categories 1, 4, and 7, while others used the whole scale. Thus the inclusion of more than three or five response options may require gradations of discrimination beyond those that some respondents are capable of making. When this is the case, the reliability may not be increased (Masters 1974). With respect to response options, the issue of whether the inclusion of a neutral option (e.g., "not sure," "I don't know") impacts on the validity of the attitude measurement has also been debated. Moreover, it must be recognized that the "uncertain" category covers both a "neutral" position and an "undecided" position, where the student does not wish to assess level of affect. Thus, some argue that the use of a neutral response option enables respondents to disguise their true attitudes. Others contend that removal of the neutral category increases the proportion of omitted responses. Obviously, if these options are used in such ways, validity suffers.

Cronbach (1942, 1946, 1950) provides evidence concerned with these and related issues. Moreover, the location of the "neutral" category following the "agree" and "disagree" categories rather than between them decreases the proportion of neutral responses and increases the proportion of "disagree" responses and as a consequence generally increases the reliability of a scale.

Stability estimates require that some period of time should elapse between the occasions on which responses are solicited or behaviors are observed. Reliability coefficients obtained by analysis of variance are used to examine the extent of the relationship between the assessments of attitude made both by two or more raters and at two or more points in time (see *Reliability in Educational and Psychological Measurement*).

Where estimates of an index of reliability fall below 0.70, and over 50 percent of the variance of individual scores on attitude measures must be attributable to error, it is generally considered inappropriate to undertake further analyses of the data. However, sometimes in combination with other related measures in latent variable models, meaningful analyses can be undertaken with scales of lower reliability.

8.2 External Validity of Attitude Measures

Adams (1982) suggests there are three basic types of validity that pertain to attitude measurement: content, predictive, and construct. "Content validity" applies only when attitudes are an intended outcome of the process of schooling. "Predictive validity" applies only when attitudes are being used to predict other characteristics or behaviors of students or teachers. However, the crux of the validity of an attitude scale is its "construct validity."

Attitudes are hypothetical constructs developed by social psychologists or educators (hence the term "construct validity"). Their existence is inferred from what people say or do. The estimation of construct validity of an attitude measure requires an understanding on the part of the instrument developer or researcher of: (a) the definitions of the attitude and the target; (b) the way in which the attitude fits into some larger conceptual framework; and (c) a set of hypotheses based on the relationship between the attitude and the other constructs within the conceptual framework.

Consider, for example, the attitude toward science of secondary school students. First, attitudes toward science must be defined. Second, attitudes toward science must be placed within a larger conceptual framework. (For an account of such developmental work in a major research study, see Keeves 1992).Constructs within that framework may include occupation(s) of parent(s) (e.g., science vs. nonscience), aptitude for science, selection of science courses, hobbies, and science achievement. Third, hypotheses relating constructs within that framework must be stated and tested. It may be hypothesized that the attitudes toward science of students whose parents were scientists would be more positive than the attitudes of students whose parents were artists. Similarly, it may be hypothesized that the attitudes toward science of students who engaged in scientific hobbies would be more positive than the attitudes of students who did not engage in such hobbies. In general, the more the hypotheses are supported by the data, the more valid the measure of attitude.

8.3 The Distribution of Scores

With increasing interest in multivariate analysis it is important that attitudinal measures should be associated with underlying normal distributions of scores, and that the scores included in analysis should conform to a normal distribution. In cases where such distributions do not pertain, with indexes of skewness and kurtosis in excess of ± 2.0, then it is generally considered inappropriate to employ maximum likelihood analytical procedures, such as are available in LISREL (Jöreskog and Sörbom 1989). Moreover, the commonly employed significance tests are likely to be invalid. Carefully constructed Likert and semantic differential scales generally provide highly satisfactory measures in this regard. In certain cases where the distribution of scores is non-normal, the data may be transformed using the logarithmic or arcsin transformations (Snedecor and Cochran 1967). Alternatively, where the data show a high degree of skewness, the values may be normalized, as the procedure is commonly referred to, or more accurately, transformed using the probit transformation (Fisher and Yates 1963). However, such transformations of data should not be undertaken without sound theoretical grounds for doing so, and without expert statistical guidance.

The advantages of employing interval scaled attitudinal data from the use of Rasch scaling procedures have yet to be fully explored.

9. Practical Problems in Attitude Measurement

As might be expected, there are several response problems inherent in attitude measurement. Among the most prevalent are "social desirability," "acquiescence," "multidimensionality," and the "treatment of non-responses." All influence the reliability and validity of attitude measurement. Cronbach (1942, 1946, 1950) has carried out a series of seminal studies into these and other related issues.

9.1 Social Desirability

As the term implies, "social desirability" refers to the subjects responding according to the way in which they think the investigator or society expects them to respond, rather than the way they feel. With respect to behavioral measures, natural settings are less likely to evoke social desirability than are contrived settings. With respect to self-report measures, making the purpose of the investigation or the nature of a correct response less obvious (so-called "disguised" instruments) will also reduce social desirability. Procedures for estimating social desirability are available (Lunnenborg and Lunnenborg 1964).

9.2 Acquiescence

Acquiescence refers to the tendency for respondents to agree with whatever statement is made (Cronbach 1970). This tendency is particularly evident in young children (Sabers et al. 1974). The effect of response sets on actual responses can be minimized in several ways. In preparing self-report measures an equal number of positive and negative statements can be written. In addition, these statements can be randomly placed on the instrument. Furthermore, relatively short self-report measures decrease the likelihood that a response set will be formed.

9.3 The Treatment of Nonresponses

A major problem involved in attitude measurement occurs when the person being measured chooses not to respond to one or more items. In cognitive measurement, a nonresponse is commonly counted as incorrect. The total score, then, is based on the number of correct responses: a total which may be corrected for the number of items omitted (see *Multiple Choice Tests, Guessing in*).

In attitude measurement, such a possibility does not generally exist because it is not possible to infer absence of knowledge from an omission. On a five-point Likert scale, for example, a nonresponse would contribute nothing to the total score. In contrast, a strongly disagreed response to a positively worded item typically counts for one point or the lowest coded score which is assigned.

In general, there are two approaches to dealing with nonresponses. First, the mean score of the person on the remaining items can be substituted for the nonresponses. This substitution permits the computation of a total score for the entire attitude scale, and is equivalent to merely using the mean response on the remaining items as the person's score. However, this assumes that the omitted item is equivalent to the remaining items for which responses were obtained. This may or may not be so. Second, if a respondent omits only one item, or perhaps less than 20 percent of the items in a scale, then an omission would seem to indicate uncertainty in responding and it can be argued that assigning a neutral response is appropriately used in compensating for the missing data. When a respondent fails to provide responses to at least 80 percent of the items, then it would seem most appropriate to exclude that respondent from consideration and to employ missing data correlations to estimate relationships on the assumption that the respondent for whom data are missing is typical of the remainder of the group who did respond. However, this assumption may be false.

10. The Present and Future of Attitude Measurement in Education

Attitude measurement has become a common part of research into schools and schooling throughout the world. In a study of classrooms in eight countries, Anderson et al. (1989) used measures of attitudes toward school and specific subject matter. Likewise, in a study of 2,000 primary school children in the United Kingdom, Mortimore et al. (1988) measured student attitudes as well as these students' perceptions, which were assumed to have an affective component, of how they were seen by their teachers, their peers, and themselves. Similarly, Tomic and Van der Sijde (1989) in their study of 50 mathematics classrooms over an 8-month period included measures of students' attitudes toward mathematics and their self-image. Finally, Weinert and Schneider (1992) in their Munich Longitudinal Study on the Genesis of Individual Competencies used attitude measures to estimate self-concept of ability and attitudes toward achievement and learning.

From these and other studies several generalizations concerning attitude can be offered. First, students tend to have positive attitudes toward school and the subject matter taught in school at all grade levels. Second, the attitudes of students toward school and school subjects tend to become less favorable over their years at school. Third, students tend to like certain subjects (e.g., science, sports, reading) more than others (mathematics, writing). Fourth, the relationship between attitudes and achievement is generally moderate and positive provided the sample is not contaminated by selection bias (see *Selection Bias in Educational Research*). Fifth, attitudes tend to be influenced by appropriate changes in school programs.

In the light of what is currently known about attitudes, certain recommendations can be offered for the future. First, the measurement of attitudes should become more common in schools, particularly since they influence future participation in schooling and subject choice. It is important to monitor the impact of education on student attitudes, whether this impact is intended or unintended. Second, multiple methods should be used to assess attitudes. However, every known method of attitude measurement is associated with problems and errors. Multiple methods, therefore, are likely to produce a greater understanding of the nature of attitudes and attitude development. Third, advances in measurement are occurring and improved measurement procedures should be employed. However, construct validity needs to be established if attitude measurement is to move forward. The establishment of construct validity requires that defensible conceptual and theoretical frameworks be developed and accepted by those in the field. Moreover, it requires that the strength of the attitude measures which are constructed should be supported by moderate and strong relationships as hypothesized in conceptual and theoretical models.

See also: Measurement in Educatonal Research

References

Adams G S 1982 Attitude measurement. In: Mitzel H E (ed.) *Encyclopedia of Educational Research*, 5th edn. Free Press, New York
Allport G W 1935 Attitudes. In: Murchison C A (ed.) *Handbook of Social Psychology*. Russell and Russell, New York
Anderson L W 1981 *Assessing Affective Characteristics in the Schools*. Allyn and Bacon, Boston, Massachusetts
Anderson L W, Ryan D W, Shapiro B J 1989 (eds.) *The IEA Classroom Environment Study*. Pergamon Press, Oxford
Andrich D 1978 Scaling attitude items constructed and scored in the Likert tradition. *Educ. Psych. Meas.* 38(3): 665–80

Andrich D 1989 Constructing fundamental measurements in social psychology. In: Keats J A, Taft R, Heath R B, Lovibond S H (eds.) *Mathematical and Theoretical Systems*. Elsevier, North Holland

Bagozzi R P, Burnkrant R E 1979 Attitude organization and the attitude–behavior relationship. *J. Pers. Soc. Psych.* 37(6): 913–29

Carroll J B 1983 Studying individual differences in cognitive abilities: Through and beyond factor analysis. In: Dillon R F, Schmeck R R (eds.) *Individual Differences in Cognition*, Vol. 1. Academic Press, New York

Cook S W, Selltiz C A 1964 A multiple-indicator approach to attitude measurement. *Psych. Bull.* 62(1): 36–55

Coopersmith S 1967 *The Antecedents of Self-Esteem*. Freeman, San Francisco, California

Cronbach L J 1942 Studies of acquiescence as a factor in the true–false test. *J. Educ. Psychol.* 33: 401–15

Cronbach L J 1946 Response sets and test validity. *Educ. Psych. Meas.* 6: 475–94

Cronbach L J 1950 Further evidence on response sets and test design. *Educ. Psych. Meas.* 10: 3–31

Cronbach L J 1951 Coefficient alpha and the internal structure of tests. *Psychometrika* 16: 297–334

Cronbach L J 1970 *Essentials of Psychological Testing*, 3rd edn. Harper and Row, New York

Edwards A L 1957 *Techniques of Attitude Scale Construction*. Appleton-Century-Crofts, New York

Fishbein M, Ajzen I 1975 *Belief, Attitude, Intention, and Behavior: An Introduction to Theory and Research*. Addison-Wesley, Reading, Massachusetts

Fisher R A, Yates F 1963 *Statistical Tables for Biological, Agricultural and Medical Research*, 6th edn. Oliver and Boyd, Edinburgh

Fisher R J 1977 Toward the more comprehensive measurement of intergroup attitudes: An interview and rating scale procedure. *Canadian J. Behavioral Sciences* 9(4): 283–94

Good C V 1959 *Dictionary of Education*, 2nd edn. McGraw Hill, New York

Guttman L 1944 A basis for scaling qualitative data. *Am. Sociol. Rev.* 9: 139–50

Guttman L 1950 The problem of attitude and opinion measurement. In: Stouffer S A (ed.) *Measurement and Prediction*. Princeton University Press, Princeton, New Jersey

Guttman L 1968 A general nonmetric technique for finding the smallest coordinate space for a configuration of points. *Psychometri.* 33(4): 469–506

Heise D R, Bohrnstedt G W 1970 Validity, invalidity, and reliability. In: Borgatta E F, Bohrnstedt G W (eds.) *Sociological Methodology 1970*. Jossey-Bass, San Francisco, California

Jöreskog K G 1971 Statistical analysis of sets of congeneric tests. *Psychometri.* 36(2): 109–33

Jöreskog K G, Sörbom D 1989 *LISREL 7: A Guide to the Program and Applications*, 2nd edn. SPSS Publications, Chicago, Illinois

Kaiser H F, Caffrey J 1965 Alpha factor analysis. *Psychometrika* 30(1): 1–4

Keeves J P (ed.) 1992 *The IEA Study of Science III. Changes in Science Education and Achievement: 1970–1984*. Pergamon Press, Oxford

Kiesler C A, Collins B E, Miller N 1969 *Attitude Change: A Critical Analysis of Theoretical Approaches*. Wiley, New York

Krathwohl D R, Bloom B S, Masia B B 1964 *Taxonomy of Educational Objectives. The Classification of Educational Goals. Handbook 2: Affective Domain*. Longman, London

Likert R 1932 A technique for the measurement of attitudes. *Archives of Psychology* 140:52

Lunnenborg P W, Lunnenborg C E 1964 The relationship of social desirability to other test-taking attitudes in children. *J. Clin. Psych.* 20(4): 473–77

Masters G N 1982 A Rasch model for partial credit scoring. *Psychometri.* 47(2): 149–74

Masters J R 1974 Relationship between number of response categories and reliability of Likert-type questionnaires. *J. Educ. Meas.* 11(1): 49–53

McGuire W J 1986 The vicissitudes of attitudes and similar representational constraints in twentieth century psychology. *Eur. J. Soc. Psychol.* 16(2): 89–130

Mortimore P, Sammons P, Stoll L 1988 *School Matters*. University of California Press, Berkeley, California

Norusis M J 1990 *SPSS Base System. User's Guide*. SPSS, Chicago, Illinois

Oppenheim A N 1992 *Questionnaire Design, Interviewing and Attitude Measurement*. Pinter, London

Osgood C E 1941 Case of individual judgment processes in relation to polarization of attitudes in the culture. *J. Social Psychol.* 14: 403–18

Osgood C E, Suci G, Tannenbaum P 1957 *The Measurement of Meaning*. University of Illinois Press, Urbana, Illinois

Postlethwaite T N, Wiley D E (eds.) 1992 *The IEA Study of Science II. Science Achievement in Twenty-Three Countries*. Pergamon Press, Oxford

Sabers D, Reschly D, Meredith K 1974 *Age Differences in Degree of Acquiescence on Positively and Negatively Scored Attitude-Scale Items*. Paper presented at the Annual Meeting of the National Council for Measurement in Education, Chicago, April 1974 (ERIC Document Reproduction Service No. ED 091 446)

Sechrest L 1969 Nonreactive assessment of attitudes. In: Willims E P, Rausch H (eds.) *Naturalistic Viewpoints in Psychological Research*. Holt, Rinehart and Winston, New York

Shaw M E, Wright J M 1967 *Scales for the Measurement of Attitudes*. McGraw Hill, New York

Snedecor G W, Cochran W G 1967 *Statistical Methods*, 6th edn. Iowa State University Press, Ames, Iowa

Tesser A, Shaffer D R 1990 Attitudes and attitude change. *Ann. Rev. Psychol.* 41: 479–523

Thorndike R L 1982 *Applied Psychometrics*. Houghton Mifflin, Boston, Massachusetts

Thurstone L L 1928 Attitudes can be measured. *Am. J. Soc.* 33: 529–54

Thurstone L L 1959 *The Measurement of Values*. University of Chicago Press, Chicago, Illinois

Tomic W, Van der Sijde P C 1989 *Changing Teaching for Better Learning*. Swets and Zeitlinger, Amsterdam

Weinert F E, Schneider W (eds.) 1992 *The Munich Longitudinal Study on the Genesis of Individual Competencies (LOGIC)*. Max-Planck-Institute for Psychological Research, Munich

Wicker A W 1969 Attitudes versus actions: The relationship of verbal and overt behavioral responses to attitude objects. *J. Soc. Issues* 25(4): 41–78

Wilson M 1991 Comparing attitude across different countries. In: Wilson M (ed.) *Objective Measurement Theory into Practice*, Vol. 2. Ablex, Norwood, New Jersey

Classroom Environments

B. J. Fraser

The environment, climate, atmosphere, tone, ethos, or ambience of a classroom is believed to exert a powerful influence on student behavior, attitudes, and achievement. Although classroom environment is a somewhat subtle concept, remarkable progress has been made over the last quarter of the twentieth century in its conceptualization and assessment, which has led to an increased understanding of its determinants and effects.

1. An Historical Perspective on the Assessment of Classroom Environments

Murray (1938) introduced the term "alpha press" to describe the environment as assessed by a detached observer and "beta press" to describe the environment as perceived by those who inhabit it. Over the years, both observational instruments and questionnaires have been used to study the classroom environment.

Several structured observation schedules for coding classroom communication and events have been reviewed by Rosenshine and Stevens (1986) and Good and Brophy (1991). One of the most widely-known is Flander's Interaction Analysis System (FIAS) which records classroom behavior at three-second intervals using 10 categories (e.g., praising and encouraging, asking questions, student-initiated talk). Medley and Mitzel constructed an omnibus instrument called OSCAR (Observation Schedule And Record) which includes 14 categories (e.g., pupil leadership activities, manifest teacher hostility, emotional climate, verbal emphasis, and social organization). Other systematic observation schemes are the Emmer Observation System, the Brophy–Good Dyadic Interaction System, and Blumenfeld and Miller's method of coding vocabulary (Good and Brophy 1991).

Since the 1970s, numerous questionnaires have been developed to assess student perceptions of their classroom environments (Fraser 1986, Fraser and Walberg 1991). Advantages claimed for questionnaires are that they can be more economical than classroom observation techniques; they are based on students' experiences over many lessons; they involve the pooled judgments of all students in a class; they can be more important than observed behaviors because they are the determinants of student behavior; and they have been found to account for more variance in student learning outcomes than have directly observed variables.

One of the most widely used questionnaires, the Learning Environment Inventory, was developed as part of the research and evaluation activities of

Harvard Project Physics (Welch and Walberg 1972). About the same time, Moos began developing numerous social climate scales which ultimately resulted in the development of the well-known Classroom Environment Scale (Moos and Trickett 1987). Both of these questionnaires built upon the theoretical, conceptual, and measurement foundations laid by pioneers such as Lewin (1936), Murray (1938), and their followers (e.g., Stern 1970). Furthermore, research using these instruments was influenced by prior studies using structured observation instruments.

A more recent approach to studying educational environments involves the application of techniques of naturalistic inquiry, ethnography, and case study. In the 1990s there is a growing acceptance of a combination of qualitative and quantitative methods (based on observation or student perceptions) in the study of classroom environment (Fraser and Tobin 1991).

2. A Summary of Questionnaires for Assessing Classroom Environments

Table 1 summarizes several questionnaires commonly used to assess student perceptions of classroom learning environment. Each questionnaire is suitable for convenient group administration, can be scored either by hand or computer, and has been shown to be reliable in extensive field trials. All questionnaires include multiple variables or scales. For example, the My Class Inventory contains five scales: cohesiveness, friction, satisfaction, difficulty, and competitiveness. A distinctive feature of most of these instruments is that, in addition to a form that measures perceptions of actual classroom environment, there is another form to measure perceptions of preferred classroom environment. The preferred forms are concerned with goals and value orientations and measure perceptions of the ideal classroom environment.

Table 1 includes the name of each scale contained in each instrument, the school level (elementary, secondary, or higher education) for which each instrument is suited, the number of items contained in each scale, and the classification of each scale according to Moos's (1974) scheme for classifying human environments. Moos's three basic dimensions are: Relationship (which identify the nature and intensity of personal relationships within the environment and assess the extent to which people are involved in the environment and support and help each other); Personal Development (which assess basic directions along which personal growth and self-enhancement tend to occur); and System Maintenance and System Change (which involve the extent to which the environment is

Table 1
Overview of scales contained in seven classroom environment instruments (LEI, CES, ICEQ, MCI, CUCEI, SLEI, and QTI)

Instrument	Level	Items per scale	Scale classified according to Moos's Scheme		
			Relationship dimensions	Personal development dimensions	System maintenance and change dimensions
Learning Environment Inventory (LEI)	secondary	7	cohesiveness friction favoritism cliqueness satisfaction apathy	speed difficulty competitiveness	diversity formality material environment goal direction disorganization democracy
Classroom Environment Scale (CES)	secondary	10	involvement affiliation teacher support	task orientation competition	order and organization rule clarity teacher control innovation
Individualized Classroom Environment Questionnaire (ICEQ)	secondary	10	personalization participation	independence investigation	differentiation
My class Inventory (MCI)	elementary	6–9	cohesiveness friction satisfaction	difficulty competitiveness	
College and University Classroom Environment Inventory (CUCEI)	higher education	7	personalization involvement student cohesiveness satisfaction	task orientation	innovation individualization
Science Laboratory Environment Inventory (SLEI)	upper secondary higher education	7	student cohesiveness	open-endedness integration	rule clarity material environment
Questionnaire on Teacher Interaction (QTI)	secondary elementary	8-10	helpful/friendly understanding dissatisfied admonishing		leadership student responsibility and freedom uncertain strict

orderly, clear in expectations, maintains control, and is responsive to change).

As mentioned above, the development of the Learning Environment Inventory (LEI) began in the late 1960s in conjunction with the evaluation and research on Harvard Project Physics (Fraser et al. 1982). The LEI contains 105 statements (seven per scale) with response alternatives of "Strongly Disagree," "Disagree," "Agree," and "Strongly Agree." The scoring direction (or polarity) is reversed for some items. A typical item contained in the "Cohesiveness" scale is: "All students know each other very well."

The Classroom Environment Scale (CES) grew out of a comprehensive program of research involving perceptual measures of a variety of human environments including psychiatric hospitals, prisons, university residences, and work milieus (Moos 1974). Moos and Trickett's (1987) final version contains nine scales with 10 true–false items in each scale. Published materials include a test manual, a questionnaire, an answer sheet, and a transparent hand scoring key. A typical item in the CES is: "The teacher takes a personal interest in the students" (Teacher Support).

The Individualized Classroom Environment Questionnaire (ICEQ) differs from other classroom environment scales in that it assesses those dimensions which distinguish individualized classrooms from conventional ones. The final published version (Fraser 1990) contains 50 items with an equal number of items belonging to each of the five scales. Each item is responded to on a five-point scale with the alternatives of "Almost Never," "Seldom," "Sometimes," "Often," and "Very Often." A typical item is: "Different students use different books, equipment, and materials" (Differentiation). The published form consists of a handbook and test master sets from which unlimited numbers of copies of the questionnaires and response sheets may be made.

The LEI has been simplified to form the My Class Inventory (MCI) which is suitable for children in the 8–12 years age range (Fraser et al. 1982) and students in the junior high school, especially those who might experience reading difficulties with the LEI. The MCI differs from the LEI in four ways. First, in order to minimize fatigue among younger children, the MCI contains only five of the LEI's original 15 scales. Second, item wording has been simplified to enhance readability. Third, the LEI's four-point response format has been reduced to a two-point (Yes–No) response format. Fourth, students answer on the questionnaire itself instead of on a separate response sheet to avoid errors in transferring responses from one place to another. The final form contains 38 items. A typical item is: "Children are always fighting with each other" (Friction).

The College and University Classroom Environment Inventory (CUCEI) was developed for small classes (but not for lectures or laboratory classes) (Fraser and Treagust 1986) as a result of the fact that little work had been done in higher education classrooms parallel to the traditions of classroom environment research at the secondary and elementary school levels. The final form of the CUCEI contains seven-item scales. Each item has four responses ("Strongly Agree," "Agree," "Disagree," "Strongly Disagree") and polarity is reversed for approximately half the items. A typical item is: "Activities in this class are clearly and carefully planned" (Task Orientation).

An instrument specifically suited to assessing the environment of science laboratory classes at the senior high school or higher education levels was developed (Fraser et al. 1992) as a result of the critical importance and uniqueness of laboratory settings in science education. The Science Laboratory Environment Inventory (SLEI) has five scales and the response alternatives for each item are "Almost Never," "Seldom," "Sometimes," "Often," and "Very Often." A typical item includes: "We know the results that we are supposed to get before we commence a laboratory activity" (Open-endedness). A noteworthy feature of the validation procedures employed is that the SLEI was field tested simultaneously in six countries (the US, Canada, England, Israel, Australia, and Nigeria).

In the Netherlands a learning environment questionnaire was developed to enable teacher educators to give preservice and inservice teachers advice about the nature and quality of the interaction between teachers and students (Wubbels and Levy 1994). Drawing upon a theoretical model of proximity (Cooperation–Opposition) and influence (Dominance–Submission), the Questionnaire of Teacher Interaction (QTI) was developed to assess eight scales: Leadership, Helpful/Friendly, Understanding, Student Responsibility and Freedom, Uncertain, Dissatisfied, Admonishing, and Strict Behavior. The QTI has 77 items altogether (approximately 10 per scale), and each item is responded to on a 5-point scale ranging from Never to Always. A typical item is "she or he gets angry" (Admonishing behavior). The validity and reliability of the QTI have been established for secondary school students in the Netherlands, the United States, and Australia (Wubbels and Levy 1994).

3. Classroom Environment Research

The strongest tradition in classroom environment research in several countries has involved investigation of associations between students' cognitive and affective learning outcomes and their perceptions of their classroom environments (Fraser 1993). Numerous studies have shown that student perceptions account for appreciable amounts of variance in learning outcomes often beyond that which can be attributed to student background characteristics. For example, better student achievement on a variety of outcome measures was found consistently in classes perceived as having greater cohesiveness and goal direction, and less disorganization and friction (Haertel et al. 1981)

Classroom environment measures were employed as dependent variables in curriculum evaluation studies, investigations of differences between student and teacher perceptions of classroom environment and studies involving other independent variables (e.g. different subject matters). The significance of curriculum evaluation studies is that classroom environment differed markedly between curricula, even when various achievement outcome measures showed negligible differences. Research involving teachers and students informs educators that teachers are likely to perceive the classroom environment more favorably than their students in the same classrooms. Research studies involving the use of classroom environment as a criterion variable have identified how the classroom environment varies with such factors as teacher personality, class size, grade level, subject matter, the nature of the school-level environment, and the type of school.

4. Practical Uses of Classroom Environment Information

Knowledge of student perceptions can be employed as a basis for reflection upon, discussion of, and systematic attempts to improve classroom environments. For example, Fraser and Fisher's (1986) attempt to improve classroom environments made use of the CES with a class of 22 Grade 9 boys and girls of mixed ability studying science at a government school in Tasmania. The procedure incorporated five fundamental steps.

First, the actual and preferred forms of the CES were administered to all students in the class. Second, the teacher was provided with profiles representing the class means of students' actual and preferred environment scores. Third, the teacher engaged in private reflection and informal discussion about the profiles in order to provide a basis for a decision about whether an attempt would be made to change the environment in terms of some of the CES's dimensions. In fact, the teacher decided to introduce an intervention aimed at increasing the levels of teacher support and order and organization in the classroom. Fourth, the teacher used the intervention for approximately two months. For example, enhancing teacher support involved the teacher moving around the class more to mix with students, providing assistance to students and talking with them more than previously. Fifth, the actual form of the scales was readministered at the end of the intervention to see whether students were perceiving their classroom environment differently from before.

The results showed that some change in student perceptions occurred during the time of the intervention. Pretest–posttest differences were statistically significant only for teacher support, task orientation, and order and organization. These findings are noteworthy because two of the dimensions on which appreciable changes were recorded were those on which the teacher had attempted to promote change. Also, there appears to be a side effect in that the intervention could have resulted in the classroom becoming more task oriented than the students would have preferred. Overall, this case study suggests the potential usefulness of teachers employing classroom environment instruments to provide meaningful information about their classrooms and a tangible basis to guide improvements in classroom environments.

5. Future Research

Assessment involving students' perceptions of classrooms can involve either individual students' perceptions or the intersubjective perceptions of all students in the same class. This distinction in past classroom environment research has often been important when choosing an appropriate unit of statistical analysis (e.g., individual student scores or class mean scores;

see Fraser 1986). The advances in multilevel analysis mean that more sophisticated techniques are available for analyzing the typical data (e.g., with students nested within classes) found in much research on classroom environments.

Although only limited progress has been made toward the desirable goal of combining quantitative and qualitative methods within the same study, the fruitfulness of this objective is illustrated in several studies (Tobin et al. 1990, Fraser and Tobin 1991). For example, in a study of higher-level cognitive learning, six researchers intensively studied the Grade 10 science classes of two teachers over a 10-week period (Tobin et al. 1990). Each lesson was observed by several researchers, interviewing of students and teachers took place on a daily basis, and students' written work was examined. The study also involved quantitative information from questionnaires assessing student perceptions of their classroom environments. An important finding was that students' perceptions of the environment within each classroom were consistent with the observers' field records of the patterns of learning activities and engagements in each classroom. For example, the high level of personalization perceived in one teacher's classroom matched the large proportion of time that she spent in small-group activities during which she constantly moved about the classroom interacting with students.

6. Conclusion

Positive classroom environments are generally assumed to be educationally desirable ends in their own right. Moreover, comprehensive evidence from past research establishes that classroom environments have a potent influence on how well students achieve a range of desired educational outcomes. Consequently, educators need not feel that they must choose between striving to achieve constructive classroom environments and attempting to enhance student achievement of cognitive and affective aims. Rather, constructive educational climates can be viewed both as means to valuable ends and as worthy ends in themselves.

References

Fraser B J 1986 *Classroom Environment*. Croom Helm, London

Fraser B J 1990 *Individualized Classroom Environment Questionnaire*. Australian Council for Educational Research, Melbourne

Fraser B J 1993 Classroom and school climate. In: Gabel D (ed.) 1993 *Handbook of Research on Science Teaching and Learning*. Macmillan, New York

Fraser B J, Anderson G J, Walberg H J 1982 *Assessment of Learning Environments: Manual for Learning Environment Inventory (LEI) and My Class Inventory (MCI)* (3rd version). Western Australian Institute of Technology, Perth

Fraser B J, Fisher D L 1986 Using short forms of classroom climate instruments to assess and improve classroom psychosocial environment. *J. Res. Sci. Teach.* 5: 387–413

Fraser B J, Treagust D F 1986 Validity and use of an instrument for assessing classroom psychosocial environment in higher education. *High. Educ.* 15: 37–57

Fraser B J, Tobin K 1991 Combining qualitative and quantitative methods in classroom environment research. In: Fraser B J, Walberg H J (eds.) 1991 *Educational Environments: Evaluation, Antecedents and Consequences.* Pergamon Press, Oxford

Fraser B J, Walberg H J (eds.) 1991 *Educational Environments: Evaluation, Antecedents and Consequences.* Pergamon Press, Oxford

Fraser B J, Giddings G J, McRobbie C J 1992 Science laboratory classroom environments at schools and universities: A cross-national study. Paper presented at the annual meeting of the National Association for Research in Science Teaching, Boston, Massachusetts

Good T L, Brophy J 1991 *Looking in Classrooms*, 5th edn. Harper Collins, New York

Haertel G D, Walberg H J, Haertel E H 1981 Sociopsychological environments and learning: A quantitative synthesis. *Br. Educ. Res. J.* 7: 27–36

Lewin K 1936 *Principles of Topological Psychology.* McGraw, New York

Moos R H 1974 *The Social Climate Scales: An Overview.* Consulting Psychologists Press, Palo Alto, California

Moos R H, Trickett E J 1987 *Classroom Environment Scale Manual*, 2nd. edn. Consulting Psychologists Press, Palo Alto, California

Murray H A 1938 *Explorations in Personality.* Oxford University Press, New York

Rosenshine B, Stevens R 1986 Teaching functions. In: Wittrock M C (ed.) 1986 *Handbook of Research on Teaching*, 3rd. edn. Macmillan, New York

Stern G G 1970 *People in Context: Measuring Person-Environment Congruence in Education and Industry.* Wiley, New York

Tobin K, Kahle J B, Fraser B J (eds.) 1990 *Windows into Science Classrooms: Problems Associated with Higher-Level Cognitive Learning.* Falmer Press, London

Welch W W, Walberg H J 1972 A national experiment in curriculum evaluation. *Am. Educ. Res. J.* 9: 373–83

Wubbels T, Levy J (eds.) 1994 *Do You Know How You Look? Interpersonal Relationships in Education.* Falmer Press, London

Descriptive Scales

C. Morgenstern and J. P. Keeves

In educational research there has long been interest both in what is learned and in ways of learning. Innovations that have been introduced into schools and classrooms have involved not only the content of the curriculum, but also the methods of teaching and the climate developed in the learning environment. The Eight-Year Study in the United States, for example, was concerned with the introduction of democratic processes and the removal of authoritarian control both in the classroom and the school (Aikin 1942). One of the most effective ways of assessing the educational climate of an institution is to obtain information from students and teachers by means of descriptive or view scales. However, the investigation of the classroom or school climate has suffered from an inability to analyze appropriately multilevel data and to separate the individual and group effects. Moreover, some uncertainty has occurred with respect to issues of the reliability and validity of such scales. These largely unresolved issues have resulted in limited use of descriptive scales in educational research and a notable disregarding of the topic in reference works and texts on educational research methods. However, the review of research into classroom and school climate (Fraser 1993) may help to do something to overcome this neglect of a potentially useful tool in educational and social science research. This entry is concerned with the development of descriptive scales, issues associated with their reliability and validity, and examples of their usefulness in educational research. In particular, it focuses on the use of descriptive scales in an international context.

1. Advantages and Disadvantages of the Use of Descriptive Scales

In the systematic measurement of classroom and school environments, two alternative approaches are available. The first involves the use of low inference observation measures of student and teacher behaviors in the classroom (see, e.g., Anderson et al. 1989). The second is to employ descriptive scales. The latter have the disadvantage that they involve high inference measures of the classroom climate, and suffer the risk of serious contamination by other circumstantial factors which lead to the clustering of students with common views and other characteristics within school and classroom groups. Perhaps the most damaging of such factors are the aptitudes and attitudes of the students themselves which influence their perceptions of the environment they experience. Thus the climate measures obtained through the use of descriptive scales are likely to be confounded by other student and teacher characteristics, which are also related to the outcome measures. The influence of such characteristics that artificially distort the relationships between the descriptive scale measures and the outcome or criterion measures must be removed before their effects can be accurately estimated. As previously mentioned, this is not a trivial task with such multilevel data.

While the student and teacher characteristics also influence the behavior observed in classrooms and schools, where the observers have been trained the measurements they record represent data that are obtained in a manner that is independent of the students and is not artificially correlated with the outcome measures. The effects of the student and teacher characteristics must be allowed for in analysis, but they represent causal influences of interest in inquiry and are not factors which may have contaminated both the descriptive scale measures as well as having influenced the outcomes.

Nonetheless, Walberg and Haertel (1980) have advanced several grounds to support the use of descriptive scale measures in preference to the use of classroom observation measures. First, the observation measures are recorded for only a few points in time, while the descriptive scale measures are based on the students' experiences over a considerable period of time. Second, the data from individual students are pooled to form classroom or group measures that are more robust than observations made at only a few time points. Third, Walberg and Haertel (1980) contend that students' views are more proximal determinants of the outcome measures than are the more distal teacher and student behaviors, which are observed in classrooms, and as such are likely to have stronger effects. However, such stronger effects may also involve contamination as has been discussed above. Finally, the most obvious reason for the employment of descriptive scales is of course that they are more economical to use both in the collection and in the analysis of data.

within groups and large variation between groups. This should result in low reliability at the student within group level and high reliability at the group level. Traditional indexes of reliability, when calculated at the level of students across classroom groups, involve a confounding of these two components of a scale's reliability.

The question of the validity of such scales has been seldom addressed. A major approach to validity has been to examine the usefulness of the scales in accounting for differences in educational outcomes. However, as previously mentioned, there has been a lack of appropriate analytical procedures to separate out individual and group effects for nonexperimental data. This has generally led to individual level analyses, the results of which are commonly seriously biased when used for the detection of the effects of group level variables. Sometimes group level analyses have been employed, but the findings have been contaminated by the effects of aggregation bias (see *Multilevel Analysis*).

Occasionally the use of descriptive scales has been validated by hypothesizing that high or low scores were to be expected in particular situations where other documentary evidence indicated that particular levels of climate should exist. Hypothesized differences between groups have been tested using available data and the expected effects confirmed or rejected.

An alternative strategy of validation has been to develop descriptive scales that could also be administered to teachers and school principals as well as to students and to compare the views of students with those of teachers and principals with respect to facets of institutional climate.

In the sections that follow, brief accounts are provided of how descriptive scales were employed in several major studies, how reliabilities and validities were estimated and examined, and the use made of the scale data in the analyses carried out and reported.

2. Issues of Reliability and Validity

Since descriptive scales obtain information from individual students in classrooms or schools, there has been a natural tendency to examine initially the responses obtained from students at the individual level. This has led to the calculation of measures of reliability, both of internal consistency and test/retest reliability at the individual student level. However, descriptive scales are employed to provide information on classrooms and schools and not on individual students, and the meaningfulness of a scale depends upon its capacity to discriminate between classrooms and schools and not between students within such groups. As a consequence, indexes of reliability should appropriately be calculated at the group as well as the individual level. A good descriptive scale might be expected to have little variation between students

3. College Characteristics Index

Pace and Stern (1958) carried out seminal work that proposed and advanced the use of descriptive scales. They recognized from the outset Murray's (1938) distinction between the "alpha press" of an environment as seen by an external observer, and the "beta press" of an environment as viewed and assessed by the participants. Their work on the measurement of college environments, like all subsequent development of descriptive scales, has involved measurement of the beta press. Moreover, they employed Murray's (1938) classification of needs as a theoretical basis and model for the construction of the College Characteristics Index. Initially, 300 statements were prepared which corresponded with 30 specified needs of commonplace socially acceptable activities and to which responses of "'like–dislike'" were given. These statements comprised an Activities Index. Then a corresponding instrument was developed to describe college environments—the College Characteristics Index, again with 300 statements, organized into 30 ten-item scales for which responses of "'true–false'" were required. The statements were about college life and referred to the curriculum, methods of teaching, rules, regulations and policy. The scales on the College Characteristics Index were administered to groups of students as well as faculty in five colleges in the United States, and item discrimination indexes were calculated for each item in each of the five colleges. From this information the scales were further refined. The Activities Index scales were also administered to the students and the validities of the two sets of climate measures examined. Subsequently Stern (1970) reported that a similar High School Characteristics Index and an Organizational Climate Index were developed and were derived from the College Characteristics Index.

Scale reliabilities for both the Activities Index and the College Characteristics Index for each of the 30 scales were calculated with data collected from large samples of over 4,000 students using the Kuder Richardson formulas 20 (see *Reliability*) at the student and not the group level and average values of 0.71 and 0.65 were obtained for the Activities Index and the College Characteristics Index respectively. Scales with properties approaching a Guttman-ordered scale were sought, and it was considered that the instrument provided measures that were approximating such scales. Stern (1970 p. 27) recognized that such estimates of the reliability of these indexes measured for students across institutions would be affected adversely by high degrees of agreement within each student body. As a consequence, the estimates of reliability calculated were computed using the average of the within groups item variance. However, there was considered to be an underestimation of the "'true'" variance. In addition, the capacity of the scales in the two indexes to discriminate between schools was examined using analysis of variance procedures, and with the exception of one of the 30 Activities Indexes, highly significant differences were reported. These results countered criticisms of response distortion, social desirability and faking which might have contaminated the measures obtained with these scales.

4. Organizational Climate Description Questionnaire (OCDQ)

Halpin (1966) has described the construction and development of the Organizational Climate Description Questionnaire (OCDQ) which measured eight dimensions of the organizational climate of schools. Four dimensions referred primarily to the behavior of the teachers, and a further four to the behavior of the principal. These eight dimensions are as follows:

Teachers' behavior—disengagement (10 items); hindrance (6 items); esprit (10 items); intimacy (7 items). *Principal's behavior*—aloofness (9 items); production emphasis (7 items); thrust (9 items); consideration (6 items).

Each dimension was measured by a set of Likert-type items to which students responded in one of four categories: (a) rarely occurs, (b) sometimes occurs, (c) often occurs, and (d) very frequently occurs. The final form of the questionnaire contained 64 items and the numbers of items in each of the eight scales are given in parentheses. While the scales were initially developed from an analysis of the responses of individual students, subsequent validation was carried out using data from 71 schools (Halpin 1966). A major finding from this work was the discrimination between the openness and closedness of organizational climates.

5. First IEA Mathematics Study

Wolf (1967 p. 111) provided an account of the development of the two descriptive scales which were employed in the First International Mathematics Study of achievement in mathematics in 12 countries conducted by the International Association for the Evaluation of Educational Achievement (IEA). One scale comprised statements concerned with views about mathematics teaching. The continuum of the scale ranged from "a formalistic, mechanical manner of teaching and learning mathematics, with stress placed on the rote memorization of rules and formulae, to teaching and learning which was directed at stimulating students to think about mathematical phenomena, develop mathematical principles and processes for themselves, and to participate in the development of methods for solving problems." The other scale involved the climate of the school and school learning. The continuum ranged from "a teacher-directed, authoritarian based educational program, to an inquiry-centered system which sought to engage each student in a continuing process of discovery of ideas and principles."

Once each scale continuum had been defined, approximately 20 statements were prepared and judged by experts to be at different points along the scale, and to cover the complete range of the scale. Where judges differed in their assigned rankings for a particular scale item, that statement was modified or rejected.

Students were asked to respond "agree", "disagree", or "uncertain" to the items. As a result of field testing the items in the two scales were reduced to 11 items each and in the final Mathematics Teaching and the School and School Learning scales there were 3 and 6 items respectively for which a "disagree" response was considered a favorable response in calculating scale scores. Where the position of an item on a scale as determined by Guttman Scale Analysis differed from the judge's ranking of the item, it was rejected. In addition, where the position of an item on the scale differed markedly from country to country, it was also rejected. The scalability of the items was considered to be an important aspect of the validity of these scales. Coefficients of reproducibility were calculated for each of the scales for seven countries and at the 13-year old level, the average coefficients were 0.87 and 0.83 for the Mathematics Teaching and School and School Learning scales respectively.

Scores on the Views of Mathematics Teaching scale were correlated with achievement on the mathematics tests and at the 13-year old level all correlations were positive and small, but at the terminal secondary school level the correlations were in general negative and small. There was little evidence that students' views of mathematics teaching and thus the climates in which they learned mathematics within the schools of a country were strongly and consistently related to their level of achievement in mathematics. No information on relationships between Views of School and School Learning and mathematics achievement or other educational outcomes was reported. However, one subsequent investigation in Australia, contrasted the teaching of mathematics using published documents in two state systems and hypothesized that there would be significant differences between these systems in Views of Mathematics Teaching, but not in Views of School and School Learning. These hypotheses were confirmed by the analysis of data collected at the lower secondary school level using the scales developed in the First International Mathematics Study (Keeves 1967).

6. Learning Environment Inventory

In the evaluation of Harvard Project Physics, following an extensive factor analytic study, a Learning Environment Inventory comprising 15 scales each with 7 statements was developed for use in American high schools. The scales were labeled with the following headings: cohesiveness, diversity, formality, speed, environment, friction, goal direction, favoritism, difficulty, apathy, democratic, cliquishness, satisfaction, disorganization, and competitiveness. Together these were considered to identify the dimensions of the social environment of learning in secondary schools of the United States. Each statement that described the environment of the classroom in which the student learned required a response by a student using one of the four response categories: "strongly agree", "agree", "disagree", "strongly disagree" (Anderson and Walberg 1974).

It should be noted that the statements employed did not mention the teacher at all, and thus did not pose a threat to the teachers of the students tested as would statements that focused on specific characteristics or behaviors of a teacher. Moreover, by excluding reference to the teacher there was tacit acknowledgment that the students themselves also influenced the climate of the classroom.

Anderson and Walberg (1974) also reported three estimates of reliability, namely: (a) Cronbach alpha for students across groups; (b) test/retest for students across groups; and (c) intraclass correlation, for classroom groups. The mean values averaged across the 15 scales for the estimates of reliability were: 0.72, 0.61, and 0.74 for the Cronbach alpha, test/retest, and intraclass correlation coefficients respectively.

Anderson and Walberg (1974) reported on nine studies that examined the determinants of the learning environment. Of particular interest were the results of the evaluation study of Harvard Project Physics (HPP) in which a national random sample of physics teachers in the United States was assigned to teach the new physics course or the course that they normally taught. Analyses of the data showed that many of the hypothesized changes in classroom climate under the new curriculum had been introduced. The HPP course was seen to be less difficult, more diverse, provided a more stimulating environment for learning, and cliques and friction among class members were perceived to be less frequent among HPP students. Other studies confirmed these relationships of the effects of the curriculum on the classroom climate.

While many studies of class size fail to reveal relationships with achievement and affective outcomes, Anderson and Walberg (1974) discuss two studies which found that smaller classes were significantly higher on cohesiveness and difficulty. The former relationship was to have been expected, but the latter relationship was unexpected and would seem to imply that instruction in smaller classes was more demanding because students were unable to hide low personal productivity.

In the studies of the effects of the classroom climate on learning, reported by Anderson and Walberg (1974), the problems of units and levels of analyses were recognized but not resolved. The evidence indicated that measures of the learning environment accounted for substantial proportions of group variance averaging 34 percent in three studies with eight achievement outcomes after the effects of pretest scores had been removed. However, allowance was not made for the fact that pretest scores might have influenced views of the learning environment. The scales which generally accounted for significant variance in measures of student learning were: cohesiveness, environment, friction, cliquishness, satisfaction, disorganization, difficulty, and apathy. In general, the directions of the relationships were those expected. These studies using the Learning Environment Inventory indicated the value of the inventory in evaluation research where both the learning environment and the achievement and affective outcomes must be investigated.

7. IEA *Science Studies*

7.1 *First IEA Science Study*

In the First IEA Science Study two science descriptive scales were proposed. One scale, The Science Teaching Scale (12 items), sought to measure "the extent to which the students in a school reported that science teaching was largely from text books or from practical experience." In addition, there was the Science Laboratory Teaching Scale (8 items) which assessed "the extent to which the students reported their laboratory work to be structured or unstructured" (Postlethwaite and Choppin 1975 p. 191). In addition there was a School Behaviour Scale (12 items) which assessed "the extent to which, through the perceptions of students, the school tended to have rigid rules on the one hand or on the other a flexible and permissive ambience." These scales were Likert-type scales which were developed using two forms of analysis: (a) factor analysis to examine the dimensionality of the space involved, and (b) standard item analysis to examine the responses to each item.

It was argued that these scales were different from Likert-type attitude scales in so far as they measured the characteristics of schools and not of students. It was proposed that the correlation ratio, η^2 should be calculated for each item using the formula:

$$\eta^2 = \frac{\sigma_b^2}{\sigma_b^2 + \sigma_w^2} \qquad (1)$$

where σ_b^2 and σ_w^2 were respectively the estimates of the between and within school variance for the item. In practice, the ratios of sum of squares between groups to the total sum of squares both for each item and for each scale were to have been used to identify items and scales that discriminated effectively between schools (Postlethwaite and Choppin 1975 p. 193). In the data processing the proposed procedures were not adhered to and only student level item analyses were carried out, and the reliabilities of these three scales, so calculated, were disappointingly low. It would appear that errors in the construction and administration of the descriptive scale questionnaires resulted in such uncertain measures that the use of these scales in further analyses was largely abandoned.

7.2 *Second IEA Science Study*

The items prepared for the First IEA Science Study were available for use in the second study which was conducted in 1983–84. (For details of this work, see Keeves 1992.) Unfortunately work on the development of the descriptive scales to be used in the Second IEA Science Study had not been completed by the time final instruments had to be made available, and it was left to research workers in England, Hong Kong, Japan, and the United States to identify groups of items that cohered to form meaningful scales. These workers, in the main, employed factor analysis at both the student and teacher levels to obtain three pairs of scales that corresponded across levels for the students and teachers respectively.

7.3 *Student Descriptive Scales*

At the student level there were three scales each of which involved a set of statements to which the students indicated whether they considered that the activity involved in each statement: (a) often took place (scored 1), (b) sometimes took place (scored 0.5), and (c) never took place (scored 0). The sum of the student's scores on the individual items were divided by the number of items in the scale, multiplied by 100 and rounded to the nearest integer. The measure obtained thus indicated a student's views in terms of the frequency, expressed as a percentage with which the defined behavior occurred. The students' scores were also summed for each school or classroom sampled and divided by the number of students in the group to obtain a measure of the extent to which the students as a group perceived the behavior as taking place in their school or classroom. These data were used primarily in analyses conducted at the group or macrolevel.

The three scales associated with students' views of science teaching were defined as follows.

(a) *Teacher-directed learning (6 items)*. The students reported that the science teacher started lessons with an explanation of work to be covered and a reminder of what was taught in previous lessons, finished with a summary, explained the relevance of the work taught, conducted demonstrations and experiments, and helped students with difficulties in learning science.

(b) *Student participation (6 items)*. The students reported being able to make a choice of science topics to be studied, doing fieldwork outside the classroom, being permitted to make up problems, and working out methods and solutions to problems. In addition, the teacher used the students' ideas and suggestions in planning science lessons.

(c) *Practical work (5 items)*. The students reported doing practical work in small groups during science lessons, with written instructions, or with instructions given by the teacher. Reports of practical work were written up for homework.

In the final selection of items to form these three scales, principal components analyses were undertaken using the students' responses for data from 10 countries at the 14-year old level. Only where the factor loadings were high or moderate (above 0.30) for a particular item in all countries were items included in a scale. If an item had a low or negative factor loading in one country, scale scores were not calculated for that scale in that particular country. While the mean student level reliabilities were not high across countries (0.58, 0.59 and 0.55 for the teacher-directed learning, student participation, and practical work scales respectively) they were considered adequate for student level data and were expected to be higher for the group level data. However, scale analysis remain to be carried out at the group level.

7.4 Teaching Emphasis Scales

The three dimensions involved in the measures of "teaching emphasis corresponded to the dimensions measured at the student level using the descriptive scales considered above. Responses to these scales were obtained from the teachers of the students sampled in the study.

(a) *Emphasis on knowledge (3 items)*. The teacher considered the official curriculum or syllabus, the prescribed textbook, and external examinations to be important. This scale corresponded to the teacher-directed learning scale at the student level.

(b) *Emphasis on student needs (4 items)*. The teacher considered the needs of the students in the next grade, and when they left school to be important. In addition, the teacher frequently used small group instruction for assignments or for practical and laboratory work, and the students followed individualized programs, involving individual printed materials and individual laboratory work. This scale corresponded to the student participation scale at the student level.

(c) *Emphasis on scientific investigation (5 items)*. The teacher considered that developing the ability of the students to think scientifically and the understanding of scientific concepts to be important. Toward these ends the teacher spent much of the time teaching science in a laboratory with the students doing practical work on their own or in small groups. In assessing student performance the teacher made frequent use of project work including practical and laboratory exercises.

Each of these three scales was considered in terms of degree of importance or the frequency of occurrence reported by the teachers of a school or classroom group of students and a series of questions was asked of the teachers to provide information on their views and practices relating to these three dimensions.

As for the student descriptive scales, the items were checked by means of principal components analysis and only those items that had strong or moderate factor loadings (above 0.30) in all countries were employed in the final scales. Where items had small or negative loadings for more than one country that item

was excluded from subsequent analyses. Since the scales contained relatively few items, their reliabilities were low, the mean reliabilities across countries were 0.50, 0.35, and 0.50 for the emphasis on knowledge, emphasis on student needs, and emphasis on scientific investigation scales respectively. The indexes of reliability calculated were the Kaiser-Caffrey (1965) coefficient (Coefficient α) obtained from the principal components analyses.

7.5 Validity of the Descriptive Scales

One of the requirements for the use of descriptive scales in cross-national studies of science achievement is that they should discriminate effectively between countries with respect to the methods employed in science teaching as reported from the perspectives of both the students and the teachers. Only for the comparison of the students' views of practical work and the teachers' views of emphasis on investigation was there any indication of correspondence between students and teachers across countries. The evidence indicated that views of both practical work and an investigatory approach were generally stronger in Japan and Thailand and weaker in Italy and the Netherlands. Unfortunately data were not available to compare the views of students with those of teachers in the United Kingdom and the United States with respect to this dimension. However, there was evidence to show that for students' views of practical work across class groups and schools there was wide variation across classes and schools in the United States ($rho = 0.66$). There was much less variation across classes and schools in the United Kingdom ($rho = 0.12$) where there would appear to be a strong and widespread emphasis on practical work in schools (see *Measures of Variation* for the use of coefficient *rho*).

If the three dimensions of science teaching and learning have strong validity, they should not only differentiate consistently between countries with regard to the emphasis given to science teaching, but they should also discriminate between the schools and classrooms within each country. Consequently a significant correlation might be expected between the views of students and the views of the teachers calculated at the school or classroom level. Data were available for seven countries to enable these correlations to be calculated. Only for the correlations between students' views of practical work and teachers' views of emphasis on investigation was there any consistency in the correlations. This set of correlations, were all positive and six of the seven correlations were both positive and statistically significant with a mean value of +0.25. While the correlations recorded were only moderate, they provided evidence of the general consistency between students and their teachers with respect to their views of what happens in schools in this area of emphasis on investigation and practical work in science. Even though there was not consistency between students' and teachers' views on the other two dimensions, these scales were used in subsequent analyses.

7.6 Explanatory Power of the Descriptive Scales

The procedures employed to identify factors which could be said to influence science achievement used the variation in the predictor measures to account for variation in the achievement outcomes. Because the effects under consideration were concerned with how science was taught and learned in classrooms and schools, data were aggregated to the group level and analyzed between groups rather than between students. Where there was uniformity between groups with respect to a particular predictor variable there was little chance that this particular variable would be found to be important. Partial Least Squares Path Analysis was employed to examine the data.

(a) *Student views of science teaching.* The direct and total effects were calculated for the three measures of student views of science teaching on science achievement, after all other factors considered to be of importance had been taken into account. In seven countries, namely: England, Finland, Hungary, Italy, the Netherlands, Thailand, and the United States, the total effect of students' views were found to be important. In all countries except Italy the direct effects of this factor were found to be important. Importance involved accounting for at least 1 percent of the variance between groups in science achievement. In all cases, except in Hungary, strong views held by students on student participation had a negative effect, while strong views on practical work had a positive effect. Thus in six out of ten countries, those students who viewed their science classes as having a greater emphasis on practical work performed better than students who viewed their science classes as having little emphasis on practical work. Likewise in six countries where students viewed science teaching as involving a higher level of student participation, the students performed worse than where students considered that less emphasis was placed on student participation. The variable involving students' views on teacher-directed learning had a slight effect only in Hungary. However, this effect of perceived emphasis on teacher-directed learning on science achievement was positive.

(b) *Science teaching emphasis.* In two countries, namely Italy and Thailand, where the science teacher placed a greater emphasis on investigation, the students in the class group did better on the science achievement tests after other factors had been taken into account.

Those scales concerned with the practical work and investigatory dimension would appear to have not only satisfactory validity, but also, probably as a consequence, moderate explanatory power in the further analyses of the data.

8. Classroom Environment Measures

Since the early 1970s work has been carried out both in the United States and Australia to develop a series of classroom environment measures (Trickett and Moos 1974, Fraser 1993). Many different scales have been constructed which differ in length and purpose to focus on different aspects of the classroom environment of: (a) interpersonal relationships, (b) personal development, and (c) system maintenance and change. Consideration is given here to only two of these sets of scales.

8.1 Classroom Environment Scale

Trickett and Moos (1974) have reported on the development of scales to measure the social environment of high school classrooms in the United States. A social system perspective helped to define two sets of variables: (a) interpersonal relationship variables, which included both student–teacher and student–student relationships; and (b) organizational or system maintenance variables, which involved the authority functions of the teacher. The Classroom Environment Scale went through successive stages of refinement, during which both unsatisfactory scales and items were eliminated until nine scales remained with 10 to 12 items in each scale. The following criteria were employed in the development of the scales: (a) each item should discriminate significantly between classrooms; (b) the true–false split should be as close to 50:50 as possible; (c) there should be approximately equal numbers of items scored favorably with true or false responses, to control for acquiescence response set; and (d) each item should correlate highly with its subscale score. The nine scales in the final form of the instrument were: involvement (0.85), affiliation (0.74), support (0.84), task-orientation (0.84), competition (0.67), order and organization (0.85), rule clarity (0.74), teacher control (0.86), and innovation (0.80). The reliability coefficients for these nine scales using Cronbach's alpha and average within-classroom item variance are given in parenthesis for each scale.

In addition, the ω^2 coefficient (see *Measures of Variation*) was used to estimate the proportion of a scale's total variance that was accounted for by differences between classrooms. Values recorded ranged from 21 percent for the affiliation scale to 48 percent for the innovation scale.

8.2 Individualized Classroom Environment Questionnaire

Fraser (1990) argued that the scales developed by Trickett and Moos (1974) failed to include dimensions that were important in open or individualized classrooms and he and his co-workers built on the work of Trickett and Moos and developed five scales each containing 10 items. These scales were: personalization, participation, independence, investigation, and differentiation. The response categories employed were: "almost never, seldom, sometimes, often, and very often," and between a third and a half of the items were scored in the reverse direction. In addition, the scales were so constructed that information could be obtained in terms of "actual" and "preferred" perceptions. The average reliabilities of the actual scales and the preferred scales at the individual student level were 0.73 and 0.72 respectively. At the class level the average reliabilities were 0.83 for both the actual and preferred scales. It is evident that the class level reliabilities are noticeably higher than the student level reliabilities. The generally high reliabilities recorded are in part a consequence of the use of five instead of two or three response categories. When the same scales were administered to teachers the reliabilities for the actual and preferred scales were 0.81 and 0.83 respectively. In addition, the average test–pretest reliability for a sample of students who were administered the scales on two separate occasions for the five scales and with actual responses was 0.76.

The issues of validity have been addressed by examining the ability of the actual scales to differentiate between classrooms and the *F*-values obtained were all highly statistically significant and the average values of η^2 across the five scales was 0.29. Furthermore, the actual scales had satisfactory levels of reliability when used in translation in Indonesia and the Netherlands.

8.3 Explanatory Power of the Classroom Environment Scales

The explanatory power of both of the sets of Classroom Environment Scales developed by Trickett and Moos (1974) and Fraser (1990) was examined in a study of 116 junior high school classroom groups. The findings of this study suffer from a failure to consider the influence of both pretest and general ability on the predictor measures of the Classroom Environment Scales although a covariance adjustment was made on the criterion measures of achievement. Some significant relationships were reported for individual scales with particular outcomes from analyses at the classroom level (Fraser and Fisher 1982).

9. Conclusion

Recent developments in the analysis of multilevel data provide new opportunities for the investigation of school and classroom climates, since these analytical procedures permit the identification and separation of individual effects from group effects, after other explanatory variables have been taken appropriately into account. Nevertheless, before such investigations

can proceed considerable work is needed to construct strong descriptive scales, to examine how their reliability is best estimated, and to explore the many different aspects of validity. The construction and development of such scales would appear to have followed work on attitude scales. However, descriptive scales differ substantially from attitude scales both with respect to their content, since they are closer to the assessment of behavior than to the assessment of attitude, and with respect to level of operation since they are concerned with the measurement of the characteristics of groups rather than with the measurement of the characteristics of individuals. Furthermore, attitude scales are bipolar, whereas descriptive scales are unipolar, since behaviors range from an absence of behavior to a universal occurrence, while attitude scales range from negative to positive. It is evident that descriptive scales involve a field of educational research that is likely to develop rapidly in the future.

The initial work by Pace and Stern (1958) saw the need to ground the scales constructed on theory. Moreover Trickett and Moos (1974) give some recognition of the need to consider theoretical perspectives. However, other research workers who have developed descriptive scales and examined aspects of their reliability and validity would not seem to have been guided by theory in their work. There are many ways in which such scales can be used in educational research. First, they can be used to describe the classroom and school climate, so that comparisons can be made between classrooms and schools within a country. Second, the mean scores and ratios of homogeneity in descriptive scales can be examined at the national level to compare both national profiles and the diversity between schools in different countries. Third, hypotheses can be advanced with respect to how teaching and learning takes place in different settings and the views of students and teachers examined to determine whether they are consistent with the hypotheses advanced. Fourth, descriptive scales have a contribution to make in evaluation studies where changes are sought in methods of teaching and learning as part of an experimental or intervention program. Finally, as descriptors of the classroom and school environment they have explanatory power in studies of factors influencing educational outcomes. There is little doubt that descriptive scales which can be administered to both students and teachers warrant greater attention than they have received in the past in educational research studies.

See also: Family and Social Environmental Measures; Attitudes, Measurement of; Classroom Environments

References

Aikin W M 1942 *Adventure in American Education. Vol. 1: The Story of the Eight-Year Study.* Harper, New York

Anderson L W, Ryan D W, Shapiro B J (eds.) 1989 *The IEA Classroom Environment Study.* Pergamon Press, Oxford

Anderson G J, Walberg H J 1974 Assessing classroom learning environment. In: Marjoribanks K (ed.) 1974 *Environments for Learning.* NFER, Windsor

Fraser B J 1990 *Individualized Classroom Environment Questionnaire: Handbook and Test Master Set.* ACER, Hawthorn

Fraser B J 1993 Context: Classroom and school climate. In: Gabel D (ed.) *Handbook of Research in Science Teaching and Learning.* Macmillan, New York

Fraser B J, Fisher D 1982 Predicting students' outcomes from their perceptions of classroom psychosocial environment. *Am. Educ. Res. J.* 19(4): 498–578

Halpin A W 1966 *Theory and Research in Administration.* Macmillan, New York

Kaiser H F, Caffrey J 1965 Alpha factor analysis. *Psychometri.* 30(1): 1–4

Keeves J P 1967 Students attitudes concerning mathematics. Unpublished M.Ed. thesis, University of Melbourne, Melbourne

Keeves J P (ed.) 1992 *The IEA Study of Science III: Changes in Science Education and Achievement: 1970–84.* Pergamon Press, Oxford

Murray H A 1938 *Explorations in Personality.* Oxford University Press, New York

Pace C R, Stern G G 1958 An approach to the measurement of psychological characteristics of college environments. *J. Educ. Psychol.* 49: 269–77

Postlethwaite T N, Choppin B H 1975 The development of the IEA questionnaires and attitudinal and descriptive scales. In: Peaker G F 1975 *An Empirical Study of Education in Twenty-One Countries: A Technical Report.* Almqvist and Wiksell, Stockholm

Stern G G 1970 *People in Context.* Wiley, New York

Trickett E M, Moos R M 1974 Social environment of junior high and high-school classrooms. In: Marjoribanks K (ed.) 1974 *Environments for Learning.* NFER, Windsor

Walberg H J, Haertel G D 1980 Validity and use of educational environment assessments. *Stud. Educ. Eval.* 63: 225–318

Wolf R M 1967 Construction of descriptive and attitude scales. In: Husén T (ed.) 1967 *International Study of Achievement in Mathematics.* Almqvist and Wiksell, Stockholm

Further Reading

Fraser B J 1986 *Classroom Environment.* Croom Helm, London

Fraser B J Walberg H J (eds.) 1991 *Educational Environments: Evaluation, Antecedents and Consequences.* Pergamon Press, Oxford

Marjoribanks K 1979 *Families and their Learning Environments: An Empirical Analysis.* Routledge and Kegan Paul, London

Keeves J P 1972 *Educational environment and student achievement.* Almqvist and Wiksell, Stockholm

Measurement of Developmental Levels

M. Wilson

For the purposes of this entry, a *developmental level* is a step in a sequence postulated as part of a theory of the progression of an individual toward maturity, broadly or narrowly defined. Most educational examples are in the field of cognitive development of persons, where the measurement tasks are designed to tap into the psychological structure of cognitive processes, but there are also theories involving developmental levels in the social and organizational fields. The measurement of developmental levels, then, includes the realization of such a sequence of levels in the real world and the techniques used to guide that realization. This entry is divided into three parts. There is a description of theories that involve developmental levels, followed by a description of methods of collecting data according to such theories, which is then followed by a discussion of various measurement models that may be used to understand and guide the measurement process. It should be noted that in standard form these models are distinguished from statistical models that may be used to analyze the resulting measurements. However, recent work in multilevel models has indicated ways to integrate measurement models and analysis models

(Adams, Wilson and Wu 1996).The entry concludes with a brief discussion of future directions in the measurement of developmental levels.

The changes in the individual toward maturity may be fundamentally continuous, in which case the levels may constitute no more than convenient labels for parts of the continuum, or the progression may be fundamentally discrete, in which case the levels must be conceptualized as a systemic part of the changes that occur. These two extremes are often termed the quantitative and the qualitative views respectively. Much debate has focused on this distinction especially in the Piagetian literature where the term "stage" was used to distinguish the qualitative extreme (see Brainerd 1978, and the peer commentary that followed). In this entry, a view and a methodology are sought that span both the extremes, and the ground between.

1. Theories that Involve Developmental Levels

The most prominent historical example of a theory that involves developmental levels is that of Piaget. This has led to the advance of a number of neo-

Piagetian theories such as those of Case and K Fischer, and others outside of the cognitive area, such as the moral and social development theories of Kohlberg and Turiel. Although the Piagetian tradition has been the most prolific in its production of developmental levels, they have also appeared in other traditions, such as van Hiele levels in geometry learning (van Hiele 1986), and Gagné's (1962) learning hierarchies. Biggs and Collis (1982) have devised the Structure of the Learning Outcome (SOLO) taxonomy to classify and structure hierarchically the responses of the learner to cognitive tasks ranging from descriptive essays to mathematics problems. According to the SOLO theory, the hierarchical levels of learning are that the response can (a) incorporate just one object of the stimulus, (b) incorporate several objects of the stimulus, (c) recognize the relations among these objects, and (d) go beyond the relationship implied in the stimulus. Clearly such a scheme can be applied in a wide variety of circumstances, and its range can be extended developmentally by "stacking" one taxonomy on another where the relations of one become the objects of the next one up.

Another related movement within education which is a rich source of developmental levels is the application of a cognitive science approach to students' conceptions of subject matter. This concentrates on discovering qualitative changes in students' conceptions of a phenomenon and thus very frequently results in the delineation of a sequence of developmental levels. In Europe, this is related to "phenomenography" (Marton 1981), and is paralleled by a similar movement in the United States that has taken as one of its major techniques the study of conceptual differences between experts and novices. This latter tendency has meant that "relatively speaking, we have most knowledge of differences between beginners and experts, but less knowledge of the intermediate stages and the nature of the transitions from level to level" (Glaser et al. 1987 p. 77). As the breadth of attention moves beyond the expert and novice extremes, more discussion can be expected of developmental levels in the American research, although different theoretical perspectives and labels may obscure their recognition (cf. White 1988). More recent developments along these lines have occurred under the banner of "constructivism".

2. Measurement Methods

The ultimate aim of measurement is to gain "objectivity and simplicity" (Glaser et al. 1987 p. 64) in relating real world observations to theory. The concept of "developmental levels" may be a useful intellectual tool in this process in a range of different situations. When a developmental continuum is postulated and data are to be gathered, levels may provide a convenient way to label portions of the continuum for practical purposes, or may be used to give practical expression to a re-

searcher's doubts about the precision of measurement (i.e., as an alternative to simply reporting standard error of measurement). At the other extreme, as in much qualitative investigation, researchers may be striving to preserve the full impact of individual differences in development by avoiding standardization of the measurement process. Nevertheless, at a conceptual level, the description of some sort of hierarchical structure becomes all but inevitable as the researcher proceeds to interpretation. This structure may be more complex than that of a sequence of developmental levels; often a structure like a (mathematical) lattice would seem more appropriate. Here a sequence of developmental levels may prove useful if considered as a projection of this more complicated structure on a single dimension. In between these two extremes lie the approaches that are explicitly based on developmental levels such as those described above.

In the search for simplicity, a sequence of developmental levels can assist by allowing the classification of individual differences into two importantly different types. First, there are those individuals whose behavior is consistent with that of the sequence of levels, and who can therefore be assigned to an estimated position in the sequence. Thus, an appropriate measurement approach must have techniques for identifying and displaying systematic ordering. Second, there are those whose behavior is inconsistent with the sequence, the interpretation of which requires theory beyond that establishing the sequence. Thus, an appropriate measurement approach must have, as a characteristic, techniques for identifying such individuals.

Researchers in the cognitive and phenomenographic traditions have used a range of qualitative assessment methods to gauge an individual's position with respect to developmental levels. These include ratings of open-ended interviews, think-aloud protocols, observations of students' attempts to solve special tasks, and, in the late twentieth century, the results of students' interactions with computer programs. Piaget's *méthode clinique* is closely related to these.

Researchers working within the American tradition have tended more toward "objective" types of methods that closely resemble traditional types of tests. The most common has been labeled the "method of multiple tasks" by Fischer et al. (1984). Several tasks are developed for each level, each task is of a standardized format with a standardized method of judging success or failure, and all tasks are given to every individual for whom they are neither absurdly difficult nor absurdly easy. For assignment of individuals to levels, a decision rule, such as "highest level for which at least four tasks are judged correct out of five," must be provided. A particularly simple form of this method is the situation where there is just one task per level, in which case the decision rule takes on an equally simple form. Fischer et al. (1984) have described straightforward data summary methods to display the likely form of results from this method that would be consistent with discontinuities between levels.

A method that can be seen as a compromise between these two is the "partial credit" method. In this approach, a set of tasks is designed at which students may succeed at different levels, and a rating scheme is applied to identify the appropriate levels. It should be noted that the partial credit method shares some of the features of the phenomenographic approach through the possibility of qualitative ratings, and some of the features of the method of multiple tasks through the possibility of replication and standardization of the ratings. One possible reason why it has not been more widely used is that models for polytomous data have historically been perceived as statistically rather complicated.

These methods can be used in a number of ways depending on the researcher's aims. For example, a researcher looking for a second-order discontinuity will have to use these methods with more than one variable. A very important distinction must be made between longitudinal designs and cross-sectional ones. Although the developmental focus of "developmental levels" obviously makes the longitudinal design the more desirable, practical considerations will work to keep cross-sectional designs common. The important issue is to be aware that the consequences of these two designs for data analysis and interpretation are quite different. Fischer et al. (1984) give an example for the method of multiple tasks. The longitudinal design, since it is an extension of the cross-sectional design, can be used to address a wider variety of issues such as the characteristics of and influences on individual growth.

3. Measurement Models

Although the results of applying the methods described above can be summarized using standard tabular and graphical devices, the interpretations commonly rest on a set of ad hoc assumptions to overcome the arbitrary features of the design. For example, in an application of the method of multiple tasks to the learning of a geometry sequence, Usiskin (1982) used five tasks per level, but then had to find a way of constructing a decision rule to classify the students. His solution was to experiment with two "at least n correct within each level" rules like the one described above. He chose "n" to be either three or four and conducted extensive studies of the differing effects of these two rules on both the internal consistency of the data he had collected and of the relationships of the resulting classifications with external validation measures. These exhaustive researches resulted in a global decision as to which one of these two rules was to be used. However, it left unanswered a great many other troubling questions, such as: why should the "n" be consistent from level to level, are all items equally

representative of their levels, and, are all students who show inconsistency with the classification rule equally inconsistent? The analysis could not answer these questions, because the analysis itself was based on assumptions (i.e., that each item was an accurate indicator of level) that denied the possibilities raised in the questions.

One strategy that has been used to deflect attention from such disturbing measurement questions is to reduce the method of multiple tasks to its simplest form: use just one task per level. Here the decision rule seems incontestable: either the student is correct on that one task, and hence at least at the matching level, or the student fails the task and is somewhere below. The usual scientific principle of replication would also seem to be ignored by this strategy. Guttman's (1950) scalogram model provides a formal model of such data, although it was originally formulated for attitude scaling. This model has been used extensively in analyses of developmental levels data, but its usefulness has been criticized. Kofsky (1966) notes:

> It is also possible that the scalogram model may not be the most accurate picture of development, since it is based on the assumption that an individual can be placed on a continuum at a point that discriminates the exact skills he has mastered from those he has never been able to perform . . . A better way of describing individual growth sequences might employ probability statements about the likelihood of mastering one task once another has been or is in the process of being mastered. (pp. 202–03)

She explains this need for a probabilistic approach thus: "The fundamental operations tested may indeed be mastered in a fixed sequence, yet the variations in instruction and material from task to task may have such a strong effect on performance that the regularities are masked" (Kofsky 1966 p. 203) (see *Thurstone Scales*). An extension of the idea of a scalogram that allows for some more flexibility in the direction of complicated learning hierarchies is ordering theory (Bart and Krus 1973) (see *Partial Order Scalogram Analyses of Nonmetric Data*).

To answer these criticisms, it is necessary to go beyond the classification of responses into discrete ordinal classes and allow a probabilistic interpretation by mapping response patterns into levels. This provides some range in the difficulties of questions that represent particular levels, and allows for the possibility of transitional states when classification may be difficult (Biggs and Collis 1982). To develop such an approach it is not necessary to do away with assumptions about the psychological and measurement processes underlying the tasks. However, other strong assumptions must be made that are based on a body of pre-existing validation evidence, and that potentially allow the checking of crucial assumptions in any application. This is the way to gain the objectivity mentioned by Glaser above.

One way to accomplish this is to base measurement on a latent trait approach such as the Rasch model

(Rasch 1960, Wright and Stone 1979). The advantages of such an approach are: (a) the resulting metric provides a means of directly comparing the ability of the learner with the tasks representing the developmental levels; (b) the probabilistic formulation constitutes a framework within which response patterns can be interpreted beyond those that conform to the very restrictive rule such as the "at least n correct" rule discussed above; (c) there is no restriction in having a particular number of tasks at all levels; and (d) the probabilistic interpretation provides a scale of acceptability for response patterns, from those which are very consistent with the postulated sequence of levels to those which are very inconsistent with the sequence (see *Rasch Measurement, Theory of*).

When the method of multiple tasks is used to assess a sequence of developmental levels with dichotomous items and the data are analyzed with the Rasch approach, the resulting scale would be expected to exhibit segmentation and order (Wilson 1989b). Segmentation occurs when items representing different levels are contained in separate segments of the scale, with a nonzero distance between segments. Order occurs when the sequence is in the order predicted by the substantive theory. There are two ways that the analysis could indicate a problem. First, the item types could have been segmented, but in a different order from that predicted. This would imply that the theory itself, or perhaps its specifications for realization, are seriously flawed. The second and more common occurrence is that the two item types overlap. This can indicate that the item types do not accurately reflect the different parts of the learning sequence, or that some characteristic of the aberrant items, thought to be irrelevant, has influenced their difficulty in some way, or it can indicate a flaw in the theory. The Rasch scaling itself does not resolve which explanation is correct. The researcher must examine the context and theory for an explanation of the meaning of such discrepant results. More complex models which involve a discrimination parameter (e.g., Birnbaum and 3PL models) allow for different orderings of items at different abilities, which means that the concepts of segmentation and ordering cannot be defined. The Rasch approach also allows the investigation of person fit, which, under conditions of segmentation and order, is an assessment of which individuals are behaving consistently and inconsistently with the theoretical order. Thus, the two requirements for measuring developmental levels, as described above, can be examined in the context of Rasch models (see *Item Response Theory*). Examples of the application of the Rasch model in Piagetian contexts have been provided by Bond (1996a), Dawson (1996) and Noelting et al. (1995). Bond (1996a, 1996b) and Bond and Bunting (1996) have also provided a comprehensive argument in favor of use of the Rasch model in such contexts.

This type of application of latent trait models has been criticized as lacking in an explicit role for the psychological structure underlying the developmental sequence (Spada and Kluwe 1980). A model that allows the postulation of type and number of cognitive operations that are applied by members of certain manifest groups of persons, and includes these explicitly into the measurement model, is the Linear Logistic Test Model (LLTM) (Fischer 1974, 1977, Spada 1977). A summary of research and applications in this area is given by Spada and McGaw (1985). Another approach has been the differentiation of components of the various cognitive processes, strategies, and knowledge stores that are involved in item responses. Separate estimates of the parameters of these component processes can then be obtained and used in the Multicomponent Latent Trait Model (MLTM) (Embretson 1985). Embretson (1985) has also described a model that combines these two. Applications of these models are usually restricted to the examination of just one pair of successive developmental levels, but the importance of their theoretical contributions should not be seen as diminished by that.

Another criticism that has been made of these models is that they do not allow second-order interactions among persons and tasks, which might, for example, result in different relative difficulties of items for different persons (Spada and McGaw 1985). In one attempt to come to grips with this more difficult problem, Embretson (1985) described an extension of the MLTM that allows different components to be combined in varying ways through alternative solution strategies. A somewhat different approach was taken by Wilson (1989a), who studied the patterns of change in relative item difficulties for persons at different levels of development, and explored the consequences for developmental theories. This approach is described in greater detail in the next section. A related approach was described by Rost (1991). Mislevy and Verhelst (1990) have placed this work in the broader context of the design of psychometric models that are suitable when subjects employ different solution strategies.

With the partial credit method of measurement, the developmental structure is built into the polytomous scoring scheme. In this case, the Partial Credit Model (Masters 1982) is the member of the Rasch family that would be appropriate. Masters (1991) has described the application of this model to developmental levels in the context of a phenomenographic example. Another polytomous model that can be used is the graded response model (Samejima 1969) (see *Partial Credit Model*).

An interesting variant to this is where bundles of items are constructed, in which each bundle is composed of items logically connected to different developmental levels. An example is the "closed form" SOLO superitem (Biggs and Collis 1982) where, for each superitem, a single piece of stimulus material is used to generate a sequence of tasks, one at each successive SOLO level. There are several ways to model such a situation (Wilson 1988). LLTM-type models pertaining to this context have been developed by Adams and Wilson (Adams and Wilson 1992, Wilson and Adams 1995). These have been applied to repeated trials in an intelligent tutoring system context by Pirolli and Wilson (1992, 1993).

The models described above have been based on a continuous latent trait conceptualization of the measurement model underlying the developmental levels. This is not the only such approach. One alternative is to consider each level as a class, leading to a latent class approach where the student is assumed to conform to exactly one of some small number of discrete latent classes. Although most applications of this idea have been applied to progress from one level to another (e.g., Macready and Dayton 1980, Haertel 1984), the possibility of applying this idea in more complicated situations has also been demonstrated (Rindskopf 1983, Yamamoto 1987).

Most of the models described above are principally concerned with cross-sectional methods of data collection. Certainly, once the measurement problem has been adequately addressed with cross-sectional data, it would seem that an appropriate next step, that would allow the examination of Fischer et al.'s (1984) second-order discontinuities, is the statistical analysis (using statistical growth models and/or multivariate analysis techniques) of the data produced by the measurement. An example using a hierarchical linear model (see *Hierarchical Linear Models*) is given in Bryk and Raudenbush (1987 p. 151). However, this approach may be an oversimplification of the problem. Fischer (1987) has argued strongly for an approach to the measurement of change based on the Rasch model using a relaxed version of the LLTM. Some researchers see the need to fold the measurement problem in with the longitudinal and multivariate structural model of the data (Jöreskog and Sörbom 1979) and longitudinal factor analysis is an established area of research (Jöreskog and Sörbom 1979, Meredith and Tisak 1982, Tisak 1984). The difficulties of applying factor analysis to data from developmental levels have been discussed by Fischer (1974), and Rogosa (1985) has strongly criticized this procedure in the context of structural equation modeling. Nevertheless, advocates of this approach argue for its usefulness (Short et al. 1984), and several influential studies have been published (McCall et al. 1977, Baltes et al. 1978). Multidimensional scaling has also been applied to developmental levels data, and a survey of those applications is provided by Shoben and Ross (1987). Although these approaches tend not to emphasize the concept of developmental levels, the points debated are an important background for the measurement of change in developmental levels (see *Scaling Methods*). Recent work integrating explicit measurement models of the type discussed in this entry and statistical models of growth (Adams, Wilson and Wu 1996), may lead to some resolution of these methodological disputes.

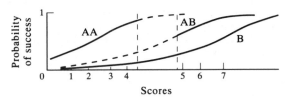

Figure 1
Saltus response curves for typical hierarchical items

4. Saltus: Measuring Across a Discontinuity

Consider a situation where it is suspected that cognitive development occurs in spurts. In particular, suppose that there are two cognitive levels, A and B, where, according to the developmental theory, the level represented by A is cognitively precedent to that represented by B, and that this ordering is nontrivial. If the levels are operationalized by a certain number of items in each, then what would the data be expected to look like? The data would be expected to "chunk" together, with subjects succeeding on most of the A items and/or most of the B items.

One way to introduce a measure of discontinuity into a logistic model is to incorporate an interaction parameter τ_{hk} into the standard equation for a Rasch model. This is called the saltus model (Wilson 1989a):

$$\text{Probability } (y_{ij} = 1 \mid \varphi_{hi} = 1) = \frac{\exp(\beta_i - \delta_j + \tau_{hk})}{1 + \exp(\beta_i - \delta_j + \tau_{hk})}$$

where y_{ij} is the response (1 representing success, 0 representing failure) of person i in level h to item j in level k, and β_i and δ_j are the usual Rasch person and item parameters respectively and where $\varphi_{hi} = 1$ indicates that person i is in level h. Note that the interaction is a group-level interaction between all persons at a certain level and all items at a certain level. Because of required identification constraints, there can be only one such parameter when there are two levels, which is labeled τ, called the "gap" between person level B and item level A, indexes a discontinuity in the underlying

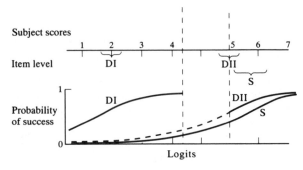

Figure 2
Saltus representation of the step from Siegler's rule I to rule II

latent trait. The larger τ, the greater the discontinuity: as τ approaches zero, the discontinuity vanishes and the Saltus model becomes a Rasch model. A possible representation of a hierarchical step is shown in Fig. 1. The gap between A and B is evident. The asymmetry of growth is expressed by the dual location of the A level item: AA labels the response curve for persons at level A, AB for persons at level B. The solid lines are the modeled probabilities, the dashed lines indicate unused portions of the curves. It should be noted that between scores 4 and 5, probabilities jump for the B items and that the relative success rates for the two item levels are not symmetrical as they would be for a Rasch model solution.

An example can be given using a re-analysis of data originally collected by Siegler (1981). He postulated a series of rules to describe development on balance beam tasks. Rule I is: Choose the side with greater weight; if weights are equal, choose neither. Rule II is: Same as I except that if weights are equal, choose the side with greater distance; if distances are also equal, choose neither. Rule III is the same as for II, but if neither the weights nor distances are equal, muddle through. Rule IV is the same as using the correct formula. For the step from Level I to Level II, which Siegler represented by item sets D and S respectively, the Saltus results are illustrated in Fig. 2. The following features of the results should be noted: (a) the large gap, as expected, between scores 4 and 5; (b) how success on S items increases considerably across the gap; and (c) how performance on D items deteriorates somewhat before returning to a high level of success. One might speculate that this last pattern might be a feature of the integration of an old skill into a new one. For the step from Levels II and III to Level IV, represented by the two item sets S and CE, the Saltus analysis is illustrated in Fig. 3. Here the gap has become smaller, and, in fact, the Saltus estimates indicate that the gap is less than one standard error in size. A contributing factor in this was the wide range of difficulty for the CE items, indicating a heterogeneity in the item set that challenges the Siegler rule classification. The effect of this on the gap is illustrated by considering

the easiest and hardest CE items, indicated in Fig. 3 as dotted curves. For these extremes, the change in success rate across the gap increases from about 0.0 to about 0.7, an increase which indicates that there are differences among the CE items which have a strong influence on the empirical results. Wilson (1989a) should be consulted for more details of this example. Mislevy and Wilson (1996) have put this approach on a sound statistical basis, and an interesting example has been published by Demetriou et al. (1993). Applications involving polytomous student responses (which allow for correspondingly more complex interpretations) have been given by Wilson and Draney (1995) and Draney, Wilson and Pirolli (1996).

5. Future Directions

The predominance of the cognitive science approach to psychology and education could transform the style of measurement that is used by the community of educational researchers and practitioners. Will the psychometric and educational measurement communities adapt to these new demands? This entry has attempted to describe the concept of "developmental level" as a common approach. For those applying cognitive science perspectives, the central idea of change in cognitive structure can lead quite naturally to developmental levels. For psychometricians, developmental levels offer a metaphor for interesting and complex models that articulate qualitative change on the basis of a quantitative substratum.

This entry has described measurement models that are presently available and that resolve problems associated with earlier nonprobabilistic approaches used in the measurement of developmental levels. But more remains to be done. There has been little attention paid in the measurement literature to the problem of individual diagnosis which is so much a feature of the work of qualitative researchers (see, e.g., Molenaar and Hoytink 1987, Wright and Stone 1979, on person fit). An important development has been the scrutiny by substantive researchers of measurement (Glaser et al. 1987). The effect of this may be seen in examples such as the close examination of the conditions under which spurts in development can be measured, by Fischer et al. (1984), and the incorporation of a cognitive science style format for measurement in the component tasks described by Embretson (1985) and Wang, Wilson and Adams (in press).

See also: Measurement in Educational Research; Rasch Measurement, Theory of

References

Adams R, Wilson M 1992 A random coefficients multinominal logit: Generalising Rasch models. Paper presented at the annual meeting of the American Educational Research Association, San Francisco, California

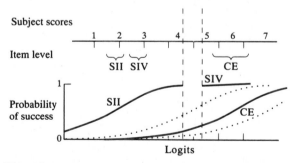

Figure 3
Saltus representation of the step from Siegler's rule II to rule IV

Adams R, Wilson M, Wu M 1996 Multilevel item response models: An approach to errors in variable regression. *Journal of Education and Behavioral Statistics*

Baltes P, Nesselroade J, Cornelius S 1978 Multivariate antecedents of structural change in development: A simulation of environmental patterns. *Mult. Beh. Res.* 13(2): 127–52

Bart W, Krus D 1973 An ordering-theoretic method to determine hierarchies among items. *Ed. Psychol. Meas.* 33(2): 291–300

Biggs J, Collis K 1982 *Evaluating the Quality of Learning: The SOLO Taxonomy*. Academic Press, New York

Bond T 1996a Piaget and measurement I: The twain really do meet. *Archives de Psychologie* 63: 71–87

Bond T 1996b Piaget and measurement II: Empirical validation of the Piagetian model. *Archives de Psychologie* 63: 155–85

Bond T, Bunting E 1996 Piaget and measurement III: Reassessing the méthode clinique. *Archives de Psychologie* 63: 231–55

Brainerd C 1978 The stage question in cognitive-developmental theory. *Behav. Brain Sci.* 1(2): 173–82

Bryk T, Raudenbush S 1987 Application of hierarchical linear models to assessing change. *Psych. Bull.* 101(1): 147–58

Dawson T 1996 Moral reasoning and evaluative reasoning about the good life: A Rasch analysis of Armon's 13-year life-span investigation. Paper presented at the 26th annual symposium of the Jean Piaget Society, Philadelphia

Demetriou A, Efklides A, Papadaki M, Papantoniou G, Economou A 1993 Structure and development of casual-experimental thought: From early adolescence to youth. *Dev. Psychol.* 29: 480–97

Draney K, Wilson M, Pirolli P 1996 Using the RCML model to investigate linear logistic test models in a complex domain. In: Engelhard G, Wilson M (eds.) *Objective Measurement III: Theory into practice*. Ablex, Norwood, New Jersey

Embretson S 1985 Multicomponent latent trait models for test design. In: Embretson S (ed.) *Test design: Developments in Psychology and Psychometrics*. Academic Press, Orlando, Florida

Fischer G 1974 *Einfuhrung in die Theorie psychologischer Tests*. Huber, Bern

Fischer G 1977 Linear logistic test models: Theory and application. In: Spada H, Kempf W (eds.) *Structural Models of Thinking and Learning*. Huber, Bern

Fischer G 1987 Applying the principles of specific objectivity and of generalisability to the measurement of change. *Psychometrika* 52(4): 565–87

Fischer K, Pipp S, Bullock D 1984 Detecting discontinuities in development: Methods and measurement. In: Emde R, Harmon R (eds.) *Continuities and Discontinuities in Development*. Plenum, New York

Gagné R 1962 The acquisition of knowledge. *Psychol. Rev.* 69(4): 355–65

Glaser R, Lesgold A, Lajoie S 1987 Toward a cognitive theory for the measurement of achievement. In: Ronning R, Glover J, Conoley J, Witt J (eds.) *The Influence of Cognitive Psychology on Testing*. LEA, Hillsdale, New Jersey

Guttman L 1950 The basis of scalogram analysis. In: Stouffer S, Guttman L, Suchman F, Lazarsfeld S, Star S, Clausen J (eds.) *Studies in Social Psychology in World War II. Vol. 4: Measurement and Prediction*. Princeton University Press, Princeton, New Jersey

Haertel E 1984 Detection of a skill dichotomy using standardized achievement test items. *J. Educ. Meas.* 21(1): 59–72

Jöreskog K, Sörbom D 1979 *Advances in Factor Analysis and Structural Equation Models*. Abt, Cambridge, Massachusetts

Kofsky E 1966 A scalogram study of classificatory development. *Child Dev.* 37: 191–204

Macready G, Dayton C 1980 The nature and use of state mastery models. *Appl. Psychol. Meas.* 4(4): 493–516

Marton F 1981 Phenomenography—describing conceptions of the world around us. *Ins. Sci.* 10(2): 177–200

Masters G 1982 A Rasch model for Partial Credit scoring. *Psychometri.* 47: 149–74

Masters G 1991 *The Measurement of Conceptual Understanding*. Australian Council for Educational Research, Hawthorn, Australia

Meredith W, Tisak J 1982 Canonical analysis of longitudinal and repeated measures data with stationary weights. *Psychometri.* 47(1): 47–67

McCall R, Eichorn D, Hogarty P 1977 Transitions in early mental development. *Mon. Soc. Res. Ch. Dev.* 42(3): 108

Mislevy R, Verhelst N 1990 Modelling item responses when different subjects employ different solution strategies. *Psychometri.* 55(2): 195–215

Mislevy R, Wilson M 1996 Marginal maximum likelihood estimation for a psychometric model of discontinuous development. *Psychometri.* 61(11): 41–71

Molenaar I, Hoytink H 1987 *The many null distributions of person fit indices*. European Meeting of the Psychometric Society, Enschede, The Netherlands

Noelting G, Coudé G, Rousseau J 1995 Rasch analysis applied to multi-domain tasks. Paper presented at the 25th annual symposium of the Jean Piaget Society, Berkeley, California

Pirolli P, Wilson M 1992 Measuring learning strategies and understanding A research framework. In: Frasson C, Gauthier G, McCalla G I (eds.) *Intelligent tutoring systems. Proceedings of the Second International Conference, Montreal*. Springer-Verlag, Berlin

Pirolli P, Wilson M 1993 Knowledge and the simultaneous conjoint measurement of activity, agents and situations. Proceedings of the Cognitive Science Society Annual Meeting, Boulder, Colorado.

Rasch G 1960 *Probabilistic models for some intelligence and attainment tests*. University of Chicago Press, Chicago, Illinois

Rindskopf D 1983 A general framework for using latent class analysis to test hierarchical and nonhierarchical learning models. *Psychometri.* 48(1): 85–97

Rogosa D 1985 Satisfying a simplex structure is simpler than it should be. *J. Ed. Stat.* 10(2): 99–107

Rost J 1991 A logistic mixture distribution for polychotomous item responses. *Br. J. Math. Stat. Psychol.* 44(1): 75–92

Samejima F 1969 Estimation of latent ability using a response pattern of graded scores. *Psychometrika Monographs Supp.* 34(4p + 2): 100

Shoben E, Ross B 1987 Structure and process in cognitive psychology using multidimensional and related techniques. In: Ronning R, Glover J, Conoley J, Witt J (eds.) *The Influence of Cognitive Psychology on Testing*. LEA, Hillsdale, New Jersey

Short R, Horn J, McArdle J 1984 Mathematical statistical

model building in analysis of developmental data. In: Emde R, Harmon R (eds.) *Continuities and Discontinuities in Development*. Ablex, Norwood, New Jersey

Siegler R 1981 Developmental sequences within and between concepts. *Monogr. Soc. Res. Child. Dev.* 46(2): 84

Spada H 1977 Logistic models of learning and thought. In: Spada H, Kempf W (eds.) *Structural Models of Thinking and Learning*. Huber, Bern

Spada H, Kluwe R 1980 Two models of intellectual development and their reference to the theory of Piaget. In: Kluwe R, Spada H (eds.) *Developmental Models of Thinking*. Academic Press, New York

Spada H, McGaw B 1985 The assessment of learning effects with linear logistic test models. In: Embretson S (ed.) *Test Design: Developments in Psychology and Education*. Academic Press, Orlando, Florida

Tisak J 1984 *Exploratory longitudinal factor analysis in multiple populations with applications to growth in intelligence*. Unpublished doctoral dissertation, Department of Psychology, University of California, Berkeley, California

Usiskin Z 1982 *Van Hiele levels and achievement in secondary school geometry*. CDASSG Project Report, University of Chicago, Chicago, Illinois

van Hiele P M 1986 *Structure and insight: A theory of mathematics education* Academic Press, Orlando, Florida

Wang W, Wilson M, Adams R in press Rasch Models for Multidimensionality Between and Within Items. In: Wilkson M, Endelhard G, Draney K (eds.) *Objective*

Measurement IV: Theory into practice. Ablex, Norwood, New Jersey

White R T 1988 *Learning Science*. Blackwell, Oxford

Wilson M 1988 Detecting and interpreting local item dependence using a family of Rasch models. *Appl. Psychol. Meas.* 12(4): 53–64

Wilson M 1989a Saltus: A psychometric model of discontinuity in development. *Psych. Bull.* 105(2): 276–89

Wilson M 1989b Empirical examination of a learning hierarchy using an Item Response Theory model. *J. Exp. Educ.* 57(4): 357–71

Wilson M, Adams R 1995 Rasch models for item bundles. *Psychometri.* 60(2): 181–98

Wilson M, Draney K in press Partial credit in a developmental context: The case for adopting a mixture model approach. In: Wilson M, Engelhard G, Dranct K (eds.) *Objective Measurement IV: Theory into practice*. Ablex, Norwood, New Jersey

Wright B, Stone M 1979 *Best Test Design*. MESA, Chicago, Illinois

Yamamoto K 1987 *A model that combines IRT and latent class models*. Unpublished doctoral dissertation, Department of Psychology, University of Illinois, Champaign-Urbana, Illinois

Further Reading

Adams R, Wilson M 1996 Formulating the Rasch model as a mixed coefficients multinomial logit. In: Engelhard G, Wilson M (eds.) 1996

Expectancy Tables in Educational Prediction

G. Morgan

An expectancy table is a tabular device designed to report, in probabilistic terms, the relationship between two or more variables. This may be taken to mean that the relationship between the variables is expressed as a table of expected probabilities of possible values (outcomes) of one of the variables, usually called the criterion, for the sets of observed combinations of values on the other variables, usually called the predictors. In other words, the table provides the conditional distribution of criterion values for different combinations of values of the predictors.

Although many formats have been used for expectancy tables, most of these have, in one way or another, specified the relationships between the variables in terms of crosstabulations, as in contingency tables. Indeed the usual starting-point in the construction of an expectancy table is a scatter plot with a superimposed grid or, equivalently, a contingency table (frequency table). In education, the units of analysis of expectancy tables are persons, and the variables

appearing in the tables represent characteristics of the persons or conditions or treatments applied to the persons. The numbers of persons or cases falling in the cells of the crosstabulations provide the primitive database of an expectancy table, but in practice most expectancy tables report the probabilistic relationship between the variables in terms of relative frequencies, conditional probabilities (proportions), or percentages.

This entry considers what is involved in constructing an expectancy table and the related technical issues.

1. Constructing an Expectancy Table

When constructing an expectancy table, the choice from the set of variables being used must be guided by substantive considerations. As a rule, only one variable from the set is chosen to be the criterion, but

Table 1
Example of a single-entry expectancy table

| Aptitude test score | Achievement test score | | | |
	20-39	40-59	60-79	80-100
80-100		0.01 (2)	0.29 (50)	0.70 (120)
60-79	0.02 (5)	0.20 (50)	0.40 (100)	0.38 (93)
40-59	0.11 (29)	0.39 (100)	0.39 (100)	0.11 (30)
20-39	0.48 (85)	0.43 (85)	0.06 (10)	0.03 (5)

which were computed by dividing each cell frequency by the total frequency of the row containing the cell. According to Table 1, the expected probability that a future applicant to the mathematics course will obtain a score on the achievement test in the score interval 60–79, given that the applicant's score on the aptitude test falls in the interval 40–59, is 0.39. Also, if the applicant's aptitude score falls in the interval 60–79, the expectancy table states that the probability that the applicant's achievement score will be greater than 59 is 0.78 (0.40+0.38).

Table 2 represents a more detailed breakdown of the data on which Table 1 was based. It is a double-entry expectancy table involving two predictors—the aptitude test score reported in Table 1 and a predictor indicating the sex of the applicants. The purpose of this expectancy table was to allow finer predictions for each of the sexes. Table 2 clearly shows that, in general, female applicants have a better chance of obtaining higher achievement scores than males for the same aptitude scores. Consequently selection decisions based on Table 2 would be more favorable to the female applicants than to the male applicants, whereas the male applicants would generally be expected to do better if decisions for them were based on Table 1 instead. Table 2 shows that by introducing a second predictor, namely the sex of the applicants, improved information about chances of success in the course can be gained for each applicant.

The above example suggests how expectancy tables could be employed to predict performance; it provides information that could subsequently be used to select applicants to courses. Typically an applicant could be selected if the applicant's score on the predictors were greater or equal to cutting scores corresponding to an appropriately chosen level of achievement on the achievement test. It is important to understand that the validity of decisions based on expectancy tables such as Tables 1 and 2 are group-dependent, and that tables should be used only with individuals or groups who are

the criterion may itself be a composite of two or more variables.

It is common to identify expectancy tables according to the number of their predictors. As examples, tables with one predictor are called single-entry expectancy tables, and tables with two predictors are called double-entry expectancy tables. Because of the problems of interpreting tables with more than two predictors, few such tables have been constructed.

In order to illustrate the concepts introduced in the foregoing discussion, two examples are presented here of expectancy tables. Table 1 is a single-entry expectancy table which reports the predictive relationship between scores on a mathematical aptitude test (the predictor) and scores on a mathematics achievement test (the criterion). The purpose of this table was to provide information that could be used to counsel and select future applicants for a university mathematics course, by providing them with measures of their likely chances of scoring satisfactorily in the course, based on their scores on the aptitude test. For this purpose, the variables were categorized as shown in Table 1; both tests allowed a maximum score of 100. Because the table was to be used in a predictive sense, the table's cell entries were expressed as conditional probabilities (raw frequencies shown in parentheses),

Table 2
Example of a double-entry expectancy table

| | Achievement test score | Aptitude test score | | | |
		20-39	40-59	60-79	80-100
Female applicants	80-100	0.05	0.18	0.45	0.76
	60-79	0.11	0.48	0.39	0.24
	40-59	0.51	0.30	0.16	
	20-39	0.33	0.04		
Male applicants	80-100		0.04	0.29	0.63
	60-79		0.28	0.42	0.35
	40-59	0.35	0.49	0.25	0.02
	20-39	0.65	0.19	0.04	

sufficiently similar to the group on which the expectancy table was based. Issues in the construction and use of expectancy tables in counseling and selection, for example, have been considered by Harmon (1989).

Perhaps one of the most important applications of expectancy tables is in test research and development, where the tables can provide a simple framework in which to report validity studies. Instead of presenting validity data in terms of correlational and regression statistics, which the nonstatistician may find difficult to understand or apply, these data have often been presented just as effectively, for most practical purposes, in tabular form as in expectancy tables. In many instances, one advantage of an expectancy table is that it can provide a picture of validity relationships rather than just a set of summary numbers.

There is no easy answer to the question of whether one, two, or more predictors should be used in an expectancy table. By and large the number of predictors is an arbitrary decision that must be rationalized on substantive grounds, and the question of ease of interpretation should be kept in mind. However, only one criterion is employed in an application of an expectancy table.

The problem of how to categorize the predictors and criterion variables is an important consideration when designing an expectancy table. Should a variable be expressed in terms of points, a dichotomy, or three or more mutually exclusive and exhaustive categories? Often the nature of a variable determines its categorization. Thus variables that are measured at the nominal level, such as the sex of individuals, come already categorized. However, variables that are measured at higher measurement levels may not suggest obvious categorizations. In these cases there is no simple answer; the purpose of the table from the point of view of the constructor and user should provide the necessary guidelines. In general, the variables should be categorized in a way that is readily understood and usable by the table's user. The point form of the variables is advantageous when computing cell entries in the expectancy table on the basis of regression analysis. However, the categorized form can often provide a more meaningful indication of the effectiveness of prediction. The use of few categories may simplify the reporting process, but it may also lead to loss of information through the aggregation of the data. The dichotomous form is useful when decisions are based on cutting scores.

As a rule, variables should not be overcategorized when there are few subjects, because the reliability of the data in an individual cell is proportional to the number of cases that fall in that cell.

The measurement units of the predictors and criterion are another important consideration. Should variables be left in their original form or expressed in terms of relative standing in the defined group? The relative standing may be expressed in terms of quantities such as percentiles and stanines. Use of the original units is recommended when the expectancy table is to apply to a single group, such as the students in a particular school or university. However, if useful comparisons are to be made between groups it is necessary to convert original units to percentages or other standardized values.

2. Technical Issues in the Construction of Expectancy Tables

Methods for constructing expectancy tables may be concrete in that they make no distributional assumptions about the variables or the relationship between variables, or they may be theoretical in that they do make distributional assumptions.

Concrete methods utilize only the observed frequencies in the cells and margins of the contingency table to construct the expectancy table. Conditional probabilities, corresponding to cells, are computed directly from the cell frequencies and the marginal frequencies. Tables 1 and 2 are examples. The advantage of a concrete approach is its mathematical simplicity; it does not entail making complex transformations of the data to accommodate statistical assumptions. It is suited to decision-making without concern for distributional assumptions. It also avoids the introduction of underlying model assumptions, which may be erroneous or unrealistic. Its major disadvantage is that without some kind of summary index, such as the correlation coefficient, which depends on statistical assumptions, it is difficult to evaluate the expectancy table or to compare it with other tables.

In contrast, the theoretical approach permits greater flexibility in the design of tables. Assumptions about the nature of the data may be varied, and different statistical techniques may be employed, in order to construct expectancy tables that serve particular purposes. Statistical techniques that have been used include those that involve the normal distribution, including regression and correlational methods and techniques based on Bayesian statistics (e.g., Novick and Jackson 1974; see *Bayesian Statistics*).

Some advantages of theoretical methods include: (a) the facility to "smooth" cell entries so that cell entries display regular progressions, free of idiosyncratic fluctuations; (b) the facility to derive results for extrapolated regions where data are very scanty; and (c) the facility to adjust variables so as to take into account restriction of range.

Of these, perhaps the one of greatest importance is the use of smoothing of data technique. Two reasons are frequently put forward for smoothing the entries in expectancy tables: (a) some cell samples may be small; and (b) the relationships between predictors and criterion may not be monotonic, because of reversals in the cell data. Reversals may occur because of sampling fluctuations. Consequently, some have suggested that before expectancy tables are used, the tables should be smoothed by statistical means rather than left in their unsmoothed forms. For example, in a counseling situation it can be argued that it would be unsound to make recommendations that capitalized on sampling reversals in the data. Research on statistical smoothing methods (e.g., Perrin and Whitney 1976) has examined methods that are based on: (a) linear and multiple regression procedures; (b) isotonic regression procedures; (c) iterative maximum likelihood procedures; and (d) noniterative minimum chi-squared procedures. Graphical approaches have also been proposed by Saupe (1991) and Solomon et al. (1989), in which smoothing is done via nomographs.

3. Conclusion

In summary, expectancy tables are simple statistical devices useful for summarizing and reporting predictive data. The information conveyed by expectancy tables enables users to see at a glance the probabilistic relationship between criterion and predictors in terms of the pattern of cell entries. Nevertheless, when constructing expectancy tables care should be exercised to warn potential users of the limitations of the inferences that can be expected from the tables. Indeed, expectancy tables are based on assumptions of one kind or another and some of these may be questionable (Wilson 1983).

References

Harmon L W 1989 Counseling. In: Linn R L (ed.) 1989 *Educational Measurement*, 3rd edn. American Council on Education. Macmillan, New York
Novick M R, Jackson P H 1974 *Statistical Methods for Educational and Psychological Research*. McGraw-Hill, New York
Perrin D W, Whitney D R 1976 Methods for smoothing expectancy tables applied to the prediction of success in college. *J. Educ. Meas.* 13(3): 223–31
Saupe J L 1991 A technique for producing a double-entry expectancy nomograph for observed proportions without distributional assumptions. Paper presented to the 1991 Annual Forum of the Association for Institutional Research
Solomon D J et al. 1989 A graphic approach for presenting expectancy of success based on two predictors. Paper presented to the 1989 Annual Meeting of the Michigan Educational Research Association
Wilson L R 1983 A critique of the expectancy formula approach: Beating a dead horse? *Psychol. Sch.* 20(2): 241–49

Further Reading

Owen D B, Li L 1980 The use of cutting scores in selection procedures. *J. Ed. Stat.* 5(2): 157–68
Schrader W B 1967 A taxonomy of expectancy tables. In: Payne D A, McMorris R F (eds.) 1967 *Educational and Psychological Measurement: Contributions to Theory and Practice*. Blaisdell, Waltham, Massachusetts

Family and School Environmental Measures

K. Marjoribanks

Families and schools are two of the most significant learning environments that influence students' school-related outcomes. In this entry, methods which have been used in educational research to measure these two environments are examined. For the analysis, the methods have been classified as involving either an environmental press approach or an interpretative mode of investigation. Some theoretical orientations for future research involving environmental measures are also presented.

1. Environmental Press Approach

In the development of a theory of personality, Murray (1938 p. 16) suggested that if the behavior of individuals is to be understood then it is necessary to devise a method of analysis which "will lead to satisfactory dynamical formulations of external environments." He proposed that an environment should be defined by the kinds of benefits or harms that it provides. The directional tendency implied in Murray's framework is designated as the press of the environment. He distinguished between the *alpha* press "which is the press that actually exists, as far as scientific discovery can determine it," and an environment's *beta* press "which is the subject's own interpretation of the phenomena that is perceived" (Murray 1938 p. 122). Studies that have used measures to assess the press of family and school learning environments are considered in the following section.

1.1 The Press of Family Environments

It was not until Bloom (1964) and a number of his doctoral students examined the environmental correlates of children's affective and cognitive characteristics, that a "school" of research emerged to assess the alpha press of family environments. Bloom defined the environment as the conditions, forces, and external stimuli that impinge on individuals. As he suggests, "such a view of the environment reduces it for analytical purposes to those aspects of the environment which are related to a particular characteristic or set of characteristics" (Bloom 1964 p. 187). In other words, the total context surrounding an individual may be defined as being composed of a number of subenvironments. If the development of a particular characteristic is to be understood, then Bloom's approach indicates that it is necessary to identify that subenvironment of press variables which potentially is associated with the characteristic.

In the initial subenvironment investigations, Dave (1964) and Wolf (1964) examined relations between family environments and measures of academic achievement and intelligence respectively. Dave defined the family environment by six press variables which were labeled as achievement press, language models, academic guidance, activeness of the family, intellectuality in the home, and work habits in the family. A semistructured home interview schedule was designed to assess the variables, and scores on the total environment measure were related to approximately 50 percent of the variance in the arithmetic problem-solving, reading, and word knowledge performance of 11-year olds. Wolf defined the intellectual environment of the home by three press variables that were labeled as press for achievement motivation, language development, and provisions for general learning. When combined into a predictor set, the measures were associated with nearly 49 percent of the variation in intelligence test scores.

In a penetrating study of family alpha environments, Keeves (1972) collected data on Australian children when they were in the final year of elementary school and in their first year of secondary school. Family contexts were assessed by three dimensions that were categorized as structural, attitudinal, and process. The three dimensions had moderate to strong associations with mathematics and science achievement and low to modest concurrent validities with the children's attitudes to mathematics and science.

In a further example of the environmental press approach, Marjoribanks (1992) investigated relationships between the alpha and beta press of family environments and the aspirations of adolescents from different Australian ethnic groups. Environment data were collected initially from the parents of 11-year old children from Anglo–Australian, English, Greek, and Southern Italian families. The alpha press of family environments was defined by parents' aspirations for their children and parents' socialization. A schedule, in the form of a semistructured parent–interview inventory, was constructed to measure these dimensions of family learning contexts. Parents' aspirations were assessed by questions such as "How much education would you like your child to receive if at all possible?" and "What kind of job would you really like your child to have?" Parents' socialization was measured by an interrelated set of components that were defined

as parents' press for independence, individualism–collectivism, English, and reading. Parents' press for independence was assessed using items that asked parents to indicate the age at which they would allow their children to undertake certain activities. In the press for individualism scale, parents were asked to react to statements such as "Even when children get married their main loyalty still belongs to their family," and "When the time comes for children to take jobs they should try and stay near their parents, even if it means giving up good opportunities." Press for English was assessed by items of the form "How often do you speak English in the home?" and "How particular are you about the way your child speaks English (e.g., good vocabulary, correct grammar)?" In the press for reading scale there were questions such as "When your child was small how often did you read to her/him?" and "How often would you help your child now with reading?" High parent socialization scores indicated that parents encouraged independence, were individualistic in their achievement orientations, and exhibited strong press for English and reading. Low socialization scores indicated that parents encouraged dependence, were collectivistic, and expressed lower press for English and reading.

In a follow-up study undertaken 5 years later, a structured questionnaire consisting of 5-point items was used to assess the 16-year olds' perceptions of their family learning environments. The schedule assessed three components of the beta press of families which were designated as adolescents' perceptions of their parents' aspirations for them, the encouragement they had received from their parents in relation to schooling, and their parents' general interest in their education. From the responses a family environment scale was formed which was defined as adolescents' perceptions of family opportunity structures.

As part of the analysis, relationships among the measures were investigated by plotting surfaces that were generated from hierarchical regression models. In the regression equations, product terms were included to test for possible interaction effects among the alpha and beta press measures, while squared terms were added to examine possible curvilinear relationships. Only one set of surfaces is presented here (see Fig. 1) and they show the relationships among parents' aspirations, adolescents' perceptions of family opportunity structures, and adolescents' realistic occupational aspirations.

The shape of the surface for Greek adolescents reflected results which indicated that initial relations between parents' and adolescents' aspirations were mediated by the association between adolescents' perceptions of family contexts and their aspirations. In contrast, parents' aspirations continued to have modest significant linear associations with realistic occupational aspirations in the Anglo–Australian group. For these latter adolescents, the shape of the surface reveals that at each value of parents' aspirations,

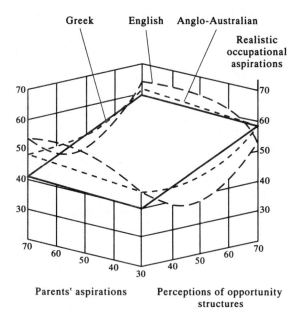

Greek   English   Anglo-Australian

Realistic occupational aspirations

Parents' aspirations   Perceptions of opportunity structures

Figure 1

Fitted-realistic occupational aspiration scores in relation to parents' aspirations and adolescents' perceptions of family opportunity structures

The importance of nonshared environmental factors suggests the need for a reconceptualization of environmental factors that focuses on experiential differences between children in the same family. That is, many environmental factors differ across families; these include socioeconomic status, parental education, and child-rearing practices. However, to the extent that these environmental factors do not differ between children growing up in the same family, they do not influence behavioral development. The critical question becomes, why are children in the same family so different from one another? The key to unlock this riddle is to study more than one child per family. This permits the study of experiential differences within a family and their associations with differences in outcome.(Plomin 1989 p. 109)

1.2 The Press of School Environments

In a review of studies that have investigated students' perceptions of school learning environments, Fraser (1986 p. 72) concludes that the research "provides consistent support for the predictive validity of student perceptions in accounting for appreciable amounts of variance in learning outcomes, often beyond that attributable to student characteristics such as pretest performance, general ability or both."

In contrast to methods that rely on observers, the perceptual approach defines classroom environments by the shared perceptions of students and sometimes by teachers' perceptions. The schedules are often referred to as high-inference measures, rather than low-inference techniques which assess specific explicit phenomena such as the number of questions asked by students in a certain section of a lesson. The strengths of the perceptual approach for assessing classroom and school environments are listed by Fraser as follows:

First, paper-and-pencil perceptual measures are more economical than classroom observation techniques which involve the expense of trained outside observers. Second, perceptual measures are based on students' experiences over many lessons, while observational data usually are restricted to a very small number of lessons. Third, perceptual measures involve the pooled judgments of all students in a class, whereas observation techniques typically involve only a single observer. Fourth, students' perceptions, because they are the determinants of student behavior more so than the real situation, can be more important than observed behaviors. Fifth, perceptual measures of classroom environment typically have been found to account for considerably more variance in student learning outcomes than have directly observed variables. (Fraser 1991 p. 4)

Four of the most commonly used perceptual measures of classrooms are the Learning Environment Inventory (LEI) (Walberg 1991), the My Class Inventory (MCI) (Fraser 1991), the Classroom Environment Scale (CES) (Moos 1991), and the Individualized Classroom Environment Questionnaire (ICEQ) (Fraser and Tobin 1991).

The Learning Environment Scale, for example, consists of 15 scales that are labeled as cohesiveness,

the beta press measure had a curvilinear association with the aspiration scores. It appears that adolescents' perceptions of family opportunity structures acted as a threshold variable in the Anglo–Australian group. That is, at low beta press levels, adolescents' perceptions had little association with occupational aspirations. After a mean level of perception scores was attained, however, adolescents' perceptions of family opportunity structures had strong associations with their occupational aspirations.

The possible complexity of relationships between family press variables and students' aspirations is shown in the regression surface for English adolescents. Parents' aspirations acted as a threshold variable, such that until a mean value of parents' aspirations was attained there were positive relations between the parental scores and adolescents' occupational aspirations. After that threshold level, however, further increments in parents' aspirations were not related to changes in realistic occupational aspirations. The surface also shows that at each level of parents' aspirations, adolescents' perceptions of family opportunity structures had a U-shaped association with their occupational aspirations.

These illustrative studies indicate that by defining family environments by press measures it is possible to enrich our understanding of differences in students' school-related outcomes. In future environmental press research, however, it will be important to address the concerns of Plomin, who has noted that:

diversity, formality, speed, material environment, friction, goal direction, favoritism, difficulty, apathy, democracy, cliquishness, satisfaction, disorganization, and competitiveness. Each scale is assessed by seven Likert-type items of the form "All students know each other very well" (cohesiveness), "Certain students in this class are responsible for petty quarrels" (friction), "Students do not have to hurry to finish their work" (speed), and "The class is well organized and efficient" (disorganization). The MCI is a simplification of the LEI, designed for children between 8 and 12 years of age. It differs, however, from the LEI in a number of ways. First, to minimize fatigue among younger children it contains only five of the original LEI scales (cohesiveness, friction, satisfaction, difficulty, and competitiveness). Item wording has also been simplified and the LEI's 4-point response format has been reduced to a Yes/No answer choice.

The Class Environment Scale assesses three general categories that are designated as the relationship, personal growth, and system maintenance dimensions. In the schedule there are 9 scales, each with 10 items using True/False responses. It has been designed to measure the actual (or real) classroom environment and the preferred (or ideal) environment. Fraser (1991 p. 8) indicates that the "ICEQ differs from other classroom environment scales in that it assesses those dimensions which distinguish individualized classrooms from conventional ones." In the ICEQ there are 50 items which are assessed by 5-point scales. It has four separate forms which measure students' and teachers' perceptions of actual and preferred environments.

From an analysis of studies that have used such perceptual measures, Fraser (1991 p. 13) concludes that "Numerous research programs have shown that student perceptions account for appreciable amounts of variance in learning outcomes, often beyond that attributable to background characteristics. The practical implication from this research is that student outcomes might be improved by creating classroom environments found empirically to be conducive to learning."

Many educators will argue that learning environments need to be examined with a greater sensitivity than can be generated from perception schedules. Researchers using such perceptual scales generally suggest, however, that the measures provide a portrayal of environments that may be enhanced by adopting other measurement methods. In the following section of the analysis, interpretative models of investigating learning environments are examined.

2. Interpretative Analyses

Increasingly, in research related to analyses of family and school learning environments, concepts and methodologies are being adopted from a number of theoretical orientations such as social phenomenology, cognitive sociology, ethnomethodology, symbolic interactionism, dramaturgical sociology, and ethogenic theories of human behavior. Although there are significant conceptual differences in the orientations, Bernstein (1977) suggests that, in general, they share common features such as an opposition to structural functionalism, a view of individuals as creators of meanings, a focus on the assumptions underlying social order (together with the treatment of social categories as being problematic), a distrust of quantification and the use of objective categories, and a focus on the transmission and acquisition of interpretative procedures.

In learning environment research these interpretative perspectives have emphasized the need to examine the processes by which members of families and schools define and manage their everyday lives. Investigations typically use variations of ethnographic methods to obtain accounts of why parents, teachers, and students perform certain acts and what social meanings they give to the actions of themselves and others. For example, in a study of inequalities in educational opportunity, Connell et al. (1982 p. 17) "talked at length with a hundred 14- and 15-year olds, their parents, their school principals, and many of their teachers. Half of those hundred students were the sons and daughters of tradesmen, factory workers, truck drivers, shop workers; the other half were the children of managers, owners of businesses, lawyers, doctors. We wanted to find out why the relationship between home and school worked so much better for one group than for the other." They conclude that:

> The evidence from our study is perfectly clear: families are very powerful institutions, and their influence over their young members registers in every part of their lives, including schooling . . . That doesn't, however, commit us to a deficit theory. One very obvious argument against it is that the same family can produce quite different educational careers for different children. (Connell et al. 1982 p. 186)

In an investigation using participant observation of first-grade classrooms, Lareau (1987) examined family–school relationships and inequalities in educational opportunities for working-class and middle-class families and concluded:

> Although the educational values of the two groups of parents did not differ, the ways in which they promoted educational success did. In the working-class community, parents turned over the responsibility for education to the teacher. Just as they depended on doctors to heal their children, they depended on teachers to educate them. In the middle-class community, however, parents saw education as a shared enterprise and scrutinized, monitored, and supplemented the school experience of their children. (Lareau 1987 p. 81)

Such interpretative investigations have provided fresh and valuable insights into the relationships between family and school learning environments and students' school-related outcomes. Howe and Eisenhart (1990 p. 2) indicate, however, that "we worry that in their eagerness to embrace qualitative methods, many educational researchers do not provide adequate and clear justifications for their methods, findings, or conclusions." Chilcott also warns that ethnographic educational research must consider the often unasked and unanswered questions, such as whether or not education is addressing the goals of society. He suggests that "without such attention to such an orientation, school ethnography will remain a mere research strategy to be employed on occasion to provide description, rather than an approach to explain educational practice from a theoretical foundation" (Chilcott 1987 p. 212).

As interpretative analyses of families and schools examine how students, parents, and teachers define and manage their everyday lives, there is a need to complement the research by investigations of the social constraints that surround individuals' learning environments. That is, if the understanding of the complexity of relationships between families, schools, and students' outcomes is to be enhanced, then investigations must use more elegant theoretical frameworks and adopt more appropriate combinations of approaches to the measurement of students' learning contexts.

3. Some Directions for Research

It is suggested by Oswald et al. that:

> The pivotal relationship between families and schools has generally been examined from two theoretical perspectives: allocation theory and socialization theory. Allocation theory stresses the differentiation of students within formal schooling (ability grouping and track placement) and characterizes the school as active and passive. Socialization theory stresses how families provide children with characteristics (linguistic traits and cognitive development) that enhance the children's performance in school. Socialization theory characterizes the family as active and the school as passive. (Oswald et al. 1988 p. 255)

They observe, however, that the two approaches often fail to examine the characteristics of schooling which may influence the actions of families with regard to their children's education. If the measurement of learning environments is to become more sensitive, then it is important to develop a theoretical orientation in which families and schools are examined, not only as places where culture and ideology are imposed upon students, but also as sites where they are produced. Such a conceptual orientation could be constructed from Max Weber's investigation of status-group competition (see Gerth and Mills 1970). In his analysis of the structure of social groups, Weber proposed that the ideal of the cultivated person accepted in a given society is the outcome of the power of the dominant social group to universalize its particular cultural ideal. A neo-Weberian perspective suggests that if certain members of social groups have the power to determine

what is valued in educational systems, then it is not surprising to find that members of subordinated social groups are disadvantaged in relation to the criteria set by the dominant group. That is, environmental measures might be constructed to assess to what extent families and schools may be viewed as teaching particular status cultures. As Aronowitz and Giroux (1988) suggest:

> White middle-class linguistic forms, modes of style, and values represent honored forms of cultural capital that are accorded a greater exchange rate in the circuits of power that define and legitimate the meaning of success in public schools. Students who represent cultural forms that rely on restricted linguistic codes, working-class or oppositional modes of dress . . . who downplay the ethos of individualism . . . who espouse a form of solidarity . . . find themselves at a decided academic, social, and ideological disadvantage in most schools. (p. 192)

This analysis of environmental measures suggests the general proposition that, if families from certain social groups have the power to decide what is "valued" in schools and society, then those favored groups have greater means of passing on to their children cultural and social capital associated with the valued goals of schooling. If such a proposition is to be examined adequately, then there is a need to bring together the theoretical orientations and measurement methods of environmental press research and interpretative models of analysis within, say, a neo-Weberian conceptual framework. Unless learning environment research becomes more sophisticated and elegant in its conceptual and measurement orientations, it is unlikely that there will be a significant advance in our understanding of the complexity of family–school environment relationships. The need to enrich that understanding is summed up by Midwinter's (1975) warning that "No matter how much you do *inside* the school, you can make virtually no impact at all without the informed support of the home" (p. 61).

References

Aronowitz S, Giroux H A 1988 Schooling culture and literacy in the age of broken dreams: A review of Bloom and Hirsch. *Harv. Educ. Rev.* 58(2): 172–94

Bernstein B B 1977 *Class, Codes and Control. Vol. 3: Towards a Theory of Educational Transmissions*, 2nd edn. Routledge and Kegan Paul, London

Bloom B S 1964 *Stability and Change in Human Characteristics.* Wiley, New York

Chilcott J H 1987 Where are you coming from and where are you going?: The reporting of ethnographic research. *Am. Educ. Res. J.* 24(2): 199–218

Connell R W, Ashenden D J, Kessler S, Dowsett G W 1982 *Making the Difference: Schools, Families and Social Division.* Allen and Unwin, Sydney

Dave R 1964 The identification and measurement of environmental process variables that are related to educational achievement. Unpublished doctoral dissertation, University of Chicago

Fraser B 1986 *Classroom Environment*. Croom Helm, London

Fraser B J 1991 Two decades of classroom environment research. In Fraser B J, Walberg H J (eds.) 1991

Fraser B J, Tobin K 1991 Combining qualitative and quantitative methods in classroom environment research. In: Fraser B J, Walberg H J (eds.) 1991

Gerth H H, Mills C W (eds.) 1970 *From Max Weber: Essays in Sociology*. Routledge and Kegan Paul, London

Howe K, Eisenhart M 1990 Standards for qualitative (and quantitative) research: A prolegomenon. *Educ. Researcher* 19(4): 2–9

Keeves J P 1972 *Educational Environment and Student Achievement*. Almqvist and Wiskell, Stockholm

Lareau A 1987 Social class differences in family–school relationships: The importance of cultural capital. *Sociol. Educ.* 60(2): 73–85

Marjoribanks K 1992 Ethnicity, families as opportunity structures, and adolescents' aspirations. *Ethnic and Racial Studies* 15(3): 381–94

Midwinter E 1975 Towards a solution of the EPA problem: The community school. In: Rushton J, Turner J D (eds.) 1975 *Education and Deprivation*. Manchester University Press, Manchester

Moos R H 1991 Connections between school, work, and family settings. In: Fraser B J, Walberg H J (eds.) 1991

Murray H A 1938 *Explorations in Personality: A Clinical and Experimental Study of Fifty Men of College Age*. Oxford University Press, New York

Oswald H, Baker D P, Stevenson D L 1988 School charter and parental management in West Germany. *Sociol. Educ.* 61(4): 255–65

Plomin R 1989 Environment and genes: Determinants of behavior. *Am. Psychol.* 44(2): 105–11

Walberg H J 1991 Educational productivity and talent development. In: Fraser B J, Walberg H J (eds.) 1991

Wolf R M 1964 The identification and measurement of environmental process variables related to intelligence. Unpublished doctoral dissertation, University of Chicago

Further Reading

Brofenbrenner U, Ceci S J 1994 Nature-Nature reconceptualization in developmental perspective: A bioecological model. *Psychol. Rev.* 101:568–86

Clifton R A, Williams T H, Clancy J 1991 The academic attainment of ethnic groups in Australia: A social psychological model. *Sociol. Educ.* 64(2): 111–26

Coleman J S 1988 Social capital in the creation of human capital. *Am. J. Sociol.* 94: S95–S120

Darling N, Steinberg, L 1993 Parenting style as context: An integrative model *Dev. Psychol.* 113(3):487–96

Fraser B J, Walberg H J (eds.) 1991 *Educational Environments*. Pergamon Press, Oxford

Hargreaves A 1996 Revisiting voice. *Educ. Researcher* 25(1):12–19

Kellaghan T, Sloan, Alvarez B, Bloom B S 1993 *Home Environments and School Learning*. Jossey-Bass, San Francisco, California

Marjoribanks K 1979 *Families and their Learning Environments: An Empirical Analysis*. Routledge and Kegan Paul, London

Marjoribanks K (ed.) 1991 *The Foundations of Students' Learning*. Pergamon Press, Oxford

Marjoribanks K 1994 Families, schools and children's learning: A study of children's learning environments. *Int. J. Educ. Res.* 21(5):439–555

Ryan B A, Adams G R (eds.) 1995 *The Family-School Connection*. Sage, Newbury Park, California

Saha L J, Keeves J P (eds.) 1991 *Schooling and Society in Australia: Sociological Perspectives*. Australian National University Press, Canberra

Item Banking

J. Umar

Availability and quick access to good quality items is usually expected by both teachers and test developers. A large collection of good items will help teachers to concentrate more on their teaching without having to spend much time on item construction. It could also ensure that only high quality items are used. When such a collection (popularly refered to as an "item bank") consists of items measuring the same thing and calibrated onto a common scale, it could help test developers in solving many of the practical testing problems. Use of a calibrated item bank could thus affect policies in educational testing and assessment. This article discusses the concept of an item bank, its rationale, practices, and the problems in its development and management.

1. What is an Item Bank?

There is no single agreement on how "item bank" is defined. It lies on a continuum from a very loose and unrestricted definition such as "any collection of test items" to "a relatively large collection of easily accessible test questions" (Millman 1984), up to a quite restrictive definition such as in Choppin (1981a): "collections of test items organized and catalogued to take into account the content of each test items and also its measurement characteristics (difficulty, reliability, validity, etc.)." In fact, an item bank could be defined differently depending upon the purpose of its uses.

Despite the different levels of restrictedness in the definitions, there is one common ground for the definitions: only "good items" are to be stored in the bank. It is differences in the levels of what is meant by "good items" that makes the definitions vary. At the basic level, an item could be taken into the bank if it is constructed properly and its content is considered valid. See Popham (1978) or Roid and Haladyna (1982) for methods of item writing and validation. This type of item bank may be useful to teachers in preparing classroom assessment, especially when a total score or a scale is not important in the interpretation.

The next level of item banking is the inclusion of "traditional" empirical validation of the items as an additional criterion in item selection. At this level, items satisfying criteria at the basic level above are pilot tested, and item selection is made based on how well they behave as expected. Here, classical psychometric properties of items such as proportion, correct correlation between item and total scores (discriminating power), and distribution of responses to items distractors (in multiple choice items), are recorded. An item bank of this level could be useful to local test developers and school districts, as well as to teachers. Many examples of item banking of this type were reported in Brzezinski and Hiscox (1984). In the past, many major test publishers tried to develop this kind of item collection in an effort to make available a sufficient number of items when several parallel forms of standardized test were to be constructed.

A higher level of item banking is a calibrated item bank. Here, items satisfying criteria of the basic level above are pilot tested in order to verify their fit to an item response model. The items which do fit the model are calibrated using a scale defined by the model. Calibration in this case involves defining the positions of individual items on a scale measuring both item difficulty and person ability. Based on this type of item bank, it is possible to design and construct a test which is expected to provide optimal information on the person's characteristic being measured, and with a high or even a desired degree of precision. Validation and calibration of items, test design and construction as well as test scoring under this level of item banking are made possible through the application of Item Response Theory (IRT). Hence, item banking of this type can not be separated from IRT itself. In fact, an item bank at this level could be considered as a model of a "measurement system." In this system, any new items intended for measuring the same attribute could be validated and calibrated onto the existing scale of the bank. Since the items are calibrated, it is possible to compare results from tests consisting of different subsets, of items from the bank. (see *Item Response Theory*)

Another way of defining levels in item banking is by looking at how a bank is organized. As previously mentioned, one of the intended features of an item bank is that the items are "easily accessible." This could mean the involvement of computers. Items stored in a computerized data base should provide greater accessibility and efficiency. In the case of a calibrated item bank, it is nearly impossible to develop and operate such an item bank without a computer. According to Hambleton (1986), the failure of the first efforts in banking test items in the late 1960s and early 1970s in the United States and the United Kingdom was due to lack of computer software and facilities, because the amount of paper and administration was tremendous. Based on the extent of computer involvement in its operation, item banking could also be classified into: (a) fully manual item banking, (b) manual item banking using item cards but with computer services used in data analysis for item validation, and (c) a fully computerized item bank. The choice of level of computerization depends upon the purpose in banking test items, local conditions and situations.

It can be concluded from the above discussion that item banks can be either unrestricted and fully manual, or calibrated and fully computerized. However, since the types are hierarchical the discussion in this entry is concerned with the development, management, and problems of the highest level of item banking, which is calibrated and fully computerized.

2. Why Item Bank?

The idea of item banking is associated with the need for making test construction easier, faster, and more efficient. In the United States, the concept of item banking has also been connected with the movements to both individualized instruction and behavioral objectives in the 1960s (Hambleton 1986). Van der Linden (1986) viewed item banking as a new practice in test development, as a product of the introduction of Item Response Theory (IRT), and the extensive use of computers in modern society. Therefore, when a large collection of good items is available to either teachers or test developers, much of the burden of test construction can be removed. The quality of tests used in the schools, for example, could be expected to be better than it could be without an item bank. When a calibrated item bank is developed under IRT, testing programs can be made more flexible and appropriate, because different groups of students can take different tests which are suitable to each of them and the results can still be compared on the same scale. Together with sophisticated computer software, application of computerized adaptive testing (Hambleton et al. 1991) could be made possible at the school or district level. Other advantages of calibrated item banking include the following (Umar 1990):

(a) The decentralization policy of a national testing program can be introduced without sacrificing comparability of results.

(b) Cost and time spent on test construction activities can be reduced dramatically.

(c) As the number of items in the bank becomes larger, the problem of security such as item leakage, becomes less important.

(d) Quality of testing programs in general can be improved because good items are easily available to users, especially teachers and local test developers.

(e) Teachers can design their own assessment instruments using relatively good items by sharing items in the bank.

(f) The best possible test for a given purpose or for a particular group of examinees can be designed.

(g) Since the basis for measurement is the item rather than the test, it facilitates a criterion-referenced interpretation.

(h) Teachers can concentrate their effort on teaching without having to spend much time on item construction.

(i) According to Choppin (1976), an item bank is suitable for countries with a large school system but with limited financial resources and psychometric expertise, because an item bank can provide a cheap but comprehensive system of educational assessment.

(j) Calibrated items can provide a systematic specification of what is important in the subject content. A curriculum can be visualized as a family of learning strands, and item calibrations (when the empirical ordering is valid) provide a curriculum map from which teaching strategies can be designed and against which rates of learning can be calculated.

(k) When an item bank is locally built, according to Millman (1984), the sense of ownership appears to be an advantage.

Choppin (1981b) also identified specific advantages of item banking for the development and operation of a system of national examinations. The advantages are classified into four categories:

(a) *Economy.* Thousands of high quality items are written by some of the finest teachers and examiners in almost every country in the world every year, and are used only once and then discarded. Under an item banking system, repeated use of items is possible.

(b) *Flexibility.* A calibrated item bank offers the facility for tailoring tests to specific applications. The tests may be long or short. Test coverage may be for a wide range of ability or focused at a particular level; covering the entire curriculum or focusing on a narrowly defined area. For any test constructed using calibrated items in a bank,

individual items can be removed or added with predictable effects on the test's characteristics. Even a fully adaptive test in which every student can be exposed to a different set of items is potentially possible, and yet the comparability of test scores still holds.

(c) *Consistency.* In an item bank where all items are calibrated onto a common scale, the measurement system has a high degree of coherence and consistency which is not obtainable from networks of standardized tests. It is possible to construct parallel tests with equal meaning for the same score regardless of with which test form the score is associated. It is also possible to construct nonparallel tests such as an easier version for schools with less advanced students.

(d) *Security.* In many countries, examinations such as national school leaving examinations and university entrance examinations play very important roles. Results from such examinations may affect an individual's future. In this situation, pirated versions of test items or leakage of test content might pose serious problems. To illustrate how the security aspect of an examination is so important in some countries, it is possible to find a country where the national examination papers are printed abroad and heavily guarded (involving the police department) until the day of the examination. There are two ways in which item banking could relax security tension. First, as the number of items becomes larger, there will be thousands of items with comprehensive coverage of the entire curricular domain stored in the bank. Of course, it is no easy matter to learn the answers to such thousands of items without understanding the background material. Hence, even when the text of all items in the bank is published, the security of the examination would no longer be a serious problem. Second, it is quite easy to construct several alternative forms of a test (without any loss of comparability of the scores) from a calibrated item bank, thereby alleviating the security problem. The particular form to be administered to a particular individual could be kept confidential until the final moment of the examination. In case of leakage of test items to one group of examinees, it would be relatively easy to substitute the test.

A number of educators and researchers have expressed reservations about item banking. For example, Baker (1986) argued that test development using item banks may not be as simple as it is claimed. Goldstein (1981) offers a number of reservations and criticisms when a calibrated item bank is built under the Rasch model. Some technical problems encountered in the establishment and operation of item banking are often considered as weaknesses or disadvantages of item banking. However, all of the reservations, criticisms, and disadvantages are problems to overcome before proper and successful item banking can take place, rather than a rejection of the idea of item banking. Such problems are discussed in a later section of this article.

3. Establishment of a Calibrated Item Bank

There are several important activities involved in the development of a calibrated item bank, namely: (a) item writing, (b) item validation and calibration, (c) item storage and retrieval, (d) linking new items to the bank, and (e) maintenance of an item bank.

3.1 Item Writing

The item writing process is a critical part of item bank development which requires both talent and skill. Unless there are a large enough number of well-trained and talented item writers, development of a calibrated item bank could not be efficient since the mortality rate of items in the validation processes may be high. Recruitment and training of item writers is clearly not an easy task, nor is it cheap. As an illustration, the following is Indonesia's scenario for the development of a national network of calibrated item banks for selected subjects taught in the lower and upper secondary schools. There are six subjects in the lower secondary school and eight subjects in the upper secondary school. For the continuity of item construction, it is planned that in each of the 27 provinces there should be at least three reasonably well-trained item writers. This means that 1,134 writers had to be recruited and trained; each of them attended a full week of intensive training on item writing using guidelines developed by the Examination Development Center. It took more than a year to implement such a training program even though courses were held twice a month with an average of 40 participants each. The cost was also enormous especially for travel since the locations are widely spread. Each item writer is assigned to construct ten items per month, hence, there are 10×3×27 or 810 new items for each subject every month. In this case, each item writer is also assigned as an item reviewer for items from other provinces. Under this scenario, it is expected that 9,720 items could be collected every year. The cost of item writing is also high even with a low cost rate, relative to many industrialized countries. This project showed that more than half of the items being collected needed revision, and that some of them even had to be dropped. In conclusion, item writing for a relatively large-scale item bank is expensive and it is more an art than simply the mastery of item writing methodology and subject matter.

The practice of item writing for item banking may vary from one place to another. Mostly, the differences are regarding (a) who constructs the items, (b) how many times the items need to be reviewed and by whom, and (c) what aspects of an item need to be reviewed. Although algorithms for generating items using a computer are available (Millman 1984), their applicability is still limited to a few content domains. In most cases, items are constructed either by teachers or subject matter specialists. It is also important to note, that sometimes there are disagreements among educators regarding what constitutes a good item. An item which is considered as good for one purpose might not be so for other purposes.

3.2 Item Validation and Calibration

It is mentioned above that item banking and Item Response Theory (IRT) are almost unseparable. Empirical validation of items in an item banking context is mostly verification of the extent to which item behavior follows a chosen IRT model. However, before empirical validation takes place, it is important to bear in mind that only good items in terms of both content validity and item construction criteria are subject to pilot testing; otherwise, a waste of resources and time would occur. The basic idea of the IRT is discussed below. Readers who are interested in the details of IRT, especially the technical aspects of it, could refer to Hambleton and Swaminathan (1985) or Hambleton et al. (1991) (see *Item Response Theory; Latent Trait Measurement Models*).

Apart from the mathematical complexities of the IRT procedure its basic idea is relatively easy to understand. It is a theory about how person variables together with item variables determine the response data when a person is responding to an item. Although there are many such variables, the theory assumes that only a few variables predominantly determine the response. In this case, it is believed that only one person variable which is the attribute to be measured by an item (e.g., proficiency in mathematics) and one or more item variables (such as its difficulty) are considered as most important. Since the individual values of both person and item variables included

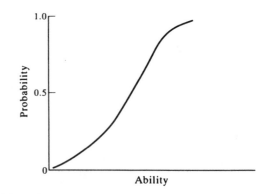

Figure 1
Theoretical item characteristic curve

in the model are unknown and to be estimated from response data, and since the model is a probabilistic one, such variables are labeled as parameters of the model. Because there is only one person parameter, namely, ability, and the performance on an item is believed to be dependent upon ability level, a curve showing the relationship between person ability and his or her performance on an item can be described. In this case, it is postulated that the curve is monotonically increasing along the ability continuum, which means the higher the ability the better the performance on the item. For a typical achievement test item with dichotomous response, the performance is represented by the correct answer. For a group of persons of a given ability level, it is represented by the proportion or probability of correct answers for that group. Since the curve describes the characteristic of an item at different levels of ability, it is called an item characteristic curve (ICC). Figure 1 shows an ICC as postulated by the theory.

Empirical validation of items under IRT is basically a verification of the extent to which an item has an empirical ICC similar to that postulated by the IRT. To obtain this information, a set of items should be tried by a large number of respondents with heterogeneous ability, and a mathematical function describing the ICC should be chosen. In this way, estimation of the values of the parameters of the ICC for each item can be made, hence, the discrepancy between the empirical and theoretical curves can be measured (for each item). Figure 2 shows the empirical curve for two items and the theoretical curve. Item 1 is considered congruent to the expected curve.

The most widely used mathematical form in describing ICC is the logistic function, which is a monotonically increasing function forming an S-shape curve. Another alternative is to use a normal ogive function. Models in IRT are usually labeled according to the number of item parameters involved. ICC for the one-parameter logistic model are given by the equation

$$P_i(\theta) = \frac{\exp(\theta - b_i)}{1 + \exp(\theta - b_i)} \quad i = 1,2,\ldots,n \quad (1)$$

where $P_i(\theta)$ is the probability that respondents with ability θ answer item i correctly; b is the item difficulty parameter; and n is the number of items in the test. The equation for the two-parameter logistic model is

$$P_i(\theta) = \frac{\exp[1.7a_i(\theta - b_i)]}{1 + \exp[1.7a_i(\theta - b_i)]} \quad i = 1,2,\ldots,n \quad (2)$$

where the additional item parameter is a, which is the item discrimination parameter. The constant 1.7 is needed to make the curve as close as possible to a normal ogive curve, which is the statistical basis of the two-parameter ICC. Another ICC model is the three-parameter logistic model whose equation is $P_i(\theta) = c_i + (1 - c_i) P_2(\theta)$ where c_i is the pseudochance-level parameter and $P_2(\theta)$ is the $P_i(\theta)$ in the two-parameter ICC.

Among the three models, the one-parameter logistic model, which is known as the Rasch model, is the most popular in item banking. It is in fact the most restricted one among the three models. However, there are some important features which are available only under the Rasch model. One of them is the possibility of estimating item parameters independently from the person's parameters, and vice versa. This provides not only better estimation of parameters even with a relatively small sample of examinees, but also provides invariance of item difficulty ordering regardless of the ability levels of examinees. This feature gives a clear and simple interpretation of the item difficulty parameter, and the concept of item calibration can be explained more readily. Under the two-parameter model, ICCs may cross to each other so that one item could be easier than another for a particular ability group but the reverse might be observed in another group of examinees.

Calibration could be defined as the construction

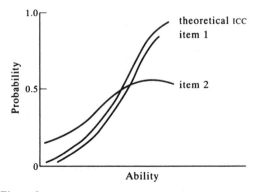

Figure 2
Empirical ICC of two items plotted against its theoretical ICC

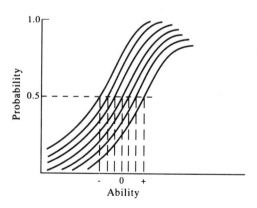

Figure 3
ICCs for a set of items fit the Rasch Model

of a scale measuring the difficulty level of items on which the location of each individual item is to be determined. The scale construction involves two main activities, namely: (a) determining the scale's origin, and (b) defining/choosing a scaling unit. The concept of calibration may be shown in a simple way if one considers a set of items which fit the Rasch model. Since under the Rasch model items may vary only in their difficulty, such a set of items will have parallel ICCs as shown in Fig. 3.

The difficulty level of an item can be defined as the point on the scale associated with the 50 percent chance for correctly answering that particular item. Items with ICCs on the right side are more difficult than the ones on the left. Calibration in this case is carried out by first defining the origin of the scale (zero point), which is arbitrary. This can be done either by defining the position of any item as the zero point, or it can be defined statistically. The second step is to determine/measure distance between the location of each item from the zero point using scaling units as defined by the mathematical formulation of the ICC. Items to the left side of the zero point have negative values with a magnitude proportional to its relative distance from the zero point. Similarly, items in the right side of the zero point have positive values. Development of a calibrated item bank is basically keeping the existing scale already defined, while new items are added continuously into the bank. An important point to note is that only fitted items are subject to calibration. Mathematical procedures for calibrating items are explained in IRT text books such as Hambleton et al. (1991) or Wright and Stone (1979). A list of IRT computer software can be found in Hambleton et al. (1991).

3.3 Linking New Items

As new items are continuously added to the bank, linking the scales obtained from new calibrations to the existing scale in the bank is an important part of item bank development. There are two important issues to be considered in this case: (a) design for ensuring a high quality and efficient link, and (b) estimation of the linking constant.

The most popular designs for linking new items to the existing bank are either using "common items" or "common persons." These designs are essentially the same because the scale for item difficulty is the same for measuring person ability. However, the common item approach is usually preferable because under this design a respondent would typically take fewer items

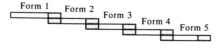

Figure 4a
Four sets of common items connecting five test forms

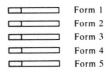

Figure 4b
One set of common items connecting five test forms

than would be necessary under the common persons design. Figures 4a and 4b show two simple ways of linking the scales obtained from five sets of items administered to five different groups of examinees (darkened areas are common items). Interested readers may refer to Wright and Stone (1979) for many possible forms of linking design.

When the Rasch model is applied, the scales obtained from separate calibrations will differ only in its origin. Hence, links can be made by simply finding a constant representing distance between origins of two different scales. Here, the scales can be transformed from one to another by simple addition or subtraction using the constant. Under the Rasch model, this linking constant can easily be estimated by calculating the difference between the means of the difficulty estimates of the common items obtained from the two groups in which they were piloted. The number of common items is the crucial part of this linking design; the greater the number of common items the better, although fewer items could be calibrated. However, if the number of common items is too small, the link might not be reliable. There have been several studies in this field but with no agreement among the results. McKinley and Reckase (1980) recommended 15 items if a concurrent calibration is made, while Wingersky and Lord (1984) recommended as few as five common items. Umar (1987) showed that five common items are acceptable and ten common items are sufficient under the Rasch model. The same research also found that the simple linking estimates under the Rasch model are quite robust against violation of the Rasch model's assumptions.

Under the two-parameter model, the linking procedure is a little more complex. Here, the scales obtained from two separate calibrations will not only differ in origin but also in scaling unit. Linking equations for both item difficulty and item discrimination under this model, complete with good numerical examples, can be found in Hambleton et al. (1991).

4. Management and Operations of an Item Bank

It is mentioned above that item banking is dependent upon information systems. The storage, cataloguing, and retrieval of items clearly require computerization, particularly in larger banks. The computation involved in parameter estimation, designing the optimal test form for a particular purpose and test scoring, taking into account the known item parameters, would otherwise be impossible. In this case, the availability of good and easy to use software is very important for practical implementation of item banking.

There are three kinds of computer software needed in item banking practice. First, a database program suitable for storage, query, retrieval, formatting a test-page layout, and printing the test paper. Ordinary database programs cannot handle achievement test items. Many items require graphical data to be inserted through either freehand drawings or optical scanning, while some other items contain mathematical or scientific symbols which are not available on the computer keyboard. In the selection of items to satisfy particular test specifications item data including the graphs and symbols should be arranged and displayed so that each item appears as on printed paper. Therefore, software specifically developed for item banking operation and management is required, however such software is still rare. Some institutions that have established and operated item banks, develop their own computer programs which are customized to their own needs so that others may have difficulty in using it without modifications.

The second type of computer software needed in item banking is statistical software for the estimation of IRT parameters and classical item analysis. Software of this type is readily available in the scientific software market but the potential users are limited since it requires technical knowledge in advanced statistics (particularly IRT). It is possible that there are institutions interested in the idea of item banking but which did not develop them due to lack of expertise in IRT.

The third type of software required by item banking is a tool for test scoring, a creative way of reporting test results, and for designing a test comprising the best possible combination of available items in the bank. Software for computerized adaptive testing can be considered to belong to this category. This type of software is usually user friendly but quite difficult to develop. Some institutions with a high level of technical expertise have developed prototype software of this type.

In addition to the computer, there are two subsystems which need to exist in item banking: a system of item production (including calibration and maintenance of items) and a system of utilization/services. For item production, it is necessary to have a continuous program of activities, carried out by full-time professionals, with an allocated budget, and using a tight schedule. It should be well-organized as opposed to an ad hoc and incidental activity.

A system of utilization or services should be developed if item banking is to be beneficial to an educational system. An example of a well-designed testing service system utilizing an advanced item bank can be seen in van Theil and Zwarts (1986). Establishment and maintenance of a sophisticated item bank is costly. In order to make the system efficient, optimal utilization should be achieved.

5. Problems in Item Banking

Since item banking is almost unseparable from IRT and computers, most problems that arise in item banking are associated with them, either directly or indirectly. The rejection of item banking is often based on reservations and the rejection of the application of IRT or the computer. Critics of the use of IRT could be best answered by efforts to develop further such a theory so that it could cope with situations that it cannot currently handle. The development of partial credit scoring under the Rasch model (Masters 1982, Masters and Evans 1986), for example, has made item banking more acceptable and beneficial because some important types of item are no longer excluded from its operations. Latest developments in computer software and hardware could also make item banking practices easier.

At the time of writing in the mid-1990s, the following problems arise in the practical implementation of item banking:

(a) Item banking requires an expensive investment especially in the beginning.

(b) Item banking requires highly specialized professionals. This is also expensive.

(c) There is a lack of powerful but easy to use software that could make advance applications by nonspecialists possible.

(d) The construction of items satisfying the IRT models is difficult. The more restricted the IRT model in use, the greater the likelihood of rejecting items, including the ones that might be good for particular purposes.

(e) The requirements of IRT are sometimes difficult to satisfy, especially for achievement test items in the social sciences.

6. Conclusion

Despite the various ways of defining an item bank, teachers and test developers could greatly benefit from establishing and utilizing a large collection of achievement test items. It can also be shown that a calibrated item bank provides flexibility, efficiency, quality of items, testing security, measurement consistency, and facilitates criterion-referenced evaluation. The recruitment and training of item writers and item reviewers is important but expensive, and the establishment of an item banking system should include systems of item production, management, and operation (computer system), and a system of utilization services. Finally, future research on item banking should be directed toward overcoming the existing problems so that its practice could be more beneficial to educational systems and more acceptable to teachers and educators.

See also: Item Sampling in Testing; Item Writing Techniques

References

Baker F B 1986 Item banking in computer-based instructional systems. *Appl. Psychol. Meas.* 10(4): 405–14
Brzezinski E J, Hiscox M D (eds.) 1984 Microcomputers and testing. *Educational Measurement: Issues and Practices* 3:4–34
Choppin B H 1976 Item banking development. In De Gruijter D N M, van der Kamp (eds.) 1976 *Advances in Psychometrics and Educational Measurement*. Wiley, London
Choppin B H 1981a Educational measurement and the item bank model. In: Lacey C, Lawton D (eds.) 1981 *Issues in Evaluation and Accountability*. Methuen, London
Choppin B H 1981b Principles of Item Banking (Unpublished training material)
Goldstein H 1981 Limitations of the Rasch model scale for educational assessment. In: Lacey C, Lawton D (eds.) 1981 *Issues in Evaluation and Accountability*. Methuen, London
Hambleton R K, Swaminathan H 1985 *Item Response Theory. Principles and Applications*. Kluwer-Nijhoff, Boston, Massachusetts
Hambleton R K 1986 The changing conception of measurement: A commentary. *Appl. Psychol. Meas.* 10: 415–21
Hambleton R K, Swaminathan H, Rogers H J 1991 *Fundamentals of Item Response Theory*. Sage, Newbury Park California
Masters G N 1982 A Rasch model for partial credit scoring. *Psychometri.* 47: 149–74
Masters G N, Evans J 1986 Banking non-dichotomously scored items. *Appl. Psychol. Meas.* 10: 355–67
McKinley R L, Reckase M D 1980 *A Successful Application of Latent Trait Theory to Tailored Achievement Testing*. Research Report 80–1. University of Missouri, Columbia, Missouri
Millman J 1984 Individualizing test construction and administration by computer. In: Berk R A (ed.) 1984 *A Guide to Criterion-referenced Test Construction*. Johns Hopkins University Press, Baltimore, Maryland
Popham W J 1978 *Criterion Reference Measurement*. Prentice-Hall, Englewood Cliffs, New Jersey
Roid G H, Haladyna T J 1982 *A Technology for Test-item Writing*. Academic Press, New York
Umar J 1987 Robustness of the simple linking procedure in item banking using the Rasch model. (Doctoral dissertation, University of California, Los Angeles)
Umar J 1990 Development of an examination system based on calibrated item bank networks. Unpublished Project Report, SIDEC, Stanford University, Stanford, California
Van der Linden W J 1986 Forewords to the special issues in item banking. *Appl. Psychol. Meas.* 10(4)
Van Theil C C, Zwarts M A 1986 Development of a testing service system. *Appl. Psychol. Meas.* 10: 371–403
Wingersky M S, Lord F M 1984 An investigation of methods for reducing sampling error in certain IRT procedures. *Appl. Psychol. Meas.* 8: 347–64
Wright B D, Stone M 1979 *Best Test Design*. MESA Press, Chicago, Illinois

Further Reading

1984 Special issues in item banking. *J. Educ. Meas.* 21(4)
1986 Special issues in item banking. *Appl. Psychol. Meas.* 10(4)
Roid G H 1989 Item writing and item banking by micro computer: An update. *Educational Measurement: Issues and Practices* 8(3): 17–20

Measurement of Social Background

J. P. Keeves and L. J. Saha

Since the early 1930s it has been increasingly recognized that in most countries differences in social background are strongly related to educational outcomes. In recognition of this relationship many countries have introduced compensatory programs to assist with the provision of educational services to those who are seen to be socially and economically disadvantaged. Underlying these developments has been the work undertaken primarily in the area of sociology concerned with the study of social stratification and social mobility and the measurement of social status. This entry is concerned with the measurement of social background and social status, and the problems encountered in the development of consistent and valid measurement.

1. Measurement Issues

Meaningful measurement requires that the properties being measured have a sound conceptual basis within an established theory, and that the operational definitions linking the theory and the scaling techniques employed yield both valid and reliable measures. However, social stratification and social mobility are fields in which there is considerable controversy. Haug (1977) has pointed out that there are at least two types of characteristics which are used to cluster persons into strata or groups that are hierarchically ordered. First, there are biologically based characteristics such as age, sex, race, and ethnic origin. Second, there are acquired characteristics such as power, wealth, and social prestige. Societies differ in the emphasis given to particular characteristics, both biological and acquired, in the process of stratification within them. Even within a given society the emphasis on these characteristics changes over time. Consequently, there is little consensus regarding which characteristics should form the basis of a general theory of social stratification. Nevertheless, the theories of Marx, that class categories are derived from the relation of a group to the means of production and thus are based on differences between ownership of property and the provision of labor, have greatly influenced thinking in this area. Another prominent view advanced by Weber is that position in society is built around the three concepts of status, power, and class, with status being related to prestige ascribed by the community, power being associated with a political context, and class having an economic basis. These three dimensions of status, power, and class are conceptually interrelated and might be expected to be highly correlated with one another. As a consequence they have provided the main foundation on which the measurement of social stratification has proceeded, particularly in industrial societies.

Two broad approaches have been employed in the investigation and measurement of social background and social status. Warner et al. (1949) have identified these two approaches, distinguishing between the approach in which an assessment is made of social standing by the observed and evaluated participation of an individual in the social system of a community, and the approach in which indexes of the status level of the individual in the community are developed using information obtained directly from the individual by either objective or subjective responses.

As a result, in undertaking the task of measuring social status it is necessary not only to consider the theoretical basis of the concepts to be employed but also how information related to an individual with respect to those concepts might be obtained. The most commonly used single indicator of a person's relative standing with respect to the concepts of status, power, and class is that of occupational status. Thus information on the social standing of an occupation can be obtained either by the use of the subjective perceptions of members of the community, or by the use of concomitant objective characteristics of the occupation associated with the level of skill required, the level of education necessary to engage in the occupation, and the income received from regular employment in the occupation. These three characteristics are interrelated insofar as economic return is determined, in part, by both level of skill and level of education, and together they form a basis for objective measurement.

2. Measurement of Occupational Status

In general, the starting point for the measurement of occupational status involves the setting up of a clas-

sification of the full range of occupations which exist in a society. Since such a large number of classified occupations exist, it is necessary to group them into categories. Once occupational categories have been formed they must be assigned to a rank order. The simplest grouping in industrialized societies is into two categories: white-collar workers and blue-collar workers. This reflects the wearing of blue denim clothing by workers in many countries especially the United States. White-collar occupations typically require a high proportion of the work to be carried out within an office. Blue-collar occupations involve a high proportion of the work being undertaken out-of-doors or away from an office desk. In most societies white-collar occupations are perceived to require a higher level of education and skill. In the main, they are more highly rewarded and are thus accorded higher status than blue-collar occupations. A more extensive categorization, again based essentially on levels of education, skill, and income, involves six categories of occupation: professional, managerial, clerical, skilled, semiskilled, and unskilled. The first three named are white-collar occupations; the last three are blue-collar occupations.

Broom et al. (1977) have identified five main approaches which have been involved in the measurement of occupations beyond the simple categorizations referred to above. First, it is possible to develop a more extensive set of occupational categories based on level of education, skill, and income and to assign integer scores to the hierarchically ordered occupational categories (Jones 1971). A second approach has been to derive socioeconomic scores for each occupation by combining average years of education and average income associated with each occupation, customarily with equal weight (e.g.: for Canada, Blishen [1958]; for New Zealand, Elley and Irving [1972]; and for the United States, Nam and Powers [1968]. A third strategy has been to carry out an auxiliary study of occupational prestige, and, using regression analysis, to estimate the weights for such characteristics as years of education and income in order to predict the prestige score for major occupations. Scores for those occupations not estimated directly may be obtained by interpolation (Duncan 1961, Pineo and Porter 1967). A fourth approach is to make direct estimates of social standing or prestige using information obtained from a single study which provides data for all occupations, or to use previous rating studies to provide some of the necessary data (Siegel 1971). A fifth procedure that has been employed is to compute scores for occupational categories from the analysis of measures obtained on several separate characteristics (for example, level of education, income, level of occupational skill) using the interrelations between the measures to generate the scores. The statistical techniques of principal components analysis, factor analysis, and canonical analysis have been employed to this end (Keeves 1972).

931

In the remainder of Sect. 2 the procedures which have been employed in selected countries are briefly described.

2.1 Australia

The starting point of the work of Broom et al. (1965) was the classified list of occupations which had been developed for use in the national census. As a first step, Broom and colleagues grouped the 342 occupational titles into 100 clusters on the basis of interrelations between occupations, and then into 16 broad categories using as the main criterion that each group should contain jobs involving the same level of skill or skill type. These 16 categories were ordered to form a prestige scale broadly in agreement with the findings of an earlier study into occupational prestige by Congalton (1963) that had produced an occupational prestige scale. Subsequently, Broom et al. (1977) extended this work using the third strategy described above, namely that of fitting an equation to prestige scores for measures of age, sex, birthplace, schooling and qualifications, housing and vehicle ownership, and interpolating for a wider set of occupations.

2.2 The United Kingdom

The first attempt in the United Kingdom to form an occupational classification was carried out for the census in 1911 when five occupational categories were defined. This classification was revised in 1971 to six classes which were: I—professional; II—intermediate occupations; III N—skilled occupations (nonmanual); III M—skilled occupations (manual); IV—partly skilled occupations; V—unskilled occupations. In addition, a stratification measure was developed by Hall and Caradog Jones (1950) based on community perceptions of occupational prestige. Initially, this scale was constructed for 30 occupational categories, and was later extended to include approximately 650 occupations (Oppenheim 1966). Subsequently, Goldthorpe and Hope (1974) grouped all the occupations in the United Kingdom census classification into 125 categories which were as homogeneous as possible with respect to both intrinsic and extrinsic rewards. They then selected a representative sample of occupational titles from each category, and in a single study obtained rankings of the prestige of each of the occupational groups. From these rankings a single scale was formed, but no attempt was made to group the final 124 categories into a smaller number of classes or strata.

2.3 The United States

In the United States, the major system of classifying occupations developed by the Bureau of Census was used as the basis for setting up measures of stratification. Edwards (1938) developed the first scale. Using education and income as criteria, he grouped together all occupations into 10 hierarchically ordered classes. Such a scale, employing income in the formation of socioeconomic groups, has become known as a scale of "socioeconomic status" (SES). This term is now widely used even where the measures employed do not strictly involve income. For the 1971 United States Census a 12-category scale was developed from Edwards's scale, but whether it retains the socioeconomic groupings of the earlier scale is open to question.

Perhaps the most frequently used measure of social stratification in the United States is the Duncan Socio-Economic Index (SEI) (Duncan 1961), which is based on occupational prestige as evaluated by public opinion, using the third strategy outlined above. However, the estimated prestige scores showed many shortcomings and Siegel (1971) sought to obtain a more secure empirical basis for the prestige ratings from a public opinion survey for as many of the major census occupations as possible.

In addition to these two measures, Miller (1991) presents four other scales for use in the United States: (a) Nam–Powers Socioeconomic Status Scores, (b) Hollingshead's Two-Factor Index of Social Position, (c) the Revised Occupational Rating Scale from Warner Meeker, and Eell's Index of Status Characteristics, and (d) Edwards's Social–Economic Group of Occupations.

2.4 Canada

The construction of measures of stratification in Canada has followed closely the work carried out in the United States. Blishen (1958) initially developed an occupational scale by combining the mean standard scores for both education and income for members of occupational groups using Canadian census classifications and data from a national census. Blishen (1967) then followed the procedures used by Duncan (1961) to obtain regression weights for education and income measures in the prediction of prestige scores. The weights obtained by Blishen for education exceeded those for income, where Duncan had obtained approximately equal weights. Furthermore, Pineo and Porter (1967) sought to obtain information on occupational prestige through a national survey. Subsequently, Pineo, Porter, and McRoberts developed an occupational classification of 16 categories for the Canadian Mobility Study, that was collapsed by McRoberts (1985) into 10 categories for the examination of mobility and attainment.

3. The Standard International Occupational Prestige Scale

Husén (1967) used an occupational scale developed at the University of Chicago with considerable success in the First Mathematics Study for the International Association for the Evaluation of Educational Achievement in 1964. One problem with this scale was that it did not allow for the societal and cultural differences between countries. Subsequently, Treiman (1977) sought to combine the many diverse scales of prestige employed in different countries into a single scheme that could be used in cross-cultural research and other comparative studies. Treiman obtained information from prestige studies in 55 countries and recoded the occupational titles according to the appropriate categories employed in the International Standard Classification of Occupations (ISCO) published by the International Labor Office in 1969. After conversion to a common standard metric, the scores obtained from the 55 countries for each occupational group were averaged across countries to obtain the international scale. Treiman claimed that the concurrent validity of the scale was high because the average coefficient obtained by correlating each country's occupational scale scores with those for the international scale with that country removed was 0.89. In addition, with the exclusion of a few developing countries and some socialist countries, the correlations between scales were unrelated to level of industrialization as measured by gross national product. In common with most of the scales in current use there are short-comings in the scales with respect to the positions of farm and rural workers. Thus for a country with a high percentage of the labor force engaged in primary industry it must be anticipated that some problems will be encountered.

4. The Occupational Power Scales

Erikson et al. (1979) have proposed an occupational scale that has been presented in detail by Goldthorpe (1980) which was developed as a class schema for the study of occupational mobility. In this scale, Classes I and II represent what has become known as the "Service Class." The Service Class comprises those with expertise who exercise power on behalf of corporate bodies, together with independent professionals and self-employed business people. Class I is the higher level and Class II the lower level of the service class. Class III comprises routine, non-manual employees associated with the service class, who do not exercise authority, or if they do, the authority is exercised within a limited field. Class IV comprises persons in self-employment with Class IVa consisting of those self-employed persons who have employees working for them; Class IVb consists of those self-employed persons who are engaged in rural occupations. Class V consists of lower level technicians and foremen, while Class VI comprises skilled manual workers. Class VII consists of some skilled and unskilled manual workers while Class VIIa comprises those not in agriculture, and Class VIIb those employed in agriculture. This class scale is now being used in cross-national studies of occupational mobility, but has not been widely used in educational research. The occupational class categorization proposed by Goldthorpe and his colleagues has a very different meaning from the scales that use concepts of socioeconomic status, prestige, and skill level of occupation. Consequently, this scale has some advantages in causal modeling where other measures of economic circumstances are also included.

5. Some Special Problems for Educational Research

There are many issues of both a methodological and substantive nature associated with the use of social background data in educational research. Although such information has been found to have considerable explanatory power, problems have been encountered that limit the usefulness of such measures.

5.1 Confidentiality of Information

During the 1970s and the 1980s there was growing awareness of the confidential nature of much of the data that were collected in large-scale surveys. The ease with which data could be stored and subsequently accessed through computerized data banks has led to widespread protest with respect to the confidentiality of personal information. In many countries research workers have had experience of data files being destroyed or mutilated. Information regarding occupation, years of education, and level of income are collected in national censuses where there is a public guarantee of confidentiality. However, in educational surveys teacher unions and parent organizations sometimes refuse permission for such data to be collected from students with respect to their parents on the grounds of invasion of privacy. Little damage is done in cases where the parent of an isolated student prevents this information being supplied in response to questionnaire items in a survey. Where the data are withheld for individual schools or groups of schools, the validity of the data that are collected is quickly cast into doubt. In some countries, for example, Japan, it is no longer possible to collect information on parental occupation from students in large-scale surveys.

5.2 Response Error in Student Reports

It has been generally accepted that most students by the age of 10 years are able to provide information on father's occupation, that some students are unable to report accurately on father's and mother's education, and that few students can provide accurate data on level of father's or mother's income. As a consequence, information on level of income is rarely sought directly from students. However, in order to obtain accurate information on parental occupation and education, students are commonly requested to check their responses with their parents on the night prior to responding to a questionnaire. This procedure is not only a courtesy to parents, informing them that such data are being sought and seeking authorization for participation in the survey, but it also helps to ensure that the data collected are accurate.

Considerable work has been carried out to study response error in student reports of parental socioeconomic characteristics (see, for example, Coleman et al. 1966, Jencks et al. 1972). Subsequently, Mason et al. (1976) developed a conceptual and analytic model and examined measurement error for White and Black students at different grade levels in the United States. For only one group, namely 12th grade White students, were the measurement errors shown to be random. It is clear that substantial bias commonly exists in such data. Nevertheless, data on socioeconomic characteristics have been found to have considerable explanatory power.

5.3 Occupational Status Scales for Women

An increasing proportion of the workforce in most countries is made up of women, and all increasing proportions of women are now engaged in occupations that were formerly the preserve of males. However, the occupational scales that have been constructed in most countries, including the Treiman scale, were developed with data from samples of adult males. These scales are not necessarily appropriate for female occupations. First, there are substantial proportions of women in many countries who are not in the labor force. These women are commonly engaged in home duties, and the reasons for their nonparticipation in the labor force differ across countries. In some countries it is only the unskilled who are not able to obtain employment. In other countries substantial numbers of the better educated women do not need to seek employment to augment the family income. Secondly, in spite of gains in female labor force participation, and educational preparation, substantial differences persist in most countries in the average earnings of men and women in the same occupational group. It is evident that women are still not ascribed the same status as men in a particular occupation. Nevertheless, valuable information is available for both prediction and explanation of student achievement in data collected from students on the occupation and level of education of their mothers as well as their fathers.

The Nam–Powers Socioeconomic Status Scores provides combined scales for men and women in the United States, in contrast to the other major scales used in that country, which provide scores for men only (Miller 1991 p. 329).

5.4 Single-parent Families

In recent decades there has been a marked increase in many countries in the incidence of divorce and the establishment of single-parent families. While this has the effect of lowering family income, its effects on intellectual development and educational achievement are more complex. In part, this is a consequence of the fact that in some countries one-parent families occur more frequently among lower socioeconomic groups, and are confounded with racial differences in countries such as the United States. Research does not show unequivocally that living in a single-parent home results in lower educational achievement (Scott-Jones 1984).

5.5 Occupational Status and Race

In many countries there has been a marked change during recent decades in the racial and ethnic composition of the labor force as a result of cross-national migration. This has also resulted in certain occupations being taken by persons from particular ethnic groups, who for a variety of reasons are assigned a lower status. As a consequence, the occupational status scales that were constructed using data from a more homogeneous population within a particular country are no longer as meaningful as they were formerly. Furthermore, in the examination of the effects of race or ethnic composition on educational outcomes it would seem necessary to control for occupational status to obtain meaningful relationships. However, such statistical control may not be fully appropriate if occupational status in the land of adoption were rather lower than it would have been in the land of origin for particular racial and ethnic groups.

5.6 Robust Measures of Occupational Status

Much effort went into developing refined measures of occupational status during the decades from 1960 to 1990. However, in studies where information with respect to the occupation of their parents is obtained from students at levels of schooling below the age of noncompulsory attendance, it is found that a simple 4-category classification: (a) professional and managerial, (b) clerical, (c) skilled blue-collar, and (d) semiskilled and unskilled worker, to which rank scaled scores of 4, 3, 2, and 1 respectively are assigned, yields just as strong relationships with educational outcomes as do more refined occupational status scales. The reason for these apparently anomalous results would appear to lie in the greater robustness of the classificatory scheme and a reduction in errors of misclassification. Generally, with a simple 4-category scale, missing data and nonresponse are best assigned to the scale value, 1 or 0, as determined by criterion scaling (Keeves 1992).

5.7 Sensitive Measures of Occupational Status

A 4-category scale is, however, of little value at levels beyond the age of compulsory schooling, because of the lack of discrimination of such a scale for father's occupation, mother's occupation, and expected occupation data. The Treiman international scale provides greater discrimination at the upper-secondary-school level and yields stronger relationships with other measures (Keeves 1992).

5.8 Differences in Relationships between Occupational Status and Achievement Outcomes in Developed and Developing Countries

The Six Subject Study conducted by the International Association for the Evaluation of Educational Achievement (IEA) in 1970–71 showed that the relationship between occupational status measures and achievement outcomes was generally greater in the more industrialized countries than in the less industrialized and developing countries (Walker 1976). Several reasons can be advanced which help to account for this difference. First, there is a lack of variance in the outcome measure in the developing countries, arising from the greater difficulty level and lower discriminating power of the tests used. Second, there is a lack of variance in the occupational status measures in the developing countries, arising from high proportions in the low-status categories and low proportions in the high-status categories. Third, there are effects of selection bias in the developing countries, with less able students from low-status homes either dropping out from school or being required to repeat grades (see *Selection Bias in Educational Research*). Fourth, there is the possibility that the occupational classification and the occupational status measure employed are conceptually inappropriate in the developing countries. Heyneman and Loxley (1983) have considered the confounding effects of selection bias and contend that this is not a plausible explanation. However, the other possible grounds for a reduced relationship remain.

5.9 Changes in the Magnitude of Relations between Measures of Social Background and Achievement Outcomes over Time

Keeves and Saha (1992) examined the magnitudes of the relationships between science achievement and measures of social background between 1970 and 1984. Data for large random samples from 10 countries were available for both occasions on a range of measures, which included father's occupation, father's education, mother's education, books in the home, use of dictionary in the home, and family size. While the measures on both occasions were similar, they were not in many cases identical. Marginally stronger relationships were recorded for 1984 than for 1970. It would appear possible that this is evidence that the effects of home background on educational achievement increased over this period of 14 years. Such a change would be consistent with the development of a more meritocratic society where education was becoming more important for the attainment of high social status. While the explanation of this stronger relationship recorded might lie in improved measurement and the use of slightly more meaningful questions, or in more variance in the outcome measure, the possibility of

greater inequalities over time in the societies being studied cannot be gainsaid.

However, Peterson (1982) contends that a marked drop in such relationships occurred in the United States in the late 1970s. Since most of the decline reported took place during a brief five-year period from 1973 to 1978, some doubt must exist regarding the quality of the samples used.

6. The Cultural Level of the Home

Floud (1961) has pointed out that the French have a phrase, *la famille éducogéne*, to describe families who provide an educative environment that reinforces the intellectual pressures exerted by the school. It is widely recognized that the educative climate of the home influences the intellectual development of the child not only during the years of schooling, but more particularly during the early years of childhood (Bloom 1964). Subsequently, Bloom (1976) argued that family background may be considered to involve three components, which are: (a) a cultural component such as the number of books in the home, visits to the theatre or museum, use of a public library; (b) a social component which comprises the parents' educational and occupational status; and (c) an economic component which refers to the family income and possessions.

In the IEA Six Subject Study in 1970–71, recognition of the cultural as well as the social component led to the development of an index of social background, which was based upon six measures: father's occupation, father's education, mother's education, use of the dictionary, number of books in the home, and family size. These six variables were weighted by criterion-scaling procedures using achievement on tests of science, reading, and word knowledge as criteria to form a composite measure assessing the sociocultural level of the home (Comber and Keeves 1973). Keeves (1972) had previously employed a similar index using five measures: family size, father's occupation, father's education, mother's occupation before marriage, and religious affiliation, combining the variables by principal components analysis. The incorporation of a scaled measure of religious affiliation led to the acceptance that the index developed involved a cultural rather than an economic emphasis. Likewise, the inclusion of mother's occupation before marriage was seen to be associated with the competence of the mother rather than being related to the contribution that she made to the total family income.

7. Educational Resources of the Home

Difficulties associated with measuring socioeconomic status, and general acceptance of the importance of the cultural level of the home, led the IEA Reading Literacy Study in 1991 to employ a variable concerned with reading resources of the home. The measures employed in the construction of this variable were: (a) number of books at home, (b) use of test language at home, and (c) home possessions (Postlethwaite and Ross 1992).

8. Conclusion

It should be noted that indexes of occupational status and socioeconomic status correlate positively and significantly with the educational outcomes of both achievement and attainment in cases where the school population has not been truncated by the removal of less able students. Even where the school population has been reduced or censored in this way these indexes are, in the main, positively related to educational outcomes. Research since the 1980s shows a clear tendency for indexes of sociocultural level to be more strongly related to educational outcomes than are indexes of occupational and socioeconomic status, and thus they have greater explanatory power. The evidence available strongly supports the contention that it is not the occupational status of the home per se that influences educational outcomes but rather the related sociocultural level of the home with its emphasis on reading and the use of language.

See also: Mobility Tables

References

Blishen B R 1958 The construction and use of an occupational scale. *Canadian J. Econ. Polit. Sci.* 24: 519–31
Blishen B R 1967 A socioeconomic index for occupations in Canada. *Canadian Rev. Soc. Anthropol.* 4: 41–53
Bloom B S 1964 *Stability and Change in Human Characteristics*. Wiley, New York
Bloom B S 1976 *Human Characteristics and School Learning*. McGraw Hill, New York
Broom L, Jones F L, Zubrzycki J 1965 An occupational classification of the Australian workforce. *Aus. N. Z. J. Sociol.* 1 (supplement)
Broom L, Duncan-Jones P, Jones F L, McDonnell P 1977 *Investigating Social Mobility*. Australian National University Press, Canberra
Coleman J S et al. 1966 *Equality of Educational Opportunity*, 2 vols. US Government Printing Office, Washington, DC
Comber L C, Keeves J P 1973 *Science Education in Nineteen Countries: An Empirical Study*. Wiley, New York
Congalton A A 1963 *Occupational Status in Australia*. University of New South Wales, School of Sociology, Kensington
Duncan O D 1961 A socioeconomic index for all occupations. In: Reiss A J (ed.) 1961 *Occupations and Social Status*. Free Press, New York
Edwards A 1938 *A Social-Economic Grouping of the Gainful Workers of the United States, Gainful Workers of 1930 in Social-Economic Groups, by Color, Nativity, Age, and Sex, and by Industry, with Comparative Statistics for 1920 and 1910*. GPO, Washington, DC
Elley W B, Irving J C 1972 A socioeconomic index for New Zealand based on levels of education and income from the 1966 Census. *N.Z. J Educ. Stud.* 7: 153–67
Erikson R, Goldthorpe J H, Portecarero L 1979 Intergenerational class mobility in three Western European societies: England, France and Sweden. *Br. J. Sociol.* 30(4): 415–41
Floud J 1961 Social class factors in educational achievement. In: Halsey A H (ed.) 1961 *Ability and Educational Opportunity*. OECD, Paris
Goldthorpe J H 1980 *Social Mobility and Class Structure in Modern Britain*. Clarendon Press, Oxford
Goldthorpe J H, Hope K 1974 *The Social Grading of Occupations: A New Approach and Scale*. Clarendon, Oxford
Hall J, Caradog Jones D 1950 Social grading of occupations. *Br. J. Sociol.* 1: 31–55
Haug M R 1977 Measurement in social stratification. *Ann. Rev. Sociol.* 3: 51–78
Heyneman S P, Loxley W A 1983 The effects of primary school quality on academic achievement across twenty-nine high- and low-income countries. *Am. J. Sociol.* 88(6): 1162–94
Husén T (ed.) 1967 *International Study of Achievement in Mathematics: A Comparison of Twelve Countries*. Almqvist and Wiksell, Stockholm
Jencks C S et al. 1972 *Inequality: A reassessment of the effect of family and schooling in America*. Basic Books, New York
Jones F L 1971 Occupational achievement in Australia and the United States: A comparative path analysis. *Am. J. Sociol.* 77: 527–39
Keeves J P 1972 *Educational Environment and Student Achievement*. Almqvist and Wiksell, Stockholm
Keeves J P (ed.) 1992 *The IEA Study of Science III. Changes in Science Education and Achievement. 1970–1984*. Pergamon, Oxford
Keeves J P, Saha L J 1992 Home background factors and educational outcomes. In: Keeves J P (ed.) 1992
Mason W M et al. 1976 Models of response error in student reports of parental socioeconomic characteristics. In: Sewell W M, Hauser R M, Featherman D L (eds.) 1976 *Schooling and Achievement in American Society*. Academic Press, New York
McRoberts H A 1985 Mobility and attainment in Canada: The effects of origin. In: Boyd M et al. 1985 *Ascription and Achievement*. Carleton University Press, Ottawa
Miller D C 1991 *Handbook of Research Design and Social Measurement*, 5th edn. Sage, Newbury Park, California
Nam C B, Powers M G 1968 Changes in relative status of workers in the United States, 1950–60. *Social Forces* 47: 158–70
Oppenheim A N 1966 *Questionnaire Design and Attitude Measurement*. Heinemann, London
Peterson P E 1982 Effect of credentials, connections, and competence on income. In: Kruskal W H (ed.) 1982 *The Social Sciences: Their Nature and Uses*. University of Chicago Press, Chicago, Illinois
Pineo P, Porter J 1967 Occupational prestige in Canada. *Canadian Rev. Sociol. Anthropol.* 4: 24–40
Postlethwaite T N, Ross K N 1992 *Effective Schools in Reading: Implications for Educational Planners*. IEA, Hamburg

Scott-Jones D 1984 Family influences on cognitive development and school achievement. *Rev. Res. Educ. II*: 259–304

Siegel P M 1971 Prestige in the American occupational structure. PhD thesis, University of Chicago

Treiman D J 1977 *Occupational Prestige in Comparative Perspective*. Academic Press, New York

Walker D A 1976 *The IEA Six Subject Survey: An Empirical Study of Education in Twenty-One Countries*. Almqvist and Wiksell, Stockholm

Warner W L, Meeker M, Eells K 1949 *Social Class in America: A Manual of Procedure for the Measurement of Social Status*. Science Research Associates, Chicago, Illinois

Models of Intelligence

J-E. Gustafsson

Research on models of intelligence has sought to determine the answers to two basic questions, namely: (a) how many dimensions are needed to describe individual differences in cognitive abilities? and (b) what are the interrelationships among the dimensions of ability? During the twentieth century these questions have been investigated by several groups of researchers, and several competing models of the structure of intelligence have been presented. Among these, one line of distinction separates models which postulate a general factor of intelligence (e.g., Burt 1949, Carroll 1993, Spearman 1904, Vernon 1961), from models which do not allow for a general factor (e.g., Cattell 1971, Gardner 1983, Guilford 1967, Thurstone 1938). Another line of distinction separates hierarchical models (e.g., Burt 1949, Carroll 1993, Horn and Cattell 1966, Vernon 1961, Sternberg 1985) from models in which all dimensions are ascribed equal generality (e.g., Gardner 1983, Guilford 1967, Thurstone 1938). Most of the models are based upon factor–analytic research, but some researchers prefer other methods of analysis.

It has proven difficult to secure evidence that firmly establishes one of these models as the superior one. This led Sternberg (1981) to conclude that the factor–analytic approach has " . . . failed because it has been too successful in supporting, or at least in failing to disconfirm, too many alternative models of intelligence" (p. 143). However, one purpose of the present entry is to present research conducted during the 1980s and 1990s which offers hope for a resolution of the problems of choice of model.

1. General Cognitive Ability

Building upon work conducted by Galton and Pearson in the late nineteenth century, Spearman (1904) suggested the first, rather crude, analytical techniques for investigating the rank of a matrix of correlations, and on the basis of empirical studies of several sets of variables, he concluded that "all branches of intellectual activity have in common one fundamental function (or

group of functions), whereas the remaining or specific elements of the activity seem in every case to be wholly different from that in all the others" (Spearman 1904 p. 284). These results were formalized in the two-factor theory of intelligence, which states that performance on a task is affected by two factors only, the g-factor, which is common to all tasks, and the s-factor which is unique to each task.

In his empirical work Spearman used small samples of variables and subjects and he often found a very good fit between the observational data and the model. But there were also deviations. For one thing it was in some cases found that the s-factors were correlated, thus giving rise to group factors. For another thing it was found that the model broke down when tests that were "too similar" were included in a battery of tests, again because of a correlation between the s-factors. These facts were readily admitted by Spearman, but they came to cause great problems for his theory when other researchers tested and rejected it.

At about the same time that Spearman published his first results on the two-factor theory, Binet and Simon (1905) published the first intelligence test. As is well-known, this test differed from previous mental tests in that it contained quite complex items, and in that it used a very varied set of items. This test proved to be most useful in practical applications, and it set a model for several generations of tests of general mental ability.

The contributions of Spearman and Binet appeared close in time so it might be thought that the Spearman model provided a theoretical basis for the Binet test. However, in spite of the fact that for both these researchers a single, general, mental ability was the focus of interest, the simultaneous appearance of their work seems to be a coincidence. They were in fact highly critical of one another: Binet did not approve of the statistical nature of Spearman's work, and Spearman argued that Binet's conception of the total score on the test as an average of several abilities was theoretically indefensible. Spearman sympathized, however, with the basic idea "of throwing many miscellaneous tests into a single pool" (Spearman 1927 p. 84) and he admitted that "Our *g* is, in fact, really obtained by this practice, with rough — much too rough — approximation" (Spearman 1927 p. 84).

The fundamental difference between the positions of Spearman and Binet is that while Spearman thought of *g* as a dimension of individual differences in its own right, Binet regarded general intelligence as being composed of several partly independent characteristics. Thus, Binet saw the test score as reflecting a mean of several different abilities while Spearman saw a test score as reflecting a unitary dimension. These two basic positions concerning the nature of general intelligence can be identified in many controversies within the field of intelligence.

Binet's work had the strongest impact on practice (Carroll 1982), however, and during the first decades of the twentieth century a large number of tests were developed. In parallel, statistical methods for test and item analysis were developed and the testing technique was accommodated to allow group testings as well. These early tests "employed a rather wide array and variety of tasks involving the understanding and manipulation of verbal and nonverbal materials and problems" (Carroll 1982 p. 36), but during the 1920s tests started to appear that purported to measure independent dimensions of ability (Carroll 1982 p. 35).

2. Primary Mental Abilities

It was not until improved factor–analytic techniques were available that viable multidimensional alternatives to Spearman's theory could be formulated. Through a generalization of the Spearman method, Thurstone extended factor analysis to encompass multiple common factors, and developed computational techniques which made it feasible to apply the method with large numbers of tests.

Thurstone (1938) applied multiple factor analysis to a test battery of 38 tests, many of which were newly developed, and found about a dozen factors, each of which accounted for performance on a subset of the factors in the battery. There was no sign of a general factor.

Most factors identified by Thurstone (1938) were replicated several times by Thurstone and his colleagues (e.g., Thurstone and Thurstone 1941) and it was possible to set up a list of six or seven easily replicable primary mental abilities (PMAs), such as: verbal comprehension (*V*), involved in understanding of language and frequently found in tests such as reading, verbal analogies, and vocabulary; word fluency (*W*), affecting the fluent production of language, and measurable by tests such as rhyming or naming words in a given category; induction (*I*), measured by tests requiring the subjects to find a rule in complex material; space (*S*), found in manipulation of geometric or spatial relations; perceptual speed (*P*), reflected in quick and accurate grasping of visual details; and

number (*N*), involved in quick and accurate arithmetic computations.

In further studies conducted during the 1940s and 1950s by Thurstone and others, the list of factorially identified primary abilities was considerably extended, partly by demonstrations that several of the original PMAs were differentiable into more narrow factors, and partly by extensions into new domains, such as perception, language, and number.

The influence of the multiple-factor approach on test construction and test use is clearly seen from about 1940 and onward, in that considerable numbers of "multifactor" batteries were published, such as the Differential Aptitude Test (DAT). These batteries contain homogeneous subtests to measure different specific abilities, and they yield profiles of scores, which may be used for purposes of diagnosis, guidance, and counseling, as well as for purposes of prediction and selection. Frequently, however, the subtest scores are also aggregated into subtotal and total scores, to represent broader areas of competence.

It would seem, however, that the multifactor batteries have not fared very well in evaluations of their power to provide differential prediction of achievements in areas that should require different profiles of abilities. On the basis of analyses of validity coefficients for the DAT and six other multitest batteries, McNemar (1964) concluded: "Aside from tests of numerical ability having differential value for predicting school grades in math, it seems safe to conclude that the worth of the multitest batteries as differential predictors of achievement in school has not been demonstrated" (p. 875). In a similar vein, Carroll (1982) speculated " . . . that a large part of whatever predictive validity the DAT and other multiple aptitude batteries have is attributable to an underlying general factor that enters into the various subtests . . ." (pp 83–84).

The rapid proliferation of mental abilities produced by Thurstone and his followers made it necessary to bring order to the multitude of factors, and from the 1950s onward much effort was devoted to this task. An example of this is the work by French and his colleagues (French 1951, French et al. 1963, Ekstrom et al. 1976) who reviewed the research, trying to determine which factors were distinct and cross-identified in several studies.

The Guilford (1967) "structure-of-intellect" (SI) model may be seen as another attempt to organize the factor–analytic findings, and to develop guidelines for further test development and research. In the SI model each test and factor is uniquely identified as a combination of levels on three facets (operations, content, and products). Guilford argued that each of the PMAs could be mapped onto the SI model, and that the model provides the guidelines necessary for constructing tests so that the other cells in the model may also be factorially identified. However, as a consequence of the assumption that the factors are orthogonal, the levels on all three facets must be identified, and a very large number of abilities must be assumed. Thus, instead of solving the problem of achieving a parsimonious description of abilities it would seem that the SI model has contributed further to the problem of proliferation of abilities.

3. The Hierarchical Approach

Ever since multiple factor analysis was invented by Thurstone it has been the dominating form of factor analysis, and it may be argued that this particular kind of factor analysis bears a large part of the responsibility for the proliferation of factors (Undheim 1981). However, yet another way to solve the problem of the multitude of factors is to allow the factors to be correlated, and then analyze the correlations among the factors with factor–analytic methods to obtain higher-order factors. Such higher-order analyses yield hierarchical models, in which factors at lower levels are subsumed under factors at higher levels. Thurstone and Thurstone (1941) conducted such an analysis of the intercorrelation among six PMAs and they did, indeed, find a general factor in the second-order analysis, which factor was most highly loaded by the *I*-factor (see *Factor Analysis*).

A more elaborate hierarchical model has been developed by Cattell and Horn (e.g., Cattell 1963, Horn 1968, Horn and Cattell 1966). The two dimensions of most central importance in this model are fluid intelligence (*Gf*) and crystallized intelligence (*Gc*), and the whole theory is often referred to as *Gf–Gc* theory. Both these dimensions reflect the capacity for abstraction, concept formation, and perception and eduction of relations. The *Gc* dimension, however, is thought to reflect individual differences associated with systematic influences of acculturation, and is central in tasks of a verbal–conceptual nature. The *Gf* dimension, in contrast, reflects effects of biological and neurological factors and factors such as incidental learning, and this dimension is most strongly shown in tasks that are new to the examinees.

In the early formulation of *Gf–Gc* theory Horn and Cattell (1966) identified some three or four additional second-order factors, such as a broad visual–spatial factor—general visualization (*Gv*)—and general speediness (*Gs*). In later research reported by Horn and colleagues (Horn and Stankov 1982) the list of second-order factors has, however, been considerably expanded, and a hierarchical model based on level of functions has been proposed. Cattell (1987) has likewise proposed an elaborate theory in hierarchical terms of the organization of abilities.

An elaborate hierarchical model based upon a most solid empirical foundation has recently been presented by Carroll (1993), who has assembled and reanalyzed almost all available matrices of correlations among tests of cognitive abilities. In the reanalyses Carroll relied upon modern forms of exploratory factor analysis and has conducted second- or third-order factor analysis followed by transformation with the Schmid–Leiman technique into an orthogonal model.

Results from reanalyses of almost 500 matrices of correlations were considered in Carroll's formulation of a "three-stratum theory" with factors of three degrees of generality: narrow, broad, and general. In this model the narrow factors at stratum I represent quite specialized abilities which largely correspond to PMAs.

The broad factors at stratum II represent moderately specialized abilities, several of which come close to the "second-order" abilities identified within the *Gf–Gc* model. Among the most well-known of these are *Gc* (or *2C* in Carroll's notation), *Gf* or *2F*, *Gv* or *2V*, and *Gs* or *2S*. The Carroll model also includes factors of general memory and learning (*2Y*), broad auditory perception (*2U*), broad retrieval ability (*2R*), and a more narrow speed factor labeled processing speed (*2T*).

At the highest level the three-stratum model also includes a general factor (*3G* in Carroll's notational system) which is general in the sense that it influences performance in each and every domain. This hierarchical model thus combines the perspective of those emphasizing several dimensions of ability with the perspective of those emphasizing one general cognitive ability.

While hierarchical models are of relatively recent origin in United States research, such models have had a strong position in the United Kingdom research following Spearman. One contributor of such a model is Burt (1949), who also made contributions to the development of factor analysis. The most influential model was, however, proposed by Vernon " . . . as a hypothetical integration of all the factorial investigations that have been carried out" (Vernon 1961 p 26).

In the Vernon model, factors of at least three degrees of generality are identified: the general factor, major group factors, and minor group factors. Among the major group factors Vernon distinguishes between verbal–numerical–educational (*v:ed*) and spatial–practical–mechanical–physical (*k:m*) ability. The *v:ed* factor subdivides into minor group factors, such as verbal and number factors and reading, spelling, linguistic, and clerical abilities, and also into fluency and divergent thinking abilities. The *k:m* factor subdivides too and this complex includes minor group factors such as perceptual, physical, psychomotor, spatial, and mechanical factors. At the level below the minor group factors the tests would be found but " . . . there is ample evidence to support the view that the group factors are almost infinitely subdivisible, depending only on the degree of detail to which the analysis is carried" (Vernon 1961 p. 26).

The Vernon model thus represents the most influential hierarchical model from the United Kingdom tradition of research while the Cattell–Horn and Carroll models represent the most elaborate and influential of the hierarchical models developed within United States research. There are obvious similarities between these models, but it may be noted that there is no group factor which corresponds to *Gf* in the Vernon model, and a stronger emphasis on the *g*-factor in the Vernon model.

One possible explanation for this is offered by results obtained in a series of studies in which competing hierarchical models were compared empirically (Gustafsson 1988, Undheim 1981). In these studies confirmatory higher-order factor–analytic techniques (LISREL, Jöreskog and Sörbom 1988) were used to test hypotheses about the arrangement of factors at different levels within a hierarchical model. The results supported a three-stratum organization of abilities close to that of the Carroll model. However, the studies also showed that there is a loading of unity of *Gf* on the *g*-factor, which implies that *Gf* is equivalent to the *g*-factor.

This latter result implies that *Gf* for reasons of parsimony should be lifted above, as it were, the other broad factors at stratum II, and that these other factors should be purged of their *g*-variance. This would leave, among other factors, a *Gc*-residual (*Gc'*) which seems to be more or less identical with the major group factor that Vernon labels *v:ed;* and it would leave a *Gv*-residual (*Gv'*) that is very similar indeed to the *k:m* factor in the Vernon model. Thus, the fact that *Gf* is identical with *g* in a sense resolves the conflict between the hierarchical models proposed by United Kingdom and United States theorists.

Since the hierarchical models include the PMAS identified in the Thurstone tradition as well, they in a sense unify several previous models that have been viewed as being quite incompatible. It must be stressed, though, that the *g*-factor identified within this model is quite different from what is obtained by most measures of general mental ability. While the former would be derived mainly from nonverbal reasoning tests, many IQ-tests have such a strong verbal bias that they should probably best be considered measures of *Gc*.

4. Alternative Taxonomic Structures

The models described so far have a strong association with a particular kind of factor analysis. However, taxonomies of abilities have also been developed on other empirical grounds than factor analysis. Three major theoretical frameworks will briefly be described: namely, Guttman's radex model; Sternberg's triarchic theory; and Gardner's theory of multiple intelligences.

4.1 The Radex Model

Multidimensional scaling takes test correlations to represent degree of similarity between the tests and constructs an *n*-dimensional space within which the tests are represented as a geometric configuration of points. Guttman (1965, 1970, Guttman and Levy 1991) formulated his "radex" (radial expansion of complexity) model partly through scaling analyses of some of the Thurstone data. The radex model involves two simultaneous orderings of tasks: one ordering according to complexity, which results in the correlational pattern known as the *simplex* pattern; and one ordering according to content, which results in the *circumplex* pattern of correlations. Guttman predicted that these patterns would combine in such a way that the less complex tests would fall closer to the center of a two-dimensional space and that the more complex tests would appear in the periphery. The content dimensions would appear as triangular areas containing, for example, verbal, figural, and numerical tests. Guttman (1965) found, however, that the less complex tests used in the Thurstone studies tended to appear toward the periphery, and that " . . . the radex seemed to represent a radial expansion of simplicity" (Snow et al. 1984 p. 58). This led Guttman to leave the notion of complexity in favor of a distinction between analytic versus achievement tests, or between rule-inferring versus rule-applying.

Guttman and Levy (1991) presented a three-dimensional model, which represents the latest version of the Guttman stuctural model. One of the dimensions represents the task requirements of the items ("inference," "application," and "learning") and another dimension represents the content of the stimulus material ("verbal," "numerical," and "geometrical"). The third dimension represents the mode of response involved in the item ("oral expression," "manual manipulation," "paper and pencil"). This three-facet model has obtained support in analyses of the WISC-R battery, but the empirical basis is as yet too limited to allow any definite conclusion about the validity of the model.

Complexity as a fundamental characteristic of tests has been focused upon in a series of studies by Snow et al. (1984), with results close to those achieved by Guttman. Their model yields a two-dimensional map of the set of tests. In the center of the radex map are complex tests (e.g., Raven, letter series, geometric analogies) which typically load on *I* and *Gf*. These tests are based upon different kinds of content but content differences seem unimportant in the complex problem-solving tasks included in these tests. However, the rest of the radex is divided into content areas (verbal, numerical, and figural) and within each content area the tests are ordered according to complexity. In the numerical domain, for example, tasks requiring application of arithmetic skills are closest to the periphery; tasks requiring more of problem solving are closer to the center; and closest to the center are highly complex tests such as arithmetic reasoning and number series. In the other content areas as well there are such progressions from less complex to more complex tasks.

4.2 Sternberg's Triarchic Theory

Sternberg (1985) has proposed a theory of intelligence which includes three subtheories: (a) a componential subtheory, which accounts for the mental mechanisms that underlie intelligent behavior; (b) a contextual subtheory, which deals with intelligence in its sociocultural context; and (c) an experiential subtheory, which specifies the situations and tasks in which intelligence is demonstrated.

The mental mechanisms that underlie intelligent performance can according to Sternberg be described in terms of three basic kinds of processing components: metacomponents, performance components, and knowledge acquisition components. Metacomponents are higher-order executive processes which plan, monitor, and evaluate the lower-order processes represented by the performance components. The number of performance components is quite large, and many, but not all, of these components are specific to narrow classes of tasks. The role of the knowledge acquisition components, finally, is to learn how the metacomponents and performance components will perform their tasks.

The experiential theory recognizes the importance of a person's previous experience of a task for the possibility of using that task in assessment of intelligence. The theory states that intelligence is best measured when the tasks or situations are either relatively novel, or in the process of becoming automatized. From the experiential theory Sternberg derives two domains of abilities: the ability to cope with novelty and the ability to automatize information processing. Tasks measuring ability to cope with novelty require the examinee to decide insightfully what information is relevant, how to put the information together, and how new information relates to old information.

The contextual subtheory argues that to understand intelligence one must also understand how thought is intelligently translated into action in different contextual settings. Thus, to test the practical aspects of intelligence everyday problems should be relied upon.

4.3 Gardner's Theory of Multiple Intelligences

Gardner (1983) has suggested a classification of abilities (or intelligences), which relies on many kinds of data on which a "subjective factor analysis" has been performed. The analysis establishes a set of criteria or "signs," as many as possible of which should be met, for distinguishing an independent intelligence. One important sign is potential isolation by brain damage, where neuropsychological evidence about consequences of lesions to a specific area of the brain is considered. The existence of idiots, savants, prodigies, and other exceptional individuals, with a highly uneven profile of abilities, may provide evidence for a particular intelligence. Other important criteria are an identifiable core operation or set of operations and a distinctive developmental history, along with a definable set of expert "end-state" performances. On the basis of an extensive review of literature from several different areas, such as developmental psychology, neuropsychology, and cross-cultural research, Gardner has proposed a list of seven intelligences.

(a) *Linguistic intelligence* includes the skills involved in reading, writing, listening, and talking. Poetry is the prime example of application of linguistic intelligence, because it involves sensitivity not only to the meaning of words but also to the order of words, to the sounds, rhythms, and inflections of words, and to different functions of language.

(b) *Logical-mathematical intelligence* enters, for example, mathematical and scientific thinking, solving logical puzzles, and in a wide range of situations met in everyday life which require analysis and judgment.

(c) *Spatial intelligence* affects the accurate perception of the visual world, transformations and modifications of initial perceptions, and recreation of visual experiences when the physical stimuli are no longer present. This intelligence is important in activities such as navigation, piloting a plane, drawing, and playing chess.

(d) *Musical intelligence* is involved in the production of music, such as singing, playing an instrument, composing, and to some extent, appreciating music.

(e) *Bodily-kinesthetic intelligence* enters into activities where the body, or different portions of it, are used, such as in dancing, athletics, acting, and surgery.

(f) *Interpersonal intelligence* is important in relations with other persons, and represents abilities to discern other persons' moods, temperaments, motivations, and intentions.

(g) *Intrapersonal intelligence*, finally, involves the ability to understand oneself, for example, to understand one's emotions and behave in ways that are appropriate to one's needs, goals, and abilities.

The theory of multiple intelligences is strongly biologically influenced and assumes, like other modular theories (e.g., Fodor 1983), the existence of independently working brain organizations. The intelligences are assumed to work in concert in the solution of a particular problem; a mathematical word problem thus involves both linguistic intelligence and logical–mathematical intelligence, and it may well involve the personal intelligences as well. However, Gardner assumes the intelligences to be independent in the sense that the level of performance achieved by one intelligence is not related to the level achieved by the other intelligences.

5. Discussion and Conclusion

The proliferation of models of intelligence has been regarded by many as a serious problem, and the difficulties involved in determining which model, if any, is the correct one have been lamented. It appears, however, that there is more reason to stress the similarities among the models than the differences. Some of the fundamental communalities among the models are discussed below.

5.1 Relations Among the Models of Intelligence

It has already been pointed out that the hierarchical models provide a framework for integrating factor-analytic models which to different degrees emphasize general and specific abilities, because the hierarchical models allow for both broad and narrow abilities. This holds in particular for those hierarchical models which operate with factors at three levels, such as the models proposed by Carroll, Gustafsson, and Vernon. In these models there is room for a general cognitive factor as proposed by Spearman, for PMAs as suggested by Thurstone, and for broad abilities of the kind demonstrated by Cattell and Horn. To the extent that the previous factor-analytic models have focused upon abilities at one or two levels only, they may be regarded as incomplete, but hardly as incorrect.

Snow et al. (1984) discussed relations between the radex model and the hierarchical factor model. They estimated the loadings of each test on the general factor, defined as the first principal factor, and showed that the factor loadings were almost perfectly related to the level of complexity of the tests, as defined by the multidimensional scaling. The content areas identified in the radex model are, of course, quite easy to identify with the broad abilities identified in the hierarchical factor model (i.e., verbal=Gc and figural=Gv). Thus, even though the representations are quite different mathematically and conceptually, a closer analysis shows the different models not only to be compatible at a general level, but also interconvertible.

The categories of abilities employed in the Sternberg theory overlap to a large extent with those employed in the other taxonomic systems. The content categories are the same as those employed by Guttman, and can thus easily be translated into dimensions in the factorial systems. Among the process categories the "componential" aspect of intelligence clearly coincides with Gf (or g). The other process categories are, however, not so easily "translated" into categories of the other taxonomic systems. This is because at least some of the tasks employed in the research are quite new, and empirical data are still lacking. It may be asked, however, to what extent the measures of ability

to cope with novelty, and the measures of the practical aspects of intelligence, are really distinguishable from Gf.

The seven intelligences proposed by Gardner represent domains of performance studied in previous work on individual differences even though some of them have been devoted less attention than others. Some of the intelligences thus seem to overlap almost perfectly with ability constructs within psychometric models. This is true for linguistic intelligence, which is very close to Gc (or $v{:}ed$) and the V-factor; and for spatial intelligence which is close to Gv (or $k{:}m$). Logical–mathematical intelligence overlaps to a large extent with Gf. Thus the Gardner intelligences seem largely compatible with the factorially identified abilities. A major difference, however, is that the "intelligences" are assumed to be uncorrelated. Gardner has suggested that the observed correlations among the psychometric abilities are due to the fact " ... that most tests of intelligence are paper-and-pencil exercises which rely heavily on linguistic and logical–mathematical abilities" (1983 p. 321). However, strong correlations are also observed for tests which are oral and manipulative (e.g., WISC and Stanford–Binet), and it also seems that linguistic and logical–mathematical abilities are highly correlated. It seems, furthermore, that Gardner is open to the possibility that logical–mathematical intelligence is important in construction and perception of analogies and metaphors which cut across different intellectual domains. Gardner (1983) thus argued that " ... it may be the particular hallmark of logical–mathematical intelligence to perceive patterns wherever they may be" (p. 290). However, if logical–mathematical intelligence is ascribed general capacities of pattern perception it implies that it must be as general an ability as is Gf and cause correlations between performances in different domains.

It thus seems that it is possible to establish logical and/or empirical relations between the hierarchical model of abilities and the other taxonomic systems. It must be stressed, however, that a considerable amount of research remains to be done until the details of the differences and similarities between the models of intelligence are understood.

5.2 Measurement of General and Specific Abilities

It is interesting to consider the implications of the hierarchical model for the measurement of intelligence. It has already been concluded that throughout the history of mental testing, measures have been obtained of a rather loosely defined general mental ability, either through use of IQ-tests of the Binet type, or through creation of composites of scores on homogeneous tests. Throughout most of the history of mental testing, specific abilities have been measured as well, as is done with the multifactor batteries. The hierarchical model includes both broad and narrow abilities, so both these practices would, in a general sense, be compatible with such a model of the structure of abilities. However, it would seem that the hierarchical model of abilities also carries much more far-reaching implications for the measurement of general and specific abilities, and in the remainder of this entry these implications are described in general and nontechnical terms.

From the hierarchical model it follows that the observed variance obtained on any test is due to a set of orthogonal factors of varying breadth. For example, of the variance in the scores on a spatial visualization (*Vz*) test 35 percent may be due to the *g*-factor; 15 percent to *Gv'* (the residual in *Gv* which remains after *g* has been partialled out), 15 percent to *Vz'* (the residual Visualization primary after *g* and *Gv'* have been partialled out), 15 percent to a test specific factor, and the remainder random error variance.

While the relative size of the contributions from these sources of variance may be influenced to a certain extent, it is quite inconceivable that any one of them could be brought up to 100 percent within a homogeneous test. This illustrates the fundamental principle that "no test measures a single factor" (Vernon 1961 p. 133). Each and every intellectual performance measure is affected by several sources of influence of different degrees of generality, and it is even theoretically impossible to achieve a truly univocal measure of a single specific ability.

From this line of reasoning it also follows that when the aim is to obtain measures of the broader abilities (i.e., g and the second-order abilities in the Cattell–Horn model) a single homogeneous test is unlikely to suffice, since the scores to a rather large extent will be influenced by narrow factors. The Raven Progressive Matrices Test is frequently cited as a good measure of the *g*-factor, and upon the suggestion of Spearman it was indeed constructed to be such a measure. However, studies indicate that only some 55 percent of the variance in this test is due to the *g*-factor, which for most theoretical and practical purposes is too low to be acceptable.

It would thus seem that the only way to estimate broad abilities is to combine information from several tests. Optimally this is done through an estimation procedure which takes into account the differential relationships between the tests and the broad abilities. Simple versions of such procedures were developed a long time ago (Spearman 1927), but they have only rarely been used in practical applications, and there is a need to develop such new procedures, which take advantage of the advances within the statistical and computational fields.

From the fact that any observed measure represents a composite of abilities it also follows that to identify uniquely a specific ability it is necessary to partial out the effects of the more general abilities. This in turn implies that even if only a certain specific ability is the focus of interest it is necessary to administer several tests, in order to allow estimation of the general and specific dimensions of ability.

In conclusion, then, the hierarchical model of ability supports the measurement of general mental ability as well as identification of specific abilities. However, in previous psychometric work it seems that general mental ability has been conceived of as a conglomerate or as an average of several more narrowly defined abilities, while in the hierarchical model the general factor is uniquely identified as an ability in its own right.

See also: Measurement in Educational Research

References

Binet A, Simon T 1905 Méthodes nouvelles pour le diagnostic du niveau intellectuel des anormaux. *L'Année Psychol.* 11: 191–244
Burt C L 1949 The structure of the mind: A review of the results of factor analysis. *Br. J. Educ. Psychol.* 19: 100–11, 176–99
Carroll J B 1982 The measurement of intelligence. In: Sternberg R J (ed.) 1982 *Handbook of Human Intelligence.* Cambridge University Press, Cambridge
Carroll J B 1993 *Human Cognitive Abilities.* Cambridge University Press, New York
Cattell R B 1963 Theory of fluid and crystallized intelligence: A critical experiment. *J. Educ. Psychol.* 54: 1–22
Cattell R B 1971 *Abilities: Their Structure, Growth and Action.* Houghton-Miffin, Boston, Massachusetts
Cattell R B 1987 *Intelligence: Its Structure, Growth and Action.* North Holland, Amsterdam
Ekstrom R B, French J W, Harman H H 1976 *Kit of Factor-referenced Cognitive Tests.* Educational Testing Service, Princeton, New Jersey
Fodor J A 1983 *The Modularity of Mind: An Essay on Faculty Psychology.* MIT Press, Cambridge, Massachusetts
French J W 1951 The description of aptitude and achievement tests in terms of rotated factors. *Psychometric Monographs* 5
French J W, Ekstrom R B, Price L A 1963 *Manual for Kit of Reference Tests for Cognitive Factors.* Educational Testing Service, Princeton, New Jersey
Gardner H 1983 *Frames of Mind: The Theory of Multiple Intelligences.* Basic Books, New York
Guilford J P 1967 *The Nature of Human Intelligence.* McGraw-Hill, New York
Gustafsson J-E 1988 Hierarchical models of the structure of cognitive abilities. In: Sternberg R J (ed.) 1988 *Advances in the Psychology of Human Intelligence*, Vol. 4. Erlbaum, Hillsdale, New Jersey
Guttman L 1965 A faceted definition of intelligence. *Stud. Psychol., Scripta Hierosolymitana.* 14: 166-81
Guttman L 1970 Integration of test design and analysis. In: *Proceedings of the 1969 Invitational Conference on Testing Problems.* Educational Testing Service, Princeton, New Jersey
Guttman L, Levy S 1991 Two structural laws for intelligence tests. *Intelligence* 15(1): 79–103
Horn J L 1968 Organization of abilities and the development of intelligence. *Psychol. Rev.* 75(3): 242–59
Horn J L, Cattell R B 1966 Refinement and test of the theory of fluid and crystallized intelligence. *J. Educ. Psychol.* 57(5): 253–70
Horn J L, Stankov L 1982 Auditory and visual factors of intelligence. *Intelligence* 6(2): 165–85

Jöreskog K G, Sörbom D 1988 LISREL 7. *A Guide to the Program and Applications*. SPSS, Chicago, Illinois

McNemar Q 1964 Lost: Our intelligence. Why? *Am. Psychol.* 19(12): 871–82

Snow R E, Kyllonen P C, Marshalek B 1984 The topography of ability and learning correlations. In: Sternberg R J (ed.) 1984 *Advances in the Psychology of Human Intelligence*, Vol. 2. Erlbaum, Hillsdale, New Jersey

Spearman C 1904 "General intelligence," objectively determined and measured. *Am. J. Psychol.* 15: 210–93

Spearman C 1927 *The Abilities of Man: Their Nature and Measurement*. Macmillan, London

Sternberg R J 1981 Nothing fails like success: The search for an intelligent paradigm for studying intelligence. *J. Educ. Psychol.* 73(2): 142–55

Sternberg R J 1985 *Beyond IQ: A Triarchic Theory of Human Intelligence*. Cambridge University Press, Cambridge

Thurstone L L 1938 Primary mental abilities. *Psychometric Monographs* 1

Thurstone L L, Thurstone T G 1941 Factorial studies of intelligence. *Psychometric Monographs* 2

Undheim J O 1981 On intelligence IV: Toward a restoration of general intelligence. *Scand. J. Psychol.* 22: 251–65

Vernon P E 1961 *The Structure of Human Abilities*, 2nd edn. Methuen, London

Personality Inventories

K. M. Miller and B. Tyler

A personality inventory is a paper-and-pencil method of measuring the personality characteristics of an individual. It is standardized, objectively scorable, and used, typically, in describing and comparing people, often with the purpose of predicting behavior in other situations. This entry considers the development of personality measures, the nature of the personality inventory, and problems of response set and validity in personality measurement. In addition, the entry describes the various types of personality inventories and lists the different personality inventories in widespread use. It concludes with a brief discussion of the use of personality inventories in the fields of education and educational research, and the conditions under which these inventories are used.

1. Development of Personality Measures

Early work in the measurement of personality tended to be clinically oriented (taking the form of a checklist of neurotic symptoms) and grew out of the need to identify individuals with emotional or mental problems—for example, screening out men unfit for war service during the First World War. Since those pioneering days, major developments have taken place, particularly from the early 1950s. Along with instruments intended specifically for the clinical field are others designed to have a wider application—measures concerned with the normal personality characteristics of normal people and providing a basis for a comprehensive description of the individual as a person. As the scope of the measures has broadened, so have their uses—for research, individual assessment, guidance, personal development and counseling, and in settings as varied as schools, public institutions, and industrial companies.

In the *Ninth Mental Measurements Yearbook*, a total of 329 personality measures (mainly questionnaires) were reviewed (Buros Institute 1985). There is currently significant research activity in the field of personality measurement—using a number of experimental measures—although, from data reported in the *Tenth* and *Eleventh Yearbooks*, there has not been a notable increase in published questionnaires.

2. Nature of the Personality Inventory

Many of the most widely used personality measures are in the form of inventories (see *Projective Testing Techniques*). These are essentially self-report questionnaires. They consist of lists of questions or statements on which respondents are asked to rate themselves by choosing alternatives on a given scale. The type of format varies. For example, in some inventories there is a forced choice between two alternatives:

"When you hear a good story, do you usually pass it on?" (*yes*) (*no*)

Sometimes a third "uncertain" alternative is allowed:

"I like to watch team games" (*yes*) (*occasionally*) (*no*)

In another, more complex format the instructions are to select from each set of four statements the one that is " *most like you*" (*M*) and the one that is " *least like you*" (*L*):

"prefers to get up early in the morning" (*M*) (*L*)
"doesn't care for popular music" (*M*) (*L*)
"has an excellent command of English" (*M*) (*L*)
"obtains a poorly balanced diet" (*M*) (*L*)

Whichever way the items are presented, the range of alternatives in any personality inventory is fixed. This is an essential requirement of an "objective" measure. Other conditions include standardized administration and instructions (making it possible for the inventory to be given in a group situation), a standard system of scoring, and normative data from an appropriate reference group which provide a basis for raw scores to be transformed into a standard form. Results are usually presented as a "profile" indicating where the individual stands (compared with the reference group) on a defined set of personality characteristics.

3. Response Set and Validity

Inevitably with a self-report questionnaire the possibility of motivational distortion arises (or, as it has been termed, "impression management"). The early clinical inventories were comprised of "face valid" items; that is, they asked obvious questions directly related to the characteristics or symptoms they were measuring. However, as the range of uses of personality measures broadened, it became evident that a person who, for example, may admit to neurotic anxiety when in the army, could be less inclined to do so when being assessed for suitability for a civilian job.

There is, in fact, research evidence to support the criticism that results can be distorted, from studies in which people were asked to adopt different "response sets" in answering an inventory. That some people may attempt to "fake good," and others to "fake bad" (e.g., a criminal pleading insanity) has led to the inclusion in some inventories of motivation distortion scales on which individuals trying to present themselves in a better (or worse) light tend to answer more items positively (or negatively) than people responding naturally. In any case, the probability of people answering questions untruthfully has probably been reduced by: (a) the move away from identifying clinical symptoms and toward measuring "normal" characteristics (although some people may still be motivated to appear more confident or more extroverted); and (b) new techniques in constructing inventories which enable the inclusion of items that do not have obvious "face" validity.

4. Types of Personality Inventories

The construction of the earliest personality inventories was based on content validity of the items—for example, by formulating questions directly from common neurotic symptoms reported in the psychiatric literature (as in Woodworth's Personal Data Sheet developed during the First World War). By definition, the items in this type of inventory are face valid. A nonclinical example of an inventory based on content validity is the Mooney Problem Check List, developed within an educational setting, the items being derived from such sources as counseling case records and statements of problems submitted by students.

Criterion-keyed inventories are constructed on an empirical basis, using the responses of contrasted groups (e.g., diagnosed "schizophrenics" vs. "normals"). This allows for the possibility of including in the questionnaire at least some items that are not face valid. The best-known example of this type of inventory is the clinically oriented Minnesota Multiphasic Personality Inventory, the scales for which are based on a standard taxonomy of psychiatric disorders. A later derivation of this instrument, the California Psychological Inventory, has been developed for use within "normal" populations.

Other inventories have used personality theories as the framework for construction. An example of this type is the Myers-Briggs Type Indicator, which is based on Jungian psychoanalytical theory.

The most rigorously empirical approach to personality measurement is based on factor analysis—a statistical technique for grouping items into relatively independent, identifiable clusters. Inventories constructed on this basis may differ from one another in two ways: (a) in identifying a small number of very complex dimensions (e.g., the Eysenck Personality Inventory) or a larger number of more unitary factors (e.g., Cattell 16 Personality Factor [16PF]); or (b) in measuring characteristics as "unipolar" dimensions, ranging from weak to strong manifestations of the particular trait (e.g., "sociability" in Gordon Personal Profile), or "bipolar" dimensions, ranging from an extreme at one end of a continuum to the opposite at the other end (e.g., "reserved" vs. "sociable" in the 16PF). Items on factorial inventories often have little or no obvious face validity.

Since the mid-1980s a trend that began in the 1960s has been growing in strength, toward the development of measures that identify a small number of broad, cross-situational variables. In particular, a five-factor classification (the "big five") has gathered support. There are several alternative models which have been used experimentally.

This approach was, in fact, foreshadowed in the mid-1950s by Cattell, who reported the existence of "second-stratum" factors or traits based on intercorrelations between the "primary" factors of the 16PF. Research during the 1960s in a number of countries (as wide ranging as Brazil, Germany, and Japan) confirmed the crosscultural application of these broader, composite traits.

For proponents of the "big five," however, the prime focus is on the five global domains established by factor analysis, although in developing a questionnaire for assessment purposes the domain scales have been broken down into a number of different "facets."

5. Some Personality Inventories in Current Use

5.1 Inventories Based Primarily on Content Validity

5.1.1 California Test of Personality (CTP; 1939, 1953)   This inventory is used with Grades kinder-

garten–3, 4–8, 7–10, and 9–14, and with adults. There are 15 measurable traits and its main application is in education—achievement and identification of problems. Over 500 research studies have been reported in the *Mental Measurements Yearbook*.

5.1.2 Mooney Problem Check List (MPCL; c.1941) This inventory is used with Grades 7–9, 9–12, 13–16, and with adults. Its main application has been in counseling, although its use has declined. In the *Mental Measurements Yearbook*, 276 research studies have been reported.

5.2 Criterion-keyed Inventories

5.2.1 Minnesota Multiphasic Personality Inventory (MMPI; 1943, 1990) This inventory is used for people aged 16 years and over. There are 10 clinical scales, 15 supplementary scales, 28 subscales, and 7 validity scales. It has been translated into over 40 languages; its main applications are clinical. For the first edition, over 5,000 research studies were reported in the *Eighth Mental Measurements Yearbook* (up to 1978; Buros Institute 1978). The *Eleventh Yearbook* notes a further 637 studies (Buros Institute 1992).

5.2.2 California Psychological Inventory (CPI; 1956, 1987) This is used for ages 13 years and upward. There are 20 scales, plus additional special purpose scales (e.g., "creative temperament") in the second edition. It has been translated into French, German, Italian, Spanish, and Dutch. It was partly derived from the MMPI for use with "normal" groups. Its main applications are occupational and educational—but it is also used in clinical assessment and prediction of delinquent behavior. In the *Mental Measurements Yearbook*, around 1,570 research studies have been reported, nearly 200 since around 1980.

5.2.3 Jesness Inventory (1962) This is used for disturbed children, adolescents aged 8–18 years, and adults. It measures 11 deviant characteristics; its main application is in predicting delinquent behavior and in the study and treatment of young offenders. A total of 32 research studies were recorded in the *Eighth Mental Measurements Yearbook* (Buros Institute 1978), but, although still available and used in relevant situations, it has not been reviewed since then.

5.3 Inventories Based on Personality Theories

5.3.1 Myers–Briggs Type Indicator (MBTI; 1943, 1989) This is used for Grades 9–16 and for adults. It measures four traits, which combine into 16 "personality types," and is based on the psychoanalytic theory of Jung. Its main applications are in education,

counseling, and occupational psychology. The *Mental Measurements Yearbook* reports over 400 research articles.

5.3.2 Edwards Personal Preference Schedule (EPPS; 1953) This is used with college-age students and with adults. It measures 15 traits and is based on Murray's theory of needs. Its main application is in occupational selection and guidance. The *Mental Measurements Yearbook* notes over 1,650 research articles.

5.3.3 Personality Research Form (Jackson; 1965, 1984) The range of use is Grade 6—college—adults. It is also based on Murray's theory of needs and has 15 dimensions, with 22 scores. There are over 400 research references in the *Mental Measurements Yearbook*.

5.4 Inventories Based on Factor Analysis

5.4.1 Guilford–Zimmerman Temperament Survey (GZTS; 1949, 1980) This is used with Grades 12–16 and with adults. It measures 10 factors, and German, Italian, and Dutch editions have been produced. Its main applications are in occupational selection, counseling, and career guidance. The *Mental Measurements Yearbook* notes 570 research articles—only a few being recent studies.

5.4.2 Sixteen Personality Factor Questionnaire (Cattell; 16PF; 1949, 1967, 1978, 1992) This is used with persons aged 16 years plus, and measures 16 factors (Motivational Distortion Scale for some forms). German, French, Spanish, Italian, and Brazilian editions have been produced. Main applications are in the occupational selection, career guidance, counseling, and clinical fields. The *Mental Measurements Yearbook* notes 1,582 research articles.

5.4.3 Junior–Senior High School Personality Questionnaire (Cattell; Jr–Sr HSPQ; 1953, 1967, 1989) This is used with persons aged 12–18 years, and measures 14 factors. Its main applications are in the educational and career guidance, and clinical fields. The *Mental Measurements Yearbook* notes 234 research articles, including 25 recent studies.

5.4.4 Children's Personality Questionnaire (Cattell; CPQ; 1959, 1975) This is used with children aged 8–12 years, and measures 14 factors. Its main applications are in educational and clinical assessment. The *Mental Measurements Yearbook* notes 133 research articles.

5.4.5 Early School Personality Questionnaire (Cattell; ESPQ; 1963) This is used with children aged 6–8 years, and measures 13 factors. Its main application is for teachers (with special training) and psychologists in schools or in a clinical setting, and tests are orally presented. The *Eighth Mental Measurements Yearbook* (Buros Institute 1978) reported 26 research studies.

5.4.6 Gordon Personal Profile and Inventory (GPPI; 1978)   This combines a version of the Gordon Personal Profile (GPP) of 1951, measuring four factors plus a composite "self-esteem" score, published together in one questionnaire with the Gordon Personal Inventory (GPI) of 1955, which also measures four factors. The questionnaires (now available in both separate and combined versions) are used with students (Grades 9–16) and adults—the main applications are in occupational, educational, and career guidance fields. The *Mental Measurements Yearbook* lists 226 research articles.

5.4.7 Maudsley Personality Inventory (Eysenck; MPI 1959)   This is suitable for college students and adults. It measures two factors, and its main applications are in guidance and clinical fields. In the *Eighth Mental Measurements Yearbook* (Buros Institute 1978) 668 research studies were reported but it had no mention in later volumes—being superseded by the Eysenck questionnaires.

5.4.8 Eysenck Personality Inventory (EPI; 1963, 1969)   A revised form of the EPI, it is used with Grades 9–16 and with adults. Two factors and a "lie scale" are incorporated in the design. Spanish, Italian, Japanese, and Serbo-Croat editions have been produced and its main applications are in occupational, guidance, counseling, and clinical fields. Over 1,050 research studies are reported in the *Mental Measurements Yearbook*.

5.4.9 Junior Eysenck Personality Inventory (JEPI; 1963)   This is used with children aged 7–15 years. As with the EPI, it measures two factors and has a "lie scale." Its main applications are in the educational and clinical fields. The *Mental Measurements Yearbook* reports 86 studies.

5.4.10 Eysenck Personality Questionnaire (EPQ; 1975)   This is a revised EPI (also still in print) and is used for ages 7–15 years, and 16 years plus. Three factors and a "lie scale" are features of its design. Its major application is clinical. The *Mental Measurements Yearbook* notes 188 research articles.

5.4.11 Comrey Personality Scale (1970)   This is for age 16 years and above. It has 10 scales and has general application. The *Mental Measurements Yearbook* reports 77 studies.

5.4.12 NEO-PI (1978, 1989)   This is based on one of the "big five" personality models and is designed for adults. It measures five global domain traits, for three of which there are six specific scales which measure facets within the domain. Developed as a device for assessing normal personality, its major use is in occupational and career counseling fields, with suggestions for applications in educational psychology and as a supplement to clinical diagnostic instruments. The *Mental Measurements Yearbook* reports 11 research studies.

5.4.13 Hogan Personality Inventory (1985)   This also embodies one of the "big five" models and is for age 18 years—adults. It is designed to obtain a broad general idea of personnel and social effectiveness, its major application being in the occupational field. It has been reviewed by the *Mental Measurements Yearbook* but no research articles have yet been reported.

6. Personality Inventories in the Educational Field

The self-report format and "normal" orientation of personality inventories measuring traits such as "sociability," "enthusiasm," "shyness," which people can recognize in themselves, makes them particularly appropriate and helpful in various aspects of guidance and counseling. On an individual basis, educational and clinical psychologists working with younger children may include an inventory as part of the assessment procedure in identifying educational, behavioral, or emotional problems, devising treatment procedures, and advising teachers and parents, and so on. With older children, adolescents, and college or university students, personality testing and "feedback" of results are likely to be an important aspect in educational and career guidance as well as in personal counseling.

In other applications the emphasis is on the group rather than the individual and personality inventories have been used, for example, to identify common problems for discussion or to stimulate personal insights in group counseling, social interaction, and sensitivity training.

7. Personality Inventories in Educational Research

With their comparative ease of group administration, their objective scoring methods, and their standard dimensions, it is not surprising that personality inventories have generated a vast amount of research in various parts of the world, covering a wide range of topics, including many related to the broad field of education. Of course, research plays a key role in the development and construction of any personality inventory, being the basis on which personal constructs or traits are postulated or identified, and the measure standardized in terms of the distribution within a given population.

While much of the applied research has been carried out in the United States, with a sizable contribution also from the United Kingdom and from other English-speaking countries, studies are also reported from countries in Europe, Asia (including India, Taiwan, and Japan), Africa, and the Middle East.

The following types of investigation using personality inventories provide some idea of the range of research topics:

(a) descriptive studies providing "profiles" of personality characteristics of selected groups from courses or disciplines as widely varied as science, religion, and acting;

(b) comparative studies investigating personality differences relating to specific variables such as different academic disciplines, sex differences, differences in cultural background (mainly within one country; e.g., American Whites, Blacks, Mexicans), athletic versus nonathletic students;

(c) studies relating personality to such variables as: (i) achievement, for example, general academic success, acquisition of specific skills such as reading, success in teacher training, cognitive problem solving, and adult education; (ii) performance under different teaching methods, for example, self-paced instruction, individualized instruction, computerized programmed learning; (iii) vocational choice; (iv) behavior aspects in school or college, for example, capacity to persevere and reasons for "dropout," disruptive behavior, and delinquency; (v) teacher variables, for example, general effectiveness in teaching, classroom management, preferences for different teaching styles; and (vi) locus of control—studies ranging from preschool and primary school children to college students;

(d) personality changes with training, for example, nursing training, T-group sensitivity training, and delinquency correctional programs.

8. Conditions for using Personality Inventories

All of the personality inventories mentioned above were developed by psychologists. In most instances, they are intended to be used by psychologists with training in general psychology, personality theory, and appropriate practical skills. Some are available to other professionals with a special interest, such as counseling, who have had training in the use of a personality inventory or who are working under the direct guidance of a qualified psychologist.

8.1 Implications of Computerized Testing

Computers have been introduced into personality measurement, as in other areas of psychometric testing. Computerized narrative reports, generated by computer from individual results, are offered for a number of the published personality inventories. These vary in complexity of interpretation, although (except in the case of very simply structured instruments) it is doubtful that a computer-generated report can bring out all the implications in the same way as a skilled and experienced user can. A computerized version of some personality inventories may be more readily obtainable without the qualifications or special training usually required. However, it is important that there are guidelines provided to assist a nonexpert reader to make appropriate use of the report, to appreciate its limitations, and to place the information in perspective.

Conditions under which specific instruments are available to nonpsychologists and the provision of training courses vary in different countries. Interested persons should contact the local test distributor or professional psychological association for information or, in countries where there are no appropriate local organizations, write for advice directly to the test publisher.

See also: Projective Testing; Vocational Interests and Aptitudes

References

Buros Institute 1978 *The Eighth Mental Measurements Yearbook*. Gryphon, Highland Park, New Jersey
Buros Institute 1985 *The Ninth Mental Measurements Yearbook*. Gryphon, Highland Park, New Jersey
Buros Institute 1989 *The Tenth Mental Measurements Yearbook*. Gryphon, Highland Park, New Jersey
Buros Institute 1992 *The Eleventh Mental Measurements Yearbook*. Gryphon, Highland Park, New Jersey

Further Reading

Anastasi A 1989 *Psychological Testing*, 6th edn. Macmillan Inc., New York
Cronbach L J 1990 *Essentials of Psychological Testing*, 5th edn. Harper and Row, New York

Practical Mathematics and Science Testing

K. C. Cheung

This entry examines modes of practical and performance assessment in mathematics and science, with emphasis on mathematical problem-solving and scientific inquiries, investigations, and explorations. Trends in school mathematics in problem-solving, assessment approaches, and the design principles employed will be presented first, followed by a similar discussion for science. The emergent trend in both subject fields in the 1990s goes beyond multiple-choice testing, and argues for an authentic and meaningful measurement of student performance. This trend agrees well with contemporary conceptions of testing validity.

1. Problem-solving in School Mathematics

First published in the 1940s, Polya's book *How to Solve It* became the Bible of mathematical problem-solving (Polya 1945). This book delineates four generic, recursive steps commonly used in mathematical problem-solving: (a) understanding the problem, (b) devising the plan, (c) carrying out the plan, and (d) reflection. Some processes and heuristic strategies described in the various editions are now commonly known as metacognitive decision-making (i.e., cognition about one's cognition). According to Polya, processes such as intuition, analogy, and reflective and inductive thinking are as important as formal deductive reasoning.

During the 1960s in the Soviet Union, a comprehensive structure of mathematical abilities was put forward by Krutetskii (Clements and Ellerton 1991). The different modes of assessment of the various types of problems were only made known to the English-speaking countries in the 1970s (Krutetskii 1976). During the same decade, mathematics educators in Western countries began to isolate pertinent process and context variables that influenced problem-solving behaviors. A notable finding is the situated (i.e., context-embedded) and generative (i.e., constructive and progressive) character of mathematical knowledge construction. As a result, problem-solving and the teaching of heuristic strategies within meaningful problem contexts became the main thrust of developments in school mathematics in the 1980s. See, for example, the *1980 Yearbook of the National Council of Teachers of Mathematics* in the United States (Krulik and Reys 1980) and the 1982 Cockcroft Report in the United Kingdom (Cockcroft 1982).

Toward the end of the 1980s there were new trends, moving beyond multiple-choice testing, arguing for an authentic and meaningful measurement of student performance. National guidelines were issued; see, for example, *Curriculum and Evaluation Standards for School Mathematics* in the United States (National Council of Teachers of Mathematics 1989) and *Mathematics for Ages 5 to 16* in the United Kingdom (United Kingdom Department of Education and Science 1988a). These statements sought to empower students to apply their mathematical knowledge and concepts, and to develop their abilities in problem-solving as well as their communication and reasoning skills.

Different types of problem have as a consequence been constructed for classroom assessment. They have included tasks that: (a) deploy different problem-solving approaches (e.g., routine exercises versus open-ended investigations set in mathematical or everyday contexts); (b) diagnose different levels of information processing (e.g., unistructural versus multistructural tasks as in Biggs and Collis's 1982 *Structure of Observed Learning Outcomes—The SOLO Taxonomy*); (c) adopt various ways of mathematical thinking (e.g., intuitive, reflective, inductive, and deductive thinking); (d) tap the various modes of cognitive functioning (e.g., iconic versus concrete–symbolic modes); and (e) utilize various types of mathematical knowledge (e.g., tacit, intuitive, and declarative knowledge). Problems may also be targeted at different stages of the problem-solving cycle; for example, problem-understanding, problem-representation, problem-execution, problem-control, and problem-evaluation (see Biggs and Collis 1991, Clements and Ellerton 1991).

Unfortunately, the teaching of problem-solving and investigation remains bedeviled by assessment difficulties. There are now developments around the world to explore the feasibility of (a) adopting criterion-referenced assessment and (b) constructing descriptive measurement scales (e.g., ILEA 1988). For example, through teacher assessment and moderation, grades are linked to descriptions of course performance and diagnostic information. One relatively unexplored question is whether students should model their problem-solving behaviors on the experts, or be taught explicitly in accordance with an effective problem-solving model. Another increasingly important area is finding means to encourage students to communicate in mathematics and talk about mathematics, particularly when they undertake open-ended investigative works in more abstract, unfamiliar problem contexts (Joffe and Foxman 1989).

2. Assessment Approaches in School Mathematics

2.1 Teaching Experiments

Influenced by Vygotsky, the Soviet researchers in the

latter half of the twentieth century have emphasized the assessment of qualitative aspects of thinking within students' "zone of proximal development." Their well-known teaching experiments, which involve combinations of pedagogical and assessment principles, probe for hunches on which to base instructional strategies for the various stages of mental development (Kantowski 1978). Within this approach, it is legitimate to give prompts during testing so that any learning that may occur in the testing situation can be observed. Unlike the Fisherian tradition of experimental design in the assessment of treatment effects, these Soviet teaching experiments are more dynamic in capturing processes as they are being formed while students are engaged in problem-solving within a social context. Furthermore, they are effective in determining optimal strategies for remediation in classroom or clinical settings. Observations, interviews, verbal and written protocols are qualitative data commonly used for the logical analyses undertaken.

2.2 The APU Assessment Framework

The practical mathematics surveys conducted by the Assessment of Performance Unit (APU) in the United Kingdom defined practical mathematics learning as mathematical knowledge gained through: (a) observations and investigations (e.g., discerning patterns and estimating quantities); (b) constructing diagrams and objects (e.g., drawing two-dimensional diagrams or building three-dimensional models); (c) concrete modeling of concepts and relationships (e.g., using square tiles and number rods to represent area and length concepts); and (d) engaging in practical situations and problem-solving in everyday life (e.g., journey planning using timetables and "best-buy" calculations using menus). Commonplace apparatuses such as dice, calculator, ruler, tape measure, protractor, compass, double pan balance, folding paper, perspex box, and mirror are used to assess number, geometry, measures, probability, and statistics concepts.

The dynamic character of the APU approach was akin to the teaching experiments described earlier, except that it was more structured for the purposes of assessment (Foxman 1987). Typically, all tasks were presented orally and students were requested to talk about the approaches, rules, and relationships involved, and the concepts and procedures deployed. The assessor's job was to observe and code the students' responses, give probes and offer help whenever necessary, and abandon a topic if the student was floundering. Thus, by adopting a communicative approach in a practical interactive setting, students' thinking processes and decision-making were externalized; conceptual and procedural deficiencies were exposed. By placing mathematical ideas in meaningful contexts, intuitive and tacit knowledge conducive to problem-solving might be tapped as well.

2.3 The SOLO Superitems

Another established way to assess mathematical problem-solving across a number of topic areas and grades is to construct superitems, each with four parts, with a common item stem targeted at the four levels of the SOLO Taxonomy (Collis and Romberg 1992). The four levels in order of progression within each mode of cognitive functioning are: (a) unistructural, (b) multistructural, (c) relational, and (d) extended abstract. Thus, the four parts constitute a cognitive learning cycle explainable in terms of some specified quality of cognitive processing. In school mathematics, the superitems generally tap the concrete–symbolic mode of cognitive functioning, although intermodal cognitive functioning such as the formal, iconic, and sensorimotor modes may be involved as well (Biggs and Collis 1991). Diagnosis and remedial work are then possible after students' responses are graded according to the SOLO levels and their attainment across topic areas determined.

2.4 Design Principles

Before constructivism became common in studies in the psychology of learning, the design of problem-solving tasks was more in line with the earlier paradigms, such as the Gestalt, associative learning, and the information-processing approaches then in vogue. Typical tasks included the matchsticks problems, Tower of Hanoi, anagram problems, jigsaw puzzles, and textbook word problems. In the 1980s an experimental approach to problem-solving was introduced, for the development of both inductive and deductive reasoning. This approach invites students to formulate appropriate rules or representation models of problem situations and apply these rules and models within boundary conditions to make decisions in particular instances in real-world settings, with due attention being paid to the nature of proof, logic, and axiomatic systems. These fundamental methods of mathematics, as espoused in the Fourth National Assessment of Educational Progress Objectives framework in the United States, cut across content areas and are argued to be central to the extension and development of mathematics and its use.

There are several important mathematics process skills worthy of practical testing (e.g., using simple measuring tools, reading tables and graphs, searching for patterns, generating hypotheses and rules, setting up mathematical models to represent situations, organizing information into tables and graphs, testing hypotheses, refining inductive rules, proving rules using logic and axiomatic systems, arguing alternatives, and communicating results). The problem contexts and investigative situations, which should be set within the students' prior mathematical experiences, involve conceptual understanding (e.g., using models, diagrams, and symbols to represent concepts) and procedural knowledge (e.g., using manipulatives and algorithms to perform operations). For younger children, storymaths, which is phrased in terms of suitably targeted language levels, may be used to promote communication skills, thinking, and problem-solving. For older children, the use of calculators is an important mathematical skill—apart from merely relieving them of the computational chores.

3. Practical Work in School Science

H E Armstrong's *heurism* was proposed in the United Kingdom at the beginning of the twentieth century (see van Praagh 1973). It is a method of science teaching that is conducted through experimental observation and deduction, with an emphasis on relating classroom activities to students' everyday and laboratory experiences. It endorses the view that learners should develop scientific mental habits and understand how discoveries are made through questioning and first-hand investigations. In the United States, Dewey believed that human understanding was related to students' actions. Hence, he eloquently advocated science learning by doing (see Dewey 1938). These two popular parallel versions of heurism, however, only developed slowly during the first half of the twentieth century. At that time, the science curriculum was very much content-based and practical work in the laboratory was mainly used as a means for the elucidation and verification of principles and laws. It was not until the late 1950s and early 1960s that waves of science curriculum reform were triggered off in Western countries (see Welch 1979). At this time, heurism again received attention.

During the 1960s and 1970s the Nuffield Foundation Science Teaching Project in the United Kingdom and SAPA (Science: A Process Approach) (see Walbesser 1968) in the United States were two exemplars of a new curriculum design. Both treated the teaching of science as inquiry and took the stance that "I do and I understand." At that time, two alternative presentations of school science were discernible: (a) as an inquiry (a process-led curriculum playing down content); (b) as a body of knowledge (a content-based curriculum playing down process skills). Because of the lack of knowledge of how learners acquire knowledge with understanding and how knowledge is constructed within a culture, this process–content dichotomy of science curriculum design and implementation led in science teaching to a serious distortion of the nature of science and its historical development as they were presented to students.

During this same period, it was common to find that school practical work was of the recipe format, seriously distorting the guiding model of a "scientist in action" into guided discovery or stage-managed heurism (Woolnough and Allsop 1985). These practices were far removed from personal discovery as espoused by Armstrong. Toward the end of the 1970s,

reviews of the goals of science education in terms of personal needs, societal issues, academic and career preparation were actively underway. The importance of the school laboratory was questioned and the appropriateness of inquiry as a focus was examined (Blosser 1981). What was found was that practical assessment was by and large neglected by the teachers, although there were some occasional attempts by science educational research workers to assess manipulative skills, such as experimental techniques and procedures, manual dexterity, and orderliness (e.g., Eglen and Kempa 1974).

The research work of the Assessment of Performance Unit throughout the early 1980s in the United Kingdom regarded students as problem-solving scientists, who should be actively inquiring, speculating, constructing, and testing knowledge in personally relevant and meaningful contexts (Cheung and Taylor 1991). Their work has illustrated the close interplay between science concepts and methods in knowledge acquisition and production. The revised 1985 science curriculum directives in the United Kingdom, *Science 5–16: A Statement of Policy* (United Kingdom Department of Education and Science 1988b) sought to realize this vision of learners as problem-solving scientists. It recommended that school science should provide opportunities for the students to make observations, deploy scientific methods, and apply science concepts to test explanations to phenomena observed, and to plan and conduct investigations in both scientific and everyday contexts. Whether methods of science can be explicitly taught or not and whether investigative tasks should be assessed holistically or in their parts remain controversial issues which need further critical analysis.

4. Assessment Approaches in School Science

4.1 The APU Assessment Framework

The assessment of practical work in science needs to delineate the interdependence of science process component skills (e.g., measuring length and time), integrative investigative skills (e.g., observation and inference making), and the general problem-solving strategies (e.g., formulating and evaluating problems). The well-researched APU Science Assessment framework defined a number of skill categories essential for the successful conduct of investigations (United Kingdom Department of Education and Science 1985). In particular, performance in the entire investigation was included as a separate category to assess how students orchestrated their process skills and deployed science concepts, prior experiences, and tacit knowledge. This was to avoid the decontextualization of process skills from the problem context and a reductionist or atomistic view of scientific inquiry. The problems investigated were drawn from an everyday or social setting and were amenable to a variety of formulations and a hypothetico–deductive mode of scientific inquiry. The aim was to initiate students into scientists' codified ways of doing science and to develop habits of applying or reworking key scientific ideas in everyday lives.

There were a variety of assessment modes, including written, individual practical, and group practical, and tasks were arranged in a circus format, where students moved from station to station. The six main categories in this framework were: (a) use of symbolic representation, (b) use of apparatus and measuring instruments, (c) observation, (d) interpretation and application, (e) planning of investigations, and (f) performance of investigations. A decade of research enabled the APU to develop a computerized item bank of appropriate tasks. The items in each category were accompanied with detailed marking schemes and national norms for the purpose of monitoring the performance of 11-, 13-, and 15-year old students in the United Kingdom. Lists of relevant science concepts at these three age levels were also delineated for the construction of assessment tasks.

The APU used checklists, written accounts, and interviews as its three basic modes of practical assessment. First, observation checklists were used to record students' activities during their investigations. The checkpoints served to document all the viable routes through the various stages of the problem-solving cycle. Therefore, performance levels were determined by reference to particular sequences and combinations of checkpoints involved in the various solution paths. Second, students' own written accounts were studied to see how they: (a) perceived a problem posed to them; (b) generated questions for investigation; (c) reformulated a problem that was open for investigation; (d) planned and set up experimental conditions; (e) carried out the plan using laboratory apparatus; (f) recorded measurements and observations; (g) organized data as graphs, tables, and charts; (h) interpreted results; and (i) applied science concepts to draw conclusions. In some cases, their evaluation of experimental design and the techniques they employed were also noted. In order that the criteria of practical performance could be made explicit, students were cued either fully or partially for the production of the written accounts. Finally, interviews were conducted to ascertain students' prior knowledge, mental models, and perspectives in order to understand the reasons behind their deployment of the science processes observed and recorded.

4.2 The SISS Assessment Framework

Before embarking on a science process skills survey in six countries, the Second Science Study (SISS) of the International Association for the Evaluation of Educational Achievement (IEA) considered a number of common approaches to practical testing; namely, teacher's continuous assessment, evaluation of stu-

dents' laboratory reports and project work, paper and pencil process tests, and a practical examination. In the First IEA Science Study the assessment of process skills was attempted through both a practical skills test and pencil-and-paper practical test items (Comber and Keeves 1973). However, because the APU had demonstrated how important it was to go to the trouble of assessing actual performance in investigations, the SISS framework focused solely on the practical examination, which measured a unique mode of performance (i.e., tapping both the cognitive and psychomotor domains), which is to a large extent distinct from the paper-and-pencil practical test items (i.e., neglecting the psychomotor domain) as were employed in the First IEA Science Study.

Again, a circus format similar to that used by the APU was adopted. Three process categories of practical work were assessed: (a) performance (e.g., observing, measuring, manipulating); (b) investigating (e.g., planning and design of experiments); and (c) reasoning (e.g., interpreting data, formulating generalizations, and building and revising models).

Since the blueprints of SISS science tests were consistent with Klopfer's (1971) science learning classification scheme, it was necessary that these process categories should match this scheme. Specifically, performance refers to the observation of objects and phenomena, description of observation, measurement of objects and changes, and skills in using common laboratory equipment. Second, investigating involves the selection of suitable tests of a hypothesis, and design of appropriate procedures for performing experiments. Last, reasoning focuses on the processing of experimental data, interpretation of experimental data and observations, and evaluation of a hypothesis under test in the light of data obtained. Practical assessment tasks with components pertaining to each of the three process categories were constructed, embracing some of the listed constituent process skills. One assessment task in the area of biology was to determine which seeds contained oil by rubbing them on paper. Another in the area of physics asked the student to use a spring scale and graduated cylinder to determine the density of a lead sinker. Detailed scoring guidelines with specified levels of performance linked with the score earned were arrived at through a consensus procedure. A plan for training the scorers was also instituted (Doran and Tamir 1992).

4.3 Design Principles

Similar to what has been discussed in the construction of mathematical problems and investigative tasks, a constructivist model of learning can likewise be used to inform the design of science assessment tasks (Cheung and Taylor 1991). Specifically, a task is designed to provide for the acquisition of certain sets of competencies and to cue selective access to the knowledge base by students. Their performance is assessed in terms of the following abilities: (a) to cope with tasks of different degrees of procedural and conceptual complexity (e.g., controlling variables in order to establish treatment effects); (b) to handle tasks requiring different problem-solving approaches (e.g., adopting a quantitative approach even though a problem is framed in an everyday context); and (c) to deploy prior alternative conceptions (e.g., challenging children's naive conceptions of animals and living things, such as the idea that a worm is not an animal). As a general guide, better quality learning outcomes are those that are associated with the more progressively differentiated, but more integrated, knowledge schemes.

Thus, a good task encourages: (a) science process component skills (e.g., identifying dependent or independent or control variables); (b) integrative process skills (e.g., carrying out observations and measurements); and (c) general problem-solving skills (e.g., evaluating design and techniques when blocked), to be called upon for inquiring, speculating, testing, and constructing knowledge. The aim is to initiate students into scientific practice and doing science. Furthermore, attention should be paid to the various claims made by students, which are informative about what they value, believe, or feel, and about how they perceive the way the world works. Hopefully, these claims can be analyzed in terms of the students' specific mental habits and prior conceptions.

During the 1980s there was in science education a worldwide trend to relate science to technology, the environment, and society. There was also an emergent call for a self-sustainable Earth. Again, in line with the guiding philosophy of viewing students as problem-solving scientists, investigative tasks were developed not merely for the purpose of illustrating science concepts and the rehearsal of experimental skills, but to engage students in applying science in their daily living and in resolving societal issues and concerns. In this way, science concepts and skills could be seen as needed resources for dealing with personally relevant problems. From this perspective, assessment would not be focused upon conceptual and procedural knowledge alone, but would be extended to include science applications, attitudes, creative and reflective thinking, and metacognitive decision-making.

5. Emergent Issues and Research Directions

The resolution of the dilemma between an assessment-led curriculum and curriculum-led assessment leads to an argument for authentic measurement and a call for a relatively long-term direct assessment of performance with due attention paid to the intrinsic educational values and meanings of learning tasks. This call necessitates a revision of the evidence needed for a consideration of testing validity, which covers both meaningful score interpretation and relevant test use (Messick 1989). Apart from a clearer explication of meanings of assessment and test measures, value implications and social consequences of practical testing are also essential considerations. Such concerns have been incorporated above when recommending an appropriate design of assessment tasks. This author advocates inculcating in students the idea that human knowledge is both personally and socially constructed.

The identification and examination of alternative conceptions, progressive development of concepts, component process skills, problem-solving, and investigative skills are now the targets of psychometric modeling. Under the rubric of "meaningful measurement," a fruitful line of research marrying cognitive science and psychometrics is now underway (Cheung 1995). For example, meaningful measurement must be defined as quantitative measurement of conceptual and procedural knowledge with qualitative interpretations that should be firmly rooted in a theory of knowing, a model for understanding learning difficulties, classroom realities, and educational objectives as specified in the program of study. The theory of knowing being referred to is a multisource, constructivist information-processing theory of knowing. This ideal, to quantify cognitive processing whenever possible, if realized, would allow cognitive hierarchies to be modeled with the resulting knowledge schemes rich in explainable cognitive and affective processing features, such as attributions, beliefs, values, attitudes, emotions, and metacognitive decision-making. Meaningful measurement is also directed toward obtaining valid test measures, because test validation in essence is scientific inquiry into score meaning—nothing more, but also nothing less (Messick 1989). The ultimate aim of meaningful measurement is to overcome learning difficulties and to promote effective intellectual development in students.

References

Biggs J B, Collis K F 1982 *Evaluating the Quality of Learning: The SOLO Taxonomy.* Academic Press, New York

Biggs J B, Collis K F 1991 Multimodal learning and the quality of intelligent behavior. In: Rowe H (ed.) 1991 *Intelligence: Reconceptualization and Measurement.* Erlbaum, Hillsdale, New Jersey

Blosser P E 1981 *A Critical Review of the Role of the Laboratory in Science Teaching.* ERIC Clearinghouse for Science, Mathematics, and Environmental Education, Columbus, Ohio (ED 206445)

Cheung K C, Taylor R 1991 Towards a humanistic constructivist model of science learning: Changing perspectives and research implications. *J. Curric. Stud.* 23(1): 21–40

Cheung K C 1995 On Meaningful Measurement: Issues of reliability and validity from a humanistic constructivist information-processing perspective. *Educ. Res. Eval.* (1):90–107

Clements M A, Ellerton N F 1991 *Polya, Krutetskii and the Restaurant Problem—Reflection on Problem Solving in School Mathematics.* Deakin University, Victoria

Cockcroft W H 1982 *Mathematics Counts: Report of Committee of Inquiry into the Teaching of Mathematics in Schools.* HMSO, London

Collis K F, Romberg T A 1992 *Collis–Romberg Mathematical Problem Solving Profiles.* Australian Council for Educational Research, Hawthorn

Comber L C, Keeves J P 1973 *Science Education in Nineteen Countries: An Empirical Study.* Wiley, New York

Dewey J 1938 *Experience and Education.* Macmillan, New York

Doran R L, Tamir P (eds.) 1992 Practical skills testing. *Stud. Educ. Eval.* 18(3): 263–406

Eglen J R, Kempa R F 1974 Assessing manipulative skills in practical chemistry. *Sch. Sci. Rev.* 56(195): 261–73

Foxman D 1987 *Assessing Practical Mathematics in Secondary Schools.* NFER-NELSON, London

Inner London Education Authority (ILEA) 1988 *Graded Assessment in Mathematics.* Macmillan, Basingstoke

Joffe L, Foxman D 1989 *Communicating Mathematical Ideas: A Practical Interactive Approach at Ages 11 and 15.* HMSO, London

Kantowski M G 1978 The teaching experiment and Soviet studies of problem solving. In: Hatfield L L (ed.) 1978 *Mathematical Problem Solving.* ERIC Information Analysis Center for Science, Mathematics, and Environment Education, Columbus, Ohio, (ED 156446)

Klopfer L E 1971 Evaluation of learning in science. In: Bloom B S, Hastings J T, Madaus G F (eds.) 1971 *Handbook on Formative and Summative Evaluation of Student Learning.* McGraw-Hill, New York

Krulik S, Reys R E (eds.) 1980 *Problem Solving in School Mathematics—1980 Yearbook of the National Council of Teachers of Mathematics.* NCTM, Reston, Virginia

Krutetskii V A 1976 *The Psychology of Mathematical Abilities in Schoolchildren.* University of Chicago Press, Chicago, Illinois

Messick S 1989 Validity. In: Linn R L (ed.) 1989 *Educational Measurement*, 3rd edn. Macmillan Inc., New York

National Council of Teachers of Mathematics 1989 *Curriculum and Evaluation Standards for School Mathematics.* NCTM, Reston, Virginia

Polya G 1945 *How to Solve It: A New Aspect of Mathematical Methods.* Princeton University Press, Princeton, New Jersey

United Kingdom Department of Education and Science 1985 *Practical Testing at Ages 11, 13 and 15: APU Science Report for Teachers No. 6.* ASE, Hatfield

United Kingdom Department of Education and Science 1988a *Mathematics for Ages 5 to 16.* HMSO, London

United Kingdom Department of Education and Science 1988b *Science 5–16: A Statement of Policy.* HMSO, London

van Praagh G 1973 *H. E. Armstrong and Science Education.* Murray, London

Walbesser H H Jr 1968 *Science: A Process Approach.* AAAS, Washington, DC

Welch W W 1979 Twenty years of science curriculum development: A look back. *Rev. Res. Educ.* 7

Woolnough B E, Allsop T 1985 *Practical Work in Science.* Cambridge University Press, Cambridge

Further Reading

American Association for the Advancement of Science (AAAS) 1989 *Science for All Americans.* AAAS, Washington, DC

National Research Council 1990 *Renewing U.S. Mathematics: A Plan for the 1990s.* National Academy Press, Washington, DC

Christofi C 1988 *Assessment and Profiling in Science.* Cassell, London

Kempa R 1986 *Assessment in Science.* Cambridge University Press, Cambridge,

Mathematical Sciences Education Board, National Research Council 1990 *Reshaping School Mathematics: A Philosophy and Framework for Curriculum.* National Academy Press, Washington, DC

National Research Council 1989 *Everybody Counts: A Report to the Nation on the Future of Mathematics Education.* Mathematical Sciences Education Board, Washington, DC

Projective Testing Techniques

J. J. Walsh

Projective techniques, while not generally considered as psychometric instruments, are widely used principally in clinical settings for descriptive and diagnostic purposes in the study of personality and adjustment. They make use of a wide variety of symbolic, pictorial, verbal, and expressive stimuli to elicit responses which are scored and interpreted by specially trained examiners. These responses are considered to be indicators of covert, latent, or unconscious aspects of personality which are not revealed by answers to self-report inventories.

The concept of projection which is inherent in these techniques refers to the process of unwittingly attributing one's own drives, needs, perceptions, attitudes, and style to others, or of giving meaning to relatively ambiguous or unstructured stimuli by drawing upon one's private desires, traits, fears, and experience. Most projective techniques are disguised tests in which the examinee is seldom aware of the psychological interpretation which will be attached to the responses.

Since the subject does not perceive the responses as revelatory of self they can be relatively free of distortion or personal censorship, and can provide data about personality dynamics of which the respondent may be unaware. Central in the theory underlying these techniques is the belief that when someone is required to interpret an unstructured or ambiguous stimulus the person draws upon those impulses, needs, conflicts, and other psychological characteristics which are dominant in that personality, and that the quality of those variables can be determined from the responses by a competent projective tester. Most of these techniques utilize psychoanalytic and organismic concepts in developing a description of the whole personality and of the interrelationships among its various aspects.

Several bases for classifying the wide array of techniques which are subsumed under the rubric of "projectives" have been proposed. One scheme (Frank 1948) differentiated the techniques on the basis of "what they require or seek to evoke from the subject." The five categories of techniques identified are: (a) constitutive, which require the imposition of a structure on some relatively unstructured material such as ink blots, modeling clay, or finger painting supplies; (b) constructive, which require the arrangement of materials such as blocks or tiles into some pattern, or which require the drawing of some specified form; (c) interpretive, which require the subject to find personal meaning in stimuli such as pictures or words; (d) cathartic which require an acting out of expressive and emotional reactions in fantasy situations such as playing with dolls; and (e) refractive, which evoke idiosyncratic variation in tasks such as handwriting. Another fivefold categorization (Lindzey 1961) utilizes the following classifications with some typical examples included: (a) association techniques —Rorschach or word association; (b) construction techniques—Thematic Apperception Test; (c) completion techniques—sentence completion, Rosenweig Picture Frustration; (d) choice or ordering techniques —Szondi, Picture Arrangement Test; and (e) expressive techniques—psychodrama, painting.

The most widely used and best-known projective technique was developed by a Swiss psychiatrist, Hermann Rorschach, who published an account of his method in 1921. In this technique the subject is asked to tell what is seen in each of 10 inkblots printed on $5\frac{1}{2} \times 9\frac{1}{2}$-inch white cards and presented in a prescribed sequence. The blots, which vary in shape and color (black, gray, red, and pastels), elicit a vast range of responses. There are no time limits, and no definite number of responses to each card is required. In current clinical practice the Rorschach is used with subjects from nursery-school age to adults. Verbatim records of responses, as well as notations for reaction time, total time per card, positions in which cards are held, emotional reactions and behavior, are made by the examiner. Following the presentation of the 10 cards the examiner conducts an inquiry in order to ascertain what elements or aspects of the blots were utilized by the subject in making responses, and to

allow for clarification of or additions to the original responses.

As the purpose of Rorschach testing shifted from diagnostic classification of subjects to an understanding of their psychodynamics, many modifications in the scoring system were introduced. Two of these (Klopfer and Kelly 1942) and (Beck 1949) are the most frequently used.

The first step in the interpretation of Rorschach responses is the calculation of the subject's scores in three categories which are referred to as location, determinants, and content. Location scores are based on the area of the blot (whole or part) which was used in formulating the response. In this category responses are classified as whole, cut-off whole, or confabulatory whole, and responses to parts of the blots are sorted into categories such as large usual, small usual, and unusual detail, or space, when a response is based on the white area of a card. Scores for the determinants category reflect the extent to which responses are based on the form, color, or perceived movement in the blots. Color responses are subdivided to allow for differentiation of responses based on shading, texture, achromatic color, and chiaroscuro responses. The content category aspects which are generally scored include human, animal, object, and abstract responses. Content responses are also frequently classified as popular or original responses, based on the relative frequency of the response in various tabulations. Additional analysis involves a comparative study of the number of responses in the various scoring categories, of the ratios of combinations of categories, and of rather complex interrelationships among categories.

While the scoring procedure is relatively systematic and objective, the interpretation of the scores and the development of the global description of the subject is necessarily qualitative and clinical. Typically, for example, emphasis on wholes is interpreted as being a characteristic of subjects with a high level of ability for conceptualization and abstraction, while responses emphasizing details are regarded as indicative of plodding, unoriginal mental processes. A preponderance of form-color responses perceived as wholes is considered as evidence of emotional control and social adaptability, while pure color responses are seen as evidence of emotional impulsiveness. Responses involving movement when combined with responses to color are viewed as evidence of creativity and a rich imaginative life, while movement responses without color reference suggest internal emotional control with a low level of effect in interpersonal relations. In developing the description of the subject's personality structure the examiner is required to integrate all the information yielded by the Rorschach protocol with all the data which are available from other sources, such as personal history, other test scores, and clinical interviews.

Many researchers have raised serious questions about the validity and the reliability of the Rorschach technique and the hypotheses which underlie its interpretation. One of the best evaluations of available evidence (Goldfried et al. 1971) concludes that this technique has its greatest validity when used as a measure of cognitive and perceptual modes, and is least satisfactory when responses are treated as fantasy productions amenable to psychoanalytic interpretation.

Some modifications of the standard Rorschach technique have substituted group administration for individual testing, and multiple-choice format instead of open-ended response. In these procedures the blots may be shown on a slide projector, standard sets of cards may be given to all subjects, or special booklets containing reproductions of the blots and the listing of choices from which responses are to be selected may be used. These modifications have not been widely adopted principally because of the loss of spontaneity in response due to the forced choice format, and the impossibility of carrying out the inquiry phase of the standard Rorschach procedure.

The Holtzman Inkblot Technique (HIT), which was published in 1961, is an effort to use blots in an approach which conforms to the technical standards for psychometric instruments. Two parallel sets of 45 cards are available for use, with a single response given to each, and scoring is completely objective. Scores on 22 variables are interpreted in terms of percentile norms which are provided for various age and clinical groups. Machine scoring and computer-generated interpretation are available options.

The Thematic Apperception Test (TAT), developed by Murray and the staff of the Harvard Psychological Clinic, is a different type of widely used projective technique. The test material consists of 30 picture cards and one blank card. Some of the pictures are appropriate for use with all subjects, but others are used with only particular age or sex groups. In the original description of the technique the use of 20 pictures administered in two sessions was recommended, but in recent practice only 10 to 14 cards are generally used. The subject is instructed to make up a story about each picture by telling what led up to the depicted scene, what is happening, what are the thoughts and feelings of the people involved, and what is the outcome of the situation. No time limits are imposed, and verbatim record of the story and of time gaps, gestures, irrelevant remarks, questions, and so on is made by the examiner.

The interpretation of the stories rests on content analysis, with the nature of the analysis varying as a function of the purpose of the testing and the psychological orientation of the examiner. Murray's scheme emphasized the identification of "needs"—forces emanating from the "hero," the character with whom the subject has identified, and of "press"—forces deriving from the environment. Examples of needs are achievement, affiliation, and aggression. Danger, criticism, and deprivation are illustrations of press. In another scheme areas such as mental approach,

imaginative processes, family dynamics, emotional reaction, and sexual adjustment may be employed as the framework for the content analysis. Sometimes the analysis may be limited to a single dimension, as in studies of achievement motivation. Regardless of whether the clinician's purpose in administering the Thematic Apperception Test is broad or limited, the material elicited by this technique is more useful for acquiring knowledge of the content of the subject's thoughts and fantasies than for understanding the personality structure or problem-solving style.

Because only two of the cards in the Thematic Apperception Test material were specifically intended for use with children, a number of additional thematic techniques have been developed for use with subjects who may be as young as 3 years of age. The most commonly used test for children between the ages of 3 and 10 is Bellak's Children's Apperception Test (CAT). The test material consists of 10 cards with animal figures in various situations, with the representation of the animals ranging from complete naturalness to total anthropomorphism. The procedures for administration are similar to those of the Thematic Apperception Test. The pictures are intended to arouse fantasies which will be useful in understanding a child's relation to important life figures, and the dynamics of the youngster's approach to such childhood experiences as feeding, oral problems generally, sibling rivalry, toilet training, aggression, and fear of loneliness. An analysis sheet which provides space for a summary of the responses in terms of 11 variables which are considered important is normally completed as an aid in preparing the interpretive report.

Bellak's assumption that children identify more readily with animals than with people was challenged by a number of researchers whose findings indicated that children's responses to human figures yielded more and richer clinical material. In 1966 the Bellaks published a modification known as CAT-H, in which human figures replaced the animal drawings, and which was recommended for use with children whose mental age is at least 10 years.

Another Thematic Apperception Test derivative which makes use of animal figures is known as the Blacky Pictures. The material consists of 11 cartoon-type drawings of Blacky—a small dog described as either male or female to agree with the sex of the subject—Blacky's parents, and a sibling named Tippy who is of unspecified sex. While the use of dogs might suggest that the test is intended for use only with children, it was developed with adults and is used with subjects from 5 years to adulthood. The content of each of the 11 cards is derived from the psychoanalytic theory of psychosexual development. Subjects respond to the cards in three ways: by telling a spontaneous story, by responding to six multiple-choice (open-ended for children) questions for each card, and by sorting the cards into "like" and "dislike" piles, with the best liked and most disliked cards being identified. The 11 variables which are of primary concern in this technique are: oral eroticism, oral sadism, anal sadism, oedipal intensity, masturbation guilt, castration anxiety (males) or penis envy (females), positive identification, sibling rivalry, guilt feelings, positive ego ideal, and love object.

Two projective techniques which make use of verbal stimuli are word association tests and sentence completion tests. Free association to words has been used by psychologists since at least 1879, when Galton reported on its use in some of his studies. Jung made use of the technique in studies designed to test Freud's theory of repression beginning about 1906. His list consisted of 100 words selected as representative of common emotional problems. It was administered by saying each word, and asking the subject to reply promptly with the first word that came to mind. The reply to each stimulus word was recorded and note was made of all unusual verbal or behavioral reactions which accompanied any response. The responses and their accompanying characteristics were then analyzed in order to identify emotional problems which were inferred from the types of stimulus words that triggered psychologically significant responses.

The first formal word association list (Kent and Rosanoff 1910) consisted of 100 stimulus words which are neutral in character and which tend to evoke similar responses from normal subjects. The Kent–Rosanoff Free Association Test is scored objectively and is interpreted on the basis of norms for the proportion of common or individual responses for various subgroups. It is used primarily as a psychiatric screening procedure. The 60-word list developed by Rapaport (Rapaport et al. 1946) consists only of nouns, many of which have significance in the psychosexual area. The purpose of the Rapaport technique is twofold: to discover impairment of thought processes and to identify significant conflict areas.

Sentence completion tests require the subject to add words, usually in writing, to a sentence stem in order to produce a complete sentence, which is often indicative of a belief, attitude, or some other residual of one's experience. Examples of such stems are: I get nervous when . . ., I would be much better if . . ., My mother . . . . While the systematic use of this technique for personality assessment dates from the late 1920s and early 1930s, the experience of American military psychologists during the Second World War served to thrust it forward as a useful clinical and research instrument in the postwar years. The technique possesses very great flexibility, and the content and structure of the stems can be varied in order to maximize the possibility of eliciting responses which are relevant to whatever particular aspect of personality is of interest. Many applications of this technique involve the construction by the researcher or clinician of stems which are germane to some immediate purpose. But a number of standardized instruments have been developed and they are the most frequently used. The prototypical

sentence completion test is generally considered to be the one developed by Rohde and Hildreth in 1940, and many of their items have been incorporated in subsequently developed instruments.

The Rotter Incomplete Sentences Blank was designed for use with college students. It consists of 40 stems to be completed in such a way as to express the subject's "real feelings." Responses are rated on a 7-point scale depending on the level of adjustment suggested by the completion, and a composite score is recommended for screening purposes. Quite a different use of the technique is exemplified by the Washington University Sentence Completion Test. This, used primarily with adult women, is designed to provide a measure of ego development based upon a conceptualization of a 7-stage process. The scoring procedure is elaborate and formalized and requires extensive practice.

One important methodological issue in the use of sentence completion tests involves the person reference, that is, first or third person, which is used in the stem. Some research has been reported showing that stems which include first person pronouns have little value as projective techniques since they are essentially self-report items, but that responses to stems containing third-person references can tap covert or latent reactions (Getzels and Walsh 1958), qualifying them as projective instruments.

A wide variety of projective techniques provides the subject with an opportunity for relatively free nonverbal self-expression. Drawing and finger painting tasks are prominent examples. While originally used as an indicator of children's intellectual capacity, the task of drawing a person has evolved into a projective technique because emotional and nonintellectual factors are reflected in the drawings. In Machover's Draw-a-person Test the subject is given paper and pencil and is asked to draw a person. When that task is completed the examinee is instructed to draw another person, this time of the opposite sex of that represented in the first drawing. The examiner notes the subject's comments and procedures while drawing, and then conducts an inquiry in which the subject is asked to make up a story about each person drawn. The analysis of the drawings takes into account such characteristics as relative size of male and female figures, placement on the page, midline emphasis, front or side view, proportions, and erasures. Significance is attached to the qualities of major parts of the body. A global personality description is developed from the analysis of the elements of the drawings. A similar technique requires the subject to draw a house, tree, and person, in that order (Buck 1948). The analysis focuses on characteristics of the drawing of the person, with the other two drawings serving principally as benchmarks.

The projective hypothesis, that significant aspects of personality and important attributes of an individual's private world can be discovered by analyzing the responses the person makes to ambiguous or affect-oriented stimuli, has spawned the development of a very wide variety of assessment techniques. The diversity in the nature of the tasks, in the purposes for which they are used and in the types of inferences which are drawn from the responses makes it impossible to reach any firm generalizations about the validity of these techniques as a class. They are the source of much controversy; they have enthusiastic users and supporters, but also caustic and unrelenting critics. They will continue to be used by clinicians who find them useful, but the projective hypothesis and the techniques associated with it are still being tested.

See also: Attitudes, Measurement of

References

Beck S J 1949 *Rorschach's Test: Basic Processes*, Vol. 1, 2nd edn. Grune and Stratton, New York

Buck J N 1948 The H-T-P technique: A qualitative and quantitative scoring method. *J. Clin. Psychol. Monogr.* 5

Frank L K 1948 *Projective Methods*. Thomas, Springfield, Illinois

Getzels J W, Walsh J J 1958 The method of paired direct and projective questionnaires in the study of attitude structure and socialization. *Psychol. Monogr.* 72(1) (whole no. 454)

Goldfried M R, Stricker G, Weiner I B 1971 *Rorschach Handbook of Clinical and Research Application*. Prentice-Hall, Englewood Cliffs, New Jersey

Kent G H, Rosanoff A J 1910 A study of association in insanity. *Am. J. Insanity* 67: 37–96, 317–90

Klopfer B, Kelly D M 1942 *The Rorschach Technique: A Manual for Projective Method of Personality Diagnosis*. World Books, New York

Lindzey G 1961 *Projective Techniques and Cross-cultural Research*. Appleton-Century-Crofts, New York

Rapaport D, Gill M, Schafer R 1946 *Diagnostic Psychological Testing: The Theory, Statistical Evaluation and Diagnostic Application of a Battery of Tests*. Yearbook, Chicago, Illinois

Further Reading

Bell J E 1948 *Projective Techniques*. Longmans Green, New York

Cronbach L J 1970 *Essentials of Psychological Testing*, 3rd edn. Harper and Row, New York

Holtzman W H, Thorpe J S, Swartz J D, Heron E W 1961 *Inkblot Perception and Personality: Holtzman Inkblot Technique*. University of Texas Press, Austin, Texas

Murstein B I 1963 *Theory and Research in Projective Techniques, Emphasizing the TAT*. Wiley, New York

Oppenheim A N 1992 *Questionnaire Design, Interviewing and Attitude Measurement*. Pinter, London

Rabin A I 1968 *Projective Techniques in Personality Assessment: A Modern Introduction*. Springer, New York

Rorschach H 1932 *Psychodiagnostik: Methodik und Ergebuisse eines Wahrnehmungsdiagnostischen Experiments*, 2nd edn. Huber, Bern

Semeonoff B 1976 *Projective Techniques*. Wiley, London

Rating Scales

R. M. Wolf

Rating scales are paper and pencil devices that are used to describe and appraise human performances or products. They are widely used in education, psychology, business, and industry for a variety of purposes. While no accurate usage figures are available, it is believed that rating scales may be the second-most widely used measurement procedure, exceeded only by teacher-made achievement tests. However, teacher-made tests, other than those simply scored right or wrong, involve the use of rating scales since student responses are typically rated on a numerical scale, in which the number of scale points is customarily the weight to be given to a question in the calculation of a total score on a test.

Most commonly, a rating scale consists of a number of trait names, perhaps somewhat further defined, and a number of categories that are used to represent varying degrees of attributes or traits. A rater is called upon to rate one or more persons or objects on attributes or traits by assigning a number, letter, adjective, or description that is judged to fit best. Rating scales were developed initially to overcome the extreme subjectivity of unstructured statements where there was a lack of a common core of content or standard of reference from person to person. Teachers and other people also face extraordinary difficulties in quantifying information produced by subjective and unstructured procedures. Rating scales attempt to overcome these deficiencies by obtaining descriptions on a common set of attributes for all raters and ratees and to have these expressed on a common scale.

This entry considers the types of rating scales that are employed in the practice of education and in educational research, the techniques used to anchor the scale categories, the research findings on the number of scale steps or categories which might be employed, the assigning of scale values to the response categories, the use of summated scales, and the reliability of such scales. In addition, the entry discusses the types of error that can occur in the use of rating scales, the analysis of errors, the training of raters and the adjustment of scale values for differences between raters. Furthermore, it considers the techniques employed in the use of ratings in data analysis and the procedures employed to compensate for missing data.

With increased emphasis in educational measurement on the use of performance measures, and the partial rejection of the widespread use of multiple choice tests, where commonly only two categories (right or wrong) are considered, the issues addressed in this entry are of marked importance in educational practice.

1. Types of Rating Scale

Guilford (1954) identified the broad categories of rating-scale types, namely, standard scales, numerical scales, graphical scales, and forced choice scales. In addition, scale items could be combined to form summated or cumulative scales. Since the issues associated with the summation of scale values differ in kind from those associated with the assigning of an appropriate single scale value, summated scales are considered separately below.

1.1 Standard Scales

In a standard scale, the response categories are defined by a verbal description or an example of a product that provides a standard. Initially, responses are simply assigned to a category, and the scaling of the categories becomes a separate issue.

1.2 Numerical Scales

In a numerical scale, an attribute or set of attributes is defined, and ordered categories, with associated scale values assigned in rank order, are employed.

1.3 Graphical Scales

In a graphical scale, which is sometimes referred to as a "visual analogue" scale, a number line is used to represent the numerical scale, indicating that there is a continuous underlying distribution. However, the graphical scale is commonly subdivided into discrete numerical categories to simplify the scoring procedures employed.

1.4 Forced Choice Ratings

The forced choice rating procedure has been developed where there are a number of attributes and where the degree or extent of possession of an attribute is difficult to determine. Thus, the response required involves simply an assessment of the presence or absence of an attribute. Alternatively, forced choice

ratings can be employed where a comparison can be made between two people or situations. It is subsequently necessary to combine the responses obtained for two or more attributes associated with an underlying trait or attribute.

One major problem in the use of these different types of rating scales is the anchoring of the scale categories (for examples, see Figs. 1, 2, and 3).

2. Anchoring of Scale Categories

The idea of a scale implies an ordering of the ratings obtained. Thus it is not only necessary to define the attribute or set of attributes under consideration, but it is also necessary to anchor the response categories to that attribute or set of attributes. Anchoring procedures relate, in part, to the type of scale employed. It is, however, important to view the anchoring procedure as distinct from both the type of scale and the nature of the attribute which must be identified and defined. Five techniques of anchoring are widely used (Nunnally 1978).

2.1 Percentage Anchoring

In the anchoring of the response categories by means of percentages, objectivity is sought by referring to the frequency of incidence of the attribute. Since a percentage scale is censored or truncated on 0 percent and 100 percent, and responses cannot be considered to be normally distributed outside the 30 to 70 percent

---

A professor rating an applicant for a fellowship is instructed to rate each candidate according to the following scale:

    Falls in the top 2 percent of students at his level of training.
    In top 10 percent, but not in top 2 percent.
    In top 25 percent, but not in top 10 percent.
    In top half, but not in top 25 percent.
    In lower half of students at his level of training.

Figure 1
Numerical scale
Source: Thorndike and Hagen 1977

Responsibility for completing work

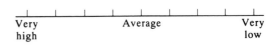

Figure 2
Graphical scale
Source: Thorndike and Hagen 1977

range, stanine scale values, or other appropriate procedures for collapsing the percentage points are commonly employed.

2.2 Agree–Disagree Anchoring

Degrees of agreement or disagreement are widely used. Such scales are, in general, readily understood where a favorable or unfavorable response is possible. There are, however, some problems associated with a "central" category, insofar as a respondent may be "undecided" and not wish to assess level of agreement or disagreement, or may hold a "neutral" position or view. This procedure is employed in Likert-type attitude scales and in descriptive scales (see *Attitudes, Measurement of; Descriptive Scales for Measuring Educational Climate*).

2.3 Bipolar Adjective Anchoring

The attribute may be considered in terms of a range of response categories which are anchored by means of bipolar adjectives. This procedure is employed in a "semantic differential scale" (see *Attitudes, Measurement of*).

2.4 Behavior Anchoring

In this type of anchoring, a specific description of behavior is provided for each response category. While there are advantages for accuracy and consistency of rating from using a specific description of behavior, it is frequently difficult to find easily specified and discrete forms of behavior that are related to a more general trait.

2.5 Product Anchoring

In this type of anchoring, an example of performance is provided that specifies the standard associated with each scale category. The choice of an example can be made by expert judgment or by consensus. It is, however, necessary for the characteristics of the attribute

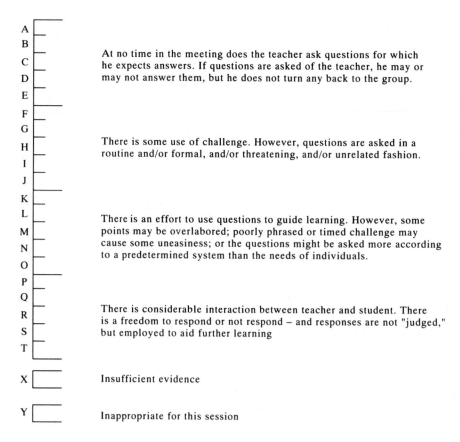

Use of "challenge"

A no time in the meeting does the teacher ask questions for which he expects answers. If questions are asked of the teacher, he may or may not answer them, but he does not turn any back to the group.

There is some use of challenge. However, questions are asked in a routine and/or formal, and/or threatening, and/or unrelated fashion.

There is an effort to use questions to guide learning. However, some points may be overlabored; poorly phrased or timed challenge may cause some uneasiness; or the questions might be asked more according to a predetermined system than the needs of individuals.

There is considerable interaction between teacher and student. There is a freedom to respond or not respond – and responses are not "judged," but employed to aid further learning

Insufficient evidence

Inappropriate for this session

Figure 3
Graphical score
Source: Jason 1962b

or set of attributes to be specified in an appropriate example so that a judgment can be made.

It is seen that the different types of anchoring which are employed are in general associated with one or more different types of scales. Thus, behavior and product anchoring relate, in general, to standard scales. Bipolar anchoring commonly relates to a graphical scale, and percentage and agree–disagree anchoring relate to numerical scales. However, variations are not uncommon.

3. Assigning of Scale Values

As the word "scale" in the title of this entry implies, ratings must be assigned to responses according to some rule involving the ordering of the attribute or set of attributes under survey. Whether the scale is a standard, numerical, or graphical scale, responses are generally obtained in categories, and while numbers are associated with the different categories for a numerical or graphical scale, it cannot be taken for granted that the numbers involve measurement along an interval scale. Several different procedures are available for assigning appropriate numbers to the different response categories in order to produce a scale.

3.1 Rank Scale Scores

The simplest scaling procedure assumes that the response categories are ordered and rank scale scores are assigned according to the rank ordering of the categories. Such a procedure is often surprisingly effective for detecting a relationship between a characteristic and a criterion measure, such as level of secondary schooling attained by a parent and the educational achievement of a child.

3.2 Criterion Scaling

In circumstances where there is no, or very limited natural ordering of categories, such as location of residence of student (inner-city, suburban, country town, rural), the categories of response may be criterion-scaled. Two types of criterion scaling are used.

3.2.1 Mean criterion scaling In this type of scaling, the group associated with each category is assigned a scale value that is equal to the mean score on a criterion measure for the group, as obtained from a one-way analysis of variance. Thus, by criterion scaling, the categorical variable involving multiple categories is replaced by a single variable which maximizes the bivariate relationship between the criterion dependent variable and the categorical variable as a predictor. There is a further advantage in this procedure. If there are missing data, such data can be considered to be an additional group in the formation of the categorical variable (Beaton 1969, Pedhazur and Kerlinger 1982).

3.2.2 Regression adjusted criterion scaling In this type of criterion scaling, the criterion variable is regressed on each of the categories associated with the categorical variable which is to be scaled (but with one category omitted or set as a dummy variable) together with one or more other strong predictor variables. The regression weights for each of the categories are then used to combine the groups associated with each category (with the dummy category assigned a zero weight) to form a categorical variable. This procedure maximizes the relationship between the criterion variable and the categorical variable so formed, after other strong predictor variables have been included in the regression equation (Peaker 1975).

3.3 Latent Variable Formation

Path-analytic procedures such as partial least-squares path analysis permit the categories associated with a categorical variable to be combined by an inward mode, equivalent to the use of regression weights, provided the weights for one category (the dummy category) are set at zero by excluding that category in the formation of the latent variable. The use of the inward mode serves to maximize the predictive power of the categorized data available. Once again missing data can be treated effectively by their inclusion as a separate category in the analysis. Generally, the inward mode is the most effective predictive procedure for combining and scaling categorized data (see *Path Analysis with Latent Variables*).

3.4 Item Response Theory (IRT) Methods

In another important development, IRT models have been employed to handle polytomous data associated with a categorical variable. Two general approaches have been advanced. With the rating scale model (see *Rating Scale Analysis*) where two or more items are combined, the differences in scale values between categories are considered to be identical across items. With the partial credit model (see *Partial Credit Model*) where two or more items are combined, the scale categories for each item are considered to differ in their locations along the combined rating scale so formed.

These procedures extend the employment of IRT methods to polytomous data, such as might be obtained from the use of rating scales. Both models assume a single underlying dimension for the variable and seek to scale the data in such a way that interval scale data are obtained for the variable so formed.

4. Summated Rating Scales

The use of single items involving a rating scale, while of value, must be considered inadequate if it is possible to employ multiple items. Multiple items have the advantages of: (a) greater reliability of the scale so formed, (b) greater precision of an individual's scale score, and (c) greater generality, because a construct with greater scope and validity can be assessed rather than a highly specific construct as indicated by an individual item. It is not essential that the rating scales that are summed should be identical in structure. It is, however, important that they should be associated with a single underlying dimension. The existence of a single dimension is usually tested using principal components analysis, after the assigning of scale values to the categories of the items. If more than one underlying dimension is expected across the items in a scale, then factor analytic procedures may be used (see *Factor Analysis*).

The reliability of a summated rating scale, where the items are assigned equal weights, is given by coefficient α (Cronbach 1951)

$$\alpha = \frac{n}{n-1} \left(1 - \frac{\sum_{i=1}^{n} s_i^2}{s_x^2} \right)$$

where n is the number of items, s_i^2 is the variance of item i, and s_x^2 is the variance of the scale x.

If, however, principal component scores are employed, the reliability is given by the Kaiser–Caffrey coefficient α (Kaiser and Caffrey 1965)

$$\alpha = \frac{n}{n-1} \left(\frac{\lambda - 1}{\lambda} \right)$$

where λ is the eigenvalue of the first principal component.

Increasing the number of items in a summated scale has the effect of increasing the reliability of the scale in accordance with the Spearman–Brown formula.

$$r_{t_n t_n} = \frac{n r_{tt}}{1 + (n-1) r_{tt}}$$

where $rt_n t_n$ = reliability of a test with n times as many items, and r_{tt} = reliability of original test.

However, increasing the number of items has a much smaller effect on the validity of a test (Gulliksen 1950) since:

$$r_{nc} = r_{tc} \sqrt{\frac{rt_n t_n}{r_{tt}}}$$

where r_{tc} = original test-criterion correlation, r_{nc} = lengthened test-criterion correlation, and r_{tt} and $rt_n t_n$ are as defined above.

It is seen that the increase in the validity is given by the square root of the increase in the reliability.

The reliability of a summated scale can be increased in two ways. First, as shown above, an increase in the number of items employed increases scale reliability. Second, increasing the number of response categories also generally increases scale reliability.

5. Number of Scale Categories

In the construction of a rating scale, an important choice has to be made regarding the number of scale categories that are employed. The range in the number of scale categories employed in practice is from 2 to 20. The greater the number of categories, the greater the discrimination involved and the more information that must be provided for effective anchoring. There is, however, a limit to the validity of the discriminations that can be made by respondents, and consideration must be given to the types of errors that arise in the use of rating scales. Gains can be made by increasing the detail provided for anchoring, and by training respondents. Generally the reliability of a rating scale increases as the number of categories increases from 2 to 20, with a rapid initial gain in reliability as the number of categories increases. However, the reliability tends to level off after 7 categories, because consistency in responding would seem likely to decline where there are many scale categories. Moreover, while the error variance increases as the number of scale categories increases, the true score variance increases at an even greater rate and the reliability tends to increase as the number of scale categories increases (Guilford 1954, Nunnally 1978). As a consequence, there is no fixed rule on the number of scale categories that should be employed. A decision must depend on the nature of the rating task, and the training given to the raters.

6. Errors and their Control

While rating scales were developed to obtain systematic descriptions and appraisals of performance and products, they often fail in this respect. There are several reasons for this. The first has to do with a rater's willingness to rate conscientiously. In some cases raters are unwilling or unable to take the necessary steps to obtain sound ratings. At best, to some raters, the making of ratings is a bother. If a rater does not take the task seriously, the ratings that are obtained are apt to be worthless. Some types of errors in the use of rating scales are of sufficient importance and occur with sufficient frequency for a classification of error types to have been made (Guilford 1954).

6.1 Errors of Leniency and Severity

Some raters under certain circumstances tend to rate with greater leniency than do others. Likewise, some raters tend to rate with greater severity. Where a consistent bias occurs, some allowance can be made through a scaling correction. However, where leniency errors occur intermittently, such errors are difficult to detect, and it is difficult for allowance to be made.

6.2 Errors of Central Tendency and Extremes

Some raters exhibit caution and tend to make ratings in the region of the center of the score distribution, while other raters seem to make greater use of the extreme categories. It is difficult to make corrections for such differences in the shape of a score distribution after the rating scale scores have been collated. However, raters are sometimes required to assign ratings in accordance with a normal distribution, provided it can be assumed that such a distribution is appropriate for the sample that they are required to assess.

6.3 The "Halo" Effect

In some cases, raters who are required to provide ratings on several attributes make a judgment of an overall kind, and permit such a judgment to influence all ratings made. Thus the ratings on certain scales may be less valid than on others, because of the transfer of a "halo" effect of global judgment to the ratings assigned to particular scales.

6.4 Errors of Contrast

Some raters show a tendency to rate highly the performance or the characteristics of persons who are similar to the rater, and to rate at a lower level those persons who are dissimilar.

6.5 Errors of Proximity

Stockford and Bissell (1949) found a tendency for adjacent attributes in a set of rating scales to correlate more highly than for distant attributes. Thus, if the attributes to be rated were presented in a different order then a very different set of ratings would be obtained.

6.6 Logical Errors

Like errors of proximity and the halo effect, where attributes appear to a rater to be logically related, then they tend to be assigned similar ratings. Thus, this type of error inflates the correlations between particular types of ratings.

7. Minimizing Errors in Rating Scales

Several steps can be taken to reduce the errors made in the use of rating scales.

7.1 Improving Scale Construction

Greater consistency and meaningfulness of ratings are obtained under circumstances where, according to Gronlund (1971): (a) attributes being rated are directly observable as behaviors; (b) categories and points in a scale are clearly defined; (c) between three and seven rating positions are provided, with raters permitted to rate at intermediate points; and (d) the characteristics or attributes are recognized as being of educational significance.

Refinements in the presentation of the stimulus variables can be achieved, which lead to a reduction of errors by defining: (a) the traits to be rated, (b) supplementing or replacing trait names with concrete definitions of the trait, and (c) elaborating traits with specific descriptions of the behaviors to be observed and rated. Improvements in the form of the response categories can be made: (a) by defining categories in terms of the percentage of a group falling in each category, (b) by defining categories in term of behavioral descriptions, or (c) by defining categories in terms of a specific example.

7.2 Employing Multiple Raters

Another way of improving the reliability of rating scale data is to combine the ratings from several raters for each item to be rated. This has been found to improve the reliability of ratings in the same way that a lengthened test will yield more reliable scores. The Spearman–Brown prophecy formula (Thorndike et al. 1991) predicts the improvement in reliability of such combined ratings almost perfectly. Thus, in situations where the ratings assigned assume considerable importance, it is desirable that multiple raters should be employed and the ratings from the several raters combined. These procedures are of course costly, and the importance of the information must be taken into consideration together with the cost involved.

7.3 Training of Raters

The third major way of improving the usefulness of rating scales is through a training program for individuals who will serve as raters. Rating scales depend heavily on the skill of the individuals who use them. Thus, a systematic program to train raters, even of relatively short duration, can yield large dividends in terms of both the reliability and validity of ratings. A typical training program would involve discussion of the rating scale with all prospective raters and a set of scheduled observations in which the prospective raters observe and rate the same ratee or product and meet to discuss and resolve differences in their ratings. Three or four such scheduled observations can result in marked improvement in inter-rater reliability. In one study (Jason 1962a), an extensive training program for raters resulted in rating scale reliabilities ranging from 0.86 to 0.93. The development of relatively inexpensive video and audio recording and playing devices have increased greatly the opportunity for training raters.

It is thus possible to standardize and stabilize the procedures to be used in many specific situations where ratings are required. Moreover, training can be more readily carried out and extended until a high level of rating performance is achieved. Training should be based on the judgments of an expert or group of experts who provide the reference standard. Guilford (1954) has listed 33 major findings from research studies of raters and their peculiarities that should be taken into consideration by persons responsible for the training and administration of raters.

7.4 Monitoring Rating Procedures

Both in the training of raters and the administration of large rating programs it is important to monitor systematically the performance of raters to ensure consistency and reproducibility of ratings. A simple index of rater performance, commonly employed either between two raters or between a single rater and a standard, is:

$$
\begin{array}{c}
\text{Coefficient of agreement} \\
\text{or} \\
\text{Proportion of agreement } (Po)
\end{array}
= 1 - \frac{\text{No. of disagreements}}{\begin{array}{c}\text{No. of agreements +}\\\text{No. of disagreements}\end{array}}
$$

Where there is perfect agreement, this coefficient is unity; and where there is total disagreement, the coefficient is zero. However, the incidence of agreements is dependent upon the number of rating categories employed. The advantage of this index is that it is readily calculated and can be used during training to monitor the degree of agreement achieved.

7.5 Assessing the Reproducibility of Ratings

Cohen (1960) proposed the use of the Kappa statistic (K) as a measure of agreement between two observers in the classification of subjects into two nominal categories. It was meant to provide an improvement on the coefficient of agreement, because it discounts the proportion of agreements which is expected to occur by chance alone (P_e). The proportion of observations for which agreement is recorded after allowance is made for chance (P_o–P_e), is divided by the maximum possible proportion (1–P_e) to provide the statistic K.

$$ K = \frac{P_o - P_e}{1 - P_e} $$

This index was subsequently extended to apply to multicategory classifications as a measure of their reproducibility, and a weighted Kappa proposed:

$$ K_w = 1 - \frac{\sum\limits_{ij} w_{ij} o_{ij}}{\sum\limits_{ij} w_{ij} e_{ij}} $$

where o_{ij} is the observed frequency in cell ij in the cross-classification of the two sets of ratings, e_{ij} is the expected frequency in cell ij due to chance, and w_{ij} is the weight given to that cell.

Maclure and Willett (1987) point out that if the weights are the squares of the cell deviations from the diagonal, the weighted Kappa is approximately equal to the product moment correlation coefficient. Moreover, under the condition of identical distributions in the marginals, the weighted Kappa is exactly equivalent to the intraclass correlation coefficient (see *Measures of Variation*). As a consequence, only the unweighted Kappa is seen as a satisfactory measure of agreement, and may be readily calculated for dichotomous categories. If the categories are polytomous and have no inherent order and the data are thus nominal, then an unweighted Kappa may be considered an appropriate measure of overall agreement. However, it is an average, and one category may account for most of the misclassification. Moreover, the unweighted Kappa calculated for a more detailed classification scheme will be lower than for a less detailed scheme. Landis and Koch (1977) have proposed the following guidelines for assessing the magnitude of the unweighted Kappa.

Value of K	Strength of agreement
< 0.00	Poor
0.00 – 0.20	Slight
0.21 – 0.40	Fair
0.41 – 0.60	Moderate
0.61 – 0.80	Substantial
0.81 – 1.00	Almost perfect

To test the statistical significance of the unweighted K, Cohen (1960) proposed an approximate standard error.

$$ se_K = \sqrt{\frac{P_o(1 - P_o)}{N(1 - P_e)^2}} $$

The weighted Kappa is a more readily calculated index than either the interclass or the intraclass correlation coefficients and continues to be employed for this reason. Kramer and Feinstein (1981) suggest that the weighted Kappa should probably be above 0.5 for an acceptable level of agreement to have been attained.

7.6 Reliability of Scaled Ratings

For the more detailed examination of scaled ratings in situations where scores are assigned and there are multiple tasks, multiple raters, and replication of ratings, analysis of variance procedures should be used to assess the reliability of the scaled ratings. The intraclass correlation coefficients calculated from an analysis of variance is superior to a weighted Kappa as a measure of reliability. A treatment of the use of analysis of variance for the examination of ratings data and the calculation of appropriate intraclass correlation coefficients as measures of reliability is provided elsewhere (see *Reliability in Educational and Psychological Measurement*). Estimates of rater and task effects obtained from an analysis of variance can also be used to compensate for systematic bias arising from differences between raters and tasks.

8. Analysis of Rating Scale Data

In most situations where rating data are being analyzed and where ordered categories and rank scaled scores are used, the scale values assigned are associated with an underlying continuous and normal distribution. Under such circumstances the analysis of these rating scale data is commonly based on the use of a product moment correlation coefficient. However, where the data are polytomous (in categories) or censored (in truncated distributions), Muthén (1984) showed that it is possible to allow for the fact that the data are associated with an underlying continuous and normal distribution by calculating a polychoric or polyserial correlation coefficient. These corrected correlation coefficients show stronger relationships than do the uncorrected product–moment correlation coefficients. They may be readily computed using the PRELIS computer program associated with LISREL 7 (Jöreskog and Sörbom 1989).

Where rating data are in nominal categories and where scale values are not assigned to the categorized data, a wide range of statistical procedures have been developed since the 1970s for the effective analysis of such data (see *Multivariate Analysis; Contingency Tables: Log-Linear Models; Correspondence Analysis of Qualitative Data; Configural Frequency Analyses of Categorized Data*).

9. Usefulness of Ratings

The picture obtained of the current status of rating scales is rather mixed. Sometimes rating scales have yielded rather disappointing results. Clearly, there are hazards and pitfalls in their development and use. There have, however, been some marked successes. Despite their limitations, there is a host of situations in which human judgments are needed. Rating scales remain one of the best means of securing these judgments.

See also: Scaling Methods; Research in Education: Epistemological Issue

References

Beaton A E 1969 Some mathematical and empirical properties of criterion scaled variables. In: Mayeske G W et al. (eds.) 1969 *A Study of Our Nation's Schools*. Office of Education, US Department of Health Education and Welfare, Washington, DC
Cohen J A 1960 A coefficient of agreement for nominal scales. *Educ. Psychol. Meas.* 20(1): 37–46
Cronbach L J 1951 Coefficient alpha and the internal structure of tests. *Psychometri.* 16: 297–334
Gronlund N E 1971 *Measurement and Evaluation in Teaching*, 2nd edn. Macmillan, New York
Guilford J P 1954 *Psychometric Methods*, 2nd edn. McGraw-Hill, New York
Gulliksen H 1950 *Theory of Mental Tests*. Wiley, New York
Jason H 1962a A study of medical teaching practices. *Journal of Medical Education* 37: 1258–84
Jason H 1962b Medical instruction observation record. In: Somon A, Boyer G (eds.) 1970 *Mirrors for Behavior*, Vol. 2. Philadelphia, Pennsylvania
Jöreskog K G, Sörbom D 1991 *LISREL 7 A Guide to the Program and Applications*, 2nd edn. SPSS Publications, Chicago, Illinois
Kaiser H F, Caffrey J 1965 Alpha factor analysis. *Psychometri.* 30(1): 1–14
Kramer M S, Feinstein A R 1981 Clinical biostatistics 54. The biostatistics of concordance. *Clinical Pharmacol. Ther.* 29(1):111–23
Landis R J, Koch G G 1977 The measurement of observer agreement for categorical data. *Biometrics* 33(1):159–74
Maclure M Willett W C 1987 Misinterpretation and misuse of the Kappa statistic. *American Journal of Epidemiology* 126(2):161–69
Muthén B O 1984 A general structural equation model with dichotomous, ordered, categorical, and continuous latent variable indicators. *Psychometri.* 49(1):115–32
Nunnally J C 1978 *Psychometric Theory*, 2nd edn. McGraw-Hill, New York
Peaker G F 1975 *An Empirical Study of Education in Twenty-One Countries: A Technical Report*. Almqvist and Wiksell, Stockholm
Pedhazur E J, Kerlinger F N 1982 *Multiple Regression in Behavioral Research*, 2nd edn. Holt, Rinehart and Winston, New York
Stockford L, Bissell H W 1949 Factors involved in establishing a merit-rating scale. *Personnel* 26:94–118
Thorndike R L, Hagen E P 1977 *Measurement and Evaluation in Psychology and Education*, 4th edn. John Wiley, New York
Thorndike R M et al. 1991 *Measurement and Evaluation in Psychology and Education*, 5th edn. Macmillan, New York

Tests and Attitude Scales, Translation of

R. K. Hambleton and A. Kanjee

For as long as psychological tests and attitude scales have existed, researchers have been interested in translating them. One reason is that it is often cheaper and faster to translate an instrument than it is to develop a new instrument for a second language group. Sometimes, too, the technical expertise to construct the required instrument does not exist in the second language group.

A second reason is that translated tests and scales allow cross-national, cross-language, and/or cross-ethnic comparative studies to take place. Such studies have become particularly popular as many countries strive to set world-class educational standards or simply to look at their own educational progress in relation to other countries. For example, over 60 countries have expressed interest in participating in the Third

International Mathematics and Science Study (TIMSS) being conducted in 1994 and 1998 by the International Association for the Evaluation of Educational Achievement (IEA).

Finally, instruments are translated to enhance fairness in assessment by enabling persons to take tests and psychological scales in their preferred languages. For example, high school students in Israel can take their college admission examinations in one of six languages. Thus, the bias in examinations scores associated with examinees being examined in their second- or third-best language is removed and examination score validity is enhanced. While an effort is made to translate the examinations properly into six languages, what translation problems remain are judged to be less serious from a validity perspective than the unfairness that would result from requiring all examination candidates to take their examinations in Hebrew.

While the reasons for translating tests and attitude scales are clear, the methods for doing the translations and establishing the equivalence of scores from the two versions of the instrument are not (Hambleton 1993). Some cross-cultural researchers have even speculated that a high percentage of research in their field is flawed to the point of being invalid because of the use of poorly translated instruments. The purposes of this entry are to review the sources of invalidity associated with translated tests and scales and to suggest solutions whenever possible. The sources of invalidity can be organized into three broad categories: cultural/language differences, technical issues and methods, and interpretation of results. For the purposes of this entry, the terms "tests," "scales," "instruments," and "assessment measures" will be used interchangeably, and "translation work" will be used in the broad sense to include adaptation work which may sometimes be needed.

1. Cultural/Language Differences Affecting Scores

Assessment and interpretation of cross-cultural results cannot be viewed in the narrow context of just the translation or adaptation of instruments. Rather, this process should be considered for all parts of the assessment process including the administration of instruments, item formats used, and the effect of speed on examinee performance. These three factors will be considered next.

1.1 Test Administration

Communication problems between examiner and examinees can prove to be a serious threat to the validity of results. Van de Vijver and Poortinga (1991) noted the communication failure experienced by Greenfield (1966, 1979) when assessing the principle of conservation among the West African Wolof people. Greenfield presented subjects with two differently shaped beakers, one tall and one broad, that contained equal amounts of water. Subjects were asked to identify the beaker which contained more water. Greenfield found that subjects frequently responded with answers that failed to show an ability to conserve, that is, many students said that the tall beaker contained more water. However, Irvine (1978) later found that in the Wolof language, "more" referred to both quantity and level, and demonstrated (by posing the question differently) that the Wolof did in fact have mastery of the principle of conservation.

One way to circumvent problems between examiner and examinees is to ensure that the instructions on the test itself are clear and self-explanatory, with minimal reliance on verbal communication (van de Vijver and Poortinga 1991). Special problems can be expected with directions for rating scales used in attitude measurement too, since they are not common in many countries. Also, test administrators should: (a) be drawn from the target communities; (b) be familiar with the culture, language, and dialects; (c) have adequate test administration skills and experience; and (d) possess some measurement expertise. Additionally, consistency in test administration across different groups can be improved by providing (basic) training to all test administrators. Training sessions should be preplanned as part of the test development process, stressing clear, unambiguous communication, the importance of following instructions, strictly following time limits, the influence of test administrators on reliability and validity, and so on.

1.2 Test Format

Differential familiarity with particular item formats presents another source of invalidity of test results in cross-cultural studies. For example, in the United States, selected response questions, especially multiple-choice questions, have been used extensively in assessment. In cross-cultural studies, it cannot be assumed that all students are as familiar with multiple-choice items as students in the United States. Nationalities that follow the United Kingdom system of education place greater emphasis on essays and short answer questions, as opposed to multiple-choice items. Thus, students from these countries are placed at a possible disadvantage as compared to their United States counterparts. Of course, when constructed response formats are emphasized or serve as the dominant mode of assessment, persons with more experience with selected response formats such as multiple-choice item formats will be placed at a disadvantage. Sometimes a balance of item formats may be the best solution to insure fairness and reduce sources of invalidity in the assessment process.

Another solution is to include only those formats with which all groups being assessed are experienced. Whenever it can be assured that examinees are not placed at a disadvantage, and when all variables of interest can still be measured, multiple-choice items or simple rating scales should be preferred. The major advantage is that multiple-choice items or simple rating scales can be objectively scored. Thus, complications in scoring associated with open-ended responses are avoided. This is especially relevant in cross-cultural studies, where it may be more difficult to translate the scoring rubrics than the test items. Also, practice items can easily be included to enable examinees to familiarize themselves with the "different" formats. In addition, extensive, unambiguous instructions including examples and exercises help to reduce differential familiarity (van de Vijver and Poortinga 1992).

A common assumption is that examinees easily grasp the meaning of pictorial stimuluses. However, pictorial stimuluses are subject to bias like any other stimuluses, as perception is strongly influenced by previous experience (Lonner 1990).

1.3 Speed

It is often assumed that examinees will work fast on "speeded" tests (van de Vijver and Poortinga 1991). However, in a study comparing Dutch and other ethnic students in the Netherlands, Van Leest and Bleichrodt (1990) found that the speed factor increased ethnic bias. Schmidtt and Crone (1991), in a differential item functioning study comparing Whites and Hispanic Americans, also found speededness to be a factor negatively affecting Hispanic examinees' performance. In a study that compared cognitive gender differences between German and United States examinees, Ellis and Weiner (1990) found no gender differences, in both American and German examinees, when speed of administration was minimized. The best solution would seem to be to minimize test speededness as a factor in cognitive test performance and attitude scales unless there is a good reason for including it.

2. Technical Issues and Methods

In this section, five technical factors which can influence the validity of translated instruments are considered: the instrument itself, selection and training of translators, the process of translation, judgmental designs for translating instruments, and empirical designs for establishing equivalence.

2.1 The Instrument Itself

If a researcher knows that he or she will be using a test or attitude scale in a different language or culture, it is advantageous to take this into account at the outset of the instrument development process. Failure to do so can introduce problems later in the translation process which will reduce the validity of the translated instrument. Choice of item formats, stimulus material for the instrument, vocabulary, sentence structure, and other aspects which might be difficult to translate well can all be taken into account in the initial instrument development to minimize problems later in translation.

For example, passages about the game of baseball which would be unfamiliar in many cultures could be rejected in favor of passages about walking through a park or other activities that would have meaning across many language and cultural groups. Units of measurement should be avoided too since they vary from one nationality to another.

With attitude scales especially, care must be taken to choose situations, vocabulary, and expressions that will translate easily across language groups and cultures. Very often these scales contain everyday expressions which enhance their meaningfulness in one language but make translations difficult. For example, an expression such as "What goes around, comes around," could be difficult to translate.

2.2 Selection and Training of Translators

The importance of obtaining the services of competent translators should be obvious. Too often, though, researchers have tried to go through the translation process with a single translator selected because he or she happened to be available. Competent translation work cannot be assumed. Also, the use of a single translator, competent or not, does not permit highly valuable discussions of independent translations across a group of competent translators.

Translators should be more than persons familiar and competent with the languages involved in the translation. They should know the cultures very well, especially the target culture (i.e., the culture of the language into which the instrument is being translated). Knowledge of the cultures involved, especially the target culture, is often essential for an effective translation. Also, subject matter knowledge in the translation of achievement tests is essential. The nuances and subtleties of a subject area will be lost on a translator unfamiliar with the subject matter. In one project, a translator translated the term "item pools," used in test development work, to "item oceans" in Japanese. Too often, translators without technical knowledge will resort to literal translations which are often problematic to target language examinees and threaten test validity.

Finally, test translators would benefit from some training in test and attitude scale construction. For example, test translators need to know that when doing translations they should not create unintentional associations that might lead test-wise examinees to the correct answers, or translate distractors in multiple-choice items unknowingly so that they have the same meaning. A test translator without any knowledge of the principles of test and scale construction could easily make test material more or less difficult unknowingly, and correspondingly lower the validity of the instrument in the target population.

2.3 Process of Translation

The problem of dialects within a language can become a threat to the validity of translated tests. It must be decided which dialect is of interest, or whether the goal is to produce a translation that could apply across dialects within a language. This problem should be resolved, used in the selection of translators, and addressed in the training of translators.

Frequency counts of words can be invaluable in producing valid translations. In general, it is best to translate words and expressions with words and expressions with approximately the same frequencies in the two languages. One additional problem is that these frequency lists of words and expressions are not always available. This is another reason for preferring translators who are familiar with both of the cultures and not just the languages.

"Decentering" is sometimes used in translating instruments. It may be that some words and expressions do not have equivalent words and expressions in the target language. It is even possible that the words and expressions do not exist in the target language. Decentering involves making revisions to the source language instrument so that equivalent material can be used in both the source and target language versions of the instrument. Such a strategy is possible when the source language instrument is under development at the same time as the target language version.

2.4 Judgmental Designs for Translating Instruments

The two most popular judgmental designs are forward translations and backward translations. With forward translations, a single translator or preferably a group of translators translate the test or attitude scale from the source language to the target language. Then, the equivalence of the two versions of the instrument is judged by another group of translators. Revisions can be made to the target version of the instrument to correct problems identified by the translators. Sometimes the validity of the judgments about the equivalence of the two versions is enhanced by also having examinees provide translators or a group of judges with their interpretations of the material on the tests and questionnaires. The basic design is weak, however, because of the high level of inferencing that must be done by the translators or the judges about the equivalence of the two versions of the instrument.

The back-translation design is the best known and most popular of the judgmental designs. In one variation, a group of translators translates the instrument from the source language to the target language. A second group of translators takes the translated instrument (in the target language) and translates it back to the source language. Then, the original version of the instrument and the back-translated version are compared and judgments are made about their equivalence. To the extent that the two versions of the instrument in the source language look similar, support is available for the equivalence of the source and target versions of the instrument. The back-translation design can be considered as a general check on translation quality that can detect at least some of the problems associated with poor translations or adaptations. It has been used successfully in many projects as a first step in assessing the quality of a translation.

Though the back-translation design is to be recommended for use in many projects, it would rarely provide a sufficient amount of evidence to support the use of a translated instrument in practice. (This design may suffice in small scale minor cross-cultural studies.) Evidence of instrument equivalence provided by a back-translation design is only one of many types of evidence that should be compiled in a translation study. One of the main shortcomings is that the comparison of instruments is carried out in the source language. It is quite possible that the translation could be poor while the evidence on the comparability of the original instrument and the back-translated instrument would suggest otherwise. This might happen if the translators used a shared set of translation rules that insured that the back-translated instrument looked like the original instrument. A second shortcoming is that the translation could be poor because it retained inappropriate aspects of the source language instrument such as the same grammatical structure and spelling. Such errors facilitate back-translations but they mask serious shortcomings in the target version of the instrument. Finally, this and other judgmental designs can be faulted because samples of the intended populations for the instruments never actually take the instruments under test-like conditions (or, for that matter, any other conditions). There is very little evidence to support the position that translators or other judges are capable of predicting the equivalence of versions of an instrument from a review, however carefully it may be done. In fact, most of the available evidence suggests that judges are not very successful at predicting test items that function differentially in two or more groups.

2.5 Empirical Designs for Establishing Equivalence

The empirical designs are of two types: those that use bilingual participants and those that use monolingual participants in the source and target languages. Designs that use bilinguals are often difficult to carry out because of the shortage of bilinguals who are equally proficient in both languages. And, when the samples taking each version of the instrument are not carefully matched on ability, only simple and not very informative statistical analyses can be carried out. For example, the relative order of item difficulty in the two versions of the instrument might be checked.

Even when an appropriate sample of bilingual participants can be found to take one or both versions of the instrument, problems remain. For one, evidence of equivalence of two versions of an instrument (such as similar item statistics, score distributions, and factor structures) in a bilingual sample of persons may not generalize to the monolingual persons in each population. For example, in a study by Hulin et al. (1982) with the *Job Descriptive Index*, they found that with a bilingual sample of participants, only 4 percent of the items in the attitude scale were identified as poorly translated. The result jumped to 30 percent of the items when monolingual samples of participants from the source and target language populations were used.

A better empirical design would involve monolinguals taking the source language version of the instrument and a second sample of monolinguals taking the target language version of the instrument. An assumption of equal ability distributions across the two groups is not usually tenable but it is still possible to compare item statistics if the analyses are carried out within an item response theory framework (Ellis 1989, Hambleton et al. 1991), or other statistical frameworks which are not based on an assumption of equal ability distributions. The advantages of this design are that samples of the source and target populations are used in the analyses and therefore findings about the equivalence of the two versions of the instrument are generalizable to the populations of interest. These studies are carried out like item bias studies (Hambleton et al. 1991). Comparisons of the item statistics in the two versions of the instrument are made controlling for any ability differences in the two groups. Items showing differences are identified and carefully studied to determine the source of the differences. Poor translation is one likely explanation.

3. Interpretation of Results

In large-scale cross-cultural studies, the purpose of the instrumentation is to provide a basis for making comparisons between various cultural/language groups, so as to understand the differences and similarities that exist (Hambleton and Bollwark 1991). Sometimes cognitive variables are of interest and other times the focus may be on the assessment of personality variables or general information. Results should be used for seeking ways of comparing groups and understanding the differences. Cross-cultural studies should not be used to support arguments about the superiority or exceptionality of nations, as if it were some sort of a horse race (Westbury 1992). In this context, to gain a better understanding when interpreting scores, other relevant factors external to the tests or assessment measures and specific to a nationality should also be considered. Curricula, educational policies, wealth, standard of living, cultural values, and so on may be essential for properly interpreting scores across cultural/language and/or national groups. Next, several of the factors which should be considered in interpreting achievement results across groups will be presented.

3.1 Similarity of Curricula

To the extent that differences in curricula exist, any achievement comparisons between different cultures will be tenuous if these curricula differences are not taken into account. Westbury (1992) notes that the results of the Second International Mathematics Study

(SIMS) indicate that students in the United States performed poorly in every grade and in every aspect of mathematics tested. When comparing performance of Japanese and United States students, major curricular differences between the two countries were noted. However, when the curricula of the two countries were similar, Westbury found no essential differences between the performance of United States and Japanese students.

In another example, Song and Ginsburg (1988) compared the early learning behavior of Korean and United States children and found that superior achievement in mathematics in Korean children could be attributed to the dual number systems taught in Korean (Chinese and English systems). In addition to other cultural factors like parental involvement and teacher–student relationship, they also found that the amount of time devoted to mathematics in Korea was greater than that in the United States.

Under these different conditions, it is not unusual to expect differences in performance. Overlooking the specific and unique national characteristics that affect the test scores can have serious consequences on the interpretation of results. Perhaps these omissions help in explaining some of the International Assessment of Educational Progress (IAEP) and IEA results.

3.2 Student Motivation

Wainer (1993) questioned whether demonstrated proficiency as measured by tests can be separated from motivation. He noted that in the recent International Assessment of Educational Progress study (Lapointe et al. 1992), all the (randomly) selected Korean students were made aware of the great honor of being chosen to represent their school and country, and thus had a responsibility to perform at their best. For United States students, on the other hand, participation in this international comparative study was just another activity.

Also, van de Vijver and Poortinga (1991) noted that it cannot be assumed that examinees will always try to achieve a high score. For example, for Black South African students, the aim in examinations is to achieve the minimum score required to pass any examination. This is because the imposed state education system is perceived by many examinees to be detrimental to Blacks, and thus students only aspire to the minimum required of them. In this context, it is not unusual to expect different levels of performance, which may have very little to do with ability.

3.3 Sociopolitical Factors

The meaning and interpretation of test scores can also differ even though the scores may be equivalent. For example, consider comparing test scores between students from developed and developing nations, or industrialized and mainly rural societies. In this context, performance of students may not be related to ability at all. Rather, it may be a reflection of the lack of access to adequate resources, or the different quality of educational services available.

The point is that, for any meaningful interpretations, the different social, political, and economic realities facing nationalities, as well as the relevance of educational opportunities in the light of these realities must be considered (Olmedo 1981). Thus it is important for test developers to be aware of those specific cultural issues that might impact on test scores. Test developers and translators familiar with the target nationality play a crucial role in this regard.

4. Emerging Issues and Research

There are no technical standards for conducting translation studies that have the support and approval of international psychology organizations whose members do cross-cultural testing and research. This is an important point because of the ever-expanding interest in translating instruments. Fortunately such a set of standards is being developed. The International Test Commission has organized an international committee of psychologists from the IEA, the European Association of Psychological Assessment, the International Association of Cross-Cultural Psychology, the International Association of Applied Psychology, and the International Union of Psychological Science to prepare a validated set of technical standards. The work of this 13-person committee which represents 6 international organizations was completed by the spring of 1994. Over 40 psychologists throughout the world have agreed to participate in the field test of the technical standards. The availability of technical standards for translating instruments should facilitate the proper translation of tests and attitude scales and the compilation of evidence to support the intended uses of these instruments.

In the 1990s, not only are more tests and attitude scales being translated than ever before, but the tests and scales are being put to important uses by national governments, such as establishing world-class performance standards. The validity of scores, therefore, from translated tests and scales must be clearly established. The consequence is that more sophisticated methodology is being used to establish equivalence. Item response theory models (see Hulin 1987) are being used to identify poorly translated items and to place scores from different translations of a test or scale on the same reporting scale. The specific details associated with model selection, test score linking designs, and identification of problematic items in the translation process still remain to be worked out. In principle, the solutions are known but considerably more experience with translated instruments, possibly involving limited sample sizes, is needed.

Structural equation models (see Jöreskog and Sörbom 1986) are being used too in the study of factor structures underlying tests and scales in multiple language groups. Such analyses are central in assessing the equivalence of instruments across cultural/language groups. Clearly, methodological advances are needed to insure that the equivalence of translated tests and scales can be adequately determined. One special problem might be the study of equivalence in factor structures across many language groups and with modest sample sizes in each.

5. Summary

To enhance the meaning of any cross-cultural research, it is important for researchers to choose carefully test administrators, use appropriate item formats, and control for the speed effect. In addition, translators who are familiar with the target group and their language, who know the content of the instrument, and who have received some training in instrument development, are the most capable persons for getting the translation job done well. Appropriately chosen judgmental designs (such as backward translations) and empirical designs and analyses (such as comparisons of results from monolingual examinees taking the instrument in their own language) can provide invaluable data bearing on the question of instrument equivalence across groups. With regard to interpretation of scores, those specific background variables that impact on performance should be carefully considered. In this regard, differing curricula, levels of motivation, and sociopolitical factors are especially important with achievement tests. Also, comparisons should not only be undertaken with emphasis on the differences. Similarities between nationalities can also provide useful and relevant information.

See also: Attitudes

References

Ellis B B 1989 Differential item functioning: Implications for test translation. *J. Appl. Psychol.* 74: 912–21
Ellis B B, Weiner S P 1990 A study of the gender differences in two countries: Implications for future research. In: Bleichrodt N, Drenth P J D (eds.) 1990 *Contemporary Issues in Cross-Cultural Psychology*. Swets and Zeitlinger, Amsterdam
Greenfield P M 1966 On culture and conservation. In: Bruner J S, Olver R R, Greenfield P M (eds.) 1966 *Studies in Cognitive Growth*. Wiley, New York
Greenfield P M 1979 Response to Wolof "magical thinking." *J. Cross-Cult. Psychol.* 10: 251–56
Hambleton R K 1993 Translating achievement tests for use in cross-national studies. *European Journal of Psychological Assessment* 9: 57–68
Hambleton R K, Bollwark J 1991 Adapting tests for use in different cultures: Technical issues and methods. *Bulletin of the International Test Commission* 18: 3–32
Hambleton R K, Swaminathan H, Rogers H J 1991 *Fundamentals of Item Response Theory*. Sage, Newbury Park, California
Hulin C L 1987 A psychometric theory of evaluations of

item and scale translations: Fidelity across languages. *J. Cross-Cult. Psychol.* 18: 115–42

Hulin C L, Drasgow F, Komocar J 1982 Application of item response theory to analysis of attitude scale translation. *J. Appl. Psychol.* 67: 818–25

Irvine J T 1978 Wolof "magical thinking": Culture and conservation revisited. *J. Cross-Cult. Psychol.* 9: 300–10

Jöreskog K G, Sörbom D 1986 LISREL8: Structural Equation Modeling with the SIMPLIS Command Language. Erlbaum, Hillsdale, New Jersey

Lapointe A E, Mead N A, Askew J M 1992 *Learning Mathematics.* Report No. 22-CAEP-01, Educational Testing Service, Princeton, New Jersey

Lonner W J 1990 An overview of cross-cultural testing and assessment. In: Brislin R W (ed.) 1990 *Applied Cross-Cultural Psychology, Vol. 14.* Sage, Newbury Park, California

Olmedo E L 1981 Testing linguistic minorities. *Am. Psychol.* 36: 1078–85

Schmitt A P, Crone C R 1991 *Alternative Mathematical Aptitude Item Types: DIF Issues.* Research Report 91–42, Educational Testing Service, Princeton, New Jersey

Song M J, Ginsburg H P 1988 The effect of the Korean number system on young children's counting: A natural experiment in numerical bilingualism. *Int. J. Psychol.* 23: 319–32

van de Vijver F J R, Poortinga Y H 1991 Testing across cultures. In: Hambleton R K, Zaal J (eds.) 1991 *Advances in Educational and Psychological Testing.* Kluwer Academic Publishers, Boston, Massachusetts

van de Vijver F J R, Poortinga Y H 1992 Testing in culturally heterogeneous populations: When are cultural loadings undesirable? *European Journal of Psychological Assessment* 8: 17–24

van Leest P F, Bleichrodt N 1990 Testing of college graduates from ethnic minority groups. In: Bleichrodt N, Drenth P J D (eds.) 1990 *Contemporary Issues in Cross-Cultural Psychology.* Swets and Zeitlinger, Amsterdam

Wainer H 1993 Measurement problems. *J. Educ. Meas.* 30: 1–21

Westbury I 1992 Comparing American and Japanese achievement: Is the United States really a low achiever? *Educ. Researcher* 21: 18–24

Test-taking Anxiety and Expectancy of Performance

F. D. Naylor

Test-taking anxiety is significant for both educators and students. In so far as it acts to distort performance it is a source of measurement error which affects both the reliability and validity of tests. How important such distortions are depends on the purposes for which test results are used. Where test-taking anxiety cuts across those purposes its presence may seriously compromise them. It is important therefore to understand the conditions under which test-taking anxiety is manifested, and its likely effects. Although it is generally considered as being detrimental to cognitive performance, there may be situations in which performance is enhanced by test-taking anxiety.

Test-taking anxiety has two major aspects: emotional and cognitive. The emotional aspect is basically a response to stress, and therefore test-taking anxiety is related to more generalized anxiety which might affect performance in any stressful context. However, the action of stress is relative to the person and the situation. For example, not all test situations are experienced as stressful, or equally stressful, by all persons. Cognitive appraisal of test situations might yield substantial differences in the degrees of stress they generate. Cognitive appraisal is itself influenced by prior conditions including subject difficulty, expectations of performance, and whether the conditions are in or out of personal control.

1. Conceptualization of Test-taking Anxiety

Mandler and Sarason's (1952) initial investigations of test-taking anxiety proposed a drive–conflict theory in which efforts to reduce anxiety were stimulated by behavior relevant to task completion, and implicit attempts to leave the testing situation through self-denigrating responses irrelevant to and interfering with task completion. Alpert and Haber (1960) formulated distinct constructs of facilitating and debilitating anxiety which suggested possibilities of conflict, the action of either separately, or no experienced anxiety. Liebert and Morris (1967) divided debilitating anxiety into worry and emotionality, and their experiments indicated that the first of these tended to interfere more with performance.

Spielberger's (1966) theory of anxiety distinguished anxiety as a trait (A-trait) and as a state (A-state). A-trait refers to individual differences in anxiety proneness, whereas A-state refers to individual differences in the actual response to a particular stressful situation. Measures of both kinds of anxiety tend to be positively correlated. High and low A-trait are inferred from the reported frequency of anxiety experiences, while differences in A-state are inferred from reports of the intensity of the experience, generally as it occurs but sometimes reminiscently.

All of these formulations imply that test-taking

anxiety interferes with performance, generally in a negative way. However, Tobias (1985) has suggested that test anxiety may be a function of poor study habits or deficient skills of test-taking which themselves have deleterious effects on performance. Attempts to alleviate test anxiety per se might ignore what could be more salient causal factors of poor performance. Gaudry and Spielberger (1971) proposed that cognitive appraisal of the test situation as threatening to self-esteem stimulates A-state which interferes with performance. A-trait and intelligence appeared to influence cognitive appraisal such that at higher levels of ability, performance appeared to be facilitated by anxiety. Presumably the threats consequent on cognitive appraisal here enhance task-directed drives (Mandler and Sarason 1952) rather than stimulating the emotional preoccupations characteristic of anxiety. However, it may also be the case that more able students tend to have better study skills and examination techniques which facilitate their performance (e.g. Tobias 1985).

Some findings (e.g., Denney 1980, Tryon 1980) suggest that although treatments of test anxiety may be efficacious, reduced or controlled anxiety does not necessarily enhance performance. Most of the treatments involved desensitization, reduction of emotional arousal, or other behavior modification techniques (Allen et al. 1980), rather than attempting cognitive change or skills development. The interference aspect of anxiety may involve unwarranted assumptions about the constancy of other relevant skills and knowledge, when it may be deficits in these which give rise to the state of worry provoking interference. Deffenbacher and Hazaleus (1985) have suggested that emotionality and worry may be related but different constructs. Worry appears consistently to correlate negatively with performance and performance expectations, while the relation of emotionality to these is less consistent (Morris et al., 1981).

2. Role of Expectancy of Performance

Expectancy is conceptualized in varying ways. There is extensive literature on teachers' expectations, but the findings in this area are not strong (Entwisle and Hayduk 1982). How they influence or relate with test-taking anxiety has not been reported, though teacher threat versus reassurance has some effect. Students' own kinds and levels of expectation are of most pertinence here.

The formulation most relevant to issues of anxiety and performance is that of Weiner (1979). He subsumes expectancy under attributions offered as explanations of behavior. Weiner et al. (1978) found that attributions of causality are internal or external, stable or unstable, and more or less controllable. Affective responses to test feedback depend on causal attribution. Thus, success attributed to external factors such as luck has affective consequences quite different

from internal attributions such as ability. Ability is more predictable than luck, and attributions based on ability are therefore more stable. Effort, by contrast with ability, for example, may be more under personal control but may also be less stable than ability. However, this is not to say that the relations between effort and performance are necessarily unstable, particularly in those cases where examination preparation is necessary.

Forsyth and McMillan (1981) investigated the three dimensions of attribution simultaneously. They hypothesized that people who attributed their outcome to controllable factors would experience more positive affective responses than those who feel they cannot control the causes of their performance. Those who succeed, and believe that internal controllable factors were the cause of their success, should be the most positive in their expectations of future success. Their results were consistent with the hypothesis, and the authors concluded that satisfying and effective educational experiences depended on causal attributions being ascribed to internal factors under the control of the student.

Test-taking anxiety may or may not be perceived as a controllable factor. This may depend on the degree of perceived threat involved. Covington and Omelich (1987), in investigating the purported interference function of test-taking anxiety, administered the same test under evaluative and nonevaluative conditions. The hypothesis that high-anxious students would retrieve more information under circumstances of reduced threat than would low-anxious students was not completely supported, particularly for complex test items. Easy-item performance provided some evidence for the interference hypothesis. Their results may also indicate the importance of mastery of content in moderating test anxiety and for enhancing performance on difficult items.

3. Control of Test-taking Anxiety

3.1 Interventions

A meta-analysis by Hembree (1988) has shown the relative importance of various approaches to the control of test-taking anxiety. Attempts to help students reporting debilitating effects of test-taking anxiety have focused on worry and emotionality either separately or together. Behavior modification techniques with particular emphasis on systematic desensitization and/or relaxation training have been commonly used to treat emotionality. Worry has been treated by techniques derived from cognitive interventions—restructuring, management, insight, and stress inoculation—and these have also been used in attempts to reduce emotionality. Most of these approaches appear effective. Group counseling approaches do not appear to be effective in reducing anxiety. Skills training in study and examination techniques appears less effective than behavioral and cognitive interventions. However, where less effective study skills or test-taking techniques are themselves contributors to anxiety, training can have positive effects.

3.2 Effects on Performance

The reduction of anxiety is not always effective in enhancing performance, even though test-taking anxiety and performance are significantly related. It is important to distinguish subject matter examinations from mental tests. In the latter case reduction in test anxiety through psychological intervention appears regularly to enhance testing performance. Study skills and examination technique appear to be salient in knowledge testing. Reducing test anxiety is not a substitute for learning. It may be that where the worry component in test anxiety results from inadequate preparation, this is the more important component in terms of effects on performance.

4. Conditions for Test-taking Anxiety

The conditions for the arousal of anxiety in the context of testing are similar to those in other contexts. Test-taking anxiety has distinctive triggers and cognitive components, but the feeling-tone is the same as anxiety in general. The two response elements of emotionality on the one hand and worry on the other express the similarities with and differences from other anxiety experiences.

The perceived threat of test and test-like situations arises from several sources. These include task difficulty, the formalities of testing, and the test's instrumental importance as a hurdle to be overcome. Difficulty refers not only to subject matter or the complexities of question or test-item construction, but also to knowledge preparation and level of ability. Anticipated difficulty as a source of anxiety may thus in part be a function of lack of preparation, which is unstable but may have been capable of control personally. On the other hand, difficulty as a consequence of low ability may be stable and beyond personal control.

Expectancies arise from test-taking history, and the circumstances which have contributed to that. The extent to which these circumstances are controllable or not indicates their potency as ongoing sources of anxiety which may not be readily or easily modified.

5. Effects of Background Variables

5.1 Sex

Sex differences in reported anxiety experiences reliably indicated that females rather than males tend to experience higher anxiety. Whether this is a real differ-

ence or merely reflects sex differences in acquiescence is not clear. Everson et al. (1991) showed that a dual factor structure, interpretable as worry and emotionality, fitted the items of the Test Anxiety Inventory (Spielberger et al. 1980). This structure did not differ for males and females, but factor means indicated higher levels of reported anxiety among females, and other results suggested that item reliabilities differed between the sexes.

An Israeli study (Furst et al. 1985) investigated sex differences in relation to type of examination (objective, physical performance, and subjective). Across all examinations women had higher emotionality and A-state scores than men, and tended to underestimate their performances, while men overestimated them. Women showed clearer and more consistent negative relationships between expectations, performance, relative success, and outcomes measures on the emotional rather than the cognitive component of anxiety.

5.2 Ethnicity

Ethnicity has not received a great deal of research attention on its relations with test-taking anxiety, but a study by Dion and Toner (1988) hypothesized that Chinese students would be most prone to exhibit high levels of test anxiety. The basis of the hypothesis lay in the stress on academic excellence to which many Asian students are subject. Dion and Toner (1988) found that test anxiety scores of Chinese students were significantly higher than those of students of Anglo or European origin. There is evidence that students of Asian origin are culturally unsympathetic to psychological counseling interventions, suggesting that they represent a distinct group with special needs.

5.3 Need for Achievement and Fear of Failure

Hembree's (1988) meta-analysis of 31 correlational studies of the relationship between need for achievement and test anxiety also showed a relationship with grade level. In the elementary grades there tended to be a negative relationship showing that the higher test-anxious had less need to achieve. The relationship became positive for high school students, and tended to zero among college students. Among seven studies of fear of failure, its relations with test anxiety remained inconclusive. Herman (1990), on the other hand, constructed a "Fear of Failure Scale" which appears to be a good predictor of academic achievement, and of the worry and emotionality components of test anxiety. Fear of failure explained more variance in the achievement variables than emotionality or worry taken separately or together. The author concluded that fear of failure was a latent trait component of test anxiety which in test conditions is manifested as a situational state component. He suggests that more research is warranted on achievement motivation and fear of failure as preconditions for test anxiety.

A Norwegian study (Gjesme 1982) of sixth graders

from Oslo suggested that test anxiety was a function of sex, the degree of general concern, engagement and involvement in the future, ability, achievement motivation, and perceived intrinsic instrumentality of schoolwork (a measure purporting to relate attitudes to present and future performance). The results showed that pupils' achievement motives and their future orientation were the two most important factors in test anxiety, with instrumentality being important in higher-order interactions. Ability and sex showed their established relations with anxiety. Girls and lower ability pupils showed greater test anxiety. It was also noted that perceived intrinsic instrumentality was negatively related to test anxiety for the girls, but not for the boys.

5.4 Self-efficacy

Bandura (1977) has theorized that a unifying construct which accounts for behavior change in various contexts is the self-efficacy expectation. This is a cognitive mechanism comprised of beliefs concerning one's capacities to perform tasks successfully. These expectations are hypothesized to affect the initiation of coping behavior, the expenditure of effort, performance, accomplishment, and persistence in overcoming obstacles. Efficacy expectations appear to be useful in predicting behavior change in clinical, vocational, and academic situations (Lent et al. 1984). How they relate to test-taking anxiety and causal attributions of academic performance has not been exhaustively studied empirically, but in so far as they relate to persistence and mastery efficacy expectations have potential importance for understanding test-taking anxiety. Lent et al. (1984) studied the relations among self-efficacy beliefs and success and persistence among students studying science and engineering. Their results indicated that strong and high-level self-efficacy expectations were positively related to performance and persistence. Smith et al. (1990) compared three theoretical models as explanations of test anxiety and performance: interference with cognitive-attentional processes by negative rumination; cognitive skills and study habits; and self-efficacy with goal-directed motivation and outcome expectations. Each contributed unique variance to test anxiety and to performance, and the authors concluded that multiple deficit formulations including all three models were needed.

6. Circumstances of Success and Failure

Success and failure experiences have substantial effects on reported levels of A-state (Gaudry and Spielberger 1971). Many experimental studies have shown that one failure experience is sufficient to elevate substantially experienced anxiety, but there appear to be no studies which deal with the anxiety

effects of anticipated failure and how these relate to previous experiences of success or failure. The attribution literature provides important clues here in its distinctions between locus of causality, stability, and controllability of circumstances. Examination outcome attributions appear to vary, inter alia, with expectancy of outcome and its confirmation. Where expectancy of success is disconfirmed by actual failure, subjects tend to increase their attributions to external unstable causes (e.g., "bad luck"), and reduce those to internal causes (e.g., ability and effort) and external stable causes (e.g., the form of testing). This may be interpreted as a defensive reaction against threat to self-esteem, which is a central cause of A-state (Spielberger 1966).

Historically the studies of Sarnoff et al. (1958), and Levy et al. (1969) of the practice in British education of ability grouping or "streaming" showed that pupils in lower streams tended to be more test anxious. The latter study suggested the possibility that the apparent correlation between test anxiety and streaming practices may have been due to pre-existing negative correlations between anxiety and ability. Australian studies reviewed by Gaudry and Spielberger (1971) indicated similar results. They argued that where students in all streams are given the same assessments on a particular curriculum, it is inevitable that those in the lower streams will have more profound failure experiences with consequent increases in test anxiety. The reviewers suggested that the lack of flexibility in the method and content of assessment appeared to be more salient than ability grouping in causing test-taking anxiety. It is still unclear how success and failure experiences influence expectations of subsequent performance, but causal attributions of performance and the beliefs constituting self-efficacy have suggestive theoretical importance. Threats to self-esteem might undermine self-efficacy additionally to stimulating A-state; and chronic failure experiences might establish a trait-like source of attributed causes of failure.

7. Mathematics: A Special Case?

The concept of mathematics anxiety has raised many issues. These include its relation to more general test-taking anxiety, to mathematics performance, disengagement with situations where mathematical skill might be required, the effects of appraisals, and attributions. Mathematics anxiety involves feelings of tension, confusion, disorganization, and helplessness when numerical manipulation is required or mathematical problems have to be solved. Dew et al. (1984) investigated the relation of mathematics anxiety to situational (state) test anxiety, mathematics performance, physiological arousal, and mathematics avoidance behavior. Their results suggested that mathematics anxiety and test anxiety were related but not identical. In terms of performance, mathematics anxiety measures did not account for performance variance much beyond what was accounted for by mathematics ability. Anxiety reduction, therefore, appeared unlikely to promote increases in performance. Mathematics anxiety showed little relation to physiological measures including heart rate and skin conductance, or to mathematics avoidance behavior.

Hunsley (1987) examined in detail the relations between mathematics and test anxiety, and particularly their capacity to predict appraisals of self and the testing situation, negative internal dialogue, and performance attributions. He concluded that even though mathematics anxiety and test anxiety are quite similar, in the context of mathematics examinations mathematics anxiety has incremental validity as a predictor of particular cognitive processes. These included importance of the examination, and performance appraisal in terms of expected grade and satisfaction with the examination. Anxiety measures were also associated with negative internal dialogue, with mathematics anxiety making a larger contribution. In terms of performance attributions only mathematics anxiety was related to blaming mathematics background for impaired test performance.

Stipek (1984) has provided important evidence on sex differences in attributions of mathematics performance among fifth and sixth graders. She found that girls more than boys were likely to attribute failure to lack of ability, and were less likely to attribute success to ability. They were also more likely to attribute performance to the difficulty of mathematics generally and to the particular test. The relation of these sex differences in attribution to sex differences in experienced mathematics anxiety does not appear to have been studied directly. However, the self-derogating attributions that appear more typical of girls, and their attributions of failure to lack of ability, are analogous to the cognitive appraisals that are sources of test-taking anxiety: threats to self-esteem and perceptions of overwhelming difficulty.

The evidence outlined here suggests that mathematics might be especially anxiety provoking, and more so among girls. Whether it is uniquely so is an interesting question which does not appear to have been studied.

8. Conclusion

Test-taking anxiety has been extensively studied since the 1950s. Its manifestations are well understood and its treatment appears to be relatively successful. Its relations with performance are complex, even though there is a pervasive finding that anxiety and performance tend to be correlated negatively. In knowledge-based examinations and testing, for example, the bases of performance may be much wider than, say, in aptitude testing. The importance of study skills and subject mastery in the former is well understood, and preparedness for examinations may well be an important moderator of test-taking anxiety.

Expectations of performance are related to its causal attributions, which may derive from many sources. These include classroom history, affective responses to previous assessments, beliefs about competencies, extent of preparedness, and so on. Affective responses to test feedback depend on whether the attributed causes of performance are internal or external, stable or unstable, and whether or not they are controllable. Failure tends to increase anxiety and tension. If it is attributed to unpreparedness, that is an internal unstable cause which is capable of being controlled. If, on the other hand, failure is attributed to lack of ability, that may be an internal stable cause which is not subject to personal control. Anxiety arising from the latter attribution may be more intractable than from the former.

The question of control leads into the issue of self-efficacy, which also appears to be an important moderator of test-taking anxiety. Beliefs that one can be successful appear to be part of overcoming the effects of test-taking anxiety and enhancing examination performance. Smith et al. (1990) concluded that theoretical formulations on the relations between anxiety and performance require understandings of the multiple deficits involved. Test-taking anxiety is not then best understood as merely debilitating emotional lability or inappropriate cognitive appraisal of the test circumstances which might be remedied by an appropriate therapeutic intervention. Rather, test-taking anxiety exists within a network of attributions of performance and self-estimates of capacities for success which themselves have to be understood if the effects of test-taking anxiety are to be moderated.

References

Allen G, Elias M, Zlotlow S 1980 Behavioral interventions for alleviating test anxiety: A methodological overview of current therapeutic practices. In: Sarason I G (ed.) 1980 *Test Anxiety: Theory, Research and Applications.* Erlbaum, Hillsdale, New Jersey

Alpert R, Haber R 1960 Anxiety in academic achievement situations. *J. Abnorm. Soc. Psychol.* 61: 207–15

Bandura A 1977 Self-efficacy: Toward a unifying theory of behavioral change. *Psychol. Rev.* 84(2): 191–215

Covington M V, Omelich C L 1987 "I knew it cold before the exam": A test of the anxiety-blockage hypothesis. *J. Educ. Psychol.* 79(4): 393–400

Deffenbacher J L, Hazaleus S L 1985 Cognitive, emotional and physiological components of test anxiety. *Cognit. Therap. Res.* 9(2): 169–86

Denney D 1980 Self-control approaches to the treatment of test anxiety. In: Sarason I G (ed.) 1980 *Test Anxiety: Theory, Research and Applications.* Erlbaum, Hillsdale, New Jersey

Dew K M K, Galassi J P, Galassi M D 1984 Math anxiety: Relation with situational test anxiety, performance, physiological arousal, and math avoidance behavior. *J. Counsel. Psychol.* 31: 580–83

Dion K L, Toner B B 1988 Ethnic differences in test anxiety. *J. Soc. Psychol.* 128(2): 165–72

Entwisle D R, Hayduk L A 1982 *Early Schooling: Cognitive and Affective Outcomes.* Johns Hopkins University Press, Baltimore, Maryland

Everson H T, Millsap R E, Rodriguez C M 1991 Isolating gender differences in text anxiety: A confirmatory factor analysis of the Test Anxiety Inventory. *Educ. Psychol. Meas.* 51(1): 243–51

Forsyth D R, McMillan J H 1981 Attributions, affect, and expectations: A test of Weiner's three-dimensional model. *J. Educ. Psychol.* 73(3): 393–403

Furst D, Tenenbaum G, Weingarten G 1985 Test anxiety, sex, and exam type. *Psychol. Rep.* 56(2): 663–68

Gaudry E, Spielberger C D 1971 *Anxiety and Educational Achievement.* Wiley Australasia, Sydney

Gjesme T 1982 Amount of manifested test anxiety in the heterogeneous classroom. *J. Psychol.* 110(2): 171–89

Hembree R 1988 Correlates, causes, effects, and treatment of test anxiety. *Rev. Educ. Res.* 58(1): 47–77

Herman W E 1990 Fear of failure as a distinctive personality trait measure of test anxiety. *J. Res. Dev. Educ.* 23(3): 180–85

Hunsley J 1987 Cognitive processes in mathematics anxiety and test anxiety: The role of appraisals, internal dialogue, and attributions. *J. Educ. Psychol.* 79(4): 388–92

Lent R W, Brown S D, Larkin K C 1984 Relation of self-efficacy expectations to academic achievement and persistence. *J. Counsel. Psychol.* 31(3): 356–62

Levy P, Gooch S, Kellmer-Pringle M L 1969 A longitudinal study of the relationship between anxiety and streaming in a progressive and a traditional junior school. *Br. J. Educ. Psychol.* 39: 166–73

Liebert R, Morris L 1967 Cognitive and emotional components of test anxiety: A distinction and some initial data. *Psychol. Rep.* 20(3): 975–78

Mandler G, Sarason S 1952 A study of anxiety and learning. *J. Abnorm. Soc. Psychol.* 47: 166–73

Morris L W, Davis M A, Hutchings C H 1981 Cognitive and emotional components of anxiety: Literature review and a revised worry-emotionality scale. *J. Educ. Psychol.* 73(4): 541–55

Sarnoff I, Lighthall F F, Waite R R, Davidson K S, Sarason S B 1958 A cross-cultural study of anxiety amongst American and English school children. *J. Educ. Psychol.* 49: 129–37

Smith R J, Arnkoff D B, Wright T L 1990 Test anxiety and academic competence: A comparison of alternative models. *J. Counsel. Psychol.* 37(3): 313–21

Spielberger C D 1966 *Anxiety and Behavior.* Academic Press, New York

Spielberger C D et al. 1980 *Preliminary (Professional) Manual for the State-trait Test Anxiety Inventory for Children.* Consulting Psychologists Press, Palo Alto, California

Stipek D J 1984 Sex differences in children's attributions for success and failure on math and spelling tests. *Sex Roles* 11(11/12): 969–81

Tobias S 1985 Test anxiety: Interference, defective skills, and cognitive capacity. *Educ. Psychol.* 20(3): 135–42

Tryon G 1980 The measurement and treatment of test anxiety. *Rev. Educ. Res.* 50(2): 353–72

Weiner B 1979 A theory of motivation for some classroom experiences. *J. Educ. Psychol.* 71(1): 3–25

Weiner B, Russell D, Lerman D 1978 Affective consequences of causal ascriptions. In: Harvey J H, Ickes W, Kidd R F (eds.) 1978 *New Directions in Attribution Research*, Vol. 2. Erlbaum, Hillsdale, New Jersey

Further Reading

Sarason I G (ed.) 1980 *Test Anxiety: Theory, Research, and Applications.* Erlbaum, Hillsdale, New Jersey

Validity of Tests

J. P. Keeves

Every achievement test involves a sample of items or tasks to which an individual or a group of individuals is required to respond in order to assess the extent to which learning has occurred. Issues concerned with the validity of a test have been widely debated and discussed, and relate to the meaningfulness of the test or whether the test measures what it purports to measure. Typically, three main aspects of validity are considered: content validity, predictive or criterion related validity, and construct validity (see *Validity*).

There are, however, questions associated with the strength of a test that seemingly go beyond these three traditional aspects of validity, or cut across them. They are concerned with a particular test and its relationships to a curriculum and to instruction in a particular field of learning. This entry considers tests and their interrelationships with the curriculum and with instruction that provide the domains from which items or tasks are selected in the development of tests. Such relationships help to assess whether the test is a meaningful instrument to measure learning with respect to that domain. Furthermore, the entry introduces several indicators that can be employed to show the extent to which a test may be considered to be a valid instrument for measuring the learning it seeks to measure.

1. Curricular Validity

The introduction of competency-test performance as a criterion for high school graduation in the United States in the late 1970s gave rise to legal challenges as to whether those states using such tests had provided students with an adequate opportunity to learn the skills being assessed. As a consequence the question of the validity of a test assumed great relevance and Jaeger (1989) reviewed and examined the issues involved. McClung (1979) in considering the opportunity provided for students to learn what the states were testing, introduced the terms "curricular validity" and "instructional validity," but such terms are readily confused with the ideas of content validity and test validity. The 1985 *Standards for Educational and Psychological Testing* issued by the American Psychological Association (APA), the American Educational Research Association (AERA), and the National Council on Measurement in Education (NCMA) stated that "content-related evidence [of validity] demonstrates the degree to which the sample of items, tasks, or questions on a test is representative of some defined universe or domain of content" (APA, AERA, NCMA 1985 p. 10).

However, Cronbach (1971 p. 443) had previously advanced the view that "validation is the process of examining the accuracy of a specific prediction or inference made from a test score." This range of views, from sampling adequacy to predictive power, as to what constitutes validity provides ample opportunity for legal debate, and little opportunity for the resolution of the theoretical, measurement, and research issues. Thus it is profitable to examine the ways in which the fairness of a test is addressed in cross-national testing programs, because such a context permits the issues to be considered without concern for the legal problems associated with administration of competency tests that influence the future livelihood of individuals.

2. Developing a Test

The first essential step in the development of any test is to define and delineate the domain from which tasks or items can be selected. A widely used strategy is to construct a table of specifications or two-way grid, with content along the vertical axis and educational objectives, behaviors, or processes along the horizontal axis. Bloom et al. (1971) presented excellent examples of two-way grids for most curriculum areas. In such grids, the *Taxonomy of Educational Objectives* (Bloom et al. 1956) provides a framework on which tasks or items can be classified with respect to the horizontal axis. However, other taxonomic classifications have been developed and are widely used in test development (see *Objective Tests in Measurement*). This table of specifications constitutes the test frame, equivalent to a sampling frame, within which items can be located and from which items can be selected either as a representative or random sample to form a specific test. Nevertheless, it is not uncommon for this two-way grid to be collapsed into one dimension only

—the content dimension—and for content alone to be taken into consideration in the construction of a test.

Irrespective of whether the frame used in the development of a test contains two or only one dimension, it is evident that not all cells of the grid are likely to be given equal weight or are likely to be equally represented by the same number of items, or by items of the same level of difficulty in any particular test. Sampling is clearly necessary, and unless items are selected as a simple random sample from a total population of items, some basis for the selection of the items must be established. Commonly, the curriculum is examined in detail and a measure of emphasis for each cell in the grid is obtained from the curriculum specifications, from the textbooks employed in the teaching of a particular subject or course, from statements of the broad content and objectives of a course, or from an estimate of the time given to instruction with respect to each cell. It is usually adequate to assess emphasis on a three-point scale (0—no or weak emphasis; 1—minor or moderate emphasis; 2—major or strong emphasis), although more elaborate rating procedures can be used. These measures of emphasis, obtained from the examination of the curriculum outlined above, provide weights for each cell of the grid used to delineate the domain. Items are then selected for inclusion in a particular test, as either a representative or random sample in proportion to the weight assigned to each cell of the grid or test frame.

Unless a procedure similar to the one described briefly above is employed in the development of a test, there is no way in which the test can be audited effectively to determine whether or not it provides a valid sampling of the items associated with the domain under consideration. However, adherence to such a procedure is not necessarily proof of the development of a valid test, although failure to follow such a procedure is likely to cast doubt on a test's validity. Indicators are clearly needed of the meaningfulness or relevance of the test with respect to both the curriculum and the students under survey.

3. Three Facets of the Curriculum

In the debate that followed the publication of the *Handbook of Formative and Summative Evaluation of Student Learning* (Bloom et al. 1971), it was recognized that the curriculum could be viewed from three distinct aspects (Keeves 1974).

First, there is the prescribed, mandated, or intended curriculum. The intended curriculum is specified or reflected in curriculum guides, course outlines, syllabi, and textbooks. In some school systems, the intended curriculum is developed at the national level. In others, it is specified and documented at the school district level, and sometimes each teacher is free to teach what is considered appropriate for the students in a particular classroom. It is rare that appropriate documentation does not exist recording what is taught to a particular group of students. However, it may be necessary, according to the policies and practices of a school system, to obtain information on the intended curriculum from a central office, from a sample of school subject coordinators, from a sample of classroom teachers, or from an inspection of the major textbooks in use in the schools.

Second, there is the translated or implemented curriculum. This aspect of the curriculum focuses on a particular school or classroom and is concerned with what has actually been taught to the students in the school or classroom. The implemented curriculum can be assessed in terms of the degree of emphasis given to a particular topic within the school or classroom, the time given to the teaching of a topic, or the proportion of the school or class group who have been exposed to the topic, since many schools and classrooms teach different sets of students using different levels or intensity of instruction. It is rare, though not unknown in some schools, for students to be taught through individualized instructional strategies, and such teaching practices should not be overlooked in attempting to assess the translated or intended curriculum. In addition, it is necessary to recognize that some of what students learn is acquired from outside the school or classroom, through general reading, the mass media, and informal instruction within the home and peer group.

The third facet of the curriculum is the attained, realized, or achieved curriculum, concerned with what students have learned as measured by the items included in a particular test. The major problem in the measurement of the achieved curriculum by means of a particular test is that every student approaches learning through exposure to a particular curriculum with some knowledge. The learning to be measured is at best relative to what is commonly an uncertain and unreliable starting point. Classical test theory does not provide a solution to this problem and as a consequence, criterion-referenced testing has been proposed as an alternative (see *Classical Test Theory; Criterion-referenced Measurement*). However, by the early 1990s, item response theory seemed to be providing the most promising approach toward the solution of this problem (see *Item Response Theory*).

The relationships between these three levels of the curriculum are shown in Fig. 1. At the first level, which involves the educational system, is the intended curriculum. The implemented curriculum is at the second level and involves the instruction that takes place in the classroom under survey. The achieved curriculum is at the third level and involves the testing of the individual student. The antecedent circumstances, conditions, and characteristics also need to be taken into consideration because they influence the three aspects of the curriculum, and their effects are mediated by the contexts of teaching and learning, namely, the system, the classroom, and the students.

These three levels of the curriculum and their ante-

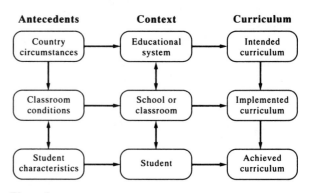

Figure 1
The context and components of the curriculum

cedents and contexts must be considered in examining the meaningfulness or strength of a particular test, and whether the items included in a test are a valid sample of the universe of items that can be derived from a particular curriculum. Furthermore, it is necessary to develop indicators that assess the extent to which a particular test has strength or validity, with respect to these three facets of the curriculum.

4. The Test and the Intended Curriculum

Three indexes have been developed to address the issue of the extent to which a test relates to a particular intended curriculum. These indexes seek to provide answers to three specific questions.

(a) To what extent do the items within the test cover the intended curriculum or syllabus?

(b) To what extent do the items in the test relate to what is taught in the intended curriculum?

(c) To what extent does a particular intended curriculum match the more general curriculum, formed by the body of content that might be taught?

It is clear, with respect to the first question, that although a test cannot, in general, cover all cells of the grid associated with a particular intended curriculum, the extent to which the test covers the curriculum is of considerable importance. The index that was developed to provide an estimate of the strength of a test, with respect to this question, has been named the "test coverage index." It gives a measure of the extent to which a particular curriculum is covered by the items included in the test. Coverage, of course, can be increased by extending the length of a test. However, it is likely that increasing the length of a test, beyond a certain point, will start to provide redundant information.

In order to answer the second question, a "test

relevance index" has been proposed. This index was developed to provide a measure of the extent to which the items included in a test are taught through a particular curriculum, or are relevant to that intended curriculum. It should be noted that even when all the items in a specific test are relevant to a particular curriculum, they may only cover a small percentage of that curriculum. The test coverage index allows for this aspect, while the test relevance index does not. The two indexes are clearly complementary.

Information to provide an answer to the third question is given by a curriculum coverage index. A classroom, school, or school system that limits itself to a very narrow range of topics or objectives is likely to achieve a high level of performance with respect to those topics or objectives, at the expense of the topics or objectives that have not been taught. Thus, although the curriculum coverage index does not provide direct information on the relationship between a test and a particular curriculum, it does provide information that is indirectly of importance, when comparisons are being made regarding performance on a particular test. In the sections that follow, an account is given as to how these three indexes of the validity of a test can be calculated.

4.1 Curriculum Ratings

The first and necessary step, to be taken before these indexes of test validity are calculated, is to obtain information with respect to the emphasis given in the curriculum to a particular cell within the content-objective grid described above. It is generally sufficient to obtain ratings on a three-point scale, namely, major or strong emphasis (2), minor or moderate emphasis (1), and no or weak emphasis (0). It is also possible to obtain information on the universality of instruction, with respect to a particular cell in the content-objective grid. Again, it is generally sufficient to obtain ratings on a three-point scale, namely, universal (2), restricted (1), and nil (0), according to whether instruction is provided to all students under survey with respect to a particular cell in the grid, or whether only some or none receive instruction with respect to the specified content or objective. Attempts have been made to combine these two aspects of instruction by extending the number of ratings beyond three, but this seems to lead to the use of the extremes by some assigners of ratings, and not by others, and thus to inconsistencies when the data from curriculum ratings are used for comparative purposes.

Information associated with these curriculum ratings is of course essential for the development of a valid test. However, the task of providing ratings for a two-way grid has proved, on several occasions, to be rather more difficult than was expected. As a consequence it would appear to be a more manageable task for teachers and curriculum experts to provide information with respect to the categories along each axis of the grid separately.

In order to explain the calculation of these three test validity indexes, a small hypothetical table is presented as Table 1. In Table 1 it should be noted that the two-way grid has been collapsed to provide only the content axis. The maximum coverage score has been assigned to each content area (Column 1) or cell in the grid. Thus each cell has been given the value of 2 as in Column 2.

Table 1
Hypothetical table for calculating curriculum validity indexes

(1)	(2)	(3)	(4)	(5)	(6)	(7)
Content area	Maximum coverage score	Curriculum emphasis score	Number of items	Item relevance score	Maximum item relevance score	Cell relevance score
A	2	2	4	(4×2)	(4×2)	2
B	2	1	3	(3×1)	(3×2)	1
C	2	2	2	(2×2)	(2×2)	2
D	2	0	1	0	2	−1
E	2	1	0	0	0	0
F	2	0	0	0	0	0
Total	12	6	10	15	20	4

Calculation of indexes

Test coverage index   = 4/6   = 0.67
Test relevance index   = 15/20 = 0.75
Curriculum coverage index = 6/12 = 0.50

4.2 Test Coverage Index

Two aspects of test coverage have to be taken into consideration. First, it is necessary to consider whether the items in the test are associated with a content area in which there is major (2), minor (1), or no (0) emphasis in a particular setting (see Column 3). Second, it is necessary to consider whether for each curriculum content area given an emphasis rating for a specific intended curriculum there is an appropriate item in the test. Where the curriculum emphasis score is 2 and there are items in the test, a cell relevance score of 2 is assigned. Where there is a cell with only a minor curriculum emphasis and there are items in the test, a score of 1 is assigned. However, if there is a cell with no emphasis on the content area and there are items in the test, a score of -1 is assigned. Where there is a cell with major or minor emphasis, but there is no item in the test, a cell relevance score of zero (0) is assigned. These cell relevance scores are recorded in Column 7 of Table 1 and the total cell relevance score is calculated. It will be seen that the cell relevance scores reflect the emphases of a particular curriculum and the test coverage index is calculated by dividing the total cell relevance score in Column 7, namely 4, by the total curriculum emphasis score in Column 3, namely 6, to give a value of 0.67.

4.3 Test Relevance Index

In Column 4 of Table 1 the number of items in the test in a particular content area is recorded. If an item lies in a content area in which, for a particular school system, the curriculum emphasis score is 2, then a value of 2 is assigned as an item relevance score, and if the curriculum emphasis score is 1, a value of 1 is assigned. For each content area the assigned item relevance score is equal to the product of the number of items associated with that content area multiplied by the curriculum emphasis score, and this product, the item relevance score, is entered in Column 5. The maximum item relevance score for a content area is entered in Column 6 and is obtained by multiplying the number of items associated with that content area by 2, which is the maximum coverage score for the cell. In Table 1 the sums for the item relevance scores and the maximum item relevance scores are calculated and are entered at the foot of Columns 5 and 6, respectively. The test relevance index gives the extent to which the items in the test are relevant to the particular curriculum under consideration, and is calculated by dividing the total item relevance score in Column 5, namely 15, by the maximum total item relevance score in Column 6, namely 20, to give the value 0.75.

4.4 Curriculum Coverage Index

For the particular curriculum under consideration, the curriculum emphasis score on a three-point scale is entered in Column 3, alongside the maximum coverage score which is entered in Column 2 in Table 1. For this fictitious set of data, the total maximum coverage score, recorded at the foot of Column 2, is 12 and the total curriculum emphasis score, recorded at the foot of Column 3, is 6. The extent to which this particular curriculum covers the complete content grid is given by the curriculum coverage index, which is calculated by dividing the total curriculum emphasis score, namely 6, by the total maximum coverage score, namely 12, to obtain a value of the index, 0.50.

4.5 Use of Indexes of Curriculum Validity of a Test

An example of the use of these three indexes of curriculum validity of a test is provided in a report of the Second Science Study of the International Association for the Evaluation of Educational Achievement (IEA) (Rosier and Keeves 1991). Although wider use of these indexes of the validity of a test with respect to the curriculum being examined is required, and while these indexes have certain shortcomings arising from the relative crudeness of the procedures involved in the calculation of the indexes, they generally appear to provide meaningful and relevant information in this cross-national study of science.

Strategies that might be used to refine and develop further such indexes of curriculum validity of a test have been explored in the United States in the Second IEA Mathematics Study (Travers 1986), in which teachers were asked to report the approximate number of class periods they spent during the school year on each of the selected topics in a list that formed the content axis of the curriculum grid employed in test construction. This information was then available to provide a measure of the intended curriculum. However, only data on the number of periods for teachers at the 10th, 25th, 50th, 75th, and 90th percentages for each of the content areas are reported (Travers 1986).

5. The Test and the Implemented Curriculum

Several studies have sought to measure the implemented curriculum with respect to items included in specific tests. The procedures employed have yielded meaningful and useful results insofar as strong relationships with achievement at a cross-national level have been reported (see Husén 1967, Comber and Keeves 1973, Keeves 1992). This work has led to the acceptance of a measure of the opportunity to learn the items included in a test as providing important and meaningful information on the relevance of the test for a particular group of students under survey. In addition, a more detailed analysis of data collected on opportunity to learn has sometimes proved to be useful in accounting for differences in achievement between students, schools, and school systems (see Rosier 1980, Keeves 1992). In addition, research workers have examined cross-national performance on individual test items with respect to the percentage of teachers of class groups who reported having taught the particular test item (see McKnight 1987).

Rating scales are generally employed to assess the opportunity that students in a particular class or school have to learn each of the items in a test. The procedure used to obtain information is to ask each teacher of a class group of students, or a group of teachers collectively in a school in which students are tested, to make an estimate of the extent to which their students have had the opportunity to learn the content of the items in the test. Thus, sometimes the ratings are assigned separately by individual teachers in a school and aggregated if a measure at the school level is required, and sometimes the ratings are made by a group of teachers acting in collaboration and after discussion, to provide a common set of ratings for the school. Two types of ratings have been widely used; namely, percentage ratings and year- or grade-level ratings. The latter type of ratings is generally used where intact class groups are under survey, and all members of the class group can be assumed to have had the same instruction with respect to a common curriculum.

5.1 Percentage Ratings

For the percentage ratings, each teacher or group of teachers is asked with reference to the group of students tested in a class or school to indicate for each item in a test what percentage of the students had the opportunity to learn the concepts tested by the item.

A.	All (100%) students	4 or	1.00
B.	More than 75% of the students	3	0.875
C.	Between 25% and 75% of the students	2	0.50
D.	Less than 25% of the students	1	0.125
E.	None (0%) of the students	0	0

Responses to this rating scale can be scored either as 4, 3, 2, 1, and 0, or alternatively with scale values at the midpoint of each range, namely, 1.00, 0.875, 0.50, 0.125, and 0 as indicated above. Whichever scoring procedure is employed, responses to individual items and by individual teachers can be aggregated to obtain a total test score for each teacher, an item score for all teachers, or a total test score for all teachers. The scores that involve the assigning of the midpoint of the range to each response category have a more readily interpretable meaning for the purposes of reporting results.

5.2 Year-level Ratings

For the year-level ratings, each teacher or group of teachers is asked, with reference to the group of students under survey, to indicate for each item the year level at which the concepts tested by the task were first taught. The categories and code values generally employed are:

A.	Two or more years earlier	1
B.	One year earlier	1
C.	Earlier during the current year	1
D.	Later during the current year or at a later year level	0
E.	Not at all	0

Responses in these categories are scored 1, 1, 1, 0, or 0, as indicated above, according to whether the students had or had not the opportunity to learn the test items.

A useful question associated with opportunity to learn and the implemented curriculum was asked in the Second IEA Science Study in Canada (Connelly et al. 1989), which involved the amount of time given to the teaching of the content required to answer a particular test item. The wording of the question used was:

The amount of time you spend teaching the students the content they need to answer the item is:
A. None
B. 15 minutes or less
C. Between 15 miniutes and 30 minutes
D. Between 30 minutes and 1 hour
E. Between 1 hour and 3 hours
F. More than 3 hours

The use of such a question is most appropriate where a teacher can respond with respect to a particular class group, where the test items relate to a specific school curriculum, and where the analysis is subsequently undertaken at the level of individual items.

Other questions apparently associated with opportunity to learn are sometimes asked. Such questions involve the proportion of students expected to answer an item correctly or the proportion of students in a class group for whom an item is considered appropriate. However, to respond to such questions requires not only a knowledge of whether or not the students under survey have had the opportunity to learn the content tested by the item, but also an assessment by the teacher of the relative difficulty of the item with respect to the ability or level of aptitude of the student group. While such measures are, no doubt, more strongly correlated with achievement outcomes than are other indexes, they appear to be assessing expected performance rather than the curriculum as implemented in schools or classrooms, and their use cannot be recommended.

It is important to recognize that in school systems where there is a centrally prescribed curriculum and where all teachers at a given grade level are expected to teach specified content, clearly identifiable relationships between measures of opportunity to learn and achievement outcomes are unlikely to exist. It is only in school systems where there are marked differences between schools or classrooms that significant relationships are likely to be observed.

6. The Test and the Achieved Curriculum

The major issue associated with the use of performance on a test as a measure of the achieved curriculum is whether a total score on the test, or a subcore on any part of the test, has the same meaning for different students and different subgroups of students, so that comparisons can be made between the relative performances of students or subgroups of students. In plain terms, the question is whether or not it is appropriate to calculate a total score. Certain analyses can be carried out to assess the meaningfulness of a total score on a test. First, the item difficulties for different subgroups may be intercorrelated and the correlations examined to determine whether the relative item difficulties are similar across subgroups. This analysis was undertaken across 10 countries with data from the First IEA Mathematics Study and strong intercorrelations were reported by Wolf (1969).

A second analysis can be undertaken to examine whether the item-remainder (total score minus item score) point biserial correlations are similar in magnitude across subgroups taking the test. The item-point biserial correlations are then correlated across subgroups to determine the extent of correspondence and whether items behave in similar ways across subgroups in discriminating between high-performing and low-performing students within a subgroup. Again Wolf (1969) has reported moderate intercorrelations across 10 countries in the First IEA Mathematics Study.

A third type of analysis involves the examination of the interrelations between subscores on a test for the different subgroups. This type of analysis was carried out by Comber and Keeves (1973) for the different subscores used in the First IEA Science Study, and moderate to strong intercorrelations between subtests were reported.

Peaker (1969) carried out a fourth type of examination with respect to the national subscore data, collected in the First IEA Mathematics Study, and reported generally moderate to high intercorrelations but with some low correlations at the preuniversity level between certain specific subscores. Furthermore, he showed that it made very little difference, in terms of the rank order of performance across countries, how the national part scores were weighted to form a national total score. Weighting schemes involving the prior judgments of the test constructors in terms of the relative numbers of items employed (or equal weights), or when following the administration of the tests the relative difficulties of the items were taken into consideration, gave rise to some divergence in rankings assigned. However, they were not large enough to produce serious discrepancies in rank orders of the total scores for the 12 countries participating in the study.

One approach that has also been used is to calculate an interitem tetrachoric correlation matrix and then to carry out a principal components or maximum likelihood factor analysis, with communalities in the diagonal, in order to investigate the factor structure of a test (Lord 1980). Where a single dominant factor is found, there is clearly strong support for the calculation of a valid total score. If, however, a more complex factor structure is observed, some ambiguities arise in obtaining a meaningful interpretation, because many different factor analytic techniques which yield different results are available for examining the data. Carroll (1983) would, however, strongly recommend the employment of oblique axes and the oblimin procedure. The ambiguities associated with the use of such techniques have given rise to the development of confirmatory factor analysis, using maximum likelihood procedures, in which the factor structure of the test is specified and an analysis is carried out to confirm or deny the existence of the hypothesized structure. Alternatively, confirmatory factor analyses can be used to choose between two or more hypothesized factor structures.

In this context, Heise and Bohrnstedt (1970) defined validity as the correlation between a measure and the true underlying variable. An index of theoretical validity is obtained as distinct from a measure of empirical validity, which involves the correlation between two observed variables. However, the estimation of theoretical validity coefficients requires a model to define the theoretical construct. The alternative, which involves the calculation of an empirical (or predictive) validity coefficient for a composite of observed measures, is quite straightforward if an appropriate criterion measure can be identified. Appropriate criterion measures are unfortunately not commonly available.

Munck (1979) examined the theoretical validity of the science achievement tests employed at the 14-year old level in the First IEA Science Study for England, Hungary, and Sweden. In these three countries, science was largely taught as the separate subjects of biology, chemistry, and physics at the time of testing in 1970, and as a consequence considerable doubt existed as to whether it was appropriate to calculate a total score from the four component tests of biology, chemistry, physics, and practical work. Reliability estimates were available for these four subscales for the three countries and could be built into the LISREL (*Li*near *S*tructural *Rel*ations Analysis) model in order to take measurement errors into consideration. For this analysis the relationship between the latent variables and the observed variance involves a simple model, in which the observed variance is the sum of the true variance and measurement error. The coefficients relating the latent trait of science achievement to the subtest true scores are then considered as validity coefficients. Analyses were initially reported for a sample of Swedish boys and subsequently for the three countries examined simultaneously. The estimated combined validity coefficients were 0.968 for physics, 0.904 for chemistry, 0.892 for biology, and 1.00 for the practical work subtest with identifiable country-specific deviations from the international pattern. The overall degree of misspecification in the international measure were: for Sweden, 0.027; for England, 0.024; and for Hungary, 0.023. This indicated a satisfactory level of fit and adequate justification for the calculation of the total score, combining across subtests, as well as the use of the total score for comparisons between countries.

7. Toward the Improvement of Measurement

The opportunity exists as a result of developmental work that has been carried out by Lord and his colleagues at Educational Testing Service (see *Item Response Theory*) and Rasch and his followers in Europe and the United States (see *Rasch Measurement, Theory of*) to construct a scale for the measurement of the achieved curriculum through the use of item response theory models. In particular, the Rasch, or one-parameter logistic function model is the most powerful but most restrictive approach. In the course of examining students' responses to items on a test in terms of these models, it is necessary to identify both test items and persons that do not fit the model, which involves a single underlying dimension. Thus, provided both items and persons fit the model involving the single hypothesized underlying dimension or latent trait, there is undeniable evidence that the test behaves as a valid measure, at least with respect to the theoretical validity of the instrument. In general, the one-parameter model may be considered reasonably robust. Consequently, it is not commonly necessary to reject more than a few items or persons that do not maintain a high level of fit to the Rasch model, when a test has been well-constructed. However, it may sometimes be necessary to reject a significant number of items and persons that do not conform to the model, when a test has not been carefully constructed and is thus not a valid measure.

The analyses carried out using the Rasch model involve the estimation of the level of difficulty of each item, which is theoretically independent of the sample of students taking the test. Under these circumstances it is possible to detect items that not only do not fit the theoretical model, but also items for which curriculum variations applying to subgroups taking the test indicate that the items do not conform to invariant levels of difficulty. An index of conformity to invariance of difficulty levels is provided by an intraclass correlation coefficient obtained from a two-way analysis of variance of item difficulty levels for the subgroups under consideration. This intraclass correlation is a further index of a test's validity. Clearly the possibilities exist for the construction of tests that involve these new approaches to measurement. However, insufficient experience is currently available to indicate whether such measurement procedures lead to the development of tests that are more meaningful and more valid with respect to specific curricula than are tests constructed using more traditional test development procedures.

Moreover, the case is "not proven" that tests that have been constructed and scaled using item response theory procedures have greater explanatory power than tests that have been constructed and scored in other ways. Ultimately, the usefulness of any procedures employed in the construction and scoring of tests rests on the strength of the relationships that can be established between test scores and other measures in prediction and explanation (see Kaplan 1964).

References

APA, AERA, NCME 1985 *Standards for Educational and Psychological Testing*. American Psychological Association, Washington, DC

Bloom B S, Hastings J F, Madaus G F 1971 *Handbook of Formative and Summative Evaluation of Student Learning*. McGraw-Hill, New York

Bloom B S, Krathwohl D R, Masia B B 1956 *Taxonomy of Educational Objectives Handbook. Vol. 1: Cognitive Domain*. McKay, New York

Carroll J B 1983 Studying individual differences in cognitive abilities: Through and beyond factor analysis. In: Dillon R F, Schmeck R R (eds.) 1983 *Individual Differences in Cognition*, Vol. 1. Academic Press, New York

Comber L C, Keeves J P 1973 *Science Education in Nineteen Countries*. Almqvist and Wiksell, Stockholm

Connelly F M, Crocker R K, Kass H 1989 *Science Education in Canada. Vol. 2: Achievement and Attitudes*. OISE Press, Toronto

Cronbach L J 1971 Test validation. In: Thorndike R L 1971 *Educational Measurement*, 2nd edn. American Council on Education, Washington, DC

Heise K, Bohrnstedt G W 1970 Validity, invalidity and reliability. In: Borgatta E G, Bohrnstedt G W (eds.) 1970 *Sociological Methodology*. Jossey-Bass, San Francisco, California

Husén T (ed.) 1967 *International Study of Achievement in Mathematics: A Comparison of 12 Countries*. Almqvist and Wiksell, Stockholm

Jaeger R M 1989 Certification of student competence. In: Linn R L 1989 *Educational Measurement*, 3rd edn. Macmillan, New York

Kaplan A 1964 *The Conduct of Inquiry*. Chandler, San Francisco, California

Keeves J P 1974 The IEA Science Project. Science achievement in three countries: Australia, the Federal Republic of Germany, and the United States. In: UNESCO 1974 *Implementation of Curricula in Science Education*. German Commission for UNESCO, Cologne

Keeves J P (ed.) 1992 *The IEA Study of Science III. Changes in Science Education and Achievement: 1970–1984*. Pergamon Press, Oxford

Lord F M 1980 *Applications of Item Response Theory to Practical Testing Problems*. Erlbaum, Hillsdale, New Jersey

McClung M S 1979 Competency testing programs: Legal and educational issues. *Fordham Law Review* 47: 651–712

McKnight C C et al. 1987 *The Underachieving Curriculum: Assessing US School Mathematics from an International Perspective*. Stipes, Champaign, Illinois

Munck I M E 1979 *Model Building in Comparative Education: Applications of the LISREL Method to Cross-national Survey Data*. Almqvist and Wiksell, Stockholm

Peaker G F 1969 How should national part scores be weighted? *Int. Rev. Educ.* 15(2): 229–37

Rosier M J 1980 *Changes in Secondary School Mathematics in Australia 1964–1978*. Australian Council for Educational Research, Hawthorn

Rosier M J, Keeves J P (eds.) 1991 *The IEA Study of Science 1. Science Education and Curricula in Twenty-Three Countries*. Pergamon Press, Oxford

Travers K J (ed.) 1986 *Second Study of Mathematics: Detailed Report United States*. Stipes, Champaign, Illinois

Wolf R M 1969 The analysis of the item data for the IEA mathematics tests. *Int. Rev. Educ.* 15(2): 237–41

Vocational Interests and Aptitudes, Measures of

J. J. Lokan

In Western societies the main source of power for most people is their occupation, because their occupation is usually their main source of money and status. In late-twentieth-century democratic societies, a strong social conscience has developed about the rights of disadvantaged and minority groups to have equality of access to life-shaping social institutions, particularly those providing educational and career opportunities. Thus, an important concern of developments in vocational interest and aptitude measurement has been that test or inventory results be used effectively and fairly, so that no individual or group is disadvantaged through their use.

That educational and career opportunities for groups who are already disadvantaged need to be widened is generally accepted. There has been considerable controversy about the ways in which the widening might best be achieved, however. This issue is discussed later in the entry. To begin with, some definitions of key terms are provided. These are followed by discussions of purposes for measuring interests and aptitudes, of ways in which interests and aptitudes may be measured and of characteristics of some of the most widely used instruments. The entry concludes with comments on the equity issues referred to above, after a brief review of topics that continue to be foci of research.

1. Definitions

When the word "vocational" is used together with terms such as "interests," "aptitudes," or even "education," it is often given connotations of courses or jobs involving lesser academic demands. For example, in the first edition of the *International Encyclopedia of Education,* Tittle referred to an educational use of vocational aptitude measures as "to select students or to assist students to select specific vocational programs such as shop or business" (1985 p. 5536). In some countries (e.g., Holland and parts of Canada) vocational schools or courses are provided for students who do not achieve or survive in the academic stream. The *Concise Oxford Dictionary* gives two meanings to "vocation": the first (from the Latin *vocare*, "to call") as a "divine call to, or sense of fitness for, a career or occupation," the second as a person's "employment, trade, profession." For the purposes of this entry the term "vocation" (and, by extension, "vocational") is given a broad connotation, having an affective component as suggested by the first dictionary definition. It is also presumed to include occupations encompassing the full range of types of work skills, not just those with less academic requirements.

While some authors use the terms "vocation" and "occupation" virtually synonymously, justifications for distinguishing between them and for attributing a broad-ranging meaning to "vocation" are provided by much of the literature in the field of vocational psychology. For example, to Crites, vocational behavior is something that is done in response to a stimulus from the occupational world and comprises all the responses an individual makes in choosing or adjusting to a job, making retirement plans, and so on (1969 p. 16). To Super, a vocation is "an occupation with commitment, distinguished primarily by its psychological as contrasted with its economic meaning; ego-involving, meaningful to the individual as an activity, not solely for its productive, distributive, or service outcome and its economic rewards" (1976 p. 10).

While "interests" have been assigned a key role in the "wise choice of a vocation" since the early twentieth century, they have been defined over those years in a variety of ways: as constellations of likes and dislikes, as patterns of behavior, as outcomes of behavior, as activities, as drives, as self-concepts, or as aspects of personality. The *Concise Oxford Dictionary* defines an interest as a "quality exciting [concern or curiosity] or holding one's attention," thus clearly imparting an affective, motivational flavor to the term. A common thread in psychological views of interests over the years is that they are a pervasive aspect of an individual's personality and are highly relevant in explaining behavior. In the introduction to a landmark early review of interest measurement by Fryer (1931), Terman wrote "Both the amount and direction of one's life accomplishments are determined largely by the factor of interest" (Terman in Fryer 1931 p.xvii). As Strong, the most prominent early figure in the field of interest measurement, expressed it: "They [interests] point to what the individual wants to do, they are reflections of what he considers satisfying" (1943 p. 19). The well-known view of Holland is summarized in the following: "[Vocational interests] represent the expression of personality in work, school subjects, hobbies, recreational activities and preferences. In short, what we have called 'vocational interests' are simply another aspect of personality." (1985 pp. 7–8).

Even more problems have been experienced with defining the term "aptitudes." In the *Concise Oxford Dictionary*, aptitude is "natural propensity or talent" or "ability to acquire a particular skill"; in turn, ability is "capacity [to do something]" or "cleverness, talent, mental power." The circularity evident in the dictionary definitions has also caused problems for psychologists: "The definition of aptitude has been beset by so many conceptual and semantic ambiguities and confusions that there is considerably less than general agreement on its meaning" (Crites 1969 p. 26). Some writers regard an ability as more generic than an aptitude, encompassing both the "degree of mastery already acquired in an activity" as well as the "specific . . . behaviors which facilitate the learning of a task and which are relatively constant over time." (Super and Crites 1962 p. 73). In this view, "ability" includes achievement, whereas "aptitude" is more akin to a trait. A more current view is that aptitude tests are tests of developed abilities, distinguished from achievement tests mainly in the purposes for which they are designed and used (Anastasi 1982).

Despite the attempts to make distinctions between the terms "ability" and "aptitude" they are found to be used interchangeably in the literature. Or, what to some authors is an ability—for example, Fleishman and Reilly (1992)—to others seems to be regarded as an aptitude. Fleishman and Reilly describe a total of 52 supposedly different abilities, in the categories cognitive, psychomotor, physical, and sensory/perceptual. By contrast, Hunter wrote that "general cognitive ability is usually measured by summing across tests of several specific aptitudes" (1986 p. 341), some of which bear resemblance to components of Fleishman and Reilly's list. For the purposes of this entry, the term "aptitude" will be assumed to include the range of human capabilities that are of potential relevance in predicting workplace performance or performance in pre-employment programs of study, regardless of academic level.

2. Purposes for Measuring Vocational Interests and Aptitudes

Why are psychologists keen to assess people's interests and capabilities? The purposes differ according to whether the question is being approached from the viewpoint of an educator/counselor or an employer's representative. The latter wishes to maximize workplace performance and efficiency, the former to provide people with information that should help them to identify careers in which they might achieve personal fulfillment. Employers are likely to place more emphasis on appropriate abilities or aptitudes, whereas counselors may give equal or even greater weighting to interests. These two perspectives of purpose are not unrelated, at least in theory—it has long been postulated that a person should be more satisfied in a job and will therefore perform its duties better if the requirements and environment of the job are compatible with the person's interests and capabilities.

3. Background: Measuring Methods and Instruments

3.1 Interests

Vocational interests have traditionally been measured with paper-and-pencil instruments. Early measures were based on the rationale of "people–similarity," which arose from the observation that people in the same job tend to have similar likes and dislikes. According to this rationale, a person will be most satisfied in a job or jobs for which the similarities between his or her interests and those of people in the job are greatest. More recently, interest measures have been based on a rationale of "activity–similarity," which assumes that if people think they like to do activities that are similar to those they would need to do on a job, then they will be satisfied with that job. Paper-and-pencil inventories of vocational interests that are in widest use usually contain either a series of statements describing work-related activities or a series of occupational titles. For such titles the respondent presumably holds beliefs about either activities or persons in the occupations or a combination of these, to which beliefs he or she reacts when completing the inventory. Some kind of measuring scale is provided by means of which respondents indicate the strength of their like or dislike of the activity or occupation. Differing methodologies are used in that some instruments rely on forced choices between clusters of two or three alternatives, some require rank ordering of larger groups of occupational titles, some use Likert scales, and others use merely Like–Dislike or Like–Indifferent–Dislike response categories.

The "big three" of interest assessment—the instruments based on the pioneering work of Strong, who published his first *Interest Blank* in 1927; Kuder, whose first *Preference Record* was published in 1934; and Holland, whose first *Vocational Preference Inventory* appeared in 1958—still dominate vocational counseling today (Borgen 1986). These instruments have continued to evolve and several new ones have appeared since the 1970s. None of the later initiatives is as innovative in its approach as Holland's work was in the 1960s. Prior to that, Strong pioneered the "empirical keying" approach, using groups of people in designated occupations compared with "Men-in-General." Kuder, on the other hand, initially developed homogeneous scales, though he did add empirically keyed occupational scales later in the *Kuder Occupational Interest Survey* (KOIS). Strong's and Kuder's inventories both required expensive research and large samples to establish their scales. Scoring is complex, generally in the 1990s requiring a computer, and yields results for a multitude of occupational scales.

By contrast, Holland's approach is characterized by simplicity—"his bent was conceptual, theoretical and practical rather than psychometric" (Borgen 1986 p. 85). Holland theorized that "in our culture most persons (and environments) can be categorized as one of six types: realistic, investigative, artistic, social, enterprising, or conventional" (1985 p. 2), and developed instruments to assess people's interests in relation to these categories. His scheme "allows a simple ordering of a person's resemblance to each of the six models [types], providing the possibility of 720 different personality patterns . . . for coping with the environment" (p. 3). The usefulness of the theory for vocational choice rests on the assumption that people will choose work "environments that allow them to exercise their skills and abilities . . . and take on agreeable problems and roles" (p. 4). Thus, realistic types seek realistic environments, and so on. Holland's inventories, the *Vocational Preference Inventory* and the *Self-Directed Search*, are easy to score and self-scoring is advocated for immediate feedback of results to respondents.

Holland's six-category scheme was found to have sufficient validity and appeal that scales called General Occupational Themes reflecting the six categories were introduced to the Strong inventory (then called the *Strong–Campbell Interest Inventory*) in 1972 and continue to be used. Further, many newer inventories feature the same or very closely related category schemes, for example, the *Harrington–O'Shea Career Decision-Making System*, Johansson's *Career Assessment Inventory*, Lamb and Prediger's *Unisex Edition of the ACT Interest Inventory* (UNIACT), and the United States Employment Service's USES Interest Inventory. Holland's scheme has not always been fully supported by research data (discussed below), but its importance is such that many authors accept it as the basis for career assessment and counseling programs (e.g., Lowman 1991). As Borgen wrote, "the amount of research generated by Holland's approach is unequaled in vocational behavior . . . due to the simplicity and elegance of his propositions, their focus on core con-

ceptual issues, and the fact that they have permitted disconfirmation" (1986 p. 89). Readers who are interested in a focused discussion of many "pros" and some "cons" for Holland's scheme are referred to the two recent special journal editions listed under "Further Reading."

3.2 Aptitudes

During the twentieth century, theories about taxonomies of human mental abilities or aptitudes have moved from the idea of a predominant single ability, or general intelligence, to the idea of several primary ability factors as proposed by Thurstone in the 1930s, to the 120 much more specific abilities allowed for in Guilford's "Structure of the Intellect" model in the 1960s, then back to the 10 or so abilities from Ekstrom's work summarized in Dunnette's (1976) review. Since that time further views have emerged in the literature—(see *Models of Intelligence*). From the point of view of vocational psychology, debate in the 1990s is not so much about the nature and organization of abilities, but rather about their role in predicting work-related performance. Some comments on this debate are made in Sect. 5.3.

A more focused strand of research on the identification of abilities or aptitudes relevant to workplace performance has been undertaken since the 1960s by industrial psychologists such as Fleishman and his colleagues. These psychologists have been concerned with physical, psychomotor, and sensory as well as cognitive abilities and have analyzed each domain at a very specific level. A major goal of their work was first to identify the abilities and then to have job experts reliably rate work tasks according to the importance of each of the abilities to the performance of the tasks. According to Peterson and Bownas (1982), 19 cognitive or perceptual abilities and 18 psychomotor or physical abilities were substantiated in this work. In Fleishman and Reilly (1992), the list has been expanded to include 52 abilities.

Vocational aptitude testing has never matched developments in theories about the nature and structure of abilities. The dominant influence on vocational aptitude measurement has remained that of Thurstone's "primary mental abilities" model. With some exceptions (such as the computer field, for which some measures claiming to be of specifically relevant aptitudes have been developed, and the clerical field for which detailed batteries have existed for some time —a good example is the *Modern Occupational Skills Tests* published in the United Kingdom by the National Foundation for Educational Research) multiaptitude batteries have reigned supreme and continue to be used extensively despite controversies in the literature about their value. The best known batteries remain the *General Aptitude Test Battery* (GATB) developed by the United States Employment Service and the *Differential Aptitude Tests* (DAT) developed by Wesman and Bennett. Both of these batteries are used in several countries besides the United States. The *Armed Services Vocational Aptitude Battery* (ASVAB) is also taken by a large number of students each year within the United States. Other less extensively used batteries based on a similar rationale include, for example, the *Employee Aptitude Survey* published in the United States and the *Differential Test Battery* published in the United Kingdom. All the batteries cited are variations on a theme, though they are designed for a range of clients.

The multiaptitude batteries usually produce between five and nine scores. The GATB, for example, yields factor scores for verbal aptitude, numerical aptitude, spatial aptitude, general learning ability (a composite of the previous three), form perception, clerical perception, motor coordination, finger dexterity, and manual dexterity. The DAT, which is advocated more for use in guidance of secondary level students than for employee selection, does not cover the sensory or motor dimensions yet still yields nine scores. As well as scales measuring verbal, numerical, general (the sum of verbal and numerical), abstract reasoning, and clerical aptitudes, the DAT includes measures of mechanical reasoning, spelling, and language usage. Most specific aptitude tests and the tests within the multiaptitude batteries are paper-and-pencil in format. Some subtests of the GATB require use of apparatus, however, and tests of psychomotor abilities or aptitudes typically involve manipulation of materials such as pegboards. A useful list of specific aptitude measures (which he calls ability measures) is included in Lowman (1991 pp. 305–06).

Although it varies from country to country and, in many cases, from area to area within countries, entry to higher level education and professional training programs is often based on a mixture of past achievement in one or more subject areas together with some indication of general "scholastic aptitude." For this purpose scholastic aptitude is usually assessed by a combination of verbal and quantitative test items, as far removed in their content from specific educational curricula as possible. The importance of a general cognitive aptitude or ability measure in assessing the potential for performance in a wide range of areas, including performance "on the job," is also recognized in the multiaptitude batteries, which usually provide for two or three of their cognitive scales to be aggregated to provide such a measure (see *Models of Intelligence* for pertinent discussion of this practice).

4. Innovations in Interest and Aptitude Measurement

4.1 Interests

A detailed discussion of innovations in interest measurement up to the mid-1980s is contained in Walsh and Osipow (1986). These include the extensive revision of widely used instruments to address issues of bias and fairness, mostly in relation to gender but also to other cultural groups or subgroups. Newer instruments such as the *Vocational Interest Inventory* of Lunneborg and the UNIACT scales of Lamb and Prediger are built on deliberate selection of items to minimize sex differences. Johansson's work with the *Career Assessment Inventory* is noteworthy for its emphasis on noncollege occupational scales. Holland also released a lower-vocabulary level version of his *Self-Directed Search* (Form E) for noncollege-bound respondents. Jackson's work in developing the *Jackson Vocational Interest Survey* in the late 1970s is recognized to be the most psychometrically sophisticated of all. Through some ingenious procedures, Jackson was able to draw on the vast occupational database of Strong's work and apply this to his own factor-based scales.

Other innovations designed to increase the acceptance and applicability of vocational interest measures to a wider cross section of the population are embodied in a range of pictorial inventories and "card sorts." These include the unisex pictorial scales of the PAYES *Vocational Interest Inventory*, developed in the United States in the 1970s by Freeberg and Vitella, and adapted for use in Australia by Lokan and Shears in the early 1980s. The scales in the PAYES VII are modeled on Roe's (1956) theoretical occupational classification scheme, have a Likert-type response method, and are designed for low-achieving adolescents. Another instrument with a similar purpose is the *Reading Free Vocational Interest Inventory*, developed by Becker in the mid-1980s, which contains sets of three illustrations of job tasks requiring forced-choice responses and makes use of a fairly narrowly defined industry-based clustering of occupations (e.g., "Automotive," "Housekeeping," "Laundry"). Perhaps the most promising work of this nature is that of Tétreau and Trahan (1988) in Canada with their *Visual Interests Test* (the TTVIT). This measure is based on Holland's RIASEC category scheme, and involves a Likert-type response method. To administer it, about 100 sex-balanced illustrations of job tasks are presented in a controlled sequence for controlled amounts of time by means of a slide projector. With 1990s technology, it would be relatively simple to transfer the presentation to a videocassette for convenience. Tétreau and Trahan have been able to demonstrate the construct validity of their scales in a wide range of countries and cultural groups.

Since the early 1980s the most significant moves in the area of interest measurement have been in the provision of more and more comprehensive interpretative materials and handbooks for counselors and clients and in the growing emphasis on the importance of appropriate test use. Vocational interest measures are used increasingly for the development of self-understanding, not just for career decision-making or job choice (Hansen 1992). Despite the large amount of technical expertise that has been devoted to debate and research on the creation of scales that are "fair," evidence suggests that differential effects reported by clients taking different inventories is minimal (Gottfredson 1986a). As was noted by Hansen (1992), researchers and instrument developers have now realized that it is more fruitful to devote their efforts to ensuring that instruments are used validly and fairly, heeding the warnings of writers such as Cole and Moss (1989) on the possible side effects of test use for individuals and society. With the proliferation of options for computer-scoring and the concomitant generation of detailed reports, together with the increasingly glossy interpretative materials being produced for hand-scored inventories, the onus on counselors to ensure that the measures are used for appropriate purposes and to assist with the interpretation of results has become stronger than ever.

4.2 Aptitudes

In comparison with interests, the field of vocational aptitude measurement is relatively stagnant. Progress has, however, been made in the application of item response modeling (IRM) techniques to the development of computer-adaptive versions of some of the aptitude batteries and specific aptitude measures (see *Item Response Theory*). Provided that the hardware is available and sufficient research effort has been devoted to establishing the test item parameters, this type of testing offers a dependable and efficient way of obtaining accurate estimates of people's aptitudes in a minimum of testing time. Further areas where innovative work is likely to be productive are referred to later in Sect. 5.

The comments made above about the proliferation of elaborate interpretative materials accompanying interest measures apply also to aptitude measures, particularly where these are part of overall career exploration systems. Actual measures of aptitudes may be used in these systems, but typically respondents are asked either for their preobtained scores on batteries such as the GATB or the DAT or to provide global self-ratings of their abilities or aptitudes and/or to rate their proficiency on a series of work-related activities. Well known examples of such systems are Holland's *Self-Directed Search* and the *Harrington–O'Shea CDM System* referred to above. Both of these instruments can be administered either by computer (not adaptively) or as paper-and-pencil tests. In either case they rely partly for their appeal on their accompanying interpretative materials, though the computerized administration and scoring allow for more detailed reporting focusing on the respondent's own scores.

4.3 Computer-assisted Guidance Systems

A review of innovations since the 1980s would not be complete without reference to computer-assisted career guidance systems. Distinction needs to be made here between systems that sort and select information about occupations and/or education and training programs and the more flexible and comprehensive systems which aim to simulate a series of guidance interviews. Many examples of the first kind of system exist, but it is the second kind that is of relevance here. Because they are costly to develop and require sophisticated programming to execute, few high-quality examples of the second kind of system are currently in operation. The most comprehensive examples are the Canadian CHOICES system, the American DISCOVER and SIGI PLUS systems, and the British PROSPECT system. A common feature of all of these systems is that they incorporate a "self-assessment" or a "self-exploration" component, key elements of which are measured or self-rated interests, aptitudes, and skills. On-screen advice is usually offered to respondents about how this kind of information should be used, together with other kinds of information in developing appropriate career choice strategies and actual career choices.

Although computer-assisted guidance systems are expensive (because of their development costs), the advent of networks of personal computers means that they can be made available at reasonable unit cost to large numbers of users. They are attractive and motivating to most respondents and are likely to be of increasing influence in guiding people's career exploration in the years to come. The major North American systems named above have influence well beyond their own shores. For example, CHOICES has been adapted for use in several European countries and an adapted version of SIGI PLUS is in use in Australia. A locally produced system is in use in Israel, and Singapore has its Jobs Orientation Backup System (JOBS) developed by the National Institute of Education. No doubt other similar developments have occurred elsewhere.

5. Research Foci

5.1 Structure of Domains

This section refers only to work on the structure of interests, as the domain of abilities or aptitudes is covered elsewhere (see *Models of Intelligence*). The derivation of justifiable classification schemes for interests and aptitudes that can be linked to justifiable classifications of occupations is fundamental to much career guidance work. Linking of categories of clients' interest and aptitude characteristics to categories of occupations is used by counselors as a strategy to focus discussion and assist with "wise" career decision-making. The rationale for such strategies has been mentioned earlier in the entry, namely that people are expected to be more satisfied with and to perform better in occupations where the incumbents have similar interests to theirs and the work tasks are suited to their capabilities.

Since computers able to cope with the calculations needed for factor analysis became widely available, many hundreds of studies have been undertaken examining the structure of interests. Many have focused on the number of underlying dimensions that can most validly be used to "cover" the interest domain and on whether the dimensions can be adequately described in two-dimensional space. The theoretical work of Holland, who proposed that an approximate hexagonal configuration would represent relationships among his six categories of interests, both in terms of order and of distances between vertices, has been highly influential in much of this work. In a recent review of about 700 such studies, Hyland and Muchinsky reported that "Those studies in which the structural validity of the [Holland's] theory has been addressed have been concerned with the correctness of the hexagon for modeling the structure of interests . . . Findings supportive of the proposed structure were reported in a large percentage of these studies" (1991 p. 75).

While findings do tend to be generally supportive, they also tend not to be fully so. A typical example is the present author's Australian work where, from data on the *Self-Directed Search* for a national random sample of adolescents, the Social and Enterprising dimensions were not clearly separated whereas from data on the *Vocational Preference Inventory* for a group of about 1,500 adult applicants for positions in the federal Department of Civil Aviation, the Realistic and Investigative dimensions were confounded (possibly due to range restriction in the applicant group). Where more than six categories emerge from factor analyses it is often because different kinds of dimensions were included in the first place. An example is Jackson's work with the *Jackson Vocational Interest Survey* (JVIS). From 34 of what Jackson called "basic interest scales" in the JVIS, a factor analysis yielded 10 dimensions—8 (similar to Roe's classification cited above) derived from activity statements related to work roles and the remaining 2 derived from statements of what most psychologists would call work "values."

In most work where six categories of interests are assumed, the order of categories in a hexagonal scheme as proposed by Holland tends to hold up, but frequently there is variation in the "distances" between the vertices in plots of the empirical relationships among the category scores. Holland (with Gottfredson 1992) has professed himself to be much less concerned if the configuration turns out to be a "mis-shapen polygon" than that practitioners find the conceptual scheme useful in their work with clients and that researchers are able to substantiate beneficial effects for clients from its use.

The predominant view in the literature is that a "two-dimensional distillation of the information derived" (Holland and Gottfredson 1992) from vocational interest measures accounts for the majority of the variance. In the late 1970s and throughout the 1980s, however, a persistent thread advocating

otherwise has arisen from the work of Gati in Israel. In the first statement of his position, Gati proposed a hierarchical model of vocational or occupational interests (he seems to use these terms interchangeably) because, in his view, "the circular-hexagonal models face[d] several theoretical and empirical problems" (1979 p. 92). One of his main concerns was the contradiction between the ordering of Enterprising, Conventional, and Realistic as adjacent on Holland's hexagon and Organization, Business, and Technology as adjacent in the circular representation for Roe's (1956) eight-category classification.

The hierarchical model of interests illustrated in Gati's 1979 article is directly analogous to Vernon's (1961) hierarchical model of abilities. There is a general interest factor at the top, two broad group factors ("soft sciences" and "hard sciences") next, followed by more specific minor groups (similar to Holland's or Roe's categories), followed by fields of occupations, and, along the bottom, specific occupations. Gati's model is based on the assumption that occupations can be characterized as collections of attributes or features—work environment characteristics such as indoors or outdoors, extent of people contact, level of independence, rewards received, and so on—attributes that most psychologists would regard as values rather than interests. He assumed "that the similarity relations among occupations can be represented by a hierarchical tree structure, and that the pattern of occupational interests is compatible with this structure" (1979 p. 93). He then presented some reanalyses of data which turned out to be equally supportive of Holland's hexagonal model as of the proposed hierarchical model, though not fully supportive of Roe's circular model.

During the 1980s Gati and colleagues published many articles, both conceptual and empirical, advocating a hierarchical structure of vocational interests —a synthesis is available (Gati 1991). Careful reading shows that these authors have continued to be concerned with work aspects that others would consider to be values rather than interests, and that much of their empirical data has come from small numbers of cases. Where inventoried interests are concerned, their work has actually demonstrated the circular model to be a better representation than the hierarchical model (Gati and Nathan 1986 p. 186). Swanson believed that Gati has overlooked the distinction between individuals' perceptions of occupations and individuals' interests, and that the hierarchical model therefore describes the former rather than the latter. She noted that Gati's claims for superiority of the hierarchical model seem "to hold true only with data obtained with the VPI, which consists solely of occupational titles as items" and that "data obtained from inventories consisting of diverse item formats . . . suggest an equal level of support for both models" (1992 p. 237). Unless a hierarchical model is demonstrated to be clearly superior, the level of acceptance and use of Holland's scheme among researchers and practitioners seems likely to be maintained. The first issue of the *Journal of Vocational Behavior* for 1996 has revitalised the interest in, and debate about, the configuration of vocational interests. The issue begins with the proposition by Tracey and Rounds (1996) that a spherical model is the most appropriate for depicting the relationships among vocational interests, based on an analysis of several hundred college and high school students' responses to an Inventory of Occupational Preferences. The third dimension in their proposed model arises from their belief that occupational prestige is an important aspect of vocational interests. Their research suggests a spherical model with a prestige dimension orthogonal to the more usual data/ideas and things/people dimensions (themselves orthogonal), linked to Holland's RIASEC categories by Prediger (1982). Reactions to Tracey and Rounds' proposal from several well-known vocational psychologists follow. Most are not convinced either that the model has been appropriately generated (e.g., Borgen and Donnay 1996) or that it could be of practical use in counseling people trying to make career choices (e.g., Hansen 1996). In an underlying observation on interest researchers' obsession with spatial configurations, one of the commentaries is headed, "Lost in Space". Much debate is certain to follow the appearance of this journal issue.

5.2 Relationships Between Domains

Lowman's potentially influential book advocating "integrative career assessment" is built on the premise of "the necessity of combining ability, interest, and other personality data to arrive at a comprehensive understanding of career dynamics" (1991 p. 177). The book contains a brief review of research concerning cross-domain relationships in the areas of abilities, personality variables, and interests, together with the lament that much more on the interactions between the domains and the implications of these for career behavior needs to be done. Interest–ability or aptitude relationships are the ones of concern in this entry. Many studies were done from the 1940s to the 1960s, but these predated modern developments in vocational interest theory. Lowman offered reasons why the early studies and even later ones found "little common variance" between the two domains and then reviewed recent research, including some of his own, which he believed had "corrected some of the early deficits" and "extended the literature" (p. 183). A good example is the work of Randahl who, by using multivariate techniques such as profile analysis of data from a large, heterogeneous sample, was able to demonstrate that "measured abilities and interests are related when examined from a typological viewpoint" (1991 p. 348), with the relationships being "strong" and "in accordance with theoretical predictions" (p. 346). Lowman believed that the research literature on cross-domain relationships is only just beginning to

emerge, and pleaded for more studies to be conducted in nonclinical, representative samples of both sexes.

5.3 Effectiveness in Prediction of Choice or Performance

The main rationale for research effort on vocational interests and aptitudes is that these variables are useful in assisting individuals with their career choices and in assisting employers with selecting employees who will be productive. Thus, research has focused and will continue to be focused on the best combinations of variables for predicting given outcomes, on whether scores should be adjusted in any way (e.g., through use of standardized scores, through use of different norm tables for different groups, or through use of differential weighting of variables for prediction of success in different courses or occupations, and so on—see Sect. 6 for further discussion of these matters), and on whether new kinds of variables and/or assessment methods will yield more useful predictions. A brief review of such research will follow.

From the 1950s to the 1970s great promise was held for research identifying different combinations or different weightings of variables for predicting success in different courses or occupations (e.g., French 1966, Horst 1957). As it turned out, "differential prediction" studies of this kind were methodologically difficult to do, and were usually not very definitive in their results. This has generally been attributed to criterion problems of overlap in measures of academic success or, in occupational contexts, of what variables and what measures to use as indicators of success (e.g., Prediger 1989). In the educational arena, course group membership (Prediger and Brandt 1991) has often been used. Generally speaking, differential prediction research, in terms of predicting levels of performance, did not live up to the hopes initially held for it. It did succeed, though, in demonstrating a substantial role for interest variables over and above aptitude variables in prediction equations (e.g., Lokan 1977).

The controversies of the 1970s about bias in prediction and whether, for example, raw scores or standardized scores on interest measures should be used as the basis for counseling students (see Weinrach 1984 for a summary of the issues and arguments), gave way by the mid-1980s to an equally vehement controversy in the literature about whether anything is achieved in the prediction of occupationally relevant performance by considering abilities or aptitudes beyond the general ability factor, "*g*". A special issue of the *Journal of Vocational Behavior* was devoted to this debate, generally claiming strong support for the importance of *g* in employment. It has been common practice to use scores on different combinations of aptitude measures to select employees for different kinds of occupations, a practice encouraged by the United States Employment Service (USES) in its specification of 66 "Occupational Aptitude Patterns" for a range of occupational areas (see Gottfredson 1986b for a discussion of this and related issues). A series of validity generalization studies and reviews was undertaken for the USES by Hunter and others in the early 1980s, leading to Hunter's assertion that "Tailoring aptitude composites to match the job does not improve on general cognitive ability in prediction except in a very small number of special cases" (1986 p. 341). The study by Ree and Earles (1991) provides an example of a recent research study on this topic.

Prediger (1987, 1989) has pointed out difficulties with the "success prediction model" and has reviewed research carried out *across* occupations (rather than *within* occupations as most commonly drawn on by Hunter). He argued that this research and research establishing different patterns of work tasks across occupations (also reviewed), together with his own substantial research on "the relevance of 14 cognitive and noncognitive abilities to six job clusters spanning the work world" (1989 p. 1) clearly implies that ability differences across occupations involve more than *g*. In other work, Prediger (1987) has argued that measures of a range of types of abilities/aptitudes are of most value in educational counseling, where a "profile similarity model" is relevant.

The research and debate mentioned in the previous two paragraphs were focused on the use of ability or aptitude measures. That measures of vocational interests can be predictive in themselves—particularly if combined with expressed vocational aspirations (Holland 1986)—or can add considerably to the prediction of course membership or area of study at secondary level has been reinforced by large-scale studies. Ainley et al. showed that "interests and aptitudes which become evident by late primary or early secondary school have a strong influence on subject choice in Years 11 and 12" (1990 p. 100). In this longitudinal research, carried out in a national random sample of several thousand Australian students, achievement in numeracy at age 10 was strongly associated with choice of physical science subjects at Year 12, and interest in Investigative activities at age 14 was associated with participation in a range of programs of study in the sciences at Year 12. Artistic interests were associated with participation in programs of study in humanities and social sciences, and in creative and performing arts. Ainley et al.'s findings with respect to Investigative interests were echoed in another longitudinal study, though on a smaller scale, by Kidd and Naylor (1991). A further survey of 20,000 upper secondary sutdents from a national random sample of almost 300 Australian schools (Ainley et al. 1994) replicated the relationships between interests, in Holland's RIASEC categories, and choice of subjects in Years 11 and 12, from the 1990 study.

In research involving over 2,000 senior high school students, Prediger and Brandt showed the usefulness of a range of interest and ability or aptitude measures for helping students identify vocational education programs in which they would be likely to experience satisfaction and success. Through a series of discriminant analyses, these researchers found that "the differentiation of vocational programs was substantial" and that "there were important program differences on each of the interest and ability measures" (1991 p. 137). Studies such as those referred to in this and the previous paragraph provide justification for Prediger's (1987) view that comparison of students' profiles of interest and ability scores with those in known educational course or occupational groups is a good basis for educational counseling.

5.4 Alternative Assessment Methods

Except in a small number of instances, for example, measures of manual dexterity involving manipulation of concrete equipment, measures of vocational interests and aptitudes have largely been paper-and-pencil in format. Since the 1980s computer administration of tests and questionnaires has become quite common, with the advantage that scoring and interpretation of results can be carried out quickly and immediately. Further, as the quality and availability of graphics packages for personal computers has improved, measures involving or depending on diagrammatic material have also been administered by computer. In these instances, however, it is the delivery of the assessment rather than the nature of the assessment method itself that has changed.

On a more innovative level, computers are being increasingly used for administering tests in an adaptive way. The progression of items administered to a respondent is determined by the pattern of his or her prior responses and is therefore tailored to his or her ability level. The statistical techniques behind this type of testing ensure that reliable estimates of respondents' abilities are achieved with exposure to a relatively small number of items, resulting in substantial savings in testing time. Adaptive testing is well suited to measures of abilities or aptitudes, where it is relatively simple to establish a hierarchy of tasks in terms of difficulty. This type of assessment method is less likely to be useful for interest measurement in which Thurstone-type scales, involving homogeneous items that are progressively harder for respondents to agree with, are more difficult to establish.

Moves for competency-based training, which has been enjoying a very high profile in many countries in the late 1980s and into the 1990s, seem likely to have some impact on vocational aptitude testing in the future in both professional and nonprofessional contexts. Going against the *g* argument referred to earlier, aptitude measures developed in the 1990s may well be more focused on tasks identified as necessary for successful completion of a training course or performance of a job. Current emphasis on performance-based assessment will probably mean less reliance on pencil-and-paper aptitude testing. Computer simulation techniques or actual tasks set up for assessment purposes, perhaps after brief training and practice periods, may become the order of the day.

6. Equity issues

In proposing new directions for interest testing in the mid-1980s, Holland wrote that "perhaps the most complex, difficult, social-emotional issue is how to insure equity in interest inventory assessments within the constraints of current beliefs, knowledge, test standards, and financial resources" (1986 p. 253). He believed the lack of consensus in the debate over use of raw versus standardized scores, referred to above, is due to lack of agreement over the purposes of career counseling in general and interest assessment in particular. He argued that the purposes of interest inventories are at least threefold: exploration (increasing the range of occupations a person will consider); reassurance (providing support for a person's vocational aspiration or potential job); and self-understanding (providing structured information for comprehending the nature of a person's interests). Holland and others (e.g., Hansen 1992) believe that the resolution of equity issues will not come from more data collection, but rather from increased awareness of the effects that taking an inventory has on different groups of respondents and increased awareness by counselors of respondents' purpose(s) for taking an inventory, together with constructively designed interpretative materials and improved use of interpretation strategies by counselors.

Equity issues in aptitude or ability measurement are probably of more import than those in interest measurement. Aptitudes, these days, are conceptualized as "developed abilities," and individuals with broader experiential backgrounds and better resourced education are better placed to develop their abilities. Systems of selection for employment and for restricted places in higher education courses are faced with the dilemma of selecting the candidates most likely to be successful, while at the same time endeavoring not to be unfair to minority groups. The debate about the usefulness of a range of aptitude measures versus reliance on measures of *g* only is relevant here, as it is well known in Western societies that many racial minorities tend to score lower on standardized tests of scholastic aptitude than the majority White group.

The most thorough investigations of equity issues in testing have been undertaken in the United States. Space does not permit more than a few cursory comments in this entry. For a thorough discussion, see the report cited below or the special journal issues on employment topics listed under Further Reading.

In an attempt to equalize employment opportunity for Hispanics and Blacks with that of all other United States citizens, the USES adopted the practice of using within-group percentile ranks on the GATB tests for employment selection decisions. This led to objections in the mid-1980s from the Civil Rights branch of the

United States Department of Justice that the practice was discriminatory against non-Hispanics and non-Blacks. The argument led to an investigation and report (Hartigan and Wigdor 1989) by a panel of experts comprising statisticians, psychologists, economists, and specialists in educational measurement. After a very thorough review the panel concluded by recommending that the practice of using within-group percentile ranks, or other approaches giving equal chances to able candidates from all groups, be continued. The main basis for their argument was that predictions based on GATB tests are inaccurate at best, often highly so, hence productivity is not likely to be greatly affected by retaining the within-group selection practices.

The review panel's recommendation was short-lived. The Civil Rights Act of 1991 (S. 1745; Public Law 102–166), signed by President Bush on 21 November 1991, "barred employers from adjusting the scores of, using different cutoff scores for, or otherwise altering the results of employment-related tests on the basis of race, color, religion, sex or national origin. This provision stemmed from concern among lawmakers in both parties that 'race norming' was leading to discrimination against qualified white applicants." (*CQ Almanac* 1991 p. 259). A month later, a window of opportunity was left open for minority students in the general ban on race-exclusive scholarships when the United States Secretary of State, Lamar Alexander, said that "schools that provided scholarships to promote student body diversity could continue to do so . . . so long as all students were eligible and race was not the only factor considered" (*CQ Almanac* 1991 p. 376). The 1991 Civil Rights Act moved the onus of arriving at equitable employment practices from the adjustment of test scores to a specially created commission, the Glass Ceiling Commission, "to study the representation of women and minorities in executive, management and senior decision-making positions . . . [and] . . . to make recommendations to help eliminate artificial barriers to the advancement of women and minorities on the job" (*CQ Almanac* 1991 p. 253). The challenge to all who wish to make use of interest and aptitude results to counsel or assign students or workers to courses or jobs in a fair way is still a very large one.

See also: Attitudes, Measurement of

References

Please note that references to published instruments cited are not given here. Sufficient detail of the names of instruments and/or authors is given in the text for bibliographic information to be obtained from reference books such as the Buros *Mental Measurements Yearbooks* published by the Buros Institute of Mental Measurements of the University of Nebraska-Lincoln or *Tests* published by the Test Corporation of America in Kansas City, Kansas.

Ainley J A, Jones W, Navaratnam K K 1990 *Subject Choice in Senior Secondary School*. Australian Government Publishing Service, Canberra

Ainley J, Robinson L, Harvey-Beavis A, Elsworth G, Fleming M 1994 *Subject Choice in Years 11 and 12*. Australian Government Publishing Services, Canberra

Anastasi A 1982 Aptitude and achievement tests: The curious case of the indestructible strawperson. In: Plake B S (ed.) 1982 *Social and Technical Issues in Testing: Implications for Test Construction and Usage*. Erlbaum, Hillsdale, New Jersey

Borgen F H 1986 New approaches to the assessment of interests. In: Walsh W B, Osipow S H (eds.) 1986

Borgen F H, Donnay D A C 1996 Slicing the vocational interest pie one more time: Comment on Tracey and Rounds. *J. Voc. Behav.* 48(1): 42–52

Cole N S, Moss P A 1989 Bias in test use. In: Linn R L (ed.) *Educational Measurement*, 3rd edn. Macmillan Inc., New York

CQ Almanac Vol. 47. 1991 Congressional Quarterly Service, Washington, DC

Crites J O 1969 *Vocational Psychology*. McGraw-Hill, New York

Dunnette M D 1976 Aptitudes, abilities and skills. In: Dunnette M D (ed.) 1976 *Handbook of Industrial and Organizational Psychology*. Rand McNally, Chicago, Illinois

Fleishman E A, Reilly M E 1992 *Handbook of Human Abilities*. Consulting Psychologists Press, Palo Alto, California

French J W 1966 The logic of and assumptions underlying differential testing. In: Anastasi A (ed.) 1966 *Testing Problems in Perspective*. American Council on Education, Washington, DC

Fryer D 1931 *The Measurement of Interests in Relation to Human Adjustment*. Holt, New York

Gati I 1979 A hierarchical model for the structure of vocational interests. *J. Voc. Behav.* 15(1): 90–106

Gati I 1991 The structure of vocational interests. *Psych. Bull.* 109(2): 309–24

Gati I, Nathan M 1986 The role of the perceived structure of occupations in vocational behavior. *J. Voc. Behav.* 29:(2) 177–93

Gottfredson L S 1986a Special groups and the beneficial use of vocational interest inventories. In: Walsh W B, Osipow S H (eds.) 1986

Gottfredson L S 1986b Occupational aptitude patterns map: Development and implications for a theory of job aptitude requirements. *J. Voc. Behav.* 29: 254–91

Hansen C 1992 Individual differences × counseling × testing = vocational psychology. Paper given at the annual meeting of American Psychological Association, Washington, DC

Hansen J-I C 1996 What goes around, comes around. *J. Voc. Behav.* 48(1) 73–76

Hartigan J A, Wigdor A K (eds.) 1989 *Fairness in Employment Testing: Validity Generalization, Minority Issues and the General Aptitude Test Battery*. National Academy Press, Washington, DC

Holland J L 1985 *Making Vocational Choices: A Theory of Vocational Personalities and Work Environments*, 2nd edn. Prentice-Hall, Englewood Cliffs, New Jersey

Holland J L 1986 New directions for interest testing. In: Plake B S, Witt J C (eds.) 1986 *The Future of Testing*. Erlbaum, Hillsdale, New Jersey

Holland J L, Gottfredson G D 1992 Studies of the hexagonal model: An evaluation (or, the perils of stalking the perfect hexagon). *J. Voc. Behav.* 40(2): 58–70

Horst P 1957 Differential prediction in college admissions. *College Board Review* 33: 19–23

Hunter J E 1986 Cognitive ability, cognitive aptitudes, job knowledge, and job performance. *J. Voc. Behav.* 29(3): 340–62

Hyland A M, Muchinsky P M 1991 Assessment of the structural validity of Holland's model with job analysis (PAQ) information. *J. App. Psych.* 76(1): 75–80

Kidd G, Naylor F 1991 The predictive power of measured interests in tertiary course choice: The case of science. *Aust. J. Educ.* 35(3): 261–72

Lokan J J 1977 The differential prediction of grades in a special vocational high school. *Meas. Eval. Guid.* 10(1): 7–16

Lowman R L 1991 *The Clinical Practice of Career Assessment: Interests, Abilities, and Personality*. American Psychological Association, Washington, DC

Peterson N G, Bownas D A 1982 Skill, task structure and performance acquisition. In: Dunnette M D, Fleishman E A (eds.) 1982 *Human Performance and Productivity. Vol. 1: Human Capability Assessment*. Erlbaum, Hillsdale, New Jersey

Prediger D J 1982 Dimensions underlying Holland's hexagon: Missing links between interests and occupations? *J. Voc. Behav.* 21: 259–287

Prediger D J 1987 *Career Counseling Validity of the ASVAB Job Cluster Scales used in DISCOVER*. American College Testing Program, Iowa City, Iowa

Prediger D J 1989 Ability differences across occupations: More than *g. J. Voc. Behav.* 34(1): 1–27

Prediger D J, Brandt W E 1991 Project CHOICE: Validity of interest and ability measures for student choice of vocational program. *Career Dev. Q.* 40(2): 132–44

Randahl G J 1991 A typological analysis of the relations between measured vocational interests and abilities. *J. Voc. Behav.* 38(3): 333–50

Ree M J, Earles J A 1991 Predicting training success: Not much more than *g. Personnel Psychology* 44(2): 321–32

Roe A 1956 *The Psychology of Occupations*. Wiley, New York

Strong E K Jr 1943 *Vocational Interests of Men and Women*. Stanford University Press, Stanford, California

Super D E 1976 *Career Education and the Meanings of Work*. United States Office of Education, Washington, DC

Super D E, Crites J O 1962 *Appraising Vocational Fitness by Means of Vocational Tests*. Harper and Row, New York

Swanson J L 1992 In search of structural validity. *J. Voc. Behav.* 40(2): 229–38

Tétreau B, Trahan M 1988 La mesure des intérêts professionels au moyen de stimuli photographiques: Le TVI. *Appl. Psychol.* 37: 51–63

Tittle C K 1985 Vocational aptitude. In: Husén T, Postlethwaite T N (eds.) 1985 *The International Encyclopedia of Education*, 1st edn. Pergamon Press, Oxford

Tracey T J G, Rounds J 1996 The spherical representation of vocational interests. *J. Voc Behav.* 48(1): 3–41

Vernon P E 1961 *The Structure of Human Abilities*, 2nd edn. Methuen, London

Walsh W B, Osipow S H (eds.) 1986 *Advances in Vocational Psychology Vol. 1: The Assessment of Interests.* Erlbaum, Hillsdale, New Jersey

Weinrach S G 1984 Determinants of vocational choice: Holland's theory. In Brown D, Brooks L (eds.) *Career Choice and Development: Applying Contemporary Theories to Practice.* Jossey-Bass, San Francisco, California

Further Reading

Journal of Counseling and Development 1984 Vol. 63(2)

(issue devoted to Computers in Counseling and Development)

Journal of Vocational Behavior 1986 Vol. 29(3) (issue devoted to The *g* Factor in Employment)

Journal of Vocational Behavior 1988 Vol. 33(3) (issue devoted to Fairness in Employment Testing)

Journal of Vocational Behavior 1992 Vol. 40(2) (issue devoted to Holland's Theory)

Journal of Vocational Behavior 1996 Vol. 48(1) (issue devoted to Research and Debate on Structure of Vocational Interests)

List of Contributors

Contributors are listed in alphabetical order together with their affiliations. Titles of articles which they have authored follow in alphabetical order, along with the respective page numbers. Where articles are co-authored, this has been indicated by an asterisk preceding the article title.

ADAMS, D. (University of Pittsburgh, Pittsburgh, Pennsylvania, USA)
Comparative Methodology in Education 31–41

ALBAN-METCALF, R. J. (Trinity and All Saints College, Leeds, UK)
Repertory Grid Technique 315–18

ALLAL, L. (University of Geneva, Geneva, Switzerland)
Generalizability Theory 737–41

ALLERUP, P. (Danish Institute for Educational Research, Copenhagen, Denmark)
Rasch Measurement Theory 863–74

ANDER, C. (National Institute for Education, Budapest, Hungary)
Galois Lattices 543–49

ANDERSON, J. (The Flinders University of South Australia, Bedford Park, South Australia, Australia)
Content and Text Analysis 340–44; *Data Banks and Data Archives* 344–49

ANDERSON, L. (University of Illinois at Chicago, Chicago, Illinois, USA)
Data Envelopment Analysis 498–503

ANDERSON, L. W. (University of South Carolina, Columbia, South Carolina, USA)
Attitudes, Measurement of 885–95

ANDRICH, D. (Murdoch University, Murdoch, Western Australia, Australia)
Essays: Equating of Marks 830–35; *Rating Scale Analysis* 874–80; *Thurstone Scales* 819–22

ANWARD, J. (Stockholm University, Stockholm, Sweden)
Semiotics in Educational Research 106–11

BALL, S. (University of Sydney, Sydney, New South Wales, Australia)
Unintended Effects in Educational Research 243–47

BALL, S. J. (University of London, London, UK)
Participant Observation 310–14

BEATON, A. E. (Boston College, Chestnut Hill, Massachusetts, USA)
Item Sampling 840–46; *Missing Scores in Survey Research* 763–66

BLEISTEIN, C. A. (Educational Testing Service, Princeton, New Jersey, USA)
Item Bias 742–49

BRYK, A. S. (University of Chicago, Chicago, Illinois, USA)
Hierarchical Linear Modeling 549–56

BURKE, G. (Monash University, Clayton, Victoria, Australia)
Census and National Survey Data 323–27

CANNELL, C. F. (University of Michigan, Ann Arbor, Michigan, USA)
Interviewing for Survey Research 361–70

CARDINET, J. (Institut Romand de Recherches et de Documentation Pédagogiques, Neuchâtel, Switzerland)
Generalizability Theory 737–41

CHEUNG, K. C. (University of Macau, Macau)
Practical Mathematics and Science Testing 949–54

† CHOPPIN, B. H. (University of California, Los Angeles, California, USA)
Objective Tests 771–75

CLANDININ, D. J. (University of Alberta, Edmonton, Alberta, Canada)
Narrative Inquiry 81–86

CONNELLY, F. M. (Ontario Institute for Studies in Education, Toronto, Ontario, Canada)
Narrative Inquiry 81–86

COOPER, M. (University of New South Wales, Kensington, New South Wales, Australia)
Nonparametric and Distribution-free Statistics 607–12

DE LANDSHEERE, G. (Université de Liège, Liège, Belgium)
History of Educational Research 8–16

DE LANDSHEERE, V. (Université de Liège, Liège, Belgium)
Taxonomies of Educational Objectives 803–12

DENZIN, N. K. (University of Illinois, Urbana, Illinois, USA)
Biographical Research Methods 55–61; *Triangulation in Educational Research* 318–22

DUNN-RANKIN, P. (University of Hawaii, Honolulu, Hawaii, USA)
*Scaling Methods 790–98

ERIKSON, R. (University of Stockholm, Stockholm, Sweden)
Mobility Tables 597–600

EVERITT, B. S. (University of London, London, UK)
Cluster Analysis 466–72; *Contingency Tables* 478–83

EVERS, C. W. (Monash University, Melbourne, Victoria, Australia)
*Research in Education: Epistemological Issues 22–31

FINN, J. D. (State University of New York, Buffalo, New York, USA)
Hypothesis Testing 556–61; *Variance and Covariance, Analysis of* 697–703

FISCHBEIN, S. (Department of Special Education, Stockholm Institute of Education, Stockholm, Sweden)
Twin Studies 162–67

FRASER, B. J. (Curtin University of Technology, Perth, Western Australia, Australia)
Classroom Environments 896–900

GALTON, M. (University of Leicester, Leicester, UK)
Classroom Observation 334–39

GERALD, D. E. (National Center for Education Statistics, United States Department of Education, Washington, DC, USA)
*Projections of Educational Statistics 643–48

GRAYSON, D. (University of Sydney, Sydney, New South Wales, Australia)
*Multitrait–Multimethod Analysis 600–07

GUBA, E. G. (Indiana University, Bloomington, Indiana, USA)
*Naturalistic and Rationalistic Enquiry 86–91

GUSTAFSSON, J-E. (University of Gothenburg, Mölndal, Sweden)
Models of Intelligence 937–44

HAIG, B. D. (University of Canterbury, Christchurch, Canterbury, New Zealand)
Feminist Research Methodology 180–85

HALL, B. L. (Ontario Institute for Studies in Education, Toronto, Ontario, Canada)
Participatory Research 198–205

HAMBLETON, R. K. (University of Massachusetts, Amherst, Massachusetts, USA)
Criterion-referenced Measurement 719–25; *Standard Setting in Criterion-referenced Tests* 798–802; **Tests and Attitude Scales, Translation of* 965–71

HÄRNQVIST, K. (University of Gothenburg, Mölndal, Sweden)
Training of Research Workers in Education 269–76

HENRY, G. (University of Liège, Liège, Belgium)
Correspondence Analysis 493–97

HERMAN, J. L. (University of California, Los Angeles, California, USA)
Item Writing Techniques 749–54

HOLLINGSWORTH, S. (Michigan State University, East Lansing, Michigan, USA)
Teachers as Researchers 247–50

HOLT, D. (University of Southampton, Southampton, UK)
Missing Data and Nonresponse 592–97

HOUSE, E. R. (University of Colorado, Boulder, Colorado, USA)
Ethics of Evaluation Studies 257–61

HUSÉN, T. (University of Stockholm, Stockholm, Sweden)
Educational History in Biographies and Autobiographies 67–70; *Educational Research and Policy-making* 251–57; *Research Paradigms in Education* 16–21

LINDMAN, H. R.   (Indiana University, Bloomington, Indiana, USA)
Bayesian Statistics 456–61

LINDSEY, J. K.   (Limburg University, Diepenbeck, Belgium)
Significance Testing 670–77

LOHNES, P. R.   (State University of New York, Buffalo, New York, USA)
Discriminant Analysis 503–08; *Factorial Modeling* 540–44

LOKAN, J. J.   (Australian Council for Educational Research, Hawthorn, Victoria, Australia)
Vocational Interests and Aptitudes, Measures of 984–94

McGAW, B.   (Australian Council for Educational Research, Hawthorn, Victoria, Australia)
Meta-analysis 371–80

McKENZIE, P. A.   (Australian Council for Educational Research, Hawthorn, Victoria, Australia)
Research in Education: Nature, Needs, and Priorities 236–43

MARJORIBANKS, K.   (University of Adelaide, Adelaide, South Australia, Australia)
Family and School Environmental Measures 918–23; *Interaction, Detection, and its Effects* 561–70

MARSH, H. W.   (University of Western Sydney, Macarthur, New South Wales, Australia)
Multitrait–Multimethod Analysis 600–07

MARTON, F.   (University of Gothenburg, Mölndal, Sweden)
Phenomenography 95–101

MASTERS, G. N.   (Australian Council for Educational Research, Hawthorn, Victoria, Australia)
Partial Credit Model 857–63

MÉRÖ, L.   (National Institute for Education, Budapest, Hungary)
Galois Lattices 543–49

MICHAEL, W. B.   (University of Southern California, Los Angeles, California, USA)
Prediction in Educational Research 412–17

MILLER, K. M.   (Miller and Tyler Ltd, London, UK)
Personality Inventories 944–48

MILLER, P. V.   (Northwestern University, Evanston, Illinois, USA)
Interviewing for Survey Research 361–70

MORGAN, G.   (Australian Council for Educational Research, Hawthorn, Victoria, Australia)
Expectancy Tables in Educational Prediction 915–18

MORGENSTERN, C.   (University of Hamburg, Hamburg, Germany)
Descriptive Scales 900–08

NAYLOR, F. D.   (University of Melbourne, Parkville, Victoria, Australia)
Test-taking Anxiety and Expectancy of Performance 971–76

NISBET, J.   (University of Aberdeen, Aberdeen, UK)
Policy-oriented Research 211–17

ÖDMAN, P-J.   (University of Stockholm, Stockholm, Sweden)
Hermeneutics 185–92

OGBU, J. U.   (University of California, Berkeley, California, USA)
Anthropological Inquiry 48–55

RAUDENBUSH, S. W.   (Michigan State University, East Lansing, Michigan, USA)
Effective Schools Research 357–61; *Hierarchical Linear Modelling* 549–56

REEVE, R. A.   (University of Illinois at Chicago, Chicago, Illinois, USA)
Secondary Data Analysis 439–44

RICHARDS, L.   (Q. S. R., P. O. Box 171, La Trobe University Post Office 3083, Australia)
Computers and Qualitative Analysis 286–90

ROGERS, H. J.   (Columbia University, New York, USA)
Multiple Choice Tests, Guessing in 766–71

ROSIER, M. J.   (University of Melbourne, Melbourne, Victoria, Australia)
Data Banks and Data Archives 344–49; *Survey Research Methods* 154–62

ROSS, K. N.   (Deakin University, Geelong, Victoria, Australia)
Sampling Errors in Survey Research 663–70; *Sampling in Survey Research* 427–38

RUSSELL, A.   (The Flinders University of South Australia, Bedford Park, South Australia, Australia)
Effects: Moderating, Mediating, and Reciprocal 508–13

RUST, K. (Westat Corporation, Rockville, Maryland, USA)
Sampling in Survey Research 427–38

SAHA, L. J. (Australian National University, Canberra, ACT, Australia)
Measurement of Social Background 930–37; *Sociometric Methods* 691–95

SÄLJÖ, R. (University of Linköping, Linköping, Sweden)
Self-report in Educational Research 101–06

SATO, N. E. (University of California, Berkeley, California, USA)
Anthropological Inquiry 48–55

SCHEUNEMAN, J. D. (Educational Testing Service, Princeton, New Jersey, USA)
Item Bias 742–49

SCHLEICHER, A. (University of Hamburg, Hamburg, Germany)
Data Management in Survey Research 349–57; *Microcomputers in Educational Survey Research* 380–86

SCHLEISMAN, J. L. (University of Minnesota, Minneapolis, Minnesota, USA)
Adaptive Testing 881–85

SELLIN, N. (University of Hamburg, Hamburg, Germany)
Multilevel Analysis 394–403; *Path Analysis with Latent Variables* 633–40

SHARPE, L. (College of St. Mark and St. John, Plymouth, UK)
Participant Verification 314–15

SHARPLEY, C. F. (Monash University, Clayton, Victoria, Australia)
Single Case Research: Measuring Change 451–55

SHYE, S. (Israel Institute of Applied Social Research, Jerusalem, Israel)
Facet theory 41–47; *Partial Order Scalogram Analysis* 613–20; *Smallest Space Analysis* 677–84

SINGER, J. D. (Harvard University, Cambridge, Massachusetts, USA)
Event History Analysis 513–19

SMITH, N. L. (Syracuse University, Syracuse, New York, USA)
Evaluation Models and Approaches 217–25

SOWDEN, S. (The Flinders University of South Australia, Bedford Park, South Australia, Australia)
Descriptive Data, Analysis of 296–306

SPEARRITT, D. (University of Sydney, Sydney, New South Wales, Australia)
Factor Analysis 528–39

SPIEL, C. (University of Vienna, Vienna, Austria)
Human Development: Research Methodology 134–38

STOCKING, M. L. (Educational Testing Service, Princeton, New Jersey, USA)
Item Response Theory 836–40

STURMAN, A. (University of Southern Queensland, Toowoomba, Queensland, Australia)
Case Study Methods 61–66

SWAMINATHAN, H. (University of Massachusetts, Amherst, Massachusetts, USA)
Latent Trait Measurement Models 851–57

TAFT, R. (Monash University, Clayton, Victoria, Australia)
Ethnographic Research Methods 71–75

TAM, HAK PING (Ohio State University, Columbus, Ohio, USA)
Log–Linear Models 571–80

TATSUOKA, M. M. (Educational Testing Service, Princeton, New Jersey, USA)
Regression Analysis of Quantified Data 648–57

THOMSON, J. D. (Australian Council for Educational Research, Hawthorn, Victoria, Australia)
Canonical Analysis 461–66

† THORNDIKE, R. L. (Columbia University, New York, USA)
Reliability 775–90

THORNDIKE, R. M. (Western Washington University, Bellingham, Washington, USA)
Correlational Methods 484–93; *Reliability* 775–90

TIMPANE, P. M. (Columbia University, New York, USA)
Politics of Educational Research 261–63

TITTLE, C. K. (City University of New York, New York, USA)
Test Bias 813–19

TROW, M. (University of California, Berkeley, California, USA)
Policy Analysis 205–11

TUIJNMAN, A. C.   (OECD, Paris, France)
Path Analysis and Linear Structural Relations Analysis 621–33; Selection Bias in Educational Research 445–51

TYLER, B.   (Miller and Tyler Ltd, London, UK)
Personality Inventories 944–48

† TYLER, R. W.   (Stanford University, Stanford, California, USA)
Evaluation: A Tylerian Perspective 225–35

UMAR, J.   (Ministry of Education and Culture, Jakarta, Indonesia)
Item Banking 923–30

VAN DER LINDEN, W. J.   (University of Twente, Enschede, The Netherlands)
Decision Theory in Educational Testing 725–30

VON EYE, A.   (Michigan State University, East Lansing, Michigan, USA)
Human Development: Research Methodology 134–38

WALBERG, H. J.   (University of Illinois at Chicago, Chicago, Illinois, USA)
*Data Envelopment Analysis 498–503; *Secondary Data Analysis 439–44*

WALKER, J. C.   (University of Canberra, Canberra, ACT, Australia)
Research in Education: Epistemological Issues 22–31

WALSH, J. J.   (Boston College, Chestnut Hill, Massachusetts, USA)
Projective Testing Techniques 954–58

WEINERT, F. E.   (Max Planck Institute for Psychological Research, Munich, Germany)
Translating Research into Practice 263–68

WEISS, D. J.   (University of Minnesota, Minneapolis, Minnesota, USA)
Adaptive Testing 881–85

WILCOX, R. R.   (University of Southern California, Los Angeles, California, USA)
Simulation as a Research Technique 150–54

WILLETT, J. B.   (Harvard University, Cambridge, Massachusetts, USA)
*Change, Measurement of 327–34; *Event History Analysis 513–19*

WILLMS, J. D.   (University of British Columbia, Vancouver, British Columbia, Canada)
Effective Schools Research 357–61

WILSON, M.   (University of California, Berkeley, California, USA)
*Measurement of Developmental Levels 908–15; *Sampling Errors in Survey Research 663–70*

WOLF, R. M.   (Columbia University, New York, USA)
Prediction in Educational Research 412–17; Q-Methodology 417–20; Quasi-experimentation 420–21; Questionnaires 422–27; Rating Scales 958–65

ZELLER, R. A.   (Bowling Green State University, Bowling Green, Ohio, USA)
Validity 822–29

ZHANG, S.   (University of Hawaii, Honolulu, Hawaii, USA)
Scaling Methods 790–98

Name Index

The Name Index has been compiled so that the reader can proceed directly to the page where an author's work is cited, or to the reference itself in the bibliography. For each name, the page numbers for the bibliographic section are given first, followed by the page number(s) in parentheses where that reference is cited in text. Where a name is referred to only in text, and not in the bibliography, the page number appears only in parentheses.

The accuracy of the spelling of authors' names has been affected by the use of different initials by some authors, or a different spelling of their name in different papers or review articles (sometimes this may arise from a transliteration process), and by those journals which give only one initial to each author.

Subject Index

The Subject Index has been compiled as a guide to the reader who is interested in locating all the references to a particular subject area within the Encyclopedia. Entries may have up to three levels of heading. Where the page numbers appear in bold italic type, this indicates a substantive discussion of the topic. Every effort has been made to index as comprehensively as possible and to standardize the terms used in the index. However, given the diverse nature of the field and the varied use of terms throughout the international community, synonyms and foreign language terms have been included with appropriate cross-references. As a further aid to the reader, cross-references have also been given to terms of related interest.